DORLAND'S
POCKET
MEDICAL
DICTIONARY

27th
EDITION

DORLAND'S
POCKET
MEDICAL
DICTIONARY

Thoroughly updated, based on
Dorland's Illustrated Medical Dictionary
with a series of 32 color plates:
The Human Body—Highlights of Structure and Function

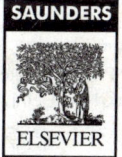

SAUNDERS

ELSEVIER

Dorland's Pocket Medical Dictionary, 27/e

Saunders
An imprint of Elsevier
The Curtis Center
170 S Independence Mall W 300E
Philadelphia, Pennsylvania 19106

© 2004 by Saunders

Original ISBN : 978-1-4160-0101-0

First Printed in India 2005
Reprinted 2006
Reprinted 2007

Indian Reprint ISBN : 978-81-8147-712-5

This edition is for sale in Bangladesh, Bhutan, India, Maldives, Nepal, Pakistan, Sri Lanka and designated countries in South-East Asia through Elsevier (Singapore) Pte. Ltd. Sale and purchase of this book outside of these countries is unauthorised by the publisher.

Published by Elsevier, a division of Reed Elsevier India Private Limited.
Sri Pratap Udyog, 274, Captain Gaur Marg, Sriniwaspuri, New Delhi - 110065 (INDIA)

Printed and bound in India by Thomson Press (I) Ltd.

PREFACE

In 1898, when *Dorland's Pocket Medical Dictionary* was first published, as the *American Pocket Medical Dictionary*, it provided a complete, compact, and up-to-date reference for medical professionals. Over a century later, the goal of the Dictionary remains the same: to provide brief, clear, accurate, current definitions for the most important and globally relevant words in medicine, while maintaining the compact size that keeps this volume portable and easily accessible.

To meet this goal, the Dictionary has been carefully examined and thoroughly updated for this new edition, its 27th, drawing extensively on the work done for the 30th edition of *Dorland's Illustrated Medical Dictionary*. In revising and updating terminology, special attention has been paid to the pharmaceutical terms, concentrating on drugs actively marketed in the United States; they have been carefully examined to ensure that they reflect the most current official prescribing information. For this edition, a large number of terms relating to complementary and alternative medicine have been added, providing the most comprehensive coverage of this field available in any small medical dictionary. The anatomical tables have been carefully checked and revised using the most recent official anatomical terminology, keeping in mind the increasing trend toward the use of English, rather than Latin, terms for many anatomical structures. Many adjectives have been added as defined terms, and other adjectival forms have been placed at the ends of the definitions of the relevant nouns, so that definitions can be found for virtually all adjectives occurring as part of compound terms elsewhere in the Dictionary.

For ease of use and a fresher look, head words and guide words are now printed in red, making them more visible. The full-color insert of anatomical structures has been doubled in size, to 32 pages, and completely redrawn, increasing the amount of detail that can be presented and also reflecting current terminology. A large section on medical etymology precedes the vocabulary section of the dictionary and explains concisely the meanings of the stems used in medical terminology; this section, too, has been thoroughly revised and updated to reflect current usage.

The result is an edition that upholds over a century of tradition, continuing to provide a compact, comprehensive, clear, and accurate guide to the language of medicine. We hope it continues to provide the help to current users that previous editions have always been to past generations.

Patricia D. Novak, PhD
Senior Lexicographer

CONTENTS

NOTES ON THE USE OF THIS DICTIONARY

Main Entries and Subentries and Their Arrangement

Terms appear as either main entries or subentries. Terms consisting of two or more words generally appear as subentries under the principal word (that is, the noun). Thus, *Addison's disease, collagen disease*, and *Raynaud's disease* appear as subentries under the main entry *disease*. Names of specific acids (e.g., *sulfuric acid*) and of enzymes (e.g., *acetyl-CoA carboxylase*) are an exception to this rule and appear as main entries under the first word of the name.

Chemical compounds having a binary name are found under the first word, so that *sodium chloride* is a subentry under *sodium*.

In all subentries, the noun (main entry) is repeated in abbreviated form (e.g., *humoral i.* under *immunity*). If the subentry is plural in form, this is indicated by adding an *'s* to the abbreviation of the main entry. Thus, under *body*, the subentry *Aschoff b's* is read *Aschoff bodies* and the entry *ketone b's* is read *ketone bodies*. Irregular and Latin plurals are spelled out, as *vasa afferentia* under *vas*.

Adjectival forms for many nouns, if not given as separate entries, are given in boldface type at the end of the entry for the noun (e.g., **allele** ... **alle′lic,** adj; **allergen** ... **allergen′ic,** adj.). In similar fashion, irregular and Latin plural forms are given on the singular forms (e.g., **epiphysis** ... pl. *epi′physes*). When, however, such forms may not be readily recognizable, they are also given as separate entries (e.g., **viscera** ... plural of *viscus*).

Syllabication

Acceptable word divisions are indicated for main entries by the use of bullets within the entry word. Not all syllable breaks are given (for example, a single vowel at the beginning or end of a word should not be separated from the rest of the word). In many cases, a word may be broken at places other than the ones shown here; for example, different pronunciations imply different syllabication.

Pronunciation

The pronunciation of words is indicated by a phonetic respelling that appears in parentheses immediately following each main entry. These phonetic respellings, devised for ease of interpretation, are presented with a minimum of diacritical markings.

The basic rules are fairly simple. An unmarked vowel ending a syllable is long; an unmarked vowel in a syllable ending with a consonant is short. A long vowel in a syllable ending with a consonant is indicated by a macron (ā, ē, ī, ō, ū), and a short vowel ending a syllable is indicated by a breve (ă, ĕ, ĭ, ŏ, ŭ). The symbol *ah* is used to represent the colorless vowel sound that occurs in many unstressed syllables (such as the *a* in *sofa*); it is also used to represent the broad *ah* sound heard in *father*.

The primary stress in a word is indicated by a single boldface accent (′) and the secondary stress by a double lightface accent (″). Unstressed syllables are followed by hyphens. Monosyllables have no stress marks.

The native pronunciations of many foreign words and proper names cannot of course be indicated by this simplified system. These are shown as closely as possible in English phonetics.

When, on successive words, the first syllables are pronounced the same way, these syllables are given in the phonetic respelling of only the first of the sequence of terms. If the stress varies or some other change occurs in the pronunciation of these syllables, the entire pronunciation is indicated in the phonetic respelling. For example:

    ich·thy·oid (ik′the-oid)
    ich·thyo·sar·co·tox·in (ik″the-o-sahr′ko-tok″sin)
    ich·thyo·sar·co·tox·ism (-tok″sizm)
    ich·thyo·si·form (ik″the-o′sĭ-form)
    ich·thy·o·sis (-sis)

Pronunciation Guide

Pronunciation of vowels is as in the following examples (for the use of breves and macrons, see the rules above):

ah	sofa	ĕ	met	ŏ	got	oi	boil
ā	mate	ī	bite	ū	fuel	o͞o	boom
ă	bat	ĭ	bit	ŭ	but	o͝o	book
ē	beam	ō	home	aw	all	ou	fowl

Pronunciation of consonants is as follows:

b	book	m	mouse	ch	chin
d	dog	n	new	ks	six
f	fog	p	park	kw	quote
g	get	r	rat	ng	sing
h	heat	s	sigh	sh	should
j	jewel, gem	t	tin	th	thin, than
k	cart, pick	w	wood	zh	measure
l	look	z	size, phase		

Abbreviations Used in This Dictionary

a.	artery (L. *arteria*)	int.	interior
adj.	adjective	L.	Latin
ant.	anterior	lat.	lateral
b.	bone	m.	muscle (L. *musculus*)
cf.	compare (L. *confer*)	n.	nerve (L. *nervus*)
e.g.	for example (L. *exempli gratia*)	pl.	plural
		post.	posterior
ext.	external	pr.	process
Fr.	French	q.v.	which see (L. *quod vide*)
Ger.	German	sing.	singular
Gr.	Greek	sup.	superior
i.e.	that is (L. *id est*)	v.	vein (L. *vena*)
inf.	inferior		

COMBINING FORMS IN MEDICAL TERMINOLOGY

The following is a list of combining forms encountered frequently in the vocabulary of medicine. A dash appended to a combining form indicates that it is not a complete word and, if the dash precedes the combining form, that it commonly appears as the terminal element of a compound. Infrequently a combining form is both preceded and followed by a dash, showing that it usually appears between two other elements. Closely related forms are shown in one entry by the use of parentheses: thus **carbo(n)**-, showing it may be either carbo-, as in *carbo*hydrate, or carbon-, as in *carbon*uria. Following each combining form, the first item of information is the Greek or Latin word, identified by [Gr.] and [L.], from which it is derived. Occasionally both a Greek and a Latin word are given. Presence of a dash before or after such an element indicates that it does not occur as an independent word in the original language. Information necessary to the understanding of the form appears next in parentheses. Then the meaning or meanings of the word are given, followed where appropriate by reference to a synonymous combining form. Finally, an example is given to illustrate use of the combining form in a compound English derivative.

a-[1] — *a-* [Gr.] (*n* is added before words beginning with a vowel) negative prefix. Cf. in-[3]. *a*metria

a-[2] — *a-* [L.] separation, away from. *a*vulsion

ab- — *ab* [L.] away from Cf. apo-. *ab*duct

abdomin- — *abdomen, abdominis* [L.] abdomen. *abdomin*oscopy

abs- — *abs* [L.] variant of ab. *abs*cess

ac- — See ad-. *ac*cretion

acanth- — *akantha* [Gr.] thorny, spiny, *acanth*ocyte

acar- — *akari* [Gr.] mite. *acar*odermatitis

acet- — *acetum* [L.] vinegar. *acet*ic acid

acid- — *acidus* [L.] sour. *acid*uric

acou- — *akouō* [Gr.] hear. *acou*stic (Also spelled acu-)

acr- — *akron* [Gr.] extremity, peak. *acr*omegaly

act- — *ago, actus* [L.] do, drive, act. re*act*ion

actin- — *aktis, aktinos* [Gr.] ray, radius, Cf. radi-. *actin*obacillus

acu- — See acou-. dys*acu*sis

ad- — *ad* [L.] (*d* changes to *c, f, g, p, s,* or *t* before words beginning with those consonants) to. *ad*renal

-ad[1] — *-ad* [L.] toward. cephal*ad*

-ad[2] — *-as, -ados* [Gr.] group, derivation from, connection with. trichomon*ad*

aden- — *adēn* [Gr.] gland. Cf. gland-. *aden*oma

adip- — *adeps, adipis* [L.] fat. Cf. lip- and stear-. *adip*ocellular

aer- — *aēr* [Gr.] air. an*aer*obiosis

af- — See ad-. *af*ferent

ag-   See ad-. agglutinant

-agogue   *agōgos* [Gr.] leading, inducing. galact*agogue*

-agra   *agra* [Gr.] catching, seizure. pod*agra*

-al[1]   *-alis* [L.] pertaining to, characterized by. arteri*al*, diarrhe*al*

-al[2]   *-alia* [L.] act, process. deni*al*

alb-   *albus* [L.] white. Cf. leuk-. *alb*iduria

alg-   *algos* [Gr.] pain. neur*alg*ia

algesi-   *algēsis* [Gr.] sense of pain. an*algesi*a, *algesi*meter

all-   *allos* [Gr.] other, different. *all*ergy

allant-   *allas, allantos* [Gr.] sausage. *allant*iasis, *allant*oid

allel-   *allēlōn* [Gr.] of one another. *allel*ic

alve-   *alveus* [L.] trough, channel, cavity. *alve*olar

ambi-   *ambi-* [L.] (*i* is dropped before words beginning with a vowel) on all sides. *ambi*dextrous

ambly-   *amblys* [Gr.] dull. *ambly*opia

ambo-   *ambo* [L.] both. *ambo*ceptor

ameb-   *amoibē* [Gr.] change. *ameb*oid

amni-   *amnion* [Gr.] bowl, membrane enveloping the fetus. *amni*ocentesis

amphi-   *amphi* [Gr.] (*i* is dropped before words beginning with a vowel) both sides. *amphi*centric

ampho-   *amphō* [Gr.] both. *ampho*teric

amygdal-   *amygdalē* [Gr.] almond. *amygdal*in, *amygdal*oid

amyl-   *amylon* [Gr.] starch. *amyl*uria

an-[1]   See a-[1]. *an*iridia

an-[2]   See ana-. *an*ode

ana-   *ana* [Gr.] (final *a* is dropped before words beginning with a vowel) up, positive. *ana*bolism

ancyl-   See ankyl-. *ancyl*ostomiasis

andr-   *anēr, andros* [Gr.] man. *andr*ogen

angi-   *angeion* [Gr.] vessel. Cf. vas-. *angi*oma

anis-   *anisos* [Gr.] unequal, uneven. *anis*ocoria

ankyl-   *ankylos* [Gr.] crooked, looped. *ankyl*osis (Also spelled ancyl-)

anomal-   *anōmalos* [Gr.] irregular. *anomal*y

ant-   See anti-. *ant*acid

ante-   *ante* [L.] before. *ante*flexion

antero-   *anterior* [L.] before. *antero*lateral

anthrac-   *anthrax* [Gr.] coal, charcoal. *anthrac*osilicosis

anthrop-   *anthrōpos* [Gr.] man, human being. *anthrop*omorphism

anti-   *anti* [Gr.] (*i* is dropped before words beginning with a vowel) against, counter. Cf. contra-. *anti*pruritic

antr-   *antron* [Gr.] cavern. *antr*ocele

ap-   See ad-. *ap*pendage

aph-   *haptō, haph-* [Gr.] touch. dys*aph*ia (See also hapt-)

apo-   *apo* [Gr.] (*o* is dropped before words beginning with a vowel) away from, detached. Cf. ab-. *apo*lipoprotein

appendic-   *appendix, appendicis* [L.] appendix. *appendic*itis

arachn-   *arachnē* [Gr.] spider. *arach*nodactyly

arch-   *archē* [Gr.] beginning, origin. *arch*enteron

arteri-   *arteria* [Gr.] (*i* is sometimes dropped) artery. *arterio*sclerosis, peri*arter*itis

arteriol-   *arteriola,* dim. of *arteria* [L.] arteriole. *arteriol*opathy

arthr-   *arthron* [Gr.] joint. Cf. articul-. *arthr*odesis

articul-   *articulus* [L.] joint. Cf. arthr-. dis*articul*ation

as-   See ad-. *as*similation

asthen-   *asthenēs* [Gr.] weak. *asthen*ocoria

astr-   *astron* [Gr.] star. *astr*ocyte

at-   See ad-. *at*tenuate

atel-   *atelēs* [Gr.] incomplete. *atel*ocardia

ather-   *athērē* [Gr.] gruel. *ather*osclerosis

atlant-   *atlas, atlantos* [Gr.] atlas. *atlant*oaxial

atm-	*atmos* [Gr.] steam, vapor. *atm*osphere
atri-	*atrium* [L.] atrium. *atri*oventricular
atroph-	*atrophos* [Gr.] ill-fed. *atrophoderma*
audi-	*audire* [L.] to hear. *audi*ometry
aur-	*auris* [L.] ear. Cf. ot-. *aur*al
aut-	*autos* [Gr.] self. *aut*oimmunity
aux-	*auxō* [Gr.] increase. *aux*otrophic
ax-	*axōn* [Gr.] or *axis* [L.] axis. *ax*olemma
axon-	*axōn* [Gr.] axis. *axon*opathy
ba-	*bainō*, *ba-* [Gr.] go, walk, stand. a*ba*sia
bacill-	*bacillus* [L.] small staff, rod. Cf. bacter-. actino*bacillo*sis
bacter-	*bactērion* [Gr.] small staff, rod. Cf. bacill-. *bacter*iophage
ball-	*ballō*, *bol-* [Gr.] throw. *ball*ismus (See also bol-)
bar-	*baros* [Gr.] weight, pressure. *bar*osinusitis
bas-	See basi-. *bas*ophil
basi-	*basis* [Gr.] base. *basi*lar (See also bas-)
bi-[1]	*bios* [Gr.] life. Cf. vit-. aero*bic*
bi-[2]	*bi-* [L.] (an *n* may be added before words beginning with a vowel) two. *bi*cornuate (See also di-[1])
bil-	*bilis* [L.] bile. Cf. chol-. *bil*iary
bin-	See bi-[2]. *bin*ocular
bis-	*bis* [L.] twice. *bis*ferious
blast-	*blastos* [Gr.] bud, child, a growing thing in its early stages. Cf. germ-. *blast*oma, mono*blast*
blenn-	*blenna* [Gr.] mucus. *blenn*orrhea
blep-	*blepō* [Gr.] look, see mono*blep*sia
blephar-	*blepharon* [Gr.] (from *blepō*; see blep-) eyelid. Cf. cili-. *blephar*oncus
bol-	See ball-. em*bol*ism
brachi-	*brachiōn* [Gr.] arm. *brachi*ocephalic
brachy-	*brachys* [Gr.] short. *brachy*dactyly
brady-	*bradys* [Gr.] slow. *brady*cardia
brom-	*brōmos* [Gr.] stench. *brom*hidrosis
bronch-	*bronchos* [Gr.] windpipe. *bronch*oscopy
bry-	*bryō* [Gr.] be full of life. em*bry*o
bucc-	*bucca* [L.] cheek. *bucc*occlusion
cac-	*kakos* [Gr.] bad, abnormal. Cf. mal-. *cac*ogeusia (See also dys-)
calc-[1]	*calx*, *calcis* [L.] stone (cf. lith-), limestone, lime. *calc*ipexy
calc-[2]	*calx*, *calcis* [L.] heel. *calc*aneodynia
calor-	*calor* [L.] heat. Cf. therm-. *calor*imeter
cancr-	*cancer*, *cancri* [L.] crab, cancer. Cf. carcin-. *cancr*oid. (Also spelled chancr-)
capit-	*caput*, *capitis* [L.] head. Cf. cephal-. de*capit*ation
capn-	*kapnos* [Gr.] smoke. *capn*ography
caps-	*capsa* [L.] (from *capio*; see cept-) container. *caps*ule
carbo(n)-	*carbo*, *carbonis* [L.] coal, charcoal. *carbo*hydrate, *carbon*ic acid
carcin-	*karkinos* [Gr.] crab, cancer. Cf. cancr-. *carcin*oma
cardi-	*kardia* [Gr.] heart. lipo*cardi*ac
cary-	See kary-. Eu*cary*otae
cata-	*kata* [Gr.] (final *a* is dropped before words beginning with a vowel) down, negative. *cat*acrotism
caud-	*cauda* [L.] tail. *caud*ad
cav-	*cavus* [L.] hollow. Cf. coel-. con*cav*e
cec-	*caecus* [L.] blind. Cf. typhl-. *cec*otomy
cel-[1]	See -cele. varico*cel*ectomy
cel-[2]	See coel-. a*cel*omate
cel-[3]	see celi-. *cel*itis
-cele	*kēlē* [Gr.] tumor, hernia. gastro*cele*
celi-	*koilia* [Gr.] belly. *celi*otomy

cell-   *cella* [L.] room, cell. Cf. cyt-. *cell*ule

cente-   *kenteō* [Gr.] to puncture. Cf. punct-. entero*centesis*

centi-   *centum* [L.] hundred. Indicates fraction in metric system. [This exemplifies the custom in the metric system of identifying fractions of units by stems from the Latin, as centimeter, decimeter, millimeter, and multiples of units by the similar stems from the Greek, as hectometer, decameter, and kilometer.] *centi*meter

centr-   *kentron* [Gr.] or *centrum* [L.] point, center. *centr*ifugal, *centr*omere

cephal-   *kephalē* [Gr.] head. Cf. capit-. en*cephal*itis, *cepha*locentesis

cept-   *capio, -cipientis, -ceptus* [L.] take, receive. re*cept*or

cer-   *kēros* [Gr.] or *cera* [L.] wax. *cer*oplasty, *cer*umen

cerat-   See kerat-. *cerat*ocricoid

cerebell-   *cerebellum*, dim. of *cerebrum* [L.] little brain. *cerebell*ifugal

cerebr-   *cerebrum* [L.] brain. *cere-brospinal

cervic-   *cervix, cervicis* [L.] neck. Cf. trachel-. *cervic*itis

chancr-   See cancr-. *chancr*oid

cheil-   *cheilos* [Gr.] lip. Cf. labi-. *cheil*oschisis

cheir-   *cheir* [Gr.] hand. Cf. man-. megalo*cheir*ia (Also spelled chir-)

chem-   *chēmeia* [Gr.] alchemy. *chem*istry, *chem*otherapy

chir-   See cheir-. *chir*opractic

chlor-   *chlōros* [Gr.] green. *chloro*phyll

chol-   *cholē* [Gr.] bile. Cf. bil-. *chol*angitis

chondr-   *chondros* [Gr.] cartilage. *chondr*omalacia

chord-   *chordē* [Gr.] string, cord. peri*chord*al

chori-   *chorion* [Gr.] membrane. *chori*ocarcinoma

chrom-   *chrōs* [Gr.] color. poly*chrom*atic

chron-   *chronos* [Gr.] time. syn*chron*ous

chrys-   *chrysos* [Gr.] gold. *chryso*derma

chy-   *cheō, chy-* [Gr.] pour. ec*chy*mosis

-cid(e)   *caedo, -cisus* [L.] cut, kill. fungi*cide*, germi*cid*al

cili-   *cilium* [L.] eyelid. Cf. blephar-. *cili*ary

cine-   See kine-. acro*cine*sis

-cipient   See cept-. ex*cipient*

circum-   *circum* [L.] around. Cf. peri-. *circum*ferential

cis-   *cis* [L.] on this side. *cis*platin

-cis-   *caedo, -cisus* [L.] cut, kill. ex*cis*ion

-clast   *klaō* [Gr.] break. osteo*clast*

clin-   *klinō* [Gr.] bend, incline, make lie down. *clino*cephaly

clus-   *claudo, -clusus* [L.] shut. mal*oclus*ion

co-   See con-. *co*hesion

cocc-   *kokkos* [Gr.] berry. gono*cocc*us

coel-   *koilos* [Gr.] hollow. Cf. cav-. *coel*oblastula. (Also spelled cel-)

-coele   See coel-. blasto*coele*

col-¹   See colon-. *col*ic

col-²   See con-. *col*lapse

colon-   *kalon* [Gr.] lower intestine. *colon*ic

colp-   *kolpos* [Gr.] hollow, vagina. Cf. sin-. *colp*itis

com-   See con-. *com*mensal

con-   *con-* [L.] (becomes co- before vowels or *h*; col- before *l*; com- before *b*, *m*, or *p*; cor- before *r*) with, together. Cf. syn-. *con*traction

coni-   *konis* [Gr.] dust. *coni*ofibrosis

contra-   *contra* [L.] against, counter. Cf. anti-. *contra*indication

copr-   *kopros* [Gr.] dung. Cf. sterc-. *copr*ophilia

cor-¹   *korē* [Gr.] doll, little image, pupil. iso*cor*ia

cor-²   See con-. *cor*relation

corpor-   *corpus, corporis* [L.] body. Cf. somat-. extra*corpor*eal

cortic-   *cortex, corticis* [L.] bark, rind. *cortic*osterone

cost-   *costa* [L.] rib. Cf. pleur-. inter*cost*al

crani-   *kranion* [Gr.] or *cranium* [L.] skull. peri*crani*um

-crasia   *krasis* [Gr.] mixture. dys*crasia*

creat-   *kreas, kreato-* [Gr.] meat, flesh. *creat*ine

-crescence   *cresco, crescentis, cretus* [L.] grow. ex*crescence*

cret-[1]   *cerno, cretus* [L.] distinguish, separate off. Cf. crin-. dis*cret*e

cret-[2]   See -crescence. ac*cret*ion

crin-   *krinō* [Gr.] distinguish, separate off. Cf. cret-[1]. endo*crin*ology

crur-   *crus, cruris* [L.] shin, leg. talo*crur*al

cry-   *kryos* [Gr.] cold. *cry*esthesia

crypt-   *kryptō* [Gr.] hide, conceal. *crypt*orchidism

cult-   *colo, cultus* [L.] tend, cultivate. *cult*ure

cune-   *cuneus* [L.] wedge. Cf. sphen-. *cune*iform

cut-   *cutis* [L.] skin. Cf. derm(at)-. sub*cut*aneous

cyan-   *kyanos* [Gr.] blue. *cyan*ophil

cycl-   *kyklos* [Gr.] circle, cycle. *cycl*ophoria

cyst-   *kystis* [Gr.] bladder. Cf. vesic-. *cyst*algia

cyt-   *kytos* [Gr.] cell. Cf. cell-. plasmo*cyt*oma

dacry-   *dakry* [Gr.] tear. *dacry*ocyst

dactyl-   *daktylos* [Gr.] finger, toe. Cf. digit-. hexa*dactyl*y

de-   *de* [L.] down from. *de*composition

deca-   *deka* [Gr.] ten. Indicates multiple in metric system. Cf. deci-. *deca*gram

deci-   *decem* [L.] ten. Indicates fraction in metric system (one-tenth). Cf. deca. *deci*bel, *deci*liter

dendr-   *dendron* [Gr.] tree. *dendr*ite

dent-   *dens, dentis* [L.] tooth. Cf. odont-. inter*dent*al

derm(at)-   *derma, dermatos* [Gr.] skin. Cf. cut-. endo*derm*, *derm*atitis

-desis   *desis* [Gr.] a binding together. arthro*desis*

desm-   *desmos* [Gr.] band, ligament: syn*desm*oplasty

deut(er)-   *deuteros* [Gr.] second. *deuter*anopia, *deut*an

dextr-   *dexter, dextr-* [L.] right-hand. ambi*dextr*ous

di-[1]   *di-* [Gr.] two. *di*morphism (See also bi-[2])

di-[2]   See dia-. *di*uresis

di-[3]   See dis-. *di*vergence

dia-   *dia* [Gr.] (*a* is dropped before words beginning with a vowel) through, apart. Cf. per-. *dia*gnosis

dicty-   *diktyon* [Gr.] net. *dicty*otene

didym-   *didymos* [Gr.] twin. Cf. gemin-. epi*didym*al

digit-   *digitus* [L.] finger, toe. Cf. dactyl-. *digit*ation

diplo-   *diploos* [Gr.] double. *diplo*myelia

dips-   *dipsa* [Gr.] thirst. poly*dips*ia, *dips*ogen

dis-   *dis-* [L.] (*s* may be dropped before a word beginning with a consonant) apart, away from. *dis*location

disc-   *diskos* [Gr.] or *discus* [L.] disk. *disc*oplacenta (Also spelled disko-)

dolich-   *dolichos* [Gr.] long. *dolicho*cephalic

dors-   *dorsum* [L.] back. *dors*oventral

drom-   *dromos* [Gr.] course. *dromo*graph

-ducent   See -duct. ad*ducent*

-duct   *duco, ducentis, ductus* [L.] lead, conduct. ovi*duct*

dur-   *durus* [L.] hard. Cf. scler-. in*dur*ation.

dynam-   *dynamis* [Gr.] power. *dyna*mometer, thermody*nam*ics

dys-   *dys-* [Gr.] bad, improper. Cf. mal-. *dys*trophy (See also cac-)

e-   *e* [L.] out from. Cf. ec- and ex-. *e*mission

ec-   *ek* [Gr.] out of. Cf. e-. *ec*centric

-ech-   *echō* [Gr.] have, hold, be. syn*ech*otomy

echin-   *echinos* [Gr.] hedgehog. *echin*ococcus

ect-   *ektos* [Gr.] outside. Cf. extra-. *ect*oderm

ectr-   *ektrōsis* [Gr.] miscarriage. *ectr*osyndactyly

ede-   *oideō* [Gr.] swell. *ede*matous

ef-   See ex-. *ef*florescent

elast-   *elasticus* [L.] elastic. *elast*ofibroma

electr-   *ēlectron* [Gr.] amber. *electr*otherapy

em-   See en-. *em*bolism, *em*pathy

-em-   *haima* [Gr.] blood. an*em*ia. (See also hem(at)-)

-emesis   *emein* [Gr.] to vomit. hyper*emesis*

en-   *en* [Gr.] (*n* changes to *m* before *b*, *p*, or *ph*) in, on. Cf. in-². *en*arthosis

encephal-   *enkephalos* [Gr.] brain. *encephal*opathy

end-   *endon* [Gr.] inside. Cf. intra-. *end*angiitis

ent-   *entos* [Gr.] inside. *ent*optic

enter-   *enteron* [Gr.] intestine. dys*entery*

entom-   *entomon* [Gr.] insect. *entom*ology

epi-   *epi* [Gr.] (*i* is dropped before words beginning with a vowel) upon, after, in addition. *epi*glottis, *ep*axial

episi-   *epision* [Gr.] pubic region. *episi*otomy

erg-   *ergon* [Gr.] work, deed. *erg*nery

erot-   *erōs*, *erōtos* [Gr.] sexual desire. *erot*omania

erythr-   *erythros* [Gr.] red. Cf. rub(r)-. *erythr*ocyte

eso-   *esō* [Gr.] inside. Cf. intra-. *eso*gastritis

esthe-   *aisthanomai*, *aisthē-* [Gr.] perceive, feel. Cf. sens-. an*esthe*sia

eu-   *eu* [Gr.] good, normal. *eu*pepsia

eury-   *eurys* [Gr.] wide. *eury*cephalic

ex-   *ex* [Gr.] or *ex* [L.] out of. Cf. e-. *ex*cretion

exo-   *exō* [Gr.] outside. Cf. extra-. *exo*skeleton

extra-   *extra* [L.] outside of, beyond. Cf. ect- and exo-. *extra*cellular. (Also written extro-)

faci-   *facies* [L.] face. Cf. prosop-. *faci*olingual

-facient   *facio*, *facientis*, *factus*, *-fectus* [L.] make. Cf. poie-. cale*facient*

-fact-   See -facient. arti*fact*

fasci-   *fascia* [L.] band. *fasci*otomy

febr-   *febris* [L.] fever. Cf. pyr-. *febr*icity

-fect-   See -facient. in*fect*ive

-ferent   *fero*, *ferentis*, *latus* [L.] bear, carry. Cf. phor-. ef*ferent*

-ferous   *ferre* [L.] to bear. lacti*ferous*

ferr-   *ferrum* [L.] iron. *ferro*protein

fet-   *fetus* [L.] fetus. *fet*oscope

fibr-   *fibra* [L.] fiber. Cf. in-¹. chondro*fibr*oma

fil-   *filum* [L.] thread. *fil*iform

fiss-   *findo*, *fissus* [L.] split. Cf. schis-. *fiss*ion

flagell-   *flagellum* [L.] whip. *flagella*tion

flav-   *flavus* [L.] yellow. Cf. xanth-. ribo*flav*in

-flect-   *flecto*, *flexus* [L.] bend, divert. de*flect*ion

-flex-   See -flect-. re*flex*ometer

flu-   *fluo*, *fluxus* [L.] flow. Cf. rhe-. *flu*id

flux-   See flu-. de*flux*ion

for-   *foro* [L.] bore. im*for*ate

-form   *forma* [L.] shape. Cf. -oid. cruci*form*

fract-   *frango*, *fractus* [L.] break. re*fract*ion

front-   *frons*, *frontis* [L.] forehead, front. naso*front*al

-fug(e)   *fugio* [L.] flee, avoid. vermi*fuge*, centri*fug*al

funct-   *fungor*, *functus* [L.] perform, serve. *funct*ion

fund-   *fundo*, *fusus* [L.] pour. in*fund*ibulum

fus-   See fund-. dif*fus*ion

galact-   *gala*, *galactos* [Gr.] milk. Cf. lact-. *galact*orrhea

gam-   *gamos* [Gr.] marriage, reproductive union. *gam*ete

gangli-   *ganglion* [Gr.] swelling, plexus. *gangli*itis

gastr-	*gastēr, gastros* [Gr.] stomach. cholangio*gastr*ostomy
ge-	*gē* [Gr.] earth. *ge*ophagia
gelat-	*gelo, gelatus* [L.] freeze, congeal. *gelat*in
gemin-	*geminus* [L.] twin, double. Cf. didym-. quadri*gemin*al
gen-¹	*gignomai, gen-, gon-* [Gr.] become, be produced, originate. endo*gen*ous
gen-²	*gennaō* [Gr.] produce, originate. cyto*gen*ic
geni-	*geneion* [Gr.] chin. *geni*al
genit-	*genitalis* [L.] belonging to birth. *genit*ourinary
ger-	*gēras* [Gr.] old age. *ger*oderma
geront-	*gerōn, gerontos* [Gr.] old man. *geront*ology
germ-	*germen, germinis* [L.] bud, a growing thing in its early stages. Cf. blast-. *germ*inal
gest-	*gero, genetis, gestus* [L.] bear, carry. con*gest*ion
gingiv-	*gingiva* [L.] gum. *gingiv*itis
gland-	*glans, glandis* [L.] acorn. Cf. aden-. uni*gland*ular
gli-	*glia* [Gr.] glue. neuro*gli*a, *gli*oma
gloss-	*glōssa* [Gr.] tongue. Cf. lingu-. tricho*gloss*ia
glott-	*glōtta* [Gr.] tongue, language. *glott*al
gluc-	See glyc(y)-. *gluc*ophore
glutin-	*gluten, glutinis* [L.] glue. ag*glutin*ation
glyc(y)-	*glykys* [Gr.] sweet. *glyc*emia, *glyc*yrrhiza (Also spelled gluc-)
gnath-	*gnathos* [Gr.] jaw. ortho*gnath*ous
gno-	*gignōsō, gnō-* [Gr.] know, discern. dia*gno*sis
gon-¹	*gonē* [Gr.] offspring, seed, genitalia. *gon*ocyte, *gon*orrhea
gon-²	*gony* [Gr.] knee. *gon*arthritis
gonad-	*gonas, gonadis* [L.] gonad. *gonad*ectomy
goni-	*gōnia* [Gr.] angle. *goni*ometer; *goni*otomy
grad-	*gradior* [L.] walk, take steps. retro*grad*e
-gram	*gramma* [Gr.] letter, drawing. cardio*gram*
gran-	*granum* [L.] grain, particle. lipo*gran*uloma
graph-	*graphō* [Gr.] scratch, write, record. angio*graph*y
grav-	*gravis* [L.] heavy. multi*grav*ida
gyn(ec)-	*gynē, gynaikos* [Gr.] woman, wife. andro*gyn*y, *gynec*ologic
gyr-	*gyros* [Gr.] ring, circle. *gyr*ospasm
haem(at)-	See hem(at)-. *Haem*aphysalis
hapl-	*haploos* [Gr.] simple, single. *hapl*otype
hapt-	*haptō* [Gr.] touch. *hapt*ics
helc-	*helkos* [Gr.] sore, ulcer. kerato*helc*osis
hem(at)-	*haima, haimatos* [Gr.] blood. Cf. sanguin-. *hem*angioma, *hemat*ocele (See also -em-) [Also written haem(at)-]
hemi-	*hēmi-* [Gr.] half. Cf. semi-. *hemi*ageusia
hepat(ic)-	*hēpar, hēpatos* [Gr.] liver. *hepat*ocele, *hepatic*olithotomy
hept(a)-	*hepta* [Gr.] seven. Cf. sept-². *hepta*chromic, *hept*ose
hered-	*heres, heredis* [L.] heir. *hered*ofamilial
heter-	*heteros* [Gr.] other, different. *heter*ochromia
hex-	*echō, hech-* [Gr.] (*hech-* added to *s* becomes *hex-*) have, hold, be. ca*hex*ia
hex(a)-	*hex* [Gr.] six. Cf. sex-¹. *hex*ose, *hexa*dactyly
hidr-	*hidros* [Gr.] sweat. hyper*hidr*osis
hist-	*histos* [Gr.] web, tissue. *hist*ocompatibility
hod-	*hodos* [Gr.] road, path. *hod*oneuromere. (See also -od- and -ode¹)
hol-	*holos* [Gr.] entire. *hol*odiastolic
hom-	*homos* [Gr.] common, same. *hom*ograft
home-	*homoios* [Gr.] like, resembling. *home*ostasis
horm-	*ormē* [Gr.] impetus, impulse. *horm*one
hyal-	*hyalos* [Gr.] glass. *hyal*oplasm

hydat-   *hydōr, hydatos* [Gr.] water. *hydat*id

hydr-   *hydōr, hydr-* [Gr.] water. Cf. lymph-. achlor*hydr*ia

hymen-   *hymēn* [Gr.] membrane. *Hymen*optera

hyp-   See hypo-. *hyp*axial

hyper-   *hyper* [Gr.] above, beyond, extreme. Cf. super-. *hyper*trophy

hypn-   *hypnos* [Gr.] sleep. *hypn*otic

hypo-   *hypo* [Gr.] (*o* is dropped before words beginning with a vowel) under, below. Cf. sub-. *hypo*calcemia

hyps-   *hypsos* [Gr.] height. *hyps*arrhythmia

hyster-   *hystera* [Gr.] womb. Cf. metr-², uter-. *hyster*opexy

iatr-   *iatros* [Gr.] physician. ped*iatr*ics

ichthy-   *ichthys* [Gr.] fish. *ichthy*osis

icter-   *ikteros* [Gr.] jaundice. *icter*ohepatitis

id-   *eidos* [Gr.] form, shape. homin*id*, dermatophyt*id*

idi-   *idios* [Gr.] peculiar, separate, distinct. *idi*osyncrasy

il-¹   See in-¹. *il*lumination

il-²   See in-². *il*legible

ile-   See ili- [ile- is commonly used to refer to the portion of the intestines known as the ileum]. *ile*ostomy

ili-   *ilium (ileum)* [L.] lower abdomen, intestines [ili- is commonly used to refer to the flaring part of the hip bone known as the ilium]. *ili*ofemoral

im-¹   See in-¹. *im*mersion

im-²   See in-². *im*perforate

in-¹   *in* [L.] (*n* changes to *l* before *l*, *m* before *b*, *m*, or *p*, and *r* before *r*) in, on. Cf. en-. *in*sertion

in-²   *in-* [L.] (*n* changes to *l* before *l*, *m* before *b*, *m*, or *p*, and *r* before *r*) negative prefix. Cf. a-¹. *in*compatible

in-³   *is, inos* [Gr.] fiber. Cf. fibr-. *in*otropic

infra-   *infra* [L.] beneath. *infra*orbital

insul-   *insula* [L.] island. *insul*in

inter-   *inter* [L.] among, between. *inter*costal

intra-   *intra* [L.] inside. Cf. end- and eso-. *intra*venous

intro-   *intro* [L.] within. *intro*spection

ir-¹   See in-¹. *ir*radiation

ir-²   See in-². *ir*reducible

irid-   *iris, iridos* [Gr.] rainbow, colored circle. *irid*ocyclitis

is-   *isos* [Gr.] equal. *is*otope

isch-   *ischein* [Gr.] to suppress. *isch*emia

ischi-   *ischion* [Gr.] hip, haunch. *ischi*opubic

-ism   *-ismos* [Gr.] noun-forming suffix. vegetarian*ism*, thigmotrop*ism*, alcohol*ism*

-itis   *-itis* [Gr.] inflammation. dermat*itis*, phleb*itis*

-ize   *-izein* [Gr.] verb-forming suffix. cauter*ize*, oxid*ize*

jact-   *iacio, iactus* [L.] throw. *jact*itation

-ject   *iacio, -iectus* [L.] throw. in*ject*ion

jejun-   *ieiunus* [L.] empty. gastro*jejun*ostomy

jug-   *iugum* [L.] yoke. con*jug*ation

junct-   *iungo, iunctus* [L.] yoke, join. con*junct*iva

juxta-   *juxta* [L.] near, close by. *juxta*glomerular

kary-   *karyon* [Gr.] nut, kernel, nucleus. Cf. nucle-. mega*kary*ocyte (Also spelled cary-)

kerat-   *keras, keratos* [Gr.] horn. *kerat*olysis (Also spelled cerat-)

kilo-   *chilioi* [Gr.] one thousand. Cf. milli-. Indicates multiple in metric system. *kilo*gram

kine-   *kineō* [Gr.] move. *kine*sthesia (Also spelled cine-)

koil-   *koilos* [Gr.] hollow. *koil*onychia

labi-   *labium* [L.] lip. Cf. cheil-. *labi*omental

lact-   *lac, lactis* [L.] milk. Cf. galact-. *lact*iferous

lal-   *laleō* [Gr.] talk, babble. glosso*lal*ia

lapar-   *lapara* [Gr.] flank. *lapar*otomy

laryng-   *larynx, laryngos* [Gr.] windpipe. *laryng*ectomy

lat-   *fero, latus* [L.] bear, carry. See -ferent. trans*lat*ion

later-   *latus, lateris* [L.] side. ventro*later*al

lecith-   *lekithos* [Gr.] yolk. iso*lecith*al

leio-   *leios* [Gr.] smooth. *leio*myoma

-lemma   *lemma* [Gr.] rind, husk. axo*lemma*

lent-   *lens, lentis* [L.] lentil. Cf. phac-. *lent*iconus

lep-   *lambanō, lēp-* [Gr.] take, seize. cata*lep*sy

lept-   *leptos* [Gr.] slender. *lept*omeninges

leuc-   See leuk-. *leuc*ine

leuk-   *leukos* [Gr.] white. Cf. alb-. *leuk*orrhea (Also spelled leuc-)

lev-   *laevus* [L.] left. *lev*ocardia, *lev*orotatory

lien-   *lien* [L.] spleen. Cf. splen-. *lien*ocele

lig-   *ligo* [L.] tie, bind. *lig*ature

lingu-   *lingua* [L.] tongue. Cf. gloss-. sub*lingu*al

lip-   *lipos* [Gr.] fat. Cf. adip-. glyco*lip*id

lith-   *lithos* [Gr.] stone. Cf. calc-[1]. nephro*lith*otomy

loc-   *locus* [L.] place. Cf. top-. *loc*omotion

log-   *legō, log-* [Gr.] speak, give an account. *log*orrhea, embryo*logy*

lumb-   *lumbus* [L.] loin. *lumb*ago

lute-   *luteus* [L.] yellow. Cf. xanth-. *lute*oma

ly-   *lyō* [Gr.] loose, dissolve. Cf. solut-. *ly*ophilization

lymph-   *lympha* [Gr.] water. cf. hydr-. *lymph*adenopathy

lys-   *lysis* [Gr.] dissolution. kerato*lys*is, *lys*ogen

macr-   *makros* [Gr.] long, large. *macr*omyeloblast

mal-   *malus* [L.] bad, abnormal. Cf. cac- and dys-. *mal*formation

malac-   *malakos* [Gr.] soft. osteo*malac*ia

mamm-   *mamma* [L.] breast. Cf. mast-. sub*mamm*ary

man-   *manus* [L.] hand. Cf. cheir-. *man*ipulation

mani-   *mania* [Gr.] mental aberration. klepto*mani*a

mast-   *mastos* [Gr.] breast. Cf. mamm-. hyper*mast*ia

mechan-   *mēchanē* [Gr.] machine. *mechan*oreceptor

medi-   *medius* [L.] middle. Cf. mes-. *medi*olateral

mega-   *megas* [Gr.] great, large. Also indicates multiple (1,000,000) in metric system. *mega*colon, *mega*volt (See also megal-)

megal-   *megas, megalou* [Gr.] great, large. acro*megaly*

mel-[1]   *melos* [Gr.] limb, member. sym*mel*ia

mel-[2]   *mēlon* [Gr.] cheek. *mel*oplasty

melan-   *melas, melanos* [Gr.] black. *melan*oglossia

men-   *mēn* [Gr.] month. dys*men*orrhea

mening-   *mēninx, mēningos* [Gr.] membrane. encephalo*mening*itis

ment-   *mens, mentis* [L.] mind. Cf. phren-, psych-, and thym-[2]. de*ment*ia

mer-   *meros* [Gr.] part. poly*mer*ic

mes-   *mesos* [Gr.] middle. Cf. medi-. *mes*oderm

meta-   *meta* [Gr.] (*a* is dropped before words beginning with a vowel) after, beyond, accompanying. *meta*carpal, *met*encephalon

metr-[1]   *metron* [Gr.] measure. audio*metr*y

metr-[2]   *metra* [Gr.] womb. Cf. hyster- and uter-. endo*metr*itis

micr-   *mikros* [Gr.] small. Also indicates fraction (one-millionth) in metric system. photo*micr*ograph, *micr*ogram

milli-   *mille* [L.] one thousand. Also indicates fraction in metric system (one-thousandth). Cf. kilo-. *milli*gram

-mimetic   *mimētikos* [Gr.] mimetic. sympatho*mimetic*

miss-   See -mittent. intro*miss*ion

mit-   *mitos* [Gr.] thread. *mit*ochondria

-mittent   *mitto, mittentis, missus* [L.] send. inter*mittent*

mne-   *mimnēskō, mnē-* [Gr.] remember. a*mne*sia

mon-   *monos* [Gr.] only, sole. *mon*oplegia

morph-   *morphē* [Gr.] form, shape. poly*morph*onuclear

mot-   *moveo, motus* [L.] move. vaso*mot*or

muc-   *mucus* [L.] mucus. *muc*ilage, *muc*ogingival, *muc*oprotein

multi-   *multus* [L.] many, much. *multi*para

my-   *mys, myos* [Gr.] muscle. leio*my*oma

-myces   *mykēs, mykētos* [Gr.] fungus. Strepto*myces*

myc(et)-   See -myces. strepto*myc*in, *myc*etoma

myel-   *myelos* [Gr.] marrow. polio*myel*itis

myring-   *myringa* [L.] membrane. *myring*otomy

myx   *myxa* [Gr.] mucus. *myx*edema

nan-   *nanos* [Gr.] dwarf. Also indicates fraction (one-billionth) in metric system. *nan*ophthalmos, *nan*ogram

narc-   *narkē* [Gr.] numbness. *narc*olepsy

nas-   *nasus* [L.] nose. Cf. rhin-. *nas*opalatine

ne-   *neos* [Gr.] new, young. *ne*onate

necr-   *nekros* [Gr.] corpse. *necr*ophilia

nephr-   *nephros* [Gr.] kidney. Cf. ren-. para*nephr*ic

neur   *neuron* [Gr.] nerve. *neur*algia

nev-   *naevus* [L.] mole. *nev*olipoma

noci-   *nocēo* [L.] to injure. *noci*ceptor

nod-   *nodus* [L.] knot. *nod*osity

nom-   *nomos* [Gr.] (from *nemō* deal out, distribute) law, custom. taxo*nom*y

non-¹   *non* [L.] not. *non*disjunction

non-²   *nona* [L.] nine. *non*apeptide

norm-   *norma* [L.] rule. *norm*otensive

nos-   *nosos* [Gr.] disease. *nos*ology

not-   *nōton* [Gr.] back. *not*ochord

nucle-   *nucleus* [L.] (from *nux, nucis* nut) kernel. Cf. kary-. *nucle*ocapsid

nutri-   *nutrio* [L.] nourish. mal*nu*trition

ob-   *ob* [L.] (*b* changes to *c* before words beginning with that consonant) against, toward. *ob*tusion

oc-   See ob-. *oc*clude

oct-   *oktō* [Gr.] or *octo* [L.] eight. *oct*igravida

ocul-   *oculus* [L.] eye. Cf. ophthalm-. *ocul*omotor

-od-   See -ode¹. esthes*od*ic

-ode¹   *hodos* [Gr.] road, path. cath*ode*. (See also hod-)

-ode²   See -oid. nemat*ode*

odont-   *odous, odontos* [Gr.] tooth. Cf. dent-. ortho*dont*ist

-odyn-   *odynē* [Gr.] pain, distress. gastr*odyn*ia

-oid   *eidos* [Gr.] form. Cf. -form. hy*oid*

-ol   See ole-. cholester*ol*

ole-   *oleum* [L.] oil. *ole*oresin

olig-   *oligos* [Gr.] few, small. *olig*ospermia

om-   *ōmos* [Gr.] shoulder. *om*ohyoid

-oma   *-ōma* [Gr.] noun-forming suffix. Used to denote a neoplasm. hepat*oma*, carcin*oma*

omphal-   *omphalos* [Gr.] navel. *omphal*ectomy

onc-   *onkos* [Gr.] bulk, mass. *onc*ogenesis

onych-	*onyx, onychos* [Gr.] claw, nail. an*onychia*
oo-	*ōon* [Gr.] egg. Cf. ov-. peri*oo*phoritis
oophor-	*ōophoros* [Gr.] bearing eggs. Cf. ovari-. *oophor*ectomy
op-	*ōps, ōp-* [Gr.] see. heter*op*sia
ophthalm-	*ophthalmos* [Gr.] eye. Cf. ocul-. ex*ophthalmos*
opisth-	*opisthen* [Gr.] behind, at the back. *opisth*otonos
or-	*os, oris* [L.] mouth. Cf. stom(at)-. ab*or*al
orb-	*orbis* [L.] circle. sub*orb*ital
orchi-	*orchis* [Gr.] testicle. Cf. test-. *orchi*opathy
organ-	*organon* [Gr.] implement, instrument. *organ*omegaly
orth-	*orthos* [Gr.] straight, right, normal. *orth*opedics
oscill-	*oscillare* [L.] to swing. *oscill*opsia
-osis	*-osis* [Gr.] noun-forming suffix. Used to denote a process, particularly a disease. dermat*osis*, acid*osis*
osm-¹	*osmē* [Gr.] odor. *osm*ophore
osm-²	*ōsmos* [Gr.] impulse. *osm*oregulation
oss-	*os, ossis* [L.] bone. Cf. ost(e)-. *oss*iferous
ost(e)-	*osteon* [Gr.] bone. Cf. oss-. en*ost*osis, *oste*oarthritis
-ostomy	*stoma* [Gr.] mouth. col*ostomy*
ot-	*ous, ōtos* [Gr.] ear. Cf. aur-. par*ot*id, *ot*otoxic
ov-	*ovum* [L.] egg. Cf. oo-. syn*ov*ia, *ov*ovegetarian
ovari-	*ovarium* [L.] ovary. Cf. oophor-, *ovari*opexy
oxy-	*oxys* [Gr.] (*y* is sometimes dropped, often denoting relationship to oxygen). sharp. *oxy*cephalic, *ox*idation
pachy-	*pachynō* [Gr.] thick. *pachy*derma
pag-	*pēgnymi, pag-* [Gr.] fix, make fast. thoraco*pag*us
palat-	*palatum* [L.] palate. Cf. uran-. *palat*orrhaphy
pale-	*palaios* [Gr.] old. *pale*ocortex
pali(n)-	*palin* [Gr.] backward, again. *palin*opsia
pan-	*pan* [Gr.] all. *pan*demic
par-¹	*pario* [L.] bear, give birth to. primi*para*
par-²	See para-. *par*occipital
para-	*para* [Gr.] (final *a* is sometimes dropped before words beginning with a vowel) beside, beyond. *para*cervical, *para*oral, *par*amnesia
part-	*pario, partus* [L.] bear, give birth to. *part*urition
path-	*pathos* [Gr.] that which one undergoes, sickness. cyto*path*ic, cardio*pathy*
pec-	*pēgnymi, pēg-* [Gr.] (*pēk-* before *t*) fix, makes fast. amylo*pec*tin (See also pex-)
ped-¹	*pais, paidos* [Gr.] child. *ped*iatrics
ped-²	*pes, pedis* [L.] foot. *ped*orthics
pell-	*pellis* [L.] skin, hide. *pell*agra
-pellent	*pello, pellentis, pulsus* [L.] drive. re*pellent*
pen-	*penomai* [Gr.] need, lack. neutro*pen*ia
pend-	*pendeo* [L.] hang down. ap*pend*ix
pent(a)-	*pente* [Gr.] five. Cf. quint-. *pent*ose, *penta*gastrin
peps-	*peptō, peps-* [Gr.] digest. eu*peps*ia
pept-	*peptō* [Gr.] digest. dys*pept*ic
per-	*per* [L.] through. Cf. dia-. *per*oral
peri-	*peri* [Gr.] around. Cf. circum-. *peri*phery
pero-	*pēros* [Gr.] maimed. *pero*melia
pet-	*peto* [L.] seek, tend toward. centri*pet*al
pex-	*pēgnymi, pēg-* [Gr.] (*pēg-* added to *s* becomes *pēx-*) fix, make fast. hepato*pexy*
pha-	*phēmi, pha-* [Gr.] say, speak. dys*pha*sia
phac-	*phakos* [Gr.] lentil, lens. Cf. lent-. *phac*osclerosis. (Also spelled phak-)
phag-	*phagein* [Gr.] eat. dys*phag*ia
phak-	See phac-. *phak*itis
phall-	*phallos* [Gr.] penis. *phall*oplasty
phan-	See phen-. *phan*erosis

pharmac-   *pharmakon* [Gr.] drug. *pharmaco*gnosy

pharyng-   *pharynx, pharyng-* [Gr.] throat. *pharyng*ocele

phen-   *phainō, phan-* [Gr.] show, be seen. phos*phene, pheno*copy

pher-   *pherō, phor-* [Gr.] bear, support. Cf. -ferent. peri*phery*

phil-   *phileō* [Gr.] like, have affinity for. eosino*phil*ia

phleb-   *phleps, phlebos* [Gr.] vein. Cf. ven-. peri*phleb*itis

phleg-   *phlogō, phlog-* [Gr.] burn, inflame. *phleg*mon

phlog-   See phleg-. *phlog*ogenic

phob-   *phobos* [Gr.] fear, dread. claustro*phob*ia

phon-   *phōne* [Gr.] sound. *phono*cardiography

phor-   See pher-. Cf. -ferent. exo*phor*ia

phos-   See phot-. *phos*phorus

phot-   *phōs, phōtos* [Gr.] light. *phot*ophobia

phrag-   *phrassō, phrag-* [Gr.] fence, wall off, stop up. Cf. sept-[1]. dia*phrag*m

phrax-   *phrassō, phrag-* [Gr.] (*phrag-* added to *s* becomes *phrax-*) fence, wall off, stop up. salpingem*phrax*is

phren-   *phrēn* [Gr.] mind, midriff. Cf. ment-. *phren*oplegia, *phren*otropic

phthi-   *phthinō* [Gr.] decay, waste away. *phthi*sis

phy-   *phyō* [Gr.] beget, bring forth, produce, be by nature. osteo*phy*te

phyl-   *phylon* [Gr.] tribe, kind. *phyl*ogeny

phylac-   *phylax* [Gr.] guard. pro*phylac*tic

-phyll   *phyllon* [Gr.] leaf. chloro*phyll*

phys-   *physaō* [Gr.] blow, inflate. *phys*ometra

physe-   *physaō, physē* [Gr.] blow, inflate. em*physe*ma

physi-   *physis* [Gr.] nature. *physi*ology

pil-   *pilus* [L.] hair. e*pil*ation

pituit-   *pituita* [L.] phlegm, rheum. *pituit*ary

placent-   *placenta* [L.] (from *plakous* [Gr.]) cake. extra*placent*al

plas-   *plassō* [Gr.] mold, shape. rhino*plas*ty

platy-   *platy-* [Gr.] broad, flat. *platy*podia

pleg-   *plēssō, pleg-* [Gr.] strike. di*pleg*ia

pleo-   *pleiōn* [Gr.] more. *pleo*morphism, *pleio*tropy (Also spelled pleio-)

plet-   *pleo, -pletus* [L.] fill. *pleth*ora

pleur-   *pleura* [Gr.] rib, side. Cf. cost-. *pleur*algia

plex-   *plēssō, plēg-* [Gr.] (*plēg-* added to *s* becomes *plēx-*) strike. apo*plex*y

plic-   *plico* [L.] fold. com*plic*ation, *plic*ate

pluri-   *plus, pluris* [L.] more. *pluri*glandular

pne-   *pneō* [Gr.] breathe. orthop*ne*a

pneum(at)-   *pneuma, pneumatos* [Gr.] breath, air. *pneum*arthrosis, *pneumat*ocele

pneumo(n)-   *pneumōn* [Gr.] lung. Cf. pulmo(n)-. *pneumo*enteritis, *pneumo*notomy

pod-   *pous, podos* [Gr.] foot. *pod*iatry

poie-   *poieō* [Gr.] make, produce. Cf. -facient. sarco*poie*tic

poikil-   *poikilos* [Gr.] spotted, mottled, varied. *poikil*oderma

pol-   *polos* [Gr.] axis of a sphere. uni*pol*ar

poli-   *polios* [Gr.] gray. *poli*omyelopathy

poly-   *polys* [Gr.] much, many. *poly*spermy

pont-   *pons, pontis* [L.] bridge. *pont*ocerebellar

por-[1]   *poros* [Gr.] passage. *por*adenitis

por-[2]   *pōros* [Gr.] callus. *por*okeratosis

posit-   *pono, positus* [L.] put, place. re*posit*or

post-   *post* [L.] after, behind in time or place. *post*natal, *post*renal

pre-   *prae* [L.] before in time or place. *pre*natal, *pre*vesical

presby- — *presbys* [Gr.] old man. *pres-byopia*

press- — *premo, pressus* [L.] press. *press*oreceptive

pro- — *pro* [Gr.] or *pro* [L.] before in time or place. *pro*hormone, *pro*labium, *pro*lapse

proct- — *prōktos* [Gr.] anus. Cf. rect-. *proct*ology

prosop- — *prosōpon* [Gr.] face. Cf. faci-. *prosop*agnosia

prot- — *prōtos* [Gr.] first. *prot*oplasm

pseud- — *pseudēs* [Gr.] false. *pseudo*-paraplegia

psych- — *psychē* [Gr.] soul, mind. Cf. ment-. *psych*osomatic

pto- — *piptō, ptō-* [Gr.] fall. neph-*ropto*sis

ptyal- — *ptyalon* [Gr.] saliva. *ptyal*ism

pub- — *pubes* [L.] adult. ischio*pub*ic. (See also puber-)

puber- — *puber* [L.] adult. *puber*ty

pulmo(n)- — *pulmo, pulmonis* [L.] lung. Cf. pneumo(n)-. cardio*pulmon*ary

puls- — *pello, pellentis, pulsus* [L.] drive. pro*puls*ion

punct- — *pungo, punctus* [L.] prick, pierce. Cf. cente-. *puncti*form

pupill- — *pupilla* [L.] girl or pupil. *pupill*ometry

pur- — *pus, puris* [L.] pus. Cf. py-. sup*pur*ation

py- — *pyon* [Gr.] pus. Cf. pur-. nephro*py*osis

pyel- — *pyelos* [Gr.] trough, basin, pelvis. nephro*pyel*itis

pykn- — *pyknos* [Gr.] thick, frequent. *pykn*ocyte

pyl- — *pylē* [Gr.] door, orifice. *pyl*ephlebitis

pyr- — *pyr* [Gr.] fire. Cf. febr-. *pyr*ogen

quadr- — *quadr-* [L.] four. Cf. tetra-. *quadr*igeminal

quint- — *quintus* [L.] fifth. Cf. pent(a)-. *quint*uplet

rachi- — *rhachis* [Gr.] spine. Cf. spin-. *rachi*odynia

radi- — *radius* [L.] ray. Cf. actin-. ir*radi*ation, *radio*carpal

re- — *re-* [L.] back, again. *re*traction

rect- — *rectum* [L.] rectum. Cf. proct-. *recto*cele

ren- — *renes* [L.] kidneys. Cf. nephr-. ad*renal*, *reno*vascular

ret- — *rete* [L.] net. *reti*form

retr- — *retro* [L.] backwards. *retro*deviation

rhabd- — *rhabdos* [Gr.] rod. *rhabdo*myolysis

rhag- — *rhēgnymi, rhag-* [Gr.] break, burst. hemor*rhage*

rhaph- — *rhaphē* [Gr.] suture. arterior*rhaphy*

rhe- — *rheos* [Gr.] flow. Cf. flu-. diar*rhea*l

rhex- — *rhēgnymi, rhēg-* [Gr.] (*rhēg-* added to *s* becomes *rhēx-*) break, burst. metror*rhexis*

rhin- — *rhis, rhinos* [Gr.] nose. Cf. nas-. *rhino*plasty

rot- — *rota* [L.] wheel. *rot*ation

rub(r)- — *ruber, rubri* [L.] red. Cf. erythr-. bili*rub*in, *rubro*spinal

racchar- — *sakcharon* [Gr.] sugar. *sacchar*ide

salping- — *salpinx, salpingos* [Gr.] tube, trumpet. *salping*itis

sangui(n)- — *sanguis, sanguinis* [L.] blood, Cf. hem(at)-. *sangui*facient, *sanguin*eous

sarc- — *sarx, sarkos* [Gr.] flesh. *sarc*oma

schis- — *schizō, schid-* [Gr.] (*schid-* before *t* or added to *s* becomes *schis-*) split. Cf. fiss-. *schis*tocyte, thoraco*schis*is (Also spelled *schiz-*)

schiz- — See schis-. *schiz*onychia

scler- — *sklēros* [Gr.] hard. Cf. dur-. *scler*osis

scop- — *skopeō* [Gr.] look at, observe. endo*scop*e

sect- — *seco, sectus* [L.] cut. Cf. tom-. *sect*ion

semi- — *semi-* [L.] half. Cf. hemi-. *semi*flexion

sens- — *sentio, sensus* [L.] perceive, feel. Cf. esthe-. *sens*ory

sep- — *sepō* [Gr.] rot, decay. *sep*sis

sept-[1] — *saepio, saeptus* [L.] fence, wall off, stop up. Cf. phrag-. *septo*nasal

sept-²   *septum* [L.] seven. Cf. hept(a)-. *sept*uplet

ser-   *serum* [L.] whey, watery substance. *ser*osynovitis

sex-¹   *sex* [L.] six. Cf. hex(a)-. *sex*tuplet

sex-²   *sexus* [L.] sex. *sex*duction

sial-   *sialon* [Gr.] saliva. *sial*adenitis

sider-   *sidéros* [Gr.] iron. *sider*oblast

sin-   *sinus* [L.] hollow, fold, Cf. colp-. *sin*obronchitis

sinistr-   *sinister* [L.] left. *sinistr*ocerebral

-sis   *-sis* [Gr.] suffix of action. amebia*sis*, psycho*sis*, diagno*sis*

sit-   *sitos* [Gr.] food. para*sit*e

solut-   *solvo, solventis, solutus* [L.] loose, dissolve, set free. Cf. ly-. dis*solut*ion

-solvent   See solut-. re*solvent*

som(at)-   *sōma, somatos* [Gr.] body. Cf. corpor-. psycho*somat*ic, chromo*som*e

somn-   *somnus* [L.] sleep. *somn*ambulism

spas-   *spaō, spas-* [Gr.] draw, pull. *spas*m, *spas*tic

spectr-   *spectrum* [L.] appearance, what is seen. micro*spectr*oscope

sperm(at)-   *sperma, spermatos* [Gr.] seed. *sperm*icide, *spermat*ozoon

spers-   *spargo, -spersus* [L.] scatter. di*spers*ion

sphen-   *sphēn* [Gr.] wedge. Cf. cune-. *sphen*oid

spher-   *sphaira* [Gr.] ball. hemi*spher*e

sphygm-   *sphygmos* [Gr.] pulsation. *sphygm*omanometer

spin-   *spina* [L.] spine. Cf. rachi-. *spin*ocerebellar

spir-   *speira* [Gr.] coil. *spir*ochete

spir(at)-   *spiro, spiratus* [L.] breathe. *spir*ometry, re*spirat*ory

splanchn-   *splanchna* [Gr.] entrails, viscera. neuro*splanchn*ic

splen-   *splēn* [Gr.] spleen. Cf. lien-. *splen*omegaly

spondyl-   *spondylos* [Gr.] vertebra. *spondyl*olisthesis

spongi-   *spongia* [L.] sponge. *spongi*oblastoma

spor-   *sporos* [Gr.] seed. *spor*ocyst, zoo*spor*e

squam-   *squama* [L.] scale. de*squam*ation

sta-   *histēmi, sta-* [Gr.] make stand, stop. hemo*sta*sis

stal-   *stellō, stal-* [Gr.] send. peri*stal*sis (See also -stol-)

staphyl-   *staphylē* [Gr.] bunch of grapes, uvula. *staphylo*coccus, *staphyl*edema

stear-   *stear, steatos* [Gr.] fat. Cf. adip-. *stear*ate

steat-   See stear-. *steat*orrhea

sten-   *stenos* [Gr.] narrow, compressed. *sten*othorax

ster-   *stereos* [Gr.] solid. chole*ster*ol

sterc-   *stercus* [L.] dung. Cf. copr-. *sterc*oroma

steth-   *stēthos* [Gr.] chest. *steth*oscope

sthen-   *sthenos* [Gr.] strength. a*sthen*ia

-stol-   *stellō, stol-* [Gr.] send. dia*stol*e

stom(at)-   *stoma, stomatos* [Gr.] mouth, orifice. Cf. or-. ana*stom*osis, *stomat*algia

strep(h)-   *strephō, strep-* (before *t*) [Gr.] twist. Cf. tors-. *strepho*symbolia, *strep*tomycin (See also stroph-)

strict-   *stringo, stringentis, strictus* [L.] draw tight, compress, cause pain. con*strict*ion

-stringent   See strict-. a*stringent*

stroph-   *strephō, stroph-* [Gr.] twist. dia*stroph*ic (See also streph-)

struct-   *struo, structus* [L.] pile up (against). ob*struct*ion

sub-   *sub* [L.] (*b* changes to *f* and *p* before words beginning with those consonants) under, below. Cf. hypo-. *sub*lingual

suf-   See sub-. *suf*fusion

sup-   See sub-. *sup*pository

super-   *super* [L.] above, beyond, extreme. Cf. hyper-. *super*motility

supra-   *supra* [L.] above. *supra*duction

sy-   See syn-. *sy*stole

sym- See syn-. *sym*biosis, *sym*metry, *sym*pathetic, *sym*physis

syn- *syn* [Gr.] (*n* disappears before *s*, changes to *l* before *l*, and changes to *m* before *b*, *m*, *p*, and *ph*) with, together. Cf. con-. *syn*arthrosis

syring- *syrinx, syringos* [Gr.] pipe, tube, fistula. *syring*ocystadenoma

ta- See ton-. ectasia

tac- *tassō, tag-* [Gr.] (*tag-* changes to *tak-* before *t*) order, arrange. a*tac*tiform

tach(y)- *tachys* [Gr.] swift. *tach*ography, *tachy*cardia

tact- *tango, tactus* [L.] touch. con*tact*

taenia *taenia* [L.] tape. *taenia*fuge (Also spelled tenia-)

tars- *tarsos* [Gr.] a broad, flat surface. *tars*orrhaphy, *tars*oclasis

tax- *tassō, tag-* [Gr.] (*tag-* added to *s* becomes *tax-*) order, arrange. a*tax*ia

tect- See teg-. pro*tect*ive

teg- *tego, tectus* [L.] cover. in*teg*ument

tel- *telos* [Gr.] end. *tel*omere

tele- *tēle* [Gr.] at a distance. *tele*ceptor

tempor- *tempus, temporis* [L.] time, temple. *tempor*omandibular

tend(in)- *tendo, tendines* [L.] tendon. *tend*ovaginal, *tendin*itis

ten(ont)- *tenōn, tenontos* [Gr.] (from *teinō* stretch) tight stretched band. *ten*odynia, *tenont*ology

tens- *tendo, tensus* [L.] stretch. Cf. ton-. ex*tens*or

terat- *teras, teratos* [Gr.] monster. *terat*oma

ter(ti)- *ter* [L.] thrice. Cf. tri-. *ter*nary, *terti*gravida

test- *testis* [L.] testicle. Cf. orchi-. *test*itis

tetr(a)- *tetra-* [L.] four. Cf. quadr-. *tetra*dactyly

thanat- *thanatos* [Gr.] death. *thanat*ognomonic

the- *tithēmi, thē-* [Gr.] put, place. syn*the*sis

thec- *thēkē* [Gr.] repository, case. *thec*ostegnosis

thel- *thēlē* [Gr.] teat, nipple. *thel*erethism, *thele*plasty

-therap- *therapeia* [Gr.] treatment. chemo*therap*y

therm- *thermē* [Gr.] heat. Cf. calor-. dia*therm*y

thi- *theion* [Gr.] sulfur. *thi*azide, *thi*ocynate

thorac- *thōrax, thōrakos* [Gr.] chest. *thorac*oplasty

-thrix See trich-. monile*thrix*

thromb- *thrombos* [Gr.] lump, clot. *thromb*ocytopenia

thym-¹ *thymos* [Gr.] thymus. *thym*oma

thym-² *thymos* [Gr.] spirit. Cf. ment-. dys*thym*ia, *thym*oleptic

thyr- *thyreos* [Gr.] shield (shaped like a door [*thyra*]). *thyr*oid

tme- *temnō, tmē-* [Gr.] cut. axono*tme*sis

toc- *tokos* [Gr.] childbirth. dys*toc*ia

tom- *temnō, tom-* [Gr.] cut. Cf. sect-. appendec*tom*y, *tom*ography

ton- *teino, ton-, ta-* [Gr.] stretch, put under tension. Cf. tens-. peri*ton*eum

top- *topos* [Gr.] place. Cf. loc-. *top*esthesia, iso*top*e

tors- *torqueo, torsus* [L.] twist. Cf. streph-. *tors*ion

tox(ic)- *toxikon* [Gr.] (from *toxon* bow) arrow poison, poison. *tox*emia, *toxic*ology

trache- *tracheia* [Gr.] windpipe. *trache*otomy

trachel- *trachēlos* [Gr.] neck. Cf. cervic-. *trachel*opexy

tract- *traho, tractus* [L.] draw, drag. pro*tract*ion

trans- *trans* [L.] through, *trans*aortic, *trans*fer

traumat- *trauma, traumatos* [Gr.] wound. *traumat*ic

tri- *treis, tria* [Gr.] or *tri-* [L.] three. *tri*laminar

trich- *thrix, trichos* [Gr.] hair. *trich*obezoar

trip- *tribō* [Gr.] rub. litho*trip*sy

trop- *trepō, trop-* [Gr.] turn, react. sito*trop*ism

troph- *trepō, troph-* [Gr.] nurture. a*troph*y

tub- *tubus* [L.] pipe. *tub*oplasty

tuber- *tuber* [L.] swelling, node. *tuber*cle

tympan- *tympanon* [Gr.] drum. *tympan*ocentesis

typ- *typos* [Gr.] (from *typto* strike) type. a*typ*ical

typh- *typhos* [Gr.] fog, stupor. *typh*us

typhl- *typhlos* [Gr.] blind. Cf. cec-. *typhl*ectasis

ul-¹ *oulē* [Gr.] scar. *ul*erythema

ul-² *oulon* [Gr.] gum. *ul*orrhagia

ultra- *ultra* [L.] beyond. *ultra*structure

uni- *unus* [L.] one. *uni*lateral

ur- *ouron* [Gr.] urine. poly*ur*ia

uran- *ouranos* [Gr.] the vault of heaven, or the roof of the mouth. Cf. palat-. *uran*ostaphyloschisis

ureter- *ourētēr* [Gr.] ureter. *uretero*graphy

urethr- *ourēthra* [Gr.] urethra. *urethr*opexy

uter- *uterus* [L.] womb. Cf. hyster- and metr-. *uter*orectal

vacc- *vacca* [L.] cow. *vacc*ine

vagin- *vagina* [L.] sheath. in*vagin*ation, *vagin*itis

varic- *varix, varicis* [L.] varicose vein. *varic*ocele

vas- *vas* [L.] vessel. Cf. angi-. *vas*cular

ven- *vena* [L.] vein. Cf. phleb-. *ven*opressor

ventr- *venter* [L.] belly. *ventr*ofixation, *ventr*iculotomy

vers- See vert-. in*vers*ion

vert- *verto, versus* [L.] turn. di*vert*iculum

vesic- *vesica* [L.] bladder. Cf. cyst-. *vesic*ovaginal

viscer- *viscus, visceris* [L.] internal organs. *viscer*omotor

vit- *vita* [L.] life. Cf. bi-¹. de*vit*alize

vivi- *vivus* [L.] alive. *vivi*parous

vuls- *vello, vulsus* [L.] pull, twitch. con*vuls*ion

xanth- *xanthos* [Gr.] yellow, blond. Cf. flav- and lute-. *xanth*ochromia

xen- *xenos* [Gr.] strange, foreign. *xen*ograft

xer- *xēros* [Gr.] dry. *xer*oderma

-yl- *hyle* [Gr.] substance. carbox*yl*

zo- *zoē* [Gr.] life or *zōon* [Gr.] animal. micro*zo*on

zyg- *zygon* [Gr.] yoke, union. *zyg*odactyly

zym- *zymē* [Gr.] ferment. en*zym*e

A

A accommodation; adenine or adenosine; alanine; ampere; anode; anterior.

A absorbance; activity (3); area; mass number.

A₂ aortic second sound.

Å angstrom.

a accommodation; atto-.

a. [L.] an′num (year); a′qua (water); arte′ria (artery).

a-¹ word element [Gr.], *without, not.*

a-² word element [L.], *separation, away from.*

a activity (2).

α (alpha, the first letter of the Greek alphabet) heavy chain of IgA; α chain of hemoglobin.

α- a prefix designating (1) the position of a substituting atom or group in a chemical compound; (2) the specific rotation of an optically active compound; (3) the orientation of an exocyclic atom or group; (4) a plasma protein migrating with the α band in electrophoresis; (5) first in a series of related entities or chemical compounds.

AA achievement age; Alcoholics Anonymous; amino acid.

AA ana (of each), used in prescription writing.

aa. [L.] arte′riae (arteries).

AAA American Association of Anatomists.

AAAS American Association for the Advancement of Science.

AABB American Association of Blood Banks.

AACP American Academy of Child Psychiatry.

AAD American Academy of Dermatology.

AADP American Academy of Denture Prosthetics.

AADR American Academy of Dental Radiology.

AADS American Association of Dental Schools.

AAE American Association of Endodontists.

AAFP American Academy of Family Physicians.

AAI American Association of Immunologists.

AAID American Academy of Implant Dentistry.

AAIN American Association of Industrial Nurses.

AAMA American Association of Medical Assistants.

AAMT American Association for Medical Transcription.

AANP American Association of Naturopathic Physicians.

AAO American Association of Orthodontists; American Academy of Ophthalmology; American Academy of Otolaryngology; American Academy of Osteopathy.

AAOP American Academy of Oral Pathology.

AAOS American Academy of Orthopaedic Surgeons.

AAP American Academy of Pediatrics; American Academy of Pedodontics; American Academy of Periodontology; American Association of Pathologists.

AAPA American Academy of Physician Assistants.

AAPMR American Academy of Physical Medicine and Rehabilitation.

AARC American Association for Respiratory Care.

AATA American Art Therapy Association.

AB [L.] Ar′tium Baccalau′reus (Bachelor of Arts).

Ab antibody.

ab [L.] preposition, *from.*

ab- word element [L.], *from; off; away from.*

abac·a·vir (ah-bak′ah-vir) a nonnucleoside reverse transcriptase inhibitor used as the sulfate salt as an antiretroviral in the treatment of human immunodeficiency virus infection.

abar·og·no·sis (a″bar-og-no′sis) baragnosis.

ab·ar·thro·sis (ab″ahr-thro′sis) abarticulation.

ab·ar·tic·u·la·tion (-ahr-tik″u-la′shun) 1. synovial joint. 2. dislocation of a joint.

aba·sia (ah-ba′zhah) inability to walk. **aba′sic, abat′ic,** adj. **a.-asta′sia,** astasia-abasia. **a. atac′tica,** abasia with uncertain movements, due to a defect of coordination. **choreic a.,** abasia due to chorea of the legs. **paralytic a.,** abasia due to paralysis of leg muscles. **paroxysmal trepidant a., spastic a.,** abasia due to spastic stiffening of the legs on attempting to stand. **a. tre′pidans,** abasia due to trembling of the legs.

abate·ment (ah-bāt′ment) decrease in severity of a pain or symptom.

ABC argon beam coagulator; aspiration biopsy cytology.

ab·cix·i·mab (ab-sik′sĭ-mab) a human-murine monoclonal antibody Fab fragment that inhibits the aggregation of platelets, used as an antithrombotic in percutaneous transluminal coronary angioplasty.

ab·do·men (ab′dah-men, ab-do′men) that part of the body lying between the thorax and the pelvis, and containing the abdominal cavity and viscera. **acute a.,** an acute intra-abdominal condition of abrupt onset, usually associated with pain due to inflammation, perforation, obstruction, infarction, or rupture of abdominal organs, and usually requiring emergency surgical intervention. **carinate a., navicular a.,** scaphoid a. **a. obsti′pum,** congenital shortness of the rectus abdominis muscle. **scaphoid a.,** one whose anterior wall is hollowed, occurring in children with cerebral disease. **surgical a.,** acute a.

ab·dom·i·nal (ab-dom′ĭ-n′l) pertaining to the abdomen.

abdomin(o)- word element [L.], *abdomen.*

ab·dom·i·no·cen·te·sis (ab-dom″ĭ-no-sen-te′sis) surgical puncture of the abdomen.

ab·dom·i·no·cys·tic (-sis′tik) pertaining to the abdomen and gallbladder.

ab·dom·i·no·hys·ter·ec·to·my (-his″ter-ek′tah-me) hysterectomy through an abdominal incision.

ab·dom·i·no·hys·ter·ot·o·my (-ot′ah-me) abdominal hysterotomy.

ab·dom·i·nos·co·py (ab-dom″ĭ-nos′kah-pe) laparoscopy.

ab·dom·i·no·vag·i·nal (ab-dom″ĭ-no-vaj′ĭ-n′l) pertaining to the abdomen and vagina.

ab·dom·i·no·ves·i·cal (-ves′ĭ-k′l) 1. abdominocystic. 2. pertaining to or connecting the abdominal cavity and urinary bladder.

ab·du·cens (ab-doo′senz) [L.] drawing away.

ab·duct (ab-dukt′) to draw away from the median plane, or (the digits) from the axial line of a limb. **abdu′cent,** adj.

ab·duc·tion (ab-duk′shun) the act of abducting; the state of being abducted.

ab·er·ran·cy (ab-er′an-se) aberration (3).

ab·er·rant (ah-ber′ant, ab′ur-ant) wandering or deviating from the usual or normal course.

ab·er·ra·tio (ab″er-a′she-o) [L.] aberration (1).

ab·er·ra·tion (-shun) 1. deviation from the normal or usual. 2. unequal refraction or focalization of a lens. 3. in cardiology, aberrant conduction. **chromatic a.,** unequal refraction of light rays of different wavelength, producing a blurred image with fringes of color. **chromosome a.,** an irregularity in the number or structure of chromosomes, usually a gain, loss, exchange, or alteration of sequence of genetic material, which often alters embryonic development. **intraventricular a.,** aberrant conduction within the ventricles of an impulse generated in the supraventricular region, excluding abnormalities due to fixed organic defects in conduction. **mental a.,** any pathological deviation from normal mental activity, usually limited to a circumscribed deviation in an otherwise adapted individual.

abeta·lipo·pro·tein·emia (a-ba″tah-lip″o-pro″te-ne′me-ah) a hereditary syndrome marked by a lack of lipoproteins that contain apolipoprotein B (chylomicrons, very-low-density lipoproteins, and low-density lipoproteins) in the blood and by acanthocytosis, hypocholesterolemia, progressive ataxic neuropathy, atypical retinitis pigmentosa, and malabsorption. **normotriglyceridemic a.,** a variant form in which apolipoprotein (apo) B-48 is present but apo B-100 is absent; chylomicrons are formed, and some fat absorption may occur.

abi·os·is (a″bi-o′sis) absence of life. **abiot′ic,** adj.

abi·ot·ro·phy (a″bi-ot′rah-fe) progressive loss of vitality of certain tissues, leading to disorders; applied to degenerative hereditary diseases of late onset, e.g., Huntington's chorea.

ab·la·tio (ab-la′she-o) [L.] ablation.

ab·la·tion (-shun) 1. separation or detachment; extirpation; eradication. 2. removal or destruction, especially by cutting.

able·pha·ria (a″blĕ-far′e-ah) cryptophthalmos. **ableph′arous,** adj.

ab·nor·mal (ab-nor′mal) not normal; contrary to the usual structure, position, condition, behavior, or rule.

ab·nor·mal·i·ty (ab″nor-mal′ĭ-te) 1. the state of being abnormal. 2. a malformation.

ab·orad (ab-or′ad) directed away from the mouth.

ab·oral (ab-or′al) opposite to, away from, or remote from the mouth.

abort (ah-bort′) 1. to arrest prematurely a disease or developmental process. 2. to cause, undergo, or experience abortion. 3. to become checked in development.

abor·ti·fa·cient (ah-bor″tĭ-fa′shent) 1. causing abortion. 2. an agent that induces abortion.

abor·tion (ah-bor′shun) 1. expulsion from the uterus of the products of conception before the fetus is viable. 2. premature stoppage of a natural or a pathological process. **artificial a.,** induced a. **complete a.,** one in which all the products of conception are expelled from the uterus and identified. **habitual a.,** spontaneous abortion occurring in three or more successive pregnancies, at about the same level of development. **incomplete a.,** that with retention of parts of the products of conception. **induced a.,** that brought on intentionally by medication or instrumentation. **inevitable a.,** a condition in which vaginal bleeding has been profuse and the cervix has become dilated, and abortion will invariably occur. **infected a.,** that associated with infection of the genital tract. **missed a.,** retention in the uterus of an abortus that has been dead for at least eight weeks. **septic a.,** that associated with serious infection of the uterus leading to generalized infection. **spontaneous a.,** that occurring naturally. **therapeutic a.,** that induced for medical considerations. **threatened a.,** a condition in which vaginal bleeding is less than in inevitable abortion and the cervix is not dilated, and abortion may or may not occur.

abor·tion·ist (ah-bor′shun-ist) one who performs abortions.

abor·tive (ah-bor′tiv) 1. incompletely developed. 2. abortifacient (1). 3. cutting short the course of a disease.

abor·tus (ah-bor′tus) a fetus weighing less than 500 g or having completed less than 20 weeks gestational age at the time of expulsion from the uterus, having no chance of survival.

abra·sio (ah-bra′se-o) [L.] abrasion. **a. cor′neae,** a rubbing off of the superficial layers of the cornea.

abra·sion (ah-bra′zhun) 1. a rubbing or scraping off through unusual or abnormal action; see also *planing.* 2. a rubbed or scraped area on skin or mucous membrane.

ab·re·ac·tion (ab″re-ak′shun) the reliving of an experience in such a way that previously repressed emotions associated with it are released.

ab·rup·tio (ab-rup′she-o) [L.] separation. **a. placen′tae,** premature detachment of the placenta.

ab·scess (ab′ses) a localized collection of pus in a cavity formed by disintegration of tissues. **amebic a.,** one caused by *Entamoeba histolytica,* usually occurring in the liver but also in the lungs, brain, and spleen. **apical a.,** a suppurative inflammatory reaction involving the tissues surrounding the apical portion of a tooth, occurring in acute and chronic forms. **appendiceal a., appendicular a.,** one resulting from perforation of an acutely inflamed appendix. **Bezold's a.,** one deep in the neck as a complication of acute mastoiditis. **brain a.,** one affecting the brain as a result of extension of an infection (e.g., otitis media) from an adjacent area, or through bloodborne infection. **Brodie's a.,** a roughly spherical region of bone destruction, filled with pus or connective tissue, usually in the metaphyseal region of long bones and caused by *Staphylococcus aureus* or *S. albus.* **cold a.,** 1. one of slow development and with little inflammation. 2. tuberculous a. **diffuse a.,** a collection of pus not enclosed by a capsule. **gas a.,** one containing gas, caused by gas-forming bacteria such as *Clostridium perfringens.* **miliary a.,** one of a set of small multiple abscesses. **Pautrier's a.,** see under *microabscess.* **peritonsillar a.,** one in the connective tissue of the tonsil capsule, from suppuration of the tonsil. **phlegmonous a.,** one associated with acute inflammation of the subcutaneous connective tissue. **ring a.,** a ring-shaped purulent infiltration at the periphery of the cornea. **shirt-stud a.,** one separated into two cavities connected by a narrow channel. **stitch a.,** one developed about a stitch or suture. **thecal a.,** one arising in a sheath, as in a tendon sheath. **tuberculous a.,** one due to infection with tubercle bacilli. **vitreous a.,** an abscess of the vitreous humor of the eye due to infection, trauma, or foreign body. **wandering a.,** one that burrows into tissues and finally points at a distance from the site of origin. **Welch's a.,** gas a.

ab·scis·sa (ab-sis′ah) the horizontal line in a graph along which are plotted the units of one of the factors considered in the study. Symbol x.

ab·scis·sion (ab-sĭ′zhun) removal by cutting.

ab·scop·al (-sko′p′l) pertaining to the effect on nonirradiated tissue resulting from irradiation of other tissue of the organism.

Ab·sid·ia (-sid′e-ah) a genus of fungi of the order Mucorales. *A. corymbi′fera* and several other species may cause mycosis in humans. *A. ramo′sa* grows on bread and decaying vegetation and causes otomycosis and sometimes mucormycosis.

ab·so·lute (ab′sah-loot) free from limitations; unlimited; uncombined.

ab·sorb (-sorb′) 1. to take in or assimilate, as to take up substances into or across tissues, e.g., the skin or intestine. 2. to react with radiation energy so as to attenuate it. 3. to retain specific wavelengths of radiation incident upon a substance, either raising its temperature or changing the energy state of its molecules.

ab·sorb·able (-sorb′ah-b′l) capable of being absorbed.

ab·sor·bance (-sor′bans) 1. in analytical chemistry, a measure of the light that a solution does not transmit compared to a pure solution. Symbol A. 2. in radiology, a measure of the ability of a medium to absorb radiation, expressed as the logarithm of the ratio of the intensity of the radiation entering the medium to that leaving it.

ab·sor·be·fa·cient (-sor″bĕ-fa′shint) 1. causing or promoting absorption. 2. absorbent (3).

ab·sor·bent (-sor′bent) 1. able to take in, or suck up and incorporate. 2. a tissue structure involved in absorption. 3. a substance that absorbs or promotes absorption.

ab·sorp·tion (-sorp′shun) 1. the uptake of substances into or across tissues. 2. in psychology, devotion of thought to one object or activity only. 3. uptake of energy by matter with which the radiation interacts. 4. in chemistry, the penetration of a substance within the inner structure of another. **intestinal a.**, the uptake from the intestinal lumen of fluids, solutes, proteins, fats, and other nutrients into the intestinal epithelial cells, blood, lymph, or interstitial fluids.

ab·sorp·tiv·i·ty (ab″sorp-tiv′ĭ-te) a measure of the amount of light absorbed by a solution.

ab·ster·gent (ab-ster′jent) 1. cleansing or detergent. 2. a cleansing agent.

ab·sti·nence (ab′stĭ-nens) a refraining from the use of or indulgence in food, stimulants, or sexual activity. **periodic a.**, rhythm method.

ab·strac·tion (ab-strak′shun) 1. the withdrawal of any ingredient from a compound. 2. malocclusion in which the occlusal plane is further from the eye-ear plane, causing lengthening of the face; cf. *attraction* (2).

abu·lia (ah-boo′le-ah) 1. loss or deficiency of will power, initiative, or drive. 2. akinetic mutism when it is less than total. **abu′lic**, adj.

abuse (ah-būs′) misuse, maltreatment, or excessive use. **child a.**, see *battered-child syndrome.* **drug a.**, substance a. **physical a.**, any act resulting in a nonaccidental physical injury. **psychoactive substance a.**, substance a. **sexual a.**, assault or other crime of a sexual nature, which need not be physical. Acts of a sexual nature are considered abuse if performed with minors or nonconsenting adults. **substance a.**, use of a substance that modifies mood or behavior in a manner characterized by a maladaptive pattern of use. See also *substance dependence,* under *dependence.*

abut·ment (ah-but′ment) a supporting structure to sustain lateral or horizontal pressure, as the anchorage tooth for a fixed or removable partial denture.

AC acromioclavicular; air conduction; alternating current; anodal closure; aortic closure.

Ac actinium.

a.c. [L.] an′te ci′bum (before meals).

ACA American College of Angiology; American College of Apothecaries.

acamp·sia (ah-kamp′se-ah) rigidity of a part or limb.

acan·tha (ah-kan′thah) 1. spine (1). 2. a spinous process of a vertebra.

acan·tha·me·bi·a·sis (ah-kan″thah-me-bi′-ah-sis) infection with *Acanthamoeba castellanii.*

Acan·tha·moe·ba (ah-kan″thah-me′bah) a genus of free-living ameboid protozoa (order Amoebida) found usually in fresh water or moist soil. Certain species, such as *A. astro-nyxis, A. castellanii, A. culbertsoni, A. hatchetti, A. polyphaga,* and *A. rhisodes,* may occur as human pathogens.

acan·thes·the·sia (a-kan″thes-the′zhah) perverted sensation of a sharp point pricking the body.

acan·thi·on (ah-kan′the-on) a point at the tip of the anterior nasal spine.

acanth(o)- word element [Gr.], *sharp spine; thorn.*

Acan·tho·ceph·a·la (ah-kan″tho-sef′ah-lah) a phylum of elongate, mostly cylindrical organisms (thorny-headed worms) parasitic in the intestines of all classes of vertebrates; in some classifications, considered to be a class of the phylum Nemathelminthes.

Acan·tho·ceph·a·lus (-sef′ah-lus) a genus of parasitic worms (phylum Acanthocephala).

Acan·tho·chei·lo·ne·ma (-ki″lo-ne′mah) a genus of long, threadlike worms. **A. per′-stans,** *Dipetalonema perstans.*

acan·tho·cyte (ah-kan′tho-sīt) a distorted erythrocyte with protoplasmic projections giving it a "thorny" appearance; seen in abetalipoproteinemia and other conditions.

acan·tho·cy·to·sis (ah-kan″tho-si-to′sis) the presence in the blood of acanthocytes, characteristic of abetalipoproteinemia and sometimes used synonymously.

acan·thol·y·sis (ak″an-thol′ĭ-sis) dissolution of the intercellular bridges of the stratum spinosum of the epidermis. **acantholyt′ic,** adj.

ac·an·tho·ma (ak″an-tho′mah, a″kan-tho′-mah) pl. *acanthomas, acantho′mata.* A tumor composed of epidermal or squamous cells.

Acan·tho·phis (ah-kan′tho-fis) a genus of snakes of the family Elapidae. *A. antarc′ticus* is the death adder of Australia and New Guinea.

ac·an·tho·sis (ak″an-tho′sis) diffuse hyperplasia and thickening of the stratum spinosum of the epidermis. **acantholyt′ic,** adj. **a. ni′gricans,** diffuse velvety acanthosis with dark pigmentation, chiefly in the axillae; it occurs in an adult form, often associated with an internal carcinoma (*malignant a. nigricans*), and in a benign, nevoid form, more or less generalized. A benign juvenile form associated with obesity, which is sometimes due to endocrine disturbance, is called *pseudoacanthosis nigricans.*

acan·thro·cy·to·sis (ah-kan″thro-si-to′sis) acanthocytosis.

acar·bia (ah-kahr′be-ah) decrease of bicarbonate in the blood.

acar·bose (a′kahr-bōs) an α-glucosidase inhibitor used in treatment of type 2 diabetes mellitus.

acar·dia (a-kahr′de-ah) congenital absence of the heart.

acar·di·us (-us) an imperfectly formed free twin fetus, lacking a heart and other body parts.

ac·a·ri·a·sis (ak″ah-ri′ah-sis) infestation with mites.

acar·i·cide (ah-kar′ĭ-sīd) 1. destructive to mites. 2. an agent that destroys mites.

acar·id (ak′ah-rid) a tick or mite of the order Acarina.

acar·i·di·a·sis (ah-kar″ĭ-di′ah-sis) acariasis.

Ac·a·ri·na (ak″ah-ri′nah) an order of arthropods (class Arachnida), including mites and ticks.

acar·i·no·sis (ah-kar″ĭ-no′sis) acariasis.

ac·a·ro·der·ma·ti·tis (ak″ah-ro-der″mah-ti′tis) any skin inflammation caused by mites (acarids). **a. urticarioi′des,** grain itch.

ac·a·rol·o·gy (ak″ah-rol′ah-je) the scientific study of mites and ticks.

Ac·a·rus (ak′ah-rus) a genus of small mites, frequent causes of skin diseases such as itch or mange. **A. folliculo′rum,** *Demodex folliculorum.* **A. scabie′i,** *Sarcoptes scabiei.* **A. si′ro,** a mite that causes vanillism in vanilla pod handlers.

acar·y·ote (ah-kār′e-ōt) akaryote.

acat·a·la·se·mia (a″kat-ah-la-se′me-ah) acatalasia.

acat·a·la·sia (a″kat-ah-la′zhah) a rare hereditary disease seen mostly in Japan and Switzerland, marked by absence of catalase; it may be associated with infections of oral structures.

acau·date (a-kaw′dāt) lacking a tail.

ACC American College of Cardiology.

ac·cel·er·a·tor (ak-sel′er-a″ter) [L.] 1. an agent or apparatus that increases the rate at which something occurs or progresses. 2. any nerve or muscle that hastens the performance of a function. 3. any of a group of chemicals used in the vulcanization of rubber or other polymerization reactions. **serum prothrombin conversion a. (SPCA),**

coagulation factor VII. **serum thrombotic a.,** a factor in serum which has procoagulant properties and the ability to induce blood coagulation.

ac·cep·tor (ak-sep′ter) a substance which unites with another substance; specifically, one that unites with hydrogen or oxygen in an oxidoreduction reaction and so enables the reaction to proceed.

ac·ces·sion·al (ak-sesh′un′l) pertaining to that which has been added or acquired.

ac·ces·so·ry (ak-ses′ah-re) supplementary; affording aid to another similar and generally more important thing.

ac·ci·den·tal (ak″sĭ-den′t′l) 1. occurring by chance, unexpectedly, or unintentionally. 2. nonessential; not innate or intrinsic.

ac·cli·ma·tion (ak″lĭ-ma′shun) the process of becoming accustomed to a new environment.

ac·com·mo·da·tion (ah-kom″ah-da′shun) adjustment, especially of the eye for seeing objects at various distances. Symbol A or a. **negative a.,** adjustment of the eye for long distances by relaxation of the ciliary muscles. **positive a.,** adjustment of the eye for short distances by contraction of the ciliary muscles.

ac·com·mo·da·tive (ah-kom′ah-da″tiv) pertaining to, of the nature of, or affecting accommodation.

ac·com·mo·dom·e·ter (ah-kom″ah-dom′ĕ-ter) an instrument for measuring accommodative capacity of the eye.

ac·couche·ment (ah-ko͞osh-maw′) [Fr.] 1. childbirth. 2. delivery. **a. forcé** for-sa′) rapid forcible delivery by one of several methods; originally, rapid dilatation of the cervix with the hands, followed by version and extraction of the fetus.

ac·cre·men·ti·tion (ak″rĕ-men-tish′un) growth by addition of similar tissue.

ac·cre·tion (ah-kre′shun) 1. growth by addition of material. 2. accumulation. 3. adherence of parts normally separated.

ac·e·bu·to·lol (as″ĕ-bu′tah-lol) a cardioselective β₁-adrenergic blocking agent with intrinsic sympathomimetic activity; used as the hydrochloride salt in the treatment of hypertension, anginia pectoris, and arrhythmias.

acel·lu·lar (a-sel′u-ler) not cellular in structure.

ace·lo·mate (ah-se′lo-māt) having no coelom or body cavity.

acen·tric (a-sen′trik) 1. not central; not located in the center. 2. lacking a centromere, so that the chromosome will not survive cell divisions.

ACEP American College of Emergency Physicians.

aceph·a·lo·cyst (a-sef'ah-lo-sist") sterile cyst.

aceph·a·lous (a-sef'ah-lus) headless.

aceph·a·lus a headless fetus.

acer·vu·line (ah-ser'vu-līn) aggregated; heaped up; said of certain glands.

ac·e·tab·u·lar (as"ĕ-tab'u-lar) pertaining to the acetabulum.

ac·e·tab·u·lec·to·my (as"ĕ-tab"u-lek'tah-me) excision of the acetabulum.

ac·e·tab·u·lo·plas·ty (as"ĕ-tab'u-lo-plas"te) plastic repair of the acetabulum.

ac·e·tab·u·lum (as"ĕ-tab'u-lum) pl. *acetabula*. [L.] the cup-shaped cavity on the lateral surface of the hip bone, receiving the head of the femur.

ac·e·tal (as'ĕ-t'l) 1. any of a class of organic compounds formed by combination of an aldehyde molecule and two alcohol molecules. 2. $CH_3CH(OC_2H_5)_2$, a colorless, volatile liquid used as a solvent and in cosmetics.

ac·et·al·de·hyde (as"et-al'dĕ-hīd") a colorless, volatile, flammable liquid used in the manufacture of acetic acid, perfumes, and flavors; it is also an intermediate in the metabolism of alcohol. It can cause irritation of mucous membranes, pneumonia, headache, and unconsciousness.

ace·ta·min·o·phen (ah-se"tah-min'o-fen) an analgesic and antipyretic with effects similar to aspirin but only weakly antiinflammatory.

ac·e·tate (as'ĕ-tāt) any salt of acetic acid.

ac·et·a·zol·a·mide (as"et-ah-zol'ah-mīd) a renal carbonic anhydrase inhibitor with uses that include treatment of glaucoma, epilepsy, familial periodic paralysis, acute mountain sickness, and uric acid renal calculi.

Ace·test (as'ĕ-test) trademark for a reagent tablet containing sodium nitroprusside, aminoacetic acid, dibasic sodium phosphate, and lactose, turning a purple color in the presence of ketone bodies in urine, blood, plasma, or serum, the intensity of the color reaction indicative of the acetoacetate or acetone concentration.

ace·tic (ah-se'tik, ah-set'ik) pertaining to vinegar or its acid; sour.

ace·tic ac·id (ah-se'tik) the two-carbon carboxylic acid, the characteristic component of vinegar; used as a solvent, menstruum, and pharmaceutic necessity. *Glacial a. a.* (anhydrous acetic acid) is used as a solvent, vesicant and caustic, and pharmaceutical necessity.

ace·to·ace·tic ac·id (ah-se"to-ah-se'tik) β-ketobutyric acid, one of the ketone bodies produced in the liver and occurring in excess in the blood and urine in ketosis.

Ace·to·bac·ter (ah-se"to-bak'ter) a genus of gram-negative, aerobic, rod-shaped bacteria (family Acetobacteraceae) made up of nonsporogenous organisms that produce acetic acid from ethanol and found in fruits, vegetables, souring juices, and alcoholic beverages.

ac·e·to·hex·a·mide (as"ĕ-to-hek'sah-mīd) an oral hypoglycemic used in the treatment of type 2 diabetes mellitus.

ac·e·to·hy·drox·am·ic ac·id (-hi"droks-am'ik) an inhibitor of bacterial urease used in the prophylaxis and treatment of certain renal calculi and the treatment of urinary tract infections caused by urease-producing bacteria.

ac·e·tone (as'ĕ-tōn) a flammable, colorless, volatile liquid with a characteristic odor, which is a solvent and antiseptic and is one of the ketone bodies produced in ketoacidosis.

ac·e·to·ni·trile (as"ĕ-to-ni'trīl) a colorless liquid with an etherlike odor used as an extractant, solvent, and intermediate; ingestion or inhalation yields cyanide as a metabolic product.

ac·e·ton·uria (as"ĕ-to-nu're-ah) ketonuria.

ace·tous (as'ĕ-tus) pertaining to, producing, or resembling acetic acid.

ac·e·tract (as'ĕ-trakt) an extract of a medicinal herb prepared using acetic acid as the solvent.

ac·e·tyl (as'ĕ-til, as'ĕ-tēl") the monovalent radical CH_3CO-, a combining form of acetic acid.

acet·y·la·tion (ah-set"ĭ-la'shun) introduction of an acetyl radical into an organic molecule.

acet·y·la·tor (ah-set'ĭ-la"ter) an organism capable of metabolic acetylation; in humans, acetylator status (fast or slow) is determined by the rate of acetylation of sulfamethazine.

ac·e·tyl·cho·line (ACh) (as"ĕ-til-, as"ĕ-tēl-ko'lēn) the acetic acid ester of choline, which is a neurotransmitter at cholinergic synapses in the central, sympathetic, and parasympathetic nervous systems; used in the form of the chloride salt as a miotic.

ac·e·tyl·cho·lin·es·ter·ase (AChE) (-ko"lĭ-nes'ter-ās) an enzyme present in the central nervous system, particularly in nervous tissue, muscle, and red cells, that catalyzes the hydrolysis of acetylcholine to choline and acetic acid.

ac·e·tyl CoA (as'ĕ-til, as'ĕ-tēl" ko-a') acetyl coenzyme A.

ac·e·tyl-CoA car·box·yl·ase (kahr-bok'sĭ-lās) a ligase that catalyzes the rate-limiting step in the synthesis of fatty acids from acetyl groups.

ac·e·tyl co·en·zyme A (ko-en′zīm) acetyl CoA; an important intermediate in the tricarboxylic acid cycle and the chief precursor of lipids and steroids; it is formed by the attachment to coenzyme A of an acetyl group during the oxidation of carbohydrates, fatty acids, or amino acids.

ac·e·tyl·cys·te·ine (as″ĕ-til-, as″ĕ-tēl-sis′te-ēn) a derivative of cysteine used as a mucolytic in various bronchopulmonary disorders and as an antidote to acetaminophen poisoning.

acet·y·lene (ah-set′ĭ-lēn) HC≡CH, a colorless, volatile, explosive gas, the simplest alkyne (unsaturated, triple-bonded hydrocarbon).

N-ac·e·tyl·ga·lac·to·sa·mine (as″ĕ-til-, as″ĕ-tēl-gal′ak-tōs′ah-mēn) the acetyl derivative of galactosamine; it is a component of structural glycosaminoglycans, glycolipids, and membrane glycoproteins.

N-ac·e·tyl·glu·co·sa·mine (-gloo-kōs′ah-mēn) the acetyl derivative of glucosamine; it is a component of structural glycosaminoglycans, glycolipids, and membrane glycoproteins.

N-ac·e·tyl·neu·ra·min·ic ac·id (-noor″ah-min′ik) the acetyl derivative of the amino sugar neuraminic acid; it occurs in many glycoproteins, glycolipids, and polysaccharides.

ac·e·tyl·sal·i·cyl·ic ac·id (ASA) (ah-se″til-sal″ĭ-sil′ik) aspirin.

ac·e·tyl·trans·fer·ase (as″ĕ-til-, as″ĕ-tēl-trans′fer-ās) any of a group of enzymes that catalyze the transfer of an acetyl group from one substance to another.

ACG American College of Gastroenterology; angiocardiography; apexcardiogram.

AcG accelerator globulin (coagulation factor V).

ACh acetylcholine.

ACHA American College of Hospital Administrators.

ach·a·la·sia (ak″ah-la′zhah) failure to relax of smooth muscle fibers at any junction of one part of the gastrointestinal tract with another, especially failure of the esophagogastric sphincter to relax with swallowing, due to degeneration of ganglion cells in the wall of the organ.

Ach·a·ti·na (ak″ah-ti′nah) a genus of very large land snails, including *A. fuli′ca*, which serves as an intermediate host of *Angiostrongylus cantonensis*.

AChE acetylcholinesterase.

achei·ria (ah-ki′re-ah) 1. congenital absence of one or both hands. 2. lack of sensation of the hands or a feeling of their absence.

achil·lo·bur·si·tis (ah-kil″o-ber-si′tis) inflammation and thickening of the bursae about the Achilles tendon.

achil·lo·dy·nia (-din′e-ah) 1. pain in the Achilles tendon. 2. achillobursitis.

ach·il·lor·rha·phy (ak″ĭ-lor′ah-fe) suturing of the Achilles tendon.

achil·lo·te·not·o·my (ah-kil″o-tĕ-not′ah-me) surgical division of the Achilles tendon.

achlor·hy·dria (a″klor-hi′dre-ah) absence of hydrochloric acid from gastric secretions. **achlorhy′dric**, adj.

acho·lia (a-ko′le-ah) lack or absence of bile secretion. **acho′lic**, adj.

acho·lu·ric (a″ko-lu′rik) not characterized by choluria.

achon·dro·gen·e·sis (a-kon″dro-jen′ĕ-sis) a hereditary disorder characterized by hypoplasia of bone, resulting in markedly shortened limbs; the head and trunk are normal.

achon·dro·pla·sia (-pla′zhah) a hereditary, congenital disorder of cartilage formation, leading to a type of dwarfism.

achon·dro·plas·tic (-plas′tik) pertaining to, or affected with, achondroplasia.

achres·tic (ah-kres′tik) not using some normal tool or process, as the inability of those with achrestic anemia to utilize vitamin B_{12}.

achro·ma·sia (ak″ro-ma′zhah) 1. lack of normal skin pigmentation. 2. the inability of tissues or cells to be stained.

achro·mat (ak′ro-mat) 1. an achromatic objective. 2. monochromat.

achro·mat·ic (ak″ro-mat′ik) 1. producing no discoloration. 2. staining with difficulty. 3. containing achromatin. 4. refracting light without decomposing it into its component colors. 5. monochromatic (2).

achro·ma·tin (ah-kro′mah-tin) the faintly staining groundwork of a cell nucleus.

achro·ma·tol·y·sis (ah-kro″mah-tol′ĭ-sis) disorganization of cell achromatin.

achro·ma·to·phil (ak″ro-mat′o-fil) 1. not easily stainable. 2. an organism or tissue that does not stain easily.

achro·ma·top·sia (ah-kro″mah-top′se-ah) monochromatic vision.

achro·ma·to·sis (ah-kro″mah-to′sis) 1. deficiency of pigmentation in the tissues. 2. lack of staining power in a cell or tissue.

achro·ma·tous (ah-kro′mah-tus) colorless.

achro·ma·tu·ria (a-kro″mah-tu′re-ah) the excretion of colorless urine.

achro·mia (ah-kro′me-ah) the lack or absence of normal color or pigmentation, as of the skin. **achro′mic**, adj.

achy·lia (ah-ki'le-ah) absence of hydrochloric acid and pepsinogens (pepsin) in the gastric juice.

achy·mia (ah-ki'me-ah) imperfect, insufficient, or absence of chyme formation.

acic·u·lar (ah-sik'u-ler) needle-shaped.

ac·id (as'id) 1. sour. 2. a chemical compound that dissociates in solution, releasing hydrogen ions and lowering the solution pH (a proton donor). An acidic solution has a pH below 7.0. Cf. *base* (3). For particular acids, see the specific names. **a. citrate dextrose (ACD),** anticoagulant citrate dextrose solution. **amino a.,** see under *amino*. **carboxylic a.,** any organic compound containing the carboxy group (—COOH), including amino and fatty acids. **fatty a.,** see under *F.* **haloid a.,** an acid which contains no oxygen in the molecule, but is composed of hydrogen and a halogen element. **hydroxy a.,** an organic acid that contains an additional hydroxyl group. **inorganic a.,** any acid containing no carbon atoms. **nucleic a.,** see under *N.* **organic a.,** an acid containing one or more carbon atoms; often specifically a carboxylic acid.

ac·i·de·mia (as″ĭ-de'me-ah) increased acidity of the blood. For those characterized by increased concentration of a specific acid, see at the acid. **organic a.,** increased concentration of one or more organic acids in the blood.

acid-fast (as'id-fast) not readily decolorized by acids after staining.

acid·ic (ah-sid'ik) of or pertaining to an acid; acid-forming.

acid·i·fi·a·ble (ah-sid″ĭ-fi'ah-b'l) capable of being made acid.

acid·i·fied (ah-sid'ĭ-fīd) having been made acid.

acid·i·fi·er (-fi-er) an agent that causes acidity; a substance used to increase gastric acidity.

acid·i·ty (-ĭ-te) the quality of being acid; the power to unite with positively charged ions or with basic substances.

ac·id li·pase (as'id li'pās) 1. cholesterol esterase. 2. a lipase with an acid pH optimum.

ac·id mal·tase (mawl'tās) a hydrolase that catalyzes the degradation of glycogen to glucose in the lysosomes; deficiency of enzyme activity results in glycogen storage disease, type II.

acid·o·phil (ah-sid'o-fil″) 1. a histologic structure, cell, or other element staining readily with acid dyes. 2. one of the hormone-producing acidophilic cells of the adenohypophysis; types include corticotrophs, lactotrophs, lipotrophs, and somatotrophs.

3. an organism that grows well in highly acid media. 4. acidophilic.

ac·i·do·phil·ic (as″ĭ-do-fil'ik) 1. easily stained with acid dyes. 2. growing best on acid media.

ac·i·do·sis (as″ĭ-do'sis) 1. the accumulation of acid and hydrogen ions or depletion of the alkaline reserve (bicarbonate content) in the blood and body tissues, decreasing the pH. 2. a pathologic condition resulting from this process. Cf. *alkalosis.* **acidot′ic,** adj. **compensated a.,** a condition in which the compensatory mechanisms have returned the pH toward normal. **diabetic a.,** metabolic acidosis produced by accumulation of ketones in uncontrolled diabetes mellitus. **hypercapnic a.,** respiratory a. **hyperchloremic a.,** metabolic acidosis accompanied by elevated plasma chloride. **lactic a.,** a metabolic acidosis occurring as a result of excess lactic acid in the blood, due to conditions causing impaired cellular respiration. **metabolic a., nonrespiratory a.,** a disturbance in which the acid-base status shifts toward the acid because of loss of base or retention of noncarbonic, or fixed (nonvolatile), acids. **renal hyperchloremia a., renal tubular a. (RTA),** metabolic acidosis resulting from impairment of renal function. **respiratory a.,** acidosis due to excess retention of carbon dioxide in the body. **starvation a.,** metabolic acidosis due to accumulation of ketone bodies which may accompany a caloric deficit. **uremic a.,** metabolic acidosis seen in chronic renal disease when the ability to excrete acid is decreased.

ac·id phos·pha·tase (as'id fos'fah-tās) a hydrolase found in mammalian liver, spleen, bone marrow, plasma and formed blood elements, and prostate gland, catalyzing the cleavage of orthophosphate from orthophosphoric monoesters under acid conditions; determination of its activity in serum is an important diagnostic test.

acid·u·lat·ed (ah-sid'u-lāt″ed) rendered acid in reaction.

acid·u·lous (-lus) somewhat acid.

ac·id·u·ria (as″ĭ-du're-ah) excess of acid in the urine. For those characterized by increased concentration of a specific acid, see at the acid. **organic a.,** excessive excretion of one or more organic acids in the urine.

ac·id·uric (as″ĭ-du'rik) capable of growing in extremely acid media; said of bacteria.

ac·i·nar (as'ĭ-nar) pertaining to or affecting one or more acini.

Ac·i·net·o·bac·ter (as″ĭ-ne″to-bak'ter) a genus of bacteria (family Neisseriaceae), consisting of aerobic, gram-negative, paired coccobacilli, it is widely distributed in nature and part of the normal mammalian flora, but can cause severe primary infections in compromised hosts. The type species, *A. calcoaceticus*, can cause fatal pneumonia.

acin·ic (ah-sin'ik) acinar.

acin·i·form (ah-sin'ĭ-form) shaped like an acinus, or grape.

acin·i·tis (as"ĭ-ni'tis) inflammation of the acini of a gland.

ac·i·nose (as'ĭ-nōs) made up of acini.

ac·i·nous (as'ĭ-nus) acinar.

ac·i·nus (as'ĭ-nus) pl. *a'cini*. [L.] a small saclike structure, particularly one in a gland; see also *alveolus*. **liver a.,** the smallest functional unit of the liver, a mass of liver parenchyma that is supplied by terminal branches of the portal vein and hepatic artery and drained by a terminal branch of the bile duct. **pancreatic a.,** one of the secretory units of the exocrine pancreas, where pancreatic juice is produced. **pulmonary a.,** terminal respiratory unit. **thyroid acini,** see under *follicle*.

ac·i·tret·in (as"e-tret'in) a second generation retinoid used in treatment of severe psoriasis.

acla·sis (ak'lah-sis) pathologic continuity of structure, as in multiple exostoses. **diaphyseal a.,** multiple exostoses.

ac·me (ak'me) the critical stage or crisis of a disease.

ac·ne (ak'ne) an inflammatory disease of the skin; often specifically, *acne vulgaris*. **bromide a.,** an acneiform eruption without comedones, one of the most constant symptoms of brominism. **common a.,** a. vulgaris. **a. conglobata, conglobate a.,** severe acne with many comedones, marked by suppuration, cysts, sinuses, and scarring. **a. cosme'tica,** a persistent, low-grade acne usually affecting the chin and cheeks of a woman who uses cosmetics. **a. deter'gicans,** aggravation of existing acne lesions by too frequent and too severe washing with comedogenic soaps and rough cloths or pads. **a. ful'minans,** a rare form affecting teenage males, marked by sudden onset of fever and eruption of highly inflammatory, tender, ulcerative, and crusted lesions on the back, chest, and face. **halogen a.,** an acneiform eruption from ingestion of the simple salts of bromine and iodine present in cold remedies, sedatives, analgesics, and vitamins. **a. indura'ta,** a progression of papular acne, with deep-seated and destructive lesions that may produce severe scarring. **a. keloid,** development of persistent hard follicular plaques along the posterior hairline of the scalp that fuse to form a thick, sclerotic,

hypertrophic, pseudokeloidal band across the occiput. **a. mecha'nica, mechanical a.,** aggravation of existing acne lesions by mechanical factors such as rubbing or stretching, as by chin straps, clothing, back packs, casts, and seats. **a. necro'tica milia'ris,** a rare and chronic form of folliculitis of the scalp, occurring principally in adults, with formation of tiny superficial pustules which are destroyed by scratching; see also *a. varioliformis*. **a. papulo'sa,** acne vulgaris with the formation of papules. **pomade a.,** acne vulgaris in blacks who groom their scalp and facial hair with greasy lubricants, marked by closed comedones on the forehead, temples, cheeks, and chin. **premenstrual a.,** acne of a cyclic nature, appearing shortly before (rarely after) the onset of menses. **a. rosa'cea,** rosacea. **tropical a., a. tropica'lis,** a severe and extensive form of acne occurring in hot, humid climates, with nodular, cystic, and pustular lesions chiefly on the back, buttocks, and thighs; conglobate abscesses frequently form, especially on the back. **a. variolifor'mis,** a rare condition with reddish-brown, papulopustular umbilicated lesions, usually on the brow and scalp; probably a deep variant of a. necrotica miliaris. **a. venena'ta,** acne produced by contact with a great variety of acnegenic chemicals, including those used in cosmetics and grooming agents and in industry. **a. vulga'ris,** chronic acne, usually occurring in adolescence, with comedones, papules, nodules, and pustules on the face, neck, and upper part of the trunk.

ac·ne·gen·ic (ak"nĕ-jen'ik) producing acne.

ac·ni·tis (ak-ni'tis) a form of papulonecrotic tuberculid occurring on the face.

ACNM American College of Nurse-Midwives.

acoe·lom·ate (a-se'lah-māt) without a coelom or body cavity; an animal lacking a body cavity.

ACOG American College of Obstetricians and Gynecologists.

ac·o·nite (ak'o-nīt) a poisonous substance from the dried tuberous root of *Aconitum napellus*, which contains aconitine and related alkaloids and causes potentially fatal ventricular fibrillation and respiratory paralysis. It is used in Chinese herbal medicine and homeopathy as an analgesic, antiinflammatory, and cardiac tonic.

acon·i·tine (ah-kon'ĭ-tin) a poisonous alkaloid, the active principle of aconite.

aco·rea (ah-kor'e-ah) absence of the pupil.

aco·ria (ah-kor'e-ah) excessive ingestion of food, not from hunger but due to loss of the sensation of satiety.

ACOS American College of Osteopathic Surgeons.

acous·tic (ah-kōōs′tik) relating to sound or hearing.

acous·tics (-tiks) the science of sound or of hearing.

acous·to·gram (-tah-gram) the graphic tracing of the curves of sounds produced by motion of a joint.

ACP American College of Physicians; acid phosphatase.

ACPS acrocephalopolysyndactyly.

ac·quired (ah-kwīrd′) incurred as a result of factors acting from or originating outside the organism; not inherited.

ac·qui·si·tion (ak″wĭ-zĭ′shun) in psychology, the period in learning during which progressive increments in response strength can be measured. Also, the process involved in such learning.

ACR American College of Radiology.

ac·ral (ak′ral) pertaining to or affecting a limb or other extremity.

Ac·re·mo·ni·um (ak″rĕ-mo′ne-um) a genus of imperfect fungi rarely isolated from human infection. *A. falcifor′me, A. kilien′se,* and *A. reci′fei* are agents of eumycotic mycetoma.

ac·ri·dine (ak′rĭ-dēn) an alkaloid from anthracene used in the synthesis of dyes and drugs.

ac·ri·vas·tine (ak″rĭ-vas′tēn) an antihistamine used in treatment of seasonal allergic rhinitis.

acr(o)- word element [Gr.], *extreme; top; extremity.*

ac·ro·ag·no·sis (ak″ro-ag-no′sis) lack of sensory recognition of a limb; lack of acrognosis.

ac·ro·an·es·the·sia (-an″es-the′zhah) anesthesia of the limbs.

ac·ro·ar·thri·tis (-ahr-thri′tis) arthritis of the limbs.

ac·ro·blast (ak′ro-blast) Golgi material in the spermatid from which the acrosome develops.

ac·ro·brachy·ceph·a·ly (ak″ro-brak″ĭ-sef′ah-le) abnormal height of the skull, with shortness of its anteroposterior dimension. **acrobrachycephal′ic,** adj.

ac·ro·cen·tric (-sen′trik) having the centromere toward one end of the replicating chromosome so that one arm is much longer than the other.

ac·ro·ceph·a·lo·poly·syn·dac·ty·ly (ACPS) (-sef″ah-lo-pol″e-sin-dak′tĭ-le) acrocephalosyndactyly with polydactyly as an additional feature. Type I is *Pfeiffer's syndrome,* and type II is *Carpenter's syndrome.*

ac·ro·ceph·a·lo·syn·dac·ty·ly (-sef″ah-lo-sin-dak′tĭ-le) any of a group of autosomal dominant syndromes in which craniostenosis is associated with acrocephaly and syndactyly. Type I is *Apert's syndrome,* type III is *Chotzen's syndrome,* and type V is *Pfeiffer's syndrome.*

ac·ro·ceph·a·ly (-sef′ah-le) oxycephaly.

ac·ro·chor·don (-kor′don) a pedunculated skin tag, occurring principally on the neck, eyelids, upper chest, and axillae in older women.

ac·ro·ci·ne·sis (-si-ne′sis) excessive motility; abnormal freedom of movement. **acrocinet′ic,** adj.

ac·ro·con·trac·ture (-kon-trak′cher) contracture of the muscles of the hand or foot.

ac·ro·cy·a·no·sis (-si″ah-no′sis) cyanosis of the limbs with discoloration of the skin of digits, wrists, and ankles, and profuse sweating and coldness of digits.

ac·ro·der·ma·ti·tis (-der″mah-ti′tis) inflammation of the skin of the hands or feet. **a. chro′nica atro′phicans,** chronic inflammation of the skin, usually of limbs, leading to sclerosis and atrophy of the skin, caused by the spirochete *Borrelia burgdorferi.* **a. conti′nua,** a variant of pustular psoriasis, with chronic inflammation of limbs that in some cases becomes generalized. **a. enteropa′thica,** a hereditary disorder due to defective zinc uptake, with a vesiculopustulous dermatitis preferentially located around orifices and on the head, elbows, knees, hands, and feet, associated with gastrointestinal disturbances, chiefly manifested by diarrhea, and total alopecia. **Hallopeau's a.,** a. continua. **infantile a., papular a. of childhood,** Gianotti-Crosti syndrome. **a. per′stans,** a. continua.

ac·ro·der·ma·to·sis (-der″mah-to′sis) pl. *acrodermato′ses.* Any disease of the skin of the limbs.

ac·ro·dol·i·cho·me·lia (-dol″ĭ-ko-me′le-ah) abnormal length of the hands and feet.

ac·ro·dyn·ia (-din′e-ah) a disease of early childhood marked by pain and swelling in, and pink coloration of, the fingers and toes and by listlessness, irritability, failure to thrive, profuse perspiration, and sometimes scarlet coloration of the cheeks and tip of the nose. Most cases are toxic neuropathies caused by exposure to mercury.

ac·ro·es·the·sia (-es-the′zhah) 1. exaggerated sensitiveness. 2. pain in the limbs.

ac·rog·no·sis (ak″rog-no′sis) sensory recognition of the limbs and of the different portions of each limb in relation to each other.

ac·ro·hy·po·ther·my (ak″ro-hi′po-ther″me) abnormal coldness of the hands and feet.

ac·ro·ker·a·to·sis (-ker″ah-to′sis) a condition in which the skin of the limbs develops horny growths.

ac·ro·ki·ne·sia (-kĭ-ne′zhah) acrocinesis. **acrokinet′ic,** adj.

acro·le·in (ak-ro′le-in) a volatile, highly toxic liquid, produced industrially and also one of the degradation products of cyclophosphamide.

ac·ro·meg·a·ly (ak″ro-meg′ah-le) abnormal enlargement of limbs, caused by hypersecretion of growth hormone after maturity.

ac·ro·meta·gen·e·sis (-met″ah-jen′ĕ-sis) undue growth of the limbs.

acro·mi·al (ah-kro′me-al) pertaining to the acromion.

ac·ro·mic·ria (ak″ro-mik′re-ah) hypoplasia of the limbs and digits, nose, and jaws.

acromi(o)- word element [Gr.], *acromion*.

acro·mio·cla·vic·u·lar (ah-kro″me-o-klah-vik′u-ler) pertaining to the acromion and clavicle.

acro·mi·on (ah-kro′me-on) the lateral extension of the spine of the scapula, forming the highest point of the shoulder.

acro·mio·nec·to·my (ah-kro″me-on-ek′tah-me) resection of the acromion.

acro·mio·plas·ty (ah-kro′me-o-plas″te) surgical removal of the anterior hook of the acromion to relieve mechanical compression of the rotator cuff during movement of the glenohumeral joint.

acrom·pha·lus (ah-krom′fah-lus) 1. bulging of the navel; sometimes a sign of umbilical hernia. 2. the center of the navel.

ac·ro·myo·to·nia (ak″ro-mi″o-to′ne-ah) contracture of the hand or foot resulting in spastic deformity.

ac·ro·neu·ro·sis (-noŏ-ro′sis) any neuropathy of the limbs.

ac·ro·os·te·ol·y·sis (-os″te-ol′ĭ-sis) osteolysis involving the distal phalanges of the fingers and toes.

ac·ro·pachy (ak′ro-pak″e) clubbing of the fingers and toes.

ac·ro·pachy·der·ma (ak″ro-pak″e-der′mah) thickening of the skin over the face, scalp, and limbs, clubbing of digits, and deformities of the long bones; usually with acromegaly.

ac·ro·pa·ral·y·sis (-pah-ral′ĭ-sis) paralysis of limbs.

ac·ro·par·es·the·sia (-par″es-the′zhah) 1. paresthesia of the digits. 2. a disease marked by attacks of tingling, numbness, and stiffness chiefly in the fingers, hands, and forearms, sometimes with pain, skin pallor, or slight cyanosis.

ac·ro·pa·thol·o·gy (-pah-thol′ah-je) pathology of diseases of limbs.

acrop·a·thy (ah-krop′ah-the) any disease of limbs. **ulcerative mutilating a.,** hereditary sensory radicular neuropathy.

ac·ro·pho·bia (ak″ro-fo′be-ah) irrational fear of heights.

ac·ro·pus·tu·lo·sis (-pus″tu-lo′sis) pustulosis of the extremities. A congenital form (*infantile a.*) is characterized by recurring episodes of small pruritic pustules on the hands and feet followed by remission.

ac·ro·scle·ro·der·ma (-skler″o-der′mah) acrosclerosis.

ac·ro·scle·ro·sis (-skler-o′sis) a combination of Raynaud's disease and scleroderma of the distal limbs, especially digits, the neck, and often the nose.

ac·ro·so·mal (ak″ro-so′mal) pertaining to the acrosome.

ac·ro·some (ak′ro-sōm) the caplike, membrane-bound structure covering the anterior portion of the head of a spermatozoon; it contains enzymes for penetrating the oocyte.

ac·ro·spi·ro·ma (ak″ro-spi-ro′mah) a tumor of the distal portion of a sweat gland.

ac·ro·tism (ak′rah-tizm) absence or imperceptibility of the pulse. **acrot′ic,** adj.

ac·ro·tropho·neu·ro·sis (ak″ro-trof″o-noŏro′sis) trophoneurotic disturbance of limbs.

acryl·a·mide (ah-kril′ah-mīd) a vinyl monomer used in the production of polymers with many industrial and research uses; the monomeric form is a neurotoxin.

acryl·ic (ah-kril′ik) pertaining to or containing polymers of acrylic acid, methacrylic acid or acrylonitrile; see also under *resin*.

acryl·ic ac·id a readily polymerizing liquid used as a monomer for acrylic polymers.

ac·ry·lo·ni·trile (ak″rĭ-lo-ni′trĭl) a colorless halogenated hydrocarbon used in the making of plastics and as a pesticide; its vapors are irritant to the respiratory tract and eyes, may cause systemic poisoning, and are carcinogenic.

ACS American Cancer Society; American Chemical Society; American College of Surgeons.

ACSM American College of Sports Medicine.

ACTH adrenocorticotropic hormone; see *corticotropin*.

ac·tin (ak′tin) a muscle protein localized in the I band of the myofibrils; acting along with myosin, it is responsible for contraction and relaxation of muscle. It occurs in globular (*G-actin*) and fibrous (*F-actin*) forms.

act·ing out (ak′ting out) the expression of unconscious feelings and fantasies in behavior; reacting to present situations as if they were the original situation that gave rise to the feelings and fantasies.

ac·tin·ic (ak-tin'ik) producing chemical action; said of rays of light beyond the violet end of the spectrum.

ac·tin·i·um **(Ac)** (ak-tin'e-um) chemical element (see *Table of Elements*), at. no. 89.

actin(o)- word element [Gr.], *ray; ray-shaped; radiation*.

ac·ti·no·bac·il·lo·sis (ak″ti-no-bas″ĭ-lo'sis) an actinomycosis-like disease of domestic animals caused by *Actinobacillus lignieresii*, in which the bacilli form radiating structures in the tissues; sometimes seen in humans.

Ac·ti·no·bac·il·lus (-bah-sil'us) a genus of potentially pathogenic schizomycetes (family Pasteurellaceae), causing granulomatous lesions.

ac·ti·no·der·ma·ti·tis (-der″mah-ti'tis) radiodermatitis.

Ac·ti·no·ma·du·ra (-mah-doo'-rah) a genus of bacteria (family Nocardiaceae), including *A. madu'rae*, the cause of actinomycotic mycetoma in which the granules in the discharged pus are white, and *A. pelletie'ri*, the cause of actinomycotic mycetoma in which the granules are red.

Ac·ti·no·my·ces (-mi'sēz) a genus of bacteria (family Actinomycetaceae). **A. israe'lii**, a species parasitic in the mouth, proliferating in necrotic tissue; it is the etiologic agent of human actinomycosis and can cause actinomycotic mycetoma. **A. naeslun'dii**, an anaerobic species that is a normal inhabitant of the oral cavity and a cause of human actinomycosis and periodontal disease.

Ac·ti·no·my·ce·ta·ceae (-mi″sah-ta'se-e) a family of bacteria (order Actinomycetales).

Ac·ti·no·my·ce·ta·les (-mi″sah-ta'lēz) an order of bacteria made up of elongated cells having a definite tendency to branch.

ac·ti·no·my·cin (-mi'sin) a family of antibiotics from various species of *Streptomyces*, which are active against bacteria and fungi; it includes the antineoplastic agent dactinomycin (actinomycin D).

ac·ti·no·my·co·sis (-mi-ko'sis) an infectious disease caused by *Actinomyces*, marked by indolent inflammatory lesions of the lymph nodes draining the mouth, by intraperitoneal abscesses, or by lung abscesses due to aspiration. **actinomycot'ic**, adj.

ac·ti·no·ther·a·py (-ther'ah-pe) phototherapy.

ac·tion (ak'shun) the accomplishment of an effect, whether mechanical or chemical, or the effect so produced. **ball-valve a.**, the intermittent obstruction caused by a free or partially attached foreign body in a tubular or cavitary structure, as by a foreign body in a bronchus, a stone in a bile duct, or a tumor in the cardiac atrium. **cumulative a.**, action of increased intensity, as the sudden and markedly increased action of a drug after administration of several doses, due to the accumulation of the drug in the body. **reflex a.**, a response, often involuntary, resulting from passage of excitation potential from a receptor to a muscle or gland over a reflex arc.

ac·ti·va·tion (ak″tĭ-va'shun) 1. the act or process of rendering active. 2. the transformation of a proenzyme into an active enzyme by the action of a kinase or another enzyme. 3. the process by which the central nervous system is stimulated into activity through the mediation of the reticular activating system. 4. the deliberate induction of a pattern of electrical activity in the brain. **allosteric a.**, increase in enzyme activity by binding of an effector at an allosteric site that affects binding or turnover at the catalytic site. **contact a.**, initiation of the intrinsic pathway of coagulation through interaction of coagulation factor XII with various electronegative surfaces. **lymphocyte a.**, stimulation of lymphocytes by antigen or mitogens resulting in macromolecular synthesis (RNA, protein, and DNA) and production of lymphokines, followed by proliferation and differentiation of the progeny into various effector and memory cells.

ac·ti·va·tor (ak'tĭ-va″ter) 1. a substance that combines with an enzyme to increase its catalytic activity. 2. a substance that stimulates the development of a specific structure in the embryo. 3. a chemical or other form of energy that causes another substance to become reactive or that induces a chemical reaction. **plasminogen a.**, any of a group of substances that have the ability to cleave plasminogen and convert it into the active form plasmin. **prothrombin a.**, any one of the substances in the extrinsic or intrinsic pathways of coagulation. **single chain urokinase-type plasminogen a. (scu-PA)**, prourokinase. **tissue plasminogen a. (TPA, t-PA)**, t-plasminogen a., an endopeptidase synthesized by endothelial cells that binds to fibrin clots and catalyzes the cleavage of plasminogen to the active form plasmin. t-PA produced by recombinant technology is used for therapeutic thrombolysis. **u-plasminogen a.**, formal name for *urokinase*. Called also *urinary plasminogen a.*

ac·tive (ak'tiv) characterized by action; not passive; not expectant.

ac·ti·vin (ak'tĭ-vin) a nonsteroidal regulator synthesized in the pituitary glands and gonads that stimulates the secretion of follicle-stimulating hormone.

ac·tiv·i·ty (ak-tiv'ĭ-te) 1. the quality or process of exerting energy or of accomplishing an effect. 2. a thermodynamic quantity that represents the effective concentration of a solute in a nonideal solution. Symbol *a.* 3. the number of disintegrations per unit time of a radioactive material. Symbol *A.* 4. the presence of recordable electrical energy in a muscle or nerve (*electrical a.*). 5. optical a. **end-plate a.,** spontaneous activity recorded close to motor end plates in normal muscle. **enzyme a.,** the catalytic effect exerted by an enzyme, expressed as units per milligram of enzyme (*specific a.*) or as molecules of substrate transformed per minute per molecule of enzyme (*molecular a.*). **intrinsic sympathomimetic a. (ISA),** the ability of a β-blocker to stimulate β-adrenergic receptors weakly during β-blockade. **optical a.,** the ability of a chemical compound to rotate the plane of polarization of plane-polarized light.

ac·to·my·o·sin (ak''to-mi'o-sin) the complex of actin and myosin occurring in muscle fibers.

acu·i·ty (ah-ku'ĭ-te) clarity or clearness, especially of vision.

acu·mi·nate (ah-ku'mĭ-nāt) sharp-pointed.

acu·point (ak'u-point) any of the specific sites for needle insertion in acupuncture; also used in other therapies, including acupressure and moxibustion. Most are areas of high electrical conductance on the body surface.

acu·pres·sure (-presh''er) the use of pressure applied, usually with the hands, at acupoints in order to release muscular tension for therapeutic purposes.

acu·punc·ture (-punk''cher) a traditional Chinese practice of piercing specific areas of the body (acupoints) along peripheral nerves with fine needles to relieve pain, to induce surgical anesthesia, and for therapeutic purposes. Other means of stimulating the acupoints, including lasers, ultrasound, and electricity, may also be used. **Korean hand a.,** a type in which the hand is considered to be a representation of the entire body, and stimulation of specific points on the hand is used to obtain effects in distant areas of the body.

acus (a'kus) a needle or needle-like process.

acute (ah-kūt') having severe symptoms and a short course.

acy·a·not·ic (a-si''ah-not'ik) characterized by absence of cyanosis.

acy·clo·vir (a-si'klo-vēr) a synthetic purine nucleoside with selective activity against herpes simplex virus; used as the base or the sodium salt in the treatment of genital and mucocutaneous herpesvirus infections.

ac·yl·ase (a'sĭ-lās) amidase (1).

ac·yl CoA (a'sil ko-a') acyl coenzyme A.

ac·yl-CoA de·hy·dro·gen·ase (de-hi'dro-jen-ās) any of several enzymes that catalyze the oxidation of acyl coenzyme A thioesters as a step in the degradation of fatty acids. Individual enzymes are specific for certain ranges of acyl chain lengths: *long-chain a.-CoA d.* (*LCAD*), *medium-chain a.-CoA d.* (*MCAD*), and *short-chain a.-CoA d.* (*SCAD*).

ac·yl co·en·zyme A (a'sil ko-en'zīm) acyl CoA; a thiol ester of a carboxylic acid, particularly a long-chain fatty acid, and coenzyme A; its formation is the first step in fatty acid oxidation.

ac·yl·glyc·er·ol (-glis'er-ol) glyceride.

*N***-ac·yl·sphin·go·sine** (-sfing'go-sēn) ceramide.

ac·yl·trans·fer·ase (-trans'fer-ās) any of a group of enzymes that catalyze the transfer of an acyl group from one substance to another.

acys·tia (a-sis'te-ah) congenital absence of the bladder.

AD [L.] au'ris dex'tra (right ear).

ad [L.] preposition, *to.*

ADA adenosine deaminase; American Dental Association; American Diabetes Association; American Dietetic Association.

adac·ty·ly (a-dak'tĭ-le) congenital absence of fingers or toes. **adac'tylous,** adj.

ad·a·man·tine (ad''ah-man'tin) pertaining to the enamel of the teeth.

ad·a·man·ti·no·ma (ad''ah-man''tĭ-no'mah) ameloblastoma.

ad·a·man·to·blast (ad''ah-man'to-blast) ameloblast.

ad·a·man·to·ma (ad''ah-man-to'mah) ameloblastoma.

adap·a·lene (ah-dap'ah-lēn) a synthetic analogue of retinoic acid used topically in the treatment of acne vulgaris.

ad·ap·ta·tion (ad''ap-ta'shun) 1. the adjustment of an organism to its environment, or the process by which it enhances such fitness. 2. the normal adjustment of the eye to variations in intensity of light. 3. the decline in the frequency of firing of a neuron, particularly of a receptor, under conditions of constant stimulation. 4. in dentistry, (*a*) the proper fitting of a denture, (*b*) the degree of proximity and interlocking of restorative material to a tooth preparation, (*c*) the exact adjustment of bands to teeth. 5. in microbiology, the adjustment of bacterial physiology to a new environment. **color a.,** 1. changes in visual perception of color with prolonged stimulation. 2. adjustment of vision to degree of brightness or color tone of illumination. **dark a.**, adaptation of the eye to vision in the dark or in reduced illumination. **genetic a.**, the natural selection of the progeny of a mutant better adapted to a new environment. **light a.**, adaptation of the eye to vision in the sunlight or in bright illumination (photopia), with reduction in the concentration of the photosensitive pigments of the eye. **phenotypic a.**, a change in the properties of an organism in response to genetic mutation or to a change in the environment.

ad·ap·tom·e·ter (ad″ap-tom′ĕ-ter) an instrument for measuring the time required for retinal adaptation, i.e., for regeneration of the visual purple; used in detecting night blindness, vitamin A deficiency, and retinitis pigmentosa. **color a.**, an instrument to demonstrate adaptation of the eye to color or light.

ADCC antibody-dependent cell-mediated cytotoxicity.

ad·der (ad′er) 1. *Vipera berus.* 2. any of many venomous snakes of the family Viperidae, such as the puff adder and European viper. **death a.**, *Acanthophis antarcticus*, an extremely venomous elapid snake of Australia and New Guinea with a short, stout body and a tail with a spine at the tip. **puff a.**, *Bitis arrietans*, an extremely venomous, brightly colored, viperine snake found in Africa and Arabia; when annoyed it inflates its stubby body and hisses loudly.

ad·dic·tion (ah-dik′shun) 1. the state of being given up to some habit or compulsion. 2. strong physiological and psychological dependence on a drug or other psychoactive substance.

ad·di·son·ism (ad′ĭ-son-izm″) addisonian syndrome.

ad·duct¹ (ah-dukt′) to draw toward the median plane or (in the digits) toward the axial line of a limb. **addu′cent**, adj.

ad·duct² (ă′dukt) inclusion complex.

ad·duc·tion (ah-duk′shun) the act of adducting; the state of being adducted.

ad·duc·tor (ah-duk′tor) [L.] that which adducts, as the adductor muscle.

adelo·mor·phous (ah-del″o-mor′fus) of indefinite form.

ad·e·nal·gia (ad″ĕ-nal′jah) pain in a gland.

aden·drit·ic (a″den-drit′ik) lacking dendrites.

ad·e·nec·to·my (ad″ĕ-nek′tah-me) excision of a gland.

ad·en·ec·to·pia (ad″ĕ-nek-to′pe-ah) malposition or displacement of a gland.

ade·nia (ah-de′ne-ah) chronic enlargement of the lymphatic glands; see also *lymphoma.*

ad·e·nine (ad′ĕ-nēn) a purine base; in plant and animal cells usually occurring complexed with ribose or deoxyribose to form adenosine and deoxyadenosine, components of nucleic acids, nucleotides, and coenzymes. A preparation is used to improve the preservation of whole blood. Symbol A. **a. arabinoside,** vidarabine.

ad·e·ni·tis (ad″ĕ-ni′tis) inflammation of a gland. **Bartholin a.**, inflammation of the greater vestibular gland (Bartholin's gland) resulting from acute infection of the gland. **cervical a.**, a condition characterized by enlarged, inflamed, and tender lymph nodes of the neck; seen in certain infectious diseases of children, such as acute throat infections. **mesenteric a.**, see under *lymphadenitis.* **vestibular a.**, chronic inflammation of the lesser vestibular glands, producing small, extremely painful ulcerations of the vestibular mucosa.

aden(o)- word element [Gr.], *gland.*

ad·e·no·ac·an·tho·ma (ad″ĕ-no-ak″an-tho′mah) adenocarcinoma in which some of the cells exhibit squamous differentiation.

ad·e·no·am·e·lo·blas·to·ma (-ah-mel″o-blas-to′mah) adenomatoid odontogenic tumor.

ad·e·no·blast (ad′ĕ-no-blast″) an embryonic cell that gives rise to glandular tissue.

ad·e·no·car·ci·no·ma (ad″ĕ-no-kahr′sĭ-no′mah) carcinoma derived from glandular tissue or in which the tumor cells form recognizable glandular structures. **acinar a.**, 1. see under *carcinoma.* 2. the most common neoplasm of the prostate, usually arising in the peripheral acini. **acinic cell a., acinous a.**, see under *carcinoma.* **bronchogenic a.**, the usual type of adenocarcinoma of the lung; cf. *bronchioloalveolar carcinoma.* **clear cell a.**, a rare malignant tumor of the female genital tract, containing tubules or small cysts; it may occur in the ovary, uterus, cervix, or vagina. One form has been linked to in utero exposure to diethylstilbestrol. **ductal a. of the prostate,** adenocarcinoma of columnar epithelium in the peripheral prostatic ducts; it may project into the urethra. **endometrioid a.**, the most common form of endometrial carcinoma, containing tumor cells differentiated into glandular tissue with little or no stroma. **gastric a.**, any of a group of common stomach cancers, usually located in the antrum; it occurs particularly in Japan, Iceland, Chile, and Finland and may be linked to certain dietary substances such as nitrosamines and benzpyrene. **a. of the lung,** a type of bronchogenic carcinoma made up of cuboidal or columnar cells in a discrete mass, usually at the periphery of the lungs. **papillary a., polypoid a.,** that in which the tumor elements are arranged as finger-like processes or as a solid spherical nodule projecting from an epithelial surface. **a. of the prostate,** acinar a. (2)

ad·e·no·cele (ad′ĕ-no-sēl″) cystadenoma.

ad·e·no·cel·lu·li·tis (ad″ĕ-no-sel″u-li′tis) inflammation of a gland and the tissue around it.

ad·e·no·cys·tic (-sis′tik) having both glandular (adenoid) and cystic elements.

ad·e·no·cys·to·ma (-sis-to′mah) cystadenoma. **papillary a. lymphomatosum,** adenolymphoma.

ad·e·no·cyte (ad′ĕ-no-sīt″) a mature secretory cell of a gland.

ad·e·no·ep·i·the·li·o·ma (ad″ĕ-no-ep″ĭ-the″le-o′mah) a tumor composed of glandular and epithelial elements.

ad·e·no·fi·bro·ma (-fi-bro′mah) a tumor composed of connective tissue containing glandular structures.

ad·e·nog·e·nous (ad″ĕ-noj′ĕ-nus) originating from glandular tissue.

ad·e·nog·ra·phy (ad″ĕ-nog′rah-fe) radiography of the glands. **adenograph′ic,** adj.

ad·e·no·hy·poph·y·sec·to·my (ad″ĕ-no-hi-pof″ĭ-sek′tah-me) excision or ablation of the adenohypophysis.

ad·e·no·hy·poph·y·sis (-hi-pof′ĭ-sis) the anterior (glandular) lobe of the pituitary gland; it secretes the anterior pituitary hormones such as growth hormone, thyrotropin, and others. **adenohypophys′eal,** adj.

ad·e·noid (ad′ĕ-noid) 1. pharyngeal tonsil. 2. pertaining to a pharyngeal tonsil. 3. resembling a gland. 4. (pl.) hypertrophy of the pharyngeal tonsils, usually seen in children.

ad·e·noid·i·tis (ad″ĕ-noid-i′tis) inflammation of the adenoids.

ad·e·no·li·po·ma (ad″ĕ-no-lĭ-po′mah) a tumor composed of both glandular and fatty tissue elements.

ad·e·no·lym·phi·tis (-lim-fi′tis) lymphadenitis.

ad·e·no·lym·pho·ma (-lim-fo′mah) a benign parotid gland tumor characterized by cystic spaces lined by tall columnar eosinophilic epithelial cells, overlying a lymphoid tissue–containing stroma.

ad·e·no·ma (ad″ĕ-no′mah) a benign epithelial tumor in which the cells form recognizable glandular structures or in which the cells are derived from glandular epithelium. **adrenocortical a.,** a benign tumor of the adrenal cortex, usually small and unilateral; most types cause endocrine symptoms. **basal cell a.,** a benign, encapsulated, slow-growing, painless salivary gland tumor of intercalated or reserve cell origin, occurring mainly in males, in the parotid gland or upper lip; *solid, canalicular, trabecular-tubular,* and *membranous* types can be distinguished histologically. **bile duct a.,** a small firm white nodule with multiple bile ducts embedded in a fibrous stroma. **bronchial a's,** tumors of low-grade malignancy situated in the submucosal tissues of large bronchi; sometimes composed of well-differentiated cells and usually circumscribed, with two histologic forms: carcinoid and cylindroma. **carcinoma ex pleomorphic a.,** see under *carcinoma.* **chromophobe a., chromophobic a.,** null-cell a. **corticotroph a.,** a pituitary adenoma made up predominantly of corticotrophs and secreting excess corticotropin. **follicular a.,** adenoma of the thyroid in which the cells are arranged in the form of follicles. **glycoprotein a.,** a pituitary adenoma that causes excessive secretion of one of the three glycoprotein hormones (follicle-stimulating hormone, luteinizing hormone, and thyrotropin). **hepatocellular a.,** a benign circumscribed tumor of the liver, usually in the right lobe, growing in a sheetlike fashion; it may be highly vascular with a tendency to hemorrhage and with areas of necrosis. **Hürthle cell a.,** see under *tumor.* **liver cell a.,** hepatocellular a. **macrofollicular a.,** a follicular adenoma composed of large follicles filled with colloid and lined with flat epithelium. **microfollicular a.,** a follicular adenoma with small, closely-packed follicles lined with epithelium. **mixed-cell a.,** a pituitary adenoma containing more than one cell type, usually making it plurihormonal. **monomorphic a.,** any of a group of benign salivary gland tumors that lack connective tissue changes and are each predominantly composed of a single cell type. **nipple a.,** a benign lesion of the breast, clinically resembling Paget's disease of the breast, consisting of ductal and stromal proliferation beneath the nipple, which presents as a mass, ulceration, or erosion, with a serous or bloody discharge. **null-cell a.,** a pituitary adenoma whose cells give negative results on tests for staining and hormone secretion, although some may contain functioning cells and be associated with a hyperpituitary state. **oncocytic a., oxyphilic a.,** 1. oncocytoma. 2. Hürthle cell adenoma.

papillary a., nipple a. **papillary cystic a.,** papillary cystadenoma. **pituitary a.,** a benign neoplasm of the anterior pituitary gland; the *endocrine-active a's* contain cells that secrete anterior pituitary hormones; the *endocrine-inactive a's* are not secretory. **pleomorphic a.,** a benign, slow-growing, epithelial tumor of the salivary gland, usually of the parotid gland, sometimes serving as a locus for development of a malignant epithelial neoplasm *(malignant pleomorphic a.).* **plurihormonal a.,** an endocrine-active adenoma that secretes two or more hormones, usually growth hormone and one or more of the glycoprotein types. **sebaceous a.,** 1. an uncommon, benign, yellow or flesh-colored, circumscribed nodule occurring on the face or scalp, generally in older men, consisting of incompletely differentiated sebaceous lobules. 2. a. sebaceum. **a. seba′ceum,** 1. cutaneous angiofibromatous proliferation, usually on the face, in association with tuberous sclerosis. 2. nevoid hyperplasia of sebaceous glands, forming multiple yellow papules or nodules of the face. **trabecular a.,** a follicular adenoma whose cells are closely packed to form cords or trabeculae, with only a few small follicles. **tubular a.,** 1. an adenoma whose cells are arranged in tubules. 2. androblastoma (1). 3. the most common type of adenomatous polyp of the colon, with tubules highly variable in size and often occurring singly. **villous a.,** an uncommon type of adenomatous polyp of the colon that is large, soft, and papillary and often premalignant.

ad·e·no·ma·la·cia (ad″ĕ-no-mah-la′shah) abnormal softening of a gland.

ad·e·no·ma·toid (ad″ĕ-no′mah-toid) resembling adenoma.

ad·e·no·ma·to·sis (ad″ĕ-no″mah-to′sis) the development of numerous adenomatous growths.

ad·e·nom·a·tous (ad″ĕ-nom′ah-tus) 1. pertaining to an adenoma. 2. pertaining to nodular hyperplasia of a gland.

ad·e·no·meg·a·ly (ad″ĕ-no-meg′ah-le) enlargement of a gland.

ad·e·no·mere (ad′ĕ-no-mēr″) the blind terminal portion of a developing gland, becoming the functional portion of the organ.

ad·e·no·myo·fi·bro·ma (ad″ĕ-no-mi″o-fi-bro′mah) a fibroma containing both glandular and muscular elements.

ad·e·no·my·o·ma (-mi-o′mah) 1. a benign tumor consisting of smooth muscle and glandular elements. 2. see *adenomyosis.*

ad·e·no·my·o·ma·to·sis (-mi″o-mah-to′sis) the formation of multiple adenomyomatous nodules in the tissues around or in the uterus.

ad·e·no·myo·me·tri·tis (-mi″o-me-tri′tis) an inflammatory lesion of the endometrium, which may lead to adenomyosis.

ad·e·no·myo·sar·co·ma (-mi″o-sahr-ko′mah) a mixed mesodermal tumor containing striated muscle cells.

ad·e·no·my·o·sis (-mi-o′sis) benign ingrowth of the endometrium into the uterine musculature, sometimes with hypertrophy of the latter; if the lesion forms a circumscribed tumorlike nodule, it is called *adenomyoma.*

ad·e·nop·a·thy (ad″ĕ-nop′ah-the) 1. adenomegaly. 2. enlargement of a lymph node. 3. lymphadenopathy.

ad·e·no·phar·yn·gi·tis (ad″ĕ-no-far″in-ji′tis) inflammation of the adenoids and pharynx, usually involving the tonsils.

ad·e·no·sar·co·ma (-sahr-ko′mah) a mixed tumor composed of both glandular and sarcomatous elements.

ad·e·no·scle·ro·sis (-sklĕ-ro′sis) hardening of a gland.

aden·o·sine (ah-den′o-sēn) a purine nucleoside consisting of adenine and ribose; a component of RNA. It is also a cardiac depressant and vasodilator used as an antiarrhythmic and as an adjunct in myocardial perfusion imaging in patients incapable of exercising adequately to undergo an exercise stress test. Symbol A. **cyclic a. monophosphate,** a cyclic nucleotide, adenosine 3′,5′-cyclic monophosphate, that serves as an intracellular, and sometimes extracellular, "second messenger" mediating the action of many peptide or amine hormones. Abbreviated 3′,5′-AMP, cAMP, and cyclic AMP. **a. diphosphate (ADP),** a nucleotide, the 5′-pyrophosphate of adenosine, involved in energy metabolism; it is produced by the hydrolysis of adenosine triphosphate (ATP) and converted back to ATP by the metabolic processes oxidative phosphorylation and substrate-level phosphorylation. **a. monophosphate (AMP),** adenylic acid; a nucleotide, the 5′-phosphate of adenosine, involved in energy metabolism and nucleotide synthesis. **a. triphosphate (ATP),** a nucleotide, the 5′-triphosphate of adenosine, involved in energy metabolism and required for RNA synthesis; it occurs in all cells and is used to store energy in the form of high-energy phosphate bonds. The free energy derived from its hydrolysis is used to drive metabolic reactions, to transport molecules against concentration gradients, and to produce mechanical motion.

aden·o·sine de·am·i·nase (ADA) (de-am′ĭ-nās) an enzyme that catalyzes the hydrolytic deamination of adenosine to form inosine, a reaction of purine metabolism. Enzyme activity is absent in many individuals with severe combined immunodeficiency.

aden·o·sine·tri·phos·pha·tase (-tri-fos'-fah-tās) an enzyme that catalyzes the hydrolysis of ATP to ADP, driving processes such as muscle contraction, maintenance of concentration gradients, membrane transport, and regulation of ion concentrations.

ad·e·no·sis (ad″ĕ-no'sis) 1. any disease of the glands. 2. the abnormal development of glandular tissue. **mammary sclerosing a., sclerosing a. of breast,** a form of disease of the breast characterized by multiple firm tender nodules, fibrous tissue, mastodynia, and sometimes small cysts.

ad·e·no·squa·mous (ad″ĕ-no-skwa'mus) having both glandular (adenoid) and squamous elements.

aden·o·syl·co·ba·la·min (AdoCbl) (ah-den″o-sil-ko-bal'ah-min) one of two metabolically active forms of cobalamin synthesized upon ingestion of vitamin B_{12}; it is the predominant form in the liver.

ad·e·no·tome (ad'ĕ-no-tōm″) an instrument for excision of adenoids.

Ad·e·no·vi·ri·dae (ad″ĕ-no-vir'ĭ-de) the adenoviruses: a family of DNA viruses with a double-stranded genome, generally with a narrow host range, and transferred by direct or indirect transmission; it includes the genus *Mastadenovirus.*

ad·e·no·vi·rus (ad'ĕ-no-vi″rus) any virus belonging to the family Adenoviridae. **adenovi'ral,** adj. **mammalian a's,** *Mastadenovirus.*

ad·e·nyl (ad'ĕ-nil) 1. the radical of adenine. 2. sometimes (incorrectly) used for *adenylyl.*

aden·yl·ate (ah-den'ĭ-lāt) the dissociated form of adenylic acid.

aden·yl·ate ki·nase (ki'nās) an enzyme that catalyzes the conversion of two molecules of ADP to AMP and ATP; it occurs predominantly in muscle, providing energy for muscle contraction.

ad·e·nyl cy·clase (ad'ĕ-nil si'klās) an enzyme that catalyzes the conversion of adenosine triphosphate (ATP) to cyclic adenosine monophosphate (cAMP) and inorganic pyrophosphate (PP$_i$). It is activated by the attachment of a hormone or neurotransmitter to a specific membrane-bound receptor.

ad·e·nyl·ic ac·id (ad″ĕ-nil'ik) phosphorylated adenosine, usually adenosine monophosphate.

aden·yl·yl (ad'ĕ-nĭ-lil) the radical of adenosine monophosphate with one OH ion removed.

ad·e·qua·cy (ad'ĕ-kwah-se) the state of being sufficient for a specific purpose. **velopharyngeal a.,** sufficient functional closure of the velum against the postpharyngeal wall so that air and hence sound cannot enter the nasopharyngeal and nasal cavities.

ad·e·quate (ad'ĕ-kwit) sufficient in quantity, quality, or amount to achieve a desired effect.

ader·mo·gen·e·sis (ah-der″mo-jen'ĕ-sis) imperfect development of skin.

ADH antidiuretic hormone.

ad·her·ence (ad-hēr'ens) the act or condition of sticking to something. **immune a.,** the adherence of antigen-antibody complexes or cells coated with antibody or complement to cells bearing complement receptors or Fc receptors. It is a sensitive detector of complement-fixing antibody.

ad·her·ent (-ent) sticking or holding fast, or having such qualities.

ad·he·sion (ad-he'zhun) 1. the property of remaining in close proximity. 2. the stable joining of parts to one another, which may occur abnormally. 3. a fibrous band or structure by which parts abnormally adhere. **interthalamic a.,** a band of gray matter joining the thalami; it develops as a secondary adhesion and is often absent. **primary a.,** healing by first intention. **secondary a.,** healing by second intention.

ad·he·si·ot·o·my (ad-he″ze-ot'ah-me) surgical division of adhesions.

ad·he·sive (ad-he'siv) 1. sticky; tenacious. 2. a substance that causes close adherence of adjoining surfaces.

adi·a·do·cho·ki·ne·sia (ah-di″ah-do″ko-kĭ-ne'zhah) a dyskinesia consisting of inability to perform the rapid alternating movements of diadochokinesia.

adi·a·pho·ria (a″di-ah-for'e-ah) nonresponse to stimuli as a result of previous exposure to similar stimuli; see also *refractory period,* under *period.*

adi·a·spi·ro·my·co·sis (ad″e-ah-spi″ro-mi-ko'sis) a pulmonary disease of many species of rodents and occasionally of humans, due to inhalation of spores of the fungi *Emmonsia parva* and *E. crescens,* and marked by huge spherules (adiaspores) in the lungs.

adi·a·spore (ad'e-ah-spor″) a spore produced by the soil fungi *Emmonsia parva* and *E. crescens;* see *adiaspiromycosis.*

adip(o)- word element [L.], *fat.*

ad·i·po·cele (ad'ĭ-po-sēl″) a hernia containing fat or fatty tissue.

ad·i·po·cel·lu·lar (ad″ĭ-po-sel'u-ler) composed of fat and connective tissue.

ad·i·po·cere (ad'ĭ-po-sēr") a waxy substance formed during decomposition of dead animal bodies, consisting mainly of insoluble salts of fatty acids. **adipocer'atous,** adj.

ad·i·po·cyte (-sīt") fat cell.

ad·i·po·gen·ic (ad"ĭ-po-jen'ik) lipogenic.

ad·i·po·ki·ne·sis (-kĭ-ne'sis) the mobilization of fat in the body. **adipokinet'ic,** adj.

ad·i·pol·y·sis (ad"ĭ-pol'ĭ-sis) lipolysis. **adipolyt'ic,** adj.

ad·i·po·ne·cro·sis (ad"ĭ-po-nĕ-kro'sis) necrosis of fatty tissue.

ad·i·po·pex·is (-pek'sis) the fixation or storing of fats. **adipopec'tic,** adj.

ad·i·pose (ad'ĭ-pōs) 1. fatty. 2. the fat present in the cells of adipose tissue.

ad·i·po·sis (ad"ĭ-po'sis) 1. obesity. 2. fatty change in an organ or tissue. **a. cerebra'lis,** cerebral adiposity. **a. doloro'sa,** a disease, usually of women, marked by painful localized fatty swellings and by various nerve lesions; death may result from pulmonary complications. **a. hepa'tica,** fatty change of the liver.

ad·i·po·si·tis (ad"ĭ-po-si'tis) panniculitis.

ad·i·pos·i·ty (ad"ĭ-pos'ĭ-te) obesity. **cerebral a.,** fatness due to cerebral disease, especially of the hypothalamus.

ad·i·po·su·ria (ad"ĭ-po-su're-ah) lipiduria.

adip·sia (ah-dip'se-ah) absence of thirst, or abnormal avoidance of drinking.

ad·i·tus (ad'ĭ-tus) pl. *a'ditus.* [L.] in anatomic nomenclature, an opening or entrance.

ad·just·ment (ah-just'ment) 1. the act or process of modification of physical parts made in response to changing conditions. 2. in psychology, the relative degree of harmony between an individual's needs and the requirements of the environment. 3. in chiropractic, any of various manual and mechanical interventions, most often applied to the spine, in which controlled and directed forces are applied to a joint to correct structural dysfunction and restore normal nerve function.

ad·ju·vant (aj"ōō-vant, ă-joo'vant) 1. assisting or aiding. 2. a substance that aids another, such as an auxiliary remedy. 3. a nonspecific stimulator of the immune response. **aluminum a.,** an aluminum-containing compound, such as aluminum hydroxide or alum, that by combining with soluble antigen forms a precipitate; slow release of the antigen from the precipitate on injection causes prolonged, strong antibody response. **Freund's a.,** a water-in-oil emulsion incorporating antigen, in the aqueous phase, into lightweight paraffin oil with the aid of an emulsifying agent. On injection, this mixture (*Freund's incomplete a.*) induces strong persistent antibody formation. The addition of killed, dried mycobacteria, e.g., *Mycobacterium butyricum,* to the oil phase (*Freund's complete a.*) elicits cell-mediated immunity (delayed hypersensitivity), as well as humoral antibody formation.

ad·ju·van·tic·i·ty (aj"ōō-van-tis'ĭ-te, ă-joo"-van-tis'ĭ-te) the ability to modify the immune response.

ad·ner·val (ad-ner'val) 1. situated near a nerve. 2. toward a nerve, said of electric current that passes through muscle toward the entrance point of a nerve.

ad·neu·ral (ad-noor'al) adnerval.

ad·nexa (ad-nek'sah) [L., pl.] appendages or accessory structures of an organ, as the appendages of the eye (*a. o'culi*), including the eyelids and lacrimal apparatus, or of the uterus (*a. u'teri*), including the uterine tubes and ligaments and ovaries.

ad·nex·al (ad-nek'sal) pertaining to adnexa.

AdoCbl adenosylcobalamin.

ad·o·les·cence (ad"o-les'ens) the period between puberty and the completion of physical growth, roughly from 11 to 19 years of age. **adoles'cent,** adj.

ad·or·al (ad-or'al) toward or near the mouth.

ADP adenosine diphosphate.

ad·re·nal (ah-dre'n'l) 1. paranephric. 2. adrenal gland. 3. pertaining to an adrenal gland.

Adren·a·lin (ah-dren'ah-lin) trademark for preparations of epinephrine.

adren·a·line (ah-dren'ah-lin) epinephrine.

adren·a·lin·uria (ah-dren"ah-lin-u're-ah) the presence of epinephrine in the urine.

adren·al·ism (ah-dren'al-izm) any disorder of adrenal function, whether decreased or increased.

adre·na·li·tis (ah-dre"nal-i'tis) inflammation of the adrenal glands.

ad·ren·er·gic (ad"ren-er'jik) 1. activated by, characteristic of, or secreting epinephrine or related substances, particularly the sympathetic nerve fibers that liberate norepinephrine at a synapse when a nerve impulse passes. 2. any agent that produces such an effect. See also under *receptor.*

adren(o)- word element [L.], *adrenal gland.*

adre·no·cep·tor (ah-dre"no-sep'ter) adrenergic receptor. **adrenocep'tive,** adj.

adre·no·cor·ti·cal (-kor'tĭ-k'l) pertaining to or arising from the adrenal cortex.

adre·no·cor·ti·co·hy·per·pla·sia (-kor"tĭ-ko-hi"per-pla'zhah) adrenal cortical hyperplasia.

adre·no·cor·ti·coid (-kor'tĭ-koid") corticosteroid.

adre·no·cor·ti·co·mi·met·ic (-kor″tĭ-ko-mi-met′ik) having effects similar to those of hormones of the adrenal cortex.

adre·no·cor·ti·co·tro·phic (-kor″tĭ-ko-tro′-fik) adrenocorticotropic.

adre·no·cor·ti·co·troph·in (-kor″tĭko-tro′-fin) corticotropin.

adre·no·cor·ti·co·tro·pic (-kor″tĭ-ko-tro′-pik) having a stimulating effect on the adrenal cortex.

adre·no·cor·ti·co·trop·in (-kor″tĭ-ko-tro′-pin) corticotropin.

adre·no·dox·in (-dok′sin) an iron-sulfur protein of the adrenal cortex that serves as an electron carrier in the biosynthesis of adrenal steroids from cholesterol.

adre·no·leu·ko·dys·tro·phy (-loo″ko-dis′-tro-fe) an X-linked disorder related to Schilder's disease, characterized by diffuse abnormality of the cerebral white matter with mental retardation and adrenal atrophy.

adre·no·lyt·ic (-lit′ik) inhibiting the action of the adrenergic nerves, or the response to epinephrine.

adre·no·med·ul·lary (-med′u-lar″e) pertaining to or originating in the adrenal medulla.

adre·no·meg·a·ly (-meg′ah-le) enlargement of one or both of the adrenal glands.

adre·no·mi·met·ic (-mi-met′ik) sympathomimetic.

adre·no·my·elo·neu·rop·a·thy (-mi″ĕ-lo-noo̅o̅-rop′ah-the) a hereditary condition related to adrenoleukodystrophy but including spinal cord degeneration and peripheral neuropathy.

adre·no·re·cep·tor (-re-sep′ter) adrenergic receptor.

adre·no·tox·in (ah-dre′no-tok″sin) any substance that is toxic to the adrenal glands.

Adri·a·my·cin (a″dre-ah-mi′sin) trademark for preparations of doxorubicin hydrochloride.

ad·sorb (ad-sorb′) to attract and retain other material on the surface; to conduct the process of adsorption.

ad·sor·bent (ad-sor′bent) 1. pertaining to or characterized by adsorption. 2. a substance that attracts other materials or particles to its surface by adsorption.

ad·sorp·tion (ad-sorp′shun) the action of a substance in attracting and holding other materials or particles on its surface.

ADTA American Dance Therapy Association.

ad·tor·sion (ad-tor′shun) intorsion.

adult (ah-dult′) having attained full growth or maturity, or an organism that has done so.

adul·te·ra·tion (ah-dul″ter-a′shun) addition of an impure, cheap, or unnecessary ingredient to cheat, cheapen, or falsify a preparation; in legal terminology, incorrect labeling, including dosage not in accordance with the label.

ad·vance·ment (ad-vans′ment) 1. surgical detachment, as of a muscle or tendon, followed by reattachment at a point further forward than the original position. 2. the surgical moving forward of the mandible in the correction of jaw deformity.

ad·ven·ti·tia (ad″ven-tish′e-ah) 1. adventitial. 2. tunica adventitia.

ad·ven·ti·tial (ad″ven-tish′al) pertaining to the tunica adventitia.

ad·ven·ti·tious (ad″ven-tish′us) 1. accidental or acquired; not natural or hereditary. 2. found out of the normal or usual place. 3. adventitial.

ad·ver·sive (ad-ver′siv) opposite; as the turning to one side in an adversive seizure.

ady·na·mia (a″di-na′me-ah) asthenia. **adynam′ic,** adj.

adys·pla·sia (a″dis-pla′zhah) severe dysplasia in which an organ or part is shrunken and sometimes ectopic, and initially appears to be absent.

A-E, AE above-elbow; see under *amputation.*

AED automatic external defibrillator.

Ae·des (a-e′dēz) a genus of mosquitoes, including approximately 600 species; some are vectors of disease, others are pests. It includes *A. aegyp′ti,* a vector of yellow fever and dengue.

aer·a·tion (ār-a′shun) 1. the exchange of carbon dioxide for oxygen by the blood in the lungs. 2. the charging of a liquid with air or gas.

aer(o)- word element [Gr.], *air; gas.*

aer·obe (ār′ōb) a microorganism that lives and grows in the presence of free oxygen. facultative a's, microorganisms that can live in the presence or absence of oxygen. obligate a's, microorganisms that require oxygen for growth.

aer·o·bic (ār-o′bik) 1. having molecular oxygen present. 2. growing, living, or occurring in the presence of molecular oxygen. 3. requiring oxygen for respiration. 4. designed to increase oxygen consumption by the body.

aero·bi·ol·o·gy (ār″o-bi-ol′o-je) the study of the distribution of microorganisms by the air.

aero·bi·o·sis (-bi-o′sis) life in the presence of molecular oxygen.

aero·cele (ār′o-sēl″) pneumatocele (1). epidural a., a collection of air between the dura mater and the wall of the spinal column.

aer·o·der·mec·ta·sia (ār″o-der″mek-ta′-zhah) subcutaneous emphysema.

aer·odon·tal·gia (-don-tal′jah) pain in the teeth due to lowered atmospheric pressure at high altitudes.

aero·em·bo·lism (-em′bo-lizm) air embolism.

aero·gen (ār′o-jen″) a gas-producing bacterium.

Aero·mo·nas (ār″o-mo′nas) a genus of schizomycetes usually found in water, some being pathogenic for fish, amphibians, reptiles, and humans.

aer·op·a·thy (ār-op′ah-the) any disease due to change in atmospheric pressure, e.g., decompression sickness.

aero·peri·to·nia (ār″o-per″ĭ-to′ne-ah) pneumoperitoneum.

aero·pha·gia (-fa′jah) excessive swallowing of air, usually an unconscious process associated with anxiety.

aero·phil·ic (-fĭl′ik) requiring air for proper growth.

aero·si·nu·si·tis (-si″nus-i′tis) barosinusitis.

aer·o·sol (ār′o-sol) a colloid system in which solid or liquid particles are suspended in a gas, especially a suspension of a drug or other substance to be dispensed in a fine spray or mist.

aero·tax·is (ār″o-tak′sis) movement of an organism in response to the presence of molecular oxygen.

aer·oti·tis (-ti′tis) barotitis.

aero·tol·er·ant (-tol′er-ant) surviving and growing in small amounts of air; said of anaerobic microorganisms.

aero·tym·pa·nal (-tim′pah-n′l) pertaining to or involving the air and the tympanum.

aes- for words beginning thus, see those beginning *es-, et-*.

Aescu·la·pi·us (es″ku-la′pe-us) [L.] the god of healing in Roman mythology; see also *caduceus* and under *staff*.

afe·brile (a-feb′ril) without fever.

af·fect (af′ekt) the external expression of emotion attached to ideas or mental representations of objects.

af·fec·tive (ah-fek′tiv) pertaining to affect.

af·fer·ent (af′er-ent) 1. conveying toward a center. 2. something that so conducts, such as a fiber or nerve.

af·fin·i·ty (ah-fin′ĭ-te) 1. attraction; a tendency to seek out or unite with another object or substance. 2. in chemistry, the tendency of two substances to form strong or weak chemical bonds forming molecules or complexes. 3. in immunology, the thermodynamic bond strength of an antigen-antibody complex. Cf. *avidity*.

afi·brin·o·gen·emia (a″fi-brin″o-jĕ-ne′-me-ah) deficiency or absence of fibrinogen (coagulation factor I) in the blood. **congenital a.,** a rare autosomal recessive hemorrhagic coagulation disorder characterized by complete incoagulability of the blood.

af·la·tox·in (af′lah-tok″sin) a toxin produced by *Aspergillus flavus* and *A. parasiticus*, molds which contaminate ground nut seedlings; it has been implicated as a cause of hepatic carcinoma in humans.

AFP alpha fetoprotein.

af·ter·birth (af′ter-birth″) the placenta and membranes delivered from the uterus after childbirth.

af·ter·brain (-brān) metencephalon.

af·ter·de·po·lar·iza·tion (af″ter-de-po″lar-ĭ-za′shun) a depolarizing afterpotential, frequently one of a series, sometimes occurring in tissues not normally excitable. It may occur before (*early a.*) or after (*delayed a.*) full repolarization.

af·ter·im·age (af′ter-im″aj) a retinal impression remaining after cessation of the stimulus causing it.

af·ter·load (-lōd″) the force against which cardiac muscle shortens: in isolated muscle, the force resisting shortening after the muscle is stimulated to contract; in the intact heart, the pressure against which the ventricle ejects blood.

af·ter·pains (-pānz″) cramplike pains following the birth of a child, due to uterine contractions.

af·ter·po·ten·tial (-po-ten″shul) the small action potential generated following termination of the spike or main potential; it has negative and (paradoxically named) positive phases, the latter being in fact more negative than the resting potential.

af·ter·taste (-tāst″) a taste continuing after the substance producing it has been removed.

AFX atypical fibroxanthoma.

AG atrial gallop.

Ag antigen; silver (L. *argen′tum*).

AGA American Gastroenterological Association.

aga·lac·tia (a″gah-lak′she-ah) absence or failure of secretion of milk.

agam·ma·glob·u·lin·emia (a-gam″ah-glob″u-lĭ-ne′me-ah) absence of all classes of immunoglobulins in the blood. See also *hypogammaglobulinemia*. **X-linked a.,** an X-linked disorder characterized by absence of circulating B lymphocytes, plasma cells, or germinal centers in lymphoid tissues, very low levels of circulating immunoglobulins, susceptibility to bacterial infection, and symptoms resembling rheumatoid arthritis; apparently due to failure of pre-B cells to differentiate into mature B cells.

agan·gli·on·ic (a-gang″gle-on′ik) pertaining to or characterized by the absence of ganglion cells.

agan·gli·on·o·sis (a-gang″gle-on-o′sis) congenital absence of parasympathetic ganglion cells.

agar (ag′ahr) a dried hydrophilic, colloidal substance extracted from various species of red algae; used in solid culture media for bacteria and other microorganisms, as a bulk laxative, in making emulsions, and as a supporting medium in procedures such as immunodiffusion and electrophoresis.

agar·ic (ah-gar′ik, ag′ah-rik) 1. any mushroom, more especially any species of *Agaricus*. 2. a preparation of rotten wood mixed with fungi or dried mushrooms.

agas·tric (a-gas′trik) having no alimentary canal.

age (āj) 1. the duration, or the measure of time, of the existence of a person or object. 2. the measure of an attribute relative to the chronological age of an average normal individual. **achievement a.,** the age of a person expressed as the chronologic age of a normal person showing the same proficiency in study. **bone a.,** osseous development shown radiographically, stated in terms of the chronological age at which the development is ordinarily attained. **chronological a.,** the measure of time elapsed since a person's birth. **fertilization a.,** the age of a conceptus defined by the time elapsed since fertilization. **gestational a.,** the age of a conceptus or pregnancy; in human clinical practice, timed from onset of the last normal menstrual period. Elsewhere the onset may be timed from estrus, coitus, artificial insemination, vaginal plug formation, fertilization, or implantation. **mental a.,** the age level of mental ability of a person as gauged by standard intelligence tests.

agen·e·sia (a″jĕ-ne′zhah) 1. imperfect development. 2. sterility or impotence.

agen·e·sis (a-jen′ĕ-sis) absence of an organ, particularly that due to nonappearance of its primordium in the embryo. **gonadal a.,** complete failure of gonadal development, as in *Turner's syndrome*. **nuclear a.,** Möbius' syndrome.

agen·i·tal·ism (a-jen′ĭ-til-izm″) 1. absence of the genitals. 2. a condition caused by failure to secrete gonadal hormones.

ageno·so·mia (ah-jen″ah-so′me-ah) congenital absence or imperfect development of the genitals and eventration of the lower part of the abdomen.

agent (a′jent) something capable of producing an effect. **adrenergic blocking a.,** one that inhibits response to sympathetic impulses by blocking the alpha (*alpha-adrenergic blocking a.*) or beta (*beta-adrenergic blocking a.*) receptor sites of effector organs. **adrenergic neuron blocking a.,** one that inhibits the release of norepinephrine from postganglionic adrenergic nerve endings. **alkylating a.,** a cytotoxic agent, e.g., a nitrogen mustard, which is highly reactive and can donate an alkyl group to another compound. Alkylating agents inhibit cell division by reacting with DNA and are used as antineoplastic agents. **blocking a.,** an agent that inhibits a biological action, such as movement of an ion across the cell membrane, passage of a neural impulse, or interaction with a specific receptor. **calcium channel blocking a.,** any of a class of drugs that inhibit the influx of calcium ions across the cell membrane or inhibit the mobilization of calcium from intracellular stores; used in the treatment of angina, cardiac arrhythmias, and hypertension. **chelating a.,** 1. a compound that combines with metal ions to form stable ring structures. 2. a substance used to reduce the concentration of free metal ion in solution by complexing it. **cholinergic blocking a.,** one that blocks or inactivates acetylcholine. **emulsifying a.,** emulsifier. **ganglionic blocking a.,** one that blocks nerve impulses at autonomic ganglionic synapses. **inotropic a.,** any of a class of agents affecting the force of muscle contraction, particularly a drug affecting the force of cardiac contraction; positive inotropic agents increase, and negative inotropic agents decrease the force of cardiac muscle contraction. **luting a.,** lute (1). **neuromuscular blocking a.,** a compound that causes paralysis of skeletal muscle by blocking neural transmission at the neuromuscular junction. **nonsteroidal antiinflammatory a.,** see under *drug*. **A. Orange,** an herbicide containing 2,4,5-T and 2,4-D and the contaminant dioxin; it is suspected of being carcinogenic and teratogenic. **oxidizing a.,** a substance capable of accepting electrons from another substance, thereby oxidizing the second substance and itself becoming reduced. **potassium channel blocking a.,** any of a class of antiarrhythmic agents that inhibit the movement of potassium ions through the potassium channels, thus prolonging repolarization of the cell membrane. **progestational a.,** progestin: any of a group of hormones secreted by the corpus luteum and placenta and, in small amounts, by the adrenal cortex, including progesterone; they induce the formation of a secretory endometrium. Agents having progestational activity are also produced synthetically. **psychoactive a., psychotropic a.,** psychoactive substance. **reducing a.,** a substance that acts as an electron donor in a chemical redox reaction. **sclerosing a.,** sclerosant; a chemical irritant injected into a vein in sclerotherapy. **sodium channel blocking a.,** any of a class of antiarrhythmic agents that prevent ectopic beats by acting on partially inactivated sodium channels to inhibit abnormal depolarizations. **surface-active a.,** a substance that exerts a change on the surface properties of a liquid, especially one that reduces its surface tension, as a detergent. **wetting a.,** a substance that lowers the surface tension of water to promote wetting.

ageu·sia (ah-goo'zhah) absence of the sense of taste. **ageu'sic,** adj.

ag·ger (aj'er) pl. *ag'geres.* [L.] an eminence or elevation.

ag·glu·ti·nant (ah-gloo'tĭ-nant) 1. promoting union by adhesion. 2. a tenacious or gluey substance that holds parts together during the healing process.

ag·glu·ti·na·tion (ah-gloo"tĭ-na'shun) 1. the action of an agglutinant substance. 2. the process of union in wound healing. 3. the clumping together in suspension of antigen-bearing cells, microorganisms, or particles in the presence of specific antibodies (agglutinins). **agglu'tinative,** adj. **cross a.,** the agglutination of particulate antigen by antibody raised against a different but related antigen; see also *group a.* **group a.,** agglutination of members of a group of biologically related organisms or corpuscles by an agglutinin specific for that group. **intravascular a.,** clumping of particulate elements within the blood vessels; used conventionally to denote red blood cell aggregation.

ag·glu·ti·na·tor (ah-gloo'tĭ-na"ter) an agglutinin.

ag·glu·ti·nin (ah-gloo'tĭ-nin) 1. antibody which aggregates a particulate antigen, e.g., bacteria, following combination with the homologous antigen. 2. any substance other than antibody, e.g., lectin, that is capable of agglutinating particles. **anti-Rh a.,** an agglutinin not normally present in human plasma, which may be produced in Rh^- mothers carrying an Rh^+ fetus or after transfusion of Rh^+ blood into an Rh^- patient. **chief a.,** major a. **cold a.,** one that acts only at relatively low temperatures (0°–20° C). **group a.,** one that has a specific action on a particular group of microorganisms. **H a.,** one that is specific for flagellar antigens of the motile strain of a microorganism. **immune a.,** any agglutinating antibody. **incomplete a.,** one that at appropriate concentrations fails to agglutinate the homologous antigen. **leukocyte a.,** one that is directed against neutrophilic and other leukocytes. **major a.,** that present at highest titer in an antiserum. **minor a., partial a.,** one present in agglutinative serum which acts on organisms and cells that are closely related to the specific antigen, but in a lower dilution. **warm a.,** an agglutinin more reactive at 37° C than at lower temperatures.

ag·glu·tin·o·gen (ag"loo-tin'o-jen) 1. any substance that, acting as an antigen, stimulates the production of agglutinin. 2. the particulate antigen used in conducting agglutination tests.

ag·glu·ti·no·phil·ic (ah-gloo"tĭ-no-fil'ik) agglutinating easily.

ag·gre·gate 1. (ag'rĕ-gāt) to crowd or cluster together. 2. (ag'rĕ-git) crowded or clustered together. 3. (ag'rĕ-git) a mass or assemblage.

ag·gre·ga·tion (ag"rĕ-ga'shun) 1. massing or clumping of materials or people together. 2. a clumped mass of material. **familial a.,** the occurrence of more cases of a given disorder in close relatives of a person with the disorder than in control families. **platelet a.,** a clumping together of platelets induced by various agents (e.g., thrombin) as part of the mechanism leading to thrombus formation.

ag·gres·sion (ah-gresh'un) behavior leading to self-assertion; it may arise from innate drives and/or a response to frustration, and may be manifested by destructive and attacking behavior, by hostility and obstructionism, or by self-expressive drive to mastery.

ag·gres·sive (ah-gres'iv) 1. characterized by aggression. 2. rapidly spreading and invasive, as a tumor. 3. characterized by or pertaining to intensive or vigorous treatment.

ag·ing (āj'ing) the gradual structural changes that occur with the passage of time, that are not due to disease or accident, and that eventually lead to death.

ag·i·ta·tion (aj"ĭ-ta'shun) excessive, purposeless cognitive and motor activity or restlessness, usually associated with a state of tension or anxiety. Called also *psychomotor a.*

aglos·sia (a-glos'e-ah) congenital absence of the tongue.

aglu·ti·tion (a"gloo-tish'un) dysphagia.

agly·ce·mia (a"gli-se'me-ah) absence of sugar from the blood.

agly·con (a-gli′kon) the noncarbohydrate group of a glycoside molecule.

agly·cone (a-gli′kōn) aglycon.

ag·ni (ug-ne′) [Sanskrit] in ayurveda, the digestive and metabolic energy created by the doshas that transforms nourishment into forms (ojas) that are used by the body and mind.

ag·no·gen·ic (ag-no-jen′ik) idiopathic.

ag·no·sia (ag-no′zhah) inability to recognize the import of sensory impressions; the varieties correspond with several senses and are distinguished as *auditory (acoustic)*, *gustatory*, *olfactory*, *tactile*, and *visual*. **face a.,** facial a., prosopagnosia. **finger a.,** loss of ability to indicate one's own or another's fingers. **time a.,** loss of comprehension of the succession and duration of events. **visual a.,** inability to recognize familiar objects by sight, usually due to a lesion in one of the visual association areas.

-agogue word element [Gr.], *something which leads or induces.*

ago·na·dism (a-go′nah-dizm) the condition of being without sex glands. **agonad′al,** adj.

ag·o·nal (ag′ah-n′l) pertaining to or occurring just before death.

ag·o·nist (ag′ah-nist) 1. one involved in a struggle or competition. 2. agonistic muscle. 3. in pharmacology, a drug that has an affinity for and stimulates physiologic activity at cell receptors normally stimulated by naturally occurring substances.

ag·o·nis·tic (ag′ŏ-nis′tik) pertaining to a struggle or competition; as an agonistic muscle, counteracted by an antagonistic muscle.

ag·o·ra·pho·bia (ag″or-ah-fo′be-ah) intense, irrational fear of open spaces, sometimes occurring in association with panic attacks.

agram·ma·tism (a-gram′ah-tizm) inability to speak grammatically because of brain injury or disease, usually with simplified sentence structure and errors in tense, number, and gender.

-agra word element [Gr.], *attack; seizure.*

agran·u·lar (a-gran′u-lar) lacking granules.

agran·u·lo·cyte (a-gran′u-lo-sīt″) nongranular leukocyte.

agran·u·lo·cy·to·sis (a-gran″u-lo-si-to′sis) a symptom complex characterized by decreased granulocytes and by lesions of the throat, other mucous membranes, gastrointestinal tract, and skin; most cases are complications of drug therapy, radiation, or exposure to chemicals.

agran·u·lo·plas·tic (-plas′tik) forming nongranular cells only; not forming granular cells.

agraph·ia (ah-graf′e-ah) impairment or loss of the ability to write. **agraph′ic,** adj.

AGS American Geriatrics Society.

AGT antiglobulin test.

ague (a′gu) 1. a chill. 2. old name for *malaria.*

agy·ria (a-ji′re-ah) a malformation in which the convolutions of the cerebral cortex are not fully formed, so that the brain surface is smooth. **agyr′ic,** adj.

AHA American Heart Association; American Hospital Association.

AHF antihemophilic factor (coagulation factor VIII).

AHG antihemophilic globulin (coagulation factor VIII).

AHP Assistant House Physician.

AHS Assistant House Surgeon.

AI aortic insufficiency; artificial insemination.

AIC Association des Infermières Canadiennes.

AICC anti-inhibitor coagulant complex.

AICD activation-induced cell death; automatic implantable cardioverter-defibrillator.

AID donor insemination (artificial insemination by donor).

aid (ād) help or assistance; by extension, applied to any device by which a function can be improved or augmented, as a hearing aid. **first a.,** the initial emergency care and treatment of an injured or ill person before definitive medical and surgical management can be secured. **hearing a.,** a device that amplifies sound to help deaf persons hear, often specifically a device worn on the body. **pharmaceutical a.,** see under *necessity.*

AIDS acquired immunodeficiency syndrome.

AIH American Institute of Homeopathy; artificial insemination by husband.

AIHA American Industrial Hygiene Association; autoimmune hemolytic anemia.

ai·lu·ro·pho·bia (i-loor″o-fo′be-ah) irrational fear of cats.

ain·hum (ān′hum, i′num) [Port.] a disease in which formation of a linear constriction around a digit, particularly the fifth toe, leads to spontaneous amputation of the distal part of the digit.

AIP acute intermittent porphyria.

air (ār) the gaseous mixture which makes up the atmosphere. **alveolar a.,** see under *gas.* **residual a.,** see under *volume.* **tidal a.,** see under *volume.*

air·borne (ār′born) suspended in, transported by, or spread by air.

air·sick·ness (-sik-nes) motion sickness due to travel by airplane.

air·way (-wa) 1. the passage by which air enters and leaves the lungs. 2. a device for securing unobstructed respiration.

esophageal obturator a., a tube inserted into the esophagus to maintain airway patency in unconscious persons for positive-pressure ventilation through the attached face mask. **conducting a.,** the upper and lower airways considered together. **laryngeal mask a.,** a device for maintaining a patent airway without tracheal intubation, consisting of a tube connected to an oval inflatable cuff that seals the larynx. **lower a.,** the airway from the inferior end of the larynx to the ends of the terminal bronchioles. **nasopharyngeal a.,** a tube inserted through a nostril, across the floor of the nose, and through the nasopharynx so that the tongue does not block air flow in an unconscious person. **oropharyngeal a.,** a tube inserted through the mouth and pharynx so that the tongue does not block air flow in an unconscious person. **upper a.,** the airway from the nares and lips to the larynx.

AIUM American Institute of Ultrasound in Medicine.

A-K, AK above-knee; see *transfemoral amputation,* under *amputation.*

akaryo·cyte (a-kar′e-o-sīt″) a non-nucleated cell, e.g., an erythrocyte.

akar·y·ote (a-kar′e-ōt) akaryocyte.

ak·a·this·ia (ak″ah-thĭ′zhah) a condition marked by motor restlessness, ranging from anxiety to inability to lie or sit quietly or to sleep, a common extrapyramidal side effect of neuroleptic drugs.

aki·ne·sia (a″kĭ-ne′zhah) absence, poverty, or loss of control of voluntary muscle movements. **a. al′gera,** a condition characterized by generalized pain associated with movement of any kind.

akin·es·the·sia (ah-kin″es-the′zhah) absence or loss of movement sense (kinesthesia).

aki·net·ic (a-kĭ-net′ik) pertaining to, characterized by, or causing akinesia.

Al aluminum.

ALA aminolevulinic acid.

Ala alanine.

ala (a′lah) pl. *a′lae.* [L.] a winglike process. **a′lar, a′late,** adj. **a. na′si,** wing of nose: the flaring cartilaginous expansion forming the outer side of each of the nares.

alac·ta·sia (a″lak-ta′zhah) malabsorption of lactose due to deficiency of lactase; see *lactase deficiency.*

al·a·nine (Ala, A) (al′ah-nēn) a nonessential amino acid occurring in proteins and also free in plasma. **β–a.,** an amino acid not found in proteins but occurring free and in some peptides; it is a precursor of acetyl CoA and an intermediate in uracil and cytosine catabolism.

al·a·nine ami·no·trans·fer·ase (ah-me″no-trans′fer-ās) alanine transaminase.

al·a·nine trans·am·i·nase (trans-am′ĭ-nās) an enzyme normally present in serum and body tissues, especially in the liver; it is released into the serum as a result of tissue injury, hence the concentration in the serum may be increased in patients with acute damage to hepatic cells.

alar (a′lar) pertaining to an ala, or wing.

alate (a′lāt) pertaining to an ala; having wings; winged.

alat·ro·flox·a·cin (ah-lat″ro-flok′sah-sin) a broad-spectrum antibacterial that is the pro-drug of trovafloxacin, to which it is rapidly converted after intravenous infusion; used as the mesylate salt.

al·ba (al′bah) [L.] white.

al·be·do (al-be′do) [L.] whiteness. **a. re′tinae,** paleness of the retina due to edema caused by transudation of fluid from the retinal capillaries.

al·ben·da·zole (al-ben′dah-zōl) a broad-spectrum anthelmintic used against many helminths and in the treatment of hydatid disease and neurocysticercosis.

al·bi·cans (al′bĭ-kans) [L.] white.

al·bi·du·ria (al″bĭ-du′re-ah) the discharge of white or pale urine.

al·bi·nism (al′bĭ-nizm) congenital absence, either total or partial, of normal pigmentation in the body (hair, skin, eyes) due to a defect in melanin synthesis. **albinot′ic,** adj. **ocular a.,** that in which skin and hair pigmentation is virtually or wholly normal, with ocular abnormalities varying by type. **oculocutaneous a. (OCA),** a human albinism occurring in ten types, all having in common decreased melanotic pigmentation of the hair, skin, and eyes, hypoplastic foveas, photophobia, nystagmus, and decreased visual acuity.

al·bi·no (al-bi′no) a person affected with albinism.

al·bi·noid·ism (al-bĭ-noid′izm) ocular or oculocutaneous hypopigmentation differing from albinism by the absence of hypoplastic foveas, nystagmus, photophobia, and, usually, decreased visual acuity.

al·bin·uria (al″bĭ-nu′re-ah) albiduria.

al·bu·gin·ea (al″bu-jin′e-ah) 1. a tough, whitish layer of fibrous tissue investing a part or organ, particularly the tunica albuginea. 2. white.

al·bu·min (al-bu′min) 1. any protein that is soluble in water and also in moderately concentrated salt solutions. 2. the major plasma protein, responsible for much of the plasma colloidal osmotic pressure and serving as a transport protein for large organic anions (e.g., fatty acids, bilirubin, some drugs) and for some hormones when their specific binding globulins are saturated. **albu′minous**, adj.

egg a., albumin of egg whites. **a. human**, a preparation of human serum albumin, used as a plasma volume expander and to increase bilirubin binding in hyperbilirubinemia. **iodinated I 125 a.**, a radiopharmaceutical used in blood and plasma volume, circulation time, and cardiac output determinations, consisting of albumin human labeled with iodine-125. **iodinated I 131 a.**, a radiopharmaceutical used in blood pool imaging and plasma volume determinations, consisting of albumin human labeled with iodine-131. **serum a.**, albumin (2).

al·bu·mi·no·cho·lia (al-bu″mĭ-no-ko′le-ah) the presence of albumin in the bile.

al·bu·mi·noid (al-bu′mĭ-noid″) 1. resembling albumin. 2. a scleroprotein. 3. an albumin-like substance, such as a scleroprotein.

al·bu·mi·nop·ty·sis (al-bu″mĭ-nop′tĭ-sis) albumin in the sputum.

al·bu·min·uria (al-bu″mĭ-nu′re-ah) presence in the urine of serum albumin, the most common kind of proteinuria. **albuminu′ric**, adj.

al·bu·ter·ol (al-bu′ter-ol) a β_2-adrenergic receptor agonist used as the base or sulfate salt as a bronchodilator.

Al·ca·lig·e·nes (al″kah-lij′ĕ-nēz) a genus of gram-negative, aerobic, rod-shaped bacteria of uncertain affiliation, found in the intestines of vertebrates and as part of the normal skin flora, and occasionally the cause of opportunistic infections. *A. faeca′lis* causes nosocomial septicemia, arising from contaminated hemodialysis or intravenous fluid, in immunocompromised patients.

al·clo·met·a·sone (al-klo-met′ah-sōn″) a synthetic corticosteroid used topically in the dipropionate form for the relief of inflammation and pruritus.

al·co·hol (al′kah-hol) 1. any of a class of organic compounds containing the hydroxyl (—OH) functional group except those in which the OH group is attached to an aromatic ring (*phenols*). Alcohols are classified as *primary*, *secondary*, or *tertiary* according to whether the carbon atom to which the OH group is attached is bonded to one, two, or three other carbon atoms and as *monohydric*, *dihydric*, or *trihydric* according to whether they contain one, two, or three OH groups; the latter two are called *diols* and *triols*, respectively. 2. ethanol. 3. a pharmaceutical preparation of ethanol, used as a disinfectant, solvent, and preservative; applied topically as a rubefacient, disinfectant, astringent, hemostatic, and coolant; and used internally in sclerotherapy and in the treatment of pain, of spasticity, and of poisoning by methyl alcohol or ethylene glycol. **absolute a.**, dehydrated a. **benzyl a.**, a colorless liquid used as a bacteriostatic in solutions for injection and topically as a local anesthetic. **cetostearyl a.**, a mixture of stearyl alcohol and cetyl alcohol used as an emulsifier. **cetyl a.**, a solid alcohol used as an emulsifying and stiffening agent. **dehydrated a.**, an extremely hygroscopic, transparent, colorless, volatile liquid, 100 per cent strength ethanol; used as a solvent and injected into nerves and ganglia for relief of pain. **denatured a.**, ethanol rendered unfit for internal use by addition of methanol or acetone. **ethyl a.**, **grain a.**, ethanol. **isopropyl a.**, a transparent, colorless, volatile liquid, used as a solvent and disinfectant, and as a topical antiseptic. **isopropyl rubbing a.**, a preparation containing between 68 and 72 per cent isopropyl alcohol in water, used as a rubefacient. **methyl a.**, a clear, colorless, flammable liquid, CH_3OH, used as a solvent. Ingestion may cause blindness or death. **polyvinyl a.**, a water-soluble synthetic polymer used as a viscosity-increasing agent in pharmaceuticals and as a lubricant and protectant in ophthalmic preparations. *n*-**propyl a.**, a colorless liquid with an alcohol-like odor; used as a solvent. **rubbing a.**, a preparation of acetone, the alcohol denaturant methyl isobutyl ketone, and 68.5 to 71.5 per cent ethanol; used as a rubefacient. **stearyl a.**, a solid alcohol prepared from stearic acid and used as an emollient and emulsifier. **wood a.**, methanol.

al·co·hol de·hy·dro·gen·ase (ADH) (de-hi′dro-jen-ās) an enzyme that catalyzes the reversible oxidation of primary or secondary alcohols to aldehydes; the reaction is the first step in the metabolism of alcohols by the liver.

al·co·hol·ic (al″kah-hol′ik) 1. pertaining to or containing alcohol. 2. a person suffering from alcoholism.

al·co·hol·ism (al′kah-hol-izm) a disorder marked by a pathological pattern of alcohol use that causes serious impairment in social or occupational functioning. It includes both alcohol abuse and alcohol dependence.

al·co·hol·y·sis (al″kah-hol′ĭ-sis) decomposition of a compound due to the incorporation and splitting of alcohol.

al·cu·ro·ni·um (al-ku-ro′ne-um) a nondepolarizing skeletal muscle relaxant used as the chloride salt.

al·dar·ic ac·id (al-dar′ik) a dicarboxylic acid resulting from oxidation of both terminal groups of an aldose to carboxyl groups.

al·de·hyde (al′dĕ-hīd) 1. any of a class of organic compounds containing the group —CHO, i.e., one with a carbonyl group (C═O) located at one end of the carbon chain. 2. a suffix used to denote a compound occurring in aldehyde conformation. 3. acetaldehyde.

al·de·hyde-ly·ase (-li′ās) any of a group of lyases that catalyze the cleavage of a C—C bond in a molecule having a carbonyl group and a hydroxyl group to form two molecules, each an aldehyde or ketone.

al·de·hyde re·duc·tase (re-duk′tās) an enzyme that catalyzes the reduction of aldoses; in one form of galactosemia, its catalysis of reduction of excess galactose in the lens of the eye results in cataract formation.

al·des·leu·kin (al″des-loo′kin) a recombinant interleukin-2 product used as an antineoplastic and biological response modifier.

al·di·carb (al′dĭ-kahrb) a carbamate pesticide used as an insecticide; in some countries, also used as a rodenticide.

al·do·lase (al′do-lās) 1. aldehyde-lyase. 2. an enzyme that acts as a catalyst in the production of dihydroxyacetone phosphate and glyceraldehyde phosphate from fructose 1,6-bisphosphate. It occurs in several isozymes, one of which is deficient in hereditary fructose intolerance.

al·don·ic ac·id (al-don′ik) a carboxylic acid resulting from oxidation of the aldehyde group of an aldose to a carboxyl group.

al·dose (al′dōs) one of two subgroups of monosaccharides, being those containing an aldehyde group (—CHO).

al·dos·ter·one (al-dos′ter-ōn) the major mineralocorticoid hormone secreted by the adrenal cortex. It promotes the retention of sodium and bicarbonate, the excretion of potassium and hydrogen ions, and the secondary retention of water. Large excesses can invoke plasma volume expansion, edema, and hypertension.

al·dos·ter·on·ism (al-dos′tĕ-ro-nizm) hyperaldosteronism; an abnormality of electrolyte balance caused by excessive secretion of aldosterone. **primary a.,** that due to oversecretion of aldosterone by an adrenal adenoma, marked by hypokalemia, alkalosis, muscular weakness, polyuria, polydipsia, and hypertension. **pseudoprimary a.,** signs and symptoms identical to those of primary aldosteronism but caused by factors other than excessive aldosterone secretion.

secondary a., that due to extra-adrenal stimulation of aldosterone secretion, usually associated with edematous states such as nephrotic syndrome, cirrhosis, heart failure, or malignant hypertension.

al·dos·ter·o·no·ma (al″do-ster″o-no′mah) a tumor, usually an adenoma, of the adrenal cortex that secretes aldosterone, causing primary aldosteronism.

al·drin (al′drin) a chlorinated hydrocarbon insecticide, closely related to dieldrin; ingestion or skin contact causes neurotoxic reactions that can be fatal.

alec·i·thal (a-les′ĭ-thal) without yolk; applied to eggs with very little yolk.

al·em·tuz·u·mab (al″em-tuz′u-mab″) a recombinant monoclonal antibody directed against the CD antigen CD52; used as an antineoplastic in the treatment of chronic lymphocytic leukemia.

alen·dro·nate (ah-len′dro-nāt) a bisphosphonate calcium-regulating agent used in the form of the sodium salt to inhibit the resorption of bone in the treatment of osteitis deformans, osteoporosis, and hypercalcemia related to malignancy.

aleu·ke·mia (a″loo-ke′me-ah) 1. leukopenia. 2. aleukemic leukemia.

aleu·ke·mic (-mik) pertaining to or characterized by leukopenia.

aleu·kia (a-loo′ke-ah) leukopenia.

aleu·ko·cy·to·sis (a-loo″ko-si-to′sis) leukopenia.

alex·ia (ah-lek′se-ah) a form of receptive aphasia in which ability to understand written language is lost as a result of a cerebral lesion. **alex′ic,** adj. **cortical a.,** a form of sensory aphasia due to lesions of the left gyrus angularis. **motor a.,** alexia in which the patient understands what he sees written or printed, but cannot read it aloud. **musical a.,** loss of the ability to read music. **optical a.,** alexia. **subcortical a.,** a form due to interruption of the connection between the optic center and the parietal lobe, including the gyrus angularis of the dominant hemisphere.

aley·dig·ism (a-li′dig-izm) absence of androgen secretion by Leydig cells.

al·fa·cal·ci·dol (al″fah-kal′sĭ-dol) a synthetic analogue of calcitriol, used in the treatment of hypocalcemia, hypophosphatemia, rickets, and osteodystrophy associated with various medical conditions.

al·fen·ta·nil (al-fen′tah-nil) an opioid analgesic of rapid onset and short duration derived from fentanyl, used as the hydrochloride salt in the induction of general anesthesia and as an adjunct in general, regional, and local anesthesia.

ALG antilymphocyte globulin.

alge- word element [Gr.], *pain.*

al·ge·sia (al-je′ze-ah) 1. pain sense. 2. excessive sensitivity to pain, a type of hyperesthesia. **alge′sic, alget′ic,** adj.

al·ge·sim·e·ter (al″jĕ-sim′ĕ-ter) an instrument for measuring sensitiveness to pain.

algesi(o)- word element [Gr.], *pain.*

al·ge·sio·gen·ic (al-je″ze-o-jen′ik) dolorific.

al·ges·the·sia (al″jes-the′zhah) 1. pain sense. 2. any painful sensation.

-algia word element [Gr.], *pain.*

al·gid (al′jid) chilly or cold.

al·gi·nate (al′jĭ-nāt) a salt of alginic acid; water-soluble alginates are useful as materials for dental impressions.

al·gin·ic ac·id (al-jin′ik) a hydrophilic colloidal carbohydrate obtained from seaweed, used as a tablet binder and emulsifying agent.

al·glu·cer·ase (al-gloo′ser-ās″) a form of β-glucocerebrosidase used to replace glucocerebrosidase (glucosylceramidase) in the treatment of the adult form of Gaucher's disease.

alg(o)- word element [Gr.], *pain.*

al·go·dys·tro·phy (al″go-dis′tro-fe) reflex sympathetic dystrophy.

al·go·gen·ic (-jen′ik) algesiogenic.

al·go·pho·bia (-fo′be-ah) irrational fear of pain.

al·go·rithm (al′go-rith′m) 1. a step-by-step method of solving a problem or making decisions, as in making a diagnosis. 2. an established mechanical procedure for solving certain mathematical problems.

ali·as·ing (a′le-as-ing) 1. introduction of an artifact or error in sampling of a periodic signal when the sampling frequency is too low to capture the signal properly. 2. in pulsed Doppler ultrasonography, an artifact occurring when the velocity of the sampled object is too great for the Doppler frequency to be determined by the system. 3. an artifact occurring in magnetic resonance imaging when a part being examined is larger than the field of view; an image of the area outside the field of view appears as an artifact inside the field of view.

al·i·cy·clic (al″ĭ-sik′lik) having the properties of both aliphatic and cyclic substances.

ali·enia (a″li-e′ne-ah) asplenia.

ali·form (al′ĭ-form) shaped like a wing.

al·i·men·ta·ry (al″ĭ-men′tah-re) pertaining to food or nutritive material, or to the organs of digestion.

al·i·men·ta·tion (al″ĭ-men-ta′shun) giving or receiving of nourishment. **rectal a.,** feeding by injection of nutriment into the rectum. **total parenteral a.,** see under *nutrition.*

ali·na·sal (al″ĭ-na′z′l) pertaining to either ala of the nose.

al·i·phat·ic (al″ĭ-fat′ik) pertaining to any member of one of the two major groups of organic compounds, those with a straight or branched chain structure.

ali·sphe·noid (-sfe′noid) 1. pertaining to the greater wing of the sphenoid. 2. a cartilage of the fetal chondrocranium on either side of the basisphenoid; later in development it forms the greater part of the great wing of the sphenoid.

al·i·tret·i·noin (-tret′ĭ-noin″) a topical antineoplastic used in the treatment of AIDS-related cutaneous Kaposi's sarcoma.

aliz·a·rin (ah-liz′ah-rin) a red crystalline dye prepared synthetically or obtained from madder; its compounds are used as indicators.

al·ka·le·mia (al″kah-le′me-ah) increased pH (abnormal alkalinity) of the blood.

al·ka·li (al′kah-li) any of a class of compounds with pH greater than 7.0, which form soluble soaps with fatty acids, turn red litmus blue, and form soluble carbonates, e.g., hydroxides or carbonates of sodium or potassium.

al·ka·line (al′kah-līn, -lin) 1. having the reactions of an alkali. 2. having a pH greater than 7.0.

al·ka·line phos·pha·tase (ALP) (fos′fah-tās) an enzyme that catalyzes the cleavage of orthophosphate from orthophosphoric monoesters under alkaline conditions. Differing forms of the enzyme occur in normal and malignant tissues. The activity in serum is useful in the clinical diagnosis of many illnesses. Deficient bone enzyme activity, an autosomal recessive trait, causes hypophosphatasia. **leukocyte a. p. (LAP),** the isozyme of alkaline phosphatase occurring in the leukocytes, specifically in the neutrophils; LAP activity is used in the differential diagnosis of neutrophilia, being lowered in chronic myelogenous leukemia but elevated in a variety of other disorders.

al·ka·lin·uria (al″kah-lĭ-nu′re-ah) an alkaline condition of the urine.

al·ka·liz·er (al′kah-li″zer) an agent that neutralizes acids or causes alkalinization.

al·ka·loid (al′kah-loid″) any of a group of organic basic substances found in plants, many of which are pharmacologically active, e.g., atropine, caffeine, morphine, nicotine, quinine, and strychnine. **ergot a's,** a group of chemically related alkaloids either derived from ergot or synthesized; some cause ergotism while others are medicinal. **vinca a's,** alkaloids produced by the common periwinkle plant (*Vinca rosea*); two, vincristine and vinblastine, are used as antineoplastic agents.

al·ka·lo·sis (al″kah-lo'sis) a pathologic condition due to accumulation of base in, or loss of acid from, the body. Cf. *acidosis.* **alkalot'ic,** adj. **altitude a.,** increased alkalinity in blood and tissues due to exposure to high altitudes. **compensated a.,** a form in which compensatory mechanisms have returned the pH toward normal. **hypochloremic a.,** metabolic alkalosis marked by hypochloremia together with hyponatremia and hypokalemia, resulting from the loss of sodium chloride and hydrochloric acid due to prolonged vomiting. **hypokalemic a.,** metabolic alkalosis associated with a low serum potassium level. **metabolic a.,** a disturbance in which the acid-base status shifts toward the alkaline side because of retention of base or loss of noncarbonic, or fixed (nonvolatile), acids. **respiratory a.,** a state due to excess loss of carbon dioxide from the body, usually as a result of hyperventilation.

al·kane (al'kān) any of a class of saturated hydrocarbons with a straight or branched chain structure, of the general formula C_nH_{2n+2}.

al·kap·ton·uria (al-kap″to-nu're-ah) an autosomal recessive aminoacidopathy with accumulation of homogentisic acid in urine (causing urine to darken on standing), ochronosis, and arthritis. **alkaptonu'ric,** adj.

al·kyl (al'k'l) the monovalent radical formed when an aliphatic hydrocarbon loses one hydrogen atom.

al·kyl·a·tion (al″kĭ-la'shun) the substitution of an alkyl group for an active hydrogen atom in an organic compound.

ALL acute lymphoblastic leukemia.

al·la·ches·the·sia (al″ah-kes-the'zhah) allesthesia.

al·lan·ti·a·sis (al″an-ti'ah-sis) sausage poisoning; botulism from improperly prepared sausages.

al·lan·to·cho·ri·on (ah-lan″to-kor'e-on) a compound membrane formed by fusion of the allantois and chorion.

al·lan·to·ic (al″an-to'ik) pertaining to the allantois.

al·lan·toid (ah-lan'toid) 1. resembling the allantois. 2. sausage-shaped.

al·lan·toi·do·an·gi·op·a·gous (al″an-toi″-do-an″je-op'ah-gus) joined by the vessels of the umbilical cord, as some twins.

al·lan·to·in (ah-lan'to-in) a crystalline substance found in allantoic fluid, fetal urine, many plants, and produced synthetically; used topically as an astringent and keratolytic.

al·lan·to·is (ah-lan'to-is) a ventral outgrowth of the embryos of reptiles, birds, and mammals. In humans, it is vestigial except that its blood vessels give rise to those of the umbilical cord.

al·lele (ah-lēl') one of two or more alternative forms of a gene at corresponding sites (loci) on homologous chromosomes, which determine alternative characters in inheritance. **allel'ic,** adj. **multiple a's,** alleles of which there are more than two alternative forms possible at any one locus.

al·le·lo·tax·is (ah-le″lo-tak'sis) development of an organ from several embryonic structures.

al·ler·gen (al'er-jen) an antigenic substance capable of producing immediate hypersensitivity (allergy). **allergen'ic,** adj. **pollen a.,** any protein antigen of weed, tree, or grass pollens capable of causing allergic asthma or rhinitis; pollen antigen extracts are used in skin testing for pollen sensitivity and in immunotherapy (desensitization) for pollen allergy.

al·ler·gy (al'er-je) a hypersensitive state acquired through exposure to a particular allergen, reexposure bringing to light an altered capacity to react. See *hypersensitivity.* **aller'gic,** adj. **atopic a.,** atopy. **bacterial a.,** specific hypersensitivity to a particular bacterial antigen. **bronchial a.,** atopic asthma; see *asthma.* **cold a.,** a condition manifested by local and systemic reactions, mediated by histamine, which is released from mast cells and basophils as a result of exposure to cold. **contact a.,** see under *dermatitis.* **delayed a.,** see under *hypersensitivity.* **drug a.,** an allergic reaction occurring as the result of unusual sensitivity to a drug. **food a., gastrointestinal a.,** allergy produced by ingested antigens in food, usually manifested by a skin reaction. **hereditary a.,** atopy. **immediate a.,** see under *hypersensitivity.* **latent a.,** that not manifested by symptoms but which may be detected by tests. **physical a.,** a condition in which the patient is sensitive to the effects of physical agents, such as heat, cold, light, etc. **pollen a.,** hay fever. **polyvalent a.,** see *pathergy* (2). **spontaneous a.,** atopy.

al·les·the·sia (al″es-the'zhah) the experiencing of a sensation, e.g., pain or touch, as occurring at a point remote from where the stimulus actually is applied.

al·le·thrin (al'ĕ-thrin) a synthetic analogue of the natural insecticide pyrethrin, used as an insecticide.

al·li·cin (al'ĭ-sin) an oily substance, extracted from garlic, which has antibacterial activity.

all(o)- word element [Gr.], *other; deviating from normal.*

al·lo·an·ti·body (al″o-an'tĭ-bod-e) isoantibody.

al·lo·an·ti·gen (-an'tĭ-jen) an antigen present in allelic forms encoded at the same gene locus in different individuals of the same species.

al·lo·chi·ria (-ki're-ah) dyschiria in which if one limb is stimulated the sensation is referred to the opposite side. **allochi'ral,** adj.

al·lo·chro·ma·sia (-kro-ma'zhah) change in color of hair or skin.

al·lo·cor·tex (-kor'teks) the older, original part of the cerebral cortex, comprising the archicortex and the paleocortex.

al·lo·dyn·ia (-din'e-ah) pain produced by a non-noxious stimulus.

al·lo·erot·i·cism (-ĕ-rot'ĭ-sizm) 1. sexual feeling directed to another person. 2. a state of maturity characterized both by direction of erotic energies to another and also by the ability to form a love relationship with that other. **alloerot'ic,** adj.

al·lo·ge·ne·ic (-jĕ-ne'ik) 1. having cell types that are antigenically distinct. 2. in transplantation biology, denoting individuals (or tissues) that are of the same species but antigenically distinct. Cf. *syngeneic* and *xenogeneic.*

al·lo·gen·ic (-jen'ik) allogeneic.

al·lo·graft (al'o-graft) a graft between individuals of the same species, but of different genotypes. Called also *homograft.*

al·lo·group (-grōōp) an allotype linkage group, especially of allotypes for the four IgG subclasses, which are closely linked and inherited as a unit.

al·lo·im·mune (al″o-ĭ-mūn') specifically immune to an allogeneic antigen.

al·lo·im·mu·ni·za·tion (-im″u-nĭ-za'shun) an immune response generated in an individual or strain of one species by an alloantigen from a different individual or strain of the same species.

al·lom·er·ism (ah-lom'er-izm) change in chemical constitution without change in crystalline form.

al·lo·mor·phism (al″o-mor'fizm) change in crystalline form without change in chemical constitution.

al·lop·a·thy (al-op'ah-the) that system of therapeutics in which diseases are treated by producing a condition incompatible with or antagonistic to the condition to be cured or alleviated. Cf. *homeopathy.* **allopath'ic,** adj.

al·lo·pla·sia (al″o-pla'zhah) heteroplasia.

al·lo·plast (al'o-plast) an inert foreign body used for implantation into tissue. **alloplas'tic,** adj.

al·lo·plas·ty (al'o-plas-te) in psychoanalytic theory, adaptation by alteration of the environment rather than one's self. **alloplas'-tic,** adj.

al·lo·pur·i·nol (al″o-pūr'ĭ-nol) an isomer of hypoxanthine, capable of inhibiting xanthine oxidase and thus of reducing serum and urinary levels of uric acid; used in prophylaxis and treatment of hyperuricemia and uric acid nephropathy and prophylaxis of renal calculus recurrence.

al·lo·re·ac·tive (-re-ak'tiv) pertaining to the immune response in reaction to a transplanted allograft.

al·lo·rhyth·mia (-rith'me-ah) irregularity of the heart beat or pulse that recurs regularly. **allorhyth'mic,** adj.

all or none (awl or nun) the heart muscle, under whatever stimulation, will contract to the fullest extent or not at all; in other muscles and in nerves, stimulation of a fiber causes an action potential to travel over the entire fiber, or not to travel at all.

al·lo·sen·si·ti·za·tion (al″o-sen″sĭ-tĭ-za'-shun) sensitization to alloantigens (isoantigens), as to Rh antigens during pregnancy.

al·lo·some (al'o-sōm) a foreign constituent of the cytoplasm which has entered from outside the cell.

al·lo·ster·ic (al″o-ster'ik) pertaining to allostery.

al·lo·ster·ism (-izm) allostery.

al·lo·ste·ry (al'o-ster″e) the condition in which binding of a substrate, product, or other effector to a subunit of a multi-subunit enzyme at a site (allosteric site) other than the functional site alters its conformation and functional properties.

al·lo·tope (-tōp) a site on the constant or nonvarying portion of an antibody molecule that can be recognized by a combining site of other antibodies.

al·lo·trans·plan·ta·tion (al″o-trans-plan-ta'-shun) allogeneic transplantation.

al·lo·tro·pic (al″o-tro'pik) 1. exhibiting allotropism. 2. concerned with others; said of a type of personality that is more preoccupied with others than with oneself.

al·lot·ro·pism (ah-lot'rah-pizm) existence of an element in two or more distinct forms, e.g., graphite and diamond.

al·lo·type (al'o-tīp) any of several allelic variants of a protein that are characterized by antigenic differences. **alloty'pic**, adj.

al·lox·an (ah-lok'san) an oxidized product of uric acid that tends to destroy the islet cells of the pancreas, thus producing diabetes (*alloxan diabetes*).

al·lyl (al'il) a univalent radical, $-CH_2=CHCH_2$.

al·mo·trip·tan (al″mo-trip'tan) a selective serotonin receptor agonist used as the malate salt in the acute treatment of migraine.

al·oe (al'o) 1. a succulent plant, of the genus *Aloe*. 2. the dried juice of leaves of various species of *Aloe*, used in various dermatologic and cosmetic preparations. **aloet'ic**, adj.

al·o·pe·cia (al″o-pe'shah) baldness; absence of hair from skin areas where it is normally present. **alope'cic**, adj. **androgenetic a.**, a progressive, diffuse, symmetric loss of scalp hair, believed due to a combination of genetic predisposition and increased response of hair follicles to androgens, in men beginning around age 30 with hair loss from the vertex and frontoparietal regions (*male pattern a.* or *male pattern baldness*), and in females beginning later with less severe hair loss in the frontocentral area of the scalp. **a. area'ta**, hair loss, usually reversible, in sharply defined areas, usually involving the beard or scalp. **cicatricial a.**, irreversible loss of hair associated with scarring, usually on the scalp. **male pattern a.**, see *androgenetic a.* **a. tota'lis**, loss of hair from the entire scalp. **traction a.**, traumatic alopecia due to continuous or prolonged traction on the hair, as applied in certain styles of hair dressing or in the habit of twisting the hair. **a. universa'lis**, loss of hair from the entire body.

ALP alkaline phosphatase.

al·pha (al'fah) α, the first letter of the Greek alphabet; see also α-.

al·pha₂-an·ti·plas·min (-an″tĭ-plaz'min) see *antiplasmin*.

al·pha₁-an·ti·tryp·sin (-an″tĭ-trip'sin) a plasma α_1-globulin produced primarily in the liver; it inhibits the activity of elastase, cathepsin G, trypsin, and other proteolytic enzymes. Deficiency is associated with development of emphysema.

al·pha fe·to·pro·tein (fe″to-pro'tēn) a plasma protein produced by the fetal liver, yolk sac, and gastrointestinal tract and also by hepatocellular carcinoma, germ cell neoplasms, other cancers, and some benign hepatic diseases in adults. The serum AFP level is used to monitor the effectiveness of cancer treatment, and the amniotic fluid AFP level is used in the prenatal diagnosis of neural tube defects.

Al·pha·her·pes·vi·ri·nae (al″fah-her″pēz-vir-i'ne) the herpes simplex–like viruses; a subfamily of the Herpesviridae, containing the genera *Simplexvirus* and *Varicellavirus*.

al·pha·lyt·ic (-lit'ik) 1. blocking α-adrenergic receptors. 2. α-blocker.

al·pha₂-mac·ro·glob·u·lin (al'fah mak'ro-glob″u-lin) α_2-macroglobulin.

al·pha·mi·met·ic (al″fah-mi-met'ik) 1. stimulating or mimicking stimulation of α-adrenergic receptors. 2. an alpha-adrenergic agent.

Al·pha·vi·rus (al'fah-vi″rus) a genus of viruses of the family Togaviridae that cause encephalitis or febrile illness with rash or arthralgia.

al·pra·zo·lam (al-pra'zo-lam) a benzodiazepine used as an antianxiety agent.

al·pros·ta·dil (al-pros'tah-dil) name for prostaglandin E₁ when used pharmaceutically as a vasodilator and platelet aggregation inhibitor; used for the treatment of patent ductus arteriosus and the diagnosis and treatment of impotence.

ALS amyotrophic lateral sclerosis; antilymphocyte serum.

al·te·plase (al'tĕ-plās) a tissue plasminogen activator produced by recombinant DNA technology; used in fibrinolytic therapy for acute myocardial infarction and as a thrombolytic in the treatment of acute ischemic stroke and pulmonary embolism.

al·ter·nans (awl-ter'nanz) [L.] 1. alternating; see *pulsus alternans*. 2. alternation. **electrical a.**, alternating variations in the amplitude of specific electrocardiographic waves over successive cardiac cycles. **mechanical a.**, alternation of the heart, particularly in contrast to electrical alternans. **pul'sus a.**, see under *pulsus*. **total a.**, pulsus alternans in which alternating beats are so weak as to be undetected, causing apparent halving of the pulse rate.

al·ter·nate (awl'ter-nĭt) 1. following in turns. 2. pertaining to every other one in a series. 3. occurring in place of another; acting as a substitute.

al·ter·nat·ing (-nāt″ing) 1. occurring in regular succession. 2. alternately direct and reversed.

al·ter·na·tion (awl″ter-na'shun) the regular succession of two opposing or different events in turn. **a. of generations**, metagenesis. **a. of the heart**, mechanical alternans; alternating variation in the intensity of the heartbeat or pulse over successive cardiac cycles of regular rhythm.

al·ter·no·bar·ic (awl-ter″no-bar′ik) pertaining to alternating or changing barometric pressures.

al·tret·amine (al-tret′ah-mēn) an antineoplastic agent used in the palliative treatment of ovarian cancer.

al·um (al′um) 1. a local astringent and styptic, prepared as an ammonium (*ammonium a.*) or potassium (*potassium a.*) compound; also used as an adjuvant in adsorbed vaccines and toxoids. 2. any member of a class of double sulfates formed on this type.

alu·mi·na (ah-loo′mĭ-nah) 1. aluminum oxide. 2. (in pharmaceuticals) aluminum hydroxide. **hydrated a.,** aluminum hydroxide.

alu·mi·no·sis (ah-loo″mĭ-no′sis) pneumoconiosis due to the presence of aluminum-bearing dust in the lungs.

alu·mi·num (Al) (ah-loo″mĭ-num) chemical element (see *Table of Elements*), at. no. 13. **a. acetate,** a salt prepared by the reaction of aluminum hydroxide and acetic acid; used in solution as an astringent. **basic a. carbonate,** see under *gel*. **a. chloride,** a topical astringent and anhidrotic. **a. chlorohydrate,** the hydrate of aluminum chloride hydroxide, astringent and anhidrotic; used as an antiperspirant and as an anhidrotic in the treatment of hyperhidrosis. **a. hydroxide,** $Al(OH)_3$, used as an antacid, and as an adjuvant in adsorbed vaccines and toxoids; see also under *gel*. **a. oxide,** Al_2O_3, occurring naturally as various minerals such as corundum; used in the production of abrasives, refractories, ceramics, catalysts, to strengthen dental ceramics, and in chromatography. **a. phosphate,** an aluminum salt used as an adjuvant in adsorbed vaccines and toxoids, with calcium sulfate and sodium silicate in dental cements, and as an antacid. **a. subacetate,** a basic acetate ester derivative used topically as an astringent. **a. sulfate,** an astringent, used topically as a local antiperspirant; also used in the preparation of aluminum subacetate topical solution.

al·ve·o·lar (al-ve′o-lar) [L. *alveolaris*] pertaining to an alveolus.

al·ve·o·late (al-ve′o-lāt) marked by honeycomb-like pits.

al·ve·o·li·tis (al-ve″o-li′tis) inflammation of a dental or pulmonary alveolus. **allergic a., extrinsic allergic a.,** hypersensitivity pneumonitis.

al·ve·o·lo·cap·il·la·ry (al-ve″o-lo-kap′ĭ-lar″e) pertaining to the pulmonary alveoli and capillaries.

al·ve·o·lo·cla·sia (-kla′zhah) disintegration or resorption of the inner wall of a tooth alveolus.

al·ve·o·lo·den·tal (-den′tal) pertaining to a tooth and its alveolus.

al·ve·o·lo·plas·ty (al-ve′o-lo-plas″te) surgical alteration of the shape and condition of the alveolar process, in preparation for denture construction.

al·ve·o·lus (al-ve′o-lus) pl. *alve′oli*. [L.] a small saclike dilatation; see also *acinus*. **dental a.,** one of the cavities or sockets of the jaw, in which the roots of the teeth are embedded. **pulmonary alveoli,** small outpocketings of the alveolar ducts and sacs and terminal bronchioles through whose walls the exchange of carbon dioxide and oxygen takes place between the alveolar air and capillary blood; see Plate 25.

al·ve·us (al′ve-us) pl. *al′vei*. [L.] a canal or trough.

alym·pho·cy·to·sis (a-lim″fo-si-to′sis) deficiency or absence of lymphocytes from the blood; lymphopenia.

alym·pho·pla·sia (-pla′zhah) failure of development of lymphoid tissue.

AM [L.] Ar′tium Magis′ter (Master of Arts).

Am americium.

AMA Aerospace Medical Association; American Medical Association; Australian Medical Association.

ama (ah′mah) [Sanskrit] in ayurveda, physical and mental toxins that are produced by poor digestion and living habits and accumulate and clog the channels of the body.

am·a·crine (am′ah-krēn) 1. without long processes. 2. see under *cell*.

amal·gam (ah-mal′gam) an alloy of two or more metals, one of which is mercury.

amal·ga·ma·tion (ah-mal′gah-ma′shun) trituration (3).

Am·a·ni·ta (am″ah-ni′tah) a genus of poisonous mushrooms; ingestion of *A. phalloi′des, A. musca′ria, A. pantheri′na, A. ver′na,* and others causes poisoning manifested by vomiting, abdominal pain, and diarrhea, followed by a period of improvement, and culminating in signs of severe hepatic, renal, and central nervous system damage. Most fatalities are due to *A. phalloides.*

aman·ta·dine (ah-man′tah-dēn) an antiviral compound used as the hydrochloride salt to treat influenza A; also used as an antidyskinetic in the treatment of parkinsonism and drug-induced extrapyramidal reactions.

amas·tia (ah-mas′te-ah) congenital absence of one or both mammary glands.

amas·ti·gote (ah-mas′tĭ-gōt) the nonflagellate, intracellular, morphologic stage in the development of certain hemoflagellates, resembling the typical adult form of *Leishmania*.

am·au·ro·sis (am″aw-ro′sis) blindness, especially that occurring without apparent lesion of the eye. **amaurot′ic,** adj. **a. conge′nita of Leber, congenital a.,** a form of hereditary blindness, occurring at or shortly after birth, associated with an atypical form of diffuse pigmentation and commonly with optic atrophy and attenuation of the retinal vessels.

am·be·no·ni·um (am″bĕ-no′ne-um) a cholinesterase inhibitor; the chloride salt is used to treat symptoms of muscular weakness and fatigue in myasthenia gravis.

am·bi·dex·trous (am″bĭ-dek′strus) able to use either hand with equal dexterity.

am·bi·lat·er·al (-lat′er-al) pertaining to or affecting both sides.

am·bi·le·vous (-le′vus) unable to use either hand with dexterity.

am·bi·o·pia (am″be-o′pe-ah) diplopia.

am·bi·sex·u·al (am″bi-sek′shoo-al) 1. bisexual. 2. pertaining to or characterized by hermaphroditism. 3. denoting sexual characteristics common to both sexes, e.g., pubic hair.

am·biv·a·lence (am-biv′ah-lens) simultaneous existence of conflicting attitudes, emotions, ideas, or wishes toward the same object. **ambiv′alent,** adj.

Am·bly·om·ma (am″ble-om′ah) a genus of hard-bodied ticks with about 100 species. *A. america′num* is the Lone Star tick, a species common from the southern United States to South America that is a vector of Rocky Mountain spotted fever. *A. cajennen′se* is found in many parts of the Americas and is a vector of São Paulo fever, a form of typhus.

am·bly·o·pia (-o′pe-ah) dimness of vision without detectable organic lesion of the eye. **amblyop′ic,** adj. **alcoholic a.,** nutritional a.; toxic a. **a. ex anop′sia,** that resulting from long disuse. **color a.,** dimness of color vision due to toxic or other influences. **nocturnal a.,** abnormal dimness of vision at night. **nutritional a.,** scotomata due to poor nutrition; seen in alcoholics, the malnourished, and those with vitamin B$_{12}$ deficiency or pernicious anemia. **tobacco a.,** nutritional a.; toxic a. **toxic a.,** that due to poisoning, as from alcohol or tobacco.

am·bly·o·scope (am′ble-o-skōp″) an instrument for training an amblyopic eye to take part in vision and for increasing fusion of the eyes.

am·bo (am′bo) ambon.

am·bo·cep·tor (am′bo-sep″ter) hemolysin, particularly its double receptors, the one combining with the blood cell, the other with complement.

am·bon (am′bon) the fibrocartilaginous ring forming the edge of the socket in which the head of a long bone is lodged.

am·bu·lant (am′bu-lant) ambulatory.

am·bu·la·to·ry (am′bu-lah-tor″e) 1. walking or able to walk; not confined to bed. 2. of a condition or a procedure, not requiring admission to a hospital.

am·cin·o·nide (am-sin′ah-nīd″) a synthetic corticosteroid used topically for the relief of inflammation and pruritus in corticosteroid-responsive dermatoses.

am·di·no·cil·lin (am-de′no-sil″in) a semisynthetic penicillin effective against many gram-negative bacteria and used in the treatment of urinary tract infections.

ame·ba (ah-me′bah) pl. *ame′bae, amebas.* [L.] a minute protozoan (class Rhizopoda, subphylum Sarcodina), occurring as a single-celled nucleated mass of protoplasm that changes shape by extending cytoplasmic processes (pseudopodia), by means of which it moves about and absorbs food; most amebae are free-living but some parasitize humans. **ame′bic,** adj.

ame·bi·a·sis (am″e-bi′ah-sis) infection with amebae, especially *Entamoeba histolytica.* **a. cu′tis,** painful ulcers with distinct borders and erythematous rims, seen in persons with active intestinal or hepatic disease. **hepatic a.,** amebic hepatitis. **intestinal a.,** amebic dysentery. **pulmonary a.,** infection of the thoracic space secondary to intestinal amebiasis, with amebic liver abscesses.

ame·bic (ah-me′bik) pertaining to or of the nature of an ameba.

ame·bi·cide (ah-me′bĭ-sīd) an agent that is destructive to amebae.

ame·bo·cyte (ah-me′bo-sīt″) ameboid cell.

ame·boid (ah-me′boid) resembling an ameba in form or movement.

am·e·bo·ma (am″e-bo′mah) a tumor-like mass caused by granulomatous reaction in the intestines in amebiasis.

ame·bu·la (ah-me′bu-lah) the motile ameboid stage of spores of certain sporozoa.

amel·a·not·ic (a″mel-ah-not′ik) pertaining to or characterized by the absence of melanin.

ame·lia (ah-me′le-ah) congenital absence of a limb or limbs.

amel·i·fi·ca·tion (ah-mel′ĭ-fĭ-ka′shun) the development of enamel cells into enamel.

am·e·lo·blast (am′ĕ-lo-blast″) a cell that takes part in forming dental enamel.

am·elo·blas·tic (am″ĕlo-blas′tik) pertaining to ameloblasts or to an ameloblastoma.

am·e·lo·blas·to·ma (-blas-to′mah) a usually benign but locally invasive neoplasm of tissue of the type characteristic of the enamel organ, but which does not differentiate to the point of enamel formation. **melanotic a.,** melanotic neuroectodermal tumor. **pituitary a.,** craniopharyngioma.

am·e·lo·den·ti·nal (-den′tĭ-nal) pertaining to the enamel and dentin of a tooth.

am·e·lo·gen·e·sis (-jen′ĕ-sis) the formation of dental enamel. **a. imperfec′ta,** a hereditary condition resulting in defective development of dental enamel, marked by a brown color of the teeth; due to improper differentiation of the ameloblasts.

am·e·lo·gen·in (-jen′in) any of several proteins secreted by ameloblasts and forming the organic matrix of tooth enamel.

am·e·lus (am′ĕ-lus) an individual exhibiting amelia.

amen·or·rhea (ah-men″o-re′ah) absence or abnormal stoppage of the menses. **amenorrhe′al,** adj. **primary a.,** failure of menstruation to occur at puberty. **secondary a.,** cessation of menstruation after it has once been established at puberty.

amen·sal·ism (a-men′sal-izm) symbiosis in which one population (or individual) is adversely affected and the other is unaffected.

amen·tia (ah-men′shah) former term for profound mental retardation.

am·er·ic·i·um (Am) (am″er-is′e-um) chemical element (see *Table of Elements*), at. no. 95.

ame·tria (a-me′tre-ah) congenital absence of the uterus.

am·e·tro·pia (am″ĕ-tro′pe-ah) a condition of the eye in which images fail to come to a proper focus on the retina, due to a discrepancy between the size and refractive powers of the eye. **ametrop′ic,** adj.

AMI acute myocardial infarction.

amic·u·lum (ah-mik′u-lum) pl. *ami′cula*. [L.] a dense surrounding coat of white fibers, as the sheath of the inferior olive and of the dentate nucleus.

am·i·dase (am′ĭ-dās) 1. any of a group of enzymes that catalyze the cleavage of carbon–nitrogen bonds in amides. 2. an enzyme that catalyzes the cleavage of the carbon–nitrogen bond of a monocarboxylic acid amide to form a monocarboxylic acid and ammonia.

am·ide (am′īd) any compound derived from ammonia by substitution of an acid radical for hydrogen, or from an acid by replacing the —OH group by —NH₂.

am·i·dine (am′ĭ-dēn) any compound containing the amidino (—C(=NH)—NH₂) group.

am·i·dine·ly·ase (-li′ās) an enzyme that catalyzes the removal of an amidino group, as from L-argininosuccinate to form fumarate and L-arginine.

am·i·do·li·gase (ah-me″do-, am″ĭ-do-li′gās) any of a group of enzymes that catalyze the transfer of the amide nitrogen from glutamine to an acceptor molecule.

am·i·fos·tine (am″ĭ-fos′tēn) a chemoprotectant used to prevent renal toxicity in cisplatin chemotherapy.

am·i·ka·cin (am″ĭ-ka′sin) a semisynthetic aminoglycoside antibiotic derived from kanamycin, used as the sulfate salt in the treatment of a wide range of infections due to aerobic gram-negative bacilli.

amil·o·ride (ah-mil′ah-rīd) a potassium-sparing diuretic used as the hydrochloride salt in the treatment of edema and hypertension and in the prevention and treatment of hypokalemia.

am·il·ox·ate (am″il-ok′sāt) an absorber of ultraviolet B radiation, used topically as a sunscreen.

amim·ia (a-mim′e-ah) loss of the power of expression by the use of signs or gestures.

am·i·na·tion (am″ĭ-na′shun) the creation of an amine, either by addition of an amino group to an organic acceptor compound or by reduction of a nitro compound.

amine (ah-mēn′, am′in) an organic compound containing nitrogen; any of a group of compounds formed from ammonia by replacement of one or more hydrogen atoms by organic radicals. **biogenic a.,** a type of amine synthesized by plants and animals and frequently involved in signaling, e.g., neurotransmitters such as acetylcholine, catecholamines, and serotonin; others are hormones or components of vitamins, phospholipids, bacteria, or ribosomes, e.g., cadaverine, choline, histamine, and spermine. **sympathomimetic a's,** amines that mimic the actions of the sympathetic nervous system, comprising the catecholamines and drugs that mimic their actions.

am·in·er·gic (am″ĭ-ner′jik) activated by, characteristic of, or secreting one of the biogenic amines.

ami·no (ah-me′no, am′ĭ-no″) the monovalent radical NH₂, when not united with an acid radical.

ami·no ac·id (ah-me′no) one of a class of organic compounds containing the amino (NH₂) and the carboxyl (COOH) groups; they occur naturally in plant and animal tissue and form the chief constituents of protein. **branched-chain a. a's,** leucine, isoleucine, and valine. **essential a. a's,** the nine α-amino acids that cannot be synthesized by humans but must be obtained from the diet. **nonessential a. a's,** the eleven α-amino acids that can be synthesized by humans and are not specifically required in the diet.

ami·no·ac·id·emia (ah-me″no-as″ĭ-de′me-ah) an excess of amino acids in the blood.

ami·no·ac·i·dop·a·thy (-as″ĭ-dop′ah-the) any of a group of disorders due to a defect in an enzymatic step in the metabolic pathway of one or more amino acids or in a protein mediator necessary for transport of certain amino acids into or out of cells.

ami·no·ac·id·u·ria (-as″ĭ-du′re-ah) an excess of amino acids in the urine.

ami·no·acy·lase (-a′sĭ-lās) an enzyme that catalyzes the hydrolytic cleavage of the acyl group from acylated L-amino acids.

ami·no·ben·zo·ate (-ben′zo-āt) p-aminobenzoate, any salt or ester of p-aminobenzoic acid; the potassium salt is used as an antifibrotic in some dermatologic disorders and various esters are used as topical sunscreens.

p-ami·no·ben·zo·ic ac·id (PABA) (-ben-zo′ik) a substance required for folic acid synthesis by many organisms; it also absorbs ultraviolet light (UVB rays) and is used (called also *aminobenzoic acid*) as a topical sunscreen.

γ-ami·no·bu·ty·rate (-bu′tĭ-rāt) the anion of γ-aminobutyric acid.

γ-ami·no·bu·tyr·ic ac·id (GABA) (-bu-tēr′ik) the principal inhibitory neurotransmitter in the brain but also occurring in several extraneural tissues, including kidney and pancreatic islet β cells. Released from presynaptic cells upon depolarization, it modulates membrane chloride permeability and inhibits postsynaptic cell firing.

ε-ami·no·ca·pro·ic ac·id (-kah-pro′ik) a nonessential amino acid that is an inhibitor of plasmin and of plasminogen activators and, indirectly, of fibrinolysis; used for treatment (as *aminocaproic acid*) of acute bleeding syndromes due to fibrinolysis and for the prevention and treatment of postsurgical hemorrhage.

ami·no·glu·teth·i·mide (-gloo-teth′ĕ-mīd) an inhibitor of cholesterol metabolism, thereby reducing adrenocortical steroid synthesis; used in the treatment of Cushing's syndrome. It also inhibits estrogen production from androgens in peripheral tissue.

ami·no·gly·co·side (-gli′ko-sīd) any of a group of antibacterial antibiotics (e.g., streptomycin, gentamicin) derived from various species of *Streptomyces* or produced synthetically; they interfere with the function of bacterial ribosomes.

p-ami·no·hip·pu·rate (-hip′u-rāt) a salt, conjugate base, or ester of p-aminohippuric acid; the sodium salt is used to measure effective renal plasma flow and to determine the functional capacity of the tubular excretory mechanism..

p-ami·no·hip·pu·ric ac·id (PAH, PAHA) (-hĭ-pūr′ik) the glycine amide of p-aminobenzoic acid, which is filtered by the renal glomeruli and secreted into the urine by the proximal tubules. See also *p-aminohippurate*.

ami·no·lev·u·lin·ate (-lev′u-lin′āt) the conjugate base of aminolevulinic acid.

ami·no·lev·u·lin·ic ac·id (ALA) (-lev′u-lin′ik) δ-aminolevulinic acid; an intermediate in the synthesis of heme; blood and urinary levels are increased in lead poisoning, and urinary levels are increased in some porphyrias. The hydrochloride salt is used as a topical photosensitizer in the treatment of nonhyperkeratotic actinic keratoses.

am·i·nol·y·sis (am″ĭ-nol′ĭ-sis) reaction with an amine, resulting in the addition of (or substitution by) an imino group —NH—.

6-ami·no·pen·i·cil·lan·ic ac·id (ah-me″no-pen″ĭ-sil-an′ik) the active nucleus common to all penicillins; it may be substituted at the 6-amino position to form the semisynthetic penicillins.

p-ami·no·phe·nol (-fe′nol) a dye intermediate and photographic developer and the parent compound of acetaminophen; it is a potent allergen that causes dermatitis, asthma, and methemoglobinemia.

am·i·noph·yl·line (am″ĭ-nof′ĭ-lin) a salt of theophylline, used as a bronchodilator and as an antidote to dipyridamole toxicity.

ami·no·quin·o·line (ah-me″no-kwin′o-lēn) a heterocyclic compound derived from quinoline by the addition of an amino group; the *4-aminoquinoline* and *8-aminoquinoline* derivatives constitute classes of antimalarials.

ami·no·sa·lic·y·late (-sah-lis′ĭ-lāt) any salt of p-aminosalicylic acid; they are antibacterials effective against mycobacteria and the sodium salt is used as a tuberculostatic.

ami·no·sal·i·cyl·ic ac·id (-sal-ĭ-sil′ik) official pharmaceutical name for *p-aminosalicylic acid*.

5-ami·no·sal·i·cyl·ic ac·id (5-ASA), mesalamine.

p-ami·no·sal·i·cyl·ic ac·id (PAS, PASA) an analogue of p-aminobenzoic acid (PABA) with antibacterial properties; used to inhibit growth and multiplication of the tubercle bacillus.

ami·no·trans·fer·ase (-trans′fer-ās) transaminase.

am·in·uria (am″ĭ-nu′re-ah) an excess of amines in the urine.

ami·o·da·rone (ah-me′o-dah-rōn″) a potassium channel blocking agent used as the hydrochloride salt in the treatment of ventricular arrhythmias.

ami·to·sis (am″ĭ-to′sis) direct cell division, i.e., the cell divides by simple cleavage of the nucleus without formation of spireme spindle figures or chromosomes. **amitot′ic**, adj.

am·i·trip·ty·line (am″ĭ-trip′tĭ-lēn) a tricyclic antidepressant with sedative effects; also used in treating enuresis, chronic pain, peptic ulcer, and bulimia nervosa.

AML acute myelogenous leukemia.

am·lex·a·nox (am-lek′sah-noks″) a topical antiulcer agent used in the treatment of recurrent aphthous stomatitis.

am·lo·di·pine (am-lo′dĭ-pēn″) a calcium channel blocking agent used as the besylate salt in the treatment of hypertension and chronic stable and vasospastic angina.

am·me·ter (am′me-ter) an instrument for measuring in amperes or subdivisions of amperes the strength of a current flowing in a circuit.

am·mo·nia (ah-mōn′yah) a colorless alkaline gas with a pungent odor and acrid taste, NH_3. Ammonia labeled with ^{13}N is used in positron emission tomography of the cardiovascular system, brain, and liver.

am·mo·ni·um (ah-mo′ne-um) the hypothetical radical, NH_4, forming salts analogous to those of the alkaline metals. **a. carbonate,** a mixture of ammonium bicarbonate (NH_4HCO_3) and ammonium carbamate ($NH_2CO_2NH_4$), used as a stimulant, as in smelling salts, and as an expectorant. **a. chloride,** a systemic and urinary acidifying agent and diuretic, also used orally as an expectorant. **a. lactate,** lactic acid neutralized with ammonium hydroxide, applied topically in the treatment of ichthyosis vulgaris and xerosis.

am·mo·ni·uria (am-mo″ne-u′re-ah) hyperammonuria.

am·mo·nol·y·sis (am″o-nol′ĭ-sis) a process analogous to hydrolysis, but in which ammonia takes the place of water.

am·ne·sia (am-ne′zhah) pathologic impairment of memory. **anterograde a.,** amnesia for events occurring subsequent to the episode precipitating the disorder. **dissociative a.,** a dissociative disorder characterized by a sudden loss of memory for important personal information and which is not due to the direct effects of a psychogenic substance or a general medical condition. **psychogenic a.,** dissociative a. **retrograde a.,** amnesia for events occurring prior to the episode precipitating the disorder. **transient global a.,** a temporary episode of short-term memory loss without other neurological impairment. **visual a.,** alexia.

am·ne·sic (am-ne′sik) affected with or characterized by amnesia.

am·nes·tic (am-nes′tik) 1. amnesic. 2. causing amnesia.

am·nio·cele (am′ne-o-sēl″) omphalocele.

am·nio·cen·te·sis (am″ne-o-sen-te′sis) surgical transabdominal or transcervical penetration of the uterus for aspiration of amniotic fluid.

am·nio·gen·e·sis (-jen′ĕ-sis) the development of the amnion.

am·nio·in·fu·sion (-in-fu′zhun) introduction of solutions into the amnion.

am·ni·on (am′ne-on) bag of waters; the extraembryonic membrane of birds, reptiles, and mammals, which lines the chorion and contains the fetus and the amniotic fluid. **amnion′ic, amniot′ic,** adj. **a. nodo′sum,** a nodular condition of the fetal surface of the amnion, observed in oligohydramnios associated with absence of the kidneys of the fetus.

am·ni·or·rhex·is (am″ne-o-rek′sis) rupture of the amnion.

am·nio·scope (am′ne-o-skōp″) an endoscope passed through the uterine cervix to visualize the fetus and amniotic fluid.

am·ni·ote (am′ne-ōt) any member of the group of vertebrates that develop an amnion, including reptiles, birds, and mammals.

am·ni·ot·ic (am″ne-ot′ik) pertaining to or developing an amnion.

am·ni·ot·o·my (am″ne-ot′ah-me) surgical rupture of the fetal membranes to induce labor.

amo·bar·bi·tal (am″o-bahr′bĭ-tal) an intermediate-acting hypnotic and sedative; also used as the sodium salt.

Amoe·ba (ah-me′bah) a genus of amebae.

amorph (a′morf) a mutant gene that produces no detectable phenotypic effect.

amor·phia (ah-mor′fe-ah) the fact or quality of being amorphous.

amor·pho·syn·the·sis (a-mor″fo-sin′thĕ-sis) defective perception of somatic sensations from one side of the body, which may be accompanied by generalized faulty awareness of spatial relationships and is often a sign of a parietal lobe lesion.

amor·phous (ah-mor′fus) 1. having no definite form; shapeless. 2. having no specific orientation of atoms. 3. in pharmacy, not crystallized.

amox·a·pine (ah-mok′sah-pēn) a tricyclic antidepressant of the dibenzoxazepine class.

amox·i·cil·lin (ah-mok″sĭ-sil′in) a semi-synthetic derivative of ampicillin effective against a broad spectrum of gram-positive and gram-negative bacteria.

AMP adenosine monophosphate. **3′,5′-AMP, cyclic AMP,** cyclic adenosine monophosphate.

am·pere (A) (am′pēr) the base SI unit of electric current strength, defined in terms of the force of attraction between two parallel conductors carrying current.

am·phet·a·mine (am-fet′ah-mēn) 1. a sympathomimetic amine with a stimulating effect on both the central and peripheral nervous systems, used in the treatment of narcolepsy and attention-deficit/hyperactivity disorder, usually as the sulfate or aspartate salt. Abuse may lead to dependence. 2. any drug closely related to amphetamine and having similar actions, e.g., methamphetamine.

amph(i)- word element [Gr.], *both; on both sides.*

am·phi·ar·thro·sis (am″fe-ahr-thro′sis) a joint permitting little motion, the opposed surfaces being connected by fibrocartilage, as between vertebrae.

Am·phib·ia (am-fib′e-ah) a class of vertebrates, including frogs, toads, newts, and salamanders, capable of living both on land and in water.

am·phi·bol·ic (am″fĭ-bol′ik) 1. uncertain; vacillating; see under *stage.* 2. see under *pathway.*

am·phi·cen·tric (-sen′trik) beginning and ending in the same vessel.

am·phi·di·ar·thro·sis (-di″ahr-thro′sis) a joint having the nature of both ginglymus and arthrodia, as that of the lower jaw. **amphidiarthro′dial,** adj.

am·phi·gon·a·dism (-go′nah-dizm) possession of both ovarian and testicular tissue.

am·phit·ri·chous (am-fit′rĭ-kus) having flagella at each end.

am·pho·cyte (am′fo-sīt) a cell staining with either acid or basic dyes.

am·pho·lyte (-līt) amphoteric electrolyte.

am·pho·phil (am′fo-fil) 1. a cell that stains readily with acid or basic dyes. 2. amphophilic.

am·pho·phil·ic (am″fo-fil′ik) staining with either acid or basic dyes.

am·phor·ic (am-for′ik) pertaining to a bottle; resembling the sound made by blowing across the neck of a bottle.

am·pho·ter·ic (am″fo-ter′ik) having opposite characters; capable of acting as both an acid and a base; capable of neutralizing either bases or acids.

am·pho·ter·i·cin B (-ter′ĭ-sin) an antibiotic derived from strains of *Streptomyces nodosus;* effective against a wide range of fungi and some species of *Leishmania.*

am·phot·o·ny (am-fot′o-ne) tonicity of the sympathetic and parasympathetic nervous systems.

am·pi·cil·lin (am″pĭ-sil′in) a semisynthetic, acid-resistant, penicillinase-sensitive penicillin used as an antibacterial against many gram-negative and gram-positive bacteria; also used as the sodium salt.

am·pli·fi·ca·tion (33000) (am″plĭ-fĭ-ka′-shun) the process of making larger, such as the increase of an auditory stimulus, as a means of improving its perception. **gene a.,** the process by which the number of copies of a gene is increased in certain cells; in humans it is most often seen in malignant cells.

am·pli·tude (am′plĭ-tood) 1. largeness, fullness; wideness in range or extent. 2. in a phenomenon that occurs in waves, the maximal deviation of a wave from the baseline. **a. of accommodation,** amount of accommodative power of the eye.

am·pren·a·vir (am-pren′ah-vir) an HIV protease inhibitor used in the treatment of HIV-1 infection.

am·pule (am′pūl) a small glass or plastic container capable of being sealed so as to preserve its contents in a sterile condition; used principally for sterile parenteral solutions.

am·pul·la (am-pul′ah) pl. *ampul′lae.* [L.] a flask-like dilatation of a tubular structure, especially of the expanded ends of the semicircular canals of the ear. **ampul′lar,** adj. **a. chy′li,** cisterna chyli. **a. duc′tus defer-en′tis,** the enlarged and tortuous distal end of the ductus deferens. **hepatopancreatic a., a. hepatopancrea′tica,** the dilatation formed by junction of the common bile and the pancreatic ducts proximal to their opening into the lumen of the duodenum. **ampul′lae lacti′ferae,** lactiferous sinuses. **ampul′lae membrana′ceae,** membranous ampullae: the dilatations at one end of each of the three semicircular ducts, anterior, lateral, and posterior. **ampul′lae os′seae,** the dilatations at one of the ends of the semicircular canals, anterior, lateral, and posterior. **phrenic a.,** a dilatation sometimes seen at the lower end of the esophagus. **rectal a., a. rec′ti,** the dilated portion of the rectum just proximal to the anal canal. **a. of Thoma,** one of the small terminal expansions of an interlobar artery in the pulp of the spleen. **a. of uterine tube,** the thin-walled, almost muscle-free, midregion of the uterine tube; its mucosa is greatly plicated. **a. of vas deferens,** a. ductus deferentis.

am·pu·ta·tion (am″pu-ta′shun) removal of a limb or other appendage of the body. **above-elbow (A-E) a.,** amputation of the upper limb between the elbow and the shoulder. **above-knee (A-K) a.,** transfemoral a. **below-elbow (B-E) a.,** amputation of the upper limb between the wrist and the elbow. **below-knee (B-K) a.,** transtibial a. **Chopart's a.,** amputation of the foot by a midtarsal disarticulation. **closed a.,** one in which flaps are made from the skin and subcutaneous tissue and sutured over the end of the bone. **a. in contiguity,** amputation at a joint. **a. in continuity,** amputation of a limb elsewhere than at a joint. **double-flap a.,** one in which two flaps are formed. **Dupuytren's a.,** amputation of the arm at the shoulder joint. **elliptic a.,** one in which the cut has an elliptical outline. **flap a.,** closed a. **flapless a.,** guillotine a. **Gritti-Stokes a.,** amputation of the leg through the knee, using an oval anterior flap. **guillotine a.,** one performed rapidly by a circular sweep of the knife and a cut of the saw, the entire cross-section being left open for dressing. **Hey's a.,** amputation of the foot between the tarsus and metatarsus. **interpelviabdominal a.,** amputation of the thigh with excision of the lateral half of the pelvis. **interscapulothoracic a.,** amputation of the arm with excision of the lateral portion of the shoulder girdle. **Larrey's a.,** amputation at the shoulder joint. **Lisfranc's a.,** 1. Dupuytren's a. 2. amputation of the foot between the metatarsus and tarsus. **oblique a.,** oval a. **open a.,** guillotine a. **oval a.,** one in which the incision consists of two reversed spirals. **Pirogoff's a.,** amputation of the foot at the ankle, part of the calcaneus being left in the stump. **pulp a.,** pulpotomy. **racket a.,** one in which there is a single longitudinal incision continuous below with a spiral incision on either side of the limb. **root a.,** removal of one or more roots from a multirooted tooth, leaving at least one root to support the crown; when only the apex of a root is involved, it is called *apicoectomy*. **spontaneous a.,** loss of a part without surgical intervention, as in diabetes mellitus. **Stokes' a.,** Gritti-Stokes a. **subperiosteal a.,** one in which the cut end of the bone is covered by periosteal flaps. **Syme's a.,** disarticulation of the foot with removal of both malleoli. **Teale's a.,** amputation with short and long rectangular flaps.

transfemoral a., amputation of the lower limb between the knee and the hip; called also *above-knee (A-A) a.* **transtibial a.,** amputation of the lower limb between the ankle and the knee. Called also *below-knee a.*

am·ri·none (am′rĭ-nōn) inamrinone.

AMRL Aerospace Medical Research Laboratories.

am·sa·crine (am′sah-krēn) an antineoplastic that inhibits DNA synthesis; used to treat some forms of leukemia.

AMTA American Music Therapy Association.

amu atomic mass unit.

amu·sia (ah-mu′ze-ah) a form of auditory agnosia in which the patient has lost the ability to recognize or produce music.

AMWA American Medical Women's Association; American Medical Writers' Association.

amy·elin·ic (a-mi″ĕ-lin′ik) unmyelinated.

amyg·da·la (ah-mig′dah-lah) 1. almond. 2. an almond-shaped structure. 3. corpus amygdaloideum.

amyg·da·lin (-lin) a glycoside (*l*-mandelonitrile-β-gentiobioside) found in bitter almonds and other members of the same family; it is split enzymatically into glucose, benzaldehyde, and hydrocyanic acid. See also *Laetrile* and *laetrile*.

amyg·da·line (-lēn″) 1. like an almond. 2. tonsillar.

amyg·da·loid (ah-mig′dah-loid) resembling an almond, or tonsil.

am·yl (am′il) the radical —C_5H_{11}. **a. nitrite,** a volatile, flammable liquid with a pungent ethereal odor. It is administered by inhalation for the treatment of cyanide poisoning, producing methemoglobin which binds cyanide, and as a diagnostic aid in tests of reserve cardiac function and diagnosis of certain heart murmurs. It is abused to produce euphoria and as a sexual stimulant.

am·y·la·ceous (am″ĭ-la′shus) composed of or resembling starch.

am·y·lase (am′ĭ-lās) an enzyme that catalyzes the hydrolysis of starch into simpler compounds. The α-*a's* occur in animals and include pancreatic and salivary amylase; the β-*a's* occur in higher plants.

amyl(o)- word element [Gr.], *starch.*

am·y·lo-1,6-glu·co·si·dase (am″ĭ-lo-glooko′sĭ-dās) a hydrolase that catalyzes the cleavage of terminal α-1,6-glucoside linkages in glycogen and similar molecules; deficiency causes glycogen storage disease, type III.

am·y·loid (am′ĭ-loid) 1. starchlike; amylaceous. 2. the pathologic, extracellular, waxy, amorphous substance deposited in amyloidosis, being composed of fibrils in bundles or in a meshwork of polypeptide chains; the two major protein types are *a. light chain (AL) protein*, occurring in immunocyte-derived amyloidosis, and *a. A (AA) protein*, occurring in reactive systemic amyloidosis.

am·y·loi·do·sis (am″ĭ-loi-do′sis) a group of conditions characterized by the accumulation of insoluble fibrillar proteins (amyloid) in various organs and tissues such that vital function is compromised. The associated disease states may be inflammatory, hereditary, or neoplastic, and deposition can be local, generalized, or systemic. The most widely used classification is based on the chemistry of the amyloid fibrils and includes immunocyte-derived (primary or AL) and reactive systemic (secondary or AA) forms. **AA a.,** reactive systemic a. **AL a.,** immunocyte-derived a. **immunocyte-derived a.,** a primary type in which the deposited fibrillar material is usually AL amyloid and deposition is most often systemic or generalized; the heart, tongue, carpal ligaments, peripheral nerves, gastrointestinal tract, and skin are usually involved. **primary a.,** that in which no obvious predisposing condition is associated; sometimes used synonymously with *immunocyte-derived a.*. **reactive systemic a.,** that in which AA amyloid is deposited, and which occurs secondary to a chronic infectious process or a chronic noninfectious inflammatory disease. It may also occur in association with certain nonlymphoid tumors and some nonimmunoglobulin-producing lymphomas. **renal a.,** amyloid deposits in the kidneys; in the primary type the fibrils are mainly AL amyloid, and in secondary types they are AA amyloid. Secondary types may accompany inflammatory disorders, chronic infectious diseases, or neoplastic diseases. **secondary a.,** reactive systemic a.

am·y·lo·pec·tin (am″ĭ-lo-pek′tin) a highly branched, water-insoluble glucan, the insoluble constituent of starch; the soluble constituent is amylose.

am·y·lo·pec·ti·no·sis (-pek″tĭ-no″sis) glycogen storage disease, type IV.

am·y·lor·rhea (-re′ah) presence of excessive starch in the stools.

am·y·lose (am′ĭ-lōs) a linear, water-soluble glucan; the soluble constituent of starch, as opposed to amylopectin.

am·y·lu·ria (am″il-u′re-ah) an excess of starch in the urine.

amyo·es·the·sia (a″mi-o-es-the′zhah) muscular anesthesia.

amyo·pla·sia (-pla′zhah) lack of muscle formation or development. **a. conge′nita,** generalized lack in the newborn of muscular development and growth, with contracture and deformity at most joints.

amyo·sta·sia (-sta′zhah) a tremor of the muscles.

amyo·to·nia (-to′ne-ah) atonic condition of the muscles.

amy·ot·ro·phy (a″mi-ot′rah-fe) muscular atrophy. **amyotro′phic,** adj. **diabetic a.,** a painful condition, associated with diabetes, with progressive wasting and weakening of muscles, usually limited to the muscles of the pelvic girdle and thigh. **neuralgic a.,** atrophy and paralysis of the muscles of the shoulder girdle, with pain across the shoulder and upper arm.

amyx·ia (ah-mik′se-ah) absence of mucus.

amyx·or·rhea (ah-mik″sah-re′ah) absence of mucus secretion.

An anode.

ANA American Nurses Association; antinuclear antibodies.

ana (an′ah) [Gr.] so much of each.

ana- word element [Gr.], *upward; again; backward; excessively.*

ana·bi·o·sis (an″ah-bi-o′sis) restoration of the vital processes after their apparent cessation; bringing back to consciousness. **anabiot′ic,** adj.

anab·o·lism (ah-nab′o-lizm) the constructive process by which living cells convert simple substances into more complex compounds, especially into living matter. **anabol′ic,** adj.

anab·o·lite (ah-nab′o-līt″) any product of anabolism.

an·acid·i·ty (an″ah-sid′ĭ-te) lack of normal acidity. **gastric a.,** achlorhydria.

ana·cli·sis (an″ah-kli′sis) physical and emotional dependence on another for protection and gratification.

ana·clit·ic (-klit′ik) 1. pertaining to anaclisis. 2. exhibiting excessive emotional dependency.

ana·crot·ic (an″ah-krot′ik) 1. pertaining to the ascending limb of a pulse tracing. 2. characterized by a notch, i.e., two waveforms in the ascending limb of the pulse tracing.

anac·ro·tism (ah-nak′rah-tizm) the presence of an anacrotic pulse.

an·adre·nal·ism (an″ah-dre′nal-izm) absence or failure of adrenal function.

an·aer·obe (an′ah-rōb) an organism that lives and grows in the absence of molecular oxygen. **facultative a's,** microorganisms that can live and grow with or without molecular oxygen. **obligate a's,** microorganisms that can grow only in the complete absence of molecular oxygen; some are killed by oxygen.

an·aer·o·bic (an″ah-ro′bik) 1. lacking molecular oxygen. 2. growing, living, or occurring in the absence of molecular oxygen; pertaining to an anaerobe.

an·aer·o·bi·o·sis (an″ah-ro″bi-o′sis) metabolic processes occurring in the absence of molecular oxygen.

an·aero·gen·ic (an″ah-ro-jen′ik) 1. producing little or no gas. 2. suppressing the formation of gas by gas-producing bacteria.

an·a·gen (an′ah-jen) the first phase of the hair cycle, during which synthesis of hair takes place.

an·ag·re·lide (an-ag′rĕ-līd) an agent used to reduce elevated platelet counts and the risk of thrombosis in the treatment of hemorrhagic thrombocythemia; used as the hydrochloride salt.

an·aku·sis (an″ah-koo′sis) total deafness.

anal (a′n′l) relating to the anus.

an·al·bu·min·emia (an″al-bu″mĭ-ne′me-ah) absence or deficiency of serum albumins.

ana·lep·tic (an″ah-lep′tik) 1. stimulating, invigorating, or restorative. 2. a drug that acts as a central nervous system stimulant, such as caffeine.

an·al·ge·sia (an″al-je′ze-ah) 1. absence of sensibility to pain. 2. the relief of pain without loss of consciousness. **continuous epidural a.,** continuous injection of an anesthetic solution into the sacral and lumbar plexuses within the epidural space to relieve the pain of childbirth; also used in general surgery to block the pain pathways below the navel. **epidural a.,** analgesia induced by introduction of the analgesic agent into the epidural space of the vertebral canal. **infiltration a.,** paralysis of the nerve endings at the site of operation by subcutaneous injection of an anesthetic. **paretic a.,** loss of the sense of pain accompanied by partial paralysis. **relative a.,** in dental anesthesia, a maintained level of conscious sedation, short of general anesthesia, in which the pain threshold is elevated; usually induced by inhalation of nitrous oxide and oxygen. **spinal a.,** analgesia produced by injection of an opioid into the subarachnoid space around the spinal cord.

an·al·ge·sic (-je′zik) 1. relieving pain. 2. pertaining to analgesia. 3. an agent that relieves pain without causing loss of consciousness. **narcotic a.,** opioid a. **nonsteroidal antiinflammatory a. (NSAIA),** see under *drug*. **opioid a.,** any of a class of

compounds that bind with the opioid receptors in the central nervous system to block the perception of pain or affect the emotional response to pain, including opium and its derivatives.

an·al·gia (an-al′jah) analgesia (1). **anal′gic,** adj.

anal·o·gous (ah-nal′ah-gus) resembling or similar in some respects, as in function or appearance, but not in origin or development.

ana·logue (an′ah-log) 1. a part or organ having the same function as another, but of different evolutionary origin. 2. a chemical compound having a structure similar to that of another but differing from it in respect to a certain component; it may have similar or opposite action metabolically.

anal·o·gy (ah-nal′ah-je) the quality of being analogous; resemblance or similarity in function or appearance, but not in origin or development.

anal·y·sand (ah-nal′ĭ-sand) one who is being psychoanalyzed.

anal·y·sis (ah-nal′ĭ-sis) pl. *anal′yses.* 1. Separation into component parts; the act of determining the component parts of a substance. 2. psychoanalysis. **analyt′ical, analyt′ical,** adj. **bite a.,** occlusal a. **blood gas a.,** the determination of oxygen and carbon dioxide concentrations and pressures with the pH of the blood by laboratory tests; the following measurements may be made: Po_2, partial pressure of oxygen in arterial blood; Pco_2, partial pressure of carbon dioxide in arterial blood; So_2, percent saturation of hemoglobin with oxygen in arterial blood; the total CO_2 content of (venous) plasma; and the pH. **gasometric a.,** analysis by measurement of the gas evolved. **gravimetric a.,** quantitative analysis in which the analyte or a derivative is determined by weighing after purification. **occlusal a.,** study of the relations of the occlusal surfaces of opposing teeth. **qualitative a.,** chemical analysis in which the presence or absence of certain compounds in a specimen is determined. **quantitative a.,** determination of the proportionate quantities of the constituents of a compound. **pulse-chase a.,** a method for examining a cellular process occurring over time by successively exposing the cells to a radioactive compound (pulse) and then to the same compound in nonradioactive form (chase). **spectroscopic a., spectrum a.,** that done by determining the wavelength(s) at which electromagnetic energy is absorbed by the sample. **transactional a.,** a type of psychotherapy based on an understanding of the interactions (transactions) between patient and therapist and between patient and others in the environment. **vector a.,** analysis of a moving force to determine both its magnitude and its direction, e.g., analysis of the scalar electrocardiogram to determine the magnitude and direction of the electromotive force for one complete cycle of the heart.

ana·lyte (an'ah-līt) a substance undergoing analysis.

ana·ly·zer (an'ah-li"zer) 1. a Nicol prism attached to a polarizing apparatus which extinguishes the ray of light polarized by the polarizer. 2. Pavlov's name for a specialized part of the nervous system which controls the reactions of the organism to changing external conditions. 3. a nervous receptor together with its central connections, by means of which sensitivity to stimulations is differentiated.

an·am·ne·sis (an"am-ne'sis) [Gr.] 1. recollection. 2. a patient case history, particularly using the patient's recollections. 3. immunologic memory.

an·am·nes·tic (an"am-nes'tik) 1. pertaining to anamnesis. 2. aiding the memory.

ana·phase (an'ah-fāz) the third stage of division of the nucleus in either meiosis or mitosis.

ana·phia (ah-na'fe-ah) tactile anesthesia.

ana·pho·ria (an"ah-for'e-ah) a tendency for the visual axes of both eyes to divert above the horizontal plane.

an·aph·ro·dis·iac (an"af-ro-diz'e-ak) 1. repressing sexual desire. 2. a drug that represses sexual desire.

ana·phy·lac·tic (an"ah-fĭ-lak'tik) pertaining to anaphylaxis.

ana·phy·lac·to·gen·e·sis (-fĭ-lak"to-jen'ĕ-sis) the production of anaphylaxis. **anaphylactogen'ic,** adj.

ana·phy·lac·toid (-fĭ-lak'toid) resembling anaphylaxis.

ana·phyl·a·tox·in (-fil'ah-tok"sin) a substance produced in blood serum during complement fixation which serves as a mediator of inflammation by inducing mast cell degranulation and histamine release; on injection into animals, it causes anaphylactic shock.

ana·phy·lax·is (-fĭ-lak'sis) anaphylactic shock; a manifestation of immediate hypersensitivity in which exposure of a sensitized individual to a specific antigen or hapten results in life-threatening respiratory distress, usually followed by vascular collapse and shock and accompanied by urticaria, pruritus, and angioedema. **active a.,** that produced by injection of a foreign protein. **antiserum a.,** passive a. **local a.,** that confined to a limited

area, e.g., cutaneous anaphylaxis. **passive a.,** that resulting in a normal person from injection of serum of a sensitized person. **passive cutaneous a.,** PCA; localized anaphylaxis passively transferred by intradermal injection of an antibody and, after a latent period (about 24 to 72 hours), intravenous injection of the homologous antigen and Evans blue dye; blueing of the skin at the site of the intradermal injection is evidence of the permeability reaction. Used in studies of antibodies causing immediate hypersensitivity reaction. **reverse a.,** that following injection of antigen, succeeded by injection of antiserum.

ana·pla·sia (-pla'zhah) dedifferentiation; loss of differentiation of cells and of their orientation to one another and to their axial framework and blood vessels, a characteristic of tumor tissue. **anaplas'tic,** adj.

Ana·plas·ma (-plaz'mah) a genus of microorganisms (family Anaplasmataceae), including *A. margina'le,* the etiologic agent of anaplasmosis.

Ana·plas·ma·ta·ce·ae (-plaz"mah-ta'se-e) a family of microorganisms (order Rickettsiales).

an·apoph·y·sis (-pof'ĭ-sis) an accessory vertebral process.

anap·tic (ah-nap'tik) marked by anaphia.

an·ar·thria (an-ahr'thre-ah) severe dysarthria resulting in speechlessness.

anas·to·mo·sis (ah-nas"tah-mo'sis) pl. *anastomo'ses.* [Gr.] 1. communication between vessels by collateral channels. 2. surgical, traumatic, or pathological formation of an opening between two normally distinct spaces or organs. **anastomot'ic,** adj. **arteriovenous a.,** one between an artery and a vein. **crucial a.,** an arterial anastomosis in the upper part of the thigh. **end-to-end a.,** 1. one connecting the end of an artery and that of some other vessel. 2. anastomosis of two sections of colon, as with partial colectomy or closure of an ileostomy. **end-to-side a.,** an anastomosis connecting the end of one vessel with the side of a larger one. **heterocladic a.,** one between branches of different arteries. **homocladic a.,** one between two branches of the same artery. **ileoanal pull-through a.,** anastomosis of an ileoanal reservoir to the anal canal by means of a short conduit of ileum pulled through the rectal cuff and sutured to the anus, allowing continent elimination of feces following colectomy. **intestinal a.,** establishment of a communication between two formerly distant portions of the intestine. **a. of Riolan,** anastomosis of the superior and inferior mesenteric arteries. **Roux-en-Y a.,** any Y-shaped anastomosis in which the small intestine is included.

anas·tro·zole (ah-nas′trah-zōl″) an antineoplastic used for treatment of advanced breast carcinoma in postmenopausal women.

anat. anatomy.

ana·tom·ic (an″ah-tom′ik) anatomical.

ana·tom·i·cal (an″ah-tom′ĭ-kal) pertaining to anatomy, or to the structure of an organism.

anat·o·my (ah-nat′ah-me) the science of the structure of living organisms. **applied a.,** anatomy as applied to diagnosis and treatment. **clinical a.,** anatomy as applied to clinical practice. **comparative a.,** comparison of the structure of different animals and plants, one with another. **developmental a.,** the field of study concerned with the changes that cells, tissues, organs, and the body as a whole undergo from fertilization of a secondary oocyte to the resulting offspring; it includes both prenatal and postnatal development. **gross a.,** that dealing with structures visible with the unaided eye. **histologic a.,** histology. **homologic a.,** the study of the related parts of the body in different animals. **macroscopic a.,** gross a. **microscopic a.,** histology. **morbid a., pathological a.,** anatomic pathology. **physiological a.,** the study of the organs with respect to their normal functions. **radiological a.,** the study of the anatomy of tissues based on their visualization on x-ray films. **special a.,** the study of particular organs or parts. **topographic a.,** the study of parts in their relation to surrounding parts. **x-ray a.,** radiological a.

ana·tro·pia (an″ah-tro′pe-ah) upward deviation of the visual axis of one eye when the other eye is fixing. **anatrop′ic,** adj.

an·chor·age (ang′ker-ij) fixation, e.g., surgical fixation of a displaced viscus or, in operative dentistry, fixation of fillings or of artificial crowns or bridges. In orthodontics, the support used for a regulating apparatus.

an·cip·i·tal (an-sip′ĭ-t′l) two-edged or two-headed.

an·co·nad (ang′ko-nad) toward the elbow or olecranon.

an·con·ag·ra (ang′kon-ag′rah) gout of the elbow.

an·co·ne·al (ang-ko′ne-al) cubital.

an·co·ni·tis (ang″ko-ni′tis) inflammation of the elbow joint.

ancyl(o)- for words beginning thus, see also those beginning *ankyl(o)-*.

An·cy·los·to·ma (an″sĭ-los′tah-mah) a genus of hookworms (family Ancylostomidae). **A. america′num,** *Necator americanus.* **A. brazilien′se,** a species parasitizing dogs and cats in tropical areas; its larvae may cause creeping eruption in humans. **A. cani′num,** the common hookworm of dogs and cats; its larvae may cause creeping eruption in humans. **A. ceylo′nicum,** *A. braziliense.* **A. duodena′le,** the common European or Old World hookworm, parasitic in the small intestine, causing hookworm disease.

an·cy·los·to·mi·a·sis (an″sĭ-los″to-mi′ah-sis) infection with hookworms; see *hookworm disease,* under *disease.*

An·cy·lo·sto·mi·dae (an″sĭ-lo-sto′mĭ-de) a family of nematode parasites having two ventrolateral cutting plates at the entrance to a large buccal capsule and small teeth at its base; the hookworms.

an·cy·roid (an′sĭ-roid) anchor-shaped.

andr(o)- word element [Gr.], *male; masculine.*

an·dro·blas·to·ma (an″dro-blas-to′mah) 1. a rare benign tumor of the testis histologically resembling the fetal testis; there are three varieties: diffuse stromal, mixed (stromal and epithelial), and tubular (epithelial). The epithelial elements contain Sertoli cells, which may produce estrogen and thus cause feminization. 2. arrhenoblastoma.

an·dro·gen (an′dro-jen) any substance, e.g., testosterone, that promotes masculinization. **adrenal a's,** the 19-carbon steroids synthesized by the adrenal cortex that function as weak steroids or steroid precursors; e.g., dehydroepiandrosterone.

an·dro·gen·e·sis (an″dro-jen′ĕ-sis) development of a zygote that contains only paternal chromosomes, as after fertilization of an oocyte whose chromosomes are absent or inactivated.

an·dro·ge·net·ic (-jĕ-net′ik) caused by androgens.

an·dro·gen·ic (an″dro-jen′ik) 1. producing masculine characteristics. 2. pertaining to an androgen.

an·drog·y·ny (an-droj′ĭ-ne) 1. sexual ambiguity, either physical or psychological. 2. female pseudohermaphroditism. **androg′ynous,** adj.

an·droid (an′droid) resembling a man.

an·dro·pause (an′dro-pawz) a variable complex of symptoms, including decreased Leydig cell numbers and androgen production, occurring in men after middle age, purported to be analogous to menopause in women.

an·dro·stane (an′dro-stān) the hydrocarbon nucleus, $C_{19}H_{32}$, from which androgens are derived.

an·dro·stane·di·ol (an″dro-stān′de-ol) an androgen implicated in the regulation of gonadotropin secretion; *a. glucuronide*, a metabolite of dihydroxytestosterone formed in the peripheral tissues, is used to estimate peripheral androgen activity.

an·dro·stene (an′dro-stēn) a cyclic hydrocarbon, $C_{19}H_{30}$, forming the nucleus of testosterone and certain other androgens.

an·dro·stene·di·ol (an″dro-stēn′di-ol) a testosterone metabolite that may contribute to gonadotropin secretion.

an·dro·stene·di·one (-di-ōn) an androgenic steroid produced by the testis, adrenal cortex, and ovary; converted metabolically to testosterone and other androgens.

an·dros·ter·one (an-dros′ter-ōn) an androgen degradation product that in some species exerts weak androgenlike effects.

-ane word termination denoting a saturated open-chain hydrocarbon (C_nH_{2n+2}).

an·ec·do·tal (an″ek-do′t'l) based on case histories rather than on controlled clinical trials.

an·echo·ic (an-ĕ-ko′ik) 1. without echoes; said of a chamber for measuring the effects of sound. 2. sonolucent.

an·ec·ta·sis (an-ek′tah-sis) congenital atelectasis due to developmental immaturity.

an·e·jac·u·la·tion failure of ejaculation of semen from the urinary meatus in sexual intercourse.

ane·mia (ah-ne′me-ah) reduction below normal of the number of erythrocytes, quantity of hemoglobin, or the volume of packed red cells in the blood; a symptom of various diseases and disorders. **ane′mic**, adj. **achrestic a.**, any of various types of megaloblastic anemia resembling pernicious anemia but unresponsive to therapy with vitamin B_{12}. **aplastic a.**, a diverse group of anemias characterized by bone marrow suppression with replacement of the hematopoietic cells by fat, which causes pancytopenia, often accompanied by granulocytopenia and thrombocytopenia. **autoimmune hemolytic a.**, AIHA; a general term covering a large group of anemias involving autoantibodies against red cell antigens; they may be idiopathic or may have any of a number of causes, including autoimmune disease, hematologic neoplasms, viral infections, or immunodeficiency disorders. **aregenerative a.**, anemia characterized by bone marrow failure, so that functional marrow cells are regenerated slowly or not at all. **Blackfan-Diamond a.**, congenital hypoplastic a. (1). **congenital hypoplastic a.**, 1. a progressive anemia of unknown etiology seen in the first year of life,

with deficiency of red cell precursors in an otherwise normally cellular bone marrow; it is unresponsive to hematinics. 2. Fanconi's syndrome (1). **congenital nonspherocytic hemolytic a.**, any of a heterogeneous group of inherited anemias characterized by shortened red cell survival, lack of spherocytosis, and normal osmotic fragility with erythrocyte membrane defects, multiple intracellular enzyme deficiencies or other defects, or unstable hemoglobins. **Cooley's a.**, thalassemia major. **drug-induced immune hemolytic a.**, immune hemolytic anemia produced by drugs, classified as the *penicillin type*, in which the drug induces the formation of specific antibodies; the *methyldopa type*, in which the drug induces the formation of anti-Rh antibodies; and the *stibophen type*, in which circulating drug-antibody complexes bind to red cells. **equine infectious a.**, a viral disease of equines, with recurring malaise and abrupt temperature rises, weight loss, edema, and anemia; transmission to humans has been suggested, in whom it causes anemia, neutropenia, and relative lymphocytosis. **Fanconi's a.**, Fanconi's syndrome (1). **hemolytic a.**, any of a group of acute or chronic anemias, inherited or acquired, characterized by shortened survival of mature erythrocytes and inability of bone marrow to compensate for the decreased life span. **hereditary iron-loading a.**, hereditary sideroblastic a. **hereditary sideroachrestic a.**, hereditary sideroblastic a. **hereditary sideroblastic a.**, an X-linked anemia characterized by ringed sideroblasts, hypochromic, microcytic erythrocytes, poikilocytosis, weakness, and later by iron overload. **hookworm a.**, hypochromic microcytic anemia resulting from infection with *Ancylostoma* or *Necator*; see also under *disease*. **hypochromic a.**, that characterized by a disproportionate reduction of red cell hemoglobin and an increased area of central pallor in the red cells. **hypoplastic a.**, that due to varying degrees of erythrocytic hypoplasia without leukopenia or thrombocytopenia. **iron deficiency a.**, a form characterized by low or absent iron stores, low serum iron concentration, low transferrin saturation, elevated transferrin, low hemoglobin concentration or hematocrit, and hypochromic, microcytic red blood cells. **macrocytic a.**, a group of anemias of varying etiologies, marked by larger than normal red cells, absence of the customary central area of pallor, and an increased mean corpuscular volume and mean corpuscular hemoglobin. **Mediterranean a.**, thalassemia major. **megaloblastic a.**, any anemia characterized by megaloblasts in the bone marrow, such as pernicious a. **microcytic a.,** that marked by decrease in size of the red cells. **myelopathic a., myelophthisic a.,** leukoerythroblastosis. **normochromic a.,** anemia in which the hemoglobin content of the red cells as measured by the MCHC is in the normal range. **normocytic a.,** that marked by a proportionate decrease in the hemoglobin content, the packed red cell volume, and the number of erythrocytes per cubic millimeter of blood. **pernicious a.,** megaloblastic anemia, most commonly affecting older adults, due to failure of the gastric mucosa to secrete adequate and potent intrinsic factor, resulting in malabsorption of vitamin B_{12}. **polar a.,** an anemic condition that occurs during exposure to low temperature; initially microcytic, but subsequently becoming normocytic. **pure red cell a.,** anemia characterized by absence of red cell precursors in the bone marrow; the congenital form is called *congenital hypoplastic a.* **refractory normoblastic a.,** refractory sideroblastic a. **refractory sideroblastic a.,** a sideroblastic anemia clinically similar to the hereditary sideroblastic form but occurring in adults and often only slowly progressive. It is unresponsive to hematinics or to withdrawal of toxic agents or drugs and may be preleukemic. **sickle cell a.,** an autosomal dominant type of hemolytic anemia, seen primarily in those of West African descent, and less often in the Mediterranean basin and a few other areas; it is caused by hemoglobin S with abnormal erythrocytes *(sickle cells)* in the blood. Homozygous individuals have the full-blown syndrome with accelerated hemolysis, increased blood viscosity and vaso-occlusion, arthralgias, acute attacks of abdominal pain, and ulcerations of the lower limbs; some have periodic attacks of *sickle cell crises.* The heterozygous condition is called *sickle cell trait* and is usually asymptomatic. **sideroachrestic a.,** sideroblastic a. **sideroblastic a.,** any of a group of anemias that may have diverse clinical manifestations; commonly characterized by large numbers of ringed sideroblasts in the bone marrow, ineffective erythropoiesis, variable proportions of hypochromic erythrocytes in the peripheral blood, and usually increased levels of tissue iron. **sideropenic a.,** a group of anemias marked by low levels of iron in the plasma; it includes iron deficiency anemia and the anemia of chronic disorders. **spur cell a.,** anemia in which the red cells have a bizarre spiculated shape and are destroyed prematurely, primarily in the spleen; it is an

acquired form occurring in severe liver disease and represents an abnormality in the cholesterol content of the red cell membrane. **toxic hemolytic a.,** that due to toxic agents, including drugs, bacterial lysins, and snake venoms.

an·en·ceph·a·ly (an″en-sef′ah-le) congenital absence of the cranial vault, with the cerebral hemispheres completely missing or reduced to small masses. **anencephal′ic,** adj.

an·er·gy (an′er-je) 1. extreme lack of energy. 2. diminished reactivity to one or more specific antigens. **aner′gic,** adj.

an·eryth·ro·pla·sia (an″ĕ-rith″ro-pla′zhah) absence of erythrocyte formation. **aneryth·ro·plas′tic,** adj.

an·eryth·ro·poi·e·sis (-poi-e′sis) deficient production of erythrocytes.

an·es·the·sia (an″es-the′zhah) 1. loss of sensation, usually by damage to a nerve or receptor. 2. loss of the ability to feel pain, caused by administration of a drug or other medical intervention. **basal a.,** narcosis produced by preliminary medication so that the inhalation of anesthetic necessary to produce surgical anesthesia is greatly reduced. **block a.,** regional a. **bulbar a.,** that due to a lesion of the pons. **caudal a.,** see under *block.* **closed circuit a.,** that produced by continuous rebreathing of a small amount of anesthetic gas in a closed system with an apparatus for removing carbon dioxide. **crossed a.,** see under *hemianesthesia.* **a. doloro′sa,** pain in an area or region that is anesthetic. **electric a.,** that induced by passage of an electric current. **endotracheal a.,** that produced by introduction of a gaseous mixture through a tube inserted into the trachea. **epidural a.,** that produced by injection of the anesthetic into the extradural space, either between the vertebral spines or into the sacral hiatus *(caudal block).* **general a.,** a state of unconsciousness and insusceptibility to pain, produced by administration of anesthetic agents by inhalation, intravenously, intramuscularly, rectally, or via the gastrointestinal tract. **infiltration a.,** local anesthesia produced by injection of the anesthetic solution in the area of terminal nerve endings. **inhalation a.,** that produced by the inhalation of vapors of a volatile liquid or gaseous anesthetic agent. **insufflation a.,** that produced by blowing a mixture of gases or vapors into the respiratory tract through a tube. **local a.,** that produced in a limited area, as by injection of a local anesthetic or by freezing with ethyl chloride. **lumbar epidural a.,** that produced by injection of the anesthetic into the epidural space at the second or third lumbar interspace. **muscular a.**, loss or lack of muscle sense. **open a.**, general inhalation anesthesia using a cone, without significant rebreathing of exhaled gases. **peripheral a.**, that due to changes in the peripheral nerves. **regional a.**, insensibility of a part induced by interrupting the sensory nerve conductivity of that region of the body; it may be produced by either *field block* or *nerve block* (see under *block*). **sacral a.**, spinal anesthesia by injection of anesthetic into the sacral canal and about the sacral nerves. **saddle block a.**, see under *block*. **spinal a.**, 1. regional anesthesia by injection of a local anesthetic into the subarachnoid space around the spinal cord. 2. loss of sensation due to a spinal lesion. **surgical a.**, that degree of anesthesia at which operation may safely be performed. **tactile a.**, loss or impairment of the sense of touch. **topical a.**, that produced by application of a local anesthetic directly to the area involved, as to the oral mucosa or the cornea. **transsacral a.**, sacral a.

an·es·the·si·ol·o·gy (an″es-the″ze-ol′ah-je) the branch of medicine which studies anesthesia and anesthetics.

an·es·thet·ic (an″es-thet′ik) 1. characterized by anesthesia; numb. 2. pertaining to or producing anesthesia. 3. an agent that produces anesthesia. **local a.**, an agent, e.g., lidocaine, procaine, or tetracaine, that produces anesthesia by paralyzing sensory nerve endings or nerve fibers at the site of application. The conduction of nerve impulses is blocked by stopping the entry of sodium into nerve cells. **topical a.**, a local anesthetic applied directly to the area to be anesthetized, usually the mucous membranes or the skin.

anes·the·tist (ah-nes′thĕ-tist) a nurse or technician trained to administer anesthetics.

an·e·to·der·ma (an″ĕ-to-der′mah) localized elastolysis producing circumscribed areas of soft, thin, wrinkled skin that often protrude in small outpouchings. **perifollicular a.**, anetoderma occurring around hair follicles not preceded by folliculitis; it may be caused by elastase-producing staphylococci, by drugs, or by endocrine factors. **postinflammatory a.**, a condition occurring usually during infancy, marked by the development of erythematous papules that enlarge to form plaques, followed by laxity of the skin resembling cutis laxa.

an·eu·ploi·dy (an″u-ploi′de) any deviation from an exact multiple of the haploid number of chromosomes, whether fewer or more.

an·eu·rysm (an′u-rizm) a sac formed by localized dilatation of the wall of an artery, a vein, or the heart. **aneurys′mal**, adj. **aortic a.**, aneurysm of the aorta. **arteriosclerotic a.**, an aneurysm arising in a large artery, usually the abdominal aorta, as a result of weakening of the wall in severe atherosclerosis. **arteriovenous a.**, abnormal communication between an artery and a vein in which the blood flows directly into a neighboring vein or is carried into the vein by a connecting sac. **atherosclerotic a.**, arteriosclerotic a. **berry a.**, a small saccular aneurysm of a cerebral artery, usually at the junction of vessels in the circle of Willis, having a narrow opening into the artery. **compound a.**, one in which some of the layers of the wall of the vessel are ruptured and some merely dilated. **dissecting a.**, one resulting from hemorrhage that causes longitudinal splitting of the arterial wall, producing a tear in the intima and establishing communication with the lumen; it usually affects the aorta (*aortic dissection*). **false a.**, 1. one in which the entire wall is injured and the blood is retained in the surrounding tissues; a sac communicating with the artery (or heart) is eventually formed. 2. pseudoaneurysm. **infected a.**, one produced by growth of microorganisms (bacteria or fungi) in the vessel wall, or infection arising within a preexisting arteriosclerotic aneurysm. **mycotic a.**, an infected aneurysm caused by fungi. **racemose a.**, dilatation and tortuous lengthening of the blood vessels. **saccular a., sacculated a.**, a distended sac affecting only part of the arterial circumference. **varicose a.**, one in which an intervening sac connects the artery with contiguous veins.

an·eu·rys·mo·plas·ty (an″u-riz′mo-plas″te) plastic repair of the affected artery in the treatment of aneurysm.

an·eu·rys·mor·rha·phy (an″u-riz-mor′ah-fe) suture of an aneurysm.

ANF antinuclear factor; see *antinuclear antibodies (ANA)*, under *antibody*.

an·gi·as·the·nia (an″je-as-the′ne-ah) loss of tone in the vascular system.

an·gi·ec·ta·sis (-ek′tah-sis) gross dilatation and often lengthening of a blood or lymph vessel. **angiectat′ic**, adj.

an·gi·ec·to·my (-ek′tah-me) excision or resection of a vessel.

an·gi·ec·to·pia (-ek-to′pe-ah) abnormal position or course of a vessel.

an·gi·i·tis (-i′tis) pl. *angii′tides*. Vasculitis. **allergic granulomatous a.**, Churg-Strauss syndrome.

an·gi·na (an-ji'nah, an'ji-nah) 1. a. pectoris. 2. spasmodic, choking, or suffocating pain. **an'ginal**, adj. **a. of effort**, stable a. pectoris; see *a. pectoris*. **herpes a., a. herpe'tica**, herpangina. **intestinal a.**, cramping abdominal pain shortly after a meal, lasting one to three hours, due to ischemia of the smooth muscle of the bowel. **a. inver'sa**, Prinzmetal's a. **Ludwig's a.**, a severe form of cellulitis of the submaxillary space and secondary involvement of the sublingual and submental spaces, usually from infection or a penetrating injury to the floor of the mouth. **a. pec'toris**, paroxysmal pain in the chest, often radiating to the arms, particularly the left, usually due to interference with the supply of oxygen to the heart muscle, and precipitated by excitement or effort. It is subdivided into *stable* and *unstable a. pectoris* based on the predictability of the frequency, duration, and causative factors for attacks. **Plaut's a.**, necrotizing ulcerative gingivostomatitis. **Prinzmetal's a.**, a variant of angina pectoris in which the attacks occur during rest, exercise capacity is well preserved, and attacks are associated electrocardiographically with elevation of the ST segment. **pseudomembranous a.**, necrotizing ulcerative gingivostomatitis. **silent a.**, an episode of coronary insufficiency in which no pain is experienced. **variant a. pectoris**, Prinzmetal's a.

angi(o)- word element [Gr.], *vessel (channel)*.

an·gio·blast (an'je-o-blast") 1. the embryonic mesenchymal tissue from which blood cells and blood vessels arise. 2. an individual vessel-forming cell. **angioblas'tic**, adj.

an·gio·blas·to·ma (an"je-o-blas-to'mah) 1. hemangioblastoma. 2. angioblastic meningioma.

an·gio·car·di·og·ra·phy (-kahr"de-og'rah-fe) radiography of the heart and great vessels after introduction of an opaque contrast medium into a blood vessel or a cardiac chamber. **equilibrium radionuclide a.**, a form of radionuclide angiocardiography in which images are taken at specific phases of the cardiac cycle over a series of several hundred cycles, with image recording set, or gated, by the occurrence of specific electrocardiographic waveforms. **first pass radionuclide a.**, a form of radionuclide angiocardiography in which a rapid sequence of images is taken immediately after administration of a bolus of radioactive material to record only the initial transit through the central circulation. **radionuclide a.**, a form

in which the contrast material is a radionuclide, usually a compound of technetium 99m.

an·gio·car·dio·ki·net·ic (-kahr"de-o-ki-net'ik) affecting the movements of the heart and blood vessels; also, an agent that affects such movements.

an·gio·car·di·tis (-kahr-di'tis) inflammation of the heart and blood vessels.

an·gio·cen·tric (-sen'trik) pertaining to lesions originating in blood vessels.

an·gio·dys·pla·sia (-dis-pla'zhah) small vascular abnormalities, such as of the intestinal tract.

an·gio·ede·ma (-ĕ-de'mah) a vascular reaction involving the deep dermis or subcutaneous or submucosal tissues, representing localized edema caused by dilatation and increased permeability of the capillaries, and characterized by the development of giant wheals. **hereditary a.**, an autosomal dominant disorder of C1 inhibitor (C1 INH), which causes uncontrolled activation of the classical complement pathway, manifested as recurrent episodes of edema of the skin and upper respiratory and gastrointestinal tracts with increased levels of several vasoactive mediators of anaphylaxis. It may be mediated by such factors as minor trauma, sudden changes in environmental temperature, and sudden emotional stress.

an·gio·en·do·the·li·o·ma (-en"do-the"le-o'mah) hemangioendothelioma.

an·gio·en·do·the·lio·ma·to·sis (-en"do-the"le-o-mah-to'sis) intravascular proliferation of tumors derived from endothelial cells.

an·gio·fi·bro·ma (-fi-bro'mah) a lesion characterized by fibrous tissue and vascular proliferation. **juvenile nasopharyngeal a.**, a benign tumor of the nasopharynx composed of fibrous connective tissue with abundant endothelium-lined vascular spaces, usually occurring during puberty in boys; nasal obstruction may become total, with adenoid speech, discomfort in swallowing, and auditory tube obstruction.

an·gio·fol·lic·u·lar (-fŏ-lik'u-ler) pertaining to a lymphoid follicle and its blood vessels.

an·gio·gen·e·sis (-jen'ĕ-sis) vasculogenesis; development of blood vessels either in the embryo or in the form of neovascularization or revascularization.

an·gio·gen·ic (-jen'ik) 1. pertaining to angiogenesis. 2. of vascular origin.

an·gi·og·ra·phy (an"je-og'rah-fe) vasography; radiography of the blood vessels after introduction of a contrast medium.

angiograph'ic, adj. **intra-arterial digital subtraction a.,** a radiologic imaging technique for arteriography that uses electronic circuitry to subtract the background of bone and soft tissue from the image of the arteries, which have been injected with contrast material. **intravenous digital subtraction a.,** a fluoroscopic imaging technique in which electronic circuitry is used to subtract the background of bone and soft tissue and provide a useful image of vessels following the injection of contrast medium. **magnetic resonance a. (MRA),** a form of magnetic resonance imaging used to study blood vessels and blood flow.

an·gio·he·mo·phil·ia (an″je-o-he″mo-fil′e-ah) von Willebrand's disease.

an·gio·hy·a·li·no·sis (-hi′ah-lĭ-no′sis) hyaline degeneration of the walls of blood vessels.

an·gi·oid (an′je-oid) resembling blood vessels.

an·gio·ker·a·to·ma (an″je-o-ker″ah-to′mah) a skin disease in which telangiectases or warty growths occur in groups, together with epidermal thickening. **a. circumscrip'tum,** a rare form with discrete papules and nodules usually localized to a small area on the leg or trunk.

an·gio·ki·net·ic (-kĭ-net′ik) vasomotor.

an·gio·leio·my·o·ma (-li″o-mi-o′mah) a leiomyoma arising from vascular smooth muscle, usually a solitary nodular, sometimes painful, subcutaneous tumor on the lower limb, particularly in middle-aged women.

an·gio·lipo·leio·my·o·ma (-lip″o-li″o-mi-o′mah) a benign tumor composed of blood vessel, adipose tissue, and smooth muscle elements, such as occurs in the kidney in association with tuberous sclerosis, where it is usually called *angiomyolipoma.*

an·gio·li·po·ma (-lĭ-po′mah) an often painful lipoma containing clusters of thin-walled proliferating blood vessels.

an·gi·ol·o·gy (an″je-ol′ah-je) the study of the vessels of the body; also, the sum of knowledge relating to the blood and lymph vessels.

an·gio·lu·poid (an″je-o-loo′poid) a rare manifestation of cutaneous sarcoidosis localized to the malar region, bridge of the nose, or around the eyes, and consisting of livid nodular regions that coalesce to form plaques.

an·gi·ol·y·sis (an″je-ol′ĭ-sis) retrogression or obliteration of blood vessels, as in embryologic development.

an·gi·o·ma (an″je-o′mah) a tumor whose cells tend to form blood vessels (hemangioma) or lymph vessels (lymphangioma); a tumor made up of blood vessels or lymph vessels.

angiom'atous, adj. **a. caverno'sum, cavernous a.,** see under *hemangioma.* **cherry a's,** bright red, circumscribed, round or oval angiomas, 2 to 6 mm in diameter, containing many vascular loops, due to a telangiectatic vascular disturbance, usually seen on the trunk but sometimes appearing on other areas of the body, as in angioma serpiginosum, and occurring in most middle-aged and older persons. **senile a's,** cherry a's. **a. serpigi·no'sum,** a skin disease marked by minute vascular points arranged in rings on the skin.

an·gi·o·ma·to·sis (an″je-o-mah-to′sis) a diseased state of the vessels with formation of multiple angiomas. **bacillary a.,** a condition seen in patients with the acquired immunodeficiency syndrome, with varying characteristics ranging from erythematous angiomatous skin lesions to more widespread disease, believed to be an opportunistic infection by a rickettsia. **cerebroretinal a.,** von Hippel-Lindau disease. **encephalofacial a., encephalotrigeminal a.,** Sturge-Weber syndrome. **a. of retina,** von Hippel's disease. **retinocerebral a.,** von Hippel-Lindau disease.

an·gio·myo·li·po·ma (-mi″o-lĭ-po′mah) a benign tumor containing vascular, adipose, and muscle elements, occurring most often as a renal tumor with smooth muscle elements (more correctly called *angiolipoleiomyoma*), usually in association with tuberous sclerosis, and considered to be a hamartoma.

an·gio·my·o·ma (-mi-o′mah) angioleiomyoma.

an·gio·myo·sar·co·ma (-mi″o-sahr-ko′mah) a tumor composed of elements of angioma, myoma, and sarcoma.

an·gio·neu·rop·a·thy (-noo-rop′ah-the) 1. angiopathic neuropathy. 2. any neuropathy affecting the blood vessels; a disorder of the vasomotor system, as angiospasm or vasomotor paralysis. **angioneuropath'ic, angioneurot·ic,** adj.

an·gio·no·ma (-no′mah) ulceration of blood vessels.

an·gio·pa·ral·y·sis (-pah-ral′ĭ-sis) vasomotor paralysis.

an·gio·pa·re·sis (-pah-re′sis) vasoparesis.

an·gi·op·a·thy (an″je-op′ah-the) any disease of the vessels. **angiopath'ic,** adj.

an·gio·plas·ty (an′je-o-plas″te) an angiographic procedure for elimination of areas of narrowing in the blood vessels. **balloon a.,** inflation and deflation of a balloon catheter inside an artery, stretching the intima and leaving a ragged interior surface, triggering a healing response and breaking up of plaque. **percutaneous transluminal a.,**

a type of balloon angioplasty in which the catheter is inserted through the skin and through the lumen of the vessel to the site of the narrowing. **percutaneous transluminal coronary a. (PTCA)**, percutaneous transluminal angioplasty to enlarge the lumen of a sclerotic coronary artery.

an·gio·poi·e·sis (an″je-o-poi-e′sis) angiogenesis. **angiopoiet′ic**, adj.

an·gio·pres·sure (an′je-o-presh″er) the application of pressure to a blood vessel to control hemorrhage.

an·gi·or·rha·phy (an″je-or′ah-fe) suture of a vessel or vessels.

an·gio·sar·co·ma (an″je-o-sahr-ko′mah) a malignant neoplasm arising from vascular endothelial cells; the term may be used generally or may denote a subtype, such as hemangiosarcoma. **hepatic a.**, a malignant liver tumor characterized by dilated sinusoids with hypertrophied or necrotic hepatocytes that leave vascular channels lined by malignant cells; it usually affects older men and has been linked to exposure to toxins.

an·gio·scle·ro·sis (-sklě-ro′sis) hardening of the walls of blood vessels. **angiosclerot′ic**, adj.

an·gio·scope (an′je-o-skōp″) 1. a fiberoptic catheter for viewing the lumen of a blood vessel. 2. a microscope for observing the capillaries.

an·gi·os·co·py (an″je-os′kah-pe) 1. use of a fiberoptic angioscope to visualize the lumen of a blood vessel. 2. visualization of capillary blood vessels with a special microscope (angioscope).

an·gio·sco·to·ma (an″je-o-sko-to′mah) a centrocecal scotoma caused by shadows of the retinal blood vessels.

an·gio·sco·tom·e·try (-sko-tom′ě-tre) the plotting or mapping of an angioscotoma; done particularly in diagnosing glaucoma.

an·gio·spasm (an′je-o-spazm″) vasospasm. **angiospas′tic**, adj.

an·gio·ste·no·sis (an″je-o-stě-no′sis) narrowing of the caliber of a vessel.

an·gi·os·te·o·sis (an″je-os″te-o′sis) ossification or calcification of a vessel.

an·gio·stron·gy·li·a·sis (an″je-o-stron″jǐ-li′ah-sis) infection with *Angiostrongylus cantonensis*.

An·gio·stron·gy·lus (-stron′jǐ-lus) a genus of nematode parasites. *A. cantonen′sis* causes eosinophilic meningitis and *A. costaricen′sis* is associated with abdominal pain, vomiting, and a lower right quadrant mass.

an·gio·te·lec·ta·sis (an″je-o-tah-lek′tah-sis) pl. *angiotelec′tases*. Dilatation of the minute arteries and veins.

an·gio·ten·sin (-ten′sin) a decapeptide hormone (a. I) formed from the plasma glycoprotein angiotensinogen by renin secreted by the juxtaglomerular apparatus. It is in turn hydrolyzed by a peptidase in the lungs to form an octapeptide (a. II), which is a powerful vasopressor and stimulator of aldosterone secretion by the adrenal cortex. This is in turn hydrolyzed to form a heptapeptide (a. III), which has less vasopressor activity but more adrenal cortex–stimulating activity.

an·gio·ten·sin·ase (-ten′sin-ās) any of a group of plasma or tissue peptidases that cleave and inactivate angiotensin.

an·gio·ten·sin·con·vert·ing en·zyme (-ten′sin kon-vert′ing en′zīm) see *peptidyldipeptidase A*.

an·gio·ten·sin·o·gen (-ten·sin′o-jen) a serum α_2-globulin secreted in the liver which, on hydrolysis by renin, gives rise to angiotensin.

an·gio·tome (an′je-o-tōm″) one of the segments of the vascular system of the embryo.

an·gio·ton·ic (an″je-o-ton′ik) increasing vascular tension.

an·gio·tro·phic (an″je-o-tro′fik) vasotrophic.

an·gle (ang′g'l) 1. the point at which two intersecting borders or surfaces converge. 2. the degree of divergence of two intersecting lines or planes. **acromial a.**, the subcutaneous bony point at which the lateral border becomes continuous with the spine of the scapula. **axial a.**, any line angle parallel with the long axis of a tooth. **cardiodiaphragmatic a.**, that formed by the junction of the shadows of the heart and diaphragm in posteroanterior radiographs of the chest. **costovertebral a.**, that formed on either side of the vertebral column between the last rib and the lumbar vertebrae. **a. of eye**, canthus. **filtration a.**, a narrow recess between the sclerocorneal junction and the attached margin of the iris, at the periphery of the anterior chamber of the eye; it is the principal exit site for the aqueous fluid. **iridial a., iridocorneal a., a. of iris**, filtration a. **line a.**, an angle formed by the junction of two planes; in dentistry, the junction of two surfaces of a tooth or of two walls of a tooth cavity. **Louis' a., Ludwig's a.**, sternal a. **optic a.**, visual a. **point a.**, one formed by the junction of three planes; in dentistry, the junction of three surfaces of a tooth, or of three walls of a tooth cavity. **a. of pubis**, subpubic a. **sternal a.**, the angle between the sternum and manubrium. **subpubic a.**, that formed by the conjoined rami of the ischial and pubic bones. **tooth a's**, those formed by two or more tooth surfaces. **venous a.**, the angle formed by junction of the internal jugular and subclavian veins. **visual a.**, the angle formed between two lines extending from the nodal point of the eye to the extremities of the object seen. **Y a.**, that between the radius fixus and the line joining the lambda and inion.

ang·strom (Å) (ang′strom) a unit of length used for atomic dimensions and light wavelengths; it is nominally equivalent to 10^{-10} meter.

an·gu·lar (ang′gu-lar) sharply bent; having corners or angles.

an·gu·la·tion (ang″gu-la′shun) 1. formation of a sharp obstructive bend, as in the intestine, ureter, or similar tubes. 2. deviation from a straight line, as in a badly set bone.

an·gu·lus (ang′gu-lus) pl. *an′guli*. [L.] angle; used in names of anatomic structures or landmarks.

an·he·do·nia (an″he-do′ne-ah) inability to experience pleasure in normally pleasurable acts.

an·hi·dro·sis (an″hĭ-dro′sis) absence or deficiency of sweating.

an·hi·drot·ic (an″hĭ-drot′ik) 1. promoting anhidrosis. 2. an agent that suppresses sweating.

an·hy·dre·mia (an″hi-dre′me-ah) deficiency of water in the blood. Cf. *dehydration* and *hypovolemia*.

an·hy·dride (an-hi′drīd) any compound derived from a substance, especially an acid, by abstraction of a molecule of water. **chromic a.**, chromic acid. **phthalic a.**, a reactive low-molecular-weight compound with various industrial uses; it causes skin irritation and its fumes cause hypersensitivity pneumonitis.

an·ic·ter·ic (an″ik-ter′ik) not associated with jaundice.

an·i·lide (an′ĭ-līd) any compound formed from aniline by substituting a radical for the hydrogen of NH_2.

an·i·line (an′ĭ-lin) the parent substance of colors or dyes derived from coal tar; it is an important cause of serious industrial poisoning associated with bone marrow depression as well as methemoglobinemia, and high doses or prolonged exposure may be carcinogenic.

an·i·lin·ism (an′ĭ-lin-izm) poisoning by exposure to aniline.

an·i·lism (an′ĭ-lizm) anilinism.

anil·i·ty (ah-nil′ĭ-te) 1. the state of existing as or like an old woman. 2. senility.

an·i·ma (an′ĭ-mah) [L.] 1. the soul. 2. in jungian terminology, the unconscious, or inner being, of the individual, as opposed to the personality presented to the world (persona); by extension, used to denote the more feminine soul or feminine component of a man's personality; cf. *animus*.

an·i·mal (an′ĭ-m'l) 1. a living organism having sensation and the power of voluntary movement and requiring for its existence oxygen and organic food; animals constitute one of the five kingdoms of living organisms. 2. of or pertaining to such an organism. **control a.**, an untreated animal otherwise identical in all respects to one that is used for purposes of experimentation, used for checking results of treatment. **hyperphagic a.**, an experimental animal in which the cells of the ventromedial nucleus of the hypothalamus have been destroyed, abolishing its awareness of the point at which it should stop eating; excessive eating and savageness characterize such an animal. **spinal a.**, one whose spinal cord has been severed, cutting off communication with the brain.

an·i·mus (an′ĭ-mus) [L.] 1. disposition. 2. ill will, hostility; animosity. 3. in jungian psychology, the masculine aspect of a woman's soul or inner being; cf. *anima* (2).

an·ion (an′i-on) a negatively charged ion. **anion′ic**, adj.

an·irid·ia (an″ĭ-rid′e-ah) congenital absence of the iris.

an·i·sa·ki·a·sis (an″ĭ-sah-ki′ah-sis) infection with the third-stage larvae of the roundworm *Anisakis marina*, which burrow into the stomach wall, producing an eosinophilic granulomatous mass. Infection is acquired by eating undercooked marine fish.

An·i·sa·kis (an″ĭ-sa′kis) a genus of nematodes that parasitize the stomachs of marine mammals and birds.

an·is·ei·ko·nia (an″is-i-ko′ne-ah) inequality of the retinal images of the two eyes.

o·an·is·i·dine (ah-nis′ĭ-dēn) a yellow to red oily aromatic amine used as an intermediate in the manufacture of azo dyes; it is an irritant and carcinogen.

an·is·in·di·one (an″is-in-di′ōn) an indanedione anticoagulant.

anis(o)- word element [Gr.], *unequal*.

an·iso·chro·mat·ic (an-i″so-kro-mat′ik) not of the same color throughout.

an·iso·co·ria (-kor′e-ah) inequality in size of the pupils of the eyes.

an·iso·cy·to·sis (-si-to′sis) presence in the blood of erythrocytes showing excessive variations in size.

an·iso·gam·ete (-gam′ēt) a gamete differing in size or structure from the one with which it unites. **anisogamet′ic**, adj.

an·isog·a·my (an″i-sog′ah-me) in the most restrictive sense, fertilization of a large motile female gamete by a small motile male gamete; often used more generally for the sexual union of two dissimilar gametes (heterogamy), particularly in lower organisms. **anisog′amous,** adj.

an·iso·kary·o·sis (an-i″so-kar″e-o′sis) inequality in the size of the nuclei of cells.

an·iso·me·tro·pia (-mĕ-tro′pe-ah) inequality in refractive power of the two eyes. **anisometrop′ic,** adj.

an·iso·pi·esis (-pi-e′sis) variation or inequality in the blood pressure as registered in different parts of the body.

an·iso·poi·ki·lo·cy·to·sis (-poi″ki-lo-si-to′-sis) the presence in the blood of erythrocytes of varying sizes and abnormal shapes.

an·iso·spore (an-i′so-spor) 1. an anisogamete of organisms reproducing by spores. 2. an asexual spore produced by heterosporous organisms.

an·isos·then·ic (an-i″sos-then′ik) not having equal power; said of muscles.

an·iso·ton·ic (an-i″so-ton′ik) 1. varying in tonicity or tension. 2. having different osmotic pressure; not isotonic.

an·iso·tro·pic (-tro′pik) 1. having unlike properties in different directions. 2. doubly refracting, or having a double polarizing power.

an·isot·ro·py (an″i-sot′rah-pe) the quality of being anisotropic.

an·is·trep·lase (an″is-trep′lās) a thrombolytic agent used to clear coronary vessel occlusions associated with myocardial infarction.

an·i·su·ria (an″i-su′re-ah) alternating oliguria and polyuria.

an·kle (ang′k'l) 1. the joint between the leg and foot. 2. the region of this joint. 3. tarsus.

ankyl(o)- word element [Gr.], *bent; crooked; in the form of a loop; adhesion.*

an·ky·lo·bleph·a·ron (ang″ki-lo-blef′ah-ron) adhesion of the ciliary edges of the eyelids to each other.

an·ky·lo·glos·sia (-glos′e-ah) tongue-tie. **a. supe′rior,** extensive adhesion of the tongue to the palate, associated with deformities of the hands and feet.

an·ky·losed (ang′ki-lōzd) fused or obliterated, as an ankylosed joint.

an·ky·lo·sis (ang″ki-lo′sis) pl. *ankylo′ses.* [Gr.] immobility and consolidation of a joint due to disease, injury, or surgical procedure. **ankylot′ic,** adj. **artificial a.,** arthrodesis. **bony a.,** union of the bones of a joint by proliferation of bone cells, resulting in complete immobility; true a. **extracapsular a.,**

that due to rigidity of structures outside the joint capsule. **false a.,** fibrous a. **fibrous a.,** reduced joint mobility due to proliferation of fibrous tissue. **intracapsular a.,** that due to disease, injury, or surgery within the joint capsule.

an·ky·rin (ang′ki-rin) a membrane protein of erythrocytes and brain that anchors spectrin to the plasma membrane at the sites of ion channels.

an·ky·roid (ang′ki-roid) hook-shaped.

an·lage (ahn-lah′gĕ, an′lāg) pl. *anla′gen.* [Ger.] primordium.

an·neal (ah-nēl′) 1. to toughen, temper, or soften a material, as a metal, by controlled heating and cooling. 2. in molecular biology, to cause the association or reassociation of single-stranded nucleic acids so that double-stranded molecules are formed, often by heating and cooling.

an·nec·tent (ah-nek′tent) connecting; joining together.

an·ne·lid (an′ĕ-lid) any member of Annelida.

An·ne·li·da (ah-nel′ĭ-dah) a phylum of metazoan invertebrates, the segmented worms, including leeches.

an·nu·lar (an′u-ler) ring-shaped.

an·nu·lo·aor·tic (an″u-lo-a-or′tik) pertaining to the aorta and the fibrous ring of the heart at the aortic orifice.

an·nu·lo·plas·ty (an′u-lo-plas″te) plastic repair of a cardiac valve.

an·nu·lor·rha·phy (an″u-lor′ah-fe) closure of a hernial ring or defect by sutures.

an·nu·lus (an′u-lus) pl. *an′nuli.* [L.] anulus.

an·ode (an′ōd) the electrode at which oxidation occurs and to which anions are attracted. **ano′dal,** adj.

an·o·dyne (an′ah-dīn) 1. relieving pain. 2. a medicine that eases pain.

anom·a·lad (ah-nom′ah-lad) sequence (2).

anom·a·ly (ah-nom′ah-le) marked deviation from normal, especially as a result of congenital or hereditary defects. **anom′alous,** adj. **Alder's a.,** an autosomal dominant condition in which leukocytes of the myelocytic series, and sometimes all leukocytes, contain coarse azurophilic granules. **Chédiak-Higashi a.,** see under *syndrome.* **congenital a.,** a developmental anomaly present at birth. **developmental a.,** 1. a structural abnormality of any type. 2. a defect resulting from imperfect embryonic development. **Ebstein's a.,** a malformation of the tricuspid valve, usually associated with an atrial septal defect. **May-Hegglin a.,** an autosomal dominant disorder of blood cell morphology, characterized by RNA-containing cytoplasmic inclusions (similar to Döhle bodies) in granulocytes, by large, poorly granulated platelets, and by thrombocytopenia. **Pelger's nuclear a.**, Pelger-Huët nuclear a. (1). **Pelger-Huët nuclear a.**, 1. a hereditary or acquired defect in which the nuclei of neutrophils and eosinophils appear rodlike, spherical, or dumbbell-shaped; the nuclear structure is coarse and lumpy. 2. an acquired condition with similar features, occurring in certain anemias and leukemias.

an·o·mer (an'o-mer) either of a pair of cyclic stereoisomers (designated α or β) of a sugar or glycoside, differing only in configuration at the reducing carbon atom. **anomer'ic**, adj.

ano·mia (ah-no'me-ah) anomic aphasia.

ano·mic (ah-no'mik) lacking a name.

an·onych·ia (an″o-nik'e-ah) congenital absence of a nail or nails.

Anoph·e·les (ah-nof'ĕ-lēz) a widely distributed genus of mosquitoes, comprising over 300 species, many of which are vectors of malaria; some are vectors of *Wuchereria bancrofti.*

an·oph·thal·mia (an″of-thal'me-ah) a developmental anomaly characterized by complete absence of the eyes (rare) or by the presence of vestigial eyes.

ano·plas·ty (a'no-plas″te) plastic or reparative surgery of the anus.

an·or·chia (an-or'ke-ah) congenital absence of one or both testes in a male.

an·or·chic (an-or'kik) anorchid.

an·or·chid (an-or'kid) lacking testes or not having testes in the scrotum.

an·or·chi·dism (an-or'kĭ-dizm″) anorchia.

an·or·chism (an-or'kizm) anorchia.

ano·rec·tic (an″o-rek'tik) 1. pertaining to anorexia. 2. an agent that diminishes the appetite.

an·orex·ia (-rek'se-ah) lack or loss of appetite for food. **a. nervo'sa**, an eating disorder usually occurring in adolescent females, characterized by refusal to maintain a normal minimal body weight, fear of gaining weight or becoming obese, disturbance of body image, undue reliance on body weight or shape for self-evaluation, and amenorrhea. The two subtypes include one characterized by dieting and exercise alone and one also characterized by binge eating and purging.

ano·rex·i·gen·ic (-rek″sĭ-jen'ik) 1. producing anorexia. 2. an agent that diminishes or controls the appetite.

an·or·gas·mia (an″or-gaz'me-ah) inability or failure to experience orgasm. **anorgas'mic**, adj.

an·or·thog·ra·phy (an″or-thog'rah-fe) agraphia.

an·or·tho·pia (-or-tho'pe-ah) asymmetrical or distorted vision.

ano·sig·moi·dos·co·py (a″no-sig″moi-dos'kah-pe) endoscopic examination of the anus, rectum, and sigmoid colon. **anosigmoidoscop'ic**, adj.

an·os·mia (an-oz'me-ah) lack of sense of smell. **anos'mic, anosmat'ic**, adj.

ano·sog·no·sia (an-o″so-no'zhah) unawareness or denial of a neurological deficit, such as hemiplegia. **anosogno'sic**, adj.

an·os·to·sis (an″os-to'sis) defective formation of bone.

an·otia (an-o'shah) congenital absence of one or both external ears.

an·ovar·ism (an-o'var-izm) absence of the ovaries.

an·ov·u·lar (an-ov'u-ler) anovulatory.

an·ov·u·la·tion (an″ov-u-la'shun) absence of ovulation.

an·ov·u·la·to·ry (an-ov'u-lah-tor″e) not accompanied by discharge of an oocyte.

anox·ia (ah-nok'se-ah) a total lack of oxygen; often used interchangeably with *hypoxia* to indicate a reduced oxygen supply to tissues. **anox'ic**, adj. **altitude a.,** see under *sickness.* **anemic a.,** that due to decrease in amount of hemoglobin or number of erythrocytes in the blood. **anoxic a.,** that due to interference with the oxygen supply. **histotoxic a.,** severe histotoxic hypoxia.

ANP atrial natriuretic peptide.

an·sa (an'sah) pl. *an'sae.* [L.] a looplike structure. **a. cervica'lis,** a nerve loop in the neck that supplies the infrahyoid muscles. **a. lenticula'ris,** a small nerve fiber tract arising in the globus pallidus and joining the anterior part of the ventral thalamic nucleus. **a. nephro'ni,** loop of Henle. **an'sae ner-vo'rum spina'lium,** loops of nerve fibers joining the ventral roots of the spinal nerves. **a. peduncula'ris,** peduncular loop; a complex grouping of nerve fibers connecting the amygdaloid nucleus, piriform area, and anterior hypothalamus, and various thalamic nuclei. **a. subcla'via, a. of Vieussens,** the subclavian loop; nerve filaments passing around the subclavian artery to form a loop connecting the middle and inferior cervical ganglia. **a. vitelli'na,** an embryonic vein from the yolk sac to the umbilical vein.

an·ser·ine (an'ser-īn) pertaining to or like a goose.

ant·ac·id (ant-as′id) counteracting acidity; an agent that so acts.

an·tag·o·nism (an-tag′o-nizm) opposition or contrariety between similar things, as between muscles, medicines, or organisms; cf. *antibiosis*.

an·tag·o·nist (an-tag′o-nist) 1. a substance that tends to nullify the action of another, as a drug that binds to a cell receptor without eliciting a biological response, blocking binding of substances that could elicit such responses. **antagonis′tic**, adj. 2. antagonistic muscle. 3. a tooth in one jaw that articulates with one in the other jaw. **α-adrenergic a.**, alpha-adrenergic blocking agent; see *adrenergic blocking agent*. **β-adrenergic a.**, beta-adrenergic blocking agent; see *adrenergic blocking agent*. **folic acid a.**, an antimetabolite, e.g., methotrexate, that interferes with DNA replication and cell division by inhibiting the enzyme dihydrofolate reductase; used in cancer chemotherapy. **H₁ receptor a.**, any of a large number of agents that block the action of histamine by competitive binding to the H₁ receptor; they also have sedative, anticholinergic, and antiemetic effects and are used for the relief of allergic symptoms, as antiemetics, as antivertigo agents, and as antidyskinetics in parkinsonism. **H₂ receptor a.**, an agent that blocks the action of histamine by competitive binding to the H₂ receptor; used to inhibit acid secretion in the treatment of peptic ulcer.

ant·al·gic (ant-al′jik) 1. counteracting or avoiding pain, as a posture or gait assumed so as to lessen pain. 2. analgesic.

ant·arth·rit·ic (ant″ahr-thrit′ik) antiarthritic.

ante- word element [L.], *before* (in time or space).

an·te·bra·chi·um (an″te-bra′ke-um) the forearm. **antebra′chial**, adj.

an·te·ce·dent (an″tĭ-se′dent) a precursor. **plasma thromboplastin a. (PTA)**, coagulation factor XI.

an·te·flex·ion (an″te-flek′shun) 1. abnormal forward bending of an organ or part. 2. the normal forward curvature of the uterus.

an·te·grade (an′tĭ-grād) anterograde.

an·te mor·tem (an′te mor′tem) [L.] before death.

an·te·mor·tem (an″te-mor′tem) [L.] occurring before death.

an·ten·na (an-ten′ah) pl. *anten′nae*. Either of the two lateral appendages on the anterior segment of the head of arthropods.

an·te·par·tal (an″te-pahr′t′l) antepartum.

an·te·par·tum (-pahr′tum) occurring before parturition, or childbirth, with reference to the mother.

an·te·py·ret·ic (-pi-ret′ik) occurring before the stage of fever.

an·te·ri·or (an-tēr′e-or) situated at or directed toward the front; opposite of posterior.

antero- word element [L.], *anterior; in front of*.

an·tero·clu·sion (an″ter-o-kloo′zhun) mesioclusion.

an·tero·grade (an′ter-o-grād″) extending or moving anteriorly.

an·tero·lat·er·al (an″ter-o-lat′er-al) situated anteriorly and to one side.

an·tero·pos·te·ri·or (-pos-tēr′e-er) directed from the front toward the back.

an·te·ver·sion (an″te-ver′zhun) the tipping forward of an entire organ or part.

ant·he·lix (ant′he-liks) the semicircular ridge on the flap of the ear, anteroinferior to the helix.

ant·hel·min·tic (ant″hel-min′tik) 1. vermifugal; destructive to worms. 2. vermicide or vermifuge; an agent destructive to worms.

an·thra·cene (an′thrah-sēn) a crystalline hydrocarbon derived from coal tar and used in the manufacture of anthracene dyes.

an·thra·cene·di·one (an″thrah-sēn-di′ōn) any of a class of derivatives of anthraquinone, some of which have antineoplastic properties.

an·thra·coid (an′thrah-koid) resembling anthrax or a carbuncle.

an·thra·co·ne·cro·sis (an″thrah-ko-nĕ-kro′sis) degeneration of tissue into a black mass.

an·thra·co·sil·i·co·sis (-sil″ĭ-ko′sis) anthracosis combined with silicosis.

an·thra·co·sis (an″thrah-ko′sis) pneumoconiosis, usually asymptomatic, due to deposition of anthracite coal dust in the lungs.

an·thra·cy·cline (-si′klēn) a class of antineoplastic antibiotics produced by *Streptomyces peucetius* and *S. coeruleorubidus*, including daunomycin and doxorubicin.

an·thra·lin (an′thrah-lin) an anthraquinone derivative used topically in psoriasis.

an·thra·quin·one (an″thrah-kwin′ōn) 1. the 9,10 quinone derivative of anthracene, used in dye manufacture. 2. any of the derivatives of this compound, some of which are dyes. They occur in aloes, cascara sagrada, senna, and rhubarb and are cathartic.

an·thrax (an′thraks) an often fatal, infectious disease of ruminants due to ingestion of spores of *Bacillus anthracis* in soil; acquired by humans through contact with contaminated wool or other animal products or by inhalation of airborne spores. **cutaneous a.**, that due to inoculation of *Bacillus anthracis* into superficial wounds or abrasions of the skin, producing a black crusted pustule on a broad zone of edema. **gastrointestinal a.**, intestinal a. **inhalational a.**, a highly fatal form due to inhalation of dust containing anthrax spores, which are transported by alveolar pneumocytes to regional lymph nodes, where they germinate; it is primarily an occupational disease seen in those who handle and sort wools and fleeces. **intestinal a.**, anthrax involving the gastrointestinal tract, caused by ingestion of poorly cooked meat contaminated by *Bacillus anthracis* spores; bowel obstruction, hemorrhage, and necrosis may result. **pulmonary a.**, inhalational a.

anthrop(o)- word element [Gr.], *man (human being)*.

an·thro·po·cen·tric (an″thro-po-sen′trik) with a human bias; considering humans the center of the universe.

an·thro·poid (an′thro-poid) resembling a human being; the anthropoid apes are tailless apes, including the chimpanzee, gibbon, gorilla, and orangutan.

An·thro·poi·dea (an″thro-poi′de-ah) a suborder of Primates, including monkeys, apes, and humans.

an·thro·pol·o·gy (an″thro-pol′o-je) the science that treats of human beings and their origins, historical and cultural development, and races.

an·thro·pom·e·try (an″thro-pom′ĕ-tre) the science dealing with measurement of the size, weight, and proportions of the human body. **anthropomet′ric**, adj.

an·thro·po·mor·phism (an″thro-po-mor′-fizm) the attribution of human characteristics to nonhuman objects.

an·thro·po·phil·ic (-fil′ik) preferring humans to other animals; said of parasites such as fungi or mosquitoes.

anti- word element [Gr.], *counteracting; effective against*.

an·ti·abor·ti·fa·cient (an″te-, an″ti-ah-bor″tĭ-fa′shent) an agent that prevents abortion or promotes pregnancy.

an·ti·ad·re·ner·gic (-ad″rĕ-ner′jik) 1. sympatholytic; opposing the effects of impulses conveyed by adrenergic postganglionic fibers of the sympathetic nervous system. 2. an agent that so acts.

an·ti·ag·glu·ti·nin (-ah-gloo′tĭ-nin) a substance that opposes the action of an agglutinin.

an·ti·ame·bic (-ah-me′bik) destroying or suppressing the growth of amebas, or an agent that does this.

an·ti·ana·phy·lax·is (-an″ah-fĭ-lak′sis) a condition in which the anaphylaxis reaction does not occur because of free antigens in the blood; the state of desensitization to antigens.

an·ti·an·dro·gen (-an′dro-jen) any substance capable of inhibiting the biological effects of androgens.

an·ti·ane·mic (-ah-ne′mik) counteracting anemia, or an agent that does this.

an·ti·an·gi·nal (-an-ji′nal) preventing or alleviating angina, or an agent that does this.

an·ti·an·ti·body (-an′tĭ-bod″e) an immunoglobulin formed in the body after administration of antibody acting as immunogen, and which interacts with the latter.

an·ti·an·xi·e·ty (-ang-zi′ĕ-te) anxiolytic; reducing anxiety.

an·ti·ar·rhyth·mic (-ah-rith′mik) 1. preventing or alleviating cardiac arrhythmias. 2. an agent that so acts.

an·ti·ar·thrit·ic (-ahr-thrit′ik) alleviating arthritis, or an agent that so acts.

an·ti·asth·mat·ic (-az-mat′ik) providing relief of asthma, or an agent that does this.

an·ti·bac·te·ri·al (-bak-tēr′e-al) destroying or suppressing growth or reproduction of bacteria; also, an agent that does this.

an·ti·bi·o·sis (-bi-o′sis) an association between two organisms that is detrimental to one of them, or between one organism and an antibiotic produced by another.

an·ti·bi·ot·ic (-bi-ot′ik) a chemical substance produced by a microorganism, which has the capacity to inhibit the growth of or to kill other microorganisms; antibiotics sufficiently nontoxic to the host are used in the treatment of infectious diseases. **broad-spectrum a.**, one effective against a wide range of bacteria. **β-lactam a.**, any of a group of antibiotics, including the cephalosporins and the penicillins, whose chemical structure contains a β-lactam ring; they inhibit synthesis of the bacterial peptidoglycan wall.

an·ti·body (Ab) (an′tĭ-bod-e) an immunoglobulin molecule that reacts with a specific antigen that induced its synthesis and with similar molecules; classified according to mode of action as agglutinin, bacteriolysin, hemolysin, opsonin, or precipitin. Antibodies are synthesized by B lymphocytes that have been activated by the binding of an antigen to a cell-surface receptor. See *immunoglobulin*. **anaphylactic a.**, IgE antibody causing anaphylaxis. **antimitochondrial a's**, circulating antibodies directed against inner mitochondrial antigens seen in almost all patients with primary biliary cirrhosis. **antinuclear a's (ANA)**, autoantibodies directed against components of the cell nucleus, e.g., DNA, RNA, and histones. **antireceptor a's**, autoantibodies against cell-surface receptors, e.g., those directed against β_2-adrenergic receptors in some patients with allergic disorders. **antisperm a. (ASA),** any of various surface-bound antibodies found on sperm after infection, trauma to the testes, or vasectomy; they interfere with the fertilization process or result in nonviable zygotes. **antithyroglobulin a's,** those directed against thyroglobulin, demonstrable in about one-third of patients with thyroiditis, Graves' disease, and thyroid carcinoma. **blocking a.,** 1. one (usually IgG) that reacts preferentially with an antigen, preventing it from reacting with a cytotropic antibody (IgE), and producing a hypersensitivity reaction. 2. incomplete a. **complement-fixing a.,** one that activates complement when reacted with antigen: IgM and IgG fix complement by the classical pathway; IgA, by the alternative pathway. **complete a.,** one that reacts with the antigen in saline, producing an agglutination or precipitation reaction. **cytophilic a.,** cytotropic a. **cytotoxic a.,** any specific antibody directed against cellular antigens that, when bound to the antigen, activates the complement pathway or activates killer cells, resulting in cell lysis. **cytotropic a.,** any of a class of antibodies that attach to tissue cells through their Fc segments to induce the release of histamine and other vasoconstrictive amines important in immediate hypersensitivity reactions. **Donath-Landsteiner a.,** an IgG antibody directed against the P blood group antigen; it binds to red cells at low temperatures and induces complement-mediated lysis on warming, and is responsible for hemolysis in paroxysmal cold hemoglobinuria. **Forssman a.,** heterophile antibody directed against the Forssman antigen. **heteroclitic a.,** antibody produced in response to immunization with one antigen but having a higher affinity for a second antigen that was not present during immunization. **heterogenetic a., heterophil a., heterophile a.,** antibody directed against heterophile antigens. Heterophile sheep erythrocyte agglutinins appear in the serum of patients with infectious mononucleosis. **immune a.,** one induced by immunization or by transfusion incompatibility, in contrast to natural antibodies. **incomplete a.,** 1. antibody that binds to erythrocytes or bacteria but does not produce agglutination. 2. a univalent antibody fragment, e.g., Fab fragment. **indium-111 antimyosin a.,** a monoclonal antibody against myosin, labeled with indium 111; it binds selectively to irreversibly damaged myocytes and is used in infarct avid scintigraphy. **monoclonal a's,** chemically and immunologically homogeneous antibodies

produced by hybridomas, used as laboratory reagents in radioimmunoassays, ELISA, and immunofluorescence assays. **natural a's,** ones that react with antigens to which the individual has had no known exposure. **neutralizing a.,** one which, on mixture with the homologous infectious agent, reduces the infectious titer. **OKT3 monoclonal a.,** a mouse monoclonal antibody directed against T3 lymphocytes and used to prevent or treat organ rejection after transplantation. **panel-reactive a. (PRA),** 1. the preexisting antibody against HLA antigens in the serum of a potential allograft recipient that reacts with a specific antigen in a panel of leukocytes, with a higher percentage indicating a higher risk of a positive crossmatch. 2. the percentage of such antibody in the recipient's blood. **P-K a's, Prausnitz-Küstner a's,** cytotropic antibodies of the immunoglobulin class IgE, responsible for cutaneous anaphylaxis. **protective a.,** one responsible for immunity to an infectious agent observed in passive immunity. **reaginic a.,** reagin. **saline a.,** complete a. **sensitizing a.,** anaphylactic a.

an·ti·cal·cu·lous (an″te-, an″ti-kal′ku-lus) suppressing the formation of calculi.

an·ti·car·io·gen·ic (-kar″e-o-jen′ik) effective in suppressing caries production.

an·ti·cho·le·litho·gen·ic (-ko″lĕ-lith″o-jen′ik) 1. preventing the formation of gallstones. 2. an agent that so acts.

an·ti·cho·les·ter·emic (-kah-les″ter-e′mik) promoting a reduction of cholesterol levels in the blood; also, any agent that so acts.

an·ti·cho·lin·er·gic (-ko″lin-er′jik) parasympatholytic; blocking the passage of impulses through the parasympathetic nerves; also, an agent that so acts.

an·ti·cho·lin·es·ter·ase (-ko″lin-es′ter-ās) cholinesterase inhibitor.

an·ti·clin·al (-kli′n′l) sloping or inclined in opposite directions.

an·ti·co·ag·u·lant (-ko-ag′u-lant) acting to suppress, delay, or nullify blood coagulation, or an agent that does this. **circulating a.,** a substance in the blood which inhibits normal blood clotting and may cause a hemorrhagic syndrome. **lupus a.,** a circulating anticoagulant that inhibits the conversion of prothrombin to thrombin; it paradoxically increases the risk of thromboembolism and is seen in some cases of systemic lupus erythematosus.

an·ti·co·ag·u·la·tion (-ko-ag″u-la′shun) 1. the prevention of coagulation. 2. the use of drugs to render the blood sufficiently incoagulable to discourage thrombosis.

an·ti·co·don (-ko′don) a triplet of nucleotides in transfer RNA that is complementary to the codon in messenger RNA which specifies the amino acid.

an·ti·com·ple·ment (-kom'plĕ-ment) a substance that counteracts a complement.

an·ti·con·vul·sant (-kon-vul'sant) inhibiting convulsions, or an agent that does this.

an·ti·con·vul·sive (-kon-vul'siv) anticonvulsant.

an·ti·cus (an-ti'kus) [L.] anterior.

an·ti-D antibody against D antigen, the most immunogenic of the Rh antigens. Commercial preparations of anti-D, $Rh_0(D)$ immune globulin, are administered to Rh-negative women following the birth of an Rh-positive baby in order to prevent maternal alloimmunization against the D antigen, which may cause hemolytic disease of the newborn in a subsequent pregnancy. Called also anti-Rh_0.

an·ti·de·pres·sant (an″te-, an″ti-de-pres'-ant) preventing or relieving depression; also, an agent that so acts. **tricyclic a.,** any of a class of drugs with particular tricyclic structure and potentiating catecholamine action; used for the treatment of depression.

an·ti·di·a·bet·ic (-di″ah-bet'ik) 1. preventing or alleviating diabetes. 2. an agent that so acts.

an·ti·di·ar·rhe·al (-di″ah-re'al) counteracting diarrhea, or an agent that does this.

an·ti·di·uret·ic (-di″u-ret'ik) 1. pertaining to or causing suppression of urine. 2. an agent that so acts.

an·ti·dote (an'tĭ-dōt) an agent that counteracts a poison. **antido'tal,** adj. **chemical a.,** one that neutralizes the poison by changing its chemical nature. **mechanical a.,** one that prevents absorption of the poison. **physiologic a.,** one that counteracts the effects of the poison by producing opposing physiologic effects.

an·ti·drom·ic (an″tĭ-drom'ik) conducting impulses in a direction opposite to the normal.

an·ti·dys·ki·net·ic (an″te-, an″ti-dis″kĭ-net'ik) relieving or preventing dyskinesia, or an agent that so acts.

an·ti·ec·ze·mat·ic (-ek″zĕ-mat'ik) alleviating eczema, or an agent that does this.

an·ti·emet·ic (-ĕ-met'ik) preventing or alleviating nausea and vomiting; also, an agent that so acts.

an·ti·es·tro·gen (-es'tro-jen) a substance capable of inhibiting the biological effects of estrogens. **antiestrogen'ic,** adj.

an·ti·feb·rile (-feb'ril) antipyretic (1).

an·ti·fi·bri·nol·y·sin (-fi″brĭ-nol'ĭ-sin) antiplasmin.

an·ti·fi·bri·no·lyt·ic (-fi″brĭ-no-lit'ik) inhibiting or preventing fibrinolysis, or an agent that does this.

an·ti·fi·brot·ic (-fi-brot'ik) causing regression of fibrosis, or an agent that so acts.

an·ti·flat·u·lent (-flat'u-lent) relieving or preventing flatulence, or an agent that does this.

an·ti·fun·gal (-fung'gal) 1. destructive to fungi, or suppressing their reproduction or growth; effective against fungal infections. 2. an agent that so acts.

an·ti·ga·lac·tic (-gah-lak'tik) 1. diminishing or stopping secretion of milk. 2. an agent with this effect.

an·ti·gen (an'tĭ-jen) any substance capable of inducing a specific immune response and of reacting with the products of that response, i.e., with specific antibody or specifically sensitized T lymphocytes, or both. Abbreviated Ag. **antigen'ic,** adj. **blood-group a's,** erythrocyte surface antigens whose antigenic differences determine blood groups. **cancer a. 125 (CA 125),** a surface glycoprotein associated with müllerian epithelial tissue; elevated serum levels are often associated with epithelial ovarian carcinoma, particularly with nonmucinous tumors, but are also seen in some other malignant and various benign pelvic disorders. **capsular a.,** one found in the capsule of a microorganism. **carcinoembryonic a. (CEA),** a cancer-specific glycoprotein antigen of colon carcinoma, also present in many adenocarcinomas of endodermal origin and in normal gastrointestinal tissues of human embryos. **CD a.,** any of a number of cell surface markers expressed by leukocytes and used to distinguish cell lineages, developmental stages, and functional subsets; such markers can be identified by monoclonal antibodies. **class I a's,** major histocompatibility antigens found on every cell except erythrocytes, recognized during graft rejection, and involved in MHC restriction. **class II a's,** major histocompatibility antigens found only on immunocompetent cells, primarily B lymphocytes and macrophages. **common acute lymphoblastic leukemia a. (CALLA),** a tumor-associated antigen occurring on lymphoblasts in about 80 per cent of patients with acute lymphoblastic leukemia (ALL) and in 40–50 per cent of patients with blastic phase chronic myelogenous leukemia (CML). **complete a.,** one which both stimulates an immune response and reacts with the products of that response. **conjugated a.,** one produced by coupling a hapten to a protein carrier molecule through covalent bonds; when it induces immunization, the resultant immune response is directed against both the hapten and the carrier. **D a.,** a red cell antigen of the Rh blood group system, important in the development of isoimmunization in Rh-negative persons exposed to the blood of Rh-positive persons. **E a.,** a red cell antigen of the Rh blood group system. **flagellar a., H antigen. Forssman a.,** a heterogenetic antigen inducing the production of antisheep hemolysin, occurring in various unrelated species, mainly in the organs but not in the erythrocytes (guinea pig, horse), but sometimes only in the erythrocytes (sheep), and occasionally in both (chicken). **H a.,** 1. a bacterial flagellar antigen important in the serological classification of enteric bacilli. 2. the precursor of the A and B blood group antigens; normal type O individuals lack the enzyme to convert it to A or B antigens. **hepatitis B core a. (HBcAg),** an antigen of the DNA core of the hepatitis B virus, indicating the presence of replicating hepatitis B virus. **hepatitis B e a. (HBeAg),** an antigen of hepatitis B virus sometimes present in the blood during acute infection, usually disappearing afterward but sometimes persisting in chronic disease. **hepatitis B surface a. (HBsAg),** a surface coat lipoprotein antigen of the hepatitis B virus, peaking with the first appearance of clinical disease symptoms. Tests for serum HBsAg are used in the diagnosis of acute or chronic hepatitis B and in testing blood products for infectivity. **heterogenetic a.,** heterophile a. **heterologous a.,** an antigen that reacts with an antibody that is not the one that induced its formation. **heterophil a., heterophile a.,** an antigen common to more than one species and whose species distribution is unrelated to its phylogenetic distribution (viz., Forssman antigen, lens protein, certain caseins, etc.). **histocompatibility a's,** genetically determined isoantigens found on the surface of nucleated cells of most tissues, which incite an immune response when grafted onto a genetically different individual and thus determine compatibility of tissues in transplantation. **HLA a's,** human leukocyte antigens. **homologous a.,** 1. the antigen inducing antibody formation. 2. isoantigen. **human leukocyte a's,** histocompatibility antigens (glycoproteins) on the surface of nucleated cells (including circulating and tissue cells) determined by a region on chromosome 6 bearing several genetic loci, designated HLA-A, -B, -C, -DP, -DQ, -DR, -MB, -MT, and -Te. They are important in cross-matching procedures and are partially responsible for

the rejection of transplanted tissues when donor and recipient HLA antigens do not match. **H-Y a.,** a histocompatibility antigen of the cell membrane, determined by a locus on the Y chromosome; it is a mediator of testicular organization (hence, sexual differentiation) in the male. **Ia a's,** one of the histocompatibility antigens governed by the I region of the major histocompatibility complex, located principally on B lymphocytes, macrophages, accessory cells, and granulocyte precursors. **Inv group a's,** Km a's. **isogeneic a.,** an antigen carried by an individual which is capable of eliciting an immune response in genetically different individuals of the same species, but not in an individual bearing it. **K a.,** a bacterial capsular antigen, a surface antigen external to the cell wall. **Km a's,** the three alloantigens found in the constant region of the κ light chains of immunoglobulins. **Ly a's, Lyt a's,** antigenic cell-surface markers of subpopulations of T lymphocytes, classified as Ly 1, 2, and 3; they are associated with helper and suppressor activities of T lymphocytes. **mumps skin test a.,** a sterile suspension of mumps virus; used as a dermal reactivity indicator. **O a.,** one occurring in the lipopolysaccharide layer of the wall of gram-negative bacteria. **oncofetal a.,** carcinoembryonic a. **organ-specific a.,** any antigen occurring only in a particular organ and serving to distinguish it from other organs; it may be limited to an organ of a single species or be characteristic of the same organ in many species. **partial a.,** hapten. **private a's,** antigens of the low frequency blood groups, probably differing from ordinary blood group systems only in their incidence. **prostate-specific a. (PSA),** an endopeptidase secreted by the epithelial cells of the prostate gland; serum levels are elevated in benign prostatic hyperplasia and prostate cancer. **public a's,** antigens of the high frequency blood groups, so called because they are found in almost all persons tested. **self-a.,** autoantigen. **T a.,** 1. tumor antigen, any of several coded for by the viral genome, and associated with transformation of infected cells by certain DNA tumor viruses. 2. see CD a. 3. an antigen present on human erythrocytes that is exposed by treatment with neuraminadase or contact with certain bacteria. **T-dependent a.,** one requiring the presence of helper cells to stimulate antibody production by B cells. **T-independent a.,** one able to trigger B cells to produce antibodies without the presence of T cells. **tumor a.,** 1. T a. (1). 2. tumor-specific a. **tumor-associated a.,** a new antigen acquired by a tumor cell line in the process of neoplastic transformation. **tumor-specific a. (TSA),** cell-surface antigens of tumors that elicit a specific immune response in the host. **Vi a.,** a K antigen of *Salmonella typhi* originally thought responsible for virulence.

an·ti·gen·emia (an″tĭ-jĕ-ne′me-ah) the presence of antigen (e.g., hepatitis B surface antigen) in the blood. **antigene′mic,** adj.

an·ti·gen·ic (an-tĭ-jen′ik) having the properties of an antigen.

an·ti·ge·nic·i·ty (an″tĭ-jĕ-nis′ĭ-te) the capacity to stimulate the production of antibodies or the capacity to react with an antibody.

an·ti·glau·co·ma (an″ti-glaw-ko′mah, -glou-ko′mah) preventing or alleviating glaucoma.

an·ti·glob·u·lin (an″te-, an″ti-glob″u-lin) an antibody directed against gamma globulin, as used in the antiglobulin test.

an·ti·he·mol·y·sin (-he-mol′ĭ-sin) any agent that opposes the action of a hemolysin.

an·ti·he·mo·phil·ic (-he″mo-fil′ik) counteracting hemophilia, or an agent that so acts.

an·ti·hem·or·rhag·ic (-hem″ah-raj′ik) exerting a hemostatic effect; counteracting hemorrhage, or an agent that does this.

an·ti·his·ta·mine (-his′tah-mēn) an agent that counteracts the action of histamine; usually used for agents blocking H_1 receptors (H_1 receptor antagonists) and used to treat allergic reactions and as components of cough and cold preparations. Agents blocking H_2 receptors, used to inhibit gastric secretion in peptic ulcer, are usually called H_2 receptor antagonists.

an·ti·his·ta·min·ic (-his-tah-min′ik) 1. counteracting the effect of histamine. 2. antihistamine.

an·ti·hy·per·cho·les·ter·ol·emic (-hi″per-ko-les″ter-ol-e′mik) effective against hypercholesterolemia, or an agent with this quality.

an·ti·hy·per·gly·ce·mic (-gli-se′mik) counteracting high levels of glucose in the blood, or an agent that so acts.

an·ti·hy·per·ka·le·mic (-kah-le′mik) effective in decreasing or preventing an excessively high blood level of potassium, or an agent that so acts.

an·ti·hy·per·lip·id·emic (-lip″ĭde′mik) promoting a reduction of lipid levels in the blood, or an agent that so acts.

an·ti·hy·per·lipo·pro·tein·emic (-lip″o-pro″tēn-e′mik) promoting a reduction of lipoprotein levels in the blood, or an agent that does this.

an·ti·hy·per·ten·sive (-ten′siv) counteracting high blood pressure, or an agent that does this.

an·ti·hy·po·gly·ce·mic (an″te-, an″ti-hi″-po-gli-se′mik) counteracting hypoglycemia, or an agent that so acts.

an·ti·hy·po·ten·sive (-ten′siv) counteracting low blood pressure, or an agent that so acts.

an·ti·in·fec·tive (-in-fek′tiv) counteracting infection, or an agent that does this.

an·ti·in·flam·ma·to·ry (-in-flam′ah-tor″e) counteracting or suppressing inflammation; also, an agent that so acts.

an·ti·leu·ko·cyt·ic (-loo″ko-sit′ik) destructive to white blood cells (leukocytes).

an·ti·li·pe·mic (-lĭ-pe′mik) antihyperlipidemic.

an·ti·lith·ic (-lith′ik) preventing the formation of calculi, or an agent that so acts.

an·ti·ly·sis (-li′sis) inhibition of lysis.

an·ti·lyt·ic (-litik) 1. pertaining to antilysis. 2. inhibiting or preventing lysis.

an·ti·ma·lar·i·al (-mah-lar′e-al) therapeutically effective against malaria, or an agent with this quality.

an·ti·mere (an′tĭ-mēr) one of the opposite corresponding parts of an organism that are symmetrical with respect to the longitudinal axis of its body.

an·ti·me·tab·o·lite (an″te-, an″ti-mĕ-tab′o-līt) a substance bearing a close structural resemblance to one required for normal physiological functioning, and exerting its effect by interfering with the utilization of the essential metabolite.

an·ti·met·he·mo·glo·bin·emic (-met-he″-mo-glo″bĭ-ne′mik) 1. promoting reduction of methemoglobin levels in the blood. 2. an agent that so acts.

an·ti·me·tro·pia (-mĕ-tro′pe-ah) hyperopia of one eye, with myopia in the other.

an·ti·mi·cro·bi·al (-mi-kro′be-al) 1. killing microorganisms or suppressing their multiplication or growth. 2. an agent with such effects.

an·ti·mon·go·lism (-mon′go-lizm) a term applied to syndromes associated with certain chromosomal abnormalities, in which some of the clinical signs, e.g., downward-slanting palpebral fissures, are variations of those seen in Down's syndrome.

an·ti·mo·ny (Sb) (an′tĭ-mo″ne) chemical element (see *Table of Elements*), at. no. 51, forming various medicinal and poisonous salts; ingestion of antimony compounds, and rarely industrial exposure to them, may produce symptoms similar to those of acute arsenic poisoning. *A. potassium tartrate* and *a.*

sodium tartrate have been used as antischisto-somals. **antimo′nial,** adj.

an·ti·mus·ca·rin·ic (an″te-, an″ti-mus′kah-rin′ik) 1. effective against the toxic effects of muscarine. 2. blocking the muscarinic receptors. 3. an agent having either such action.

an·ti·my·as·then·ic (-mi″as-then′ik) counteracting or relieving muscular weakness in myasthenia gravis, or an agent that so acts.

an·ti·my·cot·ic (-mi-kot′ik) antifungal.

an·ti·nau·se·ant (-naw′ze-ant) preventing or relieving nausea, or an agent that so acts. See also *antiemetic.*

an·ti·neo·plas·tic (-ne″o-plas′tik) 1. inhibiting or preventing development of neoplasms; checking maturation and proliferation of malignant cells. 2. an agent that so acts.

an·tin·ion (an-tin′e-on) the frontal pole of the head; the median frontal point farthest from the inion.

an·ti·no·ci·cep·tive (an″te-, an″ti-no″sī-sep′tiv) reducing sensitivity to painful stimuli.

an·ti·nu·cle·ar (-noo′kle-ar) destructive to or reactive with components of the cell nucleus.

an·ti·ox·i·dant (-ok′sĭ-dant) something added to a product to prevent or delay its deterioration by the oxygen in air.

an·ti·par·al·lel (-par′ah-lel) denoting molecules arranged side by side but in opposite directions.

an·ti·par·a·sit·ic (-par″ah-sit′ik) destructive to parasites, or an agent with this quality.

an·ti·par·kin·so·ni·an (-pahr″kin-so′ne-an) effective in treatment of parkinsonism, or an agent with this quality.

an·ti·ped·i·cu·lot·ic (-pĕ-dik″u-lot′ik) effective against lice, or an agent with this quality.

an·ti·per·i·stal·sis (-per″ĭ-stawl′sis) reversed peristalsis.

an·ti·per·i·stal·tic (-per″ĭ-stawl′tik) 1. pertaining to or causing antiperistalsis. 2. diminishing peristalsis; or an agent that so acts.

an·ti·per·spir·ant (-per′spir-ant) inhibiting or preventing perspiration, or an agent that does this.

an·ti·plas·min (-plaz′min) a substance in the blood that inhibits plasmin. The most important is α_2-*a.*, which forms stable complexes with free plasmin, is crosslinked to fibrin by factor XIII, and inhibits the binding of plasminogen to fibrin; deficiency results in tendency to severe bleeding, including hemarthrosis.

an·ti·plas·tic (-plas′tik) 1. unfavorable to healing. 2. an agent that suppresses formation of blood or other cells.

an·ti·port (an′tĭ-port) a mechanism of coupling the transport of two compounds across a membrane in opposite directions.

anti·pro·ges·tin (an″te-, an″ti-pro-jes′tin) a substance that inhibits the formation, transport, or action of progestational agents.

an·ti·pro·throm·bin (-pro-throm′bin) 1. directed against prothrombin. 2. an anticoagulant that retards the conversion of prothrombin into thrombin.

an·ti·pro·to·zo·al (-pro″tah-zo″l) lethal to protozoa, or checking their growth or reproduction; also, an agent that so acts.

an·ti·pru·rit·ic (-proo-rit′ik) preventing or relieving itching, or an agent that does this.

an·ti·pso·ri·at·ic (-sor″e-at′ik) effective against psoriasis, or an agent that so acts.

an·ti·psy·chot·ic (-si-kot′ik) effective in the treatment of psychotic disorders; also, an agent that so acts. Antipsychotics are a chemically diverse but pharmacologically similar class of drugs; besides psychotic disorders, some are also used to treat movement disorders, intractable hiccups, or severe nausea and vomiting.

an·ti·py·ret·ic (-pi-ret′ik) 1. relieving or reducing fever. 2. an agent that so acts.

an·ti·py·rine (an″te-pi′rēn) an analgesic used as a component of topical solutions for decongestion and analgesia in acute otitis media. See also *dichloralphenazone.*

an·ti·py·rot·ic (an″te-, an″ti-pi-rot′ik) 1. effective in the treatment of burns. 2. an agent with this quality.

an·ti·ret·ro·vi·ral (-ret′ro-vi″ral) effective against retroviruses, or an agent with this quality.

an·ti·rheu·mat·ic (-roo-mat′ik) 1. relieving or preventing rheumatism. 2. an agent that so acts.

an·ti·schis·to·so·mal (-shis″to-so′m′l) 1. effective against schistosomes. 2. an agent that is destructive to schistosomes.

an·ti·scor·bu·tic (-skor-bu′tik) effective in the prevention or relief of scurvy.

an·ti·se·cre·to·ry (-sĕ-kre′tah-re) 1. secretoinhibitory; inhibiting or diminishing secretion. 2. an agent that so acts, as certain drugs that inhibit or diminish gastric secretions.

an·ti·sense (an′te-, an′ti-sens) referring to the strand of a double-stranded molecule that does not directly encode the product (the *sense strand*) but is complementary to it.

an·ti·sep·sis (an″tĭ-sep′sis) 1. the prevention of sepsis by antiseptic means. 2. any procedure that reduces to a significant degree the microbial flora of skin or mucous membranes.

an·ti·sep·tic (-sep'tik) 1. pertaining to antisepsis. 2. preventing decay or putrefaction. 3. a substance that inhibits the growth and development of microorganisms without necessarily killing them.

an·ti·se·rum (an″tĭ-se″rum) a serum containing antibody(ies), obtained from an animal immunized either by injection of antigen or by infection with microorganisms containing antigen.

an·ti·si·al·a·gogue (an″te-, an″ti-si-al′ah-gog) counteracting saliva formation; also, an agent that counteracts any influence that promotes the flow of saliva. **antisialagog′ic,** adj.

an·ti·si·al·ic (-si-al′ik) checking the secretion of saliva; also, an agent that so acts.

an·ti·so·cial (-so′sh'l) 1. denoting behavior that violates the rights of others, societal mores, or the law. 2. denoting the specific personality traits seen in antisocial personality disorder.

an·ti·spas·mod·ic (-spaz-mod′ik) 1. preventing or relieving spasms. 2. an agent that so acts.

an·ti·spas·tic (-spas′tik) antispasmodic with specific reference to skeletal muscle.

an·ti·sym·pa·thet·ic (-sim″pah-thet′ik) sympatholytic.

an·ti·the·nar (-the′nar) placed opposite to the palm or sole.

an·ti·throm·bin (-throm′bin) any naturally occurring or therapeutically administered substance that neutralizes the action of thrombin and thus limits or restricts blood coagulation. **a. I,** fibrin, referring to its capacity to adsorb thrombin and thus neutralize it. **a. III,** a plasma α_2-globulin of the serpin family that inactivates thrombin and also inhibits certain coagulation factors and kallikrein. Inherited deficiency is associated with recurrent deep vein thrombosis and pulmonary emboli; the complications are prevented and treated with a preparation of antithrombin III from pooled human plasma.

an·ti·throm·bo·plas·tin (-throm″bo-plas′-tin) any agent or substance that prevents or interferes with the interaction of blood coagulation factors as they generate prothrombinase.

an·ti·throm·bot·ic (-throm-bot′ik) 1. preventing or interfering with the formation of thrombi. 2. an agent that so acts.

an·ti·thy·roid (-thi′roid) counteracting thyroid functioning, especially in its synthesis of thyroid hormones.

an·ti·tox·in (an″te-, an″ti-tok″sin) antibody produced in response to a toxin of bacterial (usually an exotoxin), animal (zootoxin),

or plant (phytotoxin) origin, which neutralizes the effects of the toxin. **an′titoxic,** adj.
botulism a., an equine antitoxin against toxins of the types A and B and/or E strains of *Clostridium botulinum.* **diphtheria a.,** equine antitoxin from horses immunized against diphtheria toxin or the toxoid. **equine a.,** an antitoxin derived from the blood of healthy horses immunized against a specific bacterial toxin. **tetanus a.,** equine antitoxin from horses that have been immunized against tetanus toxin or toxoid.

an·ti·tra·gus (an″te-tra′gus) a projection on the ear opposite the tragus.

an·ti·trich·o·mo·nal (an″te-, an″ti-trik″ah-mo′n'l) effective against *Trichomonas*; also, an agent having such effects.

α_1**-an·ti·tryp·sin** (-trip′sin) alpha$_1$-antitrypsin.

an·ti·tu·ber·cu·lin (-too-ber′ku-lin) an antibody developed after injection of tuberculin into the body.

an·ti·tu·ber·cu·lot·ic (-too-ber″ku-lot′ik) effective against tuberculosis, or an agent with this quality.

an·ti·tus·sive (-tus′iv) effective against cough, or an agent with this quality.

an·ti·ul·cer·a·tive (-ul′ser-ah-tiv) preventing ulcers or promoting their healing, or an agent that so acts.

an·ti·uro·lith·ic (-u″ro-lith′ik) 1. preventing the formation of urinary calculi. 2. an agent that so acts.

an·ti·ven·in (-ven′in) a material used in treatment of poisoning by animal venom. **black widow spider a.,** a. (*Latrodectus mactans*). **a. (Crotalidae) polyvalent,** a serum containing specific venom-neutralizing globulins, produced by immunizing horses with venoms of the fer-de-lance and the western, eastern, and tropical rattlesnakes, used for treatment of envenomation by most pit vipers throughout the world. **a. (Latrodectus mactans),** a serum containing specific venom-neutralizing globulins, prepared by immunizing horses against venom of the black widow spider (*L. mactans*). **a. (Micrurus fulvius), North American coral snake a.,** a serum containing specific venom-neutralizing globulins, produced by immunization of horses with venom of the eastern coral snake (*M. fulvius*). **polyvalent crotaline a.,** a. (Crotalidae) polyvalent.

an·ti·vi·ral (-vi′ral) destroying viruses or suppressing their replication, or an agent that so acts.

an·ti·xe·rot·ic (-ze-rot′ik) counteracting or preventing abnormal dryness.

an·tri·tis (an-tri′tis) inflammation of an antrum, chiefly of the maxillary antrum (sinus).

antr(o)- word element [L.], *chamber; cavity;* often used with specific reference to the maxillary antrum or sinus.

an·tro·cele (an′tro-sēl) cystic accumulation of fluid in the maxillary antrum.

an·tro·na·sal (an″tro-na′z'l) pertaining to the maxillary antrum and nasal fossa.

an·tro·scope (an′tro-skōp) an instrument for inspecting the maxillary antrum (sinus).

an·tros·to·my (an-tros′tah-me) the operation of making an opening into an antrum for purposes of drainage.

an·trot·o·my (an-trot′ah-me) antrostomy.

an·trum (an′trum) pl. *an′tra, antrums.* [L.] a cavity or chamber. **an′tral,** adj. **cardiac a.,** the short conical portion of the esophagus below the diaphragm, its base being continuous with the cardiac orifice of the stomach. **frontal a.,** see under *sinus.* **a. of Highmore,** maxillary sinus. **mastoid a., a. mastoi′deum,** an air space in the mastoid portion of the temporal bone communicating with the tympanic cavity and the mastoid cells. **a. maxilla′re, maxillary a.,** maxillary sinus. **pyloric a., a. pylo′ricum,** the dilated portion of the pyloric part of the stomach, between the body of the stomach and the pyloric canal. **tympanic a., a. tympa′nicum,** mastoid a.

ANUG necrotizing ulcerative gingivitis.

anu·lus (an′u-lus) pl. *an′uli.* [L.] a small ring or encircling structure; spelled also *annulus.* **a. fibro′sus, 1.** fibrous ring of heart: one of the dense fibrous rings that surround the right and left atrioventricular (tricuspid and mitral) orifices and to which are attached the atrial and ventricular muscle fibers. **2.** fibrous ring of intervertebral disk; the circumferential ringlike portion of an intervertebral disk. **a. of nuclear pore,** a circular filamentous structure surrounding a nuclear pore in the nuclear membrane of a cell. **a. of spermatozoon,** an electron-dense body at the caudal end of the neck of a spermatozoon.

an·ure·sis (an″u-re′sis) **1.** retention of urine in the bladder. **2.** anuria. **anuret′ic,** adj.

an·uria (an-u′re-ah) complete suppression of urine formation and excretion. **anu′ric,** adj.

anus (a′nus) pl. *a′ni.* The opening of the rectum on the body surface; the distal orifice of the alimentary canal. **imperforate a.,** persistence of the anal epithelial plug so that the anus is closed, either completely or partially.

an·vil (an′vil) incus; see *Table of Bones.*

an·xi·e·ty (ang-zi′ĕ-te) a feeling of apprehension, uncertainty, and fear without apparent stimulus, associated with physiological changes (tachycardia, sweating, tremor, etc.). **separation a.,** apprehension due to removal of significant persons or familiar surroundings, common in infants 12 to 24 months old; see also under *disorder.*

anx·io·lyt·ic (ang″ze-o-lit′ik) **1.** antianxiety. **2.** an antianxiety agent.

AOA American Optometric Association; American Orthopsychiatric Association; American Osteopathic Association.

aor·ta (a-or′tah) pl. *aor′tae, aortas.* [L.] the great artery arising from the left ventricle, being the main trunk from which the systemic arterial system proceeds; see *Table of Arteries* for parts of aorta, and see Plate 15. **aor′tic,** adj. **overriding a.,** a congenital anomaly occurring in tetralogy of Fallot, in which the aorta is displaced to the right so that it appears to arise from both ventricles and straddles the ventricular septal defect.

aor·ti·co·pul·mo·nary (a-or″tĭ-ko-pool′mo-nar″e) pertaining to or lying between the aorta and pulmonary artery.

aor·ti·tis (a″or-ti′tis) inflammation of the aorta.

aor·tog·ra·phy (a″or-tog′rah-fe) radiography of the aorta after introduction into it of a contrast material.

aor·top·a·thy (a″or-top′ah-the) any disease of the aorta.

aor·to·plas·ty (a-or′to-plas″te) surgical repair of the aorta.

aor·tor·rha·phy (a″or-tor′ah-fe) suture of the aorta.

aor·to·scle·ro·sis (a-or″to-sklĕ-ro′sis) sclerosis of the aorta.

aor·tot·o·my (a″or-tot′ah-me) incision of the aorta.

AOTA American Occupational Therapy Association.

AP action potential; angina pectoris; anterior pituitary (gland); anteroposterior; arterial pressure.

ap- see *apo-.*

APA American Pharmaceutical Association; American Podiatric Association; American Psychiatric Association; American Psychological Assocation.

apal·les·the·sia (ah-pal″es-the′zhah) pallanesthesia.

apan·crea (a-pan′kre-ah) absence of the pancreas.

apa·reu·nia (a″pah-roo′ne-ah) impossibility of sexual intercourse.

ap·a·thy (ap′ah-the) lack of feeling or emotion; indifference. **apathet′ic,** adj.

APC atrial premature complex; activated protein C.

APCC anti-inhibitor coagulant complex.

APD atrial premature depolarization (see *atrial premature complex*, under *complex*); pamidronate.

apel·lous (ah-pel'us) 1. skinless; not covered with skin; not cicatrized (said of a wound). 2. having no prepuce.

aper·i·stal·sis (a-per-ĭ-stahl'sis) absence of peristaltic action.

ap·er·tog·na·thia (ah-per″tog-na'the-ah) open bite.

ap·er·tu·ra (ap″er-too'rah) pl. *apertu'rae*. [L.] aperture.

ap·er·ture (ap'er-cher) opening. **piriform a.,** the anterior end of the bony nasal opening, connecting the external nose with the skull.

apex (a'peks) pl. *apexes, a'pices*. [L.] tip; the pointed end of a conical part; the top of a body, organ, or part. **ap'ical,** adj. **a. of lung,** the rounded upper extremity of either lung. **root a.,** the terminal end of the root of the tooth.

apex·car·dio·gram (a″peks-kahr'de-o-gram) the record produced by apexcardiography.

apex·car·di·og·ra·phy (-kahr″de-og'rah-fe) a method of graphically recording the pulsations of the anterior chest wall over the apex of the heart.

APHA American Public Health Association.

APhA American Pharmaceutical Association.

apha·gia (ah-fa'jah) refusal or inability to swallow.

apha·kia (ah-fa'ke-ah) absence of the lens of an eye, occurring congenitally or as a result of trauma or surgery. **apha'kic,** adj.

apha·lan·gia (a″fah-lan'jah) absence of fingers or toes.

apha·sia (ah-fa'zhah) defect or loss of the power of expression by speech, writing, or signs, or of comprehending spoken or written language, due to injury or disease of the brain centers. See also *agrammatism, dysphasia,* and *paraphasia*. **apha'sic,** adj. **amnesic a., amnestic a.,** defective recall of specific names of objects or other words, with intact abilities of comprehension and repetition. **anomic a.,** that in which recall of names is faulty. **auditory a.,** a form of receptive aphasia in which sounds are heard but convey no meaning to the mind, due to disease of the auditory center of the brain. **Broca's a.,** motor a. **conduction a.,** aphasia believed to be due to a lesion of the path between sensory and motor speech centers; spoken language is comprehended normally but words cannot be repeated correctly. **expressive a.,** motor a. **fluent a.,** a type of receptive aphasia in which speech is well articulated and grammatically correct but is lacking in content. **global a.,** total aphasia involving all the functions which go to make up speech or communication. **jargon a.,** that with utterance of meaningless phrases, either neologisms or incoherently arranged known words. **mixed a.,** global a. **motor a.,** Broca's or nonfluent aphasia; that in which the ability to speak and write is impaired, due to a lesion in the insula and surrounding operculum. **nominal a.,** anomic a. **nonfluent a.,** motor a. **receptive a.,** inability to understand written, spoken, or tactile speech symbols, due to disease of the auditory and visual word centers. **sensory a.,** receptive a. **total a.,** global a. **visual a.,** alexia. **Wernicke's a.,** receptive a.

apha·si·ol·o·gy (ah-fa″ze-ol'ah-je) the scientific study of aphasia and the specific neurologic lesions producing it.

aph·e·re·sis (af″ĕ-re'sis) withdrawal of blood from a donor, with a portion (plasma, leukocytes, platelets, etc.) being separated and retained and the remainder retransfused into the donor. It includes leukapheresis, plasmapheresis, thrombocytapheresis, etc.

apho·nia (a-fo'ne-ah) loss of voice; inability to produce vocal sounds.

aphot·ic (a-fot'ik) without light; totally dark.

aphra·sia (ah-fra'zhah) inability to speak.

aph·ro·dis·iac (af″ro-diz'e-ak) 1. arousing sexual desire. 2. a drug that arouses sexual desire.

aph·tha (af'thah) pl. *aph'thae*. [L.] (usually plural) small ulcers, especially the whitish or reddish spots in the mouth characteristic of aphthous stomatitis. **Bednar's aphthae,** symmetric excoriation of the posterior hard palate in infants. **contagious aphthae,** foot-and-mouth disease.

aph·tho·sis (af-tho'sis) a condition marked by the presence of aphthae.

aph·thous (af'thus) pertaining to, characterized by, or affected with aphthae.

Aph·tho·vi·rus (af'tho-vi″rus) foot-and-mouth disease viruses; a genus of viruses of the family Picornaviridae that cause foot-and-mouth disease.

aphy·lax·is (a″fĭ-lak'sis) absence of phylaxis or immunity. **aphylac'tic,** adj.

ap·i·cal (ap'ĭ-k'l) pertaining to an apex.

ap·i·ca·lis (ap″ĭ-ka'lis) [L.] apical.

api·cec·to·my (a″pĭ-sek'tah-me) excision of the apex of the petrous portion of the temporal bone.

api·ci·tis (a″pĭ-si'tis) inflammation of an apex, as of the lung or the root of a tooth.

api·co·ec·to·my (a″pĭ-ko-ek′tah-me) excision of the apical portion of the root of a tooth through an opening in overlying tissues of the jaw.

ap·la·nat·ic (ap″lah-nat′ik) correcting spherical aberration, as an aplanatic lens.

apla·sia (ah-pla′zhah) lack of development of an organ or tissue. **aplas′tic**, adj. **a. axia′lis extracortica′lis conge′nita,** familial centrolobar sclerosis. **a. cu′tis conge′nita,** localized failure of development of skin, most commonly of the scalp; the defects are usually covered by a thin translucent membrane or scar tissue, or may be raw, ulcerated, or covered by granulation tissue; usually lethal.

ap·nea (ap′ne-ah) cessation of breathing. **apne′ic,** adj. **central sleep a.,** sleep apnea from failure of stimulation by medullary respiratory centers. **obstructive sleep a.,** sleep apnea from collapse or obstruction of the airway during sleep, such as in the obese. **sleep a.,** transient attacks of apnea during sleep, resulting in acidosis and pulmonary arteriolar vasoconstriction and hypertension.

ap·neu·sis (ap-noo′sis) sustained effort for inhalation unrelieved by exhalation. **apneu′-stic,** adj.

ap(o)- word element [Gr.], *away from; separated; derived from.* Also, *ap-.*

apo·chro·mat (ap″o-kro′mat) an apochromatic objective.

apo·chro·mat·ic (-kro-mat′ik) free from chromatic and spherical aberrations.

apo·crine (ap′o-krin) exhibiting that type of glandular secretion in which the free end of the secreting cell is cast off along with the secretory products accumulated therein (e.g., mammary and sweat glands).

apo·en·zyme (ap″o-en′zīm) the protein component of an enzyme separable from the prosthetic group (coenzyme) but requiring the presence of the prosthetic group to form the functioning compound (holoenzyme).

apo·fer·ri·tin (-fer′ĭ-tin) an apoprotein that can bind many atoms of iron per molecule, forming ferritin, the intracellular storage form of iron.

apo·lar (a-po′ler) having neither poles nor processes; without polarity.

apo·lipo·pro·tein (ap″o-lip″o-pro′tēn) any of the protein constituents of lipoproteins, grouped by function in four classes, A, B, C, and E.

ap·o·neu·ror·rha·phy (-noo-ror′ah-fe) suture of an aponeurosis.

ap·o·neu·ro·sis (-noo-ro′sis) pl. *aponeuro′-ses.* [Gr.] a sheetlike tendinous expansion, mainly serving to connect a muscle with the parts it moves. **aponeurot′ic,** adj. **extensor a.,** see under *expansion.*

apoph·y·sis (ah-pof′ĭ-sis) pl. *apoph′yses.* [Gr.] any outgrowth or swelling, especially a bony outgrowth that has never been entirely separated from the bone of which it forms a part, such as a process, tubercle, or tuberosity. **apophys′eal,** adj.

apoph·y·si·tis (ah-pof″ĭ-si′tis) inflammation of an apophysis.

ap·o·plec·ti·form (ap″o-plek′tĭ-form) resembling apoplexy.

ap·o·plexy (ap′o-plek″se) old term for *stroke syndrome.* **adrenal a.,** sudden massive hemorrhage into the adrenal gland, occurring in Waterhouse-Friderichsen syndrome.

apo·pro·tein (ap″o-pro′tēn) the protein moiety of a molecule or complex, as of a lipoprotein.

ap·op·to·sis (ap″op-to′sis) a pattern of cell death affecting single cells, marked by shrinkage of the cell, condensation of chromatin, and fragmentation of the cell into membrane-bound bodies that are eliminated by phagocytosis. Often used synonymously with *programmed cell death.* **apoptot′ic,** adj.

apo·re·pres·sor (ap″o-re-pres′er) in genetic theory, a product of regulator genes that combines with the corepressor to form the complete repressor.

apoth·e·cary (ah-poth′ĕ-kar″e) pharmacist.

ap·pa·ra·tus (ap″ah-ră′tus) pl. *appară′tus, apparatuses.* A number of parts acting together to perform a special function. **branchial a.,** pharyngeal a. **Golgi a.,** see under *complex.* **juxtaglomerular a.,** see under *cell.* **Kirschner's a.,** a wire and stirrup apparatus for applying skeletal traction in leg fractures. **lacrimal a., a. lacrima′lis,** the lacrimal gland and ducts and associated structures. **pharyngeal a.,** the pharyngeal arches, pouches, and grooves considered as a unit. **subneural a.,** see under *cleft.* **vestibular a.,** the structures of the inner ear concerned with stimuli of equilibrium, including the semicircular canals, saccule, and utricle.

ap·pen·dage (ah-pen′dij) a subordinate portion of a structure, or an outgrowth, such as a tail. **epiploic a's,** see under *appendix.*

ap·pen·dec·to·my (ap″en-dek′tah-me) excision of the vermiform appendix.

ap·pen·dic·e·al (ap″en-dis′e-al) pertaining to an appendix.

ap·pen·di·ci·tis (ah-pen″dĭ-si′tis) inflammation of the vermiform appendix. **acute a.,** appendicitis of acute onset, requiring prompt surgery, and usually marked by pain in the right lower abdominal quadrant, referred rebound tenderness, overlying muscle spasm, and cutaneous hyperesthesia. **chronic a.,** 1. that characterized by fibrotic thickening of the organ wall due to previous acute inflammation. 2. formerly, chronic or recurrent pain in the appendiceal area, evidence of acute inflammation being absent. **fulminating a.,** that marked by sudden onset and death. **gangrenous a.,** that complicated by gangrene of the organ, due to interference of blood supply. **obstructive a.,** a common form with obstruction of the lumen, usually by a fecalith.

ap·pen·di·cos·to·my (ah-pen″dĭ-kos′tah-me) surgical creation of an opening into the vermiform appendix to irrigate or drain the large bowel.

ap·pen·di·co·ves·i·cos·to·my (-ko-ves″ĭ-kos′tah-me) surgical transference of the isolated appendix so that it can be used as a conduit for urinary diversion from the bladder to the skin in children with cloacal exstrophy or neurogenic bladder, making a route for insertion of a catheter.

ap·pen·dic·u·lar (ap″en-dik′u-lar) 1. pertaining to the vermiform appendix. 2. pertaining to an appendage.

ap·pen·dix (ah-pen′diks) pl. *appen′dices, appendixes.* [L.] 1. a supplementary, accessory, or dependent part attached to a main structure. 2. vermiform a. **epiploic appendices,** small peritoneum-covered tabs of fat attached in rows along the taeniae coli. **vermiform a.,** a wormlike diverticulum of the cecum. **xiphoid a.,** see under *process.*

ap·per·cep·tion (ap″er-sep′shun) the process of receiving, appreciating, and interpreting sensory impressions.

ap·pe·stat (ap′ĕ-stat) the brain center (probably in the hypothalamus) concerned in controlling the appetite.

ap·pla·na·tion (ap″lah-na′shun) undue flatness, as of the cornea.

ap·pla·nom·e·ter (ap″lah-nom′ĕ-ter) applanation tonometer.

ap·ple (ap′'l) 1. the edible fruit of the rosaceous tree, *Malus sylvestris;* in dried powdered form it is used as an antidiarrheal. 2. something that resembles this fruit. **Adam's a.,** laryngeal prominence.

ap·pli·ance (ah-pli′ans) in dentistry, a device used to provide a function or therapeutic effect.

ap·po·si·tion (ap″o-zish′un) juxtaposition; the placing of things in proximity; specifically, the deposition of successive layers upon those already present, as in cell walls. **apposi′tional,** adj.

ap·pre·hen·sion (ap″re-hen′shun) 1. perception and understanding. 2. anticipatory fear or anxiety.

ap·proach (ah-prōch′) in surgery, the specific procedures by which an organ or part is exposed.

ap·prox·i·ma·tion (ah-prok″sĭ-ma′shun) 1. the act or process of bringing into proximity or apposition. 2. a numerical value of limited accuracy.

ap·ra·clon·i·dine (ap″rah-klon′ĭ-dēn) an α_2-adrenergic receptor agonist used as the hydrochloride salt to reduce intraocular pressure in the treatment of open-angle glaucoma and ocular hypertension.

aprac·tag·no·sia (ah-prak″tag-no′zhah) a type of agnosia marked by inability to use objects or perform skilled motor activities.

aprax·ia (ah-prak′se-ah) loss of ability to carry out familiar purposeful movements in the absence of motor or sensory impairment, especially inability to use objects correctly. **amnestic a.,** loss of ability to carry out a movement on command due to inability to remember the command. **Bruns' a. of gait,** Bruns' frontal ataxia. **Cogan's oculomotor a., congenital oculomotor a.,** an absence or defect of horizontal eye movements so that the head must turn and the eyes exhibit nystagmus in attempts to see an object off to one side. **ideational a.,** sensory a. **innervatory a., motor a.,** impairment of skilled movements not explained by weakness of the affected parts, the patient appearing clumsy rather than weak. **sensory a.,** loss of ability to use an object due to lack of perception of its purpose.

ap·ro·bar·bi·tal (ap″ro-bahr′bĭ-tal) an intermediate-acting barbiturate, used as a sedative and hypnotic.

apro·ti·nin (ap″ro-ti′nin) an inhibitor of proteolytic enzymes used to reduce perioperative blood loss in patients undergoing cardiopulmonary bypass during coronary artery bypass graft.

APS American Physiological Society.

APTA American Physical Therapy Association.

APTT, aPTT activated partial thromboplastin time.

ap·ty·a·lism (ap-ti′ah-lizm) deficiency or absence of saliva.

APUD (*a*mine *p*recursor *u*ptake and *d*ecarboxylation) see *APUD cells,* under *cell.*

apud·o·ma (a″pud-o′mah) a tumor derived from APUD cells.

apy·o·gen·ic (a″pi-o-jen′ik) not caused by pus.

apy·ret·ic (a″pi-ret′ik) afebrile.

apy·rex·ia (a″pi-rek′se-ah) absence of fever.

AQ achievement quotient.

Aq. dest. [L.] a′qua destilla′ta (distilled water).

aq·ua (ah′kwah, ak′wah, a′kwah) [L.] water.

aq·ua·pho·bia (ak″wah-fo′be-ah) irrational fear of water.

aq·ue·duct (ak′wĕ-dukt″) any canal or passage. **cerebral a.,** a narrow channel in the midbrain connecting the third and fourth ventricles. **cochlear a.,** a small canal that interconnects the scala tympani with the subarachnoid space. **a. of Sylvius, ventricular a.,** cerebral a.

aque·ous (a′kwe-us) 1. watery; prepared with water. 2. see under *humor.*

AR alarm reaction; aortic regurgitation; artificial respiration.

Ar argon.

ara-A adenine arabinoside; see *vidarabine.*

ara-C cytarabine.

arach·ic ac·id (ah-rak′ik) arachidic acid.

ar·a·chid·ic ac·id (ar″ah-kid′ik) a saturated 20-carbon fatty acid occurring in peanut and other vegetable oils and fish oils.

arach·i·don·ic acid (ah-rak″ĭ-don′ik) a polyunsaturated 20-carbon essential fatty acid occurring in animal fats and formed by biosynthesis from linoleic acid; it is a precursor to leukotrienes, prostaglandins, and thromboxane.

Arach·ni·da (ah-rak′nĭ-dah) a class of the Arthropoda, including the spiders, scorpions, ticks, and mites.

arach·no·dac·ty·ly (ah-rak″no-dak′tĭ-le) extreme length and slenderness of fingers and toes.

arach·noid (ah-rak′noid) 1. resembling a spider's web. 2. a delicate membrane interposed between the dura mater and the pia mater, separated from the latter by the subarachnoid space.

arach·noi·dal (ar″ak-noi′d′l) pertaining to the arachnoid.

arach·noi·dea ma·ter (ar″ak-noi′de-ah ma′ter) arachnoid (2).

arach·noid·i·tis (ah-rak″noi-di′tis) inflammation of the arachnoidea mater.

arach·no·pho·bia (ah-rak″no-fo′be-ah) irrational fear of spiders.

ar·bor (ahr′bor) pl. *ar′bores.* [L.] a treelike structure or part. **a. vi′tae,** 1. (of cerebellum): treelike outlines seen in a median section of the cerebellum. 2. (of uterus): palmate folds. 3. the tree *T. occidentalis;* its leafy twigs contain the medicinal substance thuja but can be poisonous.

ar·bo·ri·za·tion (ahr″bo-rĭ-za′shun) a collection of branches, as the branching terminus of a nerve-cell process.

ar·bor·vi·rus (ahr′bor-vi″rus) arbovirus.

ar·bo·vi·rus (ahr′bo-vi″rus) any of a group of viruses, including the causative agents of yellow fever, viral encephalitides, and certain febrile infections, transmitted to humans by various mosquitoes and ticks; those transmitted by ticks are often considered in a separate category (tickborne viruses). **arbovi′ral,** adj.

ar·but·amine (ahr-bu′tah-mēn″) a synthetic catecholamine used as a diagnostic aid in cardiac stress testing in patients unable to exercise sufficiently for the test; administered as the hydrochloride salt.

ARC AIDS-related complex; American Red Cross; anomalous retinal correspondence.

arc (ahrk) 1. a structure or projected path having a curved outline. 2. a visible electrical discharge taking the outline of an arc. 3. in neurophysiology, the pathway of neural reactions. **reflex a.,** the neural arc utilized in a reflex action; an impulse travels centrally over afferent fibers to a nerve center, and the response outward to an effector organ or part over efferent fibers.

Ar·ca·no·bac·te·ri·um (ahr-ka″no-bak-tēr′e-um) a genus of irregular, rod-shaped, non–spore-forming, gram-positive bacteria. *A. haemoly′ticus* causes human infection that is manifested in adolescents as pharyngitis and a scarlatiniform rash similar to those of streptococcal infection.

arch (ahrch) a structure of bowlike or curved outline. **a. of aorta, aortic a.,** the curving portion between the ascending aorta and the descending aorta, giving rise to the brachiocephalic trunk, the left common carotid artery, and the left subclavian artery. **aortic a's,** paired vessels arching from the ventral to the dorsal aorta through the branchial arches of fishes and the pharyngeal arches of amniote embryos. In mammalian development, arches 1 and 2 disappear; 3 joins the common to the internal carotid artery; 4 becomes the arch of the aorta and joins the aorta and subclavian artery; 5 disappears; 6 forms the pulmonary arteries and, until birth, the ductus arteriosus. **branchial a's,** paired arched columns that bear the gills in lower aquatic vertebrates and which, in embryos of higher vertebrates, become modified into structures of the head and neck. In human embryos, called *pharyngeal a's.* **cervical aortic a.,** a rare anomaly in which the aortic arch has an unusually superior location. **dental a.,** the curving structure formed by the teeth in their normal position; the *inferior dental a.* is formed by the mandibular teeth, the *superior dental a.* by the maxillary teeth. **double aortic a.,** a congenital anomaly in which the aorta divides into two branches which embrace the trachea and esophagus and reunite to form the descending aorta. **a's of foot,** the longitudinal and transverse arches of the foot. **lingual a.,** a wire appliance that conforms to the lingual aspect of the dental arch, used to promote or prevent movement of the teeth in orthodontic work. **mandibular a.,** 1. the first pharyngeal arch, from which are developed the bone of the lower jaw, malleus, and incus. 2. inferior dental a. **maxillary a.,** 1. palatal a. 2. superior dental a., see *dental a.* **neural a.,** the primordium of the vertebral arch; one of the cartilaginous structures surrounding the embryonic spinal cord. **open pubic a.,** a congenital anomaly in which the pubic arch is not fused, the bodies of the pubic bones being spread apart. **oral a.,** one formed by the roof of the mouth from the teeth (or residual dental arch) on one side to those on the other. **palatal a.,** the arch formed by the roof of the mouth from the teeth on one side of the maxilla to the teeth on the other or, if the teeth are missing, from the residual dental arch on one side to that on the other. **palatoglossal a.,** the anterior of the two folds of mucous membrane on either side of the oropharynx, enclosing the palatoglossal muscle. **palatopharyngeal a.,** the posterior of the two folds of mucous membrane on either side of the oropharynx, enclosing the palatopharyngeal muscle. **palmar a's,** four arches in the palm: the *deep palmar arterial a.* formed by anastomosis of the terminal part of the radial artery with the deep branch of the ulnar, its accompanying *deep palmar venous a.,* and the *superficial palmar arterial a.* formed by anastomosis of the terminal part of the ulnar artery with the superficial palmar branch of the radial and its accompanying *superficial palmar venous a.* **pharyngeal a's,** the branchial arches in the human embryo. **plantar a.,** the arch in the foot formed by anastomosis of the lateral plantar artery with the deep plantar branch of the dorsal artery. **pubic a.,** the arch formed by the conjoined rami of the ischial and pubic bones on two sides of the body. **pulmonary a's,** the most caudal of the aortic arches, which become the pulmonary arteries. **residual dental a.,** the curved contour of the ridge remaining after tooth removal. **right aortic a.,** a congenital anomaly in which the aorta is displaced to the right and passes behind the esophagus, thus forming a vascular ring that may cause compression of the trachea and esophagus. **supraorbital a.,** the curved margin of the frontal bone forming the upper boundary of the orbit. **tarsal a's,**

two arches of the median palpebral artery, one of which supplies the upper eyelid, the other the lower. **tendinous a.,** a linear thickening of fascia over some part of a muscle. **vertebral a.,** the bony arch on the dorsal aspect of a vertebra, composed of the laminae and pedicles. **zygomatic a.,** one formed by processes of zygomatic and temporal bones.

arch-   see *archi-*.

archae(o)-   see *archi-*.

ar·chaeo·cer·e·bel·lum   (ahr″ke-o-ser″ah-bel′um)   archicerebellum.

ar·chaeo·cor·tex   (-kor′teks)   archicortex.

arch·en·ceph·a·lon   (ahrk″en-sef′ah-lon)   the primordial brain from which the midbrain and forebrain develop.

arch·en·ter·on   (ahrk-en′ter-on)   the primordial digestive cavity of those embryonic forms whose blastula becomes a gastrula by invagination.

arche(o)-   see *archi-*.

ar·che·type   (ahr′kĕ-tīp)   an ideal, original, or standard type or form.

archi-   word element [Gr.], *ancient; beginning; original; first; chief; leading.*

ar·chi·cer·e·bel·lum   (ahr″kĭ-ser″ĕ-bel′um)   the phylogenetically old part of the cerebellum, viz., the flocculonodular node and the lingula.

ar·chi·cor·tex   (-kor′teks)   that part of the cerebral cortex (pallium) that with the palaeocortex develops in association with the olfactory system and is phylogenetically older than the neocortex and lacks its layered structure.

ar·chi·neph·ron   (-nef′ron)   a unit of the pronephros.

ar·chi·pal·li·um   (-pal′e-um)   archicortex.

ar·ci·form   (ahr′sĭ-form)   arcuate.

Arc·to·staph·y·los   (ahrk″to-staf′ĭ-lōs)   a genus of North American evergreens; *A. uva-ur′si* is uva ursi (q.v.).

ar·cu·ate   (ahr′ku-āt)   arc-shaped; arranged in arches.

ar·cu·a·tion   (ahr″ku-a′shun)   a curvature, especially an abnormal curvature.

ar·cus   (ahr′kus)   pl. *ar′cus.* [L.]   arch; bow. **a. adipo′sus, a. cor′neae, a. juveni′lis,** a white or gray opaque ring in the margin of the cornea, sometimes present at birth, but usually occurring bilaterally in persons of 50 years or older as a result of cholesterol deposits in or hyalinosis of the corneal stroma.

ar·de·par·in   (ahr-de-par′in)   a low molecular weight heparin used as the sodium salt in the prophylaxis of deep venous thrombosis and pulmonary thromboembolism after knee replacement surgery.

ARDS   acute respiratory distress syndrome; adult respiratory distress syndrome.

ar·ea (ār'e-ah) pl. *a'reae, areas.* [L.] a limited space; in anatomy, a specific surface or functional region. **association a's,** areas of the cerebral cortex (excluding primary areas) connected with each other and with the neothalamus; they are responsible for higher mental and emotional processes, including memory, learning, etc. **auditory a's,** two contiguous areas of the temporal lobe in the region of the anterior transverse temporal gyrus. **Broca's motor speech a.,** an area comprising parts of the opercular and triangular portions of the inferior frontal gyrus; injury to this area may result in motor aphasia. **Brodmann's a's,** areas of the cerebral cortex distinguished by differences in arrangement of their six cellular layers; identified by numbering each area. **embryonic a.,** see under *disc.* **germinal a.,** embryonic disc. **hypophysiotropic a.,** the hypothalamic component containing neurons that secrete hormones that regulate adenohypophysial cells. **Kiesselbach's a.,** one on the anterior part of the nasal septum above the intermaxillary bone, richly supplied with capillaries, and a common site of nosebleed. **motor a.,** any area of the cerebral cortex primarily involved in stimulating muscle contractions, often specifically the primary somatomotor area. **prefrontal a.,** the cortex of the frontal lobe immediately in front of the premotor cortex, concerned chiefly with associative functions. **premotor a.,** the motor cortex of the frontal lobe immediately in front of the precentral gyrus. **primary a's,** areas of the cerebral cortex comprising the motor and sensory regions; cf. *association a's.* **primary somatomotor a.,** an area in the posterior part of the frontal lobe just anterior to the central sulcus; different regions control motor activity of specific parts of the body. **a. subcallo'sa, subcallosal a.,** a small area of cortex on the medial surface of each cerebral hemisphere. **a. of superficial cardiac dullness,** a triangular area of dullness observed on percussion of the chest, corresponding to the area of the heart not covered by lung tissue. **thymus-dependent a.,** any of the areas of the peripheral lymphoid organs populated by T lymphocytes, e.g., the paracortex in lymph nodes, the centers of the malpighian corpuscle of the spleen, and the internodal zone of Peyer's patches. **thymus-independent a.,** any of the areas of the peripheral lymphoid organs populated by B lymphocytes, e.g., the spleen lymph nodules and the lymph nodes. **vocal a.,** rima glottidis. **watershed a.,** any of several areas over the convexities of the cerebral or cerebellar hemispheres; at times of prolonged systemic hypotension they are particularly susceptible to infarction. **Wernicke's a., Wernicke's second motor speech a.,** originally a term denoting a speech center on the posterior part of the superior temporal gyrus, now used to include also the supramarginal and angular gyri.

are·flex·ia (a″re-flek'se-ah) absence of reflexes. **detrusor a.,** failure of the detrusor urinae muscle to respond to stimuli, resulting in failure to empty the bladder completely on urination.

are·gen·er·a·tive (re-jen′er-ah-tiv) characterized by absence of regeneration.

Are·na·vi·ri·dae (ah-re″nah-vir′ĭ-de) the arenaviruses; a family of RNA viruses with a pleomorphic virion and a genome consisting of two circular molecules of single-stranded RNA. The single genus is *Arenavirus.*

Are·na·vi·rus (ah-re′nah-vi″rus) arenaviruses; a genus of viruses of the family Arenaviridae that includes lymphocytic choriomeningitic (LCM) virus, Lassa virus, and viruses of the Tacaribe complex.

are·na·vi·rus (ah-re′nah-vi″rus) any virus of the family Arenaviridae.

are·o·la (ah-re′o-lah) pl. *are′olae.* [L.] 1. any minute space or interstice in a tissue. 2. a circular area of different color surrounding a central point, as that surrounding the nipple of the breast. **are′olar,** adj.

Arg arginine.

Ar·gas (ar′gas) a genus of ticks (family Argasidae), parasitic in poultry and other birds and sometimes humans.

ar·ga·sid (ahr′gah-sid) 1. a tick of the family Argasidae. 2. pertaining to a tick of the genus *Argas.*

Ar·gas·i·dae (ar-gas′ĭ-de) a family of arthropods (superfamily Ixodoidea) made up of the soft-bodied ticks.

ar·gat·ro·ban (ahr-gat′ro-ban″) an anticoagulant used in the prophylaxis and treatment of heparin-induced thrombocytopenia.

ar·gen·taf·fin (ahr-jen′taf-fin) staining with silver and chromium salts; see also under *cell.*

ar·gen·taf·fi·no·ma (ahr″jen-taf″ĭ-no′mah) a carcinoid tumor of the gastrointestinal tract formed from the argentaffin cells of the enteric canal and producing carcinoid syndrome.

ar·gi·nase (ahr′jĭ-nās) an enzyme existing primarily in the liver, which hydrolyzes arginine to form urea and ornithine in the urea cycle.

ar·gi·nine (Arg, R) (ahr′jĭ-nēn) a nonessential amino acid occurring in proteins and involved in the urea cycle, which converts ammonia to urea, and in the synthesis of creatine. Preparations of the base or the glutamate or hydrochloride salt are used in the treatment of hyperammonemia and as a diagnostic aid in the assessment of pituitary function.

ar·gi·ni·no·suc·cin·ate (ahr″jĭ-ne″no-suk′-sĭ-nāt) the anionic form of argininosuccinic acid.

ar·gi·ni·no·suc·cin·ate syn·thase (sin′thās) an enzyme that catalyzes the condensation of citrulline and aspartate, a step in the hepatic urea cycle; deficiency is an inherited disorder characterized by elevated plasma levels of citrulline and ammonia and urinary excretion of citrulline and orotic acid, often with mental retardation and neurologic abnormalities.

ar·gi·ni·no·suc·cin·ic ac·id (ASA) (-suk-sin′ik) an amino acid formed in the urea cycle.

ar·gi·ni·no·suc·cin·ic·ac·id·uria (-as″ĭ-du′re-ah) 1. an inherited aminoacidopathy due to deficiency of a urea cycle enzyme, with excessive levels of argininosuccinic acid in the blood and urine, ammonia and citrulline in blood, mental retardation, seizures, and other symptoms. 2. excretion in the urine of argininosuccinic acid.

ar·gon (Ar) (ahr′gon) chemical element (see *Table of Elements*), at. no. 18.

ar·gyr·ia (ahr-jir′e-ah) poisoning by silver or its salts; chronic argyria is marked by a permanent ashen-gray discoloration of the skin, conjunctivae, and internal organs.

ar·gy·ro·phil (ahr-ji′ro-fil) capable of binding silver salts.

ari·bo·fla·vin·o·sis (a-ri″bo-fla″vĭ-no′sis) deficiency of riboflavin in the diet, marked by angular cheilosis, nasolabial lesions, optic changes, and seborrheic dermatitis.

arm (ahrm) 1. brachium; the part of the upper limb from the shoulder to the elbow. 2. in common usage, the entire upper limb. 3. a slender part or extension that projects from a main structure. 4. chromosome a. **chromosome a.,** either of two segments of a chromosome separated by the centromere.

Ar·mil·li·fer (ahr-mil′ĭ-fer) a genus of wormlike endoparasites of reptiles; the larvae of *A. armilla′tus* and *A. monilifor′mis* are occasionally found in humans.

ar·ni·ca (ahr′nĭ-kah) the dried flower heads of the composite-flowered species *Arnica montana*; preparations are used topically for contusions, sprains, and superficial wounds, and as a counterirritant.

aro·ma·tase (ah-ro′mah-tās) an enzyme activity in the endoplasmic reticulum that

catalyzes the conversion of testosterone to the aromatic compound estradiol.

aro·ma·ther·a·py (-ther″ah-pe) the therapeutic use of essential oils extracted from plants by steam distillation or expression; used by inhalation, introduced internally, or applied topically.

ar·o·mat·ic (ar″o-mat′ik) 1. having a spicy odor. 2. in chemistry, denoting a compound containing a ring system stabilized by a closed circle of conjugated double bonds or nonbonding electron pairs, e.g., benzene or naphthalene.

arous·al (ah-rou′z′l) 1. a state of responsiveness to sensory stimulation or excitability. 2. the act or state of waking from or as if from sleep. 3. the act of stimulating to readiness or to action. **sexual a.,** physical and psychological responses to mental or physical erotic stimulation.

ar·rec·tor (ah-rek′tor) pl. *arrecto′res*. [L.] raising, or that which raises; an arrector muscle.

ar·rest (ah-rest′) cessation or stoppage, as of a function or a disease process. **cardiac a.,** sudden cessation of the pumping function of the heart with disappearance of arterial blood pressure, connoting either ventricular fibrillation or ventricular standstill. **developmental a.,** a temporary or permanent cessation of development. **epiphyseal a.,** premature interruption of longitudinal growth of bone by fusion of the epiphysis and diaphysis. **maturation a.,** interruption of the process of development, as of blood cells, before the final stage is reached. **sinus a.,** a pause in the normal cardiac rhythm due to a momentary failure of the sinus node to initiate an impulse, lasting for an interval that is not an exact multiple of the normal cardiac cycle.

arrhen(o)- word element [Gr.], *male; masculine*.

ar·rhe·no·blas·to·ma (ah-re″no-blas-to′-mah) a neoplasm of the ovary, sometimes causing defeminization and virilization.

ar·rhin·ia (ah-rin′e-ah) congenital absence of the nose.

ar·rhyth·mia (ah-rith′me-ah) variation from the normal rhythm of the heartbeat, encompassing abnormalities of rate, regularity, site of impulse origin, and sequence of activation. **arrhyth′mic,** adj. **nonphasic a.,** a form of sinus arrhythmia in which the irregularity is not linked to the phases of respiration. **sinus a.,** the physiologic cyclic variation in heart rate related to vagal impulses to the sinoatrial node; it is common, particularly in children, and is not abnormal.

ar·rhyth·mo·gen·esis (ah-rith″mo-jen′ĕ-sis) the development of an arrhythmia.

ar·rhyth·mo·gen·ic (-jen′ik) producing or promoting arrhythmia.

ARRS American Roentgen Ray Society.

ar·se·ni·a·sis (ahr″sĕ-ni′ah-sis) chronic arsenic poisoning; see *arsenic*[1].

ar·se·nic[1] **(As)** (ahr′sĕ-nik) a nonmetallic element (see *Table of Elements*), at. no. 33. Acute arsenic poisoning may result in shock and death, with skin rashes, vomiting, diarrhea, abdominal pain, muscular cramps, and swelling of the eyelids, feet, and hands; the chronic form, due to ingestion of small amounts of arsenic over long periods, is marked by skin pigmentation accompanied by scaling, hyperkeratosis of palms and soles, transverse lines on the fingernails, headache, peripheral neuropathy, and confusion. **a. trioxide,** an oxidized form of arsenic used in weed killers and rodenticides; also used as an antineoplastic in the treatment of acute promyelocytic leukemia.

ar·sen·ic[2] (ahr-sen′ik) pertaining to or containing arsenic in a pentavalent state.

ar·sine (ahr′sēn) any member of a group of volatile arsenical bases; the typical is AsH₃, a carcinogenic and very poisonous gas; some of its compounds have been used in warfare.

ART Accredited Record Technician; automated reagin test; assisted reproductive technology.

ar·te·fact (ahr′tĕ-fakt″) artifact.

Ar·te·mi·sia (ahr″tĕ-mis′e-ah) [L.] a genus of composite-flowered plants. *A. absin′thium* is common wormwood and *A. vulga′ris* (mugwort) is the source of moxa and is also used orally.

ar·te·ral·gia (ahr″ter-al′jah) pain emanating from an artery, such as headache from an inflamed temporal artery.

ar·te·ria (ahr-tēr′e-ah) pl. *arte′riae*. [L.] artery. **a. luso′ria,** an abnormally situated retroesophageal vessel, usually the subclavian artery from the aortic arch.

ar·te·ri·al (-al) pertaining to an artery or to the arteries.

ar·te·ri·ec·ta·sis (ahr-tēr″e-ek′tah-sis) dilatation and, usually, lengthening of an artery.

arteri(o)- word element [L., Gr.], *artery*.

ar·te·ri·og·ra·phy (ahr-tēr″e-og′rah-fe) angiography of an artery or arterial system. **catheter a.,** radiography of vessels after introduction of contrast material through a catheter inserted into an artery. **selective a.,** radiography of a specific vessel which is opacified by a medium introduced directly into it, usually via a catheter.

ar·te·ri·o·la (ahr-tēr″e-o′lah) pl. *arterio′lae*. [L.] arteriole.

ar·te·ri·ole (ahr-tēr′e-ōl) a minute arterial branch. **arterio′lar,** adj. **afferent glomerular a.,** a branch of an interlobular artery that goes to a renal glomerulus. **efferent glomerular a.,** one arising from a renal glomerulus, breaking up into capillaries to supply renal tubules. **postglomerular a.,** efferent glomerular a. **precapillary a.,** arterial capillary. **preglomerular a.,** afferent glomerular a. **straight a's of kidney,** see *Table of Arteries*.

ar·te·ri·o·lith (ahr-tēr′e-o-lith″) a chalky concretion in an artery.

arteriol(o)- word element [L.], *arteriole*.

ar·te·rio·lo·ne·cro·sis (ahr-tēr″e-o″lo-nĕ-kro′sis) necrosis or destruction of arterioles.

ar·te·ri·o·lop·a·thy (ahr-tēr″e-o-lop′ah-the) any disease of the arterioles.

ar·te·rio·lo·scle·ro·sis (ahr-tēr″e-o″lo-sklĕ-ro′sis) sclerosis and thickening of the walls of arterioles. The hyaline form may be associated with nephrosclerosis, the hyperplastic with malignant hypertension, nephrosclerosis, and scleroderma. **arteriolosclerot′ic,** adj.

ar·te·rio·mo·tor (ahr-tēr″e-o-mo′ter) involving or causing dilation or constriction of arteries.

ar·te·ri·op·a·thy (ahr-tēr″e-op′ah-the) any disease of an artery. **hypertensive a.,** widespread involvement of arterioles and small arteries, associated with arterial hypertension, and characterized by hypertrophy of the tunica media.

ar·te·rio·plas·ty (ahr-tēr′e-o-plas″te) surgical repair or reconstruction of an artery; applied especially to Matas' operation for aneurysm.

ar·te·ri·or·rha·phy (ahr-tēr″e-or′ah-fe) suture of an artery.

ar·te·ri·or·rhex·is (ahr-tēr″e-o-rek′sis) rupture of an artery.

ar·te·rio·scle·ro·sis (-sklĕ-ro′sis) a group of diseases characterized by thickening and loss of elasticity of the arterial walls, occurring in three forms: atherosclerosis, Mönckeberg's arteriosclerosis, and arteriolosclerosis. **arteriosclerot′ic,** adj. **Mönckeberg's a.,** arteriosclerosis with extensive deposits of calcium in the middle coat of the artery. **a. ob·li′terans,** that in which proliferation of the intima of the small vessels has caused complete obliteration of the lumen of the artery. **peripheral a.,** arteriosclerosis of the limbs.

ar·te·rio·ste·no·sis (-stĕ-no′sis) constriction of an artery.

ar·te·rio·ve·nous (-ve'nus) both arterial and venous; pertaining to or affecting an artery and a vein.

ar·ter·i·tis (ahr″ter-i'tis) pl. *arteri'tides*. Inflammation of an artery. **aortic arch a.,** Takayasu's a. **brachiocephalic a., a. brachiocepha'lica,** Takayasu's a. **coronary a.,** inflammation of the coronary arteries. **cranial a.,** giant cell a. **giant cell a.,** a chronic vascular disease of unknown origin, usually in the carotid arterial system, occurring in the elderly; it is characterized by severe headache, fever, and proliferative inflammation, often with giant cells and granulomas. Ocular involvement may cause blindness. **rheumatic a.,** generalized inflammation of arterioles and arterial capillaries occurring in rheumatic fever. **Takayasu's a.,** pulseless disease; progressive obliteration of the brachiocephalic trunk and left subclavian and left common carotid arteries, leading to loss of pulse in arms and carotids and to ischemia of brain, eyes, face, and arms. **temporal a.,** giant cell a.

ar·te·ry (ahr'tĕ-re) a vessel in which blood flows away from the heart, in the systemic circulation carrying oxygenated blood. For named arteries of the body, see *Table of Arteries* and see Plates 15–19. **arte'rial,** adj. **conducting a's,** arterial trunks characterized by large size and elasticity, such as the aorta, subclavian and common carotid arteries, and brachiocephalic and pulmonary trunks. **corkscrew a's,** small arteries in the macular region of the eye that appear markedly tortuous. **distributing a's,** most of the arteries except the conducting arteries; of muscular type, they extend from the large vessels to the arterioles. **elastic a's,** conducting a's. **end a.,** one which undergoes progressive branching without development of channels connecting with other arteries, so that if occluded it cannot supply sufficient blood to the tissue depending on it. **gonadal a's,** the ovarian arteries or the testicular arteries. **helicine a's,** small arteries that have a band of thickened intima along one side, in which longitudinal muscle fibers are embedded. They are convoluted or curled, open directly into cavernous sinuses instead of capillaries, and play a dominant role in erection of erectile tissue. See also *Table of Arteries*. **muscular a's,** 1. distributing a's. 2. see *Table of Arteries*. **nutrient a.,** any artery that supplies the marrow of a long bone. **terminal a.,** 1. end a. 2. an artery that does not divide into branches, but is directly continuous with capillaries.

ar·thral·gia (ahr-thral'jah) pain in a joint.

ar·thres·the·sia (ahr″thres-the'zhah) joint sensibility; the perception of joint motions.

ar·thrit·ic (ahr-thrit'ik) pertaining to or affected with arthritis.

ar·thri·tide (ahr'thri-tīd) a skin eruption of gouty origin.

ar·thri·tis (ahr-thri'tis) pl. *arthri'tides*. Inflammation of a joint. **acute a.,** arthritis marked by pain, heat, redness, and swelling. **chronic inflammatory a.,** inflammation of joints in chronic disorders such as rheumatoid arthritis. **a. defor'mans,** severe destruction of joints, seen in disorders such as rheumatoid arthritis. **degenerative a.,** osteoarthritis. **enteropathic a.,** arthritis associated with inflammatory bowel disease or following bacterial infection of the bowel. **hypertrophic a.,** osteoarthritis. **infectious a.,** arthritis caused by bacteria, rickettsiae, mycoplasmas, viruses, fungi, or parasites. **juvenile rheumatoid a.,** rheumatoid arthritis in children, with swelling, tenderness, and pain involving one or more joints, sometimes leading to impaired growth and development, limitation of movement, and ankylosis and flexion contractures of the joints; often accompanied by systemic manifestations. **Lyme a.,** see under *disease*. **menopausal a.,** that seen in some menopausal women, due to ovarian hormonal deficiency, and marked by pain in the small joints, shoulders, elbows, or knees. **a. mu'tilans,** severe deforming polyarthritis with gross bone and cartilage destruction, an atypical variant of rheumatoid arthritis. **rheumatoid a.,** a chronic systemic disease primarily of the joints, usually polyarticular, marked by inflammatory changes in the synovial membranes and articular structures and by atrophy and rarefaction of the bones. In late stages, deformity and ankylosis develop. **septic a., suppurative a.,** a form marked by purulent joint infiltration, chiefly due to bacterial infection but also seen in Reiter's disease. **tuberculous a.,** that secondary to tuberculosis, usually affecting a single joint, marked by chronic inflammation with effusion and destruction of contiguous bone.

arthr(o)- word element [Gr.], *joint; articulation*.

ar·thro·cen·te·sis (ahr″thro-sen-te'sis) puncture of a joint cavity with aspiration of fluid.

ar·thro·cha·la·sis (-kal'ah-sis) abnormal relaxation or flaccidity of a joint.

ar·thro·chon·dri·tis (-kon-dri'tis) inflammation of the cartilage of a joint.

ar·thro·cla·sia (-kla'zhah) surgical breaking of an ankylosis to permit a joint to move.

TABLE OF ARTERIES

Common Name*	TA Equivalent†	Origin*	Branches*	Distribution*
accompanying a. of median nerve. *See* median a.				
accompanying a. of sciatic nerve. *See* sciatic a.				
acromiothoracic a. *See* thoracoacromial a.				
alveolar a's, anterior superior	aa. alveolares superiores anteriores	infraorbital a.	dental and peridental branches	incisor and canine regions of upper jaw, maxillary sinus
alveolar a., inferior	a. alveolaris inferior	maxillary a.	dental, peridental, mental and mylohyoid branches	lower jaw, lower lip, chin
alveolar a., posterior superior	a. alveolaris superior posterior	maxillary a.	dental and peridental branches	molar and premolar regions of upper jaw, maxillary sinus, buccinator muscle
angular a.	a. angularis	facial a.		lacrimal sac, lower eyelid, nose
aorta	aorta	left ventricle		
abdominal aorta	pars abdominalis aortae	lower portion of descending aorta, from aortic hiatus of diaphragm to bifurcation into common iliac a's	inferior phrenic, lumbar, median sacral, superior and inferior mesenteric, middle suprarenal, renal, and testicular or ovarian a's, celiac trunk	
arch of aorta	arcus aortae	continuation of ascending aorta	brachiocephalic trunk, left common carotid and left subclavian a's; continues as descending (thoracic) aorta	
ascending aorta	pars ascendens aortae	proximal portion of aorta, arising from left ventricle	right and left coronary a's; continues as arch of aorta	
descending aorta. *See* thoracic aorta; abdominal aorta	pars descendens aortae	continuation of aorta from arch of aorta to division into common iliac arteries		
thoracic aorta	pars thoracica aortae	proximal portion of descending aorta, continuing from arch of aorta to aortic hiatus of diaphragm	bronchial, esophageal, pericardiac, and mediastinal branches, superior phrenic a's, posterior intercostal a's [III–XII], subcostal a's, continues as abdominal aorta	

*a. = artery; a's = (pl.) arteries.

†a. = [L.] arteria; aa. = ([L.] pl.) arteriae; r. = [L.] ramus (branch); rr. = ([L.] pl.) rami (branches).

69

TABLE OF ARTERIES *Continued*

Common Name*	TA Equivalent†	Origin*	Branches*	Distribution*
appendicular a.	a. appendicularis	ileocolic a.		vermiform appendix
arcuate a. of foot	a. arcuata pedis	dorsalis pedis a.	deep plantar branch, dorsal metatarsal a's	foot, toes
arcuate a's of kidney	aa. arcuatae renis	interlobar a.	interlobular a's, straight arterioles of kidney	parenchyma of kidney
auditory a., internal. *See* a. *of labyrinth*				
auricular a., deep	a. auricularis profunda	maxillary a.		skin of auditory canal, tympanic membrane, temporomandibular joint
auricular a., posterior	a. auricularis posterior	external carotid a.	auricular and occipital branches, stylomastoid a.	middle ear, mastoid cells, auricle, parotid gland, digastric and other muscles
axillary a.	a. axillaris	continuation of subclavian a.	subscapular branches, superior thoracic, thoracoacromial, lateral thoracic, subscapular, and anterior and posterior circumflex humeral a's	upper limb, axilla, chest, shoulder
basilar a.	a. basilaris	from junction of right and left vertebral a's	pontine branches, anterior inferior cerebellar, labyrinthine, superior cerebellar, posterior cerebral a's	brainstem, internal ear, cerebellum, posterior cerebrum
brachial a.	a. brachialis	continuation of axillary a.	superficial and deep brachial, nutrient of humerus, superior and inferior ulnar collateral, radial, ulnar a's	shoulder, arm, forearm, hand
brachial a., deep	a. profunda brachii	brachial a.	nutrient to humerus, deltoid branch, middle and radial collateral a's	humerus, muscles and skin of arm
brachial a., superficial	a. brachialis superficialis	variant brachial a., taking a more superficial course than usual	*see brachial a.*	*see brachial a.*
brachiocephalic trunk	truncus brachiocephalicus	arch of aorta	right common carotid, right subclavian a's	right side of head and neck, right arm
buccal a.	a. buccalis	maxillary a.		buccinator muscle, oral mucous membrane

Term	Latin	Branch of	Branches	Distribution
bulbourethral a. See a. of bulb of penis				
a. of bulb of penis	a. bulbi penis	internal pudendal a.		bulbourethral gland, bulb of penis
a. of bulb of vestibule	a. bulbi vestibuli	internal pudendal a.		bulb of vestibule of vagina, greater vestibular glands
callosomarginal a.	a. callosomarginalis	anterior cerebral a.	anteromedial frontal, mediomedial frontal, posteromedial frontal, cingular branches	medial and upper lateral surfaces of cerebral hemisphere
capsular a's	rr. capsulares arteriae renalis	renal a.		renal capsule
caroticotympanic a's	aa. caroticotympanicae	internal carotid a.		tympanic cavity
carotid a., common	a. carotis communis	brachiocephalic trunk (right), arch of aorta (left)	external and internal carotid a's	see *carotid a., external* and *carotid a., internal*
carotid a., external	a. carotis externa	common carotid a.	superior thyroid, ascending pharyngeal, lingual, facial, sternocleidomastoid, occipital, posterior auricular, superficial temporal, maxillary a's	neck, face, skull
carotid a., internal	a. carotis interna	common carotid a.	caroticotympanic, ophthalmic, posterior communicating, anterior choroid, anterior cerebral, middle cerebral a's	middle ear, brain, pituitary gland, orbit, choroid plexus
caudal a. See sacral a., median				
cecal a., anterior	a. caecalis anterior	ileocolic a.		cecum
cecal a., posterior	a. caecalis posterior	ileocolic a.		cecum
celiac trunk	truncus coeliacus	abdominal aorta	left gastric, common hepatic, splenic a's	esophagus, stomach, duodenum, spleen, pancreas, liver, gallbladder
central a's, anterolateral	aa. centrales anterolaterales	middle cerebral a.	medial and lateral branches	anterior lenticular and caudate nuclei and internal capsule of brain
central a's, anteromedial, of anterior cerebral a.	aa. centrales anteromediales arteriae cerebri anterioris	anterior cerebral a.		anterior and medial corpus striatum
central a's, anteromedial, of anterior communicating a.	aa. centrales anteromediales arteriae communicantis anterioris	anterior communicating a.		corpus callosum, septum pellucidum, lentiform and caudate nuclei
central a., long		anterior cerebral a.		

Common Name*	TA Equivalent†	Origin*	Branches*	Distribution*
central a.'s, posterolateral	aa. centrales posterolaterales	posterior cerebral a.		cerebral peduncle, posterior thalamus, colliculi, pineal and medial geniculate bodies
central a.'s, postcromedial, of posterior cerebral a.	aa. centrales posteromediales arteriae cerebri posterioris	posterior cerebral a.		anterior thalamus, lateral wall of third ventricle, globus pallidus
central a.'s, postcromedial, of posterior communicating a.	aa. centrales posteromediales arteriae communicantis posterioris	posterior communicating a.		medial thalamic surface and walls of third ventricle
central a., short		anterior cerebral a.		
central a. of retina	a. centralis retinae	ophthalmic a.		retina
a. of central sulcus	a. sulci centralis	middle cerebral a.		cortex of either side of central sulcus
cerebellar a., anterior inferior	a. inferior anterior cerebelli	basilar a.	posterior, spinal (usually), and labyrinthine (usually) a's	lower anterior cerebellum, lower and lateral parts of pons, (sometimes) upper part of medulla oblongata
cerebellar a., posterior inferior	a. inferior posterior cerebelli	vertebral a.	medial and lateral	lower part of cerebellum, medulla, choroid plexus of fourth ventricle
cerebellar a., superior	a. superior cerebelli	basilar a.		upper part of cerebellum, midbrain, pineal body, choroid plexus of third ventricle
cerebral a.'s	aa. cerebri	internal carotid a., basilar a.		cerebral hemispheres
cerebral a., anterior	a. cerebri anterior	internal carotid a.	*precommunical part:* antero-medial central, long and short central, anterior communicating a's; *postcommunical part:* medial frontobasal, callosomarginal, paracentral, precuneal, parietooccipital a's	orbital, frontal, and parietal cortex, corpus callosum, corpus striatum, internal capsule, choroid plexus of lateral ventricle

cerebral a., middle	a. cerebri media	internal carotid a.	*sphenoidal part:* anterolateral central a.; *insular part:* insular, lateral frontobasilar, temporal a's; *terminal* or *cortical part:* a's of sulcus, parietal a's, a. of angular gyri	orbital, frontal, parietal, and temporal cortex, corpus striatum, internal capsule
cerebral a., posterior	a. cerebri posterior	terminal bifurcation of basilar a.	*precommunical part:* posteromedial central a's; *postcommunical part:* posterolateral central a's, medial and lateral posterior choroidal, peduncular branches; *terminal* or *cortical part:* lateral and medial occipital a's	occipital and temporal cortex, choroid plexus of lateral and third ventricles, diencephalon, midbrain, visual area of cerebral cortex and other structures associated with the visual pathway
cervical a., ascending	a. cervicalis ascendens	inferior thyroid a.		muscles of neck, vertebrae, vertebral canal
cervical a., deep	a. cervicalis profunda	costocervical trunk		deep neck muscles
cervical a., transverse	a. transversa cervicis	subclavian a.	deep and superficial branches	root of neck, muscles of scapula
choroidal a., anterior	a. choroidea anterior	internal carotid or middle cerebral a.	many small branches	interior of brain, including choroid plexus of lateral ventricle and adjacent parts
ciliary a's, anterior	aa. ciliares anteriores	ophthalmic and lacrimal a's	episcleral and anterior conjunctival a's	iris, conjunctiva
ciliary a's, long posterior	aa. ciliares posteriores longae	ophthalmic a.		iris, ciliary processes
ciliary a's, short posterior	aa. ciliares posteriores breves	ophthalmic a.		choroid coat of eye
circumflex a.	ramus circumflexus arteriae coronariae sinistrae	left coronary a.	atrial, atrial anastomotic, atrioventricular, intermediate atrial, left marginal, and left posterior ventricular branches	left ventricle, left atrium
circumflex femoral a., lateral	a. circumflexa femoris lateralis	deep femoral a.	ascending, descending, and transverse branches	hip joint, thigh muscles
circumflex femoral a., medial	a. circumflexa femoris medialis	deep femoral a.	acetabular, ascending, deep, superficial, and transverse branches	hip joint, thigh muscles
circumflex humeral a., anterior	a. circumflexa humeri anterior	axillary a.		shoulder joint and head of humerus, long tendon of biceps, tendon of greater pectoral muscle
circumflex humeral a., posterior	a. circumflexa humeri posterior	axillary a.		deltoid, shoulder joint, teres minor and triceps muscles

Common Name*	TA Equivalent†	Origin*	Branches*	Distribution*
circumflex iliac a., deep	a. circumflexa ilium profunda	external iliac a.	ascending branches	iliac region, abdominal wall, groin
circumflex iliac a., superficial	a. circumflexa ilium superficialis	femoral a.		groin, abdominal wall
circumflex a. of scapula	a. circumflexa scapulae	subscapular a.		inferolateral muscles of scapula
coccygeal a. *See* sacral a., median				
colic a., accessory superior. *See* colic a., middle				
colic a., inferior right. *See* ileocolic a.				
colic a., left	a. colica sinistra	inferior mesenteric a.		descending colon
colic a., middle	a. colica media	superior mesenteric a.		transverse colon
colic a., right	a. colica dextra	superior mesenteric a.		ascending colon
collateral a., inferior ulnar	a. collateralis ulnaris inferior	brachial a.		arm muscles at back of elbow
collateral a., middle	a. collateralis media	deep brachial a.		triceps muscle, elbow joint
collateral a., radial	a. collateralis radialis	deep brachial a.		brachioradial and brachial muscles
collateral a., superior ulnar	a. collateralis ulnaris superior	brachial a.		elbow joint, triceps muscle
communicating a., anterior	a. communicans anterior	precommunical part of anterior cerebral a.		interconnects anterior cerebral a's
communicating a., posterior	a. communicans posterior	interconnects internal carotid and posterior cerebral a's	branches to optic chiasm, oculomotor nerve, thalamus, hypothalamus, and tail of caudate nucleus	
conjunctival a's, anterior	aa. conjunctivales anteriores	anterior ciliary a's		conjunctiva
conjunctival a's, posterior	aa. conjunctivales posteriores	medial palpebral a.		lacrimal caruncle, conjunctiva
coronary a., left	a. coronaria sinistra	left aortic sinus	anterior interventricular and circumflex branches	left ventricle, left atrium
coronary a., left anterior descending	ramus interventricularis anterior arteriae coronariae sinistrae	left coronary a.	conus a., lateral and interventricular septal branches	ventricles, interventricular septum
coronary a., posterior descending	ramus interventricularis posterior arteriae coronariae dextrae	right coronary a.	interventricular septal	diaphragmatic surface of ventricles, part of interventricular septum

Common Name	NA Term	Origin	Branches	Distribution
coronary a., right	a. coronaria dextra	right aortic sinus	conus a., atrial, atrioventricular node, intermediate atrial, posterior interventricular, right marginal, and sinoatrial node branches	right ventricle, right atrium
cortical radiate a's. *See* interlobular a's of kidney				
costocervical trunk	truncus costocervicalis	subclavian a.	deep cervical and highest intercostal a's	deep neck muscles, first two intercostal spaces, vertebral column, back muscles
cremasteric a.	a. cremasterica	inferior epigastric a.		cremaster muscle, coverings of spermatic cord
cystic a.	a. cystica	right branch of proper hepatic a.		gallbladder
deep a. of clitoris	a. profunda clitoridis	internal pudendal a.		clitoris
deep a. of penis	a. profunda penis	internal pudendal a.		corpus cavernosum penis
deferential a. *See* a. of ductus deferens				
deltoid a.	1. ramus deltoideus arteriae profundae brachii 2. ramus deltoideus arteriae thoracoacromialis	deep brachial a. thoracoacromial a.		brachialis and deltoid muscles deltoid and pectoralis major muscles
dental a's. *See* alveolar a's.				
digital a's, collateral. *See* digital a's, proper palmar				
digital a's, common palmar	aa. digitales palmares communes	superficial palmar arch	proper palmar digital a's	fingers
digital a's, common plantar	aa. digitales plantares communes	plantar metatarsal a's	proper plantar digital a's	toes
digital a's, proper palmar	aa. digitales palmares propriae	common palmar digital a's		fingers
digital a's, proper plantar	aa. digitales plantares propriae	common plantar digital a's		toes
digital a's of foot, common. *See* metatarsal a's, plantar				
digital a's of foot, dorsal	aa. digitales dorsales pedis	dorsal metatarsal a's		dorsum of toes
digital a's of hand, dorsal	aa. digitales dorsales manus	dorsal metacarpal a's		dorsum of fingers
dorsal a. of clitoris	a. dorsalis clitoridis	internal pudendal a.		clitoris

Common Name*	TA Equivalent†	Origin*	Branches*	Distribution*
dorsal a. of foot. *See* dorsalis pedis a.				
dorsal a. of nose	a. dorsalis nasi	ophthalmic a.	lacrimal	dorsum of nose
dorsal a. of penis	a. dorsalis penis	internal pudendal a.		glans, corona, and prepuce of penis
dorsalis pedis a.	a. dorsalis pedis	continuation of anterior tibial a.	lateral and medial tarsal, arcuate, and deep plantar a's	foot, toes
a. of ductus deferens	a. ductus deferentis	umbilical a.	ureteral artery	ureter, ductus deferens, seminal vesicles, testes
epigastric a., inferior	a. epigastrica inferior	external iliac a.	pubic branch, cremasteric a., a. of round ligament of uterus	abdominal wall
epigastric a., superficial	a. epigastrica superficialis	femoral a.		abdominal wall, groin
epigastric a., superior	a. epigastrica superior	internal thoracic a.		abdominal wall, diaphragm
episcleral a's	aa. episclerales	anterior ciliary a.		iris, ciliary processes
ethmoidal a., anterior	a. ethmoidalis anterior	ophthalmic a.	anterior meningeal, anterior septal, anterior lateral nasal branches	dura mater, nose, frontal sinus, anterior ethmoidal cells
ethmoidal a., posterior	a. ethmoidalis posterior	ophthalmic a.		posterior ethmoidal cells, dura mater, nose
facial a.	a. facialis	external carotid a.	ascending palatine, submental, inferior and superior labial, septal, lateral nasal, and angular a's; tonsillar and glandular branches	face, tonsil, palate, submandibular gland
facial a., transverse	a. transversa faciei	superficial temporal a.		parotid region
fallopian a. *See* uterine a.				
femoral a.	a. femoralis	continuation of external iliac a.	superficial epigastric, superficial circumflex iliac, external pudendal, deep femoral, and descending genicular a's	lower abdominal wall, external genitalia, lower limb
femoral a., deep	a. profunda femoris	femoral a.	medial and lateral circumflex a. of thigh, perforating a's	thigh muscles, hip joint, gluteal muscles, femur
fibular a. *See* peroneal a.				

frontal a. *See* supratrochlear a.				
frontobasal a., lateral	a. frontobasalis lateralis	middle cerebral a.		cortex of lateroinferior frontal lobe
frontobasal a., medial	a. frontobasalis medialis	anterior cerebral a.		cortex of medioinferior frontal lobe
funicular a. *See* testicular a.				
gastric a., left	a. gastrica sinistra	celiac trunk	esophageal branches	esophagus, lesser curvature of stomach
gastric a., posterior	a. gastrica posterior	splenic a.		posterior gastric wall
gastric a., right	a. gastrica dextra	common hepatic a.		lesser curvature of stomach
gastric a's, short	aa. gastricae breves	splenic a.		upper part of stomach
gastroduodenal a.	a. gastroduodenalis	common hepatic a.	supraduodenal and posterior superior pancreaticoduodenal a's	stomach, duodenum, pancreas, greater omentum
gastroepiploic a., left. *See* gastroomental a., left				
gastroepiploic a., right. *See* gastroomental a., right				
gastroomental a., left	a. gastroomentalis sinistra	splenic a.	gastric and omental branches	stomach, greater omentum
gastroomental a., right	a. gastroomentalis dextra	gastroduodenal a.	gastric and omental branches	stomach, greater omentum
genicular a., descending	a. descendens genus	femoral a.	saphenous, articular branches	knee joint, upper and medial leg
genicular a., lateral inferior	a. inferior lateralis genus	popliteal a.		knee joint
genicular a., lateral superior	a. superior lateralis genus	popliteal a.		knee joint, femur, patella, contiguous muscles
genicular a., medial inferior	a. inferior medialis genus	popliteal a.		knee joint
genicular a., medial superior	a. superior medialis genus	popliteal a.		knee joint, femur, patella, contiguous muscles
genicular a., middle	a. media genus	popliteal a.		knee joint, cruciate ligaments, patellar synovial and alar folds
gluteal a., inferior	a. glutea inferior	internal iliac a.	sciatic a.	buttock, back of thigh
gluteal a., superior	a. glutea superior	internal iliac a.	superficial and deep branches	buttocks
helicine a's of penis	aa. helicinae penis	deep and dorsal a's of penis	superficial and deep branches	erectile tissue of penis
helicine a's of uterus	rami helicinae arteriae uterinae	uterine a.		uterine muscle
hemorrhoidal a's. *See* rectal a's				
hepatic a., common	a. hepatica communis	celiac trunk	right gastric, gastroduodenal, proper hepatic a's	stomach, pancreas, duodenum, liver, gallbladder, greater omentum

TABLE OF ARTERIES *Continued*

Common Name*	TA Equivalent†	Origin*	Branches*	Distribution*
hepatic a., proper	a. hepatica propria	common hepatic a.	right and left branches	liver, gallbladder
hyaloid a.	a. hyaloidea	central a. of retina		fetal lens (usually not present after birth)
hypogastric a. *See iliac a., internal*				
hypophysial a., inferior	a. hypophysialis inferior	internal carotid a.		pituitary gland
hypophysial a., superior	a. hypophysialis superior	internal carotid a.		pituitary gland
ileal a's	aa. ileales	superior mesenteric a.		ileum
ileocolic a.	a. ileocolica	superior mesenteric a.	anterior and posterior cecal and appendicular a's, colic (ascending) and ileal branches	ileum, cecum, vermiform appendix, ascending colon
iliac a., common	a. iliaca communis	abdominal aorta	internal and external iliac a's	pelvis, abdominal wall, lower limb
iliac a., external	a. iliaca externa	common iliac a.	inferior epigastric, deep circumflex iliac a's	abdominal wall, external genitalia, lower limb
iliac a., internal	a. iliaca interna	continuation of common iliac a.	iliolumbar, obturator, superior and inferior gluteal, umbilical, inferior vesical, uterine, middle rectal, and internal pudendal a's	wall and viscera of pelvis, buttock, reproductive organs, medial aspect of thigh
iliolumbar a.	a. iliolumbalis	internal iliac a.	iliac and lumbar branches, lateral sacral a's	pelvic muscles and bones, fifth lumbar segment, sacrum
infraorbital a.	a. infraorbitalis	maxillary a.	anterior superior alveolar a's	maxilla, maxillary sinus, upper teeth, lower eyelid, cheek, nose
innominate a. *See brachiocephalic trunk*				
insular a's	aa. insulares	insular part of middle cerebral a.		cortex of insula
intercostal a., first posterior	a. intercostalis posterior prima	highest intercostal a.	dorsal and spinal branches	upper thoracic wall
intercostal a., highest	a. intercostalis suprema	costocervical trunk	first and second posterior intercostal a's	upper thoracic wall
intercostal a's, posterior (III-XI)		thoracic aorta	dorsal, spinal, lateral and medial cutaneous collateral, and lateral mammary branches	thoracic wall
intercostal a., second posterior	a. intercostalis posterior secunda	highest intercostal a.	dorsal and spinal branches	upper thoracic wall
interlobar a's of kidney	aa. interlobares renis	lobar branches of segmental a's	arcuate a's	parenchyma of kidney

78

interlobular a's of kidney	aa. corticales radiatae	arcuate a's of kidney		renal glomeruli
interlobular a's of liver	aa. interlobulares hepatis	right or left branch of proper hepatic a.	between lobules of liver	walls of interlobular veins and the accompanying bile ducts
interosseous a's, anterior	a. interossea anterior	common interosseous a.	median a.	deep parts of front of forearm
interosseous a., common	a. interossea communis	ulnar a.	anterior and posterior interosseous a's	antecubital fossa
interosseous a's, posterior	a. interossea posterior	common interosseous a.	recurrent interosseous a.	deep parts of back of forearm
interosseous a's, recurrent	a. interossea recurrens	posterior or common interosseous a.		back of elbow joint
interventricular a's, anterior. *See* coronary a., left anterior descending				
intestinal a's			vessels arising from superior mesenteric a. and supplying intestines; they include pancreaticoduodenal, jejunal, ileal, ileocolic, and colic a's	
intrarenal a's. *See* renal a's				
jejunal a's	aa. jejunales	superior mesenteric a.		jejunum
a's of kidney. *See* renal a's				
a's of knee. *See* genicular a's				
labial a's, inferior	a. labialis inferior	facial a.		lower lip
labial a's, superior	a. labialis superior	facial a.	septal and alar branches	upper lip and nose
labyrinthine a.	a. labyrinthi	basilar or anterior inferior cerebellar a.	vestibular and cochlear branches	internal ear
lacrimal a.	a. lacrimalis	ophthalmic a.	lateral palpebral a's, and recurrent meningeal branch	lacrimal gland, eyelids, conjunctiva
laryngeal a., inferior	a. laryngea inferior	inferior thyroid a.		larynx, trachea, esophagus
laryngeal a., superior	a. laryngea superior	superior thyroid a.		larynx
lingual a.	a. lingualis	external carotid a.	suprahyoid, sublingual, dorsal lingual, deep lingual branches	tongue, sublingual gland, tonsil, epiglottis
lingual a., deep	a. profunda linguae	lingual a.		tongue
lingular a.	a. lingularis	left pulmonary a.	superior and inferior lingular a's	lingular segments of superior lobe of left lung
lingular a., inferior	a. lingularis inferior	lingular a.		inferior lingular segment of superior lobe of left lung
lingular a., superior	a. lingularis superior	lingular a.		superior lingular segment of superior lobe of left lung

Common Name*	TA Equivalent†	Origin*	Branches*	Distribution*
lobar a.'s, inferior	aa. lobares inferiores	the branches of each pulmonary a. that supply the inferior lobe of the corresponding lung, consisting of the superior, anterior basal, lateral basal, medial basal, and posterior basal segmental a's		
lobar a., middle	a. lobaris media	right pulmonary a.	lateral and medial segmental a's	middle lobe of right lung
lobar a.'s, superior	aa. lobares superiores	the branches of each pulmonary a. that supply the superior lobe of the corresponding lung, consisting of the apical, anterior, and posterior segmental a's		
lumbar a.'s	aa. lumbales	abdominal aorta	dorsal and spinal branches	posterior abdominal wall, renal capsule
lumbar a.'s, lowest	aa. lumbales imae	median sacral a.		sacrum, glutus maximus muscle
malleolar a., lateral anterior	a. malleolaris anterior lateralis	anterior tibial a.		ankle joint
malleolar a., medial anterior	a. malleolaris anterior medialis	anterior tibial a.		ankle joint
mammary a., external. See thoracic a., lateral				
mammary a., internal. See thoracic a., internal				
mandibular a. See alveolar a., inferior				
marginal a. of colon	a. marginalis coli	branches from superior and inferior mesenteric a's	runs along inner perimeter of large intestine from ileocolic junction to rectum and gives off straight arteries that supply intestinal wall	
masseteric a.	a. masseterica	maxillary a.		masseter muscle
maxillary a.	a. maxillaris	external carotid a.	pterygoid branches; deep auricular, anterior tympanic, middle meningeal, masseteric, deep temporal, buccal, posterior superior alveolar, infraorbital, descending palatine, and sphenopalatine a's, and a. of pterygoid canal	both jaws, teeth, muscles of mastication, ear, meninges, nose, paranasal sinuses, palate
maxillary a., external. See facial a.				
maxillary a., internal. See maxillary a.				

median a.	a. comitans nervi mediani	anterior interosseous a.		median nerve, muscles of front of forearm
meningeal a., middle	a. meningea media	maxillary a.	frontal, parietal, lacrimal anastomotic, accessory meningeal, and petrosal branches, and superior tympanic a.	cranial bones, dura mater
meningeal a., posterior	a. meningea posterior	ascending pharyngeal a.		bones and dura mater of posterior cranial fossa
mesencephalic a's	aa. mesencephalicae	basilar a.		cerebral peduncle
mesenteric a., inferior	a. mesenterica inferior	abdominal aorta	left colic, sigmoid, and superior rectal a's	descending colon, rectum
mesenteric a., superior	a. mesenterica superior	abdominal aorta	inferior pancreaticoduodenal, jejunal, ileal, ileocolic, right and middle colic a's	small intestine, proximal half of colon
metacarpal a's, dorsal	aa. metacarpales dorsales	dorsal carpal rete and radial a.	dorsal digital a's	dorsum of fingers
metacarpal a's, palmar	aa. metacarpales palmares	deep palmar arch		deep parts of metacarpus
metatarsal a's, dorsal	aa. metatarsales dorsales	arcuate a. of foot	dorsal digital a's	dorsum of foot, including toes
metatarsal a's, plantar	aa. metatarsales plantares	plantar arch	perforating branches, common and proper plantar digital a's	plantar surface of toes
muscular a's	aa. musculares	branches of the ophthalmic a. consisting of a superior and an inferior group; the latter gives origin to the ciliary a's		
musculophrenic a.	a. musculophrenica	internal thoracic a.		diaphragm, abdominal and thoracic walls
nasal a., dorsal. See dorsal a. of nose				
nasal a's, posterior lateral	aa. nasales posteriores laterales	sphenopalatine a.		frontal, maxillary, ethmoidal, and sphenoidal sinuses
nutrient a's of femur	aa. nutriciae femoris	third perforating a.		femur
nutrient a's of fibula	aa. nutriciae fibulae	fibular a.		fibula
nutrient a's of humerus	aa. nutriciae humeri	brachial and deep brachial a's		humerus
nutrient a's of tibia	aa. nutriciae tibiae	posterior tibial a.		tibia
obturator a.	a. obturatoria	internal iliac a.	pubic, acetabular, anterior, and posterior branches	pelvic muscles, hip joint
obturator a., accessory	a. obturatoria accessoria	variant obturator a., arising from inferior epigastric instead of internal iliac a.		
occipital a.	a. occipitalis	external carotid a.	auricular, meningeal, mastoid, descending, occipital, and sternocleidomastoid branches	muscles of neck and scalp, meninges, mastoid cells

Common Name*	TA Equivalent†	Origin*	Branches*	Distribution*
occipital a., lateral	a. occipitalis lateralis	posterior cerebral a.	anterior temporal, middle intermediate temporal, and posterior temporal branches, and lateral occipital a.	anterior, medial, intermediate, and posterior parts of temporal lobe
occipital a., middle	a. occipitalis medialis	posterior cerebral a.	dorsal corpus callosum, parietal, parieto-occipital, calcarine, occipito-temporal branches	dorsum of corpus callosum, precuneus, cuneus, lingual gyrus, posterior part of lateral surface of occipital lobe
ophthalmic a.	a. ophthalmica	internal carotid a.	lacrimal and supraorbital a's, central a. of retina, ciliary, posterior and anterior ethmoidal, palpebral, supratrochlear, and dorsal nasal a's	eye, orbit, adjacent facial structures
ovarian a.	a. ovarica	abdominal aorta	ureteral and tubal branches	ureter, ovary, uterine tube
palatine a., ascending	a. palatina ascendens	facial a.		soft palate, wall of pharynx, tonsil, auditory tube
palatine a., descending	a. palatina descendens	maxillary a.	greater and lesser palatine a's	soft and hard palates, tonsil
palatine a., greater	a. palatina major	descending palatine a.		hard palate
palatine a's, lesser	aa. palatinae minores	descending palatine a.		soft palate, tonsil
palpebral a's, lateral	aa. palpebrales laterales	lacrimal a.		eyelids, conjunctiva
palpebral a's, medial	aa. palpebrales mediales	ophthalmic a.		eyelids
pancreatic a., caudal	a. caudae pancreatis	splenic a.	posterior conjuctival a's	
pancreatic a., dorsal	a. pancreatica dorsalis	splenic a.	supplies branches to tail of pancreas, and accessory spleen (if present)	neck and body of pancreas
pancreatic a., great	a. pancreatica magna	splenic a.	inferior pancreatic a.	body and tail of pancreas
pancreatic a., inferior	a. pancreatica inferior	dorsal pancreatic a.	right and left branches anastomose with other pancreatic arteries	pancreas
pancreaticoduodenal a., anterior superior	a. pancreaticoduodenalis superior anterior	gastroduodenal a.	pancreatic and duodenal branches	pancreas, duodenum
pancreaticoduodenal a's, inferior	aa. pancreaticoduodenales inferiores	superior mesenteric a.	anterior and posterior branches	pancreas, duodenum
pancreaticoduodenal a., posterior superior	a. pancreaticoduodenalis superior posterior	gastroduodenal a.	pancreatic and duodenal branches	pancreas, duodenum
paracentral a.	a. paracentralis	anterior cerebral a.		cerebral cortex and medial central sulcus
paramedian a's. *See central a's, posteromedial, of posterior cerebral a.*				

Term	Latin	Origin	Branches	Distribution
parietal a., anterior	a. parietalis anterior	middle cerebral a.		anterior parietal lobe
parietal a., posterior	a. parietalis posterior	middle cerebral a.		posterior temporal lobe
perforating a's	aa. perforantes	deep femoral a.		adductor, hamstring, and gluteal muscles, femur
perforating radiate a's	aa. perforantes radiatae	interlobular a's of kidney		perforate renal capsule
pericardiacophrenic a.	a. pericardiacophrenica	internal thoracic a		pericardium, diaphragm, pleura
perineal a.	a. perinealis	internal pudendal a.	nutrient a's	perineum, skin of external genitalia
peroneal a.	a. fibularis	posterior tibial a.	perforating, communicating, calcaneal, and lateral and medial malleolar branches, calcaneal rete	lateral side and back of ankle, deep calf muscles
pharyngeal a., ascending	a. pharyngea ascendens	external carotid a.	posterior meningeal, pharyngeal, inferior tympanic branches	pharynx, soft palate, ear, meninges
phrenic a., great. See phrenic a., inferior.				
phrenic a., inferior	a. phrenica inferior	abdominal aorta	superior suprarenal a's	diaphragm, suprarenal gland
phrenic a's, superior	aa. phrenicae superiores	thoracic aorta		upper surface of vertebral portion of diaphragm
plantar a., deep	a. plantaris profunda	dorsalis pedis a.		sole of foot to help form plantar arch
plantar a., lateral	a. plantaris lateralis	posterior tibial a.	plantar arch, plantar metatarsal a's; deep and superficial branches	sole of foot, toes
plantar a., medial	a. plantaris medialis	posterior tibial a.		sole of foot, toes
pontine a's	aa. pontis	basilar a.		pons and adjacent areas of brain
popliteal a.	a. poplitea	continuation of femoral a.	lateral and medial superior genicular, middle genicular, sural, lateral and medial inferior genicular, anterior and posterior tibial a's; articular rete of knee, patellar rete	knee and calf
a. of postcentral sulcus	a. sulci postcentralis	middle cerebral a.		cortex on either side of postcentral sulcus
a. of precentral sulcus	a. sulci precentralis	middle cerebral a.		cortex on either side of precentral sulcus
precuneal a.	a. precunealis	anterior cerebral		inferior precuneus
prepancreatic a.	a. prepancreatica	splenic a., anterior superior pancreaticoduodenal a.		between the neck and uncinate process of pancreas
princeps pollicis a.	a. princeps pollicis	radial a.	radialis indicis a.	sides and palmar aspect of thumb

TABLE OF ARTERIES *Continued*

Common Name*	TA Equivalent†	Origin*	Branches*	Distribution*
principal a. of thumb. *See* princeps pollicis a.				
a. of pterygoid canal	a. canalis pterygoidei	maxillary a.	pterygoid	roof of pharynx, auditory tube
pudendal a., deep external	a. pudenda externa profunda	femoral a.	anterior scrotal or anterior labial branches, inguinal branches	external genitalia, upper medial thigh
pudendal a., internal	a. pudenda interna	internal iliac a.	posterior scrotal or posterior labial branches, inferior rectal, perineal, urethral a's, a. of bulb of penis or vestibule, deep a. and dorsal a. of penis or clitoris	external genitalia, anal canal, perineum
pudendal a., superficial external	a. pudenda externa superficialis	femoral a.		external genitalia
pulmonary a., left	a. pulmonalis sinistra	pulmonary trunk	numerous branches named according to segments of lung to which they distribute unaerated blood	left lung
pulmonary a., right	a. pulmonalis dextra	pulmonary trunk	numerous branches named according to segments of lung to which they distribute unaerated blood	right lung
pulmonary trunk	truncus pulmonalis	right ventricle	right and left pulmonary a's	conveys unaerated blood toward lungs
radial a.	a. radialis	brachial a.	palmar carpal, superficial palmar and dorsal carpal branches; recurrent radial a., princeps pollicis a., deep palmar arch	forearm, wrist, hand
radial a., collateral. *See* collateral a., radial				
radial a. of index finger. *See* radialis indicis a.				
radialis indicis a.	a. radialis indicis	princeps pollicis a.		index finger
radiate a's of kidney. *See* interlobular a's of kidney				
ranine a. *See* lingual a., deep				
rectal a., inferior	a. rectalis inferior	internal pudendal a.		rectum, anal canal

rectal a., middle	a. rectalis media	internal iliac a.		rectum, prostate, seminal vesicles, vagina
rectal a., superior	a. rectalis superior	inferior mesenteric a.		rectum
recurrent a., anterior tibial	a. recurrens tibialis anterior	anterior tibial a.		anterior tibial muscle and long extensor muscle of toes; knee joint, contiguous fascia and skin
recurrent a., posterior tibial	a. recurrens tibialis posterior	anterior tibial a.		knee
recurrent a., radial	a. recurrens radialis	radial a.		brachioradial and brachial muscles, elbow region
recurrent a., ulnar	a. recurrens ulnaris	ulnar a.		elbow region
renal a.	a. renalis	abdominal aorta	anterior and posterior branches, ureteral branches, inferior suprarenal a.	kidney, suprarenal gland, ureter
renal a's. *See* arcuate, interlobar, *and* interlobular a's of kidney *and* straight arterioles of kidney				
retroduodenal a's	aa. retroduodenales	first branch of gastroduodenal a.		bile duct, duodenum, head of pancreas
a. of round ligament of uterus	a. ligamenti teretis uteri	inferior epigastric a.		round ligament of uterus
sacral a's, lateral	aa. sacrales laterales	iliolumbar a.	spinal branches	structures about coccyx and sacrum
sacral a., median	a. sacralis mediana	central continuation of abdominal aorta, beyond origin of common iliac a's	lowest lumbar a.	sacrum, coccyx, rectum
scapular a., dorsal	a. dorsalis scapulae	subclavian a., or may be deep branch of transverse cervical a.		rhomboid, latissimus dorsi, trapezius muscles
scapular a., transverse. *See* suprascapular a.				
sciatic a.	a. comitans nervi ischiadici	inferior gluteal a.		accompanies sciatic nerve
segmental a's of kidney	aa. segmentorum renalium	a group of arteries originating from the anterior or posterior branch of the renal a., consisting of anterior inferior, anterior superior, and posterior segmental a's; each supplies the corresponding renal segment		

TABLE OF ARTERIES *Continued*

Common Name*	TA Equivalent†	Origin*	Branches*	Distribution*
segmental a's of left lung	aa. segmentales pulmonis sinistri	branches of the left pulmonary a. that supply segments of the left lung; variable but often including lingular a's and anterior, apical, posterior, superior, anterior basal, lateral basal, medial basal, and posterior basal segmental a's, named for the segment supplied		
segmental a's of liver	aa. segmentorum hepaticorum	a group of arteries originating from the right or left branch of the proper hepatic a., consisting of anterior, posterior, medial, and lateral segmental a's; each supplies the corresponding region of the liver		
segmental a's of right lung	aa. segmentales pulmonis dextri	branches of the right pulmonary a. that supply segments of the right lung; variable but often including anterior, apical, medial, lateral, posterior, superior, anterior basal, lateral basal, medial basal, and posterior basal segmental a's, named for the segment supplied		
septal a's, anterior	rami interventriculares septales arteriae coronariae sinistrae	anterior interventricular branch of left coronary a.		anterior interventricular septum
septal a's, posterior	rami interventriculares septales arteriae coronariae dextrae	posterior interventricular branch of right coronary a.		posterior interventricular septum
sigmoid a's	aa. sigmoideae	inferior mesenteric a.		sigmoid colon
spermatic a., external. *See* cremasteric a.				
spermatic a., internal. *See* testicular a.				
sphenopalatine a.	a. sphenopalatina	maxillary a.	posterior lateral nasal a. and posterior septal branches	structures adjoining nasal cavity, nasopharynx

spinal a's	rami spinales arteriae vertebralis	transverse part of vertebral a.		spinal cord, meninges, vertebral bodies, intervertebral disks
spinal a., anterior	a. spinalis anterior	vertebral a.		spinal cord
spinal a., posterior	a. spinalis posterior	posterior inferior cerebellar a. (usually)		spinal cord
splenic a.	a. splenica	celiac trunk	pancreatic and splenic branches, prepancreatic, left gastro-omental, short gastric a's	spleen, pancreas, stomach, greater omentum
straight arterioles (or a's) of kidney	arteriolae rectae renis	arcuate a's of kidney		renal pyramids
stylomastoid a.	a. stylomastoidea	posterior auricular a.	mastoid and stapedial branches, posterior tympanica	tympanic cavity walls, mastoid cells, stapedius muscle
subclavian a.	a. subclavia	brachiocephalic trunk (right), arch of aorta (left)	vertebral, internal thoracic a's, thyrocervical and costocervical trunks	neck, thoracic wall, spinal cord, brain, meninges, upper limb
subcostal a.	a. subcostalis	thoracic aorta	dorsal and spinal branches	upper posterior abdominal wall
sublingual a.	a. sublingualis	lingual a.		sublingual gland
submental a.	a. submentalis	facial a.		tissues under chin
subscapular a.	a. subscapularis	axillary a.	thoracodorsal and circumflex scapular a's	scapular and shoulder region
supraduodenal a.	a. supraduodenalis	gastroduodenal a.	duodenal branch	superior part of duodenum
supraorbital a.	a. supraorbitalis	ophthalmic a.	superficial, deep, diploic branches	forehead, superior muscles of orbit, upper eyelid, frontal sinus
suprarenal a., inferior	a. suprarenalis inferior	renal a.		suprarenal gland
suprarenal a., middle	a. suprarenalis media	abdominal aorta		suprarenal gland
suprarenal a's, superior	aa. suprarenales superiores	inferior phrenic a.		suprarenal gland
suprascapular a.	a. suprascapularis	thyrocervical trunk	acromial branch	clavicular, deltoid, and scapular regions
supratrochlear a.	a. supratrochlearis	ophthalmic a.		anterior scalp
sural a's	aa. surales	popliteal a.		popliteal space, calf
sylvian a. See cerebral a., middle				
a. to tail of pancreas. See pancreatic a., caudal				
tarsal a., lateral	a. tarsalis lateralis	dorsalis pedis a.		tarsus
tarsal a's, medial	aa. tarsales mediales	dorsalis pedis a.		side of foot

TABLE OF ARTERIES *Continued*

Common Name*	TA Equivalent†	Origin*	Branches*	Distribution*
temporal a., anterior	r. temporalis anterior arteriae cerebri mediae	middle cerebral a.		cortex of anterior temporal lobe
temporal a., anterior deep	a. temporalis profunda anterior	maxillary a.	to zygomatic bone and greater wing of sphenoid bone	temporal muscle, and anastomoses with middle temporal a.
temporal a., middle	1. a. temporalis media 2. r. temporalis medius arteriae cerebri mediae	1. superficial temporal a. 2. middle cerebral a.		1. temporal region 2. cortex of temporal lobe
temporal a., posterior	r. temporalis posterior arteriae cerebri mediae	middle cerebral a.		cortex of posterior temporal lobe
temporal a., posterior deep	a. temporalis profunda posterior	maxillary a.		temporal muscle, and anastomoses with middle temporal a.
temporal a., superficial	a. temporalis superficialis	external carotid a.	parotid, auricular, and occipital branches; transverse facial, zygomaticoorbital, middle temporal a's	parotid and temporal regions
testicular a.	a. testicularis	abdominal aorta	ureteral and epididymal branches	ureter, epididymis, testis
thoracic a., internal	a. thoracica interna	subclavian a.	mediastinal, thymic, bronchial, tracheal, sternal, perforating, medial mammary, lateral costal and anterior intercostal branches; pericardiacophrenic, musculophrenic, superior epigastric a's	anterior thoracic wall, mediastinal structures, diaphragm
thoracic a., lateral	a. thoracica lateralis	axillary a.	mammary branches	pectoral muscles, mammary gland
thoracic a., superior	a. thoracica superior	axillary a.		axillary aspect of chest wall
thoracoacromial a.	a. thoracoacromialis	axillary a.	clavicular, pectoral, deltoid, and acromial branches	deltoid, clavicular, thoracic regions
thoracodorsal a.	a. thoracodorsalis	subscapular a.		subscapular and teres muscles
thyrocervical trunk	truncus thyrocervicalis	subclavian a.	inferior thyroid, suprascapular and transverse cervical a's	deep neck, including thyroid gland, scapular region
thyroid a., inferior	a. thyroidea inferior	thyrocervical trunk	pharyngeal, esophageal, tracheal branches; inferior laryngeal, ascending cervical a's	thyroid gland and adjacent structures
thyroid a., lowest. *See* thyroidea ima a.				

88

thyroid a., superior	a. thyroidea superior	external carotid a.	hyoid, sternocleidomastoid, superior laryngeal, cricothyroid, muscular, and glandular branches	thyroid gland and adjacent structures
thyroidea ima a.	a. thyroidea ima	arch of aorta, brachiocephalic trunk, or right common carotid, internal mammary, subclavian, or inferior thyroid a.		thyroid gland
tibial a., anterior	a. tibialis anterior	popliteal a.	posterior and anterior tibial recurrent a's, lateral and medial anterior malleolar a's, lateral and medial malleolar retes	leg, ankle, foot
tibial a., posterior	a. tibialis posterior	popliteal a.	fibular circumflex branch; peroneal, medial plantar, lateral plantar a's	leg, foot
transverse a. of face. *See* facial a., transverse				
transverse a. of neck. *See* cervical a., transverse				
tympanic a., anterior	a. tympanica anterior	maxillary a.		tympanic cavity
tympanic a., inferior	a. tympanica inferior	ascending pharyngeal a.		tympanic cavity
tympanic a., posterior	a. tympanica posterior	stylomastoid a.		tympanic cavity
tympanic a., superior	a. tympanica superior	middle meningeal a.		tympanic cavity
ulnar a.	a. ulnaris	brachial a.	palmar carpal, dorsal carpal, and deep palmar branches; ulnar recurrent and common interosseous a's, superficial palmar arch	forearm, wrist, hand
ulnar a., collateral. *See* collateral a., inferior ulnar, *and* collateral a., superior ulnar				
umbilical a.	a. umbilicalis	internal iliac a.	a. of ductus deferens, superior vesical a's	ductus deferens, seminal vesicles, testes, urinary bladder, ureter
urethral a.	a. urethralis	internal pudendal a.		urethra
uterine a.	a. uterina	internal iliac a.	ovarian and tubal branches; vaginal a.	uterus, vagina, round ligament of uterus, uterine tube, ovary
vaginal a.	a. vaginalis	uterine a.		vagina, fundus of bladder

Common Name*	TA Equivalent†	Origin*	Branches*	Distribution*
vertebral a.	a. vertebralis	subclavian a.	*transverse part:* spinal and muscular branches; *intracranial part:* anterior spinal a., and posterior inferior cerebellar a. and its branches	muscles of neck, vertebrae, spinal cord, cerebellum, interior of cerebrum
vesical a., inferior	a. vesicalis inferior	internal iliac a.	prostatic	bladder, prostate, seminal vesicles, lower ureter
vesical a's, superior	aa. vesicales superiores	umbilical a.		bladder, urachus, lower ureter
zygomaticoorbital a.	a. zygomaticoorbitalis	superficial temporal a.		lateral side of orbit

ar·thro·de·sis (-de′sis) the surgical fixation of a joint by a procedure designed to accomplish fusion of the joint surfaces by promoting the proliferation of bone cells; called also *artificial ankylosis*.

ar·thro·dia (ahr-thro′de-ah) a synovial joint which allows a gliding motion. **arthro′dial,** adj.

ar·thro·dys·pla·sia (ahr″thro-dis-pla′zhah) hereditary deformity of various joints.

ar·thro·em·py·e·sis (-em″pi-e′sis) suppuration within a joint.

ar·throg·ra·phy (ahr-throg′rah-fe) radiography of a joint after injection of opaque contrast material. **air a.,** pneumarthrography.

ar·thro·gry·po·sis (ahr″thro-grĭ-po′sis) persistent flexure of a joint.

ar·thro·lith (ahr′thro-lith) calculous deposit within a joint.

ar·throl·o·gy (ahr-throl′ah-je) the study of or the sum of knowledge regarding the joints and ligaments.

ar·thro·neu·ral·gia (ahr″thro-noo-ral′jah) pain in or around a joint.

ar·thro·oph·thal·mop·a·thy (-of″thal-mop′ah-the) an association of degenerative joint disease and eye disease.

ar·throp·a·thy (ahr-throp′ah-the) any joint disease. **arthropath′ic,** adj. **Charcot's a.,** neuropathic a. **chondrocalcific a.,** progressive polyarthritis with joint swelling and bony enlargement, most commonly in the small joints of the hand but also affecting other joints, characterized radiographically by narrowing of the joint space with subchondral erosions and sclerosis and frequently chondrocalcinosis. **neuropathic a.,** chronic progressive degeneration of the stress-bearing portion of a joint, with hypertrophic changes at the periphery; it is associated with neurologic disorders involving loss of sensation in the joint. **osteopulmonary a.,** clubbing of fingers and toes and enlargement of ends of the long bones, in cardiac or pulmonary disease.

ar·thro·plas·ty (ahr′thro-plas″te) joint replacement; plastic repair of a joint.

Ar·throp·o·da (ahr-throp′o-dah) the largest phylum of animals, composed of bilaterally symmetrical organisms with hard, segmented bodies bearing jointed legs, including, among other related forms, arachnids, crustaceans, and insects, many species of which are parasites or are vectors of disease-causing organisms.

ar·thro·py·o·sis (ahr″thro-pi-o′sis) formation of pus in a joint cavity.

ar·thro·scle·ro·sis (-sklĕ-ro′sis) stiffening or hardening of the joints.

ar·thro·scope (ahr′thro-skōp) an endoscope for examining the interior of a joint and for performing diagnostic and therapeutic procedures within the joint.

ar·thros·co·py (ahr-thros′kah-pe) examination of the interior of a joint with an arthroscope.

ar·thro·sis (ahr-thro′sis) 1. joint. 2. arthropathy.

ar·thros·to·my (ahr-thros′tah-me) surgical creation of an opening into a joint, as for drainage.

ar·thro·syn·o·vi·tis (ahr″thro-sin″o-vi′tis) inflammation of the synovial membrane of a joint.

ar·tic·u·lar (ahr-tik′u-ler) pertaining to a joint.

ar·tic·u·la·re (ahr-tik″u-lar′e) the point of intersection of the dorsal contours of the articular process of the mandible and the temporal bone.

ar·tic·u·late¹ (ahr-tik′u-lāt) 1. to pronounce clearly and distinctly. 2. to make speech sounds by manipulation of the vocal organs. 3. to express in coherent verbal form. 4. to divide into or unite so as to form a joint. 5. in dentistry, to adjust or place the teeth in their proper relation to each other in making an artificial denture.

ar·tic·u·late² (ahr-tik′u-lit) 1. divided into distinct, meaningful syllables or words. 2. endowed with the power of speech. 3. characterized by the use of clear, meaningful language. 4. divided into or united by joints.

ar·tic·u·la·tio (ahr-tik″u-la′she-o) pl. *articulatio′nes.* [L.] 1. articulation. 2. synovial joint.

ar·tic·u·la·tion (-la′shun) 1. a joint or place of junction between two different parts or objects. 2. enunciation of words and sentences. 3. in dentistry: (a) the contact relationship of the occlusal surfaces of the teeth while in action; (b) the arrangement of artificial teeth so as to accommodate the various positions of the mouth and to serve the purpose of the natural teeth which they are to replace.

ar·tic·u·lo (ahr-tik′u-lo) [L.] at the moment, or crisis. **a. mor′tis,** at the point or moment of death.

ar·ti·fact (ahr′tĭ-fakt″) any artificial (man-made) product; anything not naturally present, but introduced by some external source.

ary·ep·i·glot·tic (ar″e-ep″ĭ-glot′ik) arytenoepiglottic.

ARVO Association for Research in Vision and Ophthalmology.

aryl- in organic chemistry, a prefix denoting a radical derived from an aromatic compound by removal of a hydrogen atom.

ar·yl·for·mam·i·dase (ar″il-for-mam′ĭ-dās) an enzyme that catalyzes the hydrolytic cleavage of formylkynurenine in the catabolism of tryptophan; it also acts on other formyl aromatic amines.

ar·y·te·no·ep·i·glot·tic (ar-it″ĕ-no-ep″ĭ-glot′ik) pertaining to the arytenoid cartilage and to the epiglottis.

ar·y·te·noid (ar″ĭ-te′noid) shaped like a jug or pitcher, as arytenoid cartilage.

ar·y·te·noi·do·pexy (ar″ĭ-te-noi′do-pek″se) surgical fixation of arytenoid cartilage or muscle.

AS¹ [L.] au′ris sinis′tra (left ear).

AS² aortic stenosis; arteriosclerosis.

As arsenic.

ASA acetylsalicylic acid; American Society of Anesthesiologists; American Standards Association; American Surgical Association; argininosuccinic acid; antisperm antibody.

5-ASA mesalamine (5-aminosalicylic acid).

asa·na (ah-sah′nah) [Sanskrit] any of the postures used in hatha yoga for the purpose of achieving balance, promoting physical health, and attaining mental relaxation.

as·bes·tos (as-bes′tos) a fibrous incombustible magnesium and calcium silicate used in thermal insulation; its dust causes asbestosis and acts as an epigenetic carcinogen for pleural mesothelioma. It is divided into two main classes: *amphibole a.*, less widely used and more highly carcinogenic and including amosite and crocidolite, and *serpentine a.*, including chrysotile.

as·bes·to·sis (as″bes-to′sis) pneumoconiosis caused by inhaled asbestos fibers, characterized by interstitial fibrosis, sometimes followed by pleural mesothelioma and bronchogenic carcinoma.

as·ca·ri·a·sis (as″kah-ri′ah-sis) infection with the roundworm *Ascaris lumbricoides*. After ingestion, the larvae migrate first to the lungs then to the intestine.

as·car·i·cide (as-kar′ĭ-sīd″) an agent that destroys ascarids. **ascarici′dal**, adj.

as·ca·rid (as′kah-rid) any of the phasmid nematodes of the Ascaridoidea, which includes the genera *Ascaridia*, *Ascaris*, and *Toxocara*.

As·ca·ris (-ris) a genus of nematode parasites of the large intestine. *A. lumbricoi′des* causes ascariasis.

as·ca·ris (-ris) a nematode of the genus *Ascaris*.

as·cend·ing (ah-send′ing) having an upward course.

as·cer·tain·ment (ă″ser-tān′ment) in genetics, the method by which persons with a trait are selected or discovered by an investigator.

ASCH American Society of Clinical Hypnosis.

Asc·hel·min·thes (ask″hel-minth′ēz) a phylum of unsegmented, bilaterally symmetrical, pseudocoelomate, mostly vermiform animals whose bodies are almost entirely covered with a cuticle, and which possess a complete digestive tract lacking definite muscular walls.

ASCI American Society for Clinical Investigation.

as·ci·tes (ah-si′tēz) effusion and accumulation of serous fluid in the abdominal cavity. **ascit′ic**, adj. **chyliform a., chylous a.,** the presence of chyle in the peritoneal cavity owing to anomalies, injuries, or obstruction of the thoracic duct.

ASCLT American Society of Clinical Laboratory Technicians.

As·co·my·ce·tes (as″ko-mi-se′tēz) in some systems of classification, a class of fungi of the division Eumycota; see *Ascomycotina*.

As·co·my·co·ti·na (-mi″ko-ti′nah) a subdivision of fungi of the division Dikaryomycota (or in some classifications the Eumycota; in others it is considered a class, Ascomycetes, in the Eumycota) characterized by formation of an ascus in which sexual spores are produced; it includes the yeasts, mildews, and cheese, jelly, and fruit molds.

ascor·bic ac·id (ah-skor′bik) vitamin C, a water-soluble vitamin found in many vegetables and fruits, and an essential element in the diet of humans and many other animals; deficiency produces scurvy and poor wound repair. It is used as an antiscorbutic and nutritional supplement, in the treatment of iron-deficiency anemia and chronic iron toxicity, and in the labeling of red blood cells with sodium chromate Cr 51.

ASCP American Society of Clinical Pathologists.

ASCVD arteriosclerotic cardiovascular disease.

-ase suffix used in enzyme names, affixed to a stem indicating the substrate (luciferase), the general nature of the substrate (proteinase), the reaction catalyzed (hydrolase), or a combination of these (transaminase).

as·e·ma·sia (as″ĕ-ma′zhah) asemia.

ase·mia (a-se′me-ah) aphasia with inability to employ or to understand either speech or signs.

asep·sis (a-sep′sis) 1. freedom from infection. 2. the prevention of contact with microorganisms.

asep·tic (-tik) free from infection or septic material.

asex·u·al (a-sek′shoo-al) having no sex; not sexual; not pertaining to sex.

ASH American Society of Hematology; asymmetrical septal hypertrophy.

ASHA American School Health Association; American Speech and Hearing Association.

ASHD arteriosclerotic heart disease; see *ischemic heart disease*, under *disease*.

ASHP American Society of Hospital Pharmacists.

asi·a·lia (a″si-a′le-ah) aptyalism.

asid·er·o·sis (a″sid-er-o′sis) deficiency of iron reserve of the body.

ASII American Science Information Institute.

ASIM American Society of Internal Medicine.

-asis word element, *state; condition*.

Asn asparagine.

ASO arteriosclerosis obliterans.

aso·ma·tog·no·sia (ah-so″mah-tog-no′zhah) lack of awareness of the condition of all or part of one's body.

ASP American Society of Parasitologists.

Asp aspartic acid.

as·par·a·gin·ase (as-par′ah-jin-ās″) an enzyme that catalyzes the deamination of asparagine; a preparation is used as an antineoplastic agent in acute lymphoblastic leukemia to reduce availability of asparagine to tumor cells.

as·par·a·gine (as-par′ah-jēn, as-par′ah-jin) the β-amide of aspartic acid, a nonessential amino acid occurring in proteins; used in bacterial culture media. Symbols Asn and N.

as·par·tame (ah-spahr′tām, as′pahr-tām″) an artificial sweetener about 200 times as sweet as sucrose and used as a low-calorie sweetener.

as·par·tate (ah-spahr′tāt) a salt of aspartic acid, or aspartic acid in dissociated form.

as·par·tate trans·am·i·nase (AST, ASAT) (trans-am′ĭ-nās) an enzyme normally present in body tissues, especially in the heart and liver; it is released into the serum as the result of tissue injury, hence the concentration in the serum (SGOT) may be increased in disorders such as myocardial infarction or acute damage to hepatic cells.

as·par·tic ac·id (ah-spahr′tik) a nonessential, natural dibasic amino acid occurring in proteins and also an excitatory neurotransmitter in the central nervous system. Symbols Asp and D.

as·pect (as′pekt) that part of a surface facing in any designated direction. **dorsal a.,** that surface of a body viewed from the back (human anatomy) or from above (veterinary anatomy). **ventral a.,** that surface of a body viewed from the front (human anatomy) or from below (veterinary anatomy).

as·per·gil·lo·ma (as″per-jil-o′mah) the most common kind of fungus ball, caused by *Aspergillus* in a bronchus or lung cavity.

as·per·gil·lo·sis (-o′sis) a disease caused by species of *Aspergillus*, marked by inflammatory granulomatous lesions in the skin, ear, orbit, nasal sinuses, lungs, bones, and meninges.

as·per·gil·lo·tox·i·co·sis (as″per-jil″o-tok″sĭ-ko′sis) mycotoxicosis caused by *Aspergillus.*

As·per·gil·lus (as″per-jil′us) a genus of fungi (molds), various species of which are endoparasitic and opportunistic pathogens, and some of which produce antibiotics; it includes *A. clava′tus, A. fla′vus, A. fumiga′tus, A. ni′dulans, A. ni′ger, A. ochra′ceus,* and *A. ter′reus.*

asper·ma·to·gen·e·sis (a-sper″mah-to-jen′ĕ-sis) failure in a male of production of spermatozoa.

asper·mia (ah-sper′me-ah) 1. aspermatogenesis. 2. anejaculation.

as·phyx·ia (as-fik′se-ah) pathological changes caused by lack of oxygen in respired air, resulting in hypoxia and hypercapnia. **as·phyx′ial,** adj. **fetal a.,** asphyxia in utero due to hypoxia. **a. neonato′rum,** respiratory failure in the newborn; see also *respiratory distress syndrome of newborn,* under *syndrome.* **traumatic a.,** that due to sudden or severe compression of the thorax or upper abdomen, or both.

as·phyx·i·a·tion (as-fix″e-a′shun) suffocation; the stoppage of respiration.

as·pi·ra·tion (as″pi-ra′shun) 1. the drawing of a foreign substance, such as the gastric contents, into the respiratory tract during inhalation. 2. removal by suction, as the removal of fluid or gas from a body cavity or the procurement of biopsy specimens. **meconium a.,** aspiration of meconium by the fetus or newborn, which may result in atelectasis, emphysema, pneumothorax, or pneumonia. **microsurgical epididymal sperm a. (MESA),** retrieval of sperm from the epididymis using microsurgical techniques, done in men with obstructive azoospermia. **vacuum a.,** removal of the uterine contents by application of a vacuum through a hollow curet or a cannula introduced into the uterus.

as·pi·rin (as'pǐ-rin) acetylsalicylic acid, a nonsteroidal antiinflammatory drug having analgesic, antipyretic, antiinflammatory, and antirheumatic activity; also an inhibitor of platelet aggregation.

as·ple·nia (a-sple'ne-ah) absence of the spleen. **functional a.,** impaired reticuloendothelial function of the spleen, as seen in children with sickle cell anemia.

ASRT American Society of Radiologic Technologists.

as·say (as'a) determination of the amount of a particular constituent of a mixture, or of the potency of a drug. **biological a.,** bioassay. **CH50 a.,** a test of total complement activity as the capacity of serum to lyse a standard preparation of sheep red blood cells coated with antisheep erythrocyte antibody. The reciprocal of the dilution of serum that lyses 50 per cent of the erythrocytes is the whole complement titer in CH50 units per milliliter of serum. **enzyme-linked immunosorbent a.,** see *ELISA.* **microbiological a.,** assay by the use of microorganisms. **microcytotoxicity a.,** one using the pattern of lysis of peripheral blood lymphocytes in the presence of complement and typing sera to type serologically defined HLA antigens (HLA-A, -B, and -C antigens). **radioimmunoprecipitation a. (RIPA),** immunoprecipitation conducted with radiolabeled antibody or antigen. **radioligand a.,** any assay procedure that uses radioisotopic labeling and biologically specific binding of reagents. **stem cell a.,** a measurement of the potency of antineoplastic drugs, based on their ability to retard the growth of cultures of human tumor cells.

as·ser·tive·ness (ah-ser'tiv-nes) the quality or state of bold or confident self-expression, neither aggressive nor submissive.

as·sim·i·la·tion (ah-sim"ĭ-la'shun) 1. psychologically, absorption of new experiences into existing psychologic make-up. 2. anabolism.

as·sis·tant (ah-sis'tant) one who aids or helps another; an auxiliary. **physician a.,** see under *physician.*

as·so·ci·at·ed (ah-so'she-āt"ed) connected; accompanying; joined with another or others.

as·so·ci·a·tion (ah-so"se-a'shun) 1. a state in which two attributes occur together either more or less often than expected by chance. 2. a term applied to those regions of the brain that link the primary motor and sensory cortices; see *association areas,* under *area.* 3. the occurrence together of two or more phenotypic characteristics more often than

would be expected by chance. 4. a connection between ideas or feelings, especially between conscious thoughts and elements of the unconscious, or the formation of such a connection. **CHARGE a.,** a syndrome of associated defects including coloboma of the eye, heart anomaly, choanal atresia, retardation, and genital and ear anomalies, and often including facial palsy, cleft palate, and dysphagia. **free a.,** verbal expression of one's ideas as they arrive spontaneously; a method used in psychoanalysis.

as·sor·ta·tive (ah-sor'tah-tiv) characterized by or pertaining to selection on the basis of likeness or kind.

as·sor·tive (ah-sor'tiv) assortative.

as·sort·ment (ah-sort'ment) the random distribution of nonhomologous chromosomes to daughter cells in metaphase of the first meiotic division.

AST aspartate transaminase.

asta·sia (as-ta'zhah) motor incoordination with inability to stand. **astat'ic,** adj. **a.-aba'-sia,** inability to stand or walk although the legs are otherwise under control.

as·ta·tine (as'tah-tēn) chemical element (see *Table of Elements*), at. no. 85, symbol At.

aste·a·to·sis (as"te-ah-to'sis) any disease in which persistent dry scaling of the skin suggests scantiness or absence of sebum. **asteatot'ic,** adj.

as·ter (as'ter) [L.] a system of microtubules arranged in starlike rays around each pair of centrioles during mitosis.

as·te·ri·on (as-tēr'e-on) pl. *aste'ria.* [Gr.] the point on the skull at the junction of occipital, parietal, and temporal bones.

as·ter·ix·is (as"ter-ik'sis) a motor disturbance marked by intermittent lapses of an assumed posture as a result of intermittency of sustained contraction of groups of muscles; called *liver flap* because of its occurrence in hepatic coma, but observed also in other conditions.

aster·nal (a-ster'n'l) 1. not joined to the sternum. 2. lacking a sternum.

as·ter·oid (as'ter-oid) star-shaped.

as·the·nia (as-the'ne-ah) lack or loss of strength and energy; weakness. **neurocirculatory a.,** a syndrome of breathlessness, fear of effort, a sense of fatigue, precordial pain, and palpitation, generally considered to be a particular presentation of an anxiety disorder. **tropical anhidrotic a.,** a condition due to generalized anhidrosis in conditions of high temperature, characterized by a tendency to overfatigability, irritability, anorexia, inability to concentrate, and drowsiness, with headache and vertigo.

asthen(o)- word element [Gr.], *weak; weakness.*

as·the·no·co·ria (as-the″no-kor′e-ah) sluggishness of the pupillary light reflex; seen in hypoadrenalism.

as·the·no·pia (as″thĕ-no′pe-ah) weakness or easy fatigue of the eye, with pain in the eyes, headache, dimness of vision, etc. **asthenop′ic,** adj. **accommodative a.,** asthenopia due to strain of the ciliary muscle. **muscular a.,** asthenopia due to weakness of external ocular muscles.

as·the·no·sper·mia (as″thĕ-no-sper′me-ah) asthenozoospermia.

as·the·no·zo·o·sper·mia (-zo″o-sper′me-ah) reduced motility or vitality of spermatozoa.

as·thma (az′mah) recurrent attacks of paroxysmal dyspnea, with wheezing due to spasmodic contraction of the bronchi. It is usually either an allergic manifestation (*allergic* or *extrinsic a.)* or secondary to a chronic or recurrent condition (*intrinsic a.).* **asthmat′ic,** adj. **bronchial a.,** asthma.

astig·ma·tism (ah-stig′mah-tizm) ametropia caused by differences in curvature in different meridians of the refractive surfaces of the eye so that light rays are not sharply focused on the retina. **astigmat′ic,** adj. **compound a.,** that complicated with hypermetropia or myopia in all meridians. **corneal a.,** that due to irregularity in the curvature or refracting power of the cornea. **irregular a.,** that in which the curvature varies in different parts of the same meridian or in which refraction in successive meridians differs irregularly. **mixed a.,** that in which one principal meridian is myopic and the other hyperopic. **myopic a.,** that in which the light rays are brought to a focus in front of the retina. **regular a.,** that in which the refractive power of the eye shows a uniform increase or decrease from one meridian to another.

as·trag·a·lus (as-trag′ah-lus) talus; see *Table of Bones.* **astrag′alar,** adj.

as·tral (as′tral) of or relating to an aster.

as·tra·pho·bia (as″trah-fo′be-ah) irrational fear of thunder and lightning.

astrin·gen·cy (ah-strin′jen-se) the quality of being astringent.

astrin·gent (ah-strin′jent) 1. causing contraction, usually locally after topical application. 2. an agent that so acts.

as·tro·blast (as′tro-blast) an embryonic cell that develops into an astrocyte.

as·tro·blas·to·ma (as″tro-blas-to′mah) an astrocytoma of Grade II; its cells resemble astroblasts, with abundant cytoplasm and two or three nuclei.

as·tro·cyte (as′tro-sīt) a neuroglial cell of ectodermal origin, characterized by fibrous, protoplasmic, or plasmatofibrous processes. Collectively called *astroglia.*

as·tro·cy·to·ma (as″tro-si-to′mah) a tumor composed of astrocytes; the most common type of primary brain tumor and also found throughout the central nervous system, classified on the basis of histology or in order of malignancy (Grades I–IV).

as·trog·lia (as-trog′le-ah) 1. astrocytes. 2. the astrocytes considered as tissue.

As·tro·vi·rus (as′tro-vi″rus) an unofficial name for a group of RNA viruses with a single-stranded genome about the same size as that of the picornaviruses; they cause gastroenteritis in humans and other animals and hepatitis in ducklings.

as·tro·vi·rus (as′tro-vi″rus) any virus belonging to the group *Astrovirus.*

asym·me·try (a-sim′ĕ-tre) lack or absence of symmetry; dissimilarity in corresponding parts or organs on opposite sides of the body which are normally alike. In chemistry, lack of symmetry in the special arrangements of the atoms and radicals within the molecule or crystal. **asymmet′rical,** adj.

asyn·chro·nism (a-sing′krah-nizm) asynchrony.

asyn·chro·ny 1. lack of synchronism; disturbance of coordination. 2. occurrence at distinct times of events normally synchronous; disturbance of coordination. **asyn′chronous,** adj.

asyn·cli·tism (ah-sing′klĭ-tizm) 1. oblique presentation of the fetal head in labor, called *anterior a.* when the anterior parietal bone is designated the point of presentation, and *posterior a.* when the posterior parietal bone is so designated. 2. maturation at different times of the nucleus and cytoplasm of blood cells.

asyn·de·sis (ah-sin′dĕ-sis) a language disorder in which related elements of a sentence cannot be welded together as a whole.

asyn·ech·ia (a″sin-ek′e-ah) absence of continuity of structure.

asyn·er·gy (a-sin′er-je) lack of coordination among parts or organs normally acting in unison.

asys·to·le (a-sis′to-le) cardiac standstill or arrest; absence of heartbeat. **asystol′ic,** adj.

AT atrial tachycardia.

At astatine.

atac·ti·form (ah-tak′tĭ-form) resembling ataxia.

at·a·vism (at'ah-vizm) apparent inheritance of a characteristic from remote rather than immediate ancestors. **atavis'tic,** adj.

atax·ia (ah-tak'se-ah) failure of muscular coordination; irregularity of muscular action. **atac'tic, atax'ic,** adj. **Bruns' frontal a.,** a disturbance of equilibrium and gait due to a lesion in the frontal lobe, characterized by assumption of a broad-based gait with the feet flat on the ground and a tendency to retropulsion. **Friedreich's a.,** hereditary sclerosis of the dorsal and lateral columns of the spine, usually beginning in childhood or youth; it is attended with ataxia, speech impairment, scoliosis, peculiar movements, paralysis, and often hypertrophic cardiomyopathy. **locomotor a.,** tabes dorsalis. **motor a.,** inability to control the coordinate movements of the muscles. **sensory a.,** ataxia due to loss of proprioception (joint position sensation) between the motor cortex and peripheral nerves, resulting in poorly judged movements, the incoordination becoming aggravated when the eyes are closed. **a.-telangiectasia,** a severe autosomal recessive progressive cerebellar ataxia, associated with oculocutaneous telangiectasia, abnormal eye movements, sinopulmonary disease, and immunodeficiency.

at·e·lec·ta·sis (at'ah-lek'tah-sis) incomplete expansion of the lungs at birth, or collapse of the adult lung. **atelectat'ic,** adj. **absorption a., acquired a.,** obstructive atelectasis; that caused by an obstruction of the airway that prevents intake of air, e.g., secretions, foreign body, tumor, or external pressure. **congenital a.,** that present at birth *(primary a.)* or immediately thereafter *(secondary a.)*. **lobar a.,** that affecting only one lobe of the lung. **lobular a.,** that affecting only a lobule of the lung. **obstructive a.,** acquired a. **segmental a.,** that affecting one segment of a lung. **tympanic membrane a.,** a complication of chronic serous otitis media, with viscous fluid in the middle ear and thinning of the tympanic membrane, which adheres to middle ear structures; there is usually conductive deafness.

ate·lia (ah-te'le-ah) imperfect or incomplete development. **ateliot'ic,** adj.

atel(o)- word element [Gr.], *incomplete; imperfectly developed.*

at·e·lo·car·dia (at''ĕ-lo-kahr'de-ah) imperfect development of the heart.

aten·o·lol (ah-ten'ah-lol) a cardioselective β_1-adrenergic blocking agent used in the treatment of hypertension and chronic angina pectoris and the prophylaxis and treatment of myocardial infarction and cardiac arrhythmias.

ATG antithymocyte globulin.

athe·lia (ah-the'le-ah) congenital absence of the nipples.

ath·er·ec·to·my (ath''er-ek'tah-me) the removal of atherosclerotic plaque from an artery using a rotary cutter inside a special catheter guided radiographically; it does not extend to the tunica intima as endarterectomy does.

ather·mic (a-ther'mik) without rise of temperature; afebrile; apyretic.

ather·mo·sys·tal·tic (ah-ther''mo-sis-tahl'-tik) not contracting under the action of cold or heat; said of skeletal muscle.

ath·ero·em·bo·lus (ath''er-o-em'bo-lus) pl. *atheroem'boli.* An embolus composed of cholesterol or its esters or of fragments of atheromatous plaques, typically lodging in small arteries.

ath·ero·gen·e·sis (-jen'ĕ-sis) formation of atheromatous lesions in arterial walls. **atherogen'ic,** adj.

ath·er·o·ma (ath''er-o'mah) a mass or plaque of degenerated thickened arterial intima, occurring in atherosclerosis.

ath·er·o·ma·to·sis (ath''er-o-mah-to'sis) diffuse atheromatous arterial disease.

ath·ero·scle·ro·sis (-sklĕ-ro'sis) a form of arteriosclerosis in which atheromas containing cholesterol, lipoid material, and lipophages are formed within the intima and inner media of large and medium-sized arteries. **atherosclerot·ic,** adj.

ath·e·to·sis (ath''ĕ-to'sis) repetitive involuntary, slow, sinuous, writhing movements, especially severe in the hands.

athrep·sia (ah-threp'se-ah) marasmus. **athrep'tic,** adj.

athym·ia (ah-thīm'e-ah) 1. dementia. 2. absence of functioning thymus tissue.

athy·ria (ah-thi're-ah) 1. hypothyroidism. 2. complete absence of thyroid function. **athyrot'ic,** adj.

ATL adult T-cell leukemia/lymphoma.

at·lan·tad (at-lan'tad) toward the atlas.

at·lan·tal (at-lan't'l) pertaining to the atlas.

at·lan·to·ax·i·al (at-lan''to-ak'se-al) pertaining to the atlas and the axis.

at·lan·to·oc·cip·i·tal (-ok-sip'ĭ-t'l) pertaining to the atlas and the occiput.

at·las (at'las) the first cervical vertebra; see *Table of Bones.*

at·lo·ax·oid (at''lo-ak'soid) atlantoaxial.

atm atmosphere (3).

at·mos·phere (at'mos-fēr) 1. the entire gaseous envelope surrounding the earth and subject to the earth's gravitational field.

2. the air or climate in a particular place.
3. a unit of pressure, being that exerted by the earth's atmosphere at sea level; equal to 1.01325×10^5 pascals (approximately 760 mm Hg). Abbreviated atm.

at·mos·pher·ic (at″mos-fer′ik) of or pertaining to the atmosphere.

at no atomic number.

ato·cia (a-to′shah) sterility in the female.

at·om (at′om) the smallest particle of an element with all the properties of the element; it consists of a positively charged nucleus (made up of protons and neutrons) and negatively charged electrons, which move in orbits about the nucleus. **atom′ic**, adj.

at·om·i·za·tion (at″om-ĭ-za′shun) nebulization.

at·om·iz·er (at′om-i″zer) nebulizer.

at·o·ny (at′ah-ne) lack of normal tone or strength; flaccidity. **aton′ic**, adj.

atop·ic (a-top′ik, ah-top′ik) 1. ectopic. 2. pertaining to atopy; allergic.

atop·og·no·sia (ah-top″og-no′zhah) loss of the power of topognosia (ability to correctly locate a sensation).

at·o·py (at′ah-pe) a genetic predisposition toward the development of immediate hypersensitivity reactions against common environmental antigens (atopic allergy), most commonly manifested as allergic rhinitis but also as bronchial asthma, atopic dermatitis, or food allergy.

ator·va·stat·in (ah-tor″vah-stat′in) an antihyperlipidemic agent that acts by inhibiting cholesterol synthesis, used as the calcium salt in the treatment of hypercholesterolemia and other forms of dyslipidemia.

ato·va·quone (ah-to′vah-kwōn) an antibiotic used in treatment of mild to moderate *Pneumocystis carinii* pneumonia and the prophylaxis and treatment of falciparum malaria.

atox·ic (a-tok′sik) not poisonous; not due to a poison.

ATP adenosine triphosphate.

ATPase adenosinetriphosphatase.

atra·cu·rium (at″rah-kūr′e-um) a non-depolarizing neuromuscular blocking agent of intermediate duration, used as the besylate salt as an adjunct to general anesthesia.

atrans·fer·ri·ne·mia (a-trans″fer-ĭ-ne′-me-ah) absence of circulating iron-binding protein (transferrin).

atrau·mat·ic (a″traw-mat′ik) not producing injury or damage.

atre·sia (ah-tre′zhah) congenital absence or closure of a normal body opening or tubular structure. **atret′ic**, adj. **anal a., a. a′ni,** imperforate anus. **aortic a.,** congenital absence of the aortic orifice. **biliary a.,** obliteration or hypoplasia of part of the bile ducts due to arrested fetal development, causing persistent jaundice and liver damage ranging from biliary stasis to biliary cirrhosis, with splenomegaly as portal hypertension progresses. **follicular a.,** degeneration and resorption of an ovarian follicle before it reaches maturity and ruptures. **laryngeal a.,** congenital lack of the normal opening into the larynx. **mitral a.,** congenital obliteration of the mitral orifice, often associated with hypoplastic left heart syndrome or transposition on great vessels. **prepyloric a.,** pyloric atresia; congenital membranous obstruction of the gastric outlet, with vomiting of gastric contents only. **pulmonary a.,** congenital severe narrowing or obstruction of the pulmonary orifice, with cardiomegaly, reduced pulmonary vascularity, and right ventricular atrophy. It is usually associated with tetralogy of Fallot, transposition of great vessels, or other cardiovascular anomalies. **pyloric a.,** prepyloric a. **tricuspid a.,** congenital absence of the tricuspid orifice, circulation being made possible by the presence of an atrial septal defect. **urethral a.,** imperforation of the urethra.

atri·al (a′tre-al) pertaining to an atrium.

atrio·his·i·an (a″tre-o-his′e-an) connecting the atrium and the bundle of His.

atrio·meg·a·ly (-meg′ah-le) abnormal enlargement of an atrium of the heart.

atrio·sep·tal (sep′t′l) pertaining to or occurring in the interatrial septum.

atrio·sep·to·pexy (-sep′to-pek″se) surgical correction of a defect in the interatrial septum.

atrio·sep·to·plas·ty (-sep′to-plas″te) plastic repair of the interatrial septum.

atrio·ven·tric·u·lar (-ven-trik′u-ler) pertaining to both an atrium and a ventricle of the heart.

atri·o·ven·tric·u·la·ris   com·mu·nis (-ven-trik″u-la′ris kŏ-mu′nis) a congenital cardiac anomaly in which the endocardial cushions fail to fuse, the ostium primum persists, the atrioventricular canal is undivided, a single atrioventricular valve has anterior and posterior cusps, and there is a defect of the membranous interventricular septum.

atri·um (a′tre-um) pl. *a′tria*. [L.] a chamber; in anatomy, a chamber affording entrance to another structure or organ, especially the upper, smaller cavity (*a. cordis*) on either side of the heart, which receives blood from the pulmonary veins (*left a.*) or venae cavae (*right a.*) and delivers it to the ventricle on the same side. **a′trial,** adj. **common a.,** the single atrium found in a form of three-chambered heart.

atro·phic (a-tro′fik) pertaining to or characterized by atrophy.

at·ro·pho·der·ma (at″ro-fo-der′mah) atrophy of the skin.

at·ro·phy (at′ro-fe) 1. a wasting away; a diminution in the size of a cell, tissue, organ, or part. 2. to undergo or cause atrophy. **acute yellow a.,** the shrunken, yellow liver which is a complication, usually fatal, of fulminant hepatitis with massive hepatic necrosis. **Aran-Duchenne muscular a.,** spinal muscular a. **bone a.,** resorption of bone evident in both external form and internal density. **Duchenne-Aran muscular a.,** spinal muscular a. **healed yellow a.,** macronodular cirrhosis. **Leber's hereditary optic a.,** see under *neuropathy*. **lobar a.,** Pick's disease (1). **myelopathic muscular a.,** muscular atrophy due to lesion of the spinal cord, as in spinal muscular atrophy. **olivopontocerebellar a.,** any of a group of progressive hereditary disorders involving degeneration of the cerebellar cortex, middle peduncles, ventral pontine surface, and olivary nuclei. They occur in the young to middle-aged and are characterized by ataxia, dysarthria, and tremors similar to those of parkinsonism. **optic a.,** atrophy of the optic disk due to degeneration of the nerve fibers of the optic nerve and optic tract. **peroneal a., peroneal muscular a.,** Charcot-Marie-Tooth disease. **physiologic a.,** that affecting certain organs in all individuals as part of the normal aging process. **senile a. of skin,** the mild atrophic changes in the dermis and epidermis that occur naturally with aging. **spinal muscular a.,** progressive degeneration of the motor cells of the spinal cord, beginning usually in the small muscles of the hands, but in some cases (scapulohumeral type) in the upper arm and shoulder muscles, and progressing slowly to the leg muscles. **Sudeck's a.,** post-traumatic osteoporosis.

at·ro·pine (at′ro-pēn) an anticholinergic and antispasmodic alkaloid used as the sulfate salt to relax smooth muscles and increase and regulate the heart rate by blocking the vagus nerve, and to act as a preanesthetic antisialagogue, an antidote for various toxic and anticholinesterase agents and as an antisecretory, mydriatic, and cycloplegic.

ATS American Thoracic Society; antitetanic serum.

at·tack (ah-tak′) an episode or onset of illness. **Adams-Stokes a.,** an episode of syncope in Adams-Stokes syndrome. **drop a.,** sudden loss of balance without loss of consciousness, usually seen in elderly women. **panic a.,** an episode of acute intense anxiety, the essential feature of panic disorder. **transient ischemic a. (TIA),** a brief attack (an hour or less) of cerebral dysfunction of vascular origin, without lasting neurological effect. **vagal a., vasovagal a.,** a transient vascular and neurogenic reaction marked by pallor, nausea, sweating, bradycardia, and rapid fall in arterial blood pressure, which may result in syncope.

at·ta·pul·gite (at″ah-pul′jīt) a hydrated silicate of aluminum and magnesium, a clay mineral that is the main ingredient of fuller's earth; *activated a.* is a heat-treated form that is used in the treatment of diarrhea.

at·tend·ing (ah-ten′ding) 1. attending physician. 2. being or pertaining to such a physician.

at·ten·u·ate (ah-ten′u-āt) 1. to render thin. 2. to render less virulent.

at·ten·u·a·tion (ah-ten″u-a′shun) the act of thinning or weakening, as *(a)* the alteration of virulence of a pathogenic microorganism by passage through another host species, decreasing the virulence of the organism for the native host and increasing it for the new host, or *(b)* the process by which a beam of radiation is reduced in energy when passed through tissue or other material.

at·tic (at′ik) epitympanic recess.

at·ti·co·an·trot·o·my (at″ĭ-ko-an-trot′ah-me) surgical exposure of the attic and mastoid antrum.

at·ti·tude (at′ĭ-tōōd) 1. a position of the body; in obstetrics, the relation of the various parts of the fetal body. 2. a pattern of mental views established by cumulative prior experience.

atto- word element [Danish], *eighteen*; used in naming units of measurement to designate an amount one quintillionth (10^{-18}) the size of the unit to which it is joined; symbol a.

at·trac·tion (ah-trak′shun) 1. the force, act, or process that draws one body toward another. 2. malocclusion in which the occlusal plane is closer than normal to the eye-ear plane, causing shortening of the face; cf. *abstraction* (3). **capillary a.,** the force which causes a liquid to rise in a fine-caliber tube.

at wt atomic weight.

atyp·ia (a-tip′e-ah) deviation from the normal. **koilocytotic a.,** vacuolization and nuclear abnormalities of cells of the stratified squamous epithelium of the uterine cervix; it may be premalignant.

atyp·i·cal (-ĭ-k'l) irregular; not conformable to the type; in microbiology, applied specifically to strains of unusual type.

AU [L.] aures unitas, both ears together; auris uterque, each ear.

Au gold (L. *au'rum*).

audi(o)- word element [L.], *hearing.*

au·dio·gen·ic (aw"de-o-jen'ik) produced by sound.

au·di·ol·o·gy (aw"de-ol'ah-je) the study of impaired hearing that cannot be improved by medication or surgical therapy.

au·di·om·e·try (aw"de-om'ĭ-tre) measurement of the acuity of hearing for the various frequencies of sound waves. **audiomet'ric,** adj. **Békésy a.,** that in which the patient, by pressing a signal button, traces monaural thresholds for pure tones: the intensity of the tone decreases as long as the button is depressed and increases when it is released; both continuous and interrupted tones are used. **cortical a.,** an objective method of determining auditory acuity by recording and averaging electric potentials evoked from the cortex of the brain in response to stimulation by pure tones. **electrocochleographic a.,** measurement of electrical potentials from the middle ear or external auditory canal (cochlear microphonics and eighth nerve action potentials) in response to acoustic stimuli. **electrodermal a.,** audiometry in which the subject is conditioned by harmless electric shock to pure tones, thereafter anticipating a shock when hearing a pure tone; the anticipation results in a brief electrodermal response, which is recorded; the lowest intensity at which the response is elicited is taken to be the hearing threshold. **localization a.,** a technique for measuring the capacity to locate the source of a pure tone received binaurally in a sound field. **pure tone a.,** audiometry utilizing pure tones that are relatively free of noise and overtones.

au·di·tion (aw-dish'un) hearing. **chromatic a.,** color hearing.

au·di·to·ry (aw'dĭ-tor"e) 1. aural or otic; pertaining to the ear. 2. pertaining to hearing.

aug·men·ta·tion (awg"men-ta'shun) an adding on, or the resulting condition.

AUL acute undifferentiated leukemia.

au·la (aw'lah) the red areola formed around a vaccination vesicle.

au·ra (aw'rah) pl. *auras* or *au'rae.* [L.] a subjective sensation or motor phenomenon that precedes and marks the onset of a neurological condition, particularly an epileptic seizure (*epileptic a.*) or migraine (*migraine a.*). **epileptic a.,** a type of simple partial seizure, experienced as a subjective sensation or motor phenomenon, that sometimes signals an approaching generalized or complex partial seizure. **vertiginous a.,** a sensory seizure affecting the vestibular sense, causing a feeling of vertigo.

au·ral (aw'r'l) 1. auditory (1). 2. pertaining to an aura.

au·ran·o·fin (aw-ran'ah-fin) a gold-containing compound used in the treatment of active rheumatoid arthritis.

au·ric (aw'rik) pertaining to or containing gold.

au·ri·cle (aw'rĭ-k'l) 1. pinna; the flap of the ear. 2. the ear-shaped appendage of either atrium of the heart. 3. formerly, the atrium of the heart.

au·ric·u·la (aw-rik'u-lah) pl. *auri'culae.* [L.] auricle.

au·ric·u·lar (aw-rik'u-lar) 1. pertaining to an auricle. 2. pertaining to the ear.

au·ric·u·la·re (aw-rik'u-lar'e) a point at the top of the opening of the external auditory meatus.

au·ric·u·la·ris (aw-rik"u-lar'is) [L.] pertaining to the ear; auricular.

au·ris (aw'ris) [L.] ear.

au·ri·scope (aw'rĭ-skōp) otoscope.

au·ro·thio·glu·cose (aw"ro-thi"o-gloo'kōs) a monovalent gold salt used in treating rheumatoid arthritis.

aus·cul·ta·tion (aws"kul-ta'shun) listening for sounds within the body, chiefly to ascertain the condition of the thoracic or abdominal viscera and to detect pregnancy; it may be performed with the unaided ear (*direct* or *immediate a.*) or with a stethoscope (*mediate a.*). **auscul'tatory,** adj.

au·te·cic (aw-te'sik) autoecious.

au·te·cious (aw-te'shus) autoecious.

au·tism (aw'tizm) 1. autistic disorder. 2. autistic thinking. **infantile a.,** autistic disorder.

au·tis·tic (aw-tis'tik) characterized by or pertaining to autism.

aut(o)- word element [Gr.], *self.*

au·to·ag·glu·ti·na·tion (aw"to-ah-gloo"tĭ-na'shun) 1. clumping or agglutination of an individual's cells by his own serum, as in autohemagglutination. 2. agglutination of particulate antigens, e.g., bacteria, that does not involve antibody.

au·to·ag·glu·ti·nin (-ah-gloo'tĭ-nin) a factor in serum capable of causing clumping together of the subject's own cellular elements.

au·to·am·pu·ta·tion (-am″pu-ta′shun) spontaneous detachment from the body and elimination of an appendage or an abnormal growth, such as a polyp.

au·to·an·ti·body (-an′tĭ-bod″e) an antibody formed in response to, and reacting against, an antigenic constituent of one's own tissues.

au·to·an·ti·gen (-an′tĭ-jen) an antigen that despite being a normal tissue constituent is the target of a humoral or cell-mediated immune response, as in autoimmune disease.

au·to·ca·tal·y·sis (-kah-tal′ĭ-sis) catalysis in which a product of the reaction hastens the catalysis.

au·toch·tho·nous (aw-tok′thah-nus) 1. originating in the same area in which it is found. 2. denoting a tissue graft to a new site on the same individual.

au·toc·la·sis (aw-tok′lah-sis) destruction of a part by influences within itself, as by autoimmune processes.

au·to·clave (aw′to-klāv) a self-locking apparatus for the sterilization of materials by steam under pressure.

Au·to·clip (-klip″) trademark for a stainless steel surgical clip inserted by means of a mechanical applier that automatically feeds a series of clips for wound closing.

au·to·coid (-koid) local hormone.

au·to·crine (-krin) denoting a mode of hormone action in which a hormone binds to receptors on and affects the function of the cell type that produced it.

au·to·di·ges·tion (aw″to-di-jes′chun) self-digestion; autolysis; especially, digestion of the stomach wall and contiguous structures after death.

au·toe·cious (aw-te′shus) pertaining to parasitic fungi that pass through their life cycle in the same host.

au·to·ec·zem·a·ti·za·tion (aw″to-ek-zem″-ah-tĭ-za′shun) the spread, at first locally and later more generally, of lesions from an originally circumscribed focus of eczema.

au·to·erot·i·cism (aw″to-ĕ-rot′ĭ-sizm) sexual self-gratification or arousal without the participation of another person. **autoerot′ic,** adj.

au·tog·a·my (aw-tog′ah-me) 1. self-fertilization; fertilization by union of two chromatin masses derived from the same primary nucleus within a cell. 2. reproduction in which the two gametes are derived from division of a single mother cell.

au·to·gen·e·sis (aw″to-jen′ĕ-sis) self-generation; origination within the organism. **autogenet′ic,** adj.

au·tog·e·nous (aw-toj′ĕ-nus) autologous.

au·to·graft (aw′to-graft) a tissue graft transferred from one part of the patient's body to another part.

au·to·he·mag·glu·ti·na·tion (aw″to-he″mah-gloo″tĭ-na′shun) hemagglutination caused by a factor produced in the subject's own body.

au·to·he·mag·glu·ti·nin (-he″mah-gloo′tĭ-nin) a hemagglutinin produced in the subject's own body.

au·to·he·mol·y·sin (-he-mol′ĭ-sin) a hemolysin produced in the body of an animal which lyses its own erythrocytes.

au·to·he·mol·y·sis (-he-mol′ĭ-sis) hemolysis of an individual's blood cells by his own serum. **autohemolyt′ic,** adj.

au·to·he·mo·ther·a·py (-he″mo-ther′ah-pe) treatment using an autotransfusion.

au·to·hyp·no·sis (-hip-no′sis) the act or process of hypnotizing oneself. **autohypnot′ic,** adj.

au·to·im·mune (-ĭ-mūn′) directed against the body's own tissue; see under *disease* and *response.*

au·to·im·mu·ni·ty (-ĭ-mu′nĭ-te) a condition characterized by a specific humoral or cell-mediated immune response against the constituents of the body's own tissues (autoantigens); it may result in hypersensitivity reactions or, if severe, in autoimmune disease.

au·to·im·mu·ni·za·tion (-im″u-nĭ-za′shun) induction in an organism of an immune response to its own tissue constituents.

au·to·in·oc·u·la·tion (-in-ok″u-la′shun) inoculation with microorganisms from one's own body.

au·to·isol·y·sin (-i-sol′ĭ-sin) a substance that lyses cells (e.g., blood cells) of the individual in which it is formed, as well as those of other members of the same species.

au·to·ker·a·to·plas·ty (-ker′ah-to-plas″te) grafting of corneal tissue from one eye to the other.

au·to·le·sion (-le′zhun) a self-inflicted injury.

au·tol·o·gous (aw-tol′ah-gus) related to self; belonging to the same organism.

au·tol·y·sin (aw-tol′ĭ-sin) a lysin originating in an organism and capable of destroying its own cells and tissues.

au·tol·y·sis (aw-tol′ĭ-sis) 1. spontaneous disintegration of cells or tissues by autologous enzymes, as occurs after death and in some pathologic conditions. 2. destruction of cells of the body by its own serum. **autolyt′ic,** adj.

au·to·mat·ic (aw″to-mat′ik) 1. spontaneous or involuntary; done by no act of the will. 2. self-moving; self-regulating.

au·to·ma·ti·ci·ty (-mah-tis′ĭ-te) 1. the state or quality of being spontaneous, involuntary, or self-regulating. 2. the capacity of a cell to initiate an impulse without an external stimulus. **triggered a.**, pacemaker activity occurring as a result of a propagated or stimulated action potential, such as an afterpotential, in cells or tissues not normally displaying spontaneous automaticity.

au·tom·a·tism (aw-tom′ah-tizm) performance of nonreflex acts without conscious volition. **command a.**, abnormal responsiveness to commands, as in hypnosis.

au·to·nom·ic (aw″to-nom′ik) not subject to voluntary control. See under *system*.

au·to·nomo·tro·pic (aw″to-nom″o-tro′pik) having an affinity for the autonomic nervous system.

au·ton·o·my (aw-ton′ah-me) the state of functioning independently, without extraneous influence. **auton′omous,** adj.

au·to·ox·i·da·tion (aw″to-ok″sĭ-da′shun) spontaneous direct combination, at normal temperatures, with molecular oxygen.

au·to·pha·gia (-fa′jah) 1. eating one's own flesh. 2. nutrition of the body by consumption of its own tissues. 3. autophagy (1).

au·to·phago·some (-fag′o-sōm) an intracytoplasmic vacuole containing elements of a cell's own cytoplasm; it fuses with a lysosome and the contents are subjected to enzymatic digestion.

au·toph·a·gy (aw-tof′ah-je) 1. lysosomal digestion of a cell's own cytoplasmic material. 2. autophagia.

au·toph·o·ny (aw-tof′ah-ne) abnormal hearing of one's own voice and respiratory sounds, usually as a result of a patulous eustachian tube.

au·to·plas·ty (aw′to-plas″te) 1. autotransplantation. 2. in psychoanalytic theory, adaptation by changing one's self rather than the external environment. **autoplas′tic,** adj.

au·top·sy (aw′top-se) postmortem examination of a body to determine the cause of death or the nature of pathological changes; necropsy.

au·to·ra·di·og·ra·phy (aw″to-ra″de-og′rah-fe) the making of a radiograph of an object or tissue by recording on a photographic plate the radiation emitted by radioactive material within the object.

au·to·reg·u·la·tion (-reg″u-la′shun) 1. the process occurring when some mechanism within a biological system detects and adjusts for changes within the system. 2. in circulatory physiology, the intrinsic tendency of an organ or tissue to maintain constant blood flow despite changes in arterial pressure, or the adjustment of blood flow through an organ in accordance with its metabolic needs. **heterometric a.,** intrinsic mechanisms controlling the strength of ventricular contractions that depend on the length of myocardial fibers at the end of diastole. **homeometric a.,** 1. intrinsic mechanisms controlling the strength of ventricular contractions that are independent of the length of myocardial fibers at the end of diastole. 2. Anrep effect.

au·to·sen·si·ti·za·tion (-sen″sĭ-tĭ-za′shun) autoimmunization. **erythrocyte a.,** autoerythrocyte sensitization; see *painful bruising syndrome,* under *syndrome.*

au·to·sep·ti·ce·mia (-sep″tĭ-se′me-ah) septicemia from poisons developed within the body.

au·to·site (aw′to-sīt) the larger, more normal member of asymmetrical conjoined twin fetuses, to which the parasite is attached.

au·to·some (-sōm) any non–sex-determining chromosome; in humans there are 22 pairs of autosomes. **autoso′mal,** adj.

au·to·sple·nec·to·my (aw″to-sple-nek′tah-me) almost complete disappearance of the spleen through progressive fibrosis and shrinkage.

au·to·sug·ges·tion (-sug-jes′chun) self-suggestion; the process by which a person induces in himself an uncritical acceptance of an idea, belief, or opinion.

au·to·to·mog·ra·phy (-tah-mog′rah-fe) a method of body section radiography involving movement of the patient instead of the x-ray tube. **autotomograph′ic,** adj.

au·to·trans·fu·sion (-trans-fu′zhun) reinfusion of a patient's own blood.

au·to·trans·plan·ta·tion (-trans″plan-ta′-shun) transfer of tissue from one part of the body to another part.

au·to·troph (aw′to-trōf) an autotrophic organism.

au·to·tro·phic (aw″to-tro′fik) self-nourishing; able to build organic constituents from carbon dioxide and inorganic salts.

au·to·vac·cine (aw′to-vak″sēn) a vaccine prepared from cultures of organisms isolated from the patient's own tissues or secretions.

au·tox·i·da·tion (aw-tok″sĭ-da′shun) autooxidation.

aux·an·og·ra·phy (awk″san-og′rah-fe) a method used for determining the most suitable medium for the cultivation of microorganisms. **auxanograph′ic,** adj.

aux·e·sis (awk-se′sis) increase in size of an organism, especially that due to growth of its individual cells rather than an increase in their number. **auxet′ic,** adj.

aux·i·lyt·ic (awk″sĭ-lit′ik) increasing the lytic or destructive power.

auxo·tro·phic (awk″so-tro′fik) 1. requiring a growth factor not required by the parental or prototype strain; said of microbial mutants. 2. requiring specific organic growth factors in addition to the carbon source present in a minimal medium.

AV, A-V atrioventricular; arteriovenous.

av avoirdupois; see *avoirdupois weight*, under *weight*.

avas·cu·lar (a-vas′ku-ler) not vascular; bloodless.

avas·cu·lar·i·za·tion (a-vas″ku-ler-ĭ-za′-shun) diversion of blood from tissues, as by ligation of vessels or tight bandaging.

aver·sive (ah-ver′siv) characterized by or giving rise to avoidance; noxious.

avi·an (a′ve-an) of or pertaining to birds.

avid·i·ty (ah-vid′ĭ-te) 1. the strength of an acid or base. 2. in immunology, an imprecise measure of the strength of antigen-antibody binding based on the rate at which the complex is formed. Cf. *affinity* (3).

avir·u·lence (a-vir′u-lens) lack of virulence; lack of competence of an infectious agent to produce pathologic effects. **avir′u·lent,** adj.

av·o·ben·zone (av″o-ben′zōn) a sunscreen that absorbs light in the UVA range.

avoid·ance (ah-void′ans) a conscious or unconscious defense mechanism consisting of refusal to encounter situations, activities, or objects that would produce anxiety or conflict.

avoid·ant (ah-void′ant) moving away from; negatively oriented.

av·oir·du·pois (av″er-dah-poiz′, av-wahr″-doo-pwah′) see under *weight*.

AVRT atrioventricular reciprocating tachycardia.

avul·sion (ah-vul′shun) the tearing away of a structure or part.

ax. axis.

axen·ic (a-zen′ik) not contaminated by or associated with any foreign organisms; used in reference to pure cultures of microorganisms or to germ-free animals. Cf. *gnotobiotic*.

ax·e·til (ak′sĕ-til″) USAN contraction for *1-acetoxyethyl*.

ax·i·al (ak′se-al) of or pertaining to the axis of a structure or part.

ax·i·a·lis (ak″se-a′lis) [L.] axial; denoting relationship to an axis or location near the long axis or central part of the body.

ax·i·a·tion (ak″se-a′shun) establishment of an axis; development of polarity in an oocyte, embryo, organ, or other body structure.

ax·il·la (ak-sil′ah) pl. *axil′lae*. [L.] the armpit. **ax′illary,** adj.

axi(o)- word element [L., Gr.], *axis*; in dentistry, the *long axis of a tooth*.

ax·ip·e·tal (ak-sip′ĭ-t′l) directed toward an axis or axon.

ax·is (ak′sis) pl. *ax′es*. [L.] 1. a line through the center of a body, or about which a structure revolves; a line around which body parts are arranged. 2. the second cervical vertebra; see *Table of Bones*. **ax′ial,** adj. **basibregmatic a.,** the vertical line from the basion to the bregma. **basicranial a.,** a line from basion to gonion. **basifacial a.,** a line from gonion to subnasal point. **binauricular a.,** a line joining the two auricular points. **celiac a.,** see under *trunk*. **dorsoventral a.,** one passing from the back to the belly surface of the body. **electrical a. of heart,** the resultant of the electromotive forces within the heart at any instant. **frontal a.,** an imaginary line running from right to left through the center of the eyeball. **a. of heart,** a line passing through the center of the base of the heart and the apex. **optic a.,** 1. visual a. 2. the hypothetical straight line passing through the centers of curvature of the front and back surfaces of a simple lens. **visual a.,** an imaginary line passing from the midpoint of the visual field to the fovea centralis.

axo·ax·on·ic (ak″so-ak-son′ik) referring to a synapse between the axon of one neuron and the axon of another.

axo·den·drit·ic (-den-drit′ik) referring to a synapse between the axon of one neuron and the dendrites of another.

axo·lem·ma (-lem′ah) the plasma membrane of an axon.

ax·ol·y·sis (ak-sol′ĭ-sis) degeneration of an axon.

ax·on (ak′son) 1. that process of a neuron by which impulses travel away from the cell body; at the terminal arborization of the axon, the impulses are transmitted to other nerve cells or to effector organs. Larger axons are covered by a myelin sheath. **ax′onal,** adj. 2. vertebral column.

ax·o·neme (ak′so-nēm) the central core of a cilium or flagellum, consisting of a central pair of filaments surrounded by nine other pairs.

axo·nop·a·thy (ak″sah-nop′ah-the) a disorder disrupting the normal functioning of the axons; in *distal a.* the disease progresses from the center toward the periphery and in *proximal a.* the disease progresses from the periphery toward the center.

ax·on·ot·me·sis (ak″son-ot-me′sis) nerve injury characterized by disruption of the axon and myelin sheath but with preservation of the connective tissue fragments, resulting in degeneration of the axon distal to the injury site; regeneration of the axon is spontaneous and of good quality. Cf. *neurapraxia* and *neurotmesis*.

axo·phage (ak′so-fāj) a glial cell occurring in excavations in the myelin in myelitis.

axo·plasm (-plazm) cytoplasm of an axon. **axoplas′mic,** adj.

axo·so·mat·ic (-so-mat′ik) referring to a synapse between the axon of one neuron and the cell body of another.

axo·style (ak′so-stīl) 1. the central supporting structure of an axopodium. 2. a supporting rod running through the body of a trichomonad and protruding posteriorly.

ax·ot·o·my (ak-sot′ah-me) transection or severing of an axon.

ayur·ve·da (i″yur′ved-ah, i″yur-va′dah) [Sanskrit] a classical system of medicine founded 5000 years ago and currently practiced in India. Its emphasis is on balance with the environment and interpersonal communication and is based on the principles that humans are microcosmic representations of the entire universe and that health is the natural end of living in harmony with the environment. Disease results from disharmony between the person and the environment, and each case of disease is a manifestation of a unique state in a unique individual, therefore requiring a unique cure. The practitioner attempts to maintain or restore the balance of the doshas, with therapies including diet; herbal, color, and sound therapies; aromatherapy; application of medicated oils to the skin and massage; and meditation. Written also *Ayurveda*. **ayurve′-dic,** adj.

azat·a·dine (ah-zat′ah-dēn) an antihistamine with anticholinergic and sedative effects, used as the maleate salt.

aza·thio·prine (az″ah-thi′o-prēn) a 6-mercaptopurine derivative used as the base or the sodium salt as an immunosuppressant for prevention of transplant rejection and for treatment of rheumatoid arthritis and various autoimmune diseases.

az·e·la·ic ac·id (az″ĕ-la′ik) a topical antibacterial used in the treatment of acne vulgaris.

azel·as·tine (ah-zel′as-tēn″) a topical antihistamine used as the hydrochloride salt in the treatment of seasonal allergic rhinitis and allergic conjunctivitis.

azeo·trope (a′ze-o-trōp′) a mixture of two substances that has a constant boiling point and cannot be separated by fractional distillation. **azeotrop′ic,** adj.

az·ith·ro·my·cin (az-ith″ro-mi′sin) a macrolide antibiotic derived from erythromycin, effective against a wide range of gram-positive, gram-negative, and anaerobic bacteria.

azoo·sper·mia (a-zo″o-sper′me-ah) lack of live spermatozoa in the semen; classified as obstructive or nonobstructive depending on whether cause is blockage of the tubules or ducts.

az·ote (az′ōt) nitrogen (in France).

az·o·te·mia (az″o-te′me-ah) uremia; an excess of urea or other nitrogenous compounds in the blood.

az·o·tu·ria (-tu′re-ah) excess of urea or other nitrogenous compounds in the urine. **azotu′ric,** adj.

AZQ diaziquone.

AZT zidovudine.

az·tre·o·nam (az′tre-o-nam″) a narrow-range monobactam antibiotic effective against aerobic gram-negative bacteria.

az·ure (azh′er) one of three metachromatic basic dyes (A, B, and C).

az·u·res·in (azh″u-rez′in) a complex combination of azure A dye and carbacrylic cationic exchange resin used as a diagnostic aid in detection of gastric secretion.

az·u·ro·phil (azh-u′ro-fil″) a tissue constituent staining with azure or a similar metachromatic thiazin dye.

az·u·ro·phil·ia (azh″u-ro-fil′e-ah) a condition in which the blood contains cells having azurophilic granules.

az·y·gog·raphy (az″ĭ-gog′rah-fe) radiography of the azygous venous system. **azygo-graph′ic,** adj.

az·y·gos (az′ĭ-gus) 1. unpaired. 2. any unpaired part, as the azygos vein.

B

B bel; boron.

b base (in nucleic acid sequences); born.

β (beta, the second letter of the Greek alphabet) β chain of hemoglobin.

β- a prefix designating (1) the position of a substituting atom or group in a chemical compound; (2) the specific rotation of an optically active compound; (3) the orientation of an exocyclic atom or group; (4) a plasma protein migrating with the β band in electrophoresis; (5) second in a series of two or more related entities or chemical compounds.

BA Bachelor of Arts.

Ba barium.

Ba·be·sia (bah-be′ze-ah) a genus of protozoa found as parasites in red blood cells and transmitted by ticks; its numerous species include *B. bige′mina*, *B. bo′vis*, and *B. ma′jor*, and cause babesiosis in both wild and domestic animals and a malarialike illness in humans.

ba·be·si·a·sis (bă″be-zi′ah-sis) 1. chronic, asymptomatic infection with protozoa of the genus *Babesia*. 2. babesiosis.

ba·be·si·o·sis (bah-be″ze-o′sis) a group of tickborne diseases due to infection with species of *Babesia*, seen in wild and domestic animals associated with anemia, hemoglobinuria, and hemoglobinemia; it may spread to humans as a zoonosis that resembles malaria.

ba·by (ba′be) infant. **blue b.,** an infant born with cyanosis due to a congenital heart lesion or atelectasis. **collodion b.,** an infant born completely covered by a collodion- or parchment-like membrane; see *lamellar exfoliation of the newborn*, under *exfoliation*.

ba·cam·pi·cil·lin (bah-kam″pĭ-sil′in) a semisynthetic penicillin of the ampicillin class; its hydrochloride salt has the same actions and uses as ampicillin.

bac·cate (bak′āt) resembling a berry.

Bac·il·la·ceae (bas″ĭ-la′se-e) a family of mostly saprophytic bacteria (order Eubacteriales), commonly found in soil and as animal parasites; members of genera *Bacillus* and *Clostridium* can cause disease in humans.

bac·il·la·ry (bas′ĭ-lar″e) pertaining to bacilli or to rodlike structures.

bacille (bah-sēl′) [Fr.] bacillus. **b. Calmette-Guérin (BCG),** *Mycobacterium bovis* rendered completely avirulent by cultivation over a long period on bile-glycerol-potato medium; see *BCG vaccine*.

ba·cil·li (bah-sil′i) plural of *bacillus*.

ba·cil·lin (bah-sil′in) an antibiotic substance isolated from strains of *Bacillus subtilis*, highly active on both gram-positive and gram-negative bacteria.

ba·cil·lu·ria (bas″ĭ-lu′re-ah) bacilli in the urine.

Ba·cil·lus (bah-sil′us) a genus of bacteria, including gram-positive, spore-forming bacteria; three species are potentially pathogenic. **B. an′thracis,** the causative agent of anthrax. **B. enteri′tidis,** *Salmonella enteritidis*. **B. mal′lei,** *Pseudomonas mallei*. **B. sub′tilis,** a common saprophytic soil and water form, often occurring as a laboratory contaminant and occasionally in apparently causal relation to pathologic processes, such as conjunctivitis. **B. wel′chii,** *Clostridium perfringens*.

ba·cil·lus (bah-sil′us) pl. *bacil′li*. [L.] 1. an organism of the genus *Bacillus*. 2. any rod-shaped bacterium. **Calmette-Guérin b.,** bacille Calmette-Guérin. **coliform bacilli,** gram-negative bacilli resembling *Escherichia coli* that are found in the intestinal tract; the term generally refers to the genera *Citrobacter*, *Edwardsiella*, *Enterobacter*, *Escherichia*, *Klebsiella*, and *Serratia*. **dysentery bacilli,** gram-negative non–spore-forming rods causing dysentery in humans; see *Shigella*. **enteric b.,** a bacillus belonging to the family Enterobacteriaceae. **tubercle b.,** *Mycobacterium tuberculosis*.

bac·i·tra·cin (bas″ĭ-tra′sin) an antibacterial polypeptide elaborated by the licheniformis group of *Bacillus subtilis* that acts by interfering with bacterial cell wall synthesis; it is effective against a wide range of gram-positive and a few gram-negative bacteria; also used as the zinc salt.

back (bak) the posterior part of the trunk from the neck to the pelvis. **angry b.,** excited skin syndrome.

back·cross (bak′kros) a mating between a heterozygote and a homozygote.

back·flow (-flo) reflux or regurgitation (1). **pyelovenous b.,** drainage from the renal pelvis into the venous system occurring under certain conditions of back pressure.

bac·lo·fen (bak'lo-fen") an analogue of γ-aminobutyric acid used to treat severe spasticity.

bac·ter·as·ci·tes (bak"ter-ah-si'tēz) bacterial infection of ascitic fluid. **monomicrobial non-neutrocytic b.,** bacterial infection of ascitic fluid with no intra-abdominal source of infection and a neutrophil count less than 250 cells/mm³. **polymicrobial b.,** bacterial infection of ascitic fluid caused by several species and resulting from bowel puncture during paracentesis.

bac·ter·e·mia (-e'me-ah) the presence of bacteria in the blood.

Bac·te·ria (bak-tēr'e-ah) in former systems of classification, a division of the kingdom Procaryotae, including all prokaryotic organisms except the blue-green algae (Cyanobacteria).

bac·te·ria (bak-tēr'e-ah) plural of *bacterium.*

bac·te·ri·al (-al) pertaining to or caused by bacteria.

bac·te·ri·ci·dal (bak-tēr"ĭ-si'd'l) destructive to bacteria.

bac·te·ri·ci·din (-din) bactericidal antibody.

bac·ter·id (bak'ter-id) a skin eruption caused by bacterial infection elsewhere in the body.

bacteri(o)- word element [Gr.], *bacteria.*

bac·te·rio·chlo·ro·phyll (bak-tēr"e-o-klor'o-fil) a form of chlorophyll produced by certain bacteria and capable of carrying out photosynthesis.

bac·te·rio·ci·din (-si'din) a bactericidal antibody.

bac·te·rio·cin (bac-tēr'e-o"-sin) any of a group of substances, e.g., colicin, released by certain bacteria that kill other strains of bacteria by inducing metabolic block.

bac·te·ri·o·cin·o·gen·ic (bak-tēr"e-o-sin"ah-jen'ik) giving rise to bacteriocin; denoting bacterial plasmids that synthesize bacteriocin.

bac·te·ri·ol·o·gy (bak-tēr"e-ol'ah-je) the scientific study of bacteria. **bacteriolog'ic, bacteriolog'ical,** adj.

bac·te·ri·ol·y·sin (-ĭ-sin) an antibacterial antibody that lyses bacterial cells.

bac·te·rio·phage (bak-tēr'e-o-fāj") a virus that lyses bacteria. **bacteriopha'gic,** adj. **temperate b.,** one whose genetic material (prophage) becomes an intimate part of the bacterial genome, persisting and being reproduced through many cell division cycles; the affected bacterial cell is known as a *lysogenic bacterium* (q.v.).

bac·te·ri·op·so·nin (bak-tēr"e-op'so-nin) an antibody that acts on bacteria.

bac·te·rio·stat·ic (bak-tēr"e-o-stat'ik) inhibiting growth or multiplication of bacteria; an agent that so acts.

bac·te·ri·um (bak-tēr'e-um) pl. *bacte'ria.* [L.] in general, any of the unicellular prokaryotic microorganisms that commonly multiply by cell division, lack a nucleus or membrane-bound organelles, and possess a cell wall; they may be aerobic or anaerobic, motile or nonmotile, free-living, saprophytic, parasitic, or pathogenic. **bacter'ial,** adj. **acid-fast b.,** one not readily decolorized by acids after staining. **coliform b.,** one of the facultative, gram-negative, rod-shaped bacteria that are normal inhabitants of the intestinal tract; see *Escherichia, Klebsiella,* and *Serratia.* **coryneform bacteria,** a group of bacteria that are morphologically similiar to organisms of the genus *Corynebacterium.* **gram-negative b.,** see *gram-negative,* under G. **gram-positive b.,** see *gram-positive,* under G. **hemophilic b.,** one that has a nutritional affinity for constituents of fresh blood or whose growth is stimulated by blood-enriched media. **lysogenic b.,** a bacterial cell that harbors in its genome the genetic material (prophage) of a temperate bacteriophage and thus reproduces the bacteriophage in cell division; occasionally the prophage develops into the mature form, replicates, lyses the bacterial cell, and is free to infect other cells.

bac·te·ri·uria (bak-tēr"e-u're-ah) [*bacteri-* + *-uria*] the presence of bacteria in the urine.

Bac·te·roi·da·ceae (bak"ter-oi-da'se-e) a family of schizomycetes (order Eubacteriales).

Bac·te·roi·des (bak"ter-oi'dēz) a genus of gram-negative, anaerobic, rod-shaped bacteria, which are normal inhabitants of the oral, respiratory, intestinal, and urogenital cavities of humans and animals; some species can cause potentially fatal abscesses and bacteremias.

bac·te·roi·des (bak"ter-oi'dēz) 1. any highly pleomorphic rod-shaped bacteria. 2. an organism of the genus *Bacteroides.*

bag (bag) sac; a flexible container. **colostomy b.,** a bag worn over the stoma to receive fecal discharge after colostomy. **ileostomy b.,** a plastic or latex bag attached to the body for collection of urine or fecal material after ileostomy or cystoplasty. **Politzer's b.,** a soft bag of rubber for inflating the auditory tube. **b. of waters,** popular name for the amniotic sac.

bag·as·so·sis (bag″ah-so′sis) hypersensitivity pneumonitis due to inhalation of dust from bagasse (the residue of cane after extraction of sugar).

BAL dimercaprol (British antilewisite).

bal·ance (bal′ans) 1. an instrument for weighing. 2. equilibrium. **acid-base b.,** a normal balance between production and excretion of acid or alkali by the body, resulting in a stable concentration of H^+ in body fluids. **analytical b.,** a balance used in the laboratory, sensitive to variations of the order of 0.05 to 0.1 mg. **fluid b.,** the state of the body in relation to ingestion and excretion of water and electrolytes. **nitrogen b.,** the state of the body in regard to ingestion and excretion of nitrogen. In *negative nitrogen b.* the amount excreted is greater than the quantity ingested; in *positive nitrogen b.* the amount excreted is smaller than the quantity ingested. **water b.,** fluid b.

bal·anced (bal′ansd) existing in or maintaining an equilibrium.

ba·lan·ic (bah-lan′ik) pertaining to the glans penis or glans clitoridis.

bal·a·ni·tis (bal″ah-ni′tis) inflammation of the glans penis. **gangrenous b.,** a rapidly destructive infection producing erosion of the glans penis and often destruction of the entire external genitals; believed to be due to a spirochete. **plasma cell b., Zoon b.,** a benign erythroplasia of the inner surface of the prepuce or the glans penis, characterized histologically by plasma cell infiltration of the dermis, and clinically by a single erythematous, moist, shiny lesion.

bal·a·no·pos·thi·tis (bal″ah-no-pos-thi′tis) inflammation of the glans penis and prepuce.

bal·an·ti·di·a·sis (bal″an-ti-di′ah-sis) infection by protozoa of the genus *Balantidium*; in humans, *B. coli* may cause diarrhea and dysentery with ulceration of the colonic mucosa.

Bal·an·tid·i·um (bal″an-tid′e-um) a genus of ciliated protozoa, including many species found in the intestine in vertebrates and invertebrates, including *B. co′li*, a common parasite of swine, rarely in humans, in whom it may cause dysentery.

bald·ness (bawld′nes) alopecia, especially of the scalp. **male pattern b.,** see *androgenetic alopecia*, under *alopecia*.

ball (bawl) a more or less spherical mass. See also *globus* and *sphere*. **fungus b.,** a tumorlike granulomatous mass formed by colonization of a fungus, usually *Aspergillus*, in a body cavity.

bal·lis·mus (bah-liz′mus) violent movements of the limbs, as in chorea, sometimes affecting only one side of the body (hemiballismus).

balm (bahm) 1. a soothing or healing medicine. 2. balsam. **lemon b., sweet b.,** a preparation of the fresh or dried herb of *Melissa officinalis*, or the volatile oil; used for nervousness and insomnia, as a homeopathic preparation for menstrual irregularities, and in folk medicine.

bal·sal·a·zide (bal-sal′ah-zīd) a prodrug of the antiinflammatory mesalamine, to which it is converted in the colon; administered orally as the sodium salt in the treatment of ulcerative colitis.

bal·sam (bawl′sam) 1. a semifluid, resinous, and fragrant liquid of vegetable origin, usually trees; often composed chiefly of resins, volatile oils, and various esters. **balsam′ic,** adj. 2. balm. **Canada b.,** an oleoresin from the balsam fir, used as a microscopic mounting medium. **b. of Peru, peruvian b.,** a thick brown liquid from the tree *Myroxylon pereirae*, used as a local protectant and rubefacient. **tolu b.,** a balsam obtained from the tree *Myrotoxylon balsamum*, used as an expectorant and pharmaceutic aid.

band (band) 1. a part, structure, or appliance that binds; for anatomical structures, see *frenulum, tenia, trabecula,* and *vinculum*. 2. in dentistry, a thin metal strip fitted around a tooth or its roots. 3. in histology, a zone of a myofibril of striated muscle. 4. in cytogenetics, a segment of a chromosome stained brighter or darker than the adjacent bands; used in identifying the chromosomes and in determining the exact extent of chromosomal abnormalities. Called *Q-b's, G-b's, C-b's, T-b's,* etc., according to the staining method used. **A b.,** the dark-staining zone of a sarcomere, whose center is traversed by the H band. **b. of Broca,** a band of nerve fibers that forms the caudal zone of the anterior perforated substance where it adjoins the optic tract. **H b.,** a pale zone sometimes seen traversing the center of the A band of a striated myofibril. **I b.,** the band within a striated myofibril, seen as a light region under the light microscope and as a dark region under polarized light. **iliotibial b.,** see under *tract*. **M b.,** the narrow dark band in the center of the H band. **matrix b.,** a thin piece of metal fitted around a tooth to supply a missing wall of a multisurface cavity to allow adequate condensation of amalgam into the cavity. **oligoclonal b's,** discrete bands of immunoglobulins with decreased electrophoretic mobility whose presence in the cerebrospinal fluid may be indicative of multiple sclerosis or other disease of the central nervous system. **Z b.,** a thin membrane in a myofibril, seen on longitudinal section as a dark line in the center of the I band; the distance between Z bands delimits the sarcomeres of striated muscle.

ban·dage (ban′daj) 1. a strip or roll of gauze or other material for wrapping or binding a body part. 2. to cover by wrapping with such material. **Ace b.,** trademark for a bandage of woven elastic material. **Barton's b.,** a double figure-of-8 bandage for fracture of the lower jaw. **demigauntlet b.,** one that covers the hand but leaves the fingers exposed. **Desault's b.,** one binding the elbow to the side, with a pad in the axilla, for fractured clavicle. **Esmarch's b.,** a rubber bandage applied upward around a limb from distal to proximal in order to expel blood from it; the limb is often elevated as the elastic pressure is applied. **gauntlet b.,** one which covers the hand and fingers like a glove. **Gibney b.,** strips of adhesive 1.2 cm wide, overlapped along the sides and back of the foot and leg to hold the foot in slight varus position and leave the dorsum of foot and anterior aspect of leg exposed. **plaster b.,** one stiffened with a paste of plaster of Paris. **pressure b.,** one for applying pressure. **roller b.,** a tightly rolled, circular bandage of varying width and materials, often commercially prepared. **Scultetus b.,** a many-tailed bandage applied with the tails overlapping each other and held in position by safety pins. **spica b.,** a figure-of-8 bandage with turns that cross one another regularly like the letter V, usually applied to anatomical areas whose dimensions vary, as the pelvis and thigh. **Velpeau's b.,** one used in immobilization of certain fractures about the upper end of the humerus and shoulder joint, binding the arm and shoulder to the chest.

ban·de·lette (ban″dĕ-let′) [Fr.] a small band.

band·ing (band′ing) 1. the act of encircling and binding with a thin strip of material. 2. in genetics, any of several techniques of staining chromosomes so that a characteristic pattern of transverse dark and light bands becomes visible, permitting identification of individual chromosome pairs.

ban·dy (band′e) bowed or bent in an outward curve.

bank (bangk) a stored supply of human material or tissues for future use by other individuals, such as a *blood b.,* *bone b.,* *eye b.,* *human-milk b.,* or *skin b.*

bar (bahr) 1. a structure having greater length than width, and often some degree of rigidity. 2. a heavy wire or wrought or cast

metal segment, longer than its width, used to connect parts of a removable partial denture. **median b.,** a fibrotic formation across the neck of the prostate gland, producing obstruction of the urethra. **Mercier's b.,** interureteric ridge. **terminal b's,** zones of epithelial cell contact, once thought to represent an accumulation of dense cementing substance, but with the electron microscope shown to be a junctional complex.

bar·ag·no·sis (bar″ag-no′sis) lack or loss of the faculty of barognosis, the conscious perception of weight.

bar·bi·tur·ate (bahr-bich′er-it) any of a class of compounds derived from barbituric acid; used for their hypnotic and sedative effects.

bar·bi·tur·ic ac·id (bahr-bĭ-tūr′ik) the parent substance of the barbiturates, not itself a central nervous system depressant.

bar·bo·tage (bahr″bo-tahzh′) [Fr.] repeated alternate injection and withdrawal of fluid with a syringe, as in gastric lavage or administration of an anesthetic agent into the subarachnoid space by alternate injection of part of the anesthetic and withdrawal of cerebrospinal fluid into the syringe.

bar·es·the·si·om·e·ter (bar″es-the″ze-om′ĕ-ter) instrument for estimating sense of weight or pressure.

bar·iat·rics (-e-ă′triks) a field of medicine encompassing the study of overweight and its causes, prevention, and treatment.

bar·ium (Ba) (bar′e-um) chemical element (see *Table of Elements*), at. no. 56. Its acid-soluble salts are poisonous; causing gastrointestinal symptoms followed by severe, sometimes fatal hypokalemia with paralysis. **b. sulfate,** a water-insoluble salt, $BaSO_4$, used as an opaque contrast medium in radiography of the digestive tract.

bark (bahrk) the rind or outer cortical cover of the woody parts of a plant, tree, or shrub. **cramp b.,** the dried bark of *Viburnum opulus,* the high bush or cranberry tree; it has been used as an antispasmodic, uterine sedative, and antiscorbutic. **elm b., slippery elm b.,** the dried inner bark of the slippery elm, *Ulmus rubra,* which is mucilaginous and demulcent. **white willow b.,** a preparation of the bark of various *Salix* species collectively known as white willow, containing salicin, a precursor of salicylic acid; used as an antiinflammatory and antipyretic. **yohimbe b.,** a preparation of the bark of *Pausinystalia yohimbe,* used for the same indications as yohimbine hydrochloride; it has also been used traditionally as an aphrodisiac and for skin diseases and obesity.

baro·cep·tor (bar″o-sep′ter) baroreceptor.

bar·og·no·sis (bar″og-no′sis) conscious perception of weight.

baro·phil·ic (bar″o-fil′ik) growing best under high atmospheric pressure; said of bacteria.

baro·re·cep·tor (-re-sep′ter) a type of interoceptor that is stimulated by pressure changes, as those in blood vessel walls.

baro·re·flex (bar′o-re″fleks) baroreceptor reflex.

baro·si·nus·itis (bar″o-si″nus-i′tis) a symptom complex due to differences in environmental atmospheric pressure and the air pressure in the paranasal sinuses.

baro·tax·is (-tak′sis) stimulation of living matter by change of atmospheric pressure.

bar·oti·tis (-ti′tis) a morbid condition of the ear due to exposure to differing atmospheric pressures. **b. me′dia,** a symptom complex due to difference between atmospheric pressure of the environment and air pressure in the middle ear.

baro·trau·ma (-traw′mah) injury due to pressure, as to structures of the ear, in high-altitude flyers, owing to differences between atmospheric and intratympanic pressures; see *barosinusitis* and *barotitis.*

bar·ri·er (bar′e-er) an obstruction. **alveolar-capillary b., alveolocapillary b.,** see under *membrane.* **blood-air b.,** alveolocapillary membrane. **blood-aqueous b.,** the physiologic mechanism that prevents exchange of materials between the chambers of the eye and the blood. **blood-brain b., blood-cerebral b.,** the selective barrier separating the blood from the parenchyma of the central nervous system. Abbreviated BBB. **blood-gas b.,** alveolocapillary membrane. **blood-testis b.,** a barrier separating the blood from the seminiferous tubules, consisting of special junctional complexes between adjacent Sertoli cells near the base of the seminiferous epithelium. **placental b.,** term sometimes used for the placental membrane, because it prevents the passage of some materials between the maternal and fetal blood.

Bar·to·nel·la (bahr″to-nel′ah) a genus of the family Bartonellaceae, including *B. bacilli·for′mis,* the etiologic agent of Carrión's disease, and *B. hen′selae,* the agent of cat-scratch disease.

Bar·to·nel·la·ceae (bahr″to-nel-a′se-e) a family of the order Rickettsiales, occurring as pathogenic parasites in the erythrocytes of humans and other animals.

bar·to·nel·li·a·sis (-i′ah-sis) bartonellosis.

bar·to·nel·lo·sis (-o′sis) an infectious disease in South America due to *Bartonella*

bacilliformis, usually transmitted by the sandfly *Phlebotomus verrucarum,* appearing in an acute, highly fatal, febrile, anemic stage (Oroya fever) followed by a nodular skin eruption (verruga peruana).

ba·sad (ba′sad) toward a base or basal aspect.

ba·sal (ba′s′l) pertaining to or situated near a base; in physiology, pertaining to the lowest possible level.

ba·sa·lis (ba-sa′lis) [L.] basal.

bas·cule (bas′kūl) [Fr.] a device working on the principle of the seesaw, so that when one end is raised the other is lowered. **cecal b.,** a form of cecal volvulus in which the cecum becomes folded across bands or adhesions that run across the ascending colon.

base (bās) 1. the lowest part or foundation of anything; see also *basis.* 2. the main ingredient of a compound. 3. in chemistry, a substance that combines with acids to form salts; a substance that dissociates to give hydroxide ions in aqueous solutions; a substance whose molecule or ion can combine with a proton (hydrogen ion); a substance capable of donating a pair of electrons (to an acid) for the formation of a coordinate covalent bond. 4. a unit of a removable dental prosthesis. 5. in genetics, a nucleotide, particularly one in a nucleic acid sequence. **buffer b.,** the sum of all the buffer anions in the blood, used as an index of the degree of metabolic disturbance in the acid-base balance. **denture b.,** the material in which the teeth of a denture are set and which rests on the supporting tissues when the denture is in place in the mouth. **nitrogenous b.,** an aromatic, nitrogen-containing molecule that serves as a proton acceptor, e.g., purine or pyrimidine. **ointment b.,** a vehicle for the medicinal substances carried in an ointment. **purine b's,** a group of chemical compounds of which purine is the base, including adenine, guanine, hypoxanthine, theobromine, uric acid, and xanthine. **pyrimidine b's,** a group of chemical compounds of which pyrimidine is the base, including uracil, thymine, and cytosine. **record b.,** baseplate. **b. of stapes,** footplate. **temporary b., trial b.,** baseplate.

base·line (bās′līn) a value representing a normal background level or an initial level of a measurable quantity and used for comparison with values representing response to an environmental stimulus or intervention.

base·plate (-plāt) a sheet of plastic material used in making trial plates for artificial dentures.

ba·si·al (ba′se-al) pertaining to the basion.

ba·sic (ba'sik) 1. pertaining to or having properties of a base. 2. capable of neutralizing acids.

ba·sic·i·ty (ba-sis'ĭ-te) 1. the quality of being a base, or basic. 2. the combining power of an acid.

Ba·sid·i·ob·o·lus (bah-sid″e-ob'o-lus) a mainly saprobic genus of fungi of the family Basidiobolaceae, including *B. rana'rum*, which causes entomophthoromycosis.

ba·sid·io·my·cete (-o-mi'sēt) an individual fungus of the Basidiomycotina.

Ba·sid·io·my·co·ti·na (-o-mi″ko-ti'nah) a subdivision of fungi (or in some systems of classification, a class) comprising the club fungi, in which spores (basidiospores) are borne on club-shaped organs (basidia).

ba·sid·i·um (bah-sid'e-um) pl. *basi'dia*. [L.] the club-shaped organ bearing the spores of Basidiomycotina.

ba·si·hy·oid (ba″sĭ-hi'oid) the body of the hyoid bone; in certain animals other than humans, either of two lateral bones that are its homologues.

bas·i·lad (bas'ĭ-lad) toward the base.

bas·i·lar (bas'ĭ-lar) pertaining to a base or basal part.

ba·si·lem·ma (ba″sĭ-lem'ah) basement membrane.

bas·i·lix·i·mab (bas″ĭ-lik'sĭ-mab) a chimeric monoclonal antibody that is an interleukin-2 receptor antagonist; used in the prophylaxis of acute organ rejection after renal transplantation.

basi(o)- word element [Gr.], *base* or *foundation; basion; chemical base.*

ba·si·on (ba'se-on) the midpoint of the anterior border of the foramen magnum.

ba·sip·e·tal (bah-sip'ĕ-t'l) descending toward the base; developing in the direction of the base, as a spore.

ba·sis (ba'sis) pl. *ba'ses*. [L.] the lower, basic, or fundamental part of an object, organ, or substance.

ba·si·sphe·noid (ba″sĭ-sfe'noid) 1. postsphenoid. 2. an embryonic bone that becomes the back part of the body of the sphenoid.

bas·ket (bas'ket) 1. a container made of material woven together, or something resembling it. 2. basket cell. **stone b.,** a tiny apparatus of several wires that can be advanced through an endoscope into a body cavity or tube, manipulated to trap a calculus or other object, and withdrawn.

bas(o)- see *basi(o)-*.

ba·so·phil (ba'so-fil) 1. any structure, cell, or histologic element staining readily with basic dyes. 2. a granular leukocyte with an irregularly shaped, relatively pale-staining nucleus that is partially constricted into two lobes, and with cytoplasm containing coarse bluish-black granules of variable size. 3. one of the hormone-producing basophilic cells of the adenohypophysis; types include *gonadotrophs* and *thyrotrophs*. **basophil'ic,** adj.

ba·so·phil·ia (ba″so-fil'e-ah) 1. abnormal increase of basophils in the blood. 2. reaction of immature erythrocytes to basic dyes, becoming blue to gray in color; stippling is seen in lead poisoning.

ba·so·phil·ic (-fil'ik) 1. pertaining to basophils. 2. staining readily with basic dyes.

ba·soph·i·lism (ba-sof'ĭ-lizm) abnormal increase of basophilic cells. **Cushing's b., pituitary b.,** see under *syndrome* (1).

ba·so·phil·o·pe·nia (ba″so-fil″o-pe'ne-ah) abnormal reduction in the number of basophils in the blood.

bath (bath) 1. a medium, e.g., water, vapor, sand, or mud, with which the body is washed or in which the body is wholly or partially immersed for therapeutic or cleansing purposes; application of such a medium to the body. 2. the equipment or apparatus in which a body or object may be immersed. **colloid b.,** one containing gelatin, starch, bran, or similar substances. **contrast b.,** alternate immersion of a body part in hot and cold water. **emollient b.,** one in an emollient liquid, e.g., a decoction of bran. **half b.,** a bath of the hips and lower part of the body. **hip b.,** sitz b. **sitz b.,** immersion of only the hips and buttocks. **sponge b.,** one in which the body is not immersed but is rubbed with a wet cloth or sponge. **whirlpool b.,** one in which the water is kept in constant motion by mechanical means.

bath(o)- see *bathy-*.

batho·rho·dop·sin (bath″o-ro-dop'sin) a transient intermediate produced upon irradiation of rhodopsin in the visual cycle.

bath·ro·ceph·a·ly (bath″ro-sef'ah-le) a developmental anomaly marked by a steplike posterior projection of the skull, caused by excessive growth of the lambdoid suture.

bathy- word element [Gr.], *deep*. Also *bath(o)-*.

bathy·pnea (bath″ip-ne'ah) deep breathing.

bat·te·ry (bat'er-e) 1. a set or series of cells that yield an electric current. 2. any set, series, or grouping of similar things, as a battery of tests.

BBBB bilateral bundle branch block.

BBT basal body temperature.

BCDF B cell differentiation factors.

BCG bacille Calmette-Guérin.

BCNU carmustine.

Bdel·lo·vib·rio (del″o-vib′re-o) a genus of small, rod-shaped or curved, actively motile bacteria that are obligate parasites on certain gram-negative bacteria, including *Pseudomonas*, *Salmonella*, and coliform bacteria.

bdel·lo·vib·rio (del″o-vib′re-o) any microorganism of the genus *Bdellovibrio*.

B-E, BE below-elbow; see under *amputation*.

Be beryllium.

bead (bēd) a small spherical structure or mass. **rachitic b's**, a series of prominences at the points where the ribs join their cartilages; seen in certain cases of rickets.

bead·ed (bēd′ed) having the appearance of beads or a string of beads.

beak·er (bēk′er) a glass cup, usually with a lip for pouring, used by chemists and pharmacists.

bear·ber·ry (ber′ber-e) 1. uva ursi. 2. *Rhamnus purshiana*.

beat (bēt) a throb or pulsation, as of the heart or of an artery. **apex b.**, the beat felt over the apex of the heart, normally in or near the fifth left intercostal space. **atrioventricular (AV) junctional escape b.**, a depolarization initiated in the atrioventricular junction when one or more impulses from the sinus node are ineffective or nonexistent. **atrioventricular (AV) junctional premature b.**, see under *complex*. **capture b's**, in atrioventricular dissociation, occasional ventricular responses to a sinus impulse that reaches the atrioventricular node in a nonrefractory phase. **ectopic b.**, a heart beat originating at some point other than the sinus node. **escape b., escaped b.**, heart beats that follow an abnormally long pause. **forced b.**, an extrasystole produced by artificial stimulation of the heart. **fusion b.**, in electrocardiography, the complex resulting when an ectopic ventricular beat coincides with normal conduction to the ventricle. **heart b.**, heartbeat. **interpolated b.**, a contraction occurring exactly between two normal beats without altering the sinus rhythm. **junctional escape b.**, atrioventricular junctional escape b. **junctional premature b.**, atrioventricular junctional premature complex. **postectopic b.**, the normal beat following an ectopic beat. **premature b.**, extrasystole. **pseudofusion b.**, an ineffective pacing stimulus delivered during the absolute refractory period following a spontaneous discharge but before sufficient charge accumulates to prevent pacemaker discharge. **reciprocal b.**, a cardiac impulse that in one cycle causes ventricular contraction, travels backward toward the atria, then reexcites the ventricles. **reentrant b.**, any of the

characteristic beats of a reentrant circuit. **retrograde b.**, a beat resulting from impulse conduction that is backward relative to the normal atrioventricular direction. **ventricular escape b.**, an ectopic beat of ventricular origin occurring in the absence of supraventricular impulse generation or conduction. **ventricular premature b. (VPB)**, see under *complex*.

be·cap·ler·min (bĕ-kap′ler-min) a recombinant platelet-derived growth factor used in the treatment of chronic severe dermal ulcers of the lower limbs in diabetes mellitus.

bec·lo·meth·a·sone (bek″lo-meth′ah-sōn) a glucocorticoid used in the dipropionate form in the treatment of bronchial asthma, seasonal and nonseasonal allergic rhinitis or other allergic or inflammatory nasal conditions, and some dermatoses, and to prevent recurrence of nasal polyps.

bec·que·rel (bek″ĕ-rel′) a unit of radioactivity, defined as the quantity of a radionuclide that undergoes one decay per second (s^{-1}). One curie equals 3.7×10^{10} becquerels. Abbreviated Bq.

bed (bed) 1. a supporting structure or tissue. 2. a couch or support for the body during sleep. **capillary b.**, the capillaries, collectively, and their volume capacity; see Plate 22. **nail b.**, matrix unguis; the area of modified epithelium beneath the nail, over which the nail plate slides forward as it grows. **vascular b.**, the sum of the blood vessels supplying an organ or region.

bed·bug (bed′bug) a bug of the genus *Cimex*.

bed·sore (bed′sōr) decubitus ulcer.

bees·wax (bēz′waks) wax derived from the honeycomb of the bee *Apis mellifera*; see *yellow wax* (unbleached b.) and *white wax*, (bleached b.) under *wax*.

be·hav·ior (be-hāv′yer) deportment or conduct; any or all of a person's total activity, especially that which is externally observable. **behav′ioral**, adj.

be·hav·ior·ism (-izm) the psychologic theory based upon objectively observable, tangible, and measurable data, rather than subjective phenomena, such as ideas and emotions.

bel (bel) a unit used to express the ratio of two powers, usually electric or acoustic powers; an increase of 1 bel in intensity approximately doubles loudness of most sounds. Symbol B. See also *decibel*.

bel·la·don·na (bel″ah-don′ah) the deadly nightshade, *Atropa belladonna*, a perennial plant containing various anticholinergic alkaloids, including atropine, hyoscyamine, and scopolamine, which are used medicinally; however, the plant or its alkaloids can cause poisoning.

bel·ly (bel′e) 1. abdomen. 2. venter (1).

bel·o·noid (bel′ah-noid) needle-shaped; styloid.

ben·a·ze·pril (ben-a′zě-pril) an angiotensin-converting enzyme inhibitor used as the hydrochloride salt in the treatment of hypertension.

bend (bend) a flexure or curve; a flexed or curved part. **varolian b.,** the third cerebral flexure in the developing fetus.

ben·dro·flu·me·thi·a·zide (ben″dro-floo″mě-thi′ah-zīd) a thiazide diuretic used to treat hypertension and edema.

bends (bendz) pain in the limbs and abdomen due to rapid reduction of air pressure; see *decompression sickness,* under *sickness.*

be·nign (bě-nīn′) not malignant; not recurrent; favorable for recovery.

ben·ox·i·nate (ben-ok′sĭ-nāt) a topical anesthetic for the eye, used as the hydrochloride salt.

ben·ser·a·zide (ben-ser′ah-zīd) an inhibitor of decarboxylation of levodopa in extracerebral tissues, used in combination with levodopa as an antiparkinsonian agent.

ben·to·qua·tam (ben′to-kwah″tam) a topical skin protectant used to prevent or reduce allergic contact dermatitis resulting from contact with urushiol (poison ivy, poison oak, poison sumac).

ben·zal·de·hyde (ben-zal′dě-hīd) an aldehyde derivative of benzene, occurring in the kernels of bitter almonds or produced synthetically; used as a pharmaceutical flavoring agent.

ben·zal·ko·ni·um chlo·ride (ben″zal-ko′ne-um) a quaternary ammonium compound used as a surface disinfectant and detergent, topical antiseptic, and antimicrobial preservative.

ben·zene (ben′zēn) a liquid hydrocarbon, C_6H_6, from coal tar; used as a solvent. It is toxic by transdermal absorption, ingestion, or inhalation; chronic exposure may cause bone marrow depression and aplasia and leukemia. **b. hexachloride (BHC),** a chlorinated hydrocarbon, $C_6H_6Cl_6$, having numerous isomers; the gamma isomer is *lindane.*

ben·ze·tho·ni·um chlo·ride (ben″zě-tho′ne-um) a quaternary ammonium compound used as a local antiseptic, pharmaceutical preservative, and detergent and disinfectant.

ben·zi·dine (ben′zĭ-dēn) a carcinogen and toxin once widely used as a test for occult blood.

ben·zin (ben′zin) petroleum benzin; see under *petroleum.*

benzine (ben′zēn) petroleum benzin; see under *petroleum.*

ben·zo·ate (ben′zo-āt) a salt of benzoic acid.

ben·zo·caine (-kān) a local anesthetic applied topically to the skin and mucous membranes; also used to suppress the gag reflex in various procedures.

ben·zo·di·az·e·pine (ben″zo-di-az′ě-pēn) any of a group of compounds having a common molecular structure and similar pharmacological activities, including antianxiety, muscle relaxing, and sedative and hypnotic effects.

ben·zo·ic ac·id (ben-zo′ik) a fungistatic compound used as a pharmaceutical and food preservative and, with salicylic acid, as a topical antifungal agent.

ben·zo·na·tate (ben-zo′nah-tāt) an antitussive that reduces the cough reflex by anesthetizing the stretch receptors in the respiratory passages, lungs, and pleura.

ben·zo·pur·pu·rine (ben″zo-pur′pu-rin) any one of a series of azo dyes of a scarlet color.

ben·zo·qui·none (-kwin′ōn) 1. a substituted benzene ring containing two carbonyl groups, usually in the *para* (1,4) position; *p*-benzoquinone is used in manufacturing and in fungicides and is toxic by inhalation and an irritant to skin and mucous membranes. 2. any of a subclass of quinones derived from or containing this structure.

ben·zo·thi·a·di·a·zine (-thi″ah-di′ah-zēn) thiazide.

ben·zo·yl (ben′zo-il) the acyl radical formed from benzoic acid, C_6H_5CO—. **b. peroxide,** a topical keratolytic and antibacterial used in the treatment of acne vulgaris.

ben·zo·yl·ec·go·nine (ben″zo-il-ek′go-nēn) the major metabolite of cocaine; detectable in the blood by laboratory testing.

benz·phet·amine (benz-fet′ah-mēn) a sympathomimetic amine used as an anorectic in the form of the hydrochloride salt.

benz·quin·amide (-kwin′ah-mīd) an antiemetic used as the hydrochloride salt to prevent and treat nausea and vomiting associated with anesthesia and surgery.

benz·thi·a·zide (-thi′ah-zīd) a thiazide diuretic used to treat edema and hypertension.

benz·tro·pine (benz′tro-pēn) an antidyskinetic used as the mesylate salt in the treatment of parkinsonism and for the control of drug-induced extrapyramidal reactions.

ben·zyl (ben′zil) the hydrocarbon radical, C_7H_7. **b. benzoate,** one of the active substances in peruvian and tolu balsams, and produced synthetically; applied topically as a scabicide.

ben·zyl·pen·i·cil·lin (ben″zil-pen″ĭ-sil′in) penicillin G.

ben·zyl·pen·i·cil·lo·yl poly·ly·sine (-o-il pol″e-li′sēn) a skin test antigen composed of a benzylpenicilloyl moiety and a polylysine carrier, used in assessing hypersensitivity to penicillin by scratch test or intradermal test.

bep·ri·dil (bep′rĭ-dil) a calcium channel blocking agent used as the hydrochloride salt in the treatment of chronic angina pectoris.

ber·ac·tant (ber-ak′tant) a modified bovine lung extract that mimics the action of pulmonary surfactant, used in the prevention and treatment of respiratory distress syndrome of the newborn.

ber·ber·ine (bur′bur-ēn) an alkaloid from species of *Berberis* and related plants, and from *Hydrastis canadensis*; it has antimicrobial activity and has been used in treatment of various infections and in ulcer dressings.

beri·beri (ber″e-ber″e) a disease due to thiamine (vitamin B_1) deficiency, marked by polyneuritis, cardiac pathology, and edema; the epidemic form occurs primarily in areas in which white (polished) rice is the staple food.

berke·li·um (Bk) (berk′le-um) chemical element (see *Table of Elements*), at. no. 97.

ber·ry (ber′e) a small fruit with a succulent pericarp. **bear b.,** bearberry.

be·ryl·li·o·sis (bah-ril″e-o′sis) a morbid condition due to exposure to fumes or fine dust of beryllium salts, with formation of granulomas, usually in the lungs and less often the skin, subcutaneous tissue, lymph nodes, liver, or other organs.

be·ryl·li·um (Be) (bah-ril′le-um) chemical element (see *Table of Elements*), at. no. 4.

bes·ti·al·i·ty (bes-te-al′ĭ-te) zoophilia (2).

bes·y·late (bes′ĭ-lāt) USAN contraction for benzenesulfonate.

be·ta (ba′tah) β, the second letter of the Greek alphabet; see also β-.

be·ta·car·o·tene (ba″tah-kar′o-tēn) see under carotene.

be·ta·his·tine (-his′tēn) a histamine analogue used as the hydrochloride salt to reduce the frequency of attacks of vertigo in Meniere's disease.

Be·ta·her·pes·vi·ri·nae (-her″pēz-vir-i′ne) the cytomegaloviruses: a subfamily of viruses of the family Herpesviridae, including the genus *Cytomegalovirus*.

be·ta·ine (be′tah-ēn) the carboxylic acid derived by oxidation of choline; it acts as a transmethylating metabolic intermediate and is used in the treatment of homocystinuria. The hydrochloride salt is used as a gastric acidifier.

be·ta·meth·a·sone (ba″tah-meth′ah-sōn) a synthetic glucocorticoid, the most active of the antiinflammatory steroids; used topically as the benzoate, dipropionate, or valerate salts as an antiinflammatory, topically or rectally as the sodium phosphate salt as an antiinflammatory, and systemically as the base or the combination of sodium phosphate and acetate salts as an antiinflammatory, as a replacement for adrenal insufficiency, and as an immunosuppressant.

be·tax·o·lol (ba-tak′so-lol) a cardioselective β-adrenergic blocking agent, used in the form of the hydrochloride salt as an antihypertensive and in the treatment of glaucoma and ocular hypertension.

be·than·e·chol (bĕ-than′ĕ-kol) a cholinergic agonist, used as the chloride salt to stimulate smooth muscle contraction of the urinary bladder in cases of postoperative, postpartum, or neurogenic atony and retention.

bex·ar·o·tene (bek-sar′ah-tēn) a retinoid used as an antineoplastic in the treatment of cutaneous T-cell lymphoma and the cutaneous lesions of T-cell lymphomas and Kaposi's sarcoma.

be·zoar (be′zor) a concretion of foreign material found in the gastrointestinal or urinary tract.

BHA butylated hydroxyanisole, an antioxidant used in foods, cosmetics, and pharmaceuticals that contain fats or oils.

BHC benzene hexachloride.

BHT butylated hydroxytoluene, an antioxidant used in foods, cosmetics, pharmaceuticals, and petroleum products.

Bi bismuth.

bi- word element [L.], *two.*

bi·acro·mi·al (bi-ah-kro′me-al) between the two acromia.

bi·au·ric·u·lar (-aw-rik′u-ler) pertaining to the auricles of both ears.

bi·ax·i·al (-ak′se-al) having, pertaining to, or occurring in two axes.

bib·lio·ther·a·py (bib″le-o-ther′ah-pe) the reading of selected books as part of the treatment of mental disorders or for mental health.

bi·ca·lu·ta·mide (bi″kah-loo′tah-mīd) an antiandrogen used in the treatment of prostatic carcinoma.

bi·cam·er·al (bi-kam′er-al) having two chambers or cavities.

bi·car·bo·nate (-kahr′bah-nāt) any salt containing the HCO_3^- anion. **blood b., plasma b.,** the bicarbonate of the blood plasma, an index of alkali reserve. **b. of soda,** sodium bicarbonate. **standard b.,** the plasma bicarbonate concentration in blood equilibrated with a specific gas mixture under specific conditions.

bi·ceps (bi′seps) a muscle having two heads.

bi·cip·i·tal (bi-sip′ĭ-t'l) having two heads; pertaining to a biceps muscle.

bi·col·lis (-kol′is) having a double cervix.

bi·con·cave (bi″kon-kāv′) having two concave surfaces.

bi·con·vex (-kon-veks′) having two convex surfaces.

bi·cor·nate (-kor′nāt) bicornuate.

bi·cor·nu·ate (-kor′nu-āt) having two horns or cornua.

bi·cus·pid (-kus′pid) 1. having two cusps. 2. pertaining to a mitral (bicuspid) valve. 3. premolar tooth.

b.i.d. [L.] bis in di′e (twice a day).

bi·der·mo·ma (bi″der-mo′mah) didermoma.

bi·fas·cic·u·lar (-fah-sik′u-lar) pertaining to two bundles, or fasciculi.

bi·fid (bi′fid) cleft into two parts or branches.

Bi·fid·o·bac·te·ri·um (bi″fid-o-bak-tēr′e-um) a genus of obligate anaerobic lactobacilli commonly occurring in the feces.

bi·fo·cal (bi-fo′-, bi′fo-k'l) 1. having two foci. 2. containing one part for near vision and another part for distant vision, as in a bifocal lens.

bi·fo·cals (bi′fo-k'lz) bifocal glasses.

bi·fo·rate (bi-for′āt) having two perforations or foramina.

bi·fur·ca·tion (bi″fer-ka′shun) 1. a division into two branches. 2. the point at which division into two branches occurs.

bi·gem·i·ny (bi-jem′ĭ-ne) 1. occurring in pairs. 2. the occurrence of two beats of the pulse in rapid succession. **bigem′inal,** adj. **atrial b.,** an arrhythmia consisting of the repetitive sequence of one atrial premature complex followed by one normal sinus impulse. **atrioventricular nodal b.,** an arrhythmia in which an atrioventricular extrasystole is followed by a normal sinus impulse in repetitive sequence. **ventricular b.,** an arrhythmia consisting of the repeated sequence of one ventricular premature complex followed by one normal beat.

bi·lat·er·al (-lat′er-al) having two sides, or pertaining to both sides.

bi·lay·er (bi′la-er) a membrane consisting of two molecular layers.

bil·ber·ry (bil′ber-e) the leaves and fruit of *Vaccinium myrtillus*, having astringent and antidiarrheal effects, used topically for inflammation, burns, and skin diseases, and orally for gout, arthritis, dermatitis, diabetes mellitus, and gastrointestinal, urinary tract, and kidney disorders.

bile (bīl) a fluid secreted by the liver, concentrated in the gallbladder, and poured into the small intestine via the bile ducts, which helps in alkalinizing the intestinal contents and plays a role in emulsification, absorption, and digestion of fat; its chief constituents are conjugated bile salts, cholesterol, phospholipid, bilirubin, and electrolytes.

bile ac·id (bīl as′id) any of the steroid acids derived from cholesterol; classified as *primary*, those synthesized in the liver, e.g., cholic and chenodeoxycholic acids, or *secondary*, those produced from primary bile acids by intestinal bacteria, e.g., deoxycholic and lithocholic acids. Most of the the bile acids are reabsorbed and returned to the liver via the enterohepatic circulation. Cf. *bile salt* under *salt*.

Bil·har·zia (bil-hahr′ze-ah) *Schistosoma*.

bil·har·zi·a·sis (bil″hahr-zi′ah-sis) schistosomiasis.

bil(i)- word element [L.], *bile*.

bil·i·a·ry (bil′e-ar″e) pertaining to the bile, to the bile ducts, or to the gallbladder.

bil·i·ra·chia (bil″ĭ-ra′ke-ah) presence of bile pigments in spinal fluid.

bil·i·ru·bin (-roo′bin) a bile pigment produced by breakdown of heme and reduction of biliverdin; it normally circulates in plasma and is taken up by liver cells and conjugated to form bilirubin diglucuronide, the water-soluble pigment excreted in bile. High concentrations of bilirubin may result in jaundice. **conjugated b., direct b.,** bilirubin that has been taken up by the liver cells and conjugated to form the water-soluble bilirubin diglucuronide. **indirect b., unconjugated b.,** the lipid-soluble form of bilirubin that circulates in loose association with the plasma proteins.

bil·i·uria (bil″ĭ-u′re-ah) bile pigments or bile salts in the urine.

bil·i·ver·din (-ver′din) a green bile pigment formed by catabolism of hemoglobin and converted to bilirubin in the liver; it may also arise from oxidation of bilirubin.

bi·loc·u·lar (bi-lok′u-ler) having two compartments.

bi·lo·ma (bi′lo-mah) an encapsulated collection of bile in the peritoneal cavity.

bi·mat·o·prost (bĭ-mat′o-prost) a synthetic prostaglandin analogue used topically in the treatment of open-angle glaucoma and ocular hypertension.

Bi·lo·phi·la (bi-lof′ĭ-lah) a genus of gram-negative, anaerobic bacteria, including *B. wadswor′thia*, which causes intra-abdominal and other infections.

bi·man·u·al (bi-man′u-al) with both hands; performed by both hands.

bi·na·ry (bi′nah-re) 1. made up of two elements or of two equal parts. 2. denoting a number system with a base of two.

bi·nau·ral (bi-naw′r'l) pertaining to both ears.

bi·nau·ric·u·lar (bin″aw-rik′u-ler) biauricular.

bind·er (bīnd′er) a girdle or large bandage for support of the abdomen or breasts, particularly one applied to the abdomen after childbirth to support the relaxed abdominal walls.

binge (binj) 1. a period of uncontrolled or excessive self-indulgent activity, particularly of eating or drinking. 2. to indulge in such activity.

bin·oc·u·lar (bĭ-nok′u-ler) 1. pertaining to both eyes. 2. having two eyepieces, as in a microscope.

bi·no·mi·al (bi-no′me-al) composed of two terms, e.g., names of organisms formed by combination of genus and species names.

bin·ov·u·lar (bin-ov′u-ler) pertaining to or derived from two distinct oocytes or ova.

bi·nu·cle·a·tion (bi″noo-kle-a′shun) formation of two nuclei within a cell through division of the nucleus without division of the cytoplasm.

bi(o)- word element [Gr.], *life; living.*

bio·am·in·er·gic (bi″o-am″in-er′jik) of or pertaining to neurons that secrete biogenic amines.

bio·as·say (bi′o-as″a) determination of the active power of a drug sample by comparing its effects on a live animal or an isolated organ preparation with those of a reference standard.

bio·avail·a·bil·i·ty (bi″o-ah-vāl″ah-bil′ĭ-te) the degree to which a drug or other substance becomes available to the target tissue after administration.

bio·chem·is·try (-kem′is-tre) the chemistry of living organisms and of vital processes. **biochem′ical,** adj.

bio·com·pat·i·ble (-kom-pat′ĭ-b'l) being harmonious with life; not having toxic or injurious effects on biological function.

bio·de·grad·a·ble (-de-grād′ah-b'l) susceptible of degradation by biological processes, as by bacterial or other enzymatic action.

bio·deg·ra·da·tion (-deg″rah-da′shun) the series of processes by which living

systems render chemicals less noxious to the environment.

bio·equiv·a·lence (-e-kwiv′ah-lens) the relationship between two preparations of the same drug in the same dosage form that have a similar bioavailability. **bioequiv′alent,** adj.

bio·eth·ics (-eth′iks) obligations of a moral nature relating to biological research and its applications.

bio·feed·back (-fēd′bak) the process of furnishing someone with information on one or more physiologic variables, such as heart rate, blood pressure, or skin temperature; this may help the person gain some voluntary control over them. **alpha b.,** presentation of continuous information on the state of the brain-wave pattern, to assist in purposeful increase in the percentage of alpha activity and thus a state of relaxation and peaceful wakefulness.

bio·fla·vo·noid (-fla′vah-noid) any of the flavonoids with biological activity in mammals.

bio·gen·e·sis (-jen′ĕ-sis) 1. origin of life, or of living organisms. 2. the theory that living organisms originate only from other living organisms.

bi·o·gen·ic (-jen′ik) having origins in biological processes.

bio·im·plant (-im′plant) a prosthesis made of biosynthetic material.

bio·in·com·pat·i·ble (-in″kom-pat′ĭ-b'l) inharmonious with life; having toxic or injurious effects on life functions.

bio·ki·net·ics (-kĭ-net′iks) 1. the science of the movements within organisms. 2. the application of therapeutic exercise in rehabilitative treatment or performance enhancement.

bi·o·log·i·cals (-loj′ĭ-k'lz) medicinal preparations made from living organisms and their products, including serums, vaccines, antigens, antitoxins, etc.

bi·ol·o·gy (bi-ol′ah-je) scientific study of living organisms. **biolog′ic, biolog′ical,** adj. **molecular b.,** study of molecular structures and events underlying biological processes, including relationships between genes and the functional characteristics they determine. **radiation b.,** scientific study of effects of ionizing radiation on living organisms.

bio·mark·er (bi′o-mahr″ker) 1. a biological molecule used as a marker for a substance or process of interest. 2. tumor marker.

bio·mass (bi′o-mas) the entire assemblage of living organisms of a particular region, considered collectively.

bio·ma·te·ri·al (bi″o-mah-tēr′e-al) a synthetic dressing with selective barrier properties, used in the treatment of burns; it consists of a liquid solvent (polyethylene glycol-400) and a powdered polymer.

bio·med·i·cine (bi″o-med′ĭ-sin) clinical medicine based on the principles of the natural sciences (biology, biochemistry, etc.). **biomed′ical**, adj.

bio·mem·brane (-mem′brān) any membrane, e.g., the cell membrane, of an organism. **biomem′branous**, adj.

bi·om·e·try (bi-om′ĕ-tre) the application of statistical methods to biological phenomena.

bio·mi·cro·scope (bi″o-mi′krah-skōp) a microscope for examining living tissue in the body.

bio·mod·u·la·tion (-mod″u-la′shun) reactive or associative adjustment of the biochemical or cellular status of an organism.

bio·mod·u·la·tor (-mod′u-la″ter) biologic reponse modifier.

bio·mol·e·cule (-mol′ĕ-kūl) a molecule produced by living cells, e.g., a protein, carbohydrate, lipid, or nucleic acid.

bi·on·ics (bi-on′iks) scientific study of functions, characteristics, and phenomena observed in the living world, and the application of knowledge gained therefrom to nonliving systems.

bio·phys·ics (bi″o-fiz′iks) the science dealing with the application of physical methods and theories to biological problems. **biophys′ical**, adj.

bio·phys·i·ol·o·gy (-fiz″e-ol′ah-je) that portion of biology including organogeny, morphology, and physiology.

bio·pros·the·sis (-pros-the′sis) a prosthesis that contains biological material. **bioprosthet′ic**, adj.

bi·op·sy (bi′op-se) removal and examination, usually microscopic, of tissue from the living body, performed to establish precise diagnosis. **aspiration b.**, biopsy in which tissue is obtained by application of suction through a needle attached to a syringe. **brush b.**, biopsy in which cells or tissue are obtained by manipulating tiny brushes against the tissue or lesion in question (e.g., through a bronchoscope) at the desired site. **cone b.**, biopsy in which an inverted cone of tissue is excised, as from the uterine cervix. **core b.**, **core needle b.**, needle biopsy with a large hollow needle that extracts a core of tissue. **endoscopic b.**, removal of tissue by appropriate instruments through an endoscope. **excisional b.**, biopsy of tissue removed by surgical cutting. **incisional b.**, biopsy of a selected portion of a lesion. **needle b.**, biopsy in which tissue is obtained

by puncture of a tumor, the tissue within the lumen of the needle being detached by rotation, and the needle withdrawn. Called also *percutaneous b.* **percutaneous b.**, needle b. **punch b.**, biopsy in which tissue is obtained by a punch. **shave b.**, biopsy of a skin lesion in which the sample is excised using a cut parallel to the surface of the surrounding skin. **stereotactic b.**, biopsy of the brain using stereotactic surgery to locate the biopsy site. **sternal b.**, biopsy of bone marrow of the sternum removed by puncture or trephining.

bio·psy·chol·o·gy (bi″o-si-kol′ah-je) psychobiology (1).

bi·op·tome (bi′op-tōm″) a cutting instrument for taking biopsy specimens.

bio·re·ver·si·ble (bi″o-re-ver′sĭ-b′l) capable of being changed back to the original biologically active chemical form by processes within the organism; said of drugs.

bio·sci·ence (-si′ens) the study of biology wherein all the applicable sciences (physics, chemistry, etc.) are applied.

bio·sta·tis·tics (-stah-tis′tiks) biometry.

bio·syn·the·sis (-sin′thĕ-sis) creation of a compound by physiologic processes in a living organism. **biosynthet′ic**, adj.

bi·o·ta (bi-ō′tah) all the living organisms of a particular area; the combined flora and fauna of a region.

bio·te·lem·e·try (bi″o-tĕ-lem′ĕ-tre) the recording and measuring of certain vital phenomena of living organisms that are situated at a distance from the measuring device.

bio·ther·a·py (-ther′ah-pe) biological therapy.

bi·ot·ic (bi-ot′ik) 1. pertaining to life or living matter. 2. pertaining to the biota.

bio·tin (bi′o-tin) a member of the vitamin B complex; it is a cofactor for several enzymes, plays a role in fatty acid and amino acid metabolism, and is used in vitro in some biochemical assays.

bio·tox·i·col·o·gy (bi″o-tok″sĭ-kol′ah-je) scientific study of poisons produced by living organisms, and treatment of conditions produced by them.

bio·trans·for·ma·tion (-trans″for-ma′shun) the series of chemical alterations of a compound (e.g., a drug) occurring within the body, as by enzymatic activity.

bio·type (bi′o-tīp) 1. a group of individuals having the same genotype. 2. any of a number of strains of a species of microorganisms having differentiable physiologic characteristics.

bi·ov·u·lar (bi-ov′u-ler) binovular.

bip·a·rous (bip'ah-rus) producing two off-spring or eggs at one time.

bi·pen·ni·form (bi-pen'ĭ-form) doubly feather-shaped; said of muscles whose fibers are arranged on each side of a tendon like barbs on a feather shaft.

bi·per·i·den (-per'ĭ-den) an antidyskinetic used as the hydrochloride and lactate salts in the treatment of parkinsonism and drug-induced extrapyramidal reactions.

bi·phen·yl (-fen'il) diphenyl. **polychlori-nated b. (PCB)**, any of a group of chlorinated derivatives of biphenyl, used as heat-transfer agents and electrical insulators; they are toxic, carcinogenic, and non-biode-gradable.

bi·po·lar (-po'lar) 1. having two poles or pertaining to both poles. 2. describing neurons that have processes at both ends. 3. pertaining to mood disorders in which both depressive episodes and manic or hypomanic episodes occur.

bi·po·ten·ti·al·i·ty (bi''po-ten''she-al'ĭ-te) ability to develop or act in either of two possible ways. **bipoten'tial**, adj.

bi·ra·mous (bi-ra'mus) having two branches.

bi·re·frin·gence (bi''-re-frin'jens) the quality of transmitting light unequally in different directions. **birefrin'gent**, adj.

birth (berth) a coming into being; act or process of being born. **complete b.**, entire separation of the infant from the maternal body (after cutting of the umbilical cord). **multiple b.**, the birth of two or more off-spring produced in the same gestation period. **postterm b.**, birth of an infant at or after 42 completed weeks (294 days) of gestation. **premature b., preterm b.**, birth of an infant before 37 completed weeks (259 days) of gestation.

birth·mark (berth'mahrk) a congenital circumscribed blemish or spot on the skin; see *nevus*.

bis·ac·o·dyl (bis-ak'ah-dil) (bis''ah-ko'dil) a contact laxative, used as the base or as a complex with tannic acid (*b. tannex*).

bis·acro·mi·al (bis''ah-kro'me-al) pertain-ing to the two acromial processes.

bi·sec·tion (bi-sek'shun) division into two parts by cutting.

bi·sex·u·al (-sek'shoo-al) 1. pertaining to or characterized by bisexuality. 2. an indi-vidual exhibiting bisexuality. 3. pertaining to or characterized by hermaphroditism. 4. pertaining to or characterized by andro-gyny.

bi·sex·u·al·i·ty (-sek''shoo-al'ĭ-te) 1. sexual attraction to persons of both sexes; exhi-bition of both homosexual and heterosexual behavior. 2. true hermaphroditism. 3. androgyny (1).

bis·fe·ri·ens (bis-fe're-enz) [L.] bisferious.

bis·fe·ri·ous (-us) having two beats.

bis·il·i·ac (-il''e-ak) pertaining to the two iliac bones or to any two corresponding points on them.

bis·muth (Bi) (biz'muth) chemical element (see *Table of Elements*), at. no. 83. Its salts have been used to treat diarrhea, nausea, and other gastrointestinal conditions. **b. subsalicylate**, a bismuth salt of salicylic acid, used in the treatment of diarrhea and gastric distress, including nausea, indigestion, and heartburn.

bis·mu·tho·sis (biz''mah-tho'sis) bismuth poisoning, with anuria, stomatitis, dermatitis, and diarrhea.

bis·o·pro·lol (bis''o-pro'lol) a cardioselec-tive beta-adrenergic blocking agent, used as the fumarate salt in the treatment of hyper-tension.

2,3-bis·phos·pho·glyc·er·ate (bis-fos''fo-glis'er-āt) an intermediate in the conversion of 3-phosphoglycerate to 2-phosphoglycerate; it also acts as an allosteric effector in the regulation of oxygen binding by hemoglobin.

bis·phos·pho·nate (bis-fos'fo-nāt) diphos-phonate.

bis·tou·ry (bis'too-re) a long, narrow, straight or curved surgical knife.

bi·sul·fate (bi-sul'fāt) an acid sulfate.

bi·tar·trate (-tahr'trāt) any salt containing the anion $C_4H_5O_6^-$ derived from tartaric acid ($C_4H_6O_6$).

bite (bīt) 1. seizure with the teeth. 2. a wound or puncture made by a living organ-ism. 3. an impression made by closure of the teeth upon some plastic material, e.g., wax. 4. occlusion (2). **closed b.**, malocclu-sion in which the incisal edges of the man-dibular anterior teeth protrude past those of the maxillary teeth. **cross b.**, crossbite. **edge-to-edge b., end-to-end b.**, occlusion in which the incisors of both jaws are closed. **open b.**, occlusion in which certain opposing teeth fail to come together when the jaws are closed; usually confined to anterior teeth. **over b.**, overbite.

bite-block (bīt'blok) occlusion rim.

bite-lock (-lok) a dental device for retain-ing occlusion rims in the same relation outside the mouth which they occupied in the mouth.

bi·tem·po·ral (bi-tem'pŏ-r'l) pertaining to both temples or temporal bones.

bite-plate (-plāt) an appliance, usually plas-tic and wire, worn in the palate as a diagnostic or therapeutic adjunct in orthodontics or prosthodontics.

bite-wing (-wing) a wing or fin attached along the center of the tooth side of a dental x-ray film and bitten on by the patient, permitting production of images of the corona of the teeth in both dental arches and their contiguous periodontal tissues.

Bi·tis (bi′tis) a genus of venomous, brightly colored, thick-bodied, viperine snakes, possessing heart-shaped heads; including the puff adder (*B. arientans*), Gaboon viper (*B. gabonica*), and rhinoceros viper (*B. nasicornis*).

bi·tol·ter·ol (bi-tol′ter-ol) a β_2-adrenergic receptor agonist, administered by inhalation in the form of the mesylate salt as a bronchodilator.

bi·tro·chan·ter·ic (bi″-tro-kan-ter′ik) pertaining to both trochanters on one femur or to both greater trochanters.

bi·tu·mi·no·sis (bi-too″mĭ-no′sis) a form of pneumoconiosis due to inhalation of dust from soft coal.

bi·u·ret (bi′u-ret) a urea derivative whose presence is detected after addition of sodium hydroxide and copper sulfate solutions by a pinkish-violet color (protein test) or a pink and finally a bluish color (urea test).

bi·va·lent (bi-va′lent) 1. divalent. 2. the structure formed by a pair of homologous chromosomes by synapsis along their length during the zygotene and pachytene stages of the first meiotic prophase.

bi·val·i·ru·din (bi-val′ĭroo-din) an anticoagulant used with aspirin in patients with unstable angina pectoris who are undergoing percutaneous transluminal coronary angioplasty.

bi·ven·tric·u·lar (bi″ven-trik′u-ler) pertaining to or affecting both ventricles of the heart.

bi·zy·go·mat·ic (bi″zi-go-mat′ik) pertaining to the two most prominent points on the two zygomatic arches.

B-K, BK below-knee; see *transtibial amputation*, under *amputation*.

Bk borkelium.

BKV BK virus.

black (blak) reflecting no light or true color; of the darkest hue.

black·head (blak′hed) open comedo.

black·out (-out) loss of vision and momentary lapse of consciousness due to diminished circulation to the brain and retina. **alcoholic b.**, anterograde amnesia experienced by alcoholics during episodes of drinking, even when not fully intoxicated; indicative of early, reversible brain damage.

black·snake (-snāk) 1. *Pseudechis porphyriacus*, a large venomous semiaquatic Australian snake whose body is black on top and red underneath. 2. *Coluber constrictor*, a nonvenomous snake found in North America.

blad·der (blad′er) 1. a membranous sac, such as one serving as receptacle for a secretion. 2. urinary bladder. **atonic neurogenic b.**, neurogenic bladder due to destruction of sensory nerve fibers from the bladder to the spinal cord, with absence of control of bladder functions and of desire to urinate, bladder overdistention, and an abnormal amount of residual urine; usually associated with tabes dorsalis or pernicious anemia. **automatic b.**, neurogenic bladder due to complete transection of the spinal cord above the sacral segments, with loss of micturition reflexes and bladder sensation, involuntary urination, and an abnormal amount of residual urine. **autonomic b.**, **autonomous b.**, neurogenic bladder due to a lesion in the sacral spinal cord, interrupting the reflex arc controlling the bladder, with loss of normal bladder sensation and reflexes, inability to initiate urination normally, and incontinence. **gall b.**, gallbladder. **ileal b.**, a neobladder made from a section of ileum. **irritable b.**, a condition of the bladder marked by increased frequency of contraction with associated desire to urinate. **motor paralytic b.**, neurogenic bladder due to impairment of motor neurons or nerves controlling the bladder; the *acute* form is marked by painful distention and inability to initiate urination, and the *chronic* form by difficulty initiating urination, straining, decreased size and force of stream, interrupted stream, and recurrent urinary tract infection. **neurogenic b.**, dysfunction of the urinary bladder caused by a lesion of the central or peripheral nervous system. **uninhibited neurogenic b.**, neurogenic bladder due to a lesion in upper motor neurons with subtotal interruption of corticospinal pathways, with urgency, frequent involuntary urination, and small-volume threshold of activity. **urinary b.**, the musculomembranous sac in the anterior part of the pelvic cavity that serves as a reservoir for urine, which it receives through the ureters and discharges through the urethra.

blast¹ (blast) 1. an immature stage in cellular development before appearance of the definitive characteristics of the cell; used also as a word termination (see *-blast*). 2. blast cell (2).

blast² (blast) the wave of air pressure produced by the detonation of high-explosive bombs or shells or by other explosions; it causes pulmonary concussion and hemorrhage (*lung blast*, *blast chest*), laceration of other thoracic and abdominal viscera, ruptured eardrums, and minor effects in the central nervous system.

-blast word element [Gr.] *a type of blast*[1].

blas·te·ma (blas-te′mah) a group of cells giving rise to a new individual (in asexual reproduction) or to an organ or part (in either normal development or in regeneration). **blaste′mic,** adj.

blast(o)- word element [Gr.], *a bud; budding.*

blas·to·coele (blas′to-sēl) the fluid-filled central segmentation cavity of the blastula. **blastocoe′lic,** adj.

blas·to·cyst (-sist) the mammalian conceptus in the postmorula stage, consisting of an embryoblast (inner cell mass) and a thin trophoblast layer enclosing a blastocyst cavity.

blas·to·cyte (-sīt) an undifferentiated embryonic cell.

blas·to·derm (-derm) the single layer of cells forming the wall of the blastula, or the cellular cap above the floor of segmented yolk in the discoblastula of telolecithal eggs. **blastoder′mal, blastoder′mic,** adj.

blas·to·gen·e·sis (blas″to-jen′ĕ-sis) 1. development of an individual from a blastema, i.e., by asexual reproduction. 2. transmission of inherited characters by the germ plasm. 3. morphological transformation of small lymphocytes into larger cells resembling blast cells on exposure to phytohemagglutinin or to antigens to which the donor is immunized. **blastogenet′ic, blastogen′ic,** adj.

blas·to·ma (blas-to′mah) pl. *blastomas, blasto′mata.* A neoplasm composed of embryonic cells derived from the blastema of an organ or tissue. **blasto′matous,** adj.

blas·to·mere (blas′to-mēr) one of the cells produced by cleavage of a zygote.

Blas·to·my·ces (blas″to-mi′sēz) a genus of pathogenic fungi growing as mycelial forms at room temperature and as yeastlike forms at body temperature; applied to the yeasts pathogenic for humans and other animals. **B. brasilien′sis,** *Paracoccidioides brasiliensis.* **B. dermati′tidis,** the agent of North American blastomycosis.

blas·to·my·co·sis (-mi-ko′sis) 1. any infection caused by a yeastlike organism. 2. a chronic infection due to *Blastomyces dermatitidis,* predominantly involving the skin, lungs, and bones. **North American b.,** blastomycosis (2). **South American b.,** paracoccidioidomycosis.

blas·to·pore (blas′to-por) the opening of the archenteron to the exterior of the embryo at the gastrula stage.

blas·tu·la (blas′tu-lah) pl. *blas′tulae.* [L.] the usually spherical structure produced by cleavage of a zygote, consisting of a single layer of cells (blastoderm) surrounding a fluid-filled cavity (blastocoele).

bleb (bleb) a large flaccid vesicle, usually at least 1 cm. in diameter.

bleed·er (blēd′er) 1. one who bleeds freely. 2. any blood vessel cut during surgery that requires clamping, ligature, or cautery.

bleed·ing (-ing) 1. the escape of blood, as from an injured vessel. 2. phlebotomy. **dysfunctional uterine b. (DUB),** bleeding from the uterus when no organic lesions are present. **implantation b.,** that occurring at the time of implantation of the blastocyst in the decidua. **occult b.,** escape of blood in such small quantity that it can be detected only by chemical test or by microscopic or spectroscopic examination.

blen·nad·e·ni·tis (blen″ad-ĕ-ni′tis) myxadenitis.

blenn(o)- word element [Gr.], *mucus.*

blen·noid (blen′oid) mucoid (1).

blen·nor·rha·gia (blen″ah-ra′jah) 1. blennorrhea. 2. gonorrhea.

blen·nor·rhea (-re′ah) any free discharge of mucus, especially a gonorrheal discharge from the urethra or vagina. **blennorrhe′al,** adj. **inclusion b.,** see under *conjunctivitis.*

blen·no·tho·rax (blen″o-thor′aks) a pleural effusion with mucus.

ble·o·my·cin (ble-o-mi′sin) a polypeptide antibiotic mixture obtained from cultures of *Streptomyces verticellus;* used as the sulfate salt as an antineoplastic.

bleph·ar·ad·e·ni·tis (blef″ar-ad″ĕ-ni′tis) inflammation of the meibomian glands.

bleph·a·ri·tis (blef″ah-ri′tis) inflammation of the eyelids. **b. angula′ris,** inflammation involving the angles of the eyelids. **b. cilia′ris, marginal b.,** a chronic inflammation of the hair follicles and sebaceous gland openings of the margins of the eyelids. **nonulcerative b., seborrheic b.,** blepharitis with seborrhea of the scalp, brows, and skin behind the ears, marked by greasy scaling, hyperemia, and thickening. **ulcerative b.,** that marked by small ulcerated areas along the eyelid margin, multiple suppurative lesions, and loss of lashes.

blephar(o)- word element [Gr.], *eyelid; eyelash.*

bleph·a·ro·ath·er·o·ma (blef″ah-ro-ath″er-o′mah) an encysted tumor or sebaceous cyst of an eyelid.

bleph·a·ro·chal·a·sis (-kal′ah-sis) hypertrophy and loss of elasticity of the skin of the upper eyelid.

bleph·a·ron·cus (blef″ah-rong′kus) a tumor on the eyelid.

bleph·a·ro·phi·mo·sis (blef″ah-ro-fĭ-mo′sis) abnormal narrowness of the palpebral fissures.

bleph·a·ro·plas·ty (blef′ah-ro-plas″te) plastic surgery of the eyelids.

bleph·a·ro·ple·gia (blef″ah-ro-ple′jah) paralysis of an eyelid.

bleph·a·rop·to·sis (blef″ah-rop-to′sis) ptosis (2).

bleph·a·ro·py·or·rhea (blef″ah-ro-pi″ah-re′ah) purulent ophthalmia.

bleph·a·ror·rha·phy (blef″ah-ror′ah-fe) 1. suture of an eyelid. 2. tarsorrhaphy.

bleph·a·ro·ste·no·sis (blef″ah-ro-stĕ-no′sis) blepharophimosis.

bleph·a·ro·syn·ech·ia (-sĭ-nek′e-ah) a growing together or adhesion of the eyelids.

bleph·a·rot·o·my (blef″ah-rot′ah-me) surgical incision of an eyelid.

blind (blīnd) [A.S.] 1. not having the sense of sight. 2. pertaining to a clinical trial or other experiment in which one or more of the groups receiving, administering, and evaluating the treatment are unaware of which treatment any particular subject is receiving.

blind·ness (blīnd′nes) lack or loss of ability to see; lack of perception of visual stimuli. **blue b., blue-yellow b.,** popular names for imperfect perception of blue and yellow tints; see *tritanopia* and *tetartanopia*. **color b.,** 1. popular name for *color vision deficiency*. 2. see *monochromatic vision*. **complete color b.,** monochromatic vision. **day b.,** hemeralopia. **flight b.,** amaurosis fugax due to high centrifugal forces encountered in aviation. **green b.,** imperfect perception of green tints; see *deuteranopia* and *protanopia*. **legal b.,** that defined by law, usually, maximal visual acuity in the better eye after correction of 20/200 with a total diameter of the visual field in that eye of 20 degrees. **letter b.,** alexia characterized by inability to recognize individual letters. **music b.,** musical alexia. **night b.,** failure or imperfection of vision at night or in dim light. **object b., psychic b.,** visual agnosia. **red b.,** popular name for protanopia. **red-green b.,** popular name for any imperfect perception of red and green tints, including all the most common types of color vision deficiency. See *deuteranomaly, deuteranopia, protanomaly,* and *protanopia*. **snow b.,** dimness of vision, usually temporary, due to glare of sun upon snow. **text b.,** alexia. **total color b.,** monochromatic vision. **word b.,** alexia.

blis·ter (blis′ter) a vesicle, especially a bulla. **blood b.,** a vesicle having bloody contents, as may be caused by a pinch or bruise. **fever b.,** see *herpes simplex*. **water b.,** one with clear watery contents.

block (blok) 1. obstruction. 2. to obstruct. 3. regional anesthesia. **ankle b.,** regional anesthesia of the foot by injection of anesthetic around the tibial nerves at the ankle. **atrioventricular b., AV b.,** impairment of conduction of cardiac impulses from the atria to the ventricles, usually due to a block in the atrioventricular junctional tissue, and generally subclassified on the basis of severity as first, second, or third degree. **Bier b.,** regional anesthesia by intravenous injection; used for surgical procedures on the arm below the elbow or leg below the knee that are done in a bloodless field maintained by a pneumatic tourniquet. **bifascicular b.,** impairment of conduction in two of the three fascicles of the bundle branches. **bilateral bundle branch b. (BBBB),** interruption of cardiac impulses through both bundle branches, clinically indistinguishable from third degree (complete) heart block. **brachial plexus b.,** regional anesthesia of the shoulder, arm, and hand by injection of anesthetic into the brachial plexus. **bundle branch b. (BBB),** interruption of conduction in one of the main bundle branches, so that the impulse first reaches one ventricle, then travels to the other. **caudal b.,** anesthesia by injection of local anesthetic into the caudal or sacral canal. **cervical plexus b.,** regional anesthesia of the neck by injection of a local anesthetic into the cervical plexus. **complete heart b.,** see *heart b.* **conduction b.,** a blockage in a nerve that prevents impulses from being conducted across a given segment although the nerve beyond is viable. **elbow b.,** regional anesthesia of the forearm and hand by injection of local anesthetic around the median, radial, and ulnar nerves at the elbow. **entrance b.,** in cardiology, a unidirectional impasse to conduction that prevents an impulse from entering a specific region of excitable tissue; part of the mechanism underlying parasystole. **epidural b.,** see under *anesthesia*. **exit b.,** in cardiology, delay or failure of an impulse to be conducted from a specific region to surrounding tissues. **fascicular b.,** any of a group of disorders of conduction localized within any combination of the three fascicles of the bundle branches or their ramifications. **femoral b.,** regional anesthesia of the posterior thigh and the leg below the knee by injection of a local anesthetic around the femoral nerve just below the inguinal ligament at the lateral border of the fossa ovalis. **field b.,** regional anesthesia by encircling the operative field with injections of a local anesthetic. **first degree heart b.,** see *heart b.*; see also *atrioventricular b.* **heart b.,**

impairment of conduction of an impulse in heart excitation; it is subclassified as *first degree* when conduction time is prolonged, *second degree(partial heart b.)* when some atrial impulses are not conducted, and *third degree (complete heart b.)* when no atrial impulses are conducted; the term and its subcategories are often used specifically for atrioventricular block. **high grade atrioventricular b.,** second or third degree atrioventricular block. **incomplete heart b.,** first or second degree heart block. **intraspinal b.,** spinal anesthesia (1). **intravenous b.,** Bier b. **lumbar plexus b.,** regional anesthesia of the anterior and medial aspects of the leg by injection of a local anesthetic into the lumbar plexus. **mental b.,** *blocking* (2). **metabolic b.,** the blocking of a biosynthetic pathway due to a genetic enzyme defect or to inhibition of an enzyme by a drug or other substance. **Mobitz type I b.,** Wenckebach b. **Mobitz type II b.,** a type of second degree atrioventricular block in which dropped beats occur periodically without previous lengthening of the P–R interval, due to a block within or below the bundle of His. **motor point b.,** interruption of impulses, by anesthesia or destruction of the nerve, at a motor point in order to relieve spasticity. **nerve b.,** regional anesthesia by injection of anesthetics close to the appropriate nerve. **paracervical b.,** regional anesthesia of the inferior hypogastric plexus and ganglia produced by injection of the local anesthetic into the lateral fornices of the vagina. **parasacral b.,** regional anesthesia produced by injection of a local anesthetic around the sacral nerves as they emerge from the sacral foramina. **paravertebral b.,** infiltration of anesthetic into an area near the vertebrae. **partial heart b.,** see *heart b.* **periinfarction b.,** disturbance of intraventricular conduction after a myocardial infarction, due to delayed conduction in the infarct region. **presacral b.,** anesthesia produced by injection of the local anesthetic into the sacral nerves on the anterior aspect of the sacrum. **pudendal b.,** anesthesia produced by blocking the pudendal nerves, accomplished by injection of the local anesthetic into the tuberosity of the ischium. **retrobulbar b.,** that performed by injection of a local anesthetic into the retrobulbar space to anesthetize and immobilize the eye. **sacral b.,** see under *anesthesia.* **saddle b.,** regional anesthesia in an area of the buttocks, perineum, and inner aspects of the thighs, by introducing the anesthetic agent low in the dural sac. **second degree heart b.,** see *heart b.;* see also *atrioventricular b.* **sinoatrial b.,** delay or absence of the atrial beat due to

partial or complete interference with the propagation of impulses from the sinoatrial node to the atria. **spinal b.,** see under *anesthesia.* **subarachnoid b.,** spinal anesthesia (1). **third degree heart b.,** see *heart b.;* see also *atrioventricular b.* **trifascicular b.,** impairment of conduction in all three fascicles of the bundle branches, a form of complete heart block. **unifascicular b.,** impairment of conduction in only one fascicle of the bundle branches. **vagal b., vagus nerve b.,** blocking of vagal impulses by injection of a solution of local anesthetic into the vagus nerve at its exit from the skull. **Wenckebach b.,** a type of second degree atrioventricular block in which one or more dropped beats occur periodically after a series of steadily increasing P–R intervals. **wrist b.,** regional anesthesia of the hand by injection of a local anesthetic around the median, radial, and ulnar nerves of the wrist.

block·ade (blok-ād′) 1. the blocking of the effect of a hormone or neurotransmitter at a cell-surface receptor by a pharmacologic antagonist bound to the receptor. 2. in histochemistry, a chemical reaction that modifies certain chemical groups and blocks a specific staining method. 3. regional anesthesia. **adrenergic b.,** selective inhibition of the response to sympathetic impulses transmitted by epinephrine or norepinephrine at alpha or beta receptor sites of an effector organ or postganglionic adrenergic neuron. **cholinergic b.,** selective inhibition of cholinergic nerve impulses at autonomic ganglionic synapses, postganglionic parasympathetic effectors, or the neuromuscular junction. **ganglionic b.,** inhibition by drugs of nerve impulse transmission at autonomic ganglionic synapses. **narcotic b.,** inhibition of the euphoric effects of narcotic drugs by the use of other drugs, such as methadone, in the treatment of addiction. **neuromuscular b.,** a failure in neuromuscular transmission that can be induced pharmacologically or may result from pathological disturbances at the myoneural junction.

block·er (blok′er) something that blocks or obstructs passage, activity, etc. **α-b.,** alpha-adrenergic blocking agent; see *adrenergic blocking agent.* **β-b.,** beta-adrenergic blocking agent; see *adrenergic blocking agent.* **calcium channel b.,** calcium channel blocking agent. **potassium channel b.,** potassium channel blocking agent. **sodium channel b.,** sodium channel blocking agent.

block·ing (-ing) 1. interruption of an afferent nerve pathway; see *block.* 2. difficulty in recollection, or interruption of a train of thought or speech, due to emotional factors, usually unconscious.

blood (blud) the fluid circulating through the heart, arteries, capillaries, and veins, carrying nutriment and oxygen to body cells, and removing waste products and carbon dioxide. It consists of the liquid portion (the plasma) and the formed elements (erythrocytes, leukocytes, and platelets). **arterial b.,** oxygenated blood, found in the pulmonary veins, the left chambers of the heart, and the systemic arteries. **citrated b.,** blood treated with sodium citrate or citric acid to prevent its coagulation. **cord b.,** that contained in umbilical vessels at time of delivery of the infant. **occult b.,** that present in such small quantities that it is detectible only by chemical tests or by spectroscopic or microscopic examination. **predonated autologous b.,** blood donated prior to surgery or other invasive procedure for use in a possible auto-transfusion. **venous b.,** blood that has given up its oxygen to the tissues and is carrying carbon dioxide back through the systemic veins for gas exchange in the lungs. **whole b.,** that from which none of the elements has been removed, sometimes specifically that drawn from a selected donor under aseptic conditions, containing citrate ion or heparin, and used as a blood replenisher.

blood group (blud groōp) 1. an erythrocytic allotype (or phenotype) defined by one or more cellular antigenic groupings controlled by allelic genes. Numerous blood group systems are now known, the most widely used in matching blood for transfusion being the ABO and Rh groups. 2. any of various other characteristics or traits of cellular or fluid components of blood, considered as the expression (phenotype or allotype) of the actions and interactions of dominant genes, and useful in medicolegal and other studies of human inheritance.

blot (blot) a technique for transferring ionic solutes onto a nitrocellulose membrane, filter, or treated paper for analysis; also used to describe the substrate containing the transferred material. For specific techniques, see under *technique.*

blot·ting (blot′ing) soaking up with or transferring to absorbent material.

blow·pipe (blo′pīp) a tube through which a current of air is forced upon a flame to concentrate and intensify the heat.

blue (bloo) 1. a color between green and indigo, produced by energy with wavelengths between 420 and 490 nm. 2. a dye or stain with this color. **aniline b.,** a mixture of the trisulfonates of triphenyl rosaniline and of diphenyl rosaniline. **brilliant cresyl b.,** an oxazin dye, usually $C_{15}H_{16}N_3OCl$, used in staining blood. **methylene b.,** dark green crystals or crystalline powder with a bronzelike luster; used in the treatment of methemoglobinemia and of cyanide poisoning, and as a bacteriologic stain and an indicator. **Prussian b.,** an amorphous blue powder, $Fe_4[Fe(CN)_6]_3$, used as a stain. **toluidine b., toluidine b. O,** the chloride salt or zinc chloride double salt of amino-dimethylaminotoluphenazthionium chloride; useful as a stain for demonstrating basophilic and metachromatic substances.

blunt (blunt) having a thick or dull edge or point; not sharp.

blur (blur) indistinctness, clouding, or fogging. **spectacle b.,** the indistinct vision with spectacles occurring after removal of contact lenses, especially non–gas-permeable lenses; it is believed to result from chronic corneal hypoxia and edema.

BMA British Medical Association.

BMI body mass index.

BMR basal metabolic rate.

BMT bone marrow transplantation.

BOA British Orthopaedic Association.

bob·bing (bob′ing) a quick, jerky, up-and-down movement. **ocular b.,** a jerky downward deviation of the eyes with slow return, seen in comatose patients and believed to be due to a pontine lesion.

body (bod′e) 1. the largest and most important part of any organ. 2. any mass or collection of material. 3. trunk (1). **acetone b's,** ketone bodies. **amygdaloid b.,** corpus amygdaloideum. **anococcygeal b.,** see under *ligament.* **aortic b's,** small neurovascular structures on either side of the aorta in the region of the aortic arch, containing chemoreceptors that play a role in reflex regulation of respiration. **b's of Arantius,** small tubercles, one at the center of the free margin of each of the three cusps of the aortic and pulmonary valves. **asbestos b's,** ferruginous bodies whose center is asbestos. **Aschoff b's,** submiliary collections of cells and leukocytes in the interstitial tissues of the heart in rheumatic myocarditis. **asteroid b.,** an irregularly star-shaped inclusion body found in the giant cells in sarcoidosis and other diseases. **Auer b's,** finely granular, lamellar bodies having acid-phosphatase activity, found in the cytoplasm of myeloblasts, myelocytes, monoblasts, and granular histiocytes, rarely in plasma cells, and virtually pathognomonic of leukemia. **Barr b.,** sex chromatin. **basal b.,** a modified centriole

body 122

that occurs at the base of a flagellum or cilium. **Cabot's ring b's,** lines in the form of loops or figures-of-8, seen in stained erythrocytes in severe anemias. **carotid b.,** a small neurovascular structure lying in the bifurcation of the right and left carotid arteries, containing chemoreceptors that monitor oxygen content in blood and help to regulate respiration. **cavernous b. of penis,** corpus cavernosum penis. **ciliary b.,** the thickened part of the vascular tunic of the eye, connecting the choroid and iris. **Cowdry type I inclusion b's,** eosinophilic nuclear inclusions of nucleic acid and protein seen in cells infected with herpes simplex or varicella-zoster virus. **Döhle's inclusion b's,** small bodies seen in the cytoplasm of neutrophils in many infectious diseases, burns, aplastic anemia, and other disorders, and after the administration of toxic agents. **Donovan's b.,** an encapsulated bacterium, *Calymmatobacterium granulomatis,* found in lesions of granuloma inguinale. **embryoid b's,** structures resembling embryos, seen in several types of germ cell tumors. **ferruginous b's,** small masses of mineral matter in the lungs resulting from deposition of calcium salts, iron salts, and protein around a central core of foreign matter. **fruiting b.,** a specialized structure, as an apothecium, which produces spores. **geniculate b., lateral,** an eminence of the metathalamus, just lateral to the medial geniculate body, marking the end of the optic tract. **geniculate b., medial,** an eminence of the metathalamus, just lateral to the superior colliculi, concerned with hearing. **Golgi b.,** see under *complex.* **Hassall's b.,** one of the formed elements of the blood; a leukocyte, erythrocyte, or platelet. **Heinz b's, Heinz-Ehrlich b's,** inclusion bodies resulting from oxidative injury to and precipitation of hemoglobin; seen in the presence of certain abnormal hemoglobins and erythrocytes with enzyme deficiencies. **hematoxylin b.,** a dense, homogeneous particle consisting of the denatured nuclear material of an injured cell, occurring in systemic lupus erythematosus; lymphocytes that ingest such particles are known as LE cells. Called also *LE b.* **hyaloid b.,** vitreous b. **immune b.,** antibody. **inclusion b's,** round, oval, or irregular-shaped bodies in the cytoplasm and nuclei of cells, as in disease due to viral infection, such as rabies, smallpox, etc. **ketone b's,** the substances acetone, acetoacetic acid, and β-hydroxybutyric acid; except for acetone (which may arise spontaneously from acetoacetic acid), they are normal metabolic

products of lipid within the liver, and are oxidized by muscles; excessive production leads to urinary secretion of these bodies, as in diabetes mellitus. **lamellar b.,** keratinosome. **LE b.,** hematoxylin b. **Leishman-Donovan b.,** amastigote. **mammillary b.,** either of the pair of small spherical masses in the interpeduncular fossa of the midbrain, forming part of the hypothalamus. **Masson b's,** cellular tissue that fills the pulmonary alveoli and alveolar ducts in rheumatic pneumonia; they may be modified Aschoff bodies. **metachromatic b's,** see under *granule.* **Negri b's,** round or oval inclusion bodies seen in the cytoplasm and sometimes in the processes of neurons of rabid animals after death. **Nissl b's,** large granular basophilic bodies found in the cytoplasm of neurons, composed of rough endoplasmic reticulum and free polyribosomes. **olivary b.,** olive (2). **pacchionian b's,** arachnoidal granulations. **para-aortic b's,** enclaves of chromaffin cells near the sympathetic ganglia along the abdominal aorta, serving as chemoreceptors responsive to oxygen, carbon dioxide, and hydrogen ion concentration and which help control respiration. **pineal b.,** a small conical structure attached by a stalk to the posterior wall of the third ventricle; it secretes melatonin. Called also *epiphysis cerebri* and *pineal gland.* **pituitary b.,** hypophysis. **polar b's,** 1. small nonfunctional cells consisting of a tiny bit of cytoplasm and a nucleus, resulting from unequal division of the primary oocyte *(first polar b.)* and, if fertilization occurs, of the secondary oocyte *(second polar b.).* 2. metachromatic granules located at the ends of bacteria. **psammoma b.,** a spherical, concentrically laminated mass of calcareous material, usually of microscopic size; such bodies occur in both benign and malignant epithelial and connective-tissue tumors, and are sometimes associated with chronic inflammation. **quadrigeminal b's,** corpora quadrigemina. **Russell b's,** globular plasma cell inclusions, representing aggregates of immunoglobulins synthesized by the cell. **sand b's,** the mass of gritty matter lying in or near the pineal body, the choroid plexus, and other parts of the brain. **b. of sternum,** the principal portion of the sternum, located between the manubrium above and the xiphoid process below. **trachoma b's,** inclusion bodies found in clusters in the cytoplasm of the epithelial cells of the conjunctiva in trachoma. **tympanic b.,** an ovoid body in the upper part of the superior bulb of the internal jugular vein, believed similar to the carotid body in structure and function. **vermiform b's,** peculiar sinuous invaginations of the plasma membrane of Kupffer cells of the liver. **vitreous b.,** the transparent gel filling the inner portion of the eyeball between the lens and retina. **Weibel-Palade b's,** rod-shaped intracytoplasmic bundles of microtubules specific for vascular endothelial cells and used as markers for endothelial cell neoplasms.

body·work (-wurk″) a general term for therapeutic methods that center on the body for the promotion of physical health and emotional and spiritual well-being, including massage, various systems of touch and manipulation, relaxation techniques, and practices designed to affect the body's energy flow.

boil (boil) furuncle. **Aleppo b., Delhi b.,** cutaneous leishmaniasis (Old World).

bo·lom·e·ter (bo-lom′ĕ-ter) an instrument for measuring minute changes in radiant heat.

bo·lus (bo′lus) 1. a rounded mass of food or pharmaceutical preparation ready to swallow, or such a mass passing through the gastrointestinal tract. 2. a concentrated mass of pharmaceutical preparation, e.g., an opaque contrast medium, given intravenously. 3. a mass of scattering material, such as wax or paraffin, placed between the radiation source and the skin to achieve a precalculated isodose pattern in the tissue irradiated.

bom·be·sin (bom′bĕ-sin) a tetradecapeptide neurotransmitter and hormone found in the brain and gut.

bond (bond) the linkage between atoms or radicals of a chemical compound, or the mark indicating the number and attachment of the valences of an atom in constitutional formulas, represented by a pair of dots or a line between atoms, e.g., H—O—H, H—C≡C—H or H:O:H, H:C:::C:H. **coordinate covalent b.,** a covalent bond in which one of the bonded atoms furnishes both of the shared electrons. **covalent b.,** a chemical bond between two atoms or radicals formed by the sharing of a pair (single bond), two pairs (double bond), or three pairs of electrons (triple bond). **disulfide b.,** a strong covalent bond, —S—S—, important in linking polypeptide chains in proteins, the linkage arising as a result of the oxidation of the sulfhydryl (SH) groups of two molecules of cysteine. **high energy b.,** a chemical bond the hydrolysis of which yields high levels of free energy; it may involve phosphate (*high energy phosphate b.*) or sulfur (*high energy sulfur b.*) or other mixed anhydride types of chemical structure. **hydrogen b.,** a weak,

primarily electrostatic, bond between a hydrogen atom bound to a highly electronegative element in a given molecule and a second highly electronegative atom in another molecule or elsewhere in the same molecule; it is usually represented by three dots, e.g., X—H•••Y. **ionic b.,** a chemical bond in which electrons are transferred from one atom to another so that one bears a negative and the other a positive charge, the attraction between these opposite charges forming the bond. **peptide b.,** a —CO—NH— linkage formed between the carboxyl group of one amino acid and the amino group of another; it is an amide linkage joining amino acids to form peptides.

bone (bōn) 1. the hard, rigid form of connective tissue constituting most of the skeleton of vertebrates, composed chiefly of calcium salts. 2. any distinct piece of the skeleton of the body. See *Table of Bones* for regional listing and alphabetical listing of common names of bones of the body, and see Plates 1 and 2. **ankle b.,** talus; see *Table of Bones.* **brittle b's,** osteogenesis imperfecta. **cancellous b.,** see *lamellar b.* **cartilage b.,** bone developing within cartilage, ossification taking place within a cartilage model. **cheek b.,** zygomatic b.; see *Table of Bones.* **collar b.,** clavicle; see *Table of Bones.* **compact b.,** see *lamellar b.* **cortical b.,** the compact bone of the shaft of a bone that surrounds the marrow cavity. **flat b.,** one whose thickness is slight, sometimes consisting of only a thin layer of compact bone, or of two layers with intervening cancellous bone and marrow; usually curved rather than flat. **funny b.,** the region of the median condyle of the humerus where it is crossed by the ulnar nerve. **heel b.,** calcaneus; see *Table of Bones.* **incisive b.,** the portion of the maxilla bearing the incisors; developmentally, it is the premaxilla, which in humans later fuses with the maxilla, but in most other vertebrates persists as a separate bone. **jaw b.,** the mandible or maxilla, especially the mandible. **jugal b.,** zygomatic b.; see *Table of Bones.* **lamellar b.,** the normal type of adult bone, organized in layers (lamellae), which may be parallel (*cancellous b.*) or concentrically arranged (*compact b.*). **lingual b.,** hyoid b.; see *Table of Bones.* **malar b.,** zygomatic b.; see *Table of Bones.* **marble b's,** osteopetrosis. **mastoid b.,** mastoid part of temporal bone; see under *part.* **pelvic b.,** hip b.; see *Table of Bones.* **petrous b.,** petrous part of temporal bone; see under *part.* **pneumatic b.,** bone that contains air-filled spaces. **premaxillary b.,** premaxilla. **pterygoid b.,** see under *process.* **rider's b.,** localized ossification

BONES, LISTED BY REGIONS OF THE BODY

Region	Name	Total Number	Region	Name	Total Number
Axial skeleton			**Upper limb (× 2)**		64
	Skull	21	Shoulder	scapula	
	(eight paired—16)			clavicle	
	nasal concha		Upper arm	humerus	
	lacrimal		Lower arm	radius	
	maxilla			ulna	
	nasal		Wrist	carpal (8)	
	palatine			(capitate)	
	parietal			(hamate)	
	temporal			(lunate)	
	zygomatic			(pisiform)	
	(five unpaired—5)			(scaphoid)	
	ethmoid			(trapezium)	
	frontal			(trapezoid)	
	occipital			(triquetral)	
	sphenoid		Hand	Metacarpal (5)	
	vomer		Fingers	Phalanges (14)	
	Ossicles of each ear	6	**Lower limb (× 2)**		62
	incus		Pelvis	Hip bone (1)	
	malleus			(ilium)	
	stapes			(ischium)	
	Lower jaw	1		(pubis)	
	mandible		Thigh	femur	
	Neck	1	Knee	patella	
	hyoid		Leg	tibia	
	Vertebral column	26		fibula	
	cervical vertebrae (7)		Ankle	tarsal (7)	
	(atlas)			(calcaneus)	
	(axis)			(cuboid)	
	thoracic vertebrae (12)			(cuneiform, medial)	
	lumbar vertebrae (5)			(cuneiform, intermediate)	
	sacrum (5 fused)			(cuneiform, lateral)	
	coccyx (4–5 fused)			(navicular)	
	Chest	1		(talus)	
	sternum		Foot	Metatarsal (5)	
	ribs (12 pairs)	24	Toes	Phalanges (14)	

Common Name*	TA Equivalent†	Region	Description*	Articulations*
astragalus. *See* talus				
atlas	atlas	neck	first cervical vertebra, ring of bone supporting the skull	with occipital b. and axis
axis	axis	neck	second cervical vertebra, with thick process (odontoid process) around which first cervical vertebra pivots	with atlas above and third cervical vertebra below
calcaneus	calcaneus	foot	the "heel bone," of irregular cuboidal shape, largest of the tarsal bones	with talus and cuboid b.
capitate b.	o. capitatum	wrist	third from thumb side of 4 bones of distal row of carpal b's	with second, third, and fourth metacarpal b's, and hamate, lunate, trapezoid, and scaphoid b's
carpal b's	oss. carpi	wrist	see *capitate, bamate, lunate, pisiform b's, scaphoid, trapezium, trapezoid, and triquetral b's*	
clavicle	clavicula	shoulder	elongated slender, curved bone (collar bone) lying horizontally at root of neck, in upper par of thorax	with sternum and ipsilateral scapula and cartilage of first rib
coccyx	o. coccygis	lower back	triangular bone formed usually by fusion of last 4 (sometimes 3 or 5) (coccygeal) vertebrae	with sacrum
concha, nasal	concha nasalis	skull	(superior, inferior, middle, and supreme) thin bony plates within the nasal cavity	with ethmoid and ipsilateral lacrimal and palatine b's and maxilla
cuboid b.	o. cuboideum	foot	pyramidal bone, on lateral side of foot, in front of calcaneus	with calcaneus, lateral cuneiform b., fourth and fifth metatarsal b's, occasionally with navicular b.
cuneiform b., intermediate	o. cuneiforme intermedium	foot	smallest of 3 cuneiform b's, located between medial and lateral cuneiform b's	with navicular, medial and lateral cuneiform b's, and second metatarsal b.
cuneiform b., lateral	o. cuneiforme laterale	foot	wedge-shaped bone at lateral side of foot, inter- mediate in size between medial and intermediate cuneiform b's	with cuboid, navicular, intermediate cuneiform b's and second, third, and fourth metatarsal b's
cuneiform b., medial	o. cuneiforme mediale	foot	largest of 3 cuneiform b's, at medial side of foot	with navicular, intermediate cuneiform, and first and second metatarsal b's
epistropheus. *See* axis				
ethmoid b.	o. ethmoidale	skull	unpaired bone in front of sphenoid b. and below frontal b., forming part of nasal septum and superior and medical conchae of nose	with sphenoid and frontal b's, vomer, and both lacrimal, nasal, and palatine b's, maxillae, and inferior nasal conchae
fabella		knee	sesamoid b. in lateral head of gastrocnemius muscle	with femur
femur	femur	thigh	longest, strongest, heaviest bone of the body (thigh b.)	proximally with hip b., distally with patella and tibia

*b. = bone; b's = (pl.) bones.
†o. = [L.] os; oss. = ([L.] pl.) ossa.

125

TABLE OF BONES *Continued*

Common Name*	TA Equivalent†	Region	Description*	Articulations*
fibula	fibula	leg	lateral and smaller of 2 bones of leg	proximally with tibia, distally with tibia and talus
frontal b.	o. frontale	skull	unpaired bone constituting anterior part of skull	with ethmoid and sphenoid b's, and both parietal, nasal, lacrimal, and zygomatic b's, and maxillae
hamate b.	o. hamatum	wrist	most medial of 4 bones of distal row of carpal b's	with fourth and fifth metacarpal b's and lunate, capitate, and triquetral b's
hip b.	o. coxae	pelvis and hip	broadest bone of skeleton, composed originally of 3 bones which become fused together in acetabulum: *ilium*, broad, flaring, upper-most portion; *ischium*, thick three-sided part behind and below acetabulum and behind obturator foramen; *pubis*, consisting of body (expanded anterior portion), inferior ramus (extending backward and fusing with ramus of ischium), and superior ramus (extending from body to acetabulum)	with femur, anteriorly with its fellow (at symphysis pubis), posteriorly with sacrum
humerus	humerus	arm	long bone of upper arm	proximally with scapula, distally with radius and ulna
hyoid b.	o. hyoideum	neck	U-shaped bone at root of tongue, between mandible and larynx	none; attached by ligaments and muscles to skull and larynx
ilium	o. ilium	pelvis	see *hip b.*	
incus	incus	ear	middle ossicle of chain in the middle ear; so named because of its resemblance to an anvil	with malleus and stapes
innominate b. *See hip b.*				
ischium	o. ischii	pelvis	see *hip b.*	
lacrimal b.	o. lacrimale	skull	thin, uneven scale of bone near rim of medial wall of each orbit	with ethmoid and frontal b's, and ipsilateral inferior nasal concha and maxilla
lunate b.	o. lunatum	wrist	second from thumb side of 4 bones of proximal row of carpal b's	with radius, and capitate, hamate, scaphoid, and triquetral b's
malleus	ear	most lateral ossicle of chain in middle ear; so named because of its resemblance to a hammer	with incus; fibrous attachment to tympanic membrane	

126

mandible	mandibula	lower jaw	horseshoe-shaped bone carrying lower teeth	with temporal b's
maxilla	maxilla	skull (upper jaw)	paired bone, below orbit and at either side of nasal cavity, carrying upper teeth	with ethmoid and frontal b's, vomer, fellow maxilla, and ipsilateral inferior nasal concha and lacrimal, nasal, palatine, and zygomatic b's
metacarpal b's	oss. metacarpi	hand	five miniature long bones of hand proper, slightly concave on palmar surface	first—trapezium and proximal phalanx of thumb; second—third metacarpal b, trapezium, trapezoid, capitate, and proximal phalanx of index finger (second digit); third—second and fourth metacarpal b's, capitate and proximal phalanx of middle finger (third digit); fourth—third and fifth metacarpal b's, capitate, hamate, and proximal phalanx of ring finger (fourth digit); fifth—fourth metacarpal b., hamate b., and proximal phalanx of little finger (fifth digit)
metatarsal b's	oss. metatarsi	foot	five miniature long bones of foot, concave on plantar and slightly convex on dorsal surface	first—medial cuneiform b., proximal phalanx of great toe, and occasionally with second metatarsal b.; second—medial, intermediate, and lateral cuneiform b's, third and occasionally with first metatarsal b., and proximal phalanx of second toe; third—lateral cuneiform b., second and fourth metatarsal b's and proximal phalanx of third toe; fourth—lateral cuneiform b., cuboid b., third and fifth metatarsal b's and proximal phalanx of fourth toe; fifth—cuboid b., fourth metatarsal b., and proximal phalanx of fifth toe
nasal b.	o. nasale	skull	paired bone, the two uniting in median plane to form bridge of nose	with frontal and ethmoid b's, fellow of opposite side, and ipsilateral maxilla
navicular b.	o. naviculare	foot	bone at medial side of tarsus, between talus and cuneiform b's	with talus and 3 cuneiform b's, occasionally with cuboid b.
occipital b.	o. occipitale	skull	unpaired bone constituting back and part of base of skull	with sphenoid b. and atlas and both parietal and temporal b's
palatine b.	o. palatinum	skull	paired bone, the two forming posterior portions of bony palate	with ethmoid and sphenoid b's, vomer, fellow of opposite side, and ipsilateral inferior nasal concha and maxilla
parietal b.	o. parietale	skull	paired bone between frontal and occipital b's, forming superior and lateral parts of skull	with frontal, occipital, sphenoid, fellow parietal, and ipsilateral temporal b's
patella	patella	knee	small, irregularly rectangular compressed (sesamoid) bone over anterior aspect of knee (knee-cap)	with femur
phalanges (proximal, middle, and distal phalanges)	oss. digitorum (phalanx proximalis, phalanx media, and phalanx distalis)	fingers and toes	miniature long bones, two only in thumb and great toe, three in each of other fingers and toes	proximal phalanx of each digit with corresponding metacarpal or metatarsal b., and phalanx distal to it; other phalanges with phalanges proximal and distal (if any) to them

127

TABLE OF BONES Continued

Common Name*	TA Equivalent†	Region	Description*	Articulations*
pisiform b.	o. pisiforme	wrist	medial and palmar of 4 bones of proximal row of carpal b's	with triquetral b.
pubic b.	o. pubis	pelvis	see hip b.	
radius	radius	forearm	lateral and shorter of 2 bones of forearm	proximally with humerus and ulna; distally with ulna and lunate and scaphoid b's
ribs	costae	chest	12 pairs of thin, narrow, curved long bones, forming posterior and lateral walls of chest	all posteriorly with thoracic vertebrae; upper 7 pairs (true ribs) with sternum; lower 5 pairs (false ribs), by costal cartilages, with rib above or (lowest 2— floating ribs) unattached anteriorly
sacrum	o. sacrum	lower back	wedge-shaped bone formed usually by fusion of 5 vertebrae below lumbar vertebrae, constituting posterior wall of pelvis	with fifth lumbar vertebra above, coccyx below, and with ilium at each side
scaphoid	o. scaphoideum	wrist	most lateral of 4 bones of proximal row of carpal b's	with radius, trapezium, trapezoid, capitate and lunate b's
scapula	scapula	shoulder	wide, thin, triangular bone (shoulder blade) opposite second to seventh ribs in upper part of back	with ipsilateral clavicle and humerus
sesamoid b's	oss. sesamoidea	chiefly hands and feet	small, flat, round bones related to joints between phalanges or between digits and metacarpal or metatarsal b's; include also 2 at knee (fabella and patella)	
sphenoid b.	o. sphenoidale	base of skull	unpaired, irregularly shaped bone, constituting part of sides and base of skull and part of lateral wall or orbit	with frontal, occipital, and ethmoid b's, vomer, and both parietal, temporal, palatine, and zygomatic b's
stapes	stapes	ear	most medial ossicle of chain in middle ear; so named because of its resemblance to a stirrup	with incus; ligamentous attachment to fenestra vestibuli
sternum	sternum	chest	elongated flat bone, forming anterior wall of chest, consisting of 3 segments: *manubrium* (topmost segment), *body* (in youth composed of 4 separate segments joined by cartilage), and *xiphoid process* (lowermost segment)	with both clavicles and upper 7 pairs of ribs
talus	talus	ankle	the "ankle bone," second largest of tarsal b's	with tibia, fibula, calcaneus, and navicular b.
tarsal b's	oss. tarsi	ankle and foot	see *calcaneus, cuboid, intermediate, lateral,* and *medial cuneiform b's, navicular b.,* and *talus*	
temporal b.	o. temporale	skull	irregularly shaped bone, one on either side, forming part of side and base of skull, and containing middle and inner ear; divided into mastoid, petrous, squamous, and tympanic parts	with occipital, sphenoid, mandible, and ipsilateral parietal and zygomatic b's

tibia	tibia	leg	medial and larger of 2 bones of lower leg (shin b.)	proximally with femur and fibula, distally with talus and fibula
trapezium	o. trapezium	wrist	most lateral of 4 bones of distal row of carpal b's	with first and second metacarpal b's and trapezoid and scaphoid b's
trapezoid b.	o. trapezoideum	wrist	second from thumb side of 4 bones of distal row of carpal b's	with second metacarpal b. and capitate, trapezium, and scaphoid b's
triquetral b.	o. triquetrum	wrist	third from thumb side of 4 bones of proximal row of carpal b's	with hamate, lunate, and pisiform b's and articular disk
turbinate b. *See* concha, nasal				
ulna	ulna	forearm	medial and longer of 2 bones of forearm	proximally with humerus and radius, distally with radius and articular disk
vertebrae (cervical, thoracic, lumbar, sacral, and coccygeal)	vertebrae (vertebrae cervicales, vertebrae thoracicae, vertebrae lumbales, vertebrae sacrales, vertebrae coccygeae)	back	separate segments of vertebral column; about 33 in the child; uppermost 24 remain separate as true, movable vertebrae; the next 5 fuse to form the sacrum; the lowermost 3–5 fuse to form the coccyx	except first cervical (atlas) and fifth lumbar, each vertebra articulates with adjoining vertebrae above and below; the first cervical articulates with the occipital b. and second cervical vertebra (axis); the fifth lumbar with the fourth lumbar vertebra and sacrum; the thoracic vertebrae articulate also with the heads of the ribs
vomer	vomer	skull	thin bone forming posterior and posteroinferior part of nasal septum	with ethmoid and sphenoid b's and both maxillae and palatine b's
zygomatic b.	o. zygomaticum	skull	bone forming hard part of cheek and lower, lateral portion of rim of each orbit	with frontal and sphenoid b's and ipsilateral maxilla and temporal b.

of the inner aspect of the lower end of the tendon of the adductor muscle of the thigh; sometimes seen in horseback riders. **semilunar b.,** lunate b.; see *Table of Bones.* **shin b.,** tibia; see *Table of Bones.* **squamous b.,** squamous part of temporal bone; see under *part.* **sutural b.,** variable and irregularly shaped bones in the sutures between the bones of the skull. **tail b.,** coccyx; see *Table of Bones.* **thigh b.,** femur; see *Table of Bones.* **turbinate b.,** any of the nasal conchae. **tympanic b.,** tympanic part of temporal bone; see under *part.* **unciform b., uncinate b.,** hamate b.; see *Table of Bones.* **wormian b.,** sutural b.

bony (bo′ne) 1. pertaining to, characterized by, resembling, or consisting of bone. 2. having an internal skeleton made of bones. 3. having prominent bones or being lean or scrawny.

Bo·oph·i·lus (bo-of′ĭ-lus) a genus of hard-bodied ticks that are vectors of babesiosis, including *B. annula′tus,* the vector of *Babesia bigemina; B. mi′croplus,* the vector of *Babesia bovis;* and *B. calcara′tus,* the vector of *Babesia major.*

boost·er (boost′er) see under *dose.*

boot (boot) an encasement for the foot; a protective casing or sheath. **Gibney's b.,** an adhesive tape support used in treatment of sprains and other painful conditions of the ankle, the tape being applied in a basketweave fashion with strips placed alternately under the sole of the foot and around the back of the leg.

bor·age (bor′ij) *Borago officinalis* or preparations of its flowers, stems, and seeds, which are used in folk medicine for a wide variety of disorders; see also under *oil.*

bo·rate (bor′āt) a salt of boric acid.

bo·rax (bor′aks) sodium borate.

bor·bo·ryg·mus (bor″bah-rig′mus) pl. *borboryg′mi.* [L.] a rumbling noise caused by propulsion of gas through the intestines.

bor·der (bor′der) a bounding line, edge, or surface. **brush b.,** a specialization of the free surface of a cell, consisting of minute cylindrical processes (microvilli) that greatly increase the surface area. **vermilion b.,** the exposed red portion of the upper and lower lips.

bor·der·line (-līn) of a phenomenon, straddling the dividing line between two categories.

Bor·de·tel·la (bor″dah-tel′ah) a genus of bacteria (family Brucellaceae), including *B. bronchisep′tica,* a common cause of bronchopneumonia in guinea pigs and other rodents, in swine, and in lower primates;

B. parapertus′sis, found occasionally in whooping cough; and *B. pertus′sis,* the cause of whooping cough in humans.

bo·ric ac·id (bor′ik) H_3BO_3; used as a buffer and weak antimicrobial, and as a pesticide to kill ants and cockroaches. See also *sodium borate.*

bo·ron (B) (bor′on) chemical element (see *Table of Elements*), at. no. 5.

Bor·rel·ia (bah-rel′e-ah) a genus of bacteria (family Spirochaetaceae), parasitic in many animals. *B. burgdor′feri* causes Lyme disease and skin disease, and numerous species cause relapsing fever.

bor·rel·i·o·sis (bah-rel″e-o′sis) infection with spirochetes of the genus *Borrelia.* **Lyme b.,** any of several diseases caused by *Borrelia burgdorferi* and having similar manifestations, including Lyme disease, acrodermatitis chronica atrophicans, and erythema chronicum migrans.

boss (bos) a rounded eminence.

bot (bot) the larva of botflies, which may be parasitic in the stomach of animals and sometimes humans.

Both·rio·ceph·a·lus (both″re-o-sef′ah-lus) *Diphyllobothrium.*

bot·ry·oid (bot′re-oid) shaped like a bunch of grapes.

bot·tle (bot′l) a hollow narrow-necked vessel of glass or other material. **wash b.,** 1. a flexible squeeze-bottle with delivery tube, or one with two tubes through the cork, so arranged that blowing into one forces a stream of liquid from the other; used in washing chemical materials. 2. one containing some washing fluid, through which gases are passed for the purpose of freeing them from impurities.

bot·u·li·form (boch′ah-lĭ-form″) sausage-shaped.

bot·u·lin (boch′u-lin) botulinum toxin.

bot·u·li·nal (boch″u-li′n′l) 1. pertaining to *Clostridium botulinum.* 2. pertaining to botulinum toxin.

bot·u·lism (boch′ah-lizm) an extremely severe type of food poisoning due to a neurotoxin (botulin) produced by *Clostridium botulinum* in improperly canned or preserved foods. **infant b.,** that affecting infants, thought to result from toxin produced in the gut by ingested organisms, rather than from preformed toxins. **wound b.,** a form resulting from infection of a wound with *Clostridium botulinum.*

bou·gie (boo-zhe′) a slender, flexible, hollow or solid, cylindrical instrument for introduction into the urethra or other tubular organ, usually for calibrating or dilating constricted areas. **bulbous b.,** one with a bulb-shaped tip. **filiform b.,** one of very slender caliber.

bound (bound) 1. restrained or confined; not free. 2. held in chemical combination.

bou·ton (boo-tahn′) [Fr.] a buttonlike swelling on an axon where it has a synapse with another neuron. **synaptic b.,** b. terminal. **b. terminal** (ter-mĭ-nahl′) *pl.* boutons′ termi-naux′. A buttonlike terminal enlargement of an axon that ends in relation to another neuron at a synapse.

bo·vine (bo′vīn) pertaining to, characteristic of, or derived from cattle.

bow (bo) an arched or curved appliance or device.

bow·el (bou′el) the intestine.

bow·en·oid (bo′ĕ-noid) pertaining to or resembling the lesions of Bowen's disease.

bowl (bōl) a rounded, more or less hemispherical open container. **mastoid b., mastoidectomy b.,** the hollow bony defect in the temporal bone created by open mastoidectomy.

bow·leg (bo′leg) genu varum; an outward curvature of one or both legs near the knee.

BP 1. blood pressure. 2. *British Pharmacopoeia,* a publication of the General Medical Council, describing and establishing standards for medicines, preparations, materials, and articles used in the practice of medicine, surgery, or midwifery.

bp base pair.

BPA British Paediatric Association.

BPIG bacterial polysaccharide immune globulin.

Bq becquerel.

Br bromine.

brace (brās) an orthopedic appliance or apparatus (an orthosis) used to support, align, or hold parts of the body in correct position; also, usually in the plural, an orthodontic appliance for correction of malaligned teeth.

bra·chi·al (bra′ke-al) pertaining to the upper limb.

bra·chi·al·gia (bra″ke-al′jah) pain in the arm.

brachi(o)- word element [L., Gr.], *arm.*

bra·chio·ce·phal·ic (bra″ke-o-sĕ-fal′ik) pertaining to the arm and head.

bra·chio·cu·bi·tal (-ku′bĭ-t′l) pertaining to the arm and elbow or forearm.

bra·chi·um (bra′ke-um) pl. *bra′chia.* [L.] arm (1,3). **b. colli′culi inferio′ris,** fibers of the auditory pathway connecting the inferior quadrigeminal body to the medial geniculate body. **b. colli′culi superio′ris,** fibers

connecting the optic tract and lateral geniculate body with the superior quadrigeminal body. **b. op′ticum,** one of the processes extending from the corpora quadrigemina to the optic thalamus.

brachy- word element [Gr.], *short.*

brachy·ba·sia (brak″e-ba′zhah) a slow, shuffling, short-stepped gait.

brachy·dac·ty·ly (-dak′tĭ-le) abnormal shortness of fingers and toes.

brach·yg·na·thia (brak″ig-na′the-ah) abnormal shortness of the lower jaw.

brachy·pha·lan·gia (brak″e-fah-lan′jah) abnormal shortness of one or more of the phalanges.

brachy·ther·a·py (-ther′ah-pe) treatment with ionizing radiation whose source is applied to the surface of the body or within the body a short distance from the area being treated.

brady- word element [Gr.], *slow.*

brady·ar·rhyth·mia (brad″e-ah-rith′me-ah) any disturbance in the heart rhythm in which the heart rate is abnormally slowed.

brady·car·dia (-kahr′de-ah) slowness of the heartbeat, as evidenced by slowing of the pulse rate to less than 60. **bradycar′diac,** adj.

brady·dys·rhyth·mia (-dis-rith′me-ah) an abnormal heart rhythm with rate less than 60 beats per minute in an adult; *bradyarrhythmia* is usually used instead.

brady·es·the·sia (-es-the′zhah) slowness or dullness of perception.

brady·ki·ne·sia (-kĭ-ne′zhah) abnormal slowness of movement. **bradykinet′ic,** adj.

brady·ki·nin (-ki′nin) a nonapeptide kinin formed from HMW kininogen by the action of kallikrein; it is a very powerful vasodilator and increases capillary permeability; in addition, it constricts smooth muscle and stimulates pain receptors.

brady·pnea (brad-ip-ne′ah) abnormal slowness of breathing.

brady·sphyg·mia (brad″e-sfig′me-ah) abnormal slowness of the pulse, usually linked to bradycardia.

brady·tachy·car·dia (-tak″ĭ-kahr′de-ah) alternating attacks of bradycardia and tachycardia.

brady·to·cia (-to′she-ah) slow parturition.

brain (brān) encephalon; that part of the central nervous system contained within the cranium, comprising the prosencephalon (forebrain), mesencephalon (midbrain), and rhombencephalon (hindbrain); it develops from the anterior part of the embryonic neural tube. See also *cerebrum.* **split b.,** one in which the connections between the hemispheres have been disrupted or severed; used to provide access to the third ventricle or to control epilepsy.

brain·stem (brān'stem″) the stemlike portion of the brain connecting the cerebral hemispheres with the spinal cord, and comprising the pons, medulla oblongata, and midbrain; considered by some to include the diencephalon.

brain·wash·ing (brān'wahsh″ing) any systematic effort aimed at instilling certain attitudes and beliefs in a person against their will, usually beliefs in conflict with prior beliefs and knowledge.

bran (bran) the meal derived from the outer covering of a cereal grain; a source of dietary fiber.

branch (branch) ramus; a division or offshoot from a main stem, especially of blood vessels, nerves, or lymphatics. **bundle b.,** a branch of the bundle of His.

branch·er en·zyme (branch'er en'zīm) see under *enzyme.*

bran·chi·al (brang'ke-al) pertaining to or resembling gills of a fish or derivatives of homologous parts in higher forms.

Bran·ha·mel·la (bran″hah-mel'ah) *Moraxella (Branhamella).*

brash (brash) heartburn. **water b.,** heartburn with regurgitation of sour fluid or almost tasteless saliva into the mouth.

break·down (brāk'doun) 1. the act or process of ceasing to function. 2. an often sudden collapse in health. 3. loss of self-control. **nervous b.,** a nonspecific, popular name for any type of mental disorder that interferes with the affected individual's normal activities, often implying a severe episode with sudden onset.

breast (brest) the front of the chest, especially its modified glandular structure, the mamma; see also *mammary gland,* under *gland.* **chicken b.,** pectus carinatum. **funnel b.,** pectus excavatum. **pigeon b.,** pectus carinatum.

breast-feed·ing (brest'fēd″ing) nursing; the feeding of an infant at the mother's breast.

breath (breth) the air inhaled and exhaled during ventilation. **liver b.,** fetor hepaticus.

breath·ing (brēth'ing) ventilation (1). **frog b., glossopharyngeal b.,** breathing in which air is "swallowed" into the lungs by the tongue and muscles of the pharynx, unaided by primary or ordinary accessory muscles of respiration; used by those with chronic muscle paralysis to augment their breathing. **intermittent positive pressure b.,** the active inflation of the lungs during inhalation under positive pressure from a cycling valve.

breech (brēch) the buttocks.

breg·ma (breg'mah) the point on the surface of the skull at the junction of the coronal and sagittal sutures. **bregmat′ic,** adj.

bre·tyl·i·um (brĕ-til'e-um) an adrenergic blocking agent used as the tosylate salt as an antiarrhythmic in certain cases of ventricular tachycardia or fibrillation.

brevi·col·lis (brev″ĭ-kol'is) shortness of the neck.

bridge (brij) 1. a structure connecting two separate points, including parts of an organ. 2. a fixed partial denture. 3. tarsal coalition. **cantilever b.,** a bridge having an artificial tooth attached beyond the point of anchorage of the bridge. **cytoplasmic b.,** 1. protoplasmic b. 2. see *intercellular b.* **disulfide b.,** see under *bond.* **extension b.,** cantilever b. **intercellular b.,** a misnomer for the appearance of the junction of epithelial cells at a desmosome as a result of dehydration during fixation; it was formerly thought to constitute a bridge for cytoplasmic continuity (cytoplasmic bridge). **protoplasmic b.,** a strand of protoplasm connecting two secondary spermatocytes, occurring as a result of incomplete cytokinesis.

bridge·work (brij'werk) a partial denture retained by attachments other than clasps. **fixed b.,** one retained with crowns or inlays cemented to the natural teeth. **removable b.,** one retained by attachments allowing removal.

brim (brim) the upper edge of a basin. **pelvic b.,** the upper edge of the superior strait of the pelvis.

bri·mo·ni·dine (brĭ-mo'nĭ-dēn) an α-adrenergic receptor agonist used as the tartrate salt in the treatment of open-angle glaucoma and ocular hypertension.

brin·zo·la·mide (brin-zo'lah-mīd) a carbonic anhydrase inhibitor used in the treatment of open-angle glaucoma and ocular hypertension.

brise·ment (brēz-maw') [Fr.] the breaking up or tearing of anything. **b. forcé** for-sa') the breaking up or tearing of a bony ankylosis.

brit·tle (brit'l) 1. easily broken, snapped, or cracked, especially under slight pressure. 2. easily disrupted.

BRM biologic response modifier.

broach (brōch) a fine barbed instrument for dressing a tooth canal or extracting the pulp.

bro·me·lain (bro'mĕ-lān) any of several endopeptidases that catalyze the cleavage of specific bonds in proteins. Different forms are derived from the fruit *(fruit b.)* and stem *(stem b.)* of the pineapple plant, *Ananas* *comosus.* As the concentrate *bromelains*, it is used as an antiinflammatory agent.

brom·hi·dro·sis (bro″mĭ-dro′sis) axillary (apocrine) sweat which has become foulsmelling as a result of its bacterial decomposition.

bro·mide (bro′mīd) any binary compound of bromine in which the bromine carries a negative charge (Br⁻); specifically a salt (or organic ester) of hydrobromic acid (H⁺Br⁻).

bro·mine (Br) (bro′mēn) chemical element (see *Table of Elements*), at. no. 35.

bro·mo·crip·tine (bro″mo-krip′tēn) an ergot alkaloid dopamine agonist, used as the mesylate salt to suppress prolactin secretion and thereby treat prolactinomas and endocrine disorders secondary to hyperprolactinemia; also used as an antidyskinetic in parkinsonism and a growth hormone suppressant in acromegaly.

bro·mo·di·phen·hy·dra·mine (-di″fen-hi′drah-mēn) a derivative of monoethanolamine used as the hydrochloride salt as an antihistamine.

bro·mo·men·or·rhea (-men″o-re′ah) menstruation characterized by an offensive odor.

brom·phen·ir·amine (brōm″fen-ir′ah-mēn) an antihistamine with anticholinergic and sedative effects, used as the maleate salt.

bronch·ad·e·ni·tis (brongk″ad-ĕ-ni′tis) inflammation of the bronchial glands.

bron·chi (brong′ki) plural of *bronchus.*

bron·chi·al (brong′ke-al) pertaining to or affecting one or more bronchi.

bron·chi·ec·ta·sis (brong″ke-ek′tah-sis) chronic dilatation of one or more bronchi.

bron·chil·o·quy (brong-kil′ah-kwe) bronchophony (2).

bron·chio·cele (brong′ke-o-sēl″) bronchocele.

bron·chi·ole (brong′ke-ōl) one of the finer subdivisions of the branched bronchial tree. **respiratory b's,** the final branches of the bronchioles.

bron·chio·lec·ta·sis (brong″ke-o-lek′tahsis) dilatation of the bronchioles.

bron·chi·o·li·tis (brong″ke-o-li′tis) inflammation of the bronchioles.

bron·chi·o·lus (brong-ki′o-lus) pl. *bronchi′oli.* [L.] bronchiole.

bron·chio·spasm (brong′ke-o-spazm″) bronchospasm.

bron·chi·tis (brong-ki′tis) inflammation of one or more bronchi. **bronchit′ic,** adj. **acute b.,** a short, severe attack of bronchitis, with fever and a productive cough. **chronic b.,** a type of chronic obstructive pulmonary disease with bronchial irritation, increased secretions and a productive cough lasting at least three months, two years in a row. **fibrinous b.,** bronchitis with violent cough, paroxysmal dyspnea, and expectoration of bronchial casts containing Charcot-Leyden crystals. **b. obli′terans,** that in which the smaller bronchi become filled with nodules composed of fibrinous exudate. **pseudomembranous b.,** fibrinous b.

bron·cho·al·ve·o·lar (brong″ko-al-ve′o-ler) pertaining to a bronchus and alveoli.

bron·cho·can·di·di·a·sis (-kan″dĭ-di′ah-sis) bronchopulmonary candidiasis.

bron·cho·cele (brong′ko-sēl) localized dilatation of a bronchus.

bron·cho·con·stric·tion (brong″ko-kunstrik′shun) narrowing of air passages of the lungs from smooth muscle contraction, as in asthma.

bron·cho·con·stric·tor (brong″ko-kunstrik′ter) 1. narrowing the lumina of the air passages of the lungs. 2. an agent that causes such constriction.

bron·cho·di·la·tor (-di′la-ter) 1. expanding the lumina of the air passages of the lungs. 2. an agent which causes dilatation of the bronchi.

bron·cho·esoph·a·ge·al (-ĕ-sof″ah-je′al) pertaining to or communicating with a bronchus and the esophagus.

bron·cho·esoph·a·gos·co·py (-ĕ-sof″ahgos′kah-pe) instrumental examination of the bronchi and esophagus.

bron·cho·fi·ber·scope (-fi′ber-skōp) fiberoptic bronchoscope; a flexible bronchoscope using fiberoptics.

bron·cho·fi·bros·co·py (-fi-bros′kah-pe) examination of bronchi through a bronchofiberscope.

bron·cho·gen·ic (-jen′ik) originating in bronchi.

bron·chog·ra·phy (brong-kog′rah-fe) radiography of the lungs after instillation of an opaque medium in the bronchi. **bronchograph′ic,** adj.

bron·cho·li·thi·a·sis (brong″ko-lĭ-thi′ah-sis) the presence of calculi in the lumen of the tracheobronchial tree.

bron·chol·o·gy (brong-kol′ah-je) the study and treatment of diseases of the tracheobronchial tree. **brancholog′ic,** adj.

bron·cho·ma·la·cia (brong″ko-mah-la′shah) a deficiency in the cartilaginous wall of the trachea or a bronchus that may lead to atelectasis or obstructive emphysema.

bron·cho·mo·tor (-mo′ter) affecting the caliber of the bronchi.

bron·cho·mu·co·tro·pic (-mu″ko-tro′pik) augmenting secretion by the respiratory mucosa.

bron·cho·pan·cre·at·ic (-pan″kre-at′ik) communicating with a bronchus and the pancreas, such as a fistula.

bron·choph·o·ny (brong-kof′ah-ne) 1. normal voice sounds heard over a large bronchus. 2. abnormal voice sounds heard over the lung, with the voice too clear and high-pitched, indicating solidification.

bron·cho·plas·ty (brong′ko-plas″te) plastic surgery of a bronchus; surgical closure of a bronchial fistula.

bron·cho·ple·gia (brong″ko-ple′jah) paralysis of bronchial tube muscles.

bron·cho·pleu·ral (-ploor′il) pertaining to or communicating between a bronchus and the pleura or pleural cavity.

bron·cho·pneu·mo·nia (-noo-mo′ne-ah) bronchial pneumonia; inflammation of the lungs beginning in the terminal bronchioles.

bron·cho·pul·mo·nary (-pool′mah-nar″e) pertaining to the bronchi and the lungs.

bron·chor·rha·phy (brong-kor′ah-fe) suture of a bronchus.

bron·cho·scope (brong′kah-skōp) an instrument for inspecting the interior of the tracheobronchial tree and doing diagnostic and therapeutic maneuvers such as removing specimens or foreign bodies. **bronchoscop′ic,** adj. **fiberoptic b.,** bronchofiberscope.

bron·chos·co·py (brong-kos′kah-pe) examination of the bronchi through a bronchoscope. **fiberoptic b.,** bronchofibroscopy.

bron·cho·spasm (brong′ko-spazm) bronchial spasm; spasmodic contraction of the smooth muscle of the bronchi, as in asthma.

bron·cho·spi·rom·e·try (brong″ko-spi-rom′ĕ-tre) determination of vital capacity, oxygen intake, and carbon dioxide excretion of a lung, or simultaneous measurements of the function of each lung separately. **differential b.,** measurement of the function of each lung separately.

bron·cho·ste·no·sis (-stĕ-no′sis) narrowing of a bronchial tube by scarring or other stricture.

bron·chos·to·my (brong-kos′tah-me) the surgical creation of an opening through the chest wall into a bronchus.

bron·cho·tra·che·al (brong″ko-tra′ke-il) tracheobronchial.

bron·cho·ve·sic·u·lar (-vĕ-sik′u-ler) bronchoalveolar.

bron·chus (brong′kus) pl. *bron′chi.* [L.] one of the larger passages conveying air to a lung (right or left primary bronchus) and within the lungs (lobar and segmental bronchi).

brow (brou) the forehead, or either lateral half of it.

BRS British Roentgen Society.

Bru·cel·la (broo-sel′ah) a genus of schizomycetes (family Brucellaceae). *B. abor′tus* causes infectious abortion in cattle and is the most common cause of brucellosis in humans. *B. bronchisep′tica* is another name for *Bordetella bronchiseptica. B. su′is* usually infects swine, but can also cause severe disease in humans.

bru·cel·la (broo-sel′ah) any member of the genus *Brucella.* **brucel′lar,** adj.

Bru·cel·la·ceae (broo″sel-a′se-e) a family of schizomycetes (order Eubacteriales), some genera of which are parasites of and pathogenic for warm-blooded animals, including humans and birds.

bru·cel·lo·sis (-o′sis) a generalized infection involving primarily the reticuloendothelial system, caused by species of *Brucella.*

Brug·ia (broo′jah) a genus of filarial worms, including *B. mala′yi,* a species similar to, and often found in association with, *Wuchereria bancrofti,* which causes human filariasis and elephantiasis throughout Southeast Asia, the China Sea, and eastern India.

bruise (brooz) contusion.

bruit (brwe, broot) 1. a sound or murmur heard in auscultation, especially an abnormal one. 2. sound (3). **aneurysmal b.,** a blowing sound heard over an aneurysm. **placental b.,** see under *souffle.*

brux·ism (bruk′sizm) grinding of the teeth, especially during sleep.

BS Bachelor of Surgery; Bachelor of Science; breath sounds; blood sugar.

BSF B lymphocyte stimulatory factor.

BTU British thermal unit.

bu·bo (bu′bo) an enlarged and inflamed lymph node, particularly in the axilla or groin, due to such infections as plague, syphilis, gonorrhea, lymphogranuloma venereum, and tuberculosis. **bubon′ic,** adj. **climatic b.,** lymphogranuloma venereum.

bu·bono·cele (bu-bon′ah-sēl) inguinal or femoral hernia forming a swelling in the groin.

buc·ca (buk′ah) [L.] cheek (1). **buc′cal,** adj.

bucc(o)- word element [L.], cheek.

buc·co·clu·sion (buk″o-kloo′zhun) malocclusion in which the dental arch or a quadrant or group of teeth is buccal to the normal.

buc·co·ver·sion (-ver′zhun) position of a tooth lying buccally to the line of occlusion.

buck·ling (buk′ling) the process or an instance of becoming crumpled or warped. **scleral b.,** a technique for repair of a detached retina, in which indentations or infoldings of the sclera are made over the tears in the retina to promote adherence of the retina to the choroid.

bu·cli·zine (bu′klĭ-zēn) an antihistamine, used as the hydrochloride salt as an antinauseant in the management of motion sickness.

bud (bud) 1. a structure on a plant, often round, that encloses an undeveloped flower or leaf. 2. any small part of the embryo or adult metazoon more or less resembling the bud of a plant and presumed to have potential for growth and differentiation. **end b.,** caudal eminence. **limb b.,** a swelling on the trunk of an embryo that becomes a limb. **periosteal b.,** vascular connective tissue from the periosteum growing through apertures in the periosteal bone collar into the cartilage matrix of the primary center of ossification. **tail b.,** 1. in animals having a tail, the primordium that forms it. 2. caudal eminence. **taste b.,** one of the end organs of the gustatory nerve containing the receptor surfaces for the sense of taste. **ureteric b.,** an outgrowth of the mesonephric duct giving rise to all but the nephrons of the permanent kidney.

bu·des·o·nide (bu-des′ah-nīd) an antiinflammatory glucocorticoid used to treat allergic rhinitis, bronchial asthma, nasal inflammation, ulcerative colitis, and Crohn's disease.

buf·fer (buf′er) 1. a chemical system that prevents changes in hydrogen ion concentration. 2. a physical or physiological system that tends to maintain constancy.

buffy (buf′e) of the color buff; light yellowish pink to yellow, including orange-yellow to yellow-brown.

bulb (bulb) a rounded mass or enlargement. **bul′bar,** adj. **b. of aorta,** the enlargement of the aorta at its point of origin from the heart. **b. of corpus spongiosum,** b. of penis. **b. of hair,** the bulbous expansion at the proximal end of a hair in which the hair shaft is generated. **olfactory b.,** the bulblike expansion of the olfactory tract on the under surface of the frontal lobe of each cerebral hemisphere; the olfactory nerves enter it. **onion b.,** in neuropathology, a collection of overlapping Schwann cells resembling the bulb of an onion, encircling an axon that has become demyelinated; seen when an axon has repeatedly become demyelinated and remyelinated. **b. of penis, b. of urethra,** the enlarged proximal part of the corpus spongiosum. **b. of vestibule of vagina, vestibulovaginal b.,** a body consisting of paired masses of erectile tissue, one on either side of the vaginal opening.

bul·bar (bul′ber) 1. pertaining to a bulb. 2. pertaining to or involving the medulla oblongata.

bul·bi·tis (bul-bi′tis) inflammation of the bulb of the penis.

bul·bo·cav·er·no·sus (bul″bo-kav″er-no′sus) bulbocavernous muscle; see *Table of Muscles.*

bul·bo·cav·er·nous (-kav′er-nus) pertaining to the bulb of the penis or to the bulbocavernous muscle.

bul·bo·spi·ral (-spi′ral) pertaining to the root of the aorta (bulbus aortae) and having a spiral course; said of certain bundles of cardiac muscle fibers.

bul·bo·spon·gi·o·sus (-spon″je-o′sus) bulbocavernous muscle; see *Table of Muscles.*

bul·bo·ure·thral (-u-re′thral) pertaining to the bulb of the penis (bulb of urethra).

bul·bous (bul′bus) 1. bulbar. 2. shaped like, bearing, or arising from a bulb.

bul·bus (bul′bus) pl. *bul′bi.* [L.] bulb.

bu·lim·ia (boo-le′me-ah) [Gr.] episodic binge eating usually followed by behavior designed to negate the caloric intake of the ingested food, most commonly purging behaviors such as self-induced vomiting or laxative abuse but sometimes other methods such as excessive exercise or fasting. **bulim′ic,** adj. **b. nervo′sa,** an eating disorder occurring mainly in girls and young women, characterized by episodic binge eating followed by purging or other behaviors designed to prevent weight gain and by excessive influence of body shape and size on the patient's sense of self-worth. Bingeing episodes involve intake of quantifiably excessive quantities of food within a short, discrete period and a sense of loss of control over food intake during these periods. Unlike anorexia nervosa, no extreme weight loss occurs.

bul·la (bul′ah) pl. *bul′lae.* [L.] 1. a blister; a circumscribed, fluid-containing, elevated lesion of the skin, usually more than 5 mm in diameter. 2. a rounded, projecting anatomical structure. **bul′late, bul′lous,** adj.

bul·lec·to·my (bŭ-lek′tah-me) excision of giant bullae from the lung in emphysema to improve pulmonary function.

bul·lo·sis (bul-o′sis) the production of, or a condition characterized by, bullous lesions.

bul·lous (bul′us) pertaining to or characterized by bullae.

bu·met·a·nide (bu-met′ah-nīd) a loop diuretic used in the treatment of edema, including that associated with congestive heart failure or hepatic or renal disease, and hypertension.

BUN blood urea nitrogen; see *urea nitrogen.*

bun·dle (bun′d'l) a collection of fibers or strands, as of muscle fibers, or a fasciculus or band of nerve fibers. **atrioventricular b.,**

AV **b.**, bundle of His. **common b.**, the undivided portion of the bundle of His, from its origin at the atrioventricular node to the point of division into the right and left bundle branches. **b. of His**, a band of atypical cardiac muscle fibers connecting the atria with the ventricles of the heart, occurring as a trunk and two bundle branches; it propagates the atrial contraction rhythm to the ventricles, and its interruption produces heart block. The term is sometimes used specifically to denote only the trunk of the bundle. **medial forebrain b.**, a group of nerve fibers containing the midbrain tegmentum and elements of the limbic system. **Thorel's b.**, a bundle of muscle fibers in the human heart connecting the sinoatrial and atrioventricular nodes.

bun·dle branch (branch) see under *branch*.

bun·ion (bun'yun) an abnormal prominence on the inner aspect of the first metatarsal head, with bursal formation, and resulting in displacement of the great toe. **tailor's b.**, bunionette.

bun·ion·ette (bun″yun-et′) enlargement of the lateral aspect of the fifth metatarsal head.

Bun·ya·vi·ri·dae (bun″yah-vir′ĭ-de) the bunyaviruses: a family of RNA viruses whose genome comprises three molecules of circular negative-sense single-stranded RNA; it includes the genera *Bunyavirus, Hantavirus, Nairovirus,* and *Phlebovirus.*

Bun·ya·vi·rus (bun'yah-vi″rus) a genus of viruses of the family Bunyaviridae usually transmitted by the bite of an infected mosquito; human pathogens cause febrile disease and encephalitis. Important pathogenic species include Bunyamwera, Bwamba, California encephalitis, Guama, Jamestown Canyon, LaCrosse, Oropouche, and Tahyna viruses.

bun·ya·vi·rus (bun'yah-vi″rus) any virus of the family Bunyaviridae.

bu·piv·a·caine (bu-piv′ah-kān) a local anesthetic, used as the hydrochloride for local infiltration, peripheral nerve block, and retrobulbar, subarachnoid, sympathetic, caudal, or epidural block.

bu·pre·nor·phine (bu″prĕ-nor′fēn) a synthetic opioid agonist-antagonist derived from thebaine, used as the hydrochloride salt as an analgesic and as an anesthesia adjunct.

bu·pro·pi·on (bu-pro′pe-on) a monocyclic compound structurally similar to amphetamine, used as the hydrochloride salt as an antidepressant and as an aid in smoking cessation.

bur (bur) a form of drill used for creating openings in bone or similar hard material.

bur·bu·lence (bur′bu-lens″) gaseousness; a group of symptoms of intestinal origin, including a feeling of fullness, bloating or distention, borborygmus, and flatulence.

bu·ret (bu-ret′) a graduated glass tube used to deliver a measured amount of liquid.

Burk·hol·de·ria (burk″hol-der′e-ah) a genus of gram-negative bacteria of the family Pseudomonadaceae, comprising pathogens formerly classified in the genus *Pseudomonas. B. cepa'cia* (the type species) is an opportunistic pathogen, causing various nosocomial infections, and *B. pseudomal'lei* causes melioidosis.

burn (burn) injury to tissues caused by the contact with heat, flame, chemicals, electricity, or radiation. First degree burns show redness; second degree burns show vesication; third degree burns show necrosis through the entire skin. Burns of the *first* and *second degree* are partial-thickness burns, those of the *third degree* are full-thickness burns. **first-degree b.**, a burn that affects the epidermis only, causing erythema without blistering. **fourth-degree b.**, a burn that extends deeply into the subcutaneous tissue; it may involve muscle, fascia, or bone. **full-thickness b.**, third-degree b. **partial-thickness b.**, second-degree b. **second-degree b.**, a burn that affects the epidermis and the dermis, classified as *superficial* (involving the epidermis and the papillary dermis) or *deep* (extending into the reticular dermis). Called also *partial thickness b.* **third-degree b.**, a burn that destroys both the epidermis and the dermis, often also involving the subcutaneous tissue. Called also *full-thickness b.*

burn·er (bur′ner) the part of a lamp, stove, or furnace from which the flame issues. **Bunsen b.**, a gas burner in which the gas is mixed with air before ignition, in order to give complete oxidation.

bur·nish·ing (bur′nish-ing) a dental procedure somewhat related to polishing and abrading.

burr (bur) bur.

bur·sa (bur′sah) pl. *bur'sae*. [L.] a fluid-filled sac or saclike cavity situated in places in tissues where friction would otherwise occur. **bur'sal**, adj. **b. of Achilles tendon**, one between the calcaneal tendon and the back of the calcaneus. **anserine b.**, one between the tendons of the sartorius, gracilis, and semitendinosus muscles, and the tibial collateral ligaments. **Calori's b.**, one between the trachea and the arch of the aorta. **Fleischmann's b.**, one beneath the tongue. **His b.**, the dilatation at the end of the archenteron. **Luschka's b.**, pharyngeal b. **omental b.**, the lesser sac of the peritoneum. **pharyngeal b.,** an inconstant blind sac located above the pharyngeal tonsil in the midline of the posterior wall of the nasopharynx; it represents persistence of an embryonic communication between the anterior tip of the notochord and the roof of the pharynx. **popliteal b.,** a prolongation of the synovial tendon sheath of the popliteus muscle outside the knee joint into the popliteal space. **prepatellar b.,** one of the bursae in front of the patella; it may be subcutaneous, subfascial, or subtendinous in location. **subacromial b.,** one between the acromion and the insertion of the supraspinatus muscle, extending between the deltoid and greater tubercle of the humerus. **subdeltoid b.,** one between the deltoid and the shoulder joint capsule, usually connected to the subacromial bursa. **subtendinous iliac b.,** one at the point of insertion of the iliopsoas muscle into the lesser trochanter. **synovial b.,** a closed synovial sac interposed between surfaces that glide upon each other; it may be subcutaneous, submuscular, subfascial, or subtendinous in nature.

bur·si·tis (bur-si′tis) inflammation of a bursa; specific types of bursitis are named according to the bursa affected, e.g., prepatellar bursitis, subacromial bursitis, etc. **calcific b.,** see under *tendinitis.* **ischiogluteal b.,** inflammation of the bursa over the ischial tuberosity, characterized by sudden onset of excruciating pain over the center of the buttock and down the back of the leg. **subacromial b., subdeltoid b.,** see *calcific tendinitis,* under *tendinitis.* **Tornwaldt's b.,** chronic inflammation of the pharyngeal bursa.

bur·sot·o·my (bur-sot′ah-me) incision of a bursa.

bu·spi·rone (bu-spi′rōn) an antianxiety agent used as the hydrochloride salt in the treatment of anxiety disorders and the short-term relief of anxiety symptoms.

bu·sul·fan (bu-sul′fan) an antineoplastic used in treating chronic granulocytic leukemia, polycythemia vera, myeloid metaplasia, and myeloproliferative syndrome; also used in lieu of whole body irradiation in bone marrow transplantation.

bu·ta·bar·bi·tal (bu″tah-bahr′bĭ-tal) an intermediate-acting barbiturate used for preoperative sedation; used also as the sodium salt.

bu·tal·bi·tal (bu-tal′bĭ-tal) a short- to intermediate-acting barbiturate used as a sedative in combination with an analgesic in the treatment of headache.

bu·tam·ben (bu-tam′ben) a topical anesthetic, used as the base or picrate salt.

bu·tane (bu′tān) an aliphatic hydrocarbon from petroleum, occurring as a colorless flammable gas; used in pharmacy as an aerosol propellant.

butch·er's broom (booch′erz) the European evergreen *Ruscus aculeatus* or preparations of its rhizome, which are used in the treatment of hemorrhoids and venous insufficiency.

bu·ten·a·fine (bu-ten′ah-fēn) a topical antifungal used as the hydrochloride salt in the treatment of tinea pedis, tinea corporis, and tinea cruris.

bu·to·con·a·zole (bu″to-kon′ah-zōl) an imidazole antifungal used as the nitrate salt in the treatment of vulvovaginal candidiasis.

bu·tor·pha·nol (bu-tor′fah-nōl) a synthetic opioid used as the tartrate salt as an analgesic and anesthesia adjunct.

but·tocks (but′oks) the two fleshy prominences formed by the gluteal muscles on the lower part of the back.

but·ton (but′n) 1. a knoblike elevation or structure. 2. a spool- or disk-shaped device used in surgery for construction of intestinal anastomosis. **Jaboulay b.,** a device used for lateral intestinal anastomosis. **mescal b's,** transverse slices of the flowering heads of a Mexican cactus, *Lophophora williamsii,* whose major active principle is mescaline. **Murphy's b.,** a metallic device used for connecting the ends of a divided intestine. **skin b.,** a connector or stretch of tubing covered with a velour fabric, designed to encourage tissue ingrowth where it passes through the skin.

bu·tyl (bu′t′l) a hydrocarbon radical, C_4H_9.

bu·ty·rate (bu′tĭ-rāt) a salt, ester, or anionic form of butyric acid.

bu·tyr·ic ac·id (bu-tēr′ik) 1. any four-carbon carboxylic acid, either *n*-butyric acid or isobutyric acid. 2. *n*-butyric acid, occurring in butter, particularly rancid butter, and in much animal fat.

bu·ty·roid (bu′tĭ-roid) resembling or having the consistency of butter.

bu·ty·ro·phe·none (bu″tĭ-ro-fe′nōn) any of a class of structurally related antipsychotic agents, including haloperidol.

BVAD biventricular assist device.

by·pass (bi′pas) an auxiliary flow; a shunt; a surgically created pathway circumventing the normal anatomical pathway, such as in an artery or the intestine. **cardiopulmonary b.,** diversion of the flow of blood to the heart directly to the aorta, via a pump oxygenator, avoiding both the heart and the lungs; a form of extracorporeal circulation used in heart surgery. **coronary artery b.,** a section of vein or other conduit grafted between the aorta and a coronary artery distal to an obstructive lesion in the latter. **gastric b.,** gastrojejunostomy in which the stomach is transected high on the body, the proximal remnant being joined to a loop of jejunum in end-to-side anastomosis.

bys·si·no·sis (bis″ĭ-no′sis) brown lung; pulmonary disease due to inhalation of the dust of cotton or other textiles. **byssinot′ic,** adj.

C

C canine (tooth); carbon; large calorie; cathode; Celsius (scale); clonus; complement; compliance; contraction; coulomb; cytosine or cytidine; cylindrical lens; color sense; cervical vertebrae (C1 to C7).

C capacitance; clearance (subscripts denote the substance, e.g., C_I or C_{In}, inulin clearance); heat capacity.

c small calorie; centi-.

c molar concentration; the velocity of light in a vacuum.

χ² (chi, the twenty-second letter of the Greek alphabet) chi-squared; see *chi-square test,* under *test,* and *chi-square distribution,* under *distribution.*

CA cardiac arrest; coronary artery.

CA 125 cancer antigen 125.

Ca calcium.

Ca²⁺-ATP·ase (a-te-pe′ās) a membrane-bound enzyme that hydrolyzes ATP to provide energy to drive the cellular calcium pump.

ca·ber·go·line (cah-ber′go-lēn) a dopamine receptor agonist used in the treatment of hyperprolactinemia.

CABG coronary artery bypass graft.

ca·chec·tic (kah-kek′tik) pertaining to or characterized by cachexia.

ca·chec·tin (-tin) former name for *tumor necrosis factor α.*

ca·chet (kă-sha′) a disk-shaped wafer or capsule enclosing a dose of medicine.

ca·chex·ia (kah-kek′se-ah) a profound and marked state of constitutional disorder; general ill health and malnutrition. **cachec′-tic,** adj. **c. hypophysiopri′va,** the train of symptoms resulting from total deprivation of pituitary function, including loss of sexual function, bradycardia, hypothermia, and coma. **malarial c.,** the physical signs resulting from antecedent attacks of severe malaria, including anemia, sallow skin, yellow sclera, splenomegaly, hepatomegaly, and, in children, retardation of growth and puberty. **pituitary c.,** see *panhypopituitarism.*

cach·in·na·tion (kak″ĭ-na′shun) excessive, hysterical laughter.

cac(o)- word element [Gr.], *bad; ill.*

cac·o·dyl·ic ac·id (kak″o-dil′ik) dimethyl arsinic acid, a highly toxic herbicide.

caco·geu·sia (-goo′zhah) a parageusia consisting of a bad taste not related to ingestion of specific substances, or associated with gustatory stimuli usually considered to be pleasant.

caco·me·lia (-me′le-ah) dysmelia.

CAD coronary artery disease.

ca·dav·er (kah-dav′er) a dead body; generally applied to a human body preserved for anatomical study. **cadav′eric, cadav′erous,** adj.

ca·dav·er·ine (-in) a foul-smelling nitrogenous base, pentamethylenediamine, produced by decarboxylation of lysine. It is produced in decaying protein material by the action of bacteria, particularly species of *Vibrio.*

cad·mi·um (Cd) (kad′me-um) chemical element (see *Table of Elements*), at. no. 48. Cadmium and its salts are poisonous; inhalation of cadmium fumes or dust causes pneumoconiosis, and ingestion of foods contaminated by cadmium-plated containers causes violent gastrointestinal symptoms.

ca·du·ce·us (kah-doo′shus) [L.] the wand of Hermes or Mercury; used as a symbol of the medical profession and as the emblem of the Medical Corps of the U.S. Army. See also *staff of Aesculapius.*

cae- for words beginning thus, see those beginning *ce-.*

caf·feine (kă-fēn′, kaf′ēn) a xanthine found in coffee, tea, chocolate, and colas; it is a central nervous system stimulant, diuretic, striated muscle stimulant, and acts on the cardiovascular system. As the base or the citrate salt, it is used as a central nervous system stimulant and as an adjunct in treating neonatal apnea; as the base it is also used in the treatment of vascular headaches and as an adjunct to analgesics.

caf·fein·ism (kaf′ēn-izm) a morbid condition resulting from ingestion of excessive amounts of caffeine; characteristics include insomnia, restlessness, excitement, tachycardia, tremors, and diuresis.

cage (kāj) a box or enclosure. **rib c., thoracic c.,** the bony structure enclosing the thorax, consisting of the ribs, vertebral column, and sternum.

CAH congenital adrenal hyperplasia.

caj·e·put (kaj′ĕ-poot) the tree *Melaleuca. leucaden′dron,* whose fresh leaves and twigs yield cajeput oil.

cal calorie.

cal·a·mine (kal′ah-mīn) a preparation of zinc oxide and the coloring agent ferric oxide; used topically as a protectant.

cal·a·mus (kal′ah-mus) a reed or reedlike structure. **c. scripto′rius,** the lowest portion of the floor of the fourth ventricle, situated between the restiform bodies.

cal·ca·ne·al (kal-ka′ne-al) pertaining to the calcaneus.

cal·ca·neo·apoph·y·si·tis (kal-ka″ne-o-ah-pof″ĭ-si′tis) inflammation of the posterior part of the calcaneus, marked by pain and swelling.

cal·ca·neo·as·trag·a·loid (-ah-strag′ah-loid) pertaining to the calcaneus and astragalus.

cal·ca·ne·odyn·ia (-din′e-ah) pain in the heel.

cal·ca·ne·us (kal-ka′ne-us) pl. *calca′nei.* [L.] see *Table of Bones.* **calca′neal, calca′nean,** adj.

cal·car (kal′kar) 1. spur. 2. a spur-shaped structure. **c. a′vis,** the lower of the two medial elevations in the posterior horn of the lateral cerebral ventricle, produced by the lateral extension of the calcarine sulcus.

cal·car·e·ous (kal-kār′e-us) pertaining to or containing lime; chalky.

cal·ca·rine (kal′kah-rin) 1. spur-shaped. 2. pertaining to a calcar.

cal·ce·mia (kal-se′me-ah) hypercalcemia.

cal·ci·bil·ia (kal″sĭ-bil′e-ah) presence of calcium in the bile.

cal·cif·e·di·ol (kal″sif-ĕ-di′ol) see *25-hydroxycholecalciferol.*

cal·cif·er·ol (kal-sif′er-ol) 1. a compound having vitamin D activity, e.g., cholecalciferol or ergocalciferol. 2. ergocalciferol.

cal·cif·ic (-ik) forming lime.

cal·ci·fi·ca·tion (kal″sĭ-fĭ-ka′shun) the deposit of calcium salts in a tissue. **dystrophic**

c., the deposition of calcium in abnormal tissue, such as scar tissue or atherosclerotic plaques, without abnormalities of blood calcium. **eggshell c.,** deposition of a thin layer of calcium around a thoracic lymph node, often seen in silicosis. **Mönckeberg's c.,** see under *arteriosclerosis.*

cal·ci·no·sis (-no′sis) a condition characterized by abnormal deposition of calcium salts in the tissues. **c. circumscrip′ta,** localized deposition of calcium in small nodules in subcutaneous tissues or muscle. **c. universa′lis,** widespread deposition of calcium in nodules or plaques in the dermis, panniculus, and muscles.

cal·ci·pex·is (-pek′sis) calcipexy.

cal·ci·pexy (kal′sĭ-pek″se) fixation of calcium in the tissues. **calcipec′tic, calcipex′ic,** adj.

cal·ci·phy·lax·is (kal″sĭ-fĭ-lak′sis) a condition of induced hypersensitivity characterized by formation of calcified tissue in response to administration of a challenging agent.

cal·ci·po·tri·ene (-po-tri′ēn) a synthetic derivative of vitamin D_3 (cholecalciferol), applied topically in the treatment of psoriasis.

cal·ci·priv·ia (-priv′e-ah) deprivation or loss of calcium. **calcipri′vic,** adj.

cal·ci·to·nin (-to′nin) a polypeptide hormone secreted by C cells of the thyroid gland, and sometimes of the thymus and parathyroids, which lowers calcium and phosphate concentration in plasma and inhibits bone resorption. Preparations (*c.-human, c.-salmon*) are used in the treatment of osteitis deformans, postmenopausal osteoporosis, and hypercalcemia.

cal·ci·tri·ol (kal″sĭ-tri′ol) 1. see *dihydroxycholecalciferol.* 2. a preparation of this compound, used in the treatment of hypocalcemia, hypophosphatemia, rickets, and osteodystrophy associated with a variety of disorders.

cal·ci·um (Ca) (kal′se-um) chemical element (see *Table of Elements*), at. no. 20. Calcium phosphate salts form the dense hard material of teeth and bones. The calcium 2^+ ion is involved in many physiologic processes. A normal blood calcium level is essential for normal function of the heart, nerves, and muscles. It is involved in blood coagulation (in which connection it is called *coagulation factor IV*). Various calcium salts, including the acetate, carbonate, chloride, glubionate, gluceptate, gluconate, lactate, lactobionate, and phosphate salts, are used as calcium replenishers and supplements. **c. carbonate,**

an insoluble salt, $CaCO_3$, occurring naturally in shells, limestone, and chalk and also used in more purified forms; used as an antacid and calcium replenisher and in the treatment of osteoporosis. **c. chloride,** a salt, $CaCl_2 2H_2O$, used in the treatment of hypocalcemia, electrolyte depletion, and hyperkalemia, and as a treatment adjunct in cardiac arrest and in magnesium poisoning. **c. citrate,** a calcium replenisher also used in the treatment of hyperphosphatemia in renal osteodystrophy. **c. glubionate,** a calcium replenisher, used as a nutritional supplement and for the treatment of hypocalcemia. **c. gluceptate,** a calcium salt used in the treatment and prophylaxis of hypocalcemia and as a electrolyte replenisher. **c. gluconate,** a calcium salt used to treat or prevent hypercalcemia, nutritional deficiency, and hyperkalemia; also used as a treatment adjunct in cardiac arrest. **c. hydroxide,** a salt, $Ca(OH)_2$, used in solution as a topical astringent. **c. oxalate,** a salt of oxalic acid, which in excess in the urine may lead to formation of oxalate calculi. **c. oxide,** lime (1). **c. phosphate,** a salt containing calcium and the phosphate radical: *dibasic* and *tribasic c. phosphate* are used as sources of calcium. **c. polycarbophil,** a calcium salt of a hydrophilic resin of the polycarboxylic type; a bulk laxative. **c. pyrophosphate,** the pyrophosphate salt of calcium, used as a polishing agent in dentifrices. Crystals of the dihydrate form occur in the joints in calcium pyrophosphate deposition disease. **c. sulfate,** the sulfate salt of calcium, $CaSO_4$, occurring in the anhydrous form and in a hydrated form (*gypsum*, q.v.), which upon being calcined forms *plaster of Paris.*

cal·co·spher·ite (kal″ko-sfēr′ĭt) one of the tiny round bodies formed during calcification by chemical union of calcium particles and albuminous matter of cells.

cal·cu·lo·sis (kal″ku-lo′sis) lithiasis.

cal·cu·lus (kal′ku-lus) pl. *cal′culi.* [L.] an abnormal concretion, usually composed of mineral salts, occurring within the animal body. **cal′culous,** adj. **biliary c.,** gallstone. **dental c.,** calcium phosphate and carbonate, with organic matter, deposited on tooth surfaces. **lung c.,** one formed in the bronchi by accretion about an inorganic nucleus, or from calcified portions of lung tissue or adjacent lymph nodes. **oxalate c.,** a urinary calculus made of calcium oxalate; some have tiny sharp spines and others are smooth. **renal c.,** one in the kidney. **salivary c.,** 1. sialolith. 2. supragingival c. **struvite c.,** a urinary calculus of crystals of struvite

(magnesium ammonium phosphate). **supra-gingival c.,** that covering the coronal surface of the tooth to the crest of the gingival margin. **urinary c.,** one in any part of the urinary tract. **uterine c.,** uterolith; a concretion in the uterus. **vesical c.,** one in the urinary bladder.

cal·e·fa·cient (kal″ĕ-fa′shent) causing a sensation of warmth; an agent that so acts.

calf (kaf) sura; the fleshy back part of the leg below the knee.

Ca·len·du·la (kah-len′du-lah) [L.] a genus of composite-flowered plants. The dried florets of *C. officina'lis,* the pot marigold, have antimicrobial and antiinflammatory properties; they are used topically for inflammatory lesions and to promote healing and are used in homeopathy and folk medicine.

cal·fac·tant (kal-fak′tant) a pulmonary surfactant from calf lung, used in the prophylaxis and treatment of neonatal respiratory distress syndrome.

cal·i·ber (kal′ĭ-ber) the diameter of the opening of a canal or tube.

cal·i·bra·tion (kal″ĭ-bra′shun) determination of the accuracy of an instrument, usually by measurement of its variation from a standard, to ascertain necessary correction factors.

cal·i·cec·ta·sis (kal″ĭ-sek′tah-sis) dilatation of a calix of the kidney.

Ca·li·ci·vir·i·dae (kah-lis″ĭ-vir′ĭ-de) the caliciviruses: a family of RNA viruses having a positive-sense, single-stranded RNA genome, and transmitted via infested food, by contact, or by airborne particles. The single genus is *Calicivirus.*

Ca·li·ci·vi·rus (kah-lis′ĭ-vi″rus) caliciviruses; a genus of the family Caliciviridae that includes Norwalk virus and other viruses causing acute self-limited gastroenteritis in humans.

ca·li·ci·vi·rus a member of the family Caliciviridae.

ca·lic·u·lus (kah-lik′u-lus) pl. *cali′culi.* [L.] a bud-shaped or cup-shaped structure.

cal·i·for·ni·um (Cf) (kal″ĭ-for′ne-um) chemical element (see *Table of Elements*), at. no. 98.

cal·i·pers (kal′ĭ-perz) an instrument with two bent or curved legs used for measuring thickness or diameter of a solid.

ca·lix (ka′liks) pl. *ca′lices.* [L.] calyx.

Cal·liph·o·ra (kah-lif′o-rah) a genus of flies, including the blowflies and bluebottle flies, which deposit their eggs in decaying matter, on wounds, or in body openings; the maggots are a cause of myiasis.

cal·los·i·ty (kah-los′ĭ-te) a callus (1).

cal·lo·sum (kah-lo'sum) corpus callosum. **callo'sal**, adj.

cal·lus (kal'us) [L.] 1. localized hyperplasia of the stratum corneum of the epidermis due to pressure or friction. 2. an unorganized network of woven bone formed about the ends of a broken bone, which is absorbed as repair is completed (*provisional c.*), and ultimately replaced by true bone (*definitive c.*).

cal·mod·u·lin (kal-mod'u-lin) a calcium-binding protein present in all nucleated cells; it mediates a variety of cellular reponses to calcium.

ca·lor (kal'er) [L.] heat; one of the cardinal signs of inflammation.

ca·lo·ric (kah-lor'ik) pertaining to heat or to calories.

cal·o·rie (kal'ah-re) any of several units of heat defined as the amount of heat required to raise 1 g of water 1°C at a specified temperature; the calorie used in chemistry and biochemistry is equal to 4.184 joules. Abbreviated cal. **large c.**, the calorie now used only in metabolic studies; also used to express the fuel or energy value of food. It is equivalent to the kilocalorie. Symbol C. **small c.**, calorie, when the term large calorie had broader meaning.

ca·lor·i·gen·ic (kah-lor''ĭ-jen'ik) producing or increasing production of heat or energy; increasing oxygen consumption.

cal·o·rim·e·ter (kal''ah-rim'ĕ-ter) an instrument for measuring the amount of heat produced in any system or organism.

cal·re·tic·u·lin (kal''rĕ-tik'u-lin) a calcium-binding protein in the sarcoplasmic reticulum and in the endoplasmic reticulum of nonmuscle cells; its roles include calcium homeostasis, control of viral RNA replication, lymphocyte activation, and cytotoxicity.

cal·se·ques·trin (-sĕ-kwes'trin) a calcium-binding protein rich in carboxylate side chains, occurring on the inner membrane surface of the sarcoplasmic reticulum.

cal·va·ria (kal-var'e-ah) [L.] the domelike superior portion of the cranium, comprising the superior portions of the frontal, parietal, and occipital bones.

calx (kalks) 1. lime or chalk. 2. heel.

Ca·lym·ma·to·bac·te·ri·um (kah-lim''ah-to-bak-tēr'e-um) a genus of bacteria (family Brucellaceae), composed of pleomorphic non-motile, gram-negative rods. *C. granulo'matis* causes granuloma inguinale in humans; see also *Donovan's body*, under *body*.

ca·lyx (ka'liks) pl. *ca'lyces*. A cup-shaped organ or cavity, e.g., one of the recesses of the pelvis of the kidney which enclose the pyramids. **calice'al**, adj.

CAM complementary and alternative medicine.

cam·era (kam'ah-rah) pl. *ca'merae, cameras*. [L.] 1. a box, compartment, or chamber. 2. any enclosed space or ventricle. 3. a device for converting light or other energy from an object into a visible image. **Anger c.**, the original, and by far the most commonly used, form of scintillation (or gamma) camera, so that the terms are often used interchangeably. **c. ante'rior bul'bi**, anterior chamber (of the eye). **gamma c.**, scintillation c. **c. poste'rior bul'bi**, posterior chamber (of the eye). **c. vi'trea bul'bi**, vitreous chamber. **c. o'culi**, either the anterior or the posterior chamber of the eye. **scintillation c.**, an electronic instrument that produces photographs or cathode-ray tube images of the gamma ray emissions from organs containing tracer compounds; the term is often equated with *Anger camera*, the original and most used version.

cam·i·sole (kam'ĭ-sōl) [Fr.] straitjacket; a jacketlike device for restraining the limbs, particularly the arms, of a violently disturbed patient.

cAMP cyclic adenosine monophosphate.

cam·phor (kam'fer) a ketone derived from the Asian tree *Cinnamomum camphora* or produced synthetically; used topically as an antipruritic and antiinfective and inhaled as a nasal decongestant; also used in folk medicine and in Indian medicine.

cam·pim·e·ter (kam-pim'ĕ-ter) an apparatus for mapping the central portion of the visual field on a flat surface.

cam·pot·o·my (kam-pot'ah-me) the stereotaxic surgical technique of producing a lesion in Forel's fields, beneath the thalamus, for correction of tremor in Parkinson's disease.

camp·to·cor·mia (kamp''tah-kor'me-ah) a static deformity consisting of forward flexion of the trunk.

camp·to·dac·ty·ly (-dak'tĭ-le) permanent flexion of one or more fingers.

camp·to·me·lia (-me'le-ah) bending of the limbs, producing permanent bowing or curving of the affected part. **camptome'lic**, adj.

Cam·py·lo·bac·ter (kam'pĭ-lo-bak'ter) a genus of bacteria, family Spirillaceae, made up of gram-negative, non–spore-forming, motile, spirally curved rods, which are microaerophilic to anaerobic. *C. jeju'ni*, *C. co'li*, and certain subspecies of *C. fe'tus* can cause gastroenteritis; *C. rec'tus* is associated with periodontal disease..

cam·sy·late (kam'sĭ-lāt) USAN contraction for camphorsulfonate.

ca·nal (kah-nal') a relatively narrow tubular passage or channel. **adductor c.,** a fascial tunnel in the middle third of the medial part of the thigh, containing the femoral vessels and saphenous nerve. **Alcock's c.,** pudendal c. **alimentary c.,** the musculomembranous digestive tube extending from the mouth to the anus. **anal c.,** the terminal portion of the alimentary canal, from the rectum to the anus. **Arnold's c.,** a channel in the petrous portion of the temporal bone for passage of the vagus nerve. **atrioventricular c.,** the common canal connecting the primordial atrium and ventricle; it sometimes persists as a congenital anomaly. **birth c.,** the canal through which the fetus passes in birth. **caroticotympanic c's,** tiny passages in the temporal bone connecting the carotid canal and the tympanic cavity, carrying communicating twigs between the internal carotid and tympanic plexuses. **carotid c.,** a tunnel in the petrous portion of the temporal bone that transmits the internal carotid artery to the cranial cavity. **cochlear c.,** see under *duct*. **condylar c., condyloid c.,** an occasional opening in the condylar fossa for transmission of the transverse sinus. **c. of Cuvier,** ductus venosus. **Dorello's c.,** an occasional opening in the temporal bone through which the abducens nerve and inferior petrosal sinus enter the cavernous sinus. **facial c.,** a canal for the facial nerve in the petrous portion of the temporal bone. **femoral c.,** the medial part of the femoral sheath lateral to the base of the lacunar ligament. **Gartner's c.,** a closed rudimentary duct, lying parallel to the uterine tube, into which the transverse ducts of the epoöphoron open; it is the remains of the part of the mesonephros that participates in formation of the reproductive organs. **genital c.,** any canal for the passage of ova or for copulatory use. **haversian c.,** any of the anastomosing channels of the haversian system in compact bone, containing blood and lymph vessels and nerves. **Huguier's c.,** a small canal opening into the facial canal just before its termination, transmitting the chorda tympani nerve. **Huschke's c.,** a canal formed by the tubercles of the tympanic ring, usually disappearing during childhood. **hyaloid c.,** a passage running from in front of the optic disk to the lens of the eye; in the fetus, it transmits the hyaloid artery. **hypoglossal c.,** an opening in the occipital bone, transmitting the hypoglossal nerve and a branch of the posterior meningeal artery. **incisive c's,** the small canals opening into the incisive fossa of the hard palate, transmitting the nasopalatine nerves. **infraorbital c.,** a small canal running obliquely through the floor of the orbit, transmitting the infraorbital vessels and nerve. **inguinal c.,** the oblique passage in the lower anterior abdominal wall, through which passes the round ligament of the uterus in the female, and the spermatic cord in the male. **interdental c's,** channels in the alveolar process of the mandible between the roots of the central and lateral incisors, for passage of anastomosing blood vessels between the sublingual and inferior dental arteries. **interfacial c's,** a labyrinthine system of expanded intercellular spaces between desmosomes. **medullary c.,** 1. vertebral c. 2. see under *cavity*. **nasal c., nasolacrimal c.,** a canal formed by the maxilla laterally and the lacrimal bone and inferior nasal concha medially, transmitting the nasolacrimal duct. **neurenteric c.,** a temporary communication in the embryo between the posterior part of the neural tube and the archenteron. **c. of Nuck,** a pouch of peritoneum extending into the inguinal canal, accompanying the round ligament, in the female; usually obliterated after birth. **nutrient c.,** haversian c. **optic c.,** one of the paired openings in the sphenoid bone that transmits an optic nerve and its associated ophthalmic artery. **Petit's c.,** zonular spaces. **perivascular c.,** a lymph space about a blood vessel. **portal c.,** a space within the capsule of Glisson and liver substance, containing branches of the portal vein, of the hepatic artery, and of the hepatic duct. **pterygoid c.,** a canal in the sphenoid bone transmitting the pterygoid vessels and nerves. **pterygopalatine c.,** a passage in the sphenoid and palatine bones for the greater palatine vessels and nerve. **pudendal c.,** a tunnel formed by a splitting of the obturator fascia, which encloses the pudendal vessels and nerve. **pyloric c.,** the short narrow part of the stomach extending from the gastroduodenal junction to the pyloric antrum. **root c.,** that part of the pulp cavity extending from the pulp chamber to the apical foramen. **sacculocochlear c.,** the canal connecting the saccule and cochlea. **sacral c.,** the continuation of the vertebral canal through the sacrum. **semicircular c's,** three long canals (anterior, lateral, and posterior) of the bony labyrinth, important in the sense of equilibrium. **spermatic c.,** the inguinal canal in the male. **spiral c. of cochlea,** cochlear duct. **spiral c. of modiolus,** a canal following the course of the bony spiral lamina of the cochlea and containing the spiral ganglion. **tarsal c.,** see under *sinus*. **tympanic c. of cochlea,** scala tympani. **uterine c.,** the cavity of the uterus. **vertebral c.,** the canal formed by the series of vertebral foramina together, enclosing the spinal cord and meninges. **Volkmann's c's,** canals communicating with the haversian canals, for passage of blood vessels through bone. **c. of Wirsung,** pancreatic duct. **zygomaticotemporal c.,** see under *foramen.*

can·a·lic·u·lus (kan″ah-lik′u-lus) pl. *canali′culi.* [L.] an extremely narrow tubular passage or channel. **canalic′ular,** adj. **apical c.,** one of the numerous tubular invaginations arising from the clefts between the microvilli of the proximal convoluted tubule of the kidney and extending downward into the apical cytoplasm. **bone canaliculi,** branching tubular passages radiating like wheel spokes from each bone lacuna to connect with the canaliculi of adjacent lacunae, and with the haversian canal. **cochlear c.,** a small canal in the petrous part of the temporal bone that interconnects the scala tympani with the subarachnoid space; it houses the perilymphatic duct and a small vein. **dental canaliculi,** minute channels in dentin, extending from the pulp cavity to the overlying cement and enamel. **intercellular c.,** one located between adjacent cells, such as one of the secretory capillaries, or canaliculi, of the gastric parietal cells. **intracellular canaliculi of parietal cells,** a system of canaliculi that seem to be intracellular but are formed by deep invaginations of the surface of the gastric parietal cells rather than extending into the cytoplasm of the cell. **lacrimal c.,** the short passage in the eyelid, beginning at the lacrimal point and draining tears from the lacrimal lake to the lacrimal sac. **mastoid c.,** a small channel in the temporal bone transmitting the auricular branch of the vagus nerve. **tympanic c.,** a small opening on the inferior surface of the petrous portion of the temporal bone, transmitting the tympanic branch of the glossopharyngeal nerve and a small artery.

ca·na·lis (kah-na′lis) pl. *cana′les.* [L.] a canal or channel.

can·a·li·za·tion (kan″ah-li-za′shun) 1. formation of canals, natural or pathologic. 2. surgical creation of canals for drainage. 3. recanalization. 4. in psychology, formation in the central nervous system of new pathways by repeated passage of nerve impulses.

can·cel·lous (kan-sel′us) of a reticular, spongy, or lattice-like structure.

can·cel·lus pl. *cancel′li.* [L.] the lattice-like structure in bone; any structure arranged like a lattice.

can·cer (kan′ser) a neoplastic disease the natural course of which is fatal. Cancer cells, unlike benign tumor cells, exhibit the properties of invasion and metastasis and are highly anaplastic. The term includes the two broad categories of carcinoma and sarcoma, but is often used synonymously with the former. **can′cerous,** adj. **epithelial c.,** carcinoma.

can·cer·emia (kan″ser-e′me-ah) the presence of cancer cells in the blood.

can·cer·i·gen·ic (-ĭ-jen′ik) giving rise to a malignant tumor.

can·cer·pho·bia (-fo′be-ah) irrational fear of cancer.

can·cri·form (kang′krĭ-form) resembling cancer.

can·croid (kang′kroid) resembling cancer.

can·crum (kang′krum) [L.] canker. **c. o′ris,** see *noma.* **c. puden′di,** see *noma.*

can·de·la (cd) (kan-del′ah) the base SI unit of luminous intensity.

can·de·sar·tan (kan″dĕ-sahr′tan) an angiotensin II receptor antagonist, used in the treatment of hypertension; administered orally as *c. cilexetil.*

Can·di·da (kan′dĭ-dah) a genus of yeastlike fungi that are commonly part of the normal flora of the mouth, skin, intestinal tract, and vagina, but can cause a variety of infections (see *candidiasis*). *C. al′bicans* is the usual pathogen.

can·di·dal (kan′di-d′l) pertaining to or caused by *Candida.*

can·di·di·a·sis (kan″dĭ-di′ah-sis) infection by fungi of the genus *Candida,* generally *C. albicans,* most commonly involving the skin, oral mucosa (thrush), respiratory tract, or vagina; rarely there is a systemic infection or endocarditis. **acute pseudomembranous c.,** thrush. **atrophic c.,** a type of oral candidiasis marked by erythematous pebbled patches on the hard or soft palate, buccal mucosa, and dorsal surface of the tongue. **bronchopulmonary c.,** bronchocandidiasis; that found in the respiratory tract. **chronic mucocutaneous c.,** any of various forms characterized by chronic candidiasis of oral and vaginal mucosa, skin, and nails, resistant to treatment, and sometimes familial. **oral c.,** thrush. **vaginal c., vulvovaginal c.,** candidal infection of the vagina, and usually also the vulva, commonly characterized by pruritus, creamy white discharge, vulvar erythema and swelling, and dyspareunia.

can·di·did (kan′dĭ-did) a secondary skin eruption that is the expression of hypersensitivity to infection with *Candida* elsewhere on the body.

can·di·din (-din) a skin test antigen derived from *Candida albicans,* used in testing for the development of delayed-type hypersensitivity to the microorganism.

ca·nine (ka'nīn) 1. of, pertaining to, or characteristic of a dog. 2. cuspid tooth.

ca·ni·ti·es (kah-nish'e-ēz) grayness or whiteness of the scalp hair.

can·ker (kang'ker) an ulceration, especially of the oral mucosa.

can·nab·i·noid (kah-nab'ĭ-noid) any of the principles of *Cannabis*, including tetrahydrocannabinol, cannabinol, and cannabidiol.

can·na·bis (kan'ah-bis) the dried flowering tops of hemp plants (*Cannabis sativa*), which have euphoric principles (tetrahydrocannabinols); classified as a hallucinogen and prepared as bhang, ganja, hashish, and marihuana.

can·nu·la (kan'u-lah) a tube for insertion into a vessel, duct, or cavity; during insertion its lumen is usually occupied by a trocar.

can·thi·tis (kan-thi'tis) inflammation of the canthus.

can·tho·plas·ty (kan'thah-plas"te) plastic surgery of a canthus.

can·thot·o·my (kan-thot'ah-me) incision of a canthus.

can·thus (kan'thus) pl. *can'thi*. [L.] the angle at either end of the fissure between the eyelids, lateral or medial.

can·ti·le·ver (kan"tĭ-le'ver) a projecting structure supported on only one end and carrying a load at the other end or along its length.

CAP College of American Pathologists.

cap (kap) a protective covering for the head or for a similar structure; a structure resembling such a covering. **acrosomal c.,** acrosome. **cradle c.,** crusta lactea. **duodenal c.,** the part of the duodenum adjacent to the pylorus, forming the superior flexure. **enamel c.,** the enamel organ after it covers the top of the growing tooth papilla. **head c.,** the doubled-layered caplike structure over the upper two-thirds of the acrosome of a spermatozoon, consisting of the collapsed acrosomal vesicle. **knee c.,** patella; see *Table of Bones.* **skull c.,** calvaria.

ca·pac·i·tance (C) (kah-pas'ĭ-tans) 1. the property of being able to store an electric charge. 2. the ratio of the charge stored by a capacitor to the voltage across the capacitor.

ca·pac·i·ta·tion (kah-pas"ĭ-ta'shun) the process by which spermatozoa in the ampullary portion of a uterine tube become capable of going through the acrosome reaction and fertilizing an oocyte.

ca·pac·i·ty (kah-pas'ĭ-te) the power to hold, retain, or contain, or the ability to absorb; usually expressed numerically as the measure of such ability. **forced vital c.**

(FVC), vital capacity measured when the patient is exhaling with maximal speed and effort. **functional residual c.,** the amount of air remaining at the end of normal quiet respiration. **heat c.,** the amount of heat required to raise the temperature of a specific quantity of a substance by one degree Celsius. Symbol *C.* **inspiratory c.,** the volume of gas that can be taken into the lungs in a full inhalation, starting from the resting inspiratory position; equal to the tidal volume plus the inspiratory reserve volume. **maximal breathing c.,** maximum voluntary ventilation. **thermal c.,** heat c. **total lung c.,** the amount of gas contained in the lung at the end of a maximal inhalation. **virus neutralizing c.,** the ability of a serum to inhibit the infectivity of a virus. **vital c.,** VC; the volume of gas that can be expelled from the lungs from a position of full inspiration, with no limit to duration of inspiration; equal to inspiratory capacity plus expiratory reserve volume.

cap·e·ci·ta·bine (kap"ĕ-si'tah-bēn) an antineoplastic used in the treatment of metastatic breast or colorectal carcinoma.

cap·il·lar·ec·ta·sia (kap"ĭ-lar"ek-ta'zhah) dilatation of capillaries.

Ca·pil·la·ria (kap"ĭ-lar'e-ah) a genus of parasitic nematodes, including *C. hepat'ica,* found in the liver of rats and other mammals, including humans; and *C. philippinen'sis,* found in the human intestine in the Philippines, causing severe diarrhea, malabsorption, and high mortality.

cap·il·la·ri·a·sis (kap"ĭ-lah-ri'ah-sis) infection with nematodes of the genus *Capillaria,* especially *C. philippinensis.*

cap·il·lar·i·ty (kap"ĭ-lar'ĭ-te) the action by which the surface of a liquid in contact with a solid, as in a capillary tube, is elevated or depressed.

cap·il·lary (kap'ĭ-lar"e) 1. pertaining to or resembling a hair. 2. one of the minute vessels connecting the arterioles and venules, the walls of which act as a semipermeable membrane for interchange of various substances between the blood and tissue fluid; see Plate 22. **arterial c.,** precapillary; a type of minute vessel lacking a continuous muscular coat, intermediate in structure and location between an arteriole and a capillary. **continuous c's,** one of the two major types of capillaries, found in muscle, skin, lung, central nervous system, and other tissues, characterized by the presence of an uninterrupted endothelium and a continuous basal lamina, and by fine filaments and numerous pinocytotic vesicles. **fenestrated c's,** one of the two major types of capillaries, found in the intestinal mucosa, renal glomeruli, pancreas, endocrine glands, and other tissues, and characterized by the presence of circular fenestrae or pores that penetrate the endothelium; these pores may be closed by a very thin diaphragm. **lymph c., lymphatic c.,** one of the minute vessels of the lymphatic system; see Plate 22. **secretory c.,** any of the extremely fine intercellular canaliculi situated between adjacent gland cells, being formed by the apposition of grooves in the parietal cells and opening into the gland's lumen. **venous c.,** postcapillary venule; a type of minute vessel lacking a muscular coat, intermediate in structure and location between a venule and a capillary.

cap·il·lus (kah-pil'us) pl. *capil'li.* [L.] a hair; used in the plural to designate the aggregate of hair on the scalp.

cap·i·tate (kap'ĭ-tāt) head-shaped.

cap·i·ta·tion (kap″ĭ-ta'shun) the annual fee paid to a physician or group of physicians by each participant in a health plan.

cap·i·ta·tum (-tum) [L.] the capitate bone; see *Table of Bones.*

cap·i·tel·lum (kap″ĭ-tel'um) capitulum.

cap·i·ton·nage (kap″ĭ-to-nahzh') [Fr.] closure of a cyst by applying sutures to approximate the opposing surfaces of the cavity.

ca·pit·u·lum (kah-pit'u-lum) pl. *capi'tula.* [L.] a small eminence on a bone, as on the distal end of the humerus, by which it articulates with another bone. **capit'ular,** adj.

Cap·no·cy·toph·a·ga (kap″no-si-tof'ah-gah) a genus of anaerobic, gram-negative, rod-shaped bacteria that have been implicated in the pathogenesis of periodontal disease; they closely resemble *Bacteroides ochraceus.* **C. canimor'sus,** a species that is part of the normal oral flora of dogs and cats; following a bite it may cause serious local or systemic infection or death.

cap·no·gram (kap'no-gram″) a real-time waveform record of the concentration of carbon dioxide in the respiratory gases.

cap·no·graph (-graf″) a system for monitoring the concentration of exhaled carbon dioxide.

cap·nog·ra·phy (kap-nog'rah-fe) monitoring of the concentration of exhaled carbon dioxide in order to assess physiologic status or determine the adequacy of ventilation during anesthesia.

cap·nom·e·ter (kap-nom'ĕ-ter) a device for monitoring the end-tidal partial pressure of carbon dioxide.

cap·nom·e·try (-tre) the determination of the end-tidal partial pressure of carbon dioxide.

ca·pote·ment (kah-pōt-maw') [Fr.] a splashing sound heard in dilatation of the stomach.

cap·ping (kap'ing) 1. the provision of a protective or obstructive covering. 2. the formation of a polar cap on the surface of a cell concerned with immunologic responses, occurring as a result of movement of components on the cell surface into clusters or patches that coalesce to form the cap. The process is produced by reaction of antibody with the cell membrane and appears to involve cross-linking of antigenic determinants. **pulp c.,** the covering of an exposed or nearly exposed dental pulp with some material to provide protection against external influences and to encourage healing.

cap·reo·my·cin (kap″re-o-mi'sin) a polypeptide antibiotic produced by *Streptomyces capreolus,* which is active against human strains of *Mycobacterium tuberculosis;* used as the disulfate salt.

cap·ric ac·id (kap'rik) a saturated ten-carbon fatty acid, occurring as a minor constituent in many fats and oils.

cap·ro·ate (kap'ro-āt) 1. any salt or ester of caproic acid (hexanoic acid). 2. USAN contraction for hexanoate.

ca·pro·ic ac·id (kah-pro'ik) a saturated six-carbon fatty acid occurring in butterfat and coconut and palm oils.

cap·ry·late (kap'rĭ-lāt) any salt, ester, or anionic form of caprylic acid.

ca·pryl·ic ac·id (kah-pril'ik) an eight-carbon saturated fatty acid occurring in butterfat and palm and coconut oils.

cap·sa·i·cin (kap-sa'ĭ-sin) an alkaloid irritating to the skin and mucous membranes, the active ingredient of capsicum; used as a topical counterirritant and analgesic.

cap·si·cum (kap'sĭ-kum) a plant of the genus *Capsicum,* the hot peppers, or the dried fruit derived from certain of its species (cayenne or red pepper), containing the active principle capsaicin; used as a counterirritant and analgesic and also in pepper spray.

cap·sid (kap'sid) the shell of protein that protects the nucleic acid of a virus; it is composed of structural units, or capsomers.

cap·si·tis (kap-sīt'is) inflammation of the capsule of the crystalline lens.

cap·so·mer (kap'so-mer) a morphological unit of the capsid of a virus.

cap·su·la (kap'su-lah) pl. *cap'sulae.* [L.] capsule.

cap·sule (kap′sul) 1. an enclosing structure, as a soluble container enclosing a dose of medicine. 2. a cartilaginous, fatty, fibrous, membranous structure enveloping another structure, organ, or part. **cap′sular**, adj. **adipose renal c.**, the investment of fat surrounding the fibrous capsule of the kidney, continuous at the hilum with the fat in the renal sinus. **articular c.**, joint capsule; the saclike envelope enclosing the cavity of a synovial joint. **auditory c.**, the cartilaginous capsule of the embryo that develops into the bony labyrinth of the inner ear. **bacterial c.**, an envelope of gel surrounding a bacterial cell, usually polysaccharide but sometimes polypeptide in nature; it is associated with the virulence of pathogenic bacteria. **cartilage c.**, a basophilic zone of cartilage matrix bordering on a lacuna and its enclosed cartilage cells. **external c.**, the layer of white fibers between the putamen and claustrum. **fibrous renal c.**, the connective tissue investment of the kidney, continuous through the hilum to line the renal sinus. **Glisson's c.**, the connective tissue sheath accompanying the hepatic ducts and vessels through the hepatic portal. **glomerular c., c. of glomerulus**, the globular dilatation forming the beginning of a uriniferous tubule within the kidney and surrounding the glomerulus. **internal c.**, a fanlike mass of white fibers separating the lentiform nucleus laterally from the head of the caudate nucleus, the dorsal thalamus, and the tail of the caudate nucleus medially. **joint c.**, articular c. **c. of lens**, the elastic envelope covering the lens of the eye. **optic c.**, the embryonic structure from which the sclera develops. **otic c.**, the skeletal element enclosing the inner ear mechanism. In the human embryo, it develops as cartilage at various ossification centers and becomes completely bony and unified at about the 23rd week of fetal life. **renal c's,** the investing tissue around the kidney, divided into the *fibrous renal capsule* and the *adipose renal capsule.* **Tenon's c.**, the connective tissue enveloping the posterior eyeball.

cap·su·lec·to·my (kap″su-lek′tah-me) excision of a capsule, especially a joint capsule or lens capsule.

cap·su·li·tis (-li′tis) inflammation of a capsule, as that of the lens. **adhesive c.**, adhesive inflammation between the joint capsule and the peripheral articular cartilage of the shoulder, with obliteration of the subdeltoid bursa, characterized by increasing pain, stiffness, and limitation of motion.

cap·su·lo·plas·ty (kap′sul-o-plas″te) plastic repair of a joint capsule.

cap·su·lor·rhex·is (kap″su-lo-rek′sis) the making of a continuous circular tear in the anterior capsule during cataract surgery in order to allow expression or phacoemulsification of the nucleus of the lens.

cap·su·lot·o·my (kap″su-lot′ah-me) incision of a capsule, as that of the lens, the kidney, or a joint.

cap·to·pril (kap′to-pril) an angiotensin-converting enzyme inhibitor used in the treatment of hypertension, congestive heart failure, and post–myocardial infarction left ventricular dysfunction.

cap·ture (kap′cher) 1. to seize or catch. 2. the coalescence of an atomic nucleus and a subatomic particle, usually resulting in an unstable mass. **atrial c.**, depolarization of the atria in response to a stimulus either originating elsewhere in the heart or pacemaker-induced. **ventricular c.**, depolarization of the ventricles in response to an impulse originating either in the supraventricular region or in an artificial pacemaker.

cap·ut (kap′ut) pl. *cap′ita.* [L.] the head; a general term applied to the expanded or chief extremity of an organ or part. **c. medu′sae**, dilated cutaneous veins around the umbilicus, seen mainly in the newborn and in patients with cirrhosis. **c. succeda′neum**, edema occurring in and under the fetal scalp during labor.

CAR Canadian Association of Radiologists.

car·ba·ceph·em (kahr″bah-sef′em) any of a class of antibiotics closely related to the cephalosporins in structure and use, but chemically more stable.

car·ba·chol (kahr′bah-kol) a cholinergic agonist used as a miotic and to lower intraocular pressure in the treatment of glaucoma and following cataract surgery.

car·ba·mate (kahr′bah-māt) any ester of carbamic acid.

car·ba·maz·e·pine (kahr″bah-maz′ĕ-pēn) an anticonvulsant and analgesic used in the treatment of pain associated with trigeminal neuralgia and in epilepsy manifested by certain types of seizures.

car·bam·ic ac·id (kahr-bam′ik) NH_2COOH, a compound existing only in the form of salts or esters (carbamates), amides (carbamides), and other derivatives.

car·ba·mide (kahr′bah-mīd) urea. **c. peroxide**, a compound of urea and hydrogen peroxide used as a cerumen-softening agent, dental cleanser, bleaching agent, and anti-inflammatory.

car·bam·i·no·he·mo·glo·bin (kahr-bam″ĭ-no-he′mo-glo″bin) a combination of carbon dioxide and hemoglobin, CO_2HHb, being one of the forms in which carbon dioxide exists in the blood.

car·bam·o·yl (kahr-bam′o-il) the radical NH_2CO—; see *carbamoyltransferase.*

car·bam·o·yl·trans·fer·ase (kahr-bam″o-il-trans′fer-ās) an enzyme that catalyzes the transfer of a carbamoyl group, as from carbamoylphosphate to L-ornithine to form orthophosphate and citrulline in the synthesis of urea.

car·ben·i·cil·lin (kahr″ben-ĭ-sil′in) a semisynthetic penicillin, with activity against *Pseudomonas aeruginosa* and some other gram-negative bacteria; used as the disodium salt. It is also used as *c. indanyl sodium* in the treatment of urinary tract infections and prostatitis.

car·be·ta·pen·tane (kahr-ba″tah-pen′tān) an antitussive agent used as the tannate salt in the treatment of cough associated with upper respiratory infections.

car·bi·do·pa (kahr″bĭ-do′pah) an inhibitor of decarboxylation of levodopa in extracerebral tissues, used in combination with levodopa as an antiparkinsonian agent.

car·bi·nol (kahr′bĭ-nol) 1. methyl alcohol. 2. any aromatic or fatty alcohol formed by substituting one, two, or three hydrocarbon groups for hydrogen in methanol.

car·bi·nox·amine (kahr″bin-ok′sah-mēn) an antihistamine with anticholinergic and sedative effects, used as the maleate salt.

car·bo·hy·drate (kahr″bo-hi′drāt) any of a class of aldehyde or ketone derivatives of polyhydric alcohols, so named because the hydrogen and oxygen are usually in the proportion of water, $C_n(H_2O)$; the most important comprise the starches, sugars, glycogens, celluloses, and gums.

car·bol·fuch·sin (kahr″bol-fūk′sin) a dye containing basic fuchsin and dilute phenol.

car·bol·ic ac·id (kahr-bol′ik) phenol (1).

car·bol·ism (kahr′bah-lizm) phenol poisoning; see *phenol* (1).

car·bon (C) (kahr′bon) chemical element (see *Table of Elements*), at. no. 6. **c. dioxide,** an odorless, colorless gas, CO_2, resulting from oxidation of carbon, and formed in the tissues and eliminated by the lungs; used in some pump oxygenators to maintain blood carbon dioxide tension. In solid form it is *carbon dioxide snow* (see under *snow*). **c. monoxide,** an odorless gas, CO, formed by burning carbon or organic fuels with a scanty supply of oxygen; inhalation causes central nervous system damage and asphyxiation by

combining irreversibly with blood hemoglobin. **c. tetrachloride,** a clear, colorless, volatile liquid; inhalation of its vapors can depress central nervous system activity and cause degeneration of the liver and kidneys.

car·bon·ate (kahr′bah-nāt) a salt of carbonic acid.

car·bon·ic ac·id (kahr-bon′ik) an aqueous solution of carbon dioxide, H_2CO_3.

car·bon·ic an·hy·drase (an-hi′-drās) an enzyme that catalyzes the decomposition of carbonic acid into carbon dioxide and water, facilitating the transfer of carbon dioxide from tissues to blood and from blood to alveolar air.

car·bon·yl (kahr′bah-nil) the bivalent organic radical, C:O, characteristic of aldehydes, ketones, carboxylic acids, and esters.

car·bo·pla·tin (kahr′bo-plat″in) an antineoplastic used in the treatment of carcinomas of the ovary and numerous other organs.

car·bo·prost (-prost) a synthetic analogue of dinoprost, a prostaglandin of the F type; used as the tromethamine salt as an oxytocic for termination of pregnancy and missed abortion.

γ-car·boxy·glu·ta·mic ac·id (kahr-bok″se-gloo-tam′ik) an amino acid occurring in biologically active prothrombin, and formed in the liver in the presence of vitamin K by carboxylation of glutamic acid residues in prothrombin precursor molecules.

car·boxy·he·mo·glo·bin (-he′mo-glo″bin) hemoglobin combined with carbon monoxide, which occupies the sites on the hemoglobin molecule that normally bind with oxygen and which is not readily displaced from the molecule.

car·box·yl (kahr-bok′sil) the monovalent radical —COOH, occurring in those organic acids termed carboxylic acids.

car·box·y·lase (kahr-bok′sĭ-lās) an enzyme that catalyzes the removal of carbon dioxide from the carboxyl group of alpha amino keto acids.

car·box·y·la·tion (kahr-bok″sĭ-la′shun) the addition of carbon dioxide or bicarbonate to form a carboxyl group, as to pyruvate to form oxaloacetate.

car·box·yl·es·ter·ase (kahr-bok″sil-es′ter-ās) an enzyme of wide specificity that catalyzes the hydrolytic cleavage of the ester bond in a carboxylic ester to form an alcohol and a carboxylic acid, including acting on esters of vitamin A.

car·box·yl·trans·fer·ase (-trans′fer-ās) any of a group of enzymes that catalyze the transfer of a carboxyl group from a donor to an acceptor compound.

car·box·y·ly·ase (kahr-bok″se-li′ās) any of a group of lyases that catalyze the removal of a carboxyl group; it includes the carboxylases and decarboxylases.

car·boxy·meth·yl·cel·lu·lose (-meth″il-sel′u-lōs) a substituted cellulose polymer of variable size, used as the sodium or calcium salt as a pharmaceutical suspending agent, tablet excipient, and viscosity-increasing agent; the former is also used as a laxative.

car·boxy·myo·glo·bin (-mi″ah-glo′bin) a compound formed from myoglobin on exposure to carbon monoxide.

car·boxy·pep·ti·dase (-pep′tĭ-dās) any exopeptidase that catalyzes the hydrolytic cleavage of the terminal or penultimate bond at the end of a peptide or polypeptide where the free carboxyl group occurs.

car·bun·cle (kahr′bung-k'l) a necrotizing infection of skin and subcutaneous tissues composed of a cluster of furuncles, usually due to *Staphylococcus aureus*, with multiple drainage sinuses. **carbunc′ular**, adj. **malignant c.**, anthrax.

car·ci·no·em·bry·on·ic (kahr″sĭ-no-em″-bre-on′ik) occurring both in carcinoma and in embryonic tissue; see under *antigen*.

car·cin·o·gen (kahr-sin′ah-jen) any substance which causes cancer. **carcinogen′ic**, adj. **epigenetic c.**, one that does not itself damage DNA but causes alterations that predispose to cancer. **genotoxic c.**, one that reacts directly with DNA or with macromolecules that then react with DNA.

car·ci·no·ge·nic·i·ty (kahr″sĭ-no-jĕ-nis′ĭ-te) the ability or tendency to produce cancer.

car·ci·noid (kahr′sĭ-noid) a yellow circumscribed tumor arising from enterochromaffin cells, usually in the gastrointestinal tract; the term is sometimes used to refer specifically to the gastrointestinal tumor (*argentaffinoma*).

car·ci·nol·y·sis (kahr″sĭ-nol′ĭ-sis) destruction of cancer cells. **carcinolyt′ic**, adj.

car·ci·no·ma (kahr″sĭ-no′mah) pl. *carcino-mas, carcino′mata*. A malignant new growth made up of epithelial cells tending to infiltrate surrounding tissues and to give rise to metastases. **acinar c., acinic cell c., acinous c.**, a slow-growing malignant tumor with acinic cells in small glandlike structures, usually in the pancreas or salivary glands. **adenocystic c., adenoid cystic c.**, cylindroma; carcinoma marked by cylinders or bands of hyaline or mucinous stroma separating or surrounded by nests or cords of small epithelial cells, occurring particularly in the salivary glands. **adenosquamous c.**, 1. adenoacanthoma. 2. a diverse category of bronchogenic carcinoma, with areas of glandular, squamous, and large-cell differentiation. **adnexal c.**, that arising from, or forming structures resembling, the cutaneous appendages, particularly the sweat or sebaceous glands. **adrenocortical c.**, a malignant adrenal cortical tumor that can cause endocrine disorders such as Cushing's syndrome or adrenogenital syndrome. **alveolar c.**, bronchioloalveolar c. **ameloblastic c.**, a type of ameloblastoma in which malignant epithelial transformation has occurred, with metastases usually resembling squamous cell carcinoma. **apocrine c.**, 1. carcinoma of an apocrine gland. 2. a rare breast malignancy with a ductal or acinar growth pattern and apocrine secretions. **basal cell c.**, an epithelial tumor of the skin that seldom metastasizes but has the potential for local invasion and destruction; it usually occurs as one or several small pearly nodules with central depressions on the sun-exposed skin of older adults. **bronchioloalveolar c.**, a variant type of adenocarcinoma of the lung, with columnar to cuboidal cells lining the alveolar septa and projecting into alveolar spaces. **bronchogenic c.**, any of a group of carcinomas of the lung, so called because it arises from the epithelium of the bronchial tree. **cholangiocellular c.**, a rare primary carcinoma of the liver originating in bile duct cells. **chorionic c.**, choriocarcinoma. **clear cell c.**, 1. see under *adenocarcinoma*. 2. renal cell c. **colloid c.**, mucinous c. **cribriform c.**, 1. adenoid cystic c. 2. an adenoid cystic carcinoma of the lactiferous ducts, one of the subtypes of ductal carcinoma in situ. **ductal c. in situ (DCIS)**, any of a large group of in situ carcinomas of the lactiferous ducts. **embryonal c.**, a highly malignant, primitive form of carcinoma, probably of germinal cell or teratomatous derivation, usually arising in a gonad. **c. en cuirasse**, carcinoma of the skin manifest as areas of thickening and induration over large areas of the thorax, frequently as a result of metastasis from a primary breast lesion. **endometrioid c.**, that characterized by glandular patterns resembling those of the endometrium, occurring in the uterine fundus and ovaries. **epidermoid c.**, squamous cell c. **c. ex mixed tumor, c. ex pleomorphic adenoma**, a type of malignant pleomorphic adenoma usually occurring in the salivary glands of older adults; an epithelial malignancy arises in a preexisting mixed tumor. **follicular c. of thyroid gland**, a type of thyroid gland carcinoma with many follicles. **hepatocellular c.**, primary carcinoma of the liver cells; it has been associated with chronic hepatitis B virus infection, some types of cirrhosis, and hepatitis C virus infection. **c. in si'tu,** a neoplastic entity wherein the tumor cells are still confined to the epithelium of origin, without invasion of the basement membrane; the likelihood of subsequent invasive growth is presumed to be high. **intraductal c.,** 1. any carcinoma of the epithelium of a duct. 2. ductal c. in situ. **Hürthle cell c.,** a malignant Hürthle cell tumor. **inflammatory c. of the breast,** a highly malignant carcinoma of the breast, with pink to red skin discoloration, tenderness, edema, and rapid enlargement. **large cell c.,** a bronchogenic tumor of undifferentiated (anaplastic) cells of large size. **invasive lobular c.,** an invasive type of carcinoma of the breast characterized by linear growth into desmoplastic stroma around the terminal part of the lobules of the mammary glands; usually developing from lobular carcinoma in situ. **lobular c.,** 1. terminal duct c. 2. see *lobular c. in situ.* **lobular c. in situ (LCIS),** a type of precancerous neoplasia found in the lobules of mammary glands, progressing slowly, sometimes to invasive lobular carcinoma after many years. **medullary c.,** that composed mainly of epithelial elements with little or no stroma; commonly occurring in the breast and thyroid gland. **meningeal c.,** primary or secondary carcinomatous infiltration of the meninges, particularly the pia and arachnoid. **Merkel cell c.,** a rapidly growing malignant dermal or subcutaneous tumor occurring on sun-exposed areas in middled-aged or older adults and containing irregular anastomosing trabeculae and small dense granules typical of Merkel cells. **mucinous c.,** adenocarcinoma producing significant amounts of mucin. **mucoepidermoid c.,** a malignant epithelial tumor of glandular tissue, particularly the salivary glands, characterized by acini with mucus-producing cells and by malignant squamous elements. **nasopharyngeal c.,** a malignant tumor arising in the epithelial lining of the nasopharynx, seen most often in people of Chinese ancestry. The Epstein-Barr virus has been implicated as a causative agent. **non–small cell c., non–small cell lung c. (NSCLC),** a general term comprising all lung carcinomas except small-cell carcinoma. **oat cell c.,** a form of small cell carcinoma in which the cells are round or elongated, have scanty cytoplasm, and clump poorly. **papillary c.,** carcinoma in which there are papillary excrescences. **renal cell c.,** clear cell carcinoma; carcinoma of the renal parenchyma, composed of tubular cells in varying arrangements. **scirrhous c.,** carcinoma with a hard structure owing to the formation of dense connective tissue in the stroma. **sebaceous c.,** carcinoma of the sebaceous glands, usually occurring as a hard yellow nodule on the eyelid. **c. sim'plex,** an undifferentiated carcinoma. **signet-ring cell c.,** a highly malignant mucus-secreting tumor in which the cells are anaplastic, with nuclei displaced to one side by a globule of mucus. **small cell c., small cell lung c. (SCLC),** a common, highly malignant form of bronchogenic carcinoma in the wall of a major bronchus, usually in middle-aged smokers, composed of small, oval, undifferentiated hematoxyphilic cells. **spindle cell c.,** carcinoma, usually of the squamous cell type, marked by fusiform development of rapidly proliferating cells. **squamous cell c.,** 1. an initially local carcinoma developed from squamous epithelium and characterized by cuboid cells and keratinization. 2. the form occurring in the skin, usually originating in sun-damaged areas or preexisting lesions. 3. a form of bronchogenic carcinoma, usually in middle-aged smokers, generally forming polypoid or sessile masses obstructing the bronchial airways. **terminal duct c.,** a slow-growing, locally invasive, malignant neoplasm composed of myoepithelial and ductal elements, occurring in the minor salivary glands. **transitional cell c.,** a malignant tumor arising from a transitional type of stratified epithelium, usually affecting the urinary bladder. **tubular c.,** 1. an adenocarcinoma in which the cells are arranged in the form of tubules. 2. a type of breast cancer in which small gland-like structures are formed and infiltrate the stroma, usually developing from a ductal carcinoma in situ. **verrucous c.,** a variety of locally invasive squamous cell carcinoma with a predilection for the buccal mucosa but also affecting other oral soft tissues and the larynx; sometimes used for the similar Buschke-Löwenstein tumor on the genitals.

car·ci·no·ma·to·sis (kahr″sĭ-no-mah-to′sis) the condition of widespread dissemination of cancer throughout the body.

car·ci·nom·a·tous (kahr″sĭ-nom′ah-tus) pertaining to or of the nature of cancer.

car·ci·no·sar·co·ma (kahr″sĭ-no-sahr-ko′mah) a malignant tumor composed of carcinomatous and sarcomatous tissues. **embryonal c.,** Wilms' tumor.

car·da·mom (kahr′dah-mom) 1. a plant of the species *Elettaria cardamomum* or any of various closely related plants having similar seeds. 2. a preparation of the seeds of *E. cardamomum*, used for respiratory and gastrointestinal tract disorders, as well as in traditional Chinese medicine and ayurveda.

car·dia (kahr′de-ah) 1. the cardiac opening. 2. the cardiac part of the stomach, surrounding the esophagogastric junction and distinguished by the presence of cardiac glands.

car·di·ac (-ak) 1. pertaining to the heart. 2. pertaining to the cardia.

car·di·al·gia (kahr″de-al′jah) cardiodynia.

car·di·ec·ta·sis (-ek′tah-sis) dilatation of the heart.

car·di·nal (kahr′dĭ-n′l) 1. of primary or preeminent importance. 2. in embryology, pertaining to the main venous drainage.

cardi(o)- word element [Gr.], 1. *heart.* 2. *cardiac orifice or portion of the stomach.*

car·dio·ac·cel·er·a·tor (kahr″de-o-ak-sel′er-a-ter) quickening the heart action; an agent that so acts.

car·dio·an·gi·ol·o·gy (-an″je-ol′ah-je) the medical specialty dealing with the heart and blood vessels.

car·dio·ar·te·ri·al (-ahr-tēr′e-al) pertaining to the heart and the arteries.

Car·dio·bac·te·ri·um (-bak-tēr′e-um) a genus of gram-negative, facultatively anaerobic, fermentative, rod-shaped bacteria, part of the normal flora of the nose and throat, and also isolated from the blood. **C. ho′minis,** a species that is an etiologic agent of endocarditis.

car·dio·cele (kahr′de-o-sēl″) hernial protrusion of the heart through a fissure of the diaphragm or through a wound.

car·dio·cen·te·sis (kahr″de-o-sen-te′sis) surgical puncture of the heart.

car·dio·cha·la·sia (-kah-la′zhah) relaxation or incompetence of the sphincter action of the cardiac opening of the stomach.

car·dio·cir·rho·sis (-sĭ-ro′sis) cardiac cirrhosis.

car·dio·cyte (kahr′de-o-sīt″) myocyte.

car·dio·di·a·phrag·mat·ic (-di″ah-frag-mat′ik) pertaining to the heart and the diaphragm.

car·dio·di·o·sis (kahr″de-o-di-o′sis) dilatation of the cardiac opening of the stomach.

car·dio·dy·nam·ics (-di-nam′iks) study of the forces involved in the heart's action.

car·di·odyn·ia (-din′e-ah) pain in the heart.

car·dio·esoph·a·ge·al (-ĕ-sof″ah-je′al) pertaining to the cardia of the stomach and the esophagus, as the cardioesophageal junction or sphincter.

car·dio·gen·e·sis (-jen′ĕ-sis) the development of the heart in the embryo.

car·dio·gen·ic (-jen′ik) 1. originating in the heart; caused by normal or abnormal function of the heart. 2. pertaining to cardiogenesis.

car·dio·gram (kahr′de-o-gram″) a tracing of a cardiac event made by cardiography. **apex c.,** apexcardiogram. **precordial c.,** kinetocardiogram.

car·di·og·ra·phy (kahr″de-og′rah-fe) the graphic recording of a physical or functional aspect of the heart, e.g., apexcardiography, echocardiography, electrocardiography, kinetocardiography, phonocardiography, telecardiography, and vectorcardiography. **ultrasonic c.,** echocardiography.

car·dio·in·hib·i·tor (kahr″de-o-in-hib′ĭ-ter) an agent that restrains the heart's action.

car·dio·in·hib·i·to·ry (-in-hib′ĭ-tor-e) restraining or inhibiting the movements of the heart.

car·dio·ki·net·ic (-kĭ-net′ik) 1. exciting or stimulating the heart. 2. an agent that so acts.

car·dio·ky·mog·ra·phy (-ki-mog′rah-fe) the recording of the motion of the heart by means of the electrokymograph. **cardiokymograph′ic,** adj.

car·dio·lip·in (-lip′in) a phospholipid occurring primarily in mitochondrial inner membranes and in bacterial plasma membranes; used in certain tests for syphilis.

car·di·ol·o·gy (kahr″de-ol′ah-je) the study of the heart and its functions.

car·di·ol·y·sis (-ol′ĭ-sis) the operation of freeing the heart from its adhesions to the sternal periosteum in adhesive mediastinopericarditis.

car·dio·ma·la·cia (kahr″de-o-mah-la′shah) morbid softening of the muscular substance of the heart.

car·dio·meg·a·ly (-meg′ah-le) abnormal enlargement of the heart.

car·dio·mel·a·no·sis (-mel″ah-no′sis) melanosis of the heart.

car·dio·mo·til·i·ty (-mo-til′ĭ-te) the movements of the heart; motility of the heart.

car·dio·myo·li·po·sis (-mi″o-lĭ-po′sis) fatty degeneration of the heart muscle.

car·dio·my·op·a·thy (-mi-op′ah-the) 1. a general diagnostic term designating primary noninflammatory disease of the heart. 2. more restrictively, only those disorders in which the myocardium alone is involved and in which the cause is unknown and not part of a disease affecting other organs. **cardiomyopath′ic,** adj. **alcoholic c.,** dilated cardiomyopathy in patients chronically abusing alcohol. **beer-drinkers′ c.,** cardiac dilatation and hypertrophy due to excessive beer consumption; in at least some cases it has been due to the addition of cobalt to the beer during the manufacturing process. **congestive c., dilated c.,** a progressive syndrome of ventricular dilatation, systolic contractile dysfunction, and, often, congestive heart failure, believed due to myocardial damage by factors such as alcohol or infection. **hypertrophic c. (HCM),** a form marked by ventricular hypertrophy, particularly of the left ventricle, with impaired ventricular filling due to diastolic dysfunction. **hypertrophic obstructive c. (HOCM),** a form of hypertrophic cardiomyopathy in which the location of the septal hypertrophy causes obstructive interference to left ventricular outflow. **infiltrative c.,** restrictive cardiomyopathy characterized by deposition in the heart tissue of abnormal substances, as may occur in amyloidosis, hemochromatosis, etc. **ischemic c.,** heart failure with left ventricular dilatation resulting from ischemic heart disease. **restrictive c.,** a form in which the ventricular walls are excessively rigid, impeding ventricular filling. **right ventricular c.,** a right-sided cardiomyopathy occurring particularly in young males, with dilatation of the right ventricle with partial to total replacement of its muscle by fibrous or adipose tissue, palpitations, syncope, and sometimes sudden death.

car·di·op·a·thy (kahr″de-op′ah-the) any disorder or disease of the heart.

car·dio·pho·bia (kahr″de-o-fo′be-ah) irrational dread of heart disease.

car·dio·plas·ty (kahr′de-o-plas″te) esophagogastroplasty.

car·dio·ple·gia (kahr″de-o-ple′jah) arrest of myocardial contractions, as by use of chemical compounds or cold in cardiac surgery. **cardiople′gic,** adj.

car·dio·pneu·mat·ic (-noo-mat′ik) of or pertaining to the heart and respiration.

car·dio·pro·tec·tant (-pro-tek′tant) counteracting cardiotoxicity, or an agent that so acts.

car·di·op·to·sis (kahr″de-op′tah-sis) downward displacement of the heart.

car·dio·pul·mo·nary (kahr″de-o-pool′mahnar-e) pertaining to the heart and lungs.

car·di·or·rha·phy (kahr″de-o-or′ah-fe) suture of the heart muscle.

car·di·or·rhex·is (kahr″de-o-rek′sis) rupture of the heart.

car·dio·scle·ro·sis (-sklĕ-ro′sis) fibrous induration of the heart.

car·dio·se·lec·tive (-sĕ-lek′tiv) having greater activity on heart tissue than on other tissue.

car·dio·spasm (kahr′de-o-spazm″) achalasia of the esophagus.

car·dio·ta·chom·e·ter (kahr″de-o-tah-kom′ĕ-ter) an instrument for continuously portraying or recording the heart rate.

car·dio·ther·a·py (-ther′ah-pe) the treatment of diseases of the heart.

car·dio·tho·rac·ic (-thah-ras′ik) pertaining to the heart and the thorax.

car·dio·to·cog·ra·phy (-tah-kog′rah-fe) the monitoring of the fetal heart rate and uterine contractions, as during delivery.

car·di·ot·o·my (kahr″de-ot′ah-me) 1. surgical incision of the heart. 2. surgical incision into the cardia.

car·dio·ton·ic (kahr″de-o-ton′ik) having a tonic effect on the heart; an agent that so acts.

car·dio·to·pom·e·try (-tah-pom′ĕ-tre) measurement of the area of superficial cardiac dullness observed in percussion of the chest.

car·dio·tox·ic (kahr″de-o-tok″sik) having a poisonous or deleterious effect upon the heart.

car·dio·tox·ic·i·ty (kahr″de-o-tok-sis′ĭ-te) the quality of being cardiotoxic.

car·dio·val·vu·li·tis (-val″vu-li′tis) inflammation of the heart valves.

car·dio·val·vu·lo·tome (-val′vu-lah-tōm″) an instrument for incising a heart valve.

car·dio·vas·cu·lar (-vas′ku-ler) pertaining to the heart and blood vessels.

car·dio·ver·sion (-ver′zhun) the restoration of normal rhythm of the heart by electrical shock.

car·dio·ver·ter (-ver′ter) an energy-storage capacitor-discharge type of condenser which is discharged with an inductance; it delivers a direct-current shock which restores normal rhythm of the heart. **automatic implantable c.-defibrillator,** an implantable device that detects sustained ventricular tachycardia or fibrillation and terminates it by a shock or shocks delivered directly to the atrium.

Car·dio·vi·rus (kahr′de-o-vi″rus) EMC-like viruses; a genus of viruses of the family Picornaviridae that cause encephalomyelitis and myocarditis, comprising two groups, the encephalomyocarditis (EMC) viruses and the murine encephalomyelitis viruses.

car·di·tis (kahr-di′tis) inflammation of the heart; myocarditis.

care (kār) the services rendered by members of the health professions for the benefit of a patient. **coronary c.,** see under *unit*. **critical c.,** see *intensive care unit,* under *unit*. **intensive c.,** see under *unit*. **primary c.,** the care a patient receives at first contact with the health care system, usually involving coordination of care and continuity over time. **respiratory c.,** 1. the health care profession providing, under a physician's supervision, diagnostic evaluation, therapy, monitoring, and rehabilitation of patients with cardiopul-monary disorders. 2. respiratory therapy; the diagnostic and therapeutic use of medical gases and their apparatus, and other forms of ventilatory support including cardiopulmo-nary resuscitation. **secondary c.,** treatment by specialists to whom a patient has been referred by primary care providers. **tertiary c.,** treatment given in a health care center that includes highly trained specialists and often advanced technology.

car·ies (kar′ēz, kar′e-ēz) decay, as of bone or teeth. **ca′rious,** adj. **dental c.,** a destructive process causing decalcification of the tooth enamel and leading to continued destruction of enamel and dentin, and cavitation of the tooth.

ca·ri·na (kah-ri′nah) pl. *cari′nae.* [L.] a ridgelike structure. **c. tra′cheae,** a down-ward and backward projection of the lowest tracheal cartilage, forming a ridge between the openings of the right and left principal bronchi. **c. urethra′lis vagi′nae,** the column of rugae in the lower anterior wall of the vagina, immediately below the urethra.

car·i·nate (kar′ĭ-nāt) keel-shaped; having a keellike process.

car·io·gen·e·sis (kar″e-o-jen′ĕ-sis) devel-opment of caries.

car·iso·pro·dol (kar″i-so-pro′dol) an an-algesic and skeletal muscle relaxant used to relieve symptoms of acute painful skeleto-muscular disorders.

car·min·a·tive (kahr-min′ah-tiv) 1. reliev-ing flatulence. 2. an agent that relieves flatulence.

car·mine (kahr′min) a red coloring matter used as a histologic stain. **indigo c.,** indigo-tindisulfonate sodium.

car·min·ic acid (kahr-min′ik) the active principle of carmine and cochineal, $C_{22}H_{20}O_{13}$.

car·min·o·phil (kahr-min′ah-fil) 1. easily stainable with carmine. 2. a cell or element readily taking a stain from carmine.

car·mus·tine (kahr-mus′tēn) a cytotoxic alkylating agent of the nitrosourea group, used as an antineoplastic agent.

car·ni·tine (kahr′nĭ-tēn) a betaine derivative involved in the transport of fatty acids into mitochondria, where they are metabolized.

car·ni·vore (kahr′nĭ-vor) any animal that eats primarily flesh, particularly a mammal of the order Carnivora (cats, dogs, bears, etc.). **carniv′orous,** adj.

car·no·sin·ase (kahr′no-sĭ-nās″) an enzyme that hydrolyzes carnosine (amino-acyl-L-histidine) and other dipeptides containing L-histidine into their constituent amino acids.

serum c. deficiency, an aminoacidopathy characterized by urinary excretion of carno-sine, homocarnosine in cerebrospinal fluid, and sometimes myoclonic seizures, severe mental retardation, and spasticity.

car·no·sine (-sēn) a dipeptide composed of β-alanine and histidine, found in skeletal muscle and the brain in humans; it may be a neurotransmitter.

car·no·si·ne·mia (kahr″no-sĭ-ne′me-ah) 1. excessive amounts of carnosine in the blood. 2. former name for *serum carnosinase deficiency.*

car·no·sin·u·ria (-sĭ-nu′re-ah) excessive carnosine in the urine, such as after ingestion of meat or in serum carnosinase deficiency.

car·o·tene (kar′o-tēn) one of four isomeric pigments (α-, β-, γ-, and δ-carotene), having colors from violet to red-yellow to yellow and occurring in many dark green, leafy, and yellow vegetables and yellow fruits. They are fat-soluble, unsaturated hydrocarbons that can be converted into vitamin A in the body; in humans the β- isomer (β- or beta carotene) is the major precursor of this vitamin. **beta c.,** the β- isomer of carotene; a preparation is used to prevent vitamin A deficiency and to reduce the severity of photosensitivity in patients with erythropoietic protoporphyria.

car·o·ten·emia (kar″o-tĕ-ne′me-ah) hyper-carotenemia.

ca·rot·e·noid (kah-rot′ĕ-noid) 1. any of a group of red, orange, or yellow pigmented polyisoprenoid hydrocarbons synthesized by prokaryotes and higher plants and con-centrating in animal fat when eaten; examples are β-carotene, lycopene, and xanthophyll. 2. marked by yellow color. **provitamin A c′s,** carotenoids, particularly the carotenes, that can be converted to vitamin A in the body.

car·o·te·no·sis (kar″o-tĕ-no′sis) the yellow-ish discoloration of the skin occurring in hypercarotenemia.

ca·rot·i·co·tym·pan·ic (kah-rot″ĭ-ko-tim-pan′ik) pertaining to the carotid canal and the tympanum.

ca·rot·id (kah-rot′id) pertaining to the carotid artery, the principal artery of the neck; see *Table of Arteries.*

ca·rot·i·dyn·ia (kah-rot″ĭ-din′e-ah) episodic, usually unilateral neck pain with tenderness along the course of the common carotid artery.

carp (kahrp) a fruiting body of a fungus.

car·pal (kahr′p'l) pertaining to the carpus.

car·pec·to·my (kahr-pek′tah-me) excision of a carpal bone.

car·phen·a·zine (kahr-fen′ah-zēn) an anti-psychotic agent, used as the maleate salt.

car·phol·o·gy (kahr-fol′ah-je) floccillation.

car·pi·tis (kahr-pīt′is) inflammation of the synovial membranes of the bones of the carpal joint in domestic animals, producing swelling, pain, and lameness.

car·po·ped·al (kahr″po-ped′al) pertaining to or affecting the wrist (or the hand) and the foot.

car·pop·to·sis (kahr″po-to′sis) wristdrop.

car·pus (kahr′pus) the joint between the arm and hand, made up of eight bones; the wrist.

car·ri·er (kar′e-er) 1. one who harbors disease organisms in their body without manifest symptoms, thus acting as a distributor of infection. 2. a heterozygote, i.e., one who carries a recessive gene and thus does not express the recessive phenotype but can transmit it to offspring. 3. a chemical substance that can accept electrons and then donate them to another substance (being reduced and then reoxidized). 4. a substance that carries a radioisotopic or other label; also used for a second isotope mixed with a particular isotope (see *carrier-free*). 5. transport protein. 6. in immunology, a macromolecular substance to which a hapten is coupled in order to produce an immune response against the hapten.

car·ri·er-free (-fre″) a term denoting a radioisotope of an element in pure form, i.e., undiluted with a stable isotope carrier.

car·sick·ness (kahr′sik-nes) motion sickness due to automobile or other vehicular travel.

cart (kahrt) a vehicle for conveying patients or equipment and supplies in a hospital. **crash c.,** resuscitation c. **dressing c.,** one containing all supplies necessary for changing dressings of surgical or injured patients. **resuscitation c.,** one containing all equipment for initiating emergency resuscitation.

car·te·o·lol (kahr′te-ah-lol) a beta-adrenergic blocking agent used as the hydrochloride salt in the treatment of hypertension and of glaucoma and ocular hypertension.

car·ti·lage (kahr′tĭ-lij) a specialized, fibrous connective tissue present in adults, and forming the temporary skeleton in the embryo, providing a model in which the bones develop, and constituting a part of the organism's growth mechanism; the three most important types are hyaline cartilage, elastic cartilage, and fibrocartilage. Also, a general term for a mass of such tissue in a particular site in the body. **alar c's,** the cartilages of the wings of the nose. **aortic c.,** the second costal cartilage on the right side. **arthrodial c., articular c.,** that lining the articular surface of synovial joints. **arytenoid c.,** one

of the two pyramid-shaped cartilages of the larynx. **connecting c.,** that connecting the surfaces of an immovable joint. **corniculate c.,** a nodule of cartilage at the apex of each arytenoid cartilage. **costal c.,** a bar of hyaline cartilage that attaches a rib to the sternum in the case of true ribs, or to the rib immediately above in the case of the upper false ribs. **cricoid c.,** a ringlike cartilage forming the lower and back part of the larynx. **cuneiform c.,** either of a pair of cartilages, one on either side in the aryepiglottic fold. **dentinal c.,** the substance remaining after the lime salts of dentin have been dissolved in an acid. **diarthrodial c.,** articular c. **elastic c.,** cartilage whose matrix contains yellow elastic fibers. **ensiform c.,** xiphoid process. **floating c.,** a detached portion of semilunar cartilage in the knee joint. **hyaline c.,** a flexible semitransparent substance with an opalescent tint, composed of a basophilic, fibril-containing substance with cavities in which the chondrocytes occur. **interosseous c.,** connecting c. **Jacobson's c.,** vomeronasal c. **permanent c.,** cartilage which does not normally become ossified. **precursory c.,** temporary c. **Santorini's c.,** corniculate c. **semilunar c.,** either of the two interarticular cartilages of the knee joint. **sesamoid c's,** small cartilages found in the thyrohyoid ligament (*sesamoid c. of larynx*), on either side of the nose (*sesamoid c. of nose*), and occasionally in the vocal ligaments (*sesamoid c. of vocal ligament*). **slipping rib c.,** a loosened or deformed cartilage whose slipping over an adjacent rib cartilage may produce discomfort or pain. **temporary c.,** cartilage that is being replaced by bone or that is destined to be replaced by bone. **thyroid c.,** the shield-shaped cartilage of the larynx. **tracheal c's,** see under *ring*. **triticeous c.,** a small cartilage in the thyrohyoid ligament. **vomeronasal c.,** either of the two strips of cartilage of the nasal septum supporting the vomeronasal organ. **Weitbrecht's c.,** a pad of fibrocartilage sometimes present within the articular cavity of the acromioclavicular joint. **Wrisberg's c.,** cuneiform c. **xiphoid c.,** see under *process*. **Y c.,** Y-shaped cartilage within the acetabulum, joining the ilium, ischium, and pubes. **yellow c.,** elastic c.

car·ti·lag·i·nous (kahr″tĭ-laj′ĭ-nus) consisting of or of the nature of cartilage.

car·ti·la·go (kahr″tĭ-lah′go) pl. *cartila′gines*. [L.] cartilage.

car·un·cle (kar′ung-k'l) a small fleshy eminence, often abnormal. **hymenal c's,** small elevations of the mucous membrane around the vaginal opening, being relics of the torn hymen. **lacrimal c.,** the red eminence at the medial angle of the eye. **myrtiform c's,** hymenal caruncles. **sublingual c.,** an eminence on either side of the frenulum of the tongue, on which the major sublingual duct and the submandibular duct open. **urethral c.,** a polypoid, deep red growth on the mucous membrane of the urinary meatus in women.

ca·run·cu·la (kah-rung'ku-lah) pl. *carun'culae*. [L.] caruncle.

car·ve·dil·ol (kahr've-dil''ol) a beta-adrenergic blocking agent used in the treatment of hypertension and as an adjunct in the treatment of congestive heart failure.

car·ver (kahr'ver) a tool for producing anatomic form in artificial teeth and dental restorations.

cary(o)- for words beginning thus, see those beginning *kary(o)-*.

ca·san·thra·nol (kah-san'thrah-nōl) a purified mixture of glycosides derived from *Cascara sagrada*; used as a laxative.

cas·cade (kas-kād') a series that once initiated continues to the end, each step being triggered by the preceding one, sometimes with cumulative effect. **coagulation c.,** the series of steps beginning with activation of the intrinsic or extrinsic pathways of coagulation, or of one of the related alternative pathways, and proceeding through the common pathway of coagulation to the formation of the fibrin clot.

cas·cara (kas-kar'ah) [Sp.] bark. **c. sagra'da,** dried bark of the shrub *Rhamnus purshiana*, used as a cathartic.

case (kās) an instance of a disease. **index c.,** the case of the original patient (propositus or proband) that stimulates investigation of other members of the family to discover a possible genetic factor. In epidemiology, the first case of a contagious disease. **trial c.,** a box containing lenses, arranged in pairs, a trial spectacle frame, and other devices used in testing vision.

ca·se·a·tion (ka''se-a'shun) 1. the precipitation of casein. 2. necrosis in which tissue is changed into a dry mass resembling cheese.

case his·to·ry (kās his'tah-re) the data concerning an individual, their family, and their environment, including medical history that may be useful in analyzing and diagnosing their case or for instructional purposes.

ca·sein (ka'sēn) a phosphoprotein, the principal protein of milk, the basis of curd and of cheese. NOTE: In British nomenclature casein is called *caseinogen*, and paracasein is called *casein*.

ca·sein·o·gen (ka-sēn'ah-jen) the British term for casein.

ca·se·ous (ka'se-us) resembling cheese or curd; cheesy.

case·worm (kās'werm) echinococcus.

cas·po·fun·gin (kas''po-fun'jin) an antifungal used as the acetate salt in the treatment of invasive aspergillosis.

cas·sette (kah-set') [Fr.] a light-proof housing for x-ray film, containing front and back intensifying screens, between which the film is placed; a magazine for film or magnetic tape.

cast (kast) 1. a positive copy of an object, e.g., a mold of a tube or hollow organ, formed of effused matter such as fat or cellular debris and later extruded from the organ, such as a urinary cast. 2. a positive copy of the tissues of the jaws, made in an impression, and over which denture bases or other restorations may be fabricated. 3. to form an object in a mold. 4. a stiff dressing or casing, usually made of plaster of Paris, used to immobilize body parts. 5. strabismus. **dental c.,** see *cast* (2). **hanging c.,** one applied to the arm in fracture of the shaft of the humerus, suspended by a sling looped around the neck. **renal c., urinary c.,** one formed from gelled protein in the renal tubules, molded to the shape of the tubular lumen.

cas·trate (kas'trāt) 1. to deprive of the gonads, rendering the individual incapable of reproduction. 2. a castrated individual.

cas·tra·tion (kas-tra'shun) excision of the gonads, or their destruction as by radiation or parasites. **female c.,** bilateral oophorectomy. **male c.,** bilateral orchiectomy.

ca·su·al·ty (kazh'oo-al-te) 1. an accident; an accidental wound; death or disablement from an accident; also the person so injured. 2. in the armed forces, one missing from their unit as a result of death, injury, illness, capture, because their whereabouts are unknown, or other reasons.

cas·u·is·tics (kazh-u-is'tiks) the recording and study of cases of disease.

CAT computerized axial tomography.

cata- word element [Gr.], *down; lower; under; against; along with; very.*

cata·bi·o·sis (kat''ah-bi-o'sis) the normal senescence of cells. **catabiot'ic,** adj.

ca·tab·o·lism (kah-tab'ah-lizm) any destructive process by which complex substances are converted by living cells into more simple compounds, with release of energy. **catabol'ic,** adj.

ca·tab·o·lize (-līz) to subject to catabolism; to undergo catabolism.

ca·tac·ro·tism (kah-tak′rah-tizm) a pulse anomaly in which a small additional wave or notch appears in the descending limb of the pulse tracing. **catacrot′ic**, adj.

cata·di·cro·tism (kat″ah-di′krah-tizm) a pulse anomaly in which two small additional waves or notches appear in the descending limb of the pulse tracing. **catadicrot′ic**, adj.

cat·a·gen (kat′ah-jen) the brief portion in the hair cycle in which growth (anagen) stops and resting (telogen) starts.

cata·gen·e·sis (kat″ah-jen′ĕ-sis) involution or retrogression. **catagenet′ic**, adj.

cat·a·lase (kat′ah-lās) a hemoprotein enzyme that catalyzes the decomposition of hydrogen peroxide to water and oxygen, protecting cells. It is found in almost all animal cells except certain anaerobic bacteria; genetic deficiency of the enzyme results in acatalasia. **catalat′ic**, adj.

cat·a·lep·sy (-lep″se) indefinitely prolonged maintenance of a fixed body posture; seen in severe cases of catatonic schizophrenia. The term is sometimes used to denote *cerea flexibilitas.*

ca·tal·y·sis (kah-tal′ĭ-sis) increase in the velocity of a chemical reaction or process produced by the presence of a substance that is not consumed in the net chemical reaction or process; *negative c.* denotes the slowing down or inhibition of a reaction or process by the presence of such a substance. **catalyt′ic**, adj.

cat·am·ne·sis (kat″am-ne′sis) 1. the follow-up history of a patient after he is discharged from treatment or a hospital. 2. the history of a patient after the onset of a medical or psychiatric illness. **catamnes′tic**, adj.

cata·pha·sia (kat″ah-fa′zhah) verbigeration.

cata·pho·ria (kat″ah-for′e-ah) a permanent downward turning of the visual axis of both eyes after visual functional stimuli have been removed. **cataphor′ic**, adj.

cata·phy·lax·is (-fi-lak′sis) breaking down of the body's natural defense to infection. **cataphylac′tic**, adj.

cat·a·plexy (kat′ah-plek″se) a condition marked by abrupt attacks of muscular weakness and hypotonia triggered by such emotional stimuli as mirth, anger, fear, etc., often associated with narcolepsy. **cataplec′tic**, adj.

cat·a·ract (-rakt) an opacity of the crystalline lens of the eye or its capsule. **catarac′tous**, adj. **after-c.**, a recurrent capsular cataract. **atopic c.**, cataract in those with long-standing atopic dermatitis. **black c.**, see *senile nuclear sclerotic c.* **blue c., blue dot c.**, blue punctate opacities scattered throughout the nucleus and cortex of the lens.

brown c., brunescent c., see *senile nuclear sclerotic c.* **capsular c.**, one consisting of an opacity in the lens capsule. **complicated c.**, secondary c. **congenital c.**, 1. cataract present at birth, usually bilaterally; it may be mild or severe and may or may not impair vision depending on size, density, and location. 2. developmental c. **coronary c.**, tiny white opacities in a ring around the lens, the center and periphery of the lens remaining clear. **cortical c.**, 1. developmental punctate opacity common in the cortex and present in most lenses. The cataract is white or cerulean, increases in number with age, but rarely affects vision. 2. the most common senile cataract; white, wedgelike opacities are like spokes around the periphery of the cortex. **cupuliform c.**, a senile cataract in the posterior cortex of the lens just under the capsule. **developmental c.**, a type of small cataract in youth, resulting from heredity, malnutrition, toxicity, or inflammation, seldom affecting vision. **electric c.**, one occurring after an electric shock, especially to the head. Anterior subcapsular cataracts may form and develop within days; slowly developing or stationary opacities may follow a shock not to the head. **glass-blowers' c., heat c.**, posterior subcapsular opacities caused by chronic exposure to infrared (heat) radiation. **hypermature c.**, one with a swollen, milky cortex, the result of autolysis of the lens fibers of a mature cataract. **lamellar c.**, one affecting only certain layers between the cortex and nucleus of the lens. **mature c.**, one producing swelling and opacity of the entire lens. **membranous c.**, a condition in which the lens substance has shrunk, leaving remnants of the capsule and fibrous tissue formation. **morgagnian c.**, a mature cataract in which the cortex has liquefied and the nucleus moves freely within the lens. **nuclear c.**, one in which the opacity is in the central nucleus of the eye. **overripe c.**, hypermature c. **polar c.**, one at the center of the anterior (*anterior polar c.*) or posterior (*posterior polar c.*) pole of the lens. **pyramidal c.**, a conoid anterior cataract with its apex projecting forward into the aqueous humor. **radiation c.**, one caused by ionizing radiation, e.g., x-rays, or by nonionizing radiation, e.g., infrared (heat) rays, ultraviolet rays, microwaves. **ripe c.**, mature c. **secondary c.**, one resulting from disease, e.g., iridocyclitis; degeneration, e.g., chronic glaucoma, retinal detachment; or from surgery, e.g., glaucoma filtering, retinal reattachment. **senile c.**, cataract in the elderly. **senile nuclear sclerotic c.**, slowly increasing hardening of the nucleus, usually bilateral and brown or black, with the lens becoming inelastic and unable to accommodate. **snowflake c., snowstorm c.,** one marked by gray or blue to white flaky opacities, seen in young diabetics. **total c.,** an opacity of all the fibers of a lens. **toxic c.,** that due to exposure to a toxic drug, e.g., naphthalene. **traumatic c.,** one due to injury to the eye. **zonular c.,** lamellar c.

cat·a·rac·ta (kat″ah-rak′tah) cataract. **c. brunes′cens,** brown cataract; see *senile nuclear sclerotic cataract.* **c. caeru′lea,** blue dot cataract.

ca·tarrh (kah-tahr′) inflammation of a mucous membrane, particularly of the head and throat, with free discharge of mucus. **catar′rhal,** adj.

cata·to·nia (kat″ah-to′ne-ah) a wide group of motor abnormalities, most involving extreme under- or overactivity, associated primarily with catatonic schizophrenia. **cata·ton′ic,** adj.

cata·tri·cro·tism (-tri′krot-izm) a pulse anomaly in which three small additional waves or notches appear in the descending limb of the pulse tracing. **catatricrot′ic,** adj.

cat·e·chin (kat′ĕ-kin) an astringent principle from the heartwood of *Acacia catechu* (catechu) and *Uncaria gambier* (gambir).

cat·e·chol (kat′ah-kol) 1. catechin. 2. pyrocatechol.

cat·e·chol·amine (kat″ah-kol′ah-mēn″) any of a group of sympathomimetic amines (including dopamine, epinephrine, and norepinephrine), the aromatic portion of whose molecule is catechol.

cat·e·chol·am·in·er·gic (kat″ah-kol-am″-in-er′jik) activated by or secreting catecholamines.

cat·gut (kat′gut) surgical gut.

ca·thar·sis (kah-thahr′sis) 1. purgation; a cleansing or emptying. 2. in psychiatry, the expression and discharge of repressed emotions and ideas.

ca·thar·tic (-tik) 1. causing emptying of the bowels. 2. an agent that empties the bowels. 3. producing emotional catharsis. **bulk c.,** one stimulating bowel evacuation by increasing fecal volume. **lubricant c.,** one that acts by softening the feces and reducing friction between them and the intestinal wall. **saline c.,** one that increases fluidity of intestinal contents by retention of water by osmotic forces and indirectly increases motor activity. **stimulant c.,** one that directly increases motor activity of the intestinal tract.

ca·thep·sin (kah-thep′sin) one of a number of enzymes each of which catalyzes the hydrolytic cleavage of specific peptide bonds.

cath·e·ter (kath′ĕ-ter) 1. a tubular, flexible surgical instrument that is inserted into a cavity of the body to withdraw or introduce fluid. 2. urethral c. **angiographic c.,** one through which a contrast medium is injected for visualization of the vascular system of an organ. **atherectomy c.,** one with a rotating cutter and a collecting chamber for debris, used for atherectomy and endarterectomy and inserted under radiographic guidance. **balloon c.,** one whose tip has an inflatable balloon that holds the catheter in place or can dilate the lumen of a vessel, such as in angioplastic procedures. **cardiac c.,** a long, fine catheter designed for passage, usually through a peripheral blood vessel, into the chambers of the heart under radiographic control. **cardiac c.-microphone,** phonocatheter. **central venous c.,** a long, fine catheter introduced via a large vein into the superior vena cava or right atrium for administration of parenteral fluids or medications or for measurement of central venous pressure. **condom c.,** an external urinary collection device that fits over the penis like a condom; used in the management of urinary incontinence. **DeLee c.,** one used to suction meconium and amniotic debris from the nasopharynx and oropharynx of neonates. **double-channel c., double-lumen c.,** one with two channels, one for injection and the other for fluid removal. **elbowed c.,** a urethral catheter with a sharp bend near the beak, used to get around an enlarged prostate. **electrode c.,** a cardiac catheter containing electrodes; it may be used to pace the heart or to deliver high-energy shocks. **female c.,** a short urethral catheter for passage through the female urethra. **fluid-filled c.,** an intravascular catheter connected by a saline-filled tube to an external pressure transducer; used to measure intravascular pressure. **Foley c.,** an indwelling catheter retained in the bladder by a balloon inflated with air or liquid. **Gouley c.,** a solid, curved steel urethral catheter grooved on its inferior surface so that it can pass over a guide through a urethral stricture. **Gruentzig balloon c.,** a flexible balloon catheter with a short guidewire fixed to the tip, used for dilation of arterial stenoses. **indwelling c.,** one held in position in the urethra. **pacing c.,** a cardiac catheter containing one or more electrodes on pacing wires; used as a temporary cardiac pacing lead. **prostatic c.,** elbowed c. **self-retaining c.,** indwelling c. **snare c.,** one designed to remove intracardiac catheter fragments introduced iatrogenically. **Swan-Ganz c.,** a soft, flow-directed catheter with a balloon at the tip for measuring pulmonary arterial pressures. **Tenckhoff c.,** any of several types commonly used in peritoneal dialysis, having end and side holes and one or more extraperitoneal felt cuffs making a bacteria-tight seal. **toposcopic c.,** a miniature catheter that can pass through narrow, tortuous vessels to convey chemotherapy directly to specific sites. **two-way c.,** double-lumen c. **ureteral c.,** one inserted into the ureter, either through the urethra and bladder or posteriorly via the kidney. **urethral c.,** one inserted through the urethra into the urinary bladder. **winged c.,** a urethral catheter with two projections on the end to retain it in place.

cath·e·ter·iza·tion (kath″ĕ-ter-ĭ-za′shun) passage of a catheter into a body channel or cavity. **cardiac c.,** passage of a small catheter through a vein in an arm or leg or the neck and into the heart, permitting the securing of blood samples, determination of intracardiac pressure, detection of cardiac anomalies, planning of operative approaches, and determination, implementation, or evaluation of appropriate therapy. **retrograde c.,** passage of a cardiac catheter against the direction of blood flow and into the heart. **transseptal c.,** passage of a cardiac catheter through the right atrium into the left atrium, performed to relieve valve obstruction and in techniques such as balloon mitral valvuloplasty.

ca·thex·is (kah-thek′sis) conscious or unconscious investment of psychic energy in a person, idea, or any other object. **cathec′tic,** adj.

cath·ode (kath′ōd) the electrode at which reduction occurs and to which cations are attracted. **cathod′ic,** adj.

cat·ion (kat′i-on) a positively charged ion. **cation′ic,** adj.

cau·da (kaw′dah) pl. *cau′dae.* [L.] a tail or taillike appendage. **c. equi′na,** the collection of spinal roots descending from the lower spinal cord and occupying the vertebral canal below the cord.

cau·dad (kaw′dad) directed toward the tail or distal end; opposite to cephalad.

cau·dal (kaw′d′l) 1. pertaining to a cauda. 2. situated more toward the cauda, or tail, than some specified reference point; toward the inferior (in humans) or posterior (in animals) end of the body.

cau·date (kaw′dāt) having a tail.

caul (kawl) a piece of amnion sometimes enveloping a child's head at birth.

cau·sal (kaw′z′l) pertaining to, involving, or indicating a cause.

cau·sal·gia (kaw-zal′jah) a burning pain, often with trophic skin changes, due to peripheral nerve injury.

caus·tic (kaws′tik) 1. burning or corrosive; destructive to living tissues. 2. having a burning taste. 3. an escharotic or corrosive agent.

cau·ter·ant (kaw′ter-ant) 1. any caustic material or application. 2. caustic.

cau·ter·iza·tion (kaw″ter-ĭ-za′shun) destruction of tissue with a cautery.

cau·ter·ize (kaw′ter-īz) to apply a cautery; to destroy tissue by the application of heat, cold, or a caustic agent.

cau·tery (kaw′ter-e) 1. an agent used for cauterization. 2. cauterization. **actual c.,** 1. an instrument that destroys tissue by burning. 2. the application of such an instrument. **cold c.,** cryocautery. **electric c., galvanic c.,** electrocautery. **potential c., virtual c.,** cauterization by an escharotic, without applying heat.

ca·va (ka′vah) [L.] 1. plural of *cavum.* 2. a vena cava. **ca′val,** adj.

ca·ve·o·la (ka″ve-o′lah) pl. *caveo′lae.* [L.] one of the minute pits or incuppings of the cell membrane formed during pinocytosis.

ca·ver·na (ka-ver′nah) pl. *caver′nae.* [L.] cavity (1).

cav·er·nil·o·quy (kav″er-nil′o-kwe) low-pitched pectoriloquy indicative of a pulmonary cavity.

cav·er·ni·tis (-ni′tis) inflammation of the corpora cavernosa or corpus spongiosum of the penis.

cav·er·no·sal (-no′s′l) 1. pertaining to a corpus cavernosum. 2. cavernous.

cav·er·no·sog·ra·phy (-no-sog′rah-fe) radiographic visualization of the corpus cavernosum of the penis.

cav·er·no·som·e·try (-no-som′ĕ-tre) measurement of the vascular pressure in the corpus cavernosum.

cav·er·nous (kav′er-nus) 1. pertaining to a hollow, or containing hollow spaces. 2. having a hollow sound, such as certain abnormal breath sounds.

cav·i·ta·ry (kav′ĭ-tar-e) characterized by a cavity or cavities.

cav·i·tas (kav′ĭ-tas) pl. *cavita′tes.* [L.] cavity (1).

ca·vi·tis (ka-vi′tis) inflammation of a vena cava.

cav·i·ty (kav′ĭ-te) 1. a hollow place or space, or a potential space, within the body or one of its organs. 2. in dentistry, the lesion produced by caries. **abdominal c.,** the cavity of the body between the diaphragm and pelvis, containing the abdominal organs. **absorption c's,** cavities in developing compact bone due to osteoclastic erosion, usually occurring in the areas laid down first. **amniotic c.,** the closed sac between the embryo and the amnion, containing the amniotic fluid. **cleavage c.,** blastocoele. **complex c.,** a carious lesion involving three or more surfaces of a tooth in its prepared state. **compound c.,** a carious lesion involving two surfaces of a tooth in its prepared state. **cotyloid c.,** acetabulum. **cranial c.,** the space enclosed by the bones of the cranium. **dental c.,** the carious defect (lesion) produced by destruction of enamel and dentin in a tooth. **glenoid c.,** a depression in the lateral angle of the scapula for articulation with the humerus. **marrow c., medullary c.,** the cavity in the diaphysis of a long bone containing the marrow. **nasal c.,** the proximal part of the respiratory tract, separated by the nasal septum and extending from the nares to the pharynx. **oral c.,** the cavity of the mouth, bounded by the jaw bones and associated structures (muscles and mucosa). **pelvic c.,** the space within the walls of the pelvis. **pericardial c.,** the potential space between the epicardium and the parietal layer of the serous pericardium. **peritoneal c.,** the potential space between the parietal and the visceral peritoneum. **pleural c.,** the potential space between the parietal and visceral pleurae. **pleuroperitoneal c.,** the temporarily continuous coelomic cavity in the embryo that is later partitioned by the developing diaphragm. **prepared c.,** a lesion from which all carious tissue has been removed, preparatory to filling of the tooth. **pulp c.,** the pulp-filled central chamber in the crown of a tooth. **Rosenmüller's c.,** pharyngeal recess. **serous c.,** a coelomic cavity, like that enclosed by the pericardium, peritoneum, or pleura, not communicating with the outside body, and whose lining membrane secretes a serous fluid. **sigmoid c.,** 1. either of two depressions in the head of the ulna for articulation with the humerus. 2. a depression on the distal end of the medial side of the radius for articulation with the ulna. **simple c.,** a carious lesion whose preparation involves only one tooth surface. **somatic c.,** the intraembryonic portion of the coelom. **tension c's,** cavities of the lung in which the air pressure is greater than that of the atmosphere. **thoracic c.,** the part of the ventral body cavity between the neck and the

diaphragm. **tympanic c.,** the major portion of the middle ear, consisting of a narrow air-filled cavity in the temporal bone that contains the auditory ossicles. **uterine c.,** the flattened space within the uterus communicating proximally on either side with the uterine tubes and below with the vagina. **yolk c.,** the space between the embryonic disk and the yolk of the developing ovum of some animals.

ca·vum (ka'vum) pl. *ca'va.* [L.] cavity (1). **c. sep'ti pellu'cidi,** fifth ventricle.

ca·vus (ka'vus) [L.] hollow.

cay·enne (ki-, ka-yen') capsicum.

cbc complete blood (cell) count.

Cbl cobalamin.

cc cubic centimeter.

CCK cholecystokinin.

CCNU lomustine.

CD cadaveric donor; cluster designation (see *CD antigen,* under *antigen*); curative dose.

CD₅₀ median curative dose.

Cd cadmium; caudal or coccygeal.

cd candela.

CDC Centers for Disease Control and Prevention.

Ce cerium.

CEA carcinoembryonic antigen.

ce·as·mic (se-az'mik) characterized by persistence of embryonic fissures after birth.

ce·cal (se'k'l) 1. ending in a blind passage. 2. pertaining to the cecum.

ce·cec·to·my (se-sek'tah-me) excision of the cecum.

ce·ci·tis (se-si'tis) inflammation of the cecum.

cec(o)- word element [L.], *cecum.*

ce·co·cele (se'ko-sēl) a hernia containing part of the cecum.

ce·co·co·los·to·my (se″ko-kah-los'tah-me) surgical anastomosis of the cecum and colon.

ce·co·cys·to·plas·ty (-sis'to-plas″te) augmentation cystoplasty using an isolated part of the cecum for the added segment.

ce·co·il·e·ost·o·my (-il″e-os'tah-me) ileocecostomy.

ce·co·pli·ca·tion (-pli-ka'shun) plication of the cecal wall to correct ptosis or dilatation.

ce·cor·rha·phy (se-kor'ah-fe) suture or repair of the cecum.

ce·co·sig·moid·os·to·my (se″ko-sig″moid-os'tah-me) formation, usually by surgery, of an opening between the cecum and sigmoid.

ce·cos·to·my (se-kos'tah-me) surgical creation of an artificial opening or fistula into the cecum.

ce·cot·o·my (se-kot'ah-me) typhlotomy; incision of the cecum.

ce·co·ure·ter·o·cele (se″ko-u-re′ter-o-sēl) a ureterocele in which a blind pouch or cecum extends into the submucosa of the bladder or urethra.

ce·cum (se′kum) 1. the first part of the large intestine, forming a dilated pouch distal to the ileum and proximal to the colon, and giving off the vermiform appendix. 2. cul-de-sac.

cef·a·clor (sef′ah-klor) a semisynthetic, second-generation cephalosporin effective against a wide range of gram-positive and gram-negative bacteria.

cef·a·drox·il (sef″ah-droks′il) a semisynthetic first-generation cephalosporin antibiotic effective against a wide range of gram-positive and a very limited number of gram-negative bacteria.

cef·a·man·dole (-man′dōl) a semisynthetic second-generation cephalosporin antibiotic; used primarily as *c. nafate,* the sodium salt of the cefamandole formyl ester.

ce·faz·o·lin (sĕ-faz′o-lin) a first-generation cephalosporin effective against a wide range of gram-positive and a limited range of gram-negative bacteria; used as the sodium salt.

cef·din·ir (sef′dĭ-nir) a third-generation cephalosporin effective against a wide range of bacteria.

cef·e·pime (sef′ĕpēm) a fourth-generation cephalosporin antibiotic; used as the hydrochloride salt.

ce·fix·ime (sĕ-fik′sēm) a third-generation cephalosporin effective against a wide range of bacteria, used in the treatment of otitis media, bronchitis, pharyngitis, tonsillitis, gonorrhea, and urinary tract infections.

ce·fon·i·cid (sĕ-fon′ĭ-sid) a semisynthetic, second-generation, β-lactamase–resistant cephalosporin effective against a wide range of gram-positive and gram-negative bacteria; used as the sodium salt.

cef·o·per·a·zone (sef″o-per′ah-zōn) a β-lactamase–resistant, third-generation cephalosporin effective against a wide range of aerobic and anaerobic gram-positive and gram-negative bacteria; used as the sodium salt.

cef·o·tax·ime (-tak′sēm) a semisynthetic, broad-spectrum, β-lactamase–resistant, third-generation cephalosporin effective against a wide variety of gram-negative bacteria but less active against gram-positive cocci than are the first- and second-generation cephalosporins; used as the sodium salt.

cef·o·te·tan (sef′o-te″tan) a β-lactamase–resistant second-generation cephalosporin effective against a wide range of gram-positive

and gram-negative bacteria, used as the disodium salt.

ce·fox·i·tin (sĕ-fok′sĭ-tin) a strongly β-lactamase–resistant cephamycin antibiotic, classified as a second-generation cephalosporin and especially effective against gram-negative organisms; used as the sodium salt.

cef·po·dox·ime (sef″po-dok′sēm) a β-lactamase–resistant third-generation cephalosporin effective against a wide range of gram-positive and gram-negative bacteria; used as *c. proxetil.*

cef·pro·zil (sef-pro′zil) a broad-spectrum, second-generation cephalosporin effective against a wide range of gram-positive and gram-negative bacteria.

cef·ta·zi·dime (sef′ta-zĭ-dēm) a third-generation cephalosporin effective against gram-positive and gram-negative bacteria.

cef·ti·bu·ten (sef-ti′bu-ten) a third-generation cephalosporin used in treatment of bronchitis, pharyngitis, tonsillitis, and otitis media.

cef·ti·zox·ime (sef″tĭ-zok′sēm) a semisynthetic, β-lactamase–resistant, third-generation cephalosporin effective against a wide range of gram-positive and gram-negative bacteria, used as the sodium salt.

cef·tri·ax·one (sef″tri-ak′sōn) a semisynthetic, β-lactamase–resistant, third-generation cephalosporin effective against a wide range of gram-positive and gram-negative bacteria, used as the sodium salt.

cef·u·rox·ime (sef″u-rok′sēm) a semisynthetic, β-lactamase–resistant, second-generation cephalosporin effective against a wide range of gram-positive and gram-negative bacteria; used as the sodium salt and the axetil ester.

-cele[1] word element [Gr.], *tumor, swelling.*

-cele[2] word element [Gr.], *cavity.* See also words spelled *coele.*

cel·e·cox·ib (sel″ĕ-kok′sib) a nonsteroidal antiinflammatory drug that inhibits cyclooxygenase-1 activity, used for the treatment of osteoarthritis and rheumatoid arthritis.

ce·li·ac (se′le-ak) abdominal.

ce·li·ec·to·my (se″le-ek′tah-me) excision of an abdominal organ.

celi(o)- word element [Gr.], *abdomen; through the abdominal wall.*

ce·lio·col·pot·o·my (se″le-o-kol-pot′ah-me) incision into the abdomen through the vagina.

ce·lio·gas·trot·o·my (-gas-trot′ah-me) incision through the abdominal wall into the stomach.

ce·li·o·ma (se″le-o′mah) a tumor of the abdomen.

ce·lio·myo·si·tis (se"le-o-mi"o-si'tis) inflammation of the abdominal muscles.

ce·li·op·a·thy (se"le-op'ah-the) any abdominal disease.

ce·li·os·co·py (-os'kah-pe) laparoscopy.

ce·li·ot·o·my (-ot'ah-me) incision into the abdominal cavity. **vaginal c.,** incision into the abdominal cavity through the vagina.

ce·li·tis (se-li'tis) any abdominal inflammation.

cell (sel) 1. any of the protoplasmic masses making up organized tissue, consisting of a nucleus surrounded by cytoplasm enclosed in a cell or plasma membrane. It is the fundamental, structural, and functional unit of living organisms. In some of the lower forms of life, such as bacteria, a morphological nucleus is absent, although nucleoproteins (and genes) are present. 2. a small, more or less closed space. **accessory c's,** macrophages involved in the processing and presentation of antigens, making them more immunogenic. **acid c's,** parietal c's. **acinar c., acinic c., acinous c.,** any of the cells lining an acinus, especially the zymogen-secreting cells of the pancreatic acini. **adventitial c.,** pericyte. **air c.,** 1. any minute bodily chamber filled with air, such as an alveolus of the lung. 2. a cavity containing air and surrounded by a bodily structure, usually one of the bones of the head, such as the ethmoid or mastoid. **alpha c.,** 1. a type of cell found in the periphery of the islets of Langerhans that secretes glucagon. 2. acidophil (2). **alveolar c.,** pneumonocyte; any cell of the walls of the pulmonary alveoli; often restricted to the cells of the alveolar epithelium (squamous alveolar cells and great alveolar cells) and alveolar phagocytes. **Alzheimer c's,** 1. giant astrocytes with large prominent nuclei found in the brain in hepatolenticular degeneration and hepatic coma. 2. degenerated astrocytes. **amacrine c.,** any of five types of retinal neurons that seem to lack large axons, having only processes that resemble dendrites. **ameboid c.,** a cell that shows ameboid movement. **Anichkov's c.,** a plump modified histiocyte in the inflammatory lesions of the heart (Aschoff bodies) characteristic of rheumatic fever. **APUD c's** [*a*mine *p*recursor *u*ptake and *d*ecarboxylation], a group of cells that manufacture polypeptides and biogenic amines serving as hormones or neurotransmitters. The polypeptide production is linked to the uptake of a precursor amino acid and its decarboxylation to an amine. **argentaffin c's,** enterochromaffin cells that reduce ammoniacal silver solutions without additional treatment with a reducing agent; the reducing substance is serotonin. **Arias-Stella c's,** columnar cells in the endometrial epithelium which have a hyperchromatic enlarged nucleus and which appear to be associated with chorionic tissue in an intrauterine or extrauterine site. **Askanazy c's,** large eosinophilic cells found in the thyroid gland in autoimmune thyroiditis and Hürthle cell tumors. **automatic c.,** pacemaker c. **B c's,** B lymphocytes. **band c.,** a late metamyelocyte in which the nucleus is in the form of a curved or coiled band. **basal c.,** an early keratinocyte, present in the stratum basale of the epidermis. **basal granular c's,** APUD cells located at the base of the epithelium at many places in the gastrointestinal tract. **basket c.,** a neuron of the cerebral cortex whose fibers form a basket-like nest in which a Purkinje cell rests. **beaker c.,** goblet c. **beta c.,** 1. a type of basophilic cell that makes up most of the bulk of the islets of Langerhans and secretes insulin. 2. basophil (3). **Betz c's,** large pyramidal ganglion cells forming a layer of the gray matter of the brain. **bipolar c.,** a neuron with two processes. **blast c.,** 1. blast[1] (1). 2. the least differentiated blood cell without commitment as to its particular series; it precedes a stem cell. **blood c.,** one of the formed elements of the blood; a leukocyte, erythrocyte, or platelet. **bone c.,** osteocyte. **bristle c's,** the hair cells associated with the auditory and cochlear nerves. **burr c.,** schistocyte. **cartilage c.,** chondrocyte. **CD4 c's,** a major classification of T lymphocytes, referring to those that carry CD4 antigens; most are helper cells. **CD8 c's,** a major classification of T lymphocytes, referring to those that carry the CD8 antigen, including cytotoxic T lymphocytes and suppressor cells. **chief c's,** 1. columnar or cuboidal epithelial cells that line the lower portions of the gastric glands and secrete pepsin. 2. pinealocytes. 3. the most abundant parenchymal cells of the parathyroid, being polygonal epithelial cells rich in glycogen, having granular cytoplasm and vesicular nuclei, and arranged in plates or cords; cf. *oxyphil c's.* 4. the principal chromaffin cells of the paraganglia, each of which is surrounded by supporting cells. 5. chromophobe c's. **chromaffin c's,** cells staining readily with chromium salts, especially those of the adrenal medulla and similar cells occurring in widespread accumulations throughout the body in various organs, whose cytoplasm shows fine brown granules when stained with potassium bichromate.

chromophobe c's, faintly staining cells in the adenohypophysis; some are nongranular (either nonsecretory, immature presecretory, or degenerating cells), while others have extremely small granules; they are increased in chromophobe adenomas. **Claudius c's,** cuboidal cells, which along with Böttcher's cells form the floor of the external spiral sulcus, external to the organ of Corti. **columnar c.,** an elongate epithelial cell. **committed c.,** a lymphocyte which, after contact with antigen, is obligated to follow an individual course of development leading to antibody synthesis or immunological memory. **c. of Corti,** a hair cell in the organ of Corti. **daughter c.,** one formed by division of a mother cell. **decidual c's,** connective tissue cells of the uterine mucous membrane, enlarged and specialized during pregnancy. **Deiters c's,** the outer phalangeal cells of the organ of Corti. **delta c's,** cells in the pancreatic islets that secrete somatostatin. **dendritic c's,** cells with long cytoplasmic processes in the lymph nodes and germinal centers of the spleen; such processes, which extend along lymphoid cells, retain antigen molecules for extended periods of time. **dust c.,** alveolar macrophage. **effector c.,** any cell, such as an activated lymphocyte or plasma cell, which is instrumental in causing antigen disposal accomplished by either a cell-mediated or a humoral immunological response. **enamel c.,** ameloblast. **enterochromaffin c's,** chromaffin cells of the intestinal mucosa that stain with chromium salts and are impregnable with silver; they are sites of synthesis and storage of serotonin. **epithelioid c's,** 1. large polyhedral cells of connective tissue origin. 2. highly phagocytic, modified macrophages, resembling epithelial cells, which are characteristic of granulomatous inflammation. 3. pinealocytes. **erythroid c's,** blood cells of the erythrocytic series. **ethmoid c's, ethmoidal c's, ethmoidal air c's,** ethmoidal sinuses; paranasal sinuses found in groups within the ethmoid bone and communicating with the ethmoidal infundibulum and bulla and the superior and highest meatuses; often subdivided into *anterior, middle,* and *posterior.* **eukaryotic c.,** a cell with a true nucleus; see *eukaryote.* **excitable c.,** a cell that can generate an action potential at its membrane in response to depolarization and may transmit an impulse along the membrane. **fat c.,** a connective tissue cell specialized for the synthesis and storage of fat; such cells are bloated with globules of triglycerides, the nucleus being displaced to one side and the cytoplasm

seen as a thin line around the fat droplet. **fat-storing c's of liver,** lipid-accumulating, stellate cells located in the perisinusoidal space of the liver. **foam c's,** cells with a vacuolated appearance due to the presence of complex lipids; seen notably in xanthoma. **follicle c's, follicular c's,** cells located in the epithelium of follicles, such as those of the thyroid or ovarian follicles. **follicular center c.,** any of a series of B lymphocytes occurring normally in the germinal center and pathologically in the neoplastic nodules of follicular center cell lymphoma; they are believed to be intermediate stages in the development of lymphoblasts and plasma cells and are distinguished according to size (large or small) and the presence or absence of nuclear folds or clefts (cleaved or noncleaved). **G c's,** granular enterochromaffin cells in the mucosa of the pyloric part of the stomach, a source of gastrin. **ganglion c.,** a large nerve cell, especially one of those of the spinal ganglia. **Gaucher c.,** a large cell characteristic of Gaucher's disease, with eccentrically placed nuclei and fine wavy fibrils parallel to the long axis of the cell. **germ c's,** the cells of an organism whose function it is to reproduce its kind, i.e., oocytes and spermatozoa and their immature stages. **ghost c.,** 1. a keratinized denucleated cell with an unstained, shadowy center where the nucleus has been. 2. a degenerating or fragmented erythrocyte with no hemoglobin. **giant c.,** 1. any very large cell, such as the megakaryocyte of bone marrow. 2. any of the very large, multinucleate, modified macrophages, which may be formed by coalescence of epithelioid cells or by nuclear division without cytoplasmic division of monocytes, e.g., those characteristic of granulomatous inflammation and those that form around large foreign bodies. **glial c's,** neuroglial c's. **globoid c.,** an abnormal large histiocyte found in large numbers in intracranial tissues in Krabbe's disease. **glomus c.,** 1. any of the specific cells of the carotid body, which contain many dense-cored vesicles, occurring in clusters surrounded by other cells with no cytoplasmic granules. 2. any of the modified smooth muscle cells surrounding the arterial segment of a glomeriform arteriovenous anastomosis. **goblet c.,** a unicellular mucous gland found in the epithelium of various mucous membranes, especially that of the respiratory passages and intestines. **Golgi c's,** see under *neuron.* **granular c.,** one containing granules, such as a keratinocyte in the stratum granulosum of the epidermis, when it contains a dense collection of darkly staining granules. **granule c's,** 1. diminutive cells found in the granular layers of the cerebral and cerebellar cortices. 2. small nerve cells without axons, whose bodies are in the granular layer of the olfactory bulb. **granulosa c's,** cells surrounding the graafian follicle and forming the stratum granulosum and cumulus oophorus, after ovulation becoming lutein cells. **granulosa-lutein c's,** lutein cells of the corpus luteum derived from granulosa cells. **gustatory c's,** taste c's. **hair c's,** sensory epithelial cells with long hairlike processes (kinocilia or stereocilia) found in the organ of Corti and the vestibular labyrinth. **hairy c.,** one of the abnormal large leukocytes found in the blood in hairy cell leukemia, having numerous irregular cytoplasmic villi that give the cell a flagellated or hairy appearance. **heart-disease c's, heart-failure c's, heart-lesion c's,** macrophages containing granules of iron, found in the pulmonary alveoli and sputum in congestive heart failure. **HeLa c's,** cells of the first continuously cultured carcinoma strain, descended from a human cervical carcinoma. **helmet c.,** schistocyte. **helper c's, helper T c's,** differentiated T lymphocytes which cooperate with B lymphocytes in the synthesis of antibody to many antigens; they play an integral role in immunoregulation. **Hensen c's,** tall supporting cells constituting the outer border of the organ of Corti. **hepatic c's,** the polyhedral epithelial cells that constitute the substance of an acinus of the liver. **horizontal c.,** a retinal neuron, occurring in two types, each with one long neurite and several short ones. **Hürthle c's,** Askanazy c's. **interdental c's,** cells found in the spiral limbus between the dens acustici, which secrete the tectorial membrane of the cochlear duct. **interstitial c's,** 1. Leydig c's (1). 2. large epithelioid cells in the ovarian stroma, believed to have a secretory function, derived from the theca interna of atretic ovarian follicles. 3. cells found in the perivascular areas and between the cords of pinealocytes in the pineal body. 4. fat-storing c's of liver. **interstitial c's of Cajal,** pleomorphic cells having an oval nucleus and long, branching cytoplasmic processes that interlace with processes of adjacent cells, occurring in the gastrointestinal tract and the esophagus; thought to act as pacemakers. **islet c's,** the alpha and beta cells of the islets of Langerhans. **juxtaglomerular c's,** specialized cells containing secretory granules, located in the tunica media of the afferent glomerular arterioles, thought to stimulate aldosterone secretion and to play a role in renal autoregulation. These cells secrete the enzyme renin. **K c's,** 1. killer cells; cells mediating antibody-dependent cell-mediated cytotoxicity; they are small lymphocytes without T or B cell surface markers, having cytotoxic activity against target cells coated with specific IgG antibody. 2. cells in the duodenal and jejunal mucosa that synthesize gastric inhibitory polypeptide. **killer c's,** 1. K c's (1). 2. cytotoxic T lymphocytes. **Kupffer c's,** large, stellate or pyramidal, intensely phagocytic cells lining the walls of the hepatic sinusoids and forming part of the reticuloendothelial system. **lacunar c.,** a variant of the Reed-Sternberg cell, primarily associated with the nodular sclerosis type of Hodgkin's disease. **LAK c's,** lymphokine-activated killer c's. **Langerhans c's,** stellate dendritic cells, derived from precursors in the bone marrow, containing characteristic inclusions *(Birbeck granules)* in the cytoplasm and found principally in the epidermis. They are believed to be antigen-presenting cells involved in cell-mediated immune reactions in the skin. **large cleaved c.,** see *follicular center c.* **large noncleaved c., large uncleaved c.,** see *follicular center c.* **LE c.,** a neutrophil or macrophage that has phagocytized the denatured nuclear material of an injured cell (hematoxylin body); a characteristic of lupus erythematosus, but also found in analogous connective tissue disorders. **Leydig c's,** 1. clusters of epithelioid cells constituting the endocrine tissue of the testis, which elaborate androgens, chiefly testosterone. 2. mucous cells that do not pour their secretion out over the epithelial surface. **littoral c's,** flattened cells lining the walls of lymph or blood sinuses. **luteal c's, lutein c's,** the plump, pale-staining, polyhedral cells of the corpus luteum. **lymph c.,** lymphocyte. **lymphokine-activated killer c's,** killer cells activated by interleukin-2 and having specificity for tumors refractory to NK cells. **lymphoid c's,** lymphocytes and plasma cells; cells of the immune system that react specifically with antigen and elaborate specific cell products. **mast c.,** a connective tissue cell capable of elaborating basophilic, metachromatic cytoplasmic granules that contain histamine, heparin, hyaluronic acid, slow-reacting substance of anaphylaxis, and, in some species, serotonin. **mastoid c's,** air cells of various sizes and shapes in the mastoid process of the temporal bone. **Merkel c.,** a specialized cell at or near the epithelial–dermal junction and believed to act as a touch receptor by association with the flat, disklike ending of a nerve fiber (tactile meniscus). **Mexican hat c.,** target c. (1). **microglial c.,** a cell of the microglia. **mother c.,** one that divides to form new, or daughter, cells. **mucous c's,** cells which secrete mucus or mucin. **muscle c.,** see under *fiber*. **myoid c's,** cells in the seminiferous tubules which are presumed to be contractile and to be responsible for the rhythmic shallow contractions of the tubules. **natural killer c's,** NK c's. **nerve c.,** neuron. **neuroendocrine c's,** the specialized neurons that secrete neurohormones. **neuroglia c's, neuroglial c's,** the branching, non-neural cells of the neuroglia; they are of three types: astroglia, oligodendroglia (collectively termed macroglia), and microglia. **neurosecretory c.,** any cell with neuron-like properties that secretes a biologically active substance acting on another structure, often at a distant site. **nevus c.,** a small oval or cuboidal cell with a deeply staining nucleus and scanty pale cytoplasm, sometimes containing melanin granules, possibly derived from Schwann cells or embryonal nevoblasts; they are clustered in rounded masses (*theques*) in the epidermis, and reach the dermis by a kind of centripetal extrusion. **Niemann-Pick c's,** Pick c's. **NK c's,** natural killer cells; cells capable of mediating cytotoxic reactions without themselves being specifically sensitized against the target. **null c's,** lymphocytes that lack the surface antigens characteristic of B and T lymphocytes; seen in active systemic lupus erythematosus and other disease states. **nurse c's, nursing c's,** Sertoli c's. **olfactory c's,** a set of specialized cells of the mucous membranes of the nose, which are receptors of smell. **osteoprogenitor c's,** relatively undifferentiated cells found on or near all of the free surfaces of bone, which, under certain circumstances, undergo division and transform into osteoblasts or coalesce to give rise to osteoclasts. **oxyntic c's,** parietal c's. **oxyphil c's, oxyphilic c's,** 1. acidophilic cells found, along with the more numerous chief cells, in the parathyroid glands. 2. Askanazy c's. **P c's,** poorly staining, pale, small cells almost devoid of myofibrils, mitochondria, or other organelles; they are clustered in the sinoatrial node, where they are thought to be the center of impulse generation, and in the atrioventricular node. **pacemaker c.,** a myocardial cell displaying automaticity. **packed red blood c's,** whole blood from which plasma has been removed; used therapeutically in blood transfusions. **Paget c., paget-oid c.,** a large, irregularly shaped, pale anaplastic tumor cell found in the epidermis

in Paget's disease of the nipple and in extramammary Paget's disease. **Paneth c's,** narrow, pyramidal, or columnar epithelial cells with a round or oval nucleus close to the base of the cell, occurring in the fundus of the crypts of Lieberkühn; they contain large secretory granules that may contain peptidase. **parafollicular c's,** ovoid epithelial cells located in the thyroid follicles; they secrete calcitonin. **parietal c's,** large spheroidal or pyramidal cells that are the source of gastric hydrochloric acid and are the site of intrinsic factor production. **peptic c's,** chief c's (1). **peritubular contractile c's,** myoid c's. **pheochrome c's,** chromaffin c's. **Pick c's,** round, oval, or polyhedral cells with foamy, lipid-containing cytoplasm, found in the bone marrow and spleen in Niemann-Pick disease. **pigment c.,** any cell containing pigment granules. **pillar c's,** elongated supporting cells in a double row (*inner* and *outer pillar c's*) in the organ of Corti, arranged to form the inner tunnel. **plasma c.,** spherical or ellipsoidal cells with a single nucleus containing chromatin, an area of perinuclear clearing, and generally abundant, sometimes vacuolated, cytoplasm; they are involved in the synthesis, storage, and release of antibody. **polychromatic c's, polychromatophil c's,** immature erythrocytes staining with both acid and basic stains in a diffuse mixture of blue-gray and pink. **pre-B c's,** lymphoid cells that are immature and contain cytoplasmic IgM; they develop into B lymphocytes. **pre-T c.,** a T lymphocyte precursor before undergoing induction of the maturation process in the thymus; it lacks the characteristics of a mature T lymphocyte. **prickle c.,** a cell with delicate radiating processes connecting with similar cells, being a dividing keratinocyte of the stratum spinosum (prickle cell layer) of the epidermis. **primordial germ c.,** the earliest recognizable precursor in the embryo of a germ cell; these originate extragonadally but migrate early in embryonic development to the gonads. **prokaryotic c.,** a cell without a true nucleus; see *prokaryote*. **pulmonary epithelial c's,** extremely thin nonphagocytic squamous cells with flattened nuclei, constituting the outer layer of the alveolar wall in the lungs. **Purkinje's c's,** 1. large branching neurons in the middle layer of the cerebellar cortex. 2. large, clear, tightly packed, impulse-conducting cells of the cardiac Purkinje fibers. **red c., red blood c.,** erythrocyte. **red blood c's,** official terminology for *packed red blood c's.* **Reed c's, Reed-Sternberg c's,** the giant histiocytic cells, typically multinucleate, which are the common histologic characteristic of Hodgkin's disease. **reticular c's,** the cells forming the reticular fibers of connective tissue; those forming the framework of lymph nodes, bone marrow, and spleen form part of the reticuloendothelial system and may differentiate into macrophages. **reticuloendothelial c.,** see under *system.* **Rieder c.,** see under *lymphocyte.* **Schwann c.,** any of the large nucleated cells whose cell membrane spirally enwraps the axons of myelinated peripheral neurons supplying the myelin sheath between two nodes of Ranvier. **segmented c.,** a mature granulocyte in which the nucleus is divided into definite lobes joined by a filamentous connection. **Sertoli c's,** cells in the seminiferous tubules to which the spermatids become attached and which support, protect, and apparently nourish the spermatids until they develop into mature spermatozoa. **sickle c.,** a crescentic or sickle-shaped erythrocyte, characteristic of sickle cell anemia. **small cleaved c.,** see *follicular center c.* **small noncleaved c., small uncleaved c.,** see *follicular center c.* **somatic c's,** the cells of the somatoplasm; undifferentiated body cells. **somatostatin c's,** endocrine cells of the oxyntic and pyloric glands that secrete somatostatin. **sperm c.,** spermatozoon. **spur c.,** acanthocyte. **squamous c.,** a flat, scalelike epithelial cell. **stab c., staff c.,** band c. **stellate c.,** any star-shaped cell, as a Kupffer cell or astrocyte, having many filaments extending in all directions. **stem c.,** a generalized mother cell that has pluripotency (descendants may specialize in different directions), such as an undifferentiated mesenchymal cell that is a progenitor of both red and white blood cells. **suppressor c's,** lymphoid cells, especially T lymphocytes, that inhibit humoral and cell-mediated immune responses. They play an integral role in immunoregulation, and are believed to be operative in various autoimmune and other immunological disease states. **synovial c's,** fibroblasts lying between the cartilaginous fibers in the synovial membrane of a joint. **T c's,** T lymphocytes. **target c.,** 1. an abnormally thin erythrocyte that when stained shows a dark center surrounded by a pale unstained ring and a peripheral ring of hemoglobin; seen in certain anemias, thalassemias, hemoglobinopathies, obstructive jaundice, and the postsplenectomy state. 2. any cell selectively affected by a particular agent, such as a hormone or drug. **taste c's,** cells in the taste buds that have gustatory receptors. **tendon c's,** flattened cells of connective tissue occurring in rows between the primary bundles of the tendons. **theca c's,**

theca-lutein c's, lutein cells derived from the theca interna of the graafian follicle. **transitional c's,** 1. cells in the process of changing from one type to another. 2. in the sinoatrial and atrioventricular nodes, small, slow-conducting, heterogeneous cells interposed between the P cells and Purkinje cells. **visual c's,** the neuroepithelial elements of the retina. **white c., white blood c.,** leukocyte.

cel·la (sel′ah) [L.] cell.

cel·loi·din (sĕ-loi′din) a concentrated preparation of pyroxylin, used in microscopy for embedding specimens for section cutting.

cel·lu·la (sel′u-lah) pl. *cel′lulae.* [L.] cell.

cel·lu·lar (sel′u-lar) pertaining to or composed of cells.

cel·lu·lar·i·ty (sel″u-lar′ĭ-te) the state of a tissue or other mass as regards the number of constituent cells.

cel·lule (sel′ūl) a small cell.

cel·lu·lif·u·gal (sel″u-lif′ah-g′l) directed away from a cell body.

cel·lu·lip·e·tal (-lip′ĕ-t′l) directed toward a cell body.

cel·lu·li·tis (-li′tis) inflammation of the soft or connective tissue, in which a thin, watery exudate spreads through the cleavage planes of interstitial and tissue spaces; it may lead to ulceration and abscess. **anaerobic c.,** see *clostridial anaerobic c.* and *nonclostridial anaerobic c.* **clostridial anaerobic c.,** that due to a necrotizing clostridial infection, especially by *Clostridium perfingens,* usually arising in devitalized or otherwise compromised tissue. **gangrenous c.,** that leading to death of the tissue followed by bacterial invasion and putrefaction. **nonclostridial anaerobic c.,** that usually resulting from synergism between anaerobic and aerobic bacteria and leading to progressive tissue destruction and often fatal septicemia. **pelvic c.,** parametritis.

cel·lu·lose (sel′u-lōs) a rigid, colorless, unbranched, insoluble, long-chain polysaccharide, consisting of 3000 to 5000 glucose residues and forming the structure of most plant structures and of plant cells. **absorbable c.,** oxidized c. **c. acetate,** an acetylated cellulose used as a hemodialyzer membrane. **oxidized c.,** an absorbable oxidation product of cellulose, used as a local hemostatic. **c. sodium phosphate,** an insoluble, nonabsorbable cation exchange resin prepared from cellulose; it binds calcium and is used to prevent formation of calcium-containing renal calculi.

ce·lom (se′lum) coelom.

ce·los·chi·sis (se-los′kĭ-sis) abdominal fissure.

ce·lo·so·mia (se″lo-so′me-ah) congenital fissure or absence of the sternum, with hernial protrusion of the viscera.

ce·lot·o·my (se-lot′ah-me) herniotomy.

ce·lo·zo·ic (se″lo-zo′ik) inhabiting the intestinal canal of the body; said of parasites.

ce·ment (se-ment′) 1. a substance that produces a solid union between two surfaces. 2. dental c. 3. cementum. **cemen′tal,** adj. **dental c.,** any of various bonding substances that are placed in the mouth as a viscous liquid and set to a hard mass; used in restorative and orthodontic dental procedures as luting (cementing) agents, as protective, insulating, or sedative bases, and as restorative materials.

ce·men·ti·cle (se-men′ti-k′l) a small, discrete globular mass of cementum in the region of a tooth root.

ce·men·ti·fi·ca·tion (se-men″ti-fi-ka′shun) cementogenesis.

ce·men·to·blast (se-men′to-blast) a large cuboidal cell, found between the fibers on the surface of the cementum, which is active in cementum formation.

ce·men·to·blas·to·ma (se-men″to-blas-to′mah) a rare, benign odontogenic fibroma arising from the cementum and presenting as a proliferating mass contiguous with a tooth root.

ce·men·to·cyte (se-men′to-sīt) a cell in the lacunae of cellular cementum, frequently having long processes radiating from the cell body toward the periodontal surface of the cementum.

ce·men·to·enam·el (se-men″to-e-nam″l) pertaining to the cementum and the dental enamel.

ce·men·to·gen·e·sis (-jen′e-sis) development of cementum on the root dentin of a tooth.

ce·men·to·ma (se″men-to′mah) any of a variety of benign cementum-producing tumors including cementoblastoma, cementifying fibroma, florid osseous dysplasia, and periapical cemental dysplasia, particularly the last. **gigantiform c.,** florid osseous dysplasia.

ce·men·tum (se-men′tum) the bonelike connective tissue covering the root of a tooth and assisting in tooth support.

ce·nes·the·sia (sen″es-the′zhah) somatognosis. **cenesthe′sic, cenesthe′tic,** adj.

cen(o)- word element [Gr.], 1. *new.* 2. *empty.* 3. *common.*

ce·no·site (se′no-sīt) coinosite.

cen·sor (sen′ser) the mental faculty that prevents unconscious thoughts and wishes from coming into consciousness unless disguised, as in dreams.

cen·ter (sen′ter) 1. the middle point of a body. 2. a collection of neurons in the central nervous system that are concerned with performance of a particular function. **accelerating c.,** the part of the vasomotor center involved in acceleration of the heart. **apneustic c.,** the neurons in the brain stem controlling normal respiration. **Broca's c.,** Broca's motor speech area. **cardioinhibitory c.,** the part of the vasomotor center that exerts an inhibitory influence on the heart. **c's of chondrification,** dense aggregations of embryonic mesenchymal cells at sites of future cartilage formation. **ciliospinal c.,** one in the lower cervical and upper thoracic portions of the spinal cord, involved in dilatation of the pupil. **community mental health c. (CMHC),** a mental health facility or group of affiliated agencies that provide various psychotherapeutic services to a designated geographic area. **coughing c.,** one in the medulla oblongata above the respiratory center, which controls the act of coughing. **deglutition c.,** a nerve center in the medulla oblongata that controls the function of swallowing. **C's for Disease Control and Prevention (CDC),** an agency of the U.S. Department of Health and Human Services, serving as a center for the control, prevention, and investigation of diseases. **ejaculation c.,** the reflex center in the lumbar spinal cord that regulates ejaculation of semen during sexual stimulation. **epiotic c.,** the center of ossification that forms the mastoid process. **erection c.,** a reflex center in the sacral spinal cord that regulates erection of the penis or clitoris. **feeding c.,** a group of cells in the lateral hypothalamus that when stimulated cause a sensation of hunger. **germinal c.,** the area in the center of a lymph nodule containing aggregations of actively proliferating lymphocytes. **health c.,** 1. a community health organization for creating health work and coordinating the efforts of all health agencies. 2. an educational complex consisting of a medical school and various allied health professional schools. **medullary respiratory c.,** the part of the respiratory centers that is in the medulla oblongata. **nerve c.,** center (2). **ossification c.,** any point at which the process of ossification begins in a bone; in a long bone there is a *primary center* for the diaphysis and one *secondary center* for each epiphysis. **pneumotaxic c.,** one in the upper pons that rhythmically inhibits inspiration. **reflex c.,** any center in the brain or spinal cord in which a sensory impression is changed into a motor impulse. **respiratory c's,** a series of centers (apneustic and pneumotaxic respiratory centers and dorsal and ventral respiratory groups) in the medulla and pons that coordinate respiratory movements. **satiety c.,** a group of cells in the ventromedial hypothalamus that when stimulated suppress a desire for food. **sudorific c.,** 1. a center in the anterior hypothalamus controlling diaphoresis. 2. any of several centers in the medulla oblongata or spinal cord that exercise parasympathetic control over diaphoresis. **swallowing c.,** deglutition c. **thermoregulatory c's,** hypothalamic centers regulating the conservation and dissipation of heat. **thirst c.,** a group of cells in the lateral hypothalamus that when stimulated cause a sensation of thirst. **vasomotor c's,** centers in the medulla oblongata and lower pons that regulate the caliber of blood vessels and the heart rate and contractility.

cen·tes·i·mal (sen-tes′ĭ-mal) divided into hundredths.

cen·te·sis (sen-te′sis) [Gr.] perforation or tapping, as with a trocar or needle.

-centesis word element [Gr.], *puncture and aspiration of.*

centi- word element [L.], *hundred;* used (*a*) in naming units of measurement to indicate one hundredth (10^{-2}) of the unit designated by the root with which it is combined (symbol c) and (*b*) to denote one hundred (e.g., centipede).

cen·ti·grade (sen′tĭ-grād) having 100 gradations (steps or degrees); see under *scale.*

cen·ti·gray (cGy) (-gra″) a unit of absorbed radiation dose equal to one hundredth (10^{-2}) of a gray, or 1 rad.

cen·ti·me·ter (cm) (-me″ter) one hundredth (10^{-2}) of a meter. **cubic c. (cm^3, cc),** a unit of capacity, being that of a cube each side of which measures 1 cm; equal to 1 mL.

cen·trad (sen′trad) toward a center.

cen·tral (sen′tr′l) situated at or pertaining to a center; not peripheral.

cen·tren·ce·phal·ic (sen″tren-sĕ-fal′ik) pertaining to the center of the encephalon.

centri- word element [L., Gr.], *center, a central location.* Also, *centr(o)-.*

cen·tri·ac·i·nar (sen″trĭ-as′ĭ-nar) pertaining to the central portion of one or more acini.

cen·tric (sen′trik) 1. central. 2. having a center.

cen·tric·i·put (sen-tris′ĭ-put) the central part of the upper surface of the head, located between the occiput and sinciput.

cen·trif·u·gal (sen-trif′ah-gal) efferent (1).

cen·trif·u·gate (sen-trif′ah-gāt) material subjected to centrifugation.

cen·trif·u·ga·tion (sen-trif″u-ga′shun) the process of separating lighter portions of a solution, mixture, or suspension from the heavier portions by centrifugal force.

cen·tri·fuge (sen′trĭ-fūj) 1. a machine by which centrifugation is effected. 2. to subject to centrifugation.

cen·tri·lob·u·lar (sen″trĭ-lob′u-ler) pertaining to the central portion of a lobule.

cen·tri·ole (sen′tre-ōl) either of the two cylindrical organelles located in the centrosome and containing nine triplets of microtubules arrayed around their edges; centrioles migrate to opposite poles of the cell during cell division and serve to organize the spindles. They are capable of independent replication and of migrating to form basal bodies.

cen·trip·e·tal (sen-trip′ĕ-t′l) 1. afferent (1). 2. corticipetal.

centr(o)- see *centri-.*

cen·tro·blast (sen′tro-blast″) a general term encompassing both large and small noncleaved follicular center cells.

cen·tro·ce·cal (sen″tro-se′k′l) pertaining to the central macular area and the blind spot.

cen·tro·cyte (sen′tro-sīt″) a general term encompassing both large and small cleaved follicular center cells. **centrocyt′ic,** adj.

cen·tro·mere (-mēr) the clear constricted portion of the chromosome at which the chromatids are joined and by which the chromosome is attached to the spindle during cell division. **centromer′ic,** adj.

cen·tro·nu·cle·ar (sen″tro-noo′kle-ar) having or pertaining to a centrally located nucleus.

cen·tro·scle·ro·sis (-sklĕ-ro′sis) osteosclerosis of the marrow cavity of a bone.

cen·tro·some (sen′tro-sōm) a specialized area of condensed cytoplasm containing the centrioles and playing an important part in mitosis.

cen·trum (sen′trum) pl. *cen′tra.* [L.] 1. a center. 2. the body of a vertebra.

CEP congenital erythropoietic porphyria.

ceph·a·lad (sef′ah-lad) toward the head.

ceph·al·ede·ma (-lĕ-de′mah) edema of the head.

ceph·a·lex·in (-lek′sin) a semisynthetic first-generation cephalosporin, effective against a wide range of gram-positive and a limited range of gram-negative bacteria; used as the base or the hydrochloride salt.

ceph·al·he·mat·o·cele (sef″al-he-mat′ah-sēl) a hematocele under the pericranium, communicating with one or more dural sinuses.

ceph·al·he·ma·to·ma (-he"mah-to'mah) a subperiosteal hemorrhage limited to the surface of one cranial bone; a usually benign condition seen in the newborn as a result of bone trauma.

ceph·al·hy·dro·cele (-hi'dro-sēl) a serous or watery accumulation under the pericranium.

ce·phal·ic (sĕ-fal'ik) pertaining to the head, or to the head end of the body.

cephal(o)- word element [Gr.], *head.*

ceph·a·lo·cele (sef'ah-lo-sēl) encephalocele.

ceph·a·lo·cen·te·sis (sef"ah-lo-sen-te'sis) surgical puncture of the skull.

ceph·a·lo·dac·ty·ly (-dak'tĭ-le) malformation of the head and digits.

ceph·a·lo·gram (sef'ah-lo-gram) an x-ray image of the structures of the head; cephalometric radiograph.

ceph·a·log·ra·phy (sef"ah-log'rah-fe) radiography of the head.

ceph·a·lo·gy·ric (sef"ah-lo-ji'rik) pertaining to turning motions of the head.

ceph·a·lom·e·ter (sef"ah-lom'ĕ-ter) an instrument for measuring the head; an orienting device for positioning the head for radiographic examination and measurement.

ceph·a·lom·e·try (sef"ah-lom'ĕ-tre) scientific measurement of the dimensions of the head.

ceph·a·lo·mo·tor (sef"ah-lo-mōt'er) moving the head; pertaining to motions of the head.

Ceph·a·lo·my·ia (-mi'yah) *Oestrus.*

ceph·a·lo·nia (sef"ah-lo'ne-ah) a condition in which the head is abnormally enlarged, with sclerotic hyperplasia of the brain.

ceph·a·lop·a·thy (sef"ah-lop'ah-the) any disease of the head.

ceph·a·lo·pel·vic (sef"ah-lo-pel'vik) pertaining to the relationship of the fetal head to the maternal pelvis.

ceph·a·lo·spo·rin (sef"ah-lo-spor'in) any of a group of broad-spectrum, penicillinase-resistant antibiotics from *Acremonium,* related to the penicillins in both structure and mode of action. Those used medicinally are semisynthetic derivatives of the natural antibiotic cephalosporin C. First-generation cephalosporins have a broad range of activity against gram-positive organisms and a narrow range of activity against gram-negative organisms; second-, third-, and fourth generation agents are progressively more active against gram-negative organisms and less active against gram-positive organisms.

ceph·a·lo·spo·rin·ase (-spor'in-ās) a β-lactamase preferentially acting on cephalosporins.

Ceph·a·lo·spo·ri·um (-spor'e-um) former name for *Acremonium.*

ceph·a·lo·stat (sef'ah-lo-stat") a head-positioning device which assures reproducibility of the relations between an x-ray beam, a patient's head, and an x-ray film.

ceph·a·lot·o·my (sef"ah-lot'ah-me) 1. the cutting up of the fetal head to facilitate delivery. 2. dissection of the fetal head.

ceph·a·my·cin (sef"ah-mi'sin) any of a family of natural and semisynthetic, β-lactamase–resistant antibiotics derived from various species of *Streptomyces,* generally classed as second-generation cephalosporins but more active against anaerobes.

ceph·a·pi·rin (sef"ah-pi'rin) a semisynthetic analogue of the natural antibiotic cephalosporin C, effective against a wide range of gram-negative and gram-positive bacteria; used as the sodium salt.

ceph·ra·dine (sef'rah-dēn) a semisynthetic first-generation cephalosporin, effective against a wide range of gram-positive and a limited range of gram-negative bacteria.

ce·ram·ics (sah-ram'iks) the modeling and processing of objects made of clay or similar materials. **dental c.,** the use of porcelain and similar materials in restorative dentistry.

cer·am·i·dase (ser-am'ĭ-dās) an enzyme occurring in most mammalian tissue that catalyzes the reversible acylation-deacylation of ceramides.

cer·a·mide (ser'ah-mīd) the basic unit of the sphingolipids; it is sphingosine, or a related base, attached to a long chain fatty acyl group. Ceramides are accumulated abnormally in Farber's disease. **c. trihexoside,** any of a specific family of glycosphingolipids; due to a deficiency of α-galactosidase A, they accumulate in Fabry's disease.

cerat(o)- for words beginning thus, see those beginning *kerat(o)-.*

Cer·a·to·phyl·lus (ser"ah-tof'ĭ-lus) a genus of fleas.

cer·ca·ria (ser-kar'e-ah) pl. *cerca'riae.* The final, free-swimming larval stage of a trematode parasite. **cercar'ial,** adj.

cer·clage (ser-klahzh') [Fr.] encircling of a part with a ring or loop, as for correction of an incompetent cervix uteri or fixation of adjacent ends of a fractured bone.

ce·rea flex·i·bil·i·tas (sēr'e-ah flek"sĭ-bil'ĭ-tas) [L.] a rigidity of the body in which the patient maintains whatever position he is placed in, the limbs having a heavy waxy malleability.

cer·e·bel·lar (ser"ĕ-bel'ar) pertaining to the cerebellum.

cer·e·bel·lif·u·gal (ser″ah-bel-if′ah-g′l) conducting away from the cerebellum.

cer·e·bel·lip·e·tal (-ip′ĕ-t′l) conducting toward the cerebellum.

cer·e·bel·lo·spi·nal (ser″ah-bel″o-spi′nal) proceeding from the cerebellum to the spinal cord.

cer·e·bel·lum (ser″ah-bel′um) the part of the metencephalon situated on the back of the brain stem, to which it is attached by three cerebellar peduncles on each side; it consists of a median lobe (vermis) and two lateral lobes (the hemispheres).

cer·e·bral (sĕ-re′bral, ser′ĕ-bral) pertaining to the cerebrum.

cer·e·bra·tion (ser″ah-bra′shun) functional activity of the brain.

cer·e·brif·u·gal (-brif′u-g′l) conducting or proceeding away from the cerebrum.

cer·e·brip·e·tal (-brip′ĕ-t′l) conducting or proceeding toward the cerebrum.

cer·e·bro·mac·u·lar (ser″ĕ-bro-mak′u-ler) maculocerebral; pertaining to or affecting the brain and the macula retinae.

cer·e·bro·ma·la·cia (-mah-la′shah) abnormal softening of the substance of the cerebrum.

cer·e·bro·men·in·gi·tis (-men″in-ji′tis) meningoencephalitis.

cer·e·bron·ic ac·id (ser″ĕ-bron′ik) a fatty acid found in cerebrosides such as phrenosine.

cer·e·bro·path·ia (ser″ĕ-bro-path′e-ah) [L.] cerebropathy. **c. psy′chica toxe′mica,** Korsakoff's psychosis.

cer·e·brop·a·thy (ser″ĕ-brop′ah-the) any disorder of the cerebrum; see also *encephalopathy*.

cer·e·bro·phys·i·ol·o·gy (ser″ĕ-bro-fiz″e-ol′ah-je) the physiology of the cerebrum.

cer·e·bro·pon·tile (-pon′tĭl) pertaining to the cerebrum and pons.

cer·e·bro·scle·ro·sis (-sklĕ-ro′sis) morbid hardening of the substance of the cerebrum.

cer·e·bro·side (ser′ĕ-bro-sīd″) a general designation for sphingolipids in which sphingosine is combined with galactose or glucose; found chiefly in nervous tissue.

cer·e·bro·sis (ser″ĕ-bro′sis) cerebropathy.

cer·e·bro·spi·nal (-spi′n′l) pertaining to the brain and spinal cord.

cer·e·bro·spi·nant (-spi′nant) an agent which affects the brain and spinal cord.

cer·e·brot·o·my (-brot′ah-me) encephalotomy.

cer·e·brum (ser′ĕ-brum, sĕ-re′brum) the main portion of the brain, occupying the upper part of the cranial cavity; its two hemispheres, united by the corpus callosum, form the largest part of the central nervous system in humans. The term is sometimes applied to the postembryonic forebrain and midbrain together or to the entire brain.

ce·ri·um (Ce) (sēr′e-um) chemical element (see *Table of Elements*), at. no. 58.

ce·ro·plas·ty (sēr′o-plas″te) the making of anatomical models in wax.

ce·ru·lo·plas·min (sĕ-roo″lo-plaz′min) an α_2-globulin of plasma believed to function in copper transport and its maintenance at appropriate levels in tissue; levels are decreased in Wilson's disease.

ce·ru·men (sĕ-roo′men) earwax; the waxlike substance found within the external meatus of the ear. **ceru′minal, ceru′minous,** adj.

ce·ru·min·ol·y·sis (sĕ-roo″mĭ-nol′ĭ-sis) dissolution or disintegration of cerumen in the external auditory meatus. **ceruminolyt′ic,** adj.

cer·vi·cal (ser′vĭ-k′l) 1. pertaining to the neck. 2. pertaining to the neck or cervix of any organ or structure.

cer·vi·cec·to·my (ser″vĭ-sek′tah-me) excision of the cervix uteri.

cer·vi·ci·tis (-si′tis) inflammation of the cervix uteri.

cervic(o)- word element [L.], *neck; cervix.*

cer·vi·co·bra·chi·al·gia (ser″vĭ-ko-bra″ke-al′jah) pain in the neck radiating to the arm, due to compression of nerve roots of the cervical spinal cord.

cer·vi·co·col·pi·tis (-kol-pi′tis) inflammation of the cervix uteri and vagina.

cer·vi·co·tho·rac·ic (-thah-ras′ik) pertaining to the neck and thorax.

cer·vi·co·uter·ine (-u′ter-in) of or pertaining to the uterine cervix.

cer·vi·co·ves·i·cal (-ves′ĭ-k′l) vesicocervical.

cer·vix (ser′viks) pl. *cer′vices.* [L.] 1. neck. 2. the front portion of the neck. 3. cervix uteri. **incompetent c.,** a uterine cervix abnormally prone to dilate in the second trimester of pregnancy, resulting in premature expulsion of the fetus. **c. u′teri, uterine c.,** the narrow lower end of the uterus, between the isthmus and the opening of the uterus into the vagina. **c. vesi′cae urina′riae,** the lower, constricted part of the urinary bladder, proximal to the opening of the urethra.

ce·sar·e·an (sĕ-zar′e-an) see under *section.*

CESD cholesteryl ester storage disease.

ce·si·um (Cs) (se′ze-um) chemical element (see *Table of Elements*), at. no. 55.

ces·ti·ci·dal (ses″tĭ-si′d′l) destructive to cestodes (tapeworms).

Ces·to·da (ses-to′dah) a subclass of Cestoidea comprising the true tapeworms, which have a head (scolex) and segments (proglottides).

The adults are endoparasitic in the alimentary tract and associated ducts of various vertebrate hosts; their larvae may be found in various organs and tissues.

Ces·to·da·ria (ses″to-dar′e-ah) a subclass of tapeworms, the unsegmented tapeworms of the class Cestoidea, which are endoparasitic in the intestines and coelom of various primitive fishes and rarely in reptiles.

ces·tode, ces·toid (ses′tōd, ses′toid) 1. tapeworm. 2. resembling a tapeworm.

Ces·toi·dea (ses-toi′de-ah) a class of tapeworms (phylum Platyhelminthes), characterized by the absence of a mouth or digestive tract, and by a noncuticular layer covering their bodies.

cet·al·ko·ni·um chlo·ride (set″al-ko′ne-um) a cationic quaternary ammonium surfactant used as a topical anti-infective and disinfectant.

ce·ti·ri·zine (sĕ-tir′ĭ-zēn) a nonsedating antihistamine used as the hydrochloride salt in the treatment of allergic rhinitis, chronic idiopathic urticaria, and asthma.

cet·ri·mo·ni·um bro·mide (set″rĭ-mo′ne-um) a quaternary ammonium antiseptic and detergent applied topically to the skin to cleanse wounds, as a preoperative disinfectant, and to treat seborrhea of the scalp; also used to cleanse and to store surgical instruments.

cet·ro·rel·ix (set″ro-rel′iks) a gonadotropin-releasing hormone antagonist, used as the acetate salt to inhibit premature surges of luteinizing hormone in women undergoing controlled ovarian stimulation during infertility treatment.

ce·tyl·pyr·i·din·i·um chlo·ride (se″til-pir″ĭ-din′e-um) a cationic disinfectant; used as a local antiinfective administered sublingually or applied topically to intact skin and mucous membranes, and as a preservative in pharmaceutical preparations.

cev·i·mel·ine (sĕ-vim′ah-lēn) a cholinergic agonist used as the hydrochloride salt in the treatment of xerostomia associated with Sjögren's syndrome.

CF carbolfuchsin; cardiac failure (see *heart failure*, under *failure*); Christmas factor.

Cf californium.

CFT complement fixation test; see under *fixation*.

CGS centimeter-gram-second system.

cGy centigray.

CH50 see under *assay* and *unit*.

chafe (chāf) to irritate the skin, as by rubbing together of opposing skin folds.

cha·gas·ic (chah-gas′ik) pertaining to or due to Chagas' disease.

cha·go·ma (chah-go′mah) a skin tumor occurring in Chagas' disease.

chain (chān) a collection of objects linked end to end. **branched c.,** an open chain of atoms, usually carbon, with one or more side chains attached to it. **electron transport c.,** the final common pathway of biological oxidation, the series of electron carriers in the inner mitochondrial membrane that pass electrons from reduced coenzymes to molecular oxygen via sequential redox reactions coupled to proton transport, generating energy for biological processes. **H c., heavy c.,** any of the large polypeptide chains of five classes that, paired with the light chains, make up the antibody molecule. Heavy chains bear the antigenic determinants that differentiate the immunoglobulin classes. **J c.,** a polypeptide occurring in polymeric IgM and IgA molecules. **L c., light c.,** either of the two small polypeptide chains (molecular weight 22,000) that, when linked to heavy chains by disulfide bonds, make up the antibody molecule; they are of two types, kappa and lambda, which are unrelated to immunoglobulin class differences. **open c.,** a series of atoms united in a straight line; compounds of this series are related to methane. **polypeptide c.,** the structural element of protein, consisting of a series of amino acid residues (peptides) joined together by peptide bonds. **respiratory c.,** electron transport c. **side c.,** a group of atoms attached to a larger chain or to a ring.

chak·ra (chuk′rah, shah′krah) any of the seven energy centers, located from the perineum to the crown of the head, of yoga philosophy; also used in some energy-based complementary medicine systems.

cha·la·sia (kah-la′zhah) relaxation of a bodily opening, such as the cardiac sphincter (a cause of vomiting in infants).

cha·la·zi·on (kah-la′ze-on) pl. *chalaʹzia, chalaʹzions.* [Gr.] a small eyelid mass due to inflammation of a meibomian gland.

chal·co·sis (kal-ko′sis) copper deposits in tissue.

chal·i·co·sis (kal″ĭ-ko′sis) pneumoconiosis due to inhalation of fine particles of stone.

chal·lenge (chal′enj) 1. to administer a substance to monitor for the normal physiological response. 2. in immunology, to administer an antigen to monitor the response in a sensitized person.

chal·one (kal′ōn) a group of tissue-specific water-soluble substances that are produced within a tissue and that inhibit mitosis of cells of that tissue and whose action is reversible.

cham·ae·ceph·a·ly (kam″e-sef′ah-le) the condition of having a low flat head, i.e., a cephalic index of 70 or less. **chamaecephal'ic,** adj.

cham·ber (chām'ber) an enclosed space. **anterior c. of eye,** the part of the aqueous-containing space of the eyeball between the cornea and the iris. **aqueous c.,** the part of the eyeball filled with aqueous humor; see *anterior c.* and *posterior c.* **counting c.,** the part of a hemacytometer consisting of a microscopic slide with a depression whose base is marked in grids, and into which a measured volume of a sample of blood or bacterial culture is placed and covered with a cover glass. Cells and formed blood elements in any given square can then be counted under a microscope. **diffusion c.,** an apparatus for separating a substance by means of a semipermeable membrane. **Haldane c.,** an air-tight chamber in which animals are confined for metabolic studies. **hyperbaric c.,** an enclosed space in which gas (oxygen) can be raised to greater than atmospheric pressure. **ionization c.,** an enclosure containing two or more electrodes between which an electric current may be passed when the enclosed gas is ionized by radiation; used for determining the intensity of x-rays and other rays. **posterior c. of eye,** the part of the aqueous-containing space of the eyeball between the iris and the lens. **pulp c.,** the natural cavity in the central portion of the tooth crown that is occupied by the dental pulp. **relief c.,** the recess in a denture surface that rests on the oral structures, to reduce or eliminate pressure. **Thoma-Zeiss counting c.,** a common type of counting c. **vitreous c.,** the vitreous-containing space in the eyeball, bounded anteriorly by the lens and ciliary body and posteriorly by the posterior wall of the eyeball.

cham·o·mile (kam'o-mēl, -mīl) German chamomile; the dried flower heads of the herb *Matricaria recutita,* used for inflammatory diseases of the gastrointestinal tract and as a topical counterirritant and antiinflammatory. **English c., Roman c.,** the dried flowers of the perennial herb *Chamaemelum nobile,* used as a homeopathic preparation and in folk medicine as a carminative and counterirritant.

chan·cre (shang'ker) [Fr.] 1. the primary sore of syphilis, occurring at the site of entry of the infection. 2. the primary cutaneous lesion of such diseases as sporotrichosis and tuberculosis. **hard c., hunterian c.,** chancre (1). **c. re'dux,** chancre developing on the scar of a healed primary chancre. **soft c.,** chancroid. **true c.,** chancre (1). **tuberculous c.,** a brownish red papule which develops into an indurated nodule or plaque, representing the initial cutaneous infection of the tubercle bacillus into the skin or mucosa.

chan·croid (shang'kroid) a sexually transmitted disease caused by *Haemophilus ducreyi,* characterized by a painful primary ulcer at the site of inoculation, usually on the external genitalia, associated with regional lymphadenitis. **chancroi'dal,** adj. **phagedenic c.,** chancroid with a tendency to slough. **serpiginous c.,** a variety tending to spread in curved lines.

change (chānj) an alteration. **fatty c.,** abnormal accumulation of fat within parenchymal cells. **hyaline c.,** a pale, eosinophilic, homogeneous glassy appearance seen in histologic specimens; it is a purely descriptive term and has a variety of causes.

chan·nel (chan'ĕl) that through which anything flows; a cut or groove. **gated c.,** a protein channel that opens and closes in response to signals, such as binding of a ligand (*ligand-gated c.*) or changes in the electric potential across the cell membrane (*voltage-gated c.*). **potassium c.,** a voltage-gated protein channel selective for the passage of potassium ions. **protein c.,** a watery pathway through the interstices of a protein molecule by which ions and small molecules can cross a membrane into or out of a cell by diffusion. **sodium c.,** a voltage-gated protein channel selective for the passage of sodium ions.

cha·ot·ic (ka-ot'ik) completely confused, disorganized, or irregular.

chap·er·one (shap'er-ōn) someone or something that accompanies and oversees another. **molecular c.,** any of a diverse group of proteins that oversee the correct intracellular folding and assembly of polypeptides without being components of the final structure.

chap·er·o·nin (shap''er-o'nin) any of various heat shock proteins that act as molecular chaperones in bacteria, plasmids, mitochondria, and eukaryotic cyotsol.

char·ac·ter (kar'ak-ter) 1. a quality indicative of the nature of an object or an organism. 2. in genetics, the expression of a gene or group of genes in a phenotype. 3. in psychiatry, a term used in much the same way as personality, particularly for those personality traits shaped by life experiences. **acquired c.,** a noninheritable modification produced in an animal as a result of its own activities or of environmental influences. **primary sex c's,** those characters in the male or female that are directly involved in reproduction; the gonads and their accessory structures. **secondary sex c's,** those characters specific to the male or female but not directly involved in reproduction. See also *masculinization* and *feminization*.

char·ac·ter·is·tic (kar″ak-ter-is′tik) 1. character. 2. typical of an individual or other entity. **demand c's,** behavior exhibited by the subject of an experiment in an attempt to accomplish certain goals as a result of cues communicated by the experimenter (expectations or hypothesis).

char·coal (chahr′kōl) carbon prepared by charring wood or other organic material. **activated c.,** residue of destructive distillation of various organic materials, treated to increase its adsorptive power; used as a general-purpose antidote. **animal c.,** charcoal prepared from bone; it may be purified (*purified animal c.)* by removal of materials dissolved by hot hydrochloric acid and water; adsorbent and decolorizer.

char·ley horse (chahr′le hors) soreness and stiffness in a muscle, especially the quadriceps, due to overstrain or contusion.

chart (chahrt) a record of data in graphic or tabular form. **reading c.,** a chart printed in gradually increasing type sizes, used in testing acuity of near vision. **Reuss' color c's,** charts with colored letters printed on colored backgrounds, used in testing color vision. **Snellen's c.,** a chart with block letters in gradually decreasing sizes, used in testing visual acuity.

chaste tree (chāst′ tre″) the shrub *Vitex agnus-castus* or an extract prepared from its berries and root bark, which is used for the treatment of premenstrual syndrome and menopause; also used in homeopathy.

ChB [L.] Chirur′giae Baccalau′reus (Bachelor of Surgery).

CHD coronary heart disease.

ChE cholinesterase.

check-bite (chek′bīt) a sheet of hard wax or modeling compound placed between the teeth, used to check occlusion of the teeth.

cheek (chēk) 1. the fleshy portion of either side of the face, or the fleshy mucous membrane–covered side of the oral cavity. 2. any fleshy protuberance resembling the cheek of the face. **cleft c.,** facial cleft caused by developmental failure of union between the maxillary and frontonasal processes.

cheesy (che′ze) caseous.

chei·lec·tro·pi·on (ki″lek-tro′pe-on) eversion of the lip.

chei·li·tis (ki-li′tis) inflammation of the lips. **actinic c.,** pain and swelling of the lips and development of a scaly crust on the vermilion border after exposure to actinic rays; it may be acute or chronic. **angular c.,** perlèche. **solar c.,** actinic c.

cheil(o)- word element [Gr.], *lip.*

chei·lo·gnatho·pros·o·pos·chi·sis (ki″lo-na″tho-pros″o-pos′ki-sis) congenital oblique facial cleft continuing into the upper jaw and lip.

chei·lo·plas·ty (ki′lo-plas″te) surgical repair of a defect of the lip.

chei·lor·rha·phy (ki-lor′ah-fe) suture of the lip; surgical repair of harelip.

chei·los·chi·sis (ki-los′ki-sis) harelip.

chei·lo·sis (ki-lo′sis) fissuring and dry scaling of the vermilion surface of the lips and angles of the mouth, a characteristic of riboflavin deficiency. **angular c.,** perlèche.

chei·lo·sto·ma·to·plas·ty (ki″lo-sto′mah-to-plas″te) surgical restoration of the lips and mouth.

cheir·ar·thri·tis (ki″rahr-thri′tis) inflammation of the joints of the hands and fingers.

cheir(o)- word element [Gr.], *hand.* See also words beginning *chir(o)-.*

chei·ro·kin·es·the·sia (ki″ro-kin″es-the′-zhah) the subjective perception of movements of the hand, especially in writing.

chei·ro·meg·a·ly (-meg′ah-le) megalocheiria.

chei·ro·plas·ty (ki′ro-plas″te) plastic surgery on the hand.

chei·ro·pom·pho·lyx (ki″ro-pom′fah-liks) pompholyx.

chei·ro·spasm (ki′ro-spazm) spasm of the muscles of the hand.

che·late (ke′lāt) 1. to combine with a metal in complexes in which the metal is part of a ring. 2. by extension, a chemical compound in which a metallic ion is sequestered and firmly bound into a ring within the chelating molecules. Chelates are used in chemotherapy of metal poisoning.

chem·abra·sion (kēm″-ah-bra′zhun) superficial destruction of the epidermis and the dermis by application of a cauterant to the skin; done to remove scars, tattoos, etc.

chem·ex·fo·li·a·tion (kēm″eks-fo″le-a′shun) chemabrasion.

chem·i·cal (kem′ĭ-k'l) 1. pertaining to chemistry. 2. a substance composed of chemical elements, or obtained by chemical processes.

chemi·lu·mi·nes·cence (kem″ĭ-loo″mĭ-nes′ens) luminescence produced by direct transformation of chemical energy into light energy.

chem·ist (kem′ist) 1. an expert in chemistry. 2. (British) pharmacist.

chem·is·try (kem′is-tre) the science dealing with the elements and atomic relations of matter, and of various compounds of the elements. **colloid c.,** chemistry dealing with the nature and composition of colloids.

inorganic c., that branch of chemistry dealing with compounds not occurring in the plant or animal worlds. **organic c.,** that branch of chemistry dealing with carbon-containing compounds.

chem(o)- word element [Gr.], *chemical; chemistry.*

che·mo·at·trac·tant (ke″mo-ah-trak′tant) a chemotactic agent that induces an organism or a cell (e.g., a leukocyte) to migrate toward it.

che·mo·au·to·troph (-aw′to-trōf) a chemoautotrophic microorganism.

che·mo·au·to·tro·phic (-aw″to-tro′fik) capable of synthesizing cell constituents from carbon dioxide with energy from inorganic reactions.

che·mo·cau·tery (-kaw′ter-e) cauterization by application of a caustic substance.

che·mo·dec·to·ma (-dek-to′mah) any benign, chromaffin-negative tumor of the chemoreceptor system, e.g., a carotid body tumor or glomus jugulare tumor.

che·mo·en·do·crine (-en′do-krin) chemohormonal.

che·mo·hor·mo·nal (-hor-mo′n'l) chemoendocrine; pertaining to drugs that have hormonal activity.

che·mo·kine (ke′mo-kīn) any of a group of low molecular weight cytokines identified on the basis of their ability to induce chemotaxis or chemokinesis in leukocytes (or in particular populations of leukocytes) in inflammation.

che·mo·ki·ne·sis (ke″mo-kĭ-ne′sis) increased nondirectional activity of cells due to the presence of a chemical substance.

che·mo·li·tho·tro·phic (-lith″o-tro′fik) deriving energy from the oxidation of inorganic compounds of iron, nitrogen, sulfur, or hydrogen; said of bacteria.

che·mo·nu·cle·ol·y·sis (-noo″kle-ol′ĭ-sis) dissolution of a portion of the nucleus pulposus of an intervertebral disk by injection of a proteolytic agent such as chymopapain, particularly used for treatment of a herniated intervertebral disk.

che·mo·or·gano·troph (-or′gah-no-trōf″) an organism that derives its energy and carbon from organic compounds.

che·mo·pal·li·dec·tomy (-pal″ĭ-dek′tah-me) chemical destruction of tissue of the globus pallidus.

che·mo·pro·phy·lax·is (-pro″fĭ-lak′sis) prevention of disease by means of a chemotherapeutic agent.

che·mo·re·sis·tance (-re-zis′tans) specific resistance acquired by cells to the action of certain chemicals.

che·mo·pro·tec·tant (-pro-tek′tant) providing protection, or an agent providing protection, against the toxic effects of chemotherapeutic agents.

che·mo·psy·chi·a·try (-si-ki′ah-tre) the treatment of mental and emotional disorders by drugs.

che·mo·ra·dio·ther·a·py (-ra″de-o-ther′ah-pe) combined modality therapy using chemotherapy and radiotherapy, maximizing their interaction.

che·mo·re·cep·tor (-re-sep′ter) a receptor sensitive to stimulation by chemical substances.

che·mo·sen·si·tive (-sen′sĭ-tiv) sensitive to changes in chemical composition.

che·mo·sen·sory (-sen′sah-re) relating to the perception of chemicals, as in odor detection.

che·mo·sis (ke-mo′sis) edema of the conjunctiva of the eye.

che·mo·sur·gery (ke″mo-ser′jer-e) destruction of tissue by chemical means for therapeutic purposes. **Mohs′ c.,** see under *technique.*

che·mo·syn·the·sis (-sin′thĕ-sis) the building up of chemical compounds under the influence of chemical stimulation, specifically the formation of carbohydrates from carbon dioxide and water as a result of energy derived from chemical reactions. **chemosynthet′ic,** adj.

che·mo·tax·in (-tak′sin) a substance, e.g., a complement component, that induces chemotaxis.

che·mo·tax·is (-tak′sis) taxis in response to the influence of chemical stimulation. **chemotac′tic,** adj.

che·mo·ther·a·py (-ther′ah-pe) treatment of disease by chemical agents. **adjuvant c.,** cancer chemotherapy employed after the primary tumor has been removed by some other method. **combination c.,** that combining several different agents simultaneously in order to enhance their effectiveness. **induction c.,** the use of drug therapy as the initial treatment for patients presenting with advanced cancer that cannot be treated by other means. **neoadjuvant c.,** initial use of chemotherapy in patients with localized cancer in order to decrease the tumor burden prior to treatment by other modalities. **regional c.,** chemotherapy, especially for cancer, administered as a regional perfusion.

che·mot·ic (ke-mot′ik) pertaining to or affected with chemosis.

che·mo·tro·phic (ke″mo-tro′fik) deriving energy from the oxidation of organic (chemoorganotrophic) or inorganic (chemolithotrophic) compounds; said of bacteria.

che·mot·rop·ism (ke-mot'ro-pizm) tropism due to chemical stimulation. **chemotrop'ic,** adj.

che·no·de·oxy·cho·lic ac·id (ke″no-de-ok″se-kol'ik) a primary bile acid, usually conjugated with glycine or taurine; it facilitates fat absorption and cholesterol excretion.

che·no·di·ol (ke″no-di'ol) chenodeoxycholic acid used as an anticholelithogenic agent to dissolve radiolucent, noncalcified gallstones.

cher·ub·ism (cher'ub-izm) hereditary progressive bilateral swelling at the angle of the mandible, and sometimes the entire jaw, giving a cherubic look to the face, in some cases enhanced by upturning of the eyes.

chest (chest) thorax. **flail c.,** one whose wall moves paradoxically with respiration, owing to multiple fractures of the ribs. **funnel c.,** pectus excavatum. **pigeon c.,** pectus carinatum.

chest·nut (chest'nut) a tree of the genus *Castanea* or a nut of various species; the wood and leaves of *C. dentata* (American chestnut) contain tannin and it has been used as an astringent and in pertussis. **horse c.,** the tree *Aesculus hippocastanum* or a preparation of the medicinal parts of its seeds, having antiexudative, antiinflammatory, and immunomodulatory activity and used in the treatment of chronic venous insufficiency, in homeopathy and in folk medicine.

CHF congestive heart failure.

chi, ch'i (che) qi.

chi·asm (ki'azm) a decussation or X-shaped crossing. **optic c.,** the structure in the forebrain formed by the decussation of the fibers of the optic nerve from each half of each retina.

chi·as·ma (ki-az'mah) pl. *chias'mata.* [L.] chiasm; in genetics, the points at which members of a chromosome pair are in contact during the prophase of meiosis and because of which recombination, or crossing over, occurs on separation.

chick·en·pox (chik'en-poks) varicella; a highly contagious disease caused by human herpesvirus 3, characterized by vesicular eruptions appearing over a period of a few days to a week after an incubation period of 17–21 days; usually benign in children, but in infants and adults may be accompanied by severe symptoms.

chig·ger (chig'er) the red larva of a mite of the family Trombiculidae; it attaches to a host's skin, and its bite produces a wheal with severe itching and dermatitis. Some species are vectors of the rickettsiae of scrub typhus.

chig·oe (chig'o) the flea, *Tunga penetrans,* of subtropical and tropical America and Africa; the pregnant female burrows into the skin of the feet, legs, or other part of the body, causing intense irritation and ulceration, sometimes leading to spontaneous amputation of a digit.

chil·blain (chil'blān) a recurrent localized itching, swelling, and painful erythema of the fingers, toes, or ears, caused by mild frostbite and dampness. Called also *chilblains.*

child·birth (chīld'berth) parturition; the process of giving birth to a child.

chill (chil) a sensation of cold, with convulsive shaking of the body.

Chi·lo·mas·tix (ki″lo-mas'tiks) a genus of parasitic protozoa found in the intestines of vertebrates, including *C. mesni'li,* a common species found as a commensal in the human cecum and colon.

chi·me·ra (ki-mir'ah) 1. an organism with different cell populations derived from different zygotes of the same or different species, occurring spontaneously or produced artificially. 2. a substance created from proteins or genes of two species, as by genetic engineering. **chimer'ic,** adj.

chin (chin) the anterior prominence of the lower jaw; the mentum.

chi·on·ablep·sia (ki″ah-nah-blep'se-ah) snow blindness.

chir(o)- word element [Gr.], *hand.* See also words beginning *cheir(o)-.*

chi·rop·o·dy (ki-rop'ah-de) podiatry.

chi·ro·prac·tic (ki″ro-prak'tik) a nonpharmaceutical, nonsurgical system of health care based on the self-healing capacity of the body and the primary importance of the proper function of the nervous system in the maintenance of health; therapy is aimed at removing irritants to the nervous system and restoring proper function. The most common method of treatment is by spinal manipulation and is primarily done for musculoskeletal complaints; other methods include lifestyle modification, nutritional therapy, and physiotherapy.

chi·square (ki'skwār) see under *distribution* and *test.*

chi·tin (ki'tin) an insoluble, linear polysaccharide forming the principal constituent of arthropod exoskeletons and found in some plants, particularly fungi.

CHL crown-heel length.

Chla·myd·ia (klah-mid'e-ah) a genus of the family Chlamydiaceae. Some strains of *C. psitta'ci* cause psittacosis, ornithosis, and other diseases; various strains of *C. tracho'matis* cause trachoma, inclusion conjunctivitis, urethritis, proctitis, and lymphogranuloma venereum.

Chla·myd·i·a·ceae (klah-mid″e-a′se-e) a family of bacteria (order Chlamydiales) consisting of small coccoid microorganisms that have a unique, obligately intracellular developmental cycle and are incapable of synthesizing ATP. They induce their own phagocytosis by host cells, in which they then form intracytoplasmic colonies. They are parasites of birds and mammals (including humans). The family contains a single genus, *Chlamydia.*

Chla·myd·i·al·es (klah-mid″e-a″lēz) an order of coccoid, gram-negative, parasitic microorganisms that multiply within the cytoplasm of vertebrate host cells by a unique development cycle.

chla·myd·i·o·sis (klah-mid″e-o′sis) any infection or disease caused by *Chlamydia.*

chlam·y·do·spore (klam′ĭ-do-spor″) a thick-walled intercalary or terminal asexual spore formed by the rounding-up of a cell; it is not shed.

chlo·as·ma (klo-az′mah) melasma.

chlor·ac·ne (klor-ak′ne) an acneiform eruption due to exposure to chlorine compounds.

chlo·ral (klor′al) 1. an oily liquid with a pungent, irritating odor; used in the manufacture of chloral hydrate and DDT. 2. c. hydrate. **c. hydrate,** a hypnotic and sedative, now used mainly as an adjunct to anesthesia and as a sedative for children undergoing medical and dental procedures.

chlor·am·bu·cil (klor-am′bu-sil) an alkylating agent from the nitrogen mustard group, used as an antineoplastic.

chlor·am·phen·i·col (klor″am-fen′ĭ-kol) a broad-spectrum antibiotic effective against rickettsiae, gram-positive and gram-negative bacteria, and certain spirochetes; used also as the palmitate ester and as the sodium succinate derivative.

chlor·cy·cli·zine (klor-si′klĭ-zēn) an H_1 histamine receptor antagonist with anticholinergic, antiemetic, and local anesthetic properties, used as the hydrochloride salt as an antihistaminic and antipruritic.

chlor·dane (klor′dān) a poisonous substance of the chlorinated hydrocarbon group, used as an insecticide.

chlor·di·az·ep·ox·ide (klor″di-az″ĕ-pok′sīd) a benzodiazepine used as the base or hydrochloride salt in the treatment of anxiety disorders and short-term or preoperative anxiety, for alcohol withdrawal, and as an antitremor agent.

chlor·emia (klor-e′me-ah) hyperchloremia.

chlor·hex·i·dine (klor-heks′ĭ-dēn) an antibacterial effective against a wide variety of gram-negative and gram-positive organisms; used also as the acetate ester, as a preservative for eyedrops, and as the gluconate or hydrochloride salt, as a topical anti-infective.

chlor·hy·dria (-hi′dre-ah) hyperchlorhydria.

chlo·ride (klor′īd) a salt of hydrochloric acid; any binary compound of chlorine in which the latter is the negative element.

chlor·id·or·rhea (klor″i-dor′e-ah) diarrhea with an excess of chlorides in the stool.

chlo·ri·nat·ed (klor′ĭ-nāt″ed) treated or charged with chlorine.

chlo·rine (Cl) (klor′ēn) chemical element (see *Table of Elements*), at. no. 17. It is a disinfectant, decolorant, and irritant poison, and is used for disinfecting, fumigating, and bleaching.

chlo·rite (klor′īt) a salt of chlorous acid; disinfectant and bleaching agent.

chlo·ro·form (klor′ah-form) a colorless, mobile liquid, $CHCl_3$, with an ethereal odor and sweet taste, used as a solvent; once widely used as an inhalation anesthetic and analgesic, and as an antitussive, carminative, and counterirritant. It is hepatotoxic and nephrotoxic by ingestion.

chlo·ro·labe (klor′ah-lāb) the pigment in retinal cones that is more sensitive to the green portion of the spectrum than are the other pigments (cyanolabe and erythrolabe).

chlo·ro·leu·ke·mia (klor″o-loo-ke′me-ah) chloroma.

chlo·ro·ma (klor-o′mah) a malignant, green-colored tumor arising from myeloid tissue, associated with myelogenous leukemia.

chlo·ro·phyll (klor′o-fil) any of a group of green magnesium-containing porphyrin derivatives occurring in all photosynthetic organisms; they convert light energy to reducing potential for the reduction of CO_2. Preparations of water-soluble chlorophyll salts are used as deodorizers; see *chlorophyllin.*

chlo·ro·phyl·lin (klor′o-fil-in) any of the water-soluble salts from chlorophyll; used topically and orally for deodorizing skin lesions and orally for deodorizing the urine and feces in colostomy, ileostomy, and incontinence; used particularly in the form of the copper complex.

chlo·ro·plast (-plast) any of the chlorophyll-bearing bodies of plant cells.

chlo·ro·priv·ic (klor″o-priv′ik) deprived of chlorides; due to loss of chlorides.

chlo·ro·pro·caine (-pro′kān) a local anesthetic, used as the hydrochloride salt.

chlo·rop·sia (klor-op′se-ah) defect of vision in which objects appear to have a greenish tinge.

chlo·ro·quine (klor′o-kwin) an antiamebic and anti-inflammatory used in the treatment of malaria, giardiasis, extraintestinal amebiasis, lupus erythematosus, and rheumatoid arthritis; used also as the hydrochloride and phosphate salts.

chlo·ro·thi·a·zide (klor″o-thi′ah-zīd) a thiazide diuretic used in the form of the base or the sodium salt to treat hypertension and edema.

chlo·ro·tri·an·i·sene (-tri-an′ĭ-sēn) a synthetic estrogen used to suppress lactation postpartum, for replacement therapy of estrogen deficiency, and for palliative treatment of prostatic carcinoma.

chlo·rox·ine (klor-ok′sēn) a synthetic antibacterial used in the topical treatment of dandruff and seborrheic dermatitis of the scalp.

chlor·phen·e·sin (klor-fen′ĕ-sin) an antibacterial, antifungal, and antitrichomonal agent used in the treatment of tinea pedis and other fungal and trichomonal infections of the skin and vagina. **c. carbamate,** a centrally acting skeletal muscle relaxant used in the treatment of musculoskeletal conditions characterized by skeletal muscle spasms.

chlor·phen·ir·amine (klor″fen-ir′ah-mēn) an antihistamine with sedative and anticholinergic effects; used as *c. maleate, c. polistirex,* and *c. tannate.*

chlor·pro·ma·zine (-pro′mah-zēn) a phenothiazine used in the form of the base or the hydrochloride salt as an antipsychotic, antiemetic, and presurgical sedative, and in the treatment of intractable hiccups, acute intermittent porphyria, tetanus, the manic phase of bipolar disorder, and severe behavioral problems in children.

chlor·pro·pa·mide (-pro′pah-mīd) a sulfonylurea used as a hypoglycemic in the treatment of type 2 diabetes mellitus.

chlor·tet·ra·cy·cline (-tet-rah-si′klēn) a broad-spectrum antibiotic obtained from *Streptomyces aureofaciens;* used as the hydrochloride salt.

chlor·thal·i·done (klor-thal′ĭ-dōn) a sulfonamide with similar actions to the thiazide diuretics; used in the treament of hypertension and edema.

chlor·ure·sis (klor″u-re′sis) excretion of excessive chlorides in the urine.

chlor·uret·ic (-u-ret′ik) 1. promoting chloruresis. 2. an agent that promotes the excretion of chlorides in the urine.

chlor·zox·a·zone (klor-zok′sah-zōn) a skeletal muscle relaxant used to relieve discomfort of painful musculoskeletal conditions.

ChM [L.] Chirur′giae Magis′ter (Master of Surgery).

cho·a·na (ko′ah-nah) pl. *cho′anae.* [L.] 1. infundibulum. 2. [pl.] the paired openings between the nasal cavity and the nasopharynx.

Cho·a·no·tae·nia (ko-a″no-te′ne-ah) a genus of tapeworms.

choke (chōk) 1. strangle; to interrupt respiration by obstruction or compression. 2. strangulation; the condition resulting from such an interruption. 3. (pl.) a burning sensation in the substernal region, with uncontrollable coughing, occurring during decompression.

chol·a·gogue (ko′lah-gog) an agent that stimulates gallbladder contraction to promote bile flow. **cholagog′ic,** adj.

cho·lan·ge·itis (ko-lan″je-i′tis) cholangitis.

cho·lan·gi·ec·ta·sis (-ek′tah-sis) dilatation of a bile duct.

cho·lan·gi·o·car·ci·no·ma (ko-lan″je-o-kahr″sĭ-no′mah) 1. an adenocarcinoma arising from the epithelium of the intrahepatic bile ducts and composed of epithelial cells in tubules or acini with fibrous stroma. 2. cholangiocellular carcinoma.

cho·lan·gi·o·cel·lu·lar (-sel′u-lar) of, resembling, or pertaining to cells of the cholangioles.

cho·lan·gio·en·ter·os·to·my (-en″ter-os′tah-me) surgical anastomosis of a bile duct to the intestine.

cho·lan·gio·gas·tros·to·my (-gas-tros′tah-me) anastomosis of a bile duct to the stomach.

cho·lan·gi·og·ra·phy (kol-an″je-og′rah-fe) radiography of the bile ducts.

cho·lan·gio·hep·a·to·ma (ko-lan″je-o-hep″ah-to′mah) hepatocellular carcinoma of mixed liver cell and bile duct cell origin.

cho·lan·gi·ole (ko-lan′je-ōl) one of the fine terminal elements of the bile duct system. **cholangi′olar,** adj.

cho·lan·gi·o·li·tis (ko-lan″je-o-li′is) inflammation of the cholangioles. **cholangiolit′ic,** adj.

cho·lan·gi·o·ma (-o′mah) cholangiocellular carcinoma.

cho·lan·gio·sar·co·ma (ko-lan″je-o-sahr-ko′mah) sarcoma of bile duct origin.

cho·lan·gi·os·to·my (kol″an-je-os′tah-me) fistulization of a bile duct.

cho·lan·gi·ot·o·my (-ot′ah-me) incision into a bile duct.

cho·lan·gi·tis (ko″lan-ji′tis) inflammation of a bile duct. **cholangit′ic,** adj.

cho·lano·poi·e·sis (kol″ah-no-poi-e′sis) the synthesis of bile acids or of their conjugates and salts by the liver.

cho·lano·poi·et·ic (-poi-et′ik) 1. promoting cholanopoiesis. 2. an agent that promotes cholanopoiesis.

cho·late (ko'lāt) a salt, anion, or ester of cholic acid.

chole- word element [Gr.], *bile.*

cho·le·cal·ci·fer·ol (ko″lĕ-kal-sif′er-ol) vitamin D₃; a hormone synthesized in the skin on irradiation of 7-dehydrocholesterol or obtained from the diet; it is activated when metabolized to 1,25-dihydroxychole-calciferol. It is used as an antirachitic and in the treatment of hypocalcemic tetany and hypoparathyroidism.

cho·le·cyst (ko'lĕ-sist) gallbladder.

cho·le·cyst·a·gogue (ko″lĕ-sis′tah-gog) an agent that promotes evacuation of the gall-bladder.

cho·le·cys·tal·gia (-sis-tal′jah) 1. biliary colic. 2. pain due to inflammation of the gallbladder.

cho·le·cys·tec·ta·sia (-sis″tek-ta′zhah) distention of the gallbladder.

cho·le·cys·tec·to·my (-sis-tek′tah-me) excision of the gallbladder.

cho·le·cyst·en·ter·os·to·my (-sis″ten-ter-os′tah-me) formation of a new communication between the gallbladder and the intestine.

cho·le·cys·ti·tis (-sis-ti′tis) inflammation of the gallbladder. **emphysematous c.,** that due to gas-producing organisms, marked by gas in the gallbladder lumen, often infiltrating into the gallbladder wall and surrounding tissues.

cho·le·cys·to·co·los·to·my (-sis″to-kah-los′tah-me) anastomosis of the gallbladder and colon.

cho·le·cys·to·du·o·de·nos·to·my (-doo″-o-dah-nos′tah-me) anastomosis of the gall-bladder and duodenum.

cho·le·cys·to·gas·tros·to·my (-gas-tros′-tah-me) anastomosis between the gallbladder and stomach.

cho·le·cys·to·gram (-sis′tah-gram) a radio-graph of the gallbladder.

cho·le·cys·tog·ra·phy (-sis-tog′rah-fe) radiography of the gallbladder. **cholecysto-graph′ic,** adj.

cho·le·cys·to·je·ju·nos·to·my (-sis″to-jĕ″joo-nos′tah-me) anastomosis of the gall-bladder and jejunum.

cho·le·cys·to·ki·net·ic (-kĭ-net′ik) stimulating contraction of the gallbladder.

cho·le·cys·to·ki·nin (CCK) (-ki′nin) a polypeptide hormone secreted in the small intestine that stimulates gallbladder contraction and secretion of pancreatic enzymes.

cho·le·cys·to·li·thi·a·sis (-lĭ-thi′ah-sis) the occurrence of gallstones (see *cholelithiasis*) within the gallbladder.

cho·le·cys·to·li·thot·o·my (-lĭ-thot′ah-me) incision of the gallbladder for removal of gallstones.

cho·le·cys·to·pexy (-sis′tah-pek″se) surgical suspension or fixation of the gallbladder.

cho·le·cys·tor·rha·phy (-sis-tor′ah-fe) suture or repair of the gallbladder.

cho·le·cys·tot·o·my (-sis-tot′ah-me) incision of the gallbladder.

cho·led·o·chal (ko-led′ĕ-k′l) pertaining to the common bile duct.

cho·le·do·chec·to·my (kol″ah-do-kek′tah-me) excision of part of the common bile duct.

cho·le·do·chi·tis (-ki′tis) inflammation of the common bile duct.

choledoch(o)- word element [Gr.], *common bile duct.*

cho·led·o·cho·du·o·de·nos·to·my (ko-led″o-ko-doo″o-dĕ-nos′tah-me) anastomosis of the common bile duct to the duodenum.

cho·led·o·cho·en·ter·os·to·my (-en″ter-os′tah-me) anastomosis of the bile duct to the intestine.

cho·led·o·cho·gas·tros·to·my (-gas-tros′-tah-me) anastomosis of the bile duct to the stomach.

cho·led·o·cho·je·ju·nos·to·my (-jĕ″joo-nos′tah-me) anastomosis of the bile duct to the jejunum.

cho·led·o·cho·li·thi·a·sis (-lĭ-thi′ah-sis) the occurrence of calculi (see *cholelithiasis*) in the common bile duct.

cho·led·o·cho·li·thot·o·my (-lĭ-thot′ah-me) incision into common bile duct for stone removal.

cho·led·o·cho·plas·ty (kol-ed′ah-kah-plas″te) plastic repair of the common bile duct.

cho·led·o·chor·rha·phy (kol-ed″o-kor′ah-fe) suture or repair of the common bile duct.

cho·led·o·chos·to·my (-kos′tah-me) creation of an opening into the common bile duct for drainage.

cho·led·o·chot·o·my (-kot′ah-me) incision into the common bile duct.

cho·led·o·chus (ko-led′ah-kus) common bile duct.

cho·le·ic (ko-le′ik) biliary.

cho·le·ic ac·id (ko-le′ik) any of the complexes formed between deoxycholic acid and a fatty acid or other lipid.

cho·le·lith (ko′lĕ-lith) gallstone.

cho·le·li·thi·a·sis (ko″lĕ-lĭ-thi′ah-sis) the presence or formation of gallstones.

cho·le·li·thot·o·my (-lĭ-thot′ah-me) incision of the biliary tract for removal of gallstones.

cho·le·litho·trip·sy (-lith′ah-trip″se) crushing of a gallstone.

cho·lem·e·sis (ko-lem'ĕ-sis) vomiting of bile.

cho·le·mia (ko-le'me-ah) bile or bile pigment in the blood. **chole′mic,** adj.

cho·le·peri·to·ne·um (ko″lĕ-per″ĭ-tah-ne'um) the presence of bile in the peritoneum.

cho·le·poi·e·sis (-poi-e'sis) the formation of bile in the liver. **cholepoiet′ic,** adj.

chol·era (kol'er-ah) Asiatic c.; an acute infectious disease endemic and epidemic in Asia, caused by *Vibrio cholerae,* marked by severe diarrhea with extreme fluid and electrolyte depletion, and by vomiting, muscle cramps, and prostration. **Asiatic c.,** see *cholera.* **pancreatic c.,** a condition marked by profuse watery diarrhea, hypokalemia, and usually achlorhydria, and due to an islet-cell tumor (other than beta cell) of the pancreas.

chol·er·a·gen (kol'er-ah-jen) the exotoxin produced by the cholera vibrio, thought to stimulate electrolyte and water secretion into the small intestine.

chol·e·ra·ic (kol″ah-ra'ik) of, pertaining to, or of the nature of cholera.

cho·ler·e·sis (ko-ler'ĕ-sis) the secretion of bile by the liver.

cho·ler·et·ic (ko″ler-et'ik) stimulating bile production by the liver; an agent that so acts.

chol·er·oid (kol'er-oid) resembling cholera.

cho·le·sta·sis (ko″lĕ-sta'sis) stoppage or suppression of bile flow, having intrahepatic or extrahepatic causes. **cholestat′ic,** adj.

cho·le·ste·a·to·ma (-ste″ah-to'mah) a cystlike mass lined with stratified squamous epithelium filled with desquamating debris, often including cholesterol, usually in the middle ear and mastoid region.

cho·le·ste·a·to·sis (-ste″ah-to'sis) fatty degeneration due to cholesterol esters.

cho·les·ter·ol (kah-les'ter-ol) a eukaryotic sterol that in higher animals is the precursor of bile acids and steroid hormones and a key constituent of cell membranes. Most is synthesized by the liver and other tissues, but some is absorbed from dietary sources, with each kind transported in the plasma by specific lipoproteins. It can accumulate or deposit abnormally, as in some gallstones and in atheromas. Preparations are used as emulsfiers in pharmaceuticals. **HDL c., high–density–lipoprotein c. (HDL-C),** the serum cholesterol carried on high-density lipoproteins, approximately 20 to 30 per cent of the total. **LDL c., low–density–lipoprotein c. (LDL-C),** the serum cholesterol carried on low-density lipoproteins, approximately 60 to 70 per cent of the total.

cho·les·ter·ol·emia (kah-les″ter-ol-e'me-ah) hypercholesterolemia.

cho·les·ter·ol es·ter·ase (kah-les'ter-ol es'ter-ās) acid lipase; an enzyme that catalyzes the hydrolytic cleavage of cholesterol and other sterol esters and triglycerides. Deficiency of the lysosomal enzyme causes the allelic disorders Wolman's disease and cholesteryl ester storage disease.

cho·les·ter·ol·o·sis (-o'sis) cholesterosis.

cho·les·ter·ol·uria (-u're-ah) cholesterol in the urine.

cho·les·ter·o·sis (kah-les″ter-o'sis) abnormal deposition of cholesterol in tissues.

cho·les·ter·yl (kah-les'ter-il″) the radical of cholesterol, formed by removal of the hydroxyl group.

cho·le·sty·ra·mine (ko″lĕ-sti'rah-mēn) see *cholestyramine resin,* under *resin.*

cho·le·ther·a·py (ko″lĕ-ther'ah-pe) treatment by administration of bile salts.

cho·lic ac·id (kol'ik) one of the primary bile acids in humans, usually occurring conjugated with glycine or taurine; it facilitates fat absorption and cholesterol excretion.

cho·line (ko'lēn) a quaternary amine, often classified as a member of the B vitamin complex; it occurs in phosphatidylcholine and acetylcholine, is an important methyl donor in intermediary metabolism, and prevents the deposition of fat in the liver. **c. magnesium trisalicylate,** see under *trisalicylate.* **c. salicylate,** see *salicylate.*

cho·line acet·y·lase (ko'lēn ah-set'ĭ-lās) choline acetyltransferase.

cho·line ac·e·tyl·trans·fer·ase (ko'lēn as″ĕ-tēl-trans'fer-ās) an enzyme catalyzing the synthesis of acetylcholine; it is a marker for cholinergic neurons.

cho·lin·er·gic (ko″lin-er'jik) 1. parasympathomimetic; stimulated, activated, or transmitted by choline (acetylcholine); said of the sympathetic and parasympathetic nerve fibers that liberate acetylcholine at a synapse when a nerve impulse passes. 2. an agent that produces such an effect.

cho·lin·es·ter·ase (-es'ter-ās) serum cholinesterase, pseudocholinesterase; an enzyme that catalyzes the hydrolytic cleavage of the acyl group from various esters of choline and some related compounds; determination of activity is used to test liver function, succinylcholine sensitivity, and whether organophosphate insecticide poisoning has occurred. **true c.,** acetylcholinesterase.

cho·li·no·cep·tive (ko″lin-o-sep'tiv) pertaining to the sites on effector organs that are acted upon by cholinergic transmitters.

cho·li·no·cep·tor (-sep'ter) cholinergic receptor.

cho·li·no·lyt·ic (-lit'ik) 1. blocking the action of acetylcholine, or of cholinergic agents. 2. an agent that blocks the action of acetylcholine in cholinergic areas, i.e., organs supplied by parasympathetic nerves, and voluntary muscles.

cho·li·no·mi·met·ic (-mi-met'ik) having an action similar to acetylcholine; parasympathomimetic.

chol(o)- word element [Gr.], *bile*.

chol·uria (kol-u're-ah) biluria. **cholu'ric**, adj.

cho·lyl·gly·cine (ko"lil-gli'sēn) a bile salt, the glycine conjugate of cholic acid.

cho·lyl·tau·rine (ko"lil-taw'rēn) a bile salt, the taurine conjugate of cholic acid.

chon·dral (kon'dril) pertaining to cartilage.

chon·dral·gia (kon-dral'jah) pain in a cartilage.

chon·drec·to·my (kon-drek'tah-me) surgical removal of a cartilage.

chon·dri·fi·ca·tion (kon"drĭ-fĭ-ka'shun) the formation of cartilage; transformation into cartilage.

chondri(o)- word element [Gr.], *granule*.

chon·dri·tis (kon-dri'tis) inflammation of a cartilage.

chondr(o)- word element [Gr.], *cartilage*.

chon·dro·an·gi·o·ma (kon"dro-an"je-o'mah) a benign mesenchymoma containing chondromatous and angiomatous elements.

chon·dro·blast (kon'dro-blast) an immature cartilage-producing cell.

chon·dro·blas·to·ma (kon"dro-blas-to'mah) a usually benign tumor derived from immature cartilage cells, occurring primarily in the epiphyses of adolescents.

chon·dro·cal·cif·ic (-kal-sif'ik) characterized by deposition of calcium salts in the cartilaginous structures of one or more joints.

chon·dro·cal·ci·no·sis (-kal"sĭ-no'sis) the presence of calcium salts, especially calcium pyrophosphate, in the cartilaginous structures of one or more joints.

chon·dro·cos·tal (-kos'til) pertaining to the ribs and costal cartilages.

chon·dro·cra·ni·um (-kra'ne-um) that part of the neurocranium formed by endochondral ossification and comprising the bones of the base of the skull.

chon·dro·cyte (kon'dro-sīt) one of the cells embedded in the lacunae of the cartilage matrix. **chondrocyt'ic**, adj.

chon·dro·der·ma·ti·tis (kon"dro-der"mah-ti'tis) an inflammatory process affecting cartilage and skin; usually refers to *c. nodula'ris chron'ica hel'icis*, a condition marked by a painful nodule on the helix of the ear.

chon·dro·dyn·ia (-din'e-ah) pain in a cartilage.

chon·dro·dys·pla·sia (-dis-pla'zhah) dyschondroplasia. **c. puncta'ta**, a heterogeneous group of hereditary bone dysplasias, the common characteristic of which is stippling of the epiphyses in infancy.

chon·dro·dys·tro·phia (-dis-tro'fe-ah) chondrodystrophy.

chon·dro·dys·tro·phy (-dis'trah-fe) a disorder of cartilage formation.

chon·dro·ec·to·der·mal (-ek"to-der'm'l) of or pertaining to cartilaginous and ectodermal elements.

chon·dro·epi·phys·itis (-ep"ĭ-fiz-i'tis) inflammation involving the epiphyseal cartilages.

chon·dro·fi·bro·ma (-fi-bro'mah) a fibroma with cartilaginous elements.

chon·dro·gen·e·sis (-jen'ĕ-sis) formation of cartilage.

chon·droid (kon'droid) 1. resembling cartilage. 2. hyaline cartilage.

chon·dro·i·tin sul·fate (kon-dro'ĭ-tin) 1. a glycosaminoglycan that predominates in connective tissue, particularly cartilage, bone, and blood vessels, and in the cornea. 2. a preparation of chondroitin sulfate from bovine tracheal cartilage, administered orally for the treatment of osteoarthritis and joint pain.

chon·dro·li·po·ma (kon"dro-lĭ-po'mah) a benign mesenchymoma with cartilaginous and lipomatous elements.

chon·dro·ma (kon-dro'mah) pl. *chondromas, chondro'mata*. A benign tumor or tumor-like growth of mature hyaline cartilage. It may remain centrally within the substance of a cartilage or bone (*enchondroma*) or may develop on the surface (*juxtacortical* or *periosteal c.*). **joint c.**, a mass of cartilage in the synovial membrane of a joint. **synovial c.**, a cartilaginous body formed in a synovial membrane.

chon·dro·ma·la·cia (kon"dro-mah-la'shah) abnormal softening of cartilage.

chon·dro·ma·to·sis (-mah-to'sis) formation of multiple chondromas. **synovial c.**, a rare condition in which cartilage is formed in the synovial membrane of joints, tendon sheaths, or bursae, sometimes being detached and producing a number of loose bodies.

chon·dro·mere (kon'dro-mēr) a cartilaginous vertebra of the fetal vertebral column.

chon·dro·meta·pla·sia (kon"dro-met"ah-pla'zhah) a condition characterized by metaplastic activity of the chondroblasts.

chon·dro·my·o·ma (-mi-o'mah) a benign tumor of myomatous and cartilaginous elements.

chon·dro·myx·oid (-mik′soid) of, pertaining to, or characterized by chondroid and myxoid elements.

chon·dro·myx·o·ma (-mik-so′mah) chondromyxoid fibroma.

chon·dro·myxo·sar·co·ma (-mik″so-sahr-ko′mah) a malignant mesenchymoma containing cartilaginous and myxoid elements.

chon·dro·os·se·ous (-os′e-us) composed of cartilage and bone.

chon·drop·a·thy (kon-drop′ah-the) disease of cartilage.

chon·dro·phyte (kon′dro-fīt) a cartilaginous growth at the articular end of a bone.

chon·dro·pla·sia (kon″dro-pla′zhah) the formation of cartilage by specialized cells (chondrocytes).

chon·dro·plast (kon′dro-plast) chondroblast.

chon·dro·plas·ty (-plas″te) plastic repair of cartilage.

chon·dro·po·ro·sis (kon″dro-por-o′sis) the formation of sinuses or spaces in cartilage.

chon·dro·sar·co·ma (-sar-ko′ma) a malignant tumor derived from cartilage cells or their precursors. **central c.,** one within a bone, usually not associated with a mass.

chon·dro·sis (kon-dro′sis) cartilage formation.

chon·dros·te·o·ma (kon″dros-te-o′mah) osteochondroma.

chon·dro·ster·nal (kon″dro-ster′n'l) pertaining to the costal cartilages and the sternum.

chon·dro·ster·no·plas·ty (-ster′no-plas″te) surgical correction of funnel chest.

chon·drot·o·my (kon-drot′ah-me) the dissection or surgical division of cartilage.

chon·dro·xi·phoid (kon″dro-zi′foid) pertaining to the xiphoid process.

chord (kord) cord.

chor·da (kor′dah) pl. *chor′dae.* [L.] a cord or sinew. **chor′dal,** adj. **c. dorsa′lis,** notochord. **c. mag′na,** Achilles tendon. **chor′dae ten·di′neae cor′dis,** tendinous cords connecting the two atrioventricular valves to the appropriate papillary muscles in the heart ventricles. **c. tym′pani,** a nerve originating from the intermediate nerve, distributed to the submandibular, sublingual, and lingual glands and anterior two thirds of the tongue; it is a parasympathetic and special sensory nerve.

Chor·da·ta (kor-dāt′ah) a phylum of the animal kingdom comprising all animals having a notochord during some developmental stage.

chor·date (kor′dāt) 1. an animal of the Chordata. 2. having a notochord.

chor·dee (kor′de) downward bowing of the penis, due to a congenital anomaly or to urethral infection.

chor·di·tis (kor-di′tis) inflammation of a vocal cord or spermatic cord.

chor·do·ma (kor-do′mah) a malignant tumor arising from the embryonic remains of the notochord.

Chor·do·pox·vi·ri·nae (kor″do-poks″vir-i′ne) poxviruses of vertebrates: a subfamily of viruses of the family Poxviridae, containing the poxviruses that infect vertebrates. It includes the genus *Orthopoxvirus.*

chor·do·skel·e·ton (kor″do-skel′ĕ-ton) the part of the bony skeleton formed about the notochord.

chor·dot·o·my (kor-dot′ah-me) cordotomy.

cho·rea (ko-re′ah) [L.] the ceaseless occurrence of rapid, jerky, dyskinetic, involuntary movements. **chore′ic,** adj. **acute c.,** Sydenham's c. **chronic c., chronic progressive hereditary c.,** Huntington's c. **hereditary c., Huntington's c.,** a hereditary disease marked by chronic progressive chorea and mental deterioration to dementia. **Sydenham's c.,** a self-limited disorder, occurring between the ages of 5 and 15, or during pregnancy, linked with rheumatic fever, and marked by involuntary movements that gradually become severe, affecting all motor activities.

cho·re·i·form (ko-re′ĭ-form) resembling chorea.

cho·reo·acan·tho·cy·to·sis (kor″e-o-ah-kan″tho-si-to′sis) an autosomal recessive syndrome characterized by tics, chorea, and personality changes, with acanthocytes in the blood.

cho·reo·ath·e·to·sis (-ath″ĕ-to′-sis) a condition characterized by choreic and athetoid movements. **choreoathetot′ic,** adj.

chori(o)- word element [Gr.], *membrane.*

cho·rio·ad·e·no·ma (kor″e-o-ad″ĕ-no′mah) adenoma of the chorion. **c. destru′ens,** a hydatidiform mole in which molar chorionic villi enter the myometrium or parametrium or, rarely, are transported to distant sites, most often the lungs.

cho·rio·al·lan·to·is (-ah-lan′to-is) an extra-embryonic structure formed by union of the chorion and allantois, which by means of vessels in the associated mesoderm serves in gas exchange. In reptiles and birds, it is a membrane apposed to the shell; in many mammals, it forms the placenta. **chorioallanto′ic,** adj.

cho·rio·am·ni·o·ni·tis (-am″ne-o-ni′tis) inflammation of the chorion and amnion.

cho·rio·an·gi·o·ma (-an″je-o′mah) an angioma of the chorion.

cho·rio·cap·il·la·ris (-kap″ĭ-la′ris) lamina choroidocapillaris.

cho·rio·car·ci·no·ma (-kahr″sĭ-no′mah) a malignant neoplasm of trophoblastic cells, formed by abnormal proliferation of the placental epithelium, without production of chorionic villi; most arise in the uterus.

cho·rio·cele (kor′e-o-sēl″) protrusion of the chorion through an aperture.

cho·rio·epi·the·li·o·ma (kor″e-o-ep″ĭ-the-le-o′mah) choriocarcinoma.

cho·rio·gen·e·sis (-jen′ĕ-sis) the development of the chorion.

cho·rio·gon·a·do·tro·pin (kor″e-o-go-nad″ah-tro′pin) chorionic gonadotropin. **c. alfa,** human chorionic gonadotropin (q.v.) produced by recombinant technology, used to induce ovulation and pregnancy in certain infertile, anovulatory women, and to stimulate oocyte development and maturation in patients using assisted reproductive technologies.

cho·ri·oid (kor′e-oid) choroid.

cho·ri·o·ma (kor″e-o′mah) 1. any trophoblastic proliferation, benign or malignant. 2. choriocarcinoma.

cho·rio·men·in·gi·tis (kor″e-o-men″in-ji′-tis) cerebral meningitis with lymphocytic infiltration of the choroid plexus. **lymphocytic c.,** viral meningitis, occurring in adults between the ages of 20 and 40, during the fall and winter.

cho·ri·on (kor′e-on) 1. in human embryology, the cellular, outermost extraembryonic membrane, composed of trophoblast lined with mesoderm; it develops villi, becomes vascularized by allantoic vessels, and forms the fetal part of the placenta. 2. in mammalian embryology, the cellular, outer extraembryonic membrane, not necessarily developing villi. 3. in biology, the noncellular membrane covering eggs of various animals; e.g., fish and insects. **chorion′ic,** adj. **c. frondo′sum,** the part of chorion bearing villi. **c. lae′ve,** the nonvillous, membranous part of the chorion. **shaggy c., villous c.,** c. frondosum.

cho·rio·ret·i·nal (kor″e-o-ret′ĭ-nal) pertaining to the choroid and retina.

cho·rio·ret·i·ni·tis (-ret″ĭ-ni′tis) inflammation of the choroid and retina.

cho·rio·ret·i·nop·a·thy (-ret″in-op′ah-the) a noninflammatory process involving both the choroid and retina.

cho·ris·ta (ko-ris′tah) defective development due to, or marked by, displacement of the primordium.

cho·ris·to·ma (ko″ris-to′mah) a mass of histologically normal tissue in an abnormal location.

cho·roid (ko′roid) 1. the middle, vascular coat of the eye, between the sclera and the retina. **choroid′al,** adj. 2. resembling the chorion.

cho·roi·dea (ko-roi′de-ah) choroid.

cho·roid·er·e·mia (ko-roi″der-e′me-ah) an X-linked primary choroidal degeneration which, in males, eventually leads to blindness as degeneration of the retinal pigment epithelium progresses to complete atrophy; in females, it is nonprogressive and vision is usually normal.

cho·roid·itis (kor″oid-i′tis) inflammation of the choroid.

cho·roi·do·cyc·li·tis (kor-oi″do-sik-li′tis) inflammation of the choroid and ciliary processes.

chro·maf·fin (kro-maf′in) staining strongly with chromium salts, as the chromaffin cells.

chro·maf·fi·no·ma (kro-maf″ĭ-no′mah) any tumor containing chromaffin cells, such as pheochromocytoma.

chro·maf·fi·nop·a·thy (-nop′ah-the) disease of the chromaffin system.

chro·mate (kro′māt) any salt of chromic acid.

chro·mat·ic (kro-mat′ik) 1. pertaining to color; stainable with dyes. 2. pertaining to chromatin.

chro·ma·tid (kro′mah-tid) either of two parallel, spiral filaments joined at the centromere which make up a chromosome.

chro·ma·tin (kro′mah-tin) the substance of chromosomes, the portion of the cell nucleus that stains with basic dyes. See *euchromatin* and *heterochromatin.* **sex c.,** Barr body; the persistent mass of the inactivated X chromosome in cells of normal females.

chro·ma·tin-neg·a·tive (-neg′ah-tiv) lacking sex chromatin, a characteristic of the nuclei of cells in a normal male.

chro·ma·tin-pos·i·tive (-poz′it-iv) containing sex chromatin, a characteristic of the nuclei of cells in a normal female.

chro·ma·tism (kro′mah-tizm) abnormal pigment deposits.

chromat(o)- word element [Gr.], *color; chromatin.*

chro·ma·tog·e·nous (kro″mah-toj′ĕ-nus) producing color or coloring matter.

chro·mato·gram (kro-mat′o-gram) the record produced by chromatography.

chro·mato·graph (kro-mat′o-graf) 1. the apparatus used in chromatography. 2. to analyze by chromatography.

chro·ma·tog·ra·phy (kro″mah-tog′rah-fe) a method of separating and identifying the components of a complex mixture by differential movement through a two-phase system, in which the movement is effected by a flow of a liquid or a gas (mobile phase) which percolates through an adsorbent (stationary phase) or a second liquid phase. **chromatograph′ic,** adj. **adsorption c.,** that in which the stationary phase is an adsorbent. **affinity c.,** that based on a highly specific biological interaction such as that between antigen and antibody or receptor and ligand, one such substance being immobilized and acting as the sorbent. **column c.,** that in which the various solutes of a solution are allowed to travel down an absorptive column, the individual components being absorbed by the stationary phase. **gas c. (GC),** that in which an inert gas moves the vapors of the materials to be separated through a column of inert material. **gas-liquid c. (GLC),** gas chromatography in which the stationary phase is a nonvolatile liquid coated on a solid support. **gas-solid c. (GSC),** gas chromatography in which the sorbent is an inert porous solid. **gel-filtration c., gel-permeation c.,** that in which the stationary phase consists of gel-forming hydrophilic beads containing specifically sized pores that trap and delay molecules small enough to enter them. **high-performance liquid c., high-pressure liquid c. (HPLC),** a type of automated chromatography in which the mobile phase is a liquid which is forced under high pressure through a column packed with a sorbent. **ion exchange c.,** that in which the stationary phase is an ion exchange resin. **molecular exclusion c., molecular sieve c.,** gel-filtration c. **paper c.,** that using a sheet of blotting paper, usually filter paper, for the adsorption column. **partition c.,** a method using the partition of the solutes between two liquid phases (the original solvent and the film of solvent on the adsorption column). **thin-layer c. (TLC),** chromatography through a thin layer of inert material, such as cellulose.

chro·ma·toid (kro′mah-toid) dying or staining like, or otherwise resembling, chromatin.

chro·ma·tol·y·sis (kro″mah-tol′ĭ-sis) disintegration of Nissl bodies of a neuron as a result of injury, fatigue, or exhaustion.

chro·ma·to·phil (kro-mat′o-fil) a cell or structure which stains easily. **chromatophil′ic,** adj.

chro·mato·phore (-for) any pigmentary cell or color-producing plastid.

chro·ma·top·sia (kro″mah-top′se-ah) a visual defect in which colorless objects appear to be tinged with color.

chro·ma·top·tom·e·try (kro″mah-top′tom′ĕ-tre) measurement of color perception.

chro·ma·tu·ria (kro″mah-tūr′e-ah) abnormal coloration of the urine.

chro·mes·the·sia (kro″mes-the′zhah) association of imaginary color sensations with actual sensations of taste, hearing, or smell.

chrom·hi·dro·sis (kro″mĭ-dro′sis) secretion of colored sweat.

chro·mic (kro′mik) of, pertaining to, or related to chromium. **c. phosphate P 32,** a radiolabeled phosphate salt of chromium used in the treatment of metastatic intrapleural or intraperitoneal effusions and of certain ovarian and prostate carcinomas.

chro·mic ac·id the common name for chromium trioxide (CrO_3), although the term strictly refers to the species H_2CrO_4, which exists only in aqueous solution. It is a highly toxic, corrosive, strong oxidizing agent.

chro·mid·ro·sis (kro″mĭ-dro′sis) chromhidrosis.

chro·mi·um (Cr) (kro′me-um) chemical element (see *Table of Elements*), at. no. 24. It is an essential dietary trace element, but hexavalent chromium is carcinogenic. **c. 51,** a radioactive isotope of chromium having a half-life of 27.7 days and decaying by electron capture with emission of gamma rays (0.32 MeV); it is used to label red blood cells for measurement of mass or volume, survival time, and sequestration studies, for the diagnosis of gastrointestinal bleeding, and to label platelets to study their survival. **c. trioxide,** chromic acid.

chrom(o)- word element [Gr.], *color.*

Chro·mo·bac·te·ri·um (kro″mo-bak-tēr′e-um) a genus of schizomycetes (family Rhizobiaceae) that characteristically produce a violet pigment.

chro·mo·blast (kro′mo-blast) an embryonic cell that develops into a pigment cell.

chro·mo·blas·to·my·co·sis (kro″mo-blas″to-mi-ko′sis) a chronic fungal infection of the skin, producing wartlike nodules or papillomas that may ulcerate.

chro·mo·clas·to·gen·ic (-klas″tah-jen′ik) inducing chromosomal disruption or damage.

chro·mo·cyte (kro′mo-sīt) any colored cell or pigmented corpuscle.

chro·mo·cys·tos·co·py (kro″mo-sis-tos′-kah-pe) cystoscopy of the ureteral orifices after oral administration of a dye which is excreted in the urine.

chro·mo·dac·ry·or·rhea (-dak″re-or-e′ah) the shedding of bloody tears.

chro·mo·gen (kro′mah-jen) any substance giving origin to a coloring matter.

chro·mo·gen·e·sis (kro″mo-jen′ĕ-sis) the formation of color or pigment.

chro·mo·mere (kro′mo-mēr) 1. any of the beadlike granules occurring in series along a chromonema. 2. granulomere.

chro·mo·my·co·sis (kro″mo-mi-ko′sis) chromoblastomycosis.

chro·mo·ne·ma (-ne′mah) pl. *chromone′-mata*. The central thread of a chromatid, along which lie the chromomeres. **chromone′mal**, adj.

chro·mo·phil (kro′mo-fil) any easily stainable cell or tissue. **chromophil′ic**, adj.

chro·mo·phobe (-fōb) any cell or tissue not readily stainable, such as the chromophobe cells in the adenohypophysis.

chro·mo·pho·bia (kro″mo-fo′be-ah) the quality of staining poorly with dyes. **chromopho′bic**, adj.

chro·mo·phore (kro′mo-for) any chemical group whose presence gives a decided color to a compound and which unites with certain other groups (auxochromes) to form dyes.

chro·mo·phor·ic (kro″mo-for′ik) 1. bearing color. 2. pertaining to a chromophore.

chro·mo·phose (kro′mo-fōs) sensation of color.

chro·mos·co·py (kro-mos′kah-pe) diagnosis of renal function by color of the urine after administration of dyes.

chro·mo·some (kro′mah-sōm) in animal cells, a structure in the nucleus containing a linear thread of DNA which transmits genetic information and is associated with RNA and histones; during cell division the material composing the chromosome is compactly coiled, making it visible with appropriate staining and permitting its movement in the cell with minimal entanglement; each organism of a species is normally characterized by the same number of chromosomes in its somatic cells, 46 being the number normally present in humans, including the two (XX or XY) which determine the sex of the organism. In bacterial genetics, a closed circle of double-stranded DNA which contains the genetic material of the cell and is attached to the cell membrane; the bulk of this material forms a compact bacterial nucleus. **chromoso′mal**, adj. **bivalent c.**, see *bivalent* (2). **homologous c's**, a matching pair of chromosomes, one from each parent, with the same gene loci in the same order. **Ph¹ c.**, Philadelphia c., an abnormality of chromosome 22, characterized by shortening of its long arms (the missing portion probably translocated to chromosome 9); present in marrow cells of patients with chronic granulocytic leukemia. **ring c.**, a chromosome in which both ends have been lost (deletion) and the two broken ends have reunited to form a ring-shaped figure. **sex c's**, those associated with sex determination, in mammals constituting an unequal pair, the X and the Y chromosome. **somatic c.**, autosome. **X c.**, a sex chromosome, carried by half the male gametes and all female gametes; female diploid cells have two X chromosomes. **Y c.**, a sex chromosome, carried by half the male gametes and none of the female gametes; male diploid cells have an X and a Y chromosome.

chro·nax·ie (kro′nak-se) chronaxy.

chro·naxy (kro′nak-se) the minimum time an electric current must flow at a voltage twice the rheobase to cause a muscle to contract.

chron·ic (kron′ik) persisting for a long time.

chron(o)- word element [Gr.], *time*.

chron·o·bi·ol·o·gy (kron″o-bi-ol′ah-je) the scientific study of the effect of time on living systems and of biological rhythms. **chronobiolog′ic, chronobiolog′ical**, adj.

chron·og·no·sis (kron″og-no′sis) perception of the lapse of time.

chron·o·graph (kron′ah-graf) an instrument for recording small intervals of time.

chro·no·tar·ax·is (kron″o-tar-ak′sis) disorientation in relation to time.

chro·not·ro·pism (kro-not′ro-pizm) interference with regularity of a periodical movement, such as the heart's action. **chronotro′pic**, adj.

chry·si·a·sis (krĭ-si′ah-sis) deposition of gold in living tissue.

chrys(o)- word element [Gr.], *gold*.

chryso·der·ma (kris″o-der′mah) permanent pigmentation of the skin due to gold deposit.

Chryso·my·ia (-mi′yah) a genus of flies whose larvae may be secondary invaders of wounds or internal parasites of humans.

Chrys·ops (kris′ops) a genus of small blood-sucking horse flies, including *C. disca′lis*, a vector of tularemia in the western United States, and *C. sild′cea*, an intermediate host of *Loa loa*.

chryso·tile (kris′o-tīl) the most widely used form of asbestos, a gray-green magnesium silicate in the serpentine class of asbestos; its dust may cause asbestosis or, rarely, mesotheliomas or other lung cancers.

CHS cholinesterase.

chy·lan·gi·o·ma (ki-lan″je-o′mah) a tumor of intestinal lymph vessels filled with chyle.

chyle (kīl) the milky fluid taken up by the lacteals from food in the intestine, consisting of an emulsion of lymph and triglyceride fat (chylomicrons); it passes into the veins by the thoracic duct and mixes with blood.

chyl·ec·ta·sia (ki″lek-ta′zhah) dilatation of a lacteal.

chy·le·mia (ki-le′me-ah) chyle in the blood.

chy·li·form (ki′li-form) resembling chyle.

chy·lo·cyst (ki′lo-sist) cisterna chyli.

chy·lo·me·di·as·ti·num (-me″de-as-ti′num) chyle in the mediastinum.

chy·lo·mi·cron (-mi′kron) a class of lipoproteins that transport exogenous (dietary) cholesterol and triglycerides after meals from the small intestine to tissues for degradation to chylomicron remnants.

chy·lo·mi·cro·ne·mia (-mi″kron-e′me-ah) an excess of chylomicrons in the blood.

chy·lo·peri·car·di·um (-per″ĭ-kahr′de-um) effused chyle in the pericardium.

chy·lo·peri·to·ne·um (-per″ĭ-ton-e′um) effused chyle in the peritoneal cavity.

chy·lo·pneu·mo·tho·rax (-noo″mo-thor′aks) chyle and air in the pleural cavity.

chy·lo·tho·rax (-thor′aks) pleural effusion of chyle or chylelike fluid.

chy·lous (ki′lus) pertaining to or mixed with chyle.

chy·lu·ria (kĭl-ūr′e-ah) chyle in the urine, due to obstruction between the intestinal lymphatics and the thoracic duct and rupture of renal lymphatics into the renal tubules.

chyme (kīm) the semifluid, creamy material produced by digestion of food.

chy·mi·fi·ca·tion (ki″mĭ-fĭ-ka′shun) conversion of food into chyme; gastric digestion.

chy·mo·pa·pain (ki″mo-pah-pān′) a cysteine endopeptidase from the tropical tree *Carica papaya*; it catalyzes the hydrolysis of proteins and polypeptides with a specificity similar to that of papain and is used in chemonucleolysis.

chy·mo·sin (ki′mo-sin) rennin; an enzyme that catalyzes the cleavage of casein to form soluble paracasein, which then reacts with calcium to form a curd, insoluble paracasein. It is found in the fourth stomach of the calf and other ruminants. A commercial preparation, rennet, is used for making cheese and rennet custards.

chy·mo·tryp·sin (ki″mo-trip′sin) an endopeptidase with action similar to that of trypsin, produced in the intestine by activation of chymotrypsinogen by trypsin; a product crystallized from an extract of the pancreas of the ox is used clinically for enzymatic zonulolysis and debridement.

chy·mo·tryp·sin·o·gen (-trip-sin′ŏ-jen) an inactive proenzyme secreted by the pancreas and cleaved by trypsin in the small intestine to yield chymotrypsin.

CI cardiac index; Colour Index.

Ci curie.

cib. [L.] ci′bus (food).

cic·a·trec·to·my (sik″ah-trek′tah-me) excision of a cicatrix.

cic·a·tri·cial (sik″ah-trish′il) pertaining to or of the nature of a cicatrix.

cic·a·trix (sĭ-ka′triks, sik′ah-triks) pl. *cica′trices*. [L.] scar. **vicious c.,** one causing deformity or impairing the function of a limb.

cic·a·tri·za·tion (sik″ah-trī-za′shun) the formation of a cicatrix or scar.

cic·lo·pir·ox (si″klo-pēr′oks) a broad-spectrum antifungal with activity similar to that of the imidazoles; applied topically as the olamine salt.

ci·dof·o·vir (sĭ-dof′o-vir) an antiviral nucleoside analogue used in the treatment of cytomegalovirus retinitis in patients with acquired immunodeficiency syndrome.

-cide word element [L.], *destruction or killing* (homicide); *an agent which kills or destroys* (germicide). **-ci′dal,** adj.

ci·gua·tox·in (se′gwah-tok″sin) a heat-stable toxin originating in the dinoflagellate *Gambierdiscus toxicus* as a pretoxin and then concentrated as the active form in the tissues of certain marine fish; it causes ciguatera.

ci·gua·te·ra (se″gwah-ta′rah) a form of ichthyosarcotoxism, marked by gastrointestinal and neurologic symptoms due to ingestion of tropical or subtropical marine fish that have ciguatoxin in their tissues.

ci·la·stat·in a dipeptidase inhibitor used with imipenem to decrease the metabolism of imipenem in the kidneys and increase its concentration in the urine; administered as the sodium salt.

cil·ia (sil′e-ah) sing. *cil′ium* [L.] 1. the eyelids or their outer edges. 2. the eyelashes. 3. minute hairlike processes that extend from a cell surface, composed of nine pairs of microtubules around a core of two microtubules. They beat rhythmically to move the cell or to move fluid or mucus over the surface.

cil·i·ar·ot·o·my (sil″e-er-ot′ah-me) surgical division of the ciliary zone.

cil·i·ary (sil′e-ĕ″re) pertaining to or resembling cilia; used particularly in reference to certain eye structures, as the ciliary body or muscle.

Cil·i·a·ta (sil″e-a′tah) a class of protozoa (subphylum Ciliophora) whose members possess cilia throughout the life cycle; a few species are parasitic.

cil·i·ate (sil′e-āt) 1. having cilia. 2. any individual of the Ciliophora.

cil·i·ec·to·my (sil″e-ek′tah-me) 1. excision of a portion of the ciliary body. 2. excision of the portion of the eyelid containing the roots of the lashes.

cili(o)- word element [L.], *cilia, ciliary (body)*.

Cil·i·oph·o·ra (sil″e-of′ah-rah) a phylum of protozoa whose members possess cilia during some developmental stage and usually have two kinds of nuclei (a micro- and a macro-nucleus); it includes the Kinetofragmino-phorea, Oligohymenophorea, and Polyhy-menophorea.

cil·io·spi·nal (sil″e-o-spi′n′l) pertaining to the ciliary body and the spinal cord.

cil·i·um (sil′e-um) [L.] singular of *cilia*.

cil·lo·sis (sil-o′sis) spasms of the eyelid.

cil·o·sta·zol (sĭ-lo′stah-zol) a phospho-diesterase inhibitor that inhibits platelet aggregation and causes vasodilation; used in the treatment of intermittent claudication.

cim·bia (sim′be-ah) a white band running across the ventral surface of the crus cerebri.

ci·met·i·dine (si-met′ĭ-dēn) a histamine H_2 receptor antagonist, which inhibits gas-tric acid secretion; used as the base or the monohydrochloride salt in the treatment and prophylaxis of gastric or duodenal ulcers, gastroesophageal reflux disease, upper gastro-intestinal bleeding, and conditions associated with gastric hypersecretion.

Ci·mex (si′meks) [L.] a genus of blood-sucking insects (order Hemiptera), the bed-bugs; it includes *C. boue′ti* of West Africa and South America, *C. lectula′rius*, the com-mon bedbug of temperate regions, and *C. rotunda′tus* of the tropics.

CIN cervical intraepithelial neoplasia.

cin·cho·na (sin-ko′nah) the dried bark of the stem or root of various South American trees of the genus *Cinchona*; it is the source of quinine and other alkaloids and was used as an antimalarial.

cin·cho·nism (-nizm) toxicity due to cinchona alkaloid overdosage; symptoms are tinnitus and slight deafness, photophobia and other visual disturbances, mental dullness, depression, confusion, headache, and nausea.

cine- word element [Gr.], *movement*; see also words beginning *kine-*.

cine·an·gio·car·diog·ra·phy (sin″ĕ-an″je-o-kahr″de-og′rah-fe) the photographic re-cording of fluoroscopic images of the heart and great vessels by motion picture tech-niques.

cine·an·gi·og·ra·phy (-an″je-og′rah-fe) the photographic recording of fluoroscopic images of the blood vessels by motion picture techniques.

cine·ra·di·og·ra·phy (-ra″de-og′rah-fe) the making of a motion picture record of suc-cessive images appearing on a fluoroscopic screen.

ci·ne·rea (sĭ-ne′re-ah) the gray matter of the nervous system. **cine′real**, adj.

cinesi- for words beginning thus, see those beginning *kinesi-*.

cin·gu·late (sing′gu-lāt) pertaining to a cingulum.

cin·gu·lec·to·my (sing″gu-lek′tah-me) bi-lateral extirpation of the anterior half of the cingulate gyrus.

cin·gu·lot·o·my (sing″gu-lot′ah-me) the creation of lesions in the cingulate gyrus for relief of intractable pain and in the treatment of certain psychiatric disorders.

cin·gu·lum (sing′gu-lum) pl. *cin′gula*. [L.] 1. an encircling structure or part; a girdle. 2. a bundle of association fibers encircling the corpus callosum close to the median plane, interrelating the cingulate and hippo-campal gyri. 3. the lingual lobe of an anterior tooth.

cin·gu·lum·ot·o·my (sing″gu-lum-ot′ah-me) cingulotomy.

C1 INH C1 inhibitor.

cip·ro·flox·a·cin (sip″ro-flok′sah-sin) a synthetic antibacterial effective against many gram-positive and gram-negative bacteria; used as the hydrochloride salt.

cir·ca·di·an (ser-ka′de-an) denoting a 24-hour period; see under *rhythm*.

cir·ci·nate (ser′sĭ-nāt) 1. circular. 2. ring-shaped.

cir·cle (ser′k′l) a round structure or part. **cerebral arterial c.**, c. of Willis. **Berry's c's**, charts with circles on them for testing stereoscopic vision. **defensive c.**, the coex-istence of two conditions which tend to have an antagonistic or inhibiting effect on each other. **c. of Haller**, a circle of arteries in the sclera at the site of the entrance of the optic nerve. **Minsky's c's**, a series of circles used for the graphic recording of eye lesions. **c. of Willis**, the anastomotic loop of vessels near the base of the brain.

cir·cuit (ser′kit) [L.] the round or course traversed by an electric current. **reverber-ating c.**, a neuronal pathway arranged in a circle so that impulses are recycled to cause positive feedback or reverberation. **reen-trant c.**, the circuit formed by the circulating impulse in reentry.

cir·cu·la·tion (ser″ku-la′shun) movement in a regular course, as the movement of blood through the heart and blood vessels. **collat-eral c.**, that carried on through secondary channels after obstruction of the principal channel supplying the part. **enterohepatic c.**, the cycle in which bile salts and other substances excreted by the liver are absorbed by the intestinal mucosa and returned to the liver via the portal circulation. **cir·cu·a·corpo·real c.,** circulation of blood outside the body, as through an artificial kidney or a heart-lung apparatus. **fetal c.,** that propelled by the fetal heart through the fetus, umbilical cord, and placental villi. **first c.,** primordial c. **hypophysioportal c.,** that passing from the capillaries of the median eminence of the hypothalamus into the portal vessels to the sinusoids of the adenohypophysis. **intervillous c.,** the flow of maternal blood through the intervillous space of the placenta. **lesser c.,** pulmonary c. **omphalomesenteric c.,** vitelline c. **persistent fetal c.,** pulmonary hypertension in the postnatal period secondary to right-to-left shunting of the blood through the foramen ovale and ductus arteriosus. **placental c.,** 1. the circulation of blood through the placenta during prenatal life. 2. intervillous c. **portal c.,** a general term denoting the circulation of blood through larger vessels from the capillaries of one organ to those of another; applied to the passage of blood from the gastrointestinal tract and spleen through the portal vein to the liver. **primordial c.,** the earliest circulation by which nutrient material and oxygen are conveyed to the embryo. **pulmonary c.,** the flow of blood from the right ventricle through the pulmonary artery to the lungs, where carbon dioxide is exchanged for oxygen, and back through the pulmonary vein to the left atrium. **systemic c.,** the general circulation, carrying oxygenated blood from the left ventricle to the body tissues, and returning venous blood to the right atrium. **umbilical c.,** fetal circulation through the umbilical vessels. **vitelline c.,** the circulation through the blood vessels of the yolk sac.

cir·cu·la·to·ry (ser′ku-lah-tor″e) 1. pertaining to circulation, particularly that of the blood. 2. containing blood.

cir·cu·lus (-lus) pl. *cir′culi.* [L.] a circle.

circum- word element [L.], *encircling.*

cir·cum·anal (ser″kum-a′n'l) surrounding the anus.

cir·cum·cise (ser′kum-sīz) to perform circumcision.

cir·cum·ci·sion (ser″kum-sizh′un) the removal of all or part of the foreskin of the penis in males; see also *female c.* **female c.,** any of various procedures involving either excision of a portion of the external female genitalia or infibulation. **pharaonic c.,** a type of female circumcision comprising two procedures: a radical form in which the clitoris, labia minora, and labia majora are removed and the remaining tissues approximated, and a modified form in which the prepuce and glans

of the clitoris and adjacent labia minora are removed. **Sunna c.,** a form of female circumcision in which the prepuce of the clitoris is removed.

cir·cum·duc·tion (-duk′shun) circular movement of a limb or of the eye.

cir·cum·fer·en·tial (-fer-en′shal) pertaining to a circumference; encircling; peripheral.

cir·cum·flex (serk′um-fleks) curved like a bow.

cir·cum·in·su·lar (serk″um-in′su-ler) surrounding, situated, or occurring about the insula.

cir·cum·len·tal (-len′t'l) situated or occurring around the lens.

cir·cum·pul·pal (-pul′p'l) surrounding the pulp.

cir·cum·re·nal (-re′nil) around the kidney.

cir·cum·scribed (serk′um-skrībd) bounded or limited; confined to a limited space.

cir·cum·stan·ti·al·i·ty (serk″um-stan″she-al′it-e) a disturbed pattern of speech or writing characterized by delay in getting to the point because of the interpolation of unnecessary details and irrelevant parenthetical remarks.

cir·cum·val·late (-val′āt) surrounded by a ridge or trench, as the vallate papillae.

cir·rho·sis (sĭ-ro′sis) a group of liver diseases marked by interstitial inflammation of the liver, loss of normal hepatic architecture, fibrosis, and nodular regeneration. **cirrhot′ic,** adj. **alcoholic c.,** a type in alcoholics, due to associated nutritional deficiency or chronic excessive exposure to alcohol as a hepatotoxin. **atrophic c.,** a type in which the liver is decreased in size, seen in posthepatic or postnecrotic cirrhosis and in some alcoholics. **biliary c.,** a type due to chronic bile retention after obstruction or infection of the major extra- or intrahepatic bile ducts *(secondary biliary c.),* or of unknown etiology *(primary biliary c.),* and sometimes occurring after administration of certain drugs. **cardiac c.,** fibrosis of the liver, probably following central hemorrhagic necrosis, in association with congestive heart disease. **fatty c.,** a form in which liver cells become infiltrated with fat. **Laënnec's c.,** a type associated with alcohol abuse. **macronodular c.,** a type that follows subacute hepatic necrosis due to toxic or viral hepatitis. **metabolic c.,** a type associated with metabolic diseases, such as hemochromatosis, Wilson's disease, glycogen storage disease, galactosemia, and disorders of amino acid metabolism. **portal c.,** Laënnec's c. **posthepatitic c.,** a type (usually macronodular) that is a sequel to acute hepatitis. **postnecrotic c.,** macronodular c.

cir·soid (ser'soid) resembling a varix.

cir·som·pha·los (ser-som'fah-los) caput medusae.

cis (sis) 1. in organic chemistry, having certain atoms or radicals on the same side. 2. in genetics, denoting two or more loci, especially pseudoalleles, occurring on the same chromosome of a homologous pair. Cf. *trans*. See also *cis-trans test*, under *test*.

cis- a prefix denoting on this side, the same side, or the near side.

cis·at·ra·cu·ri·um (sis"at-rah-kūr'e-um) a nondepolarizing neuromuscular blocking agent administered intravenously as the besylate salt as an adjunct to general anesthesia or during mechanical ventilation.

cis·plat·in (sis'plat-in) DDP; a platinum coordination complex capable of producing inter- and intrastrand DNA crosslinks; used as an antineoplastic.

cis·tern (sis'tern) a closed space serving as a reservoir for fluid, e.g., one of the enlarged spaces of the body containing lymph or other fluid. **cister'nal**, adj. **terminal c's**, pairs of transversely oriented channels that are confluent with the sarcotubules, which together with an intermediate T tubule constitute a triad of skeletal muscle.

cis·ter·na (sis-ter'nah) pl. *cister'nae*. [L.] cistern. **c. cerebellomedulla'ris poste'rior**, posterior cerebellomedullary cistern; the enlarged subarachnoid space between the undersurface of the cerebellum and the posterior surface of the medulla oblongata. **c. chy'li**, the dilated part of the thoracic duct at its origin in the lumbar region. **perinuclear c.**, the space separating the inner from the outer nuclear membrane.

cis·ter·nog·ra·phy (sis"ter-nog'rah-fe) radiography of the basal cistern of the brain after subarachnoid injection of a contrast medium.

cis·tron (sis'tron) the smallest unit of genetic material that must be intact to transmit genetic information; traditionally synonymous with gene.

ci·tal·o·pram (si-tal'o-pram) 1. an antidepressant compound used in the treatment of major depressive disorder, administered orally as the hydrobromide. 2. a selective serotonin reuptake inhibitor used as the hydrobromide salt as an antidepressant.

cit·rate (sit'rāt) a salt of citric acid. **c. phosphate dextrose (CPD)**, anticoagulant citrate phosphate dextrose solution. **c. phosphate dextrose adenine (CPDA-1)**, anticoagulant citrate phosphate dextrose adenine solution.

cit·ric ac·id (sit'rik) a tricarboxylic acid obtained from citrus fruits that is an intermediate in the tricarboxylic acid cycle; it chelates calcium ions and prevents blood clotting and functions as an anticoagulant for blood specimens and for stored whole blood and red cells. It is also used in the preparation of effervescent mixtures and as a synergist to enhance the action of antioxidants.

Cit·ro·bac·ter (sit'ro-bak"ter) a genus of gram-negative, facultatively anaerobic, rod-shaped bacteria of the family Enterobacteriaceae. *C. amalona'ticus*, *C. diver'sus*, and *C. freun'dii* have been associated with nosocomial infection, particularly in debilitated patients, and in neonates have caused meningitis and brain abscess.

cit·ron·el·la (si"tron-el'ah) a fragrant grass, the source of a volatile oil (citronella oil) used in perfumes and insect repellents.

cit·rul·line (sit'rul-ēn) an alpha-amino acid involved in urea production; formed from ornithine and itself converted into arginine in the urea cycle.

cit·rul·lin·emia (sit-rul"in-e'me-ah) 1. argininosuccinate synthase deficiency. 2. excess of citrulline in the blood.

cit·rul·lin·uria (-ūr'e-ah) 1. argininosuccinate synthase deficiency. 2. excessive citrulline in the urine.

CK creatine kinase.

Cl chlorine.

clad·o·spo·ri·o·sis (klad"o-spor"e-o'sis) any infection with *Cladosporium*, e.g., brain infections, chromoblastomycosis.

clad·ri·bine (kla'drĭ-bēn) a purine antimetabolite used as an antineoplastic in the treatment of hairy cell leukemia.

Clad·o·spo·ri·um (-spor'e-um) a genus of imperfect fungi. *C. carrio'nii* is a cause of chromoblastomycosis; *C. bantia'num* causes brain abscesses and sometimes meningitis.

clair·voy·ance (klār-voi'ans) [Fr.] extrasensory perception in which knowledge of objective events is acquired without the use of the senses.

clamp (klamp) a surgical device for compressing a part or structure. **rubber dam c.**, a metallic device used to retain the dam on a tooth.

clamping (klamp'ing) in the measurement of insulin secretion and action, the infusion of a glucose solution at a rate adjusted periodically to maintain a predetermined blood glucose concentration.

clap (klap) popular name for *gonorrhea*.

cla·pote·ment (klah-pōt-maw') [Fr.] a splashing sound, as in succession.

clar·if·i·cant (klaı-if'ı-kant) a substance which clears a liquid of turbidity.

cla·rith·ro·my·cin (klah-rith″ro-mi'sin) a macrolide antibiotic effective against a wide spectrum of gram-positive and gram-negative bacteria; used in the treatment of respiratory tract, skin, and soft tissue infections and of *Helicobacter pylori*–associated duodenal ulcer.

clasp (klasp) a device to hold something.

class (klas) 1. a taxonomic category subordinate to a phylum and superior to an order. 2. a subgroup of a population for which certain variables fall between specific limits.

clas·sic (klas'ik) standard, typical, or traditional.

clas·si·cal (klas'ı-k'l) classic.

clas·si·fi·ca·tion (klas″ı-fi-ka'shun) the systematic arrangement of similar entities on the basis of certain differing characteristics. **adansonian c.,** numerical taxonomy. **Angle's c.,** a classification of dental malocclusion based on the mesiodistal position of the mandibular dental arch and teeth relative to the maxillary dental arch and teeth; see under *malocclusion*. **Bergey's c.,** a system of classifying bacteria by Gram reaction, metabolism, and morphology. **Caldwell-Moloy c.,** classification of female pelves as gynecoid, android, anthropoid, and platypelloid; see under *pelvis*. **FIGO c.,** any of the classification systems established by the International Federation of Gynecology and Obstetrics for the staging of gynecological cancers. **Gell and Coombs c.,** a classification of immune mechanisms of tissue injury, comprising four types: *type I*, immediate hypersensitivity reactions, mediated by interaction of IgE antibody and antigen and release of histamine and other mediators; *type II*, antibody-mediated hypersensitivity reactions, due to antibody-antigen interactions on cell surfaces; *type III*, immune complex–mediated hypersensitivity reactions, local or general inflammatory responses due to formation of circulating immune complexes and their deposition in tissues; and *type IV* cell-mediated hypersensitivity reactions, initiated by sensitized T lymphocytes either by release of lymphokines or by T-cell–mediated cytotoxicity. **Keith-Wagener-Barker c.,** a classification of hypertension and arteriolosclerosis based on retinal changes. **Lancefield c.,** the classification of hemolytic streptococci into groups on the basis of serologic action. **New York Heart Association (NYHA) c.,** a functional and therapeutic classification for prescription of physical activity for cardiac patients. **Revised European American Lymphoma (REAL) C.,** a classification of lymphomas based on histologic criteria, dividing them into three main categories: B-cell neoplasms, T- or NK-cell neoplasms, and Hodgkin's disease.

clas·tic (klas'tik) 1. undergoing or causing division. 2. separable into parts.

clas·to·gen·ic (klas″tah-jen'ik) causing disruption or breakages, as of chromosomes.

clas·to·thrix (klas'tah-thriks) trichorrhexis nodosa.

clath·rate (klath'rāt) 1. having the shape of a lattice. 2. a clathrate compound, or pertaining or relating to a clathrate compound; see under *compound*.

clau·di·ca·tion (klaw″dĭ-ka'shun) limping; lameness. **intermittent c.,** pain, tension, and weakness in the legs on walking, which intensifies to produce lameness and is relieved by rest; it is seen in occlusive arterial disease. **jaw c.,** a complex of symptoms like those of intermittent claudication but seen in the muscles of mastication in giant cell arteritis. **neurogenic c.,** that accompanied by pain and paresthesias in the back, buttocks, and legs that is relieved by stooping, caused by mechanical disturbances due to posture or by ischemia of the cauda equina. **venous c.,** intermittent claudication due to venous stasis.

claus·tro·pho·bia (-fo'be-ah) irrational fear of being shut in, of closed places.

claus·trum (klaws'trum) pl. *claus'tra*. [L.] the thin layer of gray matter lateral to the external capsule, separating it from the white matter of the insula.

cla·va (kla'vah) gracile tubercle.

Clav·i·ceps (klav'ĭ-seps) a genus of parasitic fungi that infest various plant seeds. *C. purpu'rea* is the source of ergot.

clav·i·cle (klav'ĭ-k'l) see *Table of Bones*. **clavic'ular,** adj.

clav·i·cot·o·my (klav″ĭ-kot'ah-me) surgical division of the clavicle.

cla·vic·u·la (klah-vik'u-lah) [L.] clavicle; see *Table of Bones*.

clav·u·la·nate (klav'u-lah-nāt) a β-lactamase inhibitor used as the potassium salt in combination with penicillins in treating infections caused by β-lactamase–producing organisms.

cla·vus (kla'vus) pl. *cla'vi*. [L.] corn.

claw (klaw) a nail of an animal, particularly a carnivore, that is long and curved and has a sharp end. **cat's c.,** a woody South American vine, *Uncaria tomentosa* or a preparation of its root bark, which has antiviral, immunostimulant, and antiinflammatory properties and is used in folk medicine. **devil's c.,** a perennial herb, *Harpagophytum procumbens,* whose dried tubular secondary roots and lateral tubers are used for dyspepsia, loss of appetite, and rheumatism; also used in homeopathy for rheumatism and in folk medicine.

claw·foot (klaw′foot) a high-arched foot with the toes hyperextended at the metatarsophalangeal joint and flexed at the distal joints.

claw·hand (-hand) flexion and atrophy of the hand and fingers.

clear (klēr) 1. to remove cloudiness from microscopic specimens by the use of a clearing agent. 2. to remove a substance from the blood. 3. transparent; not cloudy, turbid, or opaque.

clear·ance (klēr′ans) 1. the act of clearing. 2. a quantitative measure of the rate at which a substance is removed from the blood, as by the kidneys, the liver, or hemodialysis; the volume of plasma cleared per unit time. Symbol *C.* 3. the space between opposed structures. **blood-urea c.,** urea c. **creatinine c.,** the volume of plasma cleared of creatinine after parenteral administration of a specified amount of the substance. **inulin c.,** an expression of the renal efficiency in eliminating inulin from the blood. **mucociliary c.,** the clearance of mucus and other materials from the airways by the cilia of the epithelial cells. **urea c.,** the volume of the blood cleared of urea per minute by either renal clearance or hemodialysis.

cleav·age (klēv′ij) 1. division into distinct parts. 2. the early successive splitting of a zygote into smaller cells (blastomeres) by mitosis.

cleaved (klēvd) split or separated, as by cutting.

cleft (kleft) a fissure, especially one occurring during embryonic development. **anal c.,** gluteal c. **branchial c.,** 1. any of the slit-like openings in the gills of fish, between the branchial arches. 2. pharyngeal groove. **facial c.,** 1. any of the clefts between the embryonic prominences that normally unite to form the face. 2. prosoposchisis; failure of union of a facial cleft, causing a developmental defect such as cleft cheek or lip. **gluteal c.,** that which separates the buttocks. **subneural c's,** evenly spaced lamella-like clefts within the primary synaptic cleft, formed by infoldings of the sarcolemma into the underlying muscle sarcolemma. **synaptic c.,** 1. a narrow extracellular cleft between the presynaptic and postsynaptic membranes. 2. synaptic trough. **visceral c.,** pharyngeal groove.

cleid(o)- word element [Gr.], *clavicle.*

clei·do·cra·ni·al (kli″do-kra′ne-il) pertaining to the clavicle and the head.

clei·dot·o·my (kli-dot′ah-me) surgical division of the clavicle of the fetus in difficult labor to facilitate delivery.

clem·as·tine (klem′as-tēn) an antihistamine with anticholinergic and sedative effects, used as the fumarate salt.

click (klik) a brief, sharp sound, especially any of the short, dry, clicking heart sounds during systole, indicative of various heart conditions.

cli·din·i·um (kli-din′e-um) an anticholinergic with pronounced antispasmodic and antisecretory effects in the gastrointestinal tract; used as the bromide salt.

cli·mac·ter·ic (kli-mak′ter-ik) 1. the syndrome of endocrine, somatic, and psychic changes occurring at menopause in women. 2. similar changes occurring in men owing to normal diminution of sexual drives with the aging process.

cli·max (kli′maks) the period of greatest intensity, as in the course of a disease (crisis), or in sexual excitement (orgasm).

clin·da·my·cin (klin″dah-mi′sin) a semisynthetic derivative of lincomycin used systemically, topically, and vaginally as an antibacterial, primarily against gram-positive bacteria; used also as the hydrochloride and phosphate salts and as the hydrochloride salt of the ester of clindamycin and palmitic acid.

clin·ic (klin′ik) 1. a clinical lecture; examination of patients before a class of students; instruction at the bedside. 2. an establishment where patients are admitted for study and treatment by a group of physicians practicing medicine together. **ambulant c.,** one for patients not confined to the bed. **dry c.,** a clinical lecture with case histories, but without patients present.

clin·i·cal (klin′ĭ-k′l) pertaining to a clinic or to the bedside; pertaining to or founded on actual observation and treatment of patients, as distinguished from theoretical or basic sciences.

cli·ni·cian (kli-nish′in) an expert clinical physician and teacher.

clin·i·co·patho·log·ic (klin″ĭ-ko-path″ah-loj′ik) pertaining to symptoms and pathology of disease.

Clin·i·stix (klin′ĭ-stiks) trademark for glucose oxidase reagent strips used to test for glucose in urine.

Clin·i·test (-test) trademark for alkaline copper sulfate reagent tablets used to test for reducing substances, e.g., sugars, in urine.

cli·no·ceph·a·ly (kli″no-sef′ah-le) congenital flatness or concavity of the vertex of the head.

cli·no·dac·ty·ly (-dak′til-e) permanent deviation or deflection of one or more fingers.

cli·noid (kli′noid) bed-shaped.

clip (klip) a metallic device for approximating the edges of a wound or for the prevention of bleeding from small individual blood vessels.

clis·e·om·e·ter (klis″e-om′ĕ-ter) an instrument for measuring the angles between the axis of the body and that of the pelvis.

clit·i·on (klit′e-on) the midpoint of the anterior border of the clivus.

clit·o·ri·dec·to·my (klit″ah-rĭ-dek′tah-me) excision of the clitoris.

clit·o·ri·dot·o·my (-dot′ah-me) incision of the clitoris; female circumcision.

clit·o·ri·meg·a·ly (-meg′ah-le) enlargement of the clitoris.

clit·o·ris (klit′ah-ris) the small, elongated, erectile body in the female, situated at the anterior angle of the rima pudendi and homologous with the penis in the male.

clit·o·rism (klit′ah-rizm) 1. hypertrophy of the clitoris. 2. persistent erection of the clitoris.

clit·o·ri·tis (klit″ah-ri′tis) inflammation of the clitoris.

clit·o·ro·plas·ty (klit′er-o-plas″te) plastic surgery of the clitoris.

cli·vog·ra·phy (kli-vog′rah-fe) radiographic visualization of the clivus, or posterior cranial fossa.

cli·vus (kli′vus) [L.] a bony surface in the posterior cranial fossa sloping upward from the foramen magnum to the dorsum sellae.

clo·a·ca (klo-a′kah) pl. *cloa′cae.* [L.] 1. a common passage for fecal, urinary, and reproductive discharge in most lower vertebrates. 2. the terminal end of the hindgut before division into rectum, bladder, and genital primordia in mammalian embryos. 3. an opening in the involucrum of a necrosed bone. **cloa′cal,** adj.

clo·a·co·gen·ic (klo″ah-ko-jen′ik) originating from the cloaca or from persisting cloacal remnants.

clo·be·ta·sol (klo-ba′tah-sol) a synthetic corticosteroid used topically as the propionate salt for the relief of inflammation and pruritus in corticosteroid-responsive dermatoses.

clock (klok) a device for measuring time. **biological c.,** the physiologic mechanism which governs the rhythmic occurrence of certain biochemical, physiologic, and behavioral phenomena in living organisms.

clo·cor·to·lone (klo-kor′to-lōn) a synthetic corticosteroid used topically as the pivalate ester for the relief of inflammation and pruritus in certain dermatoses.

clo·fi·brate (-fi′brāt) an antihyperlipidemic used to reduce serum lipids.

clomiphene (klo′mĭ-fēn) a nonsteroid estrogen analogue, used as the citrate salt to stimulate ovulation.

clo·mip·ra·mine (klo-mip′rah-mēn) a tricyclic antidepressant with anxiolytic activity, also used in obsessive-compulsive disorder, panic disorder, bulimia nervosa, cataplexy associated with narcolepsy, and chronic, severe pain; used as the hydrochloride salt.

clo·nal·i·ty (klo-nal′ĭ-te) the ability to be cloned.

clo·naz·e·pam (klo-naz′ĕ-pam) a benzodiazepine used as an anticonvulsant and as an antipanic agent.

clone (klōn) 1. the genetically identical progeny produced by the natural or artificial asexual reproduction of a single organism, cell, or gene, e.g., plant cuttings, a cell culture descended from a single cell, or genes reproduced by recombinant DNA technology. 2. to establish or produce such a line of progeny. **clo′nal,** adj.

clon·ic (klon′ik) pertaining to or of the nature of clonus.

clo·ni·dine (klo′nĭ-dēn) a centrally acting antihypertensive agent, used as the hydrochloride salt; also used in the prophylaxis of migraine and the treatment of dysmenorrhea, menopausal symptoms, opioid withdrawal, and cancer-related pain.

clon·ism (klon′izm) a succession of clonic spasms.

clo·no·gen·ic (klo″no-jen′ik) giving rise to a clone of cells.

clo·nor·chi·a·sis (klo″nor-ki′ah-sis) infection of the biliary passages with the liver fluke *Clonorchis sinensis,* causing inflammation of the biliary tree, proliferation of the biliary epithelium, and progressive portal fibrosis; extension into the liver parenchyma causes fatty changes and cirrhosis.

clono·spasm (klon′o-spazm) clonic spasm.

clo·nus (klo′nus) 1. alternate involuntary muscular contraction and relaxation in rapid succession. 2. a continuous rhythmic reflex tremor initiated by the spinal cord below an area of spinal cord injury, set in motion by reflex testing. **clon′ic,** adj. **ankle c., foot c.,** a series of abnormal reflex movements of the foot, induced by sudden dorsiflexion, causing alternate contraction and relaxation of the triceps surae muscle. **wrist c.,** spasmodic movement of the hand, induced by forcibly extending the hand at the wrist.

clo·pid·o·grel (klo-pid′o-grel) a platelet inhibitor used as an antithrombotic for the prevention of myocardial infarction, stroke, and vascular death in patients with atherosclerosis; used as the bisulfate salt.

clor·az·e·pate (klor-az′ĕ-pāt) a benzodiazepine used as the dipotassium salt as an antianxiety agent, anticonvulsant, and aid in the treatment of acute alcohol withdrawal.

Clos·trid·i·um (klos-trid′e-um) a genus of anaerobic spore-forming bacteria (family Bacillaceae). **C. bifermen′tans,** a species common in feces, sewage, and soil and associated with gas gangrene. **C. botu·li′num,** the causative agent of botulism, divided into six types (A through F) which elaborate immunologically distinct toxins. **C. diffi′cile,** a species often occurring transiently in the gut of infants, but whose toxin causes pseudomembranous enterocolitis in those receiving prolonged antibiotic therapy. **C. histoly′ticum,** a species found in feces and soil. **C. kluy′veri,** a species used in the study of both microbial synthesis and microbial oxidation of fatty acids. **C. no′vyi,** an important cause of gas gangrene. **C. oede·ma′tiens,** *C. novyi.* **C. perfrin′gens,** the most common etiologic agent of gas gangrene, distinguishable as several different types; *type A* causes human gas gangrene, colitis, and food poisoning and *type C* causes enteritis. **C. ramo′sum,** a species found in human and animal infections and feces and commonly isolated from clinical specimens. **C. sporo′genes,** a species widespread in nature, reportedly associated with pathogenic anaerobes in gangrenous infections. **C. ter′tium,** a species found in feces, sewage, and soil and present in some gangrenous infections. **C. te′tani,** a common inhabitant of soil and human and horse intestines, and the cause of tetanus in humans and domestic animals. **C. wel′chii,** British name for *C. perfringens.*

clos·trid·i·um (klos-trid′e-um) pl. *clostri′dia.* An individual of the genus *Clostridium.* **clos·trid′ial,** adj.

clot (klot) 1. coagulum; a semisolid mass, as of blood or lymph. 2. coagulate. **agony c.,** a type of antemortem clot formed in the process of dying. **antemortem c.,** one formed in the heart or in a large vessel before death but found after death. **blood c.,** a coagulum in the bloodstream formed of an aggregation of blood factors, primarily platelets, and fibrin with entrapment of cellular elements. **chicken fat c.,** a yellow-appearing blood clot, due to settling out of erythrocytes before clotting. **currant jelly c.,** a reddish

clot, due to the presence of erythrocytes enmeshed in it. **laminated c.,** a blood clot formed by successive deposits, giving it a layered appearance. **passive c.,** one formed in the sac of an aneurysm through which the blood has stopped circulating. **plastic c.,** one formed from the intima of an artery at the point of ligation, forming a permanent obstruction of the artery. **postmortem c.,** one formed in the heart or in a large blood vessel after death.

clot·ting (klot′ing) coagulation (1).

clo·trim·a·zole (klo-trim′ah-zōl) an imidazole derivative used as a broad-spectrum antifungal agent.

cloud·ing (klowd′ing) loss of clarity. **c. of consciousness,** a lowered level of consciousness marked by loss of perception or comprehension of the environment, with loss of ability to respond properly to external stimuli.

cloudy (clou′de) 1. murky; turbid; not transparent. 2. marked by indistinct streaks.

clove (klōv) the tropical tree *Syzygium aromaticum,* or its dried flower bud, which is used as a source of clove oil.

clo·ver (klo′ver) a leguminous plant with trifoliate leaves, sometimes specifically a member of the genera *Trifolium* or *Melilotus.* **red c.,** the leguminous plant *Trifolium pratense* or a preparation of its flower heads, which is used for coughs and respiratory symptoms and for chronic skin conditions; also used in traditional Chinese medicine.

clox·a·cil·lin (klok″sah-sil′in) a semisynthetic penicillin; used as the sodium salt to treat staphylococcal infections due to penicillinase-positive organisms.

clo·za·pine (klo′zah-pēn) a sedative and antipsychotic agent; used in the treatment of schizophrenia.

club·bing (klub′ing) proliferation of soft tissue around the ends of fingers or toes, without osseous change.

club·foot (-foot) a congenitally twisted foot; see *talipes.*

club·hand (-hand) a hand deformity analogous to clubfoot; talipomanus.

clump·ing (klump′ing) the aggregation of particles, such as bacteria, into irregular masses.

clu·nis (kloo′nis) pl. *clu′nes.* [L.] buttock. **clu′neal,** adj.

cly·sis (kli′sis) 1. the administration other than orally of any of several solutions to replace lost body fluid, supply nutriment, or raise blood pressure. 2. the solution so administered.

CM [L.] Chirur′giae Magis′ter (Master of Surgery).

Cm curium.

cm centimeter.

cm³ cubic centimeter.

CMA Canadian Medical Association; Certified Medical Assistant.

CMD cerebromacular degeneration.

CMHC community mental health center.

CMI cell-mediated immunity.

CMT Certified Medical Transcriptionist.

CMV cytomegalovirus.

CNA Canadian Nurses' Association.

C3 NeF C3 nephritic factor.

cne·mi·al (ne′me-il) pertaining to the shin.

Cni·da·ria (ni-dar′e-ah) a phylum of marine invertebrates including sea anemones, hydras, corals, jellyfish, and comb jellies, characterized by a radially symmetric body bearing tentacles around the mouth.

CNM Certified Nurse-Midwife; see *nurse-midwife*.

CNS central nervous system.

CO cardiac output.

Co cobalt.

COA Canadian Orthopaedic Association.

CoA coenzyme A.

co·ac·er·va·tion (ko-as″-er-va′shun) the separation of a mixture of two liquids, one or both of which are colloids, into two phases, one of which, the coacervate, contains the colloidal particles, the other being an aqueous solution, as when gum arabic is added to gelatin.

co·ad·ap·ta·tion (ko-ad″ap-ta′shun) the correlated changes in two interdependent organs.

co·ag·glu·ti·na·tion (ko″ah-gloo″tĭ-na′shun) the aggregation of particulate antigens combined with agglutinins of more than one specificity.

co·ag·u·la·bil·i·ty (ko-ag″u-lah-bil′it-e) the capability of forming or of being formed into clots.

co·ag·u·lant (ko-ag′u-lint) promoting or accelerating coagulation of blood; an agent that so acts.

co·ag·u·lase (-lās) an antigenic substance of bacterial origin, produced by staphylococci, which may be causally related to thrombus formation.

co·ag·u·late (-lāt) to undergo coagulation.

co·ag·u·la·tion (ko-ag″u-la′shun) 1. formation of a clot. 2. in surgery, the disruption of tissue by physical means to form an amorphous residuum, as in electrocoagulation and photocoagulation. 3. in colloid chemistry, the solidification of a sol into a gelatinous mass. **blood c.,** the sequential process by which the multiple coagulation factors of blood interact in the coagulation cascade,

resulting in formation of an insoluble fibrin clot. **diffuse intravascular c., disseminated intravascular c. (DIC),** a bleeding disorder characterized by reduction in the elements involved in blood clotting due to their use in widespread clotting within the vessels. In the late stages, it is marked by profuse hemorrhaging.

co·ag·u·la·tive (ko-ag′u-lah-tiv) associated with, of the nature of, or promoting a process of coagulation.

co·ag·u·lop·a·thy (ko-ag″u-lop′ah-the) any disorder of blood coagulation. **consumption c.,** disseminated intravascular coagulation.

co·ag·u·la·tor (ko-ag′u-la″ter) a surgical device that utilizes electrical current or light to stop bleeding. **argon beam c. (ABC),** a device that uses a jet of argon gas carrying electrical energy from a needle electrode recessed inside a probe to effect hemostasis in bleeding tissue.

co·ag·u·lum (ko-ag′u-lum) pl. *coagula*. [L.] clot (1).

co·a·les·cence (ko″ah-les′ens) the fusion or blending of parts.

co·a·li·tion (ko″ah-lĭ′shun) the fusion of parts that are normally separate. **tarsal c.,** the fibrous, cartilaginous, or bony fusion of two or more of the tarsal bones, often resulting in talipes planovalgus.

co·apt (ko-apt′) to approximate, as the edges of a wound.

co·ap·ta·tion (ko-ap-ta′shun) the process of approximating, or joining together.

co·arc·tate (ko-ark′tāt) 1. to press close together; contract. 2. pressed together; restrained.

co·arc·ta·tion (ko″ahrk-ta′shun) narrowing. **c. of aorta,** a local malformation marked by deformed aortic media, causing narrowing of the lumen of the vessel. **reversed c.,** Takayasu's arteritis.

coarse (kors) not fine; not microscopic.

coat (kōt) 1. tunica; a membrane or other tissue covering or lining an organ or part. 2. the layer(s) of protective protein surrounding the nucleic acid in a virus. **buffy c.,** the thin yellowish layer of leukocytes overlying the packed erythrocytes in centrifuged blood.

co·bal·a·min (ko-bal′ah-min) a compound comprising the substituted ring and nucleotide structure characteristic of vitamin B_{12}, either one lacking a ligand at the 6 position of cobalt or any substituted derivative, including cyanocobalamin, particularly one with vitamin B_{12} activity.

co·balt (Co) (ko′bawlt) chemical element (see *Table of Elements*), at. no. 27. Inhalation of the dust can cause pneumoconiosis and exposure to the powder can cause dermatitis. **c. 60,** a radioisotope of cobalt used in radiation therapy.

co·bra (ko′brah) any of several extremely poisonous elapid snakes commonly found in Africa, Asia, and India, which are capable of expanding the neck region to form a hood and have two comparatively short, erect, deep grooved fangs. Most inject venom by biting but some species, *spitting c's*, can eject a fine spray of venom several meters and cause severe eye irritation or blindness.

co·caine (ko-kān′) an alkaloid obtained from leaves of various species of *Erythroxylon* (coca plants) or produced synthetically, used as a local anesthetic; also used as the hydrochloride salt. Abuse can lead to addiction.

co·car·cin·o·gen (ko″kahr-sin′o-jen) promoter (3).

co·car·ci·no·gen·e·sis (ko-kahr″sĭ-no-jen′ĕ-sis) the development, according to one theory, of cancer only in preconditioned cells as a result of conditions favorable to its growth.

coc·ci (kok′si) plural of *coccus*.

Coc·cid·ia (kok-sid′e-ah) a subclass of parasitic protozoa comprising the orders Agamococcidiida, Protococcidiida, and Eucoccidiida.

coc·cid·ia (kok-sid′e-ah) plural of *coccidium*.

Coc·cid·i·oi·des (kok-sid″e-oi′dēz) a genus of pathogenic fungi, including *C. im′mitis*, the cause of coccidioidomycosis. **coccidioi′dal,** adj.

coc·cid·i·oi·din (-din) a sterile preparation containing byproducts of growth products of *Coccidioides immitis*, injected intracutaneously as a test for coccidioidomycosis.

coc·cid·i·oi·do·ma (-do′mah) residual pulmonary granulomatous nodules seen radiographically as solid round foci in coccidioidomycosis.

coc·cid·i·oi·do·my·co·sis (-oi″do-mi-ko′-sis) infection with *Coccidioides immitis*, a respiratory infection due to spore inhalation, varying from a coldlike condition to severe symptoms like those of influenza (*primary c.*), or sometimes a virulent, progressive granulomatous disease involving cutaneous and subcutaneous tissues, viscera, the central nervous system, and lungs (*secondary c.*).

coc·cid·i·o·sis (kok-sid″e-o′sis) infection by coccidia. In humans, applied to the presence of *Isospora hominis* or *I. belli* in stools; it is often asymptomatic, rarely causing a severe watery mucous diarrhea.

coc·cid·i·um (kok-sid′e-um) pl. *cocci′dia*. Any member of the subclass Coccidia.

coc·ci·gen·ic (kok″sĭ-jen′ik) produced by cocci.

coc·co·ba·cil·lus (kok″o-bah-sil′us) pl. *coccobacil′li*. An oval bacterial cell intermediate between the coccus and bacillus forms. **coccobac′illary,** adj.

coc·co·bac·te·ria (-bak-tēr′e-ah) a common name for spheroid bacteria, or for bacterial cocci.

coc·cus (kok′us) pl. *coc′ci*. [L.] a spherical bacterium, less than 1 μm in diameter. **coc′cal,** adj.

coc·cy·al·gia (kok″se-al′jah) coccygodynia.

coc·cyg·e·al (kok-sij′e-il) pertaining to or located in the region of the coccyx.

coc·cy·gec·to·my (kok″sĭ-jek′tah-me) excision of the coccyx.

coc·cy·go·dyn·ia (-go-din′e-ah) pain in the coccyx and neighboring region.

coc·cy·got·o·my (-got′ah-me) incision of the coccyx.

coc·cyx (kok′siks) see *Table of Bones*.

coch·i·neal (koch′ĭ-nēl) dried female insects of *Coccus cacti*, enclosing young larvae; used as a coloring agent for pharmaceuticals and as a biological stain.

coch·lea (kok′le-ah) 1. anything of a spiral form. 2. a spiral tube forming part of the inner ear, which is the essential organ of hearing. See Plate 29. **coch′lear,** adj.

coch·le·ar·i·form (kok″le-ar′ĭ-form) spoon-shaped.

coch·leo·sac·cu·lot·o·my (kok″le-o-sak″u-lot′ah-me) creation of a fistula between the saccule and cochlear duct by means of a pick introduced through the round window, in order to relieve endolymphatic hydrops.

coch·leo·top·ic (kok″le-o-top′ik) relating to the organization of the auditory pathways and auditory area of the brain.

Coch·lio·my·ia (-mi′ah) a genus of flies, including *C. hominivo′rax*, the screw-worm fly, which deposits its eggs on animal wounds; after hatching, the larvae burrow into the wound and feed on living tissue.

coc·to·la·bile (kok″tah-la′bĭl) capable of being altered or destroyed by heating.

coc·to·sta·bile (-sta′bĭl) not altered by heating to the boiling point of water.

code (kōd) 1. a set of rules for regulating conduct. 2. a system by which information can be communicated. **genetic c.,** the arrangement of nucleotides in the polynucleotide chain of a chromosome governing transmission of genetic information to proteins, i.e., determining the sequence of amino acids in the polypeptide chain making up each protein synthesized by the cell. **triplet c.,** codon.

co·deine (ko'dēn) a narcotic alkaloid obtained from opium or prepared from morphine by methylation and used as the base or as the phosphate or sulfate salt as an opioid analgesic, antitussive, and antidiarrheal.

co·dom·i·nance (ko-dom'ĭ-nins) the full expression in a heterozygote of both alleles of a pair with neither influenced by the other, as in a person with blood group AB. **codom'-inant,** adj.

co·don (ko'don) a series of three adjacent bases in one polynucleotide chain of a DNA or RNA molecule, which codes for a specific amino acid.

coe- for words beginning thus, see also those beginning *ce-*.

co·ef·fi·cient (ko"ah-fish'int) 1. an expression of the change or effect produced by variation in certain factors, or of the ratio between two different quantities. 2. a number or figure put before a chemical formula to indicate how many times the formula is to be multiplied. **absorption c.,** 1. absorptivity. 2. linear absorption c. 3. mass absorption c. **biological c.,** the amount of potential energy consumed by the body at rest. **correlation c.,** a measure of the relationship between two statistical variables, most commonly expressed as their covariance divided by the standard deviation of each. **linear absorption c.,** in radiation physics, the fraction of a beam of radiation absorbed per unit thickness of the absorber. **mass absorption c.,** in radiation physics, the linear absorption coefficient divided by the density of the absorber. **phenol c.,** a measure of the bactericidal activity of a chemical compound in relation to phenol. **sedimentation c.,** the velocity at which a particle sediments in a centrifuge relative to the applied centrifugal field, usually expressed in Svedberg units (S), equal to 10^{-13} second, which are used to characterize the size of macromolecules. **c. of thermal conductivity,** a number indicating the quantity of heat passing in a unit of time through a unit thickness of a substance when the difference in temperature is 1°C. **c. of thermal expansion,** the change in volume per unit volume of a substance produced by a 1°C temperature increase.

-coele word element [Gr.], *cavity; space.*

Coe·len·ter·a·ta (se-len"ter-a'tah) former name for a phylum of invertebrates that included the hydras, jellyfish, sea anemones, and corals, which are now assigned to the phylum Cnidaria.

coe·len·ter·ate (se-len'ter-āt) 1. pertaining or belonging to the Cnidaria. 2. any member of the Cnidaria.

coe·lo·blas·tu·la (se"lo-blas'tu-lah) the common type of blastula, consisting of a hollow sphere composed of blastomeres.

coe·lom (se'lom) body cavity, especially the cavity in the mammalian embryo between the somatopleure and splanchnopleure, which is both intra- and extraembryonic; the principal cavities of the trunk arise from the intraembryonic portion. **coelom'ic,** adj.

coe·lo·mate (sēl'ah-māt) 1. having a coelom. 2. an individual of the Eucoelomata; eucoelomate.

coe·lo·so·my (se"lah-so'me) celosomia.

coe·nu·ro·sis (se"nu-ro'sis) infection by coenurus; a rare infection in humans is manifest as cysts in the central nervous system and increased intracranial pressure.

Coe·nu·rus (se-nu'rus) a genus of tapeworm larvae, including *C. cerebra'lis,* the larva of *Multiceps multiceps,* which causes coenurosis.

coe·nu·rus (se-nu'rus) the larval stage of tapeworms of the genus *Multiceps,* a semitransparent, fluid-filled, bladderlike organism that contains multiple scoleces attached to the inner surface of its wall and that does not form brood capsules. It develops in various parts of the host body, especially in the central nervous system.

co·en·zyme (ko-en'zīm) an organic nonprotein molecule, frequently a phosphorylated derivative of a water-soluble vitamin, that binds with the protein molecule (apoenzyme) to form the active enzyme (holoenzyme). **c. A,** a coenzyme containing among its constituents pantothenic acid and a terminal thiol group that forms high-energy thioester linkages with various acids, e.g., acetic acid (acetyl CoA) and fatty acids (acyl CoA); these thioesters play a central role in the tricarboxylic acid cycle, the transfer of acetyl groups, and the oxidation of fatty acids. Abbreviated CoA and CoA-SH. **c, Q, c Q₁₀,** ubiquinone.

coeur (ker) [Fr.] heart. **c. en sabot** (on să-bo'), a heart whose shape on a radiograph resembles that of a wooden shoe; seen in tetralogy of Fallot.

co·fac·tor (ko'fak-ter) an element or principle, e.g., a coenzyme, with which another must unite in order to function. **heparin c. II,** a serine proteinase inhibitor of the serpin family that inhibits thrombin.

cog·ni·tion (kog-nish'un) that operation of the mind process by which we become aware of objects of thought and perception, including all aspects of perceiving, thinking, and remembering. **cog'nitive,** adj.

co·he·sion (ko-he'zhun) the intermolecular attractive force causing various particles of a single material to unite. **cohe'sive,** adj.

co·hort (ko'hort) 1. in epidemiology, a group of individuals sharing a common characteristic and observed over time in the group. 2. a taxonomic category approximately equivalent to a division, order, or suborder in various systems of classification.

co·hosh (ko-hosh') [Algonquian] any of various North American medicinal plants. **black c.,** the plant *Cimicifuga racemosa* or its fresh or dried root, which has estrogenic effects and is used in menopause and premenstrual syndrome; also used in folk medicine, and traditional Chinese medicine. **blue c.,** the herb *Caulophyllum thalictroides* or its fresh roots or dried rhizome and roots, which have weak estrogenic effects; used for menstrual disorders and as an antispasmodic and uterine stimulant during labor; also used in homeopathy.

coil (koil) spiral (2).

co·in·fec·tion (ko'in-fek"shun) simultaneous infection by separate pathogens, as by hepatitis B and hepatitis D viruses.

coi·no·site (koi'no-sīt) a free commensal organism.

co·i·to·pho·bia (ko"ĭ-to-fo'be-ah) irrational fear of coitus.

co·i·tus (ko'it-us) sexual connection per vaginam between male and female. **co'ital,** adj. **c. incomple'tus, c. interrup'tus,** coitus in which the penis is withdrawn from the vagina before ejaculation. **c. reserva'tus,** coitus in which ejaculation is intentionally suppressed.

Co·ke·ro·my·ces (ko"kĕ-ro-mi'sēz) a genus of fungi of the family Thamnidiaceae. *C. recurva'tus* has been isolated occasionally from cases of mucormycosis and cystitis.

col (kol) a depression in the interdental tissues just below the interproximal contact area, connecting the buccal and lingual papillae.

col·chi·cine (kol'chĭ-sēn) an alkaloid from the tree *Colchicum autumnale* (meadow saffron), used as a suppressant for gout.

cold (kōld) 1. low in temperature, in physiological activity, or in radioactivity. 2. common cold; a catarrhal disorder of the upper respiratory tract, which may be viral, a mixed infection, or an allergic reaction, and marked by acute rhinitis, slight temperature rise, and chilly sensations. **common c.,** cold (2).

cold·sore (kōld'sor) see *herpes simplex*.

co·lec·to·my (ko-lek'tah-me) excision of the colon or of a portion of it.

co·le·sev·e·lam (ko"lĕ-sev'ĕ-lam) a bile acid–binding polymer that decreases serum levels of total cholesterol, LDL cholesterol, and apolipoprotein B and increases levels of HDL cholesterol; used as the hydrochloride salt in the treatment of primary hypercholesterolemia.

co·les·ti·pol (ko-les'tĭ-pol) an anion exchange resin that binds bile acids in the intestines to form a complex that is excreted in the feces; administered in the form of the hydrochloride salt as an antihyperlipoproteinemic.

col·fos·e·ril (kol-fos'ĕ-ril) a synthetic pulmonary surfactant used as the palmitate ester, in combination with cetyl alcohol and tyloxapol, in the prophylaxis and treatment of neonatal respiratory distress syndrome.

co·li·bac·il·lo·sis (ko"lĭbas"ĭ-lo'sis) infection with *Escherichia coli.*

co·li·bac·il·lus (ko"lĭ-bah-sil'us) *Escherichia coli.*

col·ic (kol'ik) 1. acute paroxysmal abdominal pain. 2. pertaining to the colon. **appendicular c.,** vermicular c. **biliary c.,** colic due to passage of gallstones along the bile duct. **gallstone c.,** biliary c. **hepatic c.,** biliary c. **infantile c.,** benign paroxysmal abdominal pain during the first 3 months of life. **lead c.,** colic due to lead poisoning. **renal c.,** pain due to thrombosis of the renal vein or artery, dissection of the renal artery, renal infarction, intrarenal mass lesions, or passage of a stone within the collecting system. **vermicular c.,** pain in the vermiform appendix caused by catarrhal inflammation due to blockage of the outlet of the appendix.

col·i·cin (kol'ĭ-sin) a protein secreted by colicinogenic strains of *Escherichia coli* and other enteric bacteria; lethal to related, sensitive bacteria.

col·icky (kol'ik-e) pertaining to colic.

col·i·co·ple·gia (ko"lĭ-ko-ple'jah) combined lead colic and lead paralysis.

col·i·form (kol'ĭ-form) pertaining to fermentative gram-negative enteric bacilli, sometimes restricted to those fermenting lactose, e.g., *Escherichia, Klebsiella,* or *Enterobacter.*

col·i·phage (kol'ĭ-fāj) any bacteriophage that infects *Escherichia coli.*

co·li·punc·ture (-pungk"cher) colocentesis.

col·is·ti·meth·ate (ko-lis"tĭ-meth'āt) a colistin derivative; the sodium salt is used as an antibacterial.

co·lis·tin (ko-lis'tin) an antibiotic produced by *Bacillus polymyxa* var. *colistinus,* related to polymyxin and effective against many gram-negative bacteria; used as the sulfate salt.

co·lit·i·des (ko-lit'ĭ-dēz) plural of *colitis;* inflammatory disorders of the colon, collectively.

co·li·tis (ko-li′tis) inflammation of the colon; see also *enterocolitis*. **amebic c.,** colitis due to *Entamoeba histolytica;* amebic dysentery. **antibiotic-associated c.,** see under *enterocolitis*. **collagenous c.,** a type of colitis of unknown etiology characterized by deposits of collagenous material beneath the epithelium of the colon, with crampy abdominal pain and watery diarrhea. **granulomatous c.,** transmural colitis with the formation of non-caseating granulomas. **ischemic c.,** acute vascular insufficiency of the colon, affecting the portion supplied by the inferior mesenteric artery; symptoms include pain at the left iliac fossa, bloody diarrhea, low-grade fever, and abdominal distention and tenderness. **mucous c.,** former name for *irritable bowel syndrome*. **regional c., segmental c.,** transmural or granulomatous inflammatory disease of the colon; regional enteritis involving the colon. It may be associated with ulceration, strictures, or fistulas. **transmural c.,** inflammation of the full thickness of the bowel, rather than mucosal and submucosal disease, usually with the formation of noncaseating granulomas. It may be confined to the colon, segmentally or diffusely, or may be associated with small bowel disease (regional enteritis). Clinically, it may resemble ulcerative colitis, but the ulceration is often longitudinal or deep, the disease is often segmental, stricture formation is common, and fistulas, particularly in the perineum, are a frequent complication. **ulcerative c.,** chronic ulceration in the colon, chiefly of the mucosa and submucosa, manifested by cramping abdominal pain, rectal bleeding, and loose discharges of blood, pus, and mucus with scanty fecal particles.

co·li·tox·emia (ko″lĭ-tok-se′me-ah) toxemia due to infection with *Escherichia coli.*

co·li·tox·in (ko′lĭ-tok″sin) a toxin from *Escherichia coli.*

col·la·gen (kol′ah-jen) any of a family of extracellular, closely related proteins occurring as a major component of connective tissue, giving it strength and flexibility; composed of molecules of tropocollagen. **collag′enous,** adj.

col·la·ge·nase (kah-laj′ĕ-nās) an enzyme that catalyzes the hydrolysis of peptide bonds in triple helical regions of collagen.

col·lag·e·na·tion (-na′shun) the appearance of collagen in developing cartilage.

col·lag·e·ni·tis (-ni′tis) inflammatory involvement of collagen fibers in the fibrous component of connective tissue, characterized by pain, swelling, low-grade fever, and by increased erythrocyte sedimentation rate.

col·lag·e·no·blast (kah-laj′ĕ-no-blast″) a cell arising from a fibroblast and which, as it matures, is associated with collagen production; it may also form cartilage and bone by metaplasia.

col·lag·e·no·cyte (-sīt″) a mature collagen-producing cell.

col·la·gen·o·gen·ic (kah-laj″ĕ-no-jen′ik) pertaining to or characterized by collagen production; forming collagen or collagen fibers.

col·la·gen·ol·y·sis (kol″ah-jen-ol′ĭ-sis) dissolution or digestion of collagen. **collagenolyt′ic,** adj.

col·lag·e·nous (kah-laj′ah-nus) pertaining to, forming, is or producing collagen.

col·lapse (kah-laps′) 1. a state of extreme prostration and depression, with failure of circulation. 2. abnormal falling in of the walls of a part or organ. **circulatory c.,** shock (2).

col·lar (kol′er) an encircling band, generally around the neck. **cervical c.,** see under *orthosis*. **Philadelphia c.,** a type of cervical orthosis that restricts anterior-posterior cervical motion considerably but allows some normal rotation and lateral bending.

col·lar·ette (kol″er-et′) 1. a narrow rim of loosened keratin overhanging the periphery of a circumscribed skin lesion, attached to the normal surrounding skin. 2. an irregular jagged line dividing the anterior surface of the iris into two regions.

col·lat·er·al (kah-lat′er-al) 1. secondary or accessory; not direct or immediate. 2. a small side branch, as of a blood vessel or nerve.

col·lic·u·lec·to·my (kah-lik″u-lek′tah-me) excision of the seminal colliculus.

col·lic·u·li·tis (-li′tis) inflammation about the seminal colliculus.

col·lic·u·lus (kah-lik′u-lus) pl. *collĭ′culi.* [L.] a small elevation. **seminal c., c. semina′lis,** verumontanum; a portion of the male urethral crest on which are the openings of the prostatic utricle and the ejaculatory ducts.

col·li·ma·tion (kol″ĭ-ma′shun) 1. in microscopy, the process of making light rays parallel; the adjustment or aligning of optical axes. 2. in radiology, the elimination of the more divergent portion of an x-ray beam. 3. in nuclear medicine, the use of a perforated absorber to restrict the field of view of a detector and reduce scatter.

col·liq·ua·tive (kah-lik′wah-tiv) characterized by excessive liquid discharge, or by liquefaction of tissue.

col·lo·di·a·phys·e·al (kol″o-di″ah-fiz′e-il) pertaining to the neck and shaft of a long bone, especially the femur.

col·lo·di·on (kah-lo′de-on) a syrupy liquid compounded of pyroxylin, ether, and alcohol, which dries to a transparent, tenacious film; used as a topical protectant, applied to the skin to close small wounds, abrasions, and cuts, to hold surgical dressings in place, and to keep medications in contact with the skin. **flexible c.,** a preparation of camphor, castor oil, and collodion, used as a topical protectant. **salicylic acid c.,** flexible collodion containing salicylic acid; used topically as a keratolytic.

col·loid (kol′oid) 1. glutinous or resembling glue. 2. a chemical system composed of a continuous medium (continuous phase) throughout which are distributed small particles, 1 to 1000 nm in size (disperse phase), that do not settle out under the influence of gravity; the particles may be in emulsion or in suspension. The term may be used to denote either the particles or the entire system. **colloid′al,** adj. **dispersion c.,** colloid (2), sometimes specifically an unstable colloid system. **emulsion c.,** 1. lyophilic c. 2. rarely, emulsion. **lyophilic c.,** a colloid system in which the disperse phase is relatively liquid, usually comprising highly complex organic substances such as starch, which readily absorb solvent, swell, and distribute uniformly through the medium. **lyophobic c.,** an unstable colloid system in which the disperse phase particles tend to repel liquids, are easily precipitated, and cannot be redispersed with additional solvent. **stannous sulfur c.,** a sulfur colloid containing stannous ions; complexed with technetium 99m it is used in bone, liver, and spleen imaging. **suspension c.,** lyophobic c.

col·lum (kol′um) pl. *col′la.* [L.] the neck, or a necklike part. **c. distor′tum,** torticollis. **c. val′gum,** coxa valga.

col·lu·to·ry (kol′u-tor-e) mouthwash or gargle.

col·lyr·i·um (kŏ-lir′e-um) pl. *colly′ria.* [L.] a lotion for the eyes; an eye wash.

col(o)- word element [Gr.], *colon.*

col·o·bo·ma (kol″o-bo′mah) pl. *colobomas, colobo′mata.* [L.] 1. an absence or defect of tissue. 2. a defect of ocular tissue, due to failure of part of the fetal fissure to close; it may affect the choroid, ciliary body, eyelid, iris, lens, optic nerve, or retina. **bridge c.,** coloboma of the iris in which a strip of iris tissue bridges over the fissure. **Fuchs′ c.,** a small, crescent-shaped defect of the choroid at the lower edge of the optic disk. **c. lo′buli,** fissure of the ear lobe.

col·o·cen·te·sis (ko″lo-sen-te′sis) surgical puncture of the colon.

co·lo·cho·le·cys·tos·to·my (-ko″lĕ-sis-tos′tah-me) cholecystocolostomy.

co·lo·clys·ter (ko″lo-klis′ter) an enema injected into the colon through the rectum.

co·lo·co·los·to·my (-kah-los′tah-me) surgical anastomosis between two portions of the colon.

co·lo·cu·ta·ne·ous (-ku-ta′ne us) pertaining to the colon and skin, or communicating with the colon and the cutaneous surface of the body.

co·lo·cys·to·plas·ty (-sis′to-plas″te) augmentation cystoplasty using an isolated section of colon.

co·lo·fix·a·tion (-fik-sa′shun) the fixation or suspension of the colon in cases of ptosis.

co·lon (ko′lon) [L.] the part of the large intestine extending from the cecum to the rectum. See Plate 27. **ascending c.,** the portion of the colon passing cephalad from the cecum to the right colic flexure. **congenital pouch c.,** a congenital malformation in which part or all of it is replaced by a dilated pouch and there is anorectal malformation with a fistula between the colon and the genitourinary tract. **descending c.,** the portion of the colon passing caudad from the left colic flexure to the sigmoid colon. **iliac c.,** the part of the descending colon lying in the left iliac fossa and continuous with the sigmoid colon. **irritable c.,** irritable bowel syndrome. **left c.,** the distal portion of the large intestine, developed embryonically from the hindgut and functioning in the storage and elimination from the body of nonabsorbed residue of ingested material. **pelvic c.,** sigmoid c. **right c.,** the proximal portion of the large intestine, developed embryonically from the terminal portion of the midgut and functioning in absorption of ingested material. **sigmoid c.,** that portion of the left colon situated in the pelvis and extending from the descending colon to the rectum. **spastic c.,** irritable bowel syndrome. **transverse c.,** the portion of the large intestine passing transversely across the upper part of the abdomen, between the right and left colic flexures.

co·lon·ic (ko-lon′ik) 1. pertaining to the colon. 2. colon hydrotherapy.

co·lon·og·ra·phy (ko″lon-og′rah-fe) imaging of the colon, as by computed tomography or magnetic resonance imaging.

co·lon·op·a·thy (-op′ah-the) any disease or disorder of the colon.

co·lon·os·co·py (-os′kah-pe) endoscopic examination of the colon, either transabdominally during laparotomy, or transanally by means of a fiberoptic endoscope.

col·o·ny (kol′ah-ne) a discrete group of organisms, as a collection of bacteria in a culture.

co·lo·pexy (ko′lo-pek″se) surgical fixation or suspension of the colon.

co·lo·pli·ca·tion (ko″lo-pli-ka′shun) the operation of infolding or taking tucks in the wall of the colon in cases of dilatation.

co·lo·proc·tec·to·my (-prok-tek′tah-me) surgical removal of the colon and rectum.

co·lo·proc·tos·to·my (-prok-tos′tah-me) colorectostomy.

co·lo·punc·ture (ko′lo-punk″cher) colocentesis.

col·or (kul′er) 1. a property of a surface or substance due to absorption of certain light rays and reflection of others within the range of wavelengths (roughly 370–760 mμ) adequate to excite the retinal receptors. 2. radiant energy within the range of adequate chromatic stimuli of the retina, i.e., between the infrared and ultraviolet. 3. a sensory impression of one of the rainbow hues. **complementary c′s,** a pair of colors the sensory mechanisms for which are so linked that when they are mixed on the color wheel they cancel each other out, leaving neutral gray. **confusion c′s,** different colors liable to be mistakenly matched by persons with defective color vision, and hence used for detecting different types of color vision defects. **primary c′s,** a small number of fundamental colors; (a) in visual science, red, green, and blue, the colors specifically picked up by the retinal cones; (b) in painting and printing, blue, yellow, and red. **pure c.,** one whose stimulus consists of homogeneous wavelengths, with little or no admixture of wavelengths of other hues.

co·lo·rec·tos·to·my (-rek-tos′tah-me) formation of an opening between the colon and rectum.

co·lo·rec·tum (-rek′tum) the distal 10 inches (25 cm.) of the bowel, including the distal portion of the colon and the rectum, regarded as a unit. **colorec′tal,** adj.

col·or·im·e·ter (kul″er-im′ĕ-ter) an instrument for measuring color or color intensity in a solution.

co·lor·rha·phy (kol-or′ah-fe) suture of the colon.

co·lo·sig·moid·os·to·my (ko″lo-sig″moid-os′tah-me) surgical anastomosis of a formerly remote portion of the colon to the sigmoid.

co·los·to·my (kah-los′tah-me) the surgical creation of an opening between the colon and the body surface; also, the opening (stoma) so created. **dry c.,** that performed in the left colon, the discharge from the stoma

consisting of soft or formed fecal matter. **ileotransverse c.,** surgical anastomosis between the ileum and the transverse colon. **wet c.,** colostomy in (a) the right colon, the drainage from which is liquid, or (b) the left colon following anastomosis of the ureters to the sigmoid or descending colon so that urine is also expelled through the same stoma.

co·los·trum (kol-os′trum) the thin, yellow, milky fluid secreted by the mammary gland a few days before or after parturition.

co·lot·o·my (kol-ot′ah-me) incision of the colon.

co·lo·ves·i·cal (-ves′ĭ-k′l) pertaining to or communicating with the colon and bladder.

col·pal·gia (kol-pal′jah) pain in the vagina.

col·pec·ta·sia (kol″pek-ta′zhah) distention or dilatation of the vagina.

col·pec·to·my (kol-pek′tah-me) excision of the vagina.

col·peu·ry·sis (kol-pūr′ĭ-sis) dilatation of the vagina.

col·pi·tis (kol-pi′tis) inflammation of the vagina; vaginitis.

colp(o)- word element [Gr.], vagina.

col·po·cele (kol′pah-sēl) vaginal hernia.

col·po·clei·sis (kol″pah-kli′sis) surgical closure of the vaginal canal.

col·po·cys·ti·tis (-sis-ti′tis) inflammation of the vagina and bladder.

col·po·cys·to·cele (-sis′to-sēl) hernia of the bladder into the vagina.

col·po·cy·to·gram (-sīt′ah-gram) differential listing of cells observed in vaginal smears.

col·po·cy·tol·o·gy (-si-tol′ah-je) the study of cells exfoliated from the epithelium of the vagina.

col·po·hy·per·pla·sia (-hi″per-pla′zhah) excessive growth of the mucous membrane and wall of the vagina.

col·po·mi·cro·scope (-mi′kro-skōp) an instrument for microscopic examination of the tissues of the cervix in situ.

col·po·per·i·neo·plas·ty (-per″ĭ-ne′o-plas″te) plastic repair of the vagina and perineum.

col·po·per·i·ne·or·rha·phy (-per″ĭ-ne-or′ah-fe) suture of the ruptured vagina and perineum.

col·po·pexy (kol′pah-pek″se) suture of a relaxed vagina to the abdominal wall.

col·pop·to·sis (kol″pop-to′sis) vaginocele (2).

col·por·rha·gia (kol″pah-ra′jah) hemorrhage from the vagina.

col·por·rha·phy (kol-por′ah-fe) 1. suture of the vagina. 2. the operation of denuding and suturing the vaginal wall to narrow the vagina.

col·por·rhex·is (kol″por-ek′sis) laceration of the vagina.

col·po·scope (kol′pah-skōp) vaginoscope; a speculum for examining the vagina and cervix using a magnifying lens.

col·po·spasm (-spazm) vaginal spasm.

col·po·ste·no·sis (kol″po-stĕ-no′sis) contraction or narrowing of the vagina.

col·po·ste·not·o·my (-stĕ-not′ah-me) a cutting operation for stricture of the vagina.

col·po·sus·pen·sion (-sus-pen′shun) bladder neck suspension.

col·pot·o·my (kol-pot′ah-me) incision of the vagina with entry into the cul-de-sac.

col·po·xe·ro·sis (kol″po-zēr-o′sis) abnormal dryness of the vulva and vagina.

Col·ti·vi·rus (kol′tĭ-vi″rus) a genus of viruses of the family Reoviridae, containing the agent of Colorado tick fever.

col·u·mel·la (kol″u-mel′ah) pl. *columel′lae*. [L.] 1. a little column. 2. in certain fungi and protozoa, an invagination into the sporangium. **c. coch′leae,** modiolus. **c. na′si,** the fleshy external end of the nasal septum.

col·umn (kol′um) an anatomical part in the form of a pillar-like structure. **anal c's,** vertical folds of mucous membrane at the upper half of the anal canal. **anterior c.,** 1. the anterior portion of the gray substance of the spinal cord, in transverse section seen as a horn. 2. palatoglossal arch. **c's of Bertin,** renal c's. **c. of Burdach,** fasciculus cuneatus of the spinal cord. **Clarke's c.,** thoracic c. **enamel c's,** adamantine prisms. **c. of Goll,** fasciculus gracilis of the spinal cord. **gray c's,** the longitudinally oriented parts of the spinal cord in which the nerve cell bodies are found, comprising the gray substance of the spinal cord. **lateral c. of spinal cord,** the lateral portion of the spinal cord, in transverse section seen as a horn; present only in the thoracic and upper lumbar regions. **c's of Morgagni,** anal c's. **posterior c.,** 1. the posterior portion of gray substance of the spinal cord, in transverse section seen as a horn. 2. palatopharyngeal arch. **rectal c's,** anal c's. **renal c's,** inward extensions of the cortical substance of the kidney between contiguous renal pyramids. **spinal c.,** vertebral c. **thoracic c.,** a column of cells in the posterior gray column of the spinal cord, extending from the eighth cervical segment to the third or fourth lumbar segment. **vertebral c.,** the rigid structure in the midline of the back, composed of the vertebrae.

co·lum·na (ko-lum′nah) pl. *colum′nae.* [L.] column.

co·lum·nar (kah-lum′nar) having the shape of a column; arranged in or characterized by columns.

col·um·ni·za·tion (kol″um-nĭ-za′shun) support of the prolapsed uterus by tampons.

co·ly·pep·tic (ko″lĭ-pep′tik) kolypeptic.

co·ma (ko′mah) [L.] a state of profound unconsciousness from which the patient cannot be aroused, even by powerful stimuli. **co′matose,** adj. **alcoholic c.,** stupor accompanying severe alcoholic intoxication. **diabetic c.,** the coma of severe diabetic acidosis. **hepatic c.,** coma accompanying hepatic encephalopathy. **irreversible c.,** brain death. **Kussmaul's c.,** the coma and air hunger of diabetic acidosis. **metabolic c.,** the coma accompanying metabolic encephalopathy. **uremic c.,** lethargic state due to uremia. **c. vigil,** locked-in syndrome.

com·bus·tion (kom-bus′chun) rapid oxidation with emission of heat.

com·e·do (kom′ĕ-do) pl. *comedo′nes.* A plug of keratin and sebum within the dilated orifice of a hair follicle, frequently containing the bacteria *Propionobacterium acnes, Staphylococcus albus,* and *Pityrosporon ovale.* **closed c.,** whitehead; a comedo whose opening is not widely dilated, appearing as a small, flesh-colored papule; it may rupture and cause an inflammatory lesion in the dermis. **open c.,** blackhead; a comedo with a widely dilated orifice in which the pigmented impaction is visible at the skin surface.

com·e·do·gen·ic (kom″ĕ-do-jen′ik) producing comedones.

com·e·do·mas·ti·tis (-mas-ti′tis) mammary duct ectasia.

co·mes (ko′mēz) pl. *comi′tes.* [L.] an artery or vein accompanying another artery or vein or a nerve trunk.

com·frey (kom′fre) the perennial herb *Symphytum officinale,* or a preparation of its leaves and roots, which are demulcent and astringent and are used topically for bruises and sprains and to promote bone healing; also used in folk medicine.

com·men·sal (kom-men′sil) 1. living on or within another organism, and deriving benefit without harming or benefiting the host. 2. a parasite that causes no harm to the host.

com·men·sal·ism (-izm) symbiosis in which one population (or individual) is benefited and the other is neither benefited nor harmed.

com·mi·nut·ed (kom′in-ōōt″id) broken or crushed into small pieces, as a comminuted fracture.

com·mis·su·ra (kom″ĭ-su′rah) pl. *commis-su′rae.* [L.] commissure.

com·mis·sure (kom′ĭ-shoor) a site of union of corresponding parts; specifically, the sites of junction between adjacent cusps of the heart valves. **commis′sural,** adj. **anterior c.,** the band of fibers connecting the parts of the two cerebral hemispheres. **posterior c.,** a large fiber bundle crossing from one side of the cerebrum to the other, dorsal to where the aqueduct opens into the third ventricle. **Gudden's c.,** see *supraoptic c's.* **Meynert's c.,** see *supraoptic c's.* **supraoptic c's,** commissural fibers crossing the midline of the human brain dorsal to the caudal border of the optic chiasm, representing the combined commissures of Gudden and Meynert.

com·mis·su·ror·rha·phy (kom′ĭ-shoor-or′ah-fe) suture of the components of a commissure, to lessen the size of the orifice.

com·mis·sur·ot·o·my (-ot′ah-me) surgical incision or digital disruption of the components of a commissure to increase the size of the orifice; commonly done to separate adherent, thickened leaflets of a stenotic mitral valve.

com·mon (kom′en) 1. belonging to or shared by two or more entities. 2. usual; being frequent, prevalent, widespread, or habitual. 3. most frequent and best known of its kind.

com·mu·ni·ca·ble (kah-mu′nĭ-kah-b'l) capable of being transmitted from one person to another.

com·mu·ni·cans (-kans) [L.] communicating.

com·mu·ni·cat·ing (-ka″ting) 1. denoting spreading or transmission, as of a disease. 2. being connected, one with another.

com·mu·ni·ty (-te) a body of individuals living in a defined area or having a common interest or organization. **biotic c.,** an assemblage of populations living in a defined area. **therapeutic c.,** a structured mental treatment center employing group and milieu therapy and encouraging the patient to function within social norms.

co·mor·bid (ko-mor′bid) pertaining to a disease or other pathological process that occurs simultaneously with another.

com·pact (kom′pakt, kom-pakt′) dense; having a dense structure.

com·pac·tion (kom-pak′shun) 1. a complication of labor in twin births in which there is simultaneous full engagement of the leading fetal poles of both twins, so that the lesser pelvis is filled and further descent is prevented. 2. in embryology, the process during which blastomeres change their shape and align themselves tightly against each other to form the compact morula.

com·pen·sat·ed (kom′pen-sa″tid) counterbalanced; offset.

com·pen·sa·tion (kom″pen-sa′shun) 1. the counterbalancing of any defect. 2. the conscious or unconscious process by which a person attempts to make up for real or imagined physical or psychological deficiencies. 3. in cardiology, the maintenance of an adequate blood flow without distressing symptoms, accomplished by cardiac and circulatory adjustments. **dosage c.,** in genetics, the mechanism by which the effect of the two X chromosomes of the normal female is rendered identical to that of the one X chromosome of the normal male.

com·pen·sa·to·ry (kom-pen′sah-tor″e) making good a defect or loss; restoring a lost balance.

com·pe·ti·tion (kom″pě-tish′un) the phenomenon in which two structurally similar molecules "compete" for a single binding site on a third molecule. **compet′itive,** adj. **antigenic c.,** an altered response to an immunogen resulting from the simultaneous or close administration of two immunogens: the response to one is normal, while the response to the second is suppressed or diminished.

com·plaint (kom-plānt′) a disease, symptom, or disorder. **chief c.,** the symptom or group of symptoms about which the patient first consults the doctor; the presenting symptom.

com·ple·ment (kom′plĕ-ment) a heat-labile cascade system of at least 20 serum glycoproteins that interact to provide many of the effector functions of humoral immunity and inflammation, including vasodilation and increase of vascular permeability, facilitation of phagocyte activity, and lysis of certain foreign cells. It can be activated via either the *classical* or *alternative complement pathways* (qq.v.).

com·ple·men·ta·ry (kom″plĕ-men′tah-re) 1. supplying a defect, or helping to do so; making complete; accessory. 2. in biochemistry, pertaining to the specific pairing between purine and pyrimidine bases in two nucleotide strands.

com·ple·men·ta·tion (-men-ta′shun) the interaction between two sets of cellular or viral genes within a cell such that the cell can function even though each set of genes carries a mutated, nonfunctional gene.

com·plex (kom′pleks) 1. a combination of various things, e.g., a complex of symptoms; see *syndrome.* 2. sequence (2). 3. a group of interrelated ideas, mainly unconscious, that have a common emotional tone and strongly influence a person's attitudes and behavior. 4. that portion of an electrocardiogram representing the systole of an atrium or ventricle. **AIDS dementia c.,** HIV encephalopathy. **AIDS-related c. (ARC),** a complex of signs and symptoms representing a less severe stage of human immunodeficiency virus (HIV) infection, characterized by chronic generalized lymphadenopathy, fever, weight loss, prolonged diarrhea, minor opportunistic infections, cytopenia, and T-cell abnormalities of the kind associated with AIDS. **anomalous c.,** in electrocardiography, an abnormal atrial or ventricular complex resulting from aberrant conduction over accessory pathways. **antigen-antibody c.,** a complex formed by the binding of antigen to antibody. **anti-inhibitor coagulant c. (AICC),** a concentrated fraction from pooled human plasma, which includes various coagulation factors; used as an antihemorrhagic in hemophilic patients with factor VIII inhibitors. **atrial c.,** the P wave of the electrocardiogram, representing electrical activation of the atria. **atrial premature c. (APC),** a single ectopic atrial beat arising prematurely, which may be associated with structural heart disease. **atrioventricular (AV) junctional escape c.,** see under *beat.* **atrioventricular (AV) junctional premature c.,** an ectopic beat arising prematurely in the atrioventricular junction and traveling toward both the atria and ventricles if unimpeded, causing the P wave to be premature and abnormal or absent and the QRS complex to be premature. **branched-chain α-keto acid dehydrogenase c.,** a multienzyme complex that catalyzes the oxidative decarboxylation of the keto acid analogues of the branched chain amino acids; deficiency of any enzyme of the complex causes maple syrup urine disease. **calcarine c.,** calcar avis. **castration c.,** in psychoanalytic theory, unconscious thoughts and motives stemming from fear of damage to or loss of sexual organs as punishment for forbidden sexual desires. **Eisenmenger's c.,** a defect of the interventricular septum with severe pulmonary hypertension, hypertrophy of the right ventricle, and latent or overt cyanosis. **Electra c.,** the counterpart in females of the Oedipus complex, involving the daughter's love for her father and jealousy or resentment towards her mother; now rarely used since *Oedipus complex* (q.v.) has come to be applied to both sexes. **exstrophy-epispadias c.,** a spectrum of congenital defects of the anterior abdominal wall, ranging from epispadias to exstrophy of the bladder to exstrophy of cloaca. **factor IX c.,** a partially purified factor IX fraction also including factor II, VII, and X fractions, from venous human plasma. It is used in the treatment of

hemophilia B, replacement of factor VII, and treatment of anticoagulant-induced hemorrhage. **Ghon c.,** primary c. (1). **β-glycosidase c.,** the enzyme complex comprising lactase and phlorhizin hydrolase activities, occurring in the brush border membrane of the intestinal mucosa and hydrolyzing lactose as well as cellobiose and cellotriose. **Golgi c.,** Golgi apparatus; a complex cellular organelle consisting mainly of a number of flattened sacs (cisternae) and associated vesicles, involved in the synthesis of glycoproteins, lipoproteins, membrane-bound proteins, and lysosomal enzymes. The sacs form primary lysosomes and secretory vacuoles. **immune c.,** antigen-antibody c. **inclusion c.,** one in which molecules of one type are enclosed within cavities in the crystalline lattice of another substance. **inferiority c.,** unconscious feelings of inadequacy, producing timidity or, as a compensation, exaggerated aggressiveness and expression of superiority. **junctional premature c.,** atrioventricular junctional premature c. **LCMV-LASV c.,** a group of antigenically related viruses comprising the Old World arenaviruses. Lassa virus (Lassa fever) and lymphocytic choriomeningitis virus are pathogenic for humans. **Lutembacher's c.,** see under *syndrome.* **major histocompatibility c. (MHC),** the chromosomal region containing genes that control the histocompatibility antigens. In humans, it controls the HLA antigens. **membrane attack c. (MAC),** the pentamolecular complex of components C5b,6,7,8,9 formed in the final pathway of complement activation, inserting into the target cell membrane where it creates a pore and results in cytolysis. **Oedipus c.,** the feelings and conflicts occurring in a child that result from sexual attraction to the opposite-sex parent, including envious, aggressive feelings toward the same-sex parent. **pore c.,** a nuclear pore and its annulus considered together. **primary c.,** 1. the combination of a Ghon focus and a corresponding lymph node focus in primary tuberculosis in children; similar lesions are seen with other mycobacterial and fungal infections. 2. the primary cutaneous lesion at the site of skin infection, e.g., a chancre in syphilis or tuberculosis. **primary inoculation c., primary tuberculous c.,** tuberculous chancre. **pyruvate dehydrogenase c.,** a multienzyme complex that catalyzes the formation of acetyl coenzyme A from pyruvate and coenzyme A; deficiency of any component of the complex results in lacticacidemia, ataxia, and psychomotor retardation. **QRS c.,** the portion of the electrocardiogram comprising the Q, R, and S waves, together representing ventricular depolarization. **sucrase-isomaltase c.,** the enzyme complex comprising sucrase and isomaltase activities, occurring in the brush border of the intestinal mucosa and hydrolyzing maltose as well as maltotriose and some other glycosidic bonds. **symptom c.,** syndrome. **synaptonemal c.,** the structure formed by the synapsis of homologous chromosomes during the zygotene stage of meiosis I. **Tacaribe c.,** a group of antigenically related viruses comprising the New World arenaviruses, including Junin virus, the agent of Argentinian hemorrhagic fever, and Machupo virus, the agent of Bolivian hemorrhagic fever. **VATER c.,** an association of congenital anomalies consisting of *v*ertebral defects, imperforate *a*nus, *t*racheoesophageal fistula, and *r*adial and *r*enal dysplasia. **ventricular c.,** the combined QRS complex and T wave, together representing ventricular electrical activity. **ventricular premature c. (VPC),** an ectopic beat arising in the ventricles and stimulating the myocardium prematurely.

com·plex·ion (kom-plek'shun) the color and appearance of the skin of the face.

com·pli·ance (kom-pli'ans) the quality of yielding to pressure without disruption, or an expression of the ability to do so, as an expression of the distensibility of an air- or fluid-filled organ, e.g., lung or urinary bladder, in terms of unit of volume change per unit of pressure change. Symbol C.

com·pli·cat·ed (kom'plĭ-kāt″ed) involved; associated with other injuries, lesions, or diseases.

com·pli·ca·tion (kom″plĭ-ka'shun) 1. disease(s) concurrent with another disease. 2. occurrence of several diseases in the same patient.

com·po·nent (kum-po'nent) 1. a constituent element or part. 2. in neurology, a series of neurons forming a functional system for conducting the afferent and efferent impulses in the somatic and splanchnic mechanisms of the body. **M c.,** an abnormal monoclonal immunoglobulin occurring in the serum in plasma cell dyscrasias, formed by proliferating concentrations of immunoglobulin-producing cells. **plasma thromboplastin c. (PTC),** coagulation factor IX.

com·pos·ite (kom-poz'it) 1. made up of unlike parts. 2. composite resin.

com·pos men·tis (kom'pos men'tis) [L.] sound of mind; sane.

com·pound (kom'pownd) 1. made up of two or more parts or ingredients. 2. a substance made up of two or more materials. 3. in chemistry, a substance consisting of two or more elements in union. 4. to combine to form a whole; unite. **clathrate c's,** inclusion complexes in which molecules of one type are trapped within cavities of another substance, such as within a crystalline lattice structure or large molecule. **inorganic c.,** a compound of chemical elements containing no carbon atoms. **organic c.,** a compound of chemical elements containing carbon atoms. **organometallic c.,** one in which carbon is linked to a metal. **quaternary ammonium c.,** an organic compound containing a quaternary ammonium group, a nitrogen atom carrying a single positive charge bonded to four carbon atoms, e.g., choline.

com·press (kom'pres) a pad or bolster of folded linen or other material, applied with pressure; sometimes medicated, it may be wet or dry, or hot or cold.

com·pres·sion (kom-presh'un) 1. act of pressing upon or together; the state of being pressed together. 2. in embryology, the shortening or omission of certain developmental stages.

com·pul·sion (kom-pul'shun) 1. an overwhelming urge to perform an irrational act or ritual. 2. the repetitive or stereotyped action that is the object of such an urge. **compul'sive,** adj. **repetition c.,** in psychoanalytic theory, the impulse to reenact earlier emotional experiences or traumatic behavior.

co·na·tion (ko-na'shun) in psychology, the power that impels effort of any kind; the conscious tendency to act. **con'ative,** adj.

c-onc [*c*ellular *onc*ogene] a proto-oncogene that has been activated within the host so that oncogenicity results.

con·ca·nav·a·lin A (kon″kah-nav″ah-lin) a phytohemagglutinin isolated from the jack bean (*Canavalia ensiformis*); it is a hemagglutinin that agglutinates blood erythrocytes and a mitogen stimulating predominantly T cells.

con·cave (kon-kāv') rounded and somewhat depressed or hollowed out.

con·ca·vo·con·cave (kon-ka″vo-kon'kāv) concave on each of two opposite surfaces.

con·ca·vo·con·vex (-kon'veks) having one concave and one convex surface.

con·ceive (kon-sēv') 1. to become pregnant. 2. take in, grasp, or form in the mind.

con·cen·trate (kon'sin-trāt) 1. to bring to a common center; to gather at one point. 2. to increase the strength by diminishing the bulk of, as of a liquid; to condense. 3. a drug or other preparation that has been strengthened by evaporation of its nonactive parts. **activated prothrombin complex c. (APCC),**

anti-inhibitor coagulant complex. **pro-thrombin complex c. (PCC)**, factor IX complex.

con·cen·tra·tion (kon″sen-tra′shun) 1. increase in strength by evaporation. 2. the ratio of the mass or volume of a solute to the mass or volume of the solution or solvent. **hydrogen ion c.**, the degree of concentration of hydrogen ions in a solution; related inversely to the pH of the solution by the equation $[H^+] = 10^{-pH}$. **mass c.**, the mass of a constituent substance divided by the volume of the mixture, as milligrams per liter (mg/L), etc. **mean corpuscular hemoglobin c. (MCHC)**, the average hemoglobin concentration in erythrocytes. **molar c.**, the concentration of a substance expressed in terms of molarity; symbol c.

con·cen·tric (kon-sen′trik) having a common center; extending out equally in all directions from a common center.

con·cept (kon′sept) the image of a thing held in the mind.

con·cep·tion (kon-sep′shun) 1. an imprecise term denoting the formation of a viable zygote. **concep′tive**, adj. 2. concept.

con·cep·tus (-tus) the product of the union of oocyte and spermatozoon at any stage of development from fertilization until birth, including extraembryonic membranes as well as the embryo or fetus.

con·cha (kong′kah) pl. *con′chae*. [L.] a shell-shaped structure. **c. of auricle**, the hollow of the auricle of the external ear, bounded anteriorly by the tragus and posteriorly by the anthelix. **c. bullo′sa**, a cystic distention of the middle nasal concha. **inferior nasal c.**, a thin, bony plate forming the lower part of the lateral wall of the nasal cavity, and the mucous membrane covering the plate. **middle nasal c.**, the lower of two bony plates projecting from the inner wall of the ethmoid labyrinth and separating the superior from the middle meatus of the nose, and the mucous membrane covering the plate. **sphenoidal c.**, a thin curved plate of bone at the anterior and lower part of the body of the sphenoid bone, on either side, forming part of the roof of the nasal cavity. **superior nasal c.**, the upper of two bony plates projecting from the inner wall of the ethmoid labyrinth and forming the upper boundary of the superior meatus of the nose, and the mucous membrane covering the plate. **supreme nasal c.**, a thin bony plate occasionally found projecting from the inner wall of the ethmoid labyrinth, above the bony superior nasal concha, and the mucous membrane covering the plate.

con·cli·na·tion (kon″kli-na′shun) inward rotation of the upper pole of the vertical meridian of each eye.

con·com·i·tant (kon-kom′i-tant) accompanying; accessory; joined with another.

con·cor·dance (-kord′ins) in genetics, the occurrence of a given trait in both members of a twin pair. **concor′dant**, adj.

con·cres·cence (kon-kres′ens) 1. a growing together of parts originally separate. 2. in embryology, the flowing together and piling up of cells.

con·cre·tio (kon-kre′she-o) concretion. **c. cor′dis, c. pericar′dii**, adhesive pericarditis in which the pericardial cavity is obliterated.

con·cre·tion (kon-kre′shun) 1. a calculus or inorganic mass in a natural cavity or in tissue. 2. abnormal union of adjacent parts. 3. the process of becoming harder or more solid.

con·cus·sion (kon-kush′un) a violent shock or jar, or the condition resulting from such an injury. **c. of the brain**, loss of consciousness, transient or prolonged, due to a blow to the head; there may be transient amnesia, vertigo, nausea, weak pulse, and slow respiration. **c. of the labyrinth**, deafness with tinnitus due to a blow on or explosion near the ear. **pulmonary c.**, mechanical damage to the lungs caused by an explosion. **c. of the spinal cord**, transient spinal cord dysfunction caused by mechanical injury.

con·den·sa·tion (kon″den-sa′shun) 1. conversion from a gaseous to a liquid or solid phase. 2. compression (1). 3. the packing of dental filling materials into a tooth cavity. 4. a mental process in which one symbol stands for a number of components and contains all the emotions associated with them.

con·den·ser (kon-den′ser) 1. a vessel or apparatus for condensing gases or vapors. 2. a device for illuminating microscopic objects. 3. an apparatus for concentrating energy or matter. 4. a dental instrument used to pack plastic filling material into the prepared cavity of a tooth.

con·di·tion (kon-dish′un) to train; to subject to conditioning.

con·di·tion·ing (-ing) 1. learning in which a stimulus initially incapable of evoking a certain response becomes able to do so by repeated pairing with another stimulus that does evoke the response. 2. in physical medicine, improvement of the physical state with a program of exercise. **aversive c.**, learning in which punishment or other unpleasant stimulation is used to reduce the frequency of an undesirable response. **instrumental c., operant c.**, learning in which the frequency of a particular voluntary response is altered by the application of positive or negative consequences. **pavlovian c.,** conditioning (1).

con·dom (kon'dum) a sheath or cover worn over the penis during sexual activity to prevent impregnation or infection. **female c.,** a sheath worn inside the vagina, extending outward to cover the vulva; to prevent pregnancy or transmission of infection.

con·duc·tance (kon-duk'tans) the capacity for conducting or ability to convey. Symbol *G*. **airway c.,** the reciprocal of airway resistance; the airflow divided by the mouth-to-alveoli pressure difference.

con·duc·tion (-shun) conveyance of energy, as of heat, sound, or electricity. **conduc'-tive,** adj. **aberrant c.,** cardiac conduction through pathways not normally conducting cardiac impulses, particularly through ventricular tissue. **aerotympanal c.,** conduction of sound waves to the ear through the air and the tympanum. **air c.,** conduction of sound waves to the inner ear through the external auditory canal and middle ear. **anterograde c.,** transmission of a cardiac impulse in the normal direction, from the sinus node to the ventricles, particularly forward conduction through the atrioventricular node. **bone c.,** conduction of sound waves to the inner ear through the bones of the skull. **concealed c.,** incomplete penetration of a propagating impulse through the cardiac conducting system such that electrocardiograms reveal no evidence of transmission but the behavior of one or more subsequent impulses is somehow affected. **concealed retrograde c.,** retrograde conduction blocked in the atrioventricular node; it does not produce an extra P wave but leaves the node refractory to the next normal sinus beat. **decremental c.,** delay or failure of propagation of an impulse in the atrioventricular node resulting from progressive decrease in the rate of the rise and amplitude of the action potential as it spreads through the node. **retrograde c.,** transmission of a cardiac impulse backward in the ventricular to atrial direction, particularly conduction from the atrioventricular node into the atria. **saltatory c.,** the passage of a potential from node to node of a nerve fiber, rather than along the membrane.

con·duc·tiv·i·ty (kon″duk-tiv′ĭ-te) the capacity of a body to transmit a flow of electricity or heat; the conductance per unit area of the body.

con·du·it (kon'doo-it) channel. **ileal c.,** the surgical anastomosis of the ureters to one end of a detached segment of ileum, the other end

being used to form a stoma on the abdominal wall.

con·dy·lar·thro·sis (kon″dil-ar-thro′sis) a modification of the spheroidal form of synovial joint in which the articular surfaces are ellipsoidal rather than spheroid.

con·dyle (kon'dīl) a rounded projection on a bone, usually for articulation with another bone. **con'dylar,** adj.

con·dyl·i·on (kon-dil′e-on) the most lateral point on the surface of the head of the mandible.

con·dy·loid (kon'dĭ-loid) resembling a condyle or knuckle.

con·dy·lo·ma (kon″dĭ-lo′mah) pl. *condylo′mata.* An elevated lesion of the skin. **condylo′matous,** adj. **c. acumina′tum,** pl. *condylo′mata acumina′ta.* A papilloma with a central core connective tissue in a treelike structure covered with epithelium, of viral (human papillomavirus) origin, and usually occurring on the mucous membrane or skin of the external genitals or in the perianal region. **flat c.,** condyloma latum. **giant c.,** Buschke-Löwenstein tumor. **c. la'tum,** a broad, flat syphilitic condyloma on the folds of moist skin, especially about the genitals and anus.

con·dy·lot·o·my (-lot′ah-me) transection of a condyle.

con·dy·lus (kon'dil-us) pl. *con'dyli.* [L.] condyle.

cone (kōn) 1. a solid figure or body having a circular base and tapering to a point. 2. retinal c. 3. in radiology, a conical or open-ended cylindrical structure used as an aid in centering the radiation beam and as a guide to source-to-film distance. 4. in root canal therapy, a solid substance with a tapered form, usually made of gutta-percha or silver, fashioned to conform to the shape of a root canal. **c. of light,** the triangular reflection of light seen on the tympanic membrane. **retinal c.,** one of the specialized conical or flask-shaped outer segments of the visual cells, which, with the retinal rods, form the light-sensitive elements of the retina. **twin c's,** retinal cone cells in which two cells are blended.

co·nex·us (ko-nek'sus) pl. *conex'us.* [L.] connexus.

con·fab·u·la·tion (kon-fab″u-la′shun) unconscious filling in of gaps in memory by telling imaginary experiences.

con·fi·den·ti·al·i·ty (kon″fĭ-den″she-al′ĭ-te) the principle in medical ethics that the information a patient reveals to a health care provider is private and has limits on how and when it can be disclosed to a third party.

con·flict (kon′flikt) a mental struggle, often unconscious, arising from the clash of incompatible or opposing impulses, wishes, drives, or external demands. **extrapsychic c.,** that between the self and the external environment. **intrapsychic c.,** that between forces within the self.

con·flu·ence (kon′floo-ins) 1. a running together; a meeting of streams. **con′fluent,** adj. 2. in embryology, the flowing of cells, a component process of gastrulation. **c. of sinuses,** the dilated point of confluence of the superior sagittal, straight, occipital, and two transverse sinuses of the dura mater.

con·fron·ta·tion (kon″frun-ta′shun) a therapeutic technique constituting the act of facing or being made to face one's own attitudes and shortcomings, the way one is perceived, and the consequences of one's behavior, or of causing another to face these things.

con·fu·sion (kon-fu′zhun) disturbed orientation in regard to time, place, or person, sometimes accompanied by disordered consciousness.

con·ge·ner (kon′jĕ-ner) something closely related to another thing, as a member of the same genus, a muscle having the same function as another, or a chemical compound closely related to another in composition and exerting similar or antagonistic effects, or something derived from the same source or stock. **congener′ic, congen′erous,** adj.

con·gen·ic (kon-jen′ik) of or relating to a strain of animals developed from an inbred (isogenic) strain by repeated matings with animals from another stock that have a foreign gene, the final congenic strain then presumably differing from the original inbred strain by the presence of this gene.

con·gen·i·tal (kon-jen′ĭ-t′l) existing at, and usually before, birth; referring to conditions that are present at birth, regardless of their causation.

con·ges·tion (kon-jes′chun) abnormal accumulation of blood in a part. **conges′tive,** adj. **hypostatic c.,** congestion of a dependent part of the body or an organ due to gravitational forces, as in venous insufficiency. **passive c.,** that due to lack of vital power or to obstruction of escape of blood from the part. **pulmonary c.,** engorgement of pulmonary vessels with transudation of fluid into the alveolar and interstitial spaces, seen in cardiac disease, infections, and certain injuries. **venous c.,** passive c.

con·glo·ba·tion (kon″glo-ba′shun) the act of forming, or the state of being formed, into a rounded mass. **conglo′bate,** adj.

con·glu·ti·na·tion (kon-gloo″tĭ-na′shun) 1. adhesion. 2. agglutination of erythrocytes that is dependent upon both complement and antibodies.

con·i·cal (kon′ĭ-k′l) cone-shaped.

Co·nid·io·bo·lus (ko-nid″e-ob′o-lus) a genus of fungi of the family Entomophthoraceae, order Entomophthorales, having few septa in the mycelium and producing few zygospores but many chlamydospores and conidia. *C. corona′tus* and *C. incon′gruus* can cause entomophthoromycosis of the nasal mucosa and the subcutaneous tissues.

co·nid·i·um (kah-nid′e-um) pl. *conid′ia.* [L.] an asexually produced fungal spore.

co·nio·fi·bro·sis (ko″ne-o-fi-bro′sis) pneumoconiosis with overgrowth of lung connective tissue.

co·ni·o·sis (ko″ne-o′sis) a disease caused by inhalation of dust, such as byssinosis or pneumoconiosis.

co·nio·spo·ro·sis (ko″ne-o-spor-o′sis) maple bark disease.

con·iza·tion (kon″ĭ-za′shun) the removal of a cone of tissue, as in partial excision of the cervix uteri. **cold c.,** that done with a cold knife, as opposed to electrocautery, to better preserve the histologic elements.

con·joined (kon-joind′) joined together; united.

con·ju·ga·ta (kon″ju-gāt′ah) the conjugate diameter of the pelvis. **c. ve′ra pel′vis,** the true conjugate diameter of the pelvis.

con·ju·gate (kon′joo-gāt) 1. paired, or equally coupled; working in unison. 2. a conjugate diameter of the pelvic inlet; used alone usually to denote the true conjugate diameter; see *pelvic diameter*, under *diameter*. 3. the product of chemical conjugation.

con·ju·ga·tion (kon″joo-ga′shun) 1. the act of joining together. 2. in unicellular organisms, a form of sexual reproduction in which two cells join in temporary union to transfer genetic material. 3. in chemistry, the joining together of two compounds to produce another compound.

con·junc·ti·va (kon-junk′tĭ-vah) pl. *conjunc′tivae.* [L.] the delicate membrane lining the eyelids and covering the eyeball. **conjuncti′val,** adj.

con·junc·ti·vi·tis (kon-junk″tĭ-vi′tis) inflammation of the conjunctiva. **acute contagious c., acute epidemic c.,** pinkeye; a highly contagious form of conjunctivitis caused by *Haemophilus aegyptius.* **acute hemorrhagic c.,** a contagious form due to infection with enteroviruses. **allergic c.,** conjunctival inflammation, itching, tearing, and redness caused by allergens. **atopic c.,**

allergic conjunctivitis of the immediate type, due to airborne allergens such as pollens, dusts, spores, and animal hair. **gonococcal c., gonorrheal c.,** a severe form due to infection with gonococci. **granular c.,** trachoma. **inclusion c.,** conjunctivitis affecting newborn infants, caused by a strain of *Chlamydia trachomatis,* beginning as acute purulent conjunctivitis and leading to papillary hypertrophy of the palpebral conjunctiva. **neonatal c.,** ophthalmia neonatorum. **phlyctenular c.,** that marked by small vesicles surrounded by a reddened zone. **spring c., vernal c.,** a bilateral idiopathic form usually occurring in the spring in children.

con·junc·ti·vo·ma (kon-junk″tĭ-vo′mah) a tumor of the eyelid composed of conjunctival tissue.

con·junc·ti·vo·plas·ty (kon″junk-ti′vo-plas″te) plastic repair of the conjunctiva.

con·nec·tion (kah-nek′shun) 1. the act of connecting or state of being connected. 2. anything that connects; a connector.

con·nec·tive (-tiv) serving as a link or binding.

con·nec·tor (-ter) anything serving as a link between two separate objects or units, as between the bilateral parts of a removable partial denture.

con·nex·us (kŏ-nek′sus) pl. *connex′us.* [L.] a connecting structure.

co·noid (ko′noid) cone-shaped.

con·san·guin·i·ty (kon″sang-gwin′it-e) blood relationship; kinship. **consanguin′eous,** adj.

con·science (kon′shins) the nontechnical term for the moral faculty of the mind, corresponding roughly to the superego; differing in that the operations of the superego are often unconscious, unlike the ordinary conception of conscience.

con·scious (kon′shus) 1. having awareness of one's self, acts, and surroundings. 2. a state of alertness characterized by response to external stimuli. 3. in Freud's terminology, the part of the mind that is constantly within awareness.

con·scious·ness (-nes) 1. the state of being conscious. 2. subjective awareness of the aspects of cognitive processing and the content of the mind. 3. the current totality of experience of which an individual or group is aware at any time. 4. the conscious.

con·ser·va·tive (kon-serv′ah-tiv) designed to preserve health, restore function, and repair structures by nonradical methods.

con·sol·i·da·tion (kon-sol″ĭ-da′shun) solidification; the process of becoming or the

condition of being solid; said especially of the lung as it fills with exudate in pneumonia.

con·stant (kon′stint) 1. stable; not subject to change. 2. a quantity that is not subject to change. **association c.,** a measure of the extent of a reversible association between two molecular species. **Avogadro's c.,** see under *number.* **binding c.,** association c. **Michaelis c.,** a constant representing the substrate concentration at which the velocity of an enzyme-catalyzed reaction is half maximal; symbol K_M or K_m. **sedimentation c.,** see under *coefficient.*

con·sti·pa·tion (kon″stĭ-pa′shun) infrequent or difficult evacuation of feces. **constipa′ted,** adj.

con·sti·tu·tion (kon″stĭ-too′shun) 1. the make-up or functional habit of the body. **constitu′tional,** adj. 2. the arrangement of atoms in a molecule.

con·sti·tu·tive (kon-stich′u-tiv) produced constantly or in fixed amounts, regardless of environmental conditions or demand.

con·stric·tion (kon-strik′shun) 1. a narrowing or compression of a part; a stricture. **constric′tive,** adj. 2. a diminution in range of thinking or feeling, associated with diminished spontaneity.

con·sult 1. (kon-sult′) to confer with another physician about a case. 2. (kon′sult) consultation.

con·sul·ta·tion (kon″sul-ta′shun) a deliberation by two or more physicians about diagnosis or treatment in a particular case.

con·sump·tion (kon-sump′shun) 1. the act of consuming, or the process of being consumed. 2. a wasting away of the body.

con·tact (kon′takt) 1. a mutual touching of two bodies or persons. 2. an individual known to have been sufficiently near an infected person to have been exposed to the transfer of infectious material. **direct c., immediate c.,** the contact of a healthy person with a person having a communicable disease, the disease being transmitted as a result. **balancing c.,** the contact between the upper and lower occlusal surfaces of the teeth on the side opposite the working contact. **complete c.,** contact of the entire adjoining surfaces of two teeth. **indirect c., mediate c.,** that achieved through some intervening medium, as prolongation of a communicable disease through the air or by means of fomites. **occlusal c.,** contact between the upper and lower teeth when the jaws are closed. **proximal c., proximate c.,** touching of the proximal surfaces of two adjoining teeth. **working c.,** that between the upper and lower teeth on the side toward which the mandible has been moved in mastication.

con·tac·tant (kon-tak'tint) an allergen capable of inducing delayed contact-type hypersensitivity of the epidermis after contact.

con·ta·gion (kon-ta'jun) 1. the communication of disease from one individual to another. 2. a contagious disease.

con·ta·gious (-jus) capable of being transmitted from one individual to another, as a contagious disease; communicable.

con·tam·i·nant (kon-tam'in-int) something that causes contamination.

con·tam·i·na·tion (kon-tam"ĭ-na-shun) 1. the soiling or making inferior by contact or mixture. 2. the deposition of radioactive material in any place where it is not desired.

con·tent (kon'tent) that which is contained within a thing. **latent c.,** the hidden and unconscious true meaning of a symbolic representation such as a dream or fantasy. **manifest c.,** the content of a dream or fantasy as it is experienced and remembered, and in which the latent content is disguised and distorted by various mechanisms.

con·ti·gu·i·ty (kon"tĭ-gu'ĭ-te) contact or close proximity.

con·ti·nence (kon'tin-ens) the ability to control natural impulses. **con'tinent,** adj.

con·ti·nu·i·ty (kon"tĭ-nu'ĭ-te) the quality of being without interruption or separation.

con·tin·u·ous (kon-tin'u-us) not interrupted; having no interruption.

con·tour (kon'tŏŏr) [Fr.] 1. the normal outline or configuration of the body or of a part. 2. to shape a solid along certain desired lines.

contra- word element [L.], *against; opposed.*

con·tra·an·gle (kon"trah-ang'g'l) an angulation by which the working point of a surgical instrument is brought close to the long axis of its shaft.

con·tra·ap·er·ture (-ap'er-cher) a second opening made in an abscess to facilitate the discharge of its contents.

con·tra·cep·tion (-sep'shun) the prevention of conception or impregnation.

con·tra·cep·tive (-sep'tiv) 1. diminishing the likelihood of or preventing conception. 2. an agent that so acts. **barrier c.,** a contraceptive device that physically prevents spermatozoa from entering the endometrial cavity and fallopian tubes. **chemical c.,** a spermicidal agent inserted into the vagina before intercourse to prevent pregnancy. **emergency c.,** postcoital c. **intrauterine c.,** see under *device.* **oral c.,** a hormonal compound taken orally in order to block ovulation and prevent the occurrence of

pregnancy. **postcoital c.,** one that blocks or terminates pregnancy after sexual intercourse.

con·tract (kon-trakt') 1. to shorten, or reduce in size, as a muscle. 2. to acquire or incur.

con·trac·tile (kon-trak'til) able to contract in response to a suitable stimulus.

con·trac·til·i·ty (kon"trak-til'ĭ-te) capacity for becoming shorter in response to a suitable stimulus.

con·trac·tion (kon-trak'shun) a drawing together; a shortening or shrinkage. **Braxton Hicks c's,** light, usually painless, irregular uterine contractions during pregnancy, gradually increasing in intensity and frequency and becoming more rhythmic during the third trimester. **carpopedal c.,** the condition due to chronic shortening of the muscles of the fingers, toes, arms, and legs in tetany. **cicatricial c.,** the shrinkage and spontaneous closing of open skin wounds. **clonic c.,** clonus. **hourglass c.,** contraction of an organ, as the stomach or uterus, at or near the middle. **isometric c.,** muscle contraction without appreciable shortening or change in distance between its origin and insertion. **isotonic c.,** muscle contraction without appreciable change in the force of contraction; the distance between the muscle's origin and insertion becomes lessened. **lengthening c.,** a muscle contraction in which the ends of the muscle move farther apart, as when the muscle is forcibly flexed. **paradoxical c.,** contraction of a muscle caused by the passive approximation of its extremities. **postural c.,** the state of muscular tension and contraction which just suffices to maintain the posture of the body. **shortening c.,** a muscle contraction in which the ends of the muscle move closer together, as when a flexed limb is extended. **tetanic c.,** sustained muscular contraction without intervals of relaxation. **tonic c.,** tetanic c. **twitch c.,** twitch. **uterine c.,** contraction of the uterus during labor. **wound c.,** the shrinkage and spontaneous closure of open skin wounds.

con·trac·ture (-cher) abnormal shortening of muscle tissue, rendering the muscle highly resistant to passive stretching. **Dupuytren's c.,** flexion deformity of the fingers or toes, due to shortening, thickening, and fibrosis of the palmar or plantar fascia. **ischemic c.,** muscular contracture and degeneration due to interference with the circulation from pressure, or from injury or cold. **organic c.,** permanent and continuous contracture. **Volkmann's c.,** contraction of the fingers and sometimes of the wrist, or of analogous parts of the foot, with loss of power, after severe injury or improper use of a tourniquet.

con·tra·fis·sure (kon″trah-fish′er) a fracture in a part opposite the site of the blow.

con·tra·in·ci·sion (-in-sizh′un) counter-incision to promote drainage.

con·tra·in·di·ca·tion (-in″dĭ-ka′shun) any condition which renders a particular line of treatment improper or undesirable.

con·tra·lat·er·al (-lat′er-al) pertaining to, situated on, or affecting the opposite side.

con·trast (kon′trast) 1. the degree to which light and dark areas of an image differ in brightness or in optical density. 2. in radiology, the difference in optical density in a radiograph that results from a difference in radiolucency or penetrability of the subject.

con·tre·coup (kon″truh-koo′) [Fr.] denoting an injury, as to the brain, occurring at a site opposite to the point of impact.

con·trol (kon-trōl′) 1. the governing or limitation of certain objects or events. 2. a standard against which experimental observations may be evaluated. 3. the conscious restraint, regulation, or suppression of impulses, instincts, and affects. **aversive c.,** in behavior therapy, the use of unpleasant stimuli to change undesirable behavior. **birth c.,** deliberate limitation of childbearing by measures to control fertility and to prevent conception. **motor c.,** the systematic transmission of impulses from the motor cortex to motor units, resulting in coordinated muscular contractions. **stimulus c.,** any influence of the environment on behavior.

Con·trolled Sub·stan·ces Act a federal law that regulates the prescribing and dispensing of psychoactive drugs, including narcotics, hallucinogens, depressants, and stimulants.

con·tuse (kon-tooz′) to bruise; to wound by beating.

con·tu·sion (kon-too′zhun) bruise; an injury of a part without a break in the skin. **contrecoup c.,** one resulting from a blow on one side of the head with damage to the cerebral hemisphere on the opposite side by transmitted force.

co·nus (ko′nus) pl. *co′ni.* [L.] 1. a cone or cone-shaped structure. 2. posterior staphyloma of the myopic eye. **c. arterio′sus,** infundibulum; the anterosuperior portion of the right ventricle of the heart, at the entrance to the pulmonary trunk. **c. medulla′ris,** the cone-shaped lower end of the spinal cord, at the level of the upper lumbar vertebrae. **c. termina′lis,** conus medullaris. **co′ni vasculo′si,** lobules of epididymis.

con·va·les·cence (kon″vah-les′ins) the stage of recovery from an illness, operation, or injury.

con·vec·tion (kon-vek′shun) the act of conveying or transmission, specifically transmission of heat in a liquid or gas by bulk movement of heated particles to a cooler area. **convec′tive,** adj.

con·ver·gence (kon-ver′jens) 1. in evolution, the development of similar structures or organisms in unrelated taxa. 2. in embryology, the movement of cells from the periphery to the midline in gastrulation. 3. coordinated inclination of the two lines of sight towards their common point of fixation, or that point itself. 4. the exciting of a single sensory neuron by incoming impulses from multiple other neurons. **conver′gent,** adj. **negative c.,** outward deviation of the visual axes. **positive c.,** inward deviation of the visual axes.

con·ver·sion (kon-ver′zhun) an unconscious defense mechanism by which the anxiety that stems from intrapsychic conflict is converted and expressed in somatic symptoms.

con·ver·tase (kon-ver′tās) an enzyme of the complement system that activates specific components of the system.

con·ver·tin (kon-ver′tin) the activated form of coagulation factor VII.

con·vex (kon′veks) having a rounded, somewhat elevated surface. **convex′ity,** adj.

con·vexo·con·cave (kon-vek″so-kon′kāv) having one convex and one concave surface.

con·vexo·con·vex (-kon′veks) convex on two surfaces.

con·vo·lut·ed (kon″vo-loot′ed) rolled together or coiled.

con·vo·lu·tion (-loo′shun) a tortuous irregularity or elevation caused by the infolding of a structure upon itself. **Broca's c.,** the inferior frontal gyrus of the left hemisphere of the cerebrum. **Heschl's c's,** transverse temporal gyri; see *temporal gyrus,* under *gyrus.*

con·vul·sion (kon-vul′shun) 1. an involuntary contraction or series of contractions of the voluntary muscles. 2. seizure (2). **convul′sive,** adj. **central c.,** one not excited by any external cause, but due to a lesion of the central nervous system. **clonic c.,** one marked by alternating contraction and relaxation of the muscles. **essential c.,** central c. **febrile c's,** those associated with high fever, occurring in infants and children. **mimetic c., mimic c.,** facial spasm, as in jacksonian epilepsy. **puerperal c.,** involuntary spasms in women just before, during, or just after childbirth. **salaam c's,** infantile spasms. **tetanic c.,** tonic spasm with loss of consciousness. **uremic c.,** convulsion due to uremia, or retention in the blood of material that should have been eliminated by the kidneys.

co·op·er·a·tiv·i·ty (ko-op″er-ah-tiv′ĭ-te) the phenomenon of alteration in binding of subsequent ligands upon binding of an initial ligand by an enzyme, receptor, or other molecule with multiple binding sites; the affinity for further binding may be enhanced (*positive c.*) or decreased (*negative c.*).

co·or·di·na·tion (ko-or″dĭ-na′shun) the harmonious functioning of interrelated organs and parts.

COPD chronic obstructive pulmonary disease.

cope (kōp) in dentistry, the upper or cavity side of a denture flask.

cop·ing (kōp′ing) a thin, metal covering or cap, such as the plate of metal applied over the prepared crown or root of a tooth prior to attaching an artificial crown.

copi·opia (kop″e-o′pe-ah) eyestrain.

co·poly·mer (ko-pol′ĭ-mer) a polymer containing monomers of more than one kind.

cop·per (Cu) (kop′er) chemical element (see *Table of Elements*), at. no. 29. It is an essential dietary trace element, a necessary component of several enzymes, but is toxic in excess. **c. sulfate,** cupric sulfate.

cop·per·head (-hed) 1. a venomous snake (a pit viper), *Agkistrodon contortrix,* of the United States, having a brown to copper-colored body with dark bands. 2. a very venomous elapid snake, *Denisonia superba,* of Australia, Tasmania, and the Solomon Islands.

cop·ro·an·ti·body (kop″ro-an′tĭ-bod-e) an antibody (chiefly IgA) present in the intestinal tract, associated with immunity to enteric infection.

cop·ro·la·lia (-la′le-ah) the compulsive utterance of obscene words, especially words relating to feces.

cop·ro·lith (kop′ro-lith) fecalith.

cop·ro·phil·ia (kop″ro-fil′e-ah) an absorbing interest in feces or filth, particularly a paraphilia in which sexual arousal or activity is linked to feces. **coprophil′ic, coprophil′iac,** adj.

cop·ro·pho·bia (-fo′be-ah) abnormal repugnance to defecation and to feces.

cop·ro·por·phy·ria (-por-fir′e-ah) any of various types of porphyria characterized by elevated levels of coproporphyrin in the body. **hereditary c. (HCP),** a hepatic porphyria due to a defect in an enzyme involved in porphyrin synthesis, characterized by recurrent attacks of gastroenterologic and neurologic dysfunction, cutaneous photosensitivity, and excretion of coproporphyrin III in the feces and urine and of δ-aminolevulinic acid and porphobilinogen in urine.

cop·ro·por·phy·rin (-por″fĭ-rin) a porphyrin occurring as several isomers; the III isomer, an intermediate in heme biosynthesis, is excreted in the feces and urine in hereditary coproporphyria and variegate porphyria; the I isomer, a side product, is excreted in the feces and urine in congenital erythropoietic porphyria.

cop·ro·por·phy·rin·o·gen (-por″fĭ-rin′o-jen) a porphyrinogen (q.v.) formed from uroporphyrinogen and existing naturally as two isomers, types I and III.

cop·ro·por·phy·rin·uria (-ūr′e-ah) coproporphyrin in the urine.

cop·ros·ta·sis (kop-ros′tah-sis) fecal impaction.

cop·ro·zoa (kop″rah-zo′ah) protozoa found in feces outside the body, but not in the intestines.

cop·u·la (kop′u-lah) 1. any connecting part or structure. 2. a median ventral elevation on the embryonic tongue formed by union of the second pharyngeal arches and playing a role in tongue development.

cop·u·la·tion (kop″u-la′shun) sexual union; the transfer of the sperm from male to female; usually applied to the mating process in nonhuman animals.

Co·quil·let·tid·ia (ko-kwil″ĕ-tid′e-ah) a genus of large, mostly yellow, viciously biting, fresh-water mosquitoes; *C. pertur′bans* is a vector of eastern equine encephalitis in North America and *C. venezuelen′sis* is a South American species that is the vector of several arboviruses including Oropouche virus.

cor (kor) [L.] heart. **acute c. pulmonale,** acute overload of the right ventricle due to pulmonary hypertension, usually due to acute pulmonary embolism. **c. adipo′sum,** fatty heart (2). **c. bilocula′re,** a two-chambered heart with one atrium and one ventricle, and a common atrioventricular valve, due to failure of formation of the interatrial and interventricular septa. **c. bovi′num,** a greatly enlarged heart resulting from a hypertrophied or dilated left ventricle. **chronic c. pulmonale,** heart disease due to pulmonary hypertension secondary to disease of the lung or its blood vessels, with hypertrophy of the right ventricle. **c. triatria′tum,** a heart with three atrial chambers, the pulmonary veins emptying into an accessory chamber above the true left atrium and communicating with it by a small opening. **c. trilocula′re,** three-chambered heart. **c. trilocula′re bia-tria′tum,** a three-chambered heart with two atria communicating, by the tricuspid and mitral valves, with a single ventricle. **c. tri-locula′re biventricula′re,** a three-chambered heart with one atrium and two ventricles.

cor·a·cid·i·um (kor″ah-sid′e-um) pl. *cora-ci′dia.* [L.] the individual free-swimming or free-crawling, spherical, ciliated embryo of certain tapeworms, e.g., *Diphyllobothrium latum*.

cor·a·co·cla·vic·u·lar (kor″ah-ko-klah-vik′u-lar) pertaining to the coracoid process and the clavicle.

cor·a·coid (kor′ah-koid) 1. like a crow's beak. 2. the coracoid process.

cord (kord) any long, cylindrical, flexible structure. **genital c.**, in the embryo, the midline fused caudal part of the two uro-genital ridges, each containing a mesonephric and paramesonephric duct. **gubernacular c.**, a portion of the gubernaculum testis or of the round ligament of the uterus that develops in the inguinal crest and adjoining body wall. **sexual c's**, the seminiferous tubules of the early fetus. **spermatic c.**, the structure extending from the abdominal inguinal ring to the testis, comprising the pampiniform plexus, nerves, ductus deferens, testicular artery, and other vessels. **spinal c.**, that part of the central nervous system lodged in the vertebral canal, extending from the foramen magnum to the upper part of the lumbar region; see Plate 8. **umbilical c.**, the structure connecting the fetus and placenta, and containing the vessels through which fetal blood passes to and from the placenta. **vocal c's**, folds of mucous membrane in the larynx; the superior pair are called the *false vocal cords* and the inferior, the *true vocal cords*. **Willis' c's**, fibrous bands traversing the inferior angle of the superior sagittal sinus.

cor·dec·to·my (kor-dek′tah-me) excision of all or part of a cord, as of a vocal cord or the spinal cord.

cor·di·tis (kor-di′tis) chorditis.

cor·do·cen·te·sis (kor″do-sen-te′sis) percu-taneous puncture of the umbilical vein under ultrasonographic guidance to obtain a fetal blood sample.

cor·dot·o·my (kor-dot′ah-me) 1. section of a vocal cord. 2. surgical division of the lateral spinothalamic tract of the spinal cord, usually in the anterolateral quadrant. Spelled also *chordotomy*.

core- word element [Gr.], *pupil of eye*. Also *cor(o)-*.

core·cli·sis (kor″ĕ-kli′sis) iridencleisis.

cor·ec·ta·sis (kor-ek′tah-sis) dilation of the pupil.

cor·ec·tome (ko-rek′tōm) cutting instrument for iridectomy.

co·rec·to·me·di·al·y·sis (ko-rek″to-me″de-al′ĭ-sis) surgical creation of an artificial pupil by detaching the iris from the ciliary ligament.

cor·ec·to·pia (kor″ek-to′pe-ah) abnormal location of the pupil of the eye.

core·di·al·y·sis (ko″re-di-al′ĭ-sis) surgical separation of the external margin of the iris from the ciliary body.

co·rel·y·sis (ko-rel′ĭ-sis) operative destruc-tion of the pupil; especially detachment of adhesions of the pupillary margin of the iris from the lens.

cor·e·mor·pho·sis (ko″re-mor-fo′sis) surgi-cal formation of an artificial pupil.

cor·eo·plas·ty (ko′re-o-plas″te) any plastic operation on the pupil.

co·re·pres·sor (ko″re-pres′er) in genetic theory, a small molecule that combines with an aporepressor to form the complete repressor.

co·ri·um (kor′e-um) dermis.

corn (korn) a horny induration and thickening of the stratum corneum of the epidermis, caused by friction and pressure and forming a conical mass pointing down into the dermis, producing pain and irritation. **hard c.**, one usually located on the outside of the little toe or the upper surfaces of the other toes. **soft c.**, one between the toes, kept softened by moisture, often leading to painful inflam-mation under the corn.

cor·nea (kor′ne-ah) the transparent anterior part of the eye. See Plate 30. **cor′neal**, adj. **conical c.**, keratoconus.

cor·neo·scle·ra (kor″ne-o-skler′ah) the cornea and sclera regarded as one organ.

cor·ne·ous (kor′ne-us) 1. horny. 2. ke-ratinous.

cor·nic·u·late (kor-nik′u-lāt) shaped like a small horn.

cor·nic·u·lum (-lum) [L.] corniculate carti-lage.

cor·ni·fi·ca·tion (kor″nĭ-fĭ-ka′shun) 1. keratinization. 2. conversion of epithelium to the stratified squamous type.

cor·nu (kor′noo) pl. *cor′nua*. [L.] horn. **c. ammo′nis**, hippocampus. **c. cuta′neum**, cutaneous horn. **sacral c., c. sacra′le**, either of two hook-shaped processes extending down from the arch of the last sacral vertebra.

cor·nu·al (kor′nu-al) pertaining to a horn, especially to the horns of the spinal cord.

cor·nu·ate (kor′nu-āt) cornual.

cor(o)- see *core-*.

co·ro·na (kŏ-ro′nah) pl. *coro′nae, coronas*. [L.] a crown; in anatomical nomenclature, a crownlike eminence or encircling structure. **cor′onal**, adj. **c. glan′dis pe′nis**, the rounded proximal border of the glans penis. **c. radi-a′ta**, 1. the radiating crown of projection fi-bers passing from the internal capsule to every part of the cerebral cortex. 2. an investing layer of radially elongated follicle cells sur-rounding the zona pellucida. **c. ve′neris**, a ring of syphilitic sores around the forehead.

co·ro·nad (kor′ah-nad) toward the crown of the head or any corona.

cor·o·nary (kor′ŏ-nar″e) encircling like a crown; applied to vessels, ligaments, etc., especially to the arteries of the heart, and to pathologic involvement of them.

Co·ro·na·vi·ri·dae (ko-ro″nah-vir′ĭ-de) the coronaviruses: a family of RNA viruses with a positive-sense single-stranded polyadenylated RNA genome, transmitted through contact and other mechanical means. The single genus is *Coronavirus.*

Co·ro·na·vi·rus (ko-ro′nah-vi″rus) coronaviruses; a genus of viruses of the family Coronaviridae that cause respiratory disease and possibly gastroenteritis in humans and hepatitis, gastroenteritis, encephalitis, and respiratory disease in other animals.

co·ro·na·vi·rus (kŏ-ro′nah-vi″rus) any virus belonging to the family Coronaviridae.

cor·o·ner (kor′on-er) an officer who holds inquests in regard to violent, sudden, or unexplained deaths.

cor·o·noid (kor′ah-noid) 1. shaped like a crow's beak. 2. crown-shaped.

cor·o·noi·dec·to·my (kor″ah-noi-dek′tah-me) surgical removal of the coronoid process of the mandible.

co·rot·o·my (ko-rot′ah-me) iridotomy.

cor·pu·len·cy (kor′pu-lin-se) obesity.

cor·pus (kor′pus) pl. *cor′pora.* [L.] body. **c. adipo′sum buc′cae,** sucking pad. **c. al′bicans,** white fibrous tissue that replaces the regressing corpus luteum in the human ovary in the latter half of pregnancy, or soon after ovulation when pregnancy does not supervene. **c. amygdaloi′deum,** a small mass of subcortical gray matter within the tip of the temporal lobe, anterior to the inferior horn of the lateral ventricle of the brain; it is part of the limbic system. **cor′pora amyla′cea,** small hyaline masses, of unknown pathologic significance and occurring more commonly with advancing age, derived from degenerate cells or thickened secretions and found in the prostate, neuroglia, and pulmonary alveoli. **cor′pora bige′mina,** two bodies in the brain of the human fetus that later split to become the corpora quadrigemina. **c. callo′sum,** an arched mass of white matter in the depths of the longitudinal fissure, composed of transverse fibers connecting the cerebral hemispheres. **c. caverno′sum,** either of the columns of erectile tissue forming the body of the clitoris (*c. cavernosum clitoridis*) or penis (*c. cavernosum penis*). **c. hemorrha′gicum,** a blood clot formed in the cavity left by the mature ovarian follicle after its rupture during ovulation. **c. lu′teum,** a yellow glandular mass in the ovary, formed by an ovarian follicle that has matured and discharged its oocyte. **cor′pora quadrige′mina,** four rounded eminences on the posterior surface of the mesencephalon. **c. spongio′sum pe′nis,** a column of erectile tissue forming the urethral surface of the penis, in which the urethra is found. **c. stria′tum,** a subcortical mass of gray and white substance in front of and lateral to the thalamus in each cerebral hemisphere. **c. u′teri,** body of uterus: that part of the uterus above the isthmus and below the orifices of the uterine tubes. **c. vi′treum,** the vitreous body of the eye.

cor·pus·cle (kor′pus′l) any small mass or body. **corpus′cular,** adj. **blood c.,** see under *cell.* **corneal c's,** star-shaped corpuscles within the corneal spaces. **genital c.,** a type of small encapsulated nerve ending in the mucous membranes of the genital region and the skin around the nipples. **Golgi's c.,** Golgi tendon organ. **Hassall's c's,** spherical or ovoid bodies found in the medulla of the thymus, composed of concentric arrays of epithelial cells which contain keratohyalin and bundles of cytoplasmic filaments. **lamellar c., lamellated c.,** a type of large encapsulated nerve ending found throughout the body, concerned with perception of sensations. **malpighian c's,** renal c's. **Meissner's c.,** tactile c. **Pacini's c., pacinian c.,** lamellated c. **paciniform c's,** a type of rapidly adapting lamellated corpuscles responding to muscle stretch and light pressure. **red c.,** erythrocyte. **renal c's,** bodies forming the beginning of nephrons, each consisting of the glomerulus and glomerular capsule. **tactile c.,** a type of medium-sized encapsulated nerve ending in the skin, chiefly in the palms and soles. **thymus c's,** Hassall's c's. **white c.,** leukocyte.

cor·pus·cu·lum (kor-pus′ku-lum) pl. *cor-pus′cula.* [L.] corpuscle.

cor·rec·tion (kah-rek′shun) a setting right, e.g., the provision of lenses for improvement of vision, or an arbitrary adjustment made in values or devices in performance of experiments.

cor·re·la·tion (kor″ĕ-la′shun) in statistics, the degree and direction of association of variable phenomena; how well one can be predicted from the other.

cor·re·spon·dence (kor″is-pon′dins) the condition of being in agreement or conformity. **anomalous retinal c.,** a condition in which disparate points on the retinas of the two eyes come to be associated sensorially. **normal retinal c.,** the condition in which the corresponding points on the retinas of the two eyes are associated sensorially. **retinal c.,** the state concerned with the impingement of image-producing stimuli on the retinas of the two eyes.

cor·rin (kor′in) a tetrapyrrole ring system resembling the porphyrin ring system. The cobalamins contain a corrin ring system.

cor·ro·sive (kor-o′siv) producing gradual destruction, as of a metal by electrochemical reaction or of the tissues by the action of a strong acid or alkali; an agent that so acts.

cor·tex (kor′teks) pl. *cor′tices.* [L.] the outer layer of an organ or other structure, as distinguished from its inner substance. **cor′- tical,** adj. **adrenal c.,** the outer, firm layer comprising the larger part of the adrenal gland; it secretes many steroid hormones including mineralocorticoids, glucocorticoids, androgens, 17-ketosteroids, and progestins. **cerebellar c., c. cerebella′ris,** the superficial gray matter of the cerebellum. **cerebral c., c. cerebra′lis,** the convoluted layer of gray substance covering each cerebral hemisphere; see *archicortex, paleocortex,* and *neocortex.* **c. len′tis,** the softer, external part of the lens of the eye. **motor c.,** see under *area.* **provi- sional c.,** the cortex of the fetal adrenal gland that undergoes involution in early fetal life. **renal c., c. re′nis,** the outer part of the substance of the kidney, composed mainly of glomeruli and convoluted tubules. **striate c.,** the part of the occipital lobe of the cerebral cortex that is the primary receptive area for vision. **c. of thymus,** the outer part of each lobule of the thymus; it consists chiefly of closely packed lymphocytes (thymocytes) and surrounds the medulla. **visual c.,** the area of the occipital lobe of the cerebral cortex concerned with vision.

cor·ti·cate (kor′ti-kāt) having a cortex or bark.

cor·ti·cec·to·my (kor″ti-sek′tah-me) topec- tomy.

cor·ti·cif·u·gal (sif′u-gl) efferent; proceed- ing or conducting away from the cerebral cortex.

cor·ti·cip·e·tal (-sip′ĕ-t′l) proceeding or conducting toward the cerebral cortex. Cf. *afferent.*

cor·ti·co·bul·bar (kor″ti-ko-bul′ber) per- taining to or connecting the cerebral cortex and the medulla oblongata or brain stem.

cor·ti·coid (kor′ti-koid) corticosteroid.

cor·ti·co·ster·oid (-ster′oid) any of the steroids elaborated by the adrenal cortex (excluding the sex hormones) or any synthetic equivalents; divided into two major groups, the *glucocorticoids* and *mineralocorticoids;* used

clinically for hormonal replacement therapy, for suppression of ACTH secretion, as anti- inflammatory agents, and to suppress the immune response.

cor·ti·cos·ter·one (kor″ti-kos′ter-ōn) a natural corticoid with moderate glucocorti- coid activity, some mineralocorticoid activity, and actions similar to cortisol except that it is not antiinflammatory.

cor·ti·co·ten·sin (-ten′sin) a polypeptide purified from kidney extract that exhibits a vasopressor effect when given intravenously.

cor·ti·co·troph (kor′ti-ko-trōf) an acidophil of the adenohypophysis that secretes cortico- tropin.

cor·ti·co·tro·phin (kor′ti-ko-tro″fin) corti- cotropin.

cor·ti·co·tro·pin (-tro′pin) 1. a hormone secreted by the adenohypophysis, having a stimulating effect on the adrenal cortex. 2. a preparation of the hormone derived from animals, used for diagnostic testing of adreno- cortical function and as an anticonvulsant in infantile spasms.

cor·ti·lymph (kor′ti-limf″) the fluid filling the intercellular spaces of the organ of Corti, similar in composition to perilymph.

cor·ti·sol (-sol) the major natural glucocorti- coid elaborated by the adrenal cortex; it affects the metabolism of glucose, protein, and fats and has mineralocorticoid activity. See *hydro- cortisone* for therapeutic uses.

cor·ti·sone (-sōn) a natural glucocorticoid that is metabolically convertible to cortisol; the acetate ester is used as an antiinflamma- tory and immunosuppressant and for replace- ment therapy in adrenocortical insufficiency.

co·run·dum (kor-un′dum) native aluminum oxide, Al_2O_3, used in dentistry as an abrasive and polishing agent.

cor·us·ca·tion (kor″us-ka′shun) the sensa- tion as of a flash of light before the eyes.

co·rym·bi·form (ko-rim′bĭ-form) clustered; said of lesions grouped around a single, usually larger, lesion.

Co·ry·ne·bac·te·ri·a·ceae (ko-ri″ne-bak- tēr″e-a′se-e) in former systems of classifica- tion, a family of coryneform bacteria, related to the actinomycetes, which included the genera *Corynebacterium, Erysipelothrix,* and *Listeria.*

Co·ry·ne·bac·te·ri·um (-bak-tēr′e-um) a genus of bacteria including *C. ac′nes,* a species present in acne lesions, *C. diphthe′riae,* the etiologic agent of diphtheria, *C. minutis′- simum,* the etiologic agent of erythrasma, and *C. pseudodiphtheri′ticum,* a nonpathogenic species present in the respiratory tract.

co·ry·ne·form (-form) denoting or resembling organisms of the family Corynebacteriaceae.

Co·ry·nes·po·ra (kor″ĭnes′pah-rah) a widespread genus of imperfect fungi; *C. cassi′cola* is a cause of eumycotic mycetoma.

co·ry·za (ko-ri′zah) [L.] acute rhinitis.

COS Canadian Ophthalmological Society.

cos·me·sis (koz-me′sis) 1. the preservation, restoration, or bestowing of bodily beauty. 2. the surgical correction of a disfiguring physical defect.

cos·met·ic (koz-met′ik) 1. pertaining to cosmesis. 2. a beautifying substance or preparation.

cos·ta (kos′tah) [L.] 1. a rib. 2. a thin, firm, rodlike structure running along the base of the undulating membrane of certain flagellates. **cos′tal**, adj.

cos·tal·gia (kos-tal′jah) 1. pain in the ribs. 2. pain in the costal muscles.

cos·ta·lis (kos-ta′lis) [L.] costal.

cos·tive (kos′tiv) 1. pertaining to, characterized by, or producing constipation. 2. an agent that depresses intestinal motility.

cost(o)- word element [L.], *rib*.

cos·to·chon·dral (kos″to-kon′dril) pertaining to a rib and its cartilage.

cos·to·cla·vic·u·lar (-klah-vik′u-lar) pertaining to the ribs and clavicle.

cos·to·gen·ic (-jen′ik) arising from a rib, especially from a defect of the marrow of the ribs.

cos·to·scap·u·lar·is (-skap″u-la′ris) the serratus anterior muscle.

cos·to·ster·no·plas·ty (-ster′no-plas″te) surgical repair of funnel chest, a segment of rib being used to support the sternum.

cos·to·trans·ver·sec·to·my (-trans″ver-sek′to-me) excision of a part of a rib along with the transverse process of a vertebra.

cos·to·ver·te·bral (-ver′tĕ-br'l) pertaining to a rib and a vertebra.

co·syn·tro·pin (ko-sin-tro′pin) a synthetic polypeptide identical with a portion of corticotropin, having its corticotropic activity but not its allergenicity; used in the screening of adrenal insufficiency on the basis of plasma cortisol response.

co·trans·fec·tion (ko″trans-fek′shun) simultaneous transfection with two separate, unrelated nucleic acid molecules, one of which may contain a gene that is easily assayed and acts as a marker.

co·trans·port (ko-trans′port) linking of the transport of one substance across a membrane with the simultaneous transport of a different substance in the same direction.

co·tri·mox·a·zole (ko″tri-moks′ah-zōl) a combination of trimethoprim and sulfamethoxazole, an antibacterial used primarily in the treatment of urinary tract infections and *Pneumocystis carinii* pneumonia.

cot·ton (kot′n) a plant of the genus *Gossypium*, or a textile material derived from its seeds. **absorbable c.**, oxidized cellulose. **absorbent c.**, **purified c.**, cotton freed from impurities, bleached, and sterilized; used as a surgical dressing.

cot·y·le·don (kot″ĭ-le′d'n) 1. the seed leaf of the embryo of a plant. 2. any subdivision of the uterine surface of the placenta.

cot·y·loid (kot′ĭ-loid) cup-shaped.

cough (kof) 1. sudden noisy expulsion of air from lungs. 2. to produce such an expulsion. **dry c.**, cough without expectoration. **hacking c.**, a short, frequent, shallow and feeble cough. **productive c.**, cough with expectoration of material from the bronchi. **reflex c.**, cough due to irritation of some remote organ. **wet c.**, productive c. **whooping c.**, pertussis.

cou·lomb (C) (koo′lom) the SI unit of electric charge, defined as the quantity of electric charge transferred across a surface by 1 ampere in 1 second.

cou·ma·rin (koo′mah-rin) 1. a principle extracted from the tonka bean; it contains a factor, dicumarol, that inhibits hepatic synthesis of vitamin K–dependent coagulation factors, and a number of its derivatives are used as anticoagulants in treating disorders characterized by excessive clotting. 2. any of these derivatives or any synthetic compound with similar activity.

count (kount) a numerical computation or indication. **Addis c.**, determining the number of erythrocytes, leukocytes, epithelial cells, casts, and protein content in an aliquot of a 12-hour urine specimen. **blood c.**, **blood cell c.**, determining the number of formed elements in a cubic millimeter of blood; it may be a complete blood count or it may measure just one of the formed elements. **complete blood c.**, a series of tests of the peripheral blood, including the hematocrit, the amount of hemoglobin, and counts of each type of formed element. **differential leukocyte c.**, a count on a stained blood smear of the proportion of different types of leukocytes (or other cells), expressed in percentages. **platelet c.**, determination of the total number of platelets per cubic millimeter of blood; the *direct platelet c.* simply counts the cells using a microscope, and the *indirect platelet c.* determines the ratio of platelets to erythrocytes on a peripheral blood smear and computes the number of platelets from the erythrocyte count.

coun·ter (koun'ter) an instrument to compute numerical value; in radiology, a device for enumerating ionizing events. **Coulter c.,** an automatic instrument used in enumeration of formed elements in the peripheral blood. **Geiger c., Geiger-Müller c.,** an amplifying device that indicates the presence of ionizing particles, particularly β particles. **scintillation c.,** a device for detecting ionization events, permitting determination of the concentration of radioisotopes in the body or other substance.

coun·ter·cur·rent (-kur″ent) flowing in an opposite direction.

coun·ter·ex·ten·sion (koun″ter-eks-ten′-shun) traction in a proximal direction coincident with traction in opposition to it.

coun·ter·im·mu·no·elec·tro·pho·re·sis (-im″u-no-e-lek″tro-for-e′sis) immunoelectrophoresis in which the antigen and antibody migrate in opposite directions.

coun·ter·in·ci·sion (-in-si′zhun) a second incision made to promote drainage or to relieve tension on the edges of a wound.

coun·ter·ir·ri·ta·tion (-ir″ĭ-ta′shun) superficial irritation intended to relieve some other irritation.

coun·ter·open·ing (-o″pen-ing) a second incision made across an earlier one to promote drainage.

coun·ter·pul·sa·tion (-pul-sa′shun) a technique for assisting the circulation and decreasing the work of the heart, by synchronizing the force of an external pumping device with cardiac systole and diastole. **intra-aortic balloon (IAB) c.,** circulatory support provided by a balloon inserted into the thoracic aorta, inflated during diastole and deflated during systole.

coun·ter·shock (koun′ter-shok″) a high intensity direct current shock delivered to the heart to interrupt ventricular fibrillation and restore synchronous electrical activity.

coun·ter·stain (-stān) a stain applied to render the effects of another stain more discernible.

coun·ter·trac·tion (-trak″shun) traction opposed to another traction; used in reduction of fractures.

coun·ter·trans·fer·ence (koun″ter-trans-fer′ens) a transference reaction of a psychoanalyst or other psychotherapist to a patient.

coun·ter·trans·port (-trans′port) the simultaneous transport of two substances across a membrane in opposite directions, either by the same carrier or by two carriers that are biochemically linked to each other.

coup (koo) [Fr.] a blow or attack. **c. de fouet** (dĕ-fwa′), rupture of the plantaris muscle accompanied by a sharp disabling pain. **c. de sabre, en c. de sabre** (dĕ-sahb′, ahn-koo-dĕ-sahb′), a lesion of linear scleroderma on the forehead and scalp, often associated with hemiatrophy of the face.

cou·ple (kup′l) 1. to link together; join; connect. 2. two equal forces operating on an object in parallel but opposite directions. 3. an area of contact between two dissimilar metals, producing a difference in electrical potential.

coup·let (kup′let) pair (2).

coup·ling (kup′ling) 1. the joining together of two things. 2. in genetics, the occurrence on the same chromosome in a double heterozygote of the two mutant alleles of interest. 3. in cardiology, serial occurrence of a normal heartbeat followed closely by a premature beat.

co·va·lence (ko-va′lens) 1. the number of electron pairs an atom can share with other atoms. 2. one or more chemical bonds formed by sharing of electron pairs between atoms. **cova′lent,** adj.

co·var·i·ance (ko-vār′e-ins) a measure of the tendency of two random variables to vary together.

cov·er·glass (kuv′er-glas) a thin glass plate that covers a mounted microscopical object or a culture.

cov·er·slip (-slip) coverglass.

cow·per·itis (kou″per-i′tis) inflammation of Cowper's (bulbourethral) glands.

cow·pox (kou′poks) a mild eruptive disease of milk cows, confined to the udder and teats, due to cowpox virus, and transmissible to humans.

coxa (kok′sah) [L.] 1. hip. 2. hip joint. **c. mag′na,** broadening of the head and neck of the femur. **c. pla′na,** osteochondrosis of the capitular epiphysis of the femur. **c. val′ga,** deformity of the hip with increase in the angle of inclination between the neck and shaft of the femur. **c. va′ra,** deformity of the hip with decrease in the angle of inclination between the neck and shaft of the femur.

cox·al·gia (kok-sal′jah) 1. hip-joint disease. 2. pain in the hip.

cox·ar·throp·a·thy (koks″ar-throp′ah-the) hip-joint disease.

Cox·i·el·la (kok″se-el′ah) a genus of rickettsiae, including *C. burnet′ii,* the etiologic agent of Q fever.

coxo·fem·o·ral (kok″so-fem′ah-ril) pertaining to the hip and thigh.

coxo·tu·ber·cu·lo·sis (-too-berk″u-lo′sis) hip-joint disease.

cox·sack·ie·vi·rus (kok-sak'e-vi"rus) one of a group of viruses producing, in humans, a disease resembling poliomyelitis, but without paralysis.

CPD citrate phosphate dextrose; see *anticoagulant citrate phosphate dextrose solution*, under *solution*.

CPDA-1 citrate phosphate dextrose adenine; see *anticoagulant citrate phosphate dextrose adenine solution*, under *solution*.

CPDD calcium pyrophosphate deposition disease.

C Ped Certified Pedorthist.

CPK creatine kinase.

cpm counts per minute, an expression of the rate of particle emission from a radioactive material.

CPR cardiopulmonary resuscitation.

cps cycles per second; see *hertz.*

CR conditioned reflex (response).

Cr chromium.

crack (krak) an incomplete split, break, or fissure.

crack·le (krak'l) rale.

cra·dle (kra'd'l) a frame placed over the body of a bed patient for application of heat or cold or for protecting injured parts from contact with bed covers.

cramp (kramp) a painful spasmodic muscular contraction. **heat c.,** spasm with pain, weak pulse, and dilated pupils; seen in workers in intense heat. **recumbency c's,** cramping in legs and feet occurring while resting or during light sleep. **writers' c.,** a muscle cramp in the hand caused by excessive use in writing.

cra·ni·ad (kra'ne-ad) in a cranial direction; toward the anterior (in animals) or superior (in humans) end of the body.

cra·ni·al (-al) 1. pertaining to the cranium. 2. toward the head end of the body; a synonym of *superior* in humans and other bipeds.

crani(o)- word element [L.], *skull.*

cra·nio·cele (kra'ne-o-sēl") encephalocele.

cra·nio·fa·cial (kra"ne-o-fa'sh'l) pertaining to the cranium and the face.

cra·nio·fe·nes·tria (-fen-es'tre-ah) defective development of the fetal cranium, with areas in which no bone is formed.

cra·nio·la·cu·nia (-lah-ku'ne-ah) defective development of the fetal cranium, with depressed areas on the inner surface.

cra·nio·ma·la·cia (-mah-la'shah) abnormal softness of the bones of the skull.

cra·ni·om·e·try (kra"ne-om'ah-tre) the scientific measurement of the dimensions of the bones of the skull and face. **craniomet'ric,** adj.

cra·ni·op·a·thy (-op'ah-the) any disease of the skull. **metabolic c.,** a condition characterized by lesions of the calvaria with multiple metabolic changes, and by headache, obesity, and visual disorders.

cra·nio·pha·ryn·gi·o·ma (kra"ne-o-fah-rin"je-o'mah) a tumor arising from cell rests derived from the infundibulum of the hypophysis or Rathke's pouch.

cra·nio·plas·ty (kra'ne-o-plas"te) any plastic operation on the skull.

cra·nio·ra·chis·chi·sis (kra"ne-o-rah-kis'kĭ-sis) congenital fissure of the cranium and vertebral column.

cra·ni·os·chi·sis (kra"ne-os'kĭ-sis) cranium bifidum.

cra·nio·scle·ro·sis (kra"ne-o-sklĕ-ro'sis) thickening of the bones of the skull.

cra·nio·ste·no·sis (-stĕ-no'sis) deformity of the skull caused by craniosynostosis, with consequent cessation of skull growth.

cra·ni·os·to·sis (kra"ne-os-to'sis) craniosynostosis.

cra·nio·syn·os·to·sis (kra"ne-o-sin"os-to'sis) premature closure of the sutures of the skull.

cra·ni·o·ta·bes (-ta'bēz) reduction in mineralization of the skull, with abnormal softness of the bone, usually affecting the occipital and parietal bones along the lambdoidal sutures.

cra·ni·ot·o·my (kra"ne-ot'ah-me) any operation on the cranium.

cra·ni·um (kra'ne-um) pl. *cra'nia.* [L.] the skeleton of the head, variously construed as including all of the bones of the head except the mandible, or as the eight bones forming the vault lodging the brain. **cranial,** adj. **c. bi'fidum,** a congenitally incomplete skull, often with an incomplete brain.

cra·ter (kra'ter) an excavated area surrounded by an elevated margin.

cra·vat (krah-vat') a triangular bandage.

cream (krēm) 1. the fatty part of milk from which butter is prepared, or a fluid mixture of similar consistency. 2. in pharmaceutical preparations, a semisolid dosage form being either an emulsion of oil and water or an aqueous microcrystalline dispersion of a long-chain fatty acid or alcohol.

crease (krēs) a line or slight linear depression. **flexion c., palmar c.,** any of the normal grooves across the palm that accommodate flexion of the hand by separating folds of tissue. **simian c.,** a single transverse palmar crease formed by fusion of the proximal and distal palmar creases; seen in congenital disorders such as Down syndrome.

cre·a·tine (kre'ah-tin) an amino acid occurring in vertebrate tissues, particularly in muscle; phosphorylated creatine is an important storage form of high-energy phosphate. **c. phosphate,** phosphocreatine.

cre·a·tine ki·nase (ki′nās) an enzyme that catalyzes the phosphorylation of creatine by ATP to form phosphocreatine. It occurs as three isozymes (specific to brain, cardiac muscle, and skeletal muscle, respectively), each having two components composed of M (muscle) and/or B (brain) subunits. Differential determination of isozymes is used in clinical diagnosis.

cre·at·i·nine (kre-at′ĭ-nin) an anhydride of creatine, the end product of phosphocreatine metabolism; measurements of its rate of urinary excretion are used as diagnostic indicators of kidney function and muscle mass.

crem·as·ter·ic (krem″as-ter′ik) pertaining to the cremaster muscle.

cre·na (kre′nah) pl. *cre′nae.* [L.] a notch or cleft.

cre·nat·ed (kre′nāt-id) scalloped or notched.

cre·na·tion (kren-a′shun) the formation of abnormal notching around the edge of an erythrocyte; the notched appearance of an erythrocyte due to its shrinkage after suspension in a hypertonic solution.

cre·no·cyte (kre′nah-sīt) burr cell.

crep·i·ta·tion (krep″ĭ-ta′shun) a dry sound like that of grating the ends of a fractured bone. **crep′itant,** adj.

crep·i·tus (krep′ĭ-tus) 1. the discharge of flatus from the bowels. 2. crepitation. 3. crepitant rale.

cres·cent (kres′int) 1. shaped like a new moon. 2. something with this shape. **crescen′tic,** adj. **c's of Giannuzzi,** crescent-shaped patches of serous cells surrounding the mucous tubercles in seromucous glands. **myopic c.,** a crescentic staphyloma in the fundus of the eye in myopia. **sublingual c.,** the crescent-shaped area on the floor of the mouth, bounded by the lingual wall of the mandible and the base of the tongue.

cre·sol (kre′sol) a toxic, corrosive liquid with disinfectant and antiseptic actions, obtained from coal tar as a mixture of three isomeric forms and containing not more than 5 per cent phenol; used for sterilizing items.

crest (krest) a projection, or projecting structure or ridge, especially one surmounting a bone or its border. **ampullar c.,** the most prominent part of a localized thickening of the membrane lining the ampullae of the semicircular ducts. **frontal c.,** a median ridge on the internal surface of the frontal bone. **iliac c.,** the thickened, expanded upper border of the ilium. **intertrochanteric c.,** a ridge on the posterior femur connecting the greater

with the lesser trochanter. **lacrimal c., anterior,** the lateral margin of the groove on the posterior border of the frontal process of the maxilla. **lacrimal c., posterior,** a vertical ridge dividing the lateral or orbital surface of the lacrimal bone into two parts. **nasal c.,** 1. (of maxilla) a ridge, raised along the medial border of the palatine process of the maxilla, with which the vomer articulates. 2. (of palatine) a thick ridge projecting superiorly from the horizontal plate of the palatine bone and articulating with the posterior part of the vomer. **neural c.,** a cellular band dorsolateral to the embryonic neural tube that gives origin to the spinal ganglia and other structures. **occipital c., external,** a ridge sometimes extending on the external surface of the occipital bone from the external protuberance toward the foramen magnum. **occipital c., internal,** a median ridge on the internal surface of the occipital bone, extending from the midpoint of the cruciform eminence toward the foramen magnum. **palatine c.,** a transverse ridge sometimes seen on the inferior surface of the horizontal plate of the palatine bone. **pubic c.,** the thick, rough anterior border of the body of the pubic bone. **sacral c.,** any of various ridges or tubercles on the dorsal surface of the sacrum, named for their location as *median* or as *lateral* or *medial* (relative to the dorsal sacral foramina); used alone it usually denotes the median sacral crest. **seminal c.,** see under *colliculus.* **sphenoidal c.,** a median ridge on the anterior surface of the body of the sphenoid bone, articulating with the ethmoid bone. **supramastoid c.,** the superior border of the posterior root of the zygomatic process of the temporal bone. **supraventricular c.,** a ridge on the inner wall of the right ventricle, marking off the conus arteriosus. **temporal c. of frontal bone,** a ridge extending superiorly and posteriorly from the zygomatic process of the frontal bone. **turbinal c.,** 1. (of maxilla) an oblique ridge on the maxilla, articulating with the nasal concha. 2. (of palatine bone) a horizontal ridge on the internal surface of the palatine bone. **urethral c.,** a prominent longitudinal mucosal fold along the posterior wall of the female urethra, or a median elevation along the posterior wall of the male urethra between the prostatic sinuses. **c. of vestibule,** a ridge between the spherical and elliptical recesses of the vestibule, dividing posteriorly to bound the cochlear recess.

cre·tin·ism (kre′tin-izm) arrested physical and mental development with dystrophy of bones and soft tissues, due to congenital lack of thyroid secretion. **athyrotic c.,** cretinism due to thyroid aplasia or destruction of the thyroid of the fetus in utero. **endemic c.,** a form occurring in regions of severe endemic goiter, marked by deaf-mutism, spasticity, and motor dysfunction in addition to, or instead of, the usual manifestations of cretinism. **sporadic goitrous c.,** a genetic disorder in which enlargement of the thyroid gland is associated with deficient circulating thyroid hormone.

cre·tin·oid (-oid) resembling or suggestive of cretinism.

crev·ice (krev′is) fissure. **gingival c.,** the space between the cervical enamel of a tooth and the overlying unattached gingiva.

cre·vic·u·lar (krĕ-vik′u-ler) pertaining to a crevice, especially the gingival crevice.

CRH corticotropin-releasing hormone.

crib·ra·tion (krĭ-bra′shun) 1. the quality of being cribriform. 2. the process or act of sifting or passing through a sieve.

crib·ri·form (krib′rĭ-form) perforated like a sieve.

crib·rum (krib′rum) pl. *crib′ra.* [L.] lamina cribrosa of ethmoid bone.

cri·coid (kri′koid) 1. ring-shaped. 2. the cricoid cartilage.

cri·co·thy·rot·o·my (-thi-rot′ah-me) incision through the skin and cricothyroid membrane to secure a patent airway for emergency relief of upper airway obstruction.

cri·co·tra·che·ot·o·my (-tra″ke-ot′ah-me) incision of the trachea through the cricoid cartilage.

cri du chat (kre doo shah′) [Fr.] see under *syndrome.*

crin·oph·a·gy (krin-of′ah-je) the intracytoplasmic digestion of the contents (peptides, proteins) of secretory vacuoles, after the vacuoles fuse with lysosomes.

cri·sis (kri′sis) pl. *cri′ses.* [L.] 1. the turning point of a disease for better or worse; especially a sudden change, usually for the better, in the course of an acute disease. 2. a sudden paroxysmal intensification of symptoms in the course of a disease. **addisonian c., adrenal c.,** fatigue, nausea, vomiting, and weight loss accompanying an acute attack of Addison's disease. **blast c.,** a sudden, severe change in the course of chronic granulocytic leukemia with an increase in the proportion of myeloblasts. **genital c. of newborn,** estrinization of the vaginal mucosa and hyperplasia of the breast, influenced by transplacentally acquired estrogens. **hemolytic c.,** acute red cell destruction leading to jaundice, occasionally seen with sickle cell disease. **identity c.,** a period in the psychosocial development of an individual, usually occurring during adolescence, manifested by confusion over one's self, values, or perceived role expected by society. **sickle cell c.,** a broad term for several acute conditions occurring with sickle cell disease, including hemolytic crisis and vaso-occlusive crisis. **thyroid c., thyrotoxic c.,** thyroid storm; a sudden and dangerous increase of symptoms of thyrotoxicosis. **vasoocclusive c.,** severe pain due to infarctions in the bones, joints, lungs, liver, kidney, spleen, eye, or central nervous system, an acute condition seen with sickle cell anemia.

cris·ta (kris′tah) pl. *cris′tae.* [L.] crest. **cris′tae cu′tis,** dermal ridges; ridges of the skin produced by the projecting papillae of the dermis on the palm of the hand or sole of the foot, producing a fingerprint or footprint characteristic of the individual. **c. gal′li,** a thick, triangular process projecting superiorly from the cribriform plate of the ethmoid bone. **mitochondrial cristae,** numerous narrow transverse infoldings of the inner membrane of a mitochondrion.

Cri·thid·ia (krĭ-thid′e-ah) a genus of parasitic protozoa found in the digestive tract of arthropods and other invertebrates.

crit·i·cal (krit′ĭ-k'l) 1. pertaining to or of the nature of a crisis. 2. pertaining to a disease or other morbid condition in which there is danger of death. 3. in sufficient quantity as to constitute a turning point, as a critical mass.

CRL crown-rump length.

CRNA Certified Registered Nurse Anesthetist.

cRNA complementary RNA.

cro·cid·o·lite (kro-sid′o-līt) an amphibole type of asbestos that causes asbestosis as well as mesotheliomas and other cancers.

cro·mo·lyn (kro′mol-in) an inhibitor of the release of histamine and other mediators of immediate hypersensitivity from mast cells; used as the sodium salt for prophylaxis and treatment of allergic rhinitis, bronchial asthma associated with allergy, and allergen-induced inflammation of the conjunctiva or cornea, and for treatment of mastocytosis.

cross (kros) 1. a cross-shaped figure or structure. 2. any organism produced by crossbreeding; a method of crossbreeding.

cross·bite (kros′bīt) malocclusion in which the mandibular teeth are in buccal version (or complete lingual version in posterior segments) to the maxillary teeth.

cross·breed·ing (-brēd-ing) hybridization; the mating of organisms of different strains or species.

crossed (krost) shaped or arranged like a cross or the letter X.

cross-eye (kros'i) esotropia.

cross·ing over (kros'ing o'ver) the exchanging of material between homologous chromosomes during the first meiotic division, resulting in new combinations of genes.

cross-link (kros'link″) a covalent bond formed between polymer chains, either within or across chains.

cross·match·ing (-mach-ing) determination of the compatibility of the blood of a donor and that of a recipient before transfusion by placing the donor's cells in the recipient's serum and the recipient's cells in the donor's serum; absence of agglutination, hemolysis, and cytotoxicity indicates compatibility.

cross-re·ac·tiv·i·ty (kros″re-ak-tiv'ĭ-te) the degree to which an antibody participates in cross reactions.

cross-re·sis·tance (kros-re-zis'tans) multidrug resistance.

cross-tol·er·ance (kros'tol-er-ans) extension of the tolerance for a substance to others of the same class, even those to which the body has not been exposed previously.

crot·a·lid (krot'ah-lid) 1. any snake of the family Crotalidae; a pit viper. 2. of or pertaining to the family Crotalidae.

Cro·tal·i·dae (kro-tal'ĭ-de) a family of venomous snakes, the pit vipers.

cro·ta·line (kro'tah-lēn) crotalid.

Cro·ta·lus (kro'tah-lus) a genus of rattlesnakes.

cro·ta·mi·ton (krōt″ah-mi'ton) an acaricide used in the treatment of scabies and as an antipruritic.

cro·ton·ic ac·id (kro-ton'ik) an unsaturated fatty acid found in croton oil.

croup (krōōp) acute partial obstruction of the upper airway, usually in young children and caused by a viral or bacterial infection, allergy, foreign body, or new growth; characteristics include barking cough, hoarseness, and stridor. **croup'ous, croup'y,** adj. **bacterial c., membranous c., pseudomembranous c.,** bacterial tracheitis.

crown (kroun) 1. the topmost part of an organ or structure, e.g., the top of the head. 2. artificial c. **anatomical c.,** the upper, enamel-covered part of a tooth. **artificial c.,** a reproduction of a crown affixed to the remaining natural structure of a tooth. **clinical c.,** the portion of a tooth exposed beyond the gingiva. **physiological c.,** the portion of a tooth distal to the gingival crevice or to the gum margin.

crown·ing (kroun'ing) the appearance of a large segment of the fetal scalp at the vaginal orifice in childbirth.

cru·ci·ate (krōō'she-āt) cruciform.

cru·ci·ble (krōō'sĭ-b'l) a vessel for melting refractory substances.

cru·ci·form (krōō'sĭ-form) cross-shaped.

cru·ra (krōō'rah) [L.] plural of *crus.*

cru·ral (krōōr'al) pertaining to the lower limb or to a leglike structure (crus).

cru·rot·o·my (kroo-rot'ah-me) the cutting of a crus of the stapes, usually the anterior one.

crus (krus) pl. *cru'ra.* [L.] 1. leg (1). 2. a leglike part. **c. ce're bri,** a structure comprising fiber tracts descending from the cerebral cortex to form the longitudinal fascicles of the pons. **c. of clitoris,** the continuation of each corpus cavernosum of the clitoris, diverging posteriorly to be attached to the pubic arch. **crura of diaphragm,** two fibromuscular bands that arise from the lumbar vertebrae and insert into the central tendon of the diaphragm. **c. of fornix,** either of two flattened bands of white substance that unite to form the body of the fornix. **c. of penis,** the continuation of each corpus cavernosum of the penis, diverging posteriorly to be attached to the pubic arch.

crust (krust) a formed outer layer, especially of solid matter formed by drying of a bodily exudate or secretion. **milk c.,** crusta lactea.

crus·ta (krus'tah) pl. *crus'tae.* [L.] a crust. **c. lac'tea,** seborrhea of the scalp of nursing infants.

Crus·ta·cea (krus-ta'she-ah) a class of arthropods including the lobsters, crabs, shrimps, wood lice, water fleas, and barnacles.

crutch (kruch) a staff, ordinarily extending from the armpit to the ground, with a support for the hand and usually also for the arm or axilla; used to support the body in walking.

crux (kruks) pl. *cru'ces.* [L.] cross. **c. of heart,** the intersection of the walls separating the right and left sides and the atrial and ventricular heart chambers. **cru'ces pilo'- rum,** crosslike patterns formed by hair growth, the hairs lying in opposite directions.

cry·al·ge·sia (kri″al-je'ze-ah) pain on application of cold.

cry·an·es·the·sia (kri-an″es-the'zhah) loss of power of perceiving cold.

cry·es·the·sia (kri″-es-the'zhah) abnormal sensitiveness to cold.

cry·mo·dyn·ia (kri″mo-din'e-ah) rheumatic pain occurring in cold or damp weather.

cry(o)- word element [Gr.], *cold.*

cryo·ab·la·tion (kri″o-ab-la'shun) the removal of tissue by destroying it with extreme cold.

cryo·an·al·ge·sia (kri″o-an″al-je'ze-ah) the relief of pain by application of cold by cryoprobe to peripheral nerves.

cryo·an·es·the·sia (-an″es-the′zhah) local anesthesia produced by chilling the part to near freezing temperature.

cryo·bank (kri′o-bank″) a facility for freezing and preserving semen at low temperatures (usually −196.5° C.) for future use.

cryo·bi·ol·o·gy (kri″o-bi-ol′ah-je) the science dealing with the effect of low temperatures on biological systems.

cryo·cau·tery (-kaw′ter-e) [cryo- + cautery] cauterization by freezing, using a substance such as carbon dioxide snow, or a very cold instrument.

cryo·dam·age (cri′o-dam″ij) damage to tissues, cells, or other biological substrates as a result of exposure to cold.

cryo·ex·trac·tion (kri″o-eks-trak′shun) application of extremely low temperature for the removal of a cataractous lens.

cryo·ex·trac·tor (-eks-trak′ter) a cryoprobe used in cryoextraction.

cryo·fi·brin·o·gen (-fi-brin′ah-jen) an abnormal fibrinogen that precipitates at low temperatures and redissolves at 37° C.

cryo·fi·brin·o·gen·emia (-fi-brin″ah-jen-e′me-ah) the presence of cryofibrinogen in the blood.

cry·o·gen·ic (-jen′ik) producing low temperatures.

cryo·glob·u·lin (-glob′u-lin) an abnormal globulin that precipitates at low temperatures and redissolves at 37° C.

cryo·glob·u·lin·emia (-glob″u-lin-e′me-ah) the presence in the blood of cryoglobulin, which is precipitated in the microvasculature on exposure to cold.

cryo·hy·po·phys·ec·to·my (-hi″po-fiz-ek′tah-me) destruction of the pituitary gland by the application of cold.

cry·op·a·thy (kri-op′ah-the) a morbid condition caused by cold.

cryo·phil·ic (kri″o-fil′ik) psychrophilic.

cryo·pre·cip·i·tate (-pre-sip′ĭ-tāt) any precipitate that results from cooling, sometimes specifically the one rich in coagulation factor VIII obtained from cooling of blood plasma.

cryo·pres·er·va·tion (-prez″er-va′shun) maintenance of the viability of excised tissue or organs by storing at very low temperatures.

cryo·probe (kri′o-prōb) an instrument for applying extreme cold to tissue.

cryo·pro·tec·tion (kri″o-pro-tek′shun) protection, as of a tissue, cell, organism, or other substance, from cold-induced damage.

cryo·pro·tec·tive (-pro-tek′tiv) capable of protecting against injury due to freezing, as glycerol protects frozen red blood cells.

cryo·pro·tein (-pro′tēn) a blood protein that precipitates on cooling.

cry·os·co·py (kri-os′kah-pe) examination of fluids based on the principle that the freezing point of a solution varies according to the amount and nature of the solute. **cryoscop′ic,** adj.

cryo·stat (kri′o-stat) 1. a device by which temperature can be maintained at a very low level. 2. in pathology and histology, a chamber containing a microtome for sectioning frozen tissue.

cryo·sur·gery (kri″o-ser′jer-e) the destruction of tissue by application of extreme cold.

cryo·thal·a·mec·to·my (-thal″ah-mek′tah-me) destruction of a portion of the thalamus by application of extreme cold.

cryo·ther·a·py (-ther′ah-pe) the therapeutic use of cold.

crypt (kript) a blind pit or tube on a free surface. **anal c's,** see under sinus. **bony c.,** the bony compartment surrounding a developing tooth. **enamel c.,** a space bounded by dental ledges on either side and usually by the enamel organ, and filled with mesenchyma. **c's of Fuchs, c's of iris,** pitlike depressions in the iris. **c's of Lieberkühn,** intestinal glands. **Luschka's c's,** deep indentations of the gallbladder mucosa which penetrate into the muscular layer of the organ. **c. of Morgagni,** 1. the lateral expansion of the urethra in the glans penis. 2. see anal sinuses. **synovial c.,** a pouch in the synovial membrane of a joint. **c's of tongue,** deep, irregular invaginations from the surface of the lingual tonsil. **tonsillar c's,** epithelium-lined clefts in the palatine, lingual, and pharyngeal tonsils.

cryp·ta (krip′tah) pl. cryp′tae. [L.] crypt.

cryp·tes·the·sia (krip″tes-the′zhah) subconscious perception of occurrences not ordinarily perceptible to the senses.

cryp·ti·tis (krip-ti′tis) inflammation of a crypt, especially the anal crypts.

crypt(o)- word element [Gr.], concealed; crypt.

cryp·to·coc·co·sis (-kok-o′sis) infection by Cryptococcus neoformans, having a predilection for the brain and meninges but also invading the skin, lungs, and other parts.

Cryp·to·coc·cus (-kok′us) a genus of yeast-like fungi, including C. neofor′mans, the cause of cryptococcosis in humans. **cryptococ′cal,** adj.

cryp·to·de·ter·min·ant (krip″to-de-ter′mĭ-nant) hidden determinant.

cryp·to·gen·ic (krip″to-jen′ik) of obscure or doubtful origin.

cryp·to·lith (krip′to-lith) a concretion in a crypt.

cryp·to·men·or·rhea (krip″to-men″o-re′ah) the occurrence of menstrual symptoms without external bleeding, as in imperforate hymen.

cryp·toph·thal·mia (krip″tof-thal′me-ah) cryptophthalmos.

cryp·toph·thal·mos (-mos) congenital absence of the palpebral fissure, the skin extending from the forehead to the cheek, with the eye malformed or rudimentary.

cryp·toph·thal·mus (-mus) cryptophthalmos.

cryp·to·py·ic (krip′to-pi′ik) characterized by concealed suppuration.

crypt·or·chid·ism (krip-tor′kid-izm) failure of one or both testes to descend into the scrotum. **cryptor′chid,** adj.

cryp·tor·chi·do·pexy (krip-tor′kid-ah-pek″se) orchiopexy.

cryp·tor·chism (krip-tor′kizm) cryptorchidism.

cryp·to·spo·rid·i·o·sis (krip″to-spo-rid″e-o′sis) infection with protozoa of the genus *Cryptosporidium;* in the immunocompetent it is a rare self-limited diarrhea syndrome, but in the immunocompromised it is a severe syndrome of prolonged diarrhea, weight loss, fever, and abdominal pain, sometimes spreading to the trachea and bronchial tree.

Cryp·to·spo·ri·di·um (-spo-rid′e-um) a genus of parasitic protozoa found in the intestinal tracts of many different vertebrates and the etiologic agent of cryptosporidiosis in humans.

crys·tal (kris′t'l) a homogeneous angular solid of definite form, with systematically arranged elemental units. **blood c's,** hematoidin crystals in the blood. **Charcot-Leyden c's,** elongated, diamond-shaped, birefringent crystals derived from disintegrating eosinophils, seen in serous fluids such as the bronchial secretions in asthma and in stools in some cases of intestinal parasitism.

crys·tal·line (kris′tah-lēn) 1. pertaining to crystals. 2. resembling a crystal in nature or clearness.

crys·tal·lu·ria (kris″til-ūr′e-ah) excretion of crystals in the urine, causing renal irritation.

CS cesarean section; conditioned stimulus; coronary sinus.

Cs cesium.

CSAA Child Study Association of America.

CSF cerebrospinal fluid.

CSGBI Cardiac Society of Great Britain and Ireland.

CSM cerebrospinal meningitis.

C-spine cervical spine.

CT computed tomography.

CTA Canadian Tuberculosis Association.

Cte·no·ce·phal·i·des (te″no-sĕ-fal′ĭ-dēz) a genus of fleas, including *C. ca′nis,* frequently

found on dogs, which may transmit the dog tapeworm to humans, and *C. fe′lis,* commonly parasitic on cats.

C-ter·mi·nal (ter′mĭ-nal) the end of the peptide chain carrying the free alpha carboxyl group of the last amino acid, conventionally written to the right.

CTL cytotoxic T lymphocytes.

CTP cytidine triphosphate.

Cu copper (L. *cu′prum*).

cu·bi·tus (ku′bit-us) 1. elbow. 2. the upper limb distal to the humerus: the elbow, forearm, and hand. 3. ulna. **cu′bital,** adj. **c. val′gus,** deformity of the elbow in which it deviates away from the midline of the body when extended. **c. va′rus,** deformity of the elbow in which it deviates toward the midline of the body when extended.

cu·boid (kūb′oid) 1. resembling a cube. 2. cuboid bone; see *Table of Bones.*

cu·boi·dal (ku-boi′d'l) resembling a cube.

cuff (kuf) a small, bandlike structure encircling a part or object. **musculotendinous c.,** one formed by intermingled muscle and tendon fibers. **rotator c.,** a musculotendinous structure encircling and giving strength to the shoulder joint.

cuff·ing (kuf′ing) formation of a cufflike surrounding border, as of leukocytes about a blood vessel, observed in certain infections.

cul-de-sac (kul-dĕ-sak′) [Fr.] a blind pouch. **Douglas' c.-de-s.,** rectouterine excavation.

cul·do·cen·te·sis (kul″do-sen-te′sis) transvaginal puncture of Douglas' cul-de-sac for aspiration of fluid.

cul·dos·co·py (kul-dos′kah-pe) visual examination of the female viscera through an endoscope introduced into the pelvic cavity through the posterior vaginal fornix.

Cu·lex (ku′leks) a genus of mosquitoes found throughout the world, many species of which are vectors of disease-producing organisms.

cu·li·cide (ku′lĭ-sīd) an agent which destroys mosquitoes.

cu·lic·i·fuge (ku-lis′ĭ-fūj) an agent which repels mosquitoes.

cu·li·cine (ku′lĭ-sin, ku′lĭ-sīn) 1. a member of the genus *Culex* or related genera. 2. pertaining to, involving, or affecting mosquitoes of the genus *Culex* or related species.

cul·men (kul′men) pl. *cul′mina.* [L.] 1. acme or summit. 2. the portion of the anterior lobe of the cerebellum between the central lobule and the primary fissure; called also *c. cerebel′li* and *c. monti′culi.*

cul·ti·va·tion (kul″tĭ-va′shun) the propagation of living organisms, especially the growing of cells in artificial media.

cul·ture (kul′cher) 1. the propagation of microorganisms or of living tissue cells in media conducive to their growth. 2. to induce such propagation. 3. the product of such propagation. **cul′tural**, adj. **cell c.**, a growth of cells in vitro; although the cells proliferate they do not organize into tissue. **continuous flow c.**, the cultivation of bacteria in a continuous flow of fresh medium to maintain bacterial growth in logarithmic phase. **hanging-drop c.**, a culture in which the material to be cultivated is inoculated into a drop of fluid attached to a coverglass inverted over a hollow slide. **plate c.**, one grown on a medium, usually agar or gelatin, on a Petri dish. **primary c.**, a cell or tissue culture started from material taken directly from an organism, as opposed to that from an explant from an organism. **pure c.**, a culture of a single cell species, without presence of any contaminants. **slant c.**, one made on the surface of solidified medium in a tube which has been tilted to provide a greater surface area for growth. **stab c.**, one in which the medium is inoculated by thrusting a needle deep into its substance. **streak c.**, one in which the medium is inoculated by drawing an infected wire across it. **suspension c.**, a culture in which cells multiply while suspended in a suitable medium. **tissue c.**, maintenance or growth of tissue, organ primordia, or the whole or part of an organ in vitro so as to preserve its architecture and function. **type c.**, a culture of a species of microorganism usually maintained in a central collection of type or standard cultures.

cul·ture me·di·um (kul′cher mēd′e-um) any substance used to cultivate living cells.

cu·mu·la·tive (ku′mu-lah-tiv) increasing by successive additions, the total being greater than the expected sum of its parts.

cu·mu·lus (-lus) pl. *cu′muli.* [L.] a small elevation. **c. oo′phorus**, a mass of follicular cells surrounding the oocyte in the vesicular ovarian follicle.

cu·ne·ate (ku′ne-āt) cuneiform.

cu·ne·i·form (ku-ne′ĭ-form) wedge-shaped.

cu·ne·us (ku′ne-us) pl. *cu′nei.* [L.] a wedge-shaped lobule on the medial aspect of the occipital lobe of the cerebrum.

cu·nic·u·lus (ku-nik′u-lus) pl. *cuni′culi.* [L.] 1. a tunnel. 2. a burrow in the skin made by the itch mite.

cun·ni·lin·gus (kun″ĭ-ling′gus) oral stimulation of the female genitalia.

Cun·ning·ha·mel·la (kun″ing-ham-el′ah) a genus of fungi of the order Mucorales, characterized by a lack of a sporangium and by conidia that arise from a vesicle. *C.*

berthole′tiae causes opportunistic mucormycosis of the lung in immunocompromised or debilitated patients.

cup (kup) a depression or hollow. **glaucomatous c.**, a form of optic disk depression peculiar to glaucoma. **optic c.**, 1. a depression in the center of the optic disk. 2. an indentation of the distal wall of the optic vesicle, brought about by rapid marginal growth and producing a double-layered cup. **physiologic c.**, optic c. (1)

cu·po·la (koo′pah-lah) cupula.

cup·ping (kup′ing) 1. the application of a cupping glass. 2. the formation of a cup-shaped depression.

cu·pric (koo′prik) containing copper in its divalent form (=Cu), and yielding divalent ions (Cu^{2+}) in aqueous solution. **c. sulfate**, a crystalline salt of copper used as an emetic, astringent, and fungicide, as an oral antidote to phosphorus poisoning and a topical treatment of cutaneous phosphorus burns, and as a catalyst in iron deficiency anemia.

cu·pro·phane (koo′pro-fān) a membrane made of regenerated cellulose, commonly used in hemodialyzers.

cu·prous (ku′prus) pertaining to or containing monovalent copper.

cu·pru·re·sis (ku″proo-re′sis) hypercupriuria.

cu·pu·la (koo′pu-lah) pl. *cu′pulae.* [L.] a small, inverted cup or dome-shaped cap over a structure. **cu′pular**, adj.

cu·pu·li·form (-lĭ-form″) shaped like a small cup.

cu·pu·lo·li·thi·a·sis (ku″pu-lo-lĭ-thi′ah-sis) the presence of calculi in the cupula of the posterior semicircular duct.

cu·ran·de·ra (koo-ron-da′rah) [Sp.] healer; a woman who practices curanderismo.

cu·ran·de·ris·mo (koo-ron″dĕ-riz′mo) a traditional Mexican-American healing system combining various theoretical elements into a holistic approach to illness and believing that disease may have not only natural but also spiritual causes.

cu·ran·de·ro (koo-ron-da′ro) [Sp.] healer; a man who practices curanderismo.

cu·ra·re (koo-rah′re) any of a wide variety of highly toxic extracts from various botanical sources, used originally as arrow poisons in South America. An extract of the shrub *Chondodendron tomentosum* has been used as a skeletal muscle relaxant.

cu·ra·ri·mi·met·ic (koo-rah″re-mi-met′-ik) producing effects similar to those of curare.

cu·rar·iza·tion (koo″rah-rĭ-za′shun) administration of curare (usually tubocurarine) to induce muscle relaxation by its blocking activity at the myoneural junction.

cur·a·tive (kūr'ah-tiv) tending to overcome disease and promote recovery.

cure (kūr) 1. the treatment of any disease, or of a special case. 2. the successful treatment of a disease or wound. 3. a system of treating diseases. 4. a medicine effective in treating a disease.

cu·ret (ku-ret') 1. a spoon-shaped instrument for cleansing a diseased surface. 2. to use a curet.

cu·ret·tage (ku″rĕ-tahzh') [Fr.] the cleansing of a diseased surface, as with a curet. **medical c.,** induction of bleeding from the endometrium by administration and withdrawal of a progestational agent. **periapical c.,** removal with a curet of diseased periapical tissue without excision of the root tip. **suction c., vacuum c.,** removal of the uterine contents, after dilatation, by means of a hollow curet introduced into the uterus, through which suction is applied.

cu·rette·ment (-ment) curettage. **physiologic c.,** enzymatic débridement.

cu·rie (Ci) (ku're) a unit of radioactivity, defined as the quantity of any radioactive nuclide in which the number of disintegrations per second is 3.700×10^{10}.

cu·rie-hour (-owr″) a unit of dose equivalent to that obtained by exposure for one hour to radioactive material disintegrating at the rate of 3.7×10^{10} atoms per second.

cu·ri·um (Cm) (ku're-um) chemical element (see *Table of Elements*), at. no. 96.

cur·rent (kur'ent) 1. anything that flows. 2. electric c. **action c.,** the current generated in the cell membrane of a nerve or muscle by the action potential. **alternating c.,** a current which periodically flows in opposite directions. **convection c.,** a current caused by movement by convection of warmer fluid into an area of cooler fluid. **direct c.,** a current flowing in one direction only. **electric c.,** the stream of electricity that moves along a conductor. Symbol *I*. **galvanic c.,** a steady direct current, especially one produced chemically. **c. of injury,** a flow of current to (*systolic c. of injury*) or from (*diastolic c. of injury*) the injured region of an ischemic heart, due to regional alteration in transmembrane potential. **pacemaker c.,** the small net positive current flowing into certain cardiac cells, such as those of the sinoatrial node, causing them to depolarize.

cur·va·tu·ra (ker″vah-tu'rah) pl. *curvatu'rae*. [L.] curvature.

cur·va·ture (ker'vah-cher) deviation from a rectilinear direction. **greater c. of stomach,** the left or lateral and inferior border of the stomach, marking the inferior junction of the anterior and posterior surfaces. **lesser c. of stomach,** the right or medial border of the stomach, marking the superior junction of the anterior and posterior surfaces. **Pott's c.,** abnormal posterior curvature of the spine due to tuberculous caries. **spinal c.,** abnormal deviation of the vertebral column.

curve (kerv) a line which is not straight, or which describes part of a circle, especially a line that represents varying values in a graph. **Barnes' c.,** the segment of a circle whose center is the sacral promontory, its concavity being directed posteriorly. **c. of Carus,** the normal axis of the pelvic outlet. **dental c.,** c. of occlusion. **dye dilution c.,** an indicator dilution curve in which the indicator is a dye, usually indocyanine green. **growth c.,** the curve obtained by plotting increase in size or numbers against the elapsed time. **indicator dilution c.,** a graphic representation of the concentration of an indicator added in known quantity to the circulatory system and measured over time; used in studies of cardiovascular function. **isodose c's,** lines delimiting body areas receiving the same quantity of radiation in radiotherapy. **c. of occlusion,** the curve of a dentition on which the occlusal surfaces lie. **oxygen-hemoglobin dissociation c.,** a graphic curve representing the normal variation in the amount of oxygen that combines with hemoglobin as a function of the tension of oxygen and carbon dioxide. **Price-Jones c.,** a graphic curve representing the variation in the size of the red blood corpuscles. **Starling c.,** a graphic representation of cardiac output or other measure of ventricular performance as a function of ventricular filling for a given level of contractility. **strength-duration c.,** a graphic representation of the relationship between the intensity of an electric stimulus at the motor point of a muscle and the length of time it must flow to elicit a minimal contraction. **temperature c.,** a graphic tracing showing the variations in body temperature. **tension c's,** lines observed in cancellous tissue of bones, determined by the exertion of stress during development. **ventricular function c.,** Starling c.

Cur·vu·la·ria (kur-vu-lar'e-ah) a genus of imperfect fungi commonly found in soil and elsewhere; *C. luna'ta* is found in human mycetomas.

cush·ion (koosh'un) a soft or padlike part. **endocardial c's,** elevations on the atrioventricular canal of the embryonic heart which later help form the interatrial septum. **intimal c's,** longitudinal thickenings of the intima of certain arteries, e.g., the penile arteries;

they serve functionally as valves, controlling blood flow by occluding the lumen of the artery.

cusp (kusp) a pointed or rounded projection, such as on the crown of a tooth, or one of the triangular segments of a cardiac valve. **semilunar c.,** any of the semilunar segments of the aortic valve (having posterior, right, and left cusps) or the pulmonary valve (having anterior, right, and left cusps).

cus·pid (kus'pid) 1. having one cusp or point. 2. cuspid tooth.

cus·pis (kus'pis) pl. *cus'pides.* [L.] a cusp.

cu·ta·ne·ous (ku-ta'ne-us) pertaining to the skin.

cut·down (kut'doun) creation of a small incised opening, especially over a vein (*venous c.*), to facilitate venipuncture and permit passage of a needle or cannula for withdrawal of blood or administration of fluids.

cu·ti·cle (ku'tĭ-k'l) 1. a layer of more or less solid substance covering the free surface of an epithelial cell. 2. eponychium (1). 3. a horny secreted layer. **dental c.,** a film on the enamel and cementum of some teeth, external to the primary cuticle, with which it combines, deposited by the epithelial attachment as it migrates along the tooth. **enamel c., primary c.,** a film on the enamel of unerupted teeth, consisting primarily of degenerating ameloblast remnants after completion of enamel formation. **secondary c.,** dental c.

cu·tic·u·la (ku-tik'u-lah) pl. *cuti'culae.* [L.] cuticle.

cu·ti·re·ac·tion (ku″tĭ-re-ak'shun) an inflammatory or irritative reaction on the skin, occurring in certain infectious diseases, or on application or injection of a preparation of the organism causing the disease.

cu·tis (ku'tis) the skin. **c. anseri′na,** transitory elevation of the hair follicles due to contraction of the arrectores pilorum muscles; a reflection of sympathetic nerve discharge. **c. hyperelas′tica,** Ehlers-Danlos syndrome. **c. lax′a,** a group of connective tissue disorders, usually hereditary, in which the skin hangs in loose pendulous folds; believed to be associated with decreased elastic tissue formation and an abnormality in elastin formation. **c. rhomboida′lis nu′chae,** thickening of the skin of the neck with striking accentuation of its markings, giving an appearance of diamond-shaped plaques. **c. ver′ticis gyra′ta,** enlargement and thickening of the skin of the scalp, which lies in folds resembling gyri and sulci of the brain.

cu·vette (ku-vet′) [Fr.] a glass container generally having well-defined characteristics (dimensions, optical properties), to contain solutions or suspensions for study.

CV cardiovascular.

CVID common variable immunodeficiency.

CVP central venous pressure.

CVS cardiovascular system; chorionic villus sampling.

cy·an·he·mo·glo·bin (si″an-he″mo-glo′bin) a compound formed by action of hydrocyanic acid on hemoglobin.

cy·a·nide (si′ah-nīd) 1. a compound containing the cyanide group (—CN) or ion (CN⁻). 2. hydrogen cyanide.

cy·an·met·he·mo·glo·bin (si″an-met-he′-mo-glo″bin) a tightly bound complex of methemoglobin with the cyanide ion; the pigment most widely used in hemoglobinometry.

cy·an·met·myo·glo·bin (-mi′o-glo″bin) a compound formed from myoglobin by addition of the cyanide ion to yield reduction to the ferrous state.

cyan(o)- word element [Gr.], *blue.*

Cy·a·no·bac·te·ria (si″ah-no-bak-tēr′e-ah) a subgroup of bacteria comprising the blue-green bacteria (blue-green algae), which are photosynthetic and also fix nitrogen.

cy·a·no·co·bal·a·min (-ko-bal′ah-min) a cobalamin in which the substituent is a cyanide ion; it is the form of vitamin B_{12} first isolated and, although an artifact, is used to denote the vitamin; preparations are used to treat vitamin-associated deficiencies, particularly pernicious anemia and other megaloblastic anemias.

cy·a·no·labe (si′ah-no-lāb″) the name proposed for the pigment in retinal cones that is more sensitive to the blue range of the spectrum than are chlorolabe and erythrolabe.

cy·a·no·phil (si-an′ah-fil) 1. stainable with blue dyes. 2. a cell or other histologic element readily stainable with blue dyes. **cyanoph′ilous,** adj.

Cy·a·no·phy·ceae (si″ah-no-fi′se-e) Cyanobacteria.

cy·a·nop·sia (si″ah-nop′se-ah) defect of vision in which objects appear tinged with blue.

cy·a·no·sis (si″ah-no′sis) a bluish discoloration of skin and mucous membranes due to excessive concentration of reduced hemoglobin in the blood. **cyanot′ic,** adj. **central c.,** that due to arterial unsaturation, the aortic blood carrying reduced hemoglobin. **enterogenous c.,** a syndrome due to absorption of nitrites and sulfides from the intestine, marked primarily by methemoglobinemia and/or sulfhemoglobinemia with cyanosis, as well as severe enteritis, constipation or diarrhea, headache, dyspnea, dizziness, syncope, and anemia. **peripheral c.,** that due to an excessive amount of reduced hemoglobin in the venous blood as a result of extensive oxygen extraction at the capillary level. **pulmonary c.,** central cyanosis due to poor oxygenation of the blood in the lungs. **c. re′tinae,** cyanosis of the retina, observable in certain congenital cardiac defects. **shunt c.,** central cyanosis due to the mixing of unoxygenated blood with arterial blood in the heart or great vessels.

cy·ber·net·ics (si″ber-net′iks) the science of the processes of communication and control in the animal and in the machine.

cy·ca·sin (si′kah-sin) a toxic principle from the seeds of several species of *Cycas*, native to Guam; it is neoplastic to the liver, kidneys, intestine, and lungs after hydrolysis by intestinal bacteria.

cy·cla·mate (si′klah-māt) any salt of cyclamic acid; the sodium and calcium salts have been widely used as non-nutritive sugar substitutes.

cy·clan·de·late (si-klan′dĕ-lāt) an antispasmodic acting on smooth muscle; used as a vasodilator, mainly for peripheral vascular disease.

cyc·lar·thro·sis (si″klahr-thro′sis) a pivot joint.

cy·clase (si′klās) an enzyme that catalyzes the formation of a cyclic phosphodiester.

cy·cle (si′k'l) a succession or recurring series of events. **carbon c.,** the steps by which carbon (in the form of carbon dioxide) is extracted from the atmosphere by living organisms and ultimately returned to the atmosphere. It comprises a series of interconversions of carbon compounds beginning with the production of carbohydrates by plants during photosynthesis, proceeding through animal consumption, and ending and beginning again in the decomposition of the animal or plant or in the exhalation of carbon dioxide by animals. **cardiac c.,** a complete cardiac movement, or heart beat, including systole, diastole, and intervening pause. **cell c.,** the cycle of biochemical and morphological events occurring in a reproducing cell population; it consists of: the *S phase*, occurring toward the end of interphase, in which DNA is synthesized; the *G_2 phase*, a relatively quiescent period; the *M phase*, consisting of the four phases of mitosis; and the *G_1 phase* of interphase, which lasts until the *S phase* of the next cycle. **citric acid c.,** tricarboxylic acid c. **Cori c.,** the mechanism by which lactate produced by muscles is carried to the liver, converted back to glucose

via gluconeogenesis, and returned to the muscles. **-glutamyl c.,** a metabolic cycle for transporting amino acids into cells. **hair c.,** the phases of the life of a hair, consisting of anagen, catagen, and telogen. **Krebs c.,** tricarboxylic acid c. **Krebs-Henseleit c.,** urea c. **menstrual c.,** the period of the regularly recurring physiologic changes in the endometrium, occurring during the reproductive period of female humans, culminating in partial shedding of the endometrium and some bleeding per vagina (menstruating). **mosquito c.,** that period in the life of a malarial parasite that is spent in the body of the mosquito host. **nitrogen c.,** the steps by which nitrogen is extracted from the nitrates of soil and water, incorporated as amino acids and proteins in living organisms, and ultimately reconverted to nitrates: (1) conversion of nitrogen to nitrates by bacteria; (2) the extraction of the nitrates by plants and the building of amino acids and proteins by adding an amino group to the carbon compounds produced in photosynthesis; (3) the ingestion of plants by animals, and (4) the return of nitrogen to the soil in animal excretions or on the death and decomposition of plants and animals. **ornithine c.,** urea c. **ovarian c.,** the sequence of physiologic changes in the ovary involved in ovulation. **reproductive c.,** the cycle of physiologic changes in the female reproductive organs, from the time of fertilization of the oocyte through gestation and parturition. **sex c., sexual c.,** 1. the physiologic changes recurring regularly in the genital organs of nonpregnant female mammals; in humans, the menstrual cycle. 2. the period of sexual reproduction in an organism that also reproduces asexually. **tricarboxylic acid c.,** the final common pathway for the oxidation to CO_2 of fuel molecules, most of which enter as acetyl coenzyme A; it also provides intermediates for biosynthetic reactions and generates ATP by providing electrons to the electron transport chain. **urea c.,** a series of metabolic reactions in the liver, by which ammonia is converted to urea using cyclically regenerated ornithine as a carrier. **uterine c.,** the phenomena occurring in the endometrium during the menstrual cycle, preparing it for implantation of the blastocyst. **visual c.,** the cyclic interconversion of 11-*cis*-retinal and all-*trans*-retinal and association with opsins, creating an electric potential and initiating the cascade generating a sensory nerve impulse in vision.

cyc·lec·to·my (si-klek′tah-me) 1. excision of a piece of the ciliary body. 2. excision of a portion of the ciliary border of the eyelid.

cyc·lic (sik′lik) pertaining to or occurring in a cycle or cycles; applied to chemical compounds containing a ring of atoms in the nucleus.

cyc·li·tis (si-klīt′is) inflammation of the ciliary body.

cy·cli·zine (si′klĭ-zēn) an antihistamine; the hydrochloride and lactate salts are used as antinauseants and antiemetics, particularly to prevent motion sickness.

cycl(o)- word element [Gr.], *round; recurring; ciliary body of the eye.*

cy·clo·ben·za·prine (si″klo-ben′zah-prēn) a skeletal muscle relaxant, used as the hydrochloride salt.

cy·clo·cho·roid·itis (-kor″oid-i′tis) inflammation of ciliary body and choroid.

cy·clo·cryo·ther·a·py (-kri″o-ther′ah-pe) freezing of the ciliary body; done in the treatment of glaucoma.

cy·clo·di·al·y·sis (-di-al′ĭ-sis) creation of a communication between the anterior chamber of the eye and the suprachoroidal space, in glaucoma.

cy·clo·di·a·ther·my (-di′ah-ther″me) destruction of a portion of the ciliary body by diathermy.

cy·cloid (si′kloid) characterized by alternating moods of elation and depression.

cy·clo·ker·a·ti·tis (si″klo-ker″ah-ti′tis) inflammation of cornea and ciliary body.

cy·clo·oxy·gen·ase (-ok′sĭ-jen-ās) a component of prostaglandin synthase (q.v.).

cy·clo·pho·ria (-for′e-ah) heterophoria in which there is deviation of the eye from the anteroposterior axis in the absence of visual fusional stimuli. **minus c.**, incyclophoria. **plus c.**, excyclophoria.

cy·clo·phos·pha·mide (-fos′fah-mīd) a cytotoxic alkylating agent of the nitrogen mustard group; used as an antineoplastic, as an immunosuppressant to prevent transplant rejection, and to treat some diseases characterized by abnormal immune function.

cy·clo·pia (si-klo′pe-ah) a developmental anomaly marked by a single orbital fossa, with the globe absent, rudimentary, apparently normal, or duplicated, or the nose absent or present as a tubular appendix above the orbit.

cy·clo·ple·gia (si″klo-ple′jah) paralysis of the ciliary muscle; paralysis of accommodation.

cy·clo·ple·gic (-ple′jik) pertaining to, characterized by, or causing cycloplegia; or an agent that so acts.

cy·clo·pro·pane (-pro′pān) a colorless, highly inflammable and explosive gas, C_3H_6, used as an inhalation anesthetic.

Cy·clops (si′klops) a genus of minute crustaceans, species of which are hosts of *Diphyllobothrium* and *Dracunculus.*

cy·clops (si′klops) a fetus exhibiting cyclopia.

cy·clo·ro·ta·tion (si″klo-ro-ta′shun) torsion (3). **cycloro′tary,** adj.

cy·clo·ser·ine (-sĕ′rēn) an antibiotic produced by *Streptomyces orchidaceus* or obtained synthetically; used as a tuberculostatic and in treatment of urinary tract infections.

cy·clo·spo·ri·a·sis (-spah-ri′ah-sis) infection by protozoa of the genus *Cyclospora*, especially *C. cayetanen′sis*, seen especially in immunocompromised patients and occurring as recurrent gastrointestinal disease and watery diarrhea.

cy·clo·spor·in A (-spor′in) cyclosporine.

cy·clo·spor·ine (-spor′ēn) a cyclic peptide from an extract of soil fungi that selectively inhibits T cell function; used as an immunosuppressant to prevent rejection in organ transplant recipients and to treat severe psoriasis and severe rheumatoid arthritis.

cy·clo·thy·mia (si″klo-thi′me-ah) cyclothymic disorder.

cy·clot·o·my (si-klot′ah-me) incision of the ciliary muscle.

cy·clo·tro·pia (si″klo-tro′pe-ah) permanent deviation of an eye around the anteroposterior axis in the presence of visional fusional stimuli, resulting in diplopia.

cy·e·sis (si-e′sis) pregnancy. **cyet′ic,** adj.

cyl·in·der (sil′in-der) 1. a solid body shaped like a column. **cylin′drical,** adj. 2. cylindrical lens. **axis c.**, axon (1).

cyl·in·droid (sil′in-droid) 1. shaped like a cylinder. 2. a urinary cast that tapers to a slender, sometimes curled or twisting, tail.

cyl·in·dro·ma (sil″in-dro′mah) 1. adenoid cystic carcinoma. 2. a benign skin tumor on the face and scalp, consisting of cylindrical masses of epithelial cells surrounded by a thick band of hyaline material. **cylindrom′atous,** adj.

cym·bo·ceph·a·ly (sim″bo-sef′ah-le) scaphocephaly.

cy·no·pho·bia (sin″o-fo′be-ah) irrational fear of dogs.

cyp·i·o·nate (sip′e-o-nāt) USAN contraction for cyclopentanepropionate.

cy·pro·hep·ta·dine (si″pro-hep′tah-dēn) an antihistamine with anticholinergic, sedative, and serotonin-blocking effects, used as the hydrochloride salt. It is also used in migraine prophylaxis.

cyr·to·sis (sir-to′sis) 1. kyphosis. 2. distortion of the bones.

Cys cysteine.

cyst (sist) 1. bladder. 2. an abnormal closed epithelium-lined cavity in the body, containing liquid or semisolid material. 3. a stage in the life cycle of certain parasites, during which they are enveloped in a protective wall. **adventitious c.,** one formed about a foreign body or exudate. **alveolar c's,** dilatations of pulmonary alveoli, which may fuse by breakdown of their septa to form pneumatoceles. **aneurysmal bone c.,** a benign, rapidly growing, osteolytic lesion, usually of childhood, characterized by blood-filled cystic spaces lined by bony or fibrous septa. **arachnoid c.,** a fluid-filled cyst between the layers of the leptomeninges, lined with arachnoid membrane, usually in the sylvian fissure. **Baker c.,** a swelling behind the knee due to escape of synovial fluid that has become enclosed in a sac or membrane. **Blessig c's,** cystic spaces formed at the periphery of the retina. **blue dome c.,** a benign retention cyst of the breast which shows a blue color. **Boyer c.,** an enlargement of the subhyoid bursa. **branchial c.,** one arising in the lateral aspect of the neck, from epithelial remnants of a branchial cleft (pharyngeal groove), usually between the second and third pharyngeal arches. **bronchogenic c.,** a congenital cyst, usually in the mediastinum or lung, arising from anomalous budding during formation of the tracheobronchial tree, lined with bronchial epithelium that may contain secretory elements. **chocolate c.,** one having dark, syrupy contents, resulting from collection of hemosiderin following local hemorrhage. **choledochal c.,** a congenital cystic dilatation of the common bile duct, which may cause pain in the right upper quadrant, jaundice, fever, or vomiting, or be asymptomatic. **congenital preauricular c.,** one due to imperfect fusion of the first and second branchial arches in formation of the auricle, communicating with an ear pit on the surface. **dentigerous c.,** a fluid-containing odontogenic cyst surrounding the crown of an unerupted tooth. **dermoid c.,** a teratoma, usually benign, characterized by mature ectodermal elements, having a fibrous wall lined with stratified epithelium, and containing keratinous material, hair, and sometimes material such as bone, tooth, or nerve tissue; found most often in the ovary. **duplication c.,** a congenital cystic malformation of the alimentary tract, consisting of a duplication of the segment to which it is adjacent, occurring anywhere from the mouth to the anus but most frequently affecting the ileum and esophagus. **echinococcus c.,** hydatid c.

enteric c., enterogenous c., a cyst of the intestine arising or developing from a fold or pouch along the intestinal tract. **epidermal c.,** a benign cyst derived from the epidermis or the epithelium of a hair follicle; it is formed by cystic enclosures of epithelium within the dermis, filled with keratin and lipid-rich debris. **epidermal inclusion c.,** a type of epidermal cyst occurring on the head, neck, or trunk, formed by keratinizing squamous epithelium with a granular layer. **epidermoid c.,** 1. epidermal c. 2. a benign tumor formed by inclusion of epidermal elements, especially at the time of closure of the neural groove, and located in the skull, meninges, or brain. **epithelial c.,** 1. any cyst lined by keratinizing stratified squamous epithelium, found most often in the skin. 2. epidermal c. **exudation c.,** one formed by an exudate in a closed cavity. **follicular c.,** one due to occlusion of the duct of a follicle or small gland, especially one formed by enlargement of a graafian follicle as a result of accumulated transudate. **globulomaxillary c.,** one within the maxilla at the junction of the globular portion of the medial nasal process and the maxillary process. **hydatid c.,** the larval cyst stage of the tapeworms *Echinococcus granulosus* and *E. multilocularis*, containing daughter cysts with many scoleces. **keratinizing c.,** one arising in the pilosebaceous apparatus, lined by stratified squamous epithelium and containing largely macerated keratin and often sufficient sebum to render the contents greasy or rancid. **lutein c.,** a cyst of the ovary developed from a corpus luteum. **median anterior maxillary c.,** one in or near the incisive canal, arising from proliferation of epithelial remnants of the nasopalatine duct. **median palatal c.,** one in the midline of the hard palate, between the lateral palatal processes. **meibomian c.,** a cyst of the meibomian gland, sometimes applied to a chalazion. **mucus retention c.,** a mucus-containing retention cyst caused by blockage of a salivary gland duct. **multilocular c.,** 1. a cyst containing several loculi or spaces. 2. a hydatid cyst with many small irregular cavities that may contain scoleces but generally little fluid. 3. a thick-walled cyst in the kidney, found in clusters and usually unilaterally. In children it contains blastema and may develop into a Wilms tumor. **myxoid c.,** a nodular lesion usually overlying an interphalangeal finger joint, consisting of focal mucinous degeneration of collagen of the dermis; not a true cyst, it lacks an epithelial wall and does not communicate with the underlying synovial space. **Naboth's c's,**

nabothian c's, see under *follicle.* **nasoalveolar c., nasolabial c.,** a fissural cyst arising outside the bones at the junction of the globular portion of the medial nasal process, lateral nasal process, and maxillary process. **odontogenic c.,** one derived from epithelium, usually containing fluid or semisolid material, which develops during various stages of odontogenesis; nearly always enclosed within bone. **osseous hydatid c's,** hydatid cysts formed by the larvae of *Echinococcus granulosus* in bone, which may become weakened and eroded by the exuberant growth. **parasitic c.,** one forming around larval parasites (tapeworms, amebas, trichinae), such as a hydatid cyst. **periapical c.,** a periodontal cyst involving the apex of an erupted tooth. **periodontal c.,** one in the periodontal ligament and adjacent structures, usually at the apex of the tooth *(periapical c.).* **pilar c.,** an epithelial cyst of the scalp, almost identical to an epidermal cyst, arising from the outer root sheath of the hair follicle. **piliferous c., pilonidal c.,** a hair-containing sacrococcygeal dermoid cyst or sinus, often opening at a postanal dimple. **radicular c.,** an epithelium-lined sac at the apex of a tooth. **Rathke's c's, Rathke's cleft c's,** groups of epithelial cells forming small colloid-filled cysts in the pars intermedia of the pituitary gland; they are vestiges of Rathke's pouch and are closely related to craniopharyngiomas. **retention c.,** one caused by blockage of the excretory duct of a gland, so that glandular secretions are retained. **sarcosporidian c.,** sarcocyst (2). **sebaceous c.,** a retention cyst of a sebaceous gland, containing cheesy yellow material, usually on the face, neck, scalp, or trunk. **solitary bone c.,** a pathologic bone space in the metaphyses of long bones of growing children; it may be either empty or filled with fluid and have a delicate connective tissue lining. **sterile c.,** a true hydatid cyst that fails to produce brood capsules. **subchondral c.,** a bone cyst within the fused epiphysis beneath the articular plate. **sublingual c.,** ranula. **tarry c.,** 1. one resulting from hemorrhage into a corpus luteum. 2. a bloody cyst resulting from endometriosis. **tarsal c.,** chalazion. **theca-lutein c.,** a cyst of the ovary in which the cystic cavity is lined with theca interna cells. **unicameral bone c.,** solitary bone c. **wolffian c.,** a cyst of the broad ligament developed from vestiges of the mesonephros.

cys·tad·e·no·car·ci·no·ma (sis-tad″ĕ-no-kahr″sĭ-no′mah) adenocarcinoma with tumor-lined cystic cavities, usually in the ovaries.

cys·tad·e·no·ma (sis-tad″ĕ-no′mah) adenoma characterized by epithelium-lined cystic masses that contain secreted material, usually serous or mucinous, generally in the ovaries, salivary gland, or pancreas. **mucinous c.,** a multilocular, usually benign, tumor produced by ovarian epithelial cells and having mucin-filled cavities. **papillary c.,** 1. any tumor producing patterns that are both papillary and cystic. 2. a type of adenoma in which the acini are distended by fluids or outgrowths of tissue. **serous c.,** a cystic tumor of the ovary with thin, clear yellow serum and some solid tissue.

cys·tal·gia (sis-tal′jah) pain in the bladder.

γ-cys·ta·thi·o·nase (sis″tah-thi′o-nās) a pyridoxal phosphate–containing enzyme that catalyzes the hydrolysis of cystathionine to cysteine, ammonia, and α-ketoglutarate; deficiency results in cystathioninuria.

cys·ta·thi·o·nine (-nēn) a thioester of homocysteine and serine; it serves as an intermediate in the transfer of a sulfur atom from methionine to cysteine.

cys·ta·thi·o·nine β-syn·thase (sin′thās) a pyridoxal phosphate–containing lyase that catalyzes a step in the catabolism of methionine; deficiency occurs in an aminoacidopathy characterized by homocystinuria, elevated blood methionine levels, and abnormalities in the eye and the skeletal, nervous, and vascular systems.

cys·ta·thi·o·nin·u·ria (sis″tah-thi″o-ne-nu′re-ah) 1. excess of cystathionine in the urine. 2. an inherited aminoacidopathy; a defect in cystathionine metabolism causes excess in urine and body tissues.

cys·tec·ta·sia (sis″tek-ta′zhah) slitting of the membranous portion of the urethra and dilation of the bladder neck for extraction of a calculus.

cys·tec·to·my (sis-tek′tah-me) 1. excision of a cyst. 2. excision or resection of the bladder.

cys·te·ic ac·id (sis-te′ik) an intermediate product in the oxidation of cysteine to taurine.

cys·te·ine (sis-te′ēn) a sulfur-containing, nonessential amino acid produced by enzymatic or acid hydrolysis of proteins, readily oxidized to cystine; sometimes found in urine. Symbols Cys and C.

cys·tic (sis′tik) 1. pertaining to or containing cysts. 2. pertaining to the urinary bladder or to the gallbladder.

cys·ti·cer·co·sis (sis″tĭ-ser-ko′sis) infection with cysticerci. In humans, infection with the larval forms of *Taenia solium.*

Cys·ti·cer·cus (-ser′kus) a former genus of larval forms of *Taenia,* including *C. cellulo′sae,* the larva of *Taenia solium* and *C. bo'vis*, the larval form of *Taenia saginata*.

cys·ti·cer·cus pl. *cysticer'ci*. A larval form of tapeworm, consisting of a single scolex enclosed in a bladderlike cyst; cf. *hydatid cyst*.

cys·tig·er·ous (sis-tij'er-us) containing cysts.

cys·tine (sis'tēn, sis'tin) a sulfur-containing amino acid produced by digestion or acid hydrolysis of proteins, sometimes found in the urine and kidneys, and readily reduced to two molecules of cysteine.

cys·ti·no·sis (-o'sis) a hereditary disorder of cystine metabolism; the most common type appears in childhood with osteomalacia, aminoaciduria, phosphaturia, and deposition of cystine in tissues throughout the body, leading to renal failure.

cys·tin·uria (-ūr'e-ah) a hereditary amino-aciduria with excessive urinary excretion of cystine along with lysine, ornithine, and arginine, due to impaired renal tubular reabsorption.

cys·ti·tis (sis-ti'tis) inflammation of the urinary bladder. **c. follicula'ris,** that in which the bladder mucosa is studded with nodules containing lymph follicles. **c. glandula'ris,** that in which the mucosa contains mucin-secreting glands. **hemorrhagic c.,** cystitis with severe hemorrhage, a dose-limiting toxic condition with administration of ifosfamide and cyclophosphamide or a complication of bone marrow transplantation. **interstitial c.,** a bladder condition with an inflammatory lesion, usually in the vertex, and involving the entire thickness of the wall. **radiation c.,** inflammatory changes in the bladder caused by ionizing radiation.

cys·tit·o·my (sis-tit'ah-me) surgical division of the lens capsule.

cyst(o)- word element [Gr.], *sac; cyst; bladder*.

cys·to·cele (sis'to-sēl) hernial protrusion of the urinary bladder, usually through the vaginal wall.

cys·to·gas·tros·to·my (-gas-tros'tah-me) surgical anastomosis of a cyst to the stomach for drainage.

cys·to·gram (sis'to-gram) a radiograph of the bladder.

cys·tog·ra·phy (sis-tog'rah-fe) radiography of the urinary bladder. **voiding c.,** radiography of the bladder while the patient is urinating.

cys·toid (sis'toid) 1. resembling a cyst. 2. a cystlike, circumscribed collection of softened material, having no enclosing capsule.

cys·to·je·ju·nos·to·my (sis"to-jĕ"joo-nos'-tah-me) surgical anastomosis of a cyst to the jejunum.

cys·to·li·thi·a·sis (-lĭ-thi'ah-sis) formation of vesical calculi.

cys·to·li·thot·o·my (-lĭ-thot'ah-me) incision of the bladder for removal of a calculus.

cys·tom·e·ter (sis-tom'ĕ-ter) an instrument for studying the neuromuscular mechanism of the bladder by means of measurements of pressure and capacity.

cys·to·me·trog·ra·phy (sis"to-mĕ-trog'-rah-fe) the graphic recording of intravesical volumes and pressures.

cys·to·mor·phous (-mor'fus) resembling a cyst or bladder.

cys·to·pa·re·sis (-pah-re'sis) paralysis of the urinary bladder.

cys·to·pexy (sis'to-pek"se) fixation of the bladder to the abdominal wall.

cys·to·plas·ty (-plas"te) plastic repair of the bladder. **augmentation c.,** enlargement of the bladder by grafting to it a detached segment of intestine (enterocystoplasty) or stomach (gastrocystoplasty). **sigmoid c.,** augmentation cystoplasty using an isolated segment of the sigmoid colon.

cys·to·ple·gia (sis"to-ple'jah) cystoparesis.

cys·to·pros·ta·tec·to·my (-pros-tah-tek'-tah-me) surgical removal of the urinary bladder and prostate gland.

cys·top·to·sis (sis"top-to'sis) prolapse of part of the inner bladder into the urethra.

cys·to·py·eli·tis (sis"to-pi"ĕ-li'tis) pyelocystitis.

cys·tor·rha·phy (sis-tor'ah-fe) suture of the bladder.

cys·to·sar·co·ma (sis"to-sahr-ko'mah) phyllodes tumor.

cys·tos·co·py (sis-tos'kah-pe) visual examination of the urinary tract with an endoscope. **cystoscop'ic,** adj.

cys·tos·to·my (sis-tos'tah-me) surgical formation of an opening into the bladder.

cys·tot·o·my (sis-tot'ah-me) surgical incision of the urinary bladder.

cys·to·ure·ter·itis (sis"to-u-re"ter-i'tis) inflammation of the urinary bladder and ureters.

cys·to·ure·throg·ra·phy (-u"rĕ-throg'rah-fe) radiography of the urinary bladder and urethra. **chain c.,** that in which a sterile beaded metal chain is introduced via a modified catheter into the bladder and urethra; used in evaluating anatomical relationships of the bladder and urethra.

cys·to·ure·thro·scope (-ūr-ēth'rah-skōp") an endoscope for examining the posterior urethra and bladder.

cyt·a·phe·re·sis (sīt"ah-fer-e'sis) apheresis of blood cells; see *erythrocytapheresis, leukapheresis,* and *thrombocytapheresis.*

cy·tar·a·bine (ara-C) (si-tar′ah-bēn) an antimetabolite that inhibits DNA synthesis and hence has antineoplastic properties; used in the treatment of acute myelogenous and other types of leukemia and of meningitis associated with leukemia or lymphoma.

-cyte word element [Gr.], *a cell.*

cy·ti·dyl·ic ac·id (si″tĭ-dil′ik) phosphorylated cytidine, usually cytidine monophosphate.

cy·ti·dine (si′tĭ-dēn) a purine nucleoside consisting of cytosine and ribose, a constituent of RNA and important in the synthesis of a variety of lipid derivatives. Symbol C. **c. triphosphate (CTP),** an energy-rich nucleotide that acts as an activated precursor in the biosynthesis of RNA and other cellular constituents.

cyt(o)- word element [Gr.], *cell.*

cy·to·ar·chi·tec·ton·ic (si″to-ahr″kĭ-tekton′ik) pertaining to cellular structure or the arrangement of cells in tissue.

cy·to·chal·a·sin (-kal′ah-sin) any of a group of fungal metabolites that interfere with the formation of microfilaments and thus disrupt cellular processes dependent on those filaments.

cy·to·chem·is·try (-kem′is-tre) the identification and localization of the different chemical compounds and their activities within the cell.

cy·to·chrome (si′to-krōm) any of a class of hemoproteins, widely distributed in animal and plant tissues, whose main function is electron transport using the heme prosthetic group; distinguished according to their prosthetic groups, e.g., *a, b, c, d,* and P-450.

cy·to·cide (-sīd) an agent which destroys cells. **cytoci′dal,** adj.

cy·toc·la·sis (si-tok′lah-sis) the destruction of cells. **cytoclas′tic,** adj.

cy·to·dif·fer·en·ti·a·tion (si″to-dif″ĕ-ren″-she-a′shun) the development of specialized structures and functions in embryonic cells.

cy·to·dis·tal (-dis′t′l) denoting that part of an axon remote from the cell body.

cy·to·gen·e·sis (-jen′ĕ-sis) the origin and development of cells.

cy·to·ge·net·ic (-jĕ-net′ik) 1. pertaining to chromosomes. 2. pertaining to cytogenetics.

cy·to·ge·net·ics (-jĕ-net′iks) the branch of genetics devoted to cellular constituents concerned in heredity, i.e. chromosomes. **clinical c.,** the branch of cytogenetics concerned with relations between chromosomal abnormalities and pathologic conditions.

cy·to·gen·ic (si-to-jen′ik) 1. pertaining to cytogenesis. 2. forming or producing cells.

cy·tog·e·nous (si-toj′ĕ-nus) producing cells.

cy·to·gly·co·pe·nia (sit″o-gli″ko-pe′ne-ah) deficient glucose content of body or blood cells.

cy·to·his·to·gen·e·sis (-his″to-jen′ĕ-sis) the development of the structure of cells.

cy·to·his·tol·o·gy (-his-tol′ah-je) the combination of cytologic and histologic methods. **cytohistolog′ic,** adj.

cy·toid (si′toid) resembling a cell.

cy·to·kine (si′to-kīn″) a generic term for nonantibody proteins released by one cell population on contact with specific antigen, which act as intercellular mediators, as in the generation of an immune response.

cy·to·ki·ne·sis (si″to-ki-ne′sis) the division of the cytoplasm during the division of eukaryotic cells.

cy·tol·o·gy (si-tol′ah-je) the study of cells, their origin, structure, function, and pathology. **cytolog′ic,** adj. **aspiration biopsy c. (ABC),** the microscopic study of cells obtained from superficial or internal lesions by suction through a fine needle. **exfoliative c.,** microscopic examination of cells desquamated from a body surface or lesion as a means of detecting malignancy and microbiologic changes, to measure hormonal levels, etc. Such cells are obtained by aspiration, washing, smear, or scraping.

cy·tol·y·sin (si-tol′ĭ-sin) a substance or antibody that produces cytolysis.

cy·tol·y·sis (-sis) the dissolution of cells. **cytolyt′ic,** adj. **immune c.,** cell lysis produced by antibody with the participation of complement.

cy·to·ly·so·some (sit″o-li′so-sōm) autophagosome.

cy·to·me·gal·ic (-mĕ-gal′ik) pertaining to the greatly enlarged cells with intranuclear inclusions seen in cytomegalovirus infections.

Cy·to·meg·a·lo·vi·rus (-meg′ah-lo-vi″rus) human cytomegaloviruses; a genus of ubiquitous viruses of the subfamily Betaherpesvirinae (family Herpesviridae), transmitted by multiple routes.

cy·to·meg·a·lo·vi·rus (CMV) (-meg′ah-lo-vi″rus) any of a group of highly host-specific herpesviruses, infecting humans, monkeys, or rodents, producing unique large cells with intranuclear inclusions; the virus can cause a variety of clinical syndromes, collectively known as cytomegalic inclusion disease, although most infections are mild or subclinical.

cy·to·meta·pla·sia (-met″ah-pla′zhah) alteration in the function or form of cells.

cy·tom·e·ter (si-tom′ĕ-ter) a device for counting cells, either visually or automatically.

cy·tom·e·try (-tre) the characterization and measurement of cells and cellular constituents. **flow c.,** a technique for counting cells suspended in fluid as they flow one at a time past a focus of exciting light.

cy·to·mor·phol·o·gy (sīt″o-mor-fol′ah-je) the morphology of body cells.

cy·to·mor·pho·sis (-mor-fo′sis) the changes through which cells pass in development.

cy·to·path·ic (-path′ik) pertaining to or characterized by pathologic changes in cells.

cy·to·patho·gen·e·sis (-path″o-jen′ĕ-sis) production of pathologic changes in cells. **cytopathogenet′ic,** adj.

cy·to·path·o·gen·ic (-jen′ik) capable of producing pathologic changes in cells.

cy·to·pa·thol·o·gist (-pah-thol′ah-jist) an expert in cytopathology.

cy·to·pa·thol·o·gy (-pah-thol′ah-je) the study of cells in disease.

cy·to·pe·nia (-pe′ne-ah) deficiency in the number of any of the cellular elements of the blood.

cy·to·phago·cy·to·sis (-fag″o-si-to′sis) cytophagy.

cy·toph·a·gy (si-tof′ah-je) the ingestion of cells by phagocytes.

cy·to·phil·ic (sīt″ah-fil′ik) having an affinity for cells.

cy·to·phy·lax·is (-fi-lak′sis) 1. the protection of cells against cytolysis. 2. increase in cellular activity.

cy·to·pi·pette (-pi-pet′) a pipette for taking cytological smears.

cy·to·plasm (si′to-plazm) the protoplasm of a cell exclusive of that of the nucleus (nucleoplasm). **cytoplas′mic,** adj.

cy·to·pro·tec·tive (si″to-pro-tek′tiv) 1. protecting cells from noxious chemicals or other stimuli. 2. an agent that so protects.

cy·to·prox·i·mal (sīt″o-prok′si-mil) denoting that part of an axon nearer to the cell body.

cy·to·re·duc·tion (-re-duk′shun) 1. decrease in number of cells, as in a tumor. 2. debulking.

cy·to·re·duc·tive (-re-duk′tiv) reducing the number of cells.

cy·to·sine (si′to-sēn) a pyrimidine base occurring in animal and plant cells, usually condensed with ribose or deoxyribose to form the nucleosides cytidine and deoxycytidine, major constituents of nucleic acids. Symbol C. **c. arabinoside,** cytarabine.

cy·to·skel·e·ton (-skel′it-on) a conspicuous internal reinforcement in the cytoplasm of a cell, consisting of tonofibrils, filaments of the terminal web, and other microfilaments. **cytoskel′etal,** adj.

cy·to·sol (sīt′ah-sol) the liquid medium of the cytoplasm, i.e., cytoplasm minus organelles and nonmembranous insoluble components. **cytosol′ic,** adj.

cy·to·some (-sōm) the body of a cell apart from its nucleus.

cy·to·stat·ic (sīt′ah-stat′ik) 1. suppressing the growth and multiplication of cells. 2. an agent that so acts.

cy·to·stome (sīt′ah-stōm) the cell mouth; the aperture through which food enters certain protozoa.

cy·to·tax·is (sīt′ah-tak′sis) the movement and arrangement of cells with respect to a specific source of stimulation. **cytotac′tic,** adj.

cy·toth·e·sis (si-toth′is-is) restitution of cells to their normal condition.

cy·to·tox·ic·i·ty (si″to-tok-sis′ĭ-te) the degree to which an agent possesses a specific destructive action on certain cells or the possession of such action. **cy′totoxic,** adj. **antibody-dependent cell-mediated c. (ADCC),** lysis of antibody-coated target cells by effector cells with cytolytic activity and Fc receptors. **cell-mediated c.,** cytolysis of a target cell by effector lymphocytes, such as cytotoxic T lymphocytes or NK cells; it may be antibody-dependent or independent.

cy·to·tox·in (si′to-tok″sin) a toxin or antibody having a specific toxic action upon cells of special organs.

cy·to·tro·pho·blast (-tro′fo-blast) the cellular (inner) layer of the trophoblast. **cytotrophoblas′tic,** adj.

cy·to·tro·pism (si-tah′trah-pizm) 1. cell movement in response to external stimulation. 2. the tendency of viruses, bacteria, drugs, etc., to exert their effect upon certain cells of the body. **cytotro′pic,** adj.

cy·to·zo·ic (sīt″ah-zo′ik) living within or attached to cells; said of parasites.

cy·tu·ria (si-tu′re-ah) excessive or unusual cells in the urine.

D

D dalton; deciduous (tooth); density; deuterium; died; diopter; distal; dorsal vertebrae (D1–D12); dose; duration.

D. [L.] da (give); de′tur (let it be given); dex′ter (right); do′sis (dose).

2,4-D a toxic chlorphenoxy herbicide (2,4-dichlorophenoxyacetic acid), a component of Agent Orange.

ᴅ- a chemical prefix specifying the relative configuration of an enantiomer, indicating a carbohydrate with the same configuration at a specific carbon atom as ᴅ-glyceraldehyde or an amino acid having the same configuration as ᴅ-serine. Opposed to ʟ-.

d day; deci-; deoxyribose (in nucleosides and nucleotides).

d. [L.] da (give); de′tur (let it be given); dex′ter (right); do′sis (dose).

d density; diameter.

d- dextro- (right or clockwise, dextrorotatory). Opposed to *l*-.

Δ- (capital delta, the fourth letter of the Greek alphabet) position of a double bond in a carbon chain.

δ (delta, the fourth letter of the Greek alphabet) heavy chain of IgD; δ chain of hemoglobin.

δ- a prefix designating (1) the position of a substituting atom or group in a chemical compound; (2) fourth in a series of four or more related entities or chemical compounds.

Da dalton.

DAC decitabine.

da·car·ba·zine (dah-kahr′bah-zēn) a cytotoxic alkylating agent used as an antineoplastic primarily for treatment of malignant melanoma and in combination chemotherapy for Hodgkin's disease and sarcomas.

da·cliz·u·mab (dah-kliz′u-mab) an immunosuppressant used to prevent acute organ rejection in renal transplant patients.

dacry(o)- word element [Gr.], *tears* or *the lacrimal apparatus of the eye.*

dac·ryo·ad·e·nal·gia (dak″re-o-ad″in-al′jah) pain in a lacrimal gland.

dac·ryo·ad·e·nec·to·my (-ad″in-ek′tah-me) excision of a lacrimal gland.

dac·ryo·blen·nor·rhea (-blen″or-e′ah) mucous flow from the lacrimal apparatus.

dac·ryo·cyst (-sist″) the lacrimal sac.

dac·ryo·cys·tec·to·my (-sis-tek′tah-me) excision of the wall of the lacrimal sac.

dac·ryo·cys·to·blen·nor·rhea (-sis″to-blen″or-e′ah) chronic catarrhal inflammation of the lacrimal sac, with constriction of the lacrimal gland.

dac·ryo·cys·to·cele (-sis′tah-sēl) hernial protrusion of the lacrimal sac.

dac·ryo·cys·to·rhi·no·ste·no·sis (-sis″to-ri″no-stĕ-no′sis) narrowing of the duct leading from the lacrimal sac to the nasal cavity.

dac·ryo·cys·to·rhi·nos·to·my (-sis″to-ri-nos′tah-me) surgical creation of an opening between the lacrimal sac and nasal cavity.

dac·ryo·cys·to·ste·no·sis (sis″to-stĕ-no′sis) narrowing of the lacrimal sac.

dac·ryo·cys·tos·to·my (-sis-tos′tah-me) creation of a new opening into the lacrimal sac.

dac·ryo·hem·or·rhea (-he″mor-e′ah) the discharge of tears mixed with blood.

dac·ryo·lith (dak′re-o-lith″) a lacrimal calculus.

dac·ry·o·ma (dak″re-o′mah) a tumor-like swelling due to obstruction of the lacrimal duct.

dac·ry·ops (dak′re-ops) 1. a watery state of the eye. 2. distention of a lacrimal duct by contained fluid.

dac·ryo·py·o·sis (dak″re-o-pi-o′sis) suppuration of the lacrimal apparatus.

dac·ryo·scin·tig·ra·phy (-sin-tig′rah-fe) scintigraphy of the lacrimal ducts.

dac·ryo·ste·no·sis (-stin-o′sis) stricture or narrowing of a lacrimal duct.

dac·ryo·syr·inx (-sir′inks) 1. a lacrimal duct. 2. a lacrimal fistula. 3. a syringe for irrigating the lacrimal ducts.

dac·ti·no·my·cin (dak″tĭ-no-mi′sin) actinomycin D, an antibiotic derived from several species of *Streptomyces*; used as an antineoplastic.

dac·tyl (dak′til) a digit.

dactyl(o)- word element [Gr.], *a digit; a finger or toe.*

dac·ty·log·ra·phy (dak″til-og′rah-fe) the study of fingerprints.

dac·ty·lo·gry·po·sis (dak″til-o-grĭ-po′sis) permanent flexion of the fingers.

dac·ty·lol·o·gy (dak″tĭ-lol′ah-je) signing.

dac·ty·lol·y·sis (-ĭ-sis) 1. surgical correction of syndactyly. 2. loss or amputation of a digit. **d. sponta′nea,** ainhum.

dac·ty·los·co·py (dak″til-os′kah-pe) examination of fingerprints for identification.

dac·ty·lus (dak'til-us) [L.] a digit.

DAF decay accelerating factor.

dal·fo·pris·tin (dal-fo'pris-tin) a semisynthetic antibacterial used in conjunction with quinupristin against various gram-positive organisms, including vancomycin-resistant *Enterococcus faecium.*

dal·tep·a·rin (dal-tep'ah-rin) an antithrombotic used as the sodium salt in the prevention of pulmonary thromboembolism and deep venous thrombosis in at-risk abdominal surgery patients.

dal·ton (D, Da) (dawl'ton) an arbitrary unit of mass, being 1/12 the mass of the nuclide of carbon-12, equivalent to 1.657×10^{-24} g.

dam (dam) 1. a barrier to obstruct the flow of fluid. 2. a thin sheet of latex used in surgical procedures to separate certain tissues or structures. 3. rubber d. **rubber d.,** a thin sheet of latex rubber used to isolate teeth from mouth fluids during dental therapy.

damp·ing (damp'ing) steady diminution of the amplitude of successive vibrations of a specific form of energy, as of electricity.

da·nap·a·roid (dah-nap'ah-roid) an antithrombotic used as the sodium salt in the prophylaxis of pulmonary thromboembolism and deep venous thrombosis.

dan·a·zol (dah'nah-zol) an anterior pituitary suppressant used in the treatment of endometriosis, fibrocystic breast disease, and gynecomastia and the prophylaxis of attacks of hereditary angioedema.

D and C dilatation (of cervix) and curettage (of uterus).

dan·de·li·on (dan'dĕ-li″on) a weedy herb, *Taraxacum officinale,* having deeply notched leaves and brilliant yellow flowers; used for dyspepsia, loss of appetite, urinary tract infections, and liver and gallbladder complaints.

dan·der (dan'der) small scales from the hair or feathers of animals, which may be a cause of allergy in sensitive persons.

dan·druff (dan'druf) 1. dry scaly material shed from the scalp; applied to that normally shed from the scalp epidermis as well as to the excessive scaly material associated with disease. 2. seborrheic dermatitis of the scalp.

DANS 5-dimethylamino-1-naphthalenesulfonic acid; the acyl chloride is a fluorochrome employed in immunofluorescence studies of tissues and cells.

dan·tro·lene (dan'tro-lēn) a skeletal muscle relaxant, used as the sodium salt in the treatment of chronic spasticity and the treatment and prophylaxis of malignant hyperthermia.

da·pip·ra·zole (dah-pip'rah-zol) an alpha-adrenergic blocking agent used topically as the hydrochloride salt to reverse pharmacologically induced mydriasis.

dap·sone (dap'sōn) an antibacterial bacteriostatic for a broad spectrum of gram-positive and gram-negative organisms; used as a leprostatic, as a dermatitis herpetiformis suppressant, and in the prophylaxis of falciparum malaria.

dar·tos (dahr'tos) 1. dartos muscle; see *Table of Muscles.* 2. tunica dartos.

dar·win·ism (dahr'win-izm) the theory of evolution stating that change in a species over time is partly the result of a process of natural selection, which enables the species to continually adapt to its changing environment.

daugh·ter (daw'ter) 1. decay product. 2. arising from cell division, as a daughter cell.

dau·no·ru·bi·cin (daw″no-roo'bi-sin) an anthracycline (q.v.) antibiotic used as an antineoplastic; administered as the hydrochloride salt or as a liposome-encapsulated preparation of the citrate salt.

DAy Doctor of Ayurvedic Medicine.

dB, db decibel.

DBS deep brain stimulation.

DC direct current; Doctor of Chiropractic.

D & C dilatation (of cervix) and curettage (of uterus).

DCIS ductal carcinoma in situ.

DDP, *cis*-DDP cisplatin.

DDS dapsone; Doctor of Dental Surgery.

DDT dichloro-diphenyl-trichloroethane, a powerful insect poison; used in dilution as a powder or in an oily solution as a spray.

de- word element [L.], *down; from;* sometimes negative or privative, and often intensive.

de·acyl·ase (de-as'il-ās) any hydrolase that catalyzes the cleavage of an acyl group in ester or amide linkage.

dead (ded) 1. destitute of life. 2. anesthetic (1).

deaf (def) lacking the sense of hearing or not having the full power of hearing.

de·af·fer·en·ta·tion (de-af″er-en-ta'shun) the elimination or interruption of sensory nerve fibers.

deaf·ness (-nes) hearing loss; lack or loss, complete or partial, of the sense of hearing. **acoustic trauma d.,** that due to blast injury. **Alexander's d.,** congenital deafness due to cochlear aplasia, chiefly of the organ of Corti and adjacent ganglion cells, with high-frequency hearing loss results. **conduction d., conductive d.,** conductive hearing loss. **labyrinthine d.,** that due to disease of the labyrinth. **Michel's d.,** congenital deafness due to total lack of development of the inner ear. **Mondini's d.,** congenital deafness due to dysgenesis of the organ of Corti, with partial aplasia of the bony and membranous labyrinth and a resultant flattened cochlea. **nerve d., neural d.,** that due to a lesion of the auditory nerve on the central neural pathways. **pagetoid d.,** that seen in osteitis deformans of the bones of the skull. **perceptive d.,** sensorineural hearing loss. **transmission d.,** conductive hearing loss. **word d.,** auditory aphasia.

de·am·i·dase (de-am'ĭ-dās) an enzyme that splits amides to form a carboxylic acid and ammonia.

de·am·i·di·za·tion (de-am"ĭ-dĭ-za'shun) the removal of an amido group from a molecule.

de·am·i·nase (de-am'ĭ-nās) an enzyme causing deamination, or removal of the amino group from organic compounds, usually cyclic amidines.

de·am·i·na·tion (de-am"ĭ-na'shun) removal of the amino group, —NH₂, from a compound.

death (deth) the cessation of life; permanent cessation of all vital bodily functions. **activation-induced cell d. (AICD),** recognition and deletion of T lymphocytes that have been induced to proliferate by receptor-mediated activation, preventing their overgrowth. **black d.,** bubonic plague. **brain d.,** irreversible coma; irreversible brain damage as manifested by absolute unresponsiveness to all stimuli, absence of all spontaneous muscle activity, and an isoelectric electroencephalogram for 30 minutes, all in the absence of hypothermia or intoxication by central nervous system depressants. **cot d., crib d.,** sudden infant death syndrome. **programmed cell d.,** the theory that particular cells are programmed to die at specific sites and at specific stages of development. **somatic d.,** cessation of all vital cellular activity.

de·bil·i·ty (de-bil'ĭ-te) asthenia.

de·branch·er en·zyme (de-branch'er en'zīm) see under *enzyme*.

dé·bride·ment (da-brēd-maw') [Fr.] the removal of foreign material or devitalized tissue from or adjacent to a traumatic or infected lesion until surrounding healthy tissue is exposed, either by cutting (*surgical d.*) or by application of an enzyme able to lyse devitalized tissue (*enzymatic d.*).

de·bris (dĕ-bre') fragments of devitalized tissue or foreign matter. In dentistry, soft foreign material loosely attached to a tooth surface.

debt (det) something owed. **oxygen d.,** the oxygen that must be used in the oxidative energy processes after strenuous exercise to reconvert lactic acid to glucose and

decomposed ATP and creatine phosphate to their original states.

de·bulk·ing (de-bulk'ing) cytoreduction; removal of the major portion of the material composing a lesion.

de·cal·ci·fi·ca·tion (de-kal"sĭ-fĭ-ka'shun) 1. loss of calcium salts from a bone or tooth. 2. the process of removing calcareous matter.

de·can·nu·la·tion (de-kan"u-la'shun) extubation of a cannula.

de·can·ta·tion (de"kan-ta'shun) the pouring of a clear supernatant liquid from a sediment.

de·cap·i·ta·tion (de-kap"ĭ-ta'shun) the removal of the head, as of an animal, fetus, or bone.

de·cap·su·la·tion capsulectomy. **renal d.,** removal of all or part of the renal capsule.

de·car·box·y·lase (de"kahr-bok'sĭ-lās) any enzyme of the lyase class that catalyzes the removal of a carbon dioxide molecule from carboxylic acids.

de·cay (de-ka') 1. the decomposition of dead matter. 2. the process of decline, as in aging. **beta d.,** disintegration of the nucleus of an unstable radionuclide in which the mass number is unchanged, but atomic number is changed by 1, as a result of emission of a negatively or positively charged (beta) particle. **tooth d.,** dental caries.

de·ce·dent (dĕ-se'dent) a person who has recently died.

de·cel·er·a·tion (de-sel"er-a'shun) decrease in rate or speed. **early d.,** in fetal heart rate monitoring, a transient decrease in heart rate that coincides with the onset of a uterine contraction. **late d.,** in fetal heart rate monitoring, a transient decrease in heart rate occurring at or after the peak of a uterine contraction, which may indicate fetal hypoxia. **variable d's,** in fetal heart rate monitoring, a transient series of decelerations that vary in intensity, duration, and relation to uterine contraction, resulting from vagus nerve firing in response to a stimulus such as umbilical cord compression in the first stage of labor.

de·cen·ter (-sen'ter) in optics, to design or make a lens such that the visual axis does not pass through the optical center of the lens.

de·cer·e·brate (-ser'ĕ-brāt) to eliminate cerebral function by transecting the brain stem or by ligating the common carotid arteries and basilar artery at the center of the pons; an animal so prepared, or a brain-damaged person with similar neurologic signs.

de·cho·les·ter·ol·iza·tion (-kah-les″ter-ol-ĭ-za′shun) reduction of blood cholesterol levels.

deci- word element [L.], *one tenth;* used in naming units of measurement to indicate one tenth of the unit designated by the root with which it is combined (10^{-1}); symbol d.

dec·i·bel (des′ĭ-bel) a unit used to express the ratio of two powers, usually electric or acoustic powers, equal to one-tenth of a bel; one decibel equals approximately the smallest difference in acoustic power the human ear can detect.

de·cid·ua (dĕ-sid′u-ah) the endometrium of the pregnant uterus, all of which, except the deepest layer, is shed at parturition. **decid′ual,** adj. **basal d., d. basa′lis,** that portion directly underlying the chorionic sac and attached to the myometrium. **capsular d., d. capsula′ris,** that portion directly overlying the chorionic sac and facing the uterine cavity. **parietal d., d. parieta′lis,** that portion lining the uterus elsewhere than at the site of attachment of the chorionic sac.

de·cid·u·itis (dĕ-sid″u-i′tis) a bacterial disease leading to changes in the decidua.

de·cid·u·o·sis (-o′sis) the presence of decidual tissue or of tissue resembling the endometrium of pregnancy in an ectopic site.

de·cid·u·ous (dĕ-sid′u-us) falling off or shed at maturity, as the teeth of the first dentition.

dec·i·li·ter (dL) (des′ĭ-le″ter) one tenth (10^{-1}) of a liter; 100 milliliters.

de·ci·ta·bine (DAC) (de-si′tah-bēn″) a cytotoxic compound used as an antineoplastic in the treatment of acute leukemia.

dec·li·na·tion (dek″lĭ-na′shun) cyclophoria.

de·clive (de-klīv′) a slope or a slanting surface. In anatomy, the part of the vermis of the cerebellum just caudal to the primary fissure.

de·cli·vis (de-kli′vis) [L.] declive.

de·col·or·a·tion (de-kul″er-a′shun) 1. removal of color; bleaching. 2. lack or loss of color.

de·com·pen·sa·tion (de″kom-pen-sa′shun) 1. inability of the heart to maintain adequate circulation, marked by dyspnea, venous engorgement, and edema. 2. in psychiatry, failure of defense mechanisms resulting in progressive personality disintegration.

de·com·po·si·tion (de-kom″pah-zish′un) the separation of compound bodies into their constituent principles.

de·com·pres·sion (de″kom-presh′un) removal of pressure, especially from deep-sea divers and caisson workers to prevent bends, and from persons ascending to great heights. **cardiac d.,** decompression of heart.

cerebral d., relief of intracranial pressure by removal of a skull flap and incision of the dura mater. **d. of heart,** pericardiotomy with evacuation of a hematoma. **microvascular d.,** a microsurgical procedure for relief of trigeminal neuralgia. **nerve d.,** relief of pressure on a nerve by surgical removal of the constricting fibrous or bony tissue. **d. of pericardium,** decompression of heart. **d. of spinal cord,** surgical relief of pressure on the spinal cord, which may be due to hematoma, bone fragments, etc.

de·con·ges·tant (de″kon-jes′tint) 1. tending to reduce congestion or swelling. 2. an agent that so acts.

de·con·tam·i·na·tion (de″kon-tam-ĭ-na′shun) the freeing of a person or object of some contaminating substance, e.g., war gas, radioactive material, etc.

de·cor·ti·ca·tion (de-kor″tĭ-ka′shun) 1. removal of the outer covering from a plant, seed, or root. 2. removal of portions of the cortical substance of a structure or organ.

dec·re·ment (dek′rĕ-ment) 1. subtraction, or decrease; the amount by which a quantity or value is decreased. 2. the stage of decline of a disease; see *stadium decrementi.* **decremen′tal,** adj.

de·cru·des·cence (de″kroo-des′ens) diminution or abatement of the intensity of symptoms.

de·cu·bi·tus (de-ku′bĭ-tus) pl. *decu′bitus.* [L.] 1. an act of lying down; the position assumed in lying down. 2. decubitus ulcer. **decu′bital,** adj. **dorsal d.,** lying on the back. **lateral d.,** lying on one side, designated *right lateral d.* when the subject lies on the right side and *left lateral d.* when he lies on the left side. **ventral d.,** lying on the stomach.

de·cus·sa·tio (de″kah-sa′she-o) pl. *decussatio′nes.* [L.] decussation.

de·cus·sa·tion (-sa′shun) a crossing over; the intercrossing of fellow parts or structures in the form of an X. **Forel's d.,** the ventral tegmental decussation of the rubrospinal and rubroreticular tracts in the mesencephalon. **fountain d. of Meynert,** the dorsal tegmental decussation of the tectospinal tract in the mesencephalon. **pyramidal d.,** the anterior part of the lower medulla oblongata in which most of the fibers of the pyramids intersect.

de·dif·fer·en·ti·a·tion (de-dif″er-en″she-a′shun) anaplasia.

deep (dēp) situated far beneath the surface; not superficial.

de·epi·car·di·al·iza·tion (de-ep″ĭ-kahr″de-al″ĭ-za′shun) a surgical procedure for the relief of intractable angina pectoris, in which epicardial tissue is destroyed by application of a caustic agent to promote development of collateral circulation.

deet (dēt) diethyltoluamide.

def·e·ca·tion (def″ĕ-ka′shun) 1. the evacuation of fecal matter from the rectum. 2. the removal of impurities, as chemical defecation.

def·e·cog·ra·phy (def″ĕ-kog′rah-fe) the recording, by videotape or high-speed radiographs, of defecation following barium instillation into the rectum; used in the evaluation of fecal incontinence.

de·fect (de′fekt) an imperfection, failure, or absence. **defec′tive**, adj. **acquired d.**, a non-genetic imperfection arising secondarily, after birth. **aortic septal d.**, a congenital anomaly in which there is abnormal communication between the ascending aorta and pulmonary artery just above the semilunar valves. **atrial septal d's, atrioseptal d's,** congenital anomalies in which there is persistent patency of the atrial septum, owing to failure of the ostium primum or ostium secundum. **birth d.,** one present at birth, whether a morphological defect (dysmorphism) or an inborn error of metabolism. **congenital d.,** birth d. **congenital ectodermal d.,** anhidrotic ectodermal dysplasia. **cortical d.,** a benign, symptomless, circumscribed rarefaction of cortical bone, detected radiographically. **endocardial cushion d's,** a spectrum of septal defects resulting from imperfect fusion of the endocardial cushions, and ranging from persistent ostium primum to persistent common atrioventricular canal; see *atrial septal d.* and *atrioventricularis communis.* **fibrous cortical d.,** a small, asymptomatic, osteolytic, fibrous lesion occurring within the bone cortex, particularly in the metaphyseal region of long bones in childhood. **filling d.,** any localized defect in the contour of the stomach, duodenum, or intestine, as seen in the radiograph after a barium enema. **genetic d.,** see under *disease.* **luteal phase d.,** inadequate secretory transformation of the endometrium during the luteal phase of the menstrual cycle; it can cause habitual abortion. **metaphyseal fibrous d.,** 1. fibrous cortical d. 2. nonossifying fibroma. **neural tube d.,** a developmental anomaly of failure of closure of the neural tube, resulting in conditions such as anencephaly or spina bifida. **retention d.,** a defect in the power of recalling or remembering names, numbers, or events. **septal d.,** a defect in a cardiac septum resulting in an abnormal communication between the opposite chambers of the heart. **ventricular**

septal d., a congenital cardiac anomaly in which there is persistent patency of the ventricular septum in either the muscular or fibrous portions, most often due to failure of the bulbar septum to completely close the interventricular foramen

de·fem·i·ni·za·tion (de-fem″ĭ-nĭ-za′shun) loss of female sexual characteristics.

de·fense (de-fens′) behavior directed to protection of the individual from injury. **character d.,** any character trait, e.g., a mannerism, attitude, or affectation, which serves as a defense mechanism. **insanity d.,** a legal concept that a person cannot be convicted of a crime if he lacked criminal responsibility by reason of insanity at the time of commission of the crime.

de·fen·sin (de-fen′sin) any of a group of small antimicrobial cationic peptides occurring in neutrophils and macrophages.

def·er·ens (def′er-ens) [L.] deferent; see *ductus deferens.*

def·er·ent (-ent) conveying anything away, as from a center.

def·er·en·tial (-en′shal) pertaining to the ductus deferens.

def·er·en·ti·tis (def″er-en-ti′tis) inflammation of the ductus deferens.

de·fer·ox·amine (dĕ″fer-oks′ah-mēn) an iron-chelating agent isolated from *Streptomyces pilosus;* used as the mesylate salt as an antidote in iron poisoning.

def·er·ves·cence (def″er-ves′ens) the period of abatement of fever.

de·fib·ri·la·tion (de-fib″rĭ-la′shun) termination of atrial or ventricular fibrillation, usually by electroshock.

de·fib·ril·la·tor (de-fib″rĭ-la′ter) an electronic apparatus used to counteract atrial or ventricular fibrillation by application of a brief electric shock to the heart. **automatic external d. (AED),** a portable defibrillator designed to be automated such that it can be used by persons without substantial medical training who are responding to a cardiac emergency. **automatic implantable cardioverter-d.,** see under *cardioverter.*

de·fi·bri·na·tion (de-fi″brĭ-na′shun) removal of fibrin from the blood.

de·fi·brino·gen·a·tion (de″fi-brin″o-jĕ-na′shun) induced defibrination, as in thrombolytic therapy.

de·fi·cien·cy (de-fish′en-se) a lack or shortage; a condition characterized by presence of less than normal or necessary supply or competence. **color vision d.,** color blindness; any deviation from normal perception of one or more colors. **disaccharidase d.,** less than normal activity of the enzymes of the intestinal mucosa that cleave disaccharides, usually denoting a generalized deficiency of all such enzymes secondary to a disorder of the small intestine. **familial apolipoprotein C-II (apo C-II) d.,** a form of familial hyperchylomicronemia due to lack of apo C-II, a necessary cofactor for lipoprotein lipase. **familial high-density lipoprotein (HDL) d.,** any of several inherited disorders of lipoprotein and lipid metabolism that result in decreased plasma levels of HDL, particularly Tangier disease. **familial lipoprotein d.,** any inherited disorder of lipoprotein metabolism resulting in deficiency of one or more plasma lipoproteins. **isolated IgA d., IgA d., selective,** the most common immunodeficiency disorder, deficiency of IgA but normal levels of other immunoglobulin classes and normal cellular immunity; it is marked by recurrent sinopulmonary infections, allergy, gastrointestinal disease, and autoimmune diseases. **molybdenum cofactor d.,** an inherited disorder in which deficiency of the molybdenum cofactor causes deficiency of a variety of enzymes, resulting in severe neurologic abnormalities, dislocated ocular lenses, mental retardation, xanthinuria, and early death. **plasma thromboplastin antecedent d., PTA d.,** hemophilia C.

def·i·cit (def′ĭ-sit) deficiency. **oxygen d.,** see *anoxia, hypoxemia,* and *hypoxia.* **pulse d.,** the difference between the heart rate and the pulse rate in atrial fibrillation. **reversible ischemic neurologic d. (RIND),** a type of cerebral infarction whose clinical course lasts between 24 and 72 hours.

de·fin·i·tive (dĕ-fin′ĭ-tiv) 1. established with certainty. 2. in embryology, denoting acquisition of final differentiation or character. 3. in parasitology, denoting the host in which a parasite reaches the sexual stage.

de·flec·tion (de-flek′shun) deviation or movement from a straight line or given course, such as from the baseline in electrocardiography.

de·flu·vi·um (de-floo′ve-um) [L.] 1. a flowing down. 2. a disappearance.

de·flux·ion (de-fluk′shun) 1. a sudden disappearance. 2. a copious discharge, as of catarrh. 3. a falling out, as of hair.

de·form·a·bil·i·ty (de-form″ah-bil′it-e) ability of cells to change shape when passing through narrow spaces, such as erythrocytes passing through the microvasculature.

de·for·ma·tion (de″for-ma′shun) 1. in dysmorphology, a type of structural defect characterized by the abnormal form or position of a body part, caused by a nondisruptive mechanical force. 2. the process of adapting in shape or form.

de·form·i·ty (dĕ-for′mĭ-te) distortion of any part or of the body in general. **Akerlund d.,** an indentation (in addition to the niche) in the duodenal cap in the radiograph in duodenal ulcer. **Arnold-Chiari d.,** protrusion of the cerebellum and medulla oblongata down into the spinal canal through the foramen magnum. **Madelung's d.,** radial deviation of the hand secondary to overgrowth of the distal ulna or shortening of the radius. **reduction d.,** congenital absence of a portion or all of a body part, especially of the limbs. **silver fork d.,** the deformity seen in Colles' fracture. **Sprengel's d.,** congenital elevation of the scapula, due to failure of descent of the scapula to its normal thoracic position during fetal life. **Volkmann's d.,** see under *disease.*

Deg degeneration.

de·gen·er·ate¹ (de-jen′er-āt) to change from a higher to a lower form.

de·gen·er·ate² (de-jen′er-at) characterized by degeneration.

de·gen·er·a·tion (de-jen″er-a′shun) deterioration; change from a higher to a lower form, especially change of tissue to a lower or less functionally active form. **degen′erative,** adj. **ascending d.,** wallerian degeneration affecting centripetal nerve fibers and progressing toward the brain or spinal cord. **calcareous d.,** degeneration of tissue with deposit of calcareous material. **caseous d.,** caseation (2). **cerebromacular d. (CMD), cerebroretinal d.,** 1. degeneration of brain cells and of the macula retinae. 2. any lipidosis with cerebral lesions and degeneration of the macula retinae. 3. any form of neuronal ceroid-lipofuscinosis. **congenital macular d.,** hereditary macular degeneration with a cystlike lesion that in the early stages resembles egg yolk. **Crooke's hyaline d.,** Crooke's hyalinization. **descending d.,** wallerian degeneration extending peripherally along nerve fibers. **disciform macular d.,** a form of macular degeneration seen in persons over age 40, in which sclerosis involving the macula and retina is produced by hemorrhages between Bruch's membrane and the pigment epithelium. **fibrinous d.,** necrosis with deposit of fibrin within the cells of the tissue. **gray d.,** degeneration of the white substance of the spinal cord, in which it loses myelin and assumes a gray color. **hepatolenticular d.,** Wilson's disease. **hyaline d.,** a regressive change in cells in which the cytoplasm takes on a homogeneous, glassy appearance; also used loosely to describe the histologic appearance of tissues. **lattice d. of retina,** an often bilateral, usually benign asymptomatic condition, characterized by patches of fine gray or white intersecting lines in the peripheral retina, usually with numerous round punched-out areas of retinal thinning or retinal holes. **macular d.,** degenerative changes in the macula retinae. **mucoid d.,** that with deposit of myelin and lecithin in the cells. **myxomatous d.,** degeneration in which mucus accumulates in connective tissues. **spongy d. of central nervous system, spongy d. of white matter,** a rare hereditary form of leukodystrophy of early onset in which widespread demyelination and vacuolation of cerebral white matter gives it a spongy appearance; there is mental retardation, megalocephaly, atony of neck muscles, limb spasticity, and blindness, with death in infancy. **striatonigral d.,** a form of multiple system atrophy with nerve cell degeneration mainly in the region of the substantia nigra and the neostriatum; symptoms are similar to those of parkinsonism. **subacute combined d. of spinal cord,** degeneration of posterior and lateral columns of the spinal cord, with various motor and sensory disturbances; it is due to vitamin B_{12} deficiency and usually associated with pernicious anemia. **tapetoretinal d.,** degeneration of the pigmented layer of the retina. **transneuronal d.,** atrophy of certain neurons after interruption of afferent axons or death of other neurons to which they send their efferent output. **Zenker's d.,** hyaline degeneration and necrosis of striated muscle.

de·glov·ing (de-gluv′ing) intra-oral surgical exposure of the bony mandibular chin; it can be performed in the posterior region if necessary.

de·glu·ti·tion (de″gloo-tish′un) swallowing.

deg·ra·da·tion (deg″rah-da′shun) conversion of a chemical compound to one less complex, as by splitting off one or more groups of atoms.

de·gus·ta·tion (de″gus-ta′shun) tasting.

de·his·cence (de-his′ins) a splitting open. **wound d.,** separation of the layers of a surgical wound.

de·hy·dra·tase (de-hi′drah-tās) a common name for a hydro-lyase.

de·hy·drate (de-hi′drāt) to remove water from (a compound, the body, etc.).

de·hy·dra·tion (de″hi-dra′shun) 1. removal of water from a substance. 2. the condition that results from excessive loss of body water. **hypernatremic d.,** a condition in which electrolyte losses are disproportionately smaller than water losses.

7-de·hy·dro·cho·les·ter·ol (de-hi″dro-kŏ-les′ter-ol) a sterol present in skin which, on ultraviolet irradiation, produces vitamin D. **activated 7-d.,** cholecalciferol.

11-de·hy·dro·cor·ti·cos·ter·one (-kor″tĭ-kos′ter-ōn) a steroid produced by the adrenal cortex.

de·hy·dro·epi·an·dros·ter·one (DHEA) (-ep″e-an-dros′ter-ōn) a steroid secreted by the adrenal cortex, the major androgen precursor in females; often present in excessive amounts in patients with adrenal virilism.

de·hy·dro·gen·ase (de-hi′dro-jen-ās″) an enzyme that catalyzes the transfer of hydrogen or electrons from a donor, oxidizing it, to an acceptor, reducing it.

de·hy·dro·ret·i·nol (-ret′ĭ-nol) vitamin A_2, a form of vitamin A found with retinol (vitamin A_1) in freshwater fish; it has one more conjugated double bond than retinol and approximately one-third its biological activity.

de·ion·iza·tion (de-i″on-ĭ-za′shun) the production of a mineral-free state by the removal of ions.

dé·jà vu (da′zhah voo′) [Fr.] an illusion that a new situation is a repetition of a previous experience.

de·jec·tion (de-jek′shun) a mental state marked by sadness; the lowered mood characteristic of depression.

de·lac·ta·tion (de″lak-ta′shun) 1. weaning. 2. cessation of lactation.

de·lam·i·na·tion (de-lam″ĭ-na′shun) separation into layers, as of the blastoderm.

del·a·vir·dine (del″ah-vir′dēn) an antiretroviral, inhibiting reverse transcriptase; used as the mesylate salt in the treatment of HIV infection.

de·layed-re·lease (-lād′ re-lēs′) releasing a drug at a time later than that immediately following its administration.

de·lead (-led′) to induce the removal of lead from tissues and its excretion in the urine by the administration of chelating agents.

del·e·te·ri·ous (del″ĕ-tēr′e-us) injurious; harmful.

de·le·tion (dĕ-le′shun) in genetics, loss of genetic material from a chromosome.

de·lin·quent (de-lin′kwent) 1. failing to do that which is required by law or obligation. 2. a person who neglects a legal obligation. **juvenile d.,** an individual who commits a violation of the law within the jurisdiction of the juvenile court system.

del·i·ques·cence (del″ĭ-kwes′ens) dampness or liquefaction from the absorption of water from air. **deliques′cent,** adj.

de·lir·i·um (dĕ-lēr′e-um) pl. *deli′ria.* A mental disturbance of relatively short duration usually reflecting a toxic state, marked by illusions, hallucinations, delusions, excitement, restlessness, impaired memory, and incoherence. **alcohol withdrawal d.,** that caused by cessation or reduction in alcohol consumption, typically in alcoholics with many years of heavy drinking, characterized by autonomic hyperactivity, such as tachycardia, sweating, and hypertension, a coarse, irregular tremor, and delusions, vivid hallucinations, and wild, agitated behavior. **d. tre′mens,** alcohol withdrawal d.

de·liv·ery (de-liv′er-e) expulsion or extraction of the child and fetal membranes at birth. **abdominal d.,** delivery of an infant through an incision made into the intact uterus through the abdominal wall. **breech d.,** delivery in which the fetal buttocks present first. **forceps d.,** extraction of the child from the maternal passages by application of forceps to the fetal head; designated *low* or *midforceps delivery* according to the degree of engagement of the fetal head and *high* when engagement has not occurred. **postmortem d.,** delivery of a child after death of the mother. **spontaneous d.,** birth of an infant without any aid from an attendant.

del·le (del′ah) the clear area in the center of a stained erythrocyte.

del·len (del′in) saucer-shaped excavations at the periphery of the cornea, usually on the temporal side.

de·lo·mor·phous (del″o-mor′fus) having definitely formed and well-defined limits, as a cell or tissue.

del·ta (del′ah) 1. the fourth letter of the Greek alphabet; see also δ-. 2. a triangular area.

del·toid (del′toid) 1. triangular. 2. the deltoid muscle.

de·lu·sion (dĕ-loo′zhun) an idiosyncratic false belief that is firmly maintained in spite of incontrovertible and obvious proof or evidence to the contrary. **delu′sional,** adj. **bizarre d.,** one that is patently absurd, with no possible basis in fact. **d. of control,** the delusion that one's thoughts, feelings, and actions are not one's own but are being imposed by someone else or other external force. **depressive d.,** one that is congruent with a predominant depressed mood. **erotomanic d.,** one associated with erotomania. **d. of grandeur, grandiose d.,** delusional conviction of one's own importance, power, or knowledge or that one is, or has a special relationship with, a deity or a famous person. **d. of jealousy,** a delusional belief that one's spouse or lover is unfaithful, based on erroneous inferences drawn from innocent events imagined to be evidence. **mixed d.,** one in which no central theme predominates. **d. of negation, nihilistic d.,** a depressive delusion that the self or part of the self, part of the body, other persons, or the whole world has ceased to exist. **d. of persecution,** a delusion that one is being attacked, harassed, persecuted, cheated, or conspired against. **d. of reference,** a delusional conviction that ordinary events, objects, or behaviors of others have particular and unusual meanings specifically for oneself. **systematized d's,** a group of delusions organized around a common theme.

De·man·sia (de-man′se-ah) a genus of venomous snakes of the family Elapidae, including the brown snake of Australia and New Guinea.

deme (dēm) a population of very similar organisms interbreeding in nature and occupying a circumscribed area.

dem·e·ca·ri·um (dem″e-kar′e-um) an anticholinesterase agent used topically as the bromide salt in the treatment of glaucoma and accommodative esotropia.

dem·e·clo·cy·cline (dem″ĕ-klo-si′klēn) a broad-spectrum tetracycline antibiotic produced by a mutant strain of *Streptomyces aureofaciens* or semisynthetically; used as the hydrochloride salt.

de·men·tia (dĕ-men′shah) a general loss of cognitive abilities, including impairment of memory as well as one or more of the following: aphasia, apraxia, agnosia, or disturbed planning, organizing, and abstract thinking abilities. It does not include decreased cognitive functioning due to clouding of consciousness, depression, or other functional mental disorder. **Alzheimer's d.,** see under *disease.* **d. of the Alzheimer type,** dementia of insidious onset and gradually progressive course, with histopathological changes characteristic of Alzheimer's disease, categorized as *early onset* or *late onset* depending on whether or not it begins by the age of 65. **arteriosclerotic d.,** multi-infarct dementia as a result of cerebral arteriosclerosis. **Binswanger's d.,** see under *disease.* **boxer's d.,** a syndrome due to cumulative cerebral injuries in boxers, with forgetfulness, slowness in thinking, dysarthric speech, and slow uncertain movements, especially of the legs. **dialysis d.,** see under *encephalopathy.* **multi-infarct d.,** vascular d. **paralytic d., d. paraly′tica,** general paresis. **d. prae′cox,** (*obs.*) schizophrenia. **presenile d.,** that occurring in younger persons, usually age 65 or younger; since most cases are due to Alzheimer's disease, the term is sometimes used as a synonym of *dementia of the Alzheimer type, early onset,* and has also been used to denote *Alzheimer's disease.* **senile d.,** that occurring in older persons, usually over the age of 65; since most cases are due to Alzheimer's disease, the term is sometimes used as a synonym of *dementia of the Alzheimer type, late onset.* **subcortical d.,** any of a group of dementias thought to be caused by lesions particularly affecting subcortical brain structures, characterized by memory loss with slowness of information processing and of the formation of intellectual responses. **substance-induced persisting d.,** that resulting from exposure to or use or abuse of a substance (e.g., alcohol, sedatives, anticonvulsants, or lead) but persisting long after exposure ends, usually with permanent and worsening deficits. **vascular d.,** that with a stepwise deteriorating course and a patchy distribution of neurologic deficits caused by cerebrovascular disease.

de·min·er·al·iza·tion (de-min″er-al-ĭ-za′-shun) excessive elimination of mineral or organic salts from tissues of the body.

Dem·o·dex (dem′ah-deks) a genus of mites parasitic within the hair follicles of the host, including the species *D. follicolo′rum* in humans.

de·mog·ra·phy (de-mog′rah-fe) the statistical science dealing with populations, including matters of health, disease, births, and mortality.

de·mul·cent (de-mul′sint) 1. soothing; bland. 2. a soothing mucilaginous or oily medicine or application.

de·my·elin·a·tion (de-mi″ĕ-lĭ-na′shun) destruction, removal, or loss of the myelin sheath of a nerve or nerves. Called also *myelinolysis.*

de·na·sal·i·ty (de″na-zal′it-e) hyponasality.

de·na·tur·a·tion (de-na″cher-a′shun) destruction of the usual nature of a substance, as by the addition of methanol or acetone to alcohol to render it unfit for drinking, or the change in the physical properties of a substance, as a protein or nucleic acid, caused by heat or certain chemicals that alter tertiary structure.

den·dri·form (den′drĭ-form) branched, or tree-shaped.

den·drite (den′drīt) one of the threadlike extensions of the cytoplasm of a neuron; dendrites branch into treelike processes and compose most of the receptive surface of a neuron.

den·drit·ic (den-drit′ik) 1. branched like a tree. 2. pertaining to or possessing dendrites.

dendr(o)- word element [Gr.], *tree; treelike.*

Den·dro·as·pis (den″dro-as′pis) a genus of extremely venomous African snakes of the family Elapidae, related to cobras but lacking a dilatable hood. *D. angus′ticeps* is the green mamba and *D. polyle′pis* is the black mamba.

den·dro·den·drit·ic (-den-drit′ik) referring to a synapse between dendrites of two neurons.

den·dron (den′dron) dendrite.

den·dro·phago·cy·to·sis (den″dro-fag″o-si-to′sis) the absorption by microglial cells of broken portions of astrocytes.

de·ner·va·tion (de″ner-va′shun) interruption of the nerve connection to an organ or part.

den·gue (den′ge) an infectious, eruptive, febrile, viral disease of tropical areas, transmitted by *Aedes* mosquitoes, and marked by severe pains in the head, eyes, muscles, and joints, sore throat, catarrhal symptoms, and sometimes a skin eruption and painful swellings of parts.

de·ni·al (dĭ-ni′il) in psychiatry, a defense mechanism in which the existence of unpleasant internal or external realities is kept out of conscious awareness.

den·i·da·tion (den″ĭ-da′shun) degeneration and expulsion of the endometrium during the menstrual cycle.

den·i·leu·kin dif·ti·tox (den″ĭ-loo′kin dif′tĭ-toks) a genetically engineered construct combining amino acid sequences for specific diphtheria toxin fragments linked to sequences for interleukin-2 (IL-2); used as an antineoplastic.

dens (dens) pl. *den′tes.* [L.] 1. tooth. 2. a toothlike structure. 3. dens axis; the toothlike process that projects from the superior surface of the body of the axis, ascending to articulate with the atlas. **d. in den′te,** a malformed tooth caused by invagination of the crown before it is calcified, giving the appearance of a "tooth within a tooth."

den·si·tom·e·try (den″sĭ-tom′ĭ-tre) determination of variations in density by comparison with that of another material or with a certain standard.

den·si·ty (den′sit-e) 1. the quality of being compact or dense. 2. quantity per unit space, e.g., the mass of matter per unit volume. Symbol *d.* 3. the degree of darkening of exposed and processed photographic or x-ray film.

den·tal (den′t'l) pertaining to a tooth or teeth.

den·tal·gia (den-tal′jah) toothache.

den·tate (den′tāt) notched; tooth-shaped.

den·tes (den′tēz) [L.] plural of *dens*.

den·tia (den′shah) a condition relating to development or eruption of the teeth. **d. prae′cox,** premature eruption of the teeth; presence of teeth in the mouth at birth. **d. tar′da,** delayed eruption of the teeth, beyond the usual time for their appearance.

den·ti·buc·cal (den″tĭ-buk′′l) pertaining to the cheek and teeth.

den·ti·cle (den′tĭ-k′l) 1. a small toothlike process. 2. a distinct calcified mass within the pulp chamber of a tooth.

den·ti·frice (den′tĭ-fris) a preparation for cleansing and polishing the teeth; it may contain a therapeutic agent, such as fluoride, to inhibit dental caries.

den·tig·er·ous (den-tij′er-us) bearing or having teeth.

den·ti·la·bi·al (-la′be-il) pertaining to the teeth and lips.

den·tin (den′tin) the chief substance of the teeth, surrounding the tooth pulp and covered by enamel on the crown and by cementum on the roots. **den′tinal,** adj. **adventitious d.,** secondary d. **circumpulpal d.,** the inner portion of dentin, adjacent to the pulp, consisting of thinner fibrils. **cover d.,** the peripheral portion of dentin, adjacent to the enamel or cementum, consisting of coarser fibers than the circumpulpal dentin. **irregular d.,** secondary d. **mantle d.,** cover d. **opalescent d.,** dentin giving an unusual translucent or opalescent appearance to the teeth, as occurs in dentinogenesis imperfecta. **primary d.,** dentin formed before the eruption of a tooth. **secondary d.,** new dentin formed in response to stimuli associated with the normal aging process or with pathological conditions, such as caries or injury, or cavity preparation. **transparent d.,** dentin in which some dentinal tubules have become sclerotic or calcified, producing the appearance of translucency.

den·ti·no·ce·men·tal (den″tĭ-no-sĕ-men′t′l) pertaining to the dentin and the cementum.

den·ti·no·enam·el (-ĕ-nam′′l) pertaining to the dentin and the enamel.

den·ti·no·gen·e·sis (-jen′ĕ-sis) the formation of dentin. **d. imperfec′ta,** a hereditary condition marked by imperfect formation and calcification of dentin, giving the teeth a brown or blue opalescent appearance.

den·ti·no·gen·ic (-jen′ik) forming or producing dentin.

den·ti·no·ma (den″tĭ-no′mah) a tumor of odontogenic origin, composed of immature connective tissue, odontogenic epithelium, and dysplastic dentin.

den·ti·num (den-ti′num) dentin.

den·tist (den′tist) a person with a degree in dentistry and authorized to practice dentistry.

den·tis·try (den′tis-tre) 1. that branch of the healing arts concerned with the teeth, oral cavity, and associated structures, including prevention, diagnosis, and treatment of disease and restoration of defective or missing tissue. 2. the work done by dentists, e.g., the creation of restorations, crowns, and bridges, and surgical procedures performed in and about the oral cavity. **holistic d.,** dental practice that takes into account the effect of dental treatment and materials on the overall health of the individual. **operative d.,** dentistry concerned with restoration of parts of the teeth that are defective as a result of disease, trauma, or abnormal development to a state of normal function, health, and esthetics. **pediatric d.,** pedodontics. **preventive d.,** dentistry concerned with maintenance of a normal masticating mechanism by fortifying the structures of the oral cavity against damage and disease. **prosthetic d.,** prosthodontics. **restorative d.,** dentistry concerned with the restoration of existing teeth that are defective because of disease, trauma, or abnormal development to normal function, health, and appearance; it includes crowns and bridgework.

den·ti·tion (den-tish′un) the teeth in the dental arch; ordinarily used to designate the natural teeth in position in their alveoli. **deciduous d.,** see under *tooth*. **mixed d.,** the complement of teeth in the jaws after eruption of some of the permanent teeth, but before all the deciduous teeth are shed. **permanent d.,** see under *tooth*. **precocious d.,** abnormally accelerated appearance of the deciduous or permanent teeth. **primary d.,** deciduous teeth; see under *tooth*. **retarded d.,** abnormally delayed appearance of the deciduous or permanent teeth.

dent(o)- word element [L.], *tooth; toothlike*.

den·to·al·ve·o·lar (den″to-al-ve′ah-ler) pertaining to a tooth and its alveolus.

den·to·fa·cial (-fa′shil) of or pertaining to the teeth and alveolar process and the face.

den·to·tro·pic (-tro′pik) turning toward or having an affinity for tissues composing the teeth.

den·tu·lous (den′tu-lus) having natural teeth.

den·ture (den′cher) a complement of teeth, either natural or artificial; ordinarily used to designate an artificial replacement for the natural teeth and adjacent tissues. **complete d.,** an appliance replacing all the teeth of one jaw, as well as associated structures of the jaw. **implant d.,** one constructed with

denudation

240

a metal substructure embedded within the underlying soft structures of the jaws. **interim d.,** a denture to be used for a short interval of time for reasons of esthetics, mastication, occlusal support, convenience, or to condition the patient to the acceptance of an artificial substitute for missing natural teeth until more definite prosthetic dental treatment can be provided. **overlay d.,** a complete denture supported both by soft tissue (mucosa) and by a few remaining natural teeth that have been altered, as by insertion of a long or short coping, to permit the denture to fit over them. **partial d.,** a dental appliance that is removable (*removable partial d.*) or permanently attached (*fixed partial d.* or *bridge*) and replaces one or more missing teeth, receiving support and retention from underlying tissues and some or all of the remaining teeth. **provisional d.,** an interim denture used for the purpose of conditioning the patient to the acceptance of an artificial substitute for missing natural teeth. **transitional d.,** a partial denture which is to serve as a temporary prosthesis and to which teeth will be added as more teeth are lost and which will be replaced after postextraction tissue changes have occurred.

de·nu·da·tion (den″u-da′shun) the stripping or laying bare of any part.

de·odor·ant (de-o′der-int) 1. masking offensive odors. 2. an agent that so acts.

de·or·sum·duc·tion (de-or″sum-duk′shun) infraduction.

de·os·si·fi·ca·tion (de-os″ĭ-fĭ-ka′shun) loss or removal of the mineral elements of bone.

deoxy- chemical prefix designating a compound containing one less oxygen atom than the reference substance; see also words beginning *desoxy-*.

de·oxy·chol·ic ac·id (de-ok″se-ko′lik) a secondary bile acid formed from cholic acid in the intestine; it is a choleretic.

de·oxy·he·mo·glo·bin (-he″mo-glo′bin) hemoglobin not combined with oxygen, formed when oxyhemoglobin releases its oxygen to the tissues.

de·oxy·ri·bo·nu·cle·ase (DNase) (-ri″bo-noo′kle-ās) any nuclease catalyzing the cleavage of phosphate ester linkages in deoxyribonucleic acids (DNA); separated by whether they cleave internal bonds or bonds at termini.

de·oxy·ri·bo·nu·cle·ic ac·id (DNA) (-ri″bo-noo-kle′ik) the nucleic acid in which the sugar is deoxyribose; composed also of phosphoric acid and the bases adenine, guanine, cytosine, and thymine. It constitutes the primary genetic material of all cellular

organisms and the DNA viruses and occurs predominantly in the nucleus, usually as a *double helix* (q.v.), where it serves as a template for synthesis of ribonucleic acid (transcription).

de·oxy·ri·bo·nu·cleo·pro·tein (-noo′kle-o-pro″te-in) a nucleoprotein in which the sugar is D-2-deoxyribose.

de·oxy·ri·bo·nu·cleo·side (-noo′kle-o-sīd) a nucleoside having a purine or pyrimidine base bonded to deoxyribose.

de·oxy·ri·bo·nu·cleo·tide (-noo′kle-o-tīd) a nucleotide having a purine or pyrimidine base bonded to deoxyribose, which in turn is bonded to a phosphate group.

de·oxy·ri·bose (-ri′bōs) a deoxypentose found in deoxyribonucleic acids (DNA), deoxyribonucleotides, and deoxyribonucleosides.

de·oxy·ri·bo·vi·rus (-ri′bo-vi″rus) DNA virus.

de·oxy·uri·dine (-ūr′ĭ-dēn) a pyrimidine nucleoside, uracil linked to deoxyribose; its triphosphate derivative is an intermediate in the synthesis of deoxyribonucleotides.

de·pen·dence (de-pen′dens) 1. a state of relying on or requiring the aid of something. 2. a state in which there is a compulsive or chronic need, as for a drug; see *substance d.* **psychoactive substance d., substance d.,** 1. compulsive use of a substance despite significant problems resulting from such use. Although tolerance and withdrawal were previously defined as necessary and sufficient for dependence, they are currently only two of several possible criteria. 2. substance abuse.

de·pen·den·cy (-en-se) reliance on others for love, affection, mothering, comfort, security, food, warmth, shelter, protection, and the like—the so-called dependency needs.

de·pen·dent (-ent) 1. exhibiting dependence or dependency. 2. hanging down.

De·pen·do·vi·rus (dĕ-pen′do-vi″rus) adeno-associated viruses; a genus of viruses of the family Parvoviridae that require coinfection with an adenovirus or herpesvirus to provide a helper function for replication; asymptomatic human infection is common.

de·per·son·al·iza·tion (de-per″sun-al-ĭ-za′shun) alteration in the perception of self so that the usual sense of one's own reality is temporarily lost or changed; it may be a manifestation of a neurosis or another mental disorder or can occur in mild form in normal persons.

dep·i·la·tion (dep″ĭ-la′shun) epilation; removal of hair by the roots.

de·pil·a·to·ry (dĕ-pil″ah-tor″e) 1. having the power to remove hair. 2. an agent for removing or destroying hair.

de·ple·tion (-ple′shun) the act or process of emptying or removing, as of fluid from a body compartment.

de·po·lar·iza·tion (de-po″lahr-ĭ-za′shun) 1. the process or act of neutralizing polarity. 2. in electrophysiology, reversal of the resting potential in excitable cell membranes when stimulated. **atrial premature d. (APD),** see under *complex.* **ventricular premature d. (VPD),** see under *complex.*

de·po·lym·er·iza·tion (de″po-lim″er-ĭ-za′shun) the conversion of a polymer into its component monomers.

de·pos·it (de-poz′it) 1. sediment or dregs. 2. extraneous inorganic matter collected in the tissues or in an organ of the body.

de·pot (de′po, dep′o) a body area in which a substance, e.g., a drug, can be accumulated, deposited, or stored and from which it can be distributed.

ʟ-**dep·re·nyl** (dep′rĕ-nil) selegiline.

de·pres·sant (de-pres′ant) diminishing any functional activity; an agent that so acts. **cardiac d.,** an agent that depresses the rate or force of contraction of the heart.

de·pressed (de-prest′) 1. below the normal level. 2. associated with psychological depression.

de·pres·sion (de-presh′un) 1. a hollow or depressed area; downward or inward displacement. 2. a lowering or decrease of functional activity. 3. a mental state of altered mood characterized by feelings of sadness, despair, and discouragement. **depres′sive,** adj. **agitated d.,** major depressive disorder accompanied by more or less constant activity. **anaclitic d.,** impairment of an infant's physical, social, and intellectual development resulting from absence of mothering. **congenital chondrosternal d.,** congenital deformity with a deep, funnel-shaped depression in the anterior chest wall. **endogenous d.,** a type caused by an intrinsic biological or somatic process rather than an environmental influence, in contrast to a reactive depression. **major d.,** major depressive disorder. **neurotic d.,** one that is not a psychotic depression (q.v.); used sometimes broadly to indicate any depression without psychotic features and sometimes more narrowly to denote only milder forms of depression. **pacchionian d's,** small pits on the internal cranium on either side of the groove for the superior sagittal sinus, occupied by the arachnoid granulations. **psychotic d.,** strictly, major depressive disorder with psychotic features, such as hallucinations, delusions, mutism, or stupor; often used more broadly to cover all severe depressions causing gross impairment of social or occupational functioning. **reactive d., situational d.,** a usually transient depression that is precipitated by a stressful life event or other environmental factor; cf. *endogenous d.* **unipolar d.,** that unaccompanied by episodes of mania or hypomania, as in major depressive disorder or dysthymic disorder; the term is sometimes used to denote the former specifically.

de·pres·sor (de-pres′er) 1. that which causes depression, as a muscle, agent, or instrument. 2. depressor nerve.

dep·ri·va·tion (dep-rĭ-va′shun) loss or absence of parts, powers, or things that are needed. **emotional d.,** deprivation of adequate and appropriate interpersonal or environmental experience in the early development years. **sensory d.,** deprivation of usual external stimuli and the opportunity for perception.

depth (depth) distance measured perpendicularly downward from a surface. **focal d., d. of focus,** the measure of the power of a lens to yield clear images of objects at different distances.

de·rail·ment (de-rāl′ment) disordered thought or speech characteristic of schizophrenia and marked by constant jumping from one topic to another before the first is fully realized.

de·re·al·iza·tion (de-re″al-ĭ-za′shun) a loss of the sensation of the reality of one's surroundings.

de·re·ism (de′re-izm) dereistic thinking.

de·re·is·tic (de″re-is′tik) directed away from reality; not using normal logic; see under *thinking.*

de·re·pres·sion (de″re-presh′un) removal of repression, such as of an operon so that gene transcription occurs or is enhanced, with the net result frequently being elevation of the level of a specific enzyme.

de·riv·a·tive (dĕ-riv′ah-tiv) a chemical substance produced from another substance either directly or by modification or partial substitution.

derm·abra·sion (der″mah-bra′zhun) planing of the skin done by mechanical means, e.g., sandpaper, wire brushes, etc.; see *planing.*

Der·ma·cen·tor (-sen′ter) a genus of ticks that are important transmitters of disease. *D. anderso′ni* is parasitic in various wild mammals and transmits Rocky Mountain spotted fever, Colorado tick fever, and tularemia; it also can cause tick paralysis.

D. varia′bilis, the chief vector of Rocky Mountain spotted fever in the central and eastern United States, is usually parasitic in dogs but also attacks cattle, horses, rabbits, and humans.

der·mal (der′mal) pertaining to the dermis or to the skin.

Der·ma·nys·sus (-nis′us) a genus of mites. *D. galli′nae* is the bird or chicken mite, which sometimes infests humans.

der·ma·ti·tis (der″mah-ti′tis) pl. *dermati′tides.* Inflammation of the skin. **actinic d.,** dermatitis due to exposure to actinic radiation, such as that from the sun, ultraviolet waves, or x- or gamma radiation. **allergic d.,** 1. atopic d. 2. allergic contact d. **allergic contact d.,** contact dermatitis due to allergic sensitization. **ammonia d.,** diaper dermatitis attributed to skin irritation, due to the ammonia decomposition products of urine. **atopic d.,** a chronic inflammatory, pruritic, eczematous skin disorder in individuals with a hereditary predisposition to cutaneous pruritus; often accompanied by allergic rhinitis, hay fever, and asthma. **berlock d., berloque d.,** dermatitis of the neck, face, or chest, with patches or streaks, caused by exposure to perfume or other toilet articles containing bergamot oil and then to sunlight. **cercarial d.,** swimmers′ itch. **contact d.,** acute or chronic dermatitis caused by substances contacting the skin; it may involve allergic or nonallergic mechanisms. **diaper d.,** diaper rash. **d. exfoliati′va neonato′rum,** staphylococcal scalded skin syndrome. **exfoliative d.,** virtually universal erythema, desquamation, scaling, and itching of the skin, with loss of hair. **d. herpetifor′mis,** pruritic chronic dermatitis with successive groups of symmetrical, erythematous, papular, vesicular, eczematous, or bullous lesions, usually associated with asymptomatic gluten-sensitive enteropathy. **infectious eczematous d.,** a pustular eczematoid eruption arising from a primary lesion that is the source of an infectious exudate. **insect d.,** a transient skin eruption caused by the toxin-containing irritant hairs of insects such as certain moths and their caterpillars. **irritant d.,** a nonallergic type of contact dermatitis due to exposure to a substance that damages the skin. **livedoid d.,** local pain, swelling, livedoid changes, and increased temperature; due to temporary or prolonged local ischemia from vasculitis or from accidental arterial obliteration during intragluteal administration of medications. **meadow d., meadow-grass d.,** phytophotodermatitis with eruption of vesicles and bullae in streaks or other configurations, caused by exposure to sunlight after contact with meadow grass. **photoallergic contact d., photocontact d.,** allergic contact dermatitis caused by the action of sunlight on skin sensitized by contact with substances such as halogenated salicylanilides, sandalwood oil, or hexachlorophene. **phototoxic d.,** erythema followed by hyperpigmentation of sun-exposed areas of the skin, due to exposure to agents containing photosensitizing substances, such as coal tar and psoralen-containing perfumes, drugs, or plants, and then to sunlight. **poison ivy d., poison oak d., poison sumac d.,** allergic contact dermatitis due to exposure to plants of the genus *Rhus*, which contain urushiol, a skin-sensitizing agent. **radiation d.,** radiodermatitis. **rat-mite d.,** that due to a bite of the rat-mite, *Ornithonyssus bacoti.* **d. re′pens,** acrodermatitis continua. **rhus d.,** poison ivy, poison oak, or poison sumac d. **schistosome d.,** swimmer's itch. **seborrheic d., d. seborrhe′ica,** chronic pruritic dermatitis with erythema, scaling, and yellow crust on areas such as the scalp, with exfoliation of excessive dandruff. **stasis d.,** chronic eczematous dermatitis due to venous insufficiency, initially on the inner aspect of the lower leg above the internal malleolus, sometimes spreading over the lower leg, marked by edema, pigmentation, and often ulceration. **swimmers′ d.,** see under *itch.* **uncinarial d.,** ground itch. **x-ray d.,** radiodermatitis.

dermat(o)- word element [Gr.], *skin.*

der·ma·to·au·to·plas·ty (der″mah-to-aw′to-plas″te) autotransplantation of skin.

Der·ma·to·bia (der″mah-to′be-ah) a genus of botflies. The larvae of *D. ho′minis* are parasitic in the skin of humans, mammals, and birds.

der·ma·to·fi·bro·sar·co·ma (der″mah-to-fi″bro-sahr-ko′mah) a fibrosarcoma of the skin. **d. protu′berans,** a locally aggressive, bulky, protuberant, nodular, fibrotic neoplasm occurring in the dermis, usually on the trunk, often extending into the subcutaneous fat.

der·ma·to·glyph·ics (-glif′iks) the study of the patterns of ridges of the skin of the fingers, palms, toes, and soles; of interest in anthropology and law enforcement as a means of establishing identity and in medicine, both clinically and as a genetic indicator, particularly of chromosomal abnormalities.

der·ma·tog·ra·phism (der″mah-tog′rah-fizm) urticaria due to physical allergy, in which moderately firm stroking or scratching of the skin with a dull instrument produces a pale, raised welt or wheal, with a red flare on each side. **dermatograph'ic,** adj. **black d.,** black or greenish streaking of the skin caused by deposit of fine metallic particles abraded from jewelry by various dusting powders. **white d.,** linear blanching of (usually erythematous) skin of persons with atopic dermatitis in response to firm stroking with a blunt instrument.

der·ma·to·het·ero·plas·ty (der″mah-to-het′er-o-plas″te) the grafting of skin derived from an individual of another species.

der·ma·tol·o·gy (der″mah-tol′ah-je) the medical specialty concerned with the diagnosis and treatment of skin disorders.

der·ma·tol·y·sis (-tol′ĭ-sis) cutis laxa.

der·ma·tome (der′mah-tōm) 1. an instrument for cutting thin skin slices for grafting. 2. the area of skin supplied with afferent nerve fibers by a single posterior spinal root. 3. the lateral part of an embryonic somite.

der·ma·to·mere (der′mah-to-mēr″) any segment or metamere of the embryonic integument.

der·ma·to·my·co·sis (der″mah-to-mi-ko′sis) a superficial fungal infection of the skin or its appendages.

der·ma·to·my·o·ma (-mi-o′mah) leiomyoma cutis.

der·ma·to·myo·si·tis (-mi″o-si′tis) a collagen disease marked by nonsuppurative inflammation of the skin, subcutaneous tissue, and muscles, with necrosis of muscle fibers.

der·ma·to·path·ic (-path′ik) pertaining or attributable to disease of the skin, as dermatopathic lymphadenopathy.

der·ma·top·a·thy (der″mah-top′ah-the) dermopathy.

Der·ma·toph·a·goi·des (der″mah-tof″ah-goi′dēs) a genus of sarcoptiform mites, usually found on the skin of chickens. *D. pteronys′simus* is the house dust mite, an antigenic species that produces allergic asthma in atopic persons.

der·ma·to·phar·ma·col·o·gy (der″mah-to-fahr″mah-kol′ah-je) pharmacology as applied to dermatologic disorders.

der·ma·to·phi·lo·sis (-fi-lo′sis) an actinomycotic disease caused by *Dermatophilus congolensis*, affecting ruminants, horses, and sometimes humans. The human disease is marked by painless upper limb pustules that break down and form shallow red ulcers that later regress and leave scarring.

Der·ma·toph·i·lus (der″mah-tof′ĭ-lus) 1. *Tunga.* 2. a genus of pathogenic actinomycetes. *D. congolen′sis* is the etiologic agent of dermatophilosis.

der·ma·to·phyte (der′mah-to-fīt″) a fungus parasitic upon the skin, including *Microsporum, Epidermophyton,* and *Trichophyton.*

der·ma·to·phy·tid (der″mah-tof′ĭ-tid) a secondary skin eruption that is an expression of hypersensitivity to infection by a dermatophyte, especially *Epidermophyton,* occurring on an area remote from the site of infection.

der·ma·to·phy·to·sis (der″mah-to-fi-to′sis) 1. epidermomycosis; any superficial fungal infection caused by a dermatophyte and involving the stratum corneum of the skin, hair, and nails, including onychomycosis and the various forms of tinea. 2. tinea pedis.

der·ma·to·plas·ty (der′mah-to-plas″te) a plastic operation on the skin; operative replacement of destroyed or lost skin. **dermatoplas'tic,** adj.

der·ma·to·sis (der″mah-to′sis) pl. *dermato′ses.* Any skin disease, especially one not characterized by inflammation. **d. papulo′sa ni′gra,** a form of seborrheic keratosis seen chiefly in blacks, with multiple miliary pigmented papules usually on the cheek bones, but sometimes occurring more widely on the face and neck. **progressive pigmentary d.,** Schamberg's disease. **subcorneal pustular d.,** a bullous dermatosis resembling dermatitis herpetiformis, with single and grouped vesicles and sterile pustular blebs beneath the stratum corneum of the skin.

der·ma·to·zo·on (-zo′on) any animal parasite on the skin; an ectoparasite.

der·mis (der′mis) corium; the layer of the skin deep to the epidermis, consisting of a bed of vascular connective tissue, and containing the nerves and organs of sensation, the hair roots, and sebaceous and sweat glands. **der′mal, der′mic,** adj.

der·mo·blast (der′mah-blast) the part of the mesoblast that develops into the dermis.

der·moid (der′moid) 1. skinlike. 2. dermoid cyst.

der·moid·ec·to·my (der″moid-ek′tah-me) excision of a dermoid cyst.

der·mo·myo·tome (der″mo-mi′ah-tōm) all but the sclerotome of a mesodermal somite; the primordium of skeletal muscle and, perhaps, of the dermis.

der·mop·a·thy (der-mop′ah-the) any skin disorder. **diabetic d.,** any of several cutaneous manifestations of diabetes.

der·mo·syn·o·vi·tis (der″mo-sin″o-vi′tis) inflammation of skin overlying an inflamed bursa or tendon sheath.

der·mo·vas·cu·lar (-vas′ku-ler) pertaining to the blood vessels of the skin.

DES diethylstilbestrol.

de·sat·u·ra·tion (de-sach″ah-ra′shun) the process of converting a saturated compound to one that is unsaturated, such as the introduction of a double bond between carbon atoms of a fatty acid.

des·ce·me·to·cele (des″ĕ-met′o-sēl) hernia of Descemet's membrane.

des·cend·ing (de-send′ing) extending inferiorly.

des·cen·sus (de-sen′sus) pl. *descen′sus*. [L.] downward displacement or prolapse.

de·sen·si·ti·za·tion (de-sen″sĭ-tĭ-za′shun) 1. the prevention or reduction of immediate hypersensitivity reactions by administration of graded doses of allergen. 2. treatment of phobias and related disorders by intentionally exposing the patient, in imagination or in real life, to a hierarchy of emotionally distressing stimuli.

de·ser·pi·dine (de-ser′pĭ-dēn) an alkaloid of *Rauwolfia canescens*, used as an antihypertensive.

des·fer·ri·ox·amine (des-fer′e-oks′ah-mēn) deferoxamine.

des·flu·rane (des-floo′rān) an inhalational anesthetic used for induction and maintenance of general anesthesia.

des·ic·cant (des′ĭ-kant) 1. promoting dryness. 2. an agent that promotes dryness.

de·sip·ra·mine (des-ip′rah-mēn) a tricyclic antidepressant of the dibenzazepine class; used as the hydrochloride salt.

des·lan·o·side (des-lan′o-sīd) a cardiotonic glycoside obtained from lanatoside C; used where digitalis is recommended.

des·min (dez′min) a protein that polymerizes to form the intermediate filaments of muscle cells; used as a marker of these cells.

des·mi·tis (dez-mi′tis) inflammation of a ligament.

desm(o)- word element [Gr.], *ligament*.

des·mo·cra·ni·um (dez″mo-kra′ne-um) the mass of mesoderm at the cranial end of the notochord in the early embryo, forming the earliest stage of the skull.

des·mog·e·nous (dez-moj′ah-nus) of ligamentous origin.

des·mog·ra·phy (dez-mog′rah-fe) a description of ligaments.

des·moid (dez′moid) 1. fibrous or fibroid. 2. see under *tumor*. **periosteal d.**, a benign fibrous tumorlike proliferation of the periosteum, occurring particularly in the medial femoral condyle in adolescents.

des·mo·lase (dez′mo-lās) any enzyme that catalyzes the addition or removal of some chemical group to or from a substrate without hydrolysis.

des·mop·a·thy (dez-mop′ah-the) any disease of the ligaments.

des·mo·pla·sia (dez″mo-pla′zhah) the formation and development of fibrous tissue. **desmoplas′tic**, adj.

des·mo·pres·sin (des″mo-pres′in) a synthetic analogue of vasopressin, used as the acetate salt as an antidiuretic in central diabetes insipidus and in primary nocturnal enuresis, and as an antihemorrhagic in hemophilia A and von Willebrand's disease.

des·mo·some (dez′mo-sōm) a circular, dense body that forms the site of attachment between certain epithelial cells, especially those of stratified epithelium of the epidermis, which consist of local differentiations of the apposing cell membranes.

des·mot·o·my (dez-mot′ah-me) incision or division of a ligament.

des·o·ges·trel (des″o-jes′trel) a progestational agent with little androgenic activity; used in combination with an estrogen as an oral contraceptive.

des·o·nide (des′o-nīd) a synthetic corticosteroid used topically for the relief of inflammation and pruritus in corticosteroid-responsive dermatoses.

de·sorb (de-sorb′) to remove a substance from the state of absorption or adsorption.

des·ox·i·met·a·sone (des-ok″se-met′ah-sōn) a synthetic corticosteroid used topically for the relief of inflammation and pruritus in corticosteroid-responsive dermatoses.

desoxy- older form for *deoxy-*.

de·spe·ci·ate (de-spe′se-āt) to undergo despeciation; to subject to (as by chemical treatment) or to undergo loss of species antigenic characteristics.

des·qua·ma·tion (des″kwah-ma′shun) the shedding of epithelial elements, chiefly of the skin, in scales or sheets. **desquam′ative**, adj.

dest. [L.] destilla′ta (distilled).

de·sulf·hy·drase (de″sulf-hi′drās) an enzyme that removes a hydrogen sulfide molecule from a compound.

DET diethyltryptamine.

de·tach·ment (de-tach′ment) the condition of being separated or disconnected. **d. of retina, retinal d.**, separation of the inner layers of the retina from the pigment epithelium.

de·tec·tor (de-tek′ter) an instrument or apparatus for revealing the presence of something. **lie d.**, polygraph.

de·ter·gent (de-ter′jent) 1. purifying, cleansing. 2. an agent that purifies or cleanses. 3. in biochemistry, any of a class of agents, characterized by a hydrophilic polar head group attached to a nonpolar hydrocarbon chain, which reduce the surface tension of water, emulsify, and aid in the solubilization of soil.

de·ter·mi·nant (de-ter′mĭ-nent) a factor that establishes the nature of an entity or event. **antigenic d.,** the structural component of an antigen molecule responsible for its specific interaction with antibody molecules elicited by the same or related antigen. **hidden d.,** an antigenic determinant in an unexposed region of a molecule so that it is prevented from interacting with receptors on lymphocytes, or with antibody molecules, and is unable to induce an immune response; it may appear following stereochemical alterations of molecular structure.

de·ter·mi·na·tion (de-ter″mĭ-na′shun) the establishment of the exact nature of an entity or event. **embryonic d.,** the loss of pluripotentiality in any embryonic part and its start on the way to an unalterable fate. **sex d.,** the process by which the sex of an organism is fixed; associated, in humans, with the presence or absence of the Y chromosome.

de·ter·min·ism (de-ter′mĭn-izm) the theory that all phenomena are the result of antecedent conditions, nothing occurs by chance, and there is no free will.

de·tox·i·fi·ca·tion (de-tok′sĭ-fĭ-ka′shun) 1. reduction of the toxic properties of poisons. 2. treatment designed to free an addict from a drug habit. 3. in naturopathy, the elimination of toxic substances from the body, either by metabolic change or by excretion. **metabolic d.,** reduction of the toxicity of a substance by chemical changes induced in the body, producing a compound less poisonous or more readily eliminated.

de·tri·tion (de-trish′un) the wearing away, as of teeth, by friction.

de·tri·tus (de-tri′tus) particulate matter produced by or remaining after the wearing away or disintegration of a substance or tissue.

de·tru·sor (de-troo′ser) [L.] 1. a body part that pushes down. 2. detrusor urinae (detrusor muscle of the bladder); see *Table of Muscles.*

de·tu·mes·cence (de″tu-mes′ins) the subsidence of congestion and swelling.

deu·tan (doo′tan) a person exhibiting deuteranomalopia or deuteranopia.

deu·ter·anom·a·ly (doo″ter-ah-nom′ah-le) a type of anomalous trichromatic vision in which the second, green-sensitive cones have decreased sensitivity; the most common color vision deficiency. **deuteranom′alous,** adj.

deu·ter·an·o·pia (-no′pe-ah) a type of dichromatic vision with confusion of greens and reds, and retention of the sensory mechanism for two hues only—blue and yellow. **deuteranop′ic,** adj.

deu·ter·an·op·sia (-nop′se-ah) deuteranopia.

deu·te·ri·um (D) (doo-tēr′e-um) see *hydrogen.*

Deu·tero·my·ce·tes (doo″ter-o-mi-se′tēz) in some systems of classification, the Fungi Imperfecti considered as a class.

Deu·tero·my·co·ta (-mi-ko′tah) the Fungi Imperfecti; a large heterogeneous group of fungi, ordinarily treated as a division, whose sexual stage does not exist or has not yet been discovered; subclassification is in form-classes, form-orders, etc., until their sexual stage is identified.

Deu·tero·my·co·ti·na (-mi″ko-ti′nah) in some systems of classification, the Fungi Imperfecti viewed as a subdivision of the division Eumycota.

deu·ter·op·a·thy (doo″ter-op′ah-the) a disease that is secondary to another disease.

deu·tero·plasm (doo′ter-o-plazm″) the passive or inactive materials in protoplasm, especially reserve foodstuffs, such as yolk.

de·vas·cu·lar·iza·tion (de-vas″ku-ler-ĭ-za′shun) interruption of circulation of blood to a part due to obstruction of blood vessels supplying it.

de·vel·op·ment (de-vel′up-mint) the process of growth and differentiation. **developmen′tal,** adj. **cognitive d.,** the development of intelligence, conscious thought, and problem-solving ability that begins in infancy. **psychosexual d.,** 1. development of the individual's sexuality as affected by biological, cultural, and emotional influences from prenatal life onward throughout life. 2. in psychoanalysis, libidinal maturation from infancy through adulthood (including the oral, anal, and genital stages). **psychosocial d.,** the development of the personality, and the acquisition of social attitudes and skills, from infancy through maturity.

de·vi·ant (de′ve-int) 1. varying from a determinable standard. 2. a person with characteristics varying from what is considered standard or normal.

de·vi·a·tion (de″ve-a′shun) 1. variation from the regular standard or course. 2. strabismus. 3. the difference between a sample value and the mean. **complement d.,** inhibition of complement fixation or complement-mediated immune hemolysis in the presence of excess antibody. **conjugate d.,** deflection of the eyes in the same direction at the same time. **immune d.,** modification of the immune response to an antigen by previous inoculation of the same antigen. **radial d.,** 1. a hand deformity sometimes seen in rheumatoid arthritis, in which the fingers are displaced to the radial side. 2. splinting of arthritic hands into this position to correct ulnar deviation. **sexual d.,** sexual behavior or fantasy outside that which is morally, biologically, or legally sanctioned, often specifically one of the paraphilias. **standard d. (SD),** a measure of the amount by which each value deviates from the mean; equal to the square root of the variance; symbol σ. **ulnar d.,** a hand deformity of chronic rheumatoid arthritis and lupus erythematosus in which swelling of the metacarpophalangeal joints causes displacement of the fingers to the ulnar side.

de·vice (dĭvīs′) something contrived for a specific purpose. **biventricular assist d. (BVAD),** a ventricular assist device with the combined functions of both left and right ventricular assist devices. **contraceptive d.,** one used to prevent conception, such as a barrier contraceptive, an intrauterine device, or a means of preventing ovulation (e.g., birth control pill). **intrauterine d. (IUD),** a plastic or metallic device inserted in the uterus to prevent pregnancy. **ventricular assist d. (VAD),** a circulatory support device that augments the function of the left ventricle, the right ventricle, or both, by providing mechanically assisted pulsatile blood flow.

de·vi·om·e·ter (de″ve-om′ĕ-ter) an instrument for measuring the deviation in strabismus.

de·vi·tal·ize (de-vīt′il-īz) to deprive of life or vitality.

dex·a·meth·a·sone (dek″sah-meth′ah-sōn) a synthetic glucocorticoid used primarily as an antiinflammatory in various conditions, including collagen diseases and allergic states; it is the basis of a screening test in the diagnosis of Cushing's syndrome; used also as the acetate or sodium phosphate salt.

dex·brom·phen·ir·a·mine (deks″brom-fen-ir′ah-mēn) the dextrorotatory isomer of brompheniramine, used as the maleate salt as an antihistamine.

dex·chlor·phen·ir·a·mine (-klor-fen-ēr′ah-mēn) the dextrorotatory isomer of chlorpheniramine, used as the maleate salt as an antihistamine.

dex·med·e·to·mi·dine (-med-ĕ-to′mĭ-dēn) a selective α_2-adrenergic receptor agonist, used as the hydrochloride salt as a sedative for patients in intensive care units.

Dex·on (dek′son) trademark for a synthetic suture material, polyglycolic acid, a polymer that is completely absorbable and nonirritating.

dex·ra·zox·ane (-ra-zok′sān) a cardioprotectant used in chemotherapy to counteract doxorubicin-induced cardiomyopathy.

dex·ter (deks′ter) [L.] right; on the right side.

dex·trad (dek′strad) to or toward the right side.

dex·tral (-stril) pertaining to the right side.

dex·tral·i·ty (dek-stral′it-e) lateral dominance on the right side.

dex·tran (dek′stran) a high-molecular-weight polymer of D-glucose, produced by enzymes on the cell surface of certain lactic acid bacteria. Dextrans formed from sucrose by bacteria in the mouth adhere to the tooth surfaces and produce dental plaque. Uniform molecular weight dextrans from *Leuconostoc mesenteroides* preparations are used as plasma volume expanders, with specific preparations named for their average molecular weight.

dex·trano·mer (deks-tran′o-mer) small beads of highly hydrophilic dextran polymers, used in débridement of secreting wounds, such as venous stasis ulcers; the sterilized beads are poured over secreting wounds to absorb wound exudates and prevent crust formation.

dex·trin (dek′strin) 1. any one, or the mixture, of the water-soluble, intermediate polysaccharides formed during the hydrolysis of starch to sugar. 2. a preparation of such formed by boiling starch and used in pharmacy. **limit d.,** any of the small polymers remaining after exhaustive digestion of glycogen or starch by enzymes that catalyze the removal of terminal sugar residues but that cannot cleave the linkages at branch points.

α-dex·trin·ase (-ās) isomaltase, limit dextrinase; an enzyme catalyzing the cleavage of linear and branched oligoglucosides and maltose and isomaltose, completing the digestion of starch or glycogen to glucose. It occurs in the brush border of the intestinal mucosa, as a complex with sucrase; see also *sucrase-isomaltase deficiency*.

dex·tri·no·sis (dek″strĭ-no′sis) accumulation in the tissues of an abnormal polysaccharide. **limit d.,** glycogen storage disease, type III.

dex·trin·uria (dek″strin-ūr′e-ah) presence of dextrin in the urine.

dextr(o)- word element [L.], *right*.

dex·tro·am·phet·amine (dek″stro-am-fet′ah-mēn) the dextrorotatory isomer of amphetamine; used as the sulfate salt in the treatment of narcolepsy and attention-deficit/hyperactivity disorder. Abuse of this drug may lead to dependence.

dex·tro·car·dia (-kahr′de-ah) location of the heart in the right side of the thorax, the apex pointing to the right. **isolated d.,** mirror-image transposition of the heart without accompanying alteration of the abdominal viscera. **mirror-image d.,** location of the heart in the right side of the chest, the atria being transposed and the right ventricle lying anteriorly and left of the left ventricle.

dex·tro·cli·na·tion (-klĭ-na′shun) rotation of the upper poles of the vertical meridians of the eyes to the right.

dex·tro·duc·tion (-duk′shun) movement of an eye to the right.

dex·tro·gas·tria (-gas′tre-ah) displacement of the stomach to the right.

dex·tro·gy·ra·tion (-ji-ra′shun) rotation to the right.

dex·tro·man·u·al (-man′u-al) right-handed.

dex·tro·meth·or·phan (-meth-or′fan) a synthetic morphine derivative used as an antitussive; used in the form of the base or as the hydrobromide salt or sulfonated styrene-divinylbenzene (polistirex) copolymer.

dex·tro·po·si·tion (-po-zish′un) displacement to the right.

dex·tro·ro·ta·to·ry (-ro′tah-tor″e) turning the plane of polarization to the right.

dex·trose (dek′strōs) a monosaccharide, D-glucose monohydrate; used chiefly as a fluid and nutrient replenisher, and also as a diuretic and for various other clinical purposes. Known as D-*glucose* in biochemistry and physiology.

dex·tro·sin·is·tral (dek″stro-sin′is-tral) 1. extending from right to left. 2. a left-handed person trained to use the right hand.

dex·tro·ver·sion (-ver′zhun) 1. version to the right, especially movement of the eyes to the right. 2. location of the heart in the right chest, the left ventricle remaining in the normal position on the left, but lying anterior to the right ventricle.

dez·o·cine (dez′o-sēn) an opioid analgesic, having both agonist and antagonist activity, used for the short-term relief of pain.

DH delayed hypersensitivity.

DHA docosahexaenoic acid.

dha·tu (thah′too) [Sanskrit] in ayurveda, the seven physical interconnected body tissues that are produced from metabolism and energy and anchor mind and spirit: plasma, blood, muscle, fat, bone, marrow, and reproductive tissue. Each tissue, though separate, is formed from another and depends upon its predecessor for its health.

DHEA dehydroepiandrosterone.

DHF dihydrofolate or dihydrofolic acid.

DHom Doctor of Homeopathic Medicine.

DHT dihydrotestosterone.

di- word element [Gr.], *two*.

dia- word element [Gr.], *through; between; apart; across; completely.*

di·a·be·tes (di″ah-be′tēz) any disorder characterized by excessive urine excretion. When used alone, the term refers to *diabetes mellitus*. **adult-onset d. mellitus,** type 2 d. mellitus. **brittle d.,** type 1 diabetes mellitus characterized by wide, unpredictable fluctuations of blood glucose values and difficult to control. **bronze d., bronzed d.,** hemochromatosis. **central d. insipidus,** diabetes insipidus due to injury of the neurohypophyseal system, with a deficient quantity of antidiuretic hormone being released or produced, causing failure of renal tubular reabsorption of water. **gestational d., gestational d. mellitus,** that with onset or first recognition during pregnancy. **growth-onset d. mellitus,** type 1 d. mellitus. **d. insipidus,** any of several types of polyuria in which the volume of urine exceeds 3 liters per day, causing dehydration and great thirst, as well as sometimes emaciation and great hunger. **insulin-dependent d. mellitus (IDD, IDDM),** type 1 d. mellitus. **juvenile d. mellitus, juvenile-onset d. mellitus,** type 1 d. mellitus. **ketosis-prone d. mellitus,** type 1 d. mellitus. **maturity-onset d. mellitus,** type 2 d. mellitus. **d. mel′litus (DM),** a chronic syndrome of impaired carbohydrate, protein, and fat metabolism owing to insufficient secretion of insulin or to target tissue insulin resistance. It occurs in two major forms: *type 1 d. mellitus* and *type 2 d. mellitus,* which differ in etiology, pathology, genetics, age of onset, and treatment. **nephrogenic d. insipidus,** inherited or acquired diabetes insipidus caused by failure of the renal tubules to reabsorb water in response to antidiuretic hormone, without disturbance in the renal filtration and solute excretion rates. **non–insulin-dependent d. mellitus (NIDD, NIDDM),** type 2 d. mellitus. **preclinical d.,** former name for *impaired glucose tolerance.* **renal d.,** see under *glycosuria.* **subclinical d.,** former name for *impaired glucose tolerance.* **Type I d. mellitus,** type 1 d. mellitus. **type 1 d. mellitus,** one of the two major types of diabetes mellitus, characterized by abrupt onset of symptoms (often in early adolescence), insulinopenia, and dependence on exogenous insulin; it is due to lack of insulin production by the pancreatic beta cells. With inadequate control, hyperglycemia, protein wasting, and ketone body production occur; the hyperglycemia leads to overflow glycosuria, osmotic diuresis, hyperosmolarity, dehydration, and diabetic ketoacidosis, which can progress to nausea and vomiting, stupor, and potentially fatal hyperosmolar coma. The associated angiopathy of blood vessels (particularly microangiopathy) affects the retinas, kidneys, and arteriolar basement membranes. Polyuria, polydipsia, polyphagia, weight loss, paresthesias, blurred vision, and irritability also occur. **Type II d. mellitus,** type 2 d. mellitus. **type 2 d. mellitus,** one of the two major types of diabetes mellitus, peaking in onset between 50 and 60 years of age, characterized by gradual onset with few symptoms of metabolic disturbance (glycosuria and its consequences) and control by diet, with or without oral hypoglycemics but without exogenous insulin required. Basal insulin secretion is maintained at normal or reduced levels, but insulin release in response to a glucose load is delayed or reduced. Defective glucose receptors on the pancreatic beta cells may be involved. It is often accompanied by disease of blood vessels, particularly the large ones, leading to premature atherosclerosis with myocardial infarction or stroke syndrome.

di·a·bet·ic (-bet′ik) 1. pertaining to or affected with diabetes. 2. a person with diabetes.

di·a·be·tid (-bēt′id) a cutaneous manifestation of diabetes; diabetic dermopathy.

di·a·be·to·gen·ic (-bet″ah-jen′ik) producing diabetes.

di·a·be·tog·e·nous (-be-toj′ĕ-nus) caused by diabetes.

di·a·brot·ic (-brot′ik) 1. ulcerative; caustic. 2. a corrosive or escharotic substance.

di·ac·e·tyl·mor·phine (di″ah-se″til-mor′-fēn) heroin.

di·ac·la·sis (di-ak′lah-sis) osteoclasis.

di·ac·ri·sis (di-ak′rĭ-sis) 1. diagnosis. 2. a disease marked by a morbid state of the secretions. 3. a critical discharge or excretion.

di·acyl·glyc·er·ol (di-a″sil-glis′er-ol) any of various compounds of glycerol linked to two fatty acids; they are triglyceride and phospholipid degradation products and are second messengers in calcium-mediated responses to hormones.

di·ad·o·cho·ki·ne·sia (di-ad″ah-ko-kĭ-ne′zhah) the function of arresting one motor impulse and substituting one that is diametrically opposite, permitting sequential alternating movements.

di·ag·nose (di′ag-nōs) to identify or recognize a disease.

di·ag·no·sis (di″ag-no′sis) the determination of the nature of a case of a disease or the distinguishing of one disease from another. **diagnos′tic,** adj. **clinical d.,** diagnosis based on signs, symptoms, and laboratory findings during life. **differential d.,** the determination of which one of several diseases may be producing the symptoms. **physical d.,** diagnosis based on information obtained by inspection, palpation, percussion, and auscultation. **serum d.,** serodiagnosis.

Di·ag·nos·tic and Sta·tis·ti·cal Man·u·al of Men·tal Dis·or·ders (DSM), a categorical system of classification of mental disorders, published by the American Psychiatric Association, that delineates objective criteria to be used in diagnosis.

di·ag·nos·tics (di″ag-nos′tiks) the science and practice of diagnosis of disease.

di·a·gram (di′ah-gram) a graphic representation, in simplest form, of an object or concept, made up of lines and lacking pictorial elements. **vector d.,** a diagram representing the direction and magnitude of electromotive forces of the heart for one entire cycle, based on analysis of the scalar electrocardiogram.

di·a·ki·ne·sis (di″ah-kĭ-ne′sis) the stage of first meiotic prophase in which the nucleolus and nuclear envelope disappear and the spindle fibers form.

di·al·y·sance (di-al′ĭ-sans) the minute rate of net exchange of solute molecules passing through a membrane in dialysis.

di·al·y·sate (di-al′ĭ-sāt) the fluid and solutes in a dialysis process that flow through the dialyzer, do not pass through the membrane, and are discarded along with removed toxic substances after leaving the dialyzer.

di·al·y·sis (di-al′ĭ-sis) [Gr.] 1. the process of separating macromolecules from ions and low molecular weight compounds in solution by the difference in their rates of diffusion through a semipermeable membrane, through which crystalloids pass readily but colloids pass slowly or not at all. 2. hemodialysis. **dialyt′ic,** adj. **equilibrium d.,** a technique of determination of the association constant of hapten-antibody reactions. **lymph d.,** removal of urea and other elements from lymph collected from the thoracic duct, treated outside the body, and later reinfused. **peritoneal d.,** dialysis through the peritoneum, the dialyzing solution being

di·a·lyz·er (di'ah-līz"er) hemodialyzer.

di·am·e·ter (di-am'ĕ-ter) the length of a straight line passing through the center of a circle and connecting opposite points on its circumference. Symbol *d.* **anteroposterior d.,** the distance between two points located on the anterior and posterior aspects, respectively, of the structure being measured, such as the true conjugate diameter of the pelvis or occipitofrontal diameter of the skull. **Baudelocque's d.,** external conjugate d.; see *pelvic d.* **conjugate d.,** see *pelvic d.* **cranial d's,** distances measured between certain landmarks of the skull, such as *biparietal,* that between the two parietal eminences; *bitemporal,* that between the two extremities of the coronal suture; *cervicobregmatic,* that between the center of the anterior fontanel and the junction of the neck with the floor of the mouth; *frontomental,* that between the forehead and chin; *occipitofrontal,* that between the external occipital protuberance and most prominent midpoint of the frontal bone; *occipitomental,* that between the external occipital protuberance and the most prominent midpoint of the chin; *suboccipitobregmatic,* that between the lowest posterior point of the occiput and the center of the anterior fontanel. **pelvic d.,** any diameter of the pelvis, such as *diagonal conjugate,* joining the posterior surface of the pubis to the tip of the sacral promontory; *external conjugate,* joining the depression under the last lumbar spine to the upper margin of the pubis; *true (internal) conjugate,* the anteroposterior diameter of the pelvic inlet, measured from the upper margin of the pubic symphysis to the sacrovertebral angle; *oblique,* joining one sacroiliac articulation to the iliopubic eminence of the other side; *transverse* (of inlet), joining the two most widely separated points of the pelvic inlet; *transverse* (of outlet), joining the medial surfaces of the ischial tuberosities.

p-di·ami·no·di·phen·yl (di-ah-me"no-di-fen'il) benzidine.

di·am·ni·ot·ic (di"am-ne-ot'ik) having or developing within separate amniotic cavities, as diamniotic twins.

di·a·pause (-pawz) a state of inactivity and arrested development accompanied by greatly decreased metabolism, as in many eggs, insect pupae, and plant seeds; it is a mechanism for surviving adverse winter conditions.

di·a·pe·de·sis (di"ah-pĕ-de'sis) the outward passage of blood cells through intact vessel walls.

di·aph·e·met·ric (-fĕ-mĕ'trik) pertaining to measurement of the sense of touch.

di·a·pho·re·sis (-fah-re'sis) sweating, especially of a profuse type.

di·a·pho·ret·ic (-fo-ret'ik) 1. pertaining to, characterized by, or promoting sweating. 2. an agent that promotes sweating.

di·a·phragm (di'ah-fram) 1. the musculomembranous partition separating the abdominal and thoracic cavities and serving as a major muscle aiding inhalation. See *Table of Muscles.* 2. any separating membrane or structure. 3. a disk with one or more openings or with an adjustable opening, mounted in relation to a lens or source of radiation, by which part of the light or radiation may be excluded from the area. 4. a device of molded rubber or other soft plastic material, fitted over the uterine cervix before intercourse to prevent entrance of spermatozoa. **diaphragmat'ic,** adj. **contraceptive d.,** diaphragm (4). **pelvic d.,** the portion of the floor of the pelvis formed by the coccygeal and levator ani muscles and their fasciae. **polyarcuate d.,** one showing abnormal scalloping of the margins on radiographic visualization. **Potter-Bucky d.,** see under *grid.* **respiratory d.,** diaphragm (1). **urogenital d.,** traditional but no longer valid concept that fascial layers enclose the sphincter urethrae and deep transverse perineal muscles and together form a musculomembranous sheet that extends between the ischiopubic rami. **vaginal d.,** diaphragm (4).

di·a·phrag·ma (di"ah-frag'mah) pl. *diaphrag'mata.* [Gr.] diaphragm (1).

di·a·phrag·mi·tis (-frag-mi'tis) phrenitis.

di·a·phy·se·al (-fiz'e-al) pertaining to or affecting the shaft of a long bone (diaphysis).

di·a·phys·ec·to·my (-fiz-ek'tah-me) excision of part of a diaphysis.

di·aph·y·sis (di-af'ĭ-sis) pl. *diaph'yses.* [Gr.] 1. the shaft of a long bone, between the epiphyses. 2. the portion of a long bone formed from a primary center of ossification.

di·a·phys·itis (di"ah-fiz-i'tis) inflammation of a diaphysis.

di·a·poph·y·sis (di"ah-pof'ĭ-sis) an upper transverse process of a vertebra.

di·a·py·e·sis (-pi-e'sis) suppuration. **diapyet'ic,** adj.

di·ar·rhea (-re'ah) abnormally frequent evacuation of watery feces. **diarrhe'al, diarrhe'ic,** adj. **choleraic d.,** acute diarrhea that resembles that of cholera, with serous feces and circulatory collapse. **familial**

chloride d., a type of severe watery diarrhea that begins in early infancy with feces containing excessive chloride because of impairment of chloride-bicarbonate exchange in the lower colon. Affected infants have a distended abdomen, lethargy, and retarded growth and mental development. **lienteric d.,** a form in which feces contain undigested food. **osmotic d.,** that due to the presence of osmotically active nonabsorbable solutes in the intestine, e.g., magnesium sulfate. **parenteral d.,** diarrhea due to infections outside the gastrointestinal tract. **secretory d.,** watery voluminous diarrhea resulting from increased stimulation of ion and water secretion, inhibition of their absorption, or both; osmolality of the feces approximates that of plasma. **summer d.,** acute diarrhea in children during the intense heat of summer. **toxigenic d.,** the watery voluminous diarrhea caused by enterotoxins from enterotoxigenic bacteria such as *Vibrio cholerae* and enterotoxigenic strains of *Escherichia coli*. **traveler's d.,** diarrhea in travelers, especially those visiting tropical or subtropical areas where sanitation is poor; many different agents can cause it, the most common being enterotoxigenic *Escherichia coli*. **tropical d.,** see under *sprue*. **weanling d.,** diarrhea in an infant when put on food other than its mother's milk, usually due to inadequate sanitation and infection by enterotoxigenic *Escherichia coli* or rotaviruses.

di·ar·rhe·o·gen·ic (di″ah-re″o-jen′ik) giving rise to diarrhea.

di·ar·thric (di-ahr′thrik) diarticular; pertaining to or affecting two different joints.

di·ar·thro·sis (di″ahr-thro′sis) pl. *diarthro′ses.* [Gr.] a synovial joint. **diarthro′dial,** adj.

di·ar·tic·u·lar (-tik′u-ler) diarthric.

di·as·chi·sis (di-as′kĭ-sis) loss of function and electrical activity due to cerebral lesions in areas remote from the lesion but neuronally connected to it.

di·a·scope (di′ah-skōp) a glass or clear plastic plate pressed against the skin for observing changes produced in the underlying skin after the blood vessels are emptied and the skin is blanched.

di·a·stase (-stās) a mixture of starch-hydrolyzing enzymes from malt; used to convert starch into simple sugars.

di·as·ta·sis (di-as′tah-sis) 1. dislocation or separation of two normally attached bones between which there is no true joint. Also, separation beyond the normal between associated bones, as between the ribs. 2. a relatively quiescent period of slow ventricular filling during the cardiac cycle, occurring just prior to atrial systole.

di·a·ste·ma (di″ah-ste′mah) pl. *diaste′mata.* [Gr.] 1. a space or cleft. 2. a space between two adjacent teeth in the same dental arch. 3. a narrow zone in the equatorial plane through which the cytosome divides in mitosis.

di·a·stem·a·to·cra·nia (-stem″ah-to-kra′-ne-ah) congenital longitudinal fissure of the cranium.

di·a·stem·a·to·my·elia (-mi-e′le-ah) abnormal congenital division of the spinal cord by a bony spicule or fibrous band protruding from a vertebra or two, each half surrounded by a dural sac.

di·as·to·le (di-as′tah-le) the dilatation, or the period of dilatation, of the heart, especially of the ventricles. **diastol′ic,** adj.

di·a·stroph·ic (di″ah-strof′ik) bent or curved; said of structures, such as bones, deformed in such manner.

di·atax·ia (-tak′se-ah) ataxia affecting both sides of the body. **cerebral d.,** cerebral palsy with ataxia.

di·a·ther·my (di′ah-ther″me) the heating of body tissues due to their resistance to the passage of high-frequency electromagnetic radiation, electric current, or ultrasonic waves. **short wave d.,** diathermy with high-frequency current, with frequency from 10 million to 100 million cycles per second and wavelength from 30 to 3 meters.

di·ath·e·sis (di-ath′ĕ-sis) an unusual constitutional susceptibility or predisposition to a particular disease. **diathet′ic,** adj.

di·a·tom (di′ah-tom) a unicellular microscopic form of alga having a cell wall of silica.

di·a·to·ma·ceous (di″ah-to-ma′shus) composed of diatoms; said of earth composed of the siliceous skeletons of diatoms.

dia·tri·zo·ate (-tri-zo′āt) the most commonly used water-soluble, iodinated, radiopaque x-ray contrast medium; used in the form of its meglumine and sodium salts.

di·az·e·pam (di-az′ĕ-pam) a benzodiazepine used as an antianxiety agent, sedative, antipanic agent, antitremor agent, skeletal muscle relaxant, anticonvulsant, and in the management of alcohol withdrawal symptoms.

di·a·zi·quone (AZQ) (di-a′zĭ-kwon″) an alkylating agent that acts by cross-linking DNA; used as an antineoplastic in the treatment of primary brain malignancies.

diaz(o)- the group —N=N—.

di·az·o·tize (di-az′o-tīz) to introduce the diazo group into a compound.

di·az·ox·ide (di″az-ok′sīd) an antihypertensive structurally related to chlorothiazide but having no diuretic properties; used for treatment of hypertensive emergencies. Because it inhibits release of insulin, it is also used in hypoglycemia due to hyperinsulinism.

di·ba·sic (di-ba'sik) containing two replaceable hydrogen atoms, or furnishing two hydrogen ions.

di·ben·zaz·e·pine (di″ben-zaz′ĕ-pēn) any of a group of structurally related drugs including the tricyclic antidepressants clomipramine, desipramine, imipramine, and trimipramine.

di·ben·zo·cy·clo·hep·ta·di·ene (di-ben″zo-si″klo-hep″tah-di′ēn) any of a group of structurally related drugs including the tricyclic antidepressants amitriptyline, nortriptyline, and protriptyline.

di·ben·zo·di·az·e·pine (di-ben″zo-di-az′ĕ-pēn) any of a group of structurally related drugs including the antipsychotic agent clozapine.

di·ben·zox·az·e·pine (di-ben″zok-saz′ĕ-pēn) any of a class of structurally related heterocyclic drugs, including the antipsychotic loxapine and the antidepressant amoxapine.

di·ben·zox·e·pine (-zok′sĕ-pēn) any of a group of structurally related drugs including the tricyclic antidepressant doxepin.

di·both·rio·ceph·a·li·a·sis (di-both″re-o-sef″ah-li′ah-sis) diphyllobothriasis.

di·bro·mo·chlo·ro·pro·pane (di-bro″mo-klor″o-pro′pān) a colorless, halogenated, carcinogenic hydrocarbon formerly used as a pesticide, fumigant, and nematocide but now restricted in usage.

1,2-di·bro·mo·eth·ane (-eth′ān) ethylene dibromide.

di·bu·caine (di′bu-kān) a local anesthetic used topically on the skin and mucous membranes and rectally.

DIC diffuse intravascular coagulation; disseminated intravascular coagulation.

di·cen·tric (di-sen′trik) 1. pertaining to, developing from, or having two centers. 2. having two centromeres.

di·ceph·a·lus (di-sef′ah-lus) a fetus with two heads.

di·chlo·ral·phen·a·zone (di″klor′l-fen′ah-zōn) a complex of chloral hydrate and antipyrine (phenazone); used in combination with isometheptene mucate and acetaminophen in the treatment of migraine and tension headache.

o-di·chlo·ro·ben·zene (di-klor″o-ben′zēn) a solvent, fumigant, and insecticide toxic by ingestion or inhalation.

di·chlor·phen·a·mide (di″klor-fen′ah-mīd) a carbonic anhydrase inhibitor; used as an adjunct to reduce intraocular pressure in the treatment of glaucoma.

di·cho·ri·al (di-ko′re-il) dichorionic.

di·cho·ri·on·ic (di-ko″re-on′ik) having two distinct chorions; said of dizygotic twins.

di·chro·ism (di′kro-izm) the quality or condition of showing one color in reflected and another in transmitted light. **dichro′ic**, adj.

di·chro·ma·cy (di-kro′mah-se) dichromatic vision.

di·chro·mate (-māt) a salt containing the bivalent Cr_2O_7 radical.

di·chro·mat·ic (di″kro-mat′ik) pertaining to or having dichromatic vision.

di·chro·ma·tism (di-kro′mah-tizm) 1. the quality of existing in or exhibiting two different colors. 2. dichromatic vision.

di·clo·fen·ac (di-klo′fen-ak) a nonsteroidal anti-inflammatory drug used as the potassium or sodium salt in the treatment of rheumatic and nonrheumatic inflammatory conditions, and as the potassium salt to relieve pain and dysmenorrhea; also applied topically to the conjunctiva as the sodium salt to reduce ocular inflammation or photophobia after certain kinds of surgery and to the skin to treat actinic keratoses.

di·clox·a·cil·lin (di-klok″sah-sil′in) a semisynthetic penicillinase-resistant penicillin; used as the sodium salt, primarily in the treatment of infections due to penicillinase-producing staphylococci.

di·coe·lous (di-se′lus) 1. hollowed on each of two sides. 2. having two cavities.

Dic·ro·coe·li·um (dik″ro-sēl′e-um) a genus of flukes, including *D. dendri′ticum*, which has been found in human biliary passages.

di·cro·tism (di′krot-izm) the occurrence of two sphygmographic waves or elevations to one beat of the pulse. **dicrot′ic**, adj.

dic·tyo·tene (dik′te-o-tēn″) the protracted stage resembling suspended prophase in which the primary oocyte persists from late fetal life until discharged from the ovary at or after puberty.

di·cu·ma·rol (di-koo′mah-rol) a coumarin anticoagulant, which acts by inhibiting the hepatic synthesis of vitamin K–dependent coagulation factors.

di·cy·clo·mine (-si′klo-mēn) an anticholinergic, used as the hydrochloride salt as a gastrointestinal antispasmodic.

di·dan·o·sine (-dan′o-sēn) 2′3′-dideoxyinosine, an analogue of dideoxyadenosine; an antiretroviral agent used for the treatment of advanced HIV-1 infection and acquired immunodeficiency syndrome, administered orally.

2′,3′-di·de·oxy·aden·o·sine (di″de-ok″se-ah-den′o-sēn) a dideoxynucleoside in which the base is adenine, used as an antiretroviral agent in the treatment of acquired immunodeficiency syndrome.

di·de·oxy·cy·ti·dine (-si′tĭ-dēn) a dideoxynucleoside in which the base is cytosine; it is an antiretroviral agent that acts by inhibiting reverse transcriptase and is used in treating acquired immunodeficiency syndrome.

di·de·oxy·in·o·sine (-in′o-sēn) didanosine.

di·de·oxy·nu·cleo·side (-noo′kle-o-sīd) any of a group of synthetic nucleoside analogues, several of which are used as antiretroviral agents.

di·der·mo·ma (di″der-mo′mah) a teratoma composed of cells and tissues derived from two cell layers.

did·y·mi·tis (-mi′tis) orchitis.

-didymus word element [Gr.], *fetus with duplication of parts; conjoined symmetrical twins.*

die (di) a form used in the construction of something, as a positive reproduction of the form of a prepared tooth in a suitable hard substance.

di·e·cious (di-e′shus) sexually distinct; denoting species in which male and female genitals do not occur in the same individual.

di·el·drin (di-el′drin) a chlorinated insecticide; inhalation, ingestion, or skin contact may cause poisoning.

di·en·ceph·a·lon (di″en-sef′ah-lon) 1. the posterior part of the forebrain, consisting of the hypothalamus, thalamus, metathalamus, and epithalamus; the subthalamus is often recognized as a distinct division. 2. the posterior of the two brain vesicles formed by specialization in embryonic development. See also *brain stem.* **diencephal′ic,** adj.

di·en·es·trol (di″en-es′trol) a synthetic estrogen administered intravaginally in treatment of atrophic vaginitis and kraurosis vulvae.

Di·ent·amoe·ba (di-ent″ah-me′bah) a genus of amebas commonly found in the human colon and appendix, including *D. fra′gilis,* a species that has been associated with diarrhea.

di·er·e·sis (di-er′ah-sis) 1. the division or separation of parts normally united. 2. the surgical separation of parts.

di·et (di′it) the customary amount and kind of food and drink taken by a person from day to day; more narrowly, a diet planned to meet specific requirements of the individual, including or excluding certain foods. **di′etary,** adj. **acid-ash d.,** one of meat, fish, eggs, and cereals with little fruit or vegetables and no cheese or milk. **alkali-ash d.,** one of fruit, vegetables, and milk with as little as possible of meat, fish, eggs, and cereals. **balanced d.,** one containing foods which furnish all the nutritive factors in proper proportion for adequate nutrition. **bland d.,** one that is free of irritating or stimulating foods. **diabetic d.,** one prescribed in diabetes mellitus, usually limited in the amount of sugar or readily available carbohydrate. **elimination d.,** one for diagnosis of food allergy, based on sequential omission of foods that might cause the symptoms. **Feingold d.,** a controversial diet for hyperactive children which excludes artificial colors, artificial flavors, preservatives, and salicylates. **gouty d.,** one for mitigation of gout, restricting nitrogenous, especially high-purine foods, and substituting dairy products, with prohibition of wines and liquors. **high calorie d.,** one furnishing more calories than needed to maintain weight, often more than 3500–4000 calories per day. **high fat d.,** ketogenic d. **high fiber d.,** one relatively high in dietary fibers, which decreases bowel transit time and relieves constipation. **high protein d.,** one containing large amounts of protein, consisting largely of meat, fish, milk, legumes, and nuts. **ketogenic d.,** one containing large amounts of fat, with minimal amounts of protein and carbohydrate. **low calorie d.,** one containing fewer calories than needed to maintain weight, e.g., less than 1200 calories per day for an adult. **low fat d.,** one containing limited amounts of fat. **low purine d.,** one for mitigation of gout, omitting meat, fowl, and fish and substituting milk, eggs, cheese, and vegetable protein. **low residue d.,** one giving the least possible fecal residue. **low salt d., low sodium d.,** one containing very little sodium chloride; often prescribed for hypertension and edematous states. **protein-sparing d.,** one consisting only of liquid proteins or liquid mixtures of proteins, vitamins, and minerals, and containing no more than 600 calories; designed to maintain a favorable nitrogen balance. **purine-free d.,** see *low purine d.* **salt-free d.,** low salt d.

di·e·tet·ic (di″ah-tet′ik) pertaining to diet or proper food.

di·e·tet·ics (-iks) the science of diet and nutrition.

di·eth·yl·car·bam·a·zine (di-eth″il-kahr-bam′ah-zēn) an antifilarial agent, used as the citrate salt.

di·eth·yl·ene·tri·amine   pen·ta·ace·tic ac·id (DTPA) (-ēn-tri′ah-mēn pen″tah-ah-se′tik) pentetic acid.

di·eth·yl·pro·pi·on (-pro'pe-on) a sympathomimetic amine used as an anorectic in the form of the hydrochloride salt.

di·eth·yl·stil·bes·trol (DES) (-stil-bes'trol) a synthetic nonsteroidal estrogen, used as the base or the diphosphate salt for the palliative treatment of prostatic carcinoma and sometimes breast carcinoma; it is an epigenetic carcinogen and females exposed to it in utero are subject to increased risk of vaginal and cervical carcinomas.

di·eth·yl·tol·u·am·ide (-tol-u'ah-mīd) an arthropod repellent, applied to the skin and the clothing.

di·eth·yl·tryp·ta·mine (DET) (-trip'tah-mēn) a synthetic hallucinogenic substance closely related to dimethyltryptamine.

di·e·ti·tian (di''ĕ-tish'in) one skilled in the use of diet in health and disease.

di·fe·nox·in (di''fĕ-nok'sin) an antiperistaltic used as the hydrochloride salt in the treatment of diarrhea.

dif·fer·ence (dif'cr-ens) the condition or magnitude of variation between two qualities or quantities. **differen'tial,** adj. **arteriovenous oxygen d.,** the difference in the blood oxygen content between the arterial and venous systems.

dif·fer·en·ti·ate (dif''er-en'she-āt) 1. to distinguish, on the basis of differences. 2. to develop specialized form, character, or function differing from that surrounding it or from the original.

dif·fer·en·ti·a·tion (-en''she-a'shun) 1. the distinguishing of one thing from another. 2. the act or process of acquiring completely individual characters, as occurs in progressive diversification of embryonic cells and tissues. 3. increase in morphological or chemical heterogeneity.

dif·frac·tion (dĭ-frak'shun) the bending or breaking up of a ray of light into its component parts.

dif·fu·sate (dĭ-fu'zāt) material that has diffused through a membrane, such as solutes that pass out of the blood into the dialysate fluid in a dialyzer.

dif·fuse 1. (dĭ-fūs') not definitely limited or localized. 2. (dĭ-fūz') to pass through or to spread widely through a tissue or substance.

dif·fus·ible (dĭ-fūz'ĭ-b'l) susceptible of becoming widely spread.

dif·fu·sion (dĭ-fu'zhun) 1. the process of becoming diffused, or widely spread. 2. the spontaneous movement of molecules or other particles in solution, owing to their random thermal motion, to reach a uniform concentration throughout the solvent, a process requiring no addition of energy to the system.

3. in hemodialysis, the movement of solutes across semipermeable membranes down concentration gradients. 4. immunodiffusion. **double d.,** an immunodiffusion test in which both antigen and antibody diffuse into a common area so that, if the antigen and antibody are interacting, they combine to form bands of precipitate. **gel d.,** a test in which antigen and antibody diffuse toward one another through a gel medium to form a precipitate.

di·flor·a·sone (di-flor'ah-sōn) a synthetic corticosteroid used topically as the diacetate salt in the treatment of inflammation and pruritus in certain dermatoses.

di·flu·cor·to·lone (di''floo-kor'tah-lōn'') a synthetic corticosteroid used topically as the valerate salt for the relief of inflammation and pruritus in corticosteroid-responsive dermatoses.

di·flu·ni·sal (di-floo'nĭ-sal) a nonsteroidal antiinflammatory drug that lacks antipyretic activity; used in the treatment of rheumatic and nonrheumatic inflammatory disorders, gout and calcium pyrophosphate deposition disease, dysmenorrhea, and vascular headaches.

di·gas·tric (di-gas'trik) 1. having two bellies. 2. digastric muscle; see *Table of Muscles.*

di·ge·net·ic (di''jah-net'ik) having two stages of multiplication, one sexual in the mature forms, the other asexual in the larval stages.

di·ges·tion (di-jes'chun) 1. the act or process of converting food into chemical substances that can be absorbed and assimilated. 2. the subjection of a substance to prolonged heat and moisture, so as to disintegrate and soften it. **diges'tive,** adj. **artificial d.,** digestion carried on outside the body. **gastric d.,** digestion by the action of gastric juice. **gastrointestinal d.,** the gastric and intestinal digestions together. **intestinal d.,** digestion by the action of intestinal juices. **pancreatic d.,** digestion by the action of pancreatic juice. **peptic d.,** gastric d. **primary d.,** gastrointestinal d. **salivary d.,** the change of starch into maltose by the saliva.

dig·it (dij'it) a finger or toe.

dig·i·tal (dij'ĭ-t'l) 1. of, pertaining to, or performed with, a finger. 2. resembling the imprint of a finger. 3. relating to data that is represented in the form of discrete numeric symbols.

Dig·i·tal·is (dij''ĭ-tal'is) a genus of herbs. *D. lana'ta* yields digoxin and lanatoside, and the leaves of *D. purpu'rea,* the purple foxglove, furnish digitalis.

dig·i·tal·is (dij''ĭ-tal'is) 1. the dried leaf of *Digitalis purpurea;* used as a cardiotonic agent. 2. the digitalis glycosides or cardiac glycosides, collectively.

dig·i·tal·iza·tion (dij″ĭ-tal-ĭ-za′shun) the administration of digitalis or one of its glycosides in a dosage schedule designed to produce and then maintain optimal therapeutic concentrations of its cardiotonic glycosides.

dig·i·tate (dij′ĭ-tāt) having digit-like branches.

dig·i·ta·tion (-ta′shun) 1. a finger-like process. 2. surgical creation of a functioning digit by making a cleft between two adjacent metacarpal bones, after amputation of some or all of the fingers.

dig·i·to·nin (dij″ĭ-to′nin) a saponin from *Digitalis purpurea* with no cardiotonic action; used as a reagent to precipitate cholesterol.

di·gi·toxi·ge·nin (-tok″sĭ-je′nin) the steroid nucleus that is the aglycone of digitoxin.

dig·i·tox·in (-tok′sin) a cardiotonic glycoside from *Digitalis purpurea* and other *Digitalis* species; used similarly to digitalis.

dig·i·tus (dij′ĭ-tus) pl. *di′giti*. [L.] a digit.

di·glyc·er·ide (di-glis′er-īd) diacylglycerol.

di·goxi·ge·nin (dĭ-jak″sĭ-je′nin) the steroid nucleus that is the aglycone of digoxin.

di·gox·in (dĭ-jok′sin) a cardiotonic glycoside from the leaves of *Digitalis lanata*; used similarly to digitalis. **d. immune Fab (ovine),** see under *Fab*.

di·hy·dric (di-hi′drik) having two hydrogen atoms in each molecule.

di·hy·dro·co·deine (di-hi″dro-ko′dēn) an opioid analgesic and antitussive; used as the acid tartrate for the relief of moderate to moderately severe pain; administered orally.

di·hy·dro·er·got·amine (-er-got′ah-mēn) an antiadrenergic derived from ergotamine; used as d. *mesylate* as a vasoconstrictor in the treatment of migraine.

di·hy·dro·fo·late (DHF) (-fo′lāt) an ester or dissociated form of dihydrofolic acid.

di·hy·dro·fol·ic ac·id (-fo′lik) any of the folic acids in which the bicyclic pteridine structure is in the dihydro, partially reduced form; they are intermediates in folate metabolism.

di·hy·dro·py·rim·i·dine de·hy·dro·gen·ase (NADP) (-pĭ-rim′ĭ-dēn de-hi′dro-jen-ās) an enzyme catalyzing a step in the catabolism of pyrimidines; deficiency results in elevated plasma, urine, and cerebrospinal levels of pyrimidines, cerebral dysfunction in children, and hypersensitivity to 5-fluorouracil in adults.

di·hy·dro·tach·ys·te·rol (-tak-is′ter-ol) an analogue of ergocalciferol that raises serum calcium levels, used in the treatment of hypocalcemia, hypophosphatemia, rickets,

and osteodystrophy associated with a variety of disorders and the prophylaxis and treatment of postoperative or idiopathic tetany.

di·hy·dro·tes·tos·te·rone (DHT) (-tes-tos′tĕ-rōn) an androgenic hormone formed in peripheral tissue by the action of 5α-reductase on testosterone; thought to be the androgen responsible for development of male primary sex characters during embryogenesis and of male secondary sex characters at puberty, and for adult male sexual function.

di·hy·droxy (di″hi-drok′se) a molecule containing two molecules of the hydroxy (OH) radical; used also as a prefix (hydroxy-) to denote such a compound.

di·hy·droxy·ac·e·tone (di″hi-drok″se-as′ĕ-tōn) the simplest ketose, a triose; it is an isomer of glyceraldehyde. *D. phosphate* is an intermediate in glycolysis, the glycerol phosphate shuttle, and the biosynthesis of carbohydrates and lipids.

di·hy·droxy·alu·mi·num (-ah-loo′mĭ-num) an aluminum compound having two hydroxyl groups in a molecule; available as d. *amino·acetate* and d. *sodium carbonate*, which are used as antacids.

di·hy·droxy·cho·le·cal·cif·e·rol (-ko″le-kal-sif′ĕ-rol) a group of active metabolites of cholecalciferol (vitamin D₃). 1,25-Dihydroxycholecalciferol (1,25-dihydroxyvitamin D₃ or calcitriol) increases intestinal absorption of calcium and phosphate, enhances bone resorption, and prevents rickets, and, because of these activities at sites distant from the site of its synthesis, is considered to be a hormone. See also *calcitriol*.

1,25-di·hy·droxy·vi·ta·min D (-vi′tah-min) 1,25-dihydroxycholecalciferol, the corresponding dihydroxy derivative of ergocalciferol, or both collectively.

1,25-di·hy·droxy·vi·ta·min D₃ 1,25-dihydroxycholecalciferol; see *dihydroxycholecalciferol*.

di·io·do·ty·ro·sine (di″i-o″do-ti′ro-sēn) an organic iodine-containing precursor of thyroxine, liberated from thyroglobulin by hydrolysis.

di·iso·cy·anate (di-i″so-si′ah-nāt) any of a group of compounds containing two isocyanate groups (—NCO), used in the manufacture of plastics and elastomers; they can cause sensitization and are eye and respiratory system irritants.

dik·ty·o·ma (dik″te-o′mah) a medulloepithelioma of the epithelium lining the basal lamina of the ciliary body.

di·lac·er·a·tion (di-las″er-a′shun) a tearing apart, as of a cataract. In dentistry, an abnormal angulation or curve in the root or crown of a formed tooth.

dil·a·ta·tion (dil″ah-ta′shun) 1. the condition, as of an orifice or tubular structure, of being dilated or stretched beyond normal dimensions. 2. the act of dilating or stretching. **d. of the heart,** compensatory enlargement of the cavities of the heart, with thinning of its walls. **segmental d.,** dilatation of a portion of a tubular structure, such as the bowel, the segments on either side of the dilatation being of normal caliber.

di·late (di′lāt) to stretch an opening or hollow structure beyond its normal dimensions.

di·la·tion (di-la′shun) 1. the act of dilating or stretching. 2. dilatation.

di·la·tor (di-lāt′er) 1. a structure that dilates, or an instrument used to dilate. 2. dilator muscle.

dil·ti·a·zem (dil-ti′ah-zem) a calcium channel blocker that acts as a vasodilator; used as the hydrochloride salt in the treatment of angina pectoris, hypertension, and supraventricular tachycardia.

dil·u·ent (dil′oo-int) 1. causing dilution. 2. an agent that dilutes or renders less potent or irritant.

di·lu·tion (di-loo′shun) 1. reduction of concentration of an active substance by admixture of a neutral agent. 2. a substance that has undergone dilution. 3. in homeopathy, the diffusion of a given quantity of a medicinal agent in ten or one hundred times the same quantity of water. **dilu′tional,** adj. **serial d.,** a set of dilutions in a mathematical sequence, as to obtain a culture plate with a countable number of separate colonies.

di·men·hy·dri·nate (di″men-hi′dri-nāt) an antihistamine used as an antiemetic, particularly in the treatment of motion sickness.

di·mer (di′mer) 1. a compound formed by combination of two identical molecules. 2. a capsomer having two structural subunits.

di·mer·cap·rol (di″mer-kap′rol) a metal complexing agent used as an antidote to poisoning by arsenic, gold, mercury, and lead.

di·meth·i·cone (di-meth′ĭ-kōn) a silicone oil used as a skin protective. See also *simethicone*.

di·meth·yl sulf·ox·ide (DMSO) (di-meth′il sul-fok′sīd) a powerful solvent with the ability to penetrate plant and animal tissues and to preserve living cells during freezing; it is instilled into the bladder for relief of interstitial cystitis and has been proposed as a topical analgesic and antiinflammatory agent and for increasing penetrability of other substances.

di·meth·yl·tryp·ta·mine (DMT) (di-meth″il-trip′tah-mēn) a hallucinogenic substance derived from the plant *Prestonia amazonica*, which is native to parts of South America and the West Indies.

di·mor·phism (di-mor′fizm) the quality of existing in two distinct forms. **dimor′phic, dimor′phous,** adj. **sexual d.,** 1. physical or behavioral differences associated with sex. 2. having some properties of both sexes, as in the early embryo and in some hermaphrodites.

dim·ple (dim′p'l) a slight depression, as in the flesh of the cheek, chin, or sacral region. **postanal d.,** a dermal pit near the tip of the coccyx, indicative of the site of attachment of the embryonic neural tube to the skin.

di·ni·tro·o·cre·sol (DNOC) (di-ni″tro-kre′sol) a highly toxic pesticide that affects the central nervous system and energy-producing metabolic processes; metabolic rate is increased and fatal hyperpyrexia may occur.

di·ni·tro·tolu·ene (-tol′u-ēn) any of three highly toxic, possibly carcinogenic isomers used in organic synthesis and the manufacture of dyes and explosives.

di·no·flag·el·late (di″no-flaj′ĕ-lāt) 1. of or pertaining to the order Dinoflagellida. 2. any individual of the order Dinoflagellida.

Di·no·fla·gel·li·da (-flah-jel′ĭ-dah) an order of minute plantlike, chiefly marine protozoa, which are an important component of plankton. They may be present in sea water in such vast numbers that they cause a discoloration (red tide), which may result in the death of marine animals, including fish, by exhaustion of their oxygen supply. Some species secrete a powerful neurotoxin that can cause a severe toxic reaction in humans who ingest shellfish that feed on the toxin-producing organisms.

di·no·prost (di′no-prost) name for prostaglandin $F_{2\alpha}$ when used as a pharmaceutical; used as the base or the tromethamine salt as an oxytocic for induction of abortion, for evacuation of the uterus in management of missed abortion, and in treatment of hydatidiform mole.

di·no·prost·one (di″no-pros′tōn) name given to prostaglandin E_2 when used pharmaceutically; used as an oxytocic for induction of abortion or labor, to aid ripening of the cervix, and in the treatment of missed abortion or hydatidiform mole.

di·nu·cleo·tide (di-nook′le-o-tīd″) one of the cleavage products into which a polynucleotide may be split, itself composed of two mononucleotides.

Di·oc·to·phy·ma (di-ok″to-fi′mah) a genus of nematodes, including *D. rena′le*, the kidney worm, found in dogs, cattle, horses, and other animals, and rarely in humans; it is highly destructive to kidney tissue.

di·op·ter (di-op′ter) a unit for refractive power of lenses, being the reciprocal of the focal length expressed in meters; symbol D. **prism d.**, a unit of prismatic deviation, being the deflection of 1 cm. at a distance of one meter; symbol Δ.

di·op·tom·e·try (di-op-tom′ĭ-tre) the measurement of ocular accommodation and refraction.

di·op·tric (di-op′trik) pertaining to refraction or to transmitted and refracted light; refracting.

di·ov·u·la·to·ry (-ov′u-lah-to″re) discharging two oocytes in one ovarian cycle.

di·ox·ide (-ok′sīd) an oxide with two oxygen atoms.

di·ox·in (-ok′sin) any of the heterocyclic hydrocarbons present as trace contaminants in herbicides; many are oncogenic and teratogenic.

di·oxy·ben·zone (-ok″sĭ-ben′zōn) a topical sunscreening agent, absorbing UVB and some UVA light.

di·pep·ti·dase (-pep′tĭ-dās) any of a group of enzymes that catalyze the hydrolysis of the peptide linkage in a dipeptide.

Di·pet·a·lo·ne·ma (-pet″ah-lo-ne′mah) a genus of nematode parasites (superfamily Filarioidea), including *D. per′stans* and *D. streptocer′ca*, species primarily parasitic in humans, other primates serving as reservoir hosts.

di·pha·sic (-fa′zik) having two phases.

di·phen·hy·dra·mine (di″fen-hi′drah-mēn) a potent antihistamine, used as the hydrochloride salt in the treatment of allergic symptoms and for its anticholinergic, antitussive, antiemetic, antivertigo, and antidyskinetic effects, and as the hydrochloride or citrate salt as a sedative and hypnotic.

di·phen·i·dol (di-fen′ĭ-dôl) an antiemetic, used as the base or as the hydrochloride or pamoate salt in the treatment of vertigo and to control nausea and vomiting.

di·phen·ox·y·late (di″fen-ok′sĭ-lāt) an antiperistaltic derived from meperidine; the hydrochloride salt is used as an antidiarrheal.

di·phen·yl (di-fen′il) a toxic compound comprising two linked benzene rings, used as a fungistat in containers for shipping citrus fruits.

di·phen·yl·amine chlor·ar·sine (DM) (di-fen′il-ah-mēn″ klor″ahr′sēn) a toxic, irritant compound used as a war gas and, with tear gas, in riot control, as well as in some wood preserving solutions.

di·phen·yl·bu·tyl·pi·per·i·dine (di-fen″il-bu″til-pi-per′ĭ-dēn) any of a class of structurally related antipsychotic agents that includes pimozide.

di·phos·pha·ti·dyl·glyc·er·ol (di″fos-fah-ti″dil-glis′er-ol) glycerol linked to two molecules of phosphatidic acid; 1,3-diphosphatidylglycerol is cardiolipin.

di·phos·pho·nate (di-fos′fŏ-nāt) 1. a salt, ester, or anion of a dimer of phosphonic acid, structurally similar to pyrophosphate but more stable. 2. any of a group of such compounds, having affinity for sites of osteoid mineralization and used as sodium salts to inhibit bone resorption as well as complexed with technetium Tc 99m for bone imaging.

diph·the·ria (dif-thēr′e-ah) an acute infectious disease caused by *Corynebacterium diphtheriae* and its toxin, affecting the membranes of the nose, throat, or larynx, and marked by formation of a gray-white pseudomembrane, with fever, pain, and, in the laryngeal form, aphonia and respiratory obstruction. The toxin may also cause myocarditis and neuritis. **diphthe′rial, diphther′ic, diphtherit′ic,** adj.

diph·the·roid (dif′thĕ-roid) 1. resembling diphtheria or the diphtheria bacillus. 2. any member of *Corynebacterium* other than *C. diphtheriae*. 3. pseudodiphtheria.

di·phyl·lo·both·ri·a·sis (di-fil″o-both-ri′ah-sis) infection with *Diphyllobothrium*.

Di·phyl·lo·both·ri·um (-both′re-um) a genus of large tapeworms, including *D. la′tum* (broad or fish tapeworm), found in the intestine of humans, cats, dogs, and other fish-eating mammals; its first intermediate host is a crustacean and the second a fish, the infection in humans being acquired by eating inadequately cooked fish.

di·phy·odont (dif′e-o-dont″) having two dentitions, a deciduous and a permanent.

di·piv·e·frin (di-piv′ah-frin) an ester converted in the eye to epinephrine, lowering intraocular pressure by decreasing the production and increasing the outflow of aqueous humor; the hydrochloride salt is applied topically in the treatment of open-angle or secondary glaucoma.

dip·la·cu·sis (dip″lah-koo′sis) the perception of a single auditory stimulus as two separate sounds. **binaural d.**, different perception by the two ears of a single auditory stimulus. **disharmonic d.**, binaural diplacusis in which a pure tone is heard differently in the two ears. **echo d.,** binaural diplacusis in which a sound of brief duration is heard at different times in the two ears. **monaural d.,** diplacusis in which a pure tone is heard in the same ear as a split tone of two frequencies.

di·ple·gia (di-ple′jah) paralysis of like parts on either side of the body. **diple′gic,** adj.

dip·lo·ba·cil·lus (dip″lo-bah-sil′us) pl. *diplobacil′li.* A short, rod-shaped organism occurring in pairs.

Dip·lo·coc·cus (-kok′us) former name for a genus of bacteria of the tribe Streptococceae. *D. pneumo′niae* is now called *Streptococcus pneumoniae.*

dip·lo·coc·cus (-kok′us) pl. *diplococ′ci.* 1. Any of the spherical, lanceolate, or coffee-bean–shaped bacteria occurring usually in pairs as a result of incomplete separation after cell division in a single plane. 2. an organism of the genus *Diplococcus.*

dip·loë (dip′lo-e) the spongy layer between the inner and outer compact layers of the flat bones of the skull. **diploet′ic, diplo′ic,** adj.

dip·loid (dip′loid) 1. having two sets of chromosomes, as normally found in the somatic cells; in humans, the diploid number is 46. 2. an individual or cell having two full sets of homologous chromosomes.

dip·lo·my·elia (dip″lo-mi-e′le-ah) complete or incomplete duplication of the spinal cord.

di·plo·pia (dĭ-plo′pe-ah) the perception of two images of a single object. **binocular d.,** double vision in which the images of an object are formed on noncorresponding points of the retinas. **crossed d.,** diplopia in which the image belonging to the right eye is displaced to the left of the image belonging to the left eye. **direct d.,** that in which the image belonging to the right eye appears to the right of the image belonging to the left eye. **heteronymous d.,** crossed d. **homonymous d.,** direct d. **horizontal d.,** that in which the images lie in the same horizontal plane, being either direct or crossed. **monocular d.,** perception by one eye of two images of a single object. **paradoxical d.,** crossed d. **torsional d.,** that in which the upper pole of the vertical axis of one image is inclined toward or away from that of the other. **vertical d.,** that in which one image appears above the other in the same vertical plane.

dip·lo·some (dip′lo-sōm) the two centrioles of a mammalian cell.

dip·lo·tene (-tēn) the stage of the first meiotic prophase, following the pachytene, in which the two chromosomes in each bivalent begin to repel one another and a split occurs between the chromosomes.

di·pole (di′pōl) 1. a molecule having separated charges of equal and opposite sign. 2. a pair of electric charges or magnetic poles separated by a short distance.

dip·se·sis (dip-se′sis) thirst. **dipset′ic,** adj.

-dip·sia word element [Gr.], thirst.

dip·so·gen (-sah-jen) an agent or measure that induces thirst and promotes ingestion of fluids. **dipsogen′ic,** adj.

dip·so·sis (dip-so′sis) excessive thirst.

dip·stick (dip′stik) a strip of cellulose chemically impregnated to render it sensitive to protein, glucose, or other substances in the urine.

Dip·tera (dip′ter-ah) an order of insects, including flies, gnats, and mosquitoes.

dip·ter·ous (-us) 1. having two wings. 2. pertaining to insects of the order Diptera.

Dip·y·lid·i·um (dip″ĭ-lid′e-um) a genus of tapeworms. *D. cani′num,* the dog tapeworm, is parasitic in dogs and cats and is occasionally found in humans.

di·py·rid·a·mole (dī″pī-rid′ah-mōl) a platelet inhibitor and coronary vasodilator used to prevent thromboembolism associated with mechanical heart valves, to treat transient ischemic attacks, and as an adjunct in preventing myocardial reinfarction and in myocardial perfusion imaging.

di·rect (dĭ-rekt′) 1. straight; in a straight line. 2. performed immediately and without the intervention of subsidiary means.

di·rec·tor (dĭ-rek′ter) a grooved instrument for guiding a surgical instrument.

di·rith·ro·my·cin (di-rith″ro-mi′sin) a macrolide antibiotic used in the treatment of bacterial infections of the respiratory tract, streptococcal pharyngitis, and skin and soft tissue infections; administered orally.

Di·ro·fi·la·ria (di″ro-fi-lar′e-ah) a genus of filarial nematodes (superfamily Filarioidea), including *D. immit′is,* the heartworm, found in the right heart and veins of the dog, wolf, and fox.

di·ro·fil·a·ri·a·sis (-fil″ah-ri′ah-sis) infection with nematodes of genus *Dirofilaria,* common in dogs but rare in humans.

dis-¹ word element [L.], *reversal* or *separation.*

dis-² word element [Gr.], *duplication.*

dis·a·bil·i·ty (dis″ah-bil′it-e) 1. inability to function normally, physically or mentally; incapacity. 2. anything that causes disability. 3. as defined by the federal government: "inability to engage in any substantial gainful activity by reason of any medically determinable physical or mental impairment which can be expected to last or has lasted for a continuous period of not less than 12 months." **developmental d.,** a substantial handicap of indefinite duration, with onset before the age of 18 years, such as mental retardation, autism, cerebral palsy, epilepsy, or other neuropathy.

di·sac·cha·ri·dase (di-sak′ah-rĭ-dās″) an enzyme that catalyzes the hydrolysis of disaccharides.

di·sac·cha·ride (di-sak′ah-rīd) any of a class of sugars yielding two monosaccharides on hydrolysis.

di·sac·cha·rid·uria (di-sak″ah-rīd-u′re-ah) presence of excessive levels of a disaccharide in the urine, such as in a disaccharide intolerance.

dis·ar·tic·u·la·tion (dis″ahr-tik″u-la′shun) exarticulation; amputation or separation at a joint.

disc (disk) disk. **embryonic d., germinal d.,** a flat area in a blastocyst in which the first traces of the embryo are seen, visible early in the second week in human development.

dis·charge (dis-chahrj′) 1. a setting free, or liberation. 2. matter or force set free. 3. an excretion or substance evacuated. 4. release from a hospital or other course of care. 5. the passing of an action potential through a neuron, axon, or muscle fibers. **myokymic d.,** patterns of grouped or repetitive discharges of motor unit action potentials sometimes seen in myokymia. **myotonic d.,** high frequency repetitive discharges seen in myotonia and evoked by insertion of a needle electrode, percussion of a muscle, or stimulation of a muscle or its motor nerve. **periodic lateralized epileptiform d. (PLED),** a pattern of repetitive paroxysmal slow or sharp waves seen on an electroencephalogram from just one side of the brain.

dis·ci·form (dis′ĭ-form) in the form of a disk.

dis·cis·sion (dĭ-sish′un) incision, or cutting into, as of a soft cataract.

dis·cli·na·tion (dis″klin-a′shun) extorsion.

dis·co·blas·tu·la (dis″ko-blas′tūl-ah) the specialized blastula formed by cleavage of a fertilized telolecithal egg, consisting of a cellular cap (blastoderm) separated by the blastocoele from a floor of uncleaved yolk. **discoblas′tic,** adj.

dis·co·gen·ic (-jen′ik) caused by derangement of an intervertebral disk.

dis·coid (dis′koid) 1. disk-shaped. 2. a dental instrument with a disklike or circular blade. 3. a disk-shaped dental excavator designed to remove the carious dentin of a decayed tooth.

dis·con·tin·u·ous (dis″kon-tin′u-us) 1. interrupted; intermittent; marked by breaks. 2. discrete; separate. 3. lacking logical order or coherence.

dis·cop·a·thy (dis-kop′ah-the) any disease of an intervertebral disk.

dis·co·pla·cen·ta (dis″ko-plah-sen′tah) a discoid placenta.

dis·cor·dance (dis-kord′ans) the occurrence of a given trait in only one member of a twin pair. **discor′dant,** adj.

dis·crete (dis-krēt′) made up of separated parts or characterized by lesions which do not become blended.

dis·crim·i·na·tion (-krim″ĭ-na′shun) the making of a fine distinction.

dis·cus (dis′kus) pl. *dis′ci.* [L.] disk.

dis·cu·ti·ent (dis-ku′shent) scattering, or causing a disappearance; a remedy that so acts.

dis·ease (dĭ-zēz′) any deviation from or interruption of the normal structure or function of any body part, organ, or system that is manifested by a characteristic set of symptoms and signs and whose etiology, pathology, and prognosis may be known or unknown. See also entries under *syndrome.* **acquired cystic d. of kidney,** the development of cysts in the formerly noncystic failing kidney in end-stage renal disease. **Addison's d.,** bronzelike pigmentation of the skin, severe prostration, progressive anemia, low blood pressure, diarrhea, and digestive disturbance, due to adrenal hypofunction. **Albers-Schönberg d.,** osteopetrosis. **allogeneic d.,** graft-versus-host reaction occurring in immunosuppressed animals receiving injections of allogeneic lymphocytes. **Alpers' d.,** a rare disease of young children, characterized by neuronal deterioration of the cerebral cortex and elsewhere, progressive mental deterioration, motor disturbances, seizures, and early death. **alpha chain d.,** heavy chain disease characterized by plasma cell infiltration of the lamina propria of the small intestine resulting in malabsorption with diarrhea, abdominal pain, and weight loss, possibly accompanied by pulmonary involvement. **Alzheimer's d.,** progressive degenerative disease of the brain, of unknown cause; characterized by diffuse atrophy throughout the cerebral cortex with distinctive histopathological changes. **Andersen's d.,** glycogen storage d., type IV. **apatite deposition d.,** a connective tissue disorder marked by deposition of hydroxyapatite crystals in one or more joints or bursae. **Aran-Duchenne d.,** spinal muscular atrophy. **arteriosclerotic cardiovascular d. (ASCVD),** atherosclerotic involvement of arteries to the heart and to other organs, resulting in debility or death; sometimes used specifically for ischemic heart disease. **arteriosclerotic heart d.**

(ASHD), ischemic heart d. **autoimmune d.,** any of a group of disorders in which tissue injury is associated with humoral or cell-mediated responses to the body's own constituents; they may be systemic or organ-specific. **Ayerza's d.,** polycythemia vera with chronic cyanosis, dyspnea, bronchitis, bronchiectasis, hepatosplenomegaly, bone marrow hyperplasia, and pulmonary artery sclerosis. **Banti's d.,** congestive splenomegaly. **Barlow d.,** scurvy in infants. **Barraquer's d.,** partial lipodystrophy. **Basedow's d.,** Graves' d. **Batten d., Batten-Mayou d.,** 1. Vogt-Spielmeyer d. 2. more generally, any or all of the group of disorders constituting neuronal ceroid lipofuscinosis. **Bayle's d.,** general paresis. **Bazin's d.,** erythema induratum. **Bekhterev's (Bechterew's) d.,** ankylosing spondylitis. **Benson's d.,** asteroid hyalosis. **Berger's d.,** IgA glomerulonephritis. **Bernhardt's d., Bernhardt-Roth d.,** meralgia paresthetica. **Besnier-Boeck d.,** sarcoidosis. **Best's d.,** congenital macular degeneration. **Bielschowsky-Janský d.,** Janský-Bielschowsky d. **Binswanger's d.,** a degenerative dementia of presenile onset caused by demyelination of the subcortical white matter of the brain. **black d.,** a fatal disease of sheep, and sometimes of humans, in the United States and Australia, due to *Clostridium novyi*, marked by necrotic areas in the liver. **Blocq's d.,** astasia-abasia. **Blount d.,** tibia vara. **Boeck's d.,** sarcoidosis. **Bornholm d.,** epidemic pleurodynia. **Bowen's d.,** a squamous cell carcinoma in situ, often due to prolonged exposure to arsenic; usually occurring on sun-exposed areas of skin. The corresponding lesion on the glans penis is termed erythroplasia of Queyrat. **Brill's d.,** Brill-Zinsser d. **Brill-Symmers d.,** giant follicular lymphoma. **Brill-Zinsser d.,** mild recrudescence of epidemic typhus years after the initial infection, because *Rickettsia prowazekii* has persisted in body tissue in an inactive state, with humans as the reservoir. **broad beta d.,** familial dysbetalipoproteinemia; named for the electrophoretic mobility of the abnormal chylomicron and very-low-density lipoprotein remnants produced. **Busse-Buschke d.,** cryptococcosis. **Caffey's d.,** infantile cortical hyperostosis. **calcium hydroxyapatite deposition d.,** apatite deposition d. **calcium pyrophosphate deposition d. (CPDD),** an acute or chronic inflammatory arthropathy caused by deposition of calcium pyrophosphate dihydrate (CPPD) crystals in the joints, chondrocalcinosis, and crystals in the synovial fluid. Acute attacks are sometimes called *pseudogout*. **Calvé-Perthes d.,** osteochondrosis of capitular epiphysis of femur. **Camurati-Engelmann d.,** diaphyseal dysplasia. **Canavan d., Canavan-van Bogaert-Bertrand d.,** spongy degeneration of the central nervous system. **Carrión's d.,** bartonellosis. **Castleman d.,** a benign or pre-malignant condition resembling lymphoma but without recognizable malignant cells; there are isolated masses of lymphoid tissue and lymph node hyperplasia, usually in the abdominal or mediastinal area. **cat-scratch d.,** a usually benign, self-limited disease of the regional lymph nodes, caused by *Bartonella henselae* and characterized by a papule or pustule at the site of a cat scratch, subacute painful regional lymphadenitis, and mild fever. **celiac d.,** a malabsorption syndrome precipitated by ingestion of gluten-containing foods, with loss of villous structure of the proximal intestinal mucosa, bulky, frothy diarrhea, abdominal distention, flatulence, weight loss, and vitamin and electrolyte depletion. **Chagas' d.,** trypanosomiasis due to *Trypanosoma cruzi*; its course may be acute, subacute, or chronic. **Charcot-Marie-Tooth d.,** muscular atrophy of variable inheritance, beginning in the muscles supplied by the peroneal nerves and progressing to those of the hands and arms. **cholesteryl ester storage d. (CESD),** a lysosomal storage disease due to deficiency of lysosomal cholesterol esterase, variably characterized by some combination of hepatomegaly, hyperbetalipoproteinemia, and premature atherosclerosis. **Christmas d.,** hemophilia B. **chronic granulomatous d.,** frequent, severe infections of the skin, oral and intestinal mucosa, reticuloendothelial system, bones, lungs, and genitourinary tract associated with a genetically determined defect in the intracellular bactericidal function of leukocytes. **chronic obstructive pulmonary d. (COPD),** any disorder marked by persistent obstruction of bronchial air flow. **Coats' d.,** exudative retinopathy. **collagen d.,** any of a group of diseases characterized by widespread pathologic changes in connective tissue; they include lupus erythematosus, dermatomyositis, scleroderma, polyarteritis nodosa, thrombotic purpura, rheumatic fever, and rheumatoid arthritis. Cf. *collagen disorder*. **communicable d.,** a disease the causative agents of which may pass or be carried from one person to another directly or indirectly. **Concato's d.,** progressive malignant polyserositis with large effusions into the pericardium, pleura, and peritoneum. **constitutional d.,** one involving a system of organs or one with widespread symptoms. **Cori's d.,** glycogen storage d., type III. **coronary artery d. (CAD),** atherosclerosis of the coronary arteries, which may cause angina pectoris, myocardial infarction, and sudden death; risk factors include hypercholesterolemia, hypertension, smoking, diabetes mellitus, and low levels of high-density lipoproteins. **coronary heart d. (CHD),** ischemic heart d. **Cowden d.,** a hereditary disease marked by multiple ectodermal, mesodermal, and endodermal nevoid and neoplastic anomalies. **Creutzfeldt-Jakob d.,** a rare prion disease existing in sporadic, familial, and infectious forms, with onset usually in middle life, and having a wide variety of clinical and pathological features. The most commonly seen are spongiform degeneration of neurons, neuronal loss, gliosis, and amyloid plaque formation, accompanied by rapidly progressive dementia, myoclonus, motor disturbances, and encephalographic changes, with death occurring usually within a year of onset. **Crigler-Najjar d.,** see under *syndrome*. **Crohn's d.,** regional enteritis; a chronic granulomatous inflammatory disease usually in the terminal ileum with scarring and thickening of the wall, often leading to intestinal obstruction and formation of fistulas and abscesses. **Crouzon's d.,** craniofacial dysostosis. **Cruveilhier's d.,** spinal muscular atrophy. **Cushing's d.,** Cushing's syndrome in which the hyperadrenocorticism is secondary to excessive pituitary secretion of adrenocorticotropic hormone. **cystic d. of breast,** mammary dysplasia with formation of blue dome cysts. **cytomegalic inclusion d., cytomegalovirus d.,** an infection due to cytomegalovirus and marked by nuclear inclusion bodies in enlarged infected cells. In the congenital form, there is hepatosplenomegaly with cirrhosis, and microcephaly with mental or motor retardation. Acquired disease may cause a clinical state similar to infectious mononucleosis. When acquired by blood transfusion, postperfusion syndrome results. **deficiency d.,** a condition caused by dietary or metabolic deficiency, including all diseases due to an insufficient supply of essential nutrients. **degenerative joint d.,** osteoarthritis. **Dejerine's d., Dejerine-Sottas d.,** progressive hypertrophic neuropathy. **demyelinating d.,** any condition characterized by destruction of the myelin sheaths of nerves. **disappearing bone d.,** gradual resorption of a bone or group of bones, sometimes associated with multiple hemangiomas, usually in children or

young adults and following trauma. **diverticular d.,** a general term including the prediverticular state, diverticulosis, and diverticulitis. **Duchenne's d.,** 1. spinal muscular atrophy. 2. progressive bulbar paralysis. 3. tabes dorsalis. 4. Duchenne's muscular dystrophy. **Duchenne-Aran d.,** spinal muscular atrophy. **Duhring's d.,** dermatitis herpetiformis. **Dukes' d.,** a febrile disease of childhood marked by an exanthematous eruption, probably due to a virus of the Coxsackie-ECHO group. **Durand-Nicolas-Favre d.,** lymphogranuloma venereum. **Duroziez's d.,** congenital mitral stenosis. **Ebola virus d.,** fatal acute hemorrhagic fever resembling Marburg virus disease but caused by Ebola virus, seen in the Sudan and Zaire. **Ebstein's d.,** see under *anomaly*. **end-stage renal d.,** chronic irreversible renal failure. **Erb's d.,** Duchenne's muscular dystrophy. **Erb-Goldflam d.,** myasthenia gravis. **Eulenburg's d.,** paramyotonia congenita. **extrapyramidal d.,** any of a group of clinical disorders marked by abnormal involuntary movements, alterations in muscle tone, and postural disturbances; they include parkinsonism, chorea, athetosis, etc. **Fabry's d.,** an X-linked lysosomal storage disease of glycosphingolipid catabolism resulting from deficiency of α-galactosidase A and leading to accumulation of ceramide trihexoside in the cardiovascular and renal systems. **Farber's d.,** a lysosomal storage disease due to defective ceramidase and characterized by hoarseness, aphonia, dermatitis, bone and joint deformities, granulomatous reaction, and psychomotor retardation. **Fazio-Londe d.,** a rare type of progressive bulbar palsy occurring in childhood. **Feer d.,** acrodynia. **fibrocystic d. of breast,** a form of mammary dysplasia with formation of cysts of various size containing a semitransparent, turbid fluid that imparts a brown to blue color to the unopened cysts; believed due to abnormal hyperplasia of the ductal epithelium and dilatation of the ducts of the mammary gland, resulting from exaggeration and distortion of normal menstrual cycle–related breast changes. **fibrocystic d. of the pancreas,** cystic fibrosis. **fifth d.,** erythema infectiosum. **flint d.,** chalicosis. **floating beta d.,** familial dysbetalipoproteinemia. **focal d.,** a localized disease. **foot-and-mouth d.,** an acute, contagious viral disease of wild and domestic cloven-footed animals and occasionally humans, marked by vesicular eruption on the lips, buccal cavity, pharynx, legs, and feet. **Forbes' d.,** glycogen storage d., type III. **fourth d.,** Dukes' d.

fourth venereal d., granuloma inguinale. Fox-Fordyce d., a persistent and recalcitrant, itchy, papular eruption, chiefly of the axillae and pubes, due to inflammation of apocrine sweat glands. Freiberg's d., osteochondrosis of the head of the second metatarsal bone. Friedländer's d., endarteritis obliterans. Friedreich's d., paramyoclonus multiplex. functional d., see under *disorder*. Garré's d., sclerosing nonsuppurative osteomyelitis. gastroesophageal reflux d. (GERD), any condition resulting from gastroesophageal reflux, characterized by heartburn and regurgitation; see also *reflux esophagitis*. Gaucher's d., a hereditary disorder of glucocerebroside metabolism, marked by the presence of Gaucher's cells in the marrow, and by hepatosplenomegaly and erosion of the cortices of long bones and pelvis. The adult form is associated with moderate anemia and thrombocytopenia, and yellowish pigmentation of the skin; in the infantile form there is, in addition, marked central nervous system impairment; in the juvenile form there are rapidly progressive systemic manifestations but moderate central nervous system involvement. genetic d., a general term for any disorder caused by a genetic mechanism, comprising chromosome aberrations (or anomalies), mendelian (or monogenic or single-gene) disorders, and multifactorial disorders. gestational trophoblastic d., see under *neoplasia*. Gilbert d., a familial, benign elevation of bilirubin levels without evidence of liver damage or hematologic abnormalities. Gilles de la Tourette's d., see under *syndrome*. Glanzmann d., see *thrombasthenia*. glycogen storage d., any of a number of rare inborn errors of metabolism caused by defects in specific enzymes or transporters involved in the metabolism of glycogen. *type I,* glucose-6-phosphatase deficiency: a severe hepatorenal form due to deficiency of the hepatic enzyme glucose-6-phosphatase, resulting in liver and kidney involvement, with hepatomegaly, hypoglycemia, hyperuricemia, and gout. *type IA,* glycogen storage d., type I. *type IB,* a form resembling type I but additionally predisposing to infection due to neutropenia and to chronic inflammatory bowel disease; due to a defect in the transport system for glucose 6-phosphate. *type II,* a disorder due to deficiency of the lysosomal enzyme α-1,4,-glucosidase, the severe infant form resulting in generalized glycogen accumulation, with cardiomegaly, cardiorespiratory failure, and death, and a milder adult form being a gradual skeletal

myopathy that sometimes causes respiratory problems. *type III,* a form due to deficiency of debrancher enzyme (amylo-1,6-glucosidase) in muscle, liver, or both; defects in the liver enzyme are characterized by hepatomegaly and hypoglycemia while defects in the muscle enzyme are characterized by progressive muscle wasting and weakness. *type IV,* brancher enzyme deficiency; cirrhosis of the liver, hepatosplenomegaly, progressive hepatic failure, and death due to deficiency of the glycogen brancher enzyme (1,4-α-glucan branching enzyme). *type V,* muscle cramps and fatigue during exercise due to a defect in the skeletal muscle isozyme of glycogen phosphorylase (muscle phosphorylase). *type VI,* hepatomegaly, mild to moderate hypoglycemia and mild ketosis, due to deficiency of the liver isozyme of glycogen phosphorylase (hepatic phosphorylase). *type VII,* muscle weakness and cramping after exercise due to deficiency of the muscle isozyme of 6-phosphofructokinase. *type VIII,* phosphorylase *b* kinase deficiency. graft-versus-host (GVH) d., disease caused by the immune response of histoincompatible, immunocompetent donor cells against the tissue of immunocompromised host, as a complication of bone marrow transplantation, or as a result of maternal-fetal blood transfusion, or therapeutic transfusion to an immunocompromised recipient. Graves' d., an association of hyperthyroidism, goiter, and exophthalmos, with accelerated pulse rate, profuse sweating, nervous symptoms, psychic disturbances, emaciation, and elevated basal metabolism. Greenfield's d., former name for the late infantile form of metachromatic leukodystrophy. Gull's d., atrophy of the thyroid gland with myxedema. Günther d., congenital erythropoietic porphyria. H d., Hartnup d. Hailey-Hailey d., benign familial pemphigus. Hallervorden-Spatz d., an autosomal recessive disorder caused by decreased numbers of myelin sheaths of the globus pallidus and substantia nigra, with accumulation of iron pigment, progressive rigidity beginning in the legs, choreoathetoid movements, dysarthria, and mental deterioration. Hand's d., Hand-Schüller-Christian d. hand-foot-and-mouth d., a mild, highly infectious viral disease of children, with vesicular lesions in the mouth and on the hands and feet. Hand-Schüller-Christian d., a chronic, progressive form of multifocal Langerhans cell histiocytosis, sometimes with accumulation of cholesterol, characterized by the triad of calvarial bone defects, exophthalmos, and diabetes insipidus. **Hansen's d.**, leprosy. **Hartnup d.**, a hereditary disorder of intestinal and renal transport of neutral α-amino acids, marked by a pellagra-like skin rash, with transient cerebellar ataxia, constant renal aminoaciduria, and other biochemical abnormalities. **Hashimoto's d.**, a progressive disease of the thyroid gland with degeneration of its epithelial elements and replacement by lymphoid and fibrous tissue. **heavy chain d's**, a group of malignant neoplasms of lymphoplasmacytic cells marked by the presence of immunoglobulin heavy chains or heavy chain fragments; they are classified according to heavy chain type, e.g., alpha chain disease. **Heine-Medin d.**, the major form of poliomyelitis. **hemoglobin d.**, any of various hereditary molecular diseases characterized by abnormal hemoglobins in the red blood cells; the homozygous form is manifested by hemolytic anemia. **hemolytic d. of the newborn**, erythroblastosis fetalis. **hemorrhagic d. of the newborn**, a self-limited hemorrhagic disorder of the first few days of life, due to deficiency of vitamin K–dependent coagulation factors II, VII, IX, and X. **Hers' d.**, glycogen storage d., type VI. **Heubner-Herter d.**, the infantile form of celiac disease. **hip-joint d.**, tuberculosis of the hip joint. **Hippel's d.**, von Hippel's d. **Hirschsprung's d.**, congenital megacolon. **His d.**, **His-Werner d.**, trench fever. **Hodgkin's d.**, a form of malignant lymphoma marked clinically by painless, progressive enlargement of lymph nodes, spleen, and general lymphoid tissue; other symptoms may include anorexia, lassitude, weight loss, fever, pruritus, night sweats, and anemia. Reed-Sternberg cells are characteristically present. Four types have been distinguished on the basis of histopathologic criteria. **hoof-and-mouth d.**, foot-and-mouth d. **hookworm d.**, infection with the hookworm *Ancylostoma duodenale* or *Necator americanus*, whose larvae enter the body through the skin or in contaminated food or water and migrate to the small intestine where, as adults, they attach to the mucosa and ingest blood; symptoms may include abdominal pain, diarrhea, colic or nausea, and anemia. **hyaline membrane d.**, a type of respiratory distress syndrome of the newborn in which there is formation of a hyaline-like membrane lining the terminal respiratory passages; extensive atelectasis is attributed to lack of surfactant. **hydatid d.**, an infection, usually of the liver, due to larval forms of tapeworms of the genus *Echinococcus*, marked by development of expanding cysts.

hypophosphatemic bone d., an inherited disorder resembling a mild form of X-linked hypophosphatemia, similarly due to a defect in renal tubular function but usually showing osteomalacia without radiographic evidence of rickets. **immune complex d.**, local or systemic disease caused by the formation of circulating immune complexes and their deposition in tissue, due to activation of complement and to recruitment and activation of leukocytes in type III hypersensitivity reactions. **infectious d.**, one due to organisms ranging in size from viruses to parasitic worms; it may be contagious in origin, result from nosocomial organisms, or be due to endogenous microflora from the nose and throat, skin, or bowel. **inflammatory bowel d.**, any idiopathic inflammatory disease of the bowel, such as Crohn's disease and ulcerative colitis. **intercurrent d.**, one occurring during the course of another disease with which it has no connection. **iron storage d.**, hemochromatosis. **ischemic bowel d.**, ischemic colitis. **ischemic heart d. (IHD)**, any of a group of acute or chronic cardiac disabilities resulting from insufficient supply of oxygenated blood to the heart. **Jansky-Bielschowsky d.**, the late infantile form of neuronal ceroid lipofuscinosis, occurring between two and four years of age, characterized by abnormal accumulation of lipofuscin; beginning as myoclonic seizures and progressing to neurologic and retinal deterioration and death by age 8 to 12. **jumping d.**, any of several culture-specific disorders characterized by exaggerated responses to small stimuli, muscle tics including jumping, obedience even to dangerous suggestions, and sometimes coprolalia or echolalia. **juvenile Paget d.**, hyperostosis corticalis deformans juvenilis. **Kashin-Bek (Kaschin-Beck) d.**, a disabling degenerative disease of the peripheral joints and spine, endemic in northeastern Asia; believed to be caused by ingestion of cereal grains infected with the fungus *Fusarium sporotrichiella*. **Katayama d.**, schistosomiasis japonica. **Kawasaki d.**, a febrile illness usually affecting infants and young children, with conjunctival injection, changes to the oropharyngeal mucosa, changes to the peripheral extremities including edema, erythema, and desquamation, a primarily truncal polymorphous exanthem, and cervical lymphadenopathy. It is often associated with vasculitis of the large coronary vessels. **Kienböck's d.**, slowly progressive osteochondrosis of the lunate bone; it may affect other wrist bones. **kinky hair d.**, Menkes' syndrome. **Köhler's bone d.**,

1. osteochondrosis of the tarsal navicular bone in children. 2. thickening of the shaft of the second metatarsal bone and changes about its articular head, with pain in the second metatarsophalangeal joint on walking or standing. **Krabbe's d.,** a lysosomal storage disease beginning in infancy, due to deficiency of β-galactosidase. Pathologically, there is rapidly progressive cerebral demyelination and large globoid bodies (swollen with accumulated cerebroside) in the white substance. **Kufs' d.,** the adult form of neuronal ceroid lipofuscinosis, with onset prior to age 40; characterized by progressive neurologic deterioration but not blindness, excessive storage of lipofuscin, and shortened life expectancy; **Kümmell's d.,** compression fracture of vertebra, with symptoms a few weeks after injury, including spinal pain, intercostal neuralgia, lower limb motor disturbances, and kyphosis. **Kyasanur Forest d.,** a fatal viral disease of monkeys in the Kyasanur Forest of India, communicable to humans, in whom it produces hemorrhagic symptoms. **Kyrle's d.,** a chronic disorder of keratinization marked by keratotic plugs that develop in hair follicles and eccrine ducts, penetrating the epidermis and extending down into the corium, causing foreign-body reaction and pain. **Lafora's d.,** see under *epilepsy.* **Leber's d.,** 1. Leber's hereditary optic neuropathy. 2. Leber's congenital amaurosis. **legionnaires' d.,** an often fatal bacterial infection caused by *Legionella pneumophila,* not spread by person-to-person contact, characterized by high fever, gastrointestinal pain, headache, and pneumonia; there may also be involvement of the kidneys, liver, and nervous system. **Leiner's d.,** a disorder of infancy characterized by generalized seborrhea-like dermatitis and erythroderma, severe intractable diarrhea, recurrent infections, and failure to thrive. **Leriche d.,** post-traumatic osteoporosis. **Letterer-Siwe d.,** a Langerhans cell histiocytosis of early childhood, of autosomal recessive inheritance, characterized by cutaneous lesions resembling seborrheic dermatitis, hemorrhagic tendency, hepatosplenomegaly, lymphadenitis, and progressive anemia. If untreated it is rapidly fatal. Called also *acute disseminated Langerhans cell histiocytosis.* **Libman-Sacks d.,** see under *endocarditis.* **Lindau's d., Lindau-von Hippel d.,** von Hippel-Lindau d. **Little's d.,** congenital spastic stiffness of the limbs, a form of cerebral palsy due to lack of development of the pyramidal tracts. **Lobstein's d.,** see *osteogenesis imperfecta.* **Lou Gehrig d.,** amyotrophic

lateral sclerosis. **Lowe d.,** oculocerebrorenal syndrome. **Lutz-Splendore-Almeida d.,** paracoccidioidomycosis. **Lyme d.,** a recurrent multisystemic disorder caused by the spirochete *Borrelia burgdorferi,* the vectors being the ticks *Ixodes scapularis* and *I. pacificus;* usually initially characterized by lesions of erythema chronicum migrans, followed by various manifestations including arthritis of the large joints, myalgia, and neurologic and cardiac abnormalities. **lysosomal storage d.,** an inborn error of metabolism with (1) a defect in a specific lysosomal enzyme; (2) intracellular accumulation of an unmetabolized substrate; (3) clinical progression affecting multiple tissues or organs; (4) considerable phenotypic variation within a disease. **MAC d.,** *Mycobacterium avium* complex d. **McArdle d.,** glycogen storage d., type V. **mad cow d.,** bovine spongiform encephalopathy. **Madelung's d.,** 1. see under *deformity.* 2. see under *neck.* **maple bark d.,** hypersensitivity pneumonitis in logging and sawmill workers due to inhalation of spores of a mold, *Cryptostroma corticale,* growing under the maple bark. **maple syrup urine d. (MSUD),** a hereditary enzyme defect in metabolism of branched chain amino acids, marked clinically by mental and physical retardation, severe ketoacidosis, feeding difficulties, and a characteristic maple syrup odor in the urine and on the body. **Marburg virus d.,** a severe, often fatal, viral hemorrhagic fever first reported in Marburg, Germany, among laboratory workers exposed to African green monkeys. **Marchiafava-Micheli d.,** paroxysmal nocturnal hemoglobinuria. **Marie-Bamberger d.,** hypertrophic pulmonary osteoarthropathy. **Marie-Strümpell d.,** ankylosing spondylitis. **Marie-Tooth d.,** Charcot-Marie-Tooth d. **Mediterranean d.,** thalassemia major. **medullary cystic d.,** familial juvenile nephronophthisis. **Meniere's d.,** deafness, tinnitus, and dizziness, in association with nonsuppurative disease of the labyrinth. **mental d.,** see under *disorder.* **Merzbacher-Pelizaeus d.,** Pelizaeus-Merzbacher d. **metabolic d.,** one caused by a disruption of a normal metabolic pathway because of a genetically determined enzyme defect. **Meyer's d.,** adenoid vegetations of the pharynx. **Mikulicz's d.,** benign, self-limited lymphocytic infiltration and enlargement of the lacrimal and salivary glands of uncertain etiology. **Milroy d.,** hereditary permanent lymphedema of the legs due to lymphatic obstruction. **Minamata d.,** a severe neurologic disorder due to alkyl mercury poisoning, with permanent neurologic and mental disabilities or death; once prevalent among those eating contaminated seafood from Minamata Bay, Japan. **minimal change d.,** subtle alterations in kidney function demonstrable by clinical albuminuria and the presence of lipid droplets in cells of the proximal tubules, seen primarily in young children. **mixed connective tissue d.,** a combination of scleroderma, myositis, systemic lupus erythematosus, and rheumatoid arthritis, and marked serologically by the presence of antibody against extractable nuclear antigen. **Möbius d.,** ophthalmoplegic migraine. **molecular d.,** any disease in which the pathogenesis can be traced to a single molecule, usually a protein, which is either abnormal in structure or present in reduced amounts. **Mondor's d.,** phlebitis affecting the large subcutaneous veins normally crossing the lateral chest wall and breast from the epigastric or hypochondriac region to the axilla. **Monge's d.,** chronic mountain sickness. **Morquio's d., Morquio-Ullrich d.,** see under *syndrome*. **motor neuron d., motor system d.,** any disease of a motor neuron, including spinal muscular atrophy, progressive bulbar paralysis, amyotrophic lateral sclerosis, and lateral sclerosis. *Mycobacterium avium* complex d., MAC disease; systemic disease caused by infection with organisms of the *Mycobacterium avium-intracellulare* complex in patients with human immunodeficiency virus infection. **Newcastle d.,** a viral disease of birds, including domestic fowl, transmissible to humans, characterized by respiratory, gastrointestinal or pulmonary, and encephalitic symptoms. **new variant Creutzfeldt-Jakob d. (nvCJD),** a variant of Creutzfeldt-Jakob disease having a younger age of onset than is seen in Creutzfeldt-Jakob disease, and caused by the same agent that causes bovine spongiform encephalopathy. **Nicolas-Favre d.,** lymphogranuloma venereum. **Niemann's d., Niemann-Pick d.,** a lysosomal storage disease due to sphingomyelin accumulation in the reticuloendothelial system; there are five types distinguished by age of onset, amount of central nervous system involvement, and degree of enzyme deficiency. **nil d.,** minimal change d. **Norrie's d.,** an X-linked disorder consisting of bilateral blindness from retinal malformation, mental retardation, and deafness. **notifiable d.,** one required to be reported to federal, state, or local health officials when diagnosed, because of infectiousness, severity, or frequency of occurrence. **oasthouse urine d.,** methionine malabsorption syndrome. **obstructive**

small airways d., chronic bronchitis with irreversible narrowing of the bronchioles and small bronchi with hypoxia and often hypercapnia. **occupational d.,** disease due to various factors involved in one's employment. **Oguchi's d.,** a form of hereditary night blindness and fundus discoloration following light adaptation. **organic d.,** one associated with demonstrable change in a bodily organ or tissue. **Osgood-Schlatter d.,** osteochondrosis of the tuberosity of the tibia. **Osler's d.,** 1. polycythemia vera. 2. hereditary hemorrhagic telangiectasia. **Owren's d.,** parahemophilia. **Paget's d.,** 1. (of bone) osteitis deformans. 2. (of breast) an intraductal inflammatory carcinoma of the breast, involving the areola and nipple. 3. an extramammary counterpart of Paget's disease (2), usually involving the vulva, and sometimes other sites, as the perianal and axillary regions. **Parkinson's d.,** a slowly progressive form of parkinsonism, usually seen late in life, marked by masklike facies, tremor of resting muscles, slowing of voluntary movements, festinating gait, peculiar posture, muscular weakness, and sometimes excessive sweating and feelings of heat. **Parrot's d.,** see under *pseudoparalysis*. **parrot d.,** psittacosis. **Parry's d.,** Graves' d. **Pelizaeus-Merzbacher d.,** a progressive familial form of leukoencephalopathy, marked by nystagmus, ataxia, tremor, parkinsonian facies, dysarthria, and mental deterioration. **Pellegrini's d., Pellegrini-Stieda d.,** calcification of the medial collateral ligament of the knee due to trauma. **pelvic inflammatory d. (PID),** any pelvic infection involving the upper female genital tract beyond the cervix. **periodontal d.,** any disease or disorder of the periodontium. **Perthes' d.,** osteochondrosis of capitular femoral epiphysis. **Peyronie's d.,** induration of the corpora cavernosa of the penis, producing a painful fibrous chordee and penile curvature. **Pfeiffer's d.,** infectious mononucleosis. **Pick's d.,** 1. progressive atrophy of the cerebral convolutions in a limited area (lobe) of the brain, with clinical manifestations and course similar to Alzheimer's disease. 2. Niemann-Pick d. **polycystic kidney d., polycystic d. of kidneys,** either of two unrelated heritable disorders marked by cysts in both kidneys; the *autosomal dominant* or *adult* form is more common, appears in adult life, and is marked by loss of renal function that can be either rapid or slow; the *autosomal recessive* or *infantile* form is more rare, may be congenital or may appear later in childhood, and almost always progresses to renal failure. **polycystic renal d.,** polycystic kidney d. **Pompe's d.,** glycogen storage d., type II. **Pott's d.,** spinal tuberculosis. **primary electrical d.,** serious ventricular tachycardia, and sometimes ventricular fibrillation, in the absence of recognizable structural heart disease. **prion d.,** any of a group of fatal, transmissible neurodegenerative diseases, which may be sporadic, familial, or acquired, caused by abnormalities of prion protein metabolism resulting from mutations in the prion protein gene or from infection with pathogenic forms of the protein. **pulseless d.,** Takayasu's arteritis. **Raynaud's d.,** a primary or idiopathic vascular disorder, most often affecting women, marked by bilateral attacks of Raynaud's phenomenon. **Recklinghausen's d.,** 1. neurofibromatosis. 2. (of bone) osteitis fibrosa cystica generalisata. **Refsum's d.,** an inherited disorder of lipid metabolism, characterized by accumulation of phytanic acid, chronic polyneuritis, retinitis pigmentosa, cerebellar ataxia, and persistent elevation of protein in cerebrospinal fluid. **remnant removal d.,** familial dysbetalipoproteinemia. **reversible obstructive airway d.,** a condition characterized by bronchospasm reversible by intervention, as in asthma. **rheumatic heart d.,** the most important manifestation and sequel to rheumatic fever, consisting chiefly of valvular deformities. **rheumatoid d.,** a systemic condition best known by its articular involvement (rheumatoid arthritis) but emphasizing nonarticular changes, e.g., pulmonary interstitial fibrosis, pleural effusion, and lung nodules. **Ritter's d.,** dermatitis exfoliativa neonatorum. **Roger's d.,** a ventricular septal defect; the term is usually restricted to small, asymptomatic defects. **runt d.,** a graft-versus-host disease produced by immunologically competent cells in a foreign host that is unable to reject them, resulting in gross retardation of host development and in death. **Salla d.,** an inherited disorder of sialic acid metabolism characterized by accumulation of sialic acid in lysosomes and excretion in the urine, mental retardation, delayed motor development, and ataxia. **Sandhoff's d.,** a type of GM$_2$ gangliosidosis resembling Tay-Sachs disease, seen in non-Jews, marked by a progressively more rapid course, and due to a defect in hexosaminidase, both isozymes A and B. **Schamberg's d.,** a slowly progressive purpuric and pigmentary disease of the skin affecting chiefly the shins, ankles, and dorsa of the feet. **Schilder's d.,** subacute or chronic leukoencephalopathy in children and adolescents, similar to adrenoleukodystrophy; massive destruction of the white substance of the cerebral hemispheres leads to blindness, deafness, bilateral spasticity, and mental deterioration. **Schönlein's d.,** see under *purpura.* **secondary d.,** 1. one subsequent to or as a consequence of another disease. 2. one due to introduction of incompatible, immunologically competent cells into a host rendered incapable of rejecting them by heavy exposure to ionizing radiation. **self-limited d.,** one that runs a limited and definite course. **serum d.,** see under *sickness.* **severe combined immunodeficiency d. (SCID),** see under *immunodeficiency.* **sexually transmitted d.,** venereal disease; any of a diverse group of infections transmitted by sexual contact; in some this is the only important mode of transmission, and in others transmission by nonsexual means is possible. **sickle cell d.,** any disease associated with the presence of hemoglobin S. **Simmonds' d.,** see *panhypopituitarism.* **sixth d.,** exanthema subitum. **small airways d.,** chronic obstructive bronchitis with irreversible narrowing of the bronchioles and small bronchi. See also *obstructive small airways d.* **Smith-Strang d.,** methionine malabsorption syndrome. **Spielmeyer-Vogt d.,** Vogt-Spielmeyer d. **Steinert's d.,** myotonic dystrophy. **Still's d.,** juvenile rheumatoid arthritis. **storage d.,** a metabolic disorder in which a specific substance (a lipid, a protein, etc.) accumulates in certain cells in unusually large amounts. **storage pool d.,** a blood coagulation disorder due to failure of the platelets to release adenosine diphosphate (ADP) in response to aggregating agents; characterized by mild bleeding episodes, prolonged bleeding time, and reduced aggregation response to collagen or thrombin. **Strümpell's d.,** 1. hereditary lateral sclerosis with the spasticity mainly limited to the legs. 2. cerebral poliomyelitis. **Strümpell-Leichtenstern d.,** hemorrhagic encephalitis. **Strümpell-Marie d.,** ankylosing spondylitis. **Sutton's d.,** 1. halo nevus. 2. periadenitis mucosa necrotica recurrens. 3. granuloma fissuratum. **Swift's d., Swift-Feer d.,** acrodynia. **Takayasu's d.,** see under *arteritis.* **Tangier d.,** a familial disorder characterized by a deficiency of high-density lipoproteins in the blood serum, with storage of cholesteryl esters in tissues. **Tarui d.,** glycogen storage d., type VII. **Tay-Sachs d. (TSD),** the most common GM$_2$ gangliosidosis, seen almost exclusively in northeastern European Jews, characterized by infantile onset, doll-like facies, cherry-red macular spot, early blindness, hyperacusis, macrocephaly, seizures, hypotonia, and death in early childhood. **Thomsen's d.,** myotonia congenita. **thyrotoxic heart d.,** heart disease associated with hyperthyroidism, marked by atrial fibrillation, cardiac enlargement, and congestive heart failure. **transmissible neurodegenerative d.,** prion d. **trophoblastic d.,** gestational trophoblastic neoplasia. **tsutsugamushi d.,** scrub typhus. **tunnel d.,** decompression sickness. **uremic bone d.,** renal osteodystrophy. **van den Bergh's d.,** enterogenous cyanosis. **venereal d.,** sexually transmitted d. **venoocclusive d. of the liver,** symptomatic occlusion of the small hepatic venules caused by ingestion of Senecio tea or related substances, by certain chemotherapy agents, or by radiation. **vinyl chloride d.,** acro-osteolysis resulting from exposure to vinyl chloride, characterized by Raynaud's phenomenon and skin and bony changes on the limbs. **Vogt-Spielmeyer d.,** the juvenile form of neuronal ceroid lipofuscinosis with onset between ages 5 and 10 years; characterized by rapid cerebroretinal degeneration, excessive neuronal storage of lipofuscin, and death within 10 to 15 years. **Volkmann's d.,** congenital deformity of the foot due to tibiotarsal dislocation. **von Hippel's d.,** hemangiomatosis confined principally to the retina; when associated with hemangioblastoma of the cerebellum, it is known as *von Hippel-Lindau d.* **von Hippel-Lindau d.,** a hereditary condition marked by hemangiomas of the retina and hemangioblastomas of the cerebellum, sometimes with similar lesions of the spinal cord and cysts of the viscera; there may be neurologic symptoms such as seizures and mental retardation. **von Willebrand's d.,** an autosomal dominant bleeding disorder characterized by prolonged bleeding time, deficiency of von Willebrand's factor, and often impairment of adhesion of platelets on glass beads, associated with epistaxis and increased bleeding after trauma or surgery, menorrhagia, and postpartum bleeding. **Waldenström's d.,** osteochondrosis of the capitular femoral epiphysis. **Weber-Christian d.,** nodular nonsuppurative panniculitis. **Werlhof's d.,** idiopathic thrombocytopenic purpura. **Wernicke's d.,** see under *encephalopathy.* **Westphal-Strümpell d.,** hepatolenticular degeneration. **Whipple's d.,** a malabsorption syndrome marked by diarrhea, steatorrhea, skin pigmentation, arthralgia and arthritis, lymphadenopathy, central nervous system lesions, and infiltration of the intestinal mucosa with macrophages containing PAS-positive material. **Whitmore's d.,** melioidosis. **Wilson's d.,** an inherited, progressive disorder of copper metabolism, with accumulation of copper in liver, brain, kidney, cornea, and other tissues; it is characterized by cirrhosis of the liver, degenerative changes in the brain, and a pigmented ring at the outer margin of the cornea. **Wolman's d.,** a lysosomal storage disease due to deficiency of the lysosomal sterol esterase, occurring in infants, and associated with hepatosplenomegaly, adrenal steatorrhea, calcification, abdominal distention, anemia, and inanition. **woolsorter's d.,** inhalational anthrax.

dis·en·gage·ment (dis″en-gāj′ment) emergence of the fetus from the vaginal canal.

dis·equi·lib·ri·um (dis-e″kwĭ-lib′re-um) dysequilibrium. **linkage d.,** the occurrence in a population of two linked alleles at a frequency higher or lower than expected on the basis of the gene frequencies of the individual genes.

dis·ger·mi·no·ma (-jer″mĭ-no′mah) dysgerminoma.

dish (dish) a shallow vessel of glass or other material for laboratory work. **Petri d.,** a shallow glass dish for growing bacterial cultures.

dis·in·fec·tant (dis″-in-fek′tant) 1. freeing from infection. 2. an agent that disinfects, particularly one used on inanimate objects.

dis·in·fes·ta·tion (-in-fes-ta′shun) destruction of insects, rodents, or other animal forms present on the person or their clothes or in their surroundings, and which may transmit disease.

dis·in·te·grant (dis-in′tĭ-grant) an agent used in pharmaceutical preparation of tablets, which causes them to disintegrate and release their medicinal substances on contact with moisture.

dis·in·te·gra·tion (-in″tĭ-gra′shun) 1. the process of breaking up or decomposing. 2. disruption of integrative functions of personality in mental illness; disorganization of the psychic and behavioral processes.

dis·in·te·gra·tive (dis-in′tĕ-gra″tiv) 1. being reduced to components, particles, or fragments; losing cohesion or unity. 2. having disorganized psychic and behavioral processes.

dis·junc·tion (-junk′shun) 1. the act or state of being disjoined. 2. in genetics, the moving apart of bivalent chromosomes at the first anaphase of meiosis. **craniofacial d.,** Le Fort III fracture.

disk (disk) a circular or rounded flat plate. Spelled also *disc*. **articular d.**, a pad of fibrocartilage or dense fibrous tissue present in some synovial joints. **Bowman's d's**, flat, disklike plates making up striated muscle fibers. **choked d.**, papilledema. **ciliary d.**, the thin part of the ciliary body. **contained d.**, protrusion of a nucleus pulposus in which the anulus fibrosus remains intact. **cupped d.**, a pathologically depressed optic disk. **extruded d.**, herniation of the nucleus pulposus through the anulus fibrosus, with the nuclear material remaining attached to the intervertebral disk. **gelatin d.**, a disk or lamella of gelatin variously medicated, used chiefly in eye diseases. **growth d.**, epiphyseal plate. **Hensen's d.**, H band. **herniated d.**, herniation of intervertebral disk; see under *herniation*. **intervertebral d's**, layers of fibrocartilage between the bodies of adjacent vertebrae. **intra-articular d's**, fibrous structures within the capsules of diarthrodial joints. **noncontained d.**, herniation of the nucleus pulposus with rupture of the anulus fibrosus. **optic d.**, the intraocular part of the optic nerve formed by fibers converging from the retina and appearing as a pink to white disk; because there are no sensory receptors in the region, it is not sensitive to stimuli. **Placido's d.**, a disk marked with concentric circles, used in examining the cornea. **protruded d., ruptured d.**, herniation of intervertebral disk; see under *herniation*. **sequestered d.**, a free fragment of the nucleus pulposus in the spinal canal outside of the anulus fibrosus and no longer attached to the intervertebral disk. **slipped d.**, popular term for herniation of an intervertebral disk; see under *herniation*.

dis·kec·to·my (dis-kek′tah-me) excision of an intervertebral disk.

dis·ki·tis (dis-ki′tis) inflammation of a disk, particularly of an interarticular disk.

dis·kog·ra·phy (dis-kog′rah-fe) radiography of the vertebral column after injection of radiopaque material into an intervertebral disk.

dis·lo·ca·tion (dis″lo-ka′shun) displacement of a part. **complete d.**, one completely separating the surfaces of a joint. **compound d.**, one in which the joint communicates with the air through a wound. **congenital d. of the hip**, developmental dysplasia of the hip. **pathologic d.**, one due to paralysis, synovitis, infection, or other disease. **simple d.**, one in which there is no communication with the air through a wound. **subspinous d.**, dislocation of the head of the humerus into the space below the spine of the scapula.

dis·mem·ber·ment (dis-mem′ber-ment) amputation of a limb or a portion of it.

dis·oc·clude (dis″ah-klood′) to grind a tooth so that it does not touch its antagonist in the other jaw in any masticatory movements.

di·so·pyr·amide (di″so-pir′ah-mīd) a cardiac depressant with anticholinergic properties, used as the base or phosphate salt as an antiarrhythmic.

dis·or·der (dis-or′der) a derangement or abnormality of function; a morbid physical or mental state. **acute stress d.**, an anxiety disorder characterized by development of anxiety, dissociative, and other symptoms within one month following exposure to an extremely traumatic event. If persistent, it may become posttraumatic stress disorder. **adjustment d.**, maladaptive reaction to identifiable stress (e.g., divorce, illness), which is assumed to remit when the stress ceases or when the patient adapts. **affective d's**, mood d's. **amnestic d's**, mental disorders characterized by acquired impairment in the ability to learn and recall new information, sometimes accompanied by inability to recall previously learned information. **anxiety d's**, mental disorders in which anxiety and avoidance behavior predominate, i.e., panic disorder, agoraphobia, social phobia, specific phobia, obsessive-compulsive disorder, posttraumatic stress disorder, acute stress disorder, generalized anxiety disorder, and substance-induced anxiety disorder. **attention-deficit/hyperactivity d.**, a controversial childhood mental disorder with onset before age seven, and characterized by inattention (e.g., distractibility, forgetfulness, not appearing to listen), by hyperactivity and impulsivity (e.g., restlessness, excessive running or climbing, excessive talking, and other disruptive behavior), or by a combination of both types of behavior. **autistic d.**, autism; a severe pervasive developmental disorder with onset usually before three years of age and a biological basis; it is characterized by qualitative impairment in reciprocal social interaction, verbal and nonverbal communication, and capacity for symbolic play, by restricted and unusual repertoire of activities and interests, and often by cognitive impairment. **behavior d.**, conduct d. **binge-eating d.**, an eating disorder characterized by repeated episodes of binge eating, as in bulimia nervosa, but not followed by inappropriate compensatory behavior such as purging, fasting, or excessive exercise. **bipolar d's**, mood disorders with a history of manic, mixed, or hypomanic episodes, usually with present or previous history of one or more major depressive episodes; included are *bipolar I d.*, characterized by one or more manic or mixed episodes, *bipolar II d.*, characterized by one or more hypomanic episodes but no manic episodes, and *cyclothymic disorder*. The term is sometimes used in the singular to denote either bipolar I disorder, bipolar II disorder, or both. **body dysmorphic d.,** a somatoform disorder characterized by a normal-looking person's preoccupation with an imagined defect in appearance. **breathing-related sleep d.,** any of several disorders characterized by sleep disruption due to some sleep-related breathing problem, resulting in excessive sleepiness or insomnia. **brief psychotic d.,** an episode of psychotic symptoms with sudden onset, lasting less than one month. **catatonic d.,** catatonia due to the physiological effects of a general medical condition and neither better accounted for by another mental disorder nor occurring exclusively during delirium. **character d's,** personality d's. **childhood disintegrative d.,** pervasive developmental disorder characterized by marked regression in various developmental skills, including language, play, and social and motor skills, after two to ten years of initial normal development. **circadian rhythm sleep d.,** a lack of synchrony between the schedule of sleeping and waking required by the external environment and that of a person's own circadian rhythm. **collagen d.,** an inborn error of metabolism involving abnormal structure or metabolism of collagen, e.g., Marfan syndrome, cutis laxa. Cf. *collagen disease.* **communication d's,** mental disorders characterized by difficulties with speech or language, severe enough to interfere academically, occupationally, or socially. **conduct d.,** a type of disruptive behavior disorder of childhood and adolescence marked by persistent violation of the rights of others or of age-appropriate societal norms or rules. **conversion d.,** a somatoform disorder characterized by conversion symptoms (loss or alteration of voluntary motor or sensory functioning suggesting physical illness) with no physiological basis and not produced intentionally or feigned; a psychological basis is suggested by exacerbation of symptoms during psychological stress, relief from tension (primary gain), or gain of outside support or attention (secondary gains). **cyclothymic d.,** a mood disorder characterized by alternating cycles of hypomanic and depressive periods with symptoms like those of manic and major depressive episodes but of lesser severity. **delusional d.,**

a mental disorder marked by well-organized, logically consistent delusions of grandeur, persecution, or jealousy, with no other psychotic feature. There are six types: persecutory, jealous, erotomanic, somatic, grandiose, and mixed. **depersonalization d.,** a dissociative disorder characterized by intense, prolonged, or otherwise troubling feelings of detachment from one's body or thoughts, not secondary to another mental disorder. **depressive d's,** mood disorders in which depression is unaccompanied by manic or hypomanic episodes. **developmental coordination d.,** problematic or delayed development of gross and fine motor coordination skills, not due to a neurological disorder or to general mental retardation, resulting in the appearance of clumsiness. **disruptive behavior d's,** a group of mental disorders of children and adolescents consisting of behavior that violates social norms and is disruptive. **dissociative d's,** mental disorders characterized by sudden, temporary alterations in identity, memory, or consciousness, segregating normally integrated parts of one's personality from one's dominant identity. **dissociative identity d.,** a dissociative disorder characterized by the existence in an individual of two or more distinct personalities, with at least two of the personalities controlling the patient's behavior in turns. The host personality usually is totally unaware of the alternate personalities; alternate personalities may or may not have awareness of the others. **dream anxiety d.,** nightmare d. **dysthymic d.,** a mood disorder characterized by depressed feeling, loss of interest or pleasure in one's usual activities, and other symptoms typical of depression but tending to be longer in duration and less severe than in major depressive disorder. **eating d.,** abnormal feeding habits associated with psychological factors, including anorexia nervosa, bulimia nervosa, pica, and rumination disorder. **expressive language d.,** a communication disorder occurring in children and characterized by problems with the expression of language, either oral or signed. **factitious d.,** a mental disorder characterized by repeated, intentional simulation of physical or psychological signs and symptoms of illness for no apparent purpose other than obtaining treatment. **factitious d. by proxy,** a form of factitious disorder in which one person (usually a mother) intentionally fabricates or induces physical (*Munchausen syndrome by proxy*) or psychological disorders in another person under their care (usually their child) and subjects that person to needless diagnostic procedures or treatment, without any external incentives for the behavior. **female orgasmic d.**, consistently delayed or absent orgasm in a female, even after a normal phase of sexual excitement and adequate stimulation. **female sexual arousal d.**, a sexual dysfunction involving failure by a female either to attain or maintain lubrication and swelling during sexual activity, after adequate stimulation. **functional d.**, a disorder of physiological function having no known organic basis. **gender identity d.**, a disturbance of gender identification in which the affected person has an overwhelming desire to change their anatomic sex or insists that they are of the opposite sex, with persistent discomfort about their assigned sex or about filling its usual gender role. **generalized anxiety d. (GAD)**, an anxiety disorder characterized by excessive, uncontrollable worry about two or more life circumstances for six months or more. **hypoactive sexual desire d.**, a sexual dysfunction consisting of persistently or recurrently low level or absence of sexual fantasies and desire for sexual activity. **impulse control d's**, a group of mental disorders characterized by repeated failure to resist an impulse to perform some act harmful to oneself or to others. **induced psychotic d.**, shared psychotic d. **intermittent explosive d.**, an impulse control disorder characterized by multiple discrete episodes of loss of control of aggressive impulses resulting in serious assault or destruction of property that are out of proportion to any precipitating stressors. **learning d's**, a group of disorders characterized by academic functioning that is substantially below the level expected on the basis of the patient's age, intelligence, and education. **lymphoproliferative d's**, a group of malignant neoplasms arising from cells related to the common multipotential lymphoreticular cell, including lymphocytic, histiocytic, and monocytic leukemias, multiple myeloma, plasmacytoma, and Hodgkin's disease. **lymphoreticular d's**, a group of disorders of the lymphoreticular system, characterized by the proliferation of lymphocytes or lymphoid tissues. **major depressive d.**, a mood disorder characterized by the occurrence of one or more major depressive episodes and the absence of any history of manic, mixed, or hypomanic episodes. **male erectile d.**, a sexual dysfunction involving failure by a male to attain or maintain an adequate erection until completion of sexual relations. **male orgasmic d.**, consistently delayed or absent

orgasm in a male, even after a normal phase of sexual excitement and stimulation adequate for his age. **manic-depressive d.**, former name for a mood disorder now known as *bipolar I d.* or *bipolar II d.* and often called *bipolar d.* (q.v.). **mendelian d.**, a genetic disease showing a mendelian pattern of inheritance, caused by a single mutation in the structure of DNA, which causes a single basic defect with pathologic consequences. **mental d.**, any clinically significant behavioral or psychological syndrome characterized by the presence of distressing symptoms, impairment of functioning, or significantly increased risk of suffering death, pain, or other disability. **minor depressive d.**, a mood disorder closely resembling major depressive disorder and dysthymic disorder but intermediate in severity between the two. **mixed receptive-expressive language d.**, a communication disorder involving both the expression and the comprehension of language, either spoken or signed. **monogenic d.**, mendelian d. **mood d's**, mental disorders characterized by disturbances of mood manifested as one or more episodes of mania, hypomania, depression, or some combination, the two main subcategories being *bipolar disorders* and *depressive disorders*. **motor skills d.**, any disorder characterized by inadequate development of motor coordination severe enough to restrict locomotion or the ability to perform tasks, schoolwork, or other activities. **multifactorial d.**, one caused by the interaction of genetic and sometimes also nongenetic, environmental factors, e.g., diabetes mellitus. **multiple personality d.**, dissociative identity d. **myeloproliferative d's**, a group of usually neoplastic diseases possibly related histogenetically, including granulocytic leukemias, myelomonocytic leukemias, polycythemia vera, and myelofibroerythroleukemia. **neurotic d.**, neurosis. **nightmare d.**, repeated episodes of nightmares that awaken the sleeper, with full orientation and alertness and vivid recall of the dreams. **obsessive-compulsive d. (OCD)**, an anxiety disorder characterized by recurrent obsessions or compulsions, which are severe enough to interfere significantly with personal or social functioning. Cf. *obsessive-compulsive personality disorder*, under *personality*. **obsessive-compulsive personality d.**, see under *personality*. **oppositional defiant d.**, a type of disruptive behavior disorder characterized by a recurrent pattern of defiant, hostile, disobedient, and negativistic behavior directed toward those in authority. **organic mental d.**, a term formerly used to denote any mental disorder with a specifically known or presumed organic etiology. It was sometimes used synonymously with *organic mental syndrome*. **orgasmic d's,** sexual dysfunctions characterized by inhibited or premature orgasm; see *female orgasmic d., male orgasmic d.,* and *premature ejaculation*. **pain d.,** a somatoform disorder characterized by a chief complaint of severe chronic pain which is neither feigned nor intentionally produced, but in which psychological factors appear to play a major role in onset, severity, exacerbation, or maintenance. **panic d.,** an anxiety disorder characterized by attacks of panic (anxiety), fear, or terror, by feelings of unreality, or by fears of dying, or losing control, together with somatic signs such as dyspnea, choking, palpitations, dizziness, vertigo, flushing or pallor, and sweating. It may occur with or, rarely, without agoraphobia. **paranoid d.,** older term for *delusional d*. **personality d's,** a category of mental disorders characterized by enduring, inflexible, and maladaptive personality traits that deviate markedly from cultural expectations and either generate subjective distress or significantly impair functioning. For specific disorders, see under *personality*. **pervasive developmental d's,** disorders in which there is impaired development in multiple areas, including reciprocal social interactions, verbal and nonverbal communications, and imaginative activity, as in autistic disorder. **phagocytic dysfunction d's,** a group of immunodeficiency conditions characterized by disordered phagocytic activity, occurring as both *extrinsic* and *intrinsic* types. Bacterial or fungal infections may range from mild skin infection to fatal systemic infection. **phobic d's,** see *phobia*. **phonological d.,** a communication disorder characterized by failure to use age- and dialect-appropriate sounds in speaking, with errors occurring in the selection, production, or articulation of sounds. **plasma cell d's,** see under *dyscrasia*. **postconcussional d.,** see under *syndrome*. **posttraumatic stress d. (PTSD),** an anxiety disorder caused by an intensely traumatic event, characterized by mentally reexperiencing the trauma, avoidance of trauma-associated stimuli, numbing of emotional responsiveness, and hyperalertness and difficulty in sleeping, remembering, or concentrating. **premenstrual dysphoric d.,** premenstrual syndrome viewed as a psychiatric disorder. **psychoactive substance use d's,** substance use d's. **psychosomatic d.,** one in which the physical symptoms are caused or exacerbated by psychological

factors, as in migraine headaches, lower back pain, or irritable bowel syndrome. **psychotic d.,** psychosis. **reactive attachment d.,** a mental disorder of infancy or early childhood characterized by notably unusual and developmentally inappropriate social relatedness, usually associated with grossly pathological care. **rumination d.,** excessive rumination of food by infants, after a period of normal eating habits, potentially leading to death by malnutrition. **schizoaffective d.,** a mental disorder in which symptoms of a mood disorder occur along with prominent psychotic symptoms characteristic of schizophrenia. **schizophreniform d.,** a mental disorder with the signs and symptoms of schizophrenia but of less than six months' duration. **seasonal affective d. (SAD),** depression with fatigue, lethargy, oversleeping, overeating, and carbohydrate craving recurring cyclically during specific seasons, most commonly the winter months. **separation anxiety d.,** prolonged, developmentally inappropriate, excessive anxiety and distress in a child concerning removal from parents, home, or familiar surroundings. **sexual d's,** 1. any disorders involving sexual functioning, desire, or performance. 2. specifically, any such disorder that is caused at least in part by psychological factors; divided into sexual dysfunctions and paraphilias. **sexual arousal d's,** sexual dysfunctions characterized by alterations in sexual arousal; see *female sexual arousal d.* and *male erectile d*. **sexual aversion d.,** feelings of repugnance for and active avoidance of genital sexual contact with a partner, causing substantial distress or interpersonal difficulty. **sexual desire d's,** sexual dysfunctions characterized by alteration in sexual desire; see *hypoactive sexual desire d.* and *sexual aversion d*. **sexual pain d's,** sexual dysfunctions characterized by pain associated with intercourse; it includes dyspareunia and vaginismus not due to a general medical condition. **shared psychotic d.,** a delusional system that develops in one or more persons as a result of a close relationship with someone who already has a psychotic disorder with prominent delusions. **sleep d's,** chronic disorders involving sleep, either primary (dyssomnias, parasomnias) or secondary to factors including a general medical condition, mental disorder, or substance use. **sleep terror d.,** a sleep disorder of repeated episodes of pavor nocturnus. **sleepwalking d.,** a sleep disorder of the parasomnia group, consisting of repeated episodes of somnambulism. **social anxiety d.,** social phobia. **somatization d.,** a somatoform disorder characterized by multiple somatic complaints, including a combination of pain, gastrointestinal, sexual, and neurological symptoms, and not fully explainable by any known general medical condition or the direct effect of a substance, but not intentionally feigned or produced. **somatoform d's,** mental disorders characterized by symptoms suggesting physical disorders of psychogenic origin but not under voluntary control, e.g., body dysmorphic disorder, conversion disorder, hypochondriasis, pain disorder, somatization disorder, and undifferentiated somatoform disorder. **somatoform pain d.,** pain d. **speech d.,** defective ability to speak; it may be either psychogenic (see *communication d.*) or neurogenic. See also *aphasia, aphonia, dysphasia,* and *dysphonia.* **stereotypic movement d.,** a mental disorder characterized by repetitive nonfunctional motor behavior that often appears to be driven and can result in serious self-inflicted injuries. **substance-induced d's,** a subgroup of the substance-related disorders comprising a variety of behavioral or psychological anomalies resulting from ingestion of or exposure to a drug of abuse, medication, or toxin. Cf. *substance use d's.* **substance-related d's,** any of the mental disorders associated with excessive use of or exposure to psychoactive substances, including drugs of abuse, medications, and toxins. The group is divided into *substance use d's* and *substance-induced d's.* **substance use d's,** a subgroup of the substance-related disorders, in which psychoactive substance use or abuse repeatedly results in significantly adverse consequences. The group comprises *substance abuse* and *substance dependence.* **undifferentiated somatoform d.,** one or more physical complaints, not intentionally produced or feigned and persisting for at least six months, that cannot be fully explained by a general medical condition or the direct effects of a substance. **unipolar d's,** depressive d's.

dis·or·gan·iza·tion (-or″gan-ĭ-za′shun) the process of destruction of any organic tissue; any profound change in the tissues of an organ or structure which causes the loss of most or all of its proper characters.

dis·or·i·en·ta·tion (-or″e-en-ta′shun) the loss of proper bearings, or a state of mental confusion as to time, place, or identity. **spatial d.,** the inability of a pilot or other air crew member to determine spatial attitude in relation to the surface of the earth; it occurs in conditions of restricted vision, and results from vestibular illusions.

dis·pen·sa·ry (-pen′sah-re) 1. a place for dispensation of free or low cost medical treatment. 2. any place where drugs and medicines are actually dispensed.

dis·pen·sa·to·ry (-pen′sah-tor″e) a book that describes medicines and their preparation and uses. **D. of the United States of America,** a collection of monographs on unofficial drugs and drugs recognized by the United States Pharmacopeia, the British Pharmacopoeia, and the National Formulary; also on general tests, processes, reagents, and solutions of the U.S.P. and N.F., as well as drugs used in veterinary medicine.

dis·pense (-pens′) to prepare medicines for and distribute them to their users.

di·sper·my (di′sper-me) the penetration of two spermatozoa into one oocyte.

dis·perse (dis-pers′) to scatter the component parts, as of a tumor or the fine particles in a colloid system; also, the particles so dispersed.

dis·per·sion (-per′zhun) 1. the act of scattering or separating; the condition of being scattered. 2. the incorporation of the particles of one substance into the body of another, comprising solutions, suspensions, and colloid systems; used particularly for an unstable colloid system. See *colloid* (2).

dis·per·sive (-per′siv) 1. tending to become dispersed. 2. promoting dispersion.

dis·place·ment (-plās′mint) 1. removal from the normal position or place. 2. percolation. 3. a defense mechanism in which emotions, ideas, wishes, or impulses are unconsciously shifted from their original object to a more acceptable substitute. 4. in a chemical reaction, the replacement of one atom or group in a molecule by another.

dis·pro·por·tion (dis″prah-por′shun) a lack of the proper relationship between two elements or factors. **cephalopelvic d.,** a condition in which the fetal head is too large for the mother's pelvis.

dis·rup·tion (dis-rup′shun) a morphologic defect resulting from the extrinsic breakdown of, or interference with, a developmental process.

dis·rup·tive (-tiv) 1. bursting apart; rending. 2. causing confusion or disorder.

dis·sect (dĭ-sekt′, di-sekt′) 1. to cut apart, or separate. 2. to expose structures of a cadaver for anatomical study.

dis·sec·tion (dĭ-sek′shun) 1. the act of dissection. 2. a part or whole of an organism prepared by dissecting. **aortic d.,** a dissecting aneurysm of the aorta, usually the thoracic aorta. **axillary d.,** axillary lymph node d.

axillary lymph node d., surgical removal of axillary lymph nodes, done as part of radical mastectomy. **blunt d.,** dissection accomplished by separating tissues along natural cleavage lines, without cutting. **lymph node d.,** lymphadenectomy. **sharp d.,** dissection accomplished by incising tissues with a sharp edge.

dis·sem·i·nat·ed (-sem′ĭ-nāt″ed) scattered; distributed over a considerable area.

dis·so·ci·a·tion (-so″se-a′shun) 1. the act of separating or state of being separated. 2. the separation of a molecule into two or more fragments produced by the absorption of light or thermal energy or by solvation. 3. segregation of a group of mental processes from the rest of a person's usually integrated functions of consciousness, memory, perception, and sensory and motor behavior. **atrial d.,** independent beating of the left and right atria, each with normal rhythm or with one or both having an abnormal rhythm. **atrioventricular d.,** control of the atria by one pacemaker and of the ventricles by another, independent pacemaker. **electromechanical d.,** continued electrical rhythmicity of the heart in the absence of effective mechanical function.

dis·so·ci·a·tive (-so′se-a′tiv) pertaining to or tending to produce dissociation.

dis·so·lu·tion (dis″ah-loo′shun) 1. the process in which one substance is passed in another. 2. separation of a compound into its components by chemical action. 3. liquefaction. 4. death.

dis·solve (dĭ-zolv′) 1. to cause a substance to pass into solution. 2. to pass into solution.

dis·tad (dis′tad) in a distal direction.

dis·tal (-t′l) remote; farther from any point of reference.

dis·ta·lis (dis-ta′lis) [L.] distal.

dis·tance (dis′tins) the measure of space intervening between two objects or two points of reference. **focal d.,** that from the focal point to the optical center of a lens or the surface of a concave mirror. **interarch d.,** the vertical distance between the maxillary and mandibular arches under certain specified conditions of vertical dimension. **interocclusal d.,** the distance between the occluding surfaces of the maxillary and mandibular teeth with the mandible in physiologic rest position. **interocular d.,** the distance between the eyes, usually used in reference to the interpupillary distance. **working d.,** the distance between the front lens of a microscope and the object when the instrument is correctly focused.

dis·ti·chi·a·sis (dis″tĭ-ki′ah-sis) the presence of a double row of eyelashes, one or both of which are turned in against the eyeball.

dis·til·la·tion (dis″tĭ-la′shun) vaporization; the process of vaporizing and condensing a substance to purify it or to separate a volatile substance from less volatile substances. **destructive d., dry d.,** decomposition of a solid by heating in the absence of air, resulting in volatile liquid products. **fractional d.,** that attended by the successive separation of volatilizable substances in order of their respective volatility.

dis·to·clu·sion (-to-kloo′zhun) malrelation of the dental arches with the lower jaw in a distal or posterior position in relation to the upper.

dis·to·mi·a·sis (-mi′ah-sis) infection by trematodes.

dis·to·mo·lar (-mo′ler) a supernumerary molar; any tooth distal to a third molar.

dis·tor·tion (dis-tor′shun) 1. the state of being twisted out of normal shape or position. 2. in psychiatry, the conversion of material offensive to the superego into acceptable form. 3. deviation of an image from the true outline or shape of an object or structure.

dis·trac·tion (dis-trak′shun) 1. diversion of attention. 2. separation of joint surfaces without rupture of their binding ligaments and without displacement. 3. surgical separation of the two parts of a bone after the bone is transected.

dis·tress (dis-tres′) anguish or suffering. **idiopathic respiratory d. of newborn,** respiratory distress syndrome of newborn.

dis·tri·bu·tion (dis″trĭ-bu′shun) 1. the specific location or arrangement of continuing or successive objects or events in space or time. 2. the extent of a ramifying structure such as an artery or nerve and its branches. 3. the geographical range of an organism or disease. **chi-square d.,** a distribution of sample differences using observations of a random sample drawn from a normal population. **normal d.,** a continuous probability density function roughly characterizing a random variable that is the sum of a large number of independent random events; usually represented by a smooth bell-shaped curve symmetric about the mean.

dis·tur·bance (dis-tur′bans) a departure or divergence from that which is considered normal.

di·sul·fi·ram (di-sul′fĭ-ram) an antioxidant that inhibits the oxidation of the acetaldehyde metabolized from alcohol, resulting in high concentrations of acetaldehyde in the body. Used to produce aversion to alcohol in the treatment of alcoholism because extremely uncomfortable symptoms occur when its administration is followed by ingestion of alcohol.

di·ur·ese (di″u-rēs′) to bring about diuresis.

di·ure·sis (di″u-re′sis) increased excretion of urine. **osmotic d.,** that resulting from the presence of nonabsorbable or poorly absorbable, osmotically active substances in the renal tubules. **pressure d.,** increased urinary excretion of water when arterial pressure increases, a compensatory mechanism to maintain blood pressure within the normal range.

di·uret·ic (di″u-ret′ik) 1. pertaining to or causing diuresis. 2. an agent that promotes diuresis. **high-ceiling d's, loop d's,** those exerting their action on the sodium reabsorption mechanism of the thick ascending limb of the loop of Henle, resulting in excretion of urine isotonic with plasma. **osmotic d's,** a group of low-molecular-weight substances that can remain in high concentrations in renal tubules, thus contributing to osmolality of glomerular filtrate. **potassium-sparing d's,** those blocking exchange of sodium for potassium and hydrogen ions in the distal tubule, increasing sodium and chloride excretion without increasing potassium excretion. **thiazide d's,** a group of synthetic compounds that decrease reabsorption of sodium by the kidney and thereby increase loss of water and sodium; they enhance excretion of sodium and chloride equally.

di·ur·nal (di-er′nal) pertaining to or occurring during the daytime, or period of light.

di·va·lent (di-va′lent) bivalent; carrying a valence of two.

di·val·pro·ex (di-val′pro-eks) an anticonvulsant, used as *d. sodium,* a 1:1 compound of valproate sodium and valproic acid, in the treatment of migraine, manic episodes of bipolar disorder, and epileptic seizures, particularly absence seizures.

di·ver·gence (di-ver′jens) a moving apart, or inclination away from a common point. **diver′gent,** adj.

di·ver·sion (di-ver′zhun) a turning aside. **urinary d.,** surgical creation of an alternate route for urine flow to replace an absent or diseased portion of the lower urinary tract in order to preserve renal function.

di·ver·tic·u·la (di″ver-tik′u-lah) [L.] plural of *diverticulum.*

di·ver·tic·u·lar (-lar) pertaining to or resembling a diverticulum.

di·ver·tic·u·lec·to·my (di″ver-tik″u-lek′tah-me) excision of a diverticulum.

di·ver·tic·u·li·tis (-li′tis) inflammation of a diverticulum.

di·ver·tic·u·lo·sis (-lo′sis) the presence of diverticula in the absence of inflammation.

di·ver·tic·u·lum (di″ver-tik′u-lum) pl. *diverti′cula.* A circumscribed pouch or sac occurring normally or created by herniation of the lining mucous membrane through a defect in the muscular coat of a tubular organ. **allantoic d.,** the endodermal sacculation that becomes the allantois; in humans it is an outpouching of the caudal wall of the yolk sac that becomes the urachus. **ileal d., Meckel's d.,** an occasional sacculation or appendage of the ileum, derived from an unobliterated yolk stalk.

di·vi·sion (dĭ-vizh′un) 1. the act of separating into parts. 2. a section or part of a larger structure. 3. in the taxonomy of plants and fungi, a level of classification equivalent to the *phylum* of the animal kingdom. **cell d.,** fission of a cell. **direct cell d.,** see *amitosis.* **indirect cell d.,** see *meiosis* and *mitosis.* **maturation d.,** meiosis.

di·vulse (-vuls′) to pull apart forcibly.

di·vul·sion (-vul′shun) the act of separating or pulling apart.

di·zy·got·ic (di″zi-got′ik) pertaining to or derived from two separate zygotes.

diz·zi·ness (diz′e-nes) 1. a disturbed sense of relationship to space; a sensation of unsteadiness and a feeling of movement within the head; lightheadedness; dysequilibrium. 2. erroneous synonym for *vertigo.*

dL deciliter.

DL- chemical prefix (small capitals) used with D and L convention to indicate a racemic mixture of enantiomers.

dl- chemical prefix used with the *d* and *l* convention to indicate a racemic mixture of enantiomers; the prefix (±)- is used with the same meaning.

DLE discoid lupus erythematosus.

DM diabetes mellitus; diphenylamine chlorarsine.

DMD Doctor of Dental Medicine.

DMFO eflornithine.

DMRD Diploma in Medical Radio-Diagnosis (Brit.).

DMRT Diploma in Medical Radio-Therapy (Brit.).

DMSO dimethyl sulfoxide.

DNA deoxyribonucleic acid. **complementary DNA (cDNA), copy DNA,** DNA transcribed from a specific RNA through the action of the enzyme reverse transcriptase. **mitochondrial DNA (mtDNA),** the DNA of the mitochondrial chromosome, existing in several thousand copies per cell and inherited exclusively from the mother. **nuclear DNA (nDNA),** the DNA of the chromosomes found in the nucleus of a eukaryotic cell. **recombinant DNA,** DNA artificially constructed by insertion of foreign DNA into the DNA of an appropriate organism so that the foreign DNA is replicated along with the host DNA. **repetitive DNA,** nucleotide sequences occurring multiply within a genome; it is characteristic of eukaryotes and some is satellite DNA while other sequences encode genes for ribosomal RNA and histones. **satellite DNA,** short, highly repeated eukaryotic DNA sequences, usually clustered in heterochromatin and generally not transcribed. **single copy DNA (scDNA),** nucleotide sequences present once in the haploid genome, as are most of those encoding polypeptides in the eukaryotic genome. **spacer DNA,** the nucleotide sequences occurring between genes.

DNA gyrase (ji′rās) a type II DNA topoisomerase.

DNA li·gase (li′gās) a ligase that catalyzes the linkage between two free ends of double-stranded DNA chains by forming a phosphodiester bond between them, as in the repair of damaged DNA.

DNA po·lym·er·ase (pah-lim′er-ās) any of various enzymes catalyzing the template-directed incorporation of deoxyribonucleotides into a DNA chain, particularly one using a DNA template.

DNA topo·isom·er·ase (to″po-i-som′er-ās) either of two types of isomerase that catalyze the breakage, passage, and rejoining of one or both DNA strands, *type I topoisomerases* specific for single-strand passage and *type II* for double; thus altering the topology of the molecule.

DNase deoxyribonuclease.

DNOC dinitro-*o*-cresol.

DO Doctor of Osteopathy.

DOA dead on admission (arrival).

do·bu·ta·mine (do-bu′tah-mēn) a synthetic catecholamine having direct inotropic effects; used as the hydrochloride salt in the treatment of congestive heart failure and low cardiac output.

do·ce·tax·el (do″sĕ-tak′s'l) an antineoplastic agent used particularly in treating carcinoma of the breast and non–small cell lung carcinoma.

do·co·sa·hexa·eno·ic ac·id (do-ko″sah-hek″sah-e-no′ik) an omega-3, polyunsaturated, 22-carbon fatty acid found almost exclusively in fish and marine animal oils.

do·co·sa·nol (do-ko′sah-nol) an antiviral effective against lipid-enveloped viruses,

including herpes simplex virus; used in the treatment of recurrent herpes labialis.

doc·tor (dok′ter) a practitioner of medicine, as one graduated from a college of medicine, osteopathy, dentistry, chiropractic, optometry, podiatry, or veterinary medicine, and licensed to practice.

doc·u·sate (dok′u-sāt) any of a group of anionic surfactants widely used as emulsifying, wetting, and dispersing agents; the calcium, potassium, and sodium salts are used as stool softeners.

do·fet·i·lide (do-fet′ĭ-līd) an antiarrhythmic used in the treatment of atrial arrhythmias.

dol (dōl) a unit of pain intensity.

do·las·e·tron (do-las′ĕ-tron) a selective serotonin receptor antagonist, used as the mesylate salt for the prevention of nausea and vomiting associated with chemotherapy or occurring after surgery; administered orally and intravenously.

dolich(o)- word element [Gr.], *long*.

dol·i·cho·ce·phal·ic (dol″ĭ-ko-sĕ-fal′ik) long headed; having a cephalic index of 75.9 or less.

do·lor (do′lor) pl. *dolo′res*. [L.] pain; one of the cardinal signs of inflammation.

do·lor·if·ic (do″lor-if′ik) producing pain.

do·lor·im·e·ter (-im′ĕ-ter) an instrument for measuring pain in dols.

do·lor·o·gen·ic (do-lor″o-jen′ik) dolorific.

do·main (do-mān′) in immunology, any of the homology regions of heavy or light polypeptide chains of immunoglobulins.

dom·i·nance (dom′ĭ-nans) 1. the state of being dominant. 2. in genetics, the full phenotypic expression of a gene in both heterozygotes and homozygotes. 3. in coronary artery anatomy, the state of supplying the posterior diaphragmatic part of the interventricular septum and the diaphragmatic surface of the left ventricle. **incomplete d.,** failure of one gene to be completely dominant, heterozygotes showing a phenotype intermediate between the two parents. **lateral d.,** the preferential use, in voluntary motor acts, of ipsilateral members of the major paired organs of the body.

dom·i·nant (dom′ĭ-nant) 1. exerting a ruling or controlling influence. 2. in genetics, capable of expression when carried by only one of a pair of homologous chromosomes. 3. a dominant allele or trait.

do·nep·e·zil (do-nep′ĕ-zil) an acetylcholinesterase inhibitor used as the hydrochloride salt for the treatment of mild to moderate symptoms of dementia of the Alzheimer type; administered orally.

dong quai (doong kwa, -kwi) *Angelica sinensis* Chinese angelica), or its root, a preparation of which is used for gynecologic disorders.

do·nor (do'ner) 1. an organism that supplies living tissue to be used in another body, as a person who furnishes blood for transfusion, or an organ for transplantation. 2. a substance or compound that contributes part of itself to another substance (acceptor). **universal d.,** a person whose blood is type O in the ABO blood group system; such blood is sometimes used in emergency transfusion.

do·pa (do'pah) 3,4-dihydroxyphenylalanine, produced by oxidation of tyrosine by monophenol monooxygenase; it is the precursor of dopamine and an intermediate product in the biosynthesis of norepinephrine, epinephrine, and melanin. L-dopa is the naturally occurring form; see *levodopa*.

do·pa·mine (-mēn) a catecholamine formed in the body by the decarboxylation of dopa; it is an intermediate product in the synthesis of norepinephrine, and acts as a neurotransmitter in the central nervous system. The hydrochloride salt is used to correct hemodynamic balance in the treatment of shock and is also used as a cardiac stimulant.

do·pa·min·er·gic (do''pah-mēn-er'jik) activated or transmitted by dopamine; pertaining to tissues or organs affected by dopamine.

Dop·pler (dop'ler) see under *ultrasonography.* **color D.,** color flow Doppler imaging.

dor·nase al·fa (dor'nāz al'fah) recombinant human deoxyribonuclease I (DNase I) used to reduce the viscosity of sputum in cystic fibrosis.

dor·sad (dor'sad) toward the back.

dor·sal (dor's'l) 1. pertaining to the back or to any dorsum. 2. denoting a position more toward the back surface than some other object of reference; a synonym of *posterior* in human anatomy and of *superior* in the anatomy of quadrupeds.

dor·sa·lis (dor-sa'lis) [L.] dorsal.

dor·si·flex·ion (dor''sĭ-flek'shun) flexion or bending toward the extensor aspect of a limb, as of the hand or foot.

dors(o)- word element [L.], *the back; the dorsal aspect.* Also, *dorsi-.*

dor·so·ceph·a·lad (dor''so-sef'ah-lad) toward the back of the head.

dor·so·lat·er·al (-lat'er-al) pertaining to the back and the side.

dor·so·ven·tral (-ven'tral) 1. pertaining to the back and belly surfaces of a body. 2. passing from the back to the belly surface.

dor·sum (dor'sum) pl. *dor'sa.* [L.] 1. the back. 2. the aspect of an anatomical structure or part corresponding in position to the back; posterior in the human.

dor·zo·la·mide (dor-zo'lah-mīd) a carbonic acid anhydrase inhibitor, used as an antiglaucoma agent in the treatment of openangle glaucoma and ocular hypertension; applied topically to the conjunctiva as the hydrochloride salt.

dos·age (do'saj) the determination and regulation of the size, frequency, and number of doses.

dose (dōs) the quantity to be administered at one time, as a specified amount of medication or a given quantity of radiation. **absorbed d.,** that amount of energy from ionizing radiations absorbed per unit mass of matter, expressed in rads. **air d.,** see under *exposure.* **booster d.,** a dose of an active immunizing agent, usually smaller than the initial dose, given to maintain immunity. **divided d.,** fractionated d. **effective d. (ED),** that quantity of a drug that will produce the effects for which it is given. **erythema d.,** the amount of radiation which, when applied to the skin, causes temporary reddening. **fatal d.,** lethal d. **fractionated d.,** a fraction of the total quantity of a prescribed drug or radiation to be given at intervals. **infective d.,** that amount of pathogenic organisms that will cause infection in susceptible subjects. **infinitesimal d.,** see under *principle.* **lethal d.,** that quantity of an agent that will or may be sufficient to cause death. **maximum d.,** the largest dose consistent with safety. **maximum permissible d. (MPD),** the largest amount of ionizing radiation that one may safely receive in a specified period according to recommended limits in radiation protection guides. **median curative d. (CD_{50}),** a dose that abolishes symptoms in 50 per cent of test subjects. **median effective d. (ED_{50}),** a dose that produces the desired effect in 50 per cent of a population. **median immunizing d.,** the dose of vaccine or antigen sufficient to provide immunity in 50 per cent of test subjects. **median infective d. (ID_{50}),** the amount of pathogenic microorganisms that will cause infection in 50 per cent of the test subjects. **median lethal d. (LD_{50}),** the quantity of an agent that will kill 50 per cent of the test subjects; in radiology, the amount of radiation that will kill, within a specified period, 50 per cent of individuals in a large group or population. **median toxic d. (TD_{50}),** the dose that produces a toxic effect in 50 per cent of the population. **minimum d.,** the smallest dose that will produce an appreciable effect. **minimum**

lethal d. (MLD), 1. the smallest amount of toxin that will kill an experimental animal. 2. the smallest quantity of diphtheria toxin that will kill a guinea pig of 250 g weight in 4 to 5 days when injected subcutaneously. **skin d. (SD),** 1. the air dose of radiation at the skin surface, comprising primary radiation plus backscatter. 2. the absorbed dose in the skin. **threshold d.,** the minimum dose of ionizing radiation, a chemical, or a drug that will produce a detectable degree of any given effect. **threshold erythema d.,** the single skin dose that will produce in 80 per cent of those tested a faint but definite erythema within 30 days, and in the other 20 per cent, no visible reaction. Abbreviated T.E.D. **tolerance d.,** the largest quantity of an agent that may be administered without harm.

dosha (dosh′ah) according to the principle of constitution of the physical body in ayurveda, one of the three vital bioenergies (vata, pitta, kapha) condensed from the five elements; the doshas are responsible for the physical and emotional tendencies in the mind and body, and along with the seven dhatus (tissues) and three malas (waste products) make up the human body. The attributes of the doshas and their specific combination within each individual help determine the individual's physical and mental characteristics, while imbalance among the doshas is the cause of disease.

do·sim·e·try (do-sim′ĕ-tre) scientific determination of amount, rate, and distribution of radiation emitted from a source of ionizing radiation, in *biological d.* measuring the radiation-induced changes in a body or organism, and in *physical d.* measuring the levels of radiation directly with instruments.

dot (dot) a small spot or speck. **Gunn's d's,** white dots seen about the macula lutea on oblique illumination. **Maurer's d's,** irregular dots, staining red with Leishman's stain, seen in erythrocytes infected with *Plasmodium falciparum.* **Mittendorf's d.,** a congenital anomaly manifested as a small gray or white opacity just inferior and nasal to the posterior pole of the lens, representing the remains of the lenticular attachment of the hyaloid artery; it does not affect vision. **Schüffner's d's,** minute granules observed in erythrocytes infected with *Plasmodium vivax* when stained by certain methods. **Trantas' d's,** small, white calcareous-looking dots in the limbus of the conjunctiva in vernal conjunctivitis.

dou·ble blind (dub′'l blīnd′) pertaining to an experiment in which neither the subject nor the person administering treatment knows which treatment any particular subject is receiving.

douche (doosh) [Fr.] a stream of water directed against a part of the body or into a cavity. **air d.,** a current of air blown into a cavity, particularly into the tympanum to open the eustachian tube.

doug·la·si·tis (dug″lah-si′tis) inflammation of the rectouterine excavation (Douglas' cul-de-sac).

dow·el (dou″l) a peg or pin for fastening an artificial crown or core to a natural tooth root, or affixing a die to a working model for construction of a crown, inlay, or partial denture.

down-reg·u·la·tion (doun reg-u-la′shun) a decrease in the number of receptors for a chemical or drug on cell surfaces in a given area, usually due to long-term exposure to the agent.

down·stream (doun′strēm) a region of DNA or RNA that is located to the 3′ side of a gene or region of interest.

dox·a·cu·ri·um (dok″sah-ku′re-um) a long-acting neuromuscular blocking agent used as the chloride salt as a skeletal muscle relaxant during surgery and endotracheal intubation.

dox·a·pram (dok′sah-pram) a respiratory stimulant, used after anesthesia or in chronic obstructive pulmonary disease; used as the hydrochloride salt.

dox·a·zo·sin (dok-sa′zo-sin) a compound that blocks α_1-adrenergic receptors; used as *d. mesylate* in the treatment of hypertension and of benign prostatic hyperplasia.

dox·e·pin (dok′sĕ-pin) a tricyclic antidepressant of the dibenzoxepine class; also used to treat chronic pain, peptic ulcer, pruritus, and idiopathic cold urticaria, administered as the hydrochloride salt.

dox·er·cal·cif·er·ol (dok″ser-kal-sif′er-ol) a synthetic analogue of vitamin D_2, used to reduce levels of circulating parathyroid hormone in the treatment of secondary hyperparathyroidism associated with chronic renal failure.

doxo·ru·bi·cin (dok″so-roo′bĭ-sin) an antineoplastic antibiotic, produced by *Streptomyces peucetius,* which binds to DNA and inhibits nucleic acid synthesis; used as the hydrochloride salt and as a liposome-encased preparation of the hydrochloride salt.

doxy·cy·cline (dok″se-si′klēn) a semisynthetic broad-spectrum tetracycline antibiotic, active against a wide range of gram-positive and gram-negative organisms; used also as *d. calcium* and *d. hyclate.*

dox·yl·amine (dok-sil′ah-mēn) an antihistamine with anticholinergic and sedative effects, used as the succinate salt.

DP Doctor of Pharmacy; Doctor of Podiatry.

DPH Diploma in Public Health.

DPM Diploma in Psychological Medicine; Doctor of Podiatric Medicine.

DPT diphtheria-pertussis-tetanus (diphtheria and tetanus toxoids and pertussis vaccine).

DR reaction of degeneration.

dra·cun·cu·li·a·sis (drah-kung″ku-li′ah-sis) infection by nematodes of the genus *Dracunculus.*

dra·cun·cu·lo·sis (-lo′sis) dracunculiasis.

Dra·cun·cu·lus (-lus) a genus of nematode parasites, including *D. medinen′sis* (guinea worm), a threadlike worm, 30–120 cm. long, widely distributed in India, Africa, and Arabia, inhabiting subcutaneous and intermuscular tissues of humans and other animals.

drain (drān) any device by which a channel or open area may be established for exit of fluids or purulent material from a cavity, wound, or infected area. **controlled d.,** a square of gauze, filled with gauze strips, pressed into a wound, the corners of the square and ends of the strips left protruding. **Mikulicz d.,** a single layer of gauze, packed with several thick wicks of gauze, pushed into a wound cavity. **Penrose d.,** a thin rubber tube, usually 0.5 to 1 inch in diameter. **stab wound d.,** one brought out through a small puncture wound at some distance from the operative incision, to prevent infection of the operation wound.

drain·age (drān′ij) systematic withdrawal of fluids and discharges from a wound, sore, or cavity. **capillary d.,** that effected by strands of hair, surgical gut, spun glass, or other material of small caliber which acts by capillary attraction. **closed d.,** drainage of an empyema cavity carried out with protection against the entrance of outside air into the pleural cavity. **manual lymph d.,** the application of light rhythmic strokes, similar to those of effleurage, in the direction of the heart to increase the drainage of lymph from the involved structures. **open d.,** drainage of an empyema cavity through an opening in the chest wall into which one or more rubber drainage tubes are inserted, the opening not being sealed against the entrance of outside air. **postural d.,** therapeutic drainage in bronchiectasis and lung abscess by placing the patient head downward so that the trachea will be inclined below the affected area. **through d.,** that achieved by passing a perforated tube through the cavity, so that irrigation may be effected by injecting fluid into one aperture and letting it escape out of another.

dream (drēm) 1. a mental phenomenon occurring during REM sleep in which images, emotions, and thoughts are experienced with a sense of reality. 2. to experience such a phenomenon. **day d.,** wishful, purposeless reveries, without regard to reality. **wet d.,** slang for *nocturnal emission.*

dress·ing (dres′ing) any material used for covering and protecting a wound. **antiseptic d.,** gauze impregnated with antiseptic material. **occlusive d.,** one that seals a wound from contact with air or bacteria. **pressure d.,** one by which pressure is exerted on the covered area to prevent collection of fluids in underlying tissues.

drift (drift) 1. slow movement away from the normal or original position. 2. a chance variation, as in gene frequency between populations; the smaller the population, the greater are the chance random variations. **radial d.,** see under *deviation.* **ulnar d.,** see under *deviation.*

drip (drip) the slow, drop-by-drop infusion of a liquid. **postnasal d.,** drainage of excessive mucous or mucopurulent discharge from the postnasal region into the pharynx.

driv·en·ness (driv′en-nes) hyperactivity (1). **organic d.,** hyperactivity seen in brain-damaged individuals as a result of injury to and disorganization of cerebellar structures.

dromo·graph (drom′ah-graf) a recording flowmeter for measuring blood flow.

dro·mo·stan·o·lone (dro″mo-stan′o-lōn) an androgenic, anabolic steroid used as an antineoplastic agent in the palliative treatment of advanced metastatic, inoperable breast cancer in certain postmenopausal women; used as the propionate salt.

drom·o·tro·pic (-tro′pik) affecting conductivity of a nerve fiber.

dro·nab·i·nol (dro-nab′in-ol) one of the major active substances in cannabis, used as an antiemetic for cancer chemotherapy and anorexia and weight loss in AIDS; it is subject to abuse because of its psychotomimetic activity.

drop (drop) 1. a minute sphere of liquid as it hangs or falls. 2. to descend or fall. 3. a descent or falling below the usual position.

dro·per·i·dol (dro-per′ĭ-dol) a tranquilizer of the butyrophenone series, used as a preanesthetic and anesthesia adjunct, as a postoperative antiemetic, and to produce conscious sedation. In combination with fentanyl citrate, it is used as a neuroleptanalgesic.

drop·sy (drop′se) edema.

Dro·soph·i·la (dro-sof'il-ah) a genus of fruit flies. *D. melanogas'ter* is a small species used extensively in experimental genetics.

dros·pi·re·none (dros-pi'rĕ-nōn) a spironolactone analogue that acts as a progestational agent; used in combination with an estrogen component as an oral contraceptive.

drown·ing (droun'ing) suffocation and death resulting from filling of the lungs with water or other substance.

DrPH Doctor of Public Health.

drug (drug) 1. a chemical substance that affects the processes of the mind or body. 2. any chemical compound used in the diagnosis, treatment, or prevention of disease or other abnormal condition. 3. a substance used recreationally for its effects on the central nervous system, such as a narcotic. 4. to administer a drug to. **designer d.,** a new drug of abuse similar in action to an older abused drug and usually created by making a small chemical modification in the older one. **mind-altering d.,** one that produces an altered state of consciousness. **nonsteroidal antiinflammatory d. (NSAID),** any of a large, chemically heterogeneous group of drugs that inhibit the enzyme cyclooxygenase, resulting in decreased synthesis of prostaglandin and thromboxane precursors; they have analgesic, antipyretic, and antiinflammatory actions. **orphan d.,** one that has limited commercial appeal because of the rarity of the condition it is used to treat. **psychoactive d., psychotropic d.,** see under *substance.*

drug·gist (drug'ist) pharmacist.

drum (drum) tympanic membrane.

drum·stick (-stik) a nuclear lobule attached by a slender strand to the nucleus of some polymorphonuclear leukocytes of normal females but not of normal males.

drunk·en·ness (drung'ken-nes) inebriation. **sleep d.,** prolonged transition from sleep to waking, with partial alertness, disorientation, drowsiness, poor coordination, and sometimes excited or violent behavior.

dru·sen (droo'zen) [Ger.] 1. hyaline excrescences in Bruch's membrane of the eye, usually due to aging. 2. rosettes of granules occurring in the lesions of actinomycosis.

DSM *Diagnostic and Statistical Manual of Mental Disorders.*

DT diphtheria and tetanus toxoids, pediatric use; see *diphtheria toxoid,* under *toxoid.*

DTaP diphtheria and tetanus toxoids and acellular pertussis vaccine.

DTP diphtheria and tetanus toxoids and pertussis vaccine.

DTPA diethylenetriamine pentaacetic acid; see *pentetic acid.*

DUB dysfunctional uterine bleeding.

duct (dukt) a passage with well-defined walls, especially a tubular structure for the passage of excretions or secretions. **duc'tal,** adj. **aberrant d.,** any duct that is not usually present or that takes an unusual course or direction. **alveolar d's,** small passages connecting the respiratory bronchioles and alveolar sacs. **Bartholin's d.,** the larger of the sublingual ducts, which opens into the submandibular duct. **Bellini's d.,** papillary d. **bile d.,** 1. any of the passages that convey bile in and from the liver. 2. common bile d. **biliary d.,** bile d. **branchial d's,** the drawn-out branchial grooves which open into the temporary cervical sinus of the embryo. **cochlear d.,** a spiral tube in the bony canal of the cochlea, divided into the scala tympani and scala vestibuli by the lamina spiralis. **common bile d.,** the duct formed by the union of the cystic and hepatic ducts. **d's of Cuvier,** two short venous trunks in the fetus opening into the atrium of the heart; the right one becomes the superior vena cava. **cystic d.,** the passage connecting the gallbladder neck and the common bile duct. **deferent d.,** ductus deferens. **efferent d.,** any duct which gives outlet to a glandular secretion. **ejaculatory d.,** the duct formed by union of the ductus deferens and the duct of the seminal vesicle, opening into the prostatic urethra on the colliculus seminalis. **endolymphatic d.,** a canal connecting the membranous labyrinth of the ear with the endolymphatic sac. **d. of epididymis,** the single tube into which the coiled ends of the efferent ductules of the testis open; its convolutions make up most of the epididymis. **excretory d.,** one that is merely conductive and not secretory. **genital d.,** see under *canal.* **hepatic d.,** the excretory duct of the liver (*common hepatic d.*), or one of its branches in the lobes of the liver (*left* and *right hepatic d's*). **interlobular d's,** channels between different lobules of a gland. **lacrimal d.,** see under *canaliculus.* **lactiferous d's,** ducts conveying the milk secreted by the mammary lobes to and through the nipples. **Luschka's d's,** tubular structures in the wall of the gallbladder; some are connected with bile ducts, but none with the lumen of the gallbladder. **lymphatic d's,** channels for conducting lymph. **lymphatic d., left,** thoracic d. **lymphatic d., right,** a vessel draining lymph from the upper right side of the body, receiving lymph from the right subclavian, jugular, and mediastinal trunks when those vessels do not open independently into the right brachiocephalic vein. **mesonephric d.,** an embryonic duct of the mesonephros, which in the male develops into the epididymis, ductus deferens and its ampulla, seminal vesicles, and ejaculatory duct and in the female is largely obliterated. **d. of Müller, müllerian d.,** paramesonephric d. **nasolacrimal d.,** the canal conveying the tears from the lacrimal sac to the inferior meatus of the nose. **omphalomesenteric d.,** yolk stalk. **pancreatic d.,** the main excretory duct of the pancreas, which usually unites with the common bile duct before entering the duodenum. **papillary d.,** a wide terminal tubule in the renal pyramid, formed by union of several straight collecting tubules and emptying into the renal pelvis. **paramesonephric d.,** either of the paired embryonic ducts developing into the uterine tubes, uterus, and vagina in the female and becoming largely obliterated in the male. **paraurethral d's of female urethra,** inconstantly present ducts in the female, which drain a group of the urethral glands into the vestibule. **paraurethral d's of male urethra,** the ducts of the urethral glands situated in the spongy portion of the male urethra. **parotid d.,** the duct by which the parotid gland empties into the mouth. **perilymphatic d.,** cochlear aqueduct. **pronephric d.,** the duct of the pronephros, which later serves as the mesonephric duct. **d's of prostate gland, prostatic d's,** see under *ductule*. **d's of Rivinus,** the small sublingual ducts which open into the mouth on the sublingual fold. **d. of Santorini,** a small inconstant duct draining a part of the head of the pancreas into the minor duodenal papilla. **secretory d.,** a smaller duct that is tributary to an excretory duct of a gland and that also has a secretory function. **semicircular d's,** the long ducts of the membranous labyrinth of the ear. **seminal d's,** the passages for conveyance of spermatozoa and semen. **spermatic d.,** ductus deferens. **d. of Steno, Stensen's d.,** parotid d. **submandibular d., submaxillary d. of Wharton,** the duct that drains the submandibular gland and opens at the sublingual caruncle. **tear d's,** the ducts conveying the secretion of the lacrimal glands. **thoracic d.,** the canal that ascends from the cisterna chyli to the junction of the left subclavian and left internal jugular veins. **thyroglossal d., thyrolingual d.,** an embryonic duct extending between the thyroid primordium and the posterior tongue. **urogenital d's,** the paramesonephric

and mesonephric ducts. **Wharton's d.,** submandibular d. **d. of Wirsung,** pancreatic d. **wolffian d.,** mesonephric d.

duc·tile (duk'til) susceptible of being drawn out without breaking.

duc·tion (duk'shun) in ophthalmology, the rotation of an eye by the extraocular muscles around its horizontal, vertical, or anteroposterior axis.

duct·ule (duk'tūl) a minute duct. **alveolar d's,** see under *duct*. **bile d's,** 1. the small channels that connect the interlobular ductules with the right and left hepatic ducts. 2. cholangioles. **interlobular d's,** small channels between the hepatic lobules, draining into the bile ductules. **d's of prostate,** ducts from the prostate, opening into or near the prostatic sinuses on the posterior urethra.

duc·tu·lus (duk'tu-lus) pl. *duc'tuli.* [L.] ductule.

duc·tus (duk'tus) pl. *duc'tus.* [L.] duct. **d. arterio'sus,** a fetal blood vessel that joins the descending aorta and left pulmonary artery. **d. chole'dochus,** common bile duct. **d. de'ferens,** the excretory duct of the testis which joins the excretory duct of the seminal vesicle to form the ejaculatory duct. **patent d. arteriosus (PDA),** abnormal persistence of an open lumen in the ductus arteriosus after birth, flow being from the aorta to the pulmonary artery and thus recirculating arterial blood through the lungs. **d. veno'sus,** a major blood channel that develops through the embryonic liver from the left umbilical vein to the inferior vena cava.

dull (dul) not resonant on percussion.

dull·ness (dul'nes) diminished resonance on percussion; also a peculiar percussion sound which lacks the normal resonance.

dump·ing (dump'ing) see under *syndrome*.

du·o·de·nal (doo"o-de'n'l, doo-od'ah-n'l) of or pertaining to the duodenum.

du·o·de·nec·to·my (doo"o-dĕ-nek'tah-me) excision of the duodenum, total or partial.

du·o·de·ni·tis (doo-od"ĕ-ni'tis) inflammation of the duodenal mucosa.

du·o·de·no·cho·led·o·chot·o·my (doo"o-de"no-ko-led"o-kot'ah-me) incision of the duodenum and common bile duct.

du·o·de·no·en·ter·os·to·my (-en"ter-os'tah-me) anastomosis of the duodenum to some other part of the small intestine.

du·o·de·no·gas·tric (-gas'trik) going from the duodenum to the stomach.

du·o·de·no·gram (doo-o-de'no-gram) a radiograph of the duodenum.

du·o·de·no·he·pat·ic (doo-o-de"no-hĕ-pat'ik) pertaining to the duodenum and liver.

du·o·de·no·je·ju·nal (-jĕ-joo′n′l) pertaining to the duodenum and the jejunum.

du·o·de·no·je·ju·nos·to·my (-jĕ″joo-nos′-tah-me) anastomosis of the duodenum to the jejunum.

du·o·de·no·scope (doo″o-de′no-skōp) an endoscope for examining the duodenum.

du·o·de·nos·to·my (doo″o-dĕ-nos′tah-me) surgical formation of a permanent opening into the duodenum.

du·o·de·num (doo″o-de′num) the first or proximal portion of the small intestine, extending from the pylorus to the jejunum. **duode′nal**, adj.

du·pli·ca·tion (doo-plĭ-ka′shun) 1. the act or process of doubling, or the state of being doubled. 2. in genetics, the presence in the genome of additional genetic material (a chromosome or segment thereof, a gene or part thereof). 3. abnormal doubling of a part.

dupp (dup) a syllable used to represent the second heart sound in auscultation.

du·ral (dūr′l) pertaining to the dura mater.

du·ra ma·ter (doo′rah ma′ter) the outermost, toughest of the three meninges (membranes) of the brain and spinal cord.

dur·ap·a·tite (door-ap′ah-tīt) a crystalline form of hydroxyapatite used as a prosthetic aid.

du·ro·ar·ach·ni·tis (doo″ro-ar″ak-ni′tis) inflammation of the dura mater and arachnoid.

DVM Doctor of Veterinary Medicine.

dwarf (dworf) an abnormally short person. **dwarf′ish**, adj. **achondroplastic d.**, one with achondroplasia and a large head with saddle nose and brachycephaly, short limbs, and usually lordosis. **Amsterdam d.**, one with de Lange's syndrome. **ateliotic d.**, one with infantile skeleton, with persistent nonunion between epiphyses and diaphyses. **hypophysial d.**, pituitary d. **Laron d.**, one whose skeletal growth retardation is from impaired ability to synthesize insulin-like growth factor I, usually due to growth hormone receptor defects. **normal d., physiologic d.**, a person who is unusually short but not deformed. **pituitary d.**, a dwarf with hypophysial infantilism. **rachitic d.**, a person dwarfed by rickets, having a high forehead with prominent bosses, bent long bones, and Harrison's groove. **renal d.**, one whose failure to achieve normal bone maturation is due to renal failure. **true d.**, normal d.

dwarf·ism (dworf′izm) the state of being a dwarf.

Dy dysprosium.

dy·ad (di′ad) a double chromosome resulting from the halving of a tetrad.

dy·clo·nine (di′klo-nēn) a bactericidal and fungicidal local anesthetic, used topically as the hydrochloride salt.

dye (di) any colored substance containing auxochromes and thus capable of coloring substances to which it is applied; used for staining and coloring, as a test reagent, and as a therapeutic agent. **acid d., acidic d.**, one which is acidic in reaction and usually unites with positively charged ions of the material acted upon. **amphoteric d.**, one containing both reactive basic and reactive acidic groups, and staining both acidic and basic elements. **anionic d.**, acid d. **basic d.**, one which is basic in reaction and unites with negatively charged ions of the material acted upon. **cationic d.**, basic d.

dy·nam·ic (di-nam′ik) 1. pertaining to or manifesting force. 2. of or relating to energy or to objects in motion. 3. characterized by or tending to produce change.

dy·nam·ics (di-nam′iks) the scientific study of forces in action; a phase of mechanics.

dy·na·mom·e·ter (di″nah-mom′ĕ-ter) an instrument for measuring the force of muscular contraction.

dyne (dīn) a unit of force; the amount that when acting continuously upon a mass of 1 g will impart to it an acceleration of 1 cm per second per second; equal to 10^{-5} newton.

dy·ne·in (di′nēn) an ATP-splitting enzyme essential to the motility of cilia and flagella because of its interactions with microtubules.

dy·nor·phin (di-nor′fin) any of a family of opioid peptides found throughout the central and peripheral nervous systems; most are agonists at opioid receptor sites. Some are probably involved in pain regulation and others in the hypothalamic regulation of eating and drinking.

dy·phyl·line (di′fil-in) a derivative of theophylline used as a bronchodilator in the treatment of asthma, chronic bronchitis, and emphysema.

dys- prefix [Gr.], *bad; difficult; disordered.*

dys·acu·sis (dis″ah-koo′sis) 1. a hearing impairment in which the loss is not measurable in decibels, but in disturbances in discrimination of speech or tone quality, pitch, or loudness, etc. 2. a condition in which sounds produce discomfort.

dys·aphia (dis-a′fe-ah) paraphia.

dys·ar·te·ri·ot·o·ny (dis″ahr-tēr″e-ot′ah-ne) abnormality of blood pressure.

dys·ar·thria (dis-ahr′thre-ah) a speech disorder caused by disturbances of muscular control because of damage to the central or peripheral nervous system.

dys·ar·thro·sis (dis″ahr-thro′sis) 1. deformity or malformation of a joint. 2. dysarthria.

dys·au·to·no·mia (-aw-to-no′me-ah) malfunction of the autonomic nervous system. **familial d.,** an inherited disorder of childhood characterized by defective lacrimation, skin blotching, emotional instability, motor incoordination, absence of pain sensation, and hyporeflexia; occurring almost exclusively in Ashkenazi Jews.

dys·bar·ism (dis′bar-izm) any clinical syndrome due to difference between the surrounding atmospheric pressure and the total gas pressure in the tissues, fluids, and cavities of the body.

dys·ba·sia (dis-ba′zhah) difficulty in walking, especially that due to nervous lesion.

dys·be·ta·lipo·pro·tein·emia (-ba″tah-lip″o-pro″te-ne′me-ah) 1. the accumulation of abnormal β-lipoproteins in the blood. 2. familial dysbetalipoproteinemia. **familial d.,** an inherited disorder of lipoprotein metabolism caused by interaction of a defect in apolipoprotein E with genetic and environmental factors causing hypertriglyceridemia; its phenotype is that of a type III hyperlipoproteinemia.

dys·ceph·a·ly (-sef′ah-le) malformation of the cranial and facial bones.

dys·che·zia (-ke′zhah) difficult or painful defecation.

dys·chi·ria (-ki′re-ah) loss of power to tell which side of the body has been touched.

dys·chon·dro·pla·sia (dis″kon-dro-pla′-zhah) 1. enchondromatosis. 2. formerly, a general term encompassing both enchondromatosis and exostosis, which has caused their synonyms to become tangled.

dys·chro·ma·top·sia (-kro-mah-top′se-ah) disorder of color vision.

dys·chro·mia (dis-kro′me-ah) any disorder of pigmentation of skin or hair.

dys·con·trol (dis″kon-trōl′) inability to control one's behavior; see also under *syndrome.*

dys·co·ria (-kor′e-ah) abnormality in the form or shape of the pupil or in the reaction of the two pupils.

dys·cra·sia (-kra′zhah) [Gr.] a term formerly used to indicate an abnormal mixture of the four humors; in surviving usages it is now roughly synonymous with disease or pathologic condition. **plasma cell d's,** a diverse group of neoplastic diseases involving proliferation of a single clone of cells producing a serum M component (a monoclonal immunoglobulin or immunoglobulin fragment) and usually having a plasma cell morphology; it includes multiple myeloma and heavy chain diseases.

dys·ejac·u·la·tion (-e-jak″u-la′shun) 1. any failure of normal ejaculation of semen. 2. a painful, burning sensation in the groin during semen ejaculation.

dys·em·bry·o·ma (dis″em-bre-o′mah) teratoma.

dys·en·tery (dis′en-ter″e) any of a number of disorders marked by inflammation of the intestine, especially of the colon, with abdominal pain, tenesmus, and frequent stools containing blood and mucus. **dysenter′ic,** adj. **amebic d.,** amebic colitis. **bacillary d.,** dysentery caused by *Shigella.* **viral d.,** dysentery caused by a virus, occurring in epidemics and marked by acute watery diarrhea.

dys·equi·lib·ri·um (dis-e″kwi-lib′re-um) 1. any derangement of the sense of equilibrium; see also *dizziness* and *vertigo.* 2. disturbance of a state of equilibrium. Spelled also *disequilibrium.*

dys·er·gia (dis-er′jah) motor incoordination due to defect of efferent nerve impulse.

dys·es·the·sia (dis″es-the′zhah) 1. distortion of any sense, especially of the sense of touch. 2. an unpleasant abnormal sensation produced by normal stimuli. **dysesthet′ic,** adj. **auditory d.,** dysacusis (2).

dys·fi·brin·o·ge·ne·mia (dis-fi-brin″o-jĕ-ne′me-ah) the presence in the blood of abnormal fibrinogen.

dys·func·tion (dis-funk′shun) disturbance, impairment, or abnormality of functioning of an organ. **dysfunc′tional,** adj. **erectile d.,** impotence (2). **minimal brain d.,** former name for *attention-deficit/hyperactivity disorder.* **sexual d.,** any of a group of sexual disorders characterized by disturbance either of sexual desire or of the psychophysiological changes that usually characterize sexual response.

dys·gam·ma·glob·u·lin·emia (-gam″ah-glob″u-lin-e′me-ah) an immunological deficiency state marked by selective deficiencies of one or more, but not all, classes of immunoglobulins. **dysgammaglobuline′mic,** adj.

dys·gen·e·sis (-jen′ĕ-sis) defective development; malformation. **gonadal d.,** defective development of the gonads, which may be accompanied by abnormalities of the sex chromosomes; sometimes used specifically to denote Turner's syndrome.

dys·ger·mi·no·ma (-jer″mĭ-no′mah) a malignant ovarian neoplasm, thought to be derived from primordial germ cells of the sexually undifferentiated embryonic gonad; it is the counterpart of the classical testicular seminoma.

dys·geu·sia (-goo′zhah) parageusia.

dys·gna·thia (-na′the-ah) any oral abnormality extending beyond the teeth to involve the maxilla or mandible, or both. **dysgnath′ic,** adj.

dys·graph·ia (-graf′e-ah) difficulty in writing; cf. *agraphia.*

dys·he·ma·to·poi·e·sis (-he″mah-to-poi-e′sis) defective blood formation. **dyshematopoiet′ic,** adj.

dys·he·sion (-he′zhun) 1. disordered cell adherence. 2. loss of intercellular cohesion; a characteristic of malignancy.

dys·hi·dro·sis (dis″hĭ-dro′sis) 1. pompholyx. 2. any disorder of eccrine sweat glands.

dys·kary·o·sis (-kar″e-o′sis) abnormality of the nucleus of a cell. **dyskaryot′ic,** adj.

dys·ker·a·to·ma (-ker-ah-to′mah) a dyskeratotic tumor. **warty d.,** a solitary brownish red nodule with a soft, yellowish, central keratotic plug, occurring on the face, neck, scalp, or axilla, or in the mouth; histologically it resembles an individual lesion of keratosis follicularis.

dys·ker·a·to·sis (-ker-ah-to′sis) abnormal, premature, or imperfect keratinization of the keratinocytes. **dyskeratot′ic,** adj.

dys·ki·ne·sia (-kĭ-ne′zhah) distortion or impairment of voluntary movement, as in tic or spasm. **dyskinet′ic,** adj. **biliary d.,** derangement of the filling and emptying mechanism of the gallbladder. **d. inter·mit′tens,** intermittent disability of the limbs due to impaired circulation. **orofacial d.,** facial movements resembling those of tardive dyskinesia, seen in elderly, edentulous, demented patients. **primary ciliary d.,** any of a group of hereditary syndromes characterized by delayed or absent mucociliary clearance from the airways, often accompanied by lack of motion of sperm. **tardive d.,** an iatrogenic disorder of involuntary repetitive movements of facial, buccal, oral, and cervical muscles, induced by long-term use of antipsychotic agents, sometimes persisting after withdrawal of the agent.

dys·la·lia (dis-la′le-ah) paralalia.

dys·lex·ia (-lek′se-ah) impairment of ability to read, spell, and write words, despite the ability to see and recognize letters. **dyslex′ic,** adj.

dys·lip·id·e·mia (-lip″id-e′me-ah) abnormality in, or abnormal amounts of, lipids and lipoproteins in the blood.

dys·lipo·pro·tein·emia (-lip″o-pro″te-ne′me-ah) the presence of abnormal concentrations of lipoproteins or abnormal lipoproteins in the blood.

dys·ma·tur·i·ty (dis″mah-choor′it-e) 1. disordered development. 2. postmaturity syndrome. **dysmature′,** adj. **pulmonary d.,** Wilson-Mikity syndrome.

dys·me·lia (dis-mel′e-ah) anomaly of a limb or limbs resulting from a disturbance in embryonic development.

dys·men·or·rhea (dis″men-or-e′ah) painful menstruation. **dysmenorrhe′al, dysmenorrhe′ic,** adj. **primary d.,** that not associated with pelvic pathology; usually beginning in adolescence. **secondary d.,** that associated with pelvic pathology; usually beginning after 20 years of age.

dys·me·tab·o·lism (-mě-tab′o-lizm) defective metabolism.

dys·me·tria (dis-me′tre-ah) disturbance of the power to control the range of movement in muscular action.

dys·mor·phism (-mor′fizm) 1. an abnormality in morphologic development. **dysmor′phic,** adj. 2. allomorphism. 3. ability to appear in different morphological forms.

dys·my·elin·a·tion (dis-mi″ě-lin-a′shun) breakdown or defective formation of a myelin sheath, usually involving biochemical abnormalities.

dys·odon·ti·a·sis (dis″-o-don-ti′ah-sis) defective, delayed, or difficult eruption of the teeth.

dys·on·to·gen·e·sis (-on-to-jen′ě-sis) defective embryonic development. **dysontogenet′ic,** adj.

dys·orex·ia (-o-rek′se-ah) impaired or deranged appetite.

dys·os·teo·gen·e·sis (dis-os″te-o-jen′ě-sis) defective bone formation; dysostosis.

dys·os·to·sis (dis″os-to′sis) defective ossification; defect in the normal ossification of fetal cartilages. **cleidocranial d.,** a hereditary condition marked by defective ossification of the cranial bones, absence of the clavicles, and dental and vertebral anomalies. **craniofacial d.,** a hereditary condition marked by acrocephaly, exophthalmos, hypertelorism, strabismus, parrot-beaked nose, and hypoplastic maxilla. **mandibulofacial d.,** a hereditary disorder occurring in a complete form *(Franceschetti syndrome)* and a less severe form *(Treacher Collins syndrome),* with antimongoloid slant of the palpebral fissures, coloboma of the lower lid, micrognathia and hypoplasia of the zygomatic arches, and microtia. **metaphyseal d.,** a skeletal abnormality in which the epiphyses are normal and the metaphyseal tissues are replaced by masses of cartilage, producing interference with enchondral bone formation. **d. mul′tiplex,** Hurler's syndrome. **orodigitofacial d.,** orofaciodigital syndrome.

dys·pa·reu·nia (-pah-roo'ne-ah) difficult or painful sexual intercourse.

dys·pep·sia (dis-pep'se-ah) impairment of the power or function of digestion; usually applied to epigastric discomfort after meals. **dyspep'tic,** adj. **nonulcer d.,** dyspepsia with symptoms that resemble those of peptic ulcer, although no ulcer is detectable.

dys·pha·gia (-fa'jah) difficulty in swallowing.

dys·pha·sia (-fa'zhah) impairment of speech, consisting in lack of coordination and failure to arrange words in their proper order; due to a central lesion.

dys·pho·nia (-fo'ne-ah) a voice impairment or speech disorder. **dysphon'ic,** adj.

dys·pho·ria (-for'e-ah) [Gr.] disquiet; restlessness; malaise. **dysphoret'ic, dysphor'ic,** adj. **gender d.,** unhappiness with one's biological sex or its usual gender role, with the desire for the body and role of the opposite sex.

dys·pig·men·ta·tion (dis-pig″-men-ta'shun) a disorder of pigmentation of skin or hair.

dys·pla·sia (dis-pla'zhah) 1. abnormality of development. 2. in pathology, alteration in size, shape, and organization of adult cells. **dysplas'tic,** adj. **anhidrotic ectodermal d.,** an inherited disorder characterized by ectodermal dysplasia associated with aplasia or hypoplasia of the sweat glands, hypothermia, alopecia, anodontia, conical teeth, and facial abnormalities. **anteroposterior facial d.,** defective development resulting in abnormal anteroposterior relations of the maxilla and mandible to each other or to the cranial base. **arrhythmogenic right ventricular d.,** a congenital cardiomyopathy in which transmural infiltration of adipose tissue results in weakness and bulging of regions of the right ventricle and leads to ventricular tachycardia arising in the right ventricle. **bronchopulmonary d.,** a chronic lung disease of infants, possibly related to oxygen toxicity or barotrauma, characterized by bronchiolar metaplasia and interstitial fibrosis. **chondroectodermal d.,** achondroplasia with defective development of skin, hair, and teeth, polydactyly, and defect of cardiac septum. **cretinoid d.,** a developmental abnormality characteristic of cretinism, consisting of retarded ossification and smallness of the internal and sexual organs. **developmental d. of the hip (DDH),** instability of the hip joint leading to dislocation in the neonatal period; it may be associated with various neuromuscular disorders or occur in utero but occurs most commonly in neurologically normal infants and is multifactorial in origin. Formerly called *congenital dislocation of the hip.*

diaphyseal d., thickening of the cortex of the midshaft area of the long bones, progressing toward the epiphyses, and sometimes also in the flat bones. **ectodermal d.,** any of a group of hereditary disorders involving tissues and structures derived from embryonic ectoderm, including anhidrotic ectodermal dysplasia, hidrotic ectodermal dysplasia, and EEC syndrome. **epiphyseal d.,** faulty growth and ossification of the epiphyses with radiographically apparent stippling and decreased stature, not associated with thyroid disease. **fibromuscular d.,** dysplasia with fibrosis of the muscular layer of an artery wall, with collagen deposition and hyperplasia of smooth muscle, causing stenosis and hypertension; seen most often in renal arteries, it is a major cause of renovascular hypertension. **fibrous d. of bone,** thinning of the cortex of bone and replacement of bone marrow by gritty fibrous tissue containing bony spicules, causing pain, disability, and gradually increasing deformity; only one bone may be involved (*monostotic fibrous d.*), with the process later affecting several or many bones (*polyostotic fibrous d.*). **florid osseous d.,** an exuberant form of periapical cemental dysplasia resembling diffuse sclerosing osteomyelitis but not inflammatory. **hidrotic ectodermal d.,** an inherited disorder of ectodermal dysplasia with tooth abnormalities, hypotrichosis, cutaneous hyperpigmentation over joints, and hyperkeratosis of the palms and soles. **metaphyseal d.,** a disturbance in enchondral bone growth, failure of modeling causing the ends of the shafts to remain larger than normal in circumference. **oculodentodigital d.,** a rare autosomal dominant condition, characterized by bilateral microphthalmos, abnormally small nose with anteverted nostrils, hypotrichosis, dental anomalies, camptodactyly, syndactyly, and missing phalanges of the toes. **periapical cemental d.,** a nonneoplastic condition characterized by formation of areas of fibrous connective tissue, bone, and cementum around the apex of a tooth. **septo-optic d.,** a syndrome of hypoplasia of the optic disk with other ocular abnormalities, absence of the septum pellucidum, and hypopituitarism leading to growth deficiency. **spondyloepiphyseal d.,** hereditary dysplasia of the vertebrae and extremities resulting in dwarfism of the short-trunk type, often with shortened limbs due to epiphyseal abnormalities. **thanatophoric d.,** a uniformly fatal type of skeletal dysplasia presenting as extreme shortness of the limbs, thoracic cage deformity, and relative enlargement of the head.

dysp·nea (disp-ne´ah) labored or difficult breathing. **dyspne´ic,** adj. **paroxysmal nocturnal d.,** respiratory distress that awakens patients from sleep, related to posture (especially reclining at night), attributed to congestive heart failure with pulmonary edema or sometimes to chronic pulmonary disease.

dys·prax·ia (dis-prak´se-ah) partial loss of ability to perform coordinated acts.

dys·pro·si·um (Dy) (-pro´ze-um) chemical element (see *Table of Elements*), at. no. 66.

dys·ra·phism (dis-raf´izm) [*dys-* + *raphe* + *-ia*] incomplete closure of a raphe; defective fusion, particularly of the neural tube. See also *neural tube defect.*

dys·rhyth·mia (dis-rith´me-ah) 1. disturbance of rhythm. 2. an abnormal cardiac rhythm; the term *arrhythmia* is usually used, even for abnormal but regular rhythms. **dysrhyth´mic,** adj. **cerebral d., electroencephalographic d.,** a disturbance or irregularity in the rhythm of the brain waves as recorded by electroencephalography.

dys·se·ba·cea (dis″se-ba´she-ah) disorder of sebaceous follicles; specifically, a condition seen (but not exclusively) in riboflavin deficiency, marked by greasy, branny seborrhea on the midface, with erythema in the nasal folds, canthi, or other skin folds.

dys·som·nia (dis-som´ne-ah) any of various disturbances in the quality, amount, or timing of sleep.

dys·sper·mia (-sper´me-ah) impairment of the spermatozoa, or of the semen.

dys·sta·sia (-sta´zhah) difficulty in standing. **dysstat´ic,** adj.

dys·syn·er·gia (dis″sin-er´je-ah) muscular incoordination. **d. cerebella´ris myoclo´nica,** dyssynergia cerebellaris progressiva associated with myoclonus epilepsy. **d. cerebella´ris progressi´va,** a condition marked by generalized intention tremors associated with disturbance of muscle tone and of muscular coordination; due to disorder of cerebellar function. **detrusor-sphincter d.,** contraction of the urethral sphincter muscle at the same time the detrusor muscle of the bladder is contracting, resulting in obstruction of normal urinary outflow; it may accompany detrusor hyperreflexia or instability.

dys·tax·ia (dis-tak´se-ah) difficulty in controlling voluntary movements.

dys·thy·mia (-thi´me-ah) dysthymic disorder.

dys·thy·mic (-thi´mik) characterized by symptoms of mild depression.

dys·thy·roid (dis-thi´roid) denoting defective functioning of the thyroid gland.

dys·to·cia (dis-to´se-ah) abnormal labor or childbirth.

dys·to·nia (-to´ne-ah) dyskinetic movements due to disordered tonicity of muscle. **dyston´ic,** adj. **d. musculo´rum defor´mans,** a hereditary disorder marked by involuntary, irregular, clonic contortions of the muscles of the trunk and limbs, which twist the body forward and sideways grotesquely.

dys·to·pia (-to´pe-ah) malposition; displacement.

dys·tro·phia (-tro´fe-ah) [Gr.] dystrophy. **d. adiposogenita´lis,** adiposogenital dystrophy. **d. epithelia´lis cor´neae,** dystrophy of the corneal epithelium, with erosions. **d. myoto´nica,** myotonic dystrophy. **d. un´guium,** changes in the texture, structure, and/or color of the nails due to no demonstrable cause, but presumed to be attributable to some disturbance of nutrition.

dys·tropho·neu·ro·sis (-trof″o-noor-o´sis) 1. any nervous disorder due to poor nutrition. 2. impairment of nutrition due to nervous disorder.

dys·tro·phy (dis´trof-e) any disorder due to defective or faulty nutrition. **dystroph´ic,** adj. **adiposogenital d.,** a condition marked by adiposity of the feminine type, genital hypoplasia, changes in secondary sex characters, and metabolic disturbances; seen with lesions of the hypothalamus. **Becker's muscular d., Becker type muscular d.,** a form closely resembling pseudohypertrophic muscular dystrophy but having a late onset and slowly progressive course; transmitted as an X-linked recessive trait. **Duchenne's d., Duchenne's muscular d., Duchenne type muscular d.,** the most common and severe type of pseudohypertrophic muscular dystrophy; it begins in early childhood, is chronic and progressive, and is characterized by increasing weakness in the pelvic and shoulder girdles, pseudohypertrophy of muscles followed by atrophy, lordosis, and a peculiar swinging gait with the legs kept wide apart. **Emery-Dreifuss muscular d.,** a rare X-linked form of muscular dystrophy beginning early in life and involving slowly progressive weakness of the upper arm and pelvic girdle muscles, with cardiomyopathy and flexion contractures of the elbows; muscles are not hypertrophied. **facioscapulohumeral muscular d.,** a relatively benign form of muscular dystrophy, with marked atrophy of the muscles of the face, shoulder girdle, and arm. **Fukuyama type congenital muscular d.,** a form of muscular dystrophy with muscle abnormalities resembling those of Duchenne's muscular dystrophy; characterized also by mental retardation with polymicrogyria and other cerebral abnormalities. **Landouzy d., Landouzy-Dejerine d., Landouzy-Dejerine muscular d.,** facioscapulohumeral muscular d. **Leyden-Möbius muscular d., limb-girdle muscular d.,** slowly progressive muscular dystrophy, usually beginning in childhood, marked by weakness and wasting in the pelvic girdle (*pelvifemoral muscular dystrophy*) or shoulder girdle (*scapulohumeral muscular dystrophy*). **muscular d.,** a group of genetically determined, painless, degenerative myopathies marked by muscular weakness and atrophy without nervous system involvement. The three main types are *pseudohypertrophic muscular d., facioscapulohumeral muscular d.,* and *limb-girdle muscular d.* **myotonic d.,** a rare, slowly progressive, hereditary disease, marked by myotonia followed by muscular atrophy (especially of the face and neck), cataracts, hypogonadism, frontal balding, and cardiac disorders. **oculopharyngeal d., oculopharyngeal muscular d.,** a form with onset in adulthood, characterized by weakness of the external ocular and pharyngeal muscles that causes ptosis, ophthalmoplegia, and dysphagia. **pseudohypertrophic muscular d.,** a group of muscular dystrophies characterized by enlargement (pseudohypertrophy) of muscles, most commonly *Duchenne's muscular d.* or *Becker's muscular d.* **reflex sympathetic d.,** a series of changes caused by the sympathetic nervous system, marked by pallor or rubor, pain, sweating, edema, or osteoporosis, following muscle, bone, nerve, or blood vessel trauma.

dys·uria (dis-u′re-ah) painful or difficult urination. **dysu′ric,** adj.

E

E emmetropia; enzyme; exa-.

E elastance; energy; electromotive force; illumination.

e- word element [L.], *away from, without, outside.*

ϵ (epsilon, the fifth letter of the Greek alphabet) heavy chain of IgE; the ϵ chain of hemoglobin.

ϵ- a prefix designating (1) the position of a substituting atom or group in a chemical compound; (2) fifth in a series of five or more related entities or chemical compounds.

EAC an abbreviation used in studies of complement, in which E represents erythrocyte, A antibody, and C complement.

ear (ēr) the organ of hearing and of equilibrium, consisting of the external ear, the middle ear, and the internal ear. See Plate 29. **Blainville e's,** asymmetry of the ears. **Cagot e.,** one without a lower lobe. **cauliflower e.,** a partially deformed auricle due to injury and subsequent perichondritis. **diabetic e.,** mastoiditis complicating diabetes. **external e.,** the pinna and external meatus together. **glue e.,** a chronic condition marked by a collection of fluid of high viscosity in the middle ear, due to obstruction of the eustachian tube. **inner e.,** the labyrinth; the vestibule, cochlea, and semicircular canals together. **middle e.,** the cavity in the temporal bone comprising the tympanic cavity, auditory ossicles, and auditory tube. **outer e.,** external e.

ear·wax (ēr′waks) cerumen.

eat·ing (ēt′ing) the act of ingestion. **binge e.,** uncontrolled ingestion of large quantities of food in a discrete interval, often with a sense of lack of control over the activity.

ebur·na·tion (e″ber-na′shun) conversion of bone into a hard, ivory-like mass.

EBV Epstein-Barr virus.

ecau·date (e-kaw′dāt) tail-less.

ec·bol·ic (ek-bol′ik) oxytocic.

ec·cen·tric (ek-sen′trik) situated or occurring or proceeding away from a center.

ec·cen·tro·chon·dro·pla·sia (ek-sen″tro-kon″dro-pla′zhah) Morquio's syndrome.

ec·chon·dro·ma (ek″on-dro′mah) pl. *ecchondromas, ecchondro′mata.* A hyperplastic growth of cartilaginous tissue on the surface of a cartilage or projecting under the periosteum of a bone.

ec·chy·mo·ma (ek″ĭ-mo′mah) swelling due to blood extravasation.

ec·chy·mo·sis (ek″ĭ-mo′sis) pl. *ecchymo′ses.* [Gr.] a small hemorrhagic spot in the skin or a mucous membrane, larger than a petechia, forming a nonelevated, rounded, or irregular blue or purplish patch. **ecchymot′ic,** adj.

ec·crine (ek′rin) exocrine, with special reference to ordinary sweat glands.

ec·cri·sis (ek'rĭ-sis) excretion of waste products.

ec·crit·ic (ek-rit'ik) 1. promoting excretion. 2. an agent that promotes excretion.

ec·cy·e·sis (ek"si-e'sis) ectopic pregnancy.

ECF-A eosinophil chemotactic factor of anaphylaxis; a primary mediator of Type I anaphylactic hypersensitivity.

ECG electrocardiogram.

ec·go·nine (ek'go-nin) the final basic product obtained by hydrolysis of cocaine and several related alkaloids; *e. methyl ester* is the major hydrolytic metabolite of cocaine detectable in blood by laboratory testing.

Echi·na·cea (ek"ĭ-na'shah) a genus of North American flowering herbs. *E. purpu'rea* is used for colds and respiratory and urinary tract infections and for wounds and burns. *E. pal'lida* root is used for fevers and colds. *E. angustifo'lia* is used in folk medicine.

Echi·no·coc·cus (e-ki"no-kok'us) a genus of small tapeworms, including *E. granulo'sus,* usually parasitic in dogs and wolves, whose larvae (hydatids) may develop in mammals, forming hydatid tumors or cysts chiefly in the liver; and *E. multilocula'ris,* whose larvae form alveolar or multilocular cysts and whose adult forms usually parasitize the fox and wild rodents, although humans are sporadically infected.

echi·no·coc·cus pl. *echinococ'ci.* An individual organism of the genus *Echinococcus.*

echi·no·cyte (e-ki'no-sīt) burr cell.

echo (ek'o) a repeated sound, produced by reverberation of sound waves; also, the reflection of ultrasonic, radio, and radar waves. **amphoric e.,** a resonant repetition heard on auscultation of the chest, at an interval after a vocal sound. **metallic e.,** a ringing repetition of heart sounds sometimes heard in patients with pneumopericardium or pneumothorax.

echo·acou·sia (ek"o-ah-koo'zhah) the subjective experience of hearing echoes after normally heard sounds.

echo·car·di·og·ra·phy (-kahr"de-og'rah-fe) recording of the position and motion of the heart walls or internal structures of the heart by the echo obtained from beams of ultrasonic waves directed through the chest wall. **color Doppler e.,** color flow Doppler imaging. **contrast e.,** that in which the ultrasonic beam detects tiny bubbles produced by intravascular injection of a liquid or a small amount of carbon dioxide gas. **Doppler e.,** a technique for recording the flow of red blood cells through the cardiovascular system by means of Doppler ultrasonography, either continuous wave or pulsed

wave. **M-mode e.,** that recording the amplitude and rate of motion (M) in real time, yielding a monodimensional ("icepick") view of the heart. **transesophageal e. (TEE),** the introduction of a transducer attached to a fiberoptic endoscope into the esophagus to provide two-dimensional cardiographic images or Doppler information.

echo·ge·nic·i·ty (-jĕ-nis'ĭ-te) in ultrasonography, the extent to which a structure gives rise to reflections of ultrasonic waves.

echo·graph·ia (o-graf'e-ah) agraphia in which the patient can copy writing but cannot write to express ideas.

echog·ra·phy (ĕ-kog'rah-fe) ultrasonography.

echo·ki·ne·sis (ek"o-kĭ-ne'sis) echopraxia.

echo·la·lia (ek"o-la'le-ah) stereotyped repetition of another person's words and phrases.

echo·lu·cent (-loo'sint) permitting the passage of ultrasonic waves without echoes, the representative areas appearing black on the sonogram.

echop·a·thy (ĕ-kop'ah-the) automatic repetition by a patient of words or movements of others; echolalia or echopraxia.

echo·pho·no·car·di·og·ra·phy (ek"o-fo"-no-kahr"de-og'rah-fe) the combined use of echocardiography and phonocardiography.

echo·prax·ia (-prak'se-ah) stereotyped imitation of the movements of others.

echo·rang·ing (-rānj'ing) in ultrasonography, determination of the position or depth of a body structure on the basis of the time interval between the moment an ultrasonic pulse is transmitted and the moment its echo is received.

echo·thi·o·phate (ek"o-thi'o-fāt) an anticholinesterase agent used topically as the iodide salt in the treatment of glaucoma and accommodative esotropia.

echo·vi·rus (ek'o-vi"rus) an enterovirus isolated from humans, separable into many serotypes, certain of which are associated with human disease, especially aseptic meningitis.

eclamp·sia (ĕ-klamp'se-ah) convulsions and coma, rarely coma alone, occurring in a pregnant or puerperal woman, and associated with hypertension, edema, and/or proteinuria. **eclamp'tic,** adj. **uremic e.,** that due to uremia.

eclamp·to·gen·ic (ĕ-klamp"to-jen'ik) causing convulsions.

ECMO extracorporeal membrane oxygenation.

econ·a·zole (ĕ-kon'ah-zōl) an imidazole derivative used as the nitrate salt as a broad-spectrum antifungal agent.

econ·o·my (e-kon′ah-me) the management of domestic affairs. **token e.,** in behavior therapy, a program of treatment in which the patient earns tokens, exchangeable for rewards, for appropriate personal and social behavior and loses tokens for antisocial behavior.

eco·tax·is (ek′o-tak″sis) the movement or "homing" of a circulating cell, e.g., a lymphocyte, to a specific anatomical compartment.

eco·tro·pic (e″ko-tro′pik) pertaining to a virus that infects and replicates in cells from only the original host species.

ECT electroconvulsive therapy.

ec·tad (ek′tad) directed outward.

ec·ta·sia (ek-ta′zhah) dilatation, expansion, or distention. **ectat′ic,** adj. **annuloaortic e.,** dilatation of the proximal aorta and the fibrous ring of the heart at the aortic orifice, marked by aortic regurgitation, and when severe by dissecting aneurysm; often associated with Marfan's syndrome. **mammary duct e.,** benign dilatation of the collecting ducts of the mammary gland, with inspissation of gland secretion and inflammatory changes in the tissues, usually during or after menopause.

ec·teth·moid (ek-teth′moid) ethmoidal labyrinth.

ec·thy·ma (ek-thi′mah) a shallowly ulcerative form of impetigo, chiefly on the shins or forearms.

ect(o)- word element [Gr.], *external; outside.*

ec·to·an·ti·gen (ek″to-ant′ĭ-jen) 1. an antigen that seems to be loosely attached to the outside of bacteria. 2. an antigen formed in the ectoplasm (cell membrane) of a bacterium.

ec·to·blast (ek′to-blast) 1. ectoderm. 2. an external membrane; a cell wall.

ec·to·car·dia (ek″to-kahr′de-ah) congenital displacement of the heart.

ec·to·cer·vix (-ser′viks) portio vaginalis cervicis. **ectocer′vical,** adj.

ec·to·derm (ek′to-derm) the outermost of the three primitive germ layers of the embryo; from it are derived the epidermis and epidermic tissues, such as the nails, hair, and glands of the skin, the nervous system, external sense organs and mucous membrane of the mouth and anus. **ectoder′mal, ectoder′mic,** adj.

ec·to·der·mo·sis (ek″to-der-mo′sis) a disorder based on congenital maldevelopment of organs derived from the ectoderm.

ec·to·en·zyme (-en′zīm) an extracellular enzyme.

ec·tog·e·nous (ek-toj′ĭ-nus) introduced from without; arising from causes outside the organism.

ec·to·mere (ek′to-mēr) one of the blastomeres taking part in formation of the ectoderm.

ec·to·mor·phy (-mor″fe) a type of body build in which tissues derived from the ectoderm predominate; relatively slight development of both visceral and body structures, the body being linear and delicate. **ectomor′phic,** adj.

ec·to·my (ek′tah-me) [Gr.] resection.

-ectomy word element [Gr.], *excision; surgical removal.*

ec·to·pia (ek-to′pe-ah) [Gr.] malposition, especially if congenital. **e. cor′dis,** congenital displacement of the heart outside the thoracic cavity. **e. len′tis,** abnormal position of the lens of the eye. **e. pupil′lae conge′nita,** congenital displacement of the pupil.

ec·top·ic (ek-top′ik) 1. pertaining to ectopia. 2. located away from normal position. 3. arising from an abnormal site or tissue.

ec·tos·te·al (ek-tos′te-il) pertaining to or situated outside of a bone.

ec·tos·to·sis (ek″to-sto′sis) ossification beneath the perichondrium of a cartilage or the periosteum of a bone.

ec·to·thrix (ek′to-thriks) a fungus that grows inside the shaft of a hair but produces a conspicuous external sheath of spores.

ectr(o)- word element [Gr.], *miscarriage; congenital absence.*

ec·tro·dac·ty·ly (ek″tro-dak′tĭ-le) congenital absence of a digit or part of a digit.

ec·trog·e·ny (ek-troj′ĕ-ne) congenital absence or defect of a part. **ectrogen′ic,** adj.

ec·tro·me·lia (ek″tro-me′le-ah) gross hypoplasia or aplasia of one or more long bones of one or more limbs. **ectromel′ic,** adj.

ec·tro·pi·on (ek-tro′pe-on) eversion or turning outward, as of the margin of an eyelid.

ec·tro·syn·dac·ty·ly (ek″tro-sin-dak′tĭ-le) a condition in which some digits are absent and those that remain are webbed.

ec·ze·ma (ek′zĕ-mah) a pruritic papulovesicular dermatitis characterized early by erythema, edema associated with a serous exudate in the epidermis and an inflammatory infiltrate in the dermis, oozing and vesiculation, and crusting and scaling; and later by lichenification, thickening, signs of excoriations, and altered pigmentation. **eczem′atous,** adj. **asteatotic e.,** xerotic e. **e. herpe′ticum,** Kaposi's varicelliform eruption due to infection with herpes simplex virus superimposed on a preexisting skin condition. **nummular e.,** that in which the patches are coin shaped; it may be a form of neurodermatitis. **xerotic e.,** erythema, dry scaling, fine cracking, and pruritus of the skin, occurring chiefly during the winter when low humidity in heated rooms causes excessive water loss from the stratum corneum.

ec·zem·a·toid (ek-zem′ah-toid) resembling eczema.

ED effective dose.

ED$_{50}$ median effective dose.

ede·ma (ĕ-de′mah) an abnormal accumulation of fluid in intercellular spaces of the body. **edem′atous,** adj. **angioneurotic e.,** angioedema. **cardiac e.,** a manifestation of congestive heart failure, due to increased venous and capillary pressures and often associated with renal sodium retention. **cytotoxic e.,** cerebral edema caused by hypoxic injury to brain tissue and decreased functioning of the cellular sodium pump so that the cellular elements accumulate fluid. **dependent e.,** edema in lower or dependent parts of the body. **e. neonato′rum,** a disease of premature and feeble infants resembling sclerema, marked by spreading edema with cold, livid skin. **pitting e.,** that in which pressure leaves a persistent depression in the tissues. **pulmonary e.,** diffuse edema in pulmonary tissues and air spaces due to changes in hydrostatic forces in capillaries or to increased capillary permeability, with intense dyspnea. **vasogenic e.,** cerebral edema in the area around tumors, often due to increased permeability of capillary endothelial cells.

ede·ma·gen (ĕ-de′mah-jen) an irritant that elicits edema by causing capillary damage but not the cellular response of true inflammation.

eden·tia (e-den′shah) absence of the teeth.

eden·tu·lous (-tu-lus) without teeth.

ed·e·tate (ed′ĕ-tāt) USAN contraction for ethylenediaminetetraacetate, a salt of ethylenediaminetetraacetic acid (EDTA); the salts include *e. calcium disodium,* used in the diagnosis and treatment of lead poisoning, and *e. disodium,* used in the treatment of hypercalcemia because of its affinity for calcium.

edet·ic ac·id (ĕ-det′ik) ethylenediaminetetraacetic acid.

edis·y·late (ĕ-dis′ĭ-lāt) USAN contraction for 1,2-ethanedisulfonate.

ed·ro·pho·ni·um (ed″ro-fo′ne-um) a cholinergic used in the form of the chloride salt as a curare antagonist and as a diagnostic agent in myasthenia gravis.

EDTA ethylenediaminetetraacetic acid.

EDV end-diastolic volume.

ed·u·ca·ble (ej′u-kah-b′l) capable of being educated; formerly used to refer to persons

with mild mental retardation (I.Q. approximately 50–70).

Ed·ward·si·el·la (ed-wahrd″se-el′ah) a genus of gram-negative, facultatively anaerobic bacteria of the family Enterobacteriaceae; an occasional opportunistic pathogen for humans, causing diarrhea.

EEE eastern equine encephalomyelitis.

EEG electroencephalogram.

EEJ electroejaculation.

EENT eye-ear-nose-throat.

ef·a·vi·renz (ef′ah-vi″renz) an antiretroviral, inhibiting reverse transcriptase; used in the treatment of HIV infection.

ef·face·ment (ĕ-fās′ment) the obliteration of features; said of the cervix during labor when it is so changed that only the external os remains.

ef·fect (ĕ-fekt′) the result produced by an action. **Anrep e.,** abrupt elevation of aortic pressure results in a positive inotropic effect, augmented resistance to outflow in the heart. **Bayliss e.,** increased perfusion pressure and subsequent stretch of vascular smooth muscle causes muscle contraction and increased resistance, which returns blood flow to normal in spite of the elevated perfusion pressure. **Bohr e.,** increase of carbon dioxide in blood causes decreased affinity of hemoglobin for oxygen. **Doppler e.,** the relationship of the apparent frequency of waves, as of sound, light, and radio waves, to the relative motion of the source of the waves and the observer, the frequency increasing as the two approach each other and decreasing as they move apart. **experimenter e's,** demand characteristics. **Haldane e.,** increased oxygenation of hemoglobin promotes dissociation of carbon dioxide. **position e.,** in genetics, the changed effect produced by alteration of the relative positions of various genes on the chromosomes. **pressure e.,** the sum of the changes that are due to obstruction of tissue drainage by pressure. **side e.,** a consequence other than that for which an agent is used, especially an adverse effect on another organ system. **Somogyi e.,** a rebound phenomenon occurring in diabetes: overtreatment with insulin induces hypoglycemia, which initiates the release of epinephrine, ACTH, glucagon, and growth hormone, which stimulate lipolysis, gluconeogenesis, and glycogenolysis, which, in turn, result in a rebound hyperglycemia and ketosis.

ef·fec·tive·ness (ĕ-fek′tiv-nes) 1. the ability to produce a specific result or to exert a specific measurable influence. 2. the ability of an intervention to produce the desired beneficial effect in actual usage. Cf. *efficacy*.

effec'tive, adj. **relative biological e.,** an expression of the effectiveness of other types of radiation in comparison with that of gamma or x-rays; abbreviated RBE.

ef·fec·tor (ĕ-fek'ter) 1. an agent that mediates a specific effect. 2. an organ that produces an effect in response to nerve stimulation. **allosteric e.,** an enzyme inhibitor or activator that has its effect at a site other than the catalytic site of the enzyme.

ef·fem·i·na·tion (ĕ-fem″ĭ-na'shun) feminization (2).

ef·fer·ent (ef'er-ent) 1. conveying away from a center. 2. something that so conducts, as an efferent nerve.

ef·fi·ca·cy (ef'ĭ-kah-se) 1. the ability of an intervention to produce the desired beneficial effect in expert hands and under ideal circumstances. 2. the ability of a drug to produce the desired therapeutic effect.

ef·fleu·rage (ef″loo-rahzh') [Fr.] a stroking movement in massage.

ef·flo·res·cent (ef″lŏ-res'ent) becoming powdery by losing the water of crystallization.

ef·flu·vi·um (ĕ-floo've-um) pl. *efflu'via*. [L.] 1. an outflowing or shedding, as of the hair. 2. an exhalation or emanation, especially one of noxious nature.

ef·fu·sion (ĕ-fu'zhun) 1. escape of a fluid into a part; exudation or transudation. 2. effused material; an exudate or transudate. **pleural e.,** fluid in the pleural space.

ef·lor·ni·thine (DMFO) (ef-lor'nĭ-thēn″) an inhibitor of the enzyme catalyzing the decarboxylation of ornithine; used topically as the hydrochloride salt to reduce unwanted facial hair in females.

eges·tion (e-jes'chun) the casting out of undigestible material.

egg (eg) ovum.

ego (e'go) that segment of the personality dominated by the reality principle, comprising integrative and executive aspects functioning to adapt the forces and pressures of the id and superego and the requirements of external reality by conscious perception, thought, and learning.

ego·ali·en (-āl'yen) ego-dystonic.

ego·bron·choph·o·ny (e″go-brong-kof'-ah-ne) egophony.

ego·cen·tric (-sen'trik) self-centered; preoccupied with one's own interests and needs; lacking concern for others.

ego·dys·ton·ic (e′go-dis-ton'ik) denoting aspects of a person's thoughts, impulses, and behavior that are felt to be repugnant, distressing, unacceptable, or inconsistent with the self-conception.

ego·ism (e'go-izm) 1. any of several ethical doctrines describing the relationship between morality, self-interest, and behavior. 2. excessive preoccupation with oneself, self-interest with disregard for the needs of others. 3. egotism.

ego·ma·nia (e″go-ma'ne-ah) extreme self-centeredness; extreme egotism.

egoph·o·ny (e-gof'ah-ne) increased resonance of voice sounds, with a high-pitched bleating quality, heard especially over lung tissue compressed by pleural effusion.

ego·syn·ton·ic (e′go-sin-ton'ik) denoting aspects of a person's thoughts, impulses, attitudes, and behavior that are felt to be acceptable and consistent with the self-conception.

ego·tism (e'go-tizm) 1. conceit, selfishness, self-centeredness, with an inflated sense of one's importance. 2. egoism (2).

EGTA egtazic acid; a chelator similar in structure and function to EDTA (ethylenediaminetetraacetic acid) but with a higher affinity for calcium than for magnesium.

Ehr·lich·ia (ār-lik'e-ah) a genus of the tribe Ehrlichieae transmitted by ticks and causing disease in dogs, cattle, sheep, horses, and humans, including the species *E. ca'nis*, *E. chaffeen'sis*, *E. e'qui*, and *E. sennet'su*.

Ehr·lich·i·eae (ār″lĭ-ki'e-e) a tribe of rickettsiae made up of organisms adapted for existence in invertebrates, chiefly arthropods, and pathogenic for certain mammals, including humans.

ehr·lich·i·osis (ār-lik″e-o'sis) a febrile illness due to infection with bacteria of the genus *Ehrlichia*. **human granulocytic e.,** a sometimes fatal human ehrlichiosis caused by an *Ehrlichia equi*–like species, characterized by flulike symptoms and involving predominantly neutrophils. **human monocytic e.,** a sometimes fatal human ehrlichiosis caused by *Ehrlichia chaffeensis*, characterized by flulike symptoms and involving predominantly fixed tissue mononuclear phagocytes.

ei·co·nom·e·ter (i″kah-nom'ĕ-ter) eikonometer.

ei·co·sa·pen·ta·eno·ic ac·id (EPA) (i-ko″sah-pen″tah-e-no'ik) an omega-3, polyunsaturated, 20-carbon fatty acid found almost exclusively in fish and marine animal oils.

ei·det·ic (i-det'ik) denoting exact visualization of events or objects previously seen; a person having such an ability.

ei·dop·tom·e·try (i″dop-tom'ĕ-tre) measurement of the acuteness of visual perception.

ei·ko·nom·e·ter (i″kah-nom'ĕ-ter) an instrument for measuring the degree of aniseikonia.

Ei·me·ria (i-mēr′e-ah) a genus of protozoa (order Eucoccidiida) found in the epithelial cells of humans and animals.

ein·stei·ni·um (Es) (īn-sti′ne-um) chemical element (see *Table of Elements*), at. no. 99.

EIT erythrocyte iron turnover.

ejac·u·late¹ (e-jak′u-lāt) to expel suddenly, especially semen.

ejac·u·late² (e-jak′u-lat) the semen discharged in a single ejaculation in the male, consisting of the secretions of Cowper's gland, epididymis, ductus deferens, seminal vesicles, and prostate, and containing the spermatozoa.

ejac·u·la·tio (e-jak″u-la′she-o) [L.] ejaculation. **e. prae′cox,** premature ejaculation.

ejac·u·la·tion (e-jak″u-la′shun) forcible, sudden expulsion; especially expulsion of semen from the male urethra. **ejac′ulatory,** adj. **premature e.,** that consistently occurring either prior to, upon, or immediately after penetration and before it is desired. **re-tarded e.,** male orgasmic disorder. **retrograde e.,** ejaculation in which semen travels up the urethra towards the bladder instead of to the outside of the body.

ejec·tion (e-jek′shun) 1. the act of casting out or the state of being cast out, as of excretions, secretions, or other bodily fluids. 2. something cast out. 3. the discharge of blood from the heart; see under *period.*

EKG electrocardiogram.

EKY electrokymography.

elab·o·ra·tion (ě-lab″ah-ra′shun) 1. the process of producing complex substances out of simpler materials. 2. in psychiatry, an unconscious mental process of expansion and embellishment of detail, especially of a symbol or representation in a dream.

el·a·pid (el′ah-pid) 1. any snake of the family Elapidae. 2. of or pertaining to the family Elapidae.

Elap·i·dae (e-lap′ĭ-de) a family of usually terrestrial, venomous snakes, which have cylindrical tails and front fangs that are short, stout, immovable, and grooved. It includes cobras, kraits, coral snakes, Australian copperheads, Australian blacksnakes, brown snakes, tiger snakes, death adders, and mambas.

elas·tance (e-las′tans) the quality of recoiling without disruption on removal of pressure, or an expression of the measure of the ability to do so in terms of unit of volume change per unit of pressure change. Symbol *E.* It is the reciprocal of compliance.

elas·tase (e-las′tās) see *pancreatic elastase.*

elas·tic (e-las′tik) able to resist and recover from stretching, compression, or distortion applied by a force.

elas·ti·cin (e-las′tĭ-sin) elastin.

elas·tin (e-las′tin) a yellow scleroprotein, the essential constituent of elastic connective tissue; it is brittle when dry, but when moist is flexible and elastic.

elast(o)- word element [L.], *flexibility; elastin; elastic tissue.*

elas·to·fi·bro·ma (e-las″to-fi-bro′mah) a rare, benign, firm, unencapsulated tumor consisting of abundant sclerotic collagen and thick irregular elastic fibers.

elas·tol·y·sis (e″las-tol′ĭ-sis) the digestion of elastic substance or tissue. **perifollicular e.,** see under *anetoderma.*

elas·to·ma (e″las-to′mah) a tumor or focal excess of elastic tissue fibers or abnormal collagen fibers of the skin.

elas·tom·e·try (e″las-tom′ě-tre) the measurement of elasticity.

elas·tor·rhex·is (e-las″to-rek′sis) rupture of fibers composing elastic tissue.

elas·to·sis (e″las-to′sis) 1. degeneration of elastic tissue. 2. degenerative changes in the dermal connective tissue with increased amounts of elastotic material. 3. any disturbance of the dermal connective tissue. **ac-tinic e.,** premature aging of the skin and degeneration of the elastic tissue of the dermis due to prolonged exposure to sunlight. **nodular e. of Favre and Racouchot,** actinic elastosis occurring chiefly in elderly men, with giant comedones, pilosebaceous cysts, and large folds of furrowed, yellowish skin in the periorbital region. **e. per′forans serpigino′sa, perforating e.,** an elastic tissue defect, occurring alone or in association with other disorders, including Down's syndrome and Ehlers-Danlos syndrome, in which elastomas are extruded through small keratotic papules in the epidermis; the lesions are usually arranged in arcuate serpiginous clusters on the sides of the nape, face, or arms.

elas·tot·ic (e″las-tot′ik) 1. pertaining to or characterized by elastosis. 2. resembling elastic tissue; having the staining properties of elastin.

ela·tion (ě-la′shun) emotional excitement marked by acceleration of mental and bodily activity, with extreme joy and an overly optimistic attitude.

el·bow (el′bo) 1. the bend of the arm; the region around the joint connecting the arm and forearm. 2. any angular bend. **little leaguer's e.,** medial epicondylitis of the elbow due to repeated stress on the flexor muscles of the forearm, often seen in adolescent ballplayers. **miners' e.,** enlargement of the bursa over the point of the elbow, due to resting the body weight on the elbow as in mining. **pulled e.,** subluxation of the head of the radius distally under the round ligament. **tennis e.,** a painful condition of the outer elbow, due to inflammation or irritation of the extensor tendon attachment of the lateral humeral epicondyle.

electro- word element [Gr.] *electricity.*

elec·tro·acous·tic (e-lek″tro-ah-ko͞os′tik) pertaining to the interaction or interconversion of electric and acoustic phenomena.

elec·tro·acu·punc·ture (-ak″u-punk′cher) acupuncture in which the needles are stimulated electrically. **e. after Voll (EAV),** a system of diagnosis and treatment based on the measurement of the electrical characteristics of acupoints, the results being used to determine a specific remedy.

elec·tro·an·al·ge·sia (-an″al-je′ze-ah) the reduction of pain by electrical stimulation of a peripheral nerve or the dorsal column of the spinal cord.

elec·tro·bi·ol·o·gy (-bi-ol′ah-je) the study of electric phenomena in living tissue.

elec·tro·car·dio·gram (-kahr′de-o-gram″) a graphic tracing of the variations in electrical potential caused by the excitation of the heart muscle and detected at the body surface. The normal electrocardiogram is a scalar representation that shows deflections resulting from cardiac activity as changes in the magnitude of voltage and polarity over time and comprises the P wave, QRS complex, and T and U waves. Abbreviated ECG or EKG. See also *electrogram.* **scalar e.,** see *electrocardiogram.*

elec·tro·car·di·og·ra·phy (-kahr″de-og′-rah-fe) the making of graphic records of the variations in electrical potential caused by electrical activity of the heart muscle and detected at the body surface, as a method for studying the action of the heart muscle. See also *electrocardiogram* and *electrogram.* **electrocardiograph′ic,** adj.

elec·tro·cau·tery (-kaw′ter-e) an apparatus for surgical dissection and hemostasis, using heat generated by a high-voltage, high-frequency alternating current passed through an electrode.

elec·tro·chem·i·cal (-kem′ĭ-k′l) pertaining to interaction or interconversion of chemical and electrical energies.

elec·tro·co·ag·u·la·tion (-ko-ag″ŭl-a′shun) coagulation of tissue by means of an electric current.

elec·tro·coch·le·og·ra·phy (-kok″le-og′-rah-fe) measurement of electrical potentials of the eighth cranial nerve in response to acoustic stimuli applied by an electrode to the external acoustic canal, promontory, or tympanic membrane. **electrococh′leographic,** adj.

elec·tro·con·trac·til·i·ty (-kon″trak-til′it-e) contractility in response to electrical stimulation.

elec·tro·con·vul·sive (-kun-vul′siv) inducing convulsions by means of electric shock.

elec·tro·cor·ti·cog·ra·phy (-kort″ĭ-kog′-rah-fe) electroencephalography with the electrodes applied directly to the cerebral cortex.

elec·trode (e-lek′trōd) a conductor or medium by which an electric current is conducted to or from any medium, such as a cell, body, solution, or apparatus. **active e.,** in electromyography, an exploring e. **calomel e.,** one capable of both collecting and giving up chloride ions in neutral or acidic aqueous media, consisting of mercury in contact with mercurous chloride; used as a reference electrode in pH measurements. **esophageal e., esophageal pill e.,** a pill electrode that lodges in the esophagus at the level of the atrium to obtain electrograms and deliver pacing stimuli. **exploring e.,** in electrodiagnosis, that placed nearest to the site of bioelectric activity being recorded, determining the potential in that localized area. **ground e.,** one that is connected to a ground. **indifferent e.,** reference e. **needle e.,** a thin, cylindrical electrode with an outer shaft beveled to a sharp point, enclosing a wire or series of wires. **patch e.,** a tiny electrode with a blunt tip that is used in studies of membrane potentials. **pill e.,** an electrode usually encased in a gelatin capsule and attached to a flexible wire so that it can be swallowed. **recording e.,** that used to measure electric potential change in body tissue; for recording, two electrodes must be used, the *exploring e.* and the *reference e.* **reference e.,** an electrode placed at a site remote from the source of recorded activity, so that its potential is assumed to be negligible or constant. **stimulating e.,** one used to apply electric current to tissue.

elec·tro·der·mal (e-lek″tro-der′m′l) pertaining to the electrical properties of the skin, especially to changes in its resistance.

elec·tro·des·ic·ca·tion (-des″ĭ-ka′shun) destruction of tissue by dehydration, done by means of a high-frequency electric current.

elec·tro·di·a·ly·zer (-di″ah-li′zer) a blood dialyzer utilizing an applied electric field and semipermeable membranes for separating the colloids from the solution.

elec·tro·ejac·u·la·tion (EEJ) (e-lek″tro-e-jak″u-la′shun) induction of ejaculation by application of a gradually increasing electrical current delivered through a probe inserted into the rectum.

elec·tro·en·ceph·a·lo·gram (EEG) (-en-sef'ah-lo-gram") a recording of the potentials on the skull generated by currents emanating spontaneously from nerve cells in the brain, with fluctuations in potential seen as waves.

elec·tro·en·ceph·a·log·ra·phy (-en-sef'-ah-log'rah-fe) the recording of changes in electric potential in various areas of the brain by means of electrodes placed on the scalp or on or in the brain itself. **electroencephalograph'ic,** adj.

elec·tro·fo·cus·ing (-fo'kus-ing) isoelectric focusing.

elec·tro·gas·trog·ra·phy (-gas-trog'rah-fe) the recording of the electrical activity of the stomach as measured between its lumen and the body surface. **electrogastrograph'ic,** adj.

elec·tro·gen·ic (-tro-jen'ik) pertaining to a process by which net charge is transferred to a different location so that hyperpolarization occurs.

elec·tro·gram (e-lek'tro-gram) any record produced by changes in electric potential. **esophageal e.,** one recorded by an esophageal electrode, for enhanced detection of P waves and elucidation of complex arrhythmias. **His bundle e. (HBE),** an intracardiac electrogram of potentials in the lower right atrium, atrioventricular node, and His-Purkinje system, obtained by positioning intracardiac electrodes near the tricuspid valve. **intracardiac e.,** a record of changes in the electric potentials of specific cardiac loci, as measured with electrodes placed within the heart via cardiac catheters; used for loci that cannot be assessed by body surface electrodes, such as the bundle of His or other regions within the cardiac conducting system.

elec·tro·gus·tom·e·try (e-lek"tro-gus-tom'e-tre) the testing of the sense of taste by application of galvanic stimuli to the tongue.

elec·tro·he·mos·ta·sis (-he"mos'-tah-sis) arrest of hemorrhage by electrocautery.

elec·tro·hys·ter·og·ra·phy (-his"ter-og'-rah-fe) recording of changes in electric potential associated with uterine contractions.

elec·tro·im·mu·no·dif·fu·sion (-im"u-no-dī-fu'zhun) immunodiffusion accelerated by application of an electric current.

elec·tro·ky·mog·ra·phy (-ki-mog'rah-fe) the photography on x-ray film of the motion of the heart or of other moving structures that can be visualized radiographically.

elec·trol·y·sis (e"lek-trol'ĭ-sis) destruction by passage of a galvanic current, as in disintegration of a chemical compound in solution or removal of excessive hair from the body.

elec·tro·lyte (e-lek'tro-līt) a substance that dissociates into ions when fused or in solution, thus becoming capable of conducting electricity. **amphoteric e.,** ampholyte; a compound containing at least one group that can act as a base and at least one that can act as an acid.

elec·tro·mag·net (e-lek"tro-mag'net) a temporary magnet made by passing electric current through a coil of wire surrounding a core of soft iron.

elec·tro·mag·net·ic (-mag-net'ik) involving both electricity and magnetism.

elec·tro·me·chan·i·cal (-mě-kan'ĭ-k'l) pertaining to interaction or interconversion of electrical and mechanical energies.

elec·tro·mo·tive (-mo'tiv) causing electric activity to be propagated along a conductor.

elec·tro·my·og·ra·phy (EMG) (-mi-og'-rah-fe) the recording and study of the electrical properties of skeletal muscle. **electromyograph'ic,** adj.

elec·tron (e-lek'tron) an elementary particle with the unit quantum of (negative) charge, constituting the negatively charged particles arranged in orbits around the nucleus of an atom and determining all of the atom's physical and chemical properties except mass and radioactivity. **electron'ic,** adj.

elec·tro·nar·co·sis (e-lek"tro-nahr-ko'sis) treatment of psychiatric disorders by passage of an electric current through the brain, similar to electroconvulsive therapy in the tonic phase but inducing no or limited convulsions.

elec·tron-dense (e-lek'tron-dens") in electron microscopy, having a density that prevents electrons from penetrating.

elec·tro·neg·a·tive (e-lek"tro-neg'it-iv) bearing a negative electric charge.

elec·tro·neg·a·tiv·i·ty (-neg"ah-tiv'ĭ-te) the relative power of an atom or molecule to attract electrons.

elec·tro·neu·rog·ra·phy (-noor-og'rah-fe) the measurement of the conduction velocity and latency of peripheral nerves.

elec·tro·neu·ro·my·og·ra·phy (-noor"o-mi-og'rah-fe) electromyography in which the nerve of the muscle under study is stimulated by application of an electric current.

elec·tro·nys·tag·mog·ra·phy (-nis"tag-mog'rah-fe) electroencephalographic recordings of eye movements that provide objective documentation of induced and spontaneous nystagmus.

elec·tro·oc·u·lo·gram (-ok'ūl-o-gram") the electroencephalographic tracings made while moving the eyes a constant distance between two fixation points, inducing a deflection of fairly constant amplitude; abbreviated EOG.

elec·tro·ol·fac·to·gram (-ol-fak'to-gram) a recording of electrical potential changes detected by an electrode placed on the surface of the olfactory mucosa as the mucosa is subjected to an odorous stimulus. Abbreviated EOG.

elec·tro·phile (e-lek'tro-fīl) an electron acceptor. **electrophil'ic,** adj.

elec·tro·pho·re·sis (e-lek″tro-fah-re'sis) the separation of ionic solutes based on differences in their rates of migration in an applied electric field. Support media include paper, starch, agarose gel, cellulose acetate, and polyacrylamide gel, and techniques include zone, disc (discontinuous), two-dimensional, and pulsed-field. **electrophoret'ic,** adj. counter e., counterimmunoelectrophoresis.

elec·tro·pho·reto·gram (-fō-ret'o-gram) the record produced on or in a supporting medium by bands of material that have been separated by the process of electrophoresis.

elec·tro·phren·ic (-fren'ik) pertaining to electrical stimulation of the phrenic nerve or diaphragm.

elec·tro·phys·i·ol·o·gy (-fiz″e-ol'ah-je) 1. the study of the mechanisms of production of electrical phenomena, particularly in the nervous system, and their consequences in the living organism. 2. the study of the effects of electricity on physiological phenomena.

elec·tro·pos·i·tive (e-lek″tro-poz'ĭ-tiv) bearing a positive electric charge.

elec·tro·ret·in·o·graph (-ret'ĭ-no-graf) an instrument to measure the electrical response of the retina to light stimulation; abbreviated ERG.

elec·tro·scis·sion (-sizh'un) cutting of tissue by means of electric cautery.

elec·tro·scope (e-lek'tro-skōp) an instrument for measuring radiation intensity.

elec·tro·shock (-shok) shock produced by applying electric current to the brain.

elec·tro·stat·ic (e-lek″tro-stat'ik) pertaining to static electricity.

elec·tro·stri·a·to·gram (-stri-āt'ah-gram) an electroencephalogram showing differences in electric potential recorded at various levels of the corpus striatum.

elec·tro·sur·gery (-ser'jer-e) surgery performed by electrical methods; the active electrode may be a needle, bulb, or disk. **electrosur'gical,** adj.

elec·tro·tax·is (-tak'sis) taxis in response to electric stimuli.

elec·tro·ther·a·py (-ther'ah-pe) treatment of disease by means of electricity.

elec·tro·ton·ic (-ton'ik) 1. pertaining to electrotonus. 2. denoting the direct spread of current in tissues by electrical conduction, without the generation of new current by action potentials.

elec·trot·o·nus (e-lek-trot'ah-nus) the altered electrical state of a nerve or muscle cell when a constant electric current is passed through it.

elec·tro·u·re·ter·og·ra·phy (e-lek″tro-u-re″ter-og'rah-fe) electromyography in which the action potentials produced by peristalsis of the ureter are recorded.

elec·tro·va·lence (-va'lens) 1. the number of charges an atom acquires by the gain or loss of electrons in forming an ionic bond. 2. the ionic bonding resulting from such a transfer of electrons. **electrova'lent,** adj.

elec·tro·vert (e-lek'tro-vert) to apply electricity to the heart or precordium to depolarize the heart and terminate a cardiac dysrhythmia.

el·e·doi·sin (el-ĕ-doi'sin) an endecapeptide from a species of octopus (*Eledone*), which is a precursor of a large group of biologically active peptides; it has vasodilator, hypotensive, and extravascular smooth muscle stimulant properties.

el·e·i·din (el-e'ĭ-din) a substance, allied to keratin, found in the stratum lucidum of the skin.

el·e·ment (el'ĕ-ment) 1. any of the primary parts or constituents of a thing. 2. in chemistry, a simple substance that cannot be decomposed by chemical means and that is made up of atoms which are alike in their peripheral electronic configurations and so in their chemical properties and also in the number of protons in their nuclei, but which may differ in the number of neutrons in their nuclei and so in their mass number and in their radioactive properties. See *Table of Elements.* 3. in the philosophies underlying some complementary medicine systems, a member of a group of basic substances that give rise to everything that exists. five e's, 1. see under *phase.* 2. in ayurvedic tradition, the basic entities (earth, air, fire, water, and space) whose interaction gives rise to material existence. formed e's of the blood, the blood cells. trace e's, chemical elements distributed throughout the tissues in very small amounts and that are either essential in nutrition, as cobalt, copper, etc., or harmful, as selenium. transposable e., see *transposon.*

TABLE OF CHEMICAL ELEMENTS

Element (Date of Discovery)	Symbol	Atomic Number	Atomic Weight*	Valence	Specific Gravity or Density (grams/liter)	Descriptive Comment
Actinium (1899)	Ac	89	[227]	3	10.07	radioactive element associated with uranium
Aluminum (1827)	Al	13	26.9815	3	2.6989	silvery-white metal, abundant in earth's crust, but not in free form
Americium (1944)	Am	95	[243]	3,4,5,6	13.67	fourth transuranium element discovered
Antimony (prehistoric)	Sb	51	121.760	3,5	6.691	exists in 4 allotropic forms
Argon (1894)	Ar	18	39.948	0?	1.7837 g/l	colorless, odorless gas
Arsenic (1250)	As	33	74.9216	3,5	5.73 (gray)	semimetallic solid
					4.73 (black)	
					1.97 (yellow)	
Astatine (1940)	At	85	[210]	1,3,5,7		radioactive halogen
Barium (1808)	Ba	56	137.327	2	3.5	silvery-white, alkaline earth metal
Berkelium (1949)	Bk	97	[247]	3,4		fifth transuranium element discovered
Beryllium (1798)	Be	4	9.0122	2	1.848	light, steel-gray metal
Bismuth (1753)	Bi	83	208.9804	3,5	9.747	pinkish-white, crystalline, brittle metal
Bohrium (1981)	Bh	107	[264]			fifteenth transuranium element discovered
Boron (1808)	B	5	10.811	3	2.34, 2.37	crystalline or amorphous element, not occurring free in nature
Bromine (1826)	Br	35	79.904	1,3,5,7	3.12	mobile, reddish-brown liquid, volatilizing readily red vapor with disagreeable odor
Cadmium (1817)	Cd	48	112.411	2	7.59 g/l 8.65	soft, bluish-white metal
Calcium (1808)	Ca	20	40.078	2	1.55	metallic element, forming more than 3 per cent of earth's crust
Californium (1950)	Cf	98	[251]			sixth transuranium element discovered
Carbon (prehistoric)	C	6	12.0107	2,3	1.8–2.1 (amorphous)	element widely distributed in nature
				2,3,4	1.9–2.3 (graphite)	
					3.15–3.53 (diamond)	
Cerium (1803)	Ce	58	140.116	3,4	6.67–8.23	most abundant rare earth metal
Cesium (1869)	Cs	55	132.9055	1	1.873	silvery-white, soft, alkaline metal
Chlorine (1774)	Cl	17	35.4527	1,3,5,7	3.214 g/l	greenish-yellow gas of the halogen group
Chromium (1797)	Cr	24	51.9961	2,3,6	7.18–7.20	steel-gray, lustrous, hard metal
Cobalt (1735)	Co	27	58.9332	2,3	8.9	brittle, hard metal
Copper (prehistoric)	Cu	29	63.546	1,2	8.96	reddish, lustrous, malleable metal
Curium (1944)	Cm	96	[247]	3,4	13.51	third transuranium element discovered

294

Element (year discovered)	Symbol	At. no.	At. weight	Valence	Density	Description
Dubnium (1970)	Db	105	[262]			thirteenth transuranium element discovered
Dysprosium (1886)	Dy	66	162.50	3	8.536	rare earth metal with metallic bright silver luster
Einsteinium (1952)	Es	99	[252]	2,3		seventh transuranium element discovered
Element 110 (1994)		110	[269]			eighteenth transuranium element discovered
Element 111 (1994)		111	[272]			nineteenth transuranium element discovered
Erbium (1843)	Er	68	167.26	3	9.051	soft, malleable rare earth metal
Europium (1896)	Eu	63	151.964	2,3	5.259	lustrous, silvery-white rare earth metal
Fermium (1953)	Fm	100	[257]	2,3		eighth transuranium element discovered
Fluorine (1771)	F	9	18.9984	1	1.696 g/l	pale yellow, corrosive gas of the halogen group
Francium (1939)	Fr	87	[223]	1		product of alpha disintegration of actinium
Gadolinium (1880)	Gd	64	157.25	3	7.8, 7.895	lustrous, silvery-white rare earth metal
Gallium (1875)	Ga	31	69.723	2,3	5.907	beautiful, silvery-appearing metal
Germanium (1886)	Ge	32	72.61	2,4	5.323	grayish-white, brittle metal
Gold (prehistoric)	Au	79	196.9666	1,3	19.32	malleable yellow metal
Hafnium (1923)	Hf	72	178.49	4	13.29	gray metal associated with zirconium
Hassium (1984)	Hs	108	[265]			seventeenth transuranium element discovered
Helium (1895)	He	2	4.0026	0	0.177 g/l	inert gas
Holmium (1879)	Ho	67	164.9303	3	8.803	relatively soft and malleable rare earth metal
Hydrogen (1766)	H	1	1.00794	1	0.08998 g/l / 0.070	(gas) most abundant element in the universe (liquid)
Indium (1863)	In	49	114.818	1,2?,3	7.31	soft, silvery-white metal
Iodine (1811)	I	53	126.9045	1,3,5,7	4.93, 11.27 g/l	grayish-black, lustrous solid or violet-blue gas
Iridium (1803)	Ir	77	192.217	3,4	22.42	white, brittle metal of platinum family
Iron (prehistoric)	Fe	26	55.845	2,3,4,6	7.874	fourth most abundant element in earth's crust
Krypton (1898)	Kr	36	83.80	0	3.733 g/l	inert gas
Lanthanum (1839)	La	57	138.9055	3	5.98–6.186	silvery-white, ductile, rare earth metal
Lawrencium (1961)	Lr	103	[262]	3		eleventh transuranium element discovered
Lead (prehistoric)	Pb	82	207.2	2,4	11.35	bluish-white, lustrous, malleable metal
Lithium (1817)	Li	3	6.941	1	0.534	lightest of all metals
Lutetium (1907)	Lu	71	174.967	3	9.872	rare earth metal
Magnesium (1808)	Mg	12	24.3050	2	1.738	silvery-white metallic element, eighth in abundance in earth's crust
Manganese (1774)	Mn	25	54.9380	1,2,3,4,6,7	7.21–7.44	exists in 4 allotropic forms
Meitnerium (1982)	Mt	109	[268]			sixteenth transuranium element discovered
Mendelevium (1955)	Md	101	[258]	2,3		ninth transuranium element discovered

*figures in brackets represent mass number of most stable isotope.

Element (Date of Discovery)	Symbol	Atomic Number	Atomic Weight*	Valence	Specific Gravity or Density (grams/liter)	Descriptive Comment
Mercury (prehistoric)	Hg	80	200.59	1,2	13.546	heavy, silvery-white metal, liquid at ordinary temperatures
Molybdenum (1782)	Mo	42	95.94	2,3,4?,5?,6	10.22	silvery-white, very hard metal
Neodymium (1885)	Nd	60	144.24	3	6.80, 7.004	exists in 2 allotropic forms
Neon (1898)	Ne	10	20.1797	0?	0.89990 g/l	inert gas
Neptunium (1940)	Np	93	[237]	3,4,5,6	20.45	first transuranium element discovered
Nickel (1751)	Ni	28	58.6934	0,1,2,3	8.902	silvery-white, malleable metal
Niobium (1801)	Nb	41	92.9064	2,3,4?,5	8.57	shiny white, soft ductile metal
Nitrogen (1772)	N	7	14.0067	3,5	1.2506 g/l	colorless, odorless, inert element, making up 78 per cent of the air
Nobelium (1958)	No	102	[259]	2,3		tenth transuranium element discovered
Osmium (1803)	Os	76	190.23	2,3,4,8	22.57	bluish-white, hard metal of platinum family
Oxygen (1774)	O	8	15.9994	2	1.429 g/l	colorless, odorless gas, third most abundant element in the universe
Palladium (1803)	Pd	46	106.42	2,3,4	12.02	steel-white metal of the platinum family
Phosphorus (1669)	P	15	30.9738	3,5	1.82 2.20 2.25–2.69	(white) waxy solid, transparent when pure (red) (black)
Platinum (1735)	Pt	78	195.078	1?,2,3,4	21.45	silvery-white, malleable metal
Plutonium (1940)	Pu	94	[244]	3,4,5,6,7	19.84	second transuranium element discovered
Polonium (1898)	Po	84	[209]	2,4,6	9.32	very rare natural element
Potassium (1807)	K	19	39.0983	1	0.862	soft, silvery, alkali metal, seventh in abundance in earth's crust
Praseodymium (1885)	Pr	59	140.9077	3,4	6.782, 6.64	soft, silvery rare earth metal
Promethium (1941)	Pm	61	[145]	3	7.22 ± 0.02	produced by irradiation of neodymium and praseodymium; identity established in 1945
Protactinium (1917)	Pa	91	231.0359	4,5	15.37	bright lustrous metal
Radium (1898)	Ra	88	[226]	2	5.5	brilliant white, radioactive metal
Radon (1900)	Rn	86	[222]	0	9.73 g/l	heaviest known gas
Rhenium (1925)	Re	75	186.207	−1,2,3,4, 5,6,7	21.02	silvery-white lustrous metal
Rhodium (1803)	Rh	45	102.9055	−2,3,4,5	12.41	silvery-white metal of platinum family
Rubidium (1861)	Rb	37	85.4678	1,2,3,4	1.532	soft, silvery-white, alkali metal

Element (year)	Symbol	At. No.	At. Weight	Valences	Density	Description
Ruthenium (1844)	Ru	44	101.07	0,1,2,3,4,5,6,7,8	12.41	hard white metal of platinum family
Rutherfordium (1969)	Rf	104	[261]			twelfth transuranium element discovered
Samarium (1879)	Sm	62	150.36	2,3	7.536-7.40	bright silvery lustrous metal
Scandium (1879)	Sc	21	44.9559	3	2.992	soft, silvery-white metal
Seaborgium (1974)	Sg	106	[262]			fourteenth transuranium element discovered
Selenium (1817)	Se	34	78.96	2,4,6	4.79, 4.28	exists in several allotropic forms
Silicon (1823)	Si	14	28.0855	4	2.33	a relatively inert element, second in abundance in earth's crust
Silver (prehistoric)	Ag	47	107.8682	1,2	10.50	malleable, ductile metal with brilliant white luster
Sodium (1807)	Na	11	22.9898	1	0.971	most abundant of alkali metals, sixth in abundance in earth's crust
Strontium (1808)	Sr	38	87.62	2	2.54	exists in 3 allotropic forms
Sulfur (prehistoric)	S	16	32.066	2,4,6	1.957, 2.07	exists in several isotopic and many allotropic forms
Tantalum (1802)	Ta	73	180.9479	2?,3,4?,5	16.6	gray, heavy, very hard metal
Technetium (1937)	Tc	43	[98]	3?,4,6,7	11.50	first element produced artificially
Tellurium (1782)	Te	52	127.60	2,4,6	6.24	silvery-white, lustrous element
Terbium (1843)	Tb	65	158.9253	3,4	8.272	silvery-gray, malleable, ductile rare earth metal
Thallium (1861)	Tl	81	204.3833	1,3	11.85	very soft, malleable metal
Thorium (1828)	Th	90	232.0381	4	11.66	silvery-white, lustrous metal
Thulium (1879)	Tm	69	168.9342	2,3	5.75	least abundant rare earth metal
Tin (prehistoric)	Sn	50	118.710	2,4	7.31	(gray) malleable metal existing in 2 or 3 allotropic forms, changing from white to gray on cooling and back to white on warming (white)
Titanium (1791)	Ti	22	47.867	2,3,4	4.54	lustrous white metal
Tungsten (1783)	W	74	183.84	2,3,4,5,6	19.3	steel-gray to tin-white metal
Uranium (1789)	U	92	238.0289	3,4,5,6	18.95	heavy, silvery-white metal
Vanadium (1801)	V	23	50.9415	2,3,4,5	6.11	bright, white metal
Xenon (1898)	Xe	54	131.29	0?	5.887 g/l	one of the so-called rare or inert gases
Ytterbium (1878)	Yb	70	173.04	2,3	6.977, 6.54	exists in 2 allotropic forms
Yttrium (1794)	Y	39	88.9059	3	4.45	rare earth metal with silvery metallic luster
Zinc (1746)	Zn	30	65.39	2	7.133	bluish-white, lustrous metal, malleable at 100–150°C
Zirconium (1789)	Zr	40	91.224	4	6.4	grayish-white, lustrous metal

TABLE OF ELEMENTS BY ATOMIC NUMBERS

1 hydrogen	29 copper	57 lanthanum	85 astatine
2 helium	30 zinc	58 cerium	86 radon
3 lithium	31 gallium	59 praseodymium	87 francium
4 beryllium	32 germanium	60 neodymium	88 radium
5 boron	33 arsenic	61 promethium	89 actinium
6 carbon	34 selenium	62 samarium	90 thorium
7 nitrogen	35 bromine	63 europium	91 protactinium
8 oxygen	36 krypton	64 gadolinium	92 uranium
9 fluorine	37 rubidium	65 terbium	93 neptunium
10 neon	38 strontium	66 dysprosium	94 plutonium
11 sodium	39 yttrium	67 holmium	95 americium
12 magnesium	40 zirconium	68 erbium	96 curium
13 aluminum	41 niobium	69 thulium	97 berkelium
14 silicon	42 molybdenum	70 ytterbium	98 californium
15 phosphorus	43 technetium	71 lutetium	99 einsteinium
16 sulfur	44 ruthenium	72 hafnium	100 fermium
17 chlorine	45 rhodium	73 tantalum	101 mendelevium
18 argon	46 palladium	74 tungsten	102 nobelium
19 potassium	47 silver	75 rhenium	103 lawrencium
20 calcium	48 cadmium	76 osmium	104 rutherfordium
21 scandium	49 indium	77 iridium	105 dubnium
22 titanium	50 tin	78 platinum	106 seaborgium
23 vanadium	51 antimony	79 gold	107 bohrium
24 chromium	52 tellurium	80 mercury	108 hassium
25 manganese	53 iodine	81 thallium	109 meitnerium
26 iron	54 xenon	82 lead	110 element 110
27 cobalt	55 cesium	83 bismuth	111 element 111
28 nickel	56 barium	84 polonium	

el·e·men·ta·ry (el″ĕ-men′tah-re) not resolvable or divisible into simpler parts or components.

ele(o)- word element [Gr.], *oil.*

el·e·phan·ti·a·sis (el″ĕ-fan-ti′ah-sis) 1. a chronic filarial disease, usually seen in the tropics, due to infection with *Brugia malayi* or *Wuchereria bancrofti*, marked by inflammation and obstruction of the lymphatics and hypertrophy of the skin and subcutaneous tissues, chiefly affecting the legs and external genitals. 2. hypertrophy and thickening of the tissues from any cause. **e. neuromato′sa**, neurofibroma. **e. nos′tras**, that due to either chronic streptococcal erysipelas or chronic recurrent cellulitis. **e. scro′ti**, that in which the scrotum is the main seat of the disease.

el·e·phan·toid (el″ĕ-fan′toid) relating to or resembling elephantiasis.

el·e·trip·tan (el″ĕtrip′tan) a selective serotonin receptor agonist, with actions similar to those of sumatriptan, used as the hydrobromide salt in the treatment of migraine; administered orally

eleu·the·ro (ĕ-loo′thĕ-ro) Siberian ginseng.

el·e·va·tor (el′ĭ-vāt-er) an instrument for elevating tissues for removing osseous fragments or roots of teeth.

elim·i·na·tion (e-lim″ĭ-na′shun) 1. the act of expulsion or extrusion, especially expulsion from the body. 2. omission or exclusion.

ELISA (e-li′sah) Enzyme-Linked Immuno-Sorbent Assay; any enzyme immunoassay using an enzyme-labeled immunoreactant and an immunosorbent.

elix·ir (e-lik′ser) a clear, sweetened, alcohol-containing, usually hydroalcoholic liquid containing flavoring substances and sometimes active medicinal ingredients.

el·lip·to·cyte (e-lip′to-sīt) an oval or elliptical erythrocyte.

el·lip·to·cy·to·sis (e-lip″to-si-to′sis) a hereditary disorder characterized by elliptocytes, with increased red cell destruction and anemia.

elm (elm) any tree of the genus *Ulmus*; *Ulmus rubra* is the slippery elm, the source of slippery elm bark.

el·u·ate (el'u-āt) the substance separated out by, or the product of, elution or elutriation.

elu·tion (e-loo'shun) in chemistry, separation of material by washing; the process of pulverizing substances and mixing them with water in order to separate the heavier constituents, which settle out in solution, from the lighter.

elu·tri·a·tion (e-loo″tre-a'shun) purification of a substance by dissolving it in a solvent and pouring off the solution, thus separating it from the undissolved foreign material.

Em emmetropia.

ema·ci·a·tion (e-ma″she-a'shun) a wasted condition of the body.

emas·cu·la·tion (e-mas″ku-la'shun) bilateral orchiectomy.

em·balm·ing (em-bahm'ing) treatment of a dead body to retard decomposition.

em·bar·rass (em-bar'as) to impede the function of; to obstruct.

em·bed·ding (em-bed'ing) fixation of tissue in a firm medium, in order to keep it intact during cutting of thin sections.

em·bo·lec·to·my (em″bo-lek'tah-me) surgical removal of an embolus.

em·bo·li (em'bŏ-li) plural of *embolus*.

em·bol·ic (em-bol'ik) pertaining to an embolus or to embolism.

em·bol·i·form (-ĭ-form) resembling an embolus.

em·bo·lism (em'bŏ-lizm) the sudden blocking of an artery by a clot or foreign material which has been brought to its site of lodgment by the blood current. **air e.,** that due to air bubbles entering the veins from trauma, surgical procedures, or severe decompression sickness. **cerebral e.,** embolism of a cerebral artery. **coronary e.,** embolism of a coronary artery. **fat e.,** obstruction by a fat embolus, occurring especially after fractures of large bones. **miliary e.,** embolism affecting many small blood vessels. **paradoxical e.,** blockage of a systemic artery by a thrombus originating in a systemic vein that has passed through a defect in the interatrial or interventricular septum. **pulmonary e.,** obstruction of the pulmonary artery or one of its branches by an embolus.

em·bo·li·za·tion (em″bŏ-li-za'shun) 1. the process or condition of becoming an embolus. 2. therapeutic introduction of a substance into a vessel in order to occlude it.

em·bo·lus (em'bŏ-lus) pl. *em'boli*. [L.] a mass of clotted blood or other material brought by the blood from one vessel and forced into a

smaller one, obstructing the circulation. See *embolism*. **fat e.,** one composed of oil or fat. **riding e., saddle e., straddling e.,** one at the bifurcation of an artery, blocking both branches.

em·bo·ly (em'bŏ-le) invagination of the blastula to form the gastrula.

em·bra·sure (em-bra'zher) the interproximal space occlusal to the area of contact of adjacent teeth in the same dental arch.

em·bry·ec·to·my (em″bre-ek'tah-me) excision of an extrauterine embryo or fetus.

em·bryo (em'bre-o) 1. in animals, those derivatives of the zygote that eventually become the offspring, during their period of most rapid growth, i.e., from the time the long axis appears until all major structures are represented. 2. in humans, the developing organism from fertilization to the end of the eighth week. Cf. *fetus*. 3. in plants, the element of the seed that develops into a new individual. **em'bryonal, embryon'ic,** adj. **presomite e.,** the embryo at any stage before the appearance of the first somite. **previllous e.,** the embryo before the placental chorionic villi develop. **somite e.,** the embryo between the appearance of the first and the last somites.

em·bryo·blast (em'bre-o-blast″) inner cell mass; an aggregation of cells at the embryonic pole of the blastocyst, destined to form the embryo proper.

em·bryo·gen·e·sis (em″bre-o-jen'ĕ-sis) 1. the production of an embryo. 2. the development of a new individual by means of sexual reproduction, that is, from a zygote. **embryoge'netic, embryogen'ic,** adj.

em·bry·oid (em'bre-oid) resembling an embryo.

em·bryo·le·thal·i·ty (em″bre-o-le-thal'ĭ-te) embryotoxicity that causes death of the embryo.

em·bry·ol·o·gy (em″bre-ol'ah-je) the science of the origin and development of the individual from fertilization of an oocyte to the end of the eighth week of development and, by extension, during any stage of prenatal development.

em·bry·o·ma (em″bre-o'mah) a general term applied to neoplasms thought to be derived from embryonic cells or tissues, such as dermoid cysts, teratomas, embryonal carcinomas and sarcomas, and nephroblastomas. **e. of kidney,** Wilms' tumor.

em·bry·op·a·thy (em″bre-op'ah-the) a morbid condition of the embryo or a disorder resulting from abnormal embryonic development. **rubella e.,** congenital rubella syndrome.

em·bryo·plas·tic (em'bre-o-plas"tik) pertaining to or concerned in formation of an embryo.

em·bry·ot·o·my (em"bre-ot'ah-me) 1. the dismemberment of a fetus in the uterus or vagina to facilitate delivery that is impossible by natural means. 2. the dissection of embryos and fetuses.

em·bryo·tox·ic·i·ty (em"bre-o-tok-sis'i-te) toxic effects on the embryo of a substance that crosses the placental membrane.

em·bryo·tox·on (em"bre-o-tok'son) a ringlike opacity at the margin of the cornea. **anterior e.**, embryotoxon. **posterior e.**, a developmental anomaly in which there is a ringlike opacity at Schwalbe's ring, with thickening and anterior displacement of the latter; it is seen in Axenfeld's syndrome and Rieger's syndrome.

eme·das·tine (em'ĕ-das'tēn) an antihistamine applied topically to the conjunctiva as *e. difumarate* in the treatment of allergic conjunctivitis.

emed·ul·late (e-mĕ-dul'āt) to remove bone marrow.

emer·gen·cy (e-mer'jen-se) an unlooked for or sudden occurrence, often dangerous.

emer·gent (e-mer'jent) 1. coming out from a cavity or other part. 2. pertaining to an emergency.

em·ery (em'er-e) an abrasive substance consisting of corundum and various impurities, such as iron oxide.

em·e·sis (em'ĕ-sis) vomiting.

-emesis word element [Gr.], *vomiting*.

emet·ic (ĕ-met'ik) 1. causing vomiting. 2. an agent that causes vomiting.

em·e·tine (em'ĕ-tēn) an alkaloid derived from ipecac or produced synthetically; its hydrochloride salt is used as an antiamebic.

em·e·to·ca·thar·tic (em"ĕ-to-kah-thahr'tik) both emetic and cathartic, or an agent that so acts.

EMF electromotive force.

-emia word element [Gr.], *condition of the blood*.

em·i·gra·tion (em"i-gra'shun) diapedesis. **leukocyte e.**, the escape (diapedesis) of leukocytes through the walls of small blood vessels.

em·i·nence (em'i-nĕns) a projection or boss. **caudal e.**, a taillike eminence in the early embryo, the remnant of the primitive node and the precursor of hindgut, adjacent notochord and somites, and the caudal part of the spinal cord.

em·i·nen·tia (em"i-nen'shah) pl. *eminen'tiae*. [L.] eminence.

emio·cy·to·sis (e"me-o-si-to'sis) the ejection of material, e.g., insulin granules, from a cell.

em·is·sa·ry (em'i-sĕ-re) 1. affording an outlet, as an emissary vein. 2. emissary vein.

emis·sion (e-mish'un) 1. discharge (1). 2. an involuntary discharge of semen. **nocturnal e.**, reflex emission of semen during sleep. **positron e.**, a form of radioactive decay in which a positron (β^+) and neutrino are ejected from the nucleus as a proton is transformed into a neutron. Collision of the positron with an electron causes annihilation of both particles and conversion of their masses into energy in the form of two 0.511 MeV gamma rays.

em·men·a·gogue (ĕ-men'ah-gog) an agent or measure that induces menstruation. **emmenagog'ic**, adj.

em·me·nol·o·gy (em"i-nol'ah-je) the sum of knowledge about menstruation and its disorders.

em·me·tro·pia (em"ĕ-tro'pe-ah) a state of proper correlation between the refractive system of the eye and the axial length of the eyeball, rays of light entering the eye parallel to the optic axis being brought to focus exactly on the retina. Symbol E. **emmetrop'ic**, adj.

Em·mon·sia (ĕ-mon'se-ah) a genus of Fungi Imperfecti, soil saprobes; two species, *E. cres'cens* and *E. par'va*, cause adiaspiromycosis in rodents and humans.

emol·li·ent (e-mol'yent) 1. softening or soothing. 2. an agent that softens or soothes the skin, or soothes an irritated internal surface.

emo·tion (e-mo'shun) a strong feeling state, arising subjectively and directed toward a specific object, with physiological, somatic, and behavioral components. **emo'tional**, adj.

em·pa·thy (em'pah-the) intellectual and emotional awareness and understanding of another's thoughts, feelings, and behavior. **empath'ic**, adj.

em·phy·se·ma (em"fi-se'mah) 1. a pathologic accumulation of air in tissues or organs. 2. pulmonary e. **emphysem'atous**, adj. **atrophic e.**, senile e. **bullous e.**, single or multiple large cystic alveolar dilatations of lung tissue. **centriacinar e., centrilobular e.**, focal dilatations of respiratory bronchioles rather than alveoli, throughout the lung among normal lung tissue. **congenital lobar e.**, overinflation of a lung, usually in early life in one of the upper lobes, with respiratory distress. **hypoplastic e.**, pulmonary emphysema due to a developmental anomaly, with fewer and abnormally large alveoli. **infantile lobar e.**, congenital lobar e. **interlobular e.**, air in the septa between lung lobules. **interstitial e.**, air in the peribronchial and interstitial tissues of the lungs. **intestinal e.**, pneumatosis cystoides intestinalis. **mediastinal e.,** pneumomediastinum. **obstructive e.,** that associated with partial bronchial obstruction that interferes with exhalation. **panacinar e., panlobular e.,** a type characterized by enlargement of air spaces throughout the acini. **pulmonary e.,** abnormal increase in size of lung air spaces distal to the terminal bronchioles. **pulmonary interstitial e. (PIE),** a condition seen mostly in premature infants, in which air leaks from lung alveoli into interstitial spaces, often because of underlying lung disease or use of mechanical ventilation. **senile e.,** overdistention and stretching of lung tissues due to atrophic changes. **subcutaneous e.,** air or gas in subutaneous tissues, usually caused by intrathoracic injury. **surgical e.,** subcutaneous emphysema following surgery. **vesicular e.,** panacinar e.

em·pir·i·cism (em-pir'ĭ-sizm) skill or knowledge based entirely on experience. **empir'ic, empir'ical,** adj.

em·pros·thot·o·nos (em"pros-thot'ah-nos) tetanic forward flexure of the body.

em·py·e·ma (em"pi-e'mah) 1. abscess. 2. a pleural effusion containing pus. **empye'mic,** adj.

emul·gent (e-mul'jint) causing a straining or purifying process.

emul·si·fi·er (e-mul'sĭ-fi"er) an agent used to produce an emulsion.

emul·sion (e-mul'shun) a mixture of two immiscible liquids, one being dispersed throughout the other in small droplets; a colloid system in which both the dispersed phase and the dispersion medium are liquids.

emul·soid (e-mul'soid) 1. lyophilic colloid. 2. rarely, emulsion.

enal·a·pril (ĕ-nal'ah-pril) an angiotensin-converting enzyme inhibitor used as the maleate salt in the treatment of hypertension, congestive heart failure, and asymptomatic left ventricular dysfunction.

enal·a·pril·at (-pril-at") an angiotensin-converting enzyme inhibitor, the active metabolite of enalapril, used to treat hypertensive crisis and as an intravenous substitute for oral enalapril maleate.

enam·el (ĕ-nam'l) 1. the glazed surface of baked porcelain, metal, or pottery. 2. any hard, smooth, glossy coating. 3. dental enamel; the hard, thin, translucent substance covering and protecting the dentin of a tooth crown and composed almost entirely of calcium salts. **mottled e.,** dental fluorosis: hypoplasia of the dental enamel caused by drinking water with a high fluorine content during the time of tooth formation;

characterized by defective calcification that gives a white chalky appearance to the enamel, which gradually undergoes brown discoloration.

enam·el·o·ma (ĕ-nam"il-o'mah) a small spherical nodule of enamel attached to a tooth at the cervical line or on the root.

enam·e·lum (ĕ-nam'el-um) [L.] enamel.

en·an·thate (ĕ-nan'thāt) USAN contraction for *heptanoate,* the anionic form of the seven-carbon saturated fatty acid enanthic acid, which is producible by oxidation of fats.

en·an·the·ma (en"an-the'mah) pl. *enanthe'mas, enanthe'mata.* An eruption on a mucous surface.

en·an·tio·bio·sis (en-an"te-o-bi-o'sis) commensalism in which the associated organisms are mutually antagonistic.

en·an·tio·mer (en-an'te-o"mer) one of a pair of compounds having a mirror image relationship.

en·an·ti·om·er·ism (en-an"te-om'er-izm) the relationship between two stereoisomers having molecules that are mirror images of each other; they have identical chemical and physical properties in an achiral environment but form different products when reacted with other chiral molecules and exhibit optical activity. The enantiomer that rotates the plane of polarization of a beam of polarized light in the clockwise direction is indicated by the prefix (+)-, formerly *d-* or dextro-; that rotating the plane of polarization in the counterclockwise direction is indicated by the prefix (−)-, formerly *l-* or levo-.

en·an·tio·morph (en-an'te-o-morf") 1. enantiomer. 2. either of two crystals exhibiting enantiomerism.

en·ar·thro·sis (en"ahr-thro'sis) a joint in which the rounded head of one bone is received into a socket in another, as in the hip bone. **enarthro'dial,** adj.

en·cai·nide (en-ka'nīd) a sodium channel blocker that acts on the Purkinje fibers and myocardium; used as the hydrochloride salt in treatment of life-threatening arrhythmias.

en·ceph·a·lat·ro·phy (en-sef"ah-lat'ro-fe) atrophy of the brain.

en·ce·phal·ic (en"sĕ-fal'ik) 1. pertaining to the encephalon. 2. within the skull.

en·ceph·a·li·tis (en-sef"ah-li'tis) pl. *encephali'tides.* Inflammation of the brain. **acute disseminated e.,** see under *encephalomyelitis.* **equine e.,** see under *encephalomyelitis.* **hemorrhagic e.,** that in which there is inflammation of the brain with hemorrhagic foci and perivascular exudate. **herpes e.,** that caused by herpesvirus, characterized by hemorrhagic necrosis of parts of the temporal and frontal lobes. **HIV e.**, see under *encephalopathy*. **Japanese B e.**, a form of epidemic encephalitis of varying severity, caused by a flavivirus and transmitted by the bites of infected mosquitoes in eastern and southern Asia and nearby islands. **La Crosse e.**, that caused by the La Crosse virus, transmitted by *Aedes triseriatus* and occurring primarily in children. **lead e.**, see under *encephalopathy*. **postinfectious e., postvaccinal e.**, acute disseminated encephalomyelitis. **St. Louis e.**, a viral disease first observed in Illinois in 1932, closely resembling western equine encephalomyelitis clinically; it is usually transmitted by mosquitoes. **tick-borne e.**, a form of epidemic encephalitis usually spread by the bites of ticks infected with flaviviruses, sometimes accompanied by degenerative changes in other organs. **West Nile e.**, a usually mild, febrile form caused by the flavivirus West Nile virus, transmitted by *Culex* mosquitoes and first observed in Uganda; symptoms may include drowsiness, severe frontal headache, maculopapular rash, abdominal pain, loss of appetite, nausea, and generalized lymphadenopathy.

en·ceph·a·lit·o·gen·ic (en-sef″ah-lit-o-jen′ik) causing encephalitis.

En·ce·phal·i·to·zo·on (en″sĕ-fal″ĭ-to-zo′on) a genus of parasitic protozoa, causing infection mainly in immunocompromised patients; *E. cuni′culi* affects predominantly the brain and kidney, *E. hel′lem* affects the eye, and *E. intesti na′lis* affects the intestines.

en·ce·phal·i·to·zoo·no·sis (-zo″o-no′sis) infection with protozoa of the genus *Encephalitozoon*.

encephal(o)- word element [Gr.], *brain.*

en·ceph·a·lo·cele (en-sef′ah-lo-sēl″) hernia of part of the brain and meninges through a congenital, traumatic, or postsurgical cranial defect.

en·ceph·a·lo·cys·to·cele (en-sef″ah-lo-sis′to-sēl) hydroencephalocele.

en·ceph·a·log·ra·phy (en-sef″ah-log′rah-fe) radiography demonstrating the intracranial fluid-containing spaces after the withdrawal of cerebrospinal fluid and introduction of air or other gas; it includes pneumoencephalography and ventriculography.

en·ceph·a·loid (en-sef′il-oid) 1. resembling the brain or brain substance. 2. medullary carcinoma.

en·ceph·a·lo·lith (en-sef′ah-lo-lith″) a brain calculus.

en·ceph·a·lo·ma (en-sef″ah-lo′mah) 1. any swelling or tumor of the brain. 2. medullary carcinoma.

en·ceph·a·lo·ma·la·cia (en-sef″ah-lo-mah-la′shah) softening of the brain.

en·ceph·a·lo·men·in·gi·tis (-men″in-ji′tis) meningoencephalitis.

en·ceph·a·lo·me·nin·go·cele (-mĕ-ning′-go-sēl) encephalocele.

en·ceph·a·lo·mere (en-sef′ah-lo-mēr″) one of the segments making up the embryonic brain.

en·ceph·a·lom·e·ter (en-sef″ah-lom′ĕ-ter) an instrument used in locating certain of the brain regions.

en·ceph·a·lo·my·eli·tis (en-sef″ah-lo-mi″ĕ-li′tis) inflammation of the brain and spinal cord. **acute disseminated e.**, inflammation of the brain and spinal cord after infection (especially measles) or, formerly, rabies vaccination. **acute necrotizing hemorrhagic e.**, a rare, fatal postinfection or allergic demyelinating disease of the central nervous system, having a fulminating course; characterized by liquefactive destruction of the white matter and widespread necrosis of blood vessel walls. **benign myalgic e.**, chronic fatigue syndrome. **eastern equine e. (EEE)**, a viral disease of horses and mules that can be spread to humans, usually affecting children and the elderly and manifested by fever, headache, and nausea followed by drowsiness, convulsions, and coma; in the United States it occurs primarily east of the Mississippi river. **equine e.**, see *eastern equine e., western equine e.,* and *Venezuelan equine e.* **postinfectious e., postvaccinal e.**, acute disseminated e. **Venezuelan equine e. (VEE)**, a viral disease of horses and mules; the infection in humans resembles influenza, with little or no indication of nervous system involvement; the causative agent was first isolated in Venezuela. **western equine e. (WEE)**, a viral disease of horses and mules, communicable to humans, occurring chiefly as a meningoencephalitis, with little involvement of the medulla or spinal cord; observed in the United States chiefly west of the Mississippi River.

en·ceph·a·lo·my·elo·neu·rop·a·thy (-mi″-ah-lo-noo-rop′ah-the) a disease involving the brain, spinal cord, and peripheral nerves.

en·ceph·a·lo·my·elo·ra·dic·u·li·tis (-rah-dik″u-li′tis) inflammation of the brain, spinal cord, and spinal nerve roots.

en·ceph·a·lo·my·elo·ra·dic·u·lop·a·thy (-rah-dik″u-lop′ah-the) a disease involving the brain, spinal cord, and spinal nerve roots.

en·ceph·a·lo·myo·car·di·tis (-mi″o-kahr-di′tis) a viral disease marked by degenerative and inflammatory changes in skeletal and cardiac muscle and by central lesions resembling those of poliomyelitis.

en·ceph·a·lon (en-sef′ah-lon) the brain.

en·ceph·a·lop·a·thy (en-sef″ah-lop′ah-the) any degenerative brain disease. **AIDS e.**, HIV e. **anoxic e.**, hypoxic e. **biliary e.**, **bilirubin e.**, kernicterus. **bovine spongiform e.**, a transmissible spongiform encephalopathy of adult cattle, transmitted by feed containing protein in the form of meat and bone meal derived from infected animals. The etiologic agent is also the cause of new variant Creutzfeldt-Jakob disease. **boxer's e.**, **boxer's traumatic e.**, slowing of mental function, confusion, and scattered memory loss due to continual head blows absorbed in the boxing ring. **dialysis e.**, a degenerative disease of the brain associated with long-term use of hemodialysis, marked by speech disorders and constant myoclonic jerks, progressing to global dementia; it is due to high levels of aluminum in the dialysis fluid water or to aluminum-containing drugs used in treatment. **hepatic e.**, a condition, usually occurring secondarily to advanced liver disease, marked by disturbances of consciousness that may progress to deep coma (hepatic coma), psychiatric changes of varying degree, flapping tremor, and fetor hepaticus. **HIV e.**, **HIV-related e.**, AIDS encephalopathy; a progressive primary encephalopathy caused by human immunodeficiency virus type 1 infection, manifested by a variety of cognitive, motor, and behavioral abnormalities. **hypoxic e.**, encephalopathy caused by hypoxia from decreased rate of blood flow or decreased oxygen in the blood; severe cases can cause permanent brain damage within five minutes. **hypoxic-ischemic e.**, that resulting from fetal or perinatal asphyxia, characterized by feeding difficulties, lethargy, and convulsions. **lead e.**, edema and central demyelination caused by excessive ingestion of lead compounds, particularly in young children. **myoclonic e. of childhood**, a neurologic disorder of unknown etiology with onset between ages 1 and 3, characterized by myoclonus of trunk and limbs and by opsoclonus with ataxia of gait, and intention tremor; some cases have been associated with occult neuroblastoma. **subacute spongiform e.**, **transmissible spongiform e.**, prion disease. **Wernicke's e.**, an inflammatory hemorrhagic form due to thiamine deficiency, usually associated with chronic alcoholism, with paralysis of the eye muscles, diplopia, nystagmus, ataxia, and usually accompanying or followed by Korsakoff's syndrome.

en·ceph·a·lo·py·o·sis (en-sef″ah-lo-pi-o′sis) suppuration or abscess of the brain.

en·ceph·a·lor·rha·gia (-ra′jah) hemorrhage within or from the brain.

en·ceph·a·lo·sis (en-sef″ah-lo′sis) encephalopathy.

en·ceph·a·lot·o·my (en-sef″ah-lot′ah-me) incision of the brain.

en·chon·dro·ma (en″kon-dro′mah) pl. *enchondromas, enchondro′mata*. A benign growth of cartilage arising in the metaphysis of a bone. **enchondro′matous,** adj.

en·chon·dro·ma·to·sis (en-kon″dro-mah-to′sis) hamartomatous proliferation of cartilage cells within the metaphysis of several bones, causing thinning of the overlying cortex and distortion of the growth in length; it may undergo malignant transformation.

en·clave (en′klāv) tissue detached from its normal connection and enclosed within another organ.

en·co·pre·sis (en″ko-pre′sis) fecal incontinence.

en·cy·e·sis (en-si-e′sis) normal uterine pregnancy.

en·cyo·py·eli·tis (en-si″o-pi-ĕ-li′tis) dilatation and edema of the ureters and renal pelvis during normal pregnancy, but seldom with all the classic signs of inflammation.

en·cyst·ed (en-sist′id) enclosed in a sac, bladder, or cyst.

end·an·gi·itis (end-an″je-i′tis) intimitis; inflammation of the tunica intima of a vessel.

end·aor·ti·tis (end″a-or-ti′tis) inflammation of the tunica intima of the aorta.

end·ar·ter·ec·to·my (end-ahr″ter-ek′tah-me) excision of thickened atheromatous areas of the innermost coat of an artery.

end·ar·ter·i·tis (end″ahr-ter-i′tis) inflammation of the tunica intima of an artery.

end·au·ral (-aw′r'l) within the ear.

end·brain (-brān) telencephalon.

end·bulb (-bulb) a sensory nerve ending characterized by a fibrous capsule of varying thickness that is continuous with the endoneurium.

en·dem·ic (en-dem′ik) present or usually prevalent in a population at all times.

en·de·mo·ep·i·dem·ic (en″de-mo-ep″ĭ-dem′ik) endemic, but occasionally becoming epidemic.

end·er·gon·ic (end″er-gon′ik) characterized or accompanied by the absorption of energy; requiring the input of free energy.

end·foot (end′foot) bouton terminal.

end(o)- word element [Gr.], *within; inward*.

en·do·an·eu·rys·mor·rha·phy (en″do-an″-u-riz-mor′ah-fe) opening of an aneurysmal sac and suture of the orifices.

en·do·ap·pen·di·ci·tis (-ah-pen″dǐ-si′tis) inflammation of the mucous membrane of the vermiform appendix.

en·do·blast (en′do-blast) endoderm.

en·do·bron·chi·al (en″do-brong′ke-al) within a bronchus or bronchi.

en·do·bron·chi·tis (-brong-ki′tis) inflammation of the epithelial lining of the bronchi.

en·do·car·di·al (-kahr′de-al) 1. situated or occurring within the heart. 2. pertaining to the endocardium.

en·do·car·di·tis (-kahr-di′tis) exudative and proliferative inflammatory alterations of the endocardium, usually characterized by the presence of vegetations on the surface of the endocardium or in the endocardium itself, and most commonly involving a heart valve, but also affecting the inner lining of the cardiac chambers or the endocardium elsewhere. **endocardit′ic**, adj. **atypical verrucous e.**, Libman-Sacks e. **bacterial e.**, infectious endocarditis caused by various bacteria, including streptococci, staphylococci, enterococci, gonococci, and gram-negative bacilli. **infectious e.**, **infective e.**, that due to infection with microorganisms, especially bacteria and fungi; currently classified on the basis of etiology or underlying anatomy. **Libman-Sacks e.**, nonbacterial endocarditis found in association with systemic lupus erythematosus, usually occurring on the atrioventricular valves. **Löffler's e.**, **Löffler's parietal fibroplastic e.**, endocarditis associated with eosinophilia, marked by fibroplastic thickening of the endocardium, resulting in congestive heart failure, persistent tachycardia, hepatomegaly, splenomegaly, serous effusions into the pleural cavity, and edema of the limbs. **mycotic e.**, infectious endocarditis, usually subacute, due to various fungi, most commonly *Candida*, *Aspergillus*, and *Histoplasma*. **nonbacterial thrombotic e. (NBTE)**, that usually occurring in chronic debilitating disease, characterized by non-infected vegetations consisting of fibrin and other blood elements and susceptible to embolization. **prosthetic valve e.**, infectious endocarditis as a complication of implantation of a prosthetic valve in the heart; the vegetations usually occur along the line of suture. **rheumatic e.**, that associated with rheumatic fever; more accurately termed *rheumatic valvulitis* when an entire valve is involved. **rickettsial e.**, endocarditis caused by invasion of the heart valves with *Coxiella burnetii*; it is a sequela of Q fever, usually occurring in persons who have had rheumatic fever. **vegetative e.**, **verrucous e.**, endocarditis, infectious or noninfectious, the characteristic lesions of which are vegetations or verrucae on the endocardium.

en·do·car·di·um (-kahr′de-um) the endothelial lining membrane of the cavities of the heart and the connective tissue bed on which it lies.

en·do·cer·vi·ci·tis (-ser″vǐ-si′tis) inflammation of the mucous membrane of the uterine cervix.

en·do·cer·vix (-ser′viks) 1. the mucous membrane lining the canal of the cervix uteri. 2. the region of the opening of the cervix into the uterine cavity. **endocer′vical**, adj.

en·do·chon·dral (-kon′dril) situated, formed, or occurring within cartilage.

en·do·co·li·tis (-ko-li′tis) inflammation of the mucous membrane of the colon.

en·do·cra·ni·um (-kra′ne-um) the endosteal layer of the dura mater of the brain.

en·do·crine (en′do-krin, en′do-krīn) 1. secreting internally. 2. pertaining to internal secretions; hormonal. See also under *system*.

en·do·cri·nol·o·gist (en″do-krī-nol′ah-jist) a specialist in endocrinology.

en·do·cri·nol·o·gy (-nol′ah-je) 1. the study of hormones and the endocrine system. 2. a medical specialty concerned with the diagnosis and treatment of disorders of the endocrine system.

en·do·cri·nop·a·thy (-nop′ah-the) any disease due to disorder of the endocrine system. **endocrinopath′ic**, adj.

en·do·cy·to·sis (-si-to′sis) the uptake by a cell of material from the environment by invagination of its plasma membrane; it includes both phagocytosis and pinocytosis.

en·do·derm (en′do-derm) the innermost of the three primitive germ layers of the embryo; from it are derived the epithelium of the pharynx, respiratory tract (except the nose), digestive tract, bladder, and urethra. **endoder′mal**, **endoder′mic**, adj.

En·do·der·moph·y·ton (en″do-der-mof′ĭ-ton) *Trichophyton*.

en·do·don·tics (-don′tiks) the branch of dentistry concerned with the etiology, prevention, diagnosis, and treatment of conditions that affect the tooth pulp, root, and periapical tissues.

en·do·don·ti·um (-don′she-um) dental pulp.

en·do·don·tol·o·gy (-don-tol′ah-je) endodontics.

en·do·en·ter·itis (-en″ter-i′tis) inflammation of the intestinal mucosa.

en·dog·a·my (en-dog′ah-me) 1. fertilization by union of separate cells having the same genetic ancestry. 2. restriction of marriage to persons within the same community. **endog′amous**, adj.

en·dog·e·nous (en-doj'ĕ-nus) produced within or caused by factors within the organism.

en·do·la·ryn·ge·al (en"do-lah-rin'je-il) situated or occurring within the larynx.

en·do·lymph (en'do-limf) the fluid within the membranous labyrinth. **endolymphat'ic,** adj.

en·dol·y·sin (en-dol'ĭ-sin) a bactericidal substance in cells, acting directly on bacteria.

en·do·me·tri·al (en"do-me'tre-il) pertaining to the endometrium.

en·do·me·tri·oid (-me'tre-oid) resembling endometrium.

en·do·me·tri·o·ma (-me"tre-o'mah) a solitary non-neoplastic mass containing endometrial tissue.

en·do·me·tri·o·sis (-me"tre-o'sis) the aberrant occurrence of tissue containing typical endometrial granular and stromal elements, in various locations in the pelvic cavity or other areas of the body. **endometriot'ic,** adj. **e. exter'na,** endometriosis. **e. inter'na,** adenomyosis. **ovarian e.,** that involving the ovary, in the form of either small superficial islands or epithelial ("chocolate") cysts of various sizes.

en·do·me·tri·tis (-me-tri'tis) inflammation of the endometrium. **puerperal e.,** that following childbirth. **syncytial e.,** a benign tumor-like lesion with infiltration of the uterine wall by large syncytial trophoblastic cells. **tuberculous e.,** inflammation of the endometrium, usually also involving the uterine tubes, due to infection by *Mycobacterium tuberculosis,* with the presence of tubercles.

en·do·me·tri·um (-me'tre-um) pl. *endome'tria.* The mucous membrane lining the uterus.

en·do·mi·to·sis (-mi-to'sis) reproduction of nuclear elements not followed by chromosome movements and cytoplasmic division. **endomitot'ic,** adj.

en·do·morph (en'do-morf) an individual having the type of body build in which endodermal tissues predominate: soft roundness throughout, large digestive viscera, fat accumulations, large trunk and thighs, and tapering limbs.

en·do·myo·car·di·al (en"do-mi"o-kahr'de-al) pertaining to the endocardium and the myocardium.

en·do·myo·car·di·tis (-kahr-di'tis) inflammation of the endocardium and myocardium.

en·do·mys·i·um (-mis'e-um) the sheath of delicate reticular fibrils surrounding each muscle fiber.

en·do·neu·ri·tis (-noo-ri'tis) inflammation of the endoneurium.

en·do·neu·ri·um (-noor'e-um) the innermost layer of connective tissue in a peripheral nerve, forming an interstitial layer around each individual fiber outside the neurilemma. **endoneu'rial,** adj.

en·do·nu·cle·ase (-noo'kle-ās) any nuclease specifically catalyzing the hydrolysis of interior bonds of ribonucleotide or deoxyribonucleotide chains. **restriction e.,** an endonuclease that hydrolyzes DNA, cleaving it at an individual site of a specific base pattern.

en·do·pel·vic (-pel'vik) intrapelvic.

en·do·pep·ti·dase (-pep'tĭ-dās) protease; any peptidase that catalyzes the cleavage of internal bonds in a polypeptide or protein.

en·do·peri·car·di·tis (-per"ĭ-kahr-di'tis) inflammation of the endocardium and pericardium.

en·do·peri·to·ni·tis (-per"ĭ-to-ni'tis) inflammation of the serous lining of peritoneal cavity.

en·doph·thal·mi·tis (en"dof-thal-mi'tis) inflammation of the ocular cavities and their adjacent structures.

en·do·phyte (en'do-fīt) a parasitic plant organism living within its host's body.

en·do·phyt·ic (en"do-fit'ik) 1. pertaining to an endophyte. 2. growing inward; proliferating on the interior of an organ or structure.

en·do·plasm (en'do-plazm") the central portion of the cytoplasm of a cell. **endoplas'mic,** adj.

en·do·poly·ploid (en"do-pol'e-ploid) having reduplicated chromatin within an intact nucleus, with or without an increase in the number of chromosomes (applied only to cells and tissues).

en·do·pros·the·sis (-pros-the'sis) 1. a prosthesis entirely inside the body. 2. a hollow stent inserted into a bile duct to allow biliary drainage across an obstruction.

en·do·py·elot·o·my (en"do-pi"ĕ-lot'ŏ-me) incision to correct a stenosed ureteropelvic junction, cutting from within using an instrument inserted through an endoscope.

en·do·re·du·pli·ca·tion (-re-doo"plĭ-ka'-shun) replication of chromosomes without subsequent cell division.

end·or·gan (end-or'gan) one of the large encapsulated endings of sensory nerves.

en·dor·phin (en-dor'fin) any of three neuropeptides, α-, β-, and γ-*endorphins;* they are amino acid residues of β-lipotropin that bind to opiate receptors in various areas of the brain and have potent analgesic effect.

en·do·sal·pin·gi·tis (en"do-sal"pin-ji'tis) inflammation of the endosalpinx.

en·do·sal·pin·go·ma (-sal″pin-go′mah) adenomyoma of the uterine tube.

en·do·sal·pinx (-sal′pinks) the mucous membrane lining the uterine tube.

en·do·scope (en′do-skōp) an instrument for examining the interior of a hollow viscus.

en·dos·co·py (en-dos′kah-pe) visual examination by means of an endoscope. **endoscop′ic,** adj. **peroral e.,** examination of organs accessible to observation through an endoscope passed through the mouth.

en·do·skel·e·ton (en″do-skel′ĕ-ton) the cartilaginous and bony skeleton of the body, exclusive of that part of the skeleton of dermal origin.

en·dos·mo·sis (en″dos-mo′sis) inward osmosis; inward passage of liquid through a membrane of a cell or cavity. **endosmot′ic,** adj.

en·do·some (en′do-sōm) 1. in endocytosis, a vesicle that has lost its coat of clathrin. 2. a nucleolus-like, intranuclear, RNA-containing organelle of certain flagellate protozoa that persists during mitosis.

en·dos·se·ous (en-dos′e-us) endosteal (2).

en·dos·te·al (en-dos′te-al) 1. pertaining to the endosteum. 2. occurring or located within a bone.

en·dos·te·o·ma (en-dos″te-o′mah) a tumor in the medullary cavity of a bone.

en·dos·te·um (en-dos′te-um) the tissue lining the medullary cavity of a bone.

en·do·ten·din·e·um (en″do-ten-din′e-um) the delicate connective tissue separating the secondary bundles (fascicles) of a tendon.

en·do·the·lia (-the′le-ah) [Gr.] plural of *endothelium.*

en·do·the·li·al (-the′le-al) pertaining to or made up of endothelium.

en·do·the·lio·blas·to·ma (-the″le-o-blas-to′mah) a tumor derived from primitive vasoformative tissue, it includes hemangioendothelioma, angiosarcoma, lymphangioendothelioma, and lymphangiosarcoma.

en·do·the·li·o·ma (-the″le-o′mah) any tumor, particularly a benign one, arising from the endothelial lining of blood vessels.

en·do·the·li·o·ma·to·sis (-the″le-o″mah-to′sis) formation of multiple, diffuse endotheliomas.

en·do·the·li·o·sis (-the″le-o′sis) proliferation of endothelium. **glomerular capillary e.,** a renal lesion typical of eclampsia, characterized by deposition of fibrous material in and beneath the cells of the swollen glomerular capillary epithelium, occluding the capillaries.

en·do·the·li·um (-the′le-um) pl. *endothe′-lia.* The layer of epithelial cells that lines the cavities of the heart, the serous cavities, and the lumina of the blood and lymph vessels.

en·do·ther·mal (-ther′mal) endothermic.

en·do·ther·mic (-ther′mik) characterized by or accompanied by the absorption of heat.

en·do·ther·my (-ther′me) diathermy.

en·do·tho·rac·ic (-tho-ras′ik) within the thorax; situated internal to the ribs.

en·do·thrix (en′do-thriks) a dermatophyte whose growth and spore production are confined chiefly within the hair shaft.

en·do·tox·e·mia (en″do-toks-ēm′e-ah) the presence of endotoxins in the blood, which may result in shock.

en·do·tox·in (en′do-tok″sin) a heat-stable toxin present in the intact bacterial cell but not in cell-free filtrates of cultures of intact bacteria. Endotoxins are lipopolysaccharide complexes that occur in the cell wall; they are pyrogenic and increase capillary permeability. **en′dotoxic,** adj.

en·do·tra·che·al (en″do-tra′ke-al) within or through the trachea.

en·do·urol·o·gy (-ūr-ol′ah-je) the branch of urologic surgery concerned with closed procedures for visualizing or manipulating the urinary tract.

en·do·vas·cu·li·tis (-vas″ku-li′tis) endangiitis.

end plate (end plāt) a flat termination. **motor e. p.,** the discoid expansion of a terminal branch of the axon of a motor nerve fiber where it joins a skeletal muscle fiber, forming the neuromuscular junction.

en·drin (en′drin) a highly toxic insecticide of the chlorinated hydrocarbon group.

end-tidal (end-ti′dal) pertaining to or occurring at the end of exhalation of a normal tidal volume.

en·e·ma (en′ĕ-mah) [Gr.] a solution introduced into the rectum to promote evacuation of feces or as a means of introducing nutrients, medicinal substances, or opaque material for radiologic examination of the lower intestinal tract. **barium e.,** contrast e. **contrast e.,** a suspension of barium injected into the intestine as a contrast agent for radiologic examination. **double-contrast e.,** double-contrast examination (q.v.) of the intestine.

en·er·gy (en′er-je) power which may be translated into motion, overcoming resistance, or effecting physical change; the ability to do work. Symbol *E.* **free e., Gibbs free e. (G),** that equal to the maximum amount of work that can be obtained from a process occurring under conditions of fixed temperature and pressure. **kinetic e.,** the energy of motion. **nuclear e.,** energy that can be liberated by changes in the nucleus of an atom (as by fission of a heavy nucleus or fusion of light nuclei into heavier ones with accompanying loss of mass). **potential e.,** energy at rest or not manifested in actual work. **vital e.,** see under *force.*

en·er·va·tion (en″er-va′shun) 1. lack of nervous energy. 2. neurectomy.

en·flu·rane (en′floo-rān) a potent inhalational anesthetic used for induction and maintenance of general anesthesia and for analgesia during labor and painful procedures.

ENG electronystagmography.

en·gage·ment (en-gāj′mint) the entrance of the fetal head or presenting part into the superior pelvic strait.

en·gorge·ment (en-gorj′ment) 1. local congestion; distention with fluids. 2. hyperemia.

en·graft·ment (en-graft′ment) incorporation of grafted tissue into the body of the host.

en·hance·ment (en-hans′ment) 1. the act of augmenting or the state of being augmented. 2. immunologic enhancement; prolonged survival of tumor cells in animals immunized with antigens of the tumor because of "enhancing" or "facilitating" antibodies preventing an immune response against these antigens.

en·ka·tar·rha·phy (en″kah-tar′ah-fe) the operation of burying a structure by suturing together the sides of tissues adjacent to it.

en·keph·a·lin (en-kef′ah-lin) either of two pentapeptides (*leu-enkephalin* and *met-enkephalin*) occurring in the brain and spinal cord and also in the gastrointestinal tract; they have potent opiate-like effects and probably serve as neurotransmitters.

enol (e′nol) an organic compound in which one carbon of a double-bonded pair is also attached to a hydroxyl group, thus a tautomer of the ketone form; also used as a prefix or infix, often italicized.

eno·lase (e′no-lās) an enzyme that catalyzes the dehydration of 2-phosphoglycerate to form phospho*enol*pyruvate, a step in the pathway of glucose metabolism. **neuron-specific e.,** an isozyme of enolase found in normal neurons and all the cells of the neuroendocrine system; it is a marker for neuroendocrine differentiation in tumors.

en·os·to·sis (en″os-to′sis) a morbid bony growth within a bone cavity or on the internal surface of the bone cortex.

enox·a·cin (ĕ-nok′sah-sin) a synthetic antibacterial effective against many gram-positive and gram-negative bacteria.

enox·a·par·in (e-nok″sah-par′in) a low molecular weight heparin used as the sodium salt as an antithrombotic.

enox·i·mone (en-ok′sĭ-mōn) a phosphodiesterase inhibitor similar to inamrinone; used as a cardiotonic in the short-term management of congestive heart failure, administered intravenously.

en·si·form (en′sĭ-form) xiphoid (1).

en·stro·phe (en′stro-fe) entropion.

en·sul·i·zole (en-sul′-ĭ-zōl) a water-soluble absorber of ultraviolet B radiation, used topically as a sunscreen.

ENT ears, nose, and throat (otorhinolaryngology).

en·tac·a·pone (en-tak′ah-pōn) an antidyskinetic used in conjunction with levodopa and carbidopa in the treatment of idiopathic Parkinson's disease.

en·tad (en′tad) toward a center; inwardly.

ent·ame·bi·a·sis (en″tah-me-bi′ah-sis) infection by *Entamoeba*; see *amebic dysentery.*

Ent·amoe·ba (en″tah-me′bah) a genus of amebas parasitic in the intestines of vertebrates, including three species commonly parasitic in humans: *E. co′li,* found in the intestinal tract; *E. gingiva′lis (E. bucca′lis),* found in the mouth; and *E. histoly′tica,* the cause of amebic dysentery and tropical abscess of the liver.

en·ter·al (en′ter′l) enteric.

en·ter·al·gia (en″ter-al′jah) pain in the intestine.

en·ter·epip·lo·cele (-ĕ-pip′lo-sēl) enteroepiplocele.

en·ter·ic (en-ter′ik) within or pertaining to the small intestine.

en·ter·ic-coat·ed (-kōt′ed) designating a special coating applied to tablets or capsules that prevents release and absorption of active ingredients until they reach the intestine.

en·ter·i·tis (en″ter-i′tis) inflammation of the intestine, especially of the small intestine. **regional e.,** Crohn's disease.

enter(o)- word element [Gr.], *intestines.*

En·tero·bac·ter (en′ter-o-bak″ter) a genus of gram-negative, facultatively anaerobic rod-shaped bacteria of the family Enterobacteriaceae, widely distributed in nature and occurring in the intestinal tract of humans and animals. Species including *E. aero′genes, E. agglo′merans, E. cloa′cae,* and *E. gergo′viae,* are frequently the cause of nosocomial infection, arising from contaminated medical devices and personnel.

En·tero·bac·te·ri·a·ceae (en″ter-o-bak-tēr″e-a′se-e) a family of gram-negative, rod-shaped bacteria (order Eubacteriales) occurring as plant or animal parasites or as saprophytes.

en·tero·bi·a·sis (-bi'ah-sis) infection with nematodes of the genus *Enterobius*, especially *E. vermicularis*.

En·tero·bi·us (en"ter-o'be-us) a genus of intestinal nematodes (superfamily Oxyuroidea), including *E. vermicula'ris*, the seatworm or pinworm, parasitic in the upper large intestine, and occasionally in the female genitals and bladder; infection is frequent in children, sometimes causing itching.

en·tero·cele (en'ter-o-sēl") a hernia containing intestine.

en·tero·cen·te·sis (en"ter-o-sen-te'sis) surgical puncture of the intestine.

en·tero·cly·sis (en"ter-ok'lĭ-sis) the injection of liquids into the intestine.

En·tero·coc·cus (en"ter-o-kok'us) a genus of gram-positive facultatively anaerobic cocci of the family Streptococcaceae; *E. faeca'lis* and *E. fae'cium* are normal inhabitants of the human intestinal tract that occasionally cause urinary tract infections, infective endocarditis, and bacteremia; *E. a'vium* is found primarily in the feces of chickens and may be associated with appendicitis, otitis, and brain abscesses in humans.

en·tero·coc·cus (en"ter-o-kok'us) pl. *enterococ'ci*. An organism belonging to the genus *Enterococcus*.

en·tero·co·lec·to·my (-ko-lek'tah-me) resection of the intestine, including the ileum, cecum, and colon.

en·tero·co·li·tis (-ko-li'tis) inflammation of the small intestine and colon. **antibiotic-associated e.**, that in which treatment with antibiotics alters the bowel flora and results in diarrhea or pseudomembranous enterocolitis. **hemorrhagic e.**, enterocolitis characterized by hemorrhagic breakdown of the intestinal mucosa, with inflammatory cell infiltration. **necrotizing e., pseudomembranous e.**, an acute inflammation of the bowel mucosa with formation of pseudomembranous plaques overlying an area of superficial ulceration, with passage of the pseudomembranous material in the feces; it may result from shock and ischemia or be associated with antibiotic therapy.

en·tero·cu·ta·ne·ous (-ku-ta'ne-us) pertaining to or communicating with the intestine and the skin, or surface of the body.

en·tero·cyst (en'ter-o-sist") enteric cyst.

en·tero·cys·to·cele (en"ter-o-sis'to-sēl) hernia of intestine and a portion of the urinary bladder.

en·tero·cys·to·ma (-sis-to'mah) enteric cyst.

en·tero·cys·to·plas·ty (-sis'to-plas"te) the most common type of augmentation cystoplasty, using a portion of intestine for the graft.

en·tero·en·ter·os·to·my (-en"ter-os'tah-me) surgical anastomosis between two segments of the intestine.

en·tero·epip·lo·cele (-ĕ-pip'lah-sēl) hernia of the small intestine and omentum.

en·tero·gas·trone (-gas'trōn) anthelone E; a hormone of the duodenum which mediates the humoral inhibition of gastric secretion and motility produced by ingestion of fat.

en·tero·og·e·nous (en"ter-oj'ĕ-nus) 1. arising from the foregut. 2. originating within the small intestine.

en·tero·glu·ca·gon (en"ter-o-gloo'kah-gon) a glucagon-like hyperglycemic agent released by the mucosa of the upper intestine in response to the ingestion of glucose; immunologically distinct from pancreatic glucagon but with similar activities.

en·tero·og·ra·phy (en"ter-og'rah-fe) a description of the intestine.

en·tero·he·pat·ic (en"ter-o-hĕ-pat'ik) pertaining to or connecting the liver and intestine.

en·tero·hep·a·ti·tis (-hep"ah-ti'tis) inflammation of the intestine and liver.

en·tero·hep·a·to·cele (-hep'ah-to-sēl") an umbilical hernia containing intestine and liver.

en·tero·lith (en'ter-o-lith") a calculus in the intestine.

en·ter·ol·o·gy (en"ter-ol'ah-je) scientific study of the intestine.

en·ter·ol·y·sis (en"ter-ol'ĭ-sis) surgical separation of intestinal adhesions.

en·tero·me·ro·cele (en"ter-o-me'rah-sēl) femoral hernia.

en·tero·my·co·sis (-mi-ko'sis) fungal disease of the intestine.

en·tero·pa·re·sis (en"ter-o-pah-re'sis, -pă'rĭ-sis) relaxation of the intestine resulting in dilatation.

en·tero·patho·gen·e·sis (-path"o-jen'ĕ-sis) the production of disease or disorder of the intestine.

en·ter·op·a·thy (en"ter-op'ah-the) any disease of the intestine. **enteropath'ic**, adj. **gluten e.**, celiac disease.

en·tero·pep·ti·dase (en"ter-o-pep'tĭ-dās) an endopeptidase, secreted by the small intestine, which catalyzes the cleavage of trypsinogen to the active form trypsin.

en·tero·pexy (en'ter-o-pek"se) surgical fixation of the intestine to the abdominal wall.

en·tero·plas·ty (-plas"te) plastic repair of the intestine.

en·tero·ple·gia (en"ter-o-ple'jah) adynamic ileus.

en·ter·or·rha·gia (-ra'jah) intestinal hemorrhage.

en·ter·or·rhex·is (-rek'sis) rupture of the intestine.

en·tero·scope (en'ter-o-skōp") an instrument for inspecting the inside of the intestine.

en·tero·sep·sis (en"ter-o-sep'sis) sepsis developed from the intestinal contents.

en·tero·stax·is (-stak'sis) slow hemorrhage through the intestinal mucosa.

en·tero·ste·no·sis (-stě-no'sis) narrowing or stricture of the intestine.

en·ter·os·to·my (en"ter-os'tah-me) formation of a permanent opening into the intestine through the abdominal wall. **enterosto'mal,** adj.

en·tero·tox·e·mia (en"ter-o-tok-se'me-ah) a condition characterized by the presence in the blood of toxins produced in the intestines.

en·tero·tox·in (en'ter-o-tok"sin) 1. a toxin specific for the cells of the intestinal mucosa. 2. a toxin arising in the intestine. 3. an exotoxin that is protein in nature and relatively heat-stable, produced by staphylococci.

en·tero·tro·pic (en"ter-o-tro'pik) affecting the intestine.

en·tero·vag·i·nal (-vaj'ĭ-nil) pertaining to or communicating with the intestine and the vagina.

en·tero·ve·nous (-ve'nus) communicating between the intestinal lumen and the lumen of a vein.

en·tero·ves·i·cal (-ves'ĭ-k'l) pertaining to or communicating with the urinary bladder and intestine.

En·tero·vi·rus (en'ter-o-vi"rus) enteroviruses; a genus of viruses of the family Picornaviridae that preferentially inhabit the intestinal tract, with infection usually asymptomatic or mild. Human enteroviruses were originally classified as polioviruses, coxsackieviruses, or echoviruses.

en·tero·vi·rus (en'ter-o-vi"rus) any virus of the genus *Enterovirus.* **enterovi'ral,** adj.

en·tero·zo·on (en"ter-o-zo'on) pl. *enterozo'a.* An animal parasite in the intestine. **enterozo'ic,** adj.

en·thal·py (en'thal-pe) the heat content or chemical energy of a physical system; a thermodynamic function equal to the internal energy plus the product of the pressure and volume. Symbol *H.*

en·the·sis (en-the'sis) the site of attachment of a muscle or ligament to bone.

en·the·sop·a·thy (en"thě-sop'ah-the) disorder of the muscular or tendinous attachment to bone.

en·theto·bio·sis (en-thet"o-bi-o'sis) dependency on a mechanical implant, as on an artificial cardiac pacemaker.

ent(o)- word element [Gr.], *within; inner.*

en·to·blast (en'to-blast) endoderm.

en·to·cho·roid·ea (en"to-kor-oi'de-ah) the inner layer of the choroid.

en·to·cor·nea (-kor'ne-ah) Descemet's membrane.

en·to·derm (en'to-derm) endoderm. **entoder'mal, entoder'mic,** adj.

en·to·mi·on (en-to'me-on) the tip of mastoid angle of parietal bone.

en·to·mol·o·gy (en"tah-mol'ah-je) that branch of biology concerned with the study of insects.

En·to·moph·tho·ra·les (en"to-mof"thah-ra'lēz) an order of fungi of the class Zygomycetes, typically parasites of insects but also causing human infections, often in apparently immunologically and physiologically normal people.

en·to·moph·tho·ro·my·co·sis (en"to-mof"tho-ro-mi-ko'sis) any disease caused by fungi of the order Entomophthorales.

en·top·ic (en-top'ik) occurring in the proper place.

en·top·tic (en-top'tik) originating within the eye.

en·top·tos·co·py (en"top-tos'kah-pe) inspection of the interior of the eye.

en·to·ret·i·na (en"to-ret'ĭ-nah) the nervous or inner layer of the retina.

en·to·zo·on (-zo'on) pl. *entozo'a.* An internal animal parasite. **entozo'ic,** adj.

en·train (en-trān') to modulate the cardiac rhythm by gaining control of the rate of the pacemaker with an external stimulus.

en·train·ment (en-trān'ment) 1. a technique for identifying the slowest pacing necessary to terminate an arrhythmia, particularly atrial flutter. 2. the synchronization and control of cardiac rhythm by an external stimulus.

en·trap·ment (en-trap'ment) compression of a nerve or vessel by adjacent tissue.

en·tro·pi·on (en-tro'pe-on) inversion, or the turning inward, as of the margin of an eyelid.

en·tro·py (en'tro-pe) 1. the measure of that part of the heat or energy of a system not available to perform work; it increases in all natural (spontaneous and irreversible) processes. Symbol *S.* 2. the tendency of any system to move toward randomness or disorder. 3. diminished capacity for spontaneous change.

en·ty·py (en'tĭ-pe) a method of gastrulation in which the endoderm lies external to the amniotic ectoderm.

enu·cle·a·tion (e-noo″kle-a′shun) removal of an organ or other mass intact from its supporting tissues, as of the eyeball from the orbit.

en·ure·sis (en″ūr-e′sis) involuntary discharge of urine; usually referring to involuntary discharge of urine during sleep at night. **enuret′ic,** adj.

en·ve·lope (en′vĕ-lōp) 1. an encompassing structure or membrane. 2. in virology the peplos, a coat surrounding the capsid and usually furnished at least partially by the host cell. 3. in bacteriology, the cell wall and the plasma membrane considered together. **nuclear e.,** the condensed double layer of lipids and proteins enclosing the cell nucleus and separating it from the cytoplasm; its two concentric membranes, inner and outer, are separated by a perinuclear space.

en·ven·om·a·tion (en-ven″o-ma′shun) poisoning by venom.

en·vi·ron·ment (en-vi′ron-ment) the sum total of all the conditions and elements that make up the surroundings and influence the development of an individual. **environ·men′tal,** adj.

en·vy (en′ve) a desire to have another's possessions or qualities for oneself. **penis e.** (en′ve), the concept that the female envies the male his possession of a penis or, more generally, any of his characteristics.

en·za·cam·ene (en″zah-kam′ēn) an absorber of ultraviolet radiation, used topically as a sunscreen.

en·zy·got·ic (en″zi-got′ik) developed from the same zygote.

en·zyme (en′zīm) a protein that catalyzes chemical reactions of other substances without itself being destroyed or altered upon completion of the reactions. Enzymes are divided into six main groups: oxidoreductases, transferases, hydrolases, lyases, isomerases, and ligases. Symbol E. **allosteric e.,** one whose catalytic activity is altered by binding of specific ligands at sites other than the substrate binding site. **brancher e., branching e.,** 1,4-α-glucan branching enzyme: an enzyme that catalyzes the creation of branch points in glycogen (in plants, amylopectin); deficiency causes glycogen storage disease type IV. **constitutive e.,** one produced constantly, irrespective of environmental conditions or demand. **debrancher e., debranching e.,** 1. amylo-1,6-glucosidase. 2. any enzyme removing branches from macromolecules, usually polysaccharides, by cleaving at branch points. **induced e., inducible e.,** one whose production can be stimulated by another compound, often a substrate or a structurally related molecule. **proteolytic e.,** peptidase. **repressible e.,** one whose rate of production is decreased as the concentration of certain metabolites is increased. **respiratory e.,** one that is part of an electron transport (respiratory) chain.

en·zy·mop·a·thy (en″zi-mop′ah-the) an inborn error of metabolism consisting of defective or absent enzymes, as in the glycogenoses or the mucopolysaccharidoses.

EOG electro-olfactogram.

eo·sin (e′o-sin) any of a class of rose-colored stains or dyes, all being bromine derivatives of fluorescein; *eosin Y,* the sodium salt of tetrabromofluorescein, is much used in histologic and laboratory procedures.

eo·sin·o·pe·nia (e″o-sin″o-pe′ne-ah) abnormal deficiency of eosinophils in the blood.

eo·sin·o·phil (e″o-sin′o-fil) a granular leukocyte having a nucleus with two lobes connected by a thread of chromatin, and cytoplasm containing coarse, round granules of uniform size.

eo·sin·o·phil·ia (e″o-sin″o-fil′e-ah) abnormally increased eosinophils in the blood.

eo·sin·o·phil·ic (-fil′ik) 1. readily stainable with eosin. 2. pertaining to eosinophils. 3. pertaining to or characterized by eosinophilia.

eo·sin·o·philo·tac·tic (-fil″o-tak′tik) having the power of attracting eosinophils; chemotactic for eosinophils.

EP evoked potential.

ep- see *epi-.*

EPA eicosapentaenoic acid.

epac·tal (e-pak′til) supernumerary.

ep·al·lo·bi·o·sis (ep-al″o-bi-o′sis) dependency on an external life-support system, as on a heart-lung machine or hemodialyzer.

ep·ax·i·al (ep-ak′se-il) situated upon or above an axis.

epen·dy·ma (ĕ-pen′dĭ-mah) the membrane lining the cerebral ventricles and the central canal of the spine. **epen′dymal,** adj.

epen·dy·mo·blast (ĕ-pen′dĭ-mo-blast) an embryonic ependymal cell.

epen·dy·mo·cyte (-sīt) an ependymal cell.

epen·dy·mo·ma (ĕ-pen″dĭ-mo′mah) a neoplasm, usually slow growing and benign, composed of differentiated ependymal cells.

Ep·eryth·ro·zo·on (ep″ah-rith″ro-zo′on) a genus of the family Bartonellaceae; its members are of limited pathogenicity, infecting rodents, cattle, sheep, and swine.

ephapse (ĕ-faps′) electrical synapse. **ephap′-tic,** adj.

ephe·bi·at·rics (ĕ-fe″be-at′riks) the branch of medicine which deals especially with the diagnosis and treatment of diseases and problems peculiar to youth.

Ephed·ra (ĕ-fed′rah) a genus of low, branching shrubs indigenous to China and India. *E. equiseti′na* Bunge., *E. sini′ca* Stapf., *E. vulga′ris*, and other species (all called *ma huang* in China) are sources of ephedrine.

ephed·rine (ĕ-fed′rin, ef′ĕ-drin) an adrenergic extracted from several species of *Ephedra* or produced synthetically; used in the form of the hydrochloride, sulfate, or tannate salt as a bronchodilator, antiallergic, central nervous system stimulant, and antihypotensive. It has also been used in supplements, with benefits claimed to include weight loss, increased energy, and enhanced athletic performance.

ephe·lis (ĕ-fe′lis) pl. *ephe′lides*. [Gr.] a freckle.

epi- word element [Gr.]; *upon; over.*

epi·an·dros·ter·one (ep″e-an-dros′ter-ōn) an androgenic steroid less active than androsterone and excreted in small amounts in normal human urine.

epi·blast (ep′ĭ-blast) 1. the upper layer of the bilaminar embryonic disc present during the second week; it gives rise to ectoderm. 2. ectoderm. 3. ectoderm, except for the neural plate. **epiblas′tic,** adj.

epi·bleph·a·ron (ep″ĭ-blef′ah-ron) a developmental anomaly in which a horizontal fold of skin stretches across the border of the eyelid, pressing the eyelashes inward, against the eyelid.

epib·o·ly (e-pib′o-le) a process by which an outside cell layer spreads to envelope a yolk mass or deeper layer of cells.

epi·bul·bar (ep″ĭ-bul′ber) situated upon the eyeball.

epi·can·thus (-kan′thus) a vertical fold of skin on either side of the nose, sometimes covering the inner canthus; a normal characteristic in persons of certain races, but anomalous in others. **epican′thal, epican′thic,** adj.

epi·car·dia (-kahr′de-ah) the portion of the esophagus below the diaphragm.

epi·car·di·um (-kahr′de-um) the visceral pericardium.

epi·cho·ri·on (-kor′e-on) the portion of the uterine mucosa enclosing the implanted conceptus.

epi·con·dy·lal·gia (-kon″dil-al′jah) pain in the muscles or tendons attached to the epicondyle of the humerus.

epi·con·dyle (-kon′dĭl) an eminence upon a bone, above its condyle.

epi·con·dy·lus (-kon′dil-us) pl. *epicon′dyli.* [L.] epicondyle.

epi·cra·ni·um (-kra′ne-um) the muscles, skin, and aponeurosis covering the skull.

epi·cri·sis (ep′ĭ-kri″sis) a secondary crisis.

epi·crit·ic (ep″ĭ-krit′ik) determining accurately; said of cutaneous nerve fibers sensitive to fine variations of touch or temperature.

epi·cys·tot·o·my (-sis-tot′ah-me) cystotomy by the suprapubic method.

epi·cyte (ep′ĭ-sīt) cell membrane.

ep·i·dem·ic (ep″ĭ-dem′ik) occurring suddenly in numbers clearly in excess of normal expectancy.

ep·i·de·mi·ol·o·gy (-de″me-ol′ah-je) the science concerned with the study of the factors determining and influencing the frequency and distribution of disease, injury, and other health-related events and their causes in a defined human population. Also, the sum of knowledge gained in such a study.

epi·der·mi·dal·iza·tion (-der″mid-ah-lī-za′-shun) development of epidermal cells (stratified epithelium) from mucous cells (columnar epithelium).

epi·der·mis (-der′mis) pl. *epider′mides.* The outermost and nonvascular layer of the skin, derived from the embryonic ectoderm, varying in thickness from 0.07–1.4 mm. On the palmar and plantar surfaces it comprises, from within outward, five layers: (1) *basal layer* (stratum basale), composed of columnar cells arranged perpendicularly; (2) *prickle cell* or *spinous layer* (stratum spinosum), composed of flattened polyhedral cells with short processes or spines; (3) *granular layer* (stratum granulosum) composed of flattened granular cells; (4) *clear layer* (stratum lucidum), composed of several layers of clear, transparent cells in which the nuclei are indistinct or absent; and (5) *horny layer* (stratum corneum), composed of flattened, cornified, non-nucleated cells. In the epidermis of the general body surface, the clear layer is usually absent. **epider′mal, epider′mic,** adj.

epi·der·mi·tis (-der-mi′tis) inflammation of the epidermis.

epi·der·mo·dys·pla·sia (-der″mo-dis-pla′zhah) faulty development of the epidermis. **e. verrucifor′mis,** a condition due to a virus identical with or closely related to the virus of common warts, in which the lesions are red or red-violet and widespread, and tend to become malignant.

epi·der·moid (-der′moid) 1. pertaining to or resembling the epidermis. 2. epidermoid cyst.

epi·der·moi·do·ma (-der″moi-do′mah) epidermoid cyst (2).

epi·der·mol·y·sis (-der-mol′ĭ-sis) a loosened state of the epidermis with formation of blebs and bullae, occurring either spontaneously or at the site of trauma. **epidermolyt′ic,** adj. **e. bullo′sa,** a variety with development of bullae and vesicles, often at the site of trauma; in the hereditary forms, there may be severe scarring after healing, or extensive denuded areas after rupture of the lesions.

epi·der·mo·my·co·sis (-der″mo-mi-ko′sis) dermatophytosis.

Epi·der·moph·y·ton (-der-mof′ĭ-ton) a genus of fungi, including *E. flocco′sum*, which attacks skin and nails but not hair and is one of the causative agents of tinea cruris, tinea pedis (athlete's foot), and onychomycosis.

epi·der·mo·phy·to·sis (-der″mo-fi-to′sis) 1. dermatophytosis. 2. a fungal skin infection due to *Epidermophyton*.

ep·i·did·y·mis (-did′ĭ-mis) pl. *epidiy′mides*. [Gr.] an elongated cordlike structure along the posterior border of the testis; its coiled duct provides for storage, transit, and maturation of spermatozoa and is continuous with the ductus deferens. **epidid′ymal,** adj.

epi·did·y·mi·tis (-did″ĭ-mi′tis) inflammation of the epididymis.

epi·did·y·mo·or·chi·tis (-did″ĭ-mo-or-ki′tis) inflammation of the epididymis and testis.

epi·did·y·mo·vas·os·to·my (-vas-os′tah-me) vasoepididymostomy.

epi·du·ral (-dūr′il) situated upon or outside the dura mater.

epi·du·rog·ra·phy (-dūr-og′rah-fe) radiography of the spine after a radiopaque medium has been injected into the epidural space.

epi·es·tri·ol (ep″e-es′tre-ol) an estrogenic steroid found in pregnant women.

epi·gas·tri·um (ep″ĭ-gas′tre-um) the upper and middle region of the abdomen, located within the sternal angle. **epigas′tric,** adj.

epi·gas·tro·cele (-gas′tro-sēl) epigastric hernia.

epi·gen·e·sis (-jen′ĕ-sis) the development of an organism from an undifferentiated cell, consisting in the successive formation and development of organs and parts that do not preexist in the fertilized egg. **epigenet′ic,** adj.

epi·ge·net·ic (-jĕ-net′ik) 1. pertaining to epigenesis. 2. altering the activity of genes without changing their structure.

epi·glot·ti·dec·to·my (-glot″ĭ-dek′tah-me) excision of the epiglottis.

epi·glot·tis (-glot′is) the lidlike cartilaginous structure overhanging the entrance to the larynx, guarding it during swallowing; see Plate 31. **epiglot′tic,** adj.

epi·glot·ti·tis (ep″ĭ-glŏ-ti′tis) supraglottitis.

ep·i·la·tion (-la′shun) depilation.

epil·a·to·ry (e-pil′ah-tor″e) depilatory.

ep·i·lem·ma (-lem′ah) endoneurium.

ep·i·lep·sia (-lep′se-ah) [L.] epilepsy. **e. partia′lis conti′nua,** a form of status epilepticus with focal motor seizures, marked by continuous clonic movements of a limited part of the body.

ep·i·lep·sy (ep′ĭ-lep″se) any of a group of syndromes characterized by paroxysmal transient disturbances of brain function that may be manifested as episodic impairment or loss of consciousness, abnormal motor phenomena, psychic or sensory disturbances, or perturbation of the autonomic nervous system; symptoms are due to disturbance of the electrical activity of the brain. **absence e.,** that characterized by absence seizures, usually having its onset in childhood or adolescence. **focal e.,** that consisting of focal seizures. **generalized e.,** epilepsy in which the seizures are generalized; they may have a focal onset or be generalized from the beginning. **grand mal e.,** a symptomatic form of epilepsy, often preceded by an aura, characterized by sudden loss of consciousness with tonic-clonic seizures. **jacksonian e.,** epilepsy marked by focal motor seizures with unilateral clonic movements that start in one muscle group and spread systematically to adjacent groups, reflecting the march of epileptic activity through the motor cortex. **juvenile myoclonic e.,** a syndrome of sudden myoclonic jerks, occurring particularly in the morning or under periods of stress or fatigue, primarily in children and adolescents. **Lafora's myoclonic e.,** a form characterized by attacks of intermittent or continuous clonus of muscle groups, resulting in difficulties in voluntary movement, mental deterioration, and Lafora bodies in various cells. **myoclonic e.,** any form of epilepsy accompanied by myoclonus. **petit mal e.,** absence e. **photic e., photogenic e.,** reflex epilepsy in which seizures are induced by a flickering light. **posttraumatic e.,** that occurring after head injury. **psychomotor e.,** temporal lobe e. **reflex e.,** epileptic seizures occurring in response to sensory stimuli. **rotatory e.,** temporal lobe epilepsy in which the automatisms consist of rotating body movements. **sensory e.,** 1. seizures manifested by paresthesias or hallucinations of sight, smell, or taste. 2. reflex e. **somatosensory e.,** sensory epilepsy with paresthesias such as burning, tingling, or numbness. **temporal lobe e.,** a form characterized by complex partial seizures. **visual e.,** sensory epilepsy in which there are visual hallucinations.

ep·i·lep·tic (ep″ĭ-lep′tik) 1. pertaining to or affected with epilepsy. 2. a person affected with epilepsy.

ep·i·lep·ti·form (-lep′tĭ-form) 1. resembling epilepsy or its manifestations. 2. occurring in severe or sudden paroxysms.

ep·i·lep·to·gen·ic (-lep″to-jen′ik) causing an epileptic seizure.

ep·i·lep·toid (-lep′toid) epileptiform.

epi·man·dib·u·lar (-man-dib′u-ler) situated on the lower jaw.

epi·men·or·rha·gia (-men″o-ra′jah) too frequent and excessive menstruation.

ep·i·mer (ep′ĭ-mer) either of two optical isomers that differ in the configuration around one asymmetric carbon atom.

epim·er·ase (ĕ-pim′ĕ-rās″) an isomerase that catalyzes inversion of the configuration about an asymmetric carbon atom in a substrate having more than one center of asymmetry; thus epimers are interconverted.

ep·i·mere (ep′ĭ-mēr) the dorsal portion of a somite, from which is formed muscles innervated by the dorsal ramus of a spinal nerve.

epim·er·i·za·tion (ĕ-pim″er-ĭ-za′shun) the changing of one epimeric form of a compound into another, as by enzymatic action.

epi·mor·pho·sis (ep″ĭ-mor-fo′sis) the regeneration of a part of an organism by proliferation at the cut surface. **epimor′phic**, adj.

epi·mys·i·ot·omy (-mis″e-ot′ah-me) incision of the epimysium.

epi·mys·i·um (-mis′e-um) the fibrous sheath around an entire skeletal muscle. See Plate 7.

epi·neph·rine (-nef′rin) a catecholamine hormone secreted by the adrenal medulla and a central nervous system neurotransmitter released by some neurons. It is stored in chromaffin granules and is released in response to hypoglycemia, stress, and other factors. It is a potent stimulator of the sympathetic nervous system (adrenergic receptors), and a powerful vasopressor, increasing blood pressure, stimulating the heart muscle, accelerating the heart rate, and increasing cardiac output. It is used as a topical vasoconstrictor, cardiac stimulant, systemic antiallergic, bronchodilator, and topical antiglaucoma agent; for the last two uses it is also administered as the bitartrate salt. Called also *adrenaline* (Great Britain).

epi·neph·ros (-nef′ros) adrenal gland.

epi·neph·ryl bo·rate (ep″ĭ-nef′ril) epinephrine complexed with borate; applied topically to the conjunctiva in the treatment of open-angle glaucoma.

epi·neu·ri·um (-noor′e-um) the outermost layer of connective tissue of a peripheral nerve. **epineu′rial**, adj.

epi·ot·ic (ep″e-ot′ik) situated on or above the ear.

epi·phe·nom·e·non (ep″ĭ-fĕ-nom′ĕ-non) an accessory, exceptional, or accidental occurrence in the course of any disease.

epiph·o·ra (e-pif′or-ah) [Gr.] overflow of tears due to obstruction of lacrimal duct.

epi·phys·e·al (ep″ĭ-fiz′e-al) pertaining to or of the nature of an epiphysis.

epi·phys·i·al epiphyseal.

epiph·y·sis (ĕ-pif′ĭ-sis) pl. *epi′physes*. [Gr.] the expanded articular end of a long bone, developed from a secondary ossification center, which during the period of growth is either entirely cartilaginous or is separated from the shaft by a cartilaginous disk. annular e's, secondary growth centers occurring as rings at the periphery of the superior and inferior surfaces of the vertebral body. e. ce′rebri, pineal body. stippled e's, chondrodysplasia punctata.

epiph·y·si·tis (ĕ-pif″ĭ-si′tis) inflammation of an epiphysis or of the cartilage joining the epiphysis to a bone shaft.

ep·i·phyte (ep′ĭ-fit) an external plant parasite. **epiphyt′ic**, adj.

epi·pia (ep″ĭ-pi′ah) the part of the pia mater adjacent to the arachnoidea mater, as distinguished from the pia-glia. **epipi′al**, adj.

epip·lo·cele (ĕ-pip′lo-sēl) omental hernia.

epip·lo·on (ĕ-pip′lo-on) [Gr.] the omentum. **epiplo′ic**, adj.

epi·ret·i·nal (ep″ĭ-ret′ĭ-nal) overlying the retina.

epi·ru·bi·cin (-roo′bĭ-sin) an antineoplastic with action similar to doxorubicin; used in the treatment of various carcinomas, leukemia, lymphoma, and multiple myeloma.

epi·scle·ra (-skler′ah) the loose connective tissue between the sclera and the conjunctiva.

epi·scle·ral (-skler′′l) 1. overlying the sclera. 2. of or pertaining to the episclera.

epi·scle·ri·tis (-sklĕ-ri′tis) inflammation of the episcleral and adjacent tissues.

epis·io·per·i·neo·plas·ty (ĕ-piz″e-o-per″ĭ-ne′o-plas″te) plastic repair of the vulva and perineum.

epis·io·per·i·ne·or·rha·phy (-per″ĭ-ne-or′-ah-fe) suture of the vulva and perineum.

epis·i·or·rha·phy (e-piz″e-or′ah-fe) 1. suture of the labia majora. 2. suture of a lacerated perineum.

epis·io·ste·no·sis (e-piz″e-o-stĭ-no′sis) narrowing of the vulvar orifice.

epis·i·ot·o·my (e-piz″e-ot′ah-me) surgical incision into the perineum and vagina to prevent traumatic tearing during delivery.

ep·i·sode (ep′ĭ-sōd) a noteworthy happening occurring in the course of a continuous series of events. **hypomanic e.,** a period of elevated, expansive, or irritable mood resembling a manic episode but less severe. **major depressive e.,** a period marked by depressed mood or loss of interest or pleasure in virtually all activities, associated with some combination of: altered weight, appetite, or sleep patterns, psychomotor agitation or retardation, difficulty in thinking or concentration, fatigue, feelings of worthlessness and hopelessness, and thoughts of death and suicide. **manic e.,** a period of predominant mood elevation, expansiveness, or irritation together with some combination of inflated self-esteem or grandiosity, decreased need of sleep, talkativeness, flight of ideas, distractibility, hyperactivity, hypersexuality, and recklessness. **mixed e.,** a period during which the symptoms of both a major depressive episode and of a manic episode occur nearly every day, with rapidly alternating moods.

ep·i·some (-sōm) in bacterial genetics, any accessory extrachromosomal replicating genetic element that can exist either autonomously or integrated with the chromosome.

epi·spa·di·as (ep″ĭ-spa′de-as) congenital absence of the upper wall of the urethra, occurring in both sexes, but more often in the male, with the urethral opening somewhere on the dorsum of the penis. **epispa′diac, epispa′dial,** adj.

ep·i·stax·is (-stak′sis) nosebleed; hemorrhage from the nose, usually due to rupture of small vessels overlying the anterior part of the cartilaginous nasal septum.

epi·ster·num (-ster′num) a bone present in reptiles and monotremes that may be represented as part of the manubrium, or first piece of the sternum.

epi·stro·phe·us (-stro′fe-us) axis; see *Table of Bones.*

epi·ten·din·e·um (-ten-din′e-um) the fibrous sheath covering a tendon.

epi·thal·a·mus (-thal′ah-mus) the part of the diencephalon just superior and posterior to the thalamus, comprising the pineal body and adjacent structures; considered by some to include the stria medullaris.

ep·i·the·li·al (-the′le-al) pertaining to or composed of epithelium.

ep·i·the·li·al·iza·tion (-the″le-al-ĭ-za′shun) healing by the growth of epithelium over a denuded surface.

ep·i·the·li·a·lize (-the′le-al-īz″) to cover with epithelium.

ep·i·the·li·itis (-the′le-i′tis) inflammation of epithelium.

ep·i·the·li·oid (-the′le-oid) resembling epithelium.

ep·i·the·li·ol·y·sin (-the″le-ol′ĭ-sin) a cytolysin formed in the serum in response to injection of epithelial cells from a different species; it is capable of destroying epithelial cells of animals of the donor species.

ep·i·the·li·ol·y·sis (-the″le-ol′ĭ-sis) destruction of epithelial tissue. **epitheliolyt′ic,** adj.

ep·i·the·li·o·ma (-the″le-o′mah) 1. any tumor derived from epithelium. 2. loosely and incorrectly, carcinoma. **epithelio′matous,** adj. **malignant e.,** carcinoma.

ep·i·the·li·um (-the′le-um) pl. *epithe′lia.* [Gr.] the cellular covering of internal and external body surfaces, including the lining of vessels and small cavities. It consists of cells joined by small amounts of cementing substances and is classified according to the number of layers and the shape of the cells. **ciliated e.,** that bearing vibratile cilia on the free surface. **columnar e.,** epithelium whose cells are of much greater height than width. **cubical e., cuboidal e.,** that composed of cube-shaped cells. **glandular e.,** that composed of secreting cells. **laminated e.,** stratified e. **olfactory e.,** pseudostratified epithelium lining the olfactory region of the nasal cavity and containing the receptors for the sense of smell. **pseudostratified e.,** that in which the cells are so arranged that the nuclei occur at different levels, giving the appearance of being stratified. **seminiferous e.,** stratified epithelium lining the seminiferous tubules of the testis. **simple e.,** that composed of a single layer of cells. **squamous e.,** that composed of flattened platelike cells. **stratified e.,** that composed of cells arranged in layers. **transitional e.,** that characteristically found lining hollow organs that are subject to great mechanical change due to contraction and distention; originally thought to represent a transition between stratified squamous and columnar epithelium.

ep·i·tope (ep′ĭ-tōp) an antigenic determinant (see under *determinant*) of known structure.

ep·i·trich·i·um (ep″ĭ-trik′e-um) periderm (1).

epi·troch·lea (-trok′le-ah) the inner condyle of the humerus.

epi·tym·pan·ic (-tim-pan′ik) 1. situated upon or over the tympanum. 2. pertaining to the epitympanum (epitympanic recess).

epi·tym·pa·num (-tim′pah-num) epitympanic recess.

epo·e·tin (e-po′ĕ-tin) a recombinant form of human erythropoietin, used as an antianemic; in the United States the form used is *e. alfa* but *e. beta* may be used elsewhere.

ep·o·nych·i·um (ep″o-nik′e-um) 1. cuticle; the narrow band of epidermis extending from the nail wall onto the nail surface. 2. the horny fetal epidermis at the site of the future nail.

ep·oöph·o·ron (ep″o-of′ŏ-ron) a vestigial structure associated with the ovary.

ep·o·pro·sten·ol (e″po-pros′tĕ-nol) name for prostacyclin when used pharmaceutically; used in the form of the sodium salt as an inhibitor of platelet aggregation when blood contacts nonbiological systems, a pulmonary antihypertensive, and a vasodilator.

epox·ide (ĕ-pok′sīd) an organic compound containing a reactive group resulting from the union of an oxygen atom with two other atoms, usually carbon, that are themselves joined together.

epoxy (ĕ-pok′se) 1. epoxide. 2. see under *resin.*

ep·ro·sar·tan (ep″ro-sar′tan) an angiotensin II antagonist used as the mesylate salt as an antihypertensive.

EPP erythropoietic protoporphyria.

ep·ti·fib·a·tide (ep″tĭ-fib′ah-tīd) an inhibitor of platelet aggregation used for the prevention of thrombosis in patients with acute coronary syndrome or undergoing certain percutaneous coronary procedures.

epu·lis (ĕ-pu′lis) pl. *epu′lides.* [Gr.] 1. a nonspecific term used for tumors and tumorlike masses of the gingiva. 2. peripheral ossifying fibroma. **giant cell e.,** a sessile or pedunculated lesion of the gingiva, representing an inflammatory reaction to injury or hemorrhage.

equa·tion (e-kwa′zhun) an expression of equality between two parts. **Henderson-Hasselbalch e.,** a formula for calculating the pH of a buffer solution such as blood plasma.

equa·to·ri·al (e″kwah-tor′e-al) 1. pertaining to an equator. 2. occurring at the same distance from each extremity of an axis.

equi·ax·i·al (e″kwĭ-ak′se-il) having axes of the same length.

equi·li·bra·tion (e-kwil″ĭ-bra′shun) the achievement of a balance between opposing elements or forces. **occlusal e.,** modification of the occlusal stress, to produce simultaneous occlusal contacts, or to achieve harmonious occlusion.

equi·li·bri·um (e″kwĭ-lib′re-um) 1. balance; harmonious adjustment of parts. 2. sense of equilibrium. **dynamic e.,** the condition

of balance between varying, shifting, and opposing forces that is characteristic of living processes.

equil·in (ek′wil-in) an estrogen isolated from urine of pregnant horses.

equine (e′kwīn) pertaining to, characteristic of, or derived from the horse.

equi·no·val·gus (e-kwi″no-val′gus) talipes equinovalgus.

equi·no·va·rus (-va′rus) talipes equinovarus.

equi·po·ten·tial (e″kwĭ-pah-ten′shil) having similar and equal power or capability.

equiv·a·lent (e-kwiv′ah-lent) 1. having the same value; neutralizing or counterbalancing each other. 2. see under *weight.* **migraine e.,** the presence of the aura associated with a migraine but in the absence of a headache.

ER emergency room; endoplasmic reticulum; estrogen receptor.

Er erbium.

ERBF effective renal blood flow.

er·bi·um (Er) (er′be-um) chemical element (see *Table of Elements*), at. no. 68.

erec·tile (ĕ-rek′tīl) capable of erection.

erec·tion (ĕ-rek′shun) the condition of being rigid and elevated, as erectile tissue when filled with blood.

erec·tor (ĕ-rek′ter) [L.] a structure that erects, as a muscle which raises or holds up a part.

erg (erg) a unit of work or energy, being the work performed when a force of 1 dyne moves its point of operation through a distance of 1 cm; equal to 10^{-7} joule.

er·gas·to·plasm (er-gas′to-plazm) granular endoplasmic reticulum.

er·go·cal·cif·er·ol (er″go-kal-sif′er-ol) vitamin D_2; a sterol occurring in fungi and some fish oils or synthesized from ergosterol, with similar activity and metabolism to those of cholecalciferol; used as a dietary source of vitamin D and in the treatment of hypocalcemia, hypophosphatemia, rickets, and osteodystrophy associated with a variety of disorders.

er·go·loid mes·y·lates (er′go-loid) a mixture of the methanesulfonate salts of three hydrogenated ergot alkaloids; used in the treatment of mild to moderate dementia in the elderly.

er·gom·e·ter (er-gom′ĕ-ter) a dynamometer. **bicycle e.,** an apparatus for measuring the muscular, metabolic, and respiratory effects of exercise.

er·go·nom·ics (er″go-nom′iks) the science relating to humans and their work, including the factors affecting the efficient use of human energy.

er·go·no·vine (-no′vin) an alkaloid, from ergot or produced synthetically, used in the form of the maleate salt as an oxytocic and as a diagnostic aid in coronary vasospasm.

er·go·stat (er'go-stat) a machine to be worked for muscular exercise.

er·gos·te·rol (er-gos'tĕ-rol) a sterol occurring mainly in yeast and forming ergocalciferol (vitamin D_2) on ultraviolet irradiaion or electronic bombardment.

er·got (er'got) the dried sclerotium of the fungus *Claviceps purpurea*, which is developed on rye plants; ergot alkaloids are used as oxytocics and in treatment of migraine. See also *ergotism*.

er·got·amine (er-got'ah-min) an alkaloid of ergot; the tartrate salt is used for relief of migraine and cluster headaches.

er·got·ism (er'go-tizm) chronic poisoning produced by ingestion of ergot, marked by cerebrospinal symptoms, spasms, cramps, or by a kind of dry gangrene.

erog·e·nous (ĕ-roj'ĕ-nus) arousing erotic feelings.

ero·sion (ĕ-ro'zhun) an eating or gnawing away; a shallow or superficial ulceration; in dentistry, the wasting away or loss of substance of a tooth by a chemical process that does not involve known bacterial action. **ero'sive**, adj.

erot·ic (ĕ-rot'ik) 1. charged with sexual feeling. 2. pertaining to sexual desire.

er·o·tism (er'o-tizm) a sexual instinct or desire; the expression of one's instinctual energy or drive, especially the sex drive. **anal e.**, fixation of libido at (or regression to) the anal phase of infantile development; said to produce egotistic, dogmatic, stubborn, miserly character. **genital e.**, achievement and maintenance of libido at the genital phase of psychosexual development, permitting acceptance of normal adult relationships and responsibilities. **oral e.**, fixation of libido at the oral phase of infantile development; said to produce passive, insecure, sensitive character.

ero·to·gen·ic (ĕ-rot"o-jen'ik) erogenous.

ero·to·ma·nia (-ma'ne-ah) 1. a type of delusional disorder in which the subject harbors a delusion that a particular person is deeply in love with them; lack of response is rationalized, and pursuit and harassment may occur. 2. occasionally, hypersexuality. **erotoman'ic**, adj.

ero·to·pho·bia (-fo'be-ah) irrational fear of love, especially of sexual feelings and activities.

ERP endocardial resection procedure.

ERPF effective renal plasma flow.

er·ror (er'er) a defect in structure or function; a deviation. **inborn e. of metabolism,** a genetically determined biochemical disorder in which a specific enzyme defect causes a metabolic block that may have pathologic consequences at birth or in later life.

eru·cic ac·id (ĕ-roo'sik) a fatty acid occurring in rapeseed and mustard oils; because it has been linked to cardiac muscle damage, edible canola oil products are prepared from low erucic acid varieties of rapeseed plants.

eruc·ta·tion (ĕ"ruk-ta'shun) belching; casting up wind from the stomach through the mouth.

erup·tion (ĕ-rup'shun) 1. the act of breaking out, appearing, or becoming visible, as eruption of the teeth. 2. visible efflorescent lesions of the skin due to disease, with redness, prominence, or both; a rash. **erup'tive,** adj. **creeping e.,** cutaneous larva migrans. **drug e.,** an eruption or a solitary lesion caused by a drug taken internally. **fixed e.,** a circumscribed inflammatory skin lesion(s) recurring at the same site(s) over a period of months or years; each attack lasts only a few days but leaves residual pigmentation which is cumulative.

ERV expiratory reserve volume.

er·y·sip·e·las (er"ĭ-sip'ĭ-lis) a contagious disease of the skin and subcutaneous tissues due to infection with *Streptococcus pyogenes*, with redness and swelling of affected areas, constitutional symptoms, and sometimes vesicular and bullous lesions.

er·y·sip·e·loid (er"ĭ-sip'ĕ-loid) a dermatitis or cellulitis of the hand chiefly affecting fish handlers and caused by *Erysipelothrix insidiosa*.

Er·y·sip·e·lo·thrix (er"ĭ-sip'ĭ-lah-thriks") a genus of gram-positive bacteria (family Corynebacteriaceae), containing the single species *E. insidio'sa (E. rhusiopath'iae)*, the causative agent of swine erysipelas and erysipeloid.

er·y·the·ma (er"ĭ-the'mah) redness of the skin due to congestion of the capillaries. **erythem'atous, erythe'mic,** adj. **e. annula're,** a type of erythema multiforme with ring-shaped lesions. **e. annula're centri'fugum,** a chronic variant of erythema multiforme usually affecting the thighs and lower legs, with single or multiple erythematous-edematous papules that enlarge peripherally and clear in the center to produce annular lesions that may coalesce. **e. chro'nicum mi'grans,** an annular erythema due to the bite of a tick *(Ixodes);* it begins as an erythematous plaque several weeks after the bite and spreads peripherally with central clearing. See also *Lyme disease,* under *disease.* **cold e.,** a congenital hypersensitivity to cold seen in children, characterized by localized pain, widespread erythema, occasional muscle spasms, and vascular collapse on exposure to cold, and vomiting after drinking cold liquids. **epidemic arthritic e.,** Haverhill fever. **e. indura'tum,** chronic necrotizing vasculitis, usually occurring on the calves of young women; its association with tuberculosis is in dispute. **e. infectio'sum,** a mildly contagious, sometimes epidemic, disease of children between the ages of four and twelve, marked by a rose-colored, coarsely lacelike macular rash and caused by human parvovirus B19. **e. i'ris,** a type of erythema multiforme in which the lesions form concentric rings, producing a target-like appearance. **e. margina'tum,** a type of erythema multiforme in which the reddened areas are disk-shaped with elevated edges. **e. mi'grans,** 1. benign migratory glossitis. 2. e. chronicum migrans. **e. multi-for'me,** a symptom complex with highly polymorphic skin lesions, including macular papules, vesicles, and bullae; attacks are usually self-limited but recurrences are the rule. **e. nodo'sum,** an acute inflammatory skin disease marked by tender red nodules, usually on the shins, due to exudation of blood and serum. **e. nodo'sum lepro'sum,** a form of lepra reaction occurring in lepromatous and sometimes borderline leprosy, marked by the occurrence of tender, inflamed subcutaneous nodules; the reactions resemble multifocal Arthus reactions. **toxic e., e. tox'icum,** a generalized erythematous or erythematomacular eruption due to administration of a drug or to bacterial toxins or other toxic substances. **e. tox'icum neonato'rum,** a self-limited urticarial condition affecting infants in the first few days of life.

er·y·the·mo·gen·ic (er″ĭ-the″mo-jen′ik) producing erythema.

er·y·thras·ma (er″ĭ-thraz′mah) a chronic bacterial infection of the major skin folds due to *Corynebacterium minutissimum*, marked by red or brownish patches on the skin.

er·y·thre·mia (er″ĭ-thre′me-ah) polycythemia vera.

er·y·thre·mic (er″ə-thre′mik) pertaining to erythroid cells, particularly to those occurring in the blood in abnormal numbers or exhibiting abnormal development.

erythr(o)- word element [Gr.], *red; erythrocyte.*

eryth·ro·blast (ĕ-rith′ro-blast) originally, any nucleated erythrocyte, but now more generally used to designate a nucleated precursor cell in the erythrocytic series (q.v.). Four developmental stages in the series are recognized: the *proerythroblast* (q.v.), the *basophilic e.,* in which the cytoplasm is

basophilic, the nucleus is large with clumped chromatin, and the nucleoli have disappeared; the *polychromatophilic e.,* in which the nuclear chromatin shows increased clumping and the cytoplasm begins to acquire hemoglobin and takes on an acidophilic tint; and the *orthochromatic e.,* the final stage before nuclear loss, in which the nucleus is small and ultimately becomes a blue-black, homogeneous, structureless mass.

eryth·ro·blas·to·ma (ĕ-rith″ro-blas-to′mah) a tumor-like mass composed of nucleated red blood cells.

eryth·ro·blas·to·pe·nia (-blas″to-pe′ne-ah) abnormal deficiency of erythroblasts.

eryth·ro·blas·to·sis (-blas-to′sis) the presence of erythroblasts in the circulating blood. **erythroblastot'ic,** adj. **e. feta'lis, e. neonato'rum,** hemolytic anemia of the fetus or newborn due to transplacental transmission of maternally formed antibody against the fetus' erythrocytes, usually secondary to an incompatibility between the mother's Rh blood group and that of her offspring.

eryth·ro·chro·mia (-kro′me-ah) hemorrhagic, red pigmentation of the spinal fluid.

er·y·throc·la·sis (er″ĭ-throk′lah-sis) fragmentation of the red blood cells. **erythro-clas'tic,** adj.

eryth·ro·clast (ĕ-rith′ro-klast) ghost cell (2).

eryth·ro·cy·a·no·sis (ĕ-rith″ro-si″ah-no′sis) coarsely mottled bluish red discoloration on the legs and thighs, especially of girls; thought to be a circulatory reaction to exposure to cold.

eryth·ro·cy·ta·phe·re·sis (-si″tah-fĕ-re′sis) the withdrawal of blood, separation and retention of red blood cells, and retransfusion of the remainder into the donor.

eryth·ro·cyte (ĕ-rith′ro-sīt) red blood cell; corpuscle; one of the formed elements in peripheral blood. Normally, in humans, the mature form is a non-nucleated, yellowish, biconcave disk, containing hemoglobin and transporting oxygen. For immature forms, see *erythrocytic series,* under *series.* **baso-philic e.,** an abnormal erythrocyte that takes basic stains, as seen in basophilia. **hypochromic e.,** one that contains less than normal concentration of hemoglobin and as a result appears paler than normal; it is usually also microcytic. **normochromic e.,** one of normal color with a normal concentration of hemoglobin. **polychromatic e., polychromatophilic e.,** one that, on staining, shows shades of blue combined with tinges of pink. **target e.,** see under *cell.*

eryth·ro·cy·the·mia (ĕ-rith″ro-si-the′-me-ah) hypercythemia; an increase in the number of erythrocytes in the blood, as in erythrocytosis.

eryth·ro·cyt·ic (-sit′ik) 1. pertaining to, characterized by, or of the nature of erythrocytes. 2. pertaining to the erythrocytic series.

eryth·ro·cy·tol·y·sis (-si-tol′ĭ-sis) dissolution of erythrocytes and escape of the hemoglobin.

eryth·ro·cy·toph·a·gy (-si-tof′ah-je) erythrophagocytosis.

eryth·ro·cy·tor·rhex·is (-si″to-rek′sis) the escape from erythrocytes of round, shiny granules and the splitting off of particles.

eryth·ro·cy·tos·chi·sis (-si-tos′kĭ-sis) degeneration of erythrocytes into platelet-like bodies.

eryth·ro·cy·to·sis (-si-to′sis) increase in the total red cell mass secondary to any of a number of nonhematogenic systemic disorders in response to a known stimulus (*secondary polycythemia*), in contrast to primary polycythemia (*polycythemia vera*). **leukemic e.,** polycythemia vera. **stress e.,** see under *polycythemia*.

eryth·ro·der·ma (-der′mah) abnormal redness of the skin over widespread areas of the body. **erythroder′mic,** adj. **congenital ichthyosiform e.,** a generalized hereditary dermatitis with scaling, which occurs in bullous (*epidermolytic hyperkeratosis*) and nonbullous (*lamellar ichthyosis*) forms. **e. desquamati′vum,** Leiner's disease. **e. psoria′ticum,** erythrodermic psoriasis.

eryth·ro·don·tia (-don′shah) reddish brown pigmentation of the teeth.

eryth·ro·gen·e·sis (-jen′ĕ-sis) erythropoiesis. **e. imperfec′ta,** congenital hypoplastic anemia (1).

eryth·ro·gen·ic (-jen′ik) 1. producing erythrocytes. 2. producing a sensation of red. 3. erythemogenic.

er·y·throid (er′ĭ-throid) 1. of a red color; reddish. 2. pertaining to the cells of the erythrocytic series.

eryth·ro·ker·a·to·der·mia (ĕ-rith″ro-ker″-ah-to-der′me-ah) a reddening and hyperkeratosis of the skin. **e. varia′bilis,** a rare hereditary form of ichthyosis marked by transient, migratory areas of discrete, macular erythroderma as well as fixed hyperkeratotic plaques.

eryth·ro·ki·net·ics (-kĭ-net′iks) the quantitative, dynamic study of in vivo production and destruction of erythrocytes.

eryth·ro·labe (ĕ-rith′ro-lāb) the pigment in retinal cones that is more sensitive to the red range of the spectrum than are the other pigments (chlorolabe and cyanolabe).

eryth·ro·leu·ke·mia (ĕ-rith″ro-loo-ke′me-ah) a malignant blood dyscrasia, one of the myeloproliferative disorders, with atypical erythroblasts and myeloblasts in the peripheral blood.

eryth·ro·mel·al·gia (-mel-al′jah) paroxysmal, bilateral vasodilation, particularly of the limbs, with burning pain and increased skin temperature and redness.

eryth·ro·my·cin (-mi′sin) a broad-spectrum antibiotic produced by *Streptomyces erythreus;* used against gram-positive bacteria and certain gram-negative bacteria, spirochetes, some rickettsiae, *Entamoeba*, and *Mycoplasma pneumoniae;* used in the form of the gluceptate, lactobionate, stearate, and other salts.

er·y·thron (er′ĭ-thron) the circulating erythrocytes in the blood, their precursors, and all the body elements concerned in their production.

eryth·ro·neo·cy·to·sis (ĕ-rith″ro-ne″o-si-to′sis) presence of immature erythrocytes in the blood.

eryth·ro·pe·nia (-pe′ne-ah) deficiency in the number of erythrocytes.

eryth·ro·phage (ĕ-rith′ro-fāj) a phagocyte that ingests erythrocytes.

eryth·ro·phag·o·cy·to·sis (ĕ-rith″ro-fag″o-si-to′sis) phagocytosis of erythrocytes.

eryth·ro·phil (ĕ-rith′ro-fil) 1. a cell or other element that stains easily with red. 2. easily stained with red. **erythroph′ilous,** adj.

eryth·ro·pho·bia (ĕ-rith″ro-fo′be-ah) 1. irrational fear of the color red, often accompanied by fear of blood (hematophobia). 2. fear of blushing; a distressing tendency to blush frequently.

eryth·ro·phose (ĕ-rith′ro-fōz) any red phose.

eryth·ro·pla·kia (ĕ-rith″ro-pla′ke-ah) a slow-growing, erythematous, velvety red lesion with well-defined margins, occurring on a mucous membrane, most often in the oral cavity.

eryth·ro·pla·sia (-pla′zhah) a condition of the mucous membranes characterized by erythematous papular lesions. **e. of Queyrat,** a form of epithelial dysplasia, ranging in severity from mild disorientation of epithelial cells to carcinoma in situ to invasive carcinoma, manifested as a circumscribed, velvety, erythematous papular lesion on the uncircumcised glans penis, coronal sulcus, prepuce, or occasionally the vulva. The term is sometimes used for the corresponding lesion of the oral mucosa (erythroplakia).

eryth·ro·poi·e·sis (-poi-e′sis) the formation of erythrocytes. **erythropoiet′ic,** adj.

eryth·ro·poi·e·tin (-poi′ĕ-tin) a glycoprotein hormone secreted by the kidney in the adult and by the liver in the fetus, which acts on stem cells of the bone marrow to stimulate red blood cell production (erythropoiesis). **recombinant human e. (r-HuEPO),** epoetin.

eryth·ro·pros·o·pal·gia (-pros″o-pal′jah) a disorder similar to erythromelalgia, but with the redness and pain in the face.

eryth·ror·rhex·is (-rek′sis) erythrocytorrhexis.

er·y·thro·sis (er″ĭ-thro′sis) 1. reddish or purplish discoloration of the skin and mucous membranes, as in polycythemia vera. 2. hyperplasia of the hematopoietic tissue.

eryth·ro·sta·sis (ĕ-rith″ro-sta′sis) the stoppage of erythrocytes in the capillaries, as in sickle cell anemia.

Es einsteinium.

es·cape (es-kāp′) the act of becoming free. **atrioventricular junctional e., nodal e.,** one or more escape beats in which the atrioventricular node is the cardiac pacemaker. **vagal e.,** the exhaustion of or adaptation to neural chemical mediators in the regulation of systemic arterial pressure. **ventricular e.,** the occurrence of one or more ectopic beats in which a ventricular pacemaker becomes effective before the sinoatrial pacemaker; it usually occurs with slow sinus rates and often, but not necessarily, with increased vagal tone.

es·char (es′kahr) 1. a slough produced by a thermal burn, by a corrosive application, or by gangrene. 2. tache noire.

es·cha·rot·ic (es″kah-rot′ik) 1. corrosive; capable of producing an eschar. 2. a corrosive or caustic agent.

Esch·e·rich·ia (esh″ĕ-rik′e-ah) a genus of widely distributed, gram-negative bacteria (family Enterobacteriaceae), occasionally pathogenic for humans. **E. co′li,** a species constituting the greater part of the normal intestinal flora of humans and other animals; it is a frequent cause of urinary tract infections and epidemic diarrheal disease, especially in children.

Esch·e·rich·i·eae (esh″-ĕ-rik′e-e) in some taxonomic systems, a tribe of bacteria (family Enterobacteriaceae), comprising the genera *Escherichia* and *Shigella.*

es·cutch·eon (es-kuch′un) the pattern of distribution of the pubic hair.

-esis word element, *state; condition.*

es·march (es′mark) Esmarch's bandage.

es·mo·lol (es′mo-lol) a cardioselective β_1-blocker used as the hydrochloride salt as an antiarrhythmic in the short-term control of atrial fibrillation, atrial flutter, and noncompensatory sinus tachycardia.

eso- word element [Gr.], *within.*

eso·gas·tri·tis (es″o-gas-tri′tis) inflammation of the gastric mucosa.

es·o·mep·ra·zole mag·ne·si·um (-mep′-rah-zōl) a proton pump inhibitor, administered orally as the magnesium salt in the treatment of gastroesophageal reflux disease and in the treatment of duodenal ulcer associated with *Helicobacter pylori* infection.

esoph·a·ge·al (ĕ-sof″ah-je′al) of or pertaining to the esophagus.

esoph·a·gec·ta·sia (-jek-ta′zhah) dilatation of the esophagus.

esoph·a·gism (ĕ-sof′ah-jizm) spasm of the esophagus.

esoph·a·gi·tis (ĕ-sof″ah-ji′tis) inflammation of the esophagus. **chronic peptic e.,** reflux e. **pill e.,** that resulting from irritation by a pill that passes too slowly through the esophagus. **reflux e.,** severe gastroesophageal reflux with damage to the esophageal mucosa, often with erosion and ulceration, and sometimes leading to stricture, scarring, and perforation.

esoph·a·go·cele (ĕ-sof′ah-go-sēl″) abnormal distention of the esophagus; protrusion of the esophageal mucosa through a rupture in the muscular coat.

esoph·a·go·co·lo·plas·ty (ĕ-sof″ah-go-ko′lah-plas-te) excision of a portion of esophagus and its replacement by a segment of colon.

esoph·a·go·dyn·ia (-din′e-ah) pain in the esophagus.

esoph·a·go·esoph·a·gos·to·my (-ĕ-sof″-ah-gos′tah-me) anastomosis between two formerly remote parts of the esophagus.

esoph·a·go·gas·tric (-gas′trik) gastroesophageal.

esoph·a·go·gas·tro·du·od·enos·co·py (EGD) (-gas″tro-doo″od-ĕ-nos′kah-pe) endoscopic examination of the esophagus, stomach, and duodenum.

esoph·a·go·gas·tro·plas·ty (-gas′tro-plas″te) plastic repair of the esophagus and stomach.

esoph·a·go·gas·tros·to·my (-gas-tros′tah-me) anastomosis of the esophagus to the stomach.

esoph·a·go·je·ju·nos·to·my (-jĕ″joo-nos′-tah-me) anastomosis of the esophagus to the jejunum.

esoph·a·go·my·ot·o·my (-mi-ot′ah-me) incision through the muscular coat of the esophagus.

esoph·a·go·pli·ca·tion (-pli-ka′shun) infolding of the wall of an esophageal pouch.

esoph·a·go·res·pi·ra·to·ry (-res-pir′ah-to″re) pertaining to or communicating with the esophagus and respiratory tract (trachea or a bronchus).

esoph·a·gos·co·py (ĕ-sof″ah-gos′ko-pe) endoscopic examination of the esophagus.

esoph·a·go·ste·no·sis (ĕ-sof″ah-go-stĕ-no′sis) stricture of the esophagus.

esoph·a·got·o·my (ĕ-sof″ah-got′ah-me) incision of the esophagus.

esoph·a·gus (ĕ-sof′ah-gus) the musculo-membranous passage extending from the pharynx to the stomach. See Plate 31.

eso·pho·ria (es″o-for′e-ah) deviation of the visual axis toward that of the other eye in the absence of visual fusional stimuli.

eso·sphe·noid·itis (-sfe″noi-di′tis) osteomyelitis of the sphenoid bone.

eso·tro·pia (-tro′pe-ah) cross-eye; deviation of the visual axis of one eye toward that of the other eye. **esotrop′ic**, adj.

ESR erythrocyte sedimentation rate.

ESRD end-stage renal disease.

es·sence (es′ens) 1. that which is or necessarily exists as the cause of the properties of a body. 2. in traditional Chinese medicine, jing (q.v.). 3. a solution of a volatile oil in alcohol.

es·sen·tial (ĕ-sen′shil) 1. constituting the inherent part of a thing; giving a substance its peculiar and necessary qualities. 2. indispensable; required in the diet, as essential fatty acids. 3. idiopathic; having no obvious external cause.

EST electroshock therapy.

es·taz·o·lam (es-taz′o-lam) a benzodiazepine used as a sedative and hypnotic in the treatment of insomnia.

es·ter (es′ter) a compound formed from an alcohol and an acid by removal of water.

es·ter·ase (es′ter-ās) any enzyme which catalyzes the hydrolysis of an ester into its alcohol and acid.

es·ter·i·fy (es-ter′ĭ-fi) to combine with an alcohol with elimination of a molecule of water, forming an ester.

es·ter·ol·y·sis (es″ter-ol′ĭ-sis) the hydrolysis of an ester into its alcohol and acid. **esterolyt′ic**, adj.

es·the·si·ol·o·gy (es-the″ze-ol′ah-je) the scientific study or description of the sense organs and sensations.

es·the·sod·ic (es″the-zod′ik) conducting or pertaining to conduction of sensory impulses.

es·the·tics (es-thet′iks) in dentistry, a philosophy concerned especially with the appearance of a dental restoration, as achieved through its color or form.

es·ti·mate 1. (es′tĭ-mat) a rough calculation or one based on incomplete data. 2. (es′tĭ-mat) a statistic used to characterize the value of a population parameter. 3. (es′tĭ-māt) to produce or use such a calculation or statistic.

es·ti·ma·tor (es′tĭ-ma″ter) estimate (2).

es·tra·di·ol (es″trah-di′ol, es-tra′de-ol) the most potent estrogen in humans; pharmacologically, it is often used in the form of its esters e.g., *e. cypionate, e. valerate*) or as a semisynthetic derivative *(ethinyl e.)*. For properties and uses, see *estrogen*.

es·tra·mus·tine (-mus′tēn) an antineoplastic containing estradiol joined to mechlorethamine, used for palliative treatment of metastatic or progressive carcinoma of the prostate; used as *e. phosphate sodium*.

es·trin (es′trin) estrogen.

es·tri·ol (es′tre-ol) a relatively weak human estrogen (q.v.), being a metabolic product of estradiol and estrone found in high concentrations in urine, especially during pregnancy.

es·tro·gen (es′tro-jen) a generic term for estrus-producing compounds; the female sex hormones, including estradiol, estriol, and estrone. In humans, the estrogens are formed in the ovary, adrenal cortex, testis, and fetoplacental unit, and are responsible for female secondary sex characteristic development, and, during the menstrual cycle, act on the female genitalia to produce an environment suitable for fertilization, implantation, and nutrition of the early embryo. Uses for estrogens include oral contraceptives, hormone replacement therapy, advanced prostate or postmenopausal breast carcinoma treatment, and osteoporosis prophylaxis. **conjugated e's**, a mixture of the sodium salts of the sulfate esters of estrone and equilin, having the actions and uses of estrogens. **esterified e's**, a mixture of the sodium salts of esters of estrogenic substances, principally estrone; the uses are those of estrogens.

es·tro·gen·ic (es″tro-jen′ik) 1. estrus-producing; having the properties of, or similar to, an estrogen. 2. pertaining to, having the effects of, or similar to an estrogen.

es·trone (es′trōn) an estrogen isolated from pregnancy urine, human placenta, palm kernel oil, and other sources, also prepared synthetically; for properties and uses, see *estrogen*.

es·tro·phil·in (es″tro-fil′in) a cell protein that acts as a receptor for estrogen, found in estrogenic target tissue and in estrogen-dependent tumors and metastases.

es·tro·pi·pate (es′tro-pĭ-pāt) a compound of estrone sulfate and piperazine; used as an estrogen.

ESV end-systolic volume.

eta·ner·cept (e-tan′er-sept) a soluble tumor necrosis factor receptor that inactivates tumor necrosis factor, used in the treatment of rheumatoid arthritis.

eth·a·cryn·ate (eth″ah-krin′āt) a salt, ester, or the conjugate base of ethacrynic acid; the sodium salt has the same actions as the acid.

eth·a·cryn·ic ac·id (eth-ah-krin′ik) a loop diuretic used in the treatment of edema, including that associated with congestive heart failure or hepatic or renal disease, ascites, and hypertension.

etham·bu·tol (ĕ-tham′bu-tol) an antibacterial, specifically effective against *Mycobacterium;* used with one or more other antituberculous drugs in the treatment of pulmonary tuberculosis, administered as the hydrochloride salt.

eth·a·nol (eth′ah-nol) ethyl alcohol; a primary alcohol formed by microbial fermentation of carbohydrates or by synthesis from ethylene. Excessive ingestion results in acute intoxication and ingestion during pregnancy can harm the fetus. The pharmaceutical preparation is called alcohol.

eth·a·nol·amine (eth″ah-nol′ah-mēn) monoethanolamine. **e. oleate,** the oleate salt of monoethanolamine, used as a sclerosing agent in treatment of varicose veins and esophageal varices.

eth·chlor·vy·nol (eth-klor′vĭ-nol) a nonbarbiturate sedative and hypnotic, used for the short-term treatment of insomnia; administered orally.

ether (e′ther) 1. an organic compound having an oxygen atom bonded to two carbon atoms; R–O–R′. 2. $C_2H_5OC_2H_5$ *(diethyl or ethyl e.);* the first inhalational anesthetic used for surgical anesthesia, now little used because of its flammability.

ethe·re·al (ĕ-thēr′e-il) 1. pertaining to, prepared with, containing, or resembling ether. 2. evanescent; delicate.

eth·i·nyl (eth′ĭ-nil) the radical $HC{\equiv}C{-}$, derived from acetylene. **e. estradiol,** a semisynthetic derivative of estradiol; used in combination with a progestational agent as an oral contraceptive, in hormone replacement therapy, and as an antineoplastic in the treatment of advanced breast and prostate cancers.

ethi·on·am·ide (ĕ-thi″on-am′īd) an antibacterial, effective against *Mycobacterium tuberculosis;* used in the treatment of pulmonary tuberculosis.

eth·mo·fron·tal (eth″mo-frun′t′l) pertaining to the ethmoid and frontal bones.

eth·moid (eth′moid) 1. sievelike; cribriform. 2. the ethmoid bone; see *Table of Bones.* **ethmoi′dal,** adj.

eth·moid·ec·to·my (eth″moi-dek′tah-me) excision of ethmoidal cells or of a portion of the ethmoid bone.

eth·moid·ot·o·my (eth″moi-dot′ah-me) incision into the ethmoid sinus.

eth·mo·max·il·lary (eth″mo-mak′sĭ-lar-e) pertaining to the ethmoid and maxillary bones.

eth·mo·tur·bi·nal (-turb′in-il) pertaining to the superior and middle nasal conchae.

eth·nic (eth′nik) pertaining to a group sharing cultural bonds or physical characteristics.

eth·no·bi·ol·o·gy (eth″no-bi-ol′ah-je) the study of the interaction between cultural groups and the plant and animal life in their environment.

eth·no·bot·a·ny (-bot′ah-ne) the systematic study of the interactions between a culture and the plants in its environment, particularly the knowledge about and use of such plants.

eth·nol·o·gy (eth-nol′ah-je) the science dealing with the major cultural groups of humans, their descent, relationship, etc.

eth·no·med·i·cine (eth″no-med′ĭ-sin) medical systems based on the cultural beliefs and practices of specific ethnic groups. **ethnomed′ical,** adj.

eth·no·phar·ma·col·o·gy (-fahr″mah-kol′-ah-je) the systematic study of the use of medicinal plants by specific cultural groups.

ethol·o·gy (e-thol′ah-je) the scientific study of animal behavior, particularly in the natural state. **etholog′ical,** adj.

etho·pro·pa·zine (eth″o-pro′pah-zēn) an antidyskinetic used as the hydrochloride salt in the treatment of parkinsonism and for the control of drug-induced extrapyramidal reactions.

etho·sux·i·mide (-suk′sĭ-mīd) an anticonvulsant used in the treatment of seizures in absence epilepsy.

etho·to·in (eth′o-toin) an anticonvulsant used in the treatment of grand mal epilepsy and temporal lobe epilepsy.

eth·yl (eth′il) the monovalent radical, C_2H_5. **e. chloride,** a local anesthetic sprayed on intact skin to produce anesthesia by superficial freezing caused by its rapid evaporation.

eth·yl·cel·lu·lose (eth″il-sel′u-lōs) an ethyl ether of cellulose; used as a pharmaceutical tablet binder.

eth·y·lene (eth′ĭ-lēn) a colorless flammable gas, $CH_2{=}CH_2$, with a slightly sweet odor and taste; formerly used as an inhalation anesthetic. **e. dibromide,** a fumigant and gasoline additive; it is a skin and mucous membrane irritant and is carcinogenic. **e. dichloride,** a solvent, gasoline additive, and intermediate; it is irritating and toxic, and can be carcinogenic. **e. glycol,** a solvent used as an antifreeze; ingestion can cause central nervous system depression, vomiting, hypotension, coma, convulsions, and death. **e. oxide,** a gas used in manufacturing organic compounds and as a fumigant, fungicide, and sterilizing agent; it is highly irritating to the eyes and mucous membranes and is carcinogenic.

eth·y·lene·di·a·mine (eth″ĭ-lēn-di′ah-mēn) a clear liquid with an ammonialike odor and a strong alkaline reaction; complexed with theophylline it forms aminophylline.

eth·y·lene·di·a·mine·tet·ra·a·ce·tic ac·id (EDTA) (-di″ah-mēn-tet″rah-ah-se′tik) a chelating agent that binds calcium and other metals, used as an anticoagulant for preserving blood specimens; also used to treat lead poisoning and hypercalcemia (see *edetate*).

eth·yl·i·dene (eth′il-ĭ-dēn) the bivalent radical $CH_3CH=$; its chloride derivative is used as a solvent and fumigant and is toxic and irritant.

eth·yl·nor·epi·neph·rine (eth″il-nor-ep″ĭ-nef′rin) a synthetic adrenergic, used as the hydrochloride salt in treatment of bronchial asthma.

ethy·no·di·ol (ĕ-thi″no-di′ol) a progestational agent used, as the diacetate salt, in combination with an estrogen component as an oral contraceptive.

eti·do·caine (ĕ-te′do-kān) a local anesthetic used as the hydrochloride salt for infiltration anesthesia, peripheral nerve block, retrobulbar block, and epidural block.

eti·dro·nate (e-tĭ-dro′nāt) a diphosphonate compound used for treatment of osteitis deformans, heterotopic ossification, and neoplasm-associated hypercalcemia, usually as the disodium salt. Complexed with technetium 99m it is also used in bone scanning.

eti·o·la·tion (e″te-o-la′shun) 1. blanching or paleness of a plant grown in the dark due to lack of chlorophyll. 2. the process by which the skin becomes pale when deprived of sunlight.

eti·ol·o·gy (e″te-ol′ah-je) 1. the science dealing with causes of disease. 2. the cause of a disease. **etiolog′ic, etiolog′ical,** adj.

ET-NANB enterically transmitted non-A, non-B hepatitis; see *hepatitis E*, under *hepatitis*.

eto·do·lac (e-to-do′lak) a nonsteroidal antiinflammatory drug used as an analgesic and antiinflammatory, especially to treat arthritis.

etom·i·date (ĕ-tom′ĭ-dāt) a sedative-hypnotic, administered intravenously for the induction and maintenance of anesthesia.

eto·po·side (e″to-po′sīd) a semisynthetic derivative of podophyllotoxin used as the base or the phosphate salt as an antineoplastic, particularly for treating testicular tumors and small cell lung carcinoma.

Eu europium.

eu- word element [Gr.], *normal; good; well; easy.*

Eu·bac·te·ri·a·les (u″bak-tēr′e-a′lēz) in former taxonomic systems an order of schizomycetes comprising the true bacteria.

Eu·bac·te·ri·um (u-bak-tēr′e-um) a genus of bacteria of the family Propionibacteriaceae, found as saprophytes in soil and water, and normal inhabitants of human skin and cavities, occasionally causing infection of soft tissue.

eu·ca·lyp·tol (u″kah-lip′tol) the chief constituent of eucalyptus oil, also obtained from other oils, and used as a flavoring agent, expectorant, and local anesthetic.

eu·cap·nia (u-kap′ne-ah) normal carbon dioxide tension of the blood.

Eu·cary·o·tae (u-kar″e-o′te) a kingdom of organisms that includes higher plants and animals, fungi, protozoa, and most algae (except blue-green algae); it comprises all organisms made of eukaryotic cells.

eu·chlor·hy·dria (u″klor-hi′dre-ah) the presence of the normal amount of hydrochloric acid in the gastric juice.

eu·cho·lia (u-kōl′e-ah) normal condition of the bile.

eu·chro·ma·tin (u-kro′mah-tin) that state of chromatin in which it stains lightly, is genetically active, and is considered to be partially or fully uncoiled.

eu·cra·sia (u-kra′zhah) 1. a state of health; proper balance of different factors constituting a healthy state. 2. a state in which the body reacts normally to ingested or injected drugs, proteins, etc.

eu·gen·ol (u′jen-ol) a dental analgesic and antiseptic obtained from clove oil or other natural sources; applied topically to dental cavities and also used as a component of dental protectives.

eu·glob·u·lin (u-glob′ul-in) one of a class of globulins characterized by being insoluble in water but soluble in saline solutions.

eu·gly·ce·mia (u-gli-se′me-ah) normal glucose content of the blood. **euglyce′mic,** adj.

eu·gon·ic (u-gon′ik) growing luxuriantly; said of bacterial cultures.

eu·kary·on (u-kar′e-on) 1. a highly organized nucleus bounded by a nuclear membrane, a characteristic of cells of higher organisms; cf. *prokaryon.* 2. eukaryote.

eu·kary·o·sis (u″kar-e-o′sis) the state of having a true nucleus.

Eu·kary·o·tae (u-kar″e-o′te) Eucaryotae.

eu·kary·ote (u-kar′e-ōt) an organism whose cells have a true nucleus bounded by a nuclear membrane within which lie the chromosomes; eukaryotic cells also contain many membrane-bound organelles in which cellular functions are performed. The cells of higher plants and animals, fungi, protozoa, and most algae are eukaryotic. Cf. *prokaryote.*

eu·kary·ot·ic (u″kar-e-ot′ik) pertaining to a eukaryon or to a eukaryote.

eu·lam·i·nate (u-lam′ĭ-nāt) having the normal number of laminae, as certain areas of the cerebral cortex.

eu·men·or·rhea (u″men-o-re′ah) normal menstruation.

eu·me·tria (u-me′tre-ah) [Gr.] a normal condition of nerve impulse, so that a voluntary movement just reaches the intended goal; the proper range of movement.

Eu·my·co·ta (u″mi-ko′tah) in some systems of classification, a division of the Fungi, the true fungi; organisms whose trophic phase is not motile but whose reproductive cells may be motile.

eu·nuch (u′nik) a male deprived of the testes or external genitals, especially one castrated before puberty (so that male secondary sex characteristics fail to develop).

eu·nuch·oid·ism (u′nik-oi-dizm) hypogonadism in a male; deficiency of the testes or of their secretion, with deficient secondary sex characters. **female e.,** hypogonadism in which the ovaries fail to function at puberty, resulting in infertility, absence of development of secondary sex characteristics, infantile sexual organs, and excessive growth of the long bones. **hypergonadotropic e.,** see under *hypogonadism.* **hypogonadotropic e.,** see under *hypogonadism.*

eu·pep·sia (u-pep′se-ah) good digestion; the presence of a normal amount of pepsin in the gastric juice. **eupep′tic,** adj.

Eu·phor·bia (u-for′be-ah) a large genus of trees, shrubs, and herbs of the family Euphorbiaceae, whose sap is emetic and cathartic and in some species poisonous.

eu·pho·ria (u-for′e-ah) an exaggerated feeling of physical and mental well-being, especially when not justified by external reality. **euphor′ic,** adj.

eu·plas·tic (u-plas′tik) readily becoming organized; adapted to the formation of tissue, as in embryonic development or wound healing.

eu·ploid (u′ploid) 1. having a balanced set or sets of chromosomes, in any number. 2. a euploid individual or cell.

eup·nea (ūp-ne′ah) normal respiration. **eupne′ic,** adj.

eu·rhyth·mia (u-rith′me-ah) harmonious relationships in body or organ development.

eu·ro·pi·um (Eu) (u-ro′pe-um) chemical element (see *Table of Elements*), at. no. 63.

Eu·ro·ti·um (ūr-o′she-um) a genus of fungi or molds.

eury- word element [Gr.], *wide; broad.*

eu·ry·ce·phal·ic (ūr″ĭ-sĭ-fal′ik) having a wide head.

eu·ry·on (ūr′e-on) a point on either parietal bone marking either end of the greatest transverse diameter of the skull.

eu·tha·na·sia (u″thah-na′zhah) 1. an easy or painless death. 2. mercy killing; the deliberate ending of life of a person suffering from an incurable disease.

eu·ther·mic (u-ther′mik) characterized by the proper temperature; promoting warmth.

eu·to·cia (u-to′shah) normal labor, or childbirth.

eu·top·ic (u-top′ik) situated normally; arising from the normal site or tissue.

Eu·trom·bic·u·la (u″trom-bik′ūl-ah) a subgenus of *Trombicula; E. alfreddugèsi* is the most common chigger of the United States.

eu·tro·phia (u-tro′fe-ah) a state of normal (good) nutrition. **eutroph′ic,** adj.

eV electron volt.

evac·u·ant (e-vak′u-ant) 1. emptying. 2. cathartic (1, 2). 3. a remedy that empties any organ, such as a cathartic, emetic, or diuretic.

evac·u·a·tion (e-vak″u-a′shun) 1. an emptying. 2. catharsis; emptying of the bowels.

evag·i·na·tion (e-vaj″ĭ-na′shun) obtrusion of a layer or part to form a pouch.

even·tra·tion (e″ven-tra′shun) 1. herniation of intestines; see *hernia.* 2. evisceration (1). **diaphragmatic e.,** a congenital anomaly characterized by failure of muscular development of part or all of one (or occasionally both) hemidiaphragms, resulting in superior displacement of abdominal viscera and altered lung development.

ever·sion (e-ver′zhun) a turning inside out; a turning outward.

evis·cer·a·tion (e-vis″er-a′shun) 1. removal of the abdominal viscera. 2. removal of the contents of the eyeball, leaving the sclera.

evo·ca·tion (ev″ah-ka′shun) the calling forth of morphogenetic potentialities through contact with organizer material.

evo·ca·tor (ev′o-kāt″er) a chemical substance emitted by an organizer that evokes a specific morphogenetic response from competent embryonic tissue in contact with it.

evo·lu·tion (ev″ah-loo′shun) a developmental process in which an organ or organism becomes more and more complex by differentiation of its parts; a continuous and progressive change according to certain laws and by means of resident forces. **convergent e.**, the appearance of similar forms and/or functions in two or more lines not sufficiently related phylogenetically to account for the similarity. **organic e.**, the origin and development of species; the theory that existing organisms are the result of descent with modification from those of past times.

evul·sion (e-vul′shun) extraction by force.

ex- word element [L.], *away from; out of.*

exa- a word element used in naming units of measurement to designate a quantity 10^{18} (a quintillion, or million million million) times the unit to which it is joined. Symbol E.

ex·am·i·na·tion (eg-zam″ĭ-na′shun) inspection or investigation, especially as a means of diagnosing disease, qualified according to the methods used, as physical, cystoscopic, etc. **double-contrast e.**, radiologic examination of the stomach or intestine by following a high concentration of contrast medium with evacuation and injection of air or an effervescent substance to inflate the organ; the remaining light coating of contrast medium delineates the mucosal surface.

ex·an·them (eg-zan′them) 1. any eruptive disease or fever. 2. an eruption characterizing an eruptive fever.

ex·an·the·ma (eg″zan-the′mah) pl. *exanthemas, exanthem′ata.* [Gr.] exanthem. **e. su′bitum**, an acute but mild viral disease of children, with high fever for about 3 days, followed by a rash on the trunk; caused by human herpesvirus 6.

ex·an·them·a·tous (eg″zan-them′ah-tus) characterized by or of the nature of an eruption or rash.

ex·ar·tic·u·la·tion (eks″ar-tik-ūl-a′shun) disarticulation.

ex·ca·la·tion (eks″kah-la′shun) absence or exclusion of one member of a normal series, such as a vertebra.

ex·ca·va·tio (eks″kah-va′she-o) pl. *excavatio′nes.* [L.] excavation.

ex·ca·va·tion (-shun) 1. the act of hollowing out. 2. a hollowed-out space, or pouchlike cavity. **atrophic e.**, cupping of the optic disk, due to atrophy of the optic nerve fibers. **dental e.**, removal of carious material from a tooth in preparation for filling. **recto-uterine e.**, a sac formed by a fold of peritoneum dipping down between the uterus and rectum. **rectovesical e.**, the space between the rectum and bladder in the peritoneal

cavity of the male. **vesicouterine e.**, the space between the bladder and uterus in the peritoneal cavity of the female.

ex·cess (ek′ses) a surplus, an amount greater than that which is normal or that which is required. **antigen e.**, the presence of more than enough antigen to saturate all available antibody binding sites.

ex·change (eks-chānj) 1. the substitution of one thing for another. 2. to substitute one thing for another. **plasma e.**, the removal of plasma from withdrawn blood, with retransfusion of the formed elements into the donor; done for removal of circulating antibodies or abnormal plasma constituents. The plasma removed is replaced by type-specific frozen plasma or by albumin.

ex·chang·er (eks-chānj′er) an apparatus by which something may be exchanged. **heat e.**, a device placed in the circuit of extracorporeal circulation to induce rapid cooling and rewarming of blood.

ex·cip·i·ent (ek-sip′e-int) any more or less inert substance added to a drug to give suitable consistency or form to the drug; a vehicle.

ex·cise (ek-sīz′) to remove by cutting.

ex·ci·sion (ek-sizh′un) resection; removal of a portion or all of an organ or other structure. **excis′ional**, adj.

ex·ci·ta·ble (ek-sīt′ah-b'l) irritable (1).

ex·ci·ta·tion (ek″si-ta′shun) 1. irritation or stimulation. 2. the addition of energy, such as excitation of a molecule by absorption of photons. **direct e.**, electrostimulation of a muscle by placing the electrode on the muscle itself. **indirect e.**, electrostimulation of a muscle by placing the electrode on its nerve.

ex·ci·tor (ek-si′tor) a nerve which stimulates a part to greater activity.

ex·clave (eks′klāv) a detached part of an organ.

ex·clu·sion (eks-kloo′zhun) 1. a shutting out or elimination. 2. surgical isolation of a part, as of a segment of intestine, without removal from the body.

ex·coch·le·a·tion (eks″kok-le-a′shun) curettement of a cavity.

ex·co·ri·a·tion (eks-ko″re-a′shun) any superficial loss of substance, as that produced on the skin by scratching.

ex·cre·ment (eks′krĭ-mint) 1. feces. 2. excretion (2).

ex·cres·cence (eks-kres′ins) an abnormal outgrowth; a projection of morbid origin. **excres′cent**, adj.

ex·cre·ta (eks-krēt′ah) excretion (2).

ex·crete (eks-krēt′) to throw off or eliminate by a normal discharge, such as waste matter.

ex·cre·tion (eks-kre′shun) 1. the act, process, or function of excreting. 2. material that is excreted. **ex′cretory**, adj.

ex·cur·sion (eks-kur′zhun) a range of movement regularly repeated in performance of a function, e.g., excursion of the jaws in mastication. **excur′sive**, adj.

ex·cy·clo·pho·ria (ek″si-klo-for′e-ah) cyclophoria in which the upper pole of the visual axis deviates toward the temple.

ex·cy·clo·tro·pia (-tro′pe-ah) cyclotropia in which the upper pole of the visual axis deviates toward the temple.

ex·cys·ta·tion (ek″sis-ta′shun) escape from a cyst or envelope, as in that stage in the life cycle of parasites occurring after the cystic form has been swallowed by the host.

exe·mes·tane (ek″sĕ-mes′tān) an aromatase inactivator related to androstenedione; used as an antineoplastic.

ex·en·ter·a·tion (ek-sen″ter-a′shun) 1. surgical removal of the inner organs; evisceration. 2. in ophthalmology, removal of the entire contents of the orbit. **pelvic e.,** excision of the organs and adjacent structures of the pelvis.

ex·en·ter·a·tive (eks-sen′ter-ah-tiv) pertaining to or requiring exenteration, as exenterative surgery.

ex·er·cise (ek′ser-sīz) performance of physical exertion for improvement of health or correction of physical deformity. **active e.,** motion imparted to a part by voluntary contraction and relaxation of its controlling muscles. **aerobic e.,** that designed to increase oxygen consumption and improve functioning of the cardiovascular and respiratory systems. **endurance e.,** one that involves the use of several large groups of muscles and is thus dependent on the delivery of oxygen to the muscles by the cardiovascular system. **isokinetic e.,** dynamic muscle activity performed at a constant angular velocity; torque and tension remain constant while muscles shorten or lengthen. **isometric e.,** active exercise performed against stable resistance, without change in the length of the muscle. **isotonic e.,** active exercise without appreciable change in the force of muscular contraction, with shortening of the muscle. **Kegel e's,** exercises performed to strengthen the pubococcygeal muscle. **passive e.,** motion imparted to a part by another person or outside force, or produced by voluntary effort of another segment of the patient's own body. **range of motion e.,** the putting of a joint through its full range of normal movements, either actively or passively. **resistance e., resistive e.,** that performed by the patient against resistance, as from a weight.

ex·fe·ta·tion (eks″fe-ta′shun) ectopic or extrauterine pregnancy.

ex·flag·el·la·tion (eks-flaj″ĕ-la′shun) the rapid formation in the gut of the insect vector of microgametes from the microgamont in *Plasmodium* and certain other sporozoan protozoa.

ex·fo·li·a·tion (eks-fo″le-a′shun) 1. a falling off in scales or layers. 2. the removal of scales or flakes from the surface of the skin. 3. the normal loss of primary teeth after loss of their root structure. **exfo′liative**, adj. **lamellar e. of newborn,** a congenital hereditary disorder in which the infant (collodion baby) is born entirely covered with a collodion- or parchment-like membrane that peels off within 24 hours, after which there may be complete healing, or the scales may re-form and the process be repeated; in the more severe form, the infant (harlequin fetus) is entirely covered with thick, horny, armor-like scales, and is usually stillborn or dies soon after birth.

ex·ha·la·tion (eks″hah-la′shun) 1. the giving off of watery or other vapor. 2. a vapor or other substance exhaled or given off. 3. the act of breathing out.

ex·hale (eks′hāl) to breathe out.

ex·haus·tion (eg-zaws′chun) 1. a state of extreme mental or physical fatigue. 2. the state of being drained, emptied, or consumed. **heat e.,** an effect of excessive exposure to heat, marked by subnormal body temperature with dizziness, headache, nausea, and sometimes delirium and/or collapse.

ex·hi·bi·tion·ism (ek″sĭ-bish′in-izm) a paraphilia marked by recurrent sexual urges for and fantasies of exposing one's genitals to an unsuspecting stranger.

ex·hi·bi·tion·ist (ek″sĭ-bish′in-ist) a person who indulges in exhibitionism.

ex(o)- word element [Gr.], *outside; outward.*

exo·crine (ek′so-krin) 1. secreting externally via a duct. 2. denoting such a gland or its secretion.

exo·cyc·lic (ek″so-sik′lik) denoting one or more atoms attached to a ring but outside it.

exo·cy·to·sis (-si-to′sis) 1. the discharge from a cell of particles that are too large to diffuse through the wall; the opposite of endocytosis. 2. the aggregation of migrating leukocytes in the epidermis as part of the inflammatory response.

exo·de·vi·a·tion (-de″ve-a′shun) a turning outward; in ophthalmology, exotropia.

ex·odon·tics (-don′tiks) that branch of dentistry dealing with extraction of teeth.

exo·en·zyme (-en'zīm) an enzyme that acts outside the cell which secretes it.

exo·eryth·ro·cyt·ic (-ĕ-rith″ro-sit'ik) occurring outside the erythrocyte; applied to developmental stages of malarial parasites taking place in cells other than erythrocytes.

ex·og·a·my (ek-sog'ah-me) fertilization by union of elements that are not derived from the same cell.

ex·og·e·nous (ek-soj'ĕ-nus) originating outside or caused by factors outside the organism.

ex·om·pha·los (eks-om'fah-los) 1. hernia of the abdominal viscera into the umbilical cord. 2. congenital umbilical hernia.

ex·on (ek'son) the coding region in a gene.

exo·nu·cle·ase (ek″so-noo'kle-ās) any nuclease specifically catalyzing the hydrolysis of terminal bonds of deoxyribonucleotide or ribonucleotide chains, releasing mononucleotides.

exo·pep·ti·dase (-pep'tĭ-dās) any peptidase that catalyzes the cleavage of the terminal or penultimate peptide bond, releasing a single amino acid or dipeptide from the peptide chain.

Exo·phi·a·la (-fi'ah-lah) a genus of saprobic fungi; *E. werneckii* is now called *Hortaea werneckii*.

exo·pho·ria (-for'e-ah) deviation of the visual axis of one eye away from that of the other eye in the absence of visual fusional stimuli. **exophor'ic**, adj.

ex·oph·thal·mom·e·try (ek″sof-thal-mom'ĕ-tre) measurement of the extent of protrusion of the eyeball in exophthalmos. **exophthalmomet'ric**, adj.

ex·oph·thal·mos (-thal'mos) abnormal protrusion of the eye. **exophthal'mic**, adj.

exo·phyt·ic (ek″so-fit'ik) growing outward; in oncology, proliferating on the exterior or surface epithelium of an organ or other structure in which the growth originated.

exo·skel·e·ton (-skel'ĕ-ton) a hard structure formed on the outside of the body, as a crustacean's shell; in vertebrates, applied to structures produced by the epidermis, as hair, nails, hoofs, teeth, etc.

ex·os·mo·sis (ek″sos-mo'sis) osmosis or diffusion from within outward.

ex·os·to·sis (ek″sos-to'sis) 1. a benign bony growth projecting outward from a bone surface. 2. osteochondroma. **exostot'ic**, adj. **e. cartilagi'nea**, a variety of osteoma consisting of a layer of cartilage developing beneath the periosteum of a bone. **ivory e.**, compact osteoma. **multiple e's**, an inherited condition in which multiple cartilaginous or osteocartilaginous excrescences grow out from the cortical surfaces of long bones. **subungual e.**, a cartilage-capped reactive bone spur occurring on the distal phalanx, usually of the great toe.

exo·ther·mal (ek″so-ther'mal) exothermic.

exo·ther·mic (-ther'mik) marked or accompanied by evolution of heat; liberating heat or energy.

exo·tox·in (ek'so-tok″sin) a potent toxin formed and excreted by the bacterial cell, and free in the surrounding medium. **ex'otoxic**, adj. **streptococcal pyrogenic e.**, one produced by *Streptococcus pyogenes*, existing in several antigenic types and causing fever, the rash of scarlet fever, organ damage, increased blood-brain barrier permeability, and alterations in immune response.

exo·tro·pia (-tro'pe-ah) strabismus in which there is permanent deviation of the visual axis of one eye away from that of the other, resulting in diplopia. **exotro'pic**, adj.

ex·pan·der (ek-span'der) [L.] extender. **subperiosteal tissue e. (STE)**, a fillable tube inserted temporarily into the subperiosteal tissue and progressively inflated to expand the periosteal mucosa and create space for later reconstruction.

ex·pan·sion (ek-span'shun) 1. the process or state of being increased in extent, surface, or bulk. 2. a region or area of increased bulk or surface. **clonal e.**, an immunological response in which lymphocytes stimulated by antigen proliferate and amplify the population of relevant cells. **dorsal digital e.**, **extensor e.**, extensor aponeurosis; a triangular aponeurotic extension of the digital extensor tendon on the dorsum of the proximal phalanx of each digit, to which the tendons of the lumbrical and interosseous muscles are also attached, forming a movable hood around the metacarpophalangeal joint.

ex·pec·to·rant (ek-spek'ter-ant) 1. promoting expectoration. 2. an agent that promotes expectoration. **liquefying e.**, an expectorant that promotes the ejection of mucus from the respiratory tract by decreasing its viscosity.

ex·pec·to·ra·tion (ek-spek″ter-a'shun) 1. the coughing up and spitting out of material from the lungs, bronchi, and trachea. 2. sputum.

ex·per·i·ment (ek-sper'i-ment) a procedure done in order to discover or demonstrate some fact or general truth. **experimen'tal**, adj. **control e.**, one made under standard conditions, to test the correctness of other observations.

ex·pi·rate (eks'pĭ-rāt) exhaled air or gas.

ex·pi·ra·tion (eks″pĭ-ra'shun) 1. exhalation. **expi'ratory**, adj. 2. termination or death.

ex·pire (ek-spi′er) 1. to exhale. 2. to die.

ex·plant 1. (eks-plant′) to take from the body and place in an artificial medium for growth. 2. (eks′plant) tissue taken from the body and grown in an artificial medium.

ex·plo·ra·tion (eks″plor-a′shun) investigation or examination for diagnostic purposes. **explo′ratory,** adj.

ex·plo·sive (ek-splo′siv) 1. pertaining to or occurring in a sudden violent burst. 2. tending to sudden violent outbursts.

ex·po·sure (eks-po′zher) 1. the act of laying open, as surgical exposure. 2. the condition of being subjected to something, as to infectious agents, extremes of weather, or radiation, which may have a harmful effect. 3. in radiology, a measure of the amount of ionizing radiation at the surface of the irradiated object, e.g., the body. **air e.,** radiation exposure measured in a small mass of air, excluding backscatter from irradiated objects.

ex·pres·sion (eks-presh′un) 1. the aspect or appearance of the face as determined by the physical or emotional state. 2. the act of squeezing out or evacuating by pressure. 3. gene e. **gene e.,** 1. the flow of genetic information from gene to protein. 2. the process, or the regulation thereof, by which the effects of a gene are manifested. 3. the manifestation of a heritable trait.

ex·pres·siv·i·ty (eks″pres-siv′ĭ-te) in genetics, the extent to which an inherited trait is manifested by an individual.

ex·san·gui·na·tion (ek-sang″gwin-a′shun) extensive loss of blood due to internal or external hemorrhage.

ex·sic·ca·tion (ek″sĭ-ka′shun) the act of drying out; in chemistry, the deprival of a crystalline substance of its water of crystallization.

ex·sorp·tion (ek-sorp′shun) the movement of substances out of cells, especially the movement of substances out of the blood into the intestinal lumen.

ex·stro·phy (ek′stro-fe) the turning inside out of an organ. **e. of the bladder,** congenital absence of a portion of the lower anterior abdominal wall and the anterior bladder wall, with eversion of the posterior bladder wall through the defect, an open pubic arch, and widely separated ischia connected by a fibrous band. **e. of cloaca, cloacal e.,** a developmental anomaly in which two hemibladders are separated by an area of intestine with a mucosal surface, resembling a large red tumor in the midline of the lower abdomen.

ext. extract.

ex·tend·ed-re·lease (ek-stend′ed-re-lēs′) allowing a twofold or greater reduction in frequency of administration of a drug in comparison with the frequency required by a conventional dosage form.

ex·ten·der (ek-sten′der) something that enlarges or prolongs. **artificial plasma e.,** a substance that can be transfused to maintain fluid volume of the blood in event of great necessity, supplemental to the use of whole blood and plasma.

ex·ten·sion (-shun) 1. the movement by which the two ends of any jointed part are drawn away from each other. 2. the bringing of the members of a limb into or toward a straight condition. **nail e.,** extension exerted on the distal fragment of a fractured bone by means of a nail or pin (Steinmann pin) driven into the fragment.

ex·ten·sor (-ser) [L.] 1. causing extension. 2. a muscle that extends a joint.

ex·te·ri·or·ize (ek-stēr′e-ah-rīz) 1. to form a correct mental reference of the image of an object seen. 2. in psychiatry, to turn one's interest outward. 3. to transpose an internal organ to the exterior of the body.

ex·tern (ek′stern) a medical student or graduate in medicine who assists in patient care in the hospital but does not reside there.

ex·ter·nal (ek-ster′nal) situated or occurring on the outside. In anatomy, situated toward or near the outside; lateral.

ex·ter·nus (ek-ster′nus) external; in anatomy, denoting a structure farther from the center of the part or cavity.

ex·tero·cep·tor (ek″ster-o-sep′ter) a sensory nerve ending stimulated by the immediate external environment, such as those in the skin and mucous membranes. **exterocep′tive,** adj.

ex·ti·ma (eks′tĭ-mah) [L.] outermost; the outermost coat of a blood vessel.

ex·tinc·tion (eks-tink′shun) in psychology, the disappearance of a conditioned response as a result of nonreinforcement; also, the process by which the disappearance is accomplished.

ex·tor·sion (eks-tor′shun) outward rotation of the upper pole of the vertical meridian of each eye.

ex·tor·tor (eks-tor′ter) 1. an outward rotator. 2. an extraocular muscle that produces extorsion.

extra- word element [L.], *outside; beyond the scope of; in addition.*

ex·tra·ab·dom·i·nal (eks″trah-ab-dom′ĭ-nal) outside the abdomen.

ex·tra·an·a·tom·ic (-an″ah-tom′ik) not following the normal anatomic path.

ex·tra·cap·su·lar (-kap′su-lar) situated or occurring outside a capsule.

ex·tra·car·di·ac (-kahr′de-ak) outside the heart.

ex·tra·cel·lu·lar (-sel′u-lar) outside a cell or cells.

ex·tra·chro·mo·so·mal (-kro″mo-sōm′al) outside or not involving the chromosome; as in mitochondrial inheritance, which involves only mitochondrial DNA.

ex·tra·cor·po·re·al (-kor-por′e-al) situated or occurring outside the body.

ex·tract (eks′trakt) a concentrated preparation of a vegetable or animal drug.

ex·trac·tion (eks-trak′shun) 1. the process or act of pulling or drawing out. 2. the preparation of an extract. **breech e.**, extraction of an infant from the uterus in breech presentation. **flap e.**, extraction of a cataract by an incision which makes a flap of cornea. **serial e.**, the selective extraction of deciduous teeth during an extended period of time to allow autonomous adjustment. **testicular sperm e. (TESE)**, for men with obstructive azoospermia, extraction of spermatozoa directly from the testis through the skin.

ex·trac·tive (-tiv) any substance present in an organized tissue, or in a mixture in a small quantity, and requiring extraction by a special method.

ex·trac·tor (-ter) an instrument for removing a calculus or foreign body. **basket e.**, a device for removal of calculi from the upper urinary tract. **vacuum e.**, a device to assist delivery consisting of a metal traction cup that is attached to the fetus′ head; negative pressure is applied and traction is made on a chain passed through the suction tube.

ex·tra·em·bry·on·ic (eks″trah-em″bre-on′ik) external to the embryo proper, as the extraembryonic coelom or extraembryonic membranes.

ex·tra·mal·le·o·lus (-mah-le′o-lus) the external malleolus.

ex·tra·med·ul·la·ry (-med′u-lar″e) situated or occurring outside a medulla, especially the medulla oblongata.

ex·tra·mu·ral (-mūr′il) situated or occurring outside the wall of an organ or structure.

ex·tra·nu·cle·ar (-noo′kle-er) situated or occurring outside a cell nucleus.

ex·tra·oc·u·lar (-ok′u-lar) situated outside the eye.

ex·tra·pla·cen·tal (-plah-sen′til) outside of or independent of the placenta.

ex·trap·o·la·tion (ek-strap″ah-la′shun) inference of a value on the basis of that which is known or has been observed.

ex·tra·psy·chic (eks″trah-si′kik) occurring outside the mind; taking place between the mind and the external environment.

ex·tra·pul·mo·na·ry (-pool′mo-nar″e) not connected with the lungs.

ex·tra·py·ram·i·dal (-pĭ-ram″ĭ-d′l) outside the pyramidal tracts; see under *system*.

ex·tra·re·nal (-re′n′l) outside the kidney.

ex·tra·stim·u·lus (-stim′u-lus) a premature stimulus delivered, singly or in a group of several stimuli, at precise intervals during an extrasystole in order to terminate it.

ex·tra·sys·to·le (-sis′to-le) a premature cardiac contraction that is independent of the normal rhythm and arises in response to an impulse outside the sinoatrial node. **atrial e.**, atrial premature complex. **atrioventricular (AV) e.**, atrioventricular junctional premature complex. **infranodal e.**, ventricular e. **interpolated e.**, see under *beat*. **junctional e.**, atrioventricular junctional premature complex. **nodal e.**, atrioventricular e. **retrograde e.**, a premature ventricular contraction, followed by a premature atrial contraction, due to transmission of the stimulus backward, usually over the bundle of His. **ventricular e.**, ventricular premature complex.

ex·tra·thy·roi·dal (-thi-roid″l) outside or not involving the thyroid gland.

ex·tra·uter·ine (-u′ter-in) outside the uterus.

ex·trav·a·sa·tion (ek-strav″ah-za′shun) 1. a discharge or escape, as of blood, from a vessel into the tissues; blood or other substance so discharged. 2. the process of being extravasated.

ex·tra·ver·sion (ek″strah-ver′zhun) extroversion.

ex·tra·vert (eks′trah-vert) extrovert.

ex·trem·i·tas (eks-trem′ĭ-tas) pl. *extremita′tes*. [L.] extremity.

ex·trem·i·ty (eks-trem′ĭ-te) 1. the distal or terminal portion of elongated or pointed structures. 2. limb.

ex·trin·sic (eks-trin′sik) of external origin.

ex·tro·ver·sion (eks″tro-ver′zhun) 1. a turning inside out. 2. direction of one′s energies and attention outward from the self.

ex·tro·vert (eks′tro-vert) 1. a person whose interest is turned outward. 2. to turn one′s interest outward to the external world.

ex·trude (ek-strood′) 1. to force out, or to occupy a position distal to that normally occupied. 2. in dentistry, to occupy a position occlusal to that normally occupied.

ex·tu·ba·tion (eks″too-ba′shun) removal of a tube used in intubation.

ex·u·ber·ant (eg-zoo′ber-ant) copious or excessive in production; showing excessive proliferation.

ex·u·date (eks′u-dāt) a fluid with a high content of protein and cellular debris which has escaped from blood vessels and has been deposited in tissues or on tissue surfaces, usually as a result of inflammation.

ex·u·da·tion (eks"u-da'shun) 1. the escape of fluid, cells, and cellular debris from blood vessels and their deposition in or on the tissues, usually as the result of inflammation. 2. an exudate. **exu'dative,** adj.

ex·um·bil·i·ca·tion (-um-bil"ĭ-ka'shun) 1. marked protrusion of the navel. 2. umbilical hernia.

ex·u·vi·a·tion (eg-zoo've-a'shun) shedding an epithelial structure, e.g., deciduous teeth.

ex vi·vo (eks' ve'vo) outside the living body; denoting removal of an organ (e.g., the kidney) for reparative surgery, after which it is returned to the original site.

eye (i) the organ of vision; see Plate 30. **black e.,** a bruise of the tissue around the eye, marked by discoloration, swelling, and pain. **crossed e's,** esotropia. **exciting e.,** the eye that is primarily injured and from which the influences start which involve the other eye in sympathetic ophthalmia. **Klieg e.,** conjunctivitis, edema of the eyelids, lacrimation, and photophobia due to exposure to intense lights (Klieg lights). **pink e.,** acute contagious conjunctivitis. **shipyard e.,** epidemic keratoconjunctivitis. **wall e.,** 1. leukoma of the cornea. 2. exophoria.

eye·ball (i'bawl) the ball or globe of the eye.

eye·brow (-brou) 1. supercilium; the transverse elevation at the junction of the forehead and the upper eyelid. 2. supercilia; the hairs growing on this elevation.

eye·cup (-kup) 1. a small vessel for application of cleansing or medicated solution to the exposed area of the eyeball. 2. optic cup (2).

eye·glasses (-glas-ez) glasses.

eye·ground (-ground) the fundus of the eye as seen with the ophthalmoscope.

eye·lash (-lash) cilium; one of the hairs growing on the edge of an eyelid.

eye·lid (-lid) either of two movable folds (upper and lower) protecting the anterior surface of the eyeball.

eye·piece (-pēs) the lens or system of lenses of a microscope (or telescope) nearest the user's eye, serving to further magnify the image produced by the objective.

eye·strain (-strān) fatigue of the eye from overuse or from uncorrected defect in focus of the eye.

F

F Fahrenheit (scale); farad; fertility (plasmid); visual field; fluorine; formula; French (scale); phenylalanine.

F faraday; force.

F₁ first filial generation.

F₂ second filial generation.

f femto-.

f frequency (2).

Fab [fragment, *a*ntigen-*b*inding] originally, either of two identical fragments, each containing an antigen combining site, obtained by papain cleavage of the immunoglobulin IgG molecule; now generally used as an adjective to refer to an "arm" of any immunoglobulin monomer. **digoxin immune F. (ovine),** a preparation of antigen-binding fragments derived from specific antibodies produced against digoxin in sheep; used as an antidote to digoxin and digitoxin overdose.

fa·bel·la (fah-bel'ah) pl. *fabel'lae.* [L.] see *Table of Bones.*

FACD Fellow of the American College of Dentists.

face (fās) 1. the anterior, or ventral, aspect of the head from the forehead to the chin, inclusive. 2. any presenting aspect or surface. **moon f.,** the peculiar rounded face seen in various conditions, such as Cushing's syndrome, or after administration of adrenal corticoids.

face-bow (fās'bo) a device used in dentistry to record the positional relations of the maxillary arch to the temporomandibular joints and to orient dental casts in this same relationship to the opening axis of the articulator.

fac·et (fas'it) a small plane surface on a hard body, as on a bone.

fac·e·tec·to·my (fas"ě-tek'tah-me) excision of the articular facet of a vertebra.

fa·cial (fa'shul) pertaining to or directed toward the face.

-facient word element [L.], *making; causing to become.*

fa·ci·es (fa'she-ēz) pl. *fa'cies.* [L.] 1. the face. 2. surface; the outer aspect of a body part or organ. 3. expression (1). **Potter f.,** the characteristic facial appearance seen with oligohydramnios sequence, including a flattened nose, receding chin, wide interpupillary space, and large low-set ears.

fa·cil·i·ta·tion (fah-sil″ĭ-ta'shun) [L.] 1. hastening or assistance of a natural process. 2. in neurophysiology, the effect of a nerve impulse acting across a synapse and resulting in increased postsynaptic potential of subsequent impulses in that nerve fiber or in other convergent nerve fibers.

fa·cil·i·ta·tive (fah-sil'ĭ-tāt-iv) in pharmacology, denoting a reaction arising as an indirect result of drug action, as development of an infection after the normal microflora has been altered by an antibiotic.

fac·ing (fās'ing) a piece of porcelain cut to represent the outer surface of a tooth.

faci(o)- word element [L.], *face.*

fa·cio·bra·chi·al (fa″she-o-bra'ke-il) pertaining to the face and the arm.

fa·cio·lin·gual (-ling'gwil) pertaining to the face and tongue.

fa·cio·plas·ty (fa'she-o-plas″te) restorative or plastic surgery of the face.

fa·cio·ple·gia (fa″she-o-ple'jah) facial paralysis. **facio·ple'gic,** adj.

FACOG Fellow of the American College of Obstetricians and Gynecologists.

FACP Fellow of the American College of Physicians.

FACS Fellow of the American College of Surgeons.

FACSM Fellow of the American College of Sports Medicine.

fac·ti·tial (fak-tish'il) factitious.

fac·ti·tious (fak-tish'-us) artificially induced; not natural.

fac·tor (fak'ter) an agent or element that contributes to the production of a result. **accelerator f.,** coagulation f. V. **angiogenesis f.,** a substance that causes the growth of new blood vessels, found in tissues with high metabolic requirements and also released by macrophages to initiate revascularization in wound healing. **antihemophilic f. (AHF),** 1. coagulation f. VIII. 2. a preparation of factor VIII used for the prevention or treatment of hemorrhage in patients with hemophilia A and the treatment of von Willebrand disease, hypofibrinogenemia, and factor XIII deficiency, including preparations derived from human or porcine plasma or by recombinant technology. **antihemophilic f. A,** coagulation f. VIII. **antihemophilic f. B,** coagulation f. IX.

antihemophilic f. C, coagulation f. XI. **antinuclear f. (ANF),** see under *antibody.* **f. B,** a complement component that participates in the alternative complement pathway. **B cell differentiation f's (BCDF),** factors derived from T cells that stimulate B cells to differentiate into antibody-secreting cells. **B lymphocyte stimulatory f's (BSF),** a system of nomenclature for factors that stimulate B cells, replacing individual factor names with the designation BSF and an appended descriptive code. **Christmas f.,** coagulation f. IX. **C3 nephritic f. (C3 NeF),** an autoantibody that stabilizes the alternative complement pathway C3 convertase, preventing its inactivation by factor H and resulting in complete consumption of plasma C3; it is found in the serum of many patients with type II membranoproliferative glomerulonephritis. **coagulation f's,** substances in the blood that are essential to the clotting process and hence, to the maintenance of normal hemostasis. They are designated by Roman numerals, to which the notation "a" is added to indicate the activated state. See also *platelet f's.* **f. I,** fibrinogen: a high-molecular-weight plasma protein converted to fibrin by the action of thrombin. Deficiency results in afibrinogenemia or hypofibrinogenemia. **f. II,** prothrombin: a plasma protein converted to thrombin by activated factor X in the common pathway of coagulation. Deficiency leads to hypoprothrombinemia. **f. III,** tissue thromboplastin: a lipoprotein functioning in the extrinsic pathway of coagulation, activating factor X. **f. IV,** calcium. **f. V,** proaccelerin: a factor functioning in both the intrinsic and extrinsic pathways of coagulation, catalyzing the cleavage of prothrombin to thrombin. Deficiency leads to parahemophilia. **f. VII,** proconvertin: a factor functioning in the extrinsic pathway of blood coagulation, acting with factor III to activate factor X. Deficiency, either hereditary or associated with vitamin K deficiency, leads to hemorrhagic tendency. **f. VIII,** antihemophilic factor (AHF): a storage-labile factor participating in the intrinsic pathway of blood coagulation, acting as a cofactor in the activation of factor X. Deficiency, an X-linked recessive trait, causes hemophilia A. **f. IX,** a relatively storage-stable substance involved in the intrinsic pathway of blood coagulation, activating factor X. Deficiency results in the hemorrhagic syndrome hemophilia B, resembling hemophilia A; it is treated with purified preparations of the factor, either from human plasma or recombinant, or with factor IX complex. *f. X*, Stuart factor: a storage-stable factor that participates in both the intrinsic and extrinsic pathways of blood coagulation, uniting them to begin the common pathway of coagulation; as part of the *prothrombinase* complex, activated factor X activates prothrombin. Deficiency may cause a systemic coagulation disorder. The activated form is called also *thrombokinase. f. XI*, plasma thromboplastin antecedent: a stable factor involved in the intrinsic pathway of blood coagulation, activating factor IX. Deficiency results in the blood-clotting defect hemophilia C. *f. XII*, Hageman factor: a stable factor activated by contact with glass or other foreign surfaces, which initiates the intrinsic process of blood coagulation by activating factor XI. *f. XIII*, fibrin-stabilizing factor: a factor that polymerizes fibrin monomers, enabling formation of a firm blood clot. Deficiency produces a clinical hemorrhagic diathesis. **colony-stimulating f's**, a group of glycoprotein lymphokines, produced by blood monocytes, tissue macrophages, and stimulated lymphocytes and required for the differentiation of stem cells into granulocyte and monocyte cell colonies; they stimulate the production of granulocytes and macrophages and have been used experimentally as cancer agents. **f. D**, a serine protease of the alternative complement pathway that cleaves factor B bound to C3b, releasing Ba while leaving Bb bound to C3b to form the C3 convertase C3bBb. **decay accelerating f. (DAF)**, a protein of most blood cells as well as endothelial and epithelial cells, CD55; it protects the cell membranes from attack by autologous complement. **endothelial-derived relaxant f.**, endothelium-derived relaxing f. (EDRF), nitric oxide. **extrinsic f.**, cyanocobalamin. **F (fertility) f.**, F plasmid. **fibrin-stabilizing f. (FSF)**, coagulation f. XIII. **Fitzgerald f.**, high-molecular-weight kininogen. **Fletcher f.**, prekallikrein. **glucose tolerance f.**, a biologically active complex of chromium and nicotinic acid that facilitates the reaction of insulin with receptor sites on tissues. **granulocyte colony-stimulating f. (G-CSF)**, a colony-stimulating factor that stimulates the production of neutrophils from precursor cells. **granulocyte-macrophage colony-stimulating f. (GM-CSF)**, a colony-stimulating factor that binds to stem cells and most myelocytes and stimulates their differentiation into granulocytes and macrophages. **growth f.**, any substance that promotes skeletal or somatic growth, usually a mineral,

hormone, or vitamin. **f. H**, a glycoprotein that acts as an inhibitor of the alternative pathway of complement activation. **Hageman f. (HF)**, coagulation f. XII. **histamine-releasing f. (HRF)**, a lymphokine that induces the release of histamine by IgE-bound basophils in late phase allergic reaction. **homologous restriction f. (HRF)**, a regulatory protein that binds to the membrane attack complex in autologous cells, inhibiting the final stages of complement activation. **f. I**, a plasma enzyme that regulates both classical and alternative pathways of complement activation by inactivating their C3 convertases. **inhibiting f's**, factors elaborated by one body structure that inhibit release of hormones by another structure; applied to substances of unknown chemical structure, while those of established chemical identity are called *inhibiting hormones*. **insulinlike growth f's (IGF)**, insulin-like substances in serum that do not react with insulin antibodies; they are growth hormone-dependent and possess all the growth-promoting properties of the somatomedins. **intrinsic f.**, a glycoprotein secreted by the parietal cells of the gastric glands, necessary for the absorption of vitamin B_{12}. Lack of intrinsic factor, with consequent deficiency of vitamin B_{12}, results in pernicious anemia. **LE f.**, an antinuclear antibody having a sedimentation rate of 7S and reacting with leukocyte nuclei, found in the serum in systemic lupus erythematosus. **leukocyte inhibitory f. (LIF)**, a lymphokine that prevents polymorphonuclear leukocytes from migrating. **lymph node permeability f. (LNPF)**, a substance from normal lymph nodes which produces vascular permeability. **lymphocyte mitogenic f. (LMF)**, a nondialyzable heat-stable macromolecule released by lymphocytes stimulated by a specific antigen; it causes blast transformation and cell division in normal lymphocytes. **lymphocyte transforming f. (LTF)**, a lymphokine causing transformation and clonal expansion of nonsensitized lymphocytes. **myocardial depressant f. (MDF)**, a peptide formed in response to a fall in systemic blood pressure; it has a negatively inotropic effect on myocardial muscle fibers. **osteoclast activating f. (OAF)**, a lymphokine produced by lymphocytes which facilitates bone resorption. **f. P**, properdin. **platelet f's**, factors important in hemostasis which are contained in or attached to the platelets. *platelet f. 1*, adsorbed coagulation factor V from the plasma. *platelet f. 2*, an accelerator of the thrombin-fibrinogen reaction. *platelet f. 3*, a lipoprotein with roles in the activation of both coagulation factor X and prothrombin. *platelet f. 4*, an intracellular protein component of blood platelets capable of inhibiting the activity of heparin. **platelet activating f. (PAF)**, an immunologically produced substance which is a mediator of clumping and degranulation of blood platelets and of bronchoconstriction. **platelet-derived growth f.**, a substance contained in the alpha granules of blood platelets whose action contributes to the repair of damaged blood vessel walls. **R f.**, see under *plasmid*. **releasing f's**, factors elaborated in one body structure that cause release of hormones from another structure; applied to substances of unknown chemical structure, while those of established chemical identity are called *releasing hormones*. **resistance transfer f. (RTF)**, the portion of an R plasmid containing the genes for conjugation and replication. **Rh f., Rhesus f.**, genetically determined antigens present on the surface of erythrocytes; incompatibility for these antigens between mother and offspring is responsible for erythroblastosis fetalis. **rheumatoid f. (RF)**, a protein (IgM) detectable by serological tests, which is found in the serum of most patients with rheumatoid arthritis and in other related and unrelated diseases and sometimes in apparently normal persons. **risk f.**, a clearly defined occurrence or characteristic that has been associated with the increased rate of a subsequently occurring disease. **Stuart f., Stuart-Prower f.**, coagulation f. X. **tissue f.**, coagulation f. III. **transforming growth f. (TGF)**, any of several proteins secreted by transformed cells and causing growth of normal cells, although not causing transformation. **tumor necrosis f.**, either of two lymphokines that cause hemorrhagic necrosis of certain tumor cells but do not affect normal cells; they have been used as experimental anticancer agents. *Tumor necrosis factor α* (formerly *cachectin*) is produced by macrophages, eosinophils, and NK cells. *Tumor necrosis factor β*, is lymphotoxin. **vascular endothelial growth f. (VEGF), vascular permeability f. (VPF)**, a peptide factor that is a mitogen of vascular endothelial cells; it promotes tissue vascularization and is important in tumor angiogenesis. **von Willebrand's f. (vWF)**, a glycoprotein that circulates complexed to coagulation factor VIII, mediating adhesion of platelets to damaged epithelial surfaces. Deficiency results in von Willebrand's disease.

fac·ul·ta·tive (fak′ul-ta″tiv) not obligatory; pertaining to the ability to adjust to particular circumstances or to assume a particular role.

fac·ul·ty (fak′il-te) 1. a normal power or function, especially of the mind. 2. the teaching staff of an institution of learning.

FAD flavin adenine dinucleotide.

fae- for words beginning thus, see those beginning *fe-*.

fail·ure (fāl′yer) inability to perform or to function properly. **acute congestive heart f.**, rapidly occurring cardiac output deficiency marked by venocapillary congestion, hypertension, and edema. **backward heart f.**, a concept of heart failure emphasizing the causative contribution of passive engorgement of the systemic venous system, as a result of dysfunction in a ventricle and subsequent pressure increase behind it. **bone marrow f.**, failure of the hematopoietic function of the bone marrow. **congestive heart f. (CHF)**, that characterized by breathlessness and abnormal sodium and water retention, resulting in edema, with congestion of the lungs or peripheral circulation, or both. **diastolic heart f.**, heart failure due to a defect in ventricular filling caused by an abnormality in diastolic function. **forward heart f.**, a concept of heart failure that emphasizes the inadequacy of cardiac output relative to body needs and considers venous distention as secondary. **heart f.**, inability of the heart to pump blood at a rate adequate to fill tissue metabolic requirements or the ability to do so only at an elevated filling pressure; defined clinically as a syndrome of ventricular dysfunction with reduced exercise capacity and other characteristic hemodynamic, renal, neural, and hormonal responses. **high-output heart f.**, that in which cardiac output remains high; associated with hyperthyroidism, anemia, arteriovenous fistulas, beriberi, osteitis deformans, or sepsis. **kidney f.**, renal f. **left-sided heart f., left ventricular f.**, failure of adequate output by the left ventricle, marked by pulmonary congestion and edema. **low-output heart f.**, that in which cardiac output is decreased, as in most forms of heart disease, leading to manifestations of impaired peripheral circulation and vasoconstriction. **premature ovarian f.**, premature menopause. **renal f.**, inability of the kidney to excrete metabolites at normal plasma levels under normal loading, or inability to retain electrolytes when intake is normal; in the acute form, marked by uremia and usually by oliguria, with hyperkalemia and pulmonary edema. **right-sided heart f., right ventricular f.**, failure of adequate output by the right ventricle, marked by venous engorgement, hepatic enlargement, and pitting edema. **systolic heart f.**, heart failure due to a defect in the expulsion of blood that is caused by an abnormality in systolic function. **f. to thrive,** physical and developmental retardation in infants and small children, sometimes from physical illness and sometimes from psychosocial effects such as maternal deprivation.

faint (fānt) syncope.

fal·cate (fal′kāt) falciform.

fal·cial (-shal) pertaining to a falx.

fal·ci·form (-sĭ-form) sickle-shaped.

fal·cu·lar (-ku-ler) falciform.

fal·lo·pos·co·py (fah-lo-pos′kah-pe) endoscopic visualization of the uterine tubes using a nonincisional transvaginal and transuterine approach.

false-neg·a·tive (fawls′ neg′ah-tiv) 1. denoting a test result that wrongly excludes an individual from a category. 2. an individual so excluded. 3. an instance of a false-negative result.

false-pos·i·tive (pos′it-iv) 1. denoting a test result that wrongly assigns an individual to a category. 2. an individual so categorized. 3. an instance of a false-positive result.

fal·si·fi·ca·tion (fawl″sĭ-fĭ-ka′shun) lying. **retrospective f.,** unconscious distortion of past experiences to conform to present emotional needs.

falx (falks) pl. **fal′ces.** [L.] a sickle-shaped structure. **f. cerebel′li,** a fold of dura mater separating the cerebellar hemispheres. **f. ce′rebri,** the fold of dura mater in the longitudinal fissure, separating the cerebral hemispheres. **inguinal f., f. inguina′lis,** a lateral expansion of the lateral edge of the rectus abdominis which attaches to the pubic bone.

fam·ci·clo·vir (fam-si′klo-vir) a prodrug of penciclovir used in the treatment of herpes zoster, of herpes genitalis, and of mucocutaneous herpes simplex in immunocompromised patients.

fa·mil·i·al (fah-mil′e-il) occurring in more members of a family than would be expected by chance.

fam·i·ly (fam′ĭ-le) 1. a group descended from a common ancestor. 2. a taxonomic subdivision subordinate to an order (or suborder) and superior to a tribe (or subfamily).

fam·o·ti·dine (fam-o′tĭ-dēn) a histamine H_2 receptor antagonist, which inhibits gastric acid secretion; used in the treatment and prophylaxis of gastric or duodenal ulcers, gastroesophageal reflux disease, upper gastrointestinal bleeding, and conditions associated with gastric hypersecretion.

F and R force and rhythm (of pulse).

fang (fang) 1. a large canine tooth of a carnivore. 2. the envenomed tooth of a snake.

Fan·nia (fan′e-ah) a genus of flies whose larvae cause intestinal and urinary myiasis in humans.

fan·ta·sy (fan′tah-se) an imagined sequence of events that can satisfy one's unconscious wishes or express one's unconscious conflicts.

FAPHA Fellow of the American Public Health Association.

far·ad (F) (far′ad) the SI unit of electric capacitance; the capacitance of a condenser that charged with one coulomb gives a difference of potential of 1 volt.

far·a·day (F) (far′ah-da) the electric charge carried by one mole of electrons or one equivalent weight of ions, equal to 9.649×10^4 coulombs.

far·cy (fahr′se) see *glanders.*

far·sight·ed·ness (fahr-sīt′ed-nes) hyperopia.

fas·cia (fash′e-ah) pl. *fas′ciae.* [L.] a sheet or band of fibrous tissue such as lies deep to the skin or invests muscles and various body organs. **fas′cial,** adj. **f. adhe′rens,** that portion of the junctional complex of the cells of an intercalated disk that is the counterpart of the zonula adherens of epithelial cells. **f. cribro′sa,** the superficial fascia of the thigh covering the saphenous opening. **endothoracic f.,** that beneath the serous lining of the thoracic cavity. **f. profun′da,** a dense, firm, fibrous membrane investing the trunk and limbs and giving off sheaths to the various muscles. **Scarpa's f.,** the deep membranous layer of the subcutaneous abdominal fascia. **f. of Tenon,** see under *capsule.* **Tyrrell's f.,** rectovesical septum.

fas·ci·cle (fas′ĭ-k'l) 1. a small bundle or cluster, especially of nerve, tendon, or muscle fibers. 2. a tract, bundle, or group of nerve fibers that are more or less associated functionally.

fas·cic·u·lar (fah-sik′u-lar) 1. pertaining to a fasciculus. 2. fasciculated.

fas·cic·u·lat·ed (fah-sik′ūl-āt-id) clustered together or occurring in bundles, or fasciculi.

fas·cic·u·la·tion (fah-sik″u-la′shun) 1. the formation of fascicles. 2. a small local involuntary muscular contraction visible under the skin, representing spontaneous discharge of fibers innervated by a single motor nerve filament.

fas·cic·u·lus (fah-sik′u-lus) pl. *fasci′culi.* [L.] fascicle. **cuneate f. of medulla oblongata,** the continuation into the medulla oblongata of the cuneate fasciculus of spinal cord. **cuneate f. of spinal cord**, the lateral portion of the posterior funiculus of the spinal cord, composed of ascending fibers that end in the nucleus cuneatus. **gracile f. of medulla oblongata**, the continuation into the medulla oblongata of the gracile fasciculus of spinal cord. **gracile f. of spinal cord**, the median portion of the posterior funiculus of the spinal cord, composed of ascending fibers that end in the nucleus gracilis. **mammillothalamic f.**, a stout bundle of fibers from the mammillary body to the anterior nucleus of the thalamus.

fas·ci·itis (fas-e-i′tis) inflammation of a fascia. **eosinophilic f.**, inflammation of fasciae of the limbs, with eosinophilia, edema, and swelling, often after strenuous exercise. **necrotizing f.**, a gas-forming, fulminating, necrotic infection of the superficial and deep fascia, resulting in thrombosis of the subcutaneous vessels and gangrene of the underlying tissues. It is usually caused by multiple pathogens and is frequently associated with diabetes mellitus. **nodular f.**, a benign, reactive proliferation of fibroblasts in the subcutaneous tissues, commonly affecting the deep fascia, usually in young adults. **proliferative f.**, a benign reactive proliferation of fibroblasts in subcutaneous tissues, resembling nodular fasciitis but characterized also by basophilic giant cells and occurrence in the skeletal muscles in older adults. **pseudosarcomatous f.**, nodular f.

fas·ci·od·e·sis (fas″e-od′ĭ-sis) suture of a fascia to skeletal attachment.

Fas·ci·o·la (fah-si′ol-ah) a genus of flukes, including *F. hepa′tica*, the common liver fluke of herbivores, occasionally found in the human liver.

fas·ci·o·la (fah-si′o-lah) pl. *fasci′olae*. [L.] 1. a small band or striplike structure. 2. a small bandage. **fasci′olar**, adj.

fas·cio·li·a·sis (fas″e-o-li′ah-sis) infection with *Fasciola*.

fas·ci·o·lop·si·a·sis (-lop-si′ah-sis) infection with *Fasciolopsis*.

Fas·ci·o·lop·sis (-lop′sis) a genus of trematodes, including *F. bus′ki*, the largest of the intestinal flukes, found in the small intestines of residents throughout Asia.

fas·ci·ot·o·my (fas″e-ot′ah-me) incision of a fascia.

fast (fast) 1. immovable, or unchangeable; resistant to the action of a specific agent, such as a stain or destaining agent. 2. abstention from food, or from food and liquid. 3. to abstain from food, or from food and liquid.

fas·tig·i·um (fas-tij′e-um) [L.] 1. the highest point in the roof of the fourth ventricle of the brain. 2. the acme, or highest point. **fastig′ial**, adj.

fast·ing (fast′ing) abstinence from all food and drink except water for a prescribed period.

fat (fat) 1. adipose tissue, forming soft pads between organs, smoothing and rounding out body contours, and furnishing a reserve supply of energy. 2. an ester of glycerol with fatty acids, usually oleic, palmitic, or stearic acid. **polyunsaturated f.**, one containing polyunsaturated fatty acids. **saturated f.**, one containing saturated fatty acids. **unsaturated f.**, one containing unsaturated fatty acids.

fa·tal (fa′t′l) mortal; lethal; causing death.

fat·i·ga·bil·i·ty (fat″ĭ-gah-bil′it-e) easy susceptibility to fatigue.

fa·tigue (fah-tēg′) a state of increased discomfort and decreased efficiency due to prolonged or excessive exertion; loss of power or capacity to respond to stimulation. **vocal f.**, phonasthenia.

fat·ty (fat′e) pertaining to or characterized by fat.

fat·ty ac·id (fat′e) any straight chain monocarboxylic acid, especially those naturally occurring in fats. **essential f. a.**, any fatty acid that cannot be synthesized by the body and must be obtained from dietary sources, e.g., linoleic acid and linolenic acid. **free f. a's (FFA)**, nonesterified f. a's. **monounsaturated f. a's**, unsaturated fatty acids containing a single double bond, occurring predominantly as oleic acid, in peanut, olive, and canola oils. **nonesterified f. a's (NEFA)**, the fraction of plasma fatty acids not in the form of glycerol esters. **ω-3 f. a's, omega-3 f. a's**, unsaturated fatty acids in which the double bond nearest the methyl terminus is at the third carbon from the end; present in marine animal fats and some vegetable oils and shown to affect leukotriene, prostaglandin, lipoprotein, and lipid levels and composition. **ω-6 f. a's, omega-6 f. a's**, unsaturated fatty acids in which the double bond nearest the methyl terminus is at the sixth carbon from the end, present predominantly in vegetable oils. **polyunsaturated f. a's (PUFA)**, unsaturated fatty acids containing two or more double bonds, occurring predominantly as linoleic, linolenic, and arachidonic acids, in vegetable and seed oils. **saturated f. a's**, those without double bonds, occurring predominantly in animal fats and tropical oils or produced by hydrogenation of unsaturated fatty acids.

***trans*-f. a's,** stereoisomers of the naturally occurring *cis*–fatty acids, found in margarines and shortenings as artifacts after hydrogenation. **unsaturated f. a's,** those containing one or more double bonds, predominantly in most plant-derived fats.

fau·ces (faw'sēz) the passage between the throat and pharynx. **fau'cial,** adj.

fau·ci·tis (faw-si'tis) sore throat; inflammation of the fauces.

fau·na (faw'nah) the collective animal organisms of a given locality.

fa·ve·o·late (fah-ve'o-lāt) alveolate.

fa·vid (fa'vid) a secondary skin eruption due to allergy in favus.

fa·vism (fa'vizm) an acute hemolytic anemia precipitated by fava beans (ingestion, or inhalation of pollen), usually caused by deficiency of glucose-6-phosphate dehydrogenase in the erythrocytes.

fa·vus (fa'vus) a type of tinea, usually of the scalp but sometimes affecting glabrous skin, with formation of scutula, which may enlarge and coalesce to form prominent honeycomb-like masses; due to infection by the fungus *Trichophyton*, usually *T. schoenleinii*.

Fc fragment, crystallizable; a fragment by papain digestion of immunoglobulin molecules. It contains most of the antigenic determinants.

Fc′ a fragment produced in minute quantities by papain digestion of immunoglobulin molecules. It contains the principal part of the C terminal portion of two Fc fragments.

Fd the heavy chain portion of a Fab fragment produced by papain digestion of an IgG molecule.

FDI Fédération Dentaire Internationale (International Dental Association).

Fe iron (L. *fer'rum*).

fear (fēr) the unpleasant emotional state consisting of psychological and psychophysiological responses to a real external threat or danger, including agitation, alertness, tension, and mobilization of the alarm reaction.

fe·bric·i·ty (feb-ris'it-e) feverishness.

feb·ri·fa·cient (feb″rĭ-fa'shint) 1. pyrogenic. 2. pyrogen.

fe·brif·u·gal (feb-rif'u-g'l) antipyretic (1).

feb·rile (feb'ril) pertaining to or characterized by fever.

fe·cal (fe'k'l) pertaining to or of the nature of feces.

fe·ca·lith (fe'kah-lith) coprolith; an intestinal concretion formed around a center of fecal matter.

fe·cal·oid (fe'kal-oid) resembling feces.

fe·ces (fe'sēz) [L.] waste matter discharged from the intestine.

fec·u·lent (-int) 1. having dregs or sediment. 2. pertaining to or of the nature of feces.

fe·cun·da·bil·i·ty (fĕ-kun″dah-bil'ĭ-te) the probability that conception will occur in a given population of couples during a specific time period.

fe·oun·da·tion (fe″kun-da'shun) fertilization.

fe·cun·di·ty (fĕ-kun'dit-e) 1. in demography, the physiological ability to reproduce, as opposed to fertility. 2. ability to produce offspring rapidly and in large numbers.

feed·back (fēd'bak) the return of some of the output of a system as input so as to exert some control in the process; feedback is *negative* when the return exerts an inhibitory control, *positive* when it exerts a stimulatory effect.

feed-for·ward (fēd-for'ward) the anticipatory effect that one intermediate in a metabolic or endocrine control system exerts on another intermediate further along in the pathway; such effect may be positive or negative.

feed·ing (fēd'ing) the taking or giving of food. **artificial f.,** feeding of a baby with food other than mother's milk. **breast f.,** see under *B.* **forced f.,** administration of food by force to those who cannot or will not receive it.

FEF forced expiratory flow.

fe·male (fe'māl) 1. an individual organism of the sex that bears young or produces ova or eggs. 2. feminine.

fem·i·nine (fem'ĭ-nin) 1. pertaining to the female sex. 2. having qualities normally associated with females.

fel·ba·mate (fel'bah-māt″) an anticonvulsant used in the treatment of epilepsy.

fel·la·tio (fĕ-la'she-o) oral stimulation or manipulation of the penis.

fe·lo·di·pine (fĕ-lo'dĭ-pēn) a calcium channel blocker used as a vasodilator in the treatment of hypertension.

fel·on (fel'on) a purulent infection involving the pulp of the distal phalanx of a finger.

felt·work (felt'werk) a complex of closely interwoven fibers, as of nerve fibers.

fem·i·ni·za·tion (fem″ĭ-nĭ-za'shun) 1. the normal development of primary and secondary sex characters in females. 2. the induction or development of female secondary sex characters in the male. **testicular f.,** complete androgen resistance.

fem·o·ral (fem'or-al) pertaining to the femur or to the thigh.

fem·o·ro·cele (fem'ah-ro-sēl″) femoral hernia.

femto- (fem'to) word element [Danish], *fifteen;* used in naming units of measurement to indicate one quadrillionth (10^{-15}) of the unit designated by the root with which it is combined; symbol f.

fe·mur (fe'mer) pl. *fem'ora, femurs.* [L.] 1. see *Table of Bones.* 2. thigh.

fe·nes·tra (fĕ-nes'trah) pl. *fenes'trae.* [L.] a window-like opening. **f. coch'leae,** round window; an opening in the inner wall of the middle ear covered by the secondary tympanic membrane. **f. ova'lis,** f. vestibuli. **f. rotun'da,** f. cochleae. **f. vesti'buli,** oval window; an opening in the inner wall of the middle ear, closed by the base of the stapes.

fen·es·trat·ed (fen'es-trāt"ed) pierced with one or more openings.

fen·es·tra·tion (fen"es-tra'shun) 1. the act of perforating or condition of being perforated. 2. the surgical creation of a new opening in the labyrinth of the ear for restoration of hearing in otosclerosis. **aorticopulmonary f.,** aortic septal defect.

fen·flur·amine (fen-floor'ah-mēn) an amphetamine derivative, formerly used as an anorectic in the form of the hydrochloride salt.

feng shui (fung' shwa') [Chinese] the Chinese art of positioning objects based on the premise that arrangement affects the balance of yin and yang and the flow of qi within an area, which can have positive or negative effects, including effects on health.

fen·nel (fen'il) the flowering herb *Foeniculum vulgare,* or its edible seeds, which are used as a source of fennel oil.

fen·o·fi·brate (fen"o-fi'brāt) an antihyperlipidemic agent used to reduce elevated serum lipids.

fe·nol·do·pam (fe-nol'do-pam) a vasodilator used for short-term, inpatient management of severe hypertension; used as the mesylate salt.

fen·o·pro·fen (fen"o-pro'fen) a nonsteroidal antiinflammatory drug used as the calcium salt in the treatment of rheumatic and non-rheumatic inflammatory disorders, pain, dysmenorrhea, and vascular headaches.

fen·ta·nyl (fen'tah-nil) an opioid analgesic; the citrate salt is used as an adjunct to anesthesia, in the induction and maintenance of anesthesia, in combination with droperidol (or similar agent) as a neuroleptanalgesic, and in the management of chronic severe pain.

fen·u·greek (fen'u-grēk) the leguminous plant *Trigonella foenum-graecum,* or its seeds, which are used for loss of appetite and skin inflammations; also used in traditional Chinese medicine and in Indian medicine.

fer·ment (fer-ment') to undergo fermentation; used for the decomposition of carbohydrates.

fer·men·ta·tion (fer"men-ta'shun) the anaerobic enzymatic conversion of organic compounds, especially carbohydrates, to simpler compounds, especially to ethyl alcohol, producing energy in the form of ATP.

fer·mi·um (Fm) (fer'me-um) chemical element (see *Table of Elements*), at. no. 100.

fern·ing (fern'ing) the appearance of a fernlike pattern in a dried specimen of cervical mucus or vaginal fluid, an indication of the presence of estrogen.

-ferous word element [L.], *bearing; producing.*

fer·re·dox·in (fer"ĕ-dok'sin) a nonheme iron-containing protein having a very low redox potential; the ferredoxins participate in electron transport in photosynthesis, nitrogen fixation, and various other biological processes.

fer·ric (fer'ik) containing iron in its plus-three oxidation state, Fe(III) (also written Fe^{3+}). **f. chloride,** $FeCl_3 \cdot 6H_2O$; used as a reagent and as a diagnostic aid in phenylketonuria.

fer·ri·tin (-ĭ-tin) the iron-apoferritin complex, one of the chief forms in which iron is stored in the body.

fer·ro·ki·net·ics (fer"o-kĭ-net'iks) the turnover or rate of change of iron in the body; the rate at which it is cleared from the plasma and incorporated into red cells.

fer·ro·pro·tein (-pro'tēn) a protein combined with an iron-containing radical; ferroproteins are respiratory carriers.

fer·rous (fer'us) containing iron in its plus-two oxidation state, Fe(II) (sometimes designated Fe^{2+}). Various salts are used in iron deficiency, including *iron fumarate, iron gluconate,* and *iron sulfate.*

fer·ru·gi·nous (fĕ-roo'jĭ-nus) 1. containing iron or iron rust. 2. of the color of iron rust.

fer·til·i·ty (fer-til'ĭ-te) 1. the capacity to conceive or induce conception. **fer'tile,** adj. 2. see under *rate.*

fer·ti·li·za·tion (fer"tĭ-lĭ-za'shun) impregnation; union of male and female gametes to form the diploid zygote, leading to development of a new individual. **external f.,** union of the gametes outside the bodies of the originating organisms, as in most fish. **internal f.,** union of the gametes inside the body of the female, the sperm having been transferred from the body of the male by an accessory sex organ or other means. **in vitro f.,** removal of a secondary oocyte, fertilization of it in a culture medium in the laboratory, and placement of the dividing zygote into the uterus.

fer·ves·cence (fer-ves′ens) increase of fever or body temperature.

FES functional electrical stimulation.

fes·ter (fes′ter) to suppurate superficially.

fes·ti·na·tion (fes″tĭ-na′shun) an involuntary tendency to take short accelerating steps in walking.

fes·toon (fes-tōōn′) a carving in the base material of a denture that simulates the contours of the natural tissues being replaced.

fe·tal (fe′tal) of or pertaining to a fetus or the period of its development.

fe·tal·iza·tion (fe″tal-ĭ-za′shun) retention in the adult of characters that at an earlier stage of evolution were only infantile and were rapidly lost as the organism attained maturity.

fe·ta·tion (fe-ta′shun) 1. development of the fetus. 2. pregnancy.

fe·ti·cide (fēt′ĭ-sīd) the destruction of the fetus.

fet·id (fe′tid, fet′id) having a rank, disagreeable smell.

fet·ish (fet′ish) 1. a material object, such as an idol or charm, believed to have supernatural powers. 2. an inanimate object used to obtain sexual gratification.

fet·ish·ism (-izm) 1. worship of fetishes. 2. a paraphilia marked by recurrent sexual urges for and fantasies of using fetishes, usually articles of women's clothing, for sexual arousal or orgasm. **transvestic f.,** a paraphilia of heterosexual males, characterized by recurrent, intense sexual urges, arousal, or orgasm associated with fantasized or actual dressing in clothing of the opposite sex.

fet(o)- word element [L.], *fetus.*

fe·tol·o·gy (fe-tol′ah-je) the branch of medicine dealing with the fetus in utero.

fe·tom·e·try (fe-tom′ĭ-tre) measurement of the fetus, especially of its head.

fe·top·a·thy (fe-top′ah-the) a disease or disorder seen in a fetus.

α-fe·to·pro·tein (fe″to-pro′tēn) alpha fetoprotein.

fe·tor (fe′tor) stench, or offensive odor. **f. hepa′ticus,** the peculiar odor of the breath characteristic of hepatic disease.

fe·to·scope (fēt′ah-skōp) 1. a specially designed stethoscope for listening to the fetal heart beat. 2. an endoscope for viewing the fetus *in utero.*

fe·tus (fēt′us) [L.] the developing young in the uterus, specifically the unborn offspring in the postembryonic period, in humans from nine weeks after fertilization until birth. **harlequin f.,** an infant with a severe and usually lethal form of congenital ichthyosis, manifested by hyperkeratosis with rigid skin. **mummified f.,**

a dried-up and shriveled fetus. **f. papyra′ceus,** a dead fetus pressed flat by the growth of a living twin. **parasitic f.,** in asymmetrical conjoined twins, an incomplete minor fetus attached to a larger, more completely developed twin.

FEV forced expiratory volume.

fe·ver (fe′ver) 1. pyrexia; elevation of body temperature above the normal (37°C). 2. any disease characterized by elevation of body temperature. **blackwater f.,** a dangerous complication of falciparum malaria, with passage of dark red to black urine, severe toxicity, and high mortality. **boutonneuse f.,** a tickborne disease endemic in the Mediterranean area, Crimea, Africa, and India, due to infection with *Rickettsia conorii,* with chills, fever, primary skin lesion (tache noire), and rash appearing on the second to fourth day. **cat-scratch f.,** see under *disease.* **central f.,** sustained fever resulting from damage to the thermoregulatory centers of the hypothalamus. **childbed f.,** puerperal septicemia. **Colorado tick f.,** a tickborne, nonexanthematous, febrile, viral disease caused by an arenavirus and seen in the Rocky Mountain area of the United States. **continued f.,** one that varies only slightly in 24 hours. **Crimean-Congo hemorrhagic f.,** a hemorrhagic fever caused by the Crimean-Congo hemorrhagic fever virus, transmitted by ticks and by contact with blood, secretions, or fluids from infected animals or humans; it occurs in the Crimea, Central Asia, and regions of Africa. **drug f.,** febrile reaction to a therapeutic agent, such as a vaccine, antineoplastic, or antibiotic. **elephantoid f.,** a recurrent acute febrile condition occurring with filariasis; it may be associated with elephantiasis or lymphangitis. **enteric f.,** any of a group of febrile illnesses associated with enteric symptoms caused by salmonellae, especially typhoid fever and paratyphoid fever. **epidemic hemorrhagic f.,** an acute infectious disease characterized by fever, purpura, peripheral vascular collapse, and acute renal failure, caused by viruses of the genus *Hantavirus,* thought to be transmitted to humans by contact with saliva and excreta of infected rodents. **familial Mediterranean f.,** a hereditary disease usually seen in Armenians and Sephardic Jews, with short recurrent attacks of fever, pain in the abdomen, chest, or joints, and erythema like that of erysipelas; it may be complicated by amyloidosis. **Haverhill f.,** the bacillary form of rat-bite fever, due to *Streptobacillus moniliformis,* and transmitted through contaminated raw milk and its products. **hay f.,** a seasonal form of allergic rhinitis, with acute conjunctivitis, lacrimation, itching, swelling of the nasal mucosa, nasal catarrh, and attacks of sneezing, an anaphylactic or allergic reaction excited by a specific allergen (such as pollen). **hemorrhagic f's,** a group of diverse, severe viral infections seen around the world but mainly in the tropics, usually transmitted to humans by arthropod bites or contact with virus-infected rodents; they all have certain common features, including fever, hemorrhagic manifestations, thrombocytopenia, shock, and neurologic disturbances. **humidifier f.,** malaise, fever, cough, and myalgia caused by inhalation of air that has been passed through humidifiers, dehumidifiers, or air conditioners contaminated by fungi, amebas, or thermophilic actinomycetes. **intermittent f.,** an attack of malaria or other fever, with recurring fever episodes separated by times of normal temperature. **Katayama f.,** fever associated with severe schistosomal infections, accompanied by hepatosplenomegaly and by eosinophilia. **Lassa f.,** a highly fatal, acute, febrile disease seen in West Africa, caused by a virulent arenavirus and characterized by increasing prostration, sore throat, ulcerations of the mouth or throat, rash, and general aching. **metal fume f.,** a disease of welders and others working with volatilized metals, marked by sudden thirst, metallic taste in the mouth, high fever with chills, sweating, and leukocytosis. **mud f.,** a type of leptospirosis seen in workers in flooded fields and swamps in Germany and Russia. **nonseasonal hay f.,** hay f., perennial, nonseasonal allergic rhinitis. **Oroya f.,** see *Carrión's disease.* **paratyphoid f.,** paratyphoid. **parenteric f.,** a disease clinically resembling typhoid fever and paratyphoid, but not caused by *Salmonella.* **parrot f.,** psittacosis. **pharyngoconjunctival f.,** an epidemic disease due to an adenovirus, seen mainly in school children, with fever, pharyngitis, conjunctivitis, rhinitis, and enlarged cervical lymph nodes. **phlebotomus f.,** a febrile viral disease of short duration, transmitted by the sandfly *Phlebotomus papatasi,* with dengue-like symptoms, seen in Mediterranean and Middle Eastern countries. **Pontiac f.,** a self-limited disease marked by fever, cough, muscle aches, chills, headache, chest pain, confusion, and pleuritis, caused by a strain of *Legionella pneumophila.* **pretibial f.,** an infection due to a serovar of *Leptospira interrogans,* marked by a rash on the pretibial region, with lumbar and postorbital pain, malaise, coryza, and fever. **puerperal f.,** septicemia accompanied by fever, in which the focus of infection is a lesion of the mucous membrane of the parturient canal due to trauma during childbirth; usually due to a streptococcus. **Q f.,** a febrile rickettsial infection, usually respiratory, first described in Australia, caused by *Coxiella burnetii.* **rat-bite f.,** either of two clinically similar acute infectious diseases, usually transmitted through a rat bite, one form (bacillary) of which is caused by *Streptobacillus moniliformis* and the other form (spirillary) by *Spirillum minor.* **recurrent f.,** 1. relapsing f. 2. recurrent paroxysmal fever occurring in various diseases, such as malaria. **relapsing f.,** any of a group of infectious diseases due to various species of *Borrelia,* marked by alternating periods of fever and apyrexia, each lasting from five to seven days. **remittent f.,** one that shows significant variations in 24 hours but without return to normal temperature. **rheumatic f.,** a febrile disease occurring as a sequela to Group A hemolytic streptococcal infections, characterized by multiple focal inflammatory lesions of connective tissue structures, especially of the heart, blood vessels, and joints, and by Aschoff bodies in the myocardium and skin. **Rift Valley f.,** a zoonotic febrile disease with dengue-like symptoms, due to an arbovirus, transmitted to humans by mosquitoes or by contact with diseased animals; first observed in the Rift Valley, Kenya. **Rocky Mountain spotted f.,** infection with *Rickettsia rickettsii,* transmitted by ticks, marked by fever, muscle pain, and weakness followed by a macular petechial eruption that begins on the hands and feet and spreads to the trunk and face, with other symptoms in the central nervous system and elsewhere. **rose f.,** a form of hay fever caused by grass pollens released while roses or other flowers are blooming. **scarlet f.,** an acute disease caused by Group A β-hemolytic streptococci, marked by pharyngotonsillitis and a skin rash caused by an erythrogenic toxin produced by the organism; the rash is a diffuse, bright red erythema, and desquamation of the skin begins as fine scaling with eventual peeling of the palms and soles. **Sennetsu f.,** a febrile disease seen in Japan and Malaysia and caused by *Ehrlichia sennetsu,* characterized by headache, nausea, lymphocytosis, and lymphadenopathy. **septic f.,** fever due to septicemia. **South African tickbite f.,** boutonneuse f. **trench f.,** a louse-borne rickettsial disease due to *Bartonella quintana,* transmitted by the body louse, *Pediculus humanus corporis,* and characterized by intermittent fever, generalized aches and pains, particularly severe in the shins, chills, sweating, vertigo, malaise, typhus-like rash, and multiple relapses. **typhoid f.**, infection by *Salmonella typhi* chiefly involving the lymphoid follicles of the ileum, with chills, fever, headache, cough, prostration, abdominal distention, splenomegaly, and a maculopapular rash; perforation of the bowel may occur in untreated cases. **f. of unknown origin (FUO)**, a febrile illness of at least three weeks' duration (some authorities permit a shorter duration), with a temperature of at least 38.3°C on at least three occasions and failure to establish a diagnosis in spite of intensive inpatient or outpatient evaluation (three outpatient visits or three days' hospitalization). **West Nile f.**, see under *encephalitis*. **yellow f.**, an acute, infectious, mosquito-borne viral disease, endemic primarily in tropical South America and Africa, marked by fever, jaundice due to necrosis of the liver, and albuminuria.

fe·ver·few (-fu″) the dried leaves of the herb *Tanacetum parthenium*, used for migraine, arthritis, rheumatic diseases, and allergy, and for various uses in folk medicine.

fe·ver·ish (fe′ver-ish) febrile.

fex·o·fen·a·dine (fek″so-fen′ah-dēn) an antihistamine (H_1-receptor antagonist) used as the hydrochloride salt in the treatment of hay fever and chronic idiopathic urticaria.

FFA free fatty acids.

FIAC Fellow of the International Academy of Cytology.

fi·ber (fi′ber) 1. an elongated, threadlike structure. 2. nerve f. 3. dietary f. **A f's**, myelinated afferent or efferent fibers of the somatic nervous system having a diameter of 1 to 22 μm and a conduction velocity of 5 to 120 meters per second; these include the alpha, beta, delta, and gamma fibers. **accelerating f's, accelerator f's**, adrenergic fibers that transmit the impulses which accelerate the heart beat. **adrenergic f's**, nerve fibers, usually sympathetic, that liberate epinephrine or related substances as neurotransmitters. **afferent f's, afferent nerve f's**, nerve fibers that convey sensory impulses from the periphery to the central nervous system. **alpha f's**, motor and proprioceptive fibers of the A type, having conduction velocities of 70 to 120 meters per second and ranging from 13 to 22 μm in diameter. **alveolar f's**, fibers of the periodontal ligament extending from the cementum of the tooth root to the walls of the alveolus. **arcuate f's**, the bow-shaped fibers in the brain, such as those connecting adjacent

gyri in the cerebral cortex, or the external or internal arcuate fibers of the medulla oblongata. **association f.**, one of the nerve fibers connecting different cortical areas within one hemisphere. **autonomic nerve f's**, nerve fibers that innervate smooth muscle and glandular tissues, either stimulating and activating the muscle or tissue (*autonomic efferent f's*) or receiving sensory impulses from them (*autonomic afferent f's*). **B f's**, myelinated preganglionic autonomic axons having a fiber diameter of ≤ 3 μm and a conduction velocity of 3 to 15 meters per second; these include only efferent fibers. **basilar f's**, those that form the middle layer of the zona arcuata and the zona pectinata of the organ of Corti. **beta f's**, motor and proprioceptive fibers of the A type, having conduction velocities of 30 to 70 meters per second and ranging from 8 to 13 μm in diameter. **C f's**, unmyelinated postganglionic fibers of the autonomic nervous system, also the unmyelinated fibers at the dorsal roots and at free nerve endings, having a conduction velocity of 0.6 to 2.3 meters per second and a diameter of 0.3 to 1.3 μm. **collagen f's, collagenous f's**, the soft, flexible, white fibers which are the most characteristic constituent of all types of connective tissue, consisting of the protein collagen, and composed of bundles of fibrils that are in turn made up of smaller units (microfibrils), which show a characteristic crossbanding with a major periodicity of 65 nm. **commissural f.**, one of the nerve fibers which pass between the cortex of opposite hemispheres of the brain, or between two sides of the brain stem or spinal cord. **dietary f.**, that part of whole grains, vegetables, fruits, and nuts that resists digestion in the gastrointestinal tract; it consists of carbohydrate (cellulose, etc.) and lignin. **efferent f's, efferent nerve f's**, nerve fibers that convey motor impulses away from the central nervous system toward the periphery. **elastic f's**, yellowish fibers of elastic quality traversing the intercellular substance of connective tissue. **fusimotor f's**, efferent A fibers that innervate the intrafusal fibers of the muscle spindle. **gamma f's**, any A fibers that conduct at velocities of 15 to 40 meters per second and range from 3 to 7 μm in diameter, comprising the fusimotor fibers. **gray f's**, unmyelinated nerve fibers found largely in the sympathetic nerves. **insoluble f.**, that not soluble in water, composed mainly of lignin, cellulose, and hemicelluloses and primarily found in the bran layers of cereal grains. **intrafusal f's**, modified muscle fibers which, surrounded by fluid and enclosed in a connective tissue envelope, compose the muscle spindle. **Mahaim f's,** specialized tissue connecting components of the conduction system directly to the ventricular septum. **motor f's,** efferent fibers. **Müller's f's,** elongated neuroglial cells traversing all the layers of the retina, forming its principal supporting element. **muscle f.,** any of the cells of skeletal or cardiac muscle tissue. Skeletal muscle fibers are cylindrical multinucleate cells containing contracting myofibrils, across which run transverse striations. Cardiac muscle fibers have one or sometimes two nuclei, contain myofibrils, and are separated from one another by an intercalated disk; although striated, cardiac muscle fibers branch to form an interlacing network. See Plate 7. **myelinated f's,** grayish white nerve fibers whose axons are encased in a myelin sheath, which may in turn be enclosed by a neurilemma. **nerve f.,** a slender process of a neuron, especially the prolonged axon which conducts nerve impulses away from the cell; classified as either afferent or efferent according to the direction the impulses flow, and either myelinated or unmyelinated according to whether there is or is not a myelin sheath. See Plate 14. **osteogenetic f's, osteogenic f's,** precollagenous fibers formed by osteoclasts and becoming the fibrous component of bone matrix. **preganglionic f's,** the axons of preganglionic neurons. **pressor f's,** nerve fibers which, when stimulated reflexly, cause or increase vasomotor tone. **projection f., projection nerve f's,** one of the nerve fibers that connect the cerebral cortex with the subcortical centers, the brain stem, and the spinal cord. **Purkinje f's,** modified cardiac muscle fibers composed of Purkinje cells, occurring as an interlaced network in the subendothelial tissue and constituting the terminal ramifications of the cardiac conducting system. **radicular f's,** fibers in the roots of the spinal nerves. **reticular f's,** immature connective tissue fibers staining with silver, forming the reticular framework of lymphoid and myeloid tissue, and occurring in interstitial tissue of glandular organs, the papillary layer of the dermis, and elsewhere. **sensory f's,** afferent fibers. **Sharpey's f's,** 1. collagenous fibers that pass from the periosteum and are embedded in the outer circumferential and interstitial lamellae of bone. 2. terminal portions of principal fibers that insert into the cementum of a tooth. **soluble f.,** that with an affinity for water, either dissolving or swelling to form a gel;

it includes gums, pectins, mucilages, and some hemicelluloses, and is primarily found in fruits, vegetables, oats, barley, legumes, and seaweed. **somatic nerve f's,** nerve fibers that stimulate and activate skeletal muscle and somatic tissues (*somatic efferent f's*) or receive impulses from them (*somatic afferent f's*). **spindle f's,** the microtubules radiating from the centrioles during mitosis and forming a spindle-shaped configuration. **traction f's,** spindle f's. **unmyelinated f's,** nerve fibers that lack the myelin sheath. **vasomotor f's,** unmyelinated nerve fibers going chiefly to arteriolar muscles. **visceral nerve f's,** autonomic nerve f's. **white f's,** collagenous f's.

fi·ber·il·lu·mi·nat·ed (-ĭ-loo′mĭ-nāt″ed) transmitting light by bundles of glass or plastic fibers, using a lens system to transmit the image; said of endoscopes of such design.

fi·ber·op·tics (fi″ber-op′tiks) the transmission of an image along flexible bundles of glass or plastic fibers, each of which carries an element of the image.

fi·bra (fi′brah) pl. *fi′brae.* [L.] fiber.

fi·brates (fi′brāts) general term for fibric acid (q.v.) derivatives.

fi·bric ac·id (fi′brik) any of a group of compounds structurally related to clofibrate that can reduce plasma levels of triglycerides and cholesterol; used to treat hypertriglyceridemia and hypercholesterolemia.

fi·bril (fi′bril) a minute fiber or filament. **fibril′lar, fib′rillary,** adj. **collagen f's,** delicate fibrils of collagen in connective tissue, composed of molecules of tropocollagen aggregated in linear array. **dentinal f's,** component fibrils of the dentinal matrix. **muscle f.,** myofibril.

fi·bril·la (fi-bril′ah) pl. *fibril′lae.* [L.] a fibril.

fi·bril·la·tion (fi″bri-la′shun) 1. the quality of being made up of fibrils. 2. a small, local, involuntary, muscular contraction, due to spontaneous activation of single muscle cells or muscle fibers whose nerve supply has been damaged or cut off. 3. the initial degenerative changes in osteoarthritis, marked by softening of the articular cartilage and development of vertical clefts between groups of cartilage cells. **atrial f.,** atrial arrhythmia marked by rapid randomized contractions of small areas of the atrial myocardium, causing a totally irregular, and often rapid, ventricular rate. **ventricular f.,** cardiac arrhythmia marked by fibrillary contractions of the ventricular muscle due to rapid repetitive excitation of myocardial fibers without coordinated ventricular contraction and by absence of atrial activity.

fi·brin (fi'brin) an insoluble protein that is essential to clotting of blood, formed from fibrinogen by action of thrombin.

fi·bri·no·cel·lu·lar (fi"brĭ-no-sel'u-ler) made up of fibrin and cells.

fi·brin·o·gen (fi-brin'o-jen) coagulation factor I.

fi·bri·no·gen·ic (fi"brĭ-no-jen'ik) producing or causing the formation of fibrin.

fi·bri·no·ge·nol·y·sis (-jě-nol'ĭ-sis) the proteolytic destruction of fibrinogen in circulating blood. **fibrinogenolyt'ic,** adj.

fi·brino·geno·pe·nia (fi-brin"o-jen"o-pe'ne-ah) hypofibrinogenemia.

fi·brin·oid (fi'brĭ-noid) 1. resembling fibrin. 2. a homogeneous, eosinophilic, relatively acellular refractile substance with some of the staining properties of fibrin.

fi·bri·nol·y·sin (fi"brĭ-nol'ĭ-sin) 1. plasmin. 2. a preparation of proteolytic enzyme formed from profibrinolysin (plasminogen); to promote dissolution of thrombi.

fi·bri·nol·y·sis (fi"brin-ol'ĭ-sis) dissolution of fibrin by enzymatic action. **fibrinolyt'ic,** adj.

fi·bri·no·pep·tide (fi-brin"o-pep'tĭd) either of two peptides (A and B) split off from fibrinogen during coagulation by the action of thrombin.

fi·bri·no·pu·ru·lent (-pu'roo-lent) characterized by the presence of both fibrin and pus.

fi·brin·ous (fi'brin-us) pertaining to or of the nature of fibrin.

fi·brin·uria (fi"brĭ-nu're-ah) the presence of fibrin in the urine.

fibr(o)- word element [L.], *fiber; fibrous.*

fi·bro·ad·e·no·ma (fi"bro-ad"ě-no'mah) adenofibroma. **giant f. of the breast,** phyllodes tumor.

fi·bro·ad·i·pose (-ad'ĭ-pōs) both fibrous and fatty.

fi·bro·are·o·lar (-ah-re'o-ler) both fibrous and areolar.

fi·bro·blast (fi'bro-blast) 1. an immature fiber-producing cell of connective tissue capable of differentiating into chondroblast, collagenoblast, or osteoblast. 2. collagenoblast; the collagen-producing cell. They also proliferate at the site of chronic inflammation. **fibroblas'tic,** adj.

fi·bro·blas·to·ma (fi"bro-blas-to'mah) any tumor arising from fibroblasts, divided into fibromas and fibrosarcomas.

fi·bro·bron·chi·tis (-brong-ki'tis) fibrinous bronchitis.

fi·bro·cal·cif·ic (-kal-sif'ik) pertaining to or characterized by partially calcified fibrous tissue.

fi·bro·car·ci·no·ma (-kahr"sĭ-no'mah) scirrhous carcinoma.

fi·bro·car·ti·lage (-kahr'tĭ-laj) cartilage of parallel, thick, compact collagenous bundles, separated by narrow clefts containing the typical cartilage cells (chondrocytes). **fibrocartilag'inous,** adj. **elastic f.,** that containing elastic fibers. **interarticular f.,** articular disk.

fi·bro·car·ti·la·go (-kahr'tĭ-lah'go) pl. *fibrocartilag'ines.* [L.] fibrocartilage.

fi·bro·chon·dri·tis (-kon-dri'tis) inflammation of fibrocartilage.

fi·bro·col·lag·e·nous (-ko-laj'ě-nus) both fibrous and collagenous; pertaining to or composed of fibrous tissue mainly composed of collagen.

fi·bro·cys·tic (-sis'tik) characterized by an overgrowth of fibrous tissue and development of cystic spaces, especially in a gland.

fi·bro·cyte (fi'bro-sīt) fibroblast.

fi·bro·dys·pla·sia (fi"bro-dis-pla'zhah) abnormality in development of fibrous connective tissue.

fi·bro·elas·tic (-e-las'tik) both fibrous and elastic.

fi·bro·elas·to·sis (-e"las-to'sis) overgrowth of fibroelastic elements. **endocardial f.,** diffuse patchy thickening of the mural endocardium, particularly in the left ventricle, due to proliferation of collagenous and elastic tissue; often associated with congenital cardiac malformations.

fi·bro·ep·i·the·li·al (-ep"ĭ-the'le-al) having fibrous and epithelial elements.

fi·bro·ep·i·the·li·o·ma (-ep"ĭ-the"le-o'mah) a tumor composed of both fibrous and epithelial elements.

fi·bro·fol·lic·u·lo·ma (-fah-lik"-u-lo'mah) a benign tumor of the perifollicular connective tissue, occurring as one or more yellowish dome-shaped papules, usually on the face.

fi·bro·his·tio·cyt·ic (-his"te-o-sit'ik) having fibrous and histiocytic elements.

fi·broid (fi'broid) 1. having a fibrous structure; resembling a fibroma. 2. fibroma. 3. leiomyoma. 4. in the plural, a colloquial term for leiomyoma of the uterus.

fi·broid·ec·to·my (fi"broid-ek'tah-me) uterine myomectomy.

fi·bro·la·mel·lar (fi"bro-lah-mel'er) characterized by the formation of fibers of collagen in layers.

fi·bro·li·po·ma (-lĭ-po'mah) a lipoma with excessive fibrous tissue. **fibrolipo'matous,** adj.

fi·bro·ma (fi-bro'mah) pl. *fibromas, fibro'mata.* A tumor composed mainly of fibrous or fully developed connective tissue. **ameloblastic f.,** an odontogenic tumor marked by simultaneous proliferation of both epithelial and mesenchymal tissue, without formation of enamel or dentin. **cementifying f.,** a tumor of fibroblastic tissue containing masses of cementum-like tissue, usually in the mandible of older persons. **chondromyxoid f.,** a rare, benign, slowly growing tumor of bone of chondroblastic origin, usually affecting the large long bones of the lower limb. **cystic f.,** one that has undergone cystic degeneration. **f. mollus′cum,** small subcutaneous nodules scattered over the body surface; seen in some forms of neurofibromatosis. **nonossifying f., nonosteogenic f.,** a degenerative and proliferative lesion of the medullary and cortical tissues of bone. **ossifying f., ossifying f. of bone,** a benign, slow-growing, central bone tumor, usually of the jaws, especially the mandible, composed of fibrous connective tissue within which bone is formed. **perifollicular f.,** one or more small, flesh-colored, papular, follicular lesions on the head and neck. **peripheral ossifying f.,** epulis; a fibroma, usually of the gingiva, showing areas of calcification or ossification. **periungual f.,** one of multiple smooth, firm, protruding nodules occurring at the nail folds and pathognomonic of tuberous sclerosis.

fi·bro·ma·to·sis (fi-bro″mah-to′sis) 1. the presence of multiple fibromas. 2. the formation of a fibrous, tumor-like nodule arising from the deep fascia, with a tendency to local recurrence. **aggressive f.,** desmoid tumor, particularly one that is extra-abdominal. **f. gingi′vae, gingival f.,** noninflammatory fibrous hyperplasia of the gingiva manifested as a dense, diffuse, smooth or nodular overgrowth of the gingival tissues. **palmar f.,** fibromatosis of palmar fascia, resulting in Dupuytren's contracture. **plantar f.,** fibromatosis of plantar fascia, with single or multiple nodular swellings, sometimes with pain but usually without contractures.

fi·bro·mus·cu·lar (fi″bro-mus′ku-lar) composed of fibrous and muscular tissue.

fi·bro·my·itis (-mi-i′tis) inflammation of muscle with fibrous degeneration.

fi·bro·my·o·ma (-mi-o′mah) a myoma containing fibrous elements.

fi·bro·myx·o·ma (-mik-so′mah) myxofibroma.

fi·bro·myx·o·sar·co·ma (-mik″so-sahr-ko′-mah) a sarcoma containing fibromatous and myxomatous elements.

fi·bro·nec·tin (-nek′tin) an adhesive glycoprotein: one form circulates in plasma and acts as an opsonin; another is a cell-surface protein that mediates cellular adhesive interactions.

fi·bro·odon·to·ma (-o″don-to′mah) a tumor containing both fibrous and odontogenic elements.

fi·bro·pap·il·lo·ma (-pap″ĭ-lo′mah) fibroepithelial papilloma.

fi·bro·pla·sia (-pla′zhah) the formation of fibrous tissue. **fibroplas′tic,** adj. **retrolental f. (RLF),** retinopathy of prematurity.

fi·bro·sar·co·ma (-sahr-ko′mah) a malignant, locally invasive, hematogenously spreading tumor derived from collagen-producing fibroblasts that are otherwise undifferentiated. **ameloblastic f.,** an odontogenic tumor that is the malignant counterpart to an ameloblastic fibroma, within which it usually arises. **odontogenic f.,** a malignant tumor of the jaws, originating from one of the mesenchymal components of the tooth or tooth germ.

fi·brose (fi′brōs) 1. to form fibrous tissue. 2. fibrous.

fi·bro·sis (fi-bro′sis) formation of fibrous tissue. **fibrot′ic,** adj. **congenital hepatic f.,** a developmental disorder of the liver marked by formation of irregular broad bands of fibrous tissue containing multiple cysts formed by disordered terminal bile ducts, resulting in vascular constriction and portal hypertension. **cystic f., cystic f. of the pancreas,** a generalized hereditary disorder of infants, children, and young adults, with widespread dysfunction of exocrine glands, signs of chronic pulmonary disease, obstruction of pancreatic ducts by eosinophilic concretions and consequent pancreatic enzyme deficiency, and other symptoms. **endomyocardial f.,** idiopathic myocardiopathy seen endemically in parts of Africa and less often in other areas, characterized by cardiomegaly, thickening of the endocardium with dense, white fibrous tissue that often extends to involve the inner third or half of the myocardium, and congestive heart failure. **idiopathic pulmonary f.,** chronic inflammation and progressive fibrosis of the pulmonary alveolar walls, with progressive dyspnea and potentially fatal lack of oxygen or right heart failure. The acute form is called *Hamman-Rich syndrome*. **mediastinal f.,** fibrous mediastinitis; development of white, hard fibrous tissue in the upper portion of the mediastinum, sometimes obstructing the air passages and large blood vessels. **nodular subepidermal f.,** 1. benign fibrous histiocytoma. 2. a type of benign fibrous histiocytoma marked by subepidermal formation of fibrous nodules as a result of productive inflammation. **pleural f.,** fibrosis of the visceral pleura so that part or all of a lung becomes covered with a thick layer of non-expansible fibrous tissue; fibrothorax is a more extensive form.

fi·bro·si·tis (fi″bro-si′tis) inflammatory hyperplasia of the white fibrous tissue, especially of the muscle sheaths and fascial layers of the locomotor system.

fi·bro·tho·rax (-thor′aks) adhesion of the two layers of pleura, so that the lung is covered by a thick layer of nonexpansible fibrous tissue (see *dry pleurisy*). It is often a consequence of traumatic hemothorax or of pleural effusion.

fi·brous (fi′brus) composed of or containing fibers.

fi·bro·xan·tho·ma (fi″bro-zan-tho′mah) a type of xanthoma containing fibromatous elements, sometimes described as synonymous with or a subtype of either benign or malignant fibrous histiocytoma. **atypical f. (AFX),** a small cutaneous nodular neoplasm usually occurring on sun-exposed areas of the face and neck; sometimes described as related to or a subtype of either benign or malignant fibrous histiocytoma.

fi·bro·xan·tho·sar·co·ma (-zan″tho-sahr-ko′mah) malignant fibrous histiocytoma.

fib·u·la (fib′ul-ah) [L.] see *Table of Bones.*

fib·u·lar (fib′u-lar) pertaining to the fibula or to the lateral aspect of the leg; peroneal.

fib·u·lo·cal·ca·ne·al (fib″ul-o-kal-ka′ne-il) pertaining to fibula and calcaneus.

fi·cain (fi′kān) an enzyme derived from the sap of fig trees that catalyzes the cleavage of specific bonds in proteins; it enhances the agglutination of red blood cells with IgG antibodies and is therefore used in the determination of the Rh factor.

FICD Fellow of the International College of Dentists.

fi·cin (fi′sin) ficain.

FICS Fellow of the International College of Surgeons.

field (fēld) 1. an area or open space, as an operative field or visual field. 2. a range of specialization in knowledge, study, or occupation. 3. in embryology, the developing region within a range of modifying factors. **auditory f.,** the space or range within which stimuli may be perceived as sound. **individuation f.,** a region in which an organizer influences adjacent tissue to become a part of a total embryo. **morphogenetic f.,** an embryonic region out of which definite structures normally develop. **visual f. (F, vf),** the area within which stimuli will produce the sensation of sight with the eye in a straight-ahead position.

FIGLU formiminoglutamic acid.

fig·ure (fig′yer) 1. an object of particular form. 2. a number, or numeral. **mitotic f's,** stages of chromosome aggregation exhibiting a pattern characteristic of mitosis.

fi·la (fi′lah) [L.] plural of *filum.*

fil·a·ment (fil′ah-ment) a delicate fiber or thread. **actin f.,** one of the thin contractile myofilaments in a myofibril. **intermediate f's,** a class of cytoplasmic filaments that predominantly act as structural components of the cytoskeleton and also effect various movements in cellular processes. **muscle f.,** myofilament. **myosin f.,** one of the thick contractile myofilaments in a myofibril. **thick f's,** bipolar myosin filaments occurring in striated muscle. **thin f's,** actin filaments occurring, associated with troponin and tropomyosin, in striated muscle.

fil·a·men·tous (fil″ah-men′tus) composed of long, threadlike structures.

fil·a·men·tum (fil″ah-men′tum) pl. *filamen'ta.* [L.] filament.

fi·la·ria (fi-lar′e-ah) pl. *fila'riae.* [L.] a nematode worm of the superfamily Filarioidea. **fila'rial,** adj.

fi·lar·i·cide (fi-lar′i-sīd) an agent that is destructive to filariae.

Fi·lar·i·oi·dea (fi-lar″e-oi′de-ah) a superfamily or order of parasitic nematodes, the adults being threadlike worms that invade the tissues and body cavities where the female deposits microfilariae (prelarvae).

fil·gras·tim (fil-gras′tim) a human granulocyte colony-stimulating factor produced by recombinant technology; used to enhance neutrophil function, stimulating hematopoiesis and decreasing neutropenia.

fil·i·al (fil′e-al) 1. of or pertaining to a son or daughter. 2. in genetics, of or pertaining to those generations following the initial (parental) generation.

fil·i·form (fil′i-form, fi′li-form) 1. threadlike. 2. an extremely slender bougie.

fil·let (fil′et) 1. a loop, as of cord or tape, for making traction on the fetus. 2. in the nervous system, a long band of nerve fibers.

fill·ing (fil′ing) 1. material inserted in a prepared tooth cavity. 2. restoration of the crown with appropriate material after removal of carious tissue from a tooth. **complex f.,** one for a complex cavity. **composite f.,** one consisting of a composite resin. **compound f.,** one for a cavity that involves two surfaces of a tooth.

film (film) 1. a thin layer or coating. 2. a thin transparent sheet of cellulose acetate or similar material coated on one or both sides with an emulsion that is sensitive to light or radiation. **absorbable gelatin f.,** a sterile, nonantigenic, absorbable, water-insoluble sheet of gelatin, used as an aid in surgical closure and repair of defects, and as a local hemostatic. **bite-wing f.,** an x-ray film for radiography of oral structures, with a protruding tab to be held between the upper and lower teeth. **plain f.,** a radiograph made without the use of a contrast medium. **spot f.,** a radiograph of a small anatomic area obtained either by rapid exposure during fluoroscopy to provide a permanent record of a transiently observed abnormality or by limitation of radiation passing through the area to improve definition and detail of the image produced. **x-ray f.,** film sensitized to x-rays, either before or after exposure.

film badge (baj) a pack of radiographic film or films, usually worn on the body during potential exposure to radiation in order to detect and quantitate the dosage of exposure.

fi·lo·pres·sure (fi'lo-presh″er) compression of a blood vessel by a thread.

Fi·lo·vi·ri·dae (fi″lo-vir′ĭ-de) Marburg and Ebola viruses: a family of RNA viruses with enveloped filamentous virions and a negative-sense single-stranded RNA genome; the single genus is *Filovirus.*

Fi·lo·vi·rus (fi'lo-vi″rus) Marburg and Ebola viruses: a genus of viruses of the family Filoviridae that cause hemorrhagic fevers (Marburg virus disease, Ebola virus disease).

fil·ter (fil′ter) 1. a device for eliminating or separating certain elements, as (1) particles of certain size from a solution, or (2) rays of certain wavelength from a stream of radiant energy. 2. to cause such separation or elimination. **membrane f.,** a filter made up of a thin film of collodion, cellulose acetate, or other material, available in a wide range of pore sizes. **Millipore f.,** trademark for any of a variety of membrane filters.

fil·ter·a·ble (-ah-b′l) capable of passing through the pores of a filter.

fil·trate (fil′trāt) a liquid or gas that has passed through a filter.

fil·tra·tion (fil-tra′shun) passage through a filter or other material that prevents passage of certain molecules, particles, or substances.

fi·lum (fi′lum) pl. *fi′la.* [L.] a threadlike structure or part. **f. termina′le,** a slender, threadlike prolongation of the spinal cord from the conus medullaris to the back of the coccyx.

fim·bria (fim′bre-ah) pl. *fim′briae.* [L.] 1. a fringe, border, or edge; a fringelike structure. 2. pilus (2). **f. hippocam′pi,** the band of white matter along the median edge of the ventricular surface of the hippocampus.

ovarian f., the longest of the processes that make up the fimbriae of uterine tube, extending along the free border of the mesosalpinx and fused to the ovary. **fimbriae of uterine tube,** the numerous divergent fringelike processes on the distal part of the infundibulum of the uterine tube.

fim·bri·at·ed (fim′bre-āt′ed) fringed.

fim·bri·ec·to·my (fim″bre-ek′tah-me) surgical removal of the fimbriae of the uterine tube along with tubal ligation as a method of female sterilization.

fim·brio·cele (fim′bre-o-sēl″) hernia containing the fimbriae of the uterine tube.

fim·bri·o·plas·ty (fim′bre-o-plas″te) plastic surgery of the fimbriae of uterine tube.

fi·nas·te·ride (fi-nas′ter-īd) an inhibitor of 5α-reductase, used in the treatment of benign prostatic hyperplasia and as a hair growth stimulant in the treatment of androgenetic alopecia.

fin·ger (fing′ger) one of the five digits of the hand. **baseball f.,** mallet f. **clubbed f.,** a finger with clubbing. **index f.,** forefinger. **mallet f.,** partial permanent flexion of the terminal phalanx of a finger caused by an object striking the end or back of the finger, owing to rupture of the attachment of the extensor tendon. **ring f.,** the fourth digit of the hand. **webbed f's,** syndactyly of the fingers.

fin·ger·print (-print) 1. an impression of the cutaneous ridges of the fleshy distal portion of a finger. 2. in biochemistry, the characteristic pattern of a peptide after subjection to an analytical technique.

first aid (furst ād) emergency care and treatment of an injured or ill person before complete medical and surgical treatment can be secured.

fis·sion (fish′un) 1. the act of splitting. 2. asexual reproduction in which the cell divides into two *(binary f.)* or more *(multiple f.)* daughter parts, each of which becomes an individual organism. 3. nuclear fission; the splitting of the atomic nucleus, with release of energy.

fis·sip·a·rous (fi-sip′ah-rus) propagated by fission.

fis·su·la (fis′ūl-ah) [L.] a small cleft.

fis·su·ra (fis-u′rah) pl. *fissu′rae.* [L.] fissure. **f. in a′no,** anal fissure.

fis·sure (fish′er) 1. any cleft or groove, normal or otherwise, especially a deep fold in the cerebral cortex involving its entire thickness. 2. a fault in the enamel surface of a tooth. **abdominal f.,** a congenital cleft in the abdominal wall. **anal f., f. in ano,** painful lineal ulcer at the margin of the anus.

anterior median f., a longitudinal furrow along the midline of the anterior aspect of the spinal cord and medulla oblongata. **basisylvian f.,** the part of the sylvian fissure between the temporal lobe and the orbital surface of the frontal bone. **f. of Bichat,** transverse f. (2). **branchial f.,** 1. branchial cleft (1). 2. pharyngeal groove. **calcarine f.,** see under *sulcus*. **central f.,** see under *sulcus*. **collateral f.,** see under *sulcus*. **enamel f.,** fissure (2). **hippocampal f.,** see under *sulcus*. **palpebral f.,** the longitudinal opening between the eyelids. **parietooccipital f.,** see under *sulcus*. **portal f.,** porta hepatis. **posterior median f.,** see under *sulcus*. **presylvian f.,** the anterior branch of the fissure of Sylvius. **primary f. of cerebellum,** that separating the cranial and caudal lobes in the cerebellum. **f. of Rolando,** central sulcus of cerebrum. **sphenooccipital f.,** the fissure between the basilar part of the occipital bone and the sphenoid bone. **sylvian f., f. of Sylvius,** one extending laterally between the temporal and frontal lobes, and turning posteriorly between the temporal and parietal lobes. **transverse f.,** 1. porta hepatis. 2. the transverse cerebral fissure between the diencephalon and the cerebral hemispheres.

fis·tu·la (fis′tu-lah) pl. *fistulas, fis′tulae.* [L.] an abnormal passage between two internal organs or from an internal organ to the body surface. **anal f.,** one from the anus to the skin, sometimes communicating with the rectum. **arteriovenous f.,** 1. one between an artery and a vein. 2. a surgically created arteriovenous connection that provides a site of access for hemodialysis tubing. **blind f.,** one open at one end only, opening on the skin (*external blind f.*) or on an internal mucous surface (*internal blind f.*). **branchial f.,** a persistent pharyngeal groove (branchial cleft). **cerebrospinal fluid f.,** one between the subarachnoid space and a body cavity, with leakage of cerebrospinal fluid, usually as otorrhea or rhinorrhea. **colonic f.,** one connecting the colon with the body surface or another organ. **craniosinus f.,** one between the cerebral space and one of the sinuses, permitting escape of cerebrospinal fluid into the nose. **enterovesical f.,** one connecting the urinary bladder with some part of the intestines. **fecal f.,** a colonic fistula that discharges feces on the body surface. **gastric f.,** one communicating with the stomach, either pathologically or surgically created through the abdominal wall. **genitourinary f.,** one between two organs of the urogenital system or between one of those organs and some other system. **incomplete f.,** blind f. **intestinal f.,** one communicating with the intestine; sometimes surgically created through the abdominal wall. **perilymph f.,** rupture of the round window with leakage of perilymph into the middle ear, causing sensorineural hearing loss. **pulmonary arteriovenous f.,** a congenital fistula between the pulmonary arterial and venous systems, so that unoxygenated blood enters the systemic circulation. **salivary f.,** one communicating with a salivary duct. **tracheoesophageal f.,** one connecting the trachea and esophagus, either pathologically or created surgically to restore speech after laryngectomy. **umbilical f.,** one communicating with the colon or the urachus at the umbilicus.

fis·tu·la·tome (-tōm″) an instrument for cutting a fistula.

fis·tu·li·za·tion (fis″tu-lĭ-za′shun) 1. the process of becoming fistulous. 2. the surgical creation of a fistula.

fis·tu·lot·o·my (fis″tu-lot′ah-me) incision of a fistula.

fit (fit) 1. seizure (2). 2. the adaptation of one structure into another.

fix (fiks) to fasten or hold firm; see *fixation*.

fix·a·tion (fik-sa′shun) 1. the process of holding, suturing, or fastening in a fixed position. 2. the condition of being held in a fixed position. 3. in psychiatry: (*a*) arrest of development at a particular stage, or (*b*) a close suffocating attachment to another person, especially a childhood figure, such as a parent. 4. the use of a fixative to preserve histological or cytological specimens. 5. in chemistry, the process whereby a substance is removed from the gaseous or solution phase and localized. 6. in ophthalmology, direction of the gaze so that the visual image of the object falls on the fovea centralis. 7. in film processing, removal of all undeveloped salts of the film emulsion, leaving only the developed silver to form a permanent image. **complement f., f. of complement,** addition of another serum containing an antibody and the corresponding antigen to a hemolytic serum, making the complement incapable of producing hemolysis.

fix·a·tive (fik′sit-iv) an agent used in preserving a histological or pathological specimen so as to maintain the normal structure of its constituent elements.

flac·cid (flak′sid, flas′id) 1. weak, lax, and soft. 2. atonic.

fla·gel·la (flah-jel′ah) [L.] plural of *flagellum*.

fla·gel·lar (flah-jel′ar) of or relating to a flagellum.

flag·el·late (flaj'ĕ-lāt) 1. any microorganism having flagella. 2. mastigote. 3. having flagella. 4. to practice flagellation.

flag·el·la·tion (flaj"ĕ-la'shun) 1. whipping or being whipped to achieve erotic pleasure. 2. exflagellation. 3. the formation or arrangement of flagella on an organism or surface.

fla·gel·lin (flah-jel'in) a protein of bacterial flagella; it is composed of subunits in several-stranded helical arrangement.

flag·el·lo·sis (flaj"il-o'sis) infestation with flagellate protozoa.

fla·gel·lo·spore (flah-jel'o-spōr) zoospore.

fla·gel·lum (flah-jel'um) pl. *flagel'la*. [L.] a long, mobile, whiplike appendage arising from a basal body at the surface of a cell, serving as a locomotor organelle; in eukaryotic cells, flagella contain nine pairs of microtubules arrayed around a central pair; in bacteria, they contain tightly wound strands of flagellin.

flail (flāl) exhibiting abnormal or pathologic mobility, as flail chest or flail joint.

flame (flām) 1. the luminous, irregular appearance usually accompanying combustion, or an appearance resembling it. 2. to render an object sterile by exposure to a flame.

flange (flanj) a projecting border or edge; in dentistry, that part of the denture base which extends from around the embedded teeth to the border of the denture.

flank (flank) the side of the body between ribs and ilium.

flap (flap) 1. a mass of tissue for grafting, usually including skin, only partially removed from one part of the body so that it retains its own blood supply during transfer to another site. 2. an uncontrolled movement. **bone f.**, craniotomy involving elevation of a section of the skull. **free f.**, an island flap detached from the body and reattached at the distant recipient site by microvascular anastomosis. **jump f.**, one cut from the abdomen and attached to a flap of the same size on the forearm; the forearm flap is transferred later to some other part of the body to fill a defect there. **myocutaneous f.**, a compound flap of skin and muscle with adequate vascularity to permit sufficient tissue to be transferred to the recipient site. **pedicle f.**, a flap consisting of the full thickness of the skin and the subcutaneous tissue, attached by tissue through which it receives its blood supply. **rope f.**, one made by elevating a long strip of tissue from its bed except at its two ends, the cut edges then being sutured together to form a tube. **rotation f.**, a local pedicle flap whose width is increased by having the edge distal to the defect form a curved line; the flap is then rotated and a counterincision is made at the base of the curved line to increase mobility of the flap. **skin f.**, a full-thickness mass or flap of tissue containing epidermis, dermis, and subcutaneous tissue. **sliding f.**, a flap carried to its new position by a sliding technique.

flare (flār) a diffuse area of redness on the skin around the point of application of an irritant, due to a vasomotor reaction.

flask (flask) 1. a laboratory vessel, usually of glass and with a constricted neck. 2. a metal case in which materials used in making artificial dentures are placed for processing. **Erlenmeyer f.**, a conical glass flask with a broad base and narrow neck. **volumetric f.**, a narrow-necked vessel of glass calibrated to contain or deliver an exact volume at a given temperature.

flat (flat) 1. lying in one plane; having an even surface. 2. having little or no resonance. 3. slightly below the normal pitch of a musical tone.

flat·foot (flat'foot) a condition in which one or more arches of the foot have flattened out.

flat·ness (-nes) a peculiar sound lacking resonance, heard on percussing an abnormally solid part.

flat·u·lence (flat'u-lens) excessive formation of gases in the stomach or intestine.

fla·tus (fla'tus) [L.] 1. gas or air in the gastrointestinal tract. 2. gas or air expelled through the anus.

flat·worm (flat'wurm) an individual organism of the phylum Platyhelminthes.

fla·vin (fla'vin) any of a group of water-soluble yellow pigments widely distributed in animals and plants, including riboflavin and yellow enzymes. **f. adenine dinucleotide (FAD),** a coenzyme composed of riboflavin 5′-phosphate (FMN) and adenosine 5′-phosphate in pyrophosphate linkage; it forms the prosthetic group of certain enzymes, including D-amino acid oxidase and xanthine oxidase, serving as an electron carrier by being alternately oxidized (FAD) and reduced (FADH$_2$). It is important in electron transport in mitochondria. **f. mononucleotide (FMN),** riboflavin 5′-phosphate; it acts as a coenzyme for a number of oxidative enzymes, including NADH dehydrogenase, serving as an electron carrier by being alternately oxidized (FMN) and reduced (FMNH$_2$).

Fla·vi·vi·ri·dae (fla"vĭ-vir'ĭ-de) the group B arboviruses: a family of RNA viruses with a single-stranded positive-sense RNA genome; there is a single genus, *Flavivirus*.

Fla·vi·vi·rus (fla′vĭ-vi″rus) group B arboviruses: a genus of viruses of the family Flaviviridae, many members of which cause disease in humans and animals, including the agents of yellow fever, dengue, and St. Louis and other forms of encephalitis.

fla·vi·vi·rus (fla′vĭ-vi″rus) any virus of the family Flaviviridae.

flav(o)- word element [L.], *yellow*.

Fla·vo·bac·te·ri·um (fla″vo-bak-tēr′e-um) a genus of schizomycetes (family Achromobacteriaceae), characteristically producing yellow, orange, red, or yellow-brown pigmentation, found in soil and water; some species are said to be pathogenic.

fla·vo·en·zyme (-en′zīm) any enzyme containing a flavin nucleotide (FMN or FAD) as a prosthetic group.

fla·vo·noid (fla′vah-noid) any of a group of compounds containing a characteristic aromatic nucleus and widely distributed in higher plants, often as a pigment; a subgroup with biological activity in mammals is the bioflavonoids.

fla·vox·ate (fla-voks′āt) a smooth muscle relaxant; the hydrochloride salt is used in treatment of spasms of the urinary tract.

flax·seed (flak′sēd) linseed.

flea (fle) a small, wingless, bloodsucking insect; many fleas are parasitic and may act as disease carriers.

fle·cai·nide (flĕ-ka′nīd) a sodium channel blocker that decreases the rate of cardiac conduction and increases the ventricular refractory period; used as the acetate salt in the treatment of life-threatening arrhythmias.

fleece (flēs) a mass of interlacing fibrils. **f. of Stilling,** the lacework of myelinated fibers surrounding the dentate nucleus.

flesh (flesh) 1. muscular tissue. 2. skin. **goose f.,** cutis anserina. **proud f.,** exuberant amounts of soft, edematous, granulation tissue developing during healing of large surface wounds.

fleshy (flesh′e) 1. pertaining to or resembling flesh. 2. characterized by abundant flesh.

fleur·ette (floor-et′) [Fr.] a type of cell found in clusters in retinoblastomas and retinocytomas, representing differentiation of tumor cells into photoreceptors.

flex·i·bil·i·tas (flek″sĭ-bil′ĭ-tas) [L.] flexibility. **ce′rea f.,** see under *C*.

flex·i·bil·i·ty (-ĭ-te) the quality of being readily bent without tendency to break. **flex′ible,** adj. **waxy f.,** cerea flexibilitas.

flex·ion (flek′shun) the act of bending or the condition of being bent.

flex·or (flek′ser) 1. causing flexion. 2. a muscle that flexes a joint; see *Table of Muscles*. **f. retina′culum,** see entries under *retinaculum*.

flex·u·ra (flek-shoo′rah) pl. *flexu′rae*. [L.] flexure.

flex·ure (flek′sher) a bend or fold; a curvation. **caudal f.,** the bend at the aboral end of the embryo. **cephalic f.,** the curve in the midbrain of the embryo. **cervical f.,** a bend in the neural tube of the embryo at the junction of the brain and spinal cord. **cranial f.,** cephalic f. **dorsal f.,** one of the flexures in the mid-dorsal region of the embryo. **duodenojejunal f.,** the bend at the junction of duodenum and jejunum. **lumbar f.,** the ventral curvature in the lumbar region of the back. **mesencephalic f.,** cephalic f. **nuchal f.,** cervical f. **pontine f.,** a flexure of the hindbrain in the embryo. **sacral f.,** caudal f. **sigmoid f.,** see under *colon*.

flight of ideas (flīt of i-de′ahz) a nearly continuous flow of rapid speech that jumps from topic to topic, usually based on discernible associations, distractions, or plays on words, but sometimes disorganized and incoherent.

float·ers (flo′ters) "spots before the eyes"; deposits in the vitreous of the eye, usually moving about and probably representing fine aggregates of vitreous protein occurring as a benign degenerative change.

floc·cil·la·tion (flok″sĭ-la′shun) the aimless picking at bedclothes by a patient with delirium, dementia, fever, or exhaustion.

floc·cose (flok′ōs) woolly; said of bacterial growth of short, curved chains variously oriented.

floc·cu·la·tion (flok″u-la′shun) a colloid phenomenon in which the disperse phase separates in discrete, usually visible, particles rather than congealing into a continuous mass, as in coagulation.

floc·cu·lus (flok′u-lus) pl. *floc′culi*. [L.] 1. a small tuft or mass, as of wool or other fibrous material. 2. a small mass on the lower side of each cerebral hemisphere, continuous with the nodule of the vermis. **floc′cular,** adj.

flood·ing (flud′ing) a form of desensitization for treating phobias and anxieties by repeated exposure to highly distressing stimuli until the lack of reinforcement of the anxiety response causes its extinction. It is usually used for actual exposure to the stimuli, with *implosion* used for imagined exposure, but the two terms are sometimes used synonymously.

floor (flor) the inferior inner surface of a hollow organ or other space.

flo·ra (flor'ah) [L.] 1. the collective plant organisms of a given locality. 2. the bacteria and fungi, both normally occurring and pathological, found in or on an organ. **intestinal f.,** the bacteria normally within the lumen of the intestine.

flor·id (flor'id) 1. in full bloom; occurring in fully developed form. 2. having a bright red color.

flow (flo) 1. the movement of a liquid or gas. 2. the rate at which a fluid passes through an organ or part, expressed as volume per unit of time. **blood f.,** 1. circulation (of the blood). 2. circulation rate. **effective renal blood f. (ERBF),** that portion of the total blood flow through the kidneys that perfuses functional renal tissue such as the glomeruli. **effective renal plasma f. (ERPF),** the amount of plasma that perfuses the renal tubules per unit time, generally measured by the clearance rate of p-aminohippurate. **forced expiratory f. (FEF),** the rate of airflow recorded in measurements of forced vital capacity. **maximum expiratory f.,** the rate of airflow during a forced vital capacity maneuver, often specified at a given volume. **maximum midexpiratory f.,** the average rate of airflow measured between exhaled volumes of 25 and 75 per cent of the vital capacity during a forced exhalation. **peak expiratory f. (PEF),** the greatest rate of airflow that can be achieved during forced exhalation beginning with the lungs fully inflated. **renal plasma f. (RPF),** the amount of plasma that perfuses the kidneys per unit time, approximately 10 per cent greater than the effective renal plasma flow.

flower (flou'er) [Old Fr. *flor,* from L. *flos,* gen. *floris*] the blossom of a plant; preparations of the flowers of some plants are used medicinally. **passion f.,** 1. any plant of the genus *Passiflora.* 2. a preparation of the aerial parts of *P. incarnata,* having anxiolytic and sedative properties and used for anxiety and insomnia; also used in homeopathy.

flow·me·ter (flo'me-ter) an apparatus for measuring the rate of flow of liquids or gases, often named for the method employed, e.g., *ultrasound f.*

flox·uri·dine (floks-ūr'ĭ-dēn) a derivative of fluorouracil used as an antineoplastic.

fl oz fluid ounce.

flu (floo) colloquialism for *influenza.*

flu·con·a·zole (floo-kon'ah-zōl) a triazole antifungal used in the systemic treatment of candidiasis and cryptococcal meningitis.

fluc·tu·a·tion (fluk″choo-a'shun) a variation, as about a fixed value or mass; a wave-like motion.

flu·cy·to·sine (floo-si'to-sēn″) an antifungal used in the treatment of severe candidal and cryptococcal infections.

flu·dar·a·bine (floo-dar'ah-bēn) an adenine analogue and purine antimetabolite used as the phosphate salt as an antineoplastic in the treatment of chronic lymphocytic leukemia.

flu·de·oxy·glu·cose F 18 (floo″de-ok″se-gloo'kōs) radiolabeled 2-deoxy-D-glucose; used in positron emission tomography in the diagnosis of brain disorders, cardiac disease, and tumors of various organs.

flu·dro·cor·ti·sone (floo″dro-kor'tĭ-sōn) a synthetic adrenal corticoid with effects similar to those of hydrocortisone and desoxycorticosterone, administered as the acetate salt.

flu·ent (floo'int) flowing effortlessly; said of speech.

flu·id (floo'id) 1. a liquid or gas; any liquid of the body. 2. composed of molecules which freely change their relative positions without separation of the mass. **amniotic f.,** the liquid within the amnion that bathes the developing fetus and protects it from mechanical injury. **cerebrospinal f. (CSF),** the fluid contained within the ventricles of the brain, the subarachnoid space, and the central canal of the spinal cord. **follicular f.,** the fluid in a developing ovarian follicle. **interstitial f.,** the extracellular fluid bathing most tissues, excluding the fluid within the lymph and blood vessels. **intracellular f.,** the portion of the total body water with its dissolved solutes which are within the cell membranes. **prostatic f.,** the secretion of the prostate gland, which contributes to formation of the semen. **Scarpa's f.,** endolymph. **seminal f.,** semen. **synovial f.,** synovia; the transparent, viscid fluid secreted by the synovial membrane and found in joint cavities, bursae, and tendon sheaths.

flu·id·ex·tract (floo″id-ek'strakt) a liquid preparation of a vegetable drug, containing alcohol as a solvent or preservative, of such strength that each milliliter contains the therapeutic constituents of 1 g of the standard drug it represents.

fluke (flook) trematode.

flu·like (floo'līk) 1. resembling influenza. 2. having symptoms that resemble those of influenza.

flu·ma·ze·nil (floo-ma'zĕ-nil″) a benzodiazepine agonist used to reverse the effects of benzodiazepines after sedation, general anesthesia, or overdose.

flu·men (floo'men) pl. *flu'mina.* [L.] a stream. **flu'mina pilo'rum,** the lines along which the hairs of the body are arranged as they grow.

flu·nis·o·lide (floo-nis′o-līd″) a synthetic glucocorticoid used as the acetate salt in treatment of bronchial asthma and seasonal and nonseasonal allergic rhinitis.

flu·o·cin·o·lone (floo″ah-sin′ah-lōn) a synthetic corticosteroid used topically as *f. acetonide* for the relief of inflammation and pruritus in certain dermatoses.

flu·o·cin·o·nide (-nīd) a synthetic corticosteroid used topically for the relief of inflammation and pruritus in certain dermatoses.

flu·o·res·ce·in (floo-res′ēn) a fluorescing dye; its sodium salt is used as a tracer in retinal angiography and as a diagnostic aid for revealing corneal trauma and fitting contact lenses.

flu·o·res·cence (-ens) the property of emitting light while exposed to light, the wavelength of the emitted light being longer than that of the absorbed light. **fluores′cent**, adj.

flu·o·ri·da·tion (floor″ĭ-da′shun) treatment with fluorides; the addition of fluorides to a public water supply as a public health measure to reduce the incidence of dental caries.

flu·o·rim·e·ter (floo-rim′ĕ-ter) fluorometer.

flu·o·rine (F) (floor′ēn) chemical element (see *Table of Elements*), at. no. 9.

flu·o·ro·car·bon (floor′o-kahr″bən) any of the class of organic compounds consisting of carbon and fluorine only. Fluorocarbon emulsions dissolve oxygen and carbon dioxide and can be used in place of red blood cell preparations in the prevention and treatment of ischemia.

flu·o·ro·chrome (-krōm) a fluorescent compound used as a dye to mark protein with a fluorescent label.

flu·o·ro·do·pa F 18 (floor″o-do′pah) a radiolabeled compound of fluorine and levodopa, used for positron emission tomography of the cerebrum.

flu·o·rom·e·ter (floo-rom′ĕ-ter) the instrument used in fluorometry, consisting of an energy source (e.g., a mercury arc lamp or xenon lamp) to induce fluorescence, filters or monochromators for selection of the wavelength, and a detector.

flu·o·ro·meth·o·lone (floor″o-meth′ah-lōn) a synthetic glucocorticoid used topically in the treatment of corticosteroid-responsive allergic and inflammatory conditions of the eye.

flu·o·rom·e·try (floo-rom′ĕ-tre) an analytical technique for identifying and characterizing minute amounts of a substance by excitation of the substance with a beam of ultraviolet light and detection and measurement of the characteristic wavelength of fluorescent light emitted.

flu·o·ro·neph·e·lom·e·ter (floor″-o-nef″ĕ-lom′ĕ-ter) an instrument for analysis of a solution by measuring the light scattered or emitted by it.

flu·o·ro·pho·tom·e·try (-fo-tom′ĕ-tre) fluorometry. **vitreous f.,** the measurement of light given off by intravenously injected fluorescein that has leaked through the retinal vessels into the vitreous; done to detect the breakdown of the blood-retinal barrier, an early ocular change in diabetes mellitus.

flu·o·ro·quin·o·lone (-kwin′o-lōn) any of a subgroup of fluorine-substituted quinolones, having a broader spectrum of activity than nalidixic acid.

flu·o·ro·scope (floor′o-skōp) an instrument for visual observation of the form and motion of the deep structures of the body by means of x-ray shadows projected on a fluorescent screen.

flu·o·ros·co·py (floo-ros′kah-pe) examination by means of the fluoroscope.

flu·o·ro·sis (floo-ro′sis) 1. a condition due to ingestion of excessive amounts of fluorine. 2. a condition in humans due to exposure to excessive amounts of fluorine or its compounds, resulting from accidental ingestion of certain insecticides and rodenticides, chronic inhalation of industrial dusts or gases, or prolonged ingestion of water containing large amounts of fluorides; characterized by skeletal changes such as *osteofluorosis* and by *mottled enamel* when exposure occurs during enamel formation. **chronic endemic f.,** fluorosis. **dental f.,** mottled enamel.

flu·o·ro·ura·cil (5-FU) (floor″o-ūr′ah-sil) an antimetabolite activated like uracil, used as a systemic and topical antineoplastic.

flu·ox·e·tine (floo-ok′sĕ-tēn) a selective serotonin reuptake inhibitor used as the hydrochloride salt in the treatment of depression, obsessive-compulsive disorder, bulimia nervosa, and premenstrual dysphoric disorder.

flu·ox·y·mes·ter·one (floo-ok″se-mes′ter-ōn) an androgen used in the treatment of male hypogonadism and delayed male puberty and in palliation of metastatic breast carcinoma in postmenopausal women.

flu·phen·a·zine (floo-fen′ah-zēn) a phenothiazine antipsychotic, used as *f. decanoate, f. enanthate,* and *f. hydrochloride.*

flur·an·dren·o·lide (floor″an-dren′ah-līd) a synthetic corticosteroid used topically for relief of inflammation and pruritus in dermatoses.

flu·raz·e·pam (floo-raz′ĕ-pam) a benzodiazepine used as the hydrochloride salt as a sedative and hypnotic in the treatment of insomnia.

flur·bi·pro·fen (floor-bi′pro-fen) a nonsteroidal antiinflammatory drug administered orally in the treatment of arthritis and other inflammatory disorders and dysmenorrhea, and applied topically to the conjunctiva as the sodium salt to inhibit miosis during and treat inflammation following ophthalmic surgery.

flush (flush) redness, usually transient, of the face and neck.

flu·ta·mide (floo′tah-mīd) a nonsteroidal antiandrogen, used in the treatment of metastatic prostatic carcinoma.

flu·tic·a·sone (floo-tik′ah-sōn″) a synthetic corticosteroid used as the propionate salt to treat inflammation in certain dermatoses, allergic rhinitis and other inflammatory nasal conditions, nasal polyps, and asthma.

flut·ter (flut′er) a rapid vibration or pulsation. **atrial f.,** cardiac arrhythmia in which the atrial contractions are rapid (250 to 350 per minute), but regular. **diaphragmatic f.,** peculiar wavelike fibrillations of the diaphragm of unknown cause. **impure f.,** atrial flutter in which the electrocardiogram shows alternating periods of atrial flutter and fibrillation or periods not clearly one or the other. **mediastinal f.,** abnormal motility of the mediastinum during respiration. **pure f.,** atrial f. **ventricular f. (VFl),** a possible transition stage between ventricular tachycardia and ventricular fibrillation, the electrocardiogram showing rapid, uniform, regular oscillations, 250 or more per minute.

flut·ter-fi·bril·la·tion (-fĭ-brĭ-la′shun) impure flutters constantly varying in their resemblance to flutter or fibrillation, respectively.

flu·va·stat·in (floo′vah-stat″in) an inhibitor of cholesterol biosynthesis used as the sodium salt in the treatment of hyperlipidemia and to slow the progression of atherosclerosis associated with coronary heart disease.

flu·vox·amine (floo-vok′sah-mēn) a selective serotonin reuptake inhibitor, used as the maleate salt to relieve the symptoms of obsessive-compulsive disorder.

flux (fluks) 1. an excessive flow or discharge. 2. the rate of the flow of some quantity per unit area. **magnetic f. (Φ),** a quantitative measure of a magnetic field.

flux·ion (fluk′shun) a flowing; especially an abnormal or excessive flow of fluid to a part.

fly (fli) a dipterous, or two-winged, insect that is often the vector of organisms causing disease. **tsetse f.,** see *Glossina.*

Fm fermium.

FMN flavin mononucleotide.

FNH focal nodular hyperplasia.

foam (fōm) 1. a dispersion of a gas in a liquid or solid. 2. frothy saliva. 3. to produce or cause production of such a substance. **foam′y,** adj.

fo·cus (fo′kus) pl. *fo′ci.* [L.] 1. the point of convergence of light rays or sound waves. 2. the chief center of a morbid process. **fo′cal,** adj. **epileptogenic f.,** the area of the cerebral cortex responsible for causing epileptic seizures. **Ghon f.,** the principal parenchymal lesion of primary pulmonary tuberculosis in children.

fo·cus·ing (-ing) the act of converging at a point. **isoelectric f.,** electrophoresis in which the protein mixture is subjected to an electric field in a gel medium in which a pH gradient has been established; each protein then migrates until it reaches the site at which the pH is equal to its isoelectric point.

foe- for words beginning thus, see those beginning *fe-.*

fog (fog) a colloid system in which the dispersion medium is a gas and the disperse particles are liquid.

fog·ging (fog′ing) in ophthalmology, a method of determining refractive error in astigmatism, the patient being first made artificially myopic in order to relax accommodation.

foil (foil) metal in the form of an extremely thin, pliable sheet.

fo·late (fo′lāt) 1. the anionic form of folic acid. 2. more generally, any of a group of substances containing a form of pteroic acid conjugated with L-glutamic acid and having a variety of substitutions.

fold (fōld) plica; a thin, recurved margin, or doubling over. **amniotic f.,** the folded edge of the amnion where it rises over and finally encloses the embryo. **aryepiglottic f.,** a fold of mucous membrane extending on each side between the lateral border of the epiglottis and the summit of the arytenoid cartilage. **Douglas' f.,** a crescentic line marking the termination of the posterior layer of the sheath of the rectus abdominis muscle, just below the level of the iliac crest. **gastric f's,** the series of folds in the mucous membrane of the stomach. **gluteal f.,** the crease separating the buttocks from the thigh. **head f.,** a crescentic, ventral fold of the embryonic disc at the cephalic end of the developing embryo. **lacrimal f.,** a fold of mucous membrane at the lower opening of the nasolacrimal duct. **Marshall's f.,** vestigial f. of Marshall. **medullary f.,** neural f. **mesonephric f.,** see under *ridge*. **nail f.,** the fold of palmar skin around the base and sides of the nail. **neural f.,** one of the paired folds lying on either side of the neural plate that form the neural tube. **palmate f's,** a system of folds on the anterior and posterior walls of the cervical canal of the uterus. **semilunar f. of conjunctiva,** a mucous fold at the medial angle of the eye. **skin f.,** skinfold. **tail f.,** a crescentic, ventral fold of the embryonic disc at the future caudal end of the developing embryo. **ventricular f., vestibular f.,** a false vocal cord. **vestigial f. of Marshall,** a pericardial fold enclosing the remnant of the embryonic left anterior cardinal vein. **vocal f.,** the true vocal cord.

fo·li·a·ceous (fo″le·a′shus) foliate.

fo·li·ate (fo′le-it) 1. having, pertaining to, or resembling leaves. 2. consisting of thin, leaflike layers.

fo·lic ac·id (fo′lik) a water-soluble vitamin of the B complex, pteroylglutamic acid or related derivatives, which is involved in hematopoiesis and the synthesis of amino acids and DNA; its deficiency causes megaloblastic anemia. See *tetrahydrofolic acid* and *folic acid antagonist*.

fo·lie (fo-le′) [Fr.] psychosis; insanity. **f. à deux** (ah-doo′), mental disorder affecting two persons who share the same delusions; formally classified as *shared psychotic disorder*. **f. du pourquoi** (doo-poor-kwah′), psychopathologic constant questioning. **f. gémel-laire** (zha″mē-lār′), psychosis occurring simultaneously in twins.

fo·lin·ic ac·id (fo-lin′ik) leucovorin; the 5-formyl derivative of tetrahydrofolic acid; it can act as a coenzyme carrier in certain folate-mediated reactions and is used, as the calcium salt leucovorin calcium, in the treatment of some disorders of folic acid deficiency.

fo·li·um (fo′le-um) pl. *fo′lia*. [L.] a leaflike structure, especially one of the leaflike subdivisions of the cerebellar cortex.

fol·li·cle (fol′ĭ-k′l) a sac or pouchlike depression or cavity. **follic′ular,** adj. **atretic ovarian f.,** an involuted ovarian follicle. **dominant ovarian f.,** the growing ovarian follicle in a given menstrual cycle that matures completely and forms the corpus luteum. **gastric f's,** lymphoid masses in the gastric mucosa. **graafian f's,** vesicular ovarian f's; maturing ovarian follicles among whose cells fluid has begun to accumulate, leading to the formation of a single cavity and leaving the oocyte located in the cumulus oophorus.

hair f., one of the tubular invaginations of the epidermis enclosing the hairs, and from which the hairs grow. **intestinal f's,** see under *gland*. **lingual f's,** nodular masses of lymphoid tissue at the root of the tongue, constituting the lingual tonsil. **lymph f., lymphatic f.,** 1. lymph node. 2. lymphatic nodule (2). **Naboth's f's, nabothian f's,** cystlike formations due to occlusion of the lumina of glands in the mucosa of the uterine cervix, causing them to be distended with retained secretion. **ovarian f.,** the oocyte and its encasing cells, at any stage in its development. **primary ovarian f's,** immature ovarian follicles, each comprising an immature oocyte and the specialized epithelial cells (follicle cells) surrounding it. **primordial ovarian f.,** an immature ovarian follicle that has not undergone recruitment and consists of an oocyte enclosed by a single layer of cells. **sebaceous f.,** a hair follicle with a relatively large sebaceous gland, producing a relatively insignificant hair. **solitary f's,** small lymph follicles scattered throughout the mucosa and submucosa of the small intestine. **thyroid f's,** discrete, cystlike units of the thyroid gland that are lined with cuboidal epithelium and are filled with a colloid substance, about 30 to each lobule. **vesicular ovarian f's,** graafian f's.

fol·lic·u·li (fah-lik′u-li) [L.] plural of *folliculus*.

fol·lic·u·li·tis (fah-lik″u-li′tis) inflammation of a follicle. **f. bar′bae,** sycosis vulgaris. **f. decal′vans,** suppurative folliculitis leading to scarring, with permanent hair loss on the involved area. **keloidal f., f. keloida′lis,** acne keloid. **f. ulerythemato′sa reticula′ta,** a condition in which numerous, closely crowded, small atrophic areas separated by narrow ridges appear on the face, the affected area being erythematous and the skin stretched and hard. **f. variolifor′mis,** see under *acne*.

fol·lic·u·lo·sis (fah-lik″u-lo′sis) excessive development of lymph follicles.

fol·lic·u·lus (fah-lik′u-lus) pl. *folli′culi*. [L.] follicle.

fol·li·tro·pin (fol′ĭ-tro″pin) follicle-stimulating hormone; *f. alfa* and *f. beta* are forms of follitropin produced by genetically modified hamster cells and used in the treatment of infertility.

fo·men·ta·tion (fo″men-ta′shun) treatment by warm moist applications; also, the substance thus applied.

fo·mes (fo′mēz) pl. *fo′mites*. [L.] an inanimate object or material on which disease-producing agents may be conveyed.

fo·mite (fo′mīt) fomes.

fo·mi·vir·sen (fo-miv′er-sin) an antiviral agent used as the sodium salt in the treatment of cytomegalovirus retinitis associated with AIDS.

Fon·se·caea (fon″se-se′ah) a genus of imperfect fungi. *F. compac′tum* and *F. pedro′soi* cause chromoblastomycosis.

fon·ta·nel (fon″tah-nel′) fontanelle.

fon·ta·nelle (fon″tah-nel′) a soft spot, such as one of the membrane-covered spaces remaining at the junction of the sutures in the incompletely ossified skull of the fetus or infant.

fon·tic·u·lus (fon-tik′u-lus) pl. *fontic′uli*. [L.] a fontanelle.

foot (foot) 1. the distal portion of the leg, upon which an individual stands and walks; in humans, the tarsus, metatarsus, phalanges, and the surrounding tissue. 2. something resembling this structure. 3. a unit of linear measure, 12 inches, equal to 0.3048 meter. **athlete's f.**, tinea pedis. **cleft f.**, a congenitally deformed foot in which the division between the third and fourth toes extends into the metatarsal region, often with ectrodactyly. **club f.**, see *talipes*. **dangle f.**, **drop f.**, footdrop. **flat f.**, flatfoot. **immersion f.**, a condition resembling trench foot occurring in persons who have spent long periods in water. **Madura f.**, mycetoma of the foot. **march f.**, painful swelling of the foot, usually with fracture of a metatarsal bone, after excessive foot strain. **pericapillary end f.**, **perivascular f.**, **sucker f.**, a terminal expansion of the cytoplasmic process of an astrocyte against the wall of a capillary in the central nervous system. **trench f.**, a condition of the feet resembling frostbite, due to the prolonged action of water on the skin combined with circulatory disturbance due to cold and inaction.

foot·drop (foot′drop) dropping of the foot from a peroneal or tibial nerve lesion that causes paralysis of the anterior muscles of the leg.

foot·plate (-plāt) the flat portion of the stapes, which is set into the oval window on the medial wall of the middle ear.

fo·ra·men (fo-ra′men) pl. *fora′mina*. [L.] a natural opening or passage, especially one into or through a bone. **aortic f.**, aortic hiatus. **apical f. of tooth**, an opening at or near the apex of the root of a tooth, giving passage to the vascular, lymphatic, and neural structures supplying the pulp. **auditory f., external**, external acoustic meatus. **auditory f., internal**, a passage for the auditory and facial nerves in the petrous bone. **f. of Bochdalek**, pleuroperitoneal hiatus. **cecal f., f. ce′cum**, 1. a blind opening between

the frontal crest and the crista galli. 2. a small triangular expansion at the lower border of the pons, formed by the termination of the anterior median fissure of the medulla oblongata. 3. a depression on the dorsum of the tongue at the median sulcus. **cotyloid f.**, a passage between the margin of the acetabulum and the transverse ligament. **epiploic f.**, an opening connecting the two sacs of the peritoneum, below and behind the porta hepatis. **esophageal f.**, see under *hiatus*. **ethmoidal foramina, fora′mina ethmoida′lia**, small openings in the ethmoid bone at the junction of the medial wall with the roof of the orbit, the *anterior* transmitting the nasal branch of the ophthalmic nerve and the anterior ethmoid vessels, and the *posterior* transmitting the posterior ethmoid vessels. **incisive f.**, one of the openings of the incisive canals into the incisive fossa of the hard palate. **infraorbital f.**, a passage for the infraorbital nerve and artery. **interventricular f.**, a communication between the lateral and third ventricles. **intervertebral f.**, a passage for a spinal nerve and vessels that is formed by notches on pedicles of adjacent vertebrae. **jugular f.**, an opening formed by the jugular notches on the temporal and occipital bones. **f. of Key and Retzius**, an opening at the end of each lateral recess of the fourth ventricle by which the ventricular cavity communicates with the subarachnoid space. **lacerate f., anterior**, an elongated cleft between the wings of the sphenoid bone, transmitting nerves and vessels. **lacerate f., middle**, f. lacerum. **lacerate f., posterior**, jugular f. **f. la′cerum**, a gap formed at the junction of the great wing of the sphenoid bone, tip of the petrous part of the temporal bone, and basilar part of the occipital bone. **f. of Magendie**, a deficiency in the lower part of the roof of the fourth ventricle through which the ventricular cavity communicates with the subarachnoid space. **f. mag′num**, a large opening in the anterior inferior part of the occipital bone, between the cranial cavity and vertebral canal. **mastoid f.**, an opening in the temporal bone behind the mastoid process. **medullary f.**, vertebral f. **nutrient f.**, any of the passages admitting nutrient vessels to the medullary cavity of bone. **obturator f.**, the large opening between the os pubis and ischium. **olfactory foramina**, any of the many openings of the cribriform plate of the ethmoid bone. **omental f.**, epiploic f. **optic f.**, 1. (of sclera) lamina cribrosa (3). 2. (of sphenoid bone) see under *canal*. **f. ova′le**, 1. a fetal opening between the heart's atria. 2. an aperture in the great wing of the sphenoid for vessels and nerves. **palatine f., greater,** the lower opening of the greater palatine canal, found laterally on the horizontal plate of each palatine bone, transmitting a palatine nerve and artery. **palatine foramina, lesser,** the openings of the lesser palatine canals behind the palatine crest and the greater palatine foramina. **pterygopalatine f.,** 1. greater palatine f. 2. sphenopalatine f. **quadrate f.,** f. venae cavae. **f. rotun′dum os′sis sphenoida′lis,** a round opening in the great wing of sphenoid for the maxillary branch of the trigeminal nerve. **Scarpa's f.,** an opening behind each upper medial incisor, for the nasopalatine nerve. **sciatic f.,** either of two foramina, the greater and the lesser sciatic foramina, formed by the sacrotuberal and sacrospinal ligaments in the sciatic notch of the hip bone. **sphenopalatine f.,** 1. a space between the orbital and sphenoidal processes of the palatine bone, opening into the nasal cavity, and transmitting the sphenopalatine artery and nasal nerves. 2. greater palatine f. **spinous f.,** a hole in the great wing of the sphenoid for the middle meningeal artery. **stylomastoid f.,** an opening between the styloid and mastoid processes for the facial nerve and the stylomastoid artery. **supraorbital f.,** a passage in the frontal bone for the supraorbital artery and nerve; often present as a notch bridged only by fibrous tissue. **thebesian foramina,** minute openings in the walls of the right atrium through which the smallest cardiac veins empty into the heart. **thyroid f.,** 1. an inconstant opening in the thyroid cartilage, due to incomplete union of the fourth and fifth branchial cartilages. 2. obturator f. **f. ve′nae ca′vae,** an opening in the diaphragm for the inferior vena cava and some branches of the right vagus nerve. **venous f.,** 1. f. venae cavae. 2. f. of Vesalius. **vertebral f.,** the large opening in a vertebra formed by its body and arch. **f. of Vesalius,** an occasional opening medial to the foramen ovale of the sphenoid, for passage of a vein from the cavernous sinus. **Weitbrecht's f.,** a foramen in the capsule of the shoulder joint. **f. of Winslow,** epiploic f. **zygomaticofacial f.,** the opening on the anterior surface of the zygomatic bone for the zygomaticofacial nerves and vessels. **zygomaticotemporal f.,** an opening on the temporal surface of the zygomatic bone.

fo·ram·i·na (fo-ram′ĭ-nah) plural of *foramen.*

force (fors) energy or power; that which originates or arrests motion. Symbol *F.* **electromotive f.,** that which causes a flow of electricity from one place to another, giving rise to an electric current. Abbreviated EMF. Symbol *E.* **occlusal f.,** the force exerted on opposing teeth when the jaws are brought into approximation. **reserve f.,** energy above that required for normal functioning; in the heart, the power that will take care of the additional circulatory burden imposed by exertion. **van der Waals f's,** the relatively weak, short-range forces of attraction existing between atoms and molecules and arising from brief shifts of orbital electrons; it results in the attraction of nonpolar organic compounds to each other. **vital f.,** the energy that characterizes a living organism; most systems of complementary medicine seek to affect or use it.

for·ceps (fōr′seps) [L.] 1. a two-bladed instrument with a handle for compressing or grasping tissues in surgical operations, and for handling sterile dressings, etc. 2. any forcipate organ or part. **alligator f.,** strong toothed forceps having a double clamp. **artery f.,** one for grasping and compressing an artery. **axis-traction f.,** specially jointed obstetrical forceps so made that traction can be applied in the line of the pelvic axis. **bayonet f.,** a forceps whose blades are offset from the axis of the handle. **Chamberlen f.,** the original form of obstetrical forceps. **clamp f.,** a forceps-like clamp with an automatic lock, for compressing arteries, etc. **dental f.,** one for the extraction of teeth. **dressing f.,** one with scissor-like handles for grasping lint, drainage tubes, etc., used in dressing wounds. **fixation f.,** one for holding a part steady during operation. **Kocher f.,** a strong forceps for holding tissues during operation or for compressing bleeding tissue. **Levret's f.,** an obstetrical forceps curved to correspond with the curve of the parturient canal. **Löwenberg's f.,** one for removing adenoid growth. **f. ma′jor,** the terminal fibers of the corpus callosum that pass from the splenium into the occipital lobes. **f. mi′nor,** the terminal fibers of the corpus callosum that pass from the genu to the frontal lobes. **mouse-tooth f.,** one with one or more fine teeth at the tip of each blade. **obstetrical f.,** one for extracting the fetal head from the maternal passages. **Péan f.,** a clamp for hemostasis. **rongeur f.,** one for use in cutting bone. **sequestrum f.,** one with small but strong serrated jaws for removing pieces of bone forming a sequestrum. **speculum f.,** a long, slender forceps for use through a speculum. **tenaculum f.,** one having a sharp hook at the end of each jaw. **torsion f.**, one for making torsion on an artery to arrest hemorrhage. **volsella f., vulsellum f.**, one with teeth for grasping and applying traction. **Willett f.**, a vulsellum for applying scalp traction to control hemorrhage in placenta previa.

for·ci·pate (fōr′sĭ-pāt) shaped like a forceps.

fore·arm (for′ahrm) antebrachium; the part of the arm between elbow and wrist.

fore·brain (-brān) prosencephalon.

fore·con·scious (-kon-shus) preconscious.

fore·fin·ger (-fing-ger) index finger; the second finger, counting the thumb as first.

fore·foot (-foot) 1. one of the front feet of a quadruped. 2. the fore part of the foot.

fore·gut (-gut) the endodermal canal of the embryo cephalic to the junction of the yolk stalk, giving rise to the pharynx, lung, esophagus, stomach, liver, and most of the small intestine.

fore·head (-hed) frons; the part of the face above the eyes.

for·eign (for′en) in immunology, pertaining to substances not recognized as "self" and capable of inducing an immune response.

fo·ren·sic (fah-ren′zik) pertaining to or applied in legal proceedings.

fore·play (for′pla) the sexually stimulating play preceding intercourse.

fore·skin (-skin) prepuce. **hooded f.**, absence of the ventral foreskin, usually associated with hypospadias.

fore·wa·ters (-waw-terz) the part of the amniotic sac that pouches into the uterine cervix in front of the presenting part of the fetus.

fork (fork) a pronged instrument. **replication f.**, a site on a DNA molecule at which unwinding of the helices and synthesis of daughter molecules are both occurring. **tuning f.**, a device that produces harmonic vibration when its two prongs are struck; used to test hearing and bone conduction.

for·mal·de·hyde (for-mal′dĭ-hīd) a gas formerly used as a strong disinfectant; now used as an aqueous solution (see *formaldehyde solution*, under *solution*). The gas is toxic by inhalation or absorption and is carcinogenic.

for·ma·lin (for′mah-lin) formaldehyde solution.

for·mam·i·dase (for-mam′ĭ-dās) 1. an enzyme that catalyzes the hydrolytic deamination of formamide to produce formate; it also acts on similar amides. 2. arylformamidase.

for·mate (for′māt) a salt of formic acid.

for·ma·tio (for-ma′she-o) pl. *formatio′nes*. [L.] formation.

for·ma·tion (for-ma′shun) 1. the process of giving shape or form; the creation of an entity,

or of a structure of definite shape. 2. a structure of definite shape. **reaction f.**, a defense mechanism in which a person adopts conscious attitudes, interests, or feelings that are the opposites of their unconscious feelings, impulses, or wishes. **reticular f.**, any of several diffuse networks of cells and fibers in the spinal cord and brainstem; subdivided into the reticular formations of the spinal cord, medulla oblongata, mesencephalon, and pons.

for·ma·tive (for′mah-tiv) concerned in the origination and development of an organism, part, or tissue.

forme (form) pl. *formes*. [Fr.] form. **f. fruste**, (froost) pl. *formes frustes*. An atypical, especially a mild or incomplete, form, as of a disease. **f. tardive** (tahr-dēv′), a late-occurring form of a disease that usually appears at an earlier age.

for·mic ac·id (for′mik) an acid from the distillation of ants and derivable from oxalic acid and glycerin and from the oxidation of formaldehyde; its actions resemble those of acetic acid but it is much more irritating, pungent, and caustic to the skin. The acid and its sodium and calcium salts are used as food preservatives.

for·mi·ca·tion (for″mĭ-ka′shun) a sensation as if small insects were crawling on the skin.

for·mim·i·no·glu·tam·ic ac·id (FIGLU) (for-mim″ĭ-no-gloo-tam′ik) an intermediate in the catabolic pathway from histidine to glutamate; it may be excreted in the urine in liver disease, vitamin B_{12} or folic acid deficiency, or in glutamic formiminotransferase deficiency.

for·mol (for′mol) formaldehyde solution.

for·mu·la (for′mu-lah) pl. *formulas, for′mulae*. [L.] an expression, using numbers or symbols, of the composition of, or of directions for preparing, a compound, such as a medicine, or of a procedure to follow to obtain a desired result, or of a single concept. **chemical f.**, a combination of symbols used to express the chemical composition of a substance. **dental f.**, an expression in symbols of the number and arrangement of teeth in the jaws. Letters represent the various types of teeth: I, *incisor*; C, *canine*; P, *premolar*; M, *molar*. Each letter is followed by a horizontal line. Numbers above the line represent maxillary teeth; those below, mandibular teeth. The human dental formula is $I\frac{2}{2}C\frac{1}{1}M\frac{2}{2} = 10$ (one side only) for deciduous teeth, and $I\frac{2}{2}C\frac{1}{1}P\frac{2}{2}M\frac{3}{3} = 16$ (one side only) for permanent teeth. **empirical f.**, a chemical formula which expresses the proportions of the elements present in a substance. **molecular f.,** a chemical formula expressing the number of atoms of each element present in a molecule of a substance, without indicating how they are linked. **spatial f., stereochemical f.,** a chemical formula giving the number of atoms of each element present in a molecule of a substance, which atom is linked to which, the type of linkages involved, and the relative positions of the atoms in space. **structural f.,** a chemical formula showing the number of atoms of each element in a molecule, their spatial arrangement, and their linkage to each other. **vertebral f.,** an expression of the number of vertebrae in each region of the spinal column; the human vertebral formula is C7 T12 L5 S5 Cd4 = 33.

for·mu·lary (for'mu-lar″e) a collection of recipes, formulas, and prescriptions. **National F.,** see under *N.*

for·mu·late (for'mu-lāt) 1. to state in the form of a formula. 2. to prepare in accordance with a prescribed or specified method.

for·mu·la·tion (for″mu-la'shun) the act or product of formulating. **American Law Institute F.,** a section of the American Law Institute's Model Penal Code which states that "a person is not responsible for criminal conduct if at the time of such conduct as a result of mental disease or defect he lacks substantial capacity either to appreciate the criminality [wrongfulness] of his conduct or to conform his conduct to the requirements of the law."

for·myl (for'mil) the radical, HCO—, of formic acid.

for·nix (for'niks) pl. *for'nices.* [L.] 1. an archlike structure or the vaultlike space created by such a structure. 2. fornix of brain; either of a pair of arched fiber tracts that unite under the corpus callosum, so that together they comprise two columns, a body, and two crura.

fos·car·net (fos-kahr'net) a virostatic agent used as the sodium salt in the treatment of cytomegalovirus retinitis and herpes simplex in immunocompromised patients.

fos·fo·my·cin (fos-fo-mi'sin) an antibacterial agent active against a wide range of gram-positive and gram-negative bacteria, used in the treatment of urinary tract infection; administered orally as the tromethamine salt.

fo·sin·o·pril (fo-sin'o-pril) an angiotensin-converting enzyme inhibitor administered orally as the sodium salt to treat hypertension and congestive heart failure.

fos·phen·y·to·in (fos'fen-ĭ-toin″) a prodrug of phenytoin used as the sodium salt in the treatment of epilepsy, excluding petit mal epilepsy.

fos·sa (fos'ah) pl. *fos'sae.* [L.] a trench or channel; in anatomy, a hollow or depressed area. **acetabular f.,** a nonarticular area in the floor of the acetabulum. **adipose fossae,** subcutaneous spaces in the female breast which contain fat. **axillary f.,** the small hollow underneath the arm where it joins the body at the shoulder. **canine f.,** a depression on the external surface of the maxilla superolateral to the canine tooth socket. **condylar f.,** either of two pits on the lateral part of the occipital bone. **coronoid f. of humerus,** a depression in the humerus for the coronoid process of the ulna. **cranial f.,** any one of three hollows (anterior, middle, and posterior) in the base of the cranium for the lobes of the brain. **digastric f.,** 1. a depression on the inner surface of the mandible, giving attachment to the anterior belly of the digastric muscle. 2. mastoid notch. **digital f.,** 1. trochanteric f. 2. femoral ring. 3. the depression on the inside of the anterior abdominal wall lateral to the lateral umbilical fold. **duodenojejunal f.,** either of two peritoneal pockets, one behind the inferior and the other behind the superior duodenal fold. **epigastric f.,** 1. a fossa in the epigastric region. 2. epigastrium. 3. urachal f. **ethmoid f.,** the groove in the cribriform plate of the ethmoid bones, for the olfactory bulb. **hyaloid f.,** a depression in the front of the vitreous body, lodging the lens. **hypophysial f.,** a depression in the sphenoid, lodging the pituitary gland. **iliac f.,** a concave area occupying much of the inner surface of the ala of the ilium, especially anteriorly; from it arises the iliac muscle. **incisive f. of maxilla,** a slight depression on the anterior surface of the maxilla above the incisor teeth. **infraspinous f.,** the large, slightly concave area below the spinous process on the dorsal surface of the scapula. **infratemporal f.,** an irregularly shaped cavity medial or deep to the zygomatic arch. **ischioanal f., ischiorectal f.,** a potential space between the pelvic diaphragm and the skin below it; an anterior recess extends a variable distance between the pelvic and urogenital diaphragms. **Jobert's f.,** a fossa in the popliteal region bounded by the adductor magnus and the gracilis and sartorius muscles. **lacrimal f.,** a shallow depression in the roof of the orbit, lodging the lacrimal gland. **lateral cerebral f.,** sylvian fossa; in the fetus, a depression on the lateral surface of each cerebral hemisphere; it becomes the sylvian fissure and its floor becomes the insula. **mandibular f.,** a depression in the temporal bone in which the condyle of the mandible rests. **mastoid f.,** a small triangular area between the posterior wall of the external acoustic meatus and the posterior root of the zygomatic process of the temporal bone. **nasal f.,** the portion of the nasal cavity anterior to the middle meatus. **navicular f.,** 1. the vaginal vestibule between the vaginal orifice and the frenulum of the pudendal labia. 2. the lateral expansion of the urethra of the glans penis. 3. a depression on the internal pterygoid process of the sphenoid, giving attachment to the tensor veli palatini muscle. **f. ova'lis cor'dis,** a fossa in the right atrium of the heart; the remains of the fetal foramen ovale. **ovarian f.,** a shallow pouch on the posterior surface of the broad ligament, in which the ovary is located. **popliteal f.,** the depression in the posterior region of the knee. **rhomboid f.,** the floor of the fourth ventricle, made up of the dorsal surfaces of the medulla oblongata and pons. **Rosenmül-ler's f.,** pharyngeal recess. **subarcuate f. of temporal bone,** a depression in the posterior inner surface of the petrous portion of the temporal bone. **subsigmoid f.,** a fossa between the mesentery of the sigmoid flexure and that of the descending colon. **supraspi-nous f.,** a depression above the spine of the scapula. **sylvian f.,** 1. lateral cerebral f. 2. fissure of Sylvius. **tibiofemoral f.,** a space between the articular surfaces of the tibia and femur mesial or lateral to the inferior pole of the patella. **trochanteric f.,** a depression on the medial surface of the greater trochan-ter, receiving the tendon of the obturator externus muscle. **urachal f.,** one on the inner abdominal wall, between the urachus and the hypogastric artery. **Waldeyer's f.,** the two duodenal fossae regarded as one. **zygomatic f.,** infratemporal f.

fos·sette (fŏ-set') [Fr.] 1. a small depression. 2. a small, deep, corneal ulcer.

fos·su·la (fos'u-lah) pl. *fos'sulae.* [L.] a small fossa.

foun·da·tion (foun-da'shun) the structure or basis on which something is built. **den-ture f.,** the portion of the structures and tissues of the mouth available to support a denture.

four·chette (foor-shet') [Fr.] frenulum of pudendal labia.

fo·vea (fo've-ah) pl. *fo'veae.* [L.] a small pit or depression. Often used alone to indicate the central fovea of the retina. **central f. of retina,** a small pit in the center of the macula lutea, the area of clearest vision, where the retinal layers are spread aside, and light falls directly on the cones. **submandibular**

f., a depression on the medial aspect of the mandible, lodging part of the submandibular gland.

fo·ve·a·tion (fo"ve-a'shun) formation of pits on a surface as on the skin; a pitted condition.

fo·ve·o·la (fo-ve'o-lah) pl. *fove'olae.* [L.] a minute pit or depression.

Fr francium.

frac·tion (frak'shun) 1. a portion of some-thing larger. 2. in chemistry, one of the separable constituents of a substance. **frac'-tional,** adj. **ejection f.,** the proportion of the volume of blood in the ventricles at the end of diastole that is ejected during systole; it is the stroke volume divided by the end-diastolic volume, often expressed as a percen-tage. It is normally 65 ± 8 per cent; lower values indicate ventricular dysfunction. **plasma protein f.,** a preparation of serum albumin and globulin obtained by fractionat-ing source blood, plasma, or serum from healthy human donors; used as a blood volume supporter.

frac·tion·a·tion (frak"shun-a'shun) 1. in radiology, division of the total dose of radiation into small doses administered at intervals. 2. in chemistry, separation of a substance into components, as by distillation or crystallization. 3. in histology, isolation of components of living cells by differential centrifugation.

frac·ture (frak'cher) 1. the breaking of a part, especially a bone. 2. a break or rupture in a bone. **avulsion f.,** separation of a small fragment of bone cortex at the site of attach-ment of a ligament or tendon. **axial com-pression f.,** fracture of a vertebra by excessive vertical force so that pieces of it move out in horizontal directions. **Barton's f.,** frac-ture of the distal end of the radius into the wrist joint. **Bennett's f.,** fracture of the base of the first metacarpal bone running into the carpometacarpal joint, complicated by subluxation. **blow-out f.,** fracture of the orbital floor caused by a sudden increase of intraorbital pressure due to traumatic force; the orbital contents herniate into the maxillary sinus so that the inferior rectus or inferior oblique muscle may become incar-cerated in the fracture site, producing diplopia on looking up. **burst f.,** axial compression f. **capillary f.,** one that appears on a radiogram as a fine, hairlike line, the segments of bone not being separated; sometimes seen in fractures of the skull. **closed f.,** one that does not produce an open wound in the skin; cf. *open f.* **Colles' f.,** fracture of the lower end of the radius, the lower fragment being displaced backward; if the lower fragment is displaced forward, it is a *reverse Colles' fracture.* **comminuted f.,** one in which the bone is splintered or crushed. **complete f.,** one involving the entire cross section of the bone. **compound f.,** open f. **depressed f., depressed skull f.,** fracture of the skull in which a fragment is depressed. **de Quervain's f.,** fracture of the navicular bone together with a volar luxation of the lunate bone. **direct f.,** one at the site of injury. **dislocation f.,** fracture of a bone near an articulation with concomitant dislocation of that joint. **Dupuytren's f.,** Pott's f. **Duverney's f.,** fracture of the ilium just below the anterior inferior spine. **fissure f.,** a crack extending from a surface into, but not through, a long bone. **freeze f.,** see *freeze-fracturing.* **greenstick f.,** one in which one side of a bone is broken, the other being bent. **hangman's f.,** fracture through the pedicles of the axis (C2) with or without subluxation of the second cervical vertebra or the third. **impacted f.,** one in which one fragment is firmly driven into the other. **incomplete f.,** one which does not entirely destroy the continuity of the bone. **insufficiency f.,** a stress fracture that occurs during normal stress on a bone of abnormally decreased density. **intrauterine f.,** fracture of a fetal bone incurred *in utero.* **Jefferson's f.,** fracture of the atlas (first cervical vertebra). **lead pipe f.,** one in which the bone cortex is slightly compressed and bulged on one side with a slight crack on the other side of the bone. **Le Fort f.,** bilateral horizontal fracture of the maxilla. Le Fort fractures are classified as follows: *Le Fort I f.,* a horizontal segmented fracture of the alveolar process of the maxilla, in which the teeth are usually contained in the detached portion of the bone. *Le Fort II f.,* unilateral or bilateral fracture of the maxilla, in which the body of the maxilla is separated from the facial skeleton and the separated portion is pyramidal in shape; the fracture may extend through the body of the maxilla down the midline of the hard palate, through the floor of the orbit, and into the nasal cavity. *Le Fort III f.,* a fracture in which the entire maxilla and one or more facial bones are completely separated from the craniofacial skelton; such fractures are almost always accompanied by multiple fractures of the facial bones. **Monteggia's f.,** one in the proximal half of the shaft of the ulna, with dislocation of the head of the radius. **open f.,** one in which a wound through the adjacent or overlying soft tissues communicates with the site of the break. **parry f.,** Monteggia's f. **pathologic f.,** one

due to weakening of the bone structure by pathologic processes, such as neoplasia, osteomalacia, or osteomyelitis. **ping-pong f.,** a type of depressed skull fracture usually seen in young children, resembling the indentation that can be produced with the finger in a ping-pong ball; when elevated it resumes and retains its normal position. **Pott's f.,** fracture of the lower part of the fibula, with serious injury of the lower tibial articulation, usually a chipping off of a portion of the medial malleolus, or rupture of the medial ligament. **pyramidal f. (of maxilla),** Le Fort II f. **sagittal slice f.,** fracture of a vertebra breaking it in an oblong direction; the spinal column above is displaced horizontally, usually causing paraplegia. **silver fork f.,** Colles' f. **simple f.,** closed f. **Smith's f.,** reverse Colles' f. **spiral f.,** one in which the bone has been twisted apart. **spontaneous f.,** pathologic f. **sprain f.,** the separation of a tendon from its insertion, taking with it a piece of bone. **Stieda's f.,** fracture of the internal condyle of the femur. **stress f.,** that caused by unusual or repeated stress on a bone. **transverse facial f.,** Le Fort III f. **transverse maxillary f.,** a term sometimes used for horizontal maxillary fracture (Le Fort I f.). **trophic f.,** one due to nutritional (trophic) disturbance. **wedge-compression f.,** compression fracture of only the anterior part of a vertebra, leaving it wedge-shaped.

fra·gil·i·tas (frah-jil′ĭ-tas) [L.] fragility. **f. cri′nium,** a brittleness of the hair. **f. os′sium,** osteogenesis imperfecta. **f. un′guium,** abnormal brittleness of the nails.

fra·gil·i·ty (frah-jil′it-e) susceptibility, or lack of resistance, to influences capable of causing disruption of continuity or integrity. **f. of blood,** erythrocyte f. **capillary f.,** abnormal susceptibility of capillary walls to rupture. **erythrocyte f.,** susceptibility of erythrocytes to hemolysis under certain conditions. **mechanical f.,** susceptibility of certain erythrocytes to hemolysis under mechanical stress. **osmotic f.,** susceptibility of certain erythrocytes to hemolysis in increasingly hypotonic saline solutions.

frag·men·tog·ra·phy, mass (frag″men-tog′rah-fe) an instrumental method in which samples are separated by gas chromatography and the components are identified by mass spectrometry.

fram·be·sia (fram-be′zhah) yaws. **f. tro′pica,** yaws.

fram·be·si·o·ma (fram-be″ze-o′mah) mother yaw.

frame (frām) a rigid structure for giving support to or for immobilizing a part.

Balkan f., an apparatus for continuous extension in treatment of fractures of the femur, consisting of an overhead bar, with pulleys attached, by which the leg is supported in a sling. **Bradford f.,** a canvas-covered, rectangular frame of pipe; used as a bed frame in disease of the spine or thigh. **quadriplegic standing f.,** a device for supporting in the upright position a patient whose four limbs are paralyzed. **Stryker f.,** one consisting of canvas stretched on anterior and posterior frames, on which the patient can be rotated around their longitudinal axis. **trial f.,** an eyeglass frame designed to permit insertion of different lenses used in correcting refractive errors of vision.

Fran·ci·sel·la (fran″sĭ-sel′ah) a genus of microorganisms, including *F. (Pasteurella) tularen′sis,* the etiologic agent of tularemia.

fran·ci·um (Fr) (fran′se-um) chemical element (see *Table of Elements*), at. no. 87.

fra·ter·nal (frah-ter′n'l) 1. of or pertaining to brothers. 2. of twins; derived from two oocytes.

FRCP Fellow of the Royal College of Physicians.

FRCS Fellow of the Royal College of Surgeons.

freck·le (frek′l) a pigmented spot on the skin due to accumulation of melanin resulting from exposure to sunlight. **melanotic f. of Hutchinson,** lentigo maligna.

freeze-dry·ing (frēz-dri′ing) a method of tissue preparation in which the tissue specimen is frozen and then dehydrated at low temperature in a high vacuum.

freeze-etch·ing (-ech′ing) a method used to study unfixed cells by electron microscopy, in which the object to be studied is placed in 20 per cent glycerol, frozen at −100°C, and then mounted on a chilled holder.

freeze-frac·tur·ing (-frak′cher-ing) a method of preparing cells for electron-microscopical examination: a tissue specimen is frozen at −150°C, inserted into a vacuum chamber, and fractured by a microtome; a platinum carbon replica of the exposed surfaces is made, freed of the underlying specimen, and then examined.

freeze-sub·sti·tu·tion (-sub-stĭ-too′shun) a modification of freeze-drying in which the ice within the frozen tissue is replaced by alcohol or other solvents at a very low temperature.

frem·i·tus (frem′it-us) a vibration felt on palpation. **friction f.,** rub. **hydatid f.,** see under *thrill.* **rhonchal f.,** vibrations produced by passage of air through a large mucus-filled bronchus. **tactile f.,** vocal

fremitus felt on the chest wall. **tussive f.,** one felt on the chest when the patient coughs. **vocal f. (VF),** one caused by speaking, perceived on auscultation.

fre·no·plas·ty (fre′no-plas″te) the correction of an abnormally attached frenum by surgically repositioning it.

fren·u·lum (fren′u-lum) pl. *fren′ula.* [L.] a small fold of integument or mucous membrane that limits the movements of an organ or part. **f. of clitoris,** a fold formed by union of the labia minora with the clitoris. **f. of ileocecal valve,** a fold formed by the joined extremities of the ileocecal valve, partially encircling the lumen of the colon. **f. of lip,** a median fold of mucous membrane connecting the inside of each lip to the corresponding gum. **f. of prepuce of penis,** the fold under the penis connecting it with the prepuce. **f. of pudendal labia, f. puden′di,** the posterior union of the labia minora, anterior to the posterior commissure. **f. of superior medullary velum,** a band lying in the medullary velum at its attachment to the inferior colliculi. **f. of tongue,** the vertical fold of mucous membrane under the tongue, attaching it to the floor of the mouth. **f. ve′li,** f. of superior medullary velum.

fre·num (fre′num) pl. *fre′na.* [L.] a restraining structure or part; see *frenulum.* **fre′nal,** adj.

fre·quen·cy (fre′kwen-se) 1. the number of occurrences of a periodic process in a unit of time. Symbol v. 2. in statistics, the number of occurrences of a determinable entity per unit of time or of population. Symbol f. **urinary f.,** urination at short intervals without increase in daily volume or urinary output, due to reduced bladder capacity.

freud·i·an (froi′de-in) 1. pertaining to Sigmund Freud, the founder of psychoanalysis, or his psychological theories and method of psychotherapy (psychoanalytic theory and technique). 2. an adherent or user of freudian theory or methods.

fri·a·ble (fri′ah-b'l) easily pulverized or crumbled.

fric·tion (frik′shun) 1. the act of rubbing. 2. massage using a circular or back-and-forth rubbing movement, used especially for massage of deep tissues.

fri·gid·i·ty (frĭ-jid′ĭ-te) 1. coldness. 2. former name for *female sexual arousal disorder.*

frigo·la·bile (frig″o-la′bĭl) easily affected or destroyed by cold.

frigo·sta·ble (-sta′b'l) resistant to cold or low temperatures.

frit (frit) imperfectly fused material used as a basis for making glass and in the formation of porcelain teeth.

frole·ment (frōl-maw') [Fr.] a rustling sound often heard on auscultation in pericardial disease.

frons (fronz) [L.] forehead.

fron·tad (frun'tad) toward a front, or frontal aspect.

fron·tal (frun't'l) 1. pertaining to the forehead. 2. denoting a longitudinal plane of the body.

fron·ta·lis (frun-ta'lis) [L.] frontal.

fron·to·max·il·lary (frun″to-mak'sǐ-lar″e) pertaining to the frontal bone and maxilla.

fron·to·tem·por·al (-tem'por-al) pertaining to the frontal and temporal bones.

frost (frost) 1. frozen dew or vapor. 2. a deposit resembling this. **urea f.,** the appearance on the skin of salt crystals left by evaporation of the sweat in urhidrosis.

frost·bite (frost'bīt″) injury to tissues due to exposure to cold.

frot·tage (fro-tahzh') [Fr.] frotteurism.

frot·teur (fro-toor') one who practices frotteurism.

frot·teur·ism (frŏ-toor'izm) a paraphilia in which sexual arousal or orgasm is achieved by actual or fantasized rubbing up against another person, usually in a crowded place with an unsuspecting victim.

fro·zen (fro'zen) 1. turned into, covered by, or surrounded by ice. 2. very cold. 3. stiff or immobile, or rendered immobile.

fruc·to·fu·ra·nose (frook″to-fu'rah-nōs) the combining and more reactive form of fructose.

fruc·to·ki·nase (-ki'nās) an enzyme of the liver, intestine, and kidney cortex that catalyzes the transfer of a phosphate group from ATP to fructose as the initial step in its utilization. Deficiency causes essential fructosuria.

fruc·tose (frook'tōs) a sugar, $C_6H_{12}O_6$, found in honey and many sweet fruits; used as a fluid and nutrient replenisher.

fruc·tose-1,6-bis·phos·pha·tase (bis-fos'fah-tās) an enzyme catalyzing part of the route of gluconeogenesis in the liver and kidneys; deficiency causes apnea, hyperventilation, hypoglycemia, ketosis, and lactic acidosis and can be fatal in the neonatal period.

fruc·to·se·mia (frook″to-se'me-ah) the presence of fructose in the blood, as in hereditary fructose intolerance and essential fructosuria.

fruc·to·side (frook'to-sīd) a glycoside of fructose.

fruc·to·su·ria (frook″to-su're-ah) the presence of fructose in the urine. **essential f.,** a benign hereditary disorder of carbohydrate metabolism due to a defect in fructokinase and manifested only by fructose in the blood and urine.

fruc·to·syl (frook'to-sil) a radical of fructose.

FSF fibrin-stabilizing factor (coagulation factor XIII).

FSH follicle-stimulating hormone.

FSH/LH-RH follicle-stimulating hormone and luteinizing hormone–releasing hormone.

FSH-RH follicle-stimulating hormone–releasing hormone.

5-FU 5-fluorouracil; see *fluorouracil*.

fuch·sin (fūk'sin) any of several red to purple dyes, sometimes specifically *basic f.* **acid f.,** a mixture of sulfonated fuchsins; used in various complex stains. **basic f.,** a histologic stain, containing predominantly pararosaniline and rosaniline.

fuch·sin·o·phil·ia (fūk″sin-o-fil'e-ah) the property of staining readily with fuchsin dyes. **fuchsinophil'ic,** adj.

fu·cose (fu'kōs) a monosaccharide occurring as L-fucose in a number of oligo- and polysaccharides and fucosides and in the carbohydrate portion of some mucopolysaccharides and glycoproteins, including the A, B, and O blood group antigens.

α-L-fu·co·si·dase (fu-ko'sǐ-dās) an enzyme that catalyzes the hydrolysis of fucose residues from fucosides; deficiency results in fucosidosis.

fu·co·si·do·sis (fu″ko-sǐ-do'sis) a lysosomal storage disease caused by deficient enzymatic activity of fucosidase and accumulation of fucose-containing glycoconjugates in all tissues; it is marked by progressive psychomotor deterioration, growth retardation, hepatosplenomegaly, cardiomegaly, and seizures.

FUDR, FUdR floxuridine.

fu·gac·i·ty (fu-gas'it-e) a measure of the escaping tendency of a substance from one phase to another phase, or from one part of a phase to another part of the same phase.

-fugal word element [L.], *driving away; fleeing from; repelling.*

fugue (fūg) a pathological state of altered consciousness in which an individual may act and wander around as though conscious but their behavior is not directed by their complete normal personality and is not remembered after the fugue ends. **dissociative f., psychogenic f.,** a dissociative disorder characterized by an episode of sudden, unexpected travel away from home or business, with amnesia for the past and partial to total confusion about identity or assumption of a new identity.

ful·gu·rate (ful′gūr-āt) 1. to come and go like a flash of lightning. 2. to destroy by contact with electric sparks generated by a high-frequency current.

ful·mi·nate (ful′mǐ-nāt) to occur suddenly with great intensity. **ful′minant,** adj.

fu·ma·rase (fu′mah-rās) an enzyme that catalyzes the interconversion of fumarate and malate.

fu·ma·rate (fu′mah-rāt) a salt of fumaric acid.

fu·mar·ic ac·id (fu-mar′ik) an unsaturated dibasic acid, the *trans* isomer of maleic acid and an intermediate in the tricarboxylic acid cycle.

fu·mi·ga·tion (fu″mǐ-ga′shun) exposure to disinfecting fumes.

fum·ing (fūm′ing) emitting a visible vapor.

func·tio (funk′she-o) [L.] function. **f. lae′sa,** loss of function; one of the cardinal signs of inflammation.

func·tion (funk′shun) 1. the special, normal, or proper physiologic activity of an organ or part. 2. to perform such activity. 3. in mathematics, a rule that assigns to each member of one set (the domain) a value in another set (the range).

func·tion·al (funk′shun-al) 1. pertaining to a function. 2. affecting the function but not the structure.

fun·di·form (fun′dǐ-form) shaped like a loop or sling.

fun·do·pli·ca·tion (fun″do-plǐ-ka′shun) mobilization of the lower end of the esophagus and plication of the fundus of the stomach up around it.

fun·dus (fun′dus) pl. *fun′di.* [L.] the bottom or base of anything; the bottom or base of an organ, or the part of a hollow organ farthest from its mouth. **fun′dal, fun′dic,** adj. **f. of eye,** the back portion of the interior of the eyeball, visible through the pupil by use of the ophthalmoscope. **f. of gallbladder,** the inferior, dilated portion of the gallbladder. **f. of stomach,** the part of the stomach to the left and above the level of the opening of the esophagus. **f. tym′pani,** the floor of the tympanic cavity. **f. of urinary bladder,** the base or posterior surface of the urinary bladder. **f. of uterus,** the part of the uterus above the orifices of the uterine tubes.

fun·du·scope (fun′dah-skōp) ophthalmoscope. **funduscop′ic,** adj.

fun·gal (fun′g′l) fungous; pertaining to fungi.

fun·gate (fun′gāt) 1. to produce funguslike growths. 2. to grow rapidly, like a fungus.

Fun·gi (fun′ji) [L.] a kingdom of eukaryotic, heterotrophic organisms that live as saprobes or parasites, including mushrooms, yeasts, and molds; they have rigid cell walls but lack chlorophyll.

fun·gi (fun′ji) [L.] plural of *fungus.*

fun·gi·cide (fun′jǐ-sīd) an agent that destroys fungi. **fungici′dal,** adj.

fun·gi·form (-form) shaped like a fungus.

fun·gi·sta·sis (fun″jǐ-sta′sis) inhibition of the growth of fungi. **fungistat′ic,** adj.

fun·gi·stat (fun′jǐ-stat) an agent that inhibits the growth of fungi.

fun·gi·tox·ic (-tok″sik) exerting a toxic effect upon fungi.

fun·goid (fun′goid) resembling a fungus.

fun·go·ma (fun-go′mah) fungus ball.

fun·gous (fun′gus) 1. fungal. 2. fungoid.

fun·gus pl. *fun′gi.* [L.] 1. any organism belonging to the Fungi. 2. anything resembling such an organism. **dimorphic f.,** one that lives as a yeast or mold, depending on environmental conditions. **imperfect f.,** one whose perfect (sexual) stage is unknown. **perfect f.,** one for which both sexual and asexual types of spore formation are known. **true fungi,** Eumycota.

fu·nic (fu′nik) pertaining to a funis or to a funiculus.

fu·ni·cle (fu′nǐ-k′l) funiculus.

fu·nic·u·li·tis (fu-nik″u-li′tis) 1. inflammation of the spermatic cord. 2. inflammation of that portion of a spinal nerve root lying within the intervertebral canal.

fu·nic·u·lo·ep·i·did·y·mi·tis (fu-nik″u-lo-ep″ǐ-did″ǐ-mi′tis) inflammation of the spermatic cord and the epididymis.

fu·nic·u·lus (fu-nik′u-lus) pl. *funic′uli.* [L.] a cord; a cordlike structure or part. **funic′ular,** adj. **anterior f. of spinal cord,** the white substance of the spinal cord lying on either side between the anterior median fissure and the ventral root. **lateral f.,** 1. the white substance of the spinal cord lying on either side between the dorsal and ventral roots. 2. the continuation into the medulla oblongata of all the fiber tracts of the lateral funiculus of the spinal cord with exception of the lateral pyramidal tract. **posterior f. of spinal cord,** the white substance of the spinal cord lying on either side between the posterior median sulcus and the dorsal root. **f. sperma′ticus,** spermatic cord.

fu·ni·form (fu′nǐ-form) resembling a rope or cord.

fu·nis (fu′nis) any cordlike structure, particularly the umbilical cord. **fu′nic,** adj.

FUO fever of unknown origin.

fu·ra·nose (fu′rah-nōs) any sugar containing the four-carbon furan ring structure; it is a cyclic form that ketoses and aldoses may take in solution.

fu·ra·zol·i·done (fū″rah-zol′ĭ-dōn) an antibacterial and antiprotozoal effective against many gram-negative enteric organisms; used in the treatment of diarrhea and enteritis.

fur·cal (fur′k'l) shaped like a fork; forked.

fur·ca·tion (fur-ka′shun) the anatomical area of a multirooted tooth where the roots divide.

fur·fu·ra·ceous (fur″fu-ra′shus) fine and loose; said of scales resembling bran or dandruff.

fur·fu·ral (fur′fu-ral) an aromatic compound from the distillation of bran, sawdust, etc., which irritates mucous membranes and causes photosensitivity and headaches.

fu·ror (fu′ror) fury; rage. **f. epilep′ticus,** an attack of intense anger occurring in epilepsy.

fu·ro·sem·ide (fu-ro′sĕ-mīd) a loop diuretic used in the treatment of edema and hypertension.

fur·row (fur′o) a groove or sulcus. **atrioventricular f.,** the transverse groove marking off the atria of the heart from the ventricles. **digital f.,** any one of the transverse folds across the joints on the palmar surface of a finger. **genital f.,** a groove that appears on the genital tubercle of the fetus at the end of the second month. **mentolabial f.,** the hollow just above the chin. **nympholabial f.,** a groove separating the labium majus and labium minus on each side. **scleral f.,** see under *sulcus.*

fu·run·cle (fu′rung-k'l) a boil; a painful nodule formed in the skin by circumscribed inflammation of the dermis and subcutaneous tissue, enclosing a central slough or "core"; due to staphylococci entering the skin through hair follicles. **furun′cular,** adj.

fu·run·cu·lo·sis (fu-rung″ku-lo′sis) 1. the persistent sequential occurrence of furuncles over a period of weeks or months. 2. the simultaneous occurrence of a number of furuncles.

fu·run·cu·lus (fu-rung′ku-lus) pl. *furun′culi.* [L.] furuncle.

fus·cin (fu′sin) a brown pigment of the retinal epithelium.

fu·si·ble (fu′zĭ-b'l) capable of being melted.

fu·si·form (-form) shaped like a spindle; tapered at each end.

fu·si·mo·tor (fu″sĭ-mōt′er) innervating intrafusal fibers of the muscle spindle; said of motor nerve fibers of gamma motoneurons.

fu·sion (fu′zhun) 1. the act or process of melting. 2. the merging or coherence of adjacent parts or bodies. 3. the coordination of separate images of the same object in the two eyes into one. 4. the operative formation of an ankylosis or arthrosis. **anterior interbody f.,** spinal fusion in the lumbar region using a retroperitoneal approach, with immobilization by bone grafts on the anterior and lateral surfaces. **diaphyseal-epiphyseal f.,** operative establishment of bony union between the epiphysis and diaphysis of a bone. **spinal f.,** operative immobilization or ankylosis of two or more vertebrae, often with diskectomy or laminectomy.

Fu·so·bac·te·ri·um (fu″zo-bak-tēr′e-um) a genus of anaerobic gram-negative bacteria found as normal flora in the mouth and large bowel, and often in necrotic tissue, probably as secondary invaders. *F. necroph′orum* is found in abscesses of the liver, lungs, and other tissues and in chronic ulcer of the colon.

fu·so·bac·te·ri·um pl. *fusobacte′ria.* 1. A rod-shaped bacterium in which the cell is thicker in the center and tapers toward the ends. 2. an organism of the genus *Fusobacterium.*

fu·so·cel·lu·lar (-sel′u-ler) having spindle-shaped cells.

fu·so·spi·ril·lo·sis (-spi″ril-o′sis) necrotizing ulcerative gingivitis.

fu·so·spi·ro·che·tal (-spi″ro-ke′t'l) pertaining to or caused by fusobacteria and spirochetes.

fu·so·spi·ro·che·to·sis (-spi″ro-ke-to′sis) infection with fusobacteria and spirochetes.

FVC forced vital capacity.

G

G gauss; giga-; glycine; gravida; guanidine or guanosine.

G conductance; Gibbs free energy.

g gram.

g standard gravity.

γ (gamma, the third letter of the Greek alphabet) the heavy chain of IgG; the γ chain of fetal hemoglobin; formerly, microgram.

γ- a prefix designating (1) the position of a substituting atom or group in a chemical compound; (2) a plasma protein migrating with the γ band in electrophoresis; (3) third in a series of three or more related entities or chemical compounds.

Ga gallium.

GABA γ-aminobutyric acid.

GABA·er·gic (gab″ah-er′jik) transmitting or secreting γ-aminobutyric acid.

gab·a·pen·tin (-pen′tin) an anticonvulsant related to γ-aminobutyric acid (GABA), used in the treatment of partial seizures.

GAD generalized anxiety disorder.

gad·o·lin·i·um (Gd) (gad″o-lin′e-um) chemical element (see *Table of Elements*), at. no. 64. **g. 153,** an artificial isotope of gadolinium with a half-life of 241.6 days, used in dual photon absorptiometry.

gad·o·pen·te·tate di·meg·lu·mine (gad″-o-pen′tĕ-tāt di-meg′loo-mēn) a paramagnetic agent used as a contrast agent in magnetic resonance imaging of intracranial, spinal, and associated lesions.

gag (gag) 1. a surgical device for holding the mouth open. 2. to retch, or to strive to vomit.

gain (gān) to acquire, obtain, or increase. **antigen g.,** the acquisition by cells of new antigenic determinants not normally present or not normally accessible in the parent tissue. **primary g.,** the direct alleviation of anxiety by a defense mechanism; the relief from emotional conflict or tension provided by neurotic symptoms or illness. **secondary g.,** external and incidental advantage derived from an illness, such as rest, gifts, personal attention, release from responsibility, and disability benefits.

gait (gāt) the manner or style of walking. **antalgic g.,** a limp adopted so as to avoid pain on weight-bearing structures, characterized by a very short stance phase. **ataxic g.,** an unsteady, uncoordinated walk, employing a wide base and the feet thrown out. **festinating g.,** a gait in which the patient involuntarily moves with short, accelerating steps, often on tiptoe, as in parkinsonism. **helicopod g.,** a gait in which the feet describe half circles, as in some conversion disorders. **hip extensor g.,** a gait in which the heel strike is followed by throwing forward of the hip and throwing backward of the trunk and pelvis. **myopathic g.,** exaggerated alternation of lateral trunk movements with an exaggerated elevation of the hip. **paraplegic spastic g.,** spastic g. **quadriceps g.,** a gait in which at each step on the affected leg the knee hyperextends and the trunk lurches forward. **spastic g.,** a gait in which the legs are held together and move in a stiff manner, the toes seeming to drag and catch. **step-page g.,** a gait in footdrop in which the advancing leg is lifted high so that the toes can clear the ground. **stuttering g.,** one characterized by hesitancy that resembles stuttering. **tabetic g.,** an ataxic gait that accompanies tabes dorsalis. **waddling g.,** myopathic gait.

ga·lac·ta·cra·sia (gah-lak″tah-kra′zhah) abnormal condition of the breast milk.

ga·lac·ta·gogue (gah-lak′tah-gog) promoting milk flow; an agent that so acts.

ga·lac·tan (gah-lak′tan) any polymer composed of galactose residues and occurring in plants.

gal·ac·tis·chia (gal″ak-tis′ke-ah) suppression of lactation.

galact(o)- word element [Gr.], *milk.*

ga·lac·to·cele (gah-lak′to-sēl) a milk-containing, cystic enlargement of the mammary gland.

ga·lac·to·ce·re·bro·side (gah-lak″to-sĕ-re′bro-sīd) any of the cerebrosides in which the head group is galactose; they are abundant in the cell membranes of nervous tissue.

gal·ac·tog·ra·phy (gal″ak-tog′rah-fe) radiography of the mammary ducts after injection of a radiopaque substance into the duct system.

ga·lac·to·ki·nase (gah-lak″to-ki′nās) an enzyme that catalyzes the transfer of a high-energy phosphate group from a donor to D-galactose, the initial step of galactose utilization. Absence of enzyme activity results in galactokinase deficiency galactosemia.

gal·ac·toph·ly·sis (gal″ak-tof′lĭ-sis) a vesicular eruption containing milky fluid.

ga·lac·to·phore (gah-lak′to-for) 1. galactophorous. 2. a milk duct.

gal·ac·toph·o·rous (gal″ak-tof′ah-rus) lactiferous.

ga·lac·to·pla·nia (gah-lak″to-pla′ne-ah) secretion of milk in some abnormal part.

ga·lac·to·poi·et·ic (-poi-et′ik) 1. pertaining to, marked by, or promoting milk production. 2. an agent that promotes milk flow.

ga·lac·tor·rhea (-re′ah) excessive or spontaneous milk flow; persistent secretion of milk irrespective of nursing.

ga·lac·tose (gah-lak′tōs) a six-carbon aldose epimeric with glucose but less sweet, occurring naturally in both D- and L- forms (the latter in plants). It is a component of lactose and other oligosaccharides, cerebrosides and gangliosides, and glycolipids and glycoproteins.

ga·lac·tos·e·mia (gah-lak″to-se′me-ah) any of three recessive disorders of galactose metabolism causing accumulation of galactose in the blood: the *classic* form, due to deficiency of the enzyme galactose 1-phosphate uridyltransferase, is marked by cirrhosis, hepatomegaly, cataracts, and mental retardation in survivors. *Galactokinase deficiency* results in accumulation of galactitol in the lens, causing cataracts in infancy and childhood. *Galactose epimerase deficiency* results in benign accumulation of galactose 1-phosphate in the red blood cells.

ga·lac·to·si·dase (-si′dās) an enzyme that catalyzes the cleavage of terminal galactose residues from a variety of substrates; several such enzymes exist, each specific for α- or β-linked sugars and further specific for substrates, e.g., lactase.

ga·lac·to·side (gah-lak′to-sīd) a glycoside containing galactose.

gal·ac·to·sis (gal″ak-to′sis) the formation of milk by the lacteal glands.

gal·ac·tos·ta·sis (gal″ak-tos′tah-sis) 1. cessation of lactation. 2. abnormal collection of milk in the mammary glands.

ga·lac·to·syl·trans·fer·ase (gal″ak-to″sil-trans′fer-ās) any of a group of enzymes that transfer a galactose radical from a donor to an acceptor molecule.

ga·lan·ta·mine (gah-lan′tah-mēn) a reversible competitive inhibitor of acetylcholinesterase used as the hydrobromide salt in the treatment of Alzheimer's disease.

ga·lea (ga′le-ah) [L.] a helmet-shaped structure. **g. aponeuro′tica**, the aponeurosis connecting the two bellies of the occipitofrontalis muscle.

ga·len·i·cals (gah-len′ĭ-k′lz) medicines prepared according to Galen's formulas; now used to denote standard preparations containing one or several organic ingredients, as contrasted with pure chemical substances.

ga·len·ics (gah-len′iks) galenicals.

ga·leo·pho·bia (ga″le-o-fo′be-ah) ailurophobia.

gall (gawl) bile.

gal·la·mine tri·eth·io·dide (gal′ah-mēn tri″ĕ-thi′o-dīd) a quaternary ammonium compound used to induce skeletal muscle relaxation during surgery and other procedures, such as endoscopy or intubation.

gall·blad·der (gawl′blad-er) the reservoir for bile on the posteroinferior surface of the liver.

gal·li·um (Ga) (gal′e-um) chemical element (see *Table of Elements*), at. no. 31. The nitrate salt is an inhibitor of bone calcium resorption and is used to treat cancer-related hypercalcemia. **g. Ga 67 citrate**, a radiopharmaceutical imaging agent used to image neoplasms, particularly of soft tissues, and sites of inflammation and abscess.

gal·lon (gal′on) a measure of liquid volume, 4 quarts. A standard gallon (United States) is 3.785 liters; an imperial gallon (Great Britain) is 4.546 liters.

gal·lop (gal′op) a disordered rhythm of the heart; see also under *rhythm*. **atrial g.**, S₄ g. **diastolic g.**, S₃ g. **presystolic g.**, S₄ g. **S₃ g.**, an accentuated third heart sound in patients with cardiac disease characterized by pathological alterations in ventricular filling in early diastole. **S₄ g.**, an accentuated, audible fourth heart sound usually associated with cardiac disease, often that with altered ventricular compliance. **summation g.**, one in which the third and fourth sounds are superimposed, appearing as one loud sound; usually associated with cardiac disease. **ventricular g.**, S₃ g.

gall·stone (gawl′stōn) biliary calculus; a calculus formed in the gallbladder or bile duct.

GALT gut-associated lymphoid tissue.

gal·va·nism (gal′vah-nizm) 1. galvanic current. 2. the therapeutic use of this current, particularly for stimulation of nerves and muscle. **galvan′ic**, adj. **dental g.**, production of galvanic current in the oral cavity due to the presence of two or more dissimilar metals in dental restorations that are bathed in saliva, or a single metal restoration and two electrolytes, saliva and pulp tissue fluid, thus producing an electrolytic cell and an electric current. When such restorations touch each other, the current may be high enough to irritate the dental pulp and cause sharp pain. The anodic restoration or areas of a restoration are subject to electrolytic corrosion.

gal·va·no·con·trac·til·i·ty (gal″vah-no-kon″trak-til′it-e) contractility in response to a galvanic stimulus.

gal·va·nom·e·ter (gal″vah-nom′ĕ-ter) an instrument for measuring current by electromagnetic action.

gal·va·no·pal·pa·tion (gal″vah-no-pal-pa′shun) testing of nerves of the skin by galvanic current.

gam·ete (gam′ēt) 1. one of two haploid reproductive cells, male (*spermatozoon*) and female (*oocyte*), whose union is necessary in sexual reproduction to initiate the development of a new individual. 2. the malarial parasite in its sexual form in a mosquito's stomach, either male (*microgamete*) or female (*macrogamete*); the latter is fertilized by the former to develop into an ookinete. **gamet′ic**, adj.

ga·me·to·cide (gah-me′to-sīd″) an agent that destroys gametes or gametocytes.

ga·me·to·cyte (-sīt) 1. a cell capable of dividing to form gametes; an oocyte or spermatocyte. 2. the sexual form, male or female, of certain sporozoa, such as malarial plasmodia, found in the erythrocytes, which may produce gametes when ingested by the secondary host. See also *macrogametocyte* and *microgametocyte*.

gam·e·to·gen·e·sis (gah-me″to-jen′ĕ-sis) the development of the male and female sex cells, or gametes. **gametogen′ic**, adj.

gam·e·tog·o·ny (gam″ĭ-tog′ah-ne) 1. the development of merozoites of malarial plasmodia and other sporozoa into male and female gametes, which later fuse to form a zygote. 2. reproduction by means of gametes.

gam·ma (gam′ah) 1. third letter of the Greek alphabet, see also *γ*-. 2. obsolete equivalent for microgram.

gam·ma-ami·no·bu·tyr·ic ac·id (gam″ah-ah-me″no-bu-tir′ik) *γ*-aminobutyric acid.

gam·ma ben·zene hex·a·chlo·ride (gam′ah ben′zēn hek″sah-klor′īd) lindane.

gam·ma glob·u·lin (glob′u-lin) see under *globulin*.

gam·ma·glob·u·li·nop·a·thy (gam″ah-glob″u-lin-op′ah-the) gammopathy.

Gam·ma·her·pes·vi·ri·nae (-her″pēz-vir-i′ne) the lymphocyte-associated viruses: a subfamily of the Herpesviridae, members of which are specific for either B or T lymphocytes; it includes the genus *Lymphocryptovirus*.

gam·mop·a·thy (gam-op′ah-the) abnormal proliferation of the lymphoid cells producing immunoglobulins; the gammopathies include multiple myeloma, macroglobulinemia, and Hodgkin's disease.

gamo·gen·e·sis (gam″o-jen′ĕ-sis) sexual reproduction. **gamogenet′ic**, adj.

gan·ci·clo·vir (gan-si′klo-vir) a derivative of acyclovir used in the form of the base or the sodium salt in the treatment of retinitis due to cytomegalovirus.

gan·glia (gang′gle-ah) plural of *ganglion*.

gan·gli·at·ed (gang′gle-āt″ed) ganglionated.

gan·gli·form (gang′gli-form) having the form of a ganglion.

gan·gli·itis (gang″gle-i′tis) ganglionitis.

gangli(o)- word element [Gr.], *ganglion*.

gan·glio·blast (gang′gle-o-blast″) an embryonic cell of the cerebrospinal ganglia.

gan·glio·cy·to·ma (gang″gle-o-si-to′mah) ganglioneuroma.

gan·glio·form (gang′gle-ah-form″) gangliform.

gan·glio·gli·o·ma (gang″gle-o-gli-o′mah) a ganglioneuroma in the central nervous system.

gan·glio·glio·neu·ro·ma (-gli″o-noor-o′mah) ganglioneuroma.

gan·gli·o·ma (gang″gle-o′mah) ganglioneuroma.

gan·gli·on (gang′gle-on) pl. *gan′glia*, *ganglions*. [Gr.] 1. a knot, or knotlike mass; in anatomy, a group of nerve cell bodies, located outside the central nervous system; occasionally applied to certain nuclear groups within the brain or spinal cord, e.g., basal ganglia. 2. a form of benign cystic tumor on an aponeurosis or a tendon. **gan′glial**, **ganglion′ic**, adj. **aberrant g.**, a small ganglion sometimes found on a dorsal cervical nerve root between the spinal ganglia and the spinal cord. **Acrel's g.**, a cystic tumor on an extensor tendon of the wrist. **Andersch's g.**, inferior g. (1). **autonomic ganglia**, aggregations of cell bodies of neurons of the autonomic nervous system, divided into the *sympathetic* and *parasympathetic* ganglia. **basal ganglia**, see under *nucleus*. **Bidder's ganglia**, ganglia on the cardiac nerves, situated at the lower end of the atrial septum. **Bochdalek's g.**, superior dental plexus. **cardiac ganglia**, ganglia of the cardiac plexus near the arterial ligament. **carotid g.**, an occasional small enlargement in the internal carotid plexus. **celiac ganglia**, two irregularly shaped ganglia, one on each crus of the diaphragm within the celiac plexus. **cerebrospinal ganglia,** those associated with the cranial and spinal nerves. **cervical g.,** 1. any of the three ganglia (inferior, middle, and superior) of the sympathetic trunk in the neck region. 2. one near the cervix uteri. **cervicothoracic g.,** one formed by fusion of the inferior cervical and the first thoracic ganglia. **cervicouterine g.,** cervical g. (2). **ciliary g.,** a parasympathetic ganglion in the posterior part of the orbit. **Cloquet's g.,** a swelling of the nasopalatine nerve in the anterior palatine canal. **cochlear g.,** spiral g. **Corti's g.,** spiral g. **dorsal root g.,** spinal g. **Ehrenritter's g.,** superior g. (1). **false g.,** an enlargement on a nerve that does not have a true ganglionic structure. **gasserian g.,** trigeminal g. **geniculate g.,** the sensory ganglion of the facial nerve, on the geniculum of the facial nerve. **g. im'par,** the ganglion commonly found in front of the coccyx, where the sympathetic trunks of the two sides unite. **inferior g.,** 1. the lower of two ganglia on the glossopharyngeal nerve as it passes through the jugular foramen. 2. a ganglion of the vagus nerve, just below the jugular foramen. **jugular g.,** superior g. **Lee's g.,** cervical g. (2). **Ludwig's g.,** one near the right atrium of the heart, connected with the cardiac plexus. **lumbar ganglia,** the ganglia on the lumbar part of the sympathetic trunk, usually four or five on either side. **Meckel's g.,** pterygopalatine g. **Meissner's g.,** one of the small groups of nerve cells in Meissner's plexus. **mesenteric g., inferior,** a sympathetic ganglion near the origin of the inferior mesenteric artery. **mesenteric g., superior,** one or more sympathetic ganglia at the sides of, or just below, the superior mesenteric artery. **otic g.,** a parasympathetic ganglion immediately below the foramen ovale; its postganglionic fibers supply the parotid gland. **parasympathetic g.,** one of the aggregations of cell bodies of cholinergic neurons of the parasympathetic nervous system; they are located near to or within the wall of the organs being innervated. **phrenic g.,** a sympathetic ganglion often found within the phrenic plexus at its junction with the cardiac plexus. **pterygopalatine g.,** a parasympathetic ganglion in the pterygopalatine fossa; its preganglionic fibers are derived from the facial nerve via the greater petrosal nerve and the nerve of the pterygopalatine canal and its postganglionic fibers supply the lacrimal, nasal, and palatine glands. **Remak's g.,** 1. a sympathetic ganglion on the heart wall near the superior vena cava. 2. one of the sympathetic ganglia in the

diaphragmatic opening for the inferior vena cava. 3. one of the ganglia in the gastric plexus. **Ribes' g.,** a small ganglion sometimes seen in the termination of the internal carotid plexus around the anterior communicating artery of the brain. **sacral ganglia,** those of the sacral part of the sympathetic trunk, usually three or four on either side. **Scarpa's g.,** vestibular g. **semilunar g.,** 1. trigeminal g. 2. (pl.) celiac ganglia. **sensory g.,** 1. spinal g. 2. (pl.) the ganglia on the roots of the cranial nerves, containing the cell bodies of sensory neurons. 3. both of these considered together. **simple g.,** a cystic tumor in a tendon sheath. **sphenomaxillary g., sphenopalatine g.,** pterygopalatine g. **spinal g.,** one on the posterior root of each spinal nerve, composed of unipolar nerve cell bodies of the sensory neurons of the nerve. **spiral g.,** the ganglion on the cochlear nerve, located within the modiolus, sending fibers peripherally to the organ of Corti and centrally to the cochlear nuclei of the brain stem. **splanchnic g.,** one on the greater splanchnic nerve near the twelfth thoracic vertebra. **submandibular g.,** a parasympathetic ganglion located superior to the deep part of the submandibular gland, on the lateral surface of the hyoglossal muscle. **superior g.,** 1. the upper of two ganglia on the glossopharyngeal nerve as it passes through the jugular foramen. 2. a small ganglion on the vagus nerve just as it passes through the jugular foramen. **sympathetic g.,** any of the aggregations of cell bodies of adrenergic neurons of the sympathetic nervous system; they are arranged in chainlike fashion on either side of the spinal cord. **trigeminal g.,** one on the sensory root of the fifth cranial nerve in a cleft in the dura mater on the anterior surface of the petrous part of the temporal bone, giving off the ophthalmic and maxillary nerves and part of the mandibular nerve. **tympanic g.,** an enlargement on the tympanic branch of the glossopharyngeal nerve. **vagal g.,** 1. inferior g. (2). 2. superior g. (2). **ventricular g.,** Bidder's ganglia. **vestibular g.,** the sensory ganglion of the vestibular part of the eighth cranial nerve, located in the upper part of the lateral end of the internal acoustic meatus. **Wrisberg's ganglia,** cardiac ganglia. **wrist g.,** cystic enlargement of a tendon sheath on the back of the wrist.

gan·gli·on·at·ed (gang'gle-ah-nāt″ed) provided with ganglia.

gan·gli·on·ec·to·my (gang″gle-ah-nek'tah-me) excision of a ganglion.

gan·glio·neu·ro·ma (gang″gle-o-noŏ-ro′mah) a benign neoplasm composed of nerve fibers and mature ganglion cells.

gan·gli·on·ic (-on′ik) pertaining to a ganglion.

gan·gli·on·itis (gang″gle-ah-ni′tis) inflammation of a ganglion.

gan·gli·on·os·to·my (-nos′tah-me) surgical creation of an opening into a cystic tumor on a tendon sheath or aponeurosis.

gan·gli·o·pleg·ic (-ple′jik) 1. blocking transmission of impulses through the sympathetic and parasympathetic ganglia. 2. an agent that so acts.

gan·glio·side (gang′gle-o-sīd) any of a group of glycosphingolipids found in the central nervous system tissues and having the basic composition ceramide-glucose-galactose-N-acetylneuraminic acid. The form GM_1 accumulates in tissues in GM_1 gangliosidoses and the form GM_2 in GM_2 gangliosidoses.

gan·gli·o·si·do·sis (gang″gle-o-si-do′sis) pl. *gangliosido′ses*. Any of a group of lysosomal storage diseases marked by accumulation of gangliosides GM_1 or GM_2 and related glycoconjugates due to deficiency of specific lysosomal hydrolases, and by progressive psychomotor deterioration, usually beginning in infancy or childhood and usually fatal. GM_1 g., that due to deficiency of lysosomal β-galactosidase activity, with accumulation of ganglioside GM_1, glycoproteins, and keratan sulfate. GM_2 g., that due to deficiency of activity of specific hexosaminidase isozymes, with accumulation of ganglioside GM_2 and related glycoconjugates; it occurs as three biochemically distinct variants, including Sandhoff's disease and Tay-Sachs disease.

gan·grene (gang′grēn) death of tissue, usually in considerable mass, generally with loss of vascular (nutritive) supply and followed by bacterial invasion and putrefaction. **gang′renous**, adj. **diabetic g.**, moist gangrene associated with diabetes. **dry g.**, that occurring without subsequent bacterial decomposition, the tissues becoming dry and shriveled. **embolic g.**, a condition following cutting off of blood supply by embolism. **gas g.**, an acute, severe, painful condition in which the muscles and subcutaneous tissues become filled with gas and a serosanguineous exudate; due to infection of wounds by anaerobic bacteria, among which are various species of *Clostridium*. **moist g.**, that associated with proteolytic decomposition resulting from bacterial action. **symmetric g.**, gangrene of corresponding digits on both sides, due to vasomotor disturbances.

gan·gre·no·sis (gang″grin-o′sis) the development of gangrene.

gan·i·re·lix (gan″ĭ-rel′iks) a synthetic decapeptide derived from, and an antagonist to, gonadotropin-releasing hormone; used as the acetate salt in the treatment of female infertility.

gan·o·blast (gan′ah-blast) ameloblast.

gap (gap) an unoccupied interval in time; an opening or hiatus. **air-bone g.**, the lag between the audiographic curves for air- and bone-conducted stimuli, as an indication of loss of bone conduction of the ear. **anion g.**, the concentration of plasma anions not routinely measured by laboratory screening, accounting for the difference between the measured anions and cations. **auscultatory g.**, a period in which sound is not heard in the auscultatory method of sphygmomanometry. **interocclusal g.**, see under *distance*.

gar·gle (gahr′g'l) 1. a solution for rinsing mouth and throat. 2. to rinse the mouth and throat by holding a solution in the open mouth and agitating it by expulsion of air from the lungs.

gar·goyl·ism (gahr′goil-izm) Hurler's syndrome.

gar·lic (gahr′lik) the flowering plant *Allium sativum*, or its bulbous stem base, which contains the antibacterial allicin; preparations of the bulbs are used for hyperlipidemia, hypertension, and arteriosclerosis; also used in folk medicine.

gas (gas) any elastic aeriform fluid in which the molecules are separated from one another and so have free paths. **gas′eous**, adj. **alveolar g.**, the gas in the alveoli of the lungs, where gaseous exchange with the capillary blood takes place. **blood g's.**, the partial pressures of oxygen and carbon dioxide in blood; see under *analysis*. **coal g.**, a gas, poisonous because it contains carbon monoxide, produced by destructive distillation of coal; much used for domestic cooking. **laughing g.**, nitrous oxide. **tear g.**, one which produces severe lacrimation by irritating the conjunctivae.

gas·o·met·ric (gas″o-met′rik) pertaining to the measurement of gases.

gas·ter (gas′ter) [Gr.] stomach.

Gas·ter·oph·i·lus (gas″ter-of′ĭ-lus) a genus of botflies the larvae of which develop in the gastrointestinal tract of horses and may sometimes infect humans.

gas·trad·e·ni·tis (gas″trad-ĕ-ni′tis) inflammation of the stomach glands.

gas·tral·gia (gas-tral′jah) gastrodynia.

gas·trec·to·my (gas-trek′tah-me) excision of the stomach (*total g.*) or of a portion of it (*partial* or *subtotal g.*).

gas·tric (gas'trik) pertaining to, affecting, or originating in the stomach.

gas·tric·sin (gas-trik'sin) a proteolytic enzyme isolated from gastric juice; its precursor is pepsinogen but it differs from pepsin in molecular weight and in the amino acids at the N terminal.

gas·trin (gas'trin) a polypeptide hormone secreted by certain cells of the pyloric glands, which strongly stimulates secretion of gastric acid and pepsin, and weakly stimulates secretion of pancreatic enzymes and gallbladder contraction.

gas·tri·no·ma (gas"tri-no'mah) an islet cell tumor of non-beta cells that secretes gastrin; it is the usual cause of Zollinger-Ellison syndrome.

gas·tri·tis (gas-tri'tis) inflammation of the stomach. **atrophic g.,** chronic gastritis with infiltration of the lamina propria, involving the entire mucosal thickness, by inflammatory cells. **catarrhal g.,** inflammation and hypertrophy of the gastric mucosa, with excessive secretion of mucus. **eosinophilic g.,** that in which there is considerable edema and infiltration of all coats of the wall of the pyloric antrum by eosinophils. **erosive g., exfoliative g.,** that in which the gastric surface epithelium is eroded. **giant hypertrophic g.,** excessive proliferation of the gastric mucosa, producing diffuse thickening of the stomach wall. **hypertrophic g.,** gastritis with infiltration and enlargement of the glands. **polypous g.,** hypertrophic gastritis with polypoid projections of the mucosa. **pseudomembranous g.,** that in which a false membrane occurs in patches within the stomach. **superficial g.,** chronic inflammation of the lamina propria, limited to the outer third of the mucosa in the foveolar area. **toxic g.,** that due to action of a poison or corrosive agent.

gastr(o)- word element [Gr.], *stomach.*

gas·tro·anas·to·mo·sis (gas"tro-ah-nas"tah-mo'sis) gastrogastrostomy.

gas·tro·cele (gas'tro-sēl) hernial protrusion of the stomach or of a gastric pouch.

gas·troc·ne·mi·us (gas"trok-ne'me-us) see *Table of Muscles.*

gas·tro·coele (gas'tro-sēl) archenteron.

gas·tro·col·ic (gas"tro-kol'ik) pertaining to or communicating with the stomach and colon, as a fistula.

gas·tro·co·li·tis (-ko-li'tis) inflammation of the stomach and colon.

gas·tro·co·los·to·my (-kah-los'tah-me) surgical anastomosis of the stomach to the colon.

gas·tro·cu·ta·ne·ous (-ku-ta'ne-us) pertaining to the stomach and skin, or communicating with the stomach and the cutaneous surface of the body, as a gastrocutaneous fistula.

gas·tro·cys·to·plas·ty (-sis'to-plas"te) augmentation cystoplasty using a portion of the stomach.

gas·tro·di·aph·a·ny (-di-af'ah-ne) examination of the stomach by transillumination of its walls with a small electric lamp.

Gas·tro·dis·coi·des (-dis-koi'dēz) a genus of trematodes parasitic in the intestinal tract.

gas·tro·du·o·de·ni·tis (-doo"o-dĕ-ni'tis) inflammation of the stomach and duodenum.

gas·tro·du·o·de·nos·to·my (-doo"od-in-os'tah-me) surgical anastomosis of the stomach to a formerly remote part of the duodenum.

gas·tro·dyn·ia (-din'e-ah) gastralgia; pain in the stomach.

gas·tro·en·ter·al·gia (-en"ter-al'jah) pain in the stomach and intestine.

gas·tro·en·ter·i·tis (-en"ter-i'tis) inflammation of the stomach and intestine. **eosinophilic g.,** a disorder, commonly associated with intolerance to specific foods, marked by infiltration of the mucosa of the small intestine by eosinophils, with edema but without vasculitis and by eosinophilia of the peripheral blood. Symptoms depend on the site and extent of the disorder. The stomach is also frequently involved. **Norwalk g.,** gastroenteritis caused by the Norwalk virus.

gas·tro·en·tero·anas·to·mo·sis (-en"ter-o-ah-nas"tah-mo'sis) anastomosis between the stomach and small intestine.

gas·tro·en·ter·ol·o·gy (-en"ter-ol'ah-je) the study of the stomach and intestine and their diseases.

gas·tro·en·ter·op·a·thy (-en"ter-op'ah-the) any disease of the stomach and intestines. **allergic g.,** eosinophilic gastritis of children with food allergies, particularly to cows' milk.

gas·tro·en·ter·ot·o·my (-en"ter-ot'ah-me) incision into the stomach and intestine.

gas·tro·ep·i·plo·ic (-ep"ĭ-plo'ik) pertaining to the stomach and epiploon (omentum).

gas·tro·esoph·a·ge·al (-e-sof"ah-je'al) pertaining to the stomach and esophagus.

gas·tro·esoph·a·gi·tis (-ĕ-sof"ah-ji'tis) inflammation of the stomach and esophagus.

gas·tro·fi·ber·scope (-fi'ber-skōp) a fiberscope for viewing the stomach.

gas·tro·gas·tros·to·my (-gas-tros'tah-me) surgical anastomosis of two previously remote portions of the stomach.

gas·tro·ga·vage (-gah-vahzh') artificial feeding through a tube passed into the stomach.

gas·tro·he·pat·ic (-hĕ-pat′ik) pertaining to the stomach and liver.

gas·tro·hep·a·ti·tis (-hep″ah-ti′tis) inflammation of the stomach and liver.

gas·tro·il·e·al (-il′e-al) pertaining to the stomach and ileum.

gas·tro·il·e·itis (-il-e-i′tis) inflammation of the stomach and ileum.

gas·tro·il·e·os·to·my (-il″e-os′tah-me) surgical anastomosis of the stomach to the ileum.

gas·tro·in·tes·ti·nal (-in-tes′tĭ-n′l) pertaining to or communicating with the stomach and intestine.

gas·tro·je·ju·no·col·ic (-jĕ-joo″no-kol′ik) pertaining to the stomach, jejunum, and colon.

gas·tro·je·ju·nos·to·my (-jĕ″joo-nos′tah-me) 1. surgical creation of an anastomosis between the stomach and jejunum. 2. the anastomosis so created.

gas·tro·li·e·nal (-li′in-il) gastrosplenic.

gas·tro·li·thi·a·sis (-lĭ-thi′ah-sis) the presence or formation of calculi in the stomach.

gas·trol·y·sis (gas-trol′ĭ-sis) surgical division of perigastric adhesions to mobilize the stomach.

gas·tro·ma·la·cia (gas″tro-mah-la′shah) softening of the wall of the stomach.

gas·tro·meg·a·ly (-meg′ah-le) enlargement of the stomach.

gas·tro·my·co·sis (-mi-ko′sis) fungal infection of the stomach.

gas·tro·myx·or·rhea (-mik″so-re′ah) excessive secretion of mucus by the stomach.

gas·tro·pa·re·sis (gas″tro-pah-re′sis) paralysis of the stomach.

gas·trop·a·thy (gas-trop′ah-the) any disease of the stomach.

gas·tro·pexy (gas′tro-pek″se) surgical fixation of the stomach.

Gas·troph·i·lus (gas-trof′ĭ-lus) *Gasterophilus.*

gas·tro·phren·ic (gas″tro-fren′ik) pertaining to the stomach and diaphragm.

gas·tro·pli·ca·tion (gas″tro-plĭ-ka′shun) treatment of gastric dilatation by stitching a fold in the stomach wall.

gas·trop·to·sis (gas″trop-to′sis) downward displacement of the stomach.

gas·tro·py·lo·rec·to·my (gas″tro-pi″lo-rek′tah-me) excision of the pyloric part of the stomach.

gas·tror·rha·gia (-ra′jah) hemorrhage from the stomach.

gas·tror·rhea (-re′ah) excessive secretion by the glands of the stomach.

gas·tros·chi·sis (gas-tros′kĭ-sis) congenital fissure of the anterior abdominal wall.

gas·tro·scope (gas′tro-skōp) an endoscope for inspecting the interior of the stomach. **gastroscop′ic,** adj.

gas·tro·se·lec·tive (gas″tro-sĭ-lek′tiv) having an affinity for receptors involved in regulation of gastric activities.

gas·tro·spasm (gas′tro-spazm) spasm of the stomach.

gas·tro·splen·ic (gas″tro-splen′ik) pertaining to the stomach and spleen.

gas·tro·stax·is (-stak′sis) the oozing of blood from the stomach mucosa.

gas·tros·to·ga·vage (gas-tros″to-gah-vahzh′) feeding through a gastric fistula.

gas·tros·to·la·vage (-lah-vahzh′) irrigation of the stomach through a gastric fistula.

gas·tros·to·my (gas-tros′tah-me) surgical creation of an artificial opening into the stomach, or the opening so established.

gas·trot·o·my (gas-trot′ah-me) incision into the stomach.

gas·tro·to·nom·e·ter (gas″tro-to-nom′ĕ-ter) an instrument for measuring intragastric pressure.

gas·tro·tro·pic (-tro′pik) having an affinity for or exerting a special effect on the stomach.

gas·tro·tym·pa·ni·tes (-tim″pah-ni′tēz) tympanitic distention of the stomach.

gas·tru·la (gas′troo-lah) the embryo in the stage following the blastula or blastocyst; simplest type consists of two layers of cells, the ectoderm and endoderm, which have invaginated to form the archenteron and an opening, the blastopore. In human embryos the gastrula stage occurs during the third week, as the embryonic disc becomes trilaminar, establishing the ectoderm, mesoderm, and endoderm.

gas·tru·la·tion (gas″troo-la′shun) the process by which a blastula becomes a gastrula or, in forms without a true blastula, the process by which three germ cell layers are acquired. In humans, the conversion of a bilaminar to a trilaminar embryonic disc (ectoderm, mesoderm, endoderm).

gat·i·flox·a·cin (gat″ĭ-flok′sah-sin) a fluoroquinolone antibacterial effective against many gram-positive and gram-negative bacteria.

gat·ing (gāt′ing) controlling access or passage through gates or channels.

ga·to·pho·bia (gat″o-fo′be-ah) ailurophobia.

gaunt·let (gawnt′let) a bandage covering the hand and fingers like a glove.

gauss (gous) a unit of magnetic flux density, equal to 10^{-4} tesla.

gauze (gawz) a light, open-meshed fabric of muslin or similar material. **absorbable g.,** gauze made from oxidized cellulose.

absorbent g., white cotton cloth of various thread counts and weights, supplied in various lengths and widths and in different forms (rolls or folds). **petrolatum g.,** a sterile material produced by saturation of sterile absorbent gauze with sterile white petrolatum. **zinc gelatin impregnated g.,** absorbent gauze impregnated with zinc gelatin.

ga·vage (gah-vahzh′) [Fr.] 1. forced feeding, especially through a tube passed into the stomach. 2. superalimentation.

gaze (gāz) 1. to look steadily in one direction. 2. the act of looking steadily at something. **conjugate g.,** the normal movement of the two eyes simultaneously in the same direction to bring something into view.

GC gas chromatography.

G-CSF granulocyte colony-stimulating factor.

Gd gadolinium.

Ge germanium.

ge·gen·hal·ten (ga″gen-hahl′tin) [Ger.] an involuntary resistance to passive movement, as may occur in cerebral cortical disorders.

gel (jel) 1. a colloid in which the solid disperse phase forms a network in combination with the fluid continuous phase, resulting in a viscous semirigid sol. 2. to form such a compound or any similar semi-solid material. **aluminum hydroxide g.,** a suspension of aluminum hydroxide and hydrated oxide used as a gastric antacid, especially in the treatment of peptic ulcer, and in the treatment of phosphate nephrolithiasis. **aluminum phosphate g.,** an aqueous suspension of aluminum phosphate, used as an antacid and to reduce excretion of phosphates in the feces. **APF g.,** sodium fluoride and phosphoric acid g. **basic aluminum carbonate g.,** an aluminum hydroxide–aluminum carbonate gel, used as an antacid, for treatment of hyperphosphatemia in renal insufficiency, and to prevent phosphate urinary calculi. **dried aluminum hydroxide g.,** an amorphous form of aluminum hydroxide prepared by drying aluminum hydroxide gel at low temperature; used as an antacid. **sodium fluoride and phosphoric acid g.,** a gel containing sodium fluoride, hydrofluoric acid, and phosphoric acid; applied topically to the teeth as a dental caries prophylactic.

gel·a·tin (jel′ah-tin) a substance obtained by partial hydrolysis of collagen derived from skin, white connective tissue, and bones of animals; used as a suspending agent, in manufacture of capsules and suppositories, sometimes as an adjuvant protein food, and suggested for use as a plasma substitute. **zinc g.,** a preparation of zinc oxide, gelatin,

glycerin, and purified water, used as a topical skin protectant.

ge·lat·i·nous (jĕ-lat′ĭ-nus) like jelly or softened gelatin.

ge·la·tion (jĕ-la′shun) conversion of a sol into a gel.

gem·cit·a·bine (jem-sit′ah-bēn) an antineoplastic agent used as the hydrochloride salt in the treatment of pancreatic adenocarcinoma and non–small cell lung carcinoma.

Ge·mel·la (jĕ-mel′ah) [L.] a genus of aerobic or facultatively anaerobic cocci (family Streptococcaceae), occurring singly or in pairs with adjacent sides flattened; they are found as parasites of mammals.

gem·el·lol·o·gy (jem″el-ol′ah-je) the scientific study of twins and twinning.

gem·fib·ro·zil (jem-fib′ro-zil) a hypolipidemic agent used for treatment of patients with very high serum triglyceride levels (type IV hyperlipoproteinemia) who do not respond to dietary management.

gem·i·nate (jem′ĭ-nāt) paired; occurring in twos.

gem·ma·tion (jĕ-ma′shun) budding; asexual reproduction in which a portion of the cell body is thrust out and then becomes separated, forming a new individual.

gem·mule (jem′ūl) 1. a reproductive bud; the immediate product of gemmation. 2. one of the many little spinelike processes on the dendrites of a neuron.

gem·tu·zu·mab ozo·ga·mi·cin (gem-too′zoo-mab″ o″zo-kah-mi′sin) a recombinant DNA–derived monoclonal antibody conjugated with a cytotoxic antitumor antibiotic, used as an antineoplastic.

-gen word element [Gr.], *an agent that produces.*

ge·nal (je′nil) pertaining to the cheek; buccal.

gen·der (jen′der) sex; the category to which an individual is assigned on the basis of sex.

gene (jēn) the biologic unit of heredity, self-reproducing and located at a definite position (locus) on a particular chromosome. **allelic g.,** allele. **chimeric g.,** an artificial gene constructed by juxtaposition of fragments of unrelated genes or other DNA segments, which may themselves have been altered. **complementary g's,** two independent pairs of nonallelic genes, neither of which will produce its effect in the absence of the other. **dominant g.,** one that is phenotypically expressed when present in homozygotes or heterozygotes. **H g., histocompatibility g.,** one that determines the specificity of tissue antigenicity (HLA antigens), and thus the compatibility of donor and recipient in tissue transplantation and blood transfusion.

holandric g's, genes in the nonhomologous region of the Y chromosome. **immune response (Ir) g's,** genes of the major histocompatibility complex that govern the immune response to individual immunogens. **Is g's,** genes that govern the formation of suppressor T lymphocytes. **lethal g.,** one whose presence brings about the death of the organism or permits survival only under certain conditions. **mutant g.,** one that has undergone a detectable mutation. **operator g.,** one serving as a starting point for reading the genetic code, and which, through interaction with a repressor, controls the activity of structural genes associated with it in the operon. **recessive g.,** one that produces an effect in the organism only when it is homozygous. **regulator g., regulatory g.,** 1. in genetic theory, one that synthesizes repressor, a substance that through interaction with the operator gene switches off the activity of the structural genes associated with it in the operon. 2. any gene whose product affects the activity of other genes. **repressor g.,** regulator g. (1). **sex-linked g.,** one carried on a sex chromosome, especially on an X chromosome. **split g.,** a gene containing multiple exons and at least one intron. **structural g.,** one that specifies the amino acid sequence of a polypeptide chain.

gen·e·ra (jen′er-ah) plural of *genus*.

gen·er·al (jen′er-al) affecting many parts or all parts of the organism; not local.

gen·er·al·ize (-īz) 1. to spread throughout the body, as when local disease becomes systemic. 2. to form a general principle; to reason inductively.

gen·er·a·tion (jen″ĕ-ra′shun) 1. reproduction (1). 2. a class composed of all individuals removed by the same number of successive ancestors from a common predecessor, or occupying positions on the same level in a genealogical (pedigree) chart. **alternate g.,** reproduction by alternate asexual and sexual means in an animal or plant species. **asexual g.,** production of a new organism not originating from union of gametes. **first filial g.,** the first-generation offspring of two parents; symbol F_1. **parental g.,** the generation with which a particular genetic study is begun; symbol P_1. **second filial g.,** all of the offspring produced by two individuals of the first filial generation; symbol F_2. **sexual g.,** production of a new organism from the zygote formed by the union of gametes. **spontaneous g.,** the discredited concept of continuous generation of living organisms from nonliving matter.

gen·er·a·tor (jen′er-a″-tor) 1. something that produces or causes to exist. 2. a machine that converts mechanical to electrical energy. **pattern g.,** a network of neurons that produces a stereotyped form of complex movement, such as chewing or ambulation, that is almost invariable from one performance to the next. **pulse g.,** the power source for a cardiac pacemaker system, usually powered by a lithium battery, supplying impulses to the implanted electrodes, either at a fixed rate or in some programmed pattern.

ge·ner·ic (jĕ-ner′ik) 1. pertaining to a genus. 2. nonproprietary; denoting a drug name not protected by a trademark, usually descriptive of the drug's chemical structure.

gen·e·sis (jen′ĕ-sis) [Gr.] creation; origination.

-genesis word element [Gr.], *formation; development.*

ge·net·ic (jĕ-net′ik) 1. pertaining to or determined by genes. 2. pertaining to reproduction or to birth or origin.

ge·net·ics (jĕ-net′iks) the study of heredity. **biochemical g.,** the science concerned with the chemical and physical nature of genes and the mechanism by which they control the development and maintenance of the organism. **clinical g.,** the study of genetic factors influencing the occurrence of a pathologic condition.

ge·ne·to·tro·phic (jĕ-net″o-tro′fik) pertaining to genetics and nutrition; relating to problems of nutrition that are hereditary in nature, or transmitted through the genes.

ge·ni·al (jĕ-ni′al) mental (2).

gen·ic (jen′ik) pertaining to or caused by the genes.

-genic word element [Gr.], *giving rise to; causing.*

ge·nic·u·lar (jĕ-nik′u-ler) pertaining to the knee.

ge·nic·u·late (jĕ-nik′u-lāt) bent, like a knee.

ge·nic·u·lum (jĕ-nik′u-lum) pl. *genic′cula.* [L.] a little knee; used in anatomical nomenclature to designate a sharp kneelike bend in a small structure or organ.

gen·i·tal (jen′ĭ-t′l) 1. pertaining to reproduction, or to the reproductive organs. 2. (in the plural) the reproductive organs.

gen·i·ta·lia (jen″ĭ-tāl′e-ah) [L.] the reproductive organs. **ambiguous g.,** genital organs with characteristics typical of both male and female, as seen in hermaphroditism and some types of pseudohermaphroditism. **external g.,** the reproductive organs external to the body, including pudendum, clitoris, and female urethra in the female, and scrotum, penis, and male urethra in the male. **indif-ferent g.**, the reproductive organs of the embryo prior to the establishment of definitive sex. **internal g.**, the reproductive organs within the body, including ovaries, uterine tubes, uterus, and vagina in the female, and testes, epididymides, ductus deferentes, seminal vesicles, ejaculatory ducts, prostate, and bulbourethral glands in the male.

genit(o)- word element [L.], *the organs of reproduction.*

gen·i·tog·ra·phy (jen″ĭ-tog′rah-fe) radiography of the urogenital sinus and internal duct structures after injection of a contrast medium through the sinus opening.

gen·i·to·uri·nary (jen″ĭ-to-u′rĭ-nar-e) pertaining to the genital and urinary organs.

ge·no·der·ma·to·sis (je″no-der″mah-to′sis) a genetic disorder of the skin, usually generalized.

ge·nome (je′nōm) the complete set of hereditary factors contained in the haploid set of chromosomes. **genom′ic,** adj.

ge·no·tox·ic (je′no-tok″sik) damaging to DNA: applied to agents known to damage DNA, thereby causing mutations, which can result in cancer.

ge·no·type (-tīp) 1. the entire genetic constitution of an individual; also, the alleles present at one or more specific loci. 2. the type species of a genus. **genotyp′ic,** adj.

-genous word element [Gr.], *arising or resulting from; produced by.*

gen·ta·mi·cin (jen″tah-mi′sin) an aminoglycoside antibiotic complex isolated from bacteria of the genus *Micromonospora,* effective against many gram-negative bacteria as well as certain gram-positive species; used as the sulfate salt.

gen·tian (jen′shin) the dried rhizome and roots of *Gentiana lutea;* used as a bitter tonic. **g. violet,** an antibacterial, antifungal, and anthelmintic dye, applied topically in the treatment of infections of the skin and mucous membranes associated with gram-positive bacteria and molds; also used to treat blood collected in areas endemic for Chagas' disease.

gen·tian·o·phil·ic (jen″shin-o-fil′ik) staining readily with gentian violet.

gen·tian·o·pho·bic (-fo′bik) not staining with gentian violet.

ge·nu (je′nu) pl. *ge′nua.* [L.] 1. the knee. 2. any kneelike structure. **g. extror′sum,** bowleg. **g. intror′sum,** knock-knee. **g. re-curva′tum,** hyperextensibility of the knee joint. **g. val′gum,** knock-knee. **g. va′rum,** bowleg.

ge·nus (je′nus) pl. *gen′era.* [L.] a taxonomic category subordinate to a tribe (or subtribe) and superior to a species (or subgenus).

ge(o)- word element [Gr.], *the earth; the soil.*

ge·ode (je′ōd) a dilated lymph space.

geo·graph·ic (je″o-graf′ik) in pathology, of or referring to a pattern that is well demarcated, resembling outlines on a map.

geo·med·i·cine (-med′ĭ-sin) the branch of medicine dealing with the influence of climatic and environmental conditions on health.

geo·pha·gia (-fa′jah) the habitual eating of earth or clay, a form of pica.

geo·tri·cho·sis (-trĭ-ko′sis) a candidiasis-like infection due to *Geotrichum candidum,* which may attack the bronchi, lungs, mouth, or intestinal tract.

Ge·ot·ri·chum (je-ah′trĭ-kum) a genus of yeastlike fungi, including *G. can′didum,* found in the feces and in dairy products.

ge·ot·ro·pism (je-ah′trah-pizm) a tendency of growth or movement toward or away from the earth; the influence of gravity on growth.

ge·rat·ic (jĕ-rat′ik) pertaining to old age.

GERD gastroesophageal reflux disease.

ger·i·at·ric (jer″e-at′rik) 1. pertaining to elderly persons or to the aging process. 2. pertaining to geriatrics.

ger·i·at·rics (-at′riks) the department of medicine dealing especially with the problems of aging and diseases of the elderly. **dental g.,** gerodontics.

geri·odon·tics (-o-don′tiks) gerodontics.

germ (jerm) 1. a pathogenic microorganism. 2. a living substance capable of developing into an organ, part, or organism as a whole; a primordium. **dental g.,** collective tissues from which a tooth is formed. **enamel g.,** the epithelial rudiment of the enamel organ.

ger·ma·ni·um (Ge) (jer-ma′ne-um) chemical element (see *Table of Elements*), at. no. 32.

ger·mi·ci·dal (jer″mĭ-si′d′l) antimicrobial (1).

ger·mi·nal (jer′mĭ-nal) pertaining to or of the nature of a gamete (germ cell) or the primordial stage of development.

ger·mi·na·tion (jer″mĭ-na′shun) the sprouting of a seed, spore, or plant embryo. **ger′minative,** adj.

ger·mi·no·ma (jer″mĭ-no′mah) a type of germ cell tumor with large round cells with vascular nuclei, usually found in the ovary, undescended testis, anterior mediastinum, or pineal gland; in males called *seminoma* and in females called *dysgerminoma.*

ger(o)- word element [Gr.], *old age; the aged.*

ge·ro·der·ma (jer-o-der'mah) dystrophy of the skin and genitals, giving the appearance of old age.

ger·odon·tics (-don'tiks) dentistry dealing with the dental problems of older people. **gerodon'tic**, adj.

gero·ma·ras·mus (-mah-raz'mus) the emaciation sometimes characteristic of old age.

gero·mor·phism (-mor'fizm) premature senility.

geront(o)- word element [Gr.], *old age; the aged.*

ger·on·tol·o·gy (jer″on-tol'ah-je) the scientific study of aging in all its aspects.

ger·on·to·pia (jer″on-to'pe-ah) senopia.

ger·on·to·ther·a·peu·tics (jer-on″tother″ah-pu'tiks) the science of retarding and preventing many of the aspects of senescence.

gero·psy·chi·a·try (jer″o-si-ki'ah-tre) a subspecialty of psychiatry dealing with mental illness in the elderly.

ges·ta·gen (jes'tah-jen) progestational agent.

ge·stalt (gah-stawlt′, gah-shtawlt′) [Ger.] form, shape; a whole perceptual configuration. See *gestaltism.*

ge·stal·tism (gah-stawl'tizm, gah-shtawl'tizm) the theory in psychology that the objects of mind, as immediately presented to direct experience, come as complete unanalyzable wholes or forms (Gestalten) which cannot be split up into parts.

ges·ta·tion (jes-ta'shun) pregnancy. See also *gestation period,* under *period.* **gesta'tional**, adj.

ges·to·sis (jes-to'sis) pl. *gesto'ses.* Any manifestation of preeclampsia in pregnancy.

GeV gigaelectron volt; one billion (10^9) electron volts.

GFAP glial fibrillary acidic protein.

GFR glomerular filtration rate.

GH growth hormone.

ghost (gōst) a faint or shadowy figure lacking the customary substance of reality. **red cell g.**, an erythrocyte membrane that remains intact after hemolysis.

GH-RH growth hormone–releasing hormone.

GI gastrointestinal.

gi·ant·ism (ji'ant-izm) 1. gigantism. 2. excessive size, as of cells or nuclei.

Gi·ar·dia (je-ahr'de-ah) a genus of flagellate protozoa parasitic in the intestinal tract of humans and other animals, which may cause giardiasis; *G. lam'blia (G. intestina'lis)* is the species found in humans.

gi·ar·di·a·sis (je″ahr-di'ah-sis) infection of the small intestine with the protozoan *Giardia lamblia,* spread via contaminated food or water or by direct person-to-person contact;

symptoms are rare and range from nonspecific gastrointestinal discomfort to mild to profuse diarrhea, nausea, lassitude, anorexia, and weight loss.

gib·bos·i·ty (gĭ-bos'it-e) the condition of being humped; kyphosis.

gib·bus (gib'us) hump.

GIFT gamete intrafallopian transfer.

giga- word element [Gr.], *huge;* used in naming units of measurement to designate an amount one billion (10^9) times the size of the unit to which it is joined; symbol G.

gi·gan·ti·form (ji-gan'tĭ-form) very large.

gi·gan·tism (ji-gan'tizm, ji'gan-tizm) abnormal overgrowth; excessive size and stature. **cerebral g.,** gigantism in the absence of increased levels of growth hormone, attributed to a cerebral defect; infants are large, and accelerated growth continues for the first 4 or 5 years, the rate being normal thereafter. The hands and feet are large, the head large and dolichocephalic, the eyes have an antimongoloid slant, with hypertelorism. The child is clumsy, and mental retardation of varying degree is usually present. **pituitary g.,** that caused by oversecretion of growth hormone by the pituitary gland.

gi·gan·to·cel·lu·lar (ji-gan″to-sel'u-ler) pertaining to giant cells.

gi·gan·to·mas·tia (-mas'te-ah) extreme macromastia.

gin·ger (jin'jer) the leafy herb *Zingiber officinale,* or the dried rhizome, which is used as a flavoring agent, in the treatment of digestive disorders, and to prevent motion sickness.

gin·gi·va (jin'jĭ-vah, jin-ji'vah) pl. *gin'givae.* [L.] the gum; the mucous membrane, with supporting fibrous tissue, covering the toothbearing border of the jaw. **gin'gival,** adj. **alveolar g.,** the portion covering the alveolar process. **areolar g.,** the portion attached to the alveolar process by loose areolar connective tissue, lying beyond the keratinized mucosa over the alveolar process. **attached g.,** the portion that is firm, resilient, and bound to the underlying cementum and alveolar bone. **free g.,** the portion of the gingiva that surrounds the tooth and is not directly attached to the tooth surface. **marginal g.,** the portion of the free gingiva localized to the labial, buccal, lingual, and palatal aspects of the teeth; gingival margin.

gin·gi·val·ly (jin'jĭ-val″e) toward the gingiva.

gin·gi·vec·to·my (jin″jĭ-vek'tah-me) surgical excision of all loose infected and diseased gingival tissue.

gin·gi·vi·tis (-vi'tis) inflammation of the gingiva. **acute necrotizing ulcerative g.**

(ANUG), **acute ulcerative g.**, **acute ulcero-membranous g.**, necrotizing ulcerative g. **atrophic senile g.**, inflammation, and sometimes atrophy, of the gingival and oral mucosa in menopausal and postmenopausal women, believed due to altered estrogen metabolism. **fusospirochetal g.**, necrotizing ulcerative g. **herpetic g.**, infection of the gingivae by the herpes simplex virus. **necrotizing ulcerative g.**, trench mouth; a progressive painful infection, also seen in subacute and recurrent forms, marked by crateriform lesions of interdental papillae with pseudomembranous slough circumscribed by linear erythema; fetid breath; increased salivation; and spontaneous gingival hemorrhage; see also under *gingivostomatitis*. **pregnancy g.**, any of various gingival changes ranging from gingivitis to the so-called pregnancy tumor. **Vincent's g.**, necrotizing ulcerative g.

gingiv(o)- word element [L.], *gums.*

gin·gi·vo·sis (jin″ji-vo′sis) a chronic, diffuse inflammation of the gingivae, with desquamation of papillary epithelium and mucous membrane.

gin·gi·vo·sto·ma·ti·tis (jin″ji-vo-sto″mah-ti′tis) inflammation of the gingivae and oral mucosa. **herpetic g.**, that due to infection with herpes simplex virus, with redness of the oral tissues, formation of multiple vesicles and painful ulcers, and fever. **necrotizing ulcerative g.**, Plaut's or pseudomembranous angina; a type due to extension of necrotizing ulcerative gingivitis to other areas of the oral mucosa.

gin·gly·moid (jing′gli-moid) resembling a hinge; pertaining to a ginglymus.

gin·gly·mus (-mus) a joint that allows movement in but one plane, forward and backward, as does a door hinge.

gink·go (ging′ko) the dried leaves of the deciduous tree *Ginkgo biloba*, used for symptomatic relief of brain dysfunction, for intermittent claudication, and for tinnitus and vertigo of vascular origin; also used in traditional Chinese medicine and in homeopathy.

gin·seng (jin′seng) 1. any herb of the genus *Panax*, especially *P. ginseng* (Chinese g.) and *P. quinquefolius* (American g.). 2. the root of Chinese or American ginseng, used as a tonic and stimulant. 3. Siberian g. **eleuthero g.**, **Siberian g.**, the shrub *Eleutherococcus senticosus*, or a preparation of its root, which is used to improve general well-being and for various indications in traditional Chinese medicine.

gir·dle (gir′d'l) cingulum; an encircling structure or part; anything encircling a body. **pectoral g.**, shoulder g. **pelvic g.**, the encircling bony structure supporting the lower limbs. **shoulder g.**, **thoracic g.**, the encircling bony structure supporting the upper limbs.

gla·bel·la (glah-bel′ah) the area on the frontal bone above the nasion and between the eyebrows.

gla·brous (gla′brus) smooth and bare.

gla·di·o·lus (glah-di′o-lus) body of sternum.

glairy (glār′e) resembling egg white.

gland (gland) an aggregation of cells specialized to secrete or excrete materials not related to their ordinary metabolic needs. **accessory g.**, a minor mass of glandular tissue near or at some distance from a gland of similar structure. **accessory adrenal g's**, adrenal glandular tissue, usually either cortical or medullary, found in the abdomen or pelvis. **adrenal g.**, suprarenal gland; a flattened body above either kidney, consisting of a cortex and a medulla, the former elaborating steroid hormones, and the latter epinephrine and norepinephrine. **aggregate g's**, **aggregated g's**, Peyer's patches. **apocrine g.**, one whose discharged secretion contains part of the secreting cells; particularly used to denote an apocrine sweat gland. **apocrine sweat g.**, a type of large, branched, specialized sweat gland, after puberty producing a viscous secretion that is acted on by bacteria to produce a characteristic acrid odor. **axillary g's**, lymph nodes situated in the axilla. **Bartholin's g.**, greater vestibular g. **biliary g's**, **g's of biliary mucosa**, tubuloalveolar glands in the mucosa of the bile ducts and the neck of the gallbladder. **Blandin's g's**, anterior lingual g's. **bronchial g's**, seromucous glands in the mucosa and submucosa of bronchial walls. **Bruch's g's**, lymph follicles in the conjunctiva of lower lid. **Brunner's g's**, duodenal g's. **bulbocavernous g.**, **bulbourethral g.**, one of two glands embedded in the substance of the sphincter of the urethra, posterior to the membranous part of the urethra. **cardiac g's**, mucin-secreting glands of the cardiac part (cardia) of the stomach. **celiac g's**, lymph nodes anterior to the abdominal aorta. **ceruminous g's**, cerumensecreting glands in the skin of the external auditory canal. **cervical g's of uterus**, compound clefts in the wall of the uterine cervix. **ciliary g's**, sweat glands that have become arrested in their development, located at the edges of the eyelids. **circumanal g's**, specialized sweat and sebaceous glands around the anus. **closed g's**, endocrine g's. **coccygeal g.**, glomus coccygeum. **compound g., one made up of a number of smaller units whose excretory ducts combine to form ducts of progressively higher order. **Cowper's g.,** bulbourethral g. **ductless g.,** one without a duct, of internal secretion; see *endocrine g's*. **duodenal g's,** glands in the submucosa of the duodenum, opening into the glands of the small intestine. **Ebner's g's,** serous glands at the back of the tongue near the taste buds. **eccrine g., eccrine sweat g.,** one of the ordinary, or simple, sweat glands, which is of the merocrine type. **endocrine g's,** organs whose secretions (hormones) are released directly into the circulatory system; they include the pituitary, thyroid, parathyroid, and adrenal glands, the pineal body, and the gonads. **exocrine g.,** one whose secretion is discharged through a duct opening on an internal or external surface of the body. **fundic g's, fundus g's,** tubular glands in the mucosa of the fundus and body of the stomach, containing acid- and pepsin-secreting cells. **Galeati's g's,** duodenal g's. **gastric g's,** the secreting glands of the stomach, including the fundic, cardiac, and pyloric glands. **Gay's g's,** circumanal g's. **glossopalatine g's,** mucous glands at the posterior end of the smaller sublingual glands. **haversian g's,** synovial villi. **holocrine g.,** one whose discharged secretion contains the entire secreting cells. **intestinal g's,** straight tubular glands in the mucous membrane of the intestine, opening, in the small intestine, between the bases of the villi, and containing argentaffin cells. **jugular g.,** accessory lacrimal glands deep in the conjunctival connective tissue, mainly near the upper fornix. **lacrimal g.,** either of a pair of glands that secrete tears. **g's of Lieberkühn,** intestinal g's. **lingual g's,** the seromucous glands on the surface of the tongue. **lingual g's, anterior,** the deeply placed seromucous glands near the apex of the tongue. **Littre's g's,** 1. preputial g's. 2. urethral g's (male). **lymph g.,** see under *node*. **mammary g.,** the specialized gland of the skin of female mammals, which secretes milk for nourishment of the young. **meibomian g's,** sebaceous follicles between the cartilage and conjunctiva of eyelids. **merocrine g.,** one in which the secretory cells maintain their integrity throughout the secretory cycle. **mixed g's,** 1. seromucous g's. 2. glands that have both exocrine and endocrine portions. **monoptychial g.,** one in which the tubules or alveoli are lined with a single layer of secreting cells. **Morgagni's g's,** urethral g's (male). **mucous g.,** a gland that secretes mucus. **nabothian g's,** see under

follicle. **Nuhn's g's,** anterior lingual g's. **olfactory g's,** small mucous glands in the olfactory mucosa. **parathyroid g's,** small bodies in the region of the thyroid gland, developed from the endoderm of the branchial clefts, occurring in a variable number of pairs, commonly two; they secrete parathyroid hormone and are concerned chiefly with the metabolism of calcium and phosphorus. **paraurethral g's,** see *paraurethral ducts of female urethra* and *paraurethral ducts of male urethra,* under *duct.* **parotid g.,** the largest of the three paired salivary glands, located in front of the ear. **Peyer's g's,** see under *patch.* **pharyngeal g's,** mucous glands beneath the tunica mucosa of the pharynx. **pineal g.,** see under *body.* **pituitary g.,** hypophysis; the epithelial body of dual origin at the base of the brain in the sella turcica, attached by a stalk to the hypothalamus. It consists of two main lobes, the *anterior lobe* or *adenohypophysis,* secreting most of the hormones, and the *posterior lobe* or *neurohypophysis,* which stores and releases neurohormones received from the hypothalamus. **preputial g's,** small sebaceous glands of the corona of the penis and the inner surface of the prepuce, which secrete smegma. **proper gastric g's,** fundic g's. **prostate g.,** prostate. **pyloric g's,** the mucin-secreting glands of the pyloric part of the stomach. **racemose g's,** glands composed of acini arranged like grapes on a stem. **saccular g.,** one consisting of a sac or sacs, lined with glandular epithelium. **salivary g's,** glands of the oral cavity whose combined secretion constitutes the saliva, including the parotid, sublingual, and submandibular glands and numerous small glands in the tongue, lips, cheeks, and palate. **sebaceous g.,** one of the holocrine glands in the dermis that secrete sebum. **seromucous g.,** one containing both serous and mucous secreting cells. **serous g.,** a gland that secretes a watery albuminous material, commonly but not always containing enzymes. **sex g.,** gonad. **simple g.,** one with a nonbranching duct. **Skene's g's,** paraurethral ducts of female urethra. **solitary g's,** see under *follicle.* **submandibular g., submaxillary g.,** a salivary gland on the inner side of each ramus of the lower jaw. **suprarenal g.,** adrenal g. **Suzanne's g.,** a mucous gland of the mouth, beneath the alveolingual groove. **sweat g.,** a gland that secretes sweat, found in the dermis or subcutaneous tissue, opening by a duct on the body surface. The ordinary or *eccrine* sweat glands are distributed over most of the body surface, and promote cooling by evaporation of the secretion; the *apocrine* sweat glands empty into the upper portion of a hair follicle instead of directly onto the skin, and are found only in certain body areas, as around the anus and in the axilla. **target g.,** one specifically affected by a pituitary hormone. **tarsal g's, tarsoconjunctival g's,** meibomian g's. **thymus g.,** see *thymus.* **thyroid g.,** an endocrine gland consisting of two lobes, one on each side of the trachea, joined by a narrow isthmus, producing hormones (thyroxine and triiodothyronine), which require iodine for their elaboration and which are concerned in regulating metabolic rate; it also secretes calcitonin. **Tyson's g's,** preputial g's. **unicellular g.,** a single cell that functions as a gland, e.g., a goblet cell. **urethral g's,** mucous glands in the wall of the urethra. **uterine g's,** simple tubular glands found throughout the endometrium. **vesical g's,** mucous glands sometimes found in the wall of the urinary bladder, especially in the area of the trigone. **vestibular g., greater,** Bartholin's gland: either of two small reddish yellow bodies in the vestibular bulbs, one on each side of the vaginal orifice. **vestibular g's, lesser,** small mucous glands opening upon the vestibular mucous membrane between the urethral and the vaginal orifice. **Virchow's g.,** sentinel node. **vulvovaginal g.,** Bartholin's g. **Waldeyer's g's,** glands in the attached edge of the eyelid. **Weber's g's,** the tubular mucous glands of the tongue. **g's of Zeis,** modified rudimentary sebaceous glands attached directly to the eyelash follicles.

glan·ders (glan′derz) a contagious disease of horses, communicable to humans, due to *Pseudomonas mallei,* and marked by purulent inflammation of the mucous membranes and cutaneous eruption of nodules that coalesce and break down, forming deep ulcers, which may end in necrosis of cartilage and bone; the more chronic and constitutional form is known as *farcy.*

glan·di·lem·ma (glan″dĭ-lem′ah) the capsule or outer envelope of a gland.

glan·du·la (glan′du-lah) pl. *glan′dulae.* [L.] a gland.

glan·du·lar (glan′du-ler) 1. pertaining to or of the nature of a gland. 2. glanular.

glan·dule (glan′dūl) a small gland.

glans (glanz) pl. *glan′des.* [L.] a small, rounded mass or glandlike body. **g. clito′ridis, g. of clitoris,** erectile tissue on the free end of the clitoris. **g. pe′nis,** the cap-shaped expansion of the corpus spongiosum at the end of the penis.

glan·u·lar (glan′u-ler) pertaining to the glans penis or glans clitoridis.

glan·u·lo·plas·ty (glan′u-lo-plas″te) plastic surgery on a glans.

glare (glār) discomfort in the eye and depression of central vision produced when a bright light enters the field of vision, particularly when the eye is adapted to dark. It is *direct g.* when the image of the light falls on the fovea and *indirect g.* when it falls outside the fovea.

glass (glas) 1. a hard, brittle, often transparent material, usually consisting of the fused amorphous silicates of potassium or sodium, and of calcium, with silica in excess. 2. a container, usually cylindrical, made from glass. **cupping g.,** a vessel of glass from which the air has been or can be exhausted, applied to the body to draw blood to the surface.

glass·es (glas′iz) spectacles; lenses arranged in a frame holding them in the proper position before the eyes, as an aid to vision. **bifocal g.,** those with bifocal lenses. **trifocal g.,** those with trifocal lenses.

gla·tir·a·mer (glah-tir′ah-mer) an immunomodulator used as the acetate ester to reduce relapses in multiple sclerosis.

glau·co·ma (glaw-, glou-ko′mah) a group of eye diseases characterized by an increase in intraocular pressure, causing pathological changes in the optic disk and typical visual field defects. **glauco′matous,** adj. **congenital g.,** that due to defective development of the structures in and around the anterior chamber of the eye and resulting in impairment of aqueous humor; seen first at birth or up to age three. **Donders' g.,** advanced open-angle g. **infantile g.,** congenital g. **narrow-angle g.,** a form of primary glaucoma in an eye characterized by a shallow anterior chamber and a narrow angle, in which filtration is compromised as a result of the iris blocking the angle. **open-angle g.,** a form of primary glaucoma in an eye in which the angle of the anterior chamber remains open, but filtration is gradually diminished because of the tissues of the angle. **primary g.,** increased intraocular pressure occurring in an eye without previous disease.

glaze (glāz) in dentistry, a ceramic veneer added to a porcelain restoration, to simulate enamel.

GLC gas-liquid chromatography.

gle·no·hu·mer·al (gle″no-hu′mer-al) pertaining to the glenoid cavity and the humerus.

gle·noid (gle′noid) resembling a pit or socket.

glia (gli′ah) neuroglia.

glia·cyte (-sīt) a cell of the neuroglia.

gli·a·din (-din) a protein present in wheat; it contains the toxic factor associated with celiac disease.

gli·al (gli″l) of or pertaining to the neuroglia.

gli·mep·i·ride (gli-mep′ĭ-rīd) a sulfonylurea compound used as a hypoglycemic in the treatment of type 2 diabetes mellitus.

glio·blas·to·ma (gli″o-blas-to′mah) any malignant astrocytoma. **g. multifor′me**, the most malignant type of astrocytoma, composed of spongioblasts, astroblasts, and astrocytes; it usually occurs in the brain but may occur in the brain stem or spinal cord.

gli·o·ma (gli-o′mah) a tumor composed of neuroglia in any of its states of development; sometimes extended to include all intrinsic neoplasms of the brain and spinal cord, as astrocytomas, ependymomas, etc. **glio′matous**, adj. **g. re′tinae**, retinoblastoma.

gli·o·ma·to·sis (gli″o-mah-to′sis) diffuse formation of gliomas.

gli·o·sis (gli-o′sis) an excess of astroglia in damaged areas of the central nervous system.

glip·i·zide (glip′ĭ-zīd) a sulfonylurea used as a hypoglycemic in the treatment of type 2 diabetes mellitus.

glis·sade (glis-ād′) [Fr.] a gliding involuntary movement of the eye in changing the point of fixation; it is a slower, smoother movement than is a saccade. **glissad′ic**, adj.

glis·so·ni·tis (glis″ah-ni′tis) inflammation of Glisson's capsule.

glo·bi (glo′bi) plural of *globus.*

glo·bin (glo′bin) 1. the protein constituent of hemoglobin. 2. any of a group of proteins similar to the typical globin.

glo·boid (glo′boid) globe-shaped; spheroid.

glob·o·side (glob′o-sīd) a glycosphingolipid containing acetylated amino sugars and simple hexoses that accumulates in tissues in Sandhoff's disease but not in Tay-Sachs disease.

glob·ule (glob′ūl) 1. a small spherical mass or body. 2. a small spherical drop of fluid or semifluid substance. 3. a little globe or pellet, as of medicine. **glob′ular**, adj.

glob·u·lin (glob′u-lin) any of a class of proteins insoluble in water, but soluble in saline solutions (euglobulins), or water-soluble proteins (pseudoglobulins); their other physical properties resemble true globulins; see *serum g.* **α-g's**, serum globulins with the most rapid electrophoretic mobility, further subdivided into faster α_1- and slower α_2-globulins. **AC g., accelerator g.**, coagulation factor V. **alpha g's**, α-g's. **antihemophilic g. (AHG)**, coagulation factor VIII. **antilymphocyte g. (ALG)**, the gamma globulin fraction of antilymphocyte serum (q.v.), used as an immunosuppressant in organ transplantation. **antithymocyte g. (ATG)**, the gamma globulin fraction of antiserum derived from animals (e.g., rabbits) that have been immunized against human thymocytes; it causes specific destruction of T lymphocytes, used in treatment of allograft rejection. **β-g's**, globulins in plasma which, in neutral or alkaline solutions, have an electrophoretic mobility between those of the alpha and gamma globulins. **bacterial polysaccharide immune g. (BPIG)**, a human immune globulin derived from the blood plasma of adult human donors immunized with *Haemophilus influenzae* type b, pneumococcal, and meningococcal polysaccharide vaccines; used for the passive immunization of infants under 18 months of age. **beta g's**, β-g's. **cytomegalovirus immune g.**, a purified immunoglobulin derived from pooled adult human plasma selected for high titers of antibody against cytomegalovirus (CMV); used for the treatment and prophylaxis of cytomegalovirus disease in transplant recipients. **γ-g's**, **gamma g's**, serum globulins having the least rapid electrophoretic mobility; the fraction is composed almost entirely of immunoglobulins. **hepatitis B immune g.**, a specific immune globulin derived from blood plasma of human donors with high titers of antibodies against hepatitis B surface antigen; used as a passive immunizing agent. **hyperimmune g.**, any of various immunoglobulin preparations especially high in antibodies against certain specific diseases. **immune g.**, 1. immunoglobulin. 2. a concentrated preparation of gamma globulins, predominantly IgG, from a large pool of human donors; used for passive immunization against measles, hepatitis A, and varicella and for replacement therapy in patients with immunoglobulin deficiencies. **immune human serum g.**, immune g. (2). **immune g. intravenous (human),** a preparation of immune globulin suitable for intravenous administration; used in the treatment of primary and secondary immunodeficiency states, idiopathic thrombocytopenic purpura, and Kawasaki disease. **immune serum g.**, immune g. (2). **pertussis immune g.**, a specific immune globulin derived from the blood plasma of human donors immunized with pertussis vaccine; used for the prophylaxis and treatment of pertussis. **rabies immune g.**, a specific immune globulin derived from blood plasma or serum of human donors who have been immunized with rabies vaccine and have high titers of rabies antibody; used as a passive immunizing agent. **respiratory syncytial virus immune g. intravenous,** a preparation of immunoglobulin G (IgG) from pooled adult human plasma selected for high titers of antibodies against respiratory syncytial virus; used for passive immunization of infants and young children. **Rh₀(D) immune g.,** a specific immune globulin derived from human blood plasma containing antibody to the erythrocyte factor Rh₀(D); used to prevent Rh-sensitization of Rh-negative females and thus prevent erythroblastosis fetalis in subsequent pregnancies; administered within 72 hours after exposure to Rh-positive blood resulting from delivery of an Rh-positive child, abortion or miscarriage of an Rh-positive fetus, or transfusion of Rh-positive blood; also used to stimulate the platelet count in idiopathic thrombocytopenic purpura. **serum g's,** all plasma proteins except albumin, which is not a globulin, and fibrinogen, which is not in the serum; they are subdivided into α-, β-, and γ-globulins. **sex hormone–binding g. (SHBG),** a β-globulin in plasma that binds to and transports testosterone, and to a lesser degree estrogens. **specific immune g.,** a preparation of immune globulin derived from a donor pool preselected for a high antibody titer against a specific antigen. **tetanus immune g.,** a specific immune globulin derived from the blood plasma of human donors who have been immunized with tetanus toxoid; used in the prophylaxis and treatment of tetanus. **varicella-zoster immune g. (VZIG),** a specific immune globulin derived from plasma of human donors with high titers of varicella-zoster antibodies; used as a passive immunizing agent.

glo·bus (glo'bus) pl. *glo'bi.* [L.] 1. sphere. 2. a spherical structure. 3. eyeball. 4. one of the encapsulated globular masses containing bacilli, seen in smears of lepromatous leprosy lesions. **g. hyste'ricus,** subjective sensation of a lump in the throat. **g. pal'lidus,** the smaller and more medial part of the lentiform nucleus.

glo·man·gi·o·ma (glo-man″je-o′mah) glomus tumor (1).

glom·era (glom′er-ah) plural of *glomus.*

glo·mer·u·lar (glo-mer′u-ler) pertaining to or of the nature of a glomerulus, especially a renal glomerulus.

glo·mer·u·lo·ne·phri·tis (glo-mer″u-lo-nĕ-fri′tis) nephritis with inflammation of the capillary loops in the renal glomeruli. **acute g.,** an acute form characterized by proteinuria, edema, hematuria, renal failure, and hypertension, sometimes preceded by tonsillitis or febrile pharyngitis. **chronic g.,** a slowly progressive glomerulonephritis

generally leading to irreversible renal failure. **diffuse g.,** a severe form with proliferative changes in more than half the glomeruli, often with epithelial crescent formation and necrosis; often seen in advanced systemic lupus erythematosus. **IgA g.,** IgA nephropathy; a chronic form marked by a hematuria and proteinuria and by deposits of immunoglobulin A in the mesangial areas of the renal glomeruli, with subsequent reactive hyperplasia of mesangial cells. **lobular g., membranoproliferative g.,** a chronic, slowly progressive glomerulonephritis in which the glomeruli are enlarged as a result of proliferation of mesangial cells and irregular thickening of the capillary walls, which narrows the capillary lumina. **membranous g.,** a form characterized histologically by proteinaceous deposits on the glomerular capillary basement membrane or by thickening of the membrane; clinically resembling chronic glomerulonephritis, occasionally with transient nephrotic syndrome. **mesangiocapillary g.,** membranoproliferative g.

glo·mer·u·lop·a·thy (glo-mer″u-lop′ah-the) any disease of the renal glomeruli. **diabetic g.,** diabetic glomerulosclerosis.

glo·mer·u·lo·scle·ro·sis (glo-mer″u-lo-sklĕ-ro′sis) fibrosis and scarring resulting in senescence of the renal glomeruli. **diabetic g.,** intercapillary g. **focal segmental g.,** a syndrome of focal sclerosing lesions of the renal glomeruli with proteinuria, hematuria, hypertension, and nephrosis, with variable progression to end-stage renal disease. **intercapillary g.,** a degenerative complication of diabetes, manifested as albuminuria, nephrotic edema, hypertension, renal insufficiency, and retinopathy.

glo·mer·u·lus (glo-mer′u-lus) pl. *glomer′uli.* [L.] a small tuft or cluster, as of blood vessels or nerve fibers; often used alone to designate one of the renal glomeruli. **olfactory g.,** one of the small globular masses of dense neuropil in the olfactory bulb, containing the first synapse in the olfactory pathway. **renal g.,** globular tufts of capillaries, one projecting into the expanded end or capsule of each of the uriniferous tubules, which together with the glomerular capsule constitute the renal corpuscle.

glo·mus (glo′mus) pl. *glom′era.* [L.] 1. a small histologically recognizable body composed of fine arterioles connecting directly with veins, and having a rich nerve supply. 2. a specialized arteriovenous shunt occurring predominantly in the skin of the hands and feet, regulating blood flow and temperature. **glo'mera aor'tica,** aortic bodies.

g. caro′ticum, carotid body. choroid g., g. choroi′deum, an enlargement of the choroid plexus of the lateral ventricle. coccygeal g., g. coccy′geum, a collection of arteriovenous anastomoses near the tip of the coccyx, formed by the middle sacral artery. jugular g., g. jugula′re, tympanic body.

glos·sal (glos′al) lingual.

glos·sec·to·my (glos-ek′tah-me) excision of all or a portion of the tongue.

Glos·si·na (glos-i′nah) the tsetse flies, a genus of biting flies that are vectors of trypanosomes causing trypanosomiasis in humans and other animals.

glos·si·tis (glos-i′tis) inflammation of the tongue. g. area′ta exfoliati′va, benign migratory g., an inflammatory disease of the tongue characterized by multiple annular areas of desquamation of the filiform papillae, presenting as reddish lesions outlined in yellow that shift from area to area every few days. median rhomboid g., a congenital anomaly of the tongue, with a reddish patch or plaque on the midline of the dorsal surface.

gloss(o)- word element [Gr.], tongue.

glos·so·cele (glos′o-sēl) swelling and protrusion of the tongue.

glos·so·graph (-graf) an apparatus for registering tongue movements in speech.

glos·so·la·lia (glos″o-la′le-ah) gibberish that simulates coherent speech.

glos·sol·o·gy (glos-ol′ah-je) the sum of knowledge regarding the tongue.

glos·so·pal·a·tine (glos″o-pal′ah-tīn) palatoglossal.

glos·so·pha·ryn·ge·al (-fah-rin′je-al) pertaining to the tongue and pharynx.

glos·so·plas·ty (glos′o-plas″te) plastic surgery of the tongue.

glos·sor·rha·phy (glos-or′ah-fe) suture of the tongue.

glos·so·trich·ia (glos″o-trik′e-ah) hairy tongue.

glot·tis (glot′is) pl. glot′tides. [Gr.] the vocal apparatus of the larynx, consisting of the true vocal cords and the opening between them. glot′tal, adj.

glot·tog·ra·phy (glŏ-tog′rah-fe) the recording of the movements of the vocal cords during respiration and phonation.

Glu glutamic acid.

glu·ca·gon (gloo′kah-gon) a polypeptide hormone secreted by the alpha cells of the islets of Langerhans in response to hypoglycemia or to stimulation by growth hormone, which stimulates glycogenolysis in the liver; used as the hydrochloride salt as an antihypoglycemic and as an adjunct in gastrointestinal radiography.

glu·ca·gon·o·ma (gloo″kah-gon-o′mah) an islet cell tumor of the alpha cells that secretes glucagon.

glu·can (gloo′kan) any polysaccharide composed only of recurring units of glucose; a homopolymer of glucose.

glu·cep·tate (glu-sep′tāt) USAN contraction for glucoheptonate, a 7-carbon carbohydrate derivative.

glu·ci·tol (gloo′si-tol) sorbitol.

glu·co·am·y·lase (gloo″ko-am′ĭ-lās) acid maltase.

glu·co·cer·e·bro·si·dase (-ser″ĕ-bro-si′dās) glucosylceramidase.

glu·co·cer·e·bro·side (-ser′ĕ-bro-sīd″) a cerebroside with a glucose sugar.

glu·co·cor·ti·coid (-kor′tĭ-koid) 1. any of the group of corticosteroids predominantly involved in carbohydrate metabolism, and also in fat and protein metabolism and many other activities (e.g., alteration of connective tissue response to injury and inhibition of inflammatory and allergic reactions); some also exhibit varying degrees of mineralocorticoid activity. In humans, the most important glucocorticoids are cortisol (hydrocortisone) and cortisone. 2. of, pertaining to, or resembling a glucocorticoid.

glu·co·fu·ra·nose (-fu′rah-nōs) glucose in the cyclic furanose configuration, a minor constituent of glucose solutions.

glu·co·ki·nase (-ki′nās) 1. an enzyme of invertebrates and microorganisms that catalyzes the phosphorylation of glucose to glucose 6-phosphate. 2. the liver isozyme of hexokinase.

glu·co·ki·net·ic (-kĭ-net′ik) activating sugar so as to maintain the sugar level of the body.

glu·co·nate (gloo′ko-nāt) a salt, ester, or anionic form of gluconic acid.

glu·co·neo·gen·e·sis (gloo″ko-ne″o-jen′ĕ-sis) the synthesis of glucose from molecules that are not carbohydrates, such as amino and fatty acids.

glu·con·ic ac·id (gloo-kon′ik) the hexonic acid derived from glucose by oxidation of the C-1 aldehyde to a carboxyl group.

glu·co·phore (gloo′ko-for) the group of atoms in a molecule which gives the compound a sweet taste.

glu·co·py·ra·nose (-pir′ah-nōs) glucose in the cyclic pyranose configuration, the predominant form.

glu·co·reg·u·la·tion (-reg″ŭl-a′shun) regulation of glucose metabolism.

glu·co·sa·mine (gloo-ko′sah-mēn) an amino derivative of glucose, occurring in glycosaminoglycans and a variety of complex polysaccharides such as blood group substances. The sulfate salt is used as a nutritional supplement and as a popular remedy for osteoarthritis.

glu·co·san (gloo′ko-san) glucan.

glu·cose (gloo′kōs) 1. a six-carbon aldose occurring as the D- form and found as a free monosaccharide in fruits and other plants or combined in glucosides and di-, oligo-, and polysaccharides. It is the end product of carbohydrate metabolism, and is the chief source of energy for living organisms, its utilization being controlled by insulin. Excess glucose is converted to glycogen and stored in the liver and muscles for use as needed and, beyond that, is converted to fat and stored as adipose tissue. Glucose appears in the urine in diabetes mellitus. In pharmaceuticals, called *dextrose.* 2. liquid g. **liquid g.,** a thick, sweet, syrupy liquid obtained by incomplete hydrolysis of starch and consisting chiefly of dextrose, with dextrins, maltose, and water; used as a pharmaceutic aid. **g. 1-phosphate,** an intermediate in carbohydrate metabolism. **g. 6-phosphate,** an intermediate in carbohydrate metabolism.

glu·cose-6-phos·pha·tase (fos′fah-tās″) an enzyme that catalyzes the hydrolytic dephosphorylation of glucose 6-phosphate, the principal route for hepatic gluconeogenesis; deficiency causes glycogen storage disease, type I.

glu·cose-6-phos·phate de·hy·dro·gen·ase (G6PD) (-fos′fāt de-hi′dro-jen-ās) an enzyme of the pentose phosphate pathway which, with NADP+ as coenzyme, catalyzes the oxidation of glucose 6-phosphate to a lactone. Deficiency of the enzyme causes severe hemolytic anemia.

glu·co·si·dase (gloo-ko′sĭ-dās) any of a group of enzymes of the hydrolase class that hydrolyze glucose residues from glucosides; they are specific for α- or β-configurations as well as for particular substrate configurations, e.g., maltase.

glu·co·side (gloo′ko-sīd) a glycoside in which the sugar constituent is glucose.

glu·co·syl·cer·am·i·dase (gloo″ko-sil-ser-am′ĭ-dās) an enzyme that catalyzes the hydrolytic cleavage of glucose from glucocerebrosides to form ceramides in the lysosomal degradation of sphingolipids. Deficiency of enzyme activity, an autosomal recessive trait, results in Gaucher disease.

glu·cu·ron·ic ac·id (gloo-ku-ron′ik) the uronic acid derived from glucose; it is a constituent of several glycosaminoglycans and also forms conjugates (glucuronides) with drugs and toxins in their biotransformation.

β-glu·cu·ron·i·dase (gloo″ku-ron′ĭ-dās) an enzyme that attacks terminal glycosidic linkages in natural and synthetic glucuronides and that has been implicated in estrogen metabolism and cell division; it occurs in the spleen, liver, and endocrine glands; deficiency results in Sly's syndrome.

glu·cu·ron·ide (gloo-ku′ron-īd) any glycosidic compound of glucuronic acid; they are common soluble conjugates formed as a step in the metabolism and excretion of many toxins and drugs, such as phenols and alcohols.

glu·ta·mate (gloo′tah-māt) a salt of glutamic acid; in biochemistry, the term is often used interchangeably with glutamic acid.

glu·ta·mate for·mim·i·no·trans·fer·ase (for-mim″ĭ-no-trans′fer-ās) a transferase catalyzing a step in the degradation of histidine; decreased enzyme activity has been associated with urinary excretion of formiminoglutamate and mental retardation.

glu·tam·ic ac·id (gloo-tam′ik) a dibasic, nonessential amino acid widely distributed in proteins, a neurotransmitter that inhibits neural excitation in the central nervous system; its hydrochloride salt is used as a gastric acidifier. Symbols Glu and E.

glu·tam·i·nase (gloo-tam′ĭ-nās) an enzyme that catalyzes the deamination of glutamine to form glutamate and an ammonium ion; most of the latter are converted to urea via the urea cycle.

glu·ta·mine (glōōt′ah-mēn) the monoamide of glutamic acid, a nonessential amino acid occurring in proteins; it is an important carrier of urinary ammonia and is broken down in the kidney by the enzyme glutaminase. Symbols Gln and Q.

glu·ta·ral (gloo′tah-ral) glutaraldehyde.

glu·ta·ral·de·hyde (gloo″tah-ral′dĕ-hīd) a disinfectant used in aqueous solution for sterilization of non-heat–resistant equipment; also used as a tissue fixative for light and electron microscopy.

glu·tar·ic ac·id (gloo-tar′ik) a dicarboxylic acid intermediate in the metabolism of tryptophan and lysine.

glu·tar·ic·ac·i·de·mia (gloo-tar″ik-as″ĭ-de′me-ah) 1. glutaricaciduria (1). 2. an excess of glutaric acid in the blood.

glu·tar·ic·ac·id·uria (-du′re-ah) 1. an aminoacidopathy characterized by accumulation and excretion of glutaric acid; there are two types (I and II) due to different enzyme deficiencies, with a spectrum of manifestations. 2. excretion of glutaric acid in the urine.

glu·ta·thi·one (gloo″tah-thi′ōn) a tripeptide of glutamic acid, cysteine, and glycine, existing in reduced (GSH) and oxidized (GSSG) forms and functioning in various redox reactions: in the destruction of peroxides and free radicals, as a cofactor for enzymes, and in the detoxification of harmful compounds. It is also involved in the formation and maintenance of disulfide bonds in proteins and in transport of amino acids across cell membranes.

glu·ta·thi·one syn·the·tase (sin′thĕ-tās) a ligase catalyzing the formation of glutathione; deficient activity causes decreased levels of glutathione and increased levels of 5-oxoproline and cysteine. If confined to erythrocytes, the deficiency results in well-compensated hemolytic anemia; if generalized, metabolic acidosis and neurologic dysfunction may also occur.

glu·te·al (gloo′te-al) pertaining to the buttocks.

glu·ten (gloo′ten) the protein of wheat and other grains that gives to the dough its tough elastic character.

glu·teth·i·mide (gloo-teth′ĭ-mīd) a nonbarbiturate used as a hypnotic and sedative.

glu·ti·nous (gloo′tĭ-nus) adhesive; sticky.

gly·bur·ide (gli′būr-īd) a sulfonylurea used as a hypoglycemic in the treatment of type 2 diabetes mellitus.

Gly glycine.

gly·can (gli′kan) polysaccharide.

gly·ce·mia (gli-se′me-ah) the presence of glucose in the blood.

glyc·er·al·de·hyde (glis″er-al′dĕ-hīd) an aldose, the aldehyde form of the three-carbon sugar derived from the oxidation of glycerol; isomeric with dihydroxyacetone. The 3-phosphate derivative is an intermediate in the metabolism of glucose, in both the Embden-Meyerhof and pentose phosphate pathways.

gly·cer·ic acid (gli-sēr′ik) $CH_2OH·CHOH·COOH$, an intermediate product in the transformation in the body of carbohydrate to lactic acid, formed by oxidation of glycerol.

glyc·er·ide (glis′er-īd) acylglycerol; an organic acid ester of glycerol, designated, according to the number of ester linkages, as mono-, di-, or triglyceride.

glyc·er·in (-in) a clear, colorless, syrupy liquid used as a laxative, an osmotic diuretic to reduce intraocular pressure, a demulcent in cough preparations, and a humectant and solvent for drugs. Cf. *glycerol.*

glyc·er·ol (-ol) a trihydroxy sugar alcohol that is the backbone of many lipids and an important intermediate in carbohydrate and lipid metabolism. Pharmaceutical preparations are called *glycerin.*

glyc·er·ol·ize (-ol-īz) to treat with or preserve in glycerol, as in the exposure of red blood cells to glycerol solution so that glycerol diffuses into the cells before they are frozen for preservation.

glyc·er·yl (-il) the mono-, di-, or trivalent radical formed by the removal of hydrogen from one, two, or three of the hydroxy groups of glycerol. **g. monostearate,** an emulsifying agent. **g. trinitrate,** nitroglycerin.

gly·cine (G, Gly) (gli′sēn) a nonessential amino acid occurring as a constituent of proteins and functioning as an inhibitory neurotransmitter in the central nervous system; used as a gastric antacid and dietary supplement, and as a bladder irrigation in transurethral prostatectomy.

gly·co·cal·yx (gli″ko-kal′iks) the glycoprotein-polysaccharide covering that surrounds many cells.

gly·co·cho·late (-ko′lāt) a salt of glycocholic acid.

gly·co·cho·lic ac·id (-ko′lik) cholylglycine.

gly·co·con·ju·gate (-kon′joo-gat) any of the complex molecules containing glycosidic linkages, such as glycolipids, glycopeptides, oligosaccharides, or glycosaminoglycans.

gly·co·gen (gli′ko-jen) a highly branched polysaccharide of glucose chains, the chief carbohydrate storage material in animals, stored primarily in liver and muscle; it is synthesized and degraded for energy as demanded. **glycogen′ic,** adj.

gly·co·gen·e·sis (gli″ko-jen′ĕ-sis) the conversion of glucose to glycogen for storage in the liver. **glycogenet′ic,** adj.

gly·co·ge·nol·y·sis (-jĕ-nol′ĭ-sis) the splitting up of glycogen in the liver, yielding glucose. **glycogenolyt′ic,** adj.

gly·co·ge·no·sis (-jĕ-no′sis) glycogen storage disease.

gly·co·gen phos·phor·y·lase (gli′ko-jen fos-for′ĭ-lās) see *phosphorylase.*

gly·co·geu·sia (gli″ko-goo′zhah) a sweet taste in the mouth.

gly·col (gli′kol) any of a group of aliphatic dihydric alcohols, having marked hygroscopic properties and useful as solvents and plasticizers. **polyethylene g.,** see under *P.*

gly·col·ic acid (gli-kol′ik) an intermediate in the conversion of serine to glycine; it is accumulated and excreted in primary hyperoxaluria (type I).

gly·co·lip·id (gli″ko-lip′id) a lipid containing carbohydrate groups, usually galactose but also glucose, inositol, or others; while it can describe those lipids derived from either glycerol or sphingosine, with or without phosphates, the term is usually used to denote the sphingosine derivatives lacking phosphate groups (glycosphingolipids).

gly·col·y·sis (gli-kol′ĭ-sis) the anaerobic enzymatic conversion of glucose to the simpler compounds lactate or pyruvate, resulting in energy stored in the form of ATP, as occurs in muscle. **glycolyt′ic**, adj.

gly·co·neo·gen·e·sis (gli″ko-ne″o-jen′ĕ-sis) gluconeogenesis.

gly·co·pe·nia (-pe′ne-ah) a deficiency of sugar in the tissues.

gly·co·pep·tide (-pep′tīd) any of a class of peptides that contain carbohydrates, including those that contain amino sugars.

gly·co·phil·ia (-fil′e-ah) a condition in which a small amount of glucose produces hyperglycemia.

gly·co·phor·in (-for′in) any of several related proteins that can project through the thickness of the cell membrane of erythrocytes; they attach to oligosaccharides at the outer cell membrane surface and to contractile proteins (spectrin and actin) at the cytoplasmic surface.

gly·co·pro·tein (-pro′tēn) a conjugated protein covalently linked to one or more carbohydrate groups; technically those with less than 4 per cent carbohydrate but often expanded to include the mucoproteins and proteoglycans.

gly·co·pyr·ro·late (-pir′o-lāt) a synthetic anticholinergic used as a gastrointestinal antispasmodic, a preanesthetic antisialagogue, and an antiarrhythmic for anesthesia- or surgery-associated arrhythmias.

gly·cor·rhea (-re′ah) any sugary discharge from the body.

gly·cos·ami·no·gly·can (gli″kōs-ah-me″no-gli′kan) any of a group of high molecular weight linear polysaccharides with various disaccharide repeating units and usually occurring in proteoglycans, including the chondroitin sulfates, dermatan sulfates, heparan sulfate and heparin, keratan sulfates, and hyaluronic acid. Abbreviated GAG.

gly·co·se·cre·to·ry (gli″ko-se-krēt′er-e) concerned in secretion of glycogen.

gly·co·se·mia (-sēm′e-ah) glycemia.

gly·co·si·a·lia (-si-a′le-ah) sugar in the saliva.

gly·co·si·a·lor·rhea (-si″ah-lo-re′ah) excessive flow of saliva containing glucose.

gly·co·si·dase (gli-ko′sĭ-dās) any of a group of hydrolytic enzymes that catalyze the cleavage of hemiacetal bonds of glycosides. **β-g.,** 1. a glycosidase specifically cleaving β-linked sugar residues from glycosides. 2. see under *complex.*

gly·co·side (gli′ko-sīd) any compound containing a carbohydrate molecule (sugar), particularly any such natural product in plants, convertible, by hydrolytic cleavage, into a sugar and a nonsugar component (aglycone), and named specifically for the sugar contained, as glucoside (glucose), pentoside (pentose), fructoside (fructose), etc. **cardiac g.,** any of a group of glycosides occurring in certain plants (e.g., *Digitalis, Strophanthus, Urginea*), acting on the contractile force of cardiac muscle; some are used as cardiotonics and antiarrhythmics. **digitalis g.,** any of a number of cardiotonic and antiarrhythmic glycosides derived from *Digitalis purpurea* and *D. lanata*, or any drug chemically and pharmacologically related to these glycosides.

gly·co·sphingo·lip·id (gli″ko-sfing″go-lip′id) any sphingolipid in which the head group is a mono- or oligosaccharide; included are the cerebrosides, sulfatides, and gangliosides.

gly·co·stat·ic (-stat′ik) tending to maintain a constant sugar level.

gly·cos·uria (su′re-ah) the presence of glucose in the urine. **renal g.,** that due to inherited inability of the renal tubules to reabsorb glucose completely.

gly·co·syl (gli′ko-sil) a radical derived from a carbohydrate by removal of the anomeric hydroxyl group.

gly·co·syl·a·tion (gli-ko″sĭ-la′shun) the formation of linkages with glycosyl groups.

gly·co·syl·cer·am·i·dase (gli-ko″sil-sĕ-ram′ĭ-dās) an enzyme that catalyzes the hydrolytic cleavage of β-linked sugar residues from β-glycosides with large hydrophobic aglycons; such activity occurs as part of the β-glycosidase complex, along with lactase, in the intestinal brush border membrane.

gly·co·tro·pic (gli″ko-tro′pik) having an affinity for sugar; antagonizing the effects of insulin; causing hyperglycemia.

glyc·yr·rhi·za (glis″ĭ-ri′zah) licorice.

gly·ox·y·late (gli-ok′sĭ-lāt) a salt, anion, or ester of glyoxylic acid.

gly·ox·yl·ic ac·id (gli-ok-sil′ik) a keto acid formed in the conversion of glycolic acid to glycine; it is the primary precursor of oxalic acid.

gm gram.

GM-CSF granulocyte-macrophage colony-stimulating factor.

GMP guanosine monophosphate. **3',5'-GMP, cyclic GMP,** cyclic guanosine monophosphate.

gnat (nat) a small dipterous insect. In Great Britain the term is applied to mosquitoes; in America to insects smaller than mosquitoes.

gnath·i·on (na′the-on) the most outward and everted point on the profile curvature of the chin.

gnath·itis (na-thi′tis) inflammation of the jaw.

gnath(o)- word element [Gr.], *jaw.*

gnatho·dy·na·mom·e·ter (nath″o-di″nah-mom′ĕ-ter) an instrument for measuring the force exerted in closing the jaws.

gnath·ol·o·gy (nah-thol′ah-je) a science dealing with the masticatory apparatus as a whole, including morphology, anatomy, histology, physiology, pathology, and therapeutics. **gnatholog′ic,** adj.

gnath·os·chi·sis (nah-thos′kĭ-sis) cleft jaw.

Gnath·os·to·ma (nah-thos′tah-mah) a genus of nematodes parasitic in cats, swine, cattle, and sometimes humans.

gnatho·sto·mi·a·sis (nath″o-sto-mi′ah-sis) infection with the nematode *Gnathostoma spinigerum,* acquired from eating undercooked fish infected with the larvae.

gno·sia (no′se-ah) the faculty of perceiving and recognizing. **gnos′tic,** adj.

gno·to·bi·ol·o·gy (nōt″o-bi-ol′ah-je) gnotobiotics.

gno·to·bio·ta (-bi-ōt′ah) the specifically and entirely known microfauna and microflora of a specially reared laboratory animal.

gno·to·bi·ote (-bi′ōt) a specially reared laboratory animal whose microflora and microfauna are specifically known in their entirety. **gnotobiot′ic,** adj.

Gn-RH gonadotropin-releasing hormone.

goi·ter (goi′ter) enlargement of the thyroid gland, causing a swelling in the front part of the neck. **goi′trous,** adj. **aberrant g.,** goiter of a supernumerary thyroid gland. **adenomatous g.,** that caused by adenoma or multiple colloid nodules of the thyroid gland. **Basedow's g.,** a colloid goiter which has become hyperfunctioning after administration of iodine. **colloid g.,** a large, soft goiter with distended spaces filled with colloid. **diffuse toxic g.,** Graves' disease. **diving g.,** one that is movable, sometimes above and sometimes below the sternal notch. **exophthalmic g.,** one accompanied by exophthalmos. **fibrous g.,** one in which the thyroid capsule and stroma are hyperplastic. **follicular g.,** parenchymatous g. **intrathoracic g.,** one in which a portion is in the

thoracic cavity. **iodide g.,** that occurring in reaction to iodides at high concentrations, due to inhibition of iodide organification. **lingual g.,** enlargement of the upper end of the thyroglossal duct, forming a tumor at the posterior part of the dorsum of the tongue. **lymphadenoid g.,** Hashimoto's disease. **multinodular g.,** goiter with circumscribed nodules within the gland. **nontoxic g.,** that occurring sporadically and not associated with hyperthyroidism or hypothyroidism. **parenchymatous g.,** one marked by increase in follicles and proliferation of epithelium. **simple g.,** simple hyperplasia of the thyroid gland. **suffocative g.,** one which causes dyspnea by pressure. **wandering g.,** diving g.

goi·trin (goi′trin) a goitrogenic substance isolated from rutabagas and turnips.

gold (Au) (gōld) chemical element (see *Table of Elements*), at. no. 79; gold compounds (all of which are poisonous) are used in medicine, chiefly in treating arthritis. **g. 198,** a radioisotope of gold with a half-life of 2.69 days; it has been used as an intracavitary and interstitial antineoplastic and as a scintiscanning agent. **cohesive g.,** chemically pure gold that forms a solid mass when properly condensed into a tooth cavity. **g. sodium thiomalate,** a monovalent gold salt used in treatment of rheumatoid arthritis.

gol·den·seal (gōl′den-sēl″) the North American herb *Hydrastis canadensis,* or its dried rhizome, a preparation of which is used in folk medicine and in homeopathy.

go·mit·o·li (go-mit′o-li) a network of capillaries in the upper infundibular stem (of the hypothalamus) that surround terminal arterioles of the superior hypophyseal arteries and that lead into portal veins to the adenohypophysis.

gom·pho·sis (gom-fo′sis) a type of fibrous joint in which a conical process is inserted into a socket-like portion.

go·nad (go′nad) a gamete-producing gland; an ovary or testis. **gonad′al, gonad′ial,** adj. **indifferent g.,** the sexually undifferentiated gonad of the early embryo. **streak g's,** undeveloped gonadal structures in the broad ligament below the fallopian tube, composed of whorled connective-tissue stroma without germinal or secretory cells; seen most often in Turner's syndrome.

go·nad·ar·che (go″nah-dahr′ke) the onset of gonadal functioning.

go·nad·ec·to·my (go″nah-dek′tah-me) surgical removal of an ovary or testis.

go·na·do·rel·in (go-nad″ah-rel′in) synthetic luteinizing hormone–releasing hormone; used as the acetate or hydrochloride salt in the evaluation of hypogonadism and as the acetate salt in the treatment of delayed puberty, infertility, and amenorrhea.

go·na·do·tox·ic (go-nad′ah-tok″sik) having a deleterious effect on the gonads, such as radiation or a chemotherapeutic agent.

go·nado·trope (go-nad′ah-trōp) gonadotroph.

go·nado·troph (-trōf) 1. a basophilic cell of the anterior pituitary specialized to secrete follicle-stimulating hormone and luteinizing hormone. 2. a substance that stimulates the gonads.

go·na·do·tro·phic (go-nad″ah-tro′fik) gonadotropic.

go·nado·tro·pic (-tro′pik) stimulating the gonads; applied to hormones of the anterior pituitary.

go·nado·tro·pin (-tro′pin) any hormone that stimulates the gonads, especially follicle-stimulating hormone and luteinizing hormone. **chorionic g., human chorionic g. (HCG, hCG),** a glycopeptide hormone produced by the fetal placenta syncytiotrophoblasts that maintains the function of the corpus luteum during the first few weeks of pregnancy; the basis for most commonly used pregnancy tests. It is used pharmaceutically to treat certain cases of cryptorchidism and male infertility, to induce ovulation and pregnancy in certain infertile, anovulatory women, and to stimulate oocyte development and maturation in patients using assisted reproductive technologies. See also *choriogonadotropin alfa.* **human menopausal g. (hMG),** menotropins.

gon·ag·ra (go-nag′rah) gout in the knee.

go·nal·gia (go-nal′jah) pain in the knee.

gon·ar·thri·tis (gon″ahr-thri′tis) inflammation of the knee joint.

gon·ar·throc·a·ce (-ahr-throk′ah-se) tuberculous arthritis of the knee.

go·ni·om·e·ter (go″ne-om′ĕ-ter) 1. an instrument for measuring angles. 2. a plank that can be tilted at one end to any height, used in testing for labyrinthine disease. **finger g.,** one for measuring the limits of flexion and extension of the interphalangeal joints of the fingers.

go·ni·om·e·try (go″ne-om′ĕ-tre) the measurement of angles, particularly those of range of motion of a joint.

go·ni·on (go′ne-on) pl. *go′nia.* [Gr.] the most inferior, posterior, and lateral point on the external angle of the mandible. **go′nial,** adj.

go·nio·punc·ture (go″ne-o-punk′cher) insertion of a knife blade through the clear cornea, just within the limbus, across the

anterior chamber of the eye and through the opposite corneoscleral wall, in treatment of glaucoma.

go·nio·scope (go′ne-ah-skōp″) an optical instrument for examining the anterior chamber of the eye and for demonstrating ocular motility and rotation.

go·ni·ot·o·my (go′ne-ot′ah-me) an operation for glaucoma; it consists in opening Schlemm's canal under direct vision.

gon(o)- word element [Gr.], *seed; semen.*

gono·coc·ce·mia (gon″o-kok-sēm′e-ah) the presence of gonococci in the blood.

gono·coc·cus (-kok′us) pl. *gonococ′ci.* An individual of the species *Neisseria gonorrhoeae,* the etiologic agent of gonorrhea. **gonococ′cal, gonococ′cic,** adj.

gono·cyte (gon′o-sīt) primordial germ cell.

gon·or·rhea (gon″ah-re′ah) infection with *Neisseria gonorrhoeae,* most often transmitted venereally, marked in males by urethritis with pain and purulent discharge; commonly asymptomatic in females, but may extend to produce salpingitis, oophoritis, tubo-ovarian abscess, and peritonitis. Bacteremia may occur in both sexes, causing skin lesions, arthritis, and rarely meningitis or endocarditis. **gonorrhe′al,** adj.

Gony·au·lax (gon″e-aw′laks) a genus of dinoflagellates found in fresh, salt, or brackish waters, having yellow to brown chromatophores; it includes *G. catanel′la,* a poisonous species, which helps to form the destructive red tide in the ocean; see also under *poison.*

gony·camp·sis (gon″ĭ-kamp′sis) abnormal curvature of the knee.

gonyo·cele (gon′e-o-sēl″) synovitis or tuberculous arthritis of the knee.

gony·on·cus (gon″e-ong′kus) tumor of the knee.

go·se·rel·in (go′sĕ-rel″in) a synthetic gonadotropin-releasing hormone; on prolonged administration it suppresses release of gonadotropins and is used as the acetate salt to treat breast and prostate carcinomas and endometriosis and to thin the endometrium prior to endometrial ablation.

gos·sy·pol (gos′ĭ-pol) a toxin found in cottonseed and detoxified by heating; it has male antifertility properties, apparently having its effects in the seminiferous tubules.

GOT aspartate transaminase (glutamic-oxaloacetic transaminase).

go·tu ko·la (go′too ko′lah) the creeping, umbelliferous plant *Centella asiaticus* or preparations of its leaves and stems, which are used to promote wound healing and to treat the lesions of leprosy; also widely used in ayurveda, traditional Chinese medicine, and Asian folk medicine

gouge (gouj) a hollow chisel for cutting and removing bone.

goun·dou (gōōn-doo′) a sequel of yaws and endemic syphilis, marked by headache, purulent nasal discharge, and formation of bony exostoses at the side of the nose.

gout (gout) a group of disorders of purine and pyrimidine metabolism, characterized by typhi causing recurrent paroxysmal attacks of acute inflammatory arthritis usually affecting a single peripheral joint, usually responsive to colchicine, and usually followed by complete remission; hyperuricemia and uric acid urolithiasis are also present in fully developed cases. **gout′y**, adj. **latent g., masked g.,** lithemia without the typical features of gout.

GP general paresis; general practitioner.

G6PD glucose-6-phosphate dehydrogenase.

GPT glutamic-pyruvic transaminase; see *alanine transaminase.*

grac·ile (gras′il) slender or delicate.

gra·di·ent (gra′de-ent) rate of increase or decrease of a variable value, or its graphic representation. **electrochemical g.,** a difference in ion concentration between two points so that ions tend to move passively along it.

grad·u·at·ed (graj′oo-āt″id) marked by a succession of lines, steps, or degrees.

graft (graft) 1. any tissue or organ for implantation or transplantation. 2. to implant or transplant such tissues. See also *implant.* **accordion g.,** a full-thickness graft in which slits have been made so that it may be stretched to cover a larger area. **arteriovenous g.,** an arteriovenous fistula consisting of a venous autograft or xenograft or a synthetic tube grafted onto the artery and vein. **avascular g.,** a graft of tissue in which not even transient vascularization is achieved. **Blair-Brown g.,** a split-skin graft of intermediate thickness. **bone g.,** a piece of bone used to take the place of a removed bone or bony defect. **cable g.,** a nerve graft made up of several sections of nerve in the manner of a cable. **coronary artery bypass g. (CABG),** see under *bypass.* **delayed g.,** a skin graft sutured back into its bed and subsequently shifted to a new recipient site. **dermal g., dermic g.,** skin from which epidermis and subcutaneous fat have been removed; used instead of fascia in various plastic procedures. **fascia g.,** one taken from the fascia lata or the lumbar fascia. **fascicular g.,** a nerve graft in which bundles of nerve fibers are approximated and sutured separately. **full-thickness g.,** a skin graft consisting of the full thickness of the skin, with little or none of the subcutaneous tissue. **heterodermic g.,** a skin graft taken from a donor of another species. **heterologous g., heteroplastic g.,** xenograft. **homologous g., homoplastic g.,** allograft. **isogeneic g., isologous g., isoplastic g.,** syngraft. **Krause-Wolfe g.,** full-thickness g. **lamellar g.,** replacement of the superficial layers of an opaque cornea by a thin layer of clear cornea from a donor eye. **nerve g.,** replacement of an area of defective nerve with a segment from a sound one. **omental g's,** free or attached segments of omentum used to cover suture lines following gastrointestinal or colonic surgery. **pedicle g.,** see under *flap.* **penetrating g.,** a full-thickness corneal transplant. **periosteal g.,** a piece of periosteum to cover a denuded bone. **pinch g.,** a piece of skin graft about $\frac{1}{4}$ inch in diameter, obtained by elevating the skin with a needle and slicing it off with a knife. **sieve g.,** a skin graft from which tiny circular islands of skin are removed so that a larger denuded area can be covered, the sievelike portion being placed over one area, and the individual islands over surrounding or other denuded areas. **split-skin g.,** a skin graft consisting of only a portion of the skin thickness. **thick-split g.,** a skin graft cut in pieces, often including about two thirds of the full thickness of the skin. **white g.,** avascular g.

gram (g) (gram) a unit of mass in the SI system; one thousandth of a kilogram.

-gram word element [Gr.], *written; recorded.*

gram·i·ci·din (gram″ĭ-si′din) an antibacterial polypeptide produced by *Bacillus brevis*; it is applied topically in infections due to susceptible gram-positive organisms.

gram-neg·a·tive (-neg′ah-tiv) losing the stain or decolorized by alcohol in Gram's method of staining, characteristic of bacteria having a cell wall surface more complex in chemical composition than the gram-positive bacteria.

gram-pos·i·tive (-poz′it-iv) retaining the stain or resisting decolorization by alcohol in Gram's method of staining, a primary characteristic of bacteria whose cell wall is composed of peptidoglycan and teichoic acid.

gra·na (gra′nah) dense green, chlorophyll-containing bodies in chloroplasts of plant cells.

gran·di·ose (gran′de-ōs″) in psychiatry, pertaining to exaggerated belief or claims of one's importance or identity, often manifested by delusions of great wealth, power, or fame.

grand mal (grahn mal) [Fr.] see under *epilepsy.*

gran·is·e·tron (gră-nis′ĕ-tron) an antiemetic used in conjunction with cancer chemotherapy or radiotherapy, administered as the hydrochloride salt.

gran·u·la·tio (gran″u-la′she-o) pl. *granula-tio′nes.* [L.] a granule or granular mass.

gran·u·la·tion (-shun) 1. the division of a hard substance into small particles. 2. the formation in wounds of small, rounded masses of tissue during healing; also the mass so formed. **arachnoidal g's, cerebral g's,** enlarged arachnoid villi projecting into the venous sinuses and creating slight depressions on the surface of the cranium. **exuberant g's,** excessive proliferation of granulation tissue in healing wounds.

gran·ule (gran′ūl) 1. a small particle or grain. 2. a small pill made from sucrose. **acidophil g's,** granules staining with acid dyes. **acrosomal g.,** a large globule contained within a membrane-bounded acrosomal vesicle, which enlarges further to become the core of the acrosome of a spermatozoon. **alpha g's,** 1. oval granules found in blood platelets; they are lysosomes containing acid phosphatase. 2. large granules in the alpha cells of the islets of Langerhans; they secrete glucagon. 3. granules found in the acidophils of the adenohypophysis. **azurophil g.,** one staining easily with azure dyes; they are coarse reddish granules seen in many lymphocytes. **basal g.,** see under *body.* **basophil g.,** 1. any granule staining with basic dyes. 2. one of the coarse bluish-black granules found in basophils. 3. (pl.) beta g's (2). **beta g's,** 1. granules in the beta cells of the islets of Langerhans; they secrete insulin. 2. granules found in the basophils of the adenohypophysis. **Birbeck g's,** membrane-bound rod- or tennis racquet–shaped structures with a central linear density, found in the cytoplasm of Langerhans' cells. **chromaffin g's,** organelles in the chromaffin cells of the adrenal medulla, where epinephrine and norepinephrine are synthesized, stored, and released. **elementary g's,** hemoconia. **eosinophil g.,** one of the coarse round granules that stain with eosin and are found in eosinophils. **iodophil g's,** granules staining brown with iodine, seen in polymorphonuclear leukocytes in various acute infectious diseases. **keratohyalin g's,** irregularly shaped granules, representing deposits of keratohyalin on tonofibrils in the stratum granulosum of the epidermis. **lamellar g.,** keratinosome. **Langerhans g's,** Birbeck g's. **membrane-coating g.,** keratinosome. **metachromatic g.,** a granular cell inclusion present in many bacterial cells, having an avidity for basic dyes and causing irregular staining of the cell. **Nissl's g's,** see under *body.* **oxyphil g's,** acidophil g's. **pigment g's,** small masses of coloring matter in pigment cells. **proacrosomal g.,** one of the small, dense bodies found inside one of the vacuoles of the Golgi body, which fuse to form an acrosomal granule. **Schüffner's g's,** see under *dot.* **seminal g's,** the small granular bodies in the spermatic fluid. **specific atrial g's,** membrane-bound spherical granules with a dense homogeneous interior that are concentrated in the core of sarcoplasm of the atrial cardiac muscle, extending in either direction from the poles of the nucleus, usually near the Golgi complex; they are the storage site of atrial natriuretic peptide.

gran·u·lar (gran′u-lar) made up of or marked by presence of granules or grains.

gran·u·lo·ad·i·pose (gran″ūl-o-ad′ĭ-pōs) showing fatty degeneration containing granules of fat.

gran·u·lo·blast (gran′ūl-o-blast″) old name for *myeloblast.*

gran·u·lo·cyte (gran′u-lo-sīt″) granular leukocyte. **granulocyt′ic,** adj. **band-form g.,** band cell.

gran·u·lo·cy·to·pe·nia (gran″u-lo-si″-to-pe′ne-ah) reduction in the number of granular leukocytes in the blood.

gran·u·lo·cy·to·poi·e·sis (-sīt″o-poi-e′sis) granulopoiesis. **granulocytopoiet′ic,** adj.

gran·u·lo·cy·to·sis (-si-to′sis) an excess of granulocytes in the blood.

gran·u·lo·ma (gran″u-lo′mah) pl. *granulomas, granulo′mata.* An imprecise term for (1) any small nodular delimited aggregation of mononuclear inflammatory cells, or (2) such a collection of modified macrophages resembling epithelial cells, usually surrounded by a rim of lymphocytes. **actinic g.,** a round lesion with a raised border seen on skin chronically exposed to sunlight. **g. annula′re,** a benign, self-limited disease consisting of round granulomas of the dermis in groups, with papules or nodules, mainly seen in young girls. **apical g.,** modified granulation tissue containing elements of chronic inflammation, located adjacent to the root apex of a tooth with infected, necrotic pulp. **coccidioidal g.,** secondary coccidioidomycosis. **eosinophilic g.,** 1. Langerhans cell histiocytosis. 2. a disorder similar to eosinophilic gastroenteritis, with localized nodular or pedunculated lesions of the submucosa and muscle walls, especially of the pyloric area of the stomach, caused by infiltration of eosinophils, but without peripheral eosinophilia or allergic symptoms. 3. anisakiasis. **g. fissura′tum,** a firm, red, fissured, fibrotic granuloma of the gum and buccal mucosa of an edentulous alveolar ridge between the ridge and cheek; caused by an ill-fitting denture. **infectious g.,** one due to a specific microorganism, as tubercle bacilli. **g. inguina′le,** a granulomatous venereal disease, usually seen in dark-skinned people, marked by purulent ulceration of the external genitals, caused by *Calymmatobacterium granulomatis.* **lethal midline g.,** a rare lethal necrotizing granuloma that destroys the mid-face; it is nearly always preceded by long-standing nonspecific inflammation of the nose or nasal sinuses, with purulent, often bloody discharge. **lipoid g.,** xanthoma. **lipophagic g.,** granuloma with loss of subcutaneous fat. **midline g.,** lethal midline g. **paracoccidioidal g.,** paracoccidioidomycosis. **peripheral giant cell reparative g.,** giant cell epulis. **pyogenic g.,** a benign, solitary nodule resembling granulation tissue, found anywhere but often in the mouth, usually at the site of trauma as a tissue response to non-specific infection. **reticulohistiocytic g.,** a solitary reticulohistiocytoma that is not associated with systemic involvement. **sarcoid g.,** the granuloma seen with sarcoidosis. **swimming pool g.,** one that complicates injuries sustained in swimming pools, attributed to *Mycobacterium balnei,* often healing spontaneously over time. **trichophytic g.,** tinea corporis, usually on the lower legs, due to *Trichophyton* infecting hairs at the site, with raised, circumscribed, boggy granulomas, scattered or in chains; lesions are slowly absorbed, or undergo necrosis, leaving scars.

gran·u·lo·ma·to·sis (gran″u-lo″mah-to′sis) the formation of multiple granulomas. **eosinophilic g.,** Langerhans cell histiocytosis. **Langerhans cell g.,** see under *histiocytosis.* **g. sidero′tica,** a condition in which brownish nodules are seen in the enlarged spleen. **Wegener's g.,** a progressive disease, with granulomatous lesions of the respiratory tract, focal necrotizing arteriolitis and, finally, widespread inflammation of all organs of the body.

gran·u·lom·a·tous (-lom′ah-tus) containing granulomas.

gran·u·lo·mere (gran′u-lo-mēr″) the center portion of a platelet in a dry, stained blood smear, apparently filled with fine, red granules.

gran·u·lo·pe·nia (gran″u-lo-pe′ne-ah) granulocytopenia.

gran·u·lo·plas·tic (-plas′tik) forming granules.

gran·u·lo·poi·e·sis (-poi-e′sis) the formation of granulocytes. **granulopoiet′ic,** adj.

gran·u·lo·sa (gran″u-lo′sah) pertaining to cells of the cumulus oophorus.

gran·u·lo·sis (gran″u-lo′sis) the formation of granules. **g. ru′bra na′si,** redness and marked sweating confined to the nose and surrounding area of the face, with red papules and sometimes many small vesicles, seen most often in children, and usually clearing up at puberty.

grape·seed (grāp′sēd) see under *seed.*

graph (graf) a diagram or curve representing varying relationships between sets of data.

-graph word element [Gr.], *a writing or recording instrument; the record made by such an instrument.*

-graphy word element [Gr.], *writing or recording; a method of recording.* **-graph′ic,** adj.

grat·tage (grah-tahzh′) [Fr.] removal of granulations by scraping.

grav·el (grav′l) calculi occurring in small particles.

grav·id (grav′id) pregnant.

grav·i·da (grav′ĭ-dah) a pregnant woman; called *g. I (primigravida)* during the first pregnancy, *g. II (secundigravida)* during the second, and so on. Symbol G. Cf. *para.*

grav·i·do·car·di·ac (grav″ĭ-do-kahr′de-ak) pertaining to heart disease in pregnancy.

grav·i·met·ric (grav″ĭ-mĕ′trik) pertaining to measurement by weight; performed by weight, as a gravimetric method of drug assay.

grav·i·ty (grav′it-e) 1. the phenomenon by which two bodies having mass are attracted to each other. 2. the gravitational attraction near a large body having mass, particularly near or on the surface of a planet or star. **specific g.,** the ratio of the density of a substance to that of a reference substance at a specified temperature. **standard g. (g),** the acceleration due to gravity at mean sea level on earth, 9.80616 meters per second squared.

gray (gra) 1. of a hue between white and black. 2. a unit of absorbed radiation dose equal to 100 rads. Abbreviated Gy.

green (grēn) 1. a color between yellow and blue, produced by energy with wavelengths between 490 and 570 nm. 2. a dye or stain with this color. **indocyanine g.,** a dye used intravenously in determination of blood volume and flow, cardiac output, and hepatic function.

GRH growth hormone–releasing hormone.

grid (grid) 1. a grating; in radiology, a device consisting of a series of narrow lead strips closely spaced on their edges and separated by spacers of low density material; used to reduce the amount of scattered radiation reaching the x-ray film. 2. a chart with horizontal and perpendicular lines for plotting curves. **baby g.**, a direct-reading chart on infant growth. **Potter-Bucky g.**, a grid used in radiography; it prevents scattered radiation from reaching the film, thereby securing better contrast and definition, and moves during exposure so that no lines appear in the radiograph. **Wetzel g.**, a direct-reading chart for evaluating physical fitness in terms of body build, developmental level, and basal metabolism.

grief (grēf) the normal emotional response to an external and consciously recognized loss.

grip (grip) 1. grippe. 2. a grasping or seizing. **devil's g.**, epidemic pleurodynia.

grippe (grip) [Fr.] influenza.

gris·eo·ful·vin (gris″e-o-ful′vin) an antibiotic produced by *Penicillium griseofulvum*; used as an antifungal in dermatophytoses.

groin (groin) inguen.

groove (grōōv) a narrow, linear hollow or depression. **branchial g.**, pharyngeal g. **Harrison's g.**, a horizontal groove along the lower border of the thorax corresponding to the costal insertion of the diaphragm; seen in advanced rickets in children. **medullary g.**, **neural g.**, that formed by beginning invagination of the neural plate of the embryo to form the neural tube. **pharyngeal g.**, the embryonic ectodermal cleft between successive pharyngeal arches. **primitive g.**, a lengthwise median furrow in the primitive streak of the embryo.

gross (grōs) 1. coarse or large. 2. visible to the naked eye without the use of magnification.

group (grōōp) 1. an assemblage of objects having certain things in common. 2. a number of atoms forming a recognizable and usually transferable portion of a molecule. **azo g.**, a bivalent chemical group composed of two nitrogen atoms, —N:N—. **blood g.**, see under *B*. **Diagnosis-Related G's**, groupings of diagnostic categories used as a basis for hospital payment schedules by Medicare and other third party payment plans. **dorsal respiratory g.**, a part of the medullary respiratory center that controls the basic rhythm of respiration. **encounter g.**, a sensitivity group in which the members strive to gain emotional rather than intellectual insight, with emphasis on the expression of interpersonal feelings in the group situation. **prosthetic g.**, a low molecular weight, nonprotein compound that binds with a protein component (apoprotein, specifically apoenzyme) to form a protein (e.g., holoenzyme) with biological activity. **sensitivity**

training g., **T-g.**, **training g.**, a nonclinical group, not intended for persons with severe emotional problems, which focuses on self-awareness and understanding and on interpersonal interactions in an effort to develop the assets of leadership, management, counseling, or other roles. **ventral respiratory g.**, a part of the medullary respiratory center whose neurons function during strong respiration, moving voluntary muscles to control inhalation and exhalation or modify behavior of other respiratory motoneurons.

group-trans·fer (-trans′fer) denoting a chemical reaction (excluding oxidation and reduction) in which molecules exchange functional groups, a process catalyzed by enzymes called transferases.

growth (grōth) 1. a normal process of increase in size of an organism as a result of accretion of tissue similar to that originally present. 2. an abnormal formation, such as a tumor. 3. the proliferation of cells, as in a bacterial culture. **appositional g.**, growth by addition at the periphery of a particular part. **interstitial g.**, that occurring in the interior of structures already formed.

gru·mous (groo′mus) lumpy or clotted.

gry·po·sis (grĭ-po′sis) [Gr.] abnormal curvature, as of the nails.

GSC gas-solid chromatography.

GSH reduced glutathione.

GSSG oxidized glutathione.

gt. [L.] gutta (drop).

GTN gestational trophoblastic neoplasia.

GTP guanosine triphosphate.

gtt. [L.] guttae (drops).

GU genitourinary.

guai·ac (gwi′ak) a resin from the wood of trees of the genus *Guajacum*, used as a reagent and formerly in treatment of rheumatism.

guai·fen·e·sin (gwi-fen′ĕ-sin) an expectorant believed to act by reducing sputum viscosity.

gua·na·benz (gwah′nah-benz) an α_2-adrenergic agonist used in the form of the base or the acetate ester as an antihypertensive.

gua·na·drel (-drel) an adrenergic neuron blocking agent, used in the treatment of hypertension; used as the sulfate salt.

guan·eth·i·dine (gwahn-eth′ĭ-dēn) an adrenergic blocking agent, used as the monosulfate salt as an antihypertensive.

guan·fa·cine (gwahn′fah-sēn) an α_2-adrenergic agonist used in the form of the hydrochloride salt as an antihypertensive.

gua·ni·dine (gwah′nĭ-dēn) the compound $NH=C(NH_2)_2$, a strong base found in the urine as a result of protein metabolism and used in the laboratory as a protein denaturant.

The hydrochloride salt is used in the treatment of myasthenia gravis.

gua·ni·di·no·a·ce·tic ac·id (gwah″nǐ-de″no-ah-se′tik) an intermediate product formed enzymatically in the liver, pancreas, and kidney in the synthesis of creatine.

gua·nine (gwah′nēn) a purine base, in animal and plant cells usually occurring condensed with ribose or deoxyribose to form guanosine and deoxyguanosine, constituents of nucleic acids. Symbol G.

gua·no·sine (gwah′no-sēn) a purine nucleoside, guanine linked to ribose; it is a component of RNA and its nucleotides are important in metabolism. Symbol G. **cyclic g. monophosphate**, 3′,5′-GMP, cGMP, cyclic GMP; a cyclic nucleotide that acts as a second messenger similar in action to cyclic adenosine monophosphate but generally producing opposite effects on cell function. **g. monophosphate (GMP)**, a nucleotide important in metabolism and RNA synthesis. **g. triphosphate (GTP)**, an energy-rich compound involved in several metabolic reactions and an activated precursor in the synthesis of RNA.

gua·ra·na (gwah-rah′nah) [Tupi-Guarani] the Brazilian woody vine *Paullinia cupana*, or a dried paste prepared from its seeds which is used as a stimulant and tonic in folk medicine and for the treatment of headache in homeopathy.

gu·ber·nac·u·lum (goo″ber-nak′u-lum) pl. *guberna′cula*. [L.] a guiding structure. **gubernac′ular**, adj. **g. tes′tis**, the fetal ligament attached at one end to the lower end of the epididymis and testis and at its other end to the bottom of the scrotum; it is present during the descent of the testis into the scrotum and then atrophies.

guide (gīd) a device by which another object is led in its proper course.

guide·wire (gīd′wīr) a thin, usually flexible wire that can be inserted into a confined or tortuous space to act as a guide for subsequent insertion of a stiffer or bulkier instrument.

guil·lo·tine (ge′o-tēn) [Fr.] an instrument with a sliding blade for excising a tonsil or the uvula.

gul·let (gul′it) the esophagus.

gum (gum) 1. a mucilaginous excretion of various plants. 2. gingiva. **guar g.**, a gum obtained from the ground endosperms of the leguminous tree *Cyamopsis tetragonolobus*; used in pharmaceutical preparations and as a source of soluble dietary fiber. **karaya g.**, **sterculia g.**, the dried gummy exudation from *Sterculia* species, which becomes gelatinous when moisture is added; used as a bulk laxative. It is also adhesive and is used in dental adhesives and skin adhesives and protective barriers around stomas.

gum·boil (gum′boil) parulis.

gum·ma (gum′ah) pl. *gummas, gum′mata*. 1. A soft, gummy tumor, such as that occurring in tertiary syphilis. 2. late benign syphilis.

gu·na (goo′nah) [Sanskrit] according to ayurveda, any of the three attributes of the universe and self that compose mind and body: sattva (equilibrium), rajas (activity), and tamas (inertia).

gur·ney (gur′ne) a wheeled cot used in hospitals.

gus·ta·tion (gus-ta′shun) taste. **gus′tatory**, adj.

gus·tin (gus′tin) a polypeptide present in saliva and containing two zinc atoms; it is necessary for normal development of the taste buds.

gut (gut) 1. intestine. 2. the primordial digestive tube, consisting of the fore-, mid-, and hindgut. 3. surgical g. **blind g.**, cecum. **chromic g., chromicized g.**, surgical gut treated with a chromic salt to increase its resistance to absorption in tissues. **postanal g.**, a temporary extension of the embryonic gut caudal to the cloaca. **preoral g.**, Seessel's pouch. **primordial g.**, archenteron. **surgical g.**, catgut; an absorbable sterile strand made from collagen of a mammal; used in absorbable sutures. **tail g.**, postanal g.

gut·ta (gut′ah) pl. *gut′tae*. [L.] drop.

gut·ta-per·cha (gut″ah-pur′chah) the coagulated latex of a number of trees of the family Sapotaceae; used as a dental cement and in splints.

Guttat. [L.] guttatim (drop by drop).

gut·ta·tim (gah-ta′tim) [L.] drop by drop.

gut·tur·al (gut′er-il) faucial; pertaining to the throat.

Gy gray (2).

gym·nas·tics (jim-nas′tiks) systematic muscular exercise. **Swedish g.**, a system following a rigid pattern of movement, utilizing little equipment and stressing correct body posture.

Gym·no·din·i·um (jim″no-din′e-um) a genus of dinoflagellates, most species of which have many colored chromatophores, found in water; when present in great numbers, they help to form the destructive red tide in the ocean.

gynaec(o)- for words beginning thus, see those beginning *gyneco-*.

gy·nan·drism (gi-, jǐ-nan′drizm) 1. hermaphroditism. 2. female pseudohermaphroditism. 3. masculinization (2).

gy·nan·dro·blas·to·ma (gi-, jĭ-nan″dro-blas-to′mah) an ovarian tumor containing elements of both arrhenoblastoma and granulosa cell tumor.

gy·nan·dro·mor·phism (-mor′fizm) 1. the presence of chromosomes of both sexes in different tissues of the body, producing a mosaic of male and female sex characteristics. **gynandromorph′ous,** adj. 2. hermaphroditism.

gyne- see *gynec(o)-.*

gynec(o)- word element [Gr.], *woman.*

gyne·co·gen·ic (gi″nĕ-, jin″ĕ-ko-jen′ik) producing female characteristics.

gyn·e·coid (gi′nĕ-, jin′ĕ-koid) womanlike.

gy·ne·co·log·ic (gi″nĕ-, jin″ĕ-kah-loj′ik) pertaining to the female reproductive tract or to gynecology.

gy·ne·co·log·i·cal (-kah-loj′ĭ-k′l) gynecologic.

gy·ne·col·o·gist (-kol′ah-jist) a person skilled in gynecology.

gy·ne·col·o·gy (-kol′ah-je) the branch of medicine dealing with diseases of the genital tract in women.

gyne·co·mas·tia (-ko-mas′te-ah) excessive development of the male mammary glands, even to the functional state.

gyne·pho·bia (-fo′be-ah) irrational fear of or aversion to women.

gyn(o)- see *gynec(o)-.*

gyno·plas·ty (gi′-, jin′o-plas″te) plastic or reconstructive surgery of the female reproductive organs.

gyp·sum (jip′sum) native calcium sulfate dihydrate; when calcined, it becomes *plaster of Paris.*

gy·ra·tion (ji-ra′shun) revolution about a fixed center.

gy·rec·to·my (ji-rek′tah-me) excision or resection of a cerebral gyrus, or a portion of the cerebral cortex.

Gy·ren·ceph·a·la (ji″ren-sef′ah-lah) a group of higher mammals, including humans, having cerebral hemispheres marked by convolutions.

gy·ri (ji′ri) plural of *gyrus.*

gy·rose (ji′rōs) marked by curved lines or circles.

gy·ro·spasm (ji′ro-spazm) rotatory spasm of the head.

gy·rous (ji′rus) gyrose.

gy·rus (ji′rus) pl. *gy′ri.* [L.] cerebral g. **angular g.,** one arching over the superior temporal sulcus, continuous with the middle temporal gyrus. **gy′ri bre′ves in′sulae,** the short, rostrally placed gyri on the surface of the insula. **Broca's g.,** see under *convolution.* **central g., anterior,** precentral g. **central g., posterior,** postcentral g. **cerebral g.,** any of

the tortuous convolutions on the surface of the cerebral hemispheres, caused by infolding of the cortex and separated by fissures or sulci. **cingulate g.,** an arch-shaped convolution just above the corpus callosum. **g. descen′dens,** the raised area posterior to the superior and inferior occipital gyri and anterior to the lunate sulcus when that is present. **frontal g.,** any of four gyri (inferior, medial, middle, and superior) of the frontal lobe. **fusiform g.,** one on the inferior surface of the hemisphere between the inferior temporal and parahippocampal gyri, consisting of a lateral (*lateral occipitotemporal g.*) and a medial (*medial occipitotemporal g.*) part. **g. geni′culi,** a vestigial gyrus at the anterior end of the corpus callosum. **hippocampal g.,** parahippocampal g. **infracalcarine g.,** lingual g. **interlocking gyri,** small gyri in the opposing walls of the central sulcus that interlock with each other like gears. **lingual g.,** one on the occipital lobe, forming the inferior lip of the calcarine sulcus and, with the cuneus, the visual cortex. **g. lon′gus in′sulae,** the long, occipitally directed gyrus on the surface of the insula. **occipital g.,** either of the two (superior and inferior) gyri of the occipital lobe. **occipitotemporal g., lateral,** the lateral portion of the fusiform gyrus. **occipitotemporal g., medial,** the medial portion of the fusiform gyrus. **orbital gyri,** irregular gyri on the orbital surface of the frontal lobe. **parahippocampal g.,** a convolution on the inferior surface of each cerebral hemisphere, lying between the hippocampal and collateral sulci. **paraterminal g.,** a thin sheet of gray substance in front of and ventral to the genu of the corpus callosum. **postcentral g.,** the convolution of the frontal lobe between the postcentral and central sulci; the primary sensory area of the cerebral cortex. **precentral g.,** the convolution of the frontal lobe between the precentral and central sulci; the primary motor area of the cerebral cortex. **g. rec′tus,** one on the orbital surface of the frontal lobe. **supramarginal g.,** that part of the inferior parietal convolution that curves around the upper end of the sylvian fissure. **temporal g.,** any of the gyri of the temporal lobe, including the inferior, middle, superior, and transverse temporal gyri; the more prominent of the latter (*anterior transverse temporal g.*), when two exist, represents the cortical center for hearing. **gy′ri transiti′vi ce′rebri,** various small folds on the cerebral surface that are too inconstant to bear individual names.

H henry; histidine; hydrogen; hyperopia.

H enthalpy.

h hecto-; hour.

HAART highly active antiretroviral therapy.

ha·be·na (hah-be′nah) pl. *habe′nae.* [L.] any straplike anatomic structure. **habe′nal, habe′nar,** adj.

ha·ben·u·la (hah-ben′u-lah) pl. *haben′ulae.* [L.] 1. a frenulum, or reinlike structure, such as one of a set of structures in the cochlea. 2. a small eminence on the dorso-medial surface of the thalamus, just in front of the posterior commissure. **haben′ular,** adj.

hab·it (hab′it) 1. an action which has become automatic or characteristic by repetition. 2. predisposition or bodily temperament.

ha·bit·u·al (hah-bich′u-al) 1. according to or of the nature of a habit. 2. established through long use or frequent repetition.

ha·bit·u·a·tion (hah-bich″u-a′shun) 1. the gradual adaptation to a stimulus or to the environment, with a decreasing response. 2. an older term denoting sometimes toler-ance and sometimes a psychological depend-ence due to repeated consumption of a drug, with a desire to continue its use, but with little or no tendency to increase the dose.

hab·i·tus (hab′ĭ-tus) [L.] 1. attitude (2). 2. physique.

hae- for words beginning thus, see also those beginning *he-*.

Hae·ma·dip·sa (he″mah-dip′sah) a genus of leeches.

Hae·ma·phys·a·lis (he″mah-fis′ah-lis) a genus of hard-bodied ticks, species of which are important vectors of disease.

Hae·moph·i·lus (he-mof′ĭ-lus) a genus of hemophilic gram-negative bacteria (family Pasteurellaceae) including *H. aegyp′ticus,* the cause of acute contagious conjunctivitis; *H. ducrey′i,* the cause of chancroid; *H. influen′zae* (once thought to be the cause of epidemic influenza), the cause of lethal meningitis in infants; and *H. vagina′lis,* associated with, and possibly the cause of, vaginitis.

haf·ni·um (Hf) (haf′ne-um) chemical ele-ment (see *Table of Elements*), at. no. 72.

hair (hār) pilus; a threadlike structure, especially the specialized epidermal struc-ture composed of keratin and developing from a papilla sunk in the dermis, produced only by mammals and characteristic of that group of animals. Also, the aggregate of such hairs. **hair′y,** adj. **bamboo h.,** trichor-rhexis nodosa. **beaded h.,** hair marked with alternate swellings and constrictions, as in monilethrix. **burrowing h.,** one that grows horizontally beneath the surface of the skin. **club h.,** one whose root is sur-rounded by a bulbous enlargement composed of keratinized cells, preliminary to normal loss of the hair from the follicle. **ingrown h.,** one that emerges from the skin but curves and reenters it. **lanugo h.,** lanugo. **resting h.,** see *telogen.* **sensory h's,** hairlike pro-jections on the cells of sensory epithelium. **taste h's,** clumps of microvilli that form short hairlike processes projecting into the lumen of a taste pore from the peripheral ends of the taste cells. **terminal h.,** the coarse hair on various areas of the body during adult years. **twisted h.,** one which at spaced intervals is twisted through an axis of 180 degrees, being abnormally flattened at the site of twisting. **vellus h.,** vellus (1).

hal·a·tion (hal-a′shun) indistinctness of the image caused by illumination coming from the same direction as the object being viewed.

hal·az·e·pam (-az′ĕ-pam) a benzodiazepine used as an antianxiety agent.

hal·cin·o·nide (hal-sin′ah-nīd) a synthetic corticosteroid used topically as an antiinflam-matory and antipruritic.

half-life (haf′līf) the time required for the decay of half of a sample of particles of a radionuclide or elementary particles; sym-bol $t_{1/2}$ or $T_{1/2}$. **antibody h.-l.,** a measure of the mean survival time of antibody mole-cules following their formation, usually ex-pressed as the time required to eliminate 50 per cent of a known quantity of immuno-globulin from the animal body. Half-life varies from one immunoglobulin class to another. **biological h.-l.,** the time required for a living tissue, organ, or organism to eliminate one-half of a radioactive substance which has been introduced into it.

half-way house (haf′wa hous) a residence for patients (e.g., mental patients, drug addicts, alcoholics) who do not require hospi-talization but who need an intermediate degree of care until they can return to the community.

ha·lis·te·re·sis (hah-lis″tĕ-re′sis) osteo-malacia. **halisteret′ic,** adj.

hal·i·to·sis (hal″ĭ-to′sis) offensive odor of the breath.

hal·i·tus (hal′ĭ-tus) exhalation (3).

hal·lu·ci·na·tion (hah-loo″sĭ-na′shun) a sense perception (sight, touch, sound, smell, or taste) that has no basis in external stimulation. **hallu′cinative, hallu′cinatory,** adj. **haptic h.,** tactile h. **kinesthetic h.,** a hallucination involving the sense of bodily movement. **somatic h.,** a hallucination involving the perception of a physical experience with the body. **hypnagogic h.,** one occurring just at the onset of sleep. **hypnopompic h.,** one occurring during awakening. **tactile h.,** one involving the sense of touch.

hal·lu·ci·no·gen (hah-loo′sin-ah-jen″) an agent that is capable of producing hallucinations. **hallucinogen′ic,** adj.

hal·lu·ci·no·sis (hah-loo″sĭ-no′sis) a state characterized by the presence of hallucinations without other impairment of consciousness. **hallucinot′ic,** adj. **organic h.,** a term used in a former classification system, denoting an organic mental syndrome characterized by hallucinations caused by a specific organic factor and not associated with delirium.

hal·lux (hal′uks) pl. *hal′luces.* [L.] the great toe. **h. doloro′sus,** a painful condition of the great toe, usually associated with flatfoot. **h. flex′us,** h. rigidus. **h. mal′leus,** hammer toe affecting the great toe. **h. ri′gidus,** painful flexion deformity of the great toe with limitation of motion at the metatarsophalangeal joint. **h. val′gus,** angulation of the great toe toward the other toes. **h. va′rus,** angulation of the great toe away from the other toes.

hal·ma·to·gen·e·sis (hal″mah-to-jen′ĕ-sis) a sudden alteration of type from one generation to another.

ha·lo (ha′lo) 1. a luminous or colored circle, as the colored circle seen around a light in glaucoma. 2. a ring seen around the macula lutea in ophthalmoscopic examinations. 3. the imprint of the ciliary processes on the vitreous body. 4. a metal or plastic band that encircles the head or neck, providing support and stability to an orthosis. **Fick's h.,** a colored circle appearing around a light due to the wearing of contact lenses. **h. glaucomato′sus, glaucomatous h.,** peripapillary atrophy seen in severe or chronic glaucoma. **senile h.,** a zone of variable width around the optic papilla, due to exposure of various elements of the choroid as a result of senile atrophy of the pigmented epithelium.

hal·o·be·ta·sol (hal″o-ba′tah-sol) a very high potency synthetic corticosteroid used topically in the form of the propionate salt as an antiinflammatory and antipruritic.

hal·o·fan·trine (-fan′trēn) an antimalarial used as the hydrochloride salt in the treatment of acute malaria due to *Plasmodium falciparum* and *P. vivax.*

hal·o·gen (hal′o-jen) any of the nonmetallic elements of the seventh group of the periodic system: chlorine, iodine, bromine, fluorine, and astatine.

ha·lom·e·ter (hah-lom′ĕ-ter) 1. an instrument for measuring ocular halos. 2. an instrument for estimating the size of erythrocytes by measuring the halos formed around them when a beam of light shines on them and is diffracted.

hal·o·peri·dol (hal″o-per′ĭ-dol) an antipsychotic agent of the butyrophenone group with antiemetic, hypotensive, and hypothermic actions; used especially in the management of psychoses and to control vocal utterances and tics of Gilles de la Tourette's syndrome; used also as the decanoate ester in maintenance therapy for psychotic disorders.

hal·o·thane (hal′o-thān) an inhalational anesthetic used for induction and maintenance of general anesthesia.

ham·ar·tia (ham-ahr′she-ah) defect in tissue combination during development. **hamar′tial,** adj.

ham·ar·to·ma (ham″ahr-to′mah) a benign tumor-like nodule composed of an overgrowth of mature cells and tissues normally present in the affected part, but with disorganization and often with one element predominating.

ham·ate (ham′āt) shaped like a hook.

ham·mer (ham′er) 1. an instrument with a head designed for striking blows. 2. malleus; see *Table of Bones.*

ham·ster (ham′ster) a small ratlike rodent, most commonly *Cricetus cricetus,* used extensively in laboratory experiments.

ham·string (ham′string) one of the tendons bounding the popliteal space laterally and medially. **inner h.,** the tendons of gracilis, sartorius, and two other muscles of the leg. **outer h.,** tendon of biceps flexor femoris.

ham·u·lus (ham′u-lus) pl. *ham′uli.* [L.] hook. **ham′ular,** adj.

hand (hand) the distal part of the upper limb, consisting of the carpus, metacarpus, and fingers. **ape h.,** one with the thumb permanently extended. **claw h.,** see *claw-hand.* **cleft h.,** a malformation in which the division between the fingers extends into the metacarpus; often with just two large digits, one on either side of the cleft. **club h.,** see *clubhand.* **drop h.,** wristdrop. **lobster-claw h.,** cleft h. **mitten h.,** a hand in which several fingers are fused together and have a common nail. **writing h.,** in paralysis agitans, assumption of the position by which a pen is commonly held.

H and E hematoxylin-eosin (stain).

hand·ed·ness (hand'ed-nes) the preferential use of the hand of one side in voluntary motor acts.

hand·i·cap (han'dĭ-kap) any physical or mental defect, congenital or acquired, preventing or restricting a person from participating in normal life or limiting their capacity to work.

hand·piece (hand'pēs) that part of a dental engine held in the operator's hand and engaging the bur or working point while it is being revolved.

hang·nail (hang'nāl) a shred of eponychium on a proximal or lateral nail fold.

Han·ta·vi·rus (han'tah-vi"rus) a genus of viruses of the family Bunyaviridae that cause epidemic hemorrhagic fever or pneumonia; members include Hantaan, Puumala, and Seoul viruses.

hap·loid (hap'loid) 1. having half the number of chromosomes characteristically found in the somatic (diploid) cells of an organism; typical of the gametes of a species whose union restores the diploid number. 2. an individual or cell having only one member of each pair of homologous chromosomes.

hap·lo·iden·ti·cal (hap"lo-i-den'tĭ-k'l) sharing a haplotype; having the same alleles at a set of closely linked genes on one chromosome.

hap·lo·iden·ti·ty (-i-den'tit-e) the condition of being haploidentical.

hap·lo·scope (-skōp) a stereoscope for testing the visual axis.

hap·lo·type (-tīp) the group of alleles of linked genes, e.g., the HLA complex, contributed by either parent; the haploid genetic constitution contributed by either parent.

hap·ten (hap'ten) partial antigen; a specific nonprotein substance which does not itself elicit antibody formation but does elicit the immune response when coupled with a carrier protein. **hapten'ic,** adj.

hap·tic (hap'tik) tactile.

hap·tics (-tiks) the study of the sense of touch.

hap·to·glo·bin (hap"to-glo'bin) a plasma glycoprotein with alpha electrophoretic mobility that irreversibly binds free hemoglobin,

resulting in removal of the complex by the liver and preventing free hemoglobin from being lost in the urine; it has two major genetic variants, Hp 1 and Hp 2.

hare·lip (hār'lip) former name for *cleft lip.*

har·ness (hahr'nis) the combination of straps, bands, and other pieces that forms the working gear of a draft animal, or a device resembling such gear. **Pavlik h.,** a device used to correct hip dislocations in infants with developmental dysplasia of the hip, consisting of a set of straps that hold the hips in flexion and abduction.

har·le·quin (hahr'lah-kwin) 1. having a pattern of diamond shapes, particularly in bright colors. 2. coral snake.

har·vest (hahr'vest) to remove tissues or cells from a donor and preserve them for transplantation.

hash·ish (hă-shēsh') [Arabic] a preparation of the unadulterated resin scraped from the flowering tops of female hemp plants (*Cannabis sativa*), smoked or chewed for its intoxicating effects. It is far more potent than marijuana.

hash·i·tox·i·co·sis (hash"ĭ-tok"sĭ-ko'sis) hyperthyroidism in patients with Hashimoto's disease.

haus·tel·lum (haw-stel'um) pl. *haustel'la.* [L.] a hollow tube with an eversible set of five stylets, by which certain ectoparasites, e.g., bedbugs and lice, attach themselves to the host and through which blood is drawn up.

haus·tra·tion (haws-tra'shun) 1. the formation of a haustrum. 2. a haustrum.

haus·trum (haws'trum) pl. *haus'tra.* [L.] a recess. **haus'tral,** adj. **haus'tra co'li,** sacculations in the wall of the colon produced by adaptation of its length to the tenia coli, or by the arrangement of the circular muscle fibers.

HAV hepatitis A virus.

haw·kin·sin·u·ria (haw"kin-sin-u're-ah) a rare form of tyrosinemia with urinary excretion of hawkinsin, a cyclic amino acid metabolite of tyrosine.

haw·thorn (haw'thorn) a shrub or tree of the genus *Crataegus,* or a preparation of the flowers, fruit, and leaves of certain of its species, having a mechanism of action similar to that of digitalis; used to decrease output in congestive heart failure; also used in traditional Chinese medicine, homeopathy, and folk medicine.

HB hepatitis B.

Hb hemoglobin.

HBcAg hepatitis B core antigen.

HbCV *Haemophilus* b conjugate vaccine.

HBeAg hepatitis B e antigen.

HbPV *Haemophilus* b polysaccharide vaccine.

HBsAg hepatitis B surface antigen.

HBV hepatitis B virus.

HC Hospital Corps.

HCG, hCG human chorionic gonadotropin.

HCM hypertrophic cardiomyopathy.

HDCV human diploid cell (rabies) vaccine; see *rabies vaccine.*

HDL high-density lipoprotein.

HDL-C high-density-lipoprotein cholesterol.

He helium.

head (hed) caput; the upper, anterior, or proximal extremity of a structure, especially the part of an organism containing the brain and organs of special sense.

head·ache (hed′āk) pain in the head. **cluster h.,** a migraine-like disorder marked by attacks of unilateral intense pain over the eye and forehead, with flushing and watering of the eyes and nose; attacks last about an hour and occur in clusters. **exertional h.,** one occurring after exercise. **histamine h.,** cluster h. **lumbar puncture h.,** headache in the erect position, relieved by recumbency, after lumbar puncture; due to lowering of intracranial pressure by leakage of cerebrospinal fluid through the needle tract. **migraine h.,** migraine. **organic h.,** headache due to intracranial disease or other organic disease. **postcoital h.,** one occurring during or after sexual activity, usually in males. **sick h.,** migraine. **tension h.,** a type due to prolonged overwork, emotional strain, or both, affecting especially the occipital region. **toxic h.,** headache due to systemic poisoning or associated with illness. **vascular h.,** a classification for certain types of headaches, based on a proposed etiology involving abnormal functioning of the blood vessels or vascular system of the brain; included are migraine, cluster headache, toxic headache, and headache caused by elevated blood pressure.

heal (hēl) 1. to restore wounded parts or to make healthy. 2. to become well or healthy.

heal·ing (hēl′ing) a process of cure; the restoration of integrity to injured tissue. **h. by first intention,** that in which union or restoration of continuity occurs directly without intervention of granulations. **h. by second intention,** union by closure of a wound with granulations. **spiritual h.,** the use of spiritual practices, such as prayer, for the purpose of effecting a cure of or an improvement in an illness. **h. by third intention,** treatment of a grossly contaminated wound by delaying closure until after contamination has been markedly reduced and inflammation has subsided.

health (helth) a state of physical, mental, and social well-being. **public h.,** the field of medicine concerned with safeguarding and improving the health of the community as a whole.

health main·te·nance or·ga·ni·za·tion (HMO), a broad term encompassing a variety of health care delivery systems utilizing group practice and providing alternatives to the fee-for-service private practice of medicine and allied health professions.

hear·ing (hēr′ing) 1. the sense by which sounds are perceived. 2. audition; the capacity to perceive sound. **color h.,** a form of chromesthesia in which sounds cause sensations of color.

hear·ing loss (los) deafness. **conductive h. l.,** conductive deafness; that due to a defect of the sound-conducting apparatus, i.e., of the external auditory canal or middle ear. **functional h. l.,** hearing loss that lacks any organic lesion. **mixed h. l.,** hearing loss that is both conductive and sensorineural. **nonorganic h. l.,** functional h. l. **ototoxic h. l.,** that caused by ingestion of toxic substances. **paradoxic h. l.,** that in which the hearing is better during loud noise. **sensorineural h. l.,** that due to a defect in the inner ear or the acoustic nerve.

heart (hahrt) cor; the viscus of cardiac muscle that maintains the circulation of the blood; see Plate 24. **artificial h.,** a pumping mechanism that duplicates the rate, output, and blood pressure of the natural heart; it may replace the function of a part or all of the heart. **athletic h.,** hypertrophy of the heart without valvular disease, sometimes seen in athletes. **extracorporeal h.,** an artificial heart located outside the body and usually performing pumping and oxygenating functions. **fatty h.,** 1. one that has undergone fatty degeneration. 2. a condition in which fat has accumulated around and in the heart muscle. **fibroid h.,** one in which fibrous tissue replaces portions of the myocardium, such as may occur in chronic myocarditis. **horizontal h.,** a counterclockwise rotation of the electrical axis (deviation to the left) of the heart. **left h.,** the left atrium and ventricle, which propel the blood through the systemic circulation. **right h.,** the right atrium and ventricle, which propel the venous blood into the pulmonary circulation. **stone h.,** massive contraction band necrosis in an irreversibly noncompliant hypertrophied heart, occurring as a complication of cardiac surgery; believed due to low levels of ATP and to calcium overload. **three-chambered h.,** a developmental anomaly in which the heart is missing the interventricular or interatrial septum and so has only three compartments. **water-bottle h.,** a radiographic sign of pericardial effusion, in which the cardiopericardial silhouette is enlarged and assumes the shape of a flask or water bottle.

heart·beat (hahrt′bēt) a complete cardiac cycle, during which the electrical impulse is conducted and mechanical contraction occurs.

heart block (hahrt blok) impairment of conduction of an impulse in heart excitation; often applied specifically to atrioventricular block. For specific types, see under *block.*

heart·burn (hahrt′burn) pyrosis; a retrosternal sensation of burning occurring in waves and rising toward the neck; it may be accompanied by a reflux of fluid into the mouth and is often associated with gastroesophageal reflux.

heart fail·ure (hahrt fāl′yer) see under *failure.*

heart·worm (hahrt′wurm) an individual of the species *Dirofilaria immitis.*

heat (hēt) 1. the sensation of an increase in temperature. 2. the energy producing such a sensation; it exists in the form of molecular or atomic vibration and may be transferred, as a result of a gradient in temperature. Symbol Q or q. 3. to become, or to cause to become, warmer or hotter. **conductive h.,** heat transmitted by direct contact, as with a hot water bottle. **convective h.,** heat conveyed by currents of a warm medium, such as air or water. **conversive h.,** heat developed in tissues by resistance to passage of high-energy radiations. **prickly h.,** miliaria rubra.

heat·stroke (hēt′strōk″) see under *stroke.*

he·bet·ic (hĕ-bet′ik) pubertal.

heb·e·tude (heb′ĕ-tood) dullness; apathy.

hect(o)- word element [Fr.], *hundred;* used in naming units of measurements to designate an amount 100 times (10^2) the size of the unit to which it is joined; symbol h.

he·do·nism (he′din-izm) 1. pleasure-seeking behavior. 2. the doctrine that regards pleasure and happiness as the highest good. 3. the theory that the attainment of pleasure and the avoidance of pain are the prime motivators of human behavior. **hedon′ic,** adj.

heel (hēl) calx; the hindmost part of the foot. **cracked h's,** pitted keratolysis.

height (hīt) the vertical measurement of an object or body. **h. of contour,** 1. a line encircling a tooth representing its greatest circumference. 2. the line encircling a tooth in a more or less horizontal plane and passing through the surface point of greatest

radius. 3. the line encircling a tooth at its greatest bulge or diameter with respect to a selected path of insertion.

hel·coid (hel′koid) like an ulcer.

hel·i·cal (hel′ĭ-k'l) spiral (1).

hel·i·cine (hel′ĭ-sēn) spiral (1).

He·li·co·bac·ter (hel″ĭ-ko-bak′ter) a genus of gram-negative, microaerophilic bacteria of the family Spirillaceae; *H. cinae′di* causes proctitis and colitis in homosexual men and has been implicated in septicemia in neonates and immunocompromised patients; *H. pylo′ri* causes gastritis and pyloric ulcers and has been implicated in gastric carcinogenesis.

hel·i·co·pod (hel′ĭ-ko-pod″) denoting a peculiar dragging gait; see under *gait.*

hel·i·co·tre·ma (hel″ĭ-ko-tre′mah) a foramen between the scala tympani and scala vestibuli.

heli(o)- word element [Gr.], *sun.*

he·li·um (He) (hēl′e-um) chemical element (see *Table of Elements*), at. no. 2. It is obtained from natural gas. Used as a diluent for other gases, particularly with oxygen in the treatment of certain cases of respiratory obstruction, and as a vehicle for general anesthetics.

he·lix (he′liks) pl. *he′lices, helixes.* [Gr.] 1. spiral (2). 2. the superior and posterior free margin of the pinna of the ear. **α-h.,** **alpha h.,** the structural arrangement of parts of protein molecules in which a single polypeptide chain forms a right-handed helix stabilized by intrachain hydrogen bonds. **double h., Watson-Crick h.,** a representation of the structure of DNA, consisting of two coiled chains arranged antiparallel to each other, each containing information completely specifying the other chain.

hel·minth (hel′minth) a parasitic worm.

hel·min·tha·gogue (hel-min′thah-gog) anthelmintic (2).

hel·min·them·e·sis (hel″min-them′ĕ-sis) the vomiting of worms.

hel·min·thol·o·gy (hel″min-thol′ah-je) the scientific study of parasitic worms.

he·lo·ma (hēl-o′mah) corn. **h. du′rum,** hard corn. **h. mol′le,** soft corn.

he·lot·o·my (hēl-ot′ah-me) the excision or the paring of corns or calluses.

hema·cy·tom·e·ter (he″mah-si-tom′ĕ-ter) an apparatus used for making manual blood counts with a counting chamber.

he·mad·sorp·tion (hem″ad-sorp′shun) the adherence of red cells to other cells, particles, or surfaces. **hemadsor′bent,** adj.

he·mag·glu·ti·na·tion (he″mah-gloo-tĭ-na′shun) agglutination of erythrocytes.

he·mag·glu·ti·nin (-gloo'tǐ-nin) an antibody that causes agglutination of erythrocytes. **cold h.,** one which acts only at temperatures near 4° C. **warm h.,** one which acts only at temperatures near 37° C.

he·mal (he'm'l) 1. ventral to the spinal axis, where the heart and great vessels are located, as, e.g., the hemal arches. 2. hemic. 3. pertaining to blood vessels; see *vascular*.

hem·al·um (he'mah-lum) a mixture of hematoxylin and alum used as a nuclear stain.

hem·a·nal·y·sis (he"mah-nal'ǐ-sis) analysis of the blood.

hemangi(o)- word element [Gr.], *blood vessels*.

he·man·gio·ame·lo·blas·to·ma (he-man"je-o-ah-mel"o-blas-to'mah) a highly vascular ameloblastoma.

he·man·gio·blast (he-man'je-o-blast) a mesodermal cell that gives rise to both vascular endothelium and hemocytoblasts.

he·man·gio·blas·to·ma (he-man"je-o-blas-to'mah) a benign blood vessel tumor of the cerebellum, spinal cord, or retina, consisting of proliferated blood vessel cells and angioblasts.

he·man·gio·en·do·the·li·al (-en"do-the'le-al) pertaining to the vascular endothelium.

he·man·gio·en·do·the·lio·blas·to·ma (-en"do-thēl"e-o-blas-to'mah) a hemangioendothelioma with embryonic elements of mesenchymal origin.

he·man·gio·en·do·the·lio·ma (-en"do-the"le-o'mah) 1. a true neoplasm of vascular origin, with proliferation of endothelial cells around the vascular lumen. 2. hemangiosarcoma.

he·man·gio·en·do·the·lio·sar·co·ma (-en"do-the"le-o-sahr-ko'mah) hemangiosarcoma.

he·man·gi·o·ma (he-man"je-o'mah) 1. a benign tumor, usually in infants or children, made up of newly formed blood vessels and resulting from malformation of angioblastic tissue of fetal life. 2. a benign or malignant vascular tumor resembling the classic type but occurring at any age. **ameloblastic h.,** hemangioameloblastoma. **capillary h.,** 1. the most common type, having closely packed aggregations of capillaries, usually of normal caliber, separated by scant connective stroma. 2. strawberry h. **cavernous h.,** a red-blue spongy tumor with a connective tissue framework enclosing large, cavernous, vascular spaces containing blood. **sclerosing h.,** a form of benign fibrous histiocytoma having histiocytic and fibroblastic elements, numerous blood vessels, and hemosiderin deposits. **strawberry h.,** 1. a red, firm, dome-shaped hemangioma seen at birth or soon after,

usually on the head or neck, that grows rapidly and usually regresses and involutes without scarring. 2. vascular nevus. **venous h.,** a cavernous hemangioma in which the dilated vessels have thick, fibrous walls.

he·man·gio·peri·cy·to·ma (he-man"je-o-per"ǐ-si-to'mah) a tumor composed of spindle cells with a rich vascular network, which apparently arises from pericytes.

he·man·gio·sar·co·ma (-sahr-ko'mah) a malignant tumor of vascular origin, formed by proliferation of endothelial tissue lining irregular vascular channels.

he·ma·phe·re·sis (he"mah-fě-re'sis) apheresis.

he·mar·thro·sis (he"mahr-thro'sis) extravasation of blood into a joint or its synovial cavity.

he·ma·tem·e·sis (he"mah-tem'ě-sis) the vomiting of blood.

he·mat·ic (he-mat'ik) 1. hemic. 2. hematinic.

he·ma·tid·ro·sis (he"mah-tid-ro'sis) excretion of bloody sweat.

he·ma·tin (he'mah-tin) 1. the hydroxide of heme; it stimulates the synthesis of globin, inhibits the synthesis of porphyrin, and is a component of cytochromes and peroxidases; it is also used as a reagent. 2. hemin (1).

he·ma·tin·ic (he"mah-tin'ik) 1. pertaining to hematin. 2. an agent that increases the hemoglobin level and the number of erythrocytes in the blood.

he·ma·tin·uria (he"mah-tǐ-nu're-ah) the presence of hematin in the urine.

hemat(o)- word element [Gr.], *blood*. See also words beginning *hem-* and *hemo-*.

he·ma·to·cele (he'mah-to-, hem'ah-to-sēl") an effusion of blood into a cavity, especially into the tunica vaginalis testis. **parametric h., pelvic h., retrouterine h.,** a swelling formed by effusion of blood into the pouch of Douglas.

he·ma·to·che·zia (he"mah-to-ke'zhah) defecation in which feces are bloody.

he·ma·to·chy·lu·ria (-ki-lu're-ah) the discharge of blood and chyle with the urine, as seen in filaria infections.

he·ma·to·coe·lia (-sēl'e-ah) effusion of blood into the peritoneal cavity.

he·ma·to·col·po·me·tra (-kol"po-me'trah) accumulation of menstrual blood in the vagina and uterus.

he·ma·to·col·pos (-kol'pos) blood in the vagina.

he·mat·o·crit (he-mat'o-krit) the volume percentage of erythrocytes in whole blood; also, the apparatus or procedure used in its determination.

he·ma·to·gen·ic (-jen'ik) 1. hematopoietic. 2. hematogenous.

he·ma·tog·e·nous (he"mah-toj'ĕ-nus) 1. produced by or derived from the blood. 2. disseminated through the blood stream.

he·ma·toid·in (he"mah-toid'in) a hematogenous pigment apparently chemically identical with bilirubin but formed in the tissues from hemoglobin, particularly under conditions of reduced oxygen tension.

he·ma·tol·o·gy (he"mah-tol'ah-je) the branch of medical science dealing with the blood and blood-forming tissues, including morphology, physiology, and pathology.

he·ma·to·lymph·an·gi·o·ma (hem"ah-to-lim-fan"je-o'mah) a benign tumor composed of blood and lymph vessels.

he·ma·tol·y·sis (he"mah-tol'ĭ-sis) hemolysis. **hematolyt'ic**, adj.

he·ma·to·ma (he"mah-to'mah) a localized collection of extravasated blood, usually clotted, in an organ, space, or tissue. **subdural h.**, a massive blood clot beneath the dura mater that causes neurologic symptoms by pressure on the brain.

he·ma·to·me·di·as·ti·num (hem"ah-to-me"de-as-ti'num) hemomediastinum.

he·ma·to·me·tra (-me'trah) blood in the uterus.

he·ma·tom·e·try (he"mah-tom'ĕ-tre) measurement of various parameters of the blood, such as the complete blood count.

he·ma·to·my·e·lia (hem"ah-to-mi-e'le-ah) hemorrhage into the spinal cord.

he·ma·to·my·eli·tis (-mi"ĕ-li'tis) acute myelitis with bloody effusion into the spinal cord.

he·ma·to·my·elo·pore (-mi'lo-por) formation of canals in the spinal cord due to hemorrhage.

he·ma·to·pa·thol·o·gy (-pah-thol'ah-je) hemopathology.

he·ma·to·pha·gia (-fa'jah) 1. blood drinking. 2. subsisting on blood. **hematoph'agous**, adj.

he·ma·to·poi·e·sis (-poi-e'sis) the formation and development of blood cells. **extramedullary h.**, that occurring outside the bone marrow, as in the spleen, liver, and lymph nodes.

he·ma·to·poi·et·ic (-poi-et'ik) 1. pertaining to hematopoiesis. 2. an agent that promotes hematopoiesis.

he·ma·to·por·phy·rin (-por'fi-rin) an iron-free derivative of heme, a product of the decomposition of hemoglobin.

he·ma·tor·rha·chis (he"mah-tor'ah-kis) hematomyelia.

he·ma·to·sal·pinx (-sal'pinks) blood in the uterine tube.

he·ma·to·sper·mato·cele (-sper-mat'o-sēl) a spermatocele containing blood.

he·ma·to·sper·mia (-sper'me-ah) the presence of blood in the semen.

he·ma·tos·te·on (he"mah-tos'te-on) hemorrhage into the medullary cavity of a bone.

he·ma·to·tox·ic (he'mah-to-tok"sik) 1. pertaining to blood poisoning. 2. poisonous to the blood and hematopoietic system.

he·ma·to·tro·pic (-tro'pik) having a specific affinity for or exerting a specific effect on the blood or blood cells.

he·ma·tox·y·lin (he"mah-tok'sĭ-lin) an acid coloring matter from the heartwood of *Haematoxylon campechianum;* used as a histologic stain and also as an indicator.

he·ma·tu·ria (he"mah-tu're-ah) blood (erythrocytes) in the urine. **endemic h.**, urinary schistosomiasis. **essential h.**, that for which no cause has been determined. **false h.**, pseudohematuria. **renal h.**, that in which the blood comes from the kidney. **urethral h.**, that in which the blood comes from the urethra. **vesical h.**, that in which the blood comes from the bladder.

heme (hēm) an iron compound of protoporphyrin which constitutes the pigment portion or protein-free part of the hemoglobin molecule and is responsible for its oxygen-carrying properties.

hem·er·a·lo·pia (hem"er-ah-lo'pe-ah) day blindness; defective vision in bright light.

hemi- word element [Gr.], *half.*

hemi·achro·ma·top·sia (hem"e-ah"kro-mah-top'se-ah) color vision deficiency in half, or in corresponding halves, of the visual field.

hemi·ageu·sia (-ah-goo'zhah) ageusia on one side of the tongue.

hemi·amy·os·the·nia (-ah-mi"os-the'ne-ah) lack of muscular power on one side of the body.

hemi·an·al·ge·sia (-an"al-je'ze-ah) analgesia on one side of the body.

hemi·an·es·the·sia (-an"es-the'zhah) anesthesia of one side of the body. **crossed h.**, **h. crucia'ta**, loss of sensation on one side of the face and loss of pain and temperature sense on the opposite side of the body.

hemi·an·o·pia (-an-o'pe-ah) defective vision or blindness in half of the visual field of one or both eyes; loosely, scotoma in less than half of the visual field of one or both eyes. **hemianop'ic**, adj. **absolute h.**, blindness to light, color, and form in half of the visual field. **bilateral h.**, hemianopia affecting both eyes. **binasal h.**, that in which the defect is in the nasal half of the visual field in each eye. **binocular h.**, bilateral h. **bitemporal h.,** that in which the defect is in the temporal half of the visual field in each eye. **complete h.,** that affecting an entire half of the visual field in each eye. **congruous h.,** in that in which the defect is approximately the same in each eye. **crossed h.,** heteronymous h. **heteronymous h.,** that affecting both nasal or both temporal halves of the field of vision. **homonymous h.,** that affecting the nasal half of the field of vision of one eye and the temporal half of the other. **nasal h.,** that affecting the medial half of the visual field, i.e., the half nearer the nose. **quadrant h., quadrantic h.,** quadrantanopia. **temporal h.,** that affecting the lateral vertical half of the visual field, i.e., the half nearest the temple.

hemi·aprax·ia (-ah-prak′se-ah) apraxia on one side of the body only.

hemi·atax·ia (-ah-tak′se-ah) ataxia on one side of the body.

hemi·ath·e·to·sis (-ath″ĕ-to′sis) athetosis of one side of the body.

hemi·at·ro·phy (-ă′tro-fe) atrophy of one side of the body or one half of an organ or part.

hemi·ax·i·al (-ak′se-al) at any oblique angle to the long axis of the body or a part.

hemi·bal·lis·mus (-bah-liz′mus) a violent form of dyskinesia involving one side of the body, most marked in the upper limb.

hemi·blad·der (hem′e-blad″er) a half bladder, as in exstrophy of the cloaca; the urinary bladder is formed as two physically separated parts, each with its own ureter.

hemi·block (-blok) failure in conduction of cardiac impulse in either of the two main divisions of the left branch of the bundle of His; the interruption may occur in either the anterior (superior) or posterior division.

he·mic (he′mik, hem′ik) pertaining to blood.

hemi·car·dia (hem″e-kahr′de-ah) 1. a congenital anomaly characterized by the presence of only one side of a four-chambered heart. 2. either lateral half of a normal heart.

hemi·cen·trum (-sen′trum) either lateral half of a vertebral centrum.

hemi·cho·rea (-ko-re′ah) chorea affecting only one side of the body.

hemi·cra·nia (-kra′ne-ah) 1. unilateral headache. 2. incomplete anencephaly. **chronic paroxysmal h.,** a type of one-sided headache resembling a cluster headache but occurring in paroxysms of half an hour or less, several times a day, sometimes for years.

hemi·cra·ni·o·sis (-kra″ne-o′sis) hyperostosis of one side of the cranium and face.

hemi·des·mo·some (-des′mo-sōm) a structure representing half of a desmosome, found on the basal surface of some epithelial cells, forming the site of attachment between the basal surface of the cell and the basement membrane.

hemi·dia·pho·re·sis (-di″ah-fah-re′sis) hemihyperhidrosis.

hemi·dia·phragm (-di′ah-fram) one half of the diaphragm.

hemi·dys·es·the·sia (-dis″es-the′zhah) dysesthesia on one side of the body.

hemi·epi·lep·sy (-ep′ĭ-lep″se) epilepsy affecting one side of the body.

hemi·fa·cial (-fa′shil) pertaining to or affecting half of the face.

hemi·gas·trec·to·my (-gas-trek′tah-me) excision of half of the stomach.

hemi·geu·sia (-goo′zhah) hemiageusia.

hemi·glos·sec·to·my (-glos-ek′tah-me) excision of one side of the tongue.

hemi·glos·si·tis (-glos-i′tis) inflammation of one half of the tongue.

hemi·hi·dro·sis (-hi-dro′sis) sweating on one side of the body only.

hemi·hy·pal·ge·sia (-hīp″al-je′ze-ah) diminished sensitivity to pain on one side of the body.

hemi·hy·per·es·the·sia (-hi″per-es-the′zhah) increased sensitiveness of one side of the body.

hemi·hy·per·hi·dro·sis (-hi″per-hi-dro′sis) excessive perspiration on one side of the body.

hemi·hy·per·tro·phy (-hi-per′trah-fe) overgrowth of one side of the body or of a part.

hemi·hy·pes·the·sia (-hi″pes-the′zhah) diminished sensitivity on one side of the body.

hemi·hy·po·to·nia (-hi″po-to′ne-ah) diminished muscle tone of one side of the body.

hemi·in·at·ten·tion (-in-ah-ten′shun) unilateral neglect.

hemi·lam·i·nec·to·my (-lam″ĭ-nek′tah-me) removal of a vertebral lamina on one side only.

hemi·lar·yn·gec·to·my (-lar″in-jek′tah-me) excision of one lateral half of the larynx.

hemi·lat·er·al (-lat′er-al) affecting one lateral half of the body only.

hemi·me·lia (-me′le-ah) a developmental anomaly characterized by absence of all or part of the distal half of a limb.

he·min (he′min) 1. a porphyrin chelate of iron, derived from red blood cells; the chloride of heme. It is used to treat the symptoms of various porphyrias. 2. hematin (1).

hemi·ne·phrec·to·my (hem″e-nĕ-frek′tah-me) excision of part (half) of a kidney.

hemi·opia (-o′pe-ah) hemianopia. **hemiop′ic,** adj.

hemi·par·a·ple·gia (-par″ah-ple′jah) paralysis of the lower half of one side.

hemi·pa·re·sis (-pah-re′sis) paresis affecting one side of the body.

hemi·pa·ret·ic (-pah-ret′ik) 1. pertaining to hemiparesis. 2. one affected with hemiparesis.

hemi·ple·gia (-ple′jah) paralysis of one side of the body. **hemiple′gic,** adj. **alternate h.,** paralysis of one side of the face and the opposite side of the body. **cerebral h.,** that due to a brain lesion. **crossed h.,** alternate h. **facial h.,** paralysis of one side of the face. **spastic h.,** hemiplegia with spasticity of the affected muscles and increased tendon reflexes. **spinal h.,** that due to a lesion of the spinal cord.

He·mip·tera (he-mip′ter-ah) an order of insects, winged or wingless, including ordinary bugs and lice, having mouth parts adapted for piercing and sucking.

hemi·ra·chis·chi·sis (hem″e-rah-kis′kĭ-sis) rachischisis without prolapse of the spinal cord.

hemi·sec·tion (-sek′shun) 1. division into two equal parts. 2. surgical division of a multiple rooted tooth from the crown to the furcation with removal of a root and part of the crown.

hemi·spasm (hem′e-spazm) spasm affecting one side only.

hemi·sphere (hem′ĭ-sfēr) half of a spherical or roughly spherical structure or organ. **cerebellar h.,** either of two lobes of the cerebellum lateral to the vermis. **cerebral h.,** one of the paired structures forming the bulk of the human brain, which together comprise the cerebral cortex, centrum semi-ovale, basal ganglia, and rhinencephalon, and contain the lateral ventricles. **dominant h.,** that cerebral hemisphere which is more concerned than the other in the integration of sensations and the control of voluntary functions.

hemi·sphe·ri·um (hem″ĭ-sfēr′e-um) pl. *hemisphe′ria.* [L.] either cerebral hemisphere.

hemi·ver·te·bra (hem″e-ver′tĭ-brah) 1. a developmental anomaly in which one side of a vertebra is incompletely developed. 2. a vertebra which is incompletely developed on one side.

hemi·zy·gos·i·ty (-zi-gos′ĭ-te) the state of having only one of a pair of alleles transmitting a specific character. **hemizy′gous,** adj.

hem(o)- word element [Gr.], *blood.* See also words beginning *hemato-.*

he·mo·blast (he′mo-blast) blast cell.

He·moc·cult (he′mo-kult) trademark for a guaiac reagent strip test for occult blood.

he·mo·cho·ri·al (he″mo-kor′e-al) denoting a type of placenta in which maternal blood comes in direct contact with the chorion, as in humans.

he·mo·chro·ma·to·sis (-kro″mah-to′sis) a disorder of iron metabolism with excess deposition of iron in the tissues, bronze skin pigmentation, cirrhosis, and diabetes mellitus. **hemochromatot′ic,** adj.

he·mo·con·cen·tra·tion (-kon″sen-tra′shun) decrease of the fluid content of the blood, with increased concentration of formed elements.

he·mo·co·nia (-ko′ne-ah) pl. *hemoco′niae.* [L.] small bodies exhibiting brownian movement, observed in blood platelets in darkfield microscopy of a wet film of blood.

he·mo·cy·a·nin (-si′ah-nin) a blue copper-containing respiratory pigment occurring in the blood of mollusks and arthropods.

he·mo·cyte (he′mo-sīt) blood cell.

he·mo·cy·to·blast (he″mo-si′to-blast) blast cell.

he·mo·cy·tom·e·ter (-si-tom′ĕ-ter) hemacytometer.

he·mo·cy·to·trip·sis (-si″to-trip′sis) disintegration of blood cells by pressure.

he·mo·di·a·fil·tra·tion (-di″ah-fil-tra′shun) hemofiltration with a dialytic component, so that blood flow is accelerated.

he·mo·di·ag·no·sis (-di″ag-no′sis) diagnosis by examination of the blood.

he·mo·di·al·y·sis (-di-al′ĭ-sis) removal of certain elements from the blood by virtue of the difference in rates of their diffusion through a semipermeable membrane while being circulated outside the body; the process involves both diffusion and ultrafiltration.

he·mo·di·a·lyz·er (-di′ah-līz″er) an apparatus for performing hemodialysis.

he·mo·di·lu·tion (-di-loo′shun) increase in fluid content of blood, resulting in lowered concentration of formed elements.

he·mo·dy·nam·ics (-di-nam′iks) the study of the movements of blood and of the forces concerned. **hemodynam′ic,** adj.

he·mo·fil·tra·tion (-fil-tra′shun) removal of waste products from blood by passing it through extracorporeal filters.

he·mo·flag·el·late (-flaj′ĕ-lāt) any flagellate protozoan parasite of the blood; the term includes the genera *Trypanosoma* and *Leishmania.*

he·mo·fus·cin (-fūs′in) a brownish-yellow hematogenous pigment resulting from hemoglobin decomposition, sometimes seen in the urine.

he·mo·glo·bin (he′mo-glo″bin) the oxygen-carrying pigment of erythrocytes, formed by developing erythrocytes in the bone marrow; a hemoprotein made up of four different polypeptide globin chains that contain between 141 and 146 amino acids. Hemoglobin A is normal adult hemoglobin and hemoglobin F is fetal hemoglobin. Many abnormal hemoglobins have been reported; the first were given capital letters such as hemoglobin E, H, M, and S, and later ones have been named for the place of discovery. Homozygosity for hemoglobin S results in sickle cell anemia, heterozygosity in sickle cell trait. Symbol Hb. **fetal h.,** that forming more than half of the hemoglobin of the fetus, present in minimal amounts in adults and abnormally elevated in certain blood disorders. **mean corpuscular h. (MCH),** the average hemoglobin content of an erythrocyte. **muscle h.,** myoglobin. **reduced h.,** that not combined with oxygen. **h. S,** the most common abnormal hemoglobin, with valine substituted for glutamic acid at position six of the beta chain, resulting in the abnormal erythrocytes called sickle cells, and causing sickle cell anemia.

he·mo·glo·bin·emia (he″mo-glo″bin-ēm′e-ah) excessive hemoglobin in blood plasma.

he·mo·glo·bin·ol·y·sis (-ol′ĭ-sis) the splitting up of hemoglobin.

he·mo·glo·bin·om·e·ter (-om′ĕ-ter) an instrument for colorimetric determination of hemoglobin content of blood.

he·mo·glo·bin·op·a·thy (-op′ah-the) 1. a hematologic disorder due to alteration in the genetically determined molecular structure of hemoglobin, such as sickle cell anemia, hemolytic anemia, or thalassemia. 2. sometimes more specifically, a hemoglobin disorder due to alterations in a globin chain, as opposed to the reduced or absent synthesis of normal chains in thalassemia.

he·mo·glo·bin·uria (he″mo-glo″bĭ-nu′re-ah) free hemoglobin in the urine. **hemoglobinu′ric,** adj. **march h.,** that seen after prolonged exercise. **paroxysmal cold h.,** an autoimmune or postviral disease marked by episodes of hemoglobinemia and hemoglobinuria after exposure to cold, caused by complement-dependent hemolysis due to Donath-Landsteiner antibody. **paroxysmal nocturnal h. (PNH),** a chronic acquired blood cell abnormality with episodes of intravascular hemolysis and venous thrombosis. **toxic h.,** that caused by ingestion of a poison.

he·mo·ki·ne·sis (-kĭ-ne′sis) circulation. **hemokinet′ic,** adj.

he·mo·lymph (he′mo-limf″) 1. blood and lymph. 2. the bloodlike fluid of those invertebrates having open blood-vascular systems.

he·mol·y·sin (he-mol′ĭ-sin) a substance that liberates hemoglobin from erythrocytes by interrupting their structural integrity.

he·mol·y·sis (he-mol′ĭ-sis) the liberation of hemoglobin, consisting of separation of the hemoglobin from the red cells and its appearance in the plasma. **hemolyt′ic,** adj. **immune h.,** lysis by complement of erythrocytes sensitized as a consequence of interaction with specific antibody to the erythrocytes.

he·mo·lyze (he′mo-līz) 1. to subject to hemolysis. 2. to undergo hemolysis.

he·mo·me·di·as·ti·num (he″mo-me″de-as-ti′num) an effusion of blood into the mediastinum.

he·mo·me·tra (-me′trah) hematometra.

he·mo·pa·thol·o·gy (-pah-thol′ah-je) the study of diseases of the blood.

he·mop·a·thy (he-mop′ah-the) any disease of the blood. **hemopath′ic,** adj.

he·mo·per·fu·sion (he″mo-per-fu′zhun) the passing of large volumes of blood over an extracorporeal adsorbent substance in order to remove toxic substances.

he·mo·peri·car·di·um (-per″ĭ-kahr′de-um) an effusion of blood within the pericardium.

he·mo·pex·in (-pek′sin) a heme-binding serum glycoprotein.

he·mo·phago·cyte (-fag′o-sīt) a phagocyte that destroys blood cells.

he·mo·phil (hēm′o-fil) 1. an organism thriving on blood. 2. a microorganism which grows best in media containing hemoglobin.

he·mo·phil·ia (he″mo-fil′e-ah) a hereditary hemorrhagic diathesis due to deficiency of a blood coagulation factor. **h. A,** classical h.; an X-linked recessive form due to deficiency of coagulation factor VIII. **h. B,** Christmas disease; an X-linked recessive form due to deficiency of coagulation factor IX. **h. C,** an autosomal disorder due to lack of coagulation factor XI; seen predominantly in persons of Jewish ancestry and characterized by minor bleeding, mild bruising, severe prolonged postsurgical bleeding, and abnormal clotting test times. **classical h.,** h. A. **vascular h.,** von Willebrand's disease.

he·mo·phil·ic (-fil′ik) 1. having an affinity for blood; in bacteriology, growing well in culture media containing blood or having a nutritional affinity for constituents of fresh blood. 2. pertaining to or characterized by hemophilia.

he·mo·pho·bia (he″mo-fo′be-ah) irrational fear of blood.

He·moph·i·lus (he-mof′ĭ-lus) Haemophilus.

he·mo·plas·tic (he″mo-plas′tik) hematopoietic.

he·mo·pneu·mo·peri·car·di·um (-noo″mo-per″ĭ-kahr′de-um) pneumohemopericardium.

he·mo·pneu·mo·tho·rax (-noo″mo-thor′aks) pneumothorax with hemorrhagic effusion.

he·mo·pre·cip·i·tin (-pre-sip′ĭ-tin) a blood precipitin.

he·mo·pro·tein (-pro′tēn) a conjugated protein containing heme as the prosthetic group, such as catalase, cytochrome, hemoglobin, or myoglobin.

he·mop·so·nin (he″mop-so′nin) an opsonin making erythrocytes more liable to phagocytosis.

he·mop·ty·sis (he-mop′tĭ-sis) the spitting of blood or of blood-stained sputum. **parasitic h.,** infection of the lungs with flukes of the genus *Paragonimus,* with cough, spitting of blood, and slow deterioration.

hem·or·rhage (hem′ah-rij) the escape of blood from the vessels; bleeding. **hemorrhag′ic,** adj. **capillary h.,** the oozing of blood from the minute vessels. **cerebral h.,** hemorrhage into the cerebrum; see *stroke syndrome.* **concealed h.,** internal h. **Duret's h's,** small, linear hemorrhages in the midline of the brainstem and upper pons caused by traumatic downward displacement of the brainstem. **fibrinolytic h.,** that due to abnormalities of fibrinolysis. **internal h.,** that in which the extravasated blood remains within the body. **petechial h.,** subcutaneous hemorrhage occurring in minute spots. **splinter h's,** linear hemorrhages beneath the nail.

hem·or·rha·gin (hem′ah-ra′jin) a cytolysin in certain venoms and poisons which is destructive to endothelial cells and blood vessels.

he·mor·rhe·ol·o·gy (he″mo-re-ol′ah-je) the study of deformation and flow properties of cellular and plasmatic components of blood and the rheological properties of vessel structures it comes in contact with.

hem·or·rhoid (hem′ah-roid) a varicose dilatation of a vein of the superior or inferior hemorrhoidal plexus. **hemorrhoi′dal,** adj. **external h.,** one in a vein of the inferior hemorrhoidal plexus, distal to the pectinate line and covered with modified anal skin. **internal h.,** one in a vein of the superior hemorrhoidal plexus, originating above the pectinate line and covered by mucous membrane. **prolapsed h.,** an internal hemorrhoid that has descended below the pectinate line and protruded outside the anal sphincter. **strangulated h.,** an internal

hemorrhoid that has been prolapsed so long and extensively that its blood supply has become occluded by the constricting action of the anal sphincter. **thrombosed h.,** one containing clotted blood.

hem·or·rhoid·ec·to·my (hem″ah-roi-dek′tah-me) excision of hemorrhoids.

he·mo·sid·er·in (he″mo-sid′er-in) an insoluble form of tissue storage iron, visible microscopically both with and without the use of special stains.

hemosiderinuria (-u′re-ah) hemosiderin in the urine, such as in hemochromatosis.

he·mo·sid·er·o·sis (-sid″er-o′sis) a focal or general increase in tissue iron stores without associated tissue damage. **pulmonary h.,** the deposition of abnormal amounts of hemosiderin in the lungs, due to bleeding into the lung interstitium.

he·mo·sta·sis (he″mo-sta′sis, he-mos′tah-sis) 1. the arrest of bleeding by the physiological properties of vasoconstriction and coagulation or by surgical means. 2. interruption of blood flow through any vessel or to any anatomical area.

he·mo·stat (he′mo-stat) 1. a small surgical clamp for constricting blood vessels. 2. an antihemorrhagic agent.

he·mo·stat·ic (he″mo-stat′ik) 1. causing hemostasis, or an agent that so acts. 2. due to or characterized by stasis of the blood.

he·mo·tho·rax (-thor′aks) a pleural effusion containing blood.

he·mo·tox·ic (he′mo-tok″sik) hematotoxic.

he·mo·tox·in (-tok″sin) an exotoxin characterized by hemolytic activity.

hen·ry (H) (hen′re) the SI unit of electric inductance, equivalent to one weber per ampere.

HEP hepatoerythropoietic porphyria.

Hep·ad·na·vi·ri·dae (hep-ad″nah-vir′ĭ-de) the hepatitis B–like viruses: a family of DNA viruses causing infection and associated with chronic disease and neoplasia.

he·par (he′par) [Gr.] liver.

hep·a·ran sul·fate (hep′ah-ran) a glycosaminoglycan occurring in the cell membrane of most cells, consisting of a repeating disaccharide unit of glucosamine and uronic acid residues, which may be acetylated and sulfated; it accumulates in several mucopolysaccharidoses.

hep·a·rin (hep′ah-rin) a sulfated glycosaminoglycan of mixed composition, released by mast cells and by blood basophils in many tissues, especially the liver and lungs, and having potent anticoagulant properties. It also has lipotrophic properties, promoting transfer of fat from blood to the fat depots by activation of lipoprotein lipase. It is used as the calcium or sodium salt in the prophylaxis and treatment of disorders in which there is excessive or undesirable clotting and to prevent clotting during extracorporeal circulation, blood transfusion, and blood sampling.

hep·a·ri·nize (hep′ah-rin-īz″) to render blood incoagulable with heparin.

hep·a·ta·tro·phia (hep″it-ah-tro′fe-ah) atrophy of the liver.

he·pat·ic (hĕ-pat′ik) pertaining to the liver.

hepatic(o)- word element [Gr.], *hepatic duct.*

he·pat·i·co·du·o·de·nos·to·my (hĕ-pat″ĭ-ko-doo″o-dĕ-nos′tah-me) anastomosis of the hepatic duct to the duodenum.

he·pat·i·co·gas·tros·to·my (-gas-tros′tah-me) anastomosis of the hepatic duct to the stomach.

he·pat·i·co·li·thot·o·my (-lĭ-thot′ah-me) incision of the hepatic duct, with removal of calculi.

he·pat·i·cos·to·my (hĕ-pat″ĭ-kos′tah-me) fistulization of the hepatic duct.

hepat·ic phos·phor·y·lase (hĕ-pat′ik fosfor′ĭ-lās) the liver isozyme of glycogen phosphorylase; deficiency causes glycogen storage disease, type VI.

hep·a·ti·tis (hep″ah-ti′tis) pl. *hepati′tides.* Inflammation of the liver. **h. A,** a self-limited viral disease of worldwide distribution, usually transmitted by oral ingestion of infected material but sometimes transmitted parenterally; most cases are clinically inapparent or have mild flu-like symptoms; any jaundice is mild. **anicteric h.,** viral hepatitis without jaundice. **h. B,** an acute viral disease transmitted primarily parenterally, but also orally, by intimate personal contact, and from mother to neonate. Prodromal symptoms of fever, malaise, anorexia, nausea, and vomiting decline with the onset of clinical jaundice, angioedema, urticarial skin lesions, and arthritis. After 3 to 4 months most patients recover completely, but some may become carriers or remain ill chronically. **h. C,** a viral disease caused by the hepatitis C virus, commonly occurring after transfusion or parenteral drug abuse; it frequently progresses to a chronic form that is usually asymptomatic but that may involve cirrhosis. **cholangiolitic h.,** cholestatic h. (1). **cholestatic h.,** 1. inflammation of the bile ducts of the liver associated with obstructive jaundice. 2. hepatic inflammation and cholestasis resulting from reaction to drugs such as estrogens or chlorpromazines. **h. D, delta h.,** infection with hepatitis D virus, occurring either simultaneously with

or as a superinfection in hepatitis B, whose severity it may increase. **h. E,** a type transmitted by the oral-fecal route, usually via contaminated water; chronic infection does not occur but acute infection may be fatal in pregnant women. **enterically transmitted non-A, non-B h. (ET-NANB),** h. E. **h. G,** a post-transfusion disease caused by hepatitis G virus, ranging from asymptomatic infection to fulminant hepatitis. **infectious h.,** h. A. **infectious necrotic h.,** black disease. **lupoid h.,** chronic active hepatitis with autoimmune manifestations. **neonatal h.,** hepatitis of uncertain etiology occurring soon after birth and marked by prolonged persistent jaundice that may progress to cirrhosis. **non-A, non-B h.,** a syndrome of acute viral hepatitis occurring without the serologic markers of hepatitis A or B, including hepatitis C and hepatitis E. **posttransfusion h.,** viral hepatitis, now primarily hepatitis C, transmitted via transfusion of blood or blood products, especially multiple pooled donor products such as clotting factor concentrates. **serum h.,** h. B. **transfusion h.,** posttransfusion h. **viral h.,** h. A, h. B, h. C, h. D, and h. E.

hep·a·ti·za·tion (hep″ah-tĭ-za′shun) consolidation of tissue into a liverlike mass, as in the lung in lobar pneumonia. The early stage, in which pulmonary exudate is blood stained, is called *red h.* The later stage, in which red cells disintegrate and a fibrinosuppurative exudate persists, is called *gray h.*

hepat(o)- word element [Gr.], *liver.*

hep·a·to·blas·to·ma (hep″ah-to-blas-to′mah) a malignant intrahepatic tumor consisting chiefly of embryonic tissue, occurring in infants and young children.

hep·a·to·car·ci·no·ma (-kahr″sĭ-no′mah) hepatocellular carcinoma.

hep·a·to·cele (hep′ah-to-sēl) hernia of the liver.

hep·a·to·cel·lu·lar (hep″ah-to-sel′u-lar) pertaining to or affecting liver cells.

hep·a·to·cho·lan·gio·car·ci·no·ma (-kolan″je-o-kahr″sĭ-no′mah) cholangiohepatoma.

hep·a·to·cyte (hep′ah-to-sīt″) a hepatic cell.

hep·a·to·gas·tric (hep″ah-to-gas′trik) pertaining to the liver and stomach.

hep·a·to·gen·ic (-jen′ik) 1. giving rise to or forming liver tissue. 2. hepatogenous.

hep·a·tog·e·nous (hep″ah-toj′ĕ-nus) 1. produced in or originating in the liver. 2. hepatogenic.

hep·a·to·gram (hep′ah-to-gram″) a radiograph of the liver.

hep·a·toid (hep′ah-toid) resembling the liver.

hep·a·to·jug·u·lar (hep″ah-to-jug′u-ler) pertaining to the liver and jugular vein; see under *reflux*.

hep·a·to·lith (hep′ah-to-lith″) a biliary calculus in the liver.

hep·a·to·li·thi·a·sis (hep″ah-to-lĭ-thi′ah-sis) the presence of calculi in the biliary ducts of the liver.

hep·a·tol·o·gy (hep″ah-tol′ah-je) the scientific study of the liver and its diseases.

hep·a·tol·y·sin (hep″ah-tol′ĭ-sin) a cytolysin destructive to liver cells.

hep·a·tol·y·sis (hep″ah-tol′ĭ-sis) destruction of the liver cells. **hepatolyt′ic,** adj.

hep·a·to·ma (hep″ah-to′mah) 1. a tumor of the liver. 2. hepatocellular carcinoma (malignant h.).

hep·a·to·meg·a·ly (hep″ah-to-meg′ah-le) enlargement of the liver.

hep·a·to·mel·a·no·sis (-mel″ah-no′sis) melanosis of the liver.

hep·a·tom·pha·lo·cele (hep″ah-tom′fah-lo-sēl″) umbilical hernia with liver involvement in the hernial sac.

hep·a·to·pexy (hep′ah-to-pek″se) surgical fixation of a displaced liver.

hep·a·to·pneu·mon·ic (hep″ah-to-noo-mon′ik) pertaining to, affecting, or communicating with the liver and lungs.

hep·a·to·por·tal (-port′il) pertaining to the portal system of the liver.

hep·a·to·re·nal (-rĕn′il) pertaining to the liver and kidneys.

hep·a·tor·rhex·is (hep″ah-to-rek′sis) rupture of the liver.

hep·a·to·sis (hep″ah-to′sis) any functional disorder of the liver. **serous h.,** veno-occlusive disease of the liver.

hep·a·to·sple·ni·tis (hep″ah-to-splĕ-ni′tis) inflammation of the liver and spleen.

hep·a·to·sple·no·meg·a·ly (-splen″o-meg′ah-le) enlargement of the liver and spleen.

hep·a·to·tox·in (hep′ah-to-tok″sin) a toxin that destroys liver cells. **hep′atotoxic,** adj.

hept(a)- word element [Gr.], *seven*.

hep·ta·chro·mic (hep″tah-kro′mik) 1. pertaining to or exhibiting seven colors. 2. able to distinguish all seven colors of the spectrum.

-hep·ta·ene a suffix denoting a chemical compound in which there are seven conjugated double bonds.

hep·ta·no·ate (hep″tah-no′āt) enanthate.

hep·tose (hep′tōs) a sugar whose molecule contains seven carbon atoms.

herb (erb, herb) any leafy plant without a woody stem, especially one used medicinally or as a flavoring. **her′bal,** adj.

her·bal·ism (er′-, her′bal-izm) the medical use of preparations containing only plant material.

her·biv·o·rous (her-biv′ah-rus) subsisting upon plants.

he·red·i·tary (hĕ-red′ĭ-tar-e) genetically transmitted from parent to offspring.

he·red·i·ty (-te) 1. the genetic transmission of a particular quality or trait from parent to offspring. 2. the genetic constitution of an individual.

her·e·do·fa·mil·i·al (her″ĕ-do-fah-mil′e-il) occurring in certain families under circumstances that implicate a hereditary basis.

her·i·ta·bil·i·ty (her″ĭ-tah-bil′ĭ-te) the quality of being heritable; a measure of the extent to which a phenotype is influenced by the genotype.

her·maph·ro·dite (her-maf′ro-dīt) an individual with hermaphroditism.

her·maph·ro·di·tism (her-maf′ro-di-tizm″) presence in an individual of both ovarian and testicular tissues and of ambiguous morphologic criteria of sex; see also *pseudohermaphroditism.* **hermaphrodit′ic,** adj. **bilateral h.,** that in which gonadal tissue typical of both sexes occurs on each side of the body. **false h.,** pseudohermaphroditism. **lateral h.,** presence of gonadal tissue typical of one sex on one side of the body and tissue typical of the other sex on the opposite side. **transverse h.,** that in which the external genital organs are typical of one sex and the gonads typical of the other sex. **true h.,** see *hermaphroditism.*

her·met·ic (her-met′ik) impervious to air.

her·nia (her′ne-ah) [L.] protrusion of a portion of an organ or tissue through an abnormal opening. **her′nial,** adj. **abdominal h.,** one through the abdominal wall. **Barth's h.,** one between the serosa of the abdominal wall and that of a persistent vitelline duct. **Béclard's h.,** femoral hernia at the saphenous opening. **Bochdalek's h.,** congenital diaphragmatic hernia due to failure of closure of the pleuroperitoneal hiatus. **cerebral h.,** protrusion of brain substance through the cranium. **Cloquet's h.,** pectineal h. **complete h.,** one in which the sac and its contents have passed through the hernial orifice. **diaphragmatic h.,** hernia through the diaphragm. **diverticular h.,** protrusion of a congenital diverticulum of the gut. **epigastric h.,** a hernia through the linea alba above the navel. **extrasaccular h.,** sliding h. **fat h.,** hernial protrusion of peritoneal fat through the abdominal wall. **femoral h.,** protrusion of a loop of intestine into the femoral canal. **gastroesophageal h.,** hiatal hernia in which the distal esophagus and part of the stomach protrude into the thorax. **Hesselbach's h.,** femoral hernia with a pouch through the cribriform fascia. **hiatal h., hiatus h.,** protrusion of any structure through the esophageal hiatus of the diaphragm. **Holthouse's h.,** an inguinal hernia that has turned outward into the groin. **incarcerated h.,** a hernia so occluded that it cannot be returned by manipulation; it may or may not be strangulated. **incisional h.,** one occurring through an old abdominal incision. **inguinal h.,** hernia into the inguinal canal. **intermuscular h., interparietal h.,** an interstitial hernia lying between one or another of the fascial or muscular planes of the abdomen. **interstitial h.,** one in which a knuckle of intestine lies between two layers of the abdominal wall. **ischiatic h.,** hernia through the sacrosciatic foramen. **labial h.,** one into a labium majus. **mesocolic h.,** an intra-abdominal hernia in which the small intestine rotates incompletely during development and becomes trapped in the mesentery of the colon. **obturator h.,** a protrusion through the obturator foramen. **omental h.,** an abdominal hernia containing omentum. **paraduodenal h.,** mesocolic h. **para-esophageal h.,** hiatal hernia in which part or almost all of the stomach protrudes through the hiatus into the thorax to the left of the esophagus, with the gastroesophageal junction remaining in place. **pectineal h.,** a type of femoral hernia that enters the femoral canal and then perforates the aponeurosis of the pectineus muscle. **properitoneal h.,** an interstitial hernia lying between the parietal peritoneum and the transverse fascia. **reducible h.,** one that can be returned by manipulation. **retrograde h.,** herniation of two loops of intestine, the portion between the loops lying within the abdominal wall. **Richter's h.,** incarcerated or strangulated hernia in which only a portion of the circumference of the bowel wall is involved. **scrotal h.,** inguinal hernia which has passed into the scrotum. **sliding h.,** hernia of the cecum (on the right) or the sigmoid colon (on the left) in which the wall of the viscus forms a portion of the hernial sac, the remainder of the sac being formed by the parietal peritoneum. **sliding hiatal h.,** hiatal hernia in which the upper stomach and the gastroesophageal junction protrude upward into the posterior mediastinum; the protrusion, which may be fixed or intermittent, is partially covered by a peritoneal sac. **strangulated h.,** incarcerated hernia so tightly constricted as to compromise the

blood supply of the hernial sac, leading to gangrene of the sac and its contents. **synovial h.,** protrusion of the inner lining membrane through the fibrous membrane of an articular capsule. **umbilical h.,** herniation of part of the umbilicus, the defect in the abdominal wall and protruding bowel being covered with skin and subcutaneous tissue. **h. u′teri inguina′lis,** see *persistent müllerian duct syndrome,* under *syndrome.* **vaginal h.,** vaginocele; a hernia into the vagina. **ventral h.,** abdominal h.

her·ni·at·ed (her′ne-āt′ed) protruding like a hernia; enclosed in a hernia.

her·ni·a·tion (her″ne-a′shun) abnormal protrusion of an organ or other body structure through a defect or natural opening in a covering, membrane, muscle, or bone. **h. of intervertebral disk,** herniated disk; protrusion of the nucleus pulposus or anulus fibrosus of the disk, which may impinge on nerve roots. **h. of nucleus pulposus,** see *h. of intervertebral disk.* **tentorial h.,** downward displacement of the most medially placed cerebral structures through the tentorial notch, caused by a supratentorial mass.

her·nio·plas·ty (her′ne-o-plas″te) surgical repair of a hernia; sometimes specifically that using a mesh patch or plug for reinforcement. Cf. *herniorrhaphy.*

her·ni·or·rha·phy (her″ne-or′ah-fe) surgical repair of a hernia, sometimes specifically by apposition and suturing of the edges of the defect. Cf. *hernioplasty.*

her·ni·ot·o·my (her″ne-ot′ah-me) a cutting operation for the repair of hernia.

her·o·in (her′o-in) diacetylmorphine; a highly addictive morphine derivative; the importation of heroin and its salts into the United States, as well as its use in medicine, is illegal.

herp·an·gi·na (her″pan-ji′nah) herpes angina; an infectious febrile disease due to a coxsackievirus, marked by vesicular and ulcerated lesions on the fauces or soft palate.

her·pes (her′pēz) any inflammatory skin disease marked by the formation of small vesicles in clusters; the term is usually restricted to such diseases caused by herpesviruses and is used alone to refer to *h. simplex* or to *h. zoster.* **h. febri′lis,** see *h. simplex.* **genital h., h. genita′lis,** herpes simplex due to type 2 virus, primarily transmitted sexually via genital secretions and involving the genital region; in women, the vesicular stage may give rise to confluent, painful ulcerations and may be accompanied by neurologic symptoms. **h. gestatio′nis,** a variant of dermatitis herpetiformis peculiar to pregnant women, and clearing upon termination of pregnancy. **h. labia′lis,** h. febrilis affecting the vermilion border of the lips. **h. progenita′lis,** genital h. **h. sim′plex,** an acute viral disease, caused by human herpesviruses 1 and 2, marked by groups of vesicles on the skin, often on the borders of the lips or nares (*cold sores*), or on the genitals (*genital h.*); it often accompanies fever (*fever blisters, h. febrilis*). **h. zos′ter,** shingles; an acute, unilateral, self-limited inflammatory disease of cerebral ganglia and the ganglia of posterior nerve roots and peripheral nerves in a segmented distribution, believed to represent activation of latent human herpesvirus 3 in those who have been rendered partially immune after a previous attack of chickenpox, and characterized by groups of small vesicles in the cutaneous areas along the course of affected nerves, and associated with neuralgic pain. **h. zos′ter ophthal′micus,** herpes zoster involving the ophthalmic nerve, with a vesicular erythematous rash along the nerve path (forehead, eyelid, and cornea) preceded by lancinating pain; there is iridocyclitis, and corneal involvement may lead to keratitis and corneal anesthesia. **h. zos′ter o′ticus,** Ramsay Hunt syndrome (1).

her·pes·vi·rus (-vi″rus) any of a group of DNA viruses which includes the etiologic agents of herpes simplex, herpes zoster, chickenpox, infectious mononucleosis, and cytomegalic inclusion disease in humans, and of pseudorabies and other animal diseases. See accompanying table.

her·pet·ic (her-pet′ik) pertaining to or of the nature of herpes; relating to or caused by herpesviruses.

her·sage (ār-sahzh′) [Fr.] surgical separation of the fibers in a scarred area of a peripheral nerve.

hertz (Hz) (herts) the SI unit of frequency, equal to one cycle per second.

hes·per·i·din (hes-per′ĭ-din) a bioflavonoid predominant in lemons and oranges.

het·a·starch (het′ah-stahrch) an esterified amylopectin-containing starch, used as a plasma volume expander, administered by infusion.

het·er·e·cious (het″er-e′shus) parasitic on different hosts in various stages of its existence.

het·er·es·the·sia (-es-the′zhah) variation of cutaneous sensibility on adjoining areas.

het·er·er·gic (-er′jik) having different effects; said of two drugs one of which produces a particular effect and the other does not.

heter(o)- word element [Gr.], *other; dissimilar.*

het·er·ag·glu·ti·na·tion (het″er-o-ah-gloo″tĭ-na′shun) agglutination of particulate antigens of one species by agglutinins derived from another species.

het·er·o·an·ti·body (-an′tĭ-bod″e) an antibody combining with antigens originating from a species foreign to the antibody producer.

het·er·o·an·ti·gen (-an′tĭ-jen) an antigen originating from a species foreign to the antibody producer.

het·er·o·blas·tic (-blas′tik) originating in a different kind of tissue.

het·er·o·cel·lu·lar (-sel′u-ler) composed of cells of different kinds.

het·er·o·chro·ma·tin (-kro′mah-tin) that state of chromatin in which it is dark-staining, genetically inactive, and tightly coiled.

het·er·o·chro·mia (-kro′me-ah) diversity of color in a part normally of one color. **heterochro′mic,** adj. **h. i′ridis,** difference of color in the two irides, or in different areas in the same iris.

het·er·o·clad·ic (-klad′ik) pertaining to or characterized by an anastomosis between terminal branches from different arteries.

het·er·o·clit·ic (-klit′ik) irregular; said of a kind of antibody (see under *antibody*).

HUMAN HERPESVIRUSES

Virus	Associated Disease
Human herpesvirus 1	Herpes simplex
Human herpesvirus 2	Herpes simplex
Human herpesvirus 3	Chickenpox, herpes zoster
Human herpesvirus 4	Infectious mononucleosis
Human herpesvirus 5	Cytomegalic inclusion disease
Human herpesvirus 6	Exanthema subitum
Human herpesvirus 7	None known
Human herpesvirus 8	Kaposi's sarcoma, primary effusion lymphoma, multicentric plasma cell–type Castleman disease

het·ero·crine (het´er-o-krin) secreting more than one kind of matter.

het·ero·cyc·lic (het˝er-o-sik´lik) having a closed chain or ring formation including atoms of different elements.

het·ero·cy·to·tro·pic (-si˝to-tro´pik) having an affinity for cells from different species.

het·ero·der·mic (-der´mik) denoting a skin graft from an individual of another species.

het·ero·dont (het´er-o-dont˝) having teeth of different shapes, as molars, incisors, etc.

het·er·od·ro·mous (het˝er-od´ro-mus) moving, acting, or arranged in the opposite direction.

het·ero·erot·i·cism (het˝er-o-ĕ-rot´ĭ-sizm) 1. sexual feeling directed toward someone of the opposite sex. 2. alloeroticism (1). 3. a stage in which the erotic energy is directed toward objects other than oneself, specifically to those of the opposite sex. **heteroerot´ic,** adj.

het·ero·ga·met·ic (-gah-met´ik) pertaining to production of gametes containing more than one kind of sex chromosome, as in human males (XY).

het·ero·gam·e·ty (-gam´ĕ-te) the production of unlike gametes by an individual of one sex, as the production of X- and Y-bearing gametes by the human male.

het·er·og·a·my (het˝er-og´ah-me) 1. reproduction resulting from the union of two dissimilar gametes, particularly in higher organisms. 2. alternation of generations in which the two types of sexual reproduction alternate, as bisexual and parthenogenetic. **heterog´amous,** adj.

het·ero·ge·ne·ous (het˝er-o-je´ne-us) not of uniform composition, quality, or structure.

het·ero·gen·e·sis (het˝er-o-jen´ĕ-sis) 1. metagenesis. 2. asexual generation. **heterogenet´ic,** adj.

het·ero·geu·sia (-goo´zhah) any parageusia in which all gustatory stimuli are distorted in a similar way.

het·er·og·o·ny (het˝er-og´ah-ne) heterogenesis.

het·ero·graft (het´er-o-graft˝) xenograft.

het·ero·hem·ag·glu·ti·na·tion (het˝er-o-hem˝ah-gloo˝tĭ-na´shun) agglutination of erythrocytes of one species by a hemagglutinin derived from an individual of a different species.

het·ero·he·mol·y·sin (-he-mol´ĭ-sin) a hemolysin which destroys red blood cells of animals of species other than that of the animal in which it is formed; it may occur naturally or be induced by immunization.

het·ero·im·mu·ni·ty (-ĭ-mu´nĭ-te) 1. an immune state induced in an individual by immunization with cells of an animal of another species. 2. a state in which an immune response to exogenous antigen (e.g., drugs or pathogens) results in immunopathological changes. **heteroimmune´,** adj.

het·ero·ker·a·to·plas·ty (-ker´ah-to-plas˝te) grafting of corneal tissue taken from an individual of another species.

het·er·o·ki·ne·sis (-kĭ-ne´sis) differential distribution of sex chromosomes in the developing gametes of a heterogametic organism.

het·er·ol·o·gous (het˝er-ol´ah-gus) 1. made up of tissue not normal to the part. 2. xenogeneic.

het·er·ol·y·sis (het˝er-ol´ĭ-sis) lysis of the cells of one species by lysin from a different species. **heterolyt´ic,** adj.

het·ero·mer·ic (het˝er-o-mer´ik) sending processes through one of the commissures to the white matter of the opposite side of the spinal cord; said of neurons.

het·ero·meta·pla·sia (-met˝ah-pla´zhah) formation of tissue foreign to the part where it is formed.

het·ero·met·ric (-met´rik) involving or dependent on a change in size; cf. *homeometric.*

het·ero·me·tro·pia (-mĕ-tro´pe-ah) the state in which the refraction in the two eyes differs.

het·ero·mor·pho·sis (-mor-fo´sis) the development, in regeneration, of an organ or structure different from the one that was lost.

het·ero·mor·phous (-mor´fus) of abnormal shape or structure.

het·er·on·o·mous (het˝er-on´ah-mus) 1. in biology, subject to different laws of growth; specialized along different lines. 2. in psychology, subject to another's will.

het·er·on·y·mous (-ĭ-mus) standing in opposite relations.

het·ero·os·teo·plas·ty (het˝er-o-os´te-o-plas˝te) osteoplasty with bone taken from an individual of another species.

het·ero·phago·some (-fag´o-sōm) an intracytoplasmic vacuole formed by phagocytosis or pinocytosis, which becomes fused with a lysosome, subjecting its contents to enzymatic digestion.

het·er·oph·a·gy (het˝er-of´ah-je) the taking into a cell of exogenous material by phagocytosis or pinocytosis and the digestion of the ingested material after fusion of the newly formed vacuole with a lysosome.

het·ero·phil (het´er-o-fil˝) 1. a granular leukocyte represented by neutrophils in humans, but characterized in other mammals by granules which have variable sizes and staining characteristics. 2. heterophilic.

het·ero·phil·ic (het˝er-o-fil´ik) 1. having affinity for antigens or antibodies other than the one for which it is specific. 2. staining with a type of stain other than the usual one.

het·ero·pho·ria (-for'e-ah) failure of the visual axes to remain parallel after elimination of visual fusional stimuli. **heterophor'ic,** adj.

het·er·oph·thal·mia (het″er-of-thal'me-ah) difference in the direction of the visual axes, or in the color, of the two eyes.

Het·er·oph·y·es (het″er-of'e-ēz) a genus of minute trematode worms parasitic in the intestine of fish-eating mammals.

het·ero·pla·sia (het″er-o-pla'zhah) replacement of normal by abnormal tissue; malposition of normal cells. **heteroplas'tic,** adj. **progressive osseous h.,** osteoma cutis.

het·ero·ploi·dy (-ploi″de) the state of having an abnormal number of chromosomes.

het·er·op·sia (het″er-op'se-ah) unequal vision in the two eyes.

het·ero·pyk·no·sis (het″er-o-pik-no'sis) 1. the quality of showing variations in density throughout. 2. a state of differential condensation observed in different chromosomes, or in different regions of the same chromosome; it may be attenuated (*negative h.*) or accentuated (*positive h.*). **heteropyknot'ic,** adj.

het·ero·sex·u·al (-sek'shoo-al) 1. pertaining to, characteristic of, or directed toward the opposite sex. 2. one who is sexually attracted to persons of the opposite sex.

het·er·o·sis (het″er-o'sis) the existence, in the first generation hybrid, of greater vigor than is shown by either parent strain.

het·er·os·po·rous (het″er-os'po-rus) having two kinds of spores, which reproduce asexually.

het·ero·sug·ges·tion (het″er-o-sug-jes'-chun) suggestion received from another person, as opposed to autosuggestion.

het·ero·to·nia (-to'ne-ah) a state characterized by variations in tension or tone. **heteroton'ic,** adj.

het·ero·to·pia (-to'pe-ah) displacement or misplacement of parts; the presence of a tissue in an abnormal location. **heterotop'ic,** adj.

het·ero·trans·plan·ta·tion (-trans″plan-ta'shun) xenogeneic transplantation.

het·ero·tro·phic (-tro'fik) not self-sustaining; said of microorganisms requiring a reduced form of carbon for energy and synthesis.

het·ero·tro·pia (-tro'pe-ah) strabismus.

het·ero·typ·ic (-tip'ik) pertaining to, characteristic of, or belonging to a different type.

het·ero·typ·i·cal (-tip'ĭ-k'l) heterotypic.

het·er·ox·e·nous (het″er-ok'sĕ-nus) requiring more than one host to complete the life cycle.

het·ero·zy·gos·i·ty (het″er-o-zi-gos'ĭ-te) the state of possessing different alleles at a given locus in regard to a given character. **heterozy'gous,** adj.

het·ero·zy·gote (-zi'gōt) an individual having different alleles in regard to a given character. **manifesting h.,** a female heterozygous for an X-linked disorder in whom, because of unfavorable X inactivation, the trait is expressed clinically with about the same severity as in hemizygous affected males.

heu·ris·tic (hu-ris'tik) encouraging or promoting investigation; conducive to discovery.

hex(a)- word element [Gr.], *six.*

hexa·chlo·ro·phene (hek″sah-klor'o-fēn) an antibacterial effective against gram-positive organisms; used as a local antiseptic and detergent for application to the skin.

hex·ad (hek'sad) 1. a group or combination of six similar or related entities. 2. an element with a valence of six.

hexa·dac·ty·ly (hek″sah-dak'til-e) the occurrence of six digits on one hand or foot.

hex·ane (hek'sān) a saturated hydrogen obtained by distillation from petroleum.

hexo·ki·nase (hek″so-ki'nās) an enzyme that catalyzes the transfer of a high-energy phosphate group to a hexose, the initial step in the cellular utilization of free hexoses. The enzyme occurs in all tissues as various isozymes with varying specificities; the liver isozyme (type IV) is specific for glucose and is often called *glucokinase.*

hex·os·amine (hek-sōs'ah-mēn) any of a class of hexoses in which the hydroxyl group is replaced by an amino group.

hex·os·amin·i·dase (hek″sōs-ah-min'ĭ-dās) 1. any of the enzymes that cleave hexosamines or acetylated hexosamines from gangliosides or other glycosides. 2. a specific hexosaminidase acting on keratan sulfate and ganglioside GM_2 and related compounds.

hex·ose (hek'sōs) a monosaccharide containing six carbon atoms in a molecule.

hex·uron·ic ac·id (hek″su-ron'ik) any uronic acid formed by oxidation of a hexose.

hex·yl·re·sor·ci·nol (hek″sil-rĭ-sor'sĭ-nol) a substituted phenol with bactericidal properties used as an antiseptic in mouthwashes and skin wound cleansers.

HF Hageman factor (coagulation factor XII).

Hf hafnium.

Hg mercury (L. *hydrargy'rum*).

Hgb hemoglobin.

HGH, hGH human growth hormone.

HHS Department of Health and Human Services.

hi·a·tus (hi-a'tus) [L.] an opening, gap, or cleft. **hia'tal,** adj. **aortic h.,** the opening in the diaphragm through which the aorta and thoracic duct pass. **esophageal h.,** the opening in the diaphragm for the passage of the esophagus and the vagus nerves. **pleuroperitoneal h.,** foramen of Bochdalek; a posterolateral opening in the fetal diaphragm; its failure to close leaves a congenital posterolateral defect that may become a site for congenital diaphragmatic hernia. **saphenous h.,** the depression in the fascia lata bridged by the cribriform fascia and perforated by the great saphenous vein. **semilunar h.,** the groove in the ethmoid bone through which the anterior ethmoid air cells, the maxillary sinus, and sometimes the frontonasal duct drain via the ethmoid infundibulum.

hi·ber·na·tion (hi″ber-na′shun) 1. the dormant state in which certain animals pass the winter, marked by narcosis and by sharp reduction in body temperature and metabolism. 2. an analogous temporary reduction in function, such as of an organ. **artificial h.,** a state of reduced metabolism, muscle relaxation, and a twilight sleep resembling narcosis, produced by controlled inhibition of the sympathetic nervous system and causing attenuation of the homeostatic reactions of the organism. **myocardial h.,** chronic but potentially reversible cardiac dysfunction caused by chronic myocardial ischemia, persisting at least until blood flow is restored.

hi·ber·no·ma (-no′mah) a rare, benign, soft tissue tumor arising from vestiges of brown fat resembling that in certain hibernating animal species; it is a small, lobulated, nontender lesion usually occurring on the mediastinum or intrascapular region.

hic·cup (hik′up) sharp sound of inhalation with spasm of the glottis and diaphragm.

hi·drad·e·ni·tis (hi″drad-ĕ-ni′tis) inflammation of the sweat glands. **h. suppurati′va,** a severe, chronic, recurrent suppurative infection of the apocrine sweat glands.

hi·drad·e·no·car·ci·no·ma (hi-drad″ĕ-no-kahr″sĭ-no′mah) carcinoma of the sweat glands.

hi·drad·e·noid (hi-drad′ĕ-noid) resembling a sweat gland; having components resembling elements of a sweat gland.

hi·drad·e·no·ma (hi″drad-ĕ-no′mah) a benign tumor originating in sweat gland epithelium; subtypes are designated according to histologic pattern.

hidr(o)- word element [Gr.], *sweat.*

hi·dro·ac·an·tho·ma (hi″dro-ak″an-tho′mah) a benign tumor of an eccrine gland.

hi·dro·cys·to·ma (-sis-to′mah) 1. a retention cyst of a sweat gland. 2. syringocystoma.

hi·dro·poi·e·sis (-poi-e′sis) the formation of sweat. **hidropoiet′ic,** adj.

hi·drot·ic (hi-drot′ik) 1. sudoriparous. 2. diaphoretic.

high-grade (hi′grād′) occurring near the high end of a range, as of a malignancy.

hill·ock (hil′ok) a small prominence or elevation.

hi·lum (hi′lum) pl. *hi′la.* [L.] a depression or pit on an organ, giving entrance and exit to vessels and nerves. **hi′lar,** adj.

hi·lus (hi′lus) pl. *hi′li.* [L.] hilum.

hind·brain (hīnd′brān) rhombencephalon.

hind·foot (-foot) the back of the foot, comprising the region of the talus and calcaneus.

hind·gut (-gut) the embryonic structure from which the caudal intestine, chiefly the colon, is formed.

hip (hip) coxa; the region of the body around the joint between the femur and pelvis. **snapping h.,** slipping of the hip joint, sometimes with an audible snap, due to slipping of a tendinous band over the greater trochanter.

hip·po·cam·pus (hip″o-kam′pus) [L.] a curved elevation in the floor of the inferior horn of the lateral ventricle; a functional component of the limbic system, its efferent projections form the fornix. **hippocam′pal,** adj.

Hip·poc·ra·tes (hĭ-pok′rah-tēz) the Greek physician (5th century B.C.) regarded as the "Father of Medicine." Many of his writings and those of his school have survived, among which appears the Hippocratic Oath, the ethical guide of the medical profession. **hippocrat′ic,** adj.

hip·pu·ric ac·id (hĭ-pūr′ik) $C_6H_5 \cdot CO \cdot NH \cdot CH_2 \cdot COOH$, formed by conjugation of benzoic acid and glycine.

hip·pus (hip′us) abnormal exaggeration of the rhythmic contraction and dilation of the pupil, independent of changes in illumination or in fixation of the eyes.

hir·ci (hir′si) sing. *hir′cus* [L.] the hairs growing in the axilla.

hir·sut·ism (hir′soot-izm) abnormal hairiness, especially in women.

hi·ru·di·cide (hĭ-rōōd′is-īd) an agent that is destructive to leeches. **hirudici′dal,** adj.

hi·ru·din (hĭ-rōōd′in) the active principle of the buccal secretion of leeches; it prevents coagulation by acting as an antithrombin.

Hir·u·din·ea (hir″oo-din′e-ah) a class of annelids, the leeches.

Hi·ru·do (hĭ-roo′do) [L.] a genus of leeches, including *H. medicina′lis,* which have been used extensively for drawing blood.

his·ta·mine (his′tah-mēn) an amine, $C_5H_9N_3$, produced by decarboxylation of histidine, found in all body tissues. It induces capillary dilation, which increases capillary permeability and lowers blood pressure; contraction of most smooth muscle tissue; increased gastric acid secretion; and acceleration of the heart rate. It is also a mediator of immediate hypersensitivity. There are three types of cellular receptors of histamine. H_1 receptors mediate contraction of smooth muscle and capillary dilation and H_2 receptors mediate acceleration of heart rate and promotion of gastric acid secretion. Both H_1 and H_2 receptors mediate the contraction of vascular smooth muscle. H_3 receptors are believed to play a role in regulation of the release of histamine and other neurotransmitters from neurons. Histamine is used as an aid in the diagnosis of asthma and a positive control in skin testing. **histamin′ic,** adj.

his·ta·min·er·gic (his″tah-min-er′jik) pertaining to the effects of histamine at histamine receptors of target tissues.

his·ti·dase (his′tĭ-dās) an enzyme of the liver that converts histidine to urocanic acid.

his·ti·dine (his′tĭ-din, -dēn) an essential amino acid obtainable from many proteins by the action of sulfuric acid and water; it is necessary for optimal growth in infants. Its decarboxylation results in formation of histamine. Symbols His and H.

his·ti·din·emia (his″tĭ-din-e′me-ah) a hereditary aminoacidopathy marked by excessive histidine in the blood and urine due to deficient histidase activity; it is usually benign but may cause mild central nervous system dysfunction.

his·ti·din·uria (his″tĭ-dĭ-nu′re-ah) an excess of histidine in the urine, usually associated with histidinemia or pregnancy.

histi(o)- word element [Gr.], *tissue.*

his·tio·cyte (his′te-o-sīt″) macrophage. **histiocyt′ic,** adj.

his·tio·cyt·oma (his″te-o-si-to′mah) a tumor containing histiocytes (macrophages). **benign fibrous h.,** any of a group of benign neoplasms occurring in the dermis and characterized by histiocytes and fibroblasts; the term sometimes encompasses several types of neoplasms, such as dermatofibroma, nodular subepidermal fibrosis, and sclerosing hemangioma and sometimes is synonymous with one of these. **malignant fibrous h.,** any of a group of malignant neoplasms containing cells resembling histiocytes and fibroblasts.

his·tio·cy·to·sis (-si-to′sis) a condition marked by an abnormal appearance of histiocytes in the blood. **acute disseminated**

Langerhans cell h., Letterer-Siwe disease. **Langerhans cell h.,** a generic term for a group of disorders characterized by proliferation of Langerhans cells (q.v.), believed to arise from disturbances in regulation of the immune system. Lesions may be unifocal or multifocal and may involve the bone marrow, endocrine system, or lungs. **sinus h.,** a disorder of the lymph nodes in which the distended sinuses are filled by histiocytes, as a result of active multiplication of the littoral cells. **h. X,** former name for *Langerhans cell h.*

his·ti·o·gen·ic (-jen′ik) histogenous.

his·to·blast (his′to-blast) a tissue-forming cell.

his·to·chem·is·try (his″to-kem′is-tre) that branch of histology dealing with the identification of chemical components in cells and tissues. **histochem′ical,** adj.

his·to·clin·i·cal (-klin′ĭ-k′l) combining histological and clinical evaluation.

his·to·com·pa·ti·bil·i·ty (-kom-pat″ĭ-bil′it-e) that quality of being accepted and remaining functional; said of that relationship between the genotypes of donor and host in which a graft generally will not be rejected, a relationship determined by the presence of compatible HLA antigens. **histocompat′ible,** adj.

his·to·dif·fer·en·ti·a·tion (-dif″er-en″she-a′shun) the acquisition of tissue characteristics by cell groups.

his·to·gen·e·sis (-jen′ĕ-sis) the formation or development of tissues from the undifferentiated cells of the germ layers of the embryo. **histogenet′ic,** adj.

his·tog·e·nous (his-toj′ĕ-nus) formed by the tissues.

his·to·gram (his′to-gram) a graph in which values found in a statistical study are represented by vertical bars or rectangles.

his·toid (his′toid) 1. developed from but one kind of tissue. 2. like one of the tissues of the body.

his·to·in·com·pat·i·bil·i·ty (his″to-in″kom-pat″ĭ-bil′it-e) the quality of not being accepted or not remaining functional; said of that relationship between the genotypes of donor and host in which a graft generally will be rejected. **histoincompat′ible,** adj.

his·to·ki·ne·sis (-kĭ-ne′sis) movement in the tissues of the body.

his·tol·o·gy (his-tol′ah-je) that department of anatomy dealing with the minute structure, composition, and function of tissues. **histolog′ic, histolog′ical,** adj. **pathologic h.,** the science of diseased tissues.

his·tol·y·sis (his-tol´ĭ-sis) dissolution or breaking down of tissues. **histolyt´ic**, adj.

his·tone (his´tōn) a simple protein, soluble in water and insoluble in dilute ammonia, found combined as salts with acidic substances, e.g., the protein combined with nucleic acid or the globin of hemoglobin.

his·to·phys·i·ol·o·gy (his″to-fiz″e-ol´ah-je) the correlation of function with the microscopic structure of cells and tissues.

His·to·plas·ma (-plaz´mah) a genus of fungi, including *H. capsula´tum*, the cause of histoplasmosis in humans.

his·to·plas·min (-plaz´min) a skin test antigen prepared from mycelial phase *Histoplasma capsulatum;* used primarily in epidemiologic surveys and in testing for cutaneous anergy in diagnosis of immunodeficiency.

his·to·plas·mo·ma (-plaz-mo´mah) a rounded granuloma of the lung due to infection with *Histoplasma capsulatum.*

his·to·plas·mo·sis (-plaz-mo´sis) infection with *Histoplasma capsulatum*, usually asymptomatic but in the immunocompromised sometimes causing more serious symptoms such as acute pneumonia, an influenzalike illness, disseminated reticuloendothelial hyperplasia with hepatosplenomegaly and anemia, or other organ damage. **ocular h.,** disseminated choroiditis with scars in the periphery of the fundus near the optic nerve, and disciform macular lesions, probably due to *Histoplasma capsulatum* infection.

his·to·throm·bin (-throm´bin) thrombin derived from connective tissue.

his·tot·o·my (his-tot´ah-me) dissection of tissues; microtomy.

his·to·tox·ic (his´to-tok″sik) poisonous to tissue.

his·to·tro·pic (his″to-tro´pik) having affinity for tissue cells.

his·trel·in (his-trel´in) a synthetic preparation of gonadotropin-releasing hormone, used as the acetate ester in the treatment of precocious puberty.

his·tri·on·ic (his″tre-on´ik) excessively dramatic or emotional, as in histrionic personality disorder; see under *personality.*

HIV human immunodeficiency virus.

hives (hīvz) urticaria.

H⁺,K⁺-ATPase (a-te-pe´ās) a membrane-bound enzyme occurring on the surface of the parietal cells; it uses the energy derived from ATP hydrolysis to drive the exchange of ions (protons, chloride ions, and potassium ions) across the cell membrane, secreting acid into the gastric lumen.

Hl latent hyperopia.

HLA human leukocyte antigens.

Hm manifest hyperopia.

hMG menotropins (human menopausal gonadotropin).

HMO health maintenance organization.

HMSN hereditary motor and sensory neuropathy.

Ho holmium.

HOCM hypertrophic obstructive cardiomyopathy.

ho·do·neu·ro·mere (ho″do-noor´o-mēr) a segment of the embryonic trunk with its pair of nerves and their branches.

hol·an·dric (hol-an´drik) inherited exclusively through the male descent; transmitted through genes located on the Y chromosome.

hol·ism (hōl´izm) the conception of man as a functioning whole. **holis´tic**, adj.

hol·mi·um (Ho) (hōl´me-um) chemical element (see *Table of Elements*), at. no. 67.

hol(o)- word element [Gr.], *entire; whole.*

holo·blas·tic (ho″lo-blas´tik) undergoing cleavage in which the entire zygote participates; dividing completely.

holo·crine (ho´lo-krin) exhibiting glandular secretion in which the entire secretory cell laden with its secretory products is cast off.

holo·di·a·stol·ic (hōl″o-di″ah-stol´ik) pertaining to the entire diastole.

holo·en·dem·ic (-en-dem´ik) endemic at a high level in a population, affecting most of the children and so affecting the adults in the same population less often.

holo·en·zyme (-en´zīm) the active compound formed by combination of a coenzyme and an apoenzyme.

hol·og·ra·phy (hōl-og´rah-fe) the lensless recording of three-dimensional images on film by means of laser beams.

holo·phyt·ic (hōl″o-fit´ik) obtaining food like a plant; said of certain protozoa.

holo·pros·en·ceph·a·ly (-pros″en-sef´ah-le) developmental failure of cleavage of the prosencephalon with a deficit in midline facial development and with cyclopia in the severe form; sometimes due to trisomy 13.

holo·ra·chis·chi·sis (-rah-kis´kĭ-sis) fissure of the entire spinal cord.

holo·zo·ic (-zo´ik) having the nutritional characters of an animal, i.e., digesting protein.

ho·mat·ro·pine (ho-mat´ro-pēn) an anticholinergic similar to atropine; *h. hydrobromide* is used as a ophthalmic mydriatic and cycloplegic, and *h. methylbromide* is used as an inhibitor of gastric spasm and secretion.

ho·max·i·al (ho-mak´se-il) having axes of the same length.

home(o)- word element [Gr.], *similar; same; unchanging.*

ho·meo·met·ric (ho″me-o-met′rik) independent of a change in size; cf. *heterometric*.

ho·me·op·a·thy (ho″me-op′ah-the) a system of therapeutics based on the administration of minute doses of drugs which are capable of producing in healthy persons symptoms like those of the disease treated. **homeopath′ic**, adj.

ho·meo·pla·sia (ho″me-o-pla′zhah) formation of new tissue like that normal to the part. **homeoplas′tic**, adj.

ho·meo·sta·sis (-sta′sis) a tendency to equilibrium or stability in the normal physiological states of the organism. **homeostat′ic**, adj.

ho·meo·ther·a·py (-ther′ah-pe) treatment or prevention of disease with a substance similar to the causative agent of the disease.

ho·meo·ther·my (ho′me-o-ther″me) the maintenance of a constant body temperature despite changes in the environmental temperature. **homeother′mic**, adj.

hom·er·gic (hōm-er′jik) having the same effect; said of two drugs each of which produces the same overt effect.

Ho·mo (ho′mo) [L.] the genus of primates containing the single species *H. sapiens* (man).

hom(o)- 1. word element [Gr.], *same*. 2. chemical prefix indicating addition of one CH_2 group to the main compound.

ho·mo·bio·tin (ho″mo-bio-tin) a homologue of biotin having an additional CH_2 group in the side chain and acting as a biotin antagonist.

ho·mo·car·no·sine (-kahr′no-sēn) a dipeptide consisting of γ-aminobutyric acid and histidine; in humans it is found in brain tissue only.

ho·mo·cit·rul·line an irregular amino acid related to lysine.

ho·mo·cit·rul·lin·uria (-sit″rul-in-u′re-ah) excess of homocitrulline in urine, seen in hyperornithinemia-hyperammonemia-homocitrullinuria syndrome.

ho·mo·clad·ic (-klad′ik) formed between small branches of the same artery; said of such an anastomosis.

ho·mo·cys·te·ine (-sis′te-ēn) a sulfur-containing amino acid homologous with cysteine and produced by demethylation of methionine; it can form cystine or methionine.

ho·mo·cys·tine (-sis′tēn) a homologue of cystine formed from two molecules of homocysteine; it is a source of sulfur in the body.

ho·mo·cys·tin·uria (-sis″tin-u′re-ah) excessive homocystine in the urine, having various causes, some genetic; symptoms include developmental delay, failure to thrive, neurological abnormalities, and others depending on the cause. Sometimes the term refers specifically to the disorder due to lack of the enzyme cystathionine β-synthase.

ho·mo·cy·to·tro·pic (-si″to-tro′pik) having an affinity for cells of the same species.

ho·mo·dro·mous (ho-mod′rah-mus) moving or acting in the same or in the usual direction.

homoe(o)- see *home(o)-*.

ho·mo·erot·i·cism (ho″mo-ĕ-rot′ĭ-sizm) sexual feeling directed toward a member of the same sex. **homoerot′ic**, adj.

ho·mo·gam·ete (-gam′ēt) one of two gametes of the same size and structure, as the X chromosome in the human female.

ho·mo·ga·met·ic (-gah-met′ik) pertaining to production of gametes containing only one kind of sex chromosome, as in the human female.

ho·mog·e·nate (ho-moj′in-āt) material obtained by homogenization.

ho·mo·ge·ne·ous (ho″mo-je′ne-us) of uniform quality, composition, or structure throughout.

ho·mo·gen·e·sis (-jen′ĕ-sis) reproduction by the same process in each generation. **homogenet′ic**, adj.

ho·mog·e·nize (ho-moj′in-īz) to render homogeneous.

ho·mo·gen·tis·ic ac·id (ho″mo-jen-tis′ik) an aromatic hydrocarbon formed as an intermediate in the metabolism of tyrosine and phenylalanine and accumulated and excreted in the urine in alkaptonuria.

ho·mo·graft (ho′mo-graft) allograft.

homoi(o)- see *home(o)-*.

ho·mo·log·ic (ho″mŏ-loj′ik) homologous.

ho·mol·o·gous (ho-mol′ah-gus) 1. corresponding in structure, position, origin, etc. 2. allogeneic.

ho·mo·logue (hom′ah-log) 1. any homologous organ or part. 2. in chemistry, one of a series of compounds distinguished by addition of a CH_2 group in successive members.

ho·mol·y·sin (ho-mol′ĭ-sin) a lysin produced by injection into the body of an antigen derived from an individual of the same species.

ho·mon·o·mous (ho-mon′o-mus) designating homologous serial parts, such as somites.

ho·mon·y·mous (-ĭ-mus) 1. having the same or corresponding sound or name. 2. pertaining to the corresponding vertical halves of the visual fields of both eyes.

ho·mo·phil·ic (ho″mo-fil′ik) reacting only with a specific antigen.

ho·mo·plas·tic (-plas′tik) 1. allogeneic. 2. denoting organs or parts, as the wings of birds and insects, that resemble one another in structure and function but not in origin or development.

ho·mo·poly·sac·cha·ride (-pol″e-sak′ah-rīd) a polysaccharide consisting of a single recurring monosaccharide unit.

hom·or·gan·ic (hom″or-gan′ik) produced by the same organ or by homologous organs.

ho·mo·sal·ate (ho″mo-sal′āt) an ultraviolet sunscreen effective against UVB rays, applied topically to the skin.

ho·mo·sex·u·al (-sek′shoo-al) 1. pertaining to, characteristic of, or directed toward the same sex. 2. one who is sexually attracted to persons of the same sex.

ho·mo·top·ic (-top′ik) occurring at the same place upon the body.

ho·mo·type (ho′mo-tīp) a part having reversed symmetry with its mate, as the hand. **homotyp′ic,** adj.

ho·mo·va·nil·lic ac·id (ho″mo-vah-nil′ik) a major terminal urinary metabolite, converted from dopa, dopamine, and norepinephrine.

ho·mo·zy·go·sis (-zi-go′sis) the formation of a zygote by the union of gametes that have one or more identical alleles.

hook (hook) 1. a long, thin, curved instrument for traction or holding. 2. something with that shape. **palate h.,** one for raising the palate in posterior rhinoscopy. **Tyrrell's h.,** a slender hook used in eye surgery.

hook·worm (hook′werm) a nematode parasitic in the intestines of humans and other vertebrates; two important species are *Necator americanus* (American, or New World, h.) and *Ancylostoma duodenale* (Old World h.). Infection may cause serious illness; see under *disease,* and see *ground itch,* under *itch.*

hops (hops) the dried flowers and cones of *Humulus lupulus,* the hop plant, used for nervousness and insomnia.

hor·de·o·lum (hor-de′o-lum) stye; a localized, purulent, inflammatory infection of a sebaceous gland (meibomian or zeisian) of the eyelid; *external h.* occurs on the skin surface at the edge of the lid, *internal h.* on the conjunctival surface.

hor·i·zon·tal (hor″ĭ-zon′t′l) 1. parallel to the plane of the horizon. 2. occupying or confined to a single level in a hierarchy.

hor·i·zon·ta·lis (-zon-ta′lis) horizontal: denoting relationship to this orientation when the body is in the anatomical position.

hor·mi·on (hor′me-on) point of union of the sphenoid bone with the posterior border of the vomer.

hor·mone (hor′mōn) a chemical substance produced in the body which has a specific regulatory effect on the activity of certain cells or a certain organ or organs. **hormo′nal,**

adj. **adrenocortical h.,** 1. any of the corticosteroids elaborated by the adrenal cortex, the major ones being the glucocorticoids and mineralocorticoids, and including some androgens, progesterone, and perhaps estrogens. 2. corticosteroid. **adrenocorticotropic h. (ACTH),** corticotropin. **adrenomedullary h's,** substances secreted by the adrenal medulla, including epinephrine and norepinephrine. **androgenic h.,** androgen. **anterior pituitary h's,** those produced in the adenohypophysis (anterior pituitary), including corticotropin, follicle-stimulating hormone, growth hormone, luteinizing hormone, prolactin, and thyrotropin. **antidiuretic h.,** vasopressin. **cortical h.,** adrenocortical h. **corticotropin-releasing h. (CRH),** a neuropeptide elaborated mainly by the median eminence of the hypothalamus, but also by the pancreas and brain, that stimulates the secretion of corticotropin. **ectopic h.,** one released from a neoplasm or cells outside the usual source of the hormone. **eutopic h.,** one released from its usual site or from a neoplasm of that tissue. **fibroblast growth h.,** a peptide hormone secreted by the adenohypophysis that is a potent mitogen of vascular endothelial cells and a regulator of tissue vascularization. **follicle-stimulating h. (FSH),** one of the gonadotropic hormones of the adenohypophysis; it stimulates ovarian follicle growth and maturation, estrogen secretion, and endometrial changes characteristic of the first portion of the menstrual cycle in females, and stimulates spermatogenesis in males. **follicle-stimulating h.–releasing h. (FSH-RH),** luteinizing hormone–releasing h. **gonadotropic h.,** gonadotropin. **gonadotropin-releasing h. (Gn-RH),** 1. luteinizing hormone–releasing h. 2. any hypothalamic factor that stimulates release of both follicle-stimulating hormone and luteinizing hormone. **growth h. (GH),** any of several related hormones secreted by the adenohypophysis that directly influence protein, carbohydrate, and lipid metabolism and control the rate of skeletal and visceral growth; used pharmaceutically as *somatrem* and *somatropin.* **growth h.–releasing h. (GH-RH),** one elaborated by the hypothalamus, stimulating release of growth hormone from the adenohypophysis. **inhibiting h's,** hormones elaborated by one body structure that inhibit release of hormones from another structure; applied to substances of established clinical identity, while those whose chemical structure is still unknown are called *inhibiting factors.* **interstitial cell–stimulating h.,** luteinizing h. **lactation h., lactogenic h.,** prolactin. **local h.,** a substance with hormonelike properties that acts at an anatomically restricted site. **luteinizing h. (LH),** a gonadotropin of the adenohypophysis, acting with follicle-stimulating hormone in females to promote ovulation as well as secretion of androgens and progesterone. It instigates and maintains the secretory portion of the menstrual cycle and is concerned with corpus luteum formation. In males, it stimulates the development and functional activity of testicular Leydig cells. **luteinizing h.–releasing h. (LH-RH),** a glycoprotein gonadotropic hormone of the adenohypophysis that acts with follicle-stimulating hormone to promote ovulation and promotes secretion of androgen and progesterone. A preparation of the salts is used in the differential diagnosis of hypothalamic, pituitary, and gonadal dysfunction and in the treatment of some forms of infertility and hypogonadism. **melanocyte-stimulating h., melanophore-stimulating h. (MSH),** one of several peptides secreted by the anterior pituitary in humans and in the rhomboid fossa in lower vertebrates, influencing melanin formation and deposition in the body and causing color changes in the skin of amphibians, fishes, and reptiles. **neurohypophysial h's,** posterior pituitary h's. **ovarian h's,** those secreted by the ovary, such as estrogens and progestational agents. **parathyroid h.,** a polypeptide hormone secreted by the parathyroid glands, which influences calcium and phosphorus metabolism and bone formation. **placental h's,** those produced by the placenta during pregnancy, including chorionic gonadotropin and other substances having estrogenic, progestational, or adrenocorticoid activity. **plant h.,** phytohormone. **posterior pituitary h's,** those released from the neurohypophysis (posterior pituitary), including oxytocin and vasopressin. **progestational h.,** 1. progesterone. 2. see under *agent.* **releasing h's,** hormones elaborated in one structure that cause the release of hormones from another structure; applied to substances of established chemical identity, while those whose chemical structure is unknown are called *releasing factors.* **sex h's,** the estrogens and androgens considered together. **somatotrophic h., somatotropic h.,** growth h. **somatotropin-releasing h. (SRH),** growth hormone–releasing h. **steroid h's,** those that are biologically active steroids; they are secreted by the adrenal cortex, testis, ovary, and placenta and include the progestogens, glucocorticoids, mineralocorticoids, androgens, and estrogens. **thyroid h's,** thyroxine, calcitonin, and triiodothyronine; in the singular, thyroxine and/or triiodothyronine. **thyroid-stimulating h. (TSH) thyrotropic h.,** thyrotropin. **thyrotropin-releasing h. (TRH),** a tripeptide hormone of the hypothalamus, which stimulates release of thyrotropin from the adenohypophysis and also acts as a prolactin-releasing factor. It is used in diagnosis of mild hyperthyroidism and Graves' disease, and in differentiating among primary, secondary, and tertiary hypothyroidism. A synthetic preparation is called *protirelin.*

hor·mon·o·gen (hor'mon-o-jen") prohormone.

horn (horn) 1. cornu; a pointed projection such as the paired processes on the head of certain animals. 2. something shaped like the horn of an animal. **horn′y,** adj. **cicatricial h.,** a hard, dry outgrowth from a cicatrix, commonly scaly and rarely osseous. **cutaneous h.,** a horny excrescence on the skin, commonly on the face or scalp; it often overlies premalignant or malignant lesions. **h. of pulp,** an extension of the pulp into an accentuation of the roof of the pulp chamber directly under a cusp or lobe of the tooth. **h. of spinal cord,** the horn-shaped structure, anterior or posterior, seen in transverse section of the spinal cord; the anterior horn is formed by the anterior column of the cord and the posterior by the posterior column.

ho·rop·ter (hor-op'ter) the sum of all points seen in binocular vision with the eyes fixed.

hor·ror (hor′er) [L.] dread; terror. **h. auto·tox′icus,** former name for self-tolerance.

Hor·taea (hor-te′ah) a genus of Fungi Imperfecti with the sole species *H. werneckii* (formerly *Exophiala werneckii*), a halophilic, dematiaceous yeast that inhabits the soil and is the cause of tinea nigra.

hos·pice (hos′pis) a facility that provides palliative and supportive care for terminally ill patients and their families, either directly or on a consulting basis.

hos·pi·tal (hos′pĭ-t'l) an institute for the treatment of the sick. **lying-in h., maternity h.,** one for the care of obstetric patients. **open h.,** 1. a mental hospital, or section of a hospital, without locked doors or other forms of physical restraint. 2. a hospital to which physicians who are not staff members may send their own patients and supervise their treatment. **teaching h.,** one that conducts formal educational programs or courses of instruction that lead to granting of recognized certificates, diplomas, or degrees, or that are required for professional certification or licensure. **voluntary h.,** a private, not-for-profit hospital that provides uncompensated care to the poor.

hos·pi·tal·iza·tion (hos"pĭ-t'l-ĭ-za'shun) 1. the placing of a patient in a hospital for treatment. 2. the term of confinement in a hospital. **partial h.,** a psychiatric treatment program for patients who do not need full-time hospitalization, involving a special facility or an arrangement within a hospital setting to which the patient may come for treatment during the days, the nights, or the weekends only.

host (hōst) 1. an organism that harbors or nourishes another organism (the parasite). 2. the recipient of an organ or other tissue derived from another organism (the donor). **accidental h.,** one that accidentally harbors an organism that is not ordinarily parasitic in the particular species. **definitive h., final h.,** the organism in which a parasite passes its adult and sexual existence. **intermediate h.,** the organism in which a parasite passes its larval or nonsexual existence. **paratenic h.,** an animal acting as a substitute intermediate host of a parasite, usually having acquired the parasite by ingestion of the original host. **primary h.** definitive h. **reservoir h.,** reservoir (3).

hot (hot) 1. characterized by high temperature. 2. radioactive; particularly used for the presence of significantly or dangerously high levels of radioactivity.

hot line (hot līn) telephone assistance for those in need of crisis intervention, generally round-the-clock and staffed by nonprofessionals, with mental health professionals serving as advisors or in a back-up capacity.

HPL, hPL human placental lactogen.

HPLC high-performance liquid chromatography.

HPV human papillomavirus.

HRCT high-resolution computed tomography.

HRF histamine-releasing factor; homologous restriction factor.

HSAN hereditary sensory and autonomic neuropathy.

HSR homogeneously staining regions.

HSV herpes simplex virus.

5-HT 5-hydroxytryptamine; see *serotonin.*

HTLV-1 human T-lymphotropic virus 1.

HTLV-2 human T-lymphotropic virus 2.

hum (hum) a low, steady, prolonged sound. **venous h.,** a continuous blowing, singing, or humming murmur heard on auscultation over the right jugular vein in the sitting or erect position; it is an innocent sign that is obliterated on assumption of the recumbent position or on exerting pressure over the vein.

hu·mec·tant (hu-mek'tant) 1. moistening. 2. a moistening or diluent medicine.

hu·mer·us (hu'mer-us) pl. *hu'meri.* [L.] see *Table of Bones.* **hu'meral,** adj.

hu·mor (hu'mer) pl. *humors, humo'res.* [L.] any fluid or semifluid of the body. **hu'moral,** adj. **aqueous h.,** the fluid produced in the eye and filling the spaces (anterior and posterior) in front of the lens and its attachments. **ocular h.,** either of the humors (aqueous and vitreous) of the eye. **vitreous h.,** 1. the fluid portion of the vitreous body. 2. vitreous body.

hump (hump) a rounded eminence. **dowager's h.,** popular name for dorsal kyphosis caused by multiple wedge fractures of the thoracic vertebrae seen in osteoporosis.

hump·back (hump'bak) kyphosis.

hunch·back (hunch'bak) old term for KYPHOSIS, now considered offensive.

hun·ger (hung'er) a craving, as for food. **air h.,** Kussmaul's respiration.

husk (husk) an outer covering or shell, as of some fruits and seeds. **psyllium h.,** the cleaned, dried seed coat from the seeds of *Plantago* species; used as a bulk-forming laxative; also used for various purposes in ayurveda and folk medicine.

hy·a·lin (hi'ah-lin) a translucent albuminoid product of amyloid degeneration.

hy·a·line (hi'ah-līn) glassy and translucent.

hy·a·lin·i·za·tion (hi"ah-lin-ĭ-za'shun) conversion into hyalin. **Crooke's h.,** degeneration of corticotrophs of the pituitary gland, in which they lose their specific granulations and the cytoplasm becomes hyalinized; seen in Cushing's syndrome and Addison's disease.

hy·a·li·no·sis (hi"ah-lin-o'sis) hyaline degeneration.

hy·a·li·tis (hi"ah-li'tis) inflammation of the vitreous body or the vitreous (hyaloid) membrane. **asteroid h.,** see under *hyalosis.* **suppurative h.,** purulent inflammation of the vitreous body.

hyal(o)- word element [Gr.], *glassy.*

hy·al·o·gen (hi-al'o-jen) an albuminous substance occurring in cartilage, vitreous body, etc., and convertible into hyalin.

hy·a·lo·hy·pho·my·co·sis (hi"ah-lo-hi"fo-mi-ko'sis) any opportunistic type of hyphomycosis caused by mycelial fungi with colorless walls.

hy·a·loid (hi'ah-loid) hyaline.

hy·a·lo·mere (hi'ah-lo-mēr") the pale, homogeneous portion of a blood platelet in a dry, stained blood smear.

Hy·a·lom·ma (hi"ah-lom'ah) a genus of ticks found on humans and other animals in

hy·a·lo·mu·coid (hi″ah-lo-mu′koid) the mucoid of the vitreous body.

hy·a·lo·nyx·is (-nik′sis) puncturing of the vitreous body.

hy·a·lo·plasm (hi′ah-lo-plazm″) the more fluid, finely granular substance of the cytoplasm of a cell. **nuclear h.,** karyolymph.

hy·a·lo·se·ro·si·tis (hi″ah-lo-sĕr″o-si′tis) inflammation of serous membranes, with hyalinization of the serous exudate into a pearly investment of the affected organ. **progressive multiple h.,** Concato's disease.

hy·a·lo·sis (hi″ah-lo′sis) degenerative changes in the vitreous humor. **asteroid h.,** the presence of spherical or star-shaped opacities in the vitreous humor.

hy·al·o·some (hi-al′o-sōm) a structure resembling the nucleolus of a cell, but staining only slightly.

hy·al·uro·nate (hi″ah-lōō′ro-nāt) a salt, anion, or ester of hyaluronic acid. The sodium salt and a derivative of it are used as analgesics in the treatment of osteoarthritis of the knee.

hy·al·uron·ic ac·id (hi″ah-lōō-ron′ik) a glycosaminoglycan found in lubricating proteoglycans of synovial fluid, vitreous humor, cartilage, blood vessels, skin, and the umbilical cord. It is a linear chain of about 2500 repeating disaccharide units.

hy·al·uron·i·dase (hi″ah-lōō-ron′ĭ-dās) any of three enzymes that catalyze the hydrolysis of hyaluronic acid and similar glycosaminoglycans, found in snake and spider venom, in mammalian testicular and spleen tissue, and produced by various pathogenic bacteria, enabling them to spread through tissues; a preparation from mammalian testes is used to aid absorption and dispersion of other injected drugs and fluids, for hypodermoclysis, and for improving resorption of radiopaque media.

hy·brid (hi′brid) an offspring of parents of different genera, varieties, or species.

hy·brid·iza·tion (hi″brid-ĭ-za′shun) 1. crossbreeding; the act or process of producing hybrids. 2. molecular hybridization 3. formation of a heterokaryon by fusion of two somatic cells, usually of different species. 4. in chemistry, a procedure whereby orbitals of intermediate energy and desired directional character are constructed. **in situ h.,** molecular hybridization used to analyze prepared cells or histologic sections in situ in order to analyze the intracellular or intrachromosomal distribution, transcription, or other characteristics of specific nucleic acids. **molecular h.,** formation of a partially or wholly complementary nucleic acid duplex by association of single strands, in order to detect and isolate specific sequences, measure homology, or define other characteristics of one or both strands.

hy·brid·o·ma (hi″brid-o′mah) a somatic cell hybrid formed by fusion of normal lymphocytes and tumor cells.

hy·da·tid (hi′dah-tid) 1. hydatid cyst. 2. any cystlike structure. **h. of Morgagni,** 1. a cystlike remnant of the müllerian duct on the upper end of the testis. 2. one of the small pedunculated structures attached to the uterine tubes near their fimbriated end; remnants of the mesonephric ducts. **sessile h.,** h. of Morgagni (1).

hy·da·tid·i·form (hi″dah-tid′ĭ-form) resembling a hydatid cyst; see under *mole*.

hy·da·tid·o·sis (hi″dah-tĭ-do′sis) hydatid disease.

hy·da·tid·os·to·my (hi″dah-tĭ-dos′tah-me) incision and drainage of a hydatid cyst.

hy·dra·gogue (hi′drah-gog) 1. producing watery discharge, especially from the bowels. 2. a cathartic that causes watery purgation.

hy·dral·a·zine (hi-dral′ah-zēn) a peripheral vasodilator used in the form of the hydrochloride salt as an antihypertensive.

hy·dram·ni·os (hi-dram′ne-os) polyhydramnios.

hy·dran·en·ceph·a·ly (hi″dran-en-sef′ah-le) complete or almost complete absence of the cerebral hemispheres, their normal site being occupied by cerebrospinal fluid. **hydranencephal′ic,** adj.

hy·drar·thro·sis (hi″drahr-thro′sis) an accumulation of effused watery fluid in a joint cavity. **hydrarthro′dial,** adj.

hy·dra·tase (hi′drah-tās) a hydro-lyase that catalyzes a reaction in which the equilibrium lies toward hydration.

hy·drate (hi′drāt) 1. any compound of a radical with water. 2. any salt or other compound containing water of crystallization.

hy·dra·tion (hi-dra′shun) the absorption of or combination with water.

hy·drau·lics (hi-draw′liks) the science dealing with the mechanics of liquids.

hy·dra·zine (hi′drah-zēn) a toxic, irritant, carcinogenic, gaseous diamine, $H_2N \cdot NH_2$, or any of its substitution derivatives.

hy·dri·od·ic ac·id (hi″dri-od′ik) a gaseous haloid acid, HI; its aqueous solution and syrup have been used as alteratives.

hydr(o)- word element [Gr.], *hydrogen; water.*

hy·droa (hi-dro′ah) a vesicular eruption with intense itching and burning on skin exposed to sunlight.

hy·dro·al·co·hol·ic (hi″dro-al″kah-hol′ik) pertaining to or containing both water and alcohol.

hy·dro·bro·mic ac·id (-bro′mik) a gaseous haloid acid, HBr.

hy·dro·bro·mide (-bro′mīd) an addition salt of hydrobromic acid.

hy·dro·ca·ly·co·sis (hi″dro-kal″ĭ-ko′sis) a usually asymptomatic cystic dilatation of a major renal calix, lined by transitional epithelium and due to obstruction of the infundibulum.

hy·dro·car·bon (hi′dro-kahr″bon) an organic compound that contains carbon and hydrogen only. **alicyclic h.**, one that has cyclic structure and aliphatic properties. **aliphatic h.**, one in which no carbon atoms are joined to form a ring. **aromatic h.**, one that has cyclic structure and a closed conjugated system of double bonds. **chlorinated h.**, any of a group of toxic compounds used mainly as refrigerants, industrial solvents, and dry cleaning fluids, and formerly as anesthetics.

hy·dro·cele (hi′dro-sēl) a circumscribed collection of fluid, especially in the tunica vaginalis of the testis or along the spermatic cord.

hy·dro·ceph·a·lo·cele (hi″dro-sef′ah-lo-sēl″) hydroencephalocele.

hy·dro·ceph·a·lus (-sef′ah-lus) a congenital or acquired condition marked by dilatation of the cerebral ventricles, usually occurring secondarily to obstruction of the cerebrospinal fluid pathways, and accompanied by an accumulation of cerebrospinal fluid within the skull; typically, there is enlargement of the head, prominence of the forehead, brain atrophy, mental deterioration, and convulsions. **hydrocephal′ic**, adj. **communicating h.**, that in which there is free access of fluid between the ventricles of the brain and the spinal canal. **noncommunicating h.**, obstructive h. **normal-pressure h., normal-pressure occult h.**, dementia, ataxia, and urinary incontinence with enlarged ventricles associated with inadequacy of the subarachnoid spaces, but with normal cerebrospinal fluid pressure. **obstructive h.**, that due to obstruction of the flow of cerebrospinal fluid within the brain ventricles or through their exit foramina. **otitic h.**, that caused by spread of inflammation of otitis media to the cranial cavity. **posthemorrhagic h.**, hydrocephalus in an infant following intracranial hemorrhage that has distended the ventricles and obstructed normal pathways for cerebrospinal fluid. **h. ex va′cuo**, compensatory replacement by cerebrospinal fluid of the volume of tissue lost in atrophy of the brain.

hy·dro·chlo·ric ac·id (-klor′ik) hydrogen chloride in aqueous solution, HCl, a highly corrosive mineral acid; it is used as a laboratory reagent and is a constituent of gastric juice, secreted by the gastric parietal cells.

hy·dro·chlo·ride (-klor′īd) a salt of hydrochloric acid.

hy·dro·chlo·ro·thi·a·zide (-klor″o-thi′ah-zīd) a thiazide diuretic, used for treatment of hypertension and edema.

hy·dro·cho·le·cys·tis (-ko″lĕ-sis′tis) distention of the gallbladder with watery fluid.

hy·dro·cho·le·re·sis (-ko″lĕ-re′sis) choleresis with increased water output, or induction of excretion of bile relatively low in specific gravity, viscosity, and total solid content.

hy·dro·co·done (-ko′dōn) a semisynthetic opioid analgesic similar to but more active than codeine; used as the bitartrate salt or polistirex complex as an analgesic and antitussive.

hy·dro·col·loid (-kol′oid) a colloid system in which water is the dispersion medium.

hy·dro·cor·ti·sone (-kor′tĭ-sōn) the name given to natural or synthetic cortisol when it is used as a pharmaceutical. The base and its salts, including *h. acetate, h. butyrate, h. cypionate, h. probutate, h. sodium phosphate, h. sodium succinate,* and *h. valerate* are used as replacement therapy in adrenocortical insufficiency and as antiinflammatory and immunosuppressant agents in the treatment of a wide variety of disorders.

hy·dro·cy·an·ic ac·id (-si-an′ik) hydrogen cyanide; see under *hydrogen.*

hy·dro·de·lin·e·a·tion (-de-lin″e-a′shun) injection of fluid between the layers of the nucleus of the lens using a blunt needle; done to delineate the nuclear zones during cataract surgery.

hy·dro·dis·sec·tion (-di-sek′shun) injection of a small amount of fluid into the capsule of the lens for dissection and maneuverability during extracapsular or phacoemulsification surgery.

hy·dro·en·ceph·a·lo·cele (-en-sef′ah-lo-sēl) encephalocele into a distended sac containing cerebrospinal fluid.

hy·dro·flu·me·thi·a·zide (-floo″mĕ-thi′ah-zīd) a thiazide diuretic used for treatment of hypertension and edema.

hy·dro·flu·or·ic ac·id (-floor′ik) a gaseous haloid acid, HF, extremely poisonous and corrosive.

hy·dro·gen (H) (hi′dro-jen) chemical element (see *Table of Elements*), at. no. 1; it exists as the mass 1 isotope (*protium, light or ordinary h.*), mass 2 isotope (*deuterium, heavy h.*), and mass 3 isotope (*tritium*). **h. cyanide,** an extremely poisonous liquid or gas, HCN, used as a rodenticide and insecticide. **h. peroxide,** a strongly disinfectant cleansing and bleaching liquid, H_2O_2, used in dilute solution in water. **h. sulfide,** an ill-smelling, colorless, poisonous gas, H_2S.

hy·dro·ki·net·ic (hi″dro-kĭ-net′ik) relating to movement of water or other fluid, as in a whirlpool bath.

hy·dro·ki·net·ics (-kĭ-net′iks) the science treating of fluids in motion.

hy·dro·lase (hi′dro-lās) one of the six main classes of enzymes, comprising those that catalyze the hydrolytic cleavage of a compound.

hy·dro·ly·ase (hi″dro-li′ās) a lyase that catalyzes the removal of water from a substrate by breakage of a carbon-oxygen bond, leading to formation of a double bond.

hy·drol·y·sate (hi-drol′ĭ-sāt) any compound produced by hydrolysis. **protein h.,** a mixture of amino acids prepared by splitting a protein with acid, alkali, or enzyme; used as a fluid and nutrient replenisher.

hy·drol·y·sis (hi-drol′ĭ-sis) pl. *hydrol′yses*. The cleavage of a compound by the addition of water, the hydroxyl group being incorporated in one fragment and the hydrogen atom in the other. **hydrolyt′ic,** adj.

hy·dro·ma (hi-dro′mah) hygroma.

hy·dro·me·nin·go·cele (hi″dro-mě-ning′go-sēl) a meningocele forming a sac containing cerebrospinal fluid but no brain or spinal cord substance.

hy·drom·e·ter (hi-drom′ě-ter) an instrument for determining the specific gravity of a fluid.

hy·dro·me·tro·col·pos (hi″dro-me″tro-kol′pos) a collection of watery fluid in the uterus and vagina.

hy·drom·e·try (hi-drom′ĭ-tre) measurement of specific gravity with a hydrometer. **hydromet′ric,** adj.

hy·dro·mi·cro·ceph·a·ly (hi″dro-mi″kro-sef′ah-le) smallness of the head with an abnormal amount of cerebrospinal fluid.

hy·dro·mor·phone (-mor′fōn) a morphine alkaloid having opioid analgesic effects similar to but greater and of shorter duration than those of morphine; used as the hydrochloride salt as an analgesic, antitussive, and anesthesia adjunct.

hy·dro·my·elia (-mi-e′le-ah) dilatation of the central canal of the spinal cord with an abnormal accumulation of fluid.

hy·dro·my·elo·me·nin·go·cele (-mi″ě-lo-mě-ning′go-sēl) myelomeningocele containing both cerebrospinal fluid and spinal cord tissue.

hy·dro·my·o·ma (-mi-o′mah) uterine leiomyoma with cystic degeneration.

hy·dro·ne·phro·sis (-ně-fro′sis) distention of the renal pelvis and calices with urine, due to obstruction of the ureter, with atrophy of the kidney parenchyma. **hydronephrot′ic,** adj.

hy·dro·ni·um (hi-dro′ne-um) the hydrated proton H_3O^+; it is the form in which the proton (hydrogen ion, H^+) exists in aqueous solution, a combination of H^+ and H_2O.

hy·dro·peri·car·di·tis (hi″dro-per″ĭ-kahr-di′tis) pericarditis with watery effusion.

hy·dro·peri·to·ne·um (-per″ĭ-to-ne′um) ascites.

Hy·dro·phi·idae (-fi′ĭ-de) the sea snakes, a family of venomous snakes adapted for living in the ocean, found in the Indian and Pacific Oceans and characterized by an oarlike tail and immovable hollow fangs.

hy·dro·phil·ic (-fil′ik) readily absorbing moisture; hygroscopic; having strongly polar groups that readily interact with water.

hy·dro·pho·bia (-fo′be-ah) 1. irrational fear of water. 2. choking, gagging, and fear on attempts to drink in the acute neurologic phase of rabies. 3. former term for *rabies.*

hy·dro·pho·bic (-fo′bik) 1. pertaining to hydrophobia (rabies). 2. not readily absorbing water, or being adversely affected by water. 3. lacking polar groups and therefore insoluble in water.

hy·droph·thal·mos (hi″drof-thal′mos) distention of the eyeball in infantile glaucoma.

hy·drop·ic (hi-drop′ik) edematous.

hy·dro·pneu·ma·to·sis (hi″dro-noo″mah-to′sis) a collection of fluid and gas in the tissues.

hy·dro·pneu·mo·go·ny (-noo-mo′go-ne) injection of air into a joint to detect effusion.

hy·dro·pneu·mo·peri·to·ne·um (-noo″mo-per″ĭ-to-ne′um) fluid and gas in the peritoneal cavity.

hy·dro·pneu·mo·tho·rax (-thor′aks) fluid and gas within the pleural cavity.

hy·drops (hi′drops) [L.] edema. **fetal h., h. feta′lis,** gross edema of the entire body, with severe anemia, occurring in hemolytic disease of the newborn.

hy·dro·quin·one (hi″dro-kwĭ-nōn′) the reduced form of quinone, used topically as a skin depigmenting agent.

hy·dror·rhea (-re′ah) a copious watery discharge. **h. gravida′rum,** watery discharge from the vagina during pregnancy.

hy·dro·sal·pinx (-sal′pinks) a collection of watery fluid in a uterine tube, occurring as the end stage of pyosalpinx.

hy·dro·sol (hi′dro-sawl) a sol in which the dispersion medium is water.

hy·dro·stat·ics (hi″dro-stat′iks) science of equilibrium of fluids and the pressures they exert. **hydrostat′ic**, adj.

hy·dro·tax·is (-tak′sis) taxis in response to the influence of water or moisture.

hy·dro·ther·a·py (-ther′ah-pe) the application of water, usually externally, in the treatment of disease. colon h., an extension of the enema, used for cleansing and detoxification; the entire colon is irrigated with water, which may contain enzymes or herbs, introduced through the rectum.

hy·dro·thio·ne·mia (-thi″on-ēm′e-ah) hydrogen sulfide in the blood.

hy·dro·tho·rax (-thor′aks) a pleural effusion containing serous fluid.

hy·drot·ro·pism (hi-drot′tro-pizm) a growth response of a nonmotile organism to the presence of water or moisture.

hy·dro·tu·ba·tion (hi″dro-too-ba′shun) introduction into the uterine tube of hydrocortisone in saline solution followed by chymotrypsin in saline solution to maintain its patency.

hy·dro·ure·ter (-u-re′ter) distention of the ureter with urine or watery fluid, due to obstruction.

hy·drox·ide (hi-drok′sīd) any compound containing a hydroxyl group.

hy·droxo·co·bal·a·min (hi-drok″so-ko-bal′ah-min) a hydroxyl-substituted cobalamin derivative, the naturally occurring form of vitamin B_{12} and sometimes used as a source of that vitamin.

hydroxy- chemical prefix indicating the presence of the univalent radical OH.

hy·droxy·am·phet·amine (hi-drok″se-am-fet′ah-mēn) a sympathomimetic amine; its hydrobromide salt is used as a nasal decongestant, pressor, and mydriatic.

hy·droxy·ap·a·tite (-ap′ah-tīt) an inorganic calcium-containing constituent of bone matrix and teeth, imparting rigidity to these structures. Synthetic compounds with similar structure are used as calcium supplements and prosthetic aids (see *durapatite*).

hy·droxy·bu·ty·rate (-bu′tĭ-rāt) a salt or anionic form of hydroxybutyric acid.

hy·droxy·bu·tyr·ic ac·id (-bu-tir′ik) any of several hydroxy derivatives of butyric acid; *β-h.a. (3-h.a.)* is a ketone body and is elevated in the blood and urine in ketosis, and *γ-h.a. (4-h.a.)* is elevated in some body fluids in semialdehyde dehydrogenase deficiency.

4-hy·droxy·bu·tyr·ic·ac·id·uria, *γ-hy·droxy·bu·tyr·ic·ac·id·uria* (-bu-tir″ik-as″ĭ-du′re-ah) succinic semialdehyde dehydrogenase deficiency; see *succinate-semialdehyde dehydrogenase*.

hy·droxy·chlo·ro·quine (-klor′o-kwin) an antiinflammatory and antiprotozoal used as the sulfate salt in the treatment of malaria, lupus erythematosus, and rheumatoid arthritis.

25-hy·droxy·cho·le·cal·cif·e·rol (-ko″lĕ-kal-sif′er-ol) an intermediate in the hepatic activation of cholecalciferol; as the pharmaceutical preparation *calcifediol*, it is used in the treatment of hypocalcemia, hypophosphatemia, rickets, and osteodystrophy associated with various medical conditions.

hy·droxy·cor·ti·co·ste·roid (-kor″tĭ-ko-ster′oid) a corticosteroid bearing a hydroxyl substitution; *17-h's* are intermediates in the biosynthesis of steroid hormones and are accumulated and excreted abnormally in various disorders of steroidogenesis.

hy·droxy·glu·tar·ic ac·id (-gloo-tar′ik) any of several hydroxylated derivatives of glutaric acid, some of which are accumulated and excreted in specific forms of glutaricaciduria.

5-hy·droxy·in·dole·ace·tic ac·id (-in″dōl-ah-se′tik) a product of serotonin metabolism present in increased amounts in the urine in patients with carcinoid tumors.

3-hy·droxy·iso·va·ler·ic ac·id (-i″so-vah-ler′ik) a methylated form of isovaleric acid accumulated and excreted in the urine in some disorders of leucine catabolism.

hy·drox·yl (hi-drok′sil) the univalent radical OH.

hy·drox·yl·ap·a·tite (hi-drok″sil-ap′ah-tīt) hydroxyapatite.

hy·drox·y·lase (hi-drok′sĭ-lās) any of a group of enzymes that catalyze the formation of a hydroxyl group on a substrate by incorporation of one atom (monooxygenases) or two atoms (dioxygenases) of oxygen from O_2. **11β-h.,** an enzyme that catalyzes the hydroxylation of steroids at the 11 position, a step in the synthesis of steroid hormones; deficiency causes a form of congenital adrenal hyperplasia. **17α-h.,** an enzyme that catalyzes the oxidation of steroids at the 17 positions, steps in the synthesis of steroid hormones; deficiency causes a form of congenital adrenal hyperplasia and if it occurs during gestation can cause male pseudohermaphroditism. **18-h.,** an enzyme that catalyzes several steps in the biosynthesis of aldosterone from corticosteroids; deficiency causes salt wasting.

21-h., an enzyme that catalyzes the hydroxylation of steroids at the 21 position, a step in the synthesis of steroid hormones; deficiency impairs the ability to produce all glucocorticoids and causes a form of congenital adrenal hyperplasia.

hy·droxy·preg·nen·o·lone (hi-drok″se-preg-nēn′ah-lōn) an intermediate in the biosynthesis of steroid hormones, accumulated and excreted abnormally in some disorders of steroidogenesis.

hy·droxy·pro·ges·ter·one (-pro-jes′ter-ōn) 1. 17α-hydroxyprogesterone; an intermediate formed in the conversion of cholesterol to cortisol, androgens, and estrogens. 2. a synthetic preparation of the caproate ester, used in treatment of dysfunctional uterine bleeding and menstrual cycle abnormalities, and in the diagnosis of endogenous estrogen production.

hy·droxy·pro·line (-pro′lēn) a hydroxylated form of proline, occurring in collagen and other connective tissue proteins.

hy·droxy·pro·lin·e·mia (-pro″li-ne′me-ah) 1. excess of hydroxyproline in the blood. 2. a disorder of amino acid metabolism characterized by an excess of free hydroxyproline in the plasma and urine, due to a defect in the enzyme hydroxyproline oxidase; it may be associated with mental retardation.

hy·droxy·pro·pyl cel·lu·lose (-pro′pil sel′u-lōs) a partially substituted, water-soluble cellulose ether, used as a pharmaceutic aid and as a topical ophthalmic protectant and lubricant.

hy·droxy·pro·pyl meth·yl·cel·lu·lose (-pro′pil meth″il-sel′u-lōs) hypromellose.

8-hy·droxy·quin·o·line (-kwin′o-lēn) oxyquinoline.

hy·droxy·ste·roid (-ster′oid) a steroid carrying a hydroxyl group.

17β-hy·droxy·ste·roid de·hy·dro·gen·ase de·fi·cien·cy an autosomal recessive disorder of steroidogenesis due to deficiency of the testicular enzyme testosterone 17β-dehydrogenase (NADP⁺); characterized by male pseudohermaphroditism with postpubertal virilization and sometimes gynecomastia, decreased plasma testosterone, and increased androstenedione.

5-hy·droxy·tryp·ta·mine (5-HT) (-trip′tah-mēn) serotonin.

hy·droxy·urea (-u-re′ah) an antineoplastic that inhibits a step in DNA synthesis, used in treatment of chronic granulocytic leukemia, some carcinomas, malignant melanoma, and polycythemia vera. It is also used to reduce the frequency of painful sickle cell crisis.

25-hy·droxy·vi·ta·min D (-vi′tah-min) either 25-hydroxycholecalciferol, the corresponding hydroxy- derivative of ergocalciferol, or both together.

hy·droxy·zine (hi-drok′si-zēn) a central nervous system depressant having antispasmodic, antihistaminic, and antifibrillatory actions; used as *h. hydrochloride* or *h. pamoate* as an antianxiety agent, antihistamine, antiemetic, and sedative.

hy·dru·ria (hi-droor′e-ah) excretion of urine of low osmolality or low specific gravity. **hydrur′ic,** adj.

hy·giene (hi′jēn) science of health and its preservation. **hygien′ic,** adj. **oral h.,** proper care of the mouth and teeth.

hy·gien·ist (hi-jen′ist, hi″je-en′ist) a specialist in hygiene. **dental h.,** an auxiliary member of the dental profession, trained in the art of removing calcareous deposits and stains from surfaces of teeth and in providing additional services and information on prevention of oral disease.

hygr(o)- word element [Gr.], *moisture.*

hy·gro·ma (hi-gro′mah) pl. *hygromas, hygro′mata.* An accumulation of fluid in a sac, cyst, or bursa. **hygrom′atous,** adj. **h. col′li,** a watery tumor of the neck. **cystic h., h. cys′ticum,** a lymphangioma usually occurring in the neck and composed of large, multilocular, thin-walled cysts.

hy·grom·e·try (hi-grom′ĕ-tre) measurement of moisture in the atmosphere.

hy·gro·scop·ic (hi″gro-skop′ik) readily absorbing moisture.

hy·men (hi′men) the membranous fold partially or wholly occluding the external vaginal orifice. **hy′menal,** adj.

hy·me·no·lep·i·a·sis (hi″mĕ-no-lep-i′ah-sis) infection with *Hymenolepis.*

Hy·me·nol·e·pis (hi″mĕ-nol′ĕ-pis) a genus of tapeworms, including *H. na′na,* found in rodents, rats, and humans, especially children.

hy·men·ol·o·gy (-ol′ah-je) the science dealing with the membranes of the body.

Hy·men·op·tera (-op′ter-ah) an order of insects with two pairs of well-developed membranous wings, like bees and wasps.

hyo·epi·glot·tic (hi″o-ep″ĭ-glot′ik) pertaining to the hyoid bone and the epiglottis.

hyo·epi·glot·tid·e·an (-glŏ-tid′e-in) hyoepiglottic.

hyo·glos·sal (-glos′′l) pertaining to the hyoid bone and tongue or to the hyoglossus muscle.

hy·oid (hi′oid) shaped like Greek letter upsilon (υ); pertaining to the hyoid bone.

hyo·scine (hi′o-sēn) scopolamine.

hyo·scy·amine (hi″o-si′ah-mēn) an anticholinergic alkaloid that is the levorotatory component of racemic atropine and has similar actions but twice the potency; used as an antispasmodic in gastrointestinal and urinary tract disorders, as the base or hydrobromide or sulfate salt.

hyp·al·ge·sia (hi″pal-je′ze-ah) decreased pain sense. **hypalge′sic**, adj.

hyp·ana·ki·ne·sis (hĭp″an-ah-kĭ-ne′sis) hypokinesia.

hyp·ar·te·ri·al (-ahr-tēr′e-il) beneath an artery.

hyp·ax·i·al (hi-pak′se-al) ventral to the long axis of the body.

hyper- word element [Gr.], *abnormally increased; excessive.*

hy·per·ac·id (hi″per-as′id) excessively acid.

hy·per·ac·tiv·i·ty (-ak-tiv′ĭ-te) 1. excessive or abnormally increased muscular function or activity. 2. former name for *attention-deficit/hyperactivity disorder.* **hyperac′tive**, adj.

hy·per·acu·sis (-ah-koo′sis) an exceptionally acute sense of hearing, the threshold being very low.

hy·per·ad·e·no·sis (-ad″ĕ-no′sis) enlargement of glands.

hy·per·ad·i·po·sis (-ad″ĭ-po′sis) extreme fatness.

hy·per·adre·nal·ism (-ah-drēn′ah-lizm) overactivity of the adrenal glands.

hy·per·adre·no·cor·ti·cal·ism (-ah-dre″no-kor′tĭ-kahl-izm) hypersecretion by the adrenal cortex.

hy·per·adre·no·cor·ti·cism (-ah-dre″no-kor′tĭ-sizm) hyperadrenocorticalism.

hy·per·al·dos·ter·on·ism (-al-dos′tĕ-ro-nizm) aldosteronism.

hy·per·al·ge·sia (-al-je′ze-ah) abnormally increased pain sense. **hyperalge′sic**, adj.

hy·per·al·i·men·ta·tion (-al″ĭ-men-ta′shun) the ingestion or administration of a greater than optimal amount of nutrients. **parenteral h.**, total parenteral nutrition.

hy·per·al·pha·lipo·pro·tein·emia (-al″-fah-lip″o-pro″te-ne′me-ah) the presence of abnormally high levels of high-density lipoproteins in the serum.

hy·per·am·mo·ne·mia (-am″o-ne′me-ah) a metabolic disturbance marked by elevated levels of ammonia in the blood.

hy·per·am·mo·nu·ria (-am″o-nu′re-ah) excessive ammonia in the urine.

hy·per·ana·ki·ne·sia (-an″ah-kĭ-ne′zhah) hyperdynamia.

hy·per·an·dro·gen·ism (-an′dro-jen-izm) the state of having excessive secretion of androgens, as in congenital adrenal hyperplasia.

hy·per·aphia (-a′fe-ah) tactile hyperesthesia. **hyperaph′ic**, adj.

hy·per·arou·sal (-ah-rou′z′l) a state of increased psychological and physiological tension marked by such effects as reduced pain tolerance, anxiety, exaggeration of startle responses, insomnia, fatigue, and accentuation of personality traits.

hy·per·azo·te·mia (-az″o-te′me-ah) an excess of nitrogenous matter in the blood.

hy·per·bar·ic (-bar′ik) having greater than normal pressure or weight; said of gases under greater than atmospheric pressure, or of a solution of greater specific gravity than another used as a reference standard.

hy·per·bar·ism (-bar′izm) a condition due to exposure to ambient gas pressure or atmospheric pressures exceeding the pressure within the body.

hy·per·be·ta·lipo·pro·tein·emia (-ba″tah-lip″o-pro″te-ne′me-ah) increased accumulation of low-density lipoproteins in the blood.

hy·per·bil·i·ru·bin·emia (-bil″ĭ-roo″bĭ-ne′me-ah) excess of bilirubin in the blood; classified as conjugated or unconjugated, according to the predominant form of bilirubin present.

hy·per·brady·ki·nin·ism (-brad″ĭ-ki′nin-izm) a syndrome of high plasma bradykinin associated with a fall in systolic blood pressure on standing, increased diastolic pressure and heart rate, and ecchymoses of lower limbs.

hy·per·cal·ce·mia (-kal-se′me-ah) an excess of calcium in the blood. **idiopathic h.,** a condition of infants, associated with vitamin D intoxication, characterized by elevated serum calcium levels, increased density of the skeleton, mental deterioration, and nephrocalcinosis. **h. of malignancy,** abnormal elevation of serum calcium associated with malignant tumors, resulting from osteolysis caused by bone metastases or by the action of circulating cytokines released from tumor cells.

hy·per·cal·ci·uria (-kal″se-u′re-ah) excess of calcium in the urine.

hy·per·cap·nia (-kap′ne-ah) excessive carbon dioxide in the blood. **hypercap′nic**, adj.

hy·per·car·bia (-kahr′be-ah) hypercapnia.

hy·per·car·o·ten·emia (-kar″o-tĕ-ne′me-ah) excessive carotene in the blood, often with yellowing of the skin (carotenosis).

hy·per·ca·thar·sis (-kah-thahr′sis) excessive catharsis. **hypercathar′tic**, adj.

hy·per·cel·lu·lar·i·ty (-sel″u-lar′ĭ-te) abnormal increase in the number of cells present, as in bone marrow. **hypercell′ular**, adj.

hy·per·chlor·emia (-klor-e′me-ah) an excess of chlorides in the blood. **hyperchlore′mic,** adj.

hy·per·chlor·hy·dria (-klor-hi′dre-ah) excessive hydrochloric acid in gastric juice.

hy·per·cho·les·ter·ol·emia (-ko-les″ter-ol-e′me-ah) an excess of cholesterol in the blood. **hypercholesterole′mic,** adj. **familial h.,** an inherited disorder of lipoprotein metabolism due to defects in the receptor for low-density lipoprotein (LDL), with xanthomas, corneal arcus, premature corneal atherosclerosis, and a type II-a hyperlipoproteinemia biochemical phenotype with elevated plasma LDL and cholesterol.

hy·per·chro·ma·sia (-kro-ma′zhah) hyperchromatism.

hy·per·chro·ma·tism (-kro′mah-tizm) 1. excessive pigmentation. 2. degeneration of cell nuclei, which become filled with particles of pigment (chromatin). 3. increased staining capacity. **hyperchromat′ic,** adj.

hy·per·chro·mia (-kro′me-ah) 1. hyperchromatism. 2. abnormal increase in the hemoglobin content of erythrocytes.

hy·per·chy·lia (-ki′le-ah) excessive secretion of gastric juice.

hy·per·chy·lo·mi·cro·nemia (-ki″lo-mi″kro-ne′me-ah) presence in the blood of an excessive number of chylomicrons. **familial h.,** an inherited disorder of lipoprotein metabolism characterized by elevated plasma chylomicrons and triglycerides, pancreatitis, cutaneous xanthomas, and hepatosplenomegaly; it is usually due to deficiency of lipoprotein lipase or its cofactor apolipoprotein C-II.

hy·per·cry·al·ge·sia (-kri″al-je′ze-ah) hypercryesthesia.

hy·per·cry·es·the·sia (-kri″es-the′zhah) excessive sensitivity to cold.

hy·per·cu·pre·mia (-ku-pre′me-ah) an excess of copper in the blood.

hypercupriuria (-ku-pre-u′re-ah) excessive copper in the urine.

hy·per·cy·a·not·ic (-si″ah-not′ik) extremely cyanotic.

hy·per·cy·the·mia (-si-the′me-ah) erythrocythemia.

hy·per·cy·to·sis (-si-to′sis) abnormally increased number of cells, especially of leukocytes.

hy·per·di·crot·ic (-di-krot′ik) markedly dicrotic.

hy·per·dis·ten·tion (-dis-ten′shun) excessive distention.

hy·per·dy·na·mia (-di-na′me-ah) hyperactivity (1). **hyperdynam′ic,** adj.

hy·per·em·e·sis (-em′ĕ-sis) excessive vomiting. **hyperemet′ic,** adj. **h. gravida′rum,** the pernicious vomiting of pregnancy. **h. lacten′tium,** excessive vomiting in nursing babies.

hy·per·emia (-e′me-ah) engorgement; an excess of blood in a part. **hypere′mic,** adj. **active h., arterial h.,** that due to local or general relaxation of arterioles. **exercise h.,** vasodilation of the capillaries in muscles in response to the onset of exercise, proportionate to the force of the muscular contractions. **passive h.,** that due to obstruction to flow of blood from the area. **reactive h.,** that due to increase in blood flow after its temporary interruption. **venous h.,** passive h.

hy·per·eo·sin·o·phil·ia (-e″o-sin″o-fil′e-ah) extreme eosinophilia. **hypereosinophil′ic,** adj.

hy·per·equi·lib·ri·um (-e″kwĭ-lib′re-um) excessive tendency to vertigo.

hy·per·eso·pho·ria (-es″o-for′e-ah) deviation of the visual axes upward and inward.

hy·per·es·the·sia (-es-the′zhah) increased sensitivity to stimulation, particularly to touch. **hyperesthet′ic,** adj. **acoustic h., auditory h.,** hyperacusis. **cerebral h.,** that due to a cerebral lesion. **gustatory h.,** hypergeusia. **muscular h.,** muscular oversensitivity to pain or fatigue. **olfactory h.,** hyperosmia. **oneiric h.,** increased sensitivity or pain during sleep and dreams. **optic h.,** abnormal sensitivity of the eye to light. **tactile h.,** excessive sensitivity of the sense of touch.

hy·per·es·tro·gen·ism (-es′tro-jen-izm) excessive amounts of estrogens in the body.

hy·per·exo·pho·ria (-ek″so-for′e-ah) deviation of the visual axes upward and outward.

hy·per·fer·re·mia (-fĕ-re′me-ah) an excess of iron in the blood. **hyperferre′mic,** adj.

hy·per·fi·bri·no·ge·ne·mia (-fi-brin″o-jĕ-ne′me-ah) excessive fibrinogen in the blood.

hy·per·fil·tra·tion (-fil-tra′shun) an elevation in the glomerular filtration rate, often a sign of early type 1 diabetes mellitus.

hy·per·frac·tion·a·tion (-frak″shun-a′shun) a subdivision of a radiation treatment schedule with some reduction of dose per exposure so as to decrease side effects while still delivering an equal or greater total dose of radiation over the course.

hy·per·func·tion (-fungk′shun) excessive functioning of a part or organ.

hy·per·ga·lac·tia (-gah-lak′she-ah) excessive secretion of milk.

hy·per·gal·ac·to·sis (-gal″ak-to′sis) hypergalactia.

hy·per·gam·ma·glob·u·lin·emia (-gam″-ah-glob″u-lĭ-ne′me-ah) increased gamma globulins in the blood. **hypergammaglobuline′mic**, adj. **monoclonal h's**, plasma cell dyscrasias.

hy·per·gen·e·sis (-jen′ĕ-sis) excessive development. **hypergenet′ic**, adj.

hy·per·geus·es·the·sia (-go͞os″es-the-zhah) hypergeusia.

hy·per·geu·sia (-goo′zhah) abnormal acuteness of the sense of taste.

hy·per·glu·ca·gon·emia (-gloo″kah-gon-e′me-ah) abnormally high levels of glucagon in the blood.

hy·per·gly·ce·mia (-gli-se′me-ah) abnormally increased content of glucose in the blood.

hy·per·gly·ce·mic (-gli-se′mik) 1. pertaining to, characterized by, or causing hyperglycemia. 2. an agent that increases the glucose level of the blood.

hy·per·glyc·er·i·de·mia (-glis″er-i-de′me-ah) excess of glycerides in the blood.

hy·per·glyc·er·ol·emia (-glis″er-ol-e′me-ah) 1. accumulation and excretion of glycerol due to deficiency of an enzyme catalyzing its phosphorylation; the infantile form is due to a chromosomal deletion which may also involve the loci causing Duchenne muscular dystrophy or congenital adrenal hyperplasia or both. 2. excess of glycerol in the blood.

hy·per·gly·cin·e·mia (-gli″sĭ-ne′me-ah) excess of glycine in the blood or other body fluids; *ketotic h.* includes ketotic disorders secondary to a variety of organic acidemias; *nonketotic h.* is a hereditary disorder of neonatal onset, due to a defect in the glycine cleavage system, with lethargy, absence of cerebral development, seizures, myoclonic jerks, and frequently coma and respiratory failure.

hy·per·gly·cin·uria (-gli″sĭ-nu′re-ah) an excess of glycine in the urine; see *hyperglycinemia*.

hy·per·gly·co·gen·ol·y·sis (-gli″ko-jen-ol′ĭ-sis) excessive glycogenolysis, resulting in excessive glucose in the body.

hy·per·gly·cor·rha·chia (-gli″ko-ra′ke-ah) excessive sugar in the cerebrospinal fluid.

hy·per·go·nad·ism (-go′nad-izm) abnormally increased functional activity of the gonads, with accelerated growth and precocious sexual development.

hy·per·go·nado·tro·pic (-go-nad″ah-tro′pik) relating to or caused by excessive amounts of gonadotropins.

hy·per·hi·dro·sis (-hi-dro′sis) excessive perspiration. **hyperhidrot′ic**, adj. **emotional h.**, an inherited disorder of the eccrine sweat glands in which emotional stimuli cause axillary or volar sweating.

hy·per·hy·dra·tion (-hi-dra′shun) overhydration; excessive fluids in the body.

Hy·per·i·cum (hi-per′ĭ-kum) a genus of herbs, including several types of St. John's wort. **H. perfora′tum**, the species of St. John's wort whose above-ground parts are used medicinally.

hy·per·im·mune (hi″per-ĭ-mūn′) possessing very large quantities of specific antibodies in the serum.

hy·per·im·mu·no·glob·u·lin·emia (-im″u-no-glob″u-lĭ-ne′me-ah) abnormally high levels of immunoglobulins in the serum.

hy·per·in·su·lin·ism (-in′sŭ-lin-izm″) 1. excessive secretion of insulin. 2. insulin shock.

hy·per·ir·ri·ta·bil·i·ty (-ir″ĭ-tah-bil′ĭ-te) pathological responsiveness to slight stimuli.

hy·per·iso·ton·ic (-i″so-ton′ik) denoting a solution containing more than 0.45% salt, in which erythrocytes become crenated as a result of exosmosis.

hy·per·ka·le·mia (-kah-le′me-ah) an excess of potassium in the blood; hyperpotassemia. **hyperkale′mic**, adj.

hy·per·ker·a·tin·iza·tion (-ker″ah-tin″ĭ-za′shun) excessive development or retention of keratin in the epidermis.

hy·per·ker·a·to·sis (-ker″ah-to′sis) 1. hypertrophy of the stratum corneum of the skin, or any disease so characterized. 2. hypertrophy of the cornea. **epidermolytic h.**, a hereditary disease, with hyperkeratosis, blisters, and erythema; at birth the skin is entirely covered with thick, horny, armorlike plates that are soon shed, leaving a raw surface on which scales then reform. **h. follicula′ris in cu′tem pe′netrans**, Kyrle's disease.

hy·per·ke·ton·emia (-ke″to-ne′me-ah) ketonemia.

hy·per·ki·ne·mia (-kĭ-ne′me-ah) abnormally high cardiac output; increased rate of blood flow through the circulatory system. **hyperkine′mic**, adj.

hy·per·ki·ne·sia (-kĭ-ne′zhah) hyperactivity.

hy·per·ki·ne·sis (hi″per-kĭ-ne′sis) hyperactivity. **hyperkinet′ic**, adj.

hy·per·lac·ta·tion (-lak-ta′shun) lactation in greater than normal amount or for a longer than normal period.

hy·per·leu·ko·cy·to·sis (-loo″ko-si-to′sis) abnormally excessive numbers of leukocytes in the blood.

hy·per·li·pe·mia (-lĭ-pe′me-ah) hyperlipidemia. **carbohydrate-induced h.**, elevated blood lipids, particularly triglycerides, after carbohydrate ingestion; sometimes used synonymously with hyperlipoproteinemia type IV or V phenotypes, or the genetic disorders causing them. **combined fat-and carbohydrate-induced h.,** persistently elevated blood levels of very-low-density lipoproteins and chylomicrons after ingestion of fat or carbohydrates; sometimes used synonymously with a type V hyperlipoproteinemia or the genetic disorders causing it. **endogenous h.,** elevated plasma lipids derived from body stores (i.e., very-low-density lipoproteins), rather than dietary sources; used as a generic descriptor of the type IV hyperlipoproteinemia phenotype. **essential familial h.,** an inherited disorder causing a type I hyperlipoproteinemia phenotype, or the phenotype itself. **exogenous h.,** elevated plasma levels of lipoproteins derived from dietary sources (i.e., chylomicrons); used as a generic descriptor of the type I hyperlipoproteinemia phenotype. **familial fat-induced h.,** persistently elevated blood chylomicrons after fat ingestion; sometimes used synonymously with hyperlipoproteinemia type I phenotype or the genetic disorders causing it. **mixed h.,** generic designation for a hyperlipoproteinemia in which several classes of lipoproteins are elevated; usually used to denote a type V phenotype, but sometimes used for a type II-b phenotype.

hy·per·lip·id·emia (-lip″ĭ-de′me-ah) elevated concentrations of any or all of the lipids in the plasma, including hypertriglyceridemia, hypercholesterolemia, etc. **hyperlipide′mic,** adj. **combined h.,** a generic designation for a hyperlipidemia in which several classes of lipids are elevated; usually used to denote the phenotype of a type II-b hyperlipoproteinemia. **familial combined h.,** an inherited disorder of lipoprotein metabolism manifested in adulthood as hypercholesterolemia, hypertriglyceridemia, or a combination, with elevated plasma apolipoprotein B and premature coronary atherosclerosis. **mixed h.,** see under *hyperlipemia.* **remnant h.,** a form in which the accumulated lipoproteins are normally transient intermediates, chylomicron remnants, and intermediate-density lipoproteins; a generic descriptor for the type III hyperlipoproteinemia phenotype.

hy·per·lipo·pro·tein·emia (-lip″o-pro″te-ne′me-ah) an excess of lipoproteins in the blood, due to a disorder of lipoprotein metabolism; it may be acquired or familial. It has been subdivided on the basis of

biochemical phenotype, each type having a generic description and a variety of causes: *type I,* exogenous hyperlipemia; *type II-a,* hypercholesterolemia; *type II-b,* combined hyperlipidemia; *type III,* remnant hyperlipidemia; *type IV,* endogenous hyperlipemia; *type V,* mixed hyperlipemia.

hy·per·lu·cen·cy (-loo′sen-se) excessive radiolucency.

hy·per·ly·sin·emia (-li″sĭ-ne′me-ah) 1. excess of lysine in the blood. 2. an aminoacidopathy characterized by excess of lysine, and sometimes of saccharopine, in the blood and urine, possibly associated with mental retardation.

hy·per·mag·ne·se·mia (-mag″ně-se′me-ah) an abnormally large magnesium content of the blood plasma.

hy·per·mas·tia (-mas′te-ah) 1. presence of supernumerary mammary glands. 2. macromastia.

hy·per·ma·ture (-mah-choor′) past the stage of maturity.

hy·per·men·or·rhea (-men″o-re′ah) menstruation with an excessive flow but at regular intervals and of usual duration.

hy·per·me·tab·o·lism (-mě-tab′o-lizm) increased metabolism. **extrathyroidal h.,** abnormally elevated basal metabolism unassociated with thyroid disease.

hy·per·me·tria (-me′tre-ah) ataxia in which movements overreach the intended goal.

hy·per·met·rope (-me′trōp) hyperope.

hy·per·me·tro·pia (-mě-tro′pe-ah) hyperopia.

hy·per·mo·bil·i·ty (-mo-bil′ĭ-te) greater than normal range of motion in a joint. **hypermo′bile,** adj.

hy·per·morph (hi′per-morf) 1. a person who is tall but of low sitting height. 2. a mutant gene that shows an increase in the activity it influences. **hypermor′phic,** adj.

hy·per·mo·til·i·ty (hi″per-mo-til′ĭ-te) abnormally increased motility, as of the gastrointestinal tract.

hy·per·my·ot·ro·phy (-mi-ot′rah-fe) excessive development of muscular tissue.

hy·per·na·sal·i·ty (-na-zal′ĭ-te) a quality of voice in which the emission of air through the nose is excessive due to velopharyngeal insufficiency; it causes deterioration of intelligibility of speech.

hy·per·na·tre·mia (-na-tre′me-ah) an excess of sodium in the blood. **hypernatre′mic,** adj.

hy·per·neo·cy·to·sis (-ne″o-si-to′sis) hyperleukocytosis with an excessive number of immature forms.

hy·per·ne·phro·ma (-ně-fro′mah) renal cell carcinoma.

hy·per·nu·tri·tion (-noo-trish'un) hyperalimentation.

hy·per·ope (hi'per-ōp) an individual exhibiting hyperopia.

hy·per·opia (hi″per-o′pe-ah) farsightedness; a visual defect in which parallel light rays reaching the eye come to a focus behind the retina, vision being better for far objects than for near. Symbol H. **hypero′pic,** adj. **absolute h.,** that which cannot be corrected by accommodation. **axial h.,** that due to shortness of the anteroposterior diameter of the eye. **facultative h.,** that which can be entirely corrected by accommodation. **latent h.,** that degree of the total hyperopia corrected by the physiologic tone of the ciliary muscle, revealed by cycloplegic examination. **manifest h.,** that degree of the total hyperopia not corrected by the physiologic tone of the ciliary muscle, revealed by cycloplegic examination. **relative h.,** facultative h. **total h.,** manifest and latent hyperopia combined.

hy·per·or·chi·dism (-or'kid-izm) excessive functional activity of the testes.

hy·per·orex·ia (-o-rek'se-ah) excessive appetite.

hy·per·or·ni·thin·emia (-or″nĭ-thī-ne′me-ah) excess of ornithine in the plasma.

hy·per·or·tho·cy·to·sis (-or″tho-si-to′sis) hyperleukocytosis with a normal proportion of the various forms of leukocytes.

hy·per·os·mia (-oz′me-ah) increased sensitivity of smell.

hy·per·os·mo·lal·i·ty (-oz″mo-lal′ĭ-te) an increase in the osmolality of the body fluids.

hy·per·os·mo·lar·i·ty (-oz″mo-lar′ĭ-te) abnormally increased osmolar concentration.

hy·per·os·to·sis (-os-to′sis) hypertrophy of bone. **hyperostot′ic,** adj. **h. cortica′lis defor′mans juveni′lis,** an inherited disorder of limb fractures and bowing, thickening of skull bones, osteoporosis, and elevated levels of serum alkaline phosphatase and urinary hydroxyproline. **h. cortica′lis generalisa′ta,** a hereditary disorder beginning during puberty, marked chiefly by osteosclerosis of the skull, mandible, clavicles, ribs, and diaphyses of long bones, associated with elevated blood alkaline phosphatase. **h. cra′nii,** hyperostosis involving the cranial bones. **h. fronta′lis inter′na,** thickening of the inner table of the frontal bone, which may be associated with hypertrichosis and obesity, most commonly affecting women near menopause. **infantile cortical h.,** a disease of young infants, with soft tissue swelling over affected bones, fever, irritability, and periods of remission and exacerbation.

hy·per·ox·al·uria (-ok″sah-lu″re-ah) an excess of oxalates in the urine. **enteric h.,** formation of calcium oxalate calculi in the urinary tract after resection or disease of the ileum, due to excessive absorption of oxalate from the colon. **primary h.,** an inborn error of metabolism with defective glyoxylate metabolism, excessive urinary excretion of oxalate, nephrolithiasis, nephrocalcinosis, early onset of renal failure, and often a generalized deposit of calcium oxalate.

hy·per·ox·ia (-ok′se-ah) an excess of oxygen in the system. **hyperox′ic,** adj.

hy·per·par·a·site (-par′ah-sīt) a parasite that preys on a parasite. **hyperparasit′ic,** adj.

hy·per·para·thy·roid·ism (-par″ah-thi′roid-izm) excessive activity of the parathyroid glands. *Primary h.* is associated with neoplasia or hyperplasia; the excess of parathyroid hormone leads to alteration in function of bone cells, renal tubules, and gastrointestinal mucosa. *Secondary h.* occurs when the serum calcium tends to fall below normal, as in chronic renal disease, etc. *Tertiary h.* refers to that due to a parathyroid adenoma arising from secondary hyperplasia caused by chronic renal failure.

hy·per·peri·stal·sis (-per″ĭ-stawl′sis) excessively active peristalsis.

hy·per·pha·gia (-fa′jah) polyphagia. **hyperpha′gic,** adj.

hy·per·phen·yl·al·a·nin·emia (-fen″il-al″ah-nĭ-ne′me-ah) 1. any of several inherited defects in the hydroxylation of phenylalanine causing it to be accumulated and excreted; some are benign while others cause phenylketonuria, at least one type of which is unresponsive to treatment and rapidly fatal. 2. excess of phenylalanine in the blood.

hy·per·pho·ne·sis (-fo-ne′sis) intensification of the sound in auscultation or percussion.

hy·per·pho·ria (-for′e-ah) upward deviation of the visual axis of one eye in the absence of visual fusional stimuli.

hy·per·phos·pha·ta·se·mia (-fos″fah-ta-se′me-ah) high levels of alkaline phosphatase in the blood.

hy·per·phos·pha·ta·sia (-fos″fah-ta′zhah) hyperphosphatasemia.

hy·per·phos·pha·te·mia (-fos″fah-te′me-ah) an excessive amount of phosphates in the blood.

hy·per·phos·pha·tu·ria (-fos″fah-tu′re-ah) an excess of phosphates in the urine.

hy·per·pig·men·ta·tion (-pig″men-ta′shun) abnormally increased pigmentation.

hy·per·pi·tu·i·ta·rism (-pĭ-too′ĭ-ter-izm″) a condition due to pathologically increased activity of the pituitary gland, either of the basophilic cells, resulting in basophil adenoma causing compression of the pituitary gland, or of the eosinophilic cells, producing overgrowth, acromegaly, and gigantism (*true h.*).

hy·per·pla·sia (-pla′zhah) abnormal increase in the number of normal cells in normal arrangement in an organ or tissue, which increases its volume. **hyperplas′tic,** adj. **adrenal cortical h., adrenocortical h.,** hyperplasia of adrenal cortical cells, as in adrenogenital syndrome and Cushing's syndrome. **benign prostatic h.,** age-associated enlargement of the prostate resulting from proliferation of both stromal and glandular elements; it may cause urethral obstruction and compression. **C-cell h.,** a premalignant stage in the development of the familial forms of medullary thyroid carcinoma, characterized by multicentric patches of parafollicular cells (C cells). **congenital adrenal h. (CAH),** a group of inherited disorders of cortisol biosynthesis that result in compensatory hypersecretion of corticotropin and subsequent adrenal hyperplasia, excessive androgen production, and a spectrum of phenotypes. **cutaneous lymphoid h.,** a group of benign cutaneous disorders with lesions clinically and histologically resembling those of malignant lymphoma. **focal nodular h. (FNH),** a benign, firm, nodular, highly vascular tumor of the liver, resembling cirrhosis. **intravascular papillary endothelial h.,** a benign vascular tumor usually occurring as a solitary nodule of the head, neck, or finger and resembling angiosarcoma. **nodular h. of the prostate,** benign prostatic h. **verrucous h.,** a superficial, typically white, hyperplastic lesion of the oral mucosa, usually occurring in older males and believed to be a precursor to verrucous carcinoma.

hy·per·ploi·dy (hi′per-ploi″de) the state of having more than the typical number of chromosomes in unbalanced sets, as in Down syndrome.

hy·per·pnea (hi″perp-ne′ah) abnormal increase in depth and rate of respiration. **hyperpne′ic,** adj.

hy·per·po·lar·iza·tion (hi″per-po″ler-ĭ-za′shun) any increase in the amount of electrical charge separated by the cell membrane, and hence in the strength of the transmembrane potential.

hy·per·po·ne·sis (-po-ne′sis) excessive action-potential output from the motor and premotor areas of the cortex. **hyperponet′ic,** adj.

hy·per·po·sia (-po′zhah) abnormally increased ingestion of fluids for relatively brief periods.

hy·per·po·tas·se·mia (-pot″ah-se′me-ah) hyperkalemia.

hy·per·prax·ia (-prak′se-ah) abnormal activity; restlessness.

hy·per·pre·be·ta·lipo·pro·tein·emia (-pre-ba″tah-lip″o-pro″te-ne′me-ah) an excess of pre-beta lipoproteins (very-low-density lipoproteins) in the blood.

hy·per·pro·in·su·lin·emia (-pro-in″sah-lĭ-ne′me-ah) elevated levels of proinsulin or proinsulin-like material in the blood.

hy·per·pro·lac·tin·emia (-pro-lak″tĭ-ne′me-ah) increased levels of prolactin in the blood, often associated with pituitary adenoma. **hyperprolactine′mic,** adj.

hy·per·pro·lin·emia (-pro″lĭ-ne′me-ah) 1. any of several benign aminoacidopathies marked by an excess of proline in the body fluids. 2. excess of proline in the blood.

hy·per·pro·sex·ia (-pro-sek′se-ah) preoccupation with one idea to the exclusion of all others.

hy·per·pro·te·o·sis (-pro″te-o′sis) a condition due to an excess of protein in the diet.

hy·per·py·rex·ia (-pi-rek′se-ah) hyperthermia. **hyperpyrex′ial, hyperpyret′ic,** adj. **malignant h.,** see under *hyperthermia.*

hy·per·re·ac·tio lu·te·in·a·lis (-re-ak′she-o loo″te-ĭ-na′lis) bilateral ovarian enlargement during pregnancy due to the presence of numerous theca-lutein cysts, usually associated with abnormally high levels of human chorionic gonadotropin.

hy·per·re·ac·tive (-re-ak′tiv) showing a greater than normal response to stimuli.

hy·per·re·flex·ia (-re-flek′se-ah) disordered response to stimuli characterized by exaggeration of reflexes. **autonomic h.,** paroxysmal hypertension, bradycardia, forehead sweating, headache, and gooseflesh due to distention of the bladder and rectum, associated with lesions above the outflow of the splanchnic nerves. **detrusor h.,** increased contractile activity of the detrusor muscle of the bladder, resulting in urinary incontinence.

hy·per·re·nin·emia (-re″nĭ-ne′me-ah) elevated levels of renin in the blood, which may lead to aldosteronism and hypertension.

hy·per·res·o·nance (-rez′o-nans) exaggerated resonance on percussion.

hy·per·re·spon·sive (-re-spon′siv) hyperreactive.

hy·per·sal·i·va·tion (-sal″ĭ-va′shun) ptyalism.

hy·per·sar·co·sin·e·mia (-sahr″ko-sĭ-ne′me-ah) sarcosinemia.

hy·per·se·cre·tion (-se-kre′shun) excessive secretion.

hy·per·sen·si·tiv·i·ty (-sen″sĭ-tiv′ĭ-te) a state of altered reactivity in which the body reacts with an exaggerated immune response to what is perceived as a foreign substance. The hypersensitivity states and resulting reactions are usually subclassified by the Gell and Coombs classification (q.v.). **hypersen′sitive,** adj. **antibody-mediated h.,** 1. type II h.; see *Gell and Coombs classification,* under *classification.* 2. occasionally, any form of hypersensitivity in which antibodies, rather than T lymphocytes, are the primary mediators, i.e., types I–III. **cell-mediated h.,** type IV h.; see *Gell and Coombs classification,* under *classification.* **contact h.,** a type IV hypersensitivity produced by contact of the skin with a chemical substance having the properties of an antigen or hapten. **cytotoxic h.,** type II h.; see *Gell and Coombs classification,* under *classification.* **delayed h. (DH) delayed-type h. (DTH),** that which takes 24 to 72 hours to develop and is mediated by T lymphocytes rather than by antibodies; usually used to denote the subset of type IV hypersensitivity involving cytokine release and macrophage activation, as opposed to direct cytolysis, but sometimes used more broadly, even as a synonym of *type IV h.* **immediate h.,** 1. type I h.; see *Gell and Coombs classification,* under *classification.* 2. occasionally, any form of hypersensitivity mediated by antibodies and developing rapidly, generally in minutes to hours (i.e., *types I–III*), as distinguished from that mediated by T lymphocytes and macrophages and requiring days to develop (*type IV,* or *delayed h.*). **immune complex–mediated h.,** type III h.; see *Gell and Coombs classification,* under *classification.* **T cell–mediated h.,** type IV h.; see *Gell and Coombs classification,* under *classification.* **type I h.,** see *Gell and Coombs classification,* under *classification.* **type II h.,** see *Gell and Coombs classification,* under *classification.* **type III h.,** see *Gell and Coombs classification,* under *classification.* **type IV h.,** see *Gell and Coombs classification,* under *classification.*

hy·per·som·nia (-som′ne-ah) excessive sleeping or sleepiness.

hy·per·som·no·lence (-som′n -lens) hypersomnia.

hy·per·splen·ism (-splen′izm) exaggeration of the hemolytic function of the spleen, resulting in deficiency of peripheral blood elements, hypercellularity of bone marrow, and splenomegaly.

hy·per·sthe·nia (-sthe′ne-ah) great strength or tonicity. **hypersthen′ic,** adj.

hy·per·stim·u·la·tion (-stim″u-la′shun) excessive stimulation of an organ or part. **controlled ovarian h.,** monitored administration of agents designed to induce ovulation by a greater number of ovarian follicles and thus increase the probability of fertilization.

hy·per·telo·rism (-te′lor-izm) abnormally increased distance between two organs or parts. **ocular h., orbital h.,** increase in the interorbital distance, often associated with cleidocranial or craniofacial dysostosis and sometimes with mental deficiency.

hy·per·ten·sion (-ten′shun) persistently high arterial blood pressure; it may have no known cause (*essential, idiopathic,* or *primary h.*) or may be associated with other diseases (*secondary h.*). **accelerated h.,** progressive hypertension with the funduscopic vascular changes of malignant hypertension but without papilledema. **adrenal h.,** that associated with an adrenal tumor which secretes mineralocorticoids. **borderline h.,** a condition in which the arterial blood pressure is sometimes within the normotensive range and sometimes within the hypertensive range. **Goldblatt h.,** that caused experimentally by a Goldblatt kidney. **labile h.,** borderline h. **malignant h.,** a severe hypertensive state with papilledema of the ocular fundus and vascular hemorrhagic lesions, thickening of the small arteries and arterioles, left ventricular hypertrophy, and poor prognosis. **ocular h.,** persistently elevated intraocular pressure in the absence of any other signs of glaucoma; it may or may not progress to chronic simple glaucoma. **portal h.,** abnormally increased pressure in the portal circulation. **pulmonary h.,** abnormally increased pressure in the pulmonary circulation. **renal h.,** that associated with or due to renal disease with a factor of parenchymatous ischemia. **renovascular h.,** that due to occlusive disease of the renal arteries. **systemic venous h.,** elevation of systemic venous pressure, usually detected by inspection of the jugular veins.

hy·per·ten·sive (-ten′siv) 1. characterized by increased tension or pressure. 2. an agent that causes hypertension. 3. a person with hypertension.

hy·per·the·co·sis (-the-ko′sis) hyperplasia and excessive luteinization of the cells of the inner stromal layer of the ovary.

hy·per·the·lia (-the′le-ah) polythelia.

hy·per·ther·mal·ge·sia (-ther″mal-je′ze-ah) abnormal sensitivity to heat.

hy·per·ther·mia (-ther′me-ah) hyperpyrexia; greatly increased body temperature. **hyperther′mal, hyperther′mic,** adj. **malignant h.,** an autosomal dominant inherited condition affecting patients undergoing general anesthesia, marked by sudden, rapid rise in body temperature, associated with signs of increased muscle metabolism, and, usually, muscle rigidity.

hy·per·thy·mia (-thi′me-ah) 1. excessive emotionalism. 2. excessive activity, verging on hypomania. **hyperthy′mic,** adj.

hy·per·thy·mism (-thi′mizm) excessive activity of the thymus gland.

hy·per·thy·roid·ism (-thi′roid-izm) excessive thyroid gland activity, marked by increased metabolic rate, goiter, and disturbances in the autonomic nervous system and in creatine metabolism. **hyperthy′roid,** adj.

hy·per·to·nia (-to′ne-ah) a condition of excessive tone of the skeletal muscles; increased resistance of muscle to passive stretching.

hy·per·ton·ic (-ton′ik) 1. denoting increased tone or tension. 2. denoting a solution having greater osmotic pressure than the solution with which it is compared.

hy·per·to·nic·i·ty (-to-nis′ĭ-te) the state or quality of being hypertonic.

hy·per·tri·cho·sis (-trĭ-ko′sis) excessive growth of hair. Cf. *hirsutism.*

hy·per·tri·glyc·er·i·de·mia (-tri-glis″er-i-de′me-ah) an excess of triglycerides in the blood.

hy·per·tro·phy (hi-per′tro-fe) enlargement or overgrowth of an organ or part due to increase in size of its constituent cells. **hypertro′phic,** adj. **asymmetrical septal h. (ASH),** hypertrophic cardiomyopathy, sometimes specifically that in which the hypertrophy is localized to the interventricular septum. **benign prostatic h.,** see under *hyperplasia.* **ventricular h.,** hypertrophy of the myocardium of a ventricle, due to chronic pressure overload.

hy·per·tro·pia (hi″per-tro′pe-ah) strabismus in which there is permanent upward deviation of the visual axis of an eye.

hy·per·ty·ro·sin·emia (-ti″ro-sĭ-ne′me-ah) 1. an elevated concentration of tyrosine in the blood. 2. tyrosinemia.

hy·per·uri·ce·mia (-u″rĭ-se′me-ah) uricemia; an excess of uric acid in the blood. **hyperurice′mic,** adj.

hy·per·u·ri·co·su·ria (-u″rĭ-ko-su′re-ah) uricosuria; an excess of urates or uric acid in the urine.

hy·per·u·ric·uria (-u″rĭ-ku′re-ah) hyperuricosuria.

hy·per·val·i·ne·mia (-val″ĭ-ne′me-ah) 1. an aminoacidopathy characterized by elevated levels of valine in the plasma and urine with failure to thrive. 2. elevated level of valine in the plasma.

hy·per·ven·ti·la·tion (-ven″tĭ-la′shun) 1. abnormally increased pulmonary ventilation, resulting in reduction of carbon dioxide tension, which, if prolonged, may lead to alkalosis. 2. see under *syndrome.*

hy·per·vig·i·lance (-hi″per-vij′ĭ-lans) abnormally increased arousal, responsiveness to stimuli, and scanning of the environment for threats.

hy·per·vis·cos·i·ty (-vis-kos′ĭ-te) excessive viscosity, as of the blood.

hy·per·vi·ta·min·o·sis (-vi″tah-mĭ-no′sis) a condition due to ingestion of an excess of one or more vitamins; symptom complexes are associated with excessive intake of vitamins A and D. **hypervitaminot′ic,** adj.

hy·per·vo·le·mia (-vo-le′me-ah) abnormal increase in the plasma volume in the body.

hyp·es·the·sia (hi″pes-the′zhah) hypoesthesia.

hy·pha (hi′fah) pl. *hy′phae.* [L.] 1. one of the filaments composing the mycelium of a fungus. 2. branching filamentous outgrowths produced by some bacteria, sometimes forming a mycelium. **hy′phal,** adj.

hyp·he·do·nia (hip″hĕ-do′ne-ah) diminution of power of enjoyment.

hy·phe·ma (hi-fe′mah) hemorrhage within the anterior chamber of the eye.

hy·phe·mia (hi-fe′me-ah) hyphema.

hyp·hi·dro·sis (hip″hi-dro′sis) hypohidrosis.

Hy·pho·my·ce·tes (hi′fo-mi-sēt′ēz) the mycelial (hyphal) fungi, i.e., the molds.

hy·pho·my·co·sis (-mi-ko′sis) see *hyalohyphomycosis* and *phaeohyphomycosis.*

hyp·na·gog·ic (hip″nah-goj′ik) 1. hypnotic (1, 2). 2. occurring just before sleep; applied to hallucinations occurring at sleep onset.

hyp·na·gogue (hip′nah-gog) hypnotic (1, 2).

hyp·nal·gia (hip-nal′jah) pain during sleep.

hypn(o)- word element [Gr.], *sleep; hypnosis.*

hyp·no·anal·y·sis (hip″no-ah-nal′ĭ-sis) a method of psychotherapy combining psychoanalysis with hypnosis.

hyp·no·don·tics (-don′tiks) the application of hypnosis and controlled suggestion in the practice of dentistry.

hyp·no·gen·ic (-jen′ik) hypnotic (1).

hyp·noid (hip′noid) resembling hypnosis or sleep.

hyp·nol·o·gy (hip-nol′ah-je) scientific study of sleep or of hypnotism.

hyp·no·pom·pic (hip″no-pom′pik) persisting after sleep; applied to hallucinations occurring on awakening.

hyp·no·sis (hip-no′sis) an altered state of consciousness characterized by focusing of attention, suspension of disbelief, increased amenability and responsiveness to suggestions and commands, and the subjective experience of responding involuntarily.

hyp·no·ther·a·py (hip″no-ther′ah-pe) the use of hypnosis in the treatment of disease.

hyp·not·ic (hip-not′ik) 1. inducing sleep. 2. an agent that induces sleep. 3. pertaining to or of the nature of hypnosis or hypnotism.

hyp·no·tism (hip′no-tizm) the study of or the method or practice of inducing hypnosis.

hyp·no·tize (-tīz) to induce a state of hypnosis.

hy·po (hi′po) 1. colloquialism for a hypodermic inoculation or syringe. 2. sodium thiosulfate.

hyp(o)- word element [Gr.], *beneath; under; deficient.* In chemistry, a compound containing the lowest proportion of oxygen in a series of similar compounds.

hy·po·acu·sis (hi″po-ah-ku′sis) slightly diminished auditory sensitivity.

hy·po·ac·tiv·i·ty (-ak-tiv′ĭ-te) 1. abnormally diminished activity, as of peristalsis. 2. abnormally decreased motor and cognitive activity, with slowing of thought, speech, and movement. **hypoac′tive,** adj.

hy·po·adren·a·lism (-ah-dre′nal-izm) adrenal insufficiency (1).

hy·po·adre·no·cor·ti·cism (-ah-drēn″o-kort′is-izm) adrenocortical insufficiency.

hy·po·al·bu·min·o·sis (-al-bu″min-o′sis) abnormally low level of albumin.

hy·po·al·i·men·ta·tion (-al″ĭ-men-ta′shun) insufficient nourishment.

hy·po·al·pha·lipo·pro·tein·emia (-al″fah-lip″o-pro″te-ne′me-ah) 1. deficiency of high-density (alpha) lipoproteins in the blood. 2. Tangier disease.

hy·po·azo·tu·ria (-az″o-tu′re-ah) diminished nitrogenous material in the urine.

hy·po·bar·ic (-bar′ik) having less than normal pressure or weight; said of gases under less than atmospheric pressure, or to solutions of lower specific gravity than another taken as a standard of reference.

hy·po·bar·ism (-bar′izm) the condition resulting when ambient gas or atmospheric pressure is below that within the body tissues.

hy·po·bar·op·a·thy (-bar-op′ah-the) 1. the disturbances experienced in high altitudes due to reduced air pressure, as in high-altitude sickness and mountain sickness. 2. hypobarism.

hy·po·blast (hi′po-blast) the embryonic precursor to the endoderm. **hypoblas′tic,** adj.

hy·po·cal·ce·mia (hi″po-kal-se′me-ah) reduction of the blood calcium below normal. **hypocalce′mic,** adj.

hy·po·cap·nia (-kap′ne-ah) deficiency of carbon dioxide in the blood. **hypocap′nic,** adj.

hy·po·car·bia (-kahr′be-ah) hypocapnia.

hy·po·chlor·emia (-klor-ēm′e-ah) diminished chloride in the blood. **hypochlore′mic,** adj.

hy·po·chlor·hy·dria (-klor-hi′dre-ah) lack of hydrochloric acid in the gastric juice.

hy·po·chlo·rite (-klor′īt) any salt of hypochlorous acid; used as a medicinal agent with disinfectant action, particularly as a diluted solution of sodium hypochlorite.

hy·po·chlo·rous ac·id (-klor′us) an unstable compound with disinfectant and bleaching action.

hy·po·cho·les·te·re·mia (-ko-les″tĕ-re′me-ah) hypocholesterolemia.

hy·po·cho·les·ter·ol·emia (-ko-les″ter-ol-e′me-ah) diminished cholesterol in the blood. **hypocholesterole′mic,** adj.

hy·po·chon·dria (-kon′dre-ah) 1. plural of *hypochondrium.* 2. hypochondriasis.

hy·po·chon·dri·ac (-kon′dre-ak) 1. pertaining to the hypochondrium. 2. pertaining to hypochondriasis. 3. a person with hypochondriasis.

hy·po·chon·dri·a·sis (-kon-dri′ah-sis) a somatoform disorder characterized by a preoccupation with bodily functions and the interpretation of normal sensations or minor abnormalities as indications of serious problems needing medical attention. **hypochon′driac, hypochondri′acal,** adj.

hy·po·chon·dri·um (hi″po-kon′dre-um) pl. *hypochon′dria.* The upper lateral abdominal region, overlying the costal cartilages, on either side of the epigastrium. **hypochon′drial,** adj.

hy·po·chro·ma·sia (-kro-ma′zhah) 1. the condition of staining less intensely than normal. 2. hypochromia (1).

hy·po·chro·ma·tism (-kro′mat-izm) 1. abnormally deficient pigmentation, especially deficiency of chromatin in a cell nucleus. 2. hypochromia (1).

hy·po·chro·ma·to·sis (-kro″mah-to′sis) the gradual fading and disappearance of the cell nucleus (chromatin).

hy·po·chro·mia (-kro′me-ah) 1. abnormal decrease in the hemoglobin content of the erythrocytes. 2. hypochromatism (1). **hypochro′mic,** adj.

hy·po·cit·ra·tu·ria (-sĭ-tra-tu′re-ah) diminished citrates in the urine.

hy·po·com·ple·men·te·mia (-kom″plĕ-men-te′me-ah) diminution of complement levels in the blood.

hy·po·cy·clo·sis (-si-klo′sis) insufficient accommodation in the eye.

hy·po·cy·the·mia (-si-thēm′e-ah) deficiency in the number of erythrocytes in the blood.

Hy·po·der·ma (-der′mah) a genus of ox-warble or heel flies whose larvae cause disease in cattle and a form of larva migrans in humans.

hy·po·der·mi·a·sis (-der-mi′ah-sis) a creeping eruption of the skin caused by larvae of *Hypoderma*.

hy·po·der·mic (-der′mik) applied or administered beneath the skin.

hy·po·der·mis (-der′mis) 1. subcutaneous tissue. 2. the outer cellular layer of invertebrates that secretes the cuticular exoskeleton.

hy·po·der·mo·cly·sis (-der-mok′lĭ-sis) subcutaneous injection of fluids, e.g., saline solution.

hy·po·dip·sia (-dip′se-ah) abnormally diminished thirst.

hy·po·don·tia (-don′shah) partial anodontia.

hy·po·dy·na·mia (-di-nām′e-ah) abnormally diminished power. **hypodynam′ic,** adj.

hy·po·ec·cris·ia (-ĕ-kris′e-ah) abnormally diminished excretion. **hypoeccrit′ic,** adj.

hy·po·echo·ic (-ĕ-ko′ik) in ultrasonography, giving off few echoes; said of tissues or structures that reflect relatively few of the ultrasound waves directed at them.

hy·po·er·gia (-er′jah) hyposensitivity to allergens. **hypoer′gic,** adj.

hy·po·eso·pho·ria (-es″o-for′e-ah) deviation of the visual axes downward and inward.

hy·po·es·the·sia (-es-the′zhah) abnormally decreased sensitivity, particularly to touch. **hypoesthet′ic,** adj.

hy·po·exo·pho·ria (-ek″so-for′e-ah) deviation of the visual axes downward and laterally.

hy·po·fer·re·mia (-fĕ-re′me-ah) deficiency of iron in the blood.

hy·po·fer·til·i·ty (-fer-til′ĭ-te) subfertility. **hypofer′tile,** adj.

hy·po·fi·brin·o·gen·emia (-fi-brin″o-jĕ-ne′me-ah) deficiency of fibrinogen in the blood.

hy·po·ga·lac·tia (-gah-lak′she-ah) deficiency of milk secretion. **hypogalac′tous,** adj.

hy·po·gam·ma·glob·u·lin·emia (-gam″ah-glob″u-lĭ-ne′me-ah) deficiency of all classes of immunoglobulins, as in agammaglobulinemia, dysglobulinemia, and immunodeficiency. This is normal for a short period in infants but should not be prolonged. **hypogammaglobuline′mic,** adj. **common variable h.,** see under *immunodeficiency.*

hy·po·gan·gli·o·no·sis (-gang″gle-on-o′sis) lessened number of myenteric ganglion cells in the distal large bowel, with constipation; a congenital type of megacolon.

hy·po·gas·tric (-gas′trik) 1. inferior to the stomach. 2. pertaining to the hypogastrium. 3. pertaining to the internal iliac artery.

hy·po·gas·tri·um (-gas′tre-um) the pubic region, the lowest middle abdominal region.

hy·po·gas·tros·chi·sis (-gas-tros′kĭ-sis) congenital fissure of the hypogastrium.

hy·po·gen·e·sis (-jen′ĕ-sis) defective embryonic development. **hypogenet′ic,** adj.

hy·po·gen·i·tal·ism (-jen′ĭ-t'l-izm″) hypogonadism.

hy·po·geus·es·the·sia (-gōōs′es-the′zhah) hypogeusia.

hy·po·geu·sia (-goo′zhah) abnormally diminished sense of taste.

hy·po·glos·sal (hi′po-glos′al) sublingual.

hy·po·glu·ca·gon·emia (-gloo″kah-gon-e′me-ah) abnormally reduced levels of glucagon in the blood.

hy·po·gly·ce·mia (-gli-sēm′e-ah) deficiency of glucose concentration in the blood, which may lead to hypothermia, headache, and more serious neurological symptoms.

hy·po·gly·ce·mic (-gli-sēm′ik) 1. pertaining to, characterized by, or causing hypoglycemia. 2. an agent that lowers blood glucose levels.

hy·po·gly·cor·rha·chia (-gli″ko-ra′ke-ah) abnormally low sugar content in the cerebrospinal fluid.

hy·po·go·nad·ism (-go′nad-izm) decreased functional activity of the gonads, with retardation of growth, sexual development, and secondary sex characters. **hypergonadotropic h.,** that associated with high levels of gonadotropins, as in Klinefelter's syndrome. **hypogonadotropic h.,** that due to lack of gonadotropin secretion.

hy·po·go·nado·tro·pic (-go-nad″ah-tro′pik) relating to or caused by deficiency of gonadotropin.

hy·po·hi·dro·sis (-hi-dro′sis) abnormally diminished perspiration. **hypohidrot′ic,** adj.

hy·po·ka·le·mia (-kah-lēm′e-ah) abnormally low potassium levels in the blood, which may lead to neuromuscular and renal disorders.

hy·po·ka·le·mic (-kah-lēm′ik) 1. pertaining to or characterized by hypokalemia. 2. an agent that lowers blood potassium levels.

hy·po·ki·ne·sia (-kĭ-ne′zhah) abnormally diminished motor function or activity. **hypokinet′ic,** adj.

hy·po·lac·ta·sia (-lak-ta′zhah) deficiency of lactase activity in the intestines; see *lactase deficiency*.

hy·po·ley·dig·ism (-līd′ig-izm) abnormally diminished secretion of androgens by Leydig cells.

hy·po·lip·id·emic (-lip″id-ēm′ik) promoting the reduction of lipid concentrations in the serum.

hy·po·mag·ne·se·mia (-mag″nes-ēm′e-ah) abnormally low magnesium content of the blood.

hy·po·ma·nia (-ma′ne-ah) an abnormality of mood resembling mania but of lesser intensity. **hypoman′ic,** adj.

hy·po·men·or·rhea (-men″o-re′ah) diminution of menstrual flow or duration.

hy·po·mere (hi′po-mēr) 1. the ventrolateral portion of a myotome, innervated by an anterior ramus of a spinal nerve. 2. the lateral plate of mesoderm that develops into the walls of the body cavities.

hy·po·me·tria (-me′tre-ah) ataxia in which movements fall short of the intended goal.

hy·pom·ne·sia (hi″pom-ne′zhah) defective memory.

hy·po·morph (hi′po-morf) 1. a person short in standing height as compared with sitting height. 2. in genetics, a mutant gene that shows only a partial reduction in the activity it influences. **hypomor′phic,** adj.

hy·po·myx·ia (hi″po-mik′se-ah) decreased secretion of mucus.

hy·po·na·sal·i·ty (-na-zal′it-e) a quality of voice in which there is a complete lack of nasal emission of air and nasal resonance, so that the speaker sounds as if he has a cold.

hy·po·na·tre·mia (-na-trēm′e-ah) deficiency of sodium in the blood. **depletional h.,** that in which low plasma concentration of sodium is associated with low total body sodium. **dilutional h.,** that in which low plasma concentration of sodium results from loss of sodium from the body with nonosmotic retention of water.

hy·po·neo·cy·to·sis (-ne″o-si-to′sis) leukopenia with immature leukocytes in the blood.

hy·po·noia (-noi′ah) slow mental activity.

hy·po·nych·i·um (-nik′e-um) the thickened epidermis beneath the free distal end of the nail. **hyponych′ial,** adj.

hy·po·or·tho·cy·to·sis (-or″tho-si-to′sis) leukopenia with a normal proportion of the various forms of leukocytes.

hy·po·os·mot·ic (-oz-mot′ik) containing a lower concentration of osmotically active components than a standard solution.

hy·po·para·thy·roid (-par″ah-thi′roid) pertaining to or characterized by reduced function of the parathyroid glands.

hy·po·para·thy·roid·ism (-par″ah-thi′roid-izm) greatly reduced function of parathyroid glands, with hypocalcemia that may lead to tetany, hyperphosphatemia with decreased bone resorption, and other symptoms.

hy·po·per·fu·sion (-per-fu′zhun) decreased blood flow through an organ, as in hypovolemic shock; if prolonged, it may result in permanent cellular dysfunction and death.

hy·po·peri·stal·sis (-per″ĭ-stawl′sis) abnormally sluggish peristalsis.

hy·po·phar·ynx (-far′inks) laryngopharynx.

hy·po·pho·ne·sis (-fo-ne′sis) diminution of the sound in auscultation or percussion.

hy·po·pho·nia (-fo′ne-ah) a weak voice due to incoordination of the vocal muscles.

hy·po·pho·ria (-for′e-ah) downward deviation of the visual axis of one eye in the absence of visual fusional stimuli.

hy·po·phos·pha·ta·sia (-fos″fah-ta′zhah) an inborn error of metabolism with abnormally low serum alkaline phosphatase activity and phosphoethanolamine in the urine, most severe in babies before six months. Affected infants and children have rickets and adults have osteomalacia.

hy·po·phos·pha·te·mia (-fos″fah-te′me-ah) deficiency of phosphates in the blood, as may occur in rickets and osteomalacia. See also *hypophosphatasia*. **hypophosphate′mic,** adj. **familial h.,** familial hypophosphatemic rickets. **X-linked h.,** a form of familial hypophosphatemic rickets.

hy·po·phos·pha·tu·ria (-fos″fah-tu′re-ah) deficiency of phosphates in the urine.

hy·po·phos·phor·ous ac·id (-fos-for′us) a toxic, monobasic acid with strong reducing properties, H_3PO_2, which forms hypophosphites.

hy·po·phren·ic (hi″po-fren′ik) subphrenic.

hy·po·phys·e·al (-fiz′e-al) hypophysial.

hy·po·phys·ec·to·my (hi-pof″ĭ-sek′tah-me) excision of the pituitary gland (hypophysis).

hy·po·phys·i·al (hi″po-fiz′e-al) pertaining to the hypophysis.

hy·po·phys·io·por·tal (-fiz″e-o-por′t′l) denoting the portal system of the pituitary gland, in which hypothalamic venules connect with capillaries of the anterior pituitary.

hy·po·phys·io·priv·ic (-priv′ik) pertaining to deficiency of hormonal secretion of the pituitary gland (hypophysis).

hy·po·phys·io·tro·pic (-tro′pik) acting on the pituitary gland (hypophysis), as certain hormones.

hy·poph·y·sis (hi-pof′ĭ-sis) [Gr.] pituitary gland. **h. ce′rebri**, pituitary gland. **pharyngeal h.**, a mass in the pharyngeal wall with structure similar to that of the pituitary gland.

hy·po·pi·tu·i·ta·rism (hi″po-pĭ-too′ĭ-tah-rizm″) diminished hormonal secretion by the pituitary gland, especially the anterior pituitary.

hy·po·pla·sia (-pla′zhah) incomplete development or underdevelopment of an organ or tissue. **hypoplas′tic**, adj. **enamel h.**, incomplete or defective development of the enamel of the teeth; it may be hereditary or acquired. **oligomeganephronic renal h.**, oligomeganephronia.

hy·pop·nea (hi-pop′ne-ah) diminished depth and rate of respiration. **hypopne′ic**, adj.

hy·po·po·ro·sis (hi″po-por-o′sis) deficient callus formation after bone fracture.

hy·po·po·tas·se·mia (-po″tah-se′me-ah) hypokalemia.

hy·po·pros·o·dy (-pros′o-de) diminution of the normal variation of stress, pitch, and rhythm of speech.

hy·po·pty·al·ism (-ti′ah-lizm) abnormally decreased secretion of saliva.

hy·po·py·on (hi-po′pe-on) pus in the anterior chamber of the eye.

hy·po·sal·i·va·tion (hi″po-sal″ĭ-va′shun) hypoptyalism.

hy·po·se·cre·tion (-sĕ-kre′shun) diminished secretion, as by a gland.

hy·po·sen·si·tive (-sen′sĭ-tiv) 1. exhibiting abnormally decreased sensitivity. 2. less sensitive to a specific allergen after repeated and gradually increasing doses of the offending substance.

hy·pos·mia (hi-poz′me-ah) diminished sense of smell.

hy·po·so·mato·tro·pism (hi″po-so″mat-o-tro′pizm) deficient secretion of somatotropin (growth hormone), resulting in short stature.

hy·po·som·nia (-som′ne-ah) reduced time of sleep.

hy·po·spa·di·as (-spa′de-is) a developmental anomaly in which the urethra opens inferior to its normal location; usually seen in males, with the opening on the underside of the penis or on the perineum. **hypospadi′ac**, adj. **female h.**, a developmental anomaly in the female in which the urethra opens into the vagina.

hy·po·sper·ma·to·gen·e·sis (-sper″mah-to-jen′ĕ-sis) abnormally decreased production of spermatozoa.

hy·po·splen·ism (-splen′izm) diminished functioning of the spleen, resulting in an increase in peripheral blood elements.

hy·pos·ta·sis (hi-pos′tah-sis) poor or stagnant circulation in a dependent part of the body or an organ.

hy·po·stat·ic (hi″po-stat′ik) 1. pertaining to, due to, or associated with hypostasis. 2. pertaining to certain inherited traits that are particularly liable to be suppressed by other traits.

hy·pos·the·nia (hi″pos-the′ne-ah) weakness. **hyposthen′ic**, adj.

hy·po·styp·sis (hi″po-stip′sis) moderate astringency. **hypostyp′tic**, adj.

hy·po·syn·er·gia (-sĭ-ner′jah) dyssynergia.

hy·po·telo·rism (-tēl′er-izm) abnormally decreased distance between two organs or parts. **ocular h.**, **orbital h.**, abnormal decrease in the intraorbital distance.

hy·po·ten·sion (-ten′shun) abnormally low blood pressure. **orthostatic h.**, a fall in blood pressure associated with dizziness, blurred vision, and sometimes syncope, occurring upon standing or when standing motionless in a fixed position.

hy·po·ten·sive (-ten′siv) marked by low blood pressure or serving to reduce blood pressure.

hy·po·thal·a·mus (-thal′ah-mus) the part of the diencephalon forming the floor and part of the lateral wall of the third ventricle, including the optic chiasm, mammillary bodies, tuber cinereum, and infundibulum; the pituitary gland is also in this region but is physiologically distinct. Hypothalamic nuclei help activate, control, and integrate peripheral autonomic mechanisms, endocrine activities, and many somatic functions. **hypothalam′ic**, adj.

hy·poth·e·nar (hi-poth′en-ar) 1. the fleshy eminence along the ulnar side of the palm. 2. relating to this eminence.

hy·po·ther·mia (hi″po-ther′me-ah) 1. low body temperature, such as from cold weather, or from artificial induction to decrease metabolism and need for oxygen during surgical procedures. 2. a reduction of core body temperature to 32°C (95°F) or lower, as that due to exposure in cold weather or that induced as a means of decreasing metabolism of tissues and thereby the need for oxygen, as used in various surgical procedures. **hypother′mal**, **hypother′mic**, adj. **accidental h.**, unintentional reduction of the core body temperature, as in a cold environment.

hy·poth·e·sis (hi-poth′ĕ-sis) a supposition that appears to explain a group of phenomena and is advanced as a basis for further investigation. **alternative h.**, one that is compared with the null hypothesis in a statistical test. **biogenic amine h.**, the hypothesis that depression is associated with deficiency of biogenic amines, especially norepinephrine, at functionally important receptor sites in the brain and that elation is associated with excess of such amines. **jelly roll h.,** a theory explaining the formation of nerve myelin, which states that it consists of several layers of the plasma membrane of a Schwann cell wrapped spirally around the axon in a jelly roll fashion. **lattice h.,** a theory of the nature of the antigen-antibody reaction which postulates reaction between multivalent antigen and divalent antibody to give an antigen-antibody complex of a lattice-like structure. **Lyon h.,** the random and fixed inactivation (in the form of sex chromatin) of one X chromosome in mammalian cells at an early stage of embryogenesis, leading to mosaicism of paternal and maternal X chromosomes in the female. **null h.,** the particular one under investigation, which frequently asserts a lack of effect or of difference. **one gene–one polypeptide chain h.,** a gene is the DNA sequence that codes for the production of one polypeptide chain. Antibodies are an exception; separate genes for variable and constant regions are rearranged to code for a single polypeptide. **response-to-injury h.,** one explaining atherogenesis as initiating with some injury to the endothelial cells lining the artery walls, which causes endothelial dysfunction and leads to abnormal cellular interactions and initiation and progression of atherogenesis. **sliding filament h.,** the stretching of individual muscle fibers raises the number of tension-developing bridges between the sliding contractile protein elements (actin and myosin) and thus augments the force of the next muscle contraction. **Starling's h.,** the direction and rate of fluid transfer between blood plasma in the capillary and fluid in the tissue spaces depend on the hydrostatic pressure on each side of the capillary wall, on the osmotic pressure of protein in plasma and in tissue fluid, and on the properties of the capillary walls as a filtering membrane. **wobble h.,** one describing how a specific transfer RNA (tRNA) molecule can translate different codons in a messenger RNA (mRNA) template. It states that the third base of the tRNA anticodon does not have to pair with a complementary codon (as do the first two) but can form base pairs with any of several related codons.

hy·po·thy·mia (hi″po-thi′me-ah) abnormally diminished emotional tone, as in depression. **hypothy′mic,** adj.

hy·po·thy·mism (-thi′mizm) diminished thymus activity.

hy·po·thy·roid·ism (-thi′roid-izm) deficiency of thyroid activity, a cause of cretinism in children and myxedema in adults, with decreased metabolic rate, tiredness, and lethargy. **hypothy′roid,** adj.

hy·po·to·nia (-tōn′e-ah) diminished tone of the skeletal muscles.

hy·po·ton·ic (-ton′ik) 1. denoting decreased tone or tension. 2. denoting a solution having less osmotic pressure than one with which it is compared.

hy·po·tri·cho·sis (-trĭ-ko′sis) presence of less than the normal amount of hair.

hy·pot·ro·phy (hi-pah′trah-fe) abiotrophy.

hy·po·tro·pia (hi″po-tro′pe-ah) strabismus with permanent downward deviation of the visual axis of one eye.

hy·po·tym·pa·not·o·my (-tim″pah-not′ah-me) surgical opening of the hypotympanum.

hy·po·tym·pa·num (-tim′pah-num) the lower part of the cavity of the middle ear, in the temporal bone.

hy·po·uri·ce·mia (-u″rĭ-se′me-ah) diminished uric acid in the blood, along with xanthinuria, due to deficiency of xanthine oxidase, the enzyme required for conversion of hypoxanthine to xanthine and of xanthine to uric acid.

hy·po·ven·ti·la·tion (-ven″tĭ-la′shun) reduction in amount of air entering pulmonary alveoli. **primary alveolar h.,** impairment of automatic control of respiration, resulting in apnea during sleep.

hy·po·vo·le·mia (-vōl-ēm′e-ah) diminished volume of circulating blood in the body. **hypovole′mic,** adj.

hy·po·vo·lia (-vōl′e-ah) diminished water content or volume, as of extracellular fluid.

hy·po·xan·thine (-zan′thēn) a purine base formed as an intermediate in the degradation of purines and purine nucleosides to uric acid and in the salvage of free purines. Complexed with ribose it is inosine.

hy·pox·emia (hi″pok-sēm′e-ah) deficient oxygenation of the blood.

hy·pox·ia (hi-pok′se-ah) reduction of oxygen supply to a tissue below physiological levels despite adequate perfusion of the tissue by blood. **hypox′ic,** adj. **anemic h.,** that due to reduction of the oxygen-carrying capacity of the blood owing to decreased total hemoglobin or altered hemoglobin constituents. **histotoxic h.,** that due to impaired use of oxygen by tissues. **hypoxic h.,** that due to insufficient oxygen reaching the blood.

stagnant h., that due to failure to transport sufficient oxygen because of inadequate blood flow.

hy·pro·mel·lose (hi-pro′mĕ-lōs) a propylene glycol ether of methylcellulose, supplied in differing degrees of viscosity; used as a suspending and viscosity-increasing agent and tablet binder, coating, and excipient in pharmaceutical preparations, and applied topically to the conjunctiva to protect and lubricate the cornea. Called also *hydroxypropyl methylcellulose*. **h. phthalate,** a phthalic acid ester of hydroxypropyl methylcellulose, used as a coating agent for tablets and granules.

hyp·sar·rhyth·mia (hip″sah-rith′me-ah) an electroencephalographic abnormality commonly associated with jackknife seizures, with random, high-voltage slow waves and spikes spreading to all cortical areas.

hyp·so·ki·ne·sis (hip″so-kĭ-ne′sis) a backward swaying or falling when in erect posture; seen in paralysis agitans, Wilson's disease, and similar conditions.

hys·ter·al·gia (his″ter-al′jah) pain in the uterus.

hys·ter·ec·to·my (-ek′tah-me) excision of the uterus. **abdominal h.,** that performed through the abdominal wall. **cesarean h.,** cesarean section followed by removal of the uterus. **complete h.,** total h. **partial h.,** subtotal h. **radical h.,** excision of the uterus, upper vagina, and parametrium. **subtotal h.,** that in which the cervix is left in place. **total h.,** that in which the uterus and cervix are completely excised. **vaginal h.,** that performed through the vagina.

hys·te·re·sis (his″tĕ-re′sis) [Gr.] 1. a time lag in the occurrence of two associated phenomena, as between cause and effect. 2. in cardiac pacemaker terminology, the number of pulses per minute below the programmed pacing rate that the heart must drop in order to cause initiation of pacing.

hys·ter·eu·ry·sis (his″ter-u′rĕ-sis) dilation of the os uteri.

hys·ter·ia (his-ter′e-ah) a term formerly used widely in psychiatry. Its meanings have included (1) classical hysteria (now *somatization disorder*); (2) hysterical neurosis (now divided into *conversion disorder* and *dissociative disorders*); (3) anxiety hysteria; and (4) hysterical personality (now *histrionic personality*). **hyster′ic, hyster′ical,** adj. **fixation h.,** conversion disorder with symptoms based on an existing or previous organic disease or injury.

hys·ter·ics (his-ter′iks) popular term for an uncontrollable emotional outburst.

hyster(o)- word element [Gr.], *uterus; hysteria.*

hys·tero·cele (his″ter-o-sēl″) hernia of the uterus.

hys·tero·ep·i·lep·sy (his″ter-o-ep′ĭ-lep″se) hysteria with attacks imitating epileptic seizures.

hys·ter·og·ra·phy (his″ter-og′rah-fe) 1. the graphic recording of the strength of uterine contractions in labor. 2. radiography of the uterus after instillation of a contrast medium.

hys·ter·oid (his′ter-oid) resembling hysteria.

hys·tero·lith (his′ter-o-lith″) uterine calculus.

hys·ter·ol·y·sis (his″ter-ol′ĭ-sis) freeing of the uterus from adhesions.

hys·tero·myo·ma (his″ter-o-mi-o′mah) leiomyoma of the uterus.

hys·tero·myo·mec·to·my (-mi″o-mek′tah-me) uterine myomectomy.

hys·tero·my·ot·o·my (-mi-ot′ah-me) incision of the uterus for removal of a solid tumor.

hys·ter·op·a·thy (his″ter-op′ah-the) any disease of the uterus.

hys·tero·pexy (his′ter-o-pek″se) surgical fixation of a displaced uterus.

hys·ter·op·to·sis (his″ter-op-to′sis) prolapse of the uterus.

hys·ter·or·rha·phy (his″ter-or′ah-fe) 1. suture of the uterus. 2. hysteropexy.

hys·ter·or·rhex·is (his″ter-o-rek′sis) metrorrhexis.

hys·tero·sal·pin·gec·to·my (-sal″pin-jek′tah-me) excision of the uterus and uterine tubes.

hys·tero·sal·pin·gog·ra·phy (-sal″ping-gog′rah-fe) radiography of the uterus and uterine tubes.

hys·tero·sal·pin·go·ooph·o·rec·to·my (-sal″ping-go-o″of-o-rek′tah-me) excision of the uterus, uterine tubes, and ovaries.

hys·tero·sal·pin·gos·to·my (-sal″ping-gos′tah-me) anastomosis of a uterine tube to the uterus.

hys·tero·scope (his′ter-o-skōp″) an endoscope for direct visual examination of the cervical canal and uterine cavity.

hys·tero·spasm (-spazm″) spasm of the uterus.

hys·ter·ot·o·my (his″ter-ot′ah-me) incision of the uterus, performed either transabdominally (*abdominal h.*) or vaginally (*vaginal h.*).

Hz hertz.

I

I incisor; iodine; inosine (in nucleotides); isoleucine.

I electric current.

-ia word element [Gr.], *state; condition.*

IABP intra-aortic balloon pump.

IAEA International Atomic Energy Agency.

-iasis word element [Gr.], *condition; state.*

iat·ric (i-ă′trik) pertaining to medicine or to a physician.

-iatrics word element [Gr.], *medical treatment.*

iatr(o)- word element [Gr.], *medicine; physician.*

iat·ro·gen·ic (i-ă″tro-jen′ik) resulting from the activity of physicians; said of any adverse condition in a patient resulting from treatment by a physician or surgeon.

-iatry word element [Gr.], *medical treatment.*

ibu·pro·fen (i″bu-pro′fen) a nonsteroidal antiinflammatory drug used in the treatment of pain, fever, dysmenorrhea, osteoarthritis, rheumatoid arthritis, and other rheumatic and nonrheumatic inflammatory disorders, and vascular headaches.

ibu·ti·lide (ĭ-bu′tĭ-līd) a cardiac depressant used as an antiarrhythmic agent in the treatment of atrial arrhythmias; administered by intravenous infusion as the fumarate salt.

IC inspiratory capacity; irritable colon.

ICD International Classification of Diseases (of the World Health Organization); intrauterine contraceptive device.

ice (īs) the solid state of water occurring at or below 0°C and 1 atmosphere. **dry i.,** carbon dioxide snow.

ichthy(o)- word element [Gr.], *fish.*

ich·thy·oid (ik′the-oid) fishlike.

ich·thyo·sar·co·tox·in (ik″the-o-sahr′ko-tok″sin) a toxin found in the flesh of poisonous fishes.

ich·thyo·sar·co·tox·ism (-tok″sizm) poisoning from eating of poisonous fish, marked by gastrointestinal and neurological disturbances.

ich·thyo·si·form (ik″the-o′sĭ-form) resembling ichthyosis.

ich·thy·o·sis (-sis) any in a group of cutaneous disorders characterized by increased or aberrant keratinization, resulting in non-inflammatory scaling of the skin; most are genetically determined; often used to denote *i. vulgaris.* **ichthyot′ic,** adj. **i. hys′trix,** a

rare form of epidermolytic hyperkeratosis, marked by generalized, dark brown, linear verrucoid ridges somewhat like porcupine skin. **lamellar i.,** a hereditary disease present at or soon after birth, with large, quadrilateral, grayish brown scales; it may be associated with short stature, oligophrenia, spastic paralysis, genital hypoplasia, hypotrichia, and shortened life-span. **i. sim′plex,** i. vulgaris. **i. u′teri,** transformation of the columnar epithelium of the endometrium into stratified squamous epithelium. **i. vulga′ris,** hereditary ichthyosis present at or shortly after birth, with large, thick, dry scales on the neck, ears, scalp, face, and flexural surfaces.

ICN International Council of Nurses.

ICP intracranial pressure.

ICS International College of Surgeons.

ICSH interstitial cell–stimulating hormone.

ic·tal (ik′t'l) pertaining to, marked by, or due to a stroke or an acute epileptic seizure.

ICSI intracytoplasmic sperm injection.

ic·tero·gen·ic (ik″ter-o-jen′ik) causing jaundice.

ic·tero·hep·a·ti·tis (-hep″ah-ti′tis) inflammation of the liver with marked jaundice.

ic·ter·us (ik′ter-us) [L.] jaundice. **icter′ic,** adj. **i. neonato′rum,** jaundice in newborn children.

ic·tus (ik′tus) pl. *ic′tus.* [L.] a seizure, stroke, blow, or sudden attack. **ic′tal,** adj.

ICU intensive care unit.

ID₅₀ median infective dose.

id (id) in psychoanalytic theory, the innate, unconscious, primitive aspect of the personality dominated by the pleasure principle and seeking immediate gratification.

-id word element [Gr.], 1. *having the shape of, resembling.* 2. *an id reaction associated with the disorder specified by the root word.*

ida·ru·bi·cin (i″dah-roo′bĭ-sin) an anthracycline antineoplastic used as the hydrochloride salt in the treatment of acute myelogenous leukemia.

IDD, IDDM insulin-dependent diabetes mellitus; see *type 1 diabetes mellitus,* under *diabetes.*

-ide (īd) a suffix indicating a binary chemical compound.

idea (i-de′ah) a mental impression or conception. **autochthonous i.,** a persistent idea originating within the mind but seeming to have come from an outside source and often therefore felt to be of malevolent origin. **dominant i.**, one that controls or colors every action and thought. **fixed i.**, a persistent morbid impression or belief that cannot be changed by reason. **overvalued i.**, a false or exaggerated belief sustained beyond reason or logic but with less rigidity than a delusion, also often being less patently unbelievable. **i. of reference**, the incorrect idea that words and actions of others refer to oneself or the projection of the causes of one's own imaginary difficulties upon someone else.

ide·al (i-de′il) a pattern or concept of perfection. **ego i.**, the component of the superego comprising the standard of perfection unconsciously created by a person for himself.

ide·al·iza·tion (i-de″il-ĭ-za′shun) a conscious or unconscious mental mechanism in which the individual overestimates an admired aspect or attribute of another person.

ide·a·tion (i″de-a′shun) the formation of ideas or images. **idea′tional**, adj.

idée fixe (e-da′ fēks) [Fr.] fixed idea.

iden·ti·fi·ca·tion (i-den″tĭ-fĭ-ka′shun) a largely unconscious process, sometimes a defense mechanism, by which one person patterns himself after another.

iden·ti·ty (i-den′tit-e) the aggregate of characteristics by which an individual is recognized by himself and others. **gender i.**, a person's concept of himself as being male and masculine or female and feminine, or ambivalent.

ideo·ge·net·ic (i″de-o-jĕ-net′ik) related to mental processes in which images of sense impressions are used, rather than ideas ready for verbal expression.

ide·ol·o·gy (i″de-ol′ah-je, id″e-) 1. the science of the development of ideas. 2. the body of ideas characteristic of an individual or of a social unit.

ideo·mo·tion (i″de-o-mo′shun) motion or muscular action induced by a dominant idea rather than by reflex or volition.

ideo·mo·tor (-mōt′er) aroused by an idea or thought; said of involuntary motion so aroused.

idi(o)- word element [Gr.], *self; peculiar to a substance or organism.*

id·i·o·cy (id′e-ah-se) obsolete, offensive name for profound mental retardation. **amaurotic i., amaurotic familial i.**, former name for *neuronal ceroid lipofuscinosis.* **mongolian i.**, former name for *Down syndrome* or the associated mental retardation; now considered offensive.

id·io·glos·sia (id″e-o-glos′e-ah) extremely defective articulation, with the utterance of virtually unintelligible vocal sounds. **idioglot′tic**, adj.

id·io·gram (id′e-ah-gram) a drawing or photograph of the chromosomes of a particular cell.

id·io·path·ic (id″e-o-path′ik) self-originated; occurring without known cause.

id·io·ret·i·nal (-ret′ĭ-n′l) pertaining to the retina alone; applied to a visual sensation occurring without a visual stimulus.

id·io·syn·cra·sy (-sing′krah-se) 1. a habit peculiar to an individual. 2. an abnormal susceptibility to an agent (e.g., a drug) peculiar to an individual. **idiosyncrat′ic**, adj.

id·i·ot (id′e-it) obsolete, offensive name for a person with profound mental retardation. **i. savant**, a mentally retarded person with a particular mental faculty developed to an unusually high degree, as for mathematics, music, etc.

id·io·tro·phic (id″e-o-tro′fik) capable of selecting its own nourishment.

id·io·ven·tric·u·lar (-ven-trik′u-ler) pertaining to the cardiac ventricles alone.

IDL intermediate-density lipoprotein.

idox·ur·i·dine (i″doks-u′rĭ-dēn) an analogue of pyrimidine that inhibits viral DNA synthesis; used as an antiviral agent in the treatment of herpes simplex keratitis.

IDU idoxuridine.

idu·ron·ic ac·id (i″du-ron′ik) a uronic acid that is a constituent of dermatan sulfate, heparan sulfate, and heparin.

ʟ-id·uron·i·dase (i″du-ron′ĭ-dās) a hydrolase that catalyzes a step in the degradation of the glycosaminoglycans dermatan sulfate and heparan sulfate; deficiency leads to mucopolysaccharidosis I.

ifos·fa·mide (i-fos′fah-mīd) a cytotoxic alkylating agent of the nitrogen mustard group, in structure and actions similar to cyclophosphamide; used in the treatment of solid tumors of the testis, ovary, and lung as well as sarcomas.

Ig immunoglobulin of any of the five classes: IgA, IgD, IgE, IgG, and IgM.

IGF insulin-like growth factor.

IGT impaired glucose tolerance.

IHD ischemic heart disease.

IHSS idiopathic hypertrophic subaortic stenosis.

IL interleukin.

Ile isoleucine.

il·e·ac (il′e-ak) 1. of the nature of ileus. 2. ileal.

il·e·al (il′e-ahl) pertaining to the ileum.

il·e·itis (-i′tis) inflammation of the ileum. **distal i., regional i.,** Crohn's disease affecting the ileum.

ile(o)- word element [L.], *ileum.*

il·eo·a·nal (il″e-o-a′n′l) pertaining to or connecting the ileum and the anus.

il·eo·ce·cal (-se′k′l) pertaining to the ileum and cecum.

il·eo·ce·cos·to·my (-se-kos′tah-me) surgical anastomosis of the ileum to the cecum.

il·eo·col·ic (-kol′ik) pertaining to the ileum and colon.

il·eo·co·li·tis (-ko-li′tis) inflammation of the ileum and colon. **i. ulcero′sa chro′nica,** chronic ileocolitis with fever, rapid pulse, anemia, diarrhea, and right iliac pain.

il·eo·co·los·to·my (-kah-los′tah-me) surgical anastomosis of the ileum to the colon.

il·eo·cys·to·plas·ty (-sis′tah-plas″te) augmentation cystoplasty using an isolated segment of the ileum.

il·eo·cys·tos·to·my (-sis-tos′tah-me) ileovesicostomy.

il·eo·ile·os·to·my (-il″e-os′tah-me) surgical anastomosis between two parts of the ileum.

il·e·or·rha·phy (il″e-or′ah-fe) suture of the ileum.

il·eo·sig·moi·dos·to·my (il″e-o-sig″moi-dos′tah-me) surgical anastomosis of the ileum to the sigmoid colon.

il·e·os·to·my (il″e-os′tah-me) surgical creation of an opening into the ileum, with a stoma on the abdominal wall.

il·e·ot·o·my (-ot′ah-me) incision of the ileum.

il·eo·trans·verse (il″e-o-trans-vers′) pertaining to or connecting the ileum and the transverse colon.

il·eo·ves·i·cos·to·my (-ves″i-kos′tah-me) use of a section of ileum to create a channel leading from the urinary bladder upwards to the abdominal surface.

il·e·um (il′e-um) the distal portion of the small intestine, extending from the jejunum to the cecum. **duplex i.,** congenital duplication of the ileum.

il·e·us (il′e-us) intestinal obstruction. **ady-namic i.,** that due to inhibition of bowel motility. **dynamic i., hyperdynamic i.,** spastic i. **mechanical i.,** that due to mechanical causes, such as hernia, adhesions, volvulus, etc. **meconium i.,** ileus in the newborn due to blocking of the bowel with thick meconium. **occlusive i.,** mechanical i. **paralytic i., i. paraly′ticus,** adynamic i. **spastic i.,** mechanical ileus due to persistent contracture of a bowel segment. **i. sub-par′ta,** that due to pressure of the gravid uterus on the pelvic colon.

il·i·ac (il′e-ak) pertaining to the ilium.

ili(o)- word element [L.], *ilium.*

il·io·cos·tal (il″e-o-kos′t′l) connecting or pertaining to the ilium and ribs.

il·io·fem·or·al (-fem′er-al) pertaining to the ilium and femur.

il·io·lum·bar (-lum′bar) pertaining to the iliac and lumbar regions.

il·io·pec·tin·e·al (-pek-tin′e-al) pertaining to the ilium and pubes.

il·io·tib·i·al (-tib′e-al) pertaining to or extending between the ilium and tibia.

il·io·tro·chan·ter·ic (-tro-kan-ter′ik) pertaining to the ilium and a trochanter.

il·i·um (il′e-um) pl. *i′lia.* [L.] see *Table of Bones.*

ill·ness (il′nes) disease. **emotional i.,** a colloquialism for *mental disorder,* but not usually including mental retardation or mental disorders with a specific, known, organic etiology. **mental i.,** see under *disorder.*

il·lu·mi·na·tion (ĭ-loo″mĭ-na′shun) 1. the lighting up of a part, organ, or object for inspection. 2. the luminous flux per unit area of a given surface; SI unit, lux. Symbol *E.* **darkfield i., dark-ground i.,** the casting of peripheral light rays upon a microscopical object from the side, the center rays being blocked out; the object appears bright on a dark background.

il·lu·sion (ĭ-loo′zhun) a mental impression derived from misinterpretation of an actual experience. **illu′sional,** adj.

IM intramuscular.

im- a prefix, replacing *in-* before words beginning *b, m,* and *p.*

im·age (im′ahj) a picture or concept with likeness to an objective reality. **body i.,** the three-dimensional concept of one's self, recorded in the cortex by perception of everchanging body postures, and constantly changing with them. **false i.,** that formed by the deviating eye in strabismus. **mirror i.,** one with right and left relations reversed, as in the reflection of an object in a mirror. **Purkinje-Sanson mirror i's,** three reflected images of an object seen in observing the pupil of the eye: two on the posterior and anterior surfaces of the lens, one on the anterior surface of the cornea. **motor i.,** the organized cerebral model of the possible movements of the body. **real i.,** one formed where the emanating rays are collected, in which the object is pictured as being inverted. **virtual i.,** a picture from projected light rays that are intercepted before focusing.

im·age·ry (im′aj-re) 1. the formation of a mental representation of something perceived by the senses. **2.** any of a number of therapeutic techniques that use the formation of such representations to elicit changes in attitudes, behaviors, or physiologic reactions. **guided i.**, a therapeutic technique in which the patient enters a relaxed state and focuses on an image related to the issue being confronted, which the therapist uses as the basis of an interactive dialogue to help resolve the issue.

imag·ing (im′ah-jing) the production of diagnostic images, e.g., radiography, ultrasonography, or scintillation photography. **color flow Doppler i.**, a method of visualizing direction and velocity of movement using Doppler ultrasonography and coding them as colors and shades, respectively. **echo planar i.**, a technique for obtaining a magnetic resonance image in less than 50 msec. **electrostatic i.**, a method of visualizing deep structures of the body, in which an electron beam is passed through the patient and the emerging beam strikes an electrostatically charged plate, dissipating the charge according to the strength of the beam. A film is then made from the plate. **gated cardiac blood pool i.**, equilibrium radionuclide angiocardiography. **gated magnetic resonance i.**, a method for magnetic resonance imaging in which signal acquisition is gated to minimize motion or other artifacts. **hot spot i., infarct avid i.**, see under *scintigraphy*. **magnetic resonance i. (MRI)**, a method of visualizing soft tissues of the body by applying an external magnetic field that makes it possible to distinguish between hydrogen atoms in different environments. **myocardial perfusion i.**, see under *scintigraphy*. **pyrophosphate i.**, infarct avid scintigraphy. **technetium Tc 99m pyrophosphate i.**, **1.** infarct avid scintigraphy. **2.** any type of imaging using Tc 99m pyrophosphate as an imaging agent.

ima·go (ĭ-ma′go) pl. *ima′goes*, *ima′gines*. [L.] **1.** the adult or definitive form of an insect. **2.** a usually idealized, unconscious mental image of a key person in one's early life.

im·at·i·nib (ĭ-mă′tĭ-nib″) an antineoplastic used as the mesylate salt in the treatment of chronic myeloid leukemia, inhibiting an abnormal enzyme form constitutively produced in the disease.

im·bal·ance (im-bal′ans) **1.** lack of balance, such as between two opposing muscles or between electrolytes in the body. **2.** dysequilibrium (2). **autonomic i.**, defective coordination between the sympathetic and parasympathetic nervous systems, especially with respect to vasomotor activities.

sympathetic i., vagotonia. **vasomotor i.**, autonomic i.

im·bi·bi·tion (im″bĭ-bish′un) absorption of a liquid.

im·bri·cat·ed (im′brĭ-kāt″id) overlapping like shingles.

ImD₅₀ median immunizing dose.

im·id·az·ole (im″id-az′ōl) **1.** a heterocyclic organic compound in which two of five ring atoms are nitrogen; used as an insecticide. **2.** any of a class of antifungal compounds containing this structure.

im·ide (im′īd) any compound containing the bivalent group, =NH, to which are attached only acid radicals.

imido- a prefix denoting the presence of the bivalent group =NH attached to two acid radicals.

im·i·glu·cer·ase (im″ĭgloo′ser-ās) an analogue of glucosylceramidase, for which it is used as an enzyme replenisher in type 1 Gaucher's disease.

imine (ĭ-mēn′) an organic compound containing an imino group; in a *substituted imine*, a nonacyl group replaces the imino hydrogen.

imino- a prefix denoting the presence of the bivalent group =NH attached to nonacid radicals.

im·i·no ac·id (ĭ-me′no) an organic acid containing the bivalent group =NH; e.g., proline.

im·i·no·gly·cin·uria (ĭ-me″no-gli″sin-ūr′e-ah) a benign hereditary disorder of renal tubular reabsorption of glycine and the imino acids proline and hydroxyproline, with an excess of all three in urine.

im·i·no·stil·bene (im″ĭ-no-stil′bēn) a class of anticonvulsants used in the treatment of epilepsy.

im·i·pen·em (im″ĭ-pen′em) a β-lactam antibiotic with a broad spectrum of activity against both gram-positive and gram-negative organisms.

imip·ra·mine (ĭ-mip′rah-mēn) a tricyclic antidepressant of the dibenzazepine class, used as *i. hydrochloride* or *i. pamoate*.

im·i·quim·od (im″ĭ-kwim′od) a biologic response modifier used topically in the treatment of condyloma acuminatum.

im·ma·ture (im″ah-choor′) unripe or not fully developed.

im·mer·sion (ĭ-mer′zhun) **1.** the plunging of a body into a liquid. **2.** the use of the microscope with the object and object glass both covered with a liquid.

im·mis·ci·ble (ĭ-mis′ĭ-b'l) not susceptible to being mixed.

im·mo·bil·iza·tion (ĭ-mo″bil-ĭ-za′shun) the act of rendering immovable, as by a cast or splint.

im·mor·tal·iza·tion (ĭmor″tah-lĭ-za′shun) the gaining of immunity to normal limitations on growth or life span, sometimes achieved by animal cells in vitro or by tumor cells.

im·mune (ĭ-mūn′) 1. resistant to a disease because of the formation of humoral antibodies or the development of cellular immunity, or both, or from some other mechanism, as interferon activity in viral infections. 2. characterized by the development of humoral antibodies or cellular immunity, or both, following antigenic challenge. 3. produced in response to antigenic challenge, as immune serum globulin.

im·mu·ni·ty (ĭ-mu′nĭ-te) the condition of being immune; the protection against infectious disease conferred either by the immune response generated by immunization or previous infection or by other nonimmunologic factors. **acquired i.,** that occurring as a result of prior exposure to an infectious agent or its antigens *(active i.),* or of passive transfer of antibody or immune lymphoid cells *(passive i.).* **active i.,** see *acquired i.* **artificial i.,** acquired (active or passive) immunity produced by deliberate exposure to an antigen, as in vaccination. **cell-mediated i. (CMI), cellular i.,** acquired immunity in which the role of T lymphocytes is predominant. **genetic i.,** innate i. **herd i.,** the resistance of a group to attack by a disease to which a large proportion of the members are immune. **humoral i.,** acquired immunity in which the role of circulating antibodies is predominant. **inherent i., innate i.,** that determined by the genetic constitution of the individual. **maternal i.,** humoral immunity passively transferred across the placenta from mother to fetus. **natural i.,** the resistance of the normal animal to infection. **nonspecific i.,** that which does not involve humoral or cell-mediated immunity, but includes lysozyme and interferon activity, etc. **passive i.,** see *acquired i.* **specific i.,** immunity against a particular disease or antigen.

im·mu·ni·za·tion (im″u-nī-za′shun) the process of rendering a subject immune, or of becoming immune. **active i.,** stimulation with a specific antigen to induce an immune response. **passive i.,** the conferral of specific immune reactivity on previously nonimmune individuals by administration of sensitized lymphoid cells or serum from immune individuals.

im·mu·no·ad·ju·vant (im″u-no-aj′ōō-vant, -ad-joo′vant) a nonspecific stimulator of the immune response, e.g., BCG vaccine or Freund's complete and incomplete adjuvants.

im·mu·no·ad·sor·bent (-ad-sor′bint) a preparation of antigen attached to a solid support or antigen in an insoluble form, which adsorbs homologous antibodies from a mixture of immunoglobulins.

im·mu·no·as·say (-as′a) quantitative determination of antigenic substances (e.g., hormones, drugs, vitamins) by serological means, as by immunofluorescent techniques, radioimmunoassay, etc.

immunobead (im′u-no-bēd″) a minute plastic bead coated with antigen or antibody so that it aggregates or agglutinates in the presence of the corresponding antibody or antigen.

im·mu·no·bio·log·i·cal (im″u-no-bi″o-loj′ĭ-k′l) an antigenic or antibody-containing preparation derived from a pool of human donors and used for immunization and immune therapy.

im·mu·no·bi·ol·o·gy (-bi-ol′ah-je) that branch of biology dealing with immunologic effects on such phenomena as infectious disease, growth and development, recognition phenomena, hypersensitivity, heredity, aging, cancer, and transplantation.

im·mu·no·blas·tic (-blas′tik) pertaining to or involving the stem cells (immunoblasts) of lymphoid tissue.

im·mu·no·blot (im′u-no-blot″) a technique for, or the blot resulting from, analyzing or identifying proteins via antigen-antibody specific reactions, as in Western blot technique.

im·mu·no·chem·is·try (im″u-no-kem′is-tre) the study of the physical chemical basis of immune phenomena and their interactions.

im·mu·no·che·mo·ther·a·py (-ke″mo-ther′ah-pe) a combination of immunotherapy and chemotherapy.

im·mu·no·com·pe·tence (-kom′pĕ-tens) immunoresponsiveness; the capacity to develop an immune response after exposure to antigen. **immunocom′petent,** adj.

im·mu·no·com·plex (-kom′pleks) antigen-antibody complex.

im·mu·no·com·pro·mised (-kom′pro-mīzd) having the immune response attenuated by administration of immunosuppressive drugs, by irradiation, by malnutrition, or by certain disease processes (e.g., cancer).

im·mu·no·con·glu·ti·nin (-kon-gloo′tĭ-nin) antibody formed against complement components that are part of an antigen-antibody complex, especially C3.

im·mu·no·cyte (im'u-no-sīt") any cell of the lymphoid series which can react with antigen to produce antibody or to participate in cell-mediated reactions.

im·mu·no·cy·to·ad·her·ence (im"u-no-sīt"o-ad-hēr'ens) the aggregation of red cells to form rosettes around lymphocytes with surface immunoglobulins.

im·mu·no·de·fi·cien·cy (-dĕ-fish'en-se) a deficiency of immune response or a disorder characterized by deficient immune response; classified as *antibody* (B cell), *cellular* (T cell), or *combined immunodeficiency*, or *phagocytic dysfunction disorders*. **immunodefi'cient,** adj. **common variable i. (CVID),** a heterogeneous group of disorders characterized by hypogammaglobulinemia, decreased antibody production, and recurrent pyogenic infections, and often associated with hematologic and autoimmune disorders. Most patients appear to have an intrinsic defect of B cell differentiation. **severe combined i. (SCID),** a group of rare congenital disorders, ocurring in both autosomal recessive and X-linked forms; characterized by gross impairment of both humoral and cell-mediated immunity, absence of T lymphocytes, and, in some forms, lack of B lymphocytes. Immunoglobulins are usually absent and there is marked lymphocytopenia. Unless treated with bone marrow or fetal tissue transplant, infants manifest persistent diarrhea, chronic mucocutaneous candidiasis, and failure to thrive, and die from opportunistic infection.

im·mu·no·der·ma·tol·o·gy (-der"mah-tol'-ah-je) the study of immunologic phenomena as they affect skin disorders and their treatment or prophylaxis.

im·mu·no·dif·fu·sion (-dĭ-fu'zhun) any technique involving diffusion of antigen or antibody through a semisolid medium, usually agar or agarose gel, resulting in a precipitin reaction.

im·mu·no·dom·i·nance (-dom'ĭ-nans) the degree to which a subunit of an antigenic determinant is involved in binding or reacting with antibody.

im·mu·no·elec·tro·pho·re·sis (-e-lek"tro-fah-re'sis) a method of distinguishing proteins and other materials on the basis of their electrophoretic mobility and antigenic specificities. **rocket i.,** electrophoresis in which antigen migrates from a well through agar gel containing antiserum, forming cone-shaped (rocket) precipitin bands.

im·mu·no·flu·o·res·cence (-floo-res'ens) a method of determining the location of antigen (or antibody) in a tissue section or smear by the pattern of fluorescence resulting when the specimen is exposed to the specific antibody (or antigen) labeled with a fluorochrome.

im·mu·no·gen (im'ūn-ah-jen) any substance capable of eliciting an immune response.

im·mu·no·ge·net·ics (im"ūn-o-jĕ-net'iks) the study of the genetic factors controlling the individual's immune response and the transmission of those factors from generation to generation. **immunogenet'ic,** adj.

im·mu·no·ge·nic·i·ty (-jĕ-nis'it-e) the property enabling a substance to provoke an immune response, or the degree to which a substance possesses this property. **immunogen'ic,** adj.

im·mu·no·glob·u·lin (-glob'ūl-in) a protein of animal origin with known antibody activity, synthesized by lymphocytes and plasma cells and found in serum and in other body fluids and tissues; abbreviated Ig. There are five distinct classes based on structural and antigenic properties: IgA, IgD, IgE, IgG, and IgM. See accompanying table. **secretory i. A,** IgA immunoglobulin in which two IgA molecules are linked by a polypeptide (secretory piece) and by a J chain; it is the predominant immunoglobulin.

THE HUMAN IMMUNOGLOBULINS

	Mol Wt	Number of Subclasses	Function
IgM	900,000	2	Activation of classic complement pathway; opsonization
IgG	150,000	4	Activation of classic and alternative complement pathways; opsonization (IgG1 and IgG3 only); only class transferred across placenta, thus providing fetus and neonate with protection against infection
IgA	155,000 (serum IgA)	2	Activation of alternative complement pathway; secretory IgA is the predominant immunoglobulin in secretions
IgD	180,000	—	Not yet determined
IgE	190,000	—	Mediation of immediate hypersensitivity reactions

im·mu·no·glob·u·lin·op·a·thy (im″u-no-glob″u-lin-op′ah-the) gammopathy.

im·mu·no·hem·a·tol·o·gy (-hem″ah-tol′ah-je) the study of antigen-antibody reactions as they relate to blood disorders.

im·mu·no·his·to·chem·i·cal (-his″to-kem′ĭ-k'l) denoting the application of antigen-antibody interactions to histochemical techniques, as in the use of immunofluorescence.

im·mu·no·in·com·pe·tent (-in-kom′pit-int) lacking the ability or capacity to develop an immune response to antigenic challenge.

im·mu·nol·o·gy (im″u-nol′ah-je) the branch of biomedical science concerned with the response of the organism to antigenic challenge, the recognition of self and not self, and all the biological, serological, and physical chemical effects of immune phenomena. **immunolog′ic,** adj.

im·mu·no·lym·pho·scin·tig·ra·phy (im″u-no-lim″fo-sin-tig′rah-fe) immunoscintigraphy used to detect metastatic tumor in lymph nodes.

im·mu·no·mod·u·la·tion (-mod″u-la′shun) adjustment of the immune response to a desired level, as in immunopotentiation, immunosuppression, or induction of immunologic tolerance.

im·mu·no·mod·u·lat·or (-mod′u-la′ter) an agent that augments or diminishes immune responses.

im·mu·no·patho·gen·e·sis (-path″o-jen′ĕ-sis) the process of development of a disease in which an immune response or the products of an immune reaction are involved.

im·mu·no·pa·thol·o·gy (-pah-thol′ah-je) 1. the branch of biomedical science concerned with immune reactions associated with disease, whether the reactions be beneficial, without effect, or harmful. 2. the structural and functional manifestations associated with immune responses to disease. **immunopatholog′ic,** adj.

im·mu·no·phe·no·type (-fe′no-tīp) a phenotype of cells of hematopoietic neoplasms defined according to their resemblance to normal T cells and B cells.

im·mu·no·po·ten·cy (-pōt′n-se) the immunogenic capacity of an individual antigenic determinant on an antigen molecule to initiate antibody synthesis.

im·mu·no·po·ten·ti·a·tion (-po-ten″she-a′shun) accentuation of the response to an immunogen by administration of another substance.

im·mu·no·pre·cip·i·ta·tion (-pre-sip″ĭ-ta′-shun) precipitation resulting from interaction of specific antibody and antigen.

im·mu·no·pro·lif·er·a·tive (-pro-lif′ĕ-rah-tiv) characterized by the proliferation of the lymphoid cells producing immunoglobulins, as in the gammopathies.

im·mu·no·ra·di·om·e·try (-ra″de-om′ĭ-tre) the use of radiolabeled antibody (in the place of radiolabeled antigen) in radioimmunoassay techniques. **immunoradiomet′ric,** adj.

im·mu·no·reg·u·la·tion (-reg″u-la′shun) the control of specific immune responses and interactions between B and T lymphocytes and macrophages.

im·mu·no·re·spon·sive·ness (-re-spon′-siv-nes) immunocompetence.

im·mu·no·scin·tig·ra·phy (-sin-tig′rah-fe) scintigraphic imaging of a lesion using radiolabeled monoclonal antibodies or antibody fragments specific for antigen associated with the lesion.

im·mu·no·sor·bent (-sor′bent) an insoluble support for antigen or antibody used to absorb homologous antibodies or antigens, respectively, from a mixture; the antibodies or antigens so removed may then be eluted in pure form.

im·mu·no·stim·u·la·tion (-stim″u-la′shun) stimulation of an immune response, e.g., by use of BCG vaccine.

im·mu·no·sup·pres·sant (-sah-pres′ant) an agent capable of suppressing immune responses.

im·mu·no·sup·pres·sion (-sah-presh′un) prevention or diminution of the immune response, such as by radiation, antimetabolites, or specific antibody. **immunosuppres′-sive,** adj.

im·mu·no·ther·a·py (-ther′ah-pe) passive immunization of an individual by administration of preformed antibodies (serum or gamma globulin) actively produced in another individual; by extension, the term has come to include the use of immunopotentiators, replacement of immunocompetent lymphoid tissue (e.g., bone marrow or thymus), etc.

im·mu·no·tox·in (im′u-no-tok″sin) any antitoxin.

im·mu·no·trans·fu·sion (im″u-no-transfu′zhun) transfusion of blood from a donor previously rendered immune to the disease affecting the patient.

im·pact·ed (im-pak′ted) being wedged in firmly or closely, as an impacted tooth or impacted twins.

im·pac·tion (im-pak′shun) 1. the condition of being impacted. 2. in obstetrics, the indentation of any fetal parts of one twin onto the surface of its co-twin, so that the simultaneous partial engagement of both twins is permitted. **dental i.,** prevention of eruption, normal occlusion, or routine removal of a tooth because of its being locked in position by bone, dental restoration, or surfaces of adjacent teeth. **fecal i.,** a collection of hardened feces in the rectum or sigmoid.

im·pair·ment (im-pār′ment) any abnormality of, partial or complete loss of, or loss of the function of, a body part, organ, or system. **hearing i.,** hearing loss.

im·pal·pa·ble (im-pal′pah-b′l) not detectable by touch.

im·ped·ance (im-pēd′ans) obstruction or opposition to passage or flow, as of an electric current or other form of energy. Symbol Z. **acoustic i.,** an expression of the opposition to passage of sound waves, being the product of the density of a substance and the velocity of sound in it. **aortic i.,** the sum of the external factors that resist ventricular ejection.

im·per·fect (im-per′fekt) of a fungus, capable of reproducing only by means of conidia (asexual spores).

im·per·fo·rate (-per′for-āt) not open; abnormally closed.

im·per·me·a·ble (-per′me-ah-b′l) not permitting passage, as of fluid.

im·pe·ti·go (im″pě-ti′go) [L.] 1. impetigo contagiosa; a streptococcal or staphylococcal skin infection marked by vesicles that become pustular, rupture and form yellow crusts. **im·petig′inous,** adj. 2. i. bullosa. **i. bullo′sa, bullous i.,** impetigo in which the developing vesicles progress to form large bullae, which collapse and become covered with crusts. **i. contagio′sa,** impetigo (1). **i. herpetifor′-mis,** a very rare, acute dermatitis with symmetrically ringed, pustular lesions, occurring chiefly in pregnant women and associated with severe constitutional symptoms. **i. neonato′rum,** impetigo bullosa of newborn infants.

im·plant¹ (im-plant′) to insert or to graft (tissue, or inert or radioactive material) into intact tissues or a body cavity.

im·plant² (im′plant) an object or material inserted or grafted into the body for prosthetic, therapeutic, diagnostic, or experimental purposes. **cochlear i.,** a mechanical alternative to hearing for deaf persons, consisting of a microphone, signal processor, external transmitter, and implanted receiver. **endosseous i., endosteal i.,** a dental implant consisting of a blade, screw, pin, or vent, inserted into the jaw bone through the alveolar or basal bone, with a post protruding through the mucoperiosteum into the oral cavity to serve as an abutment for dentures or orthodontic appliances, or to serve in fracture fixation. **penile i.,** see under *prosthesis*. **subperiosteal i.,** a metal frame implanted under the periosteum and resting on the bone, with a post protruding into the oral cavity. **transmandibular i.,** a dental implant for patients with severe mandibular alveolar atrophy; it is fixed to the symphyseal border and traverses the mandible to attach directly to a denture, bearing the denture directly.

im·plan·ta·tion (im″plan-ta′shun) 1. attachment of the blastocyst to the epithelial lining of the uterus, its penetration through the epithelium, and, in humans, its embedding in the stratum compactum of the endometrium, occurring six or seven days after fertilization of the oocyte. 2. the insertion of an organ or tissue in a new site in the body. 3. the insertion or grafting into the body of biological, living, inert, or radioactive material.

im·plo·sion (im-plo′zhun) see *flooding*.

im·po·tence (im′po-tens) 1. lack of power. 2. specifically, lack of copulative power in the male due to failure to initiate an erection or maintain an erection until ejaculation; usually considered to be due to a physical disorder (*organic i.*) or an underlying psychological condition (*psychogenic i.*, usually called *male erectile disorder*).

im·preg·na·tion (im″preg-na′shun) 1. fertilization. 2. saturation (1).

im·pres·sio (im-pres′e-o) pl. *impressio′nes*. [L.] impression (1).

im·pres·sion (im-presh′un) 1. a slight indentation, as one produced in the surface of one organ by pressure exerted by another. 2. a negative imprint of an object made in some plastic material that later solidifies. 3. an effect produced upon the mind, body, or senses by some external stimulus or agent. **basilar i.,** 1. platybasia. 2. basilar invagination. **cardiac i.,** an impression made by the heart on another organ. **dental i.,** one made of the jaw or teeth in some plastic material, which is later filled in with plaster of Paris to produce a facsimile of the oral structures present.

im·print·ing (im′print-ing) a species-specific, rapid kind of learning during a critical period of early life in which social attachment and identification are established.

im·pulse (im′puls) 1. a sudden pushing force. 2. a sudden uncontrollable determination to act. 3. nerve i. **cardiac i.,** movement of the chest wall caused by the heart beat.

ectopic i., 1. the impulse that causes an ectopic beat. 2. a pathologic nerve impulse that begins in the middle of an axon and proceeds simultaneously towards the cell body and the periphery. **nerve i.,** the electrochemical process propagated along nerve fibers.

im·pul·sion (im-pul'shun) blind obedience to internal drives, without regard for acceptance by others or pressure from the superego; seen in children and in adults with weak defensive organization.

In indium.

in-¹ word element [L.], *in, within,* or *into.*

in-² word element [L.], *not.*

INA International Neurological Association.

in·ac·ti·va·tion (in-ak″tĭ-va'shun) the destruction of biological activity, as of a virus, by the action of heat or other agent.

in·am·ri·none (-am'rĭ-nōn) a vasodilator and positive inotropic agent used as the lactate for the short-term management of congestive heart failure.

in·an·i·mate (-an'im-it) 1. without life. 2. lacking in animation.

in·a·ni·tion (in″ah-nish'un) the exhausted state due to prolonged undernutrition; starvation.

in·ap·pe·tence (in-ap'it-ins) lack of appetite or desire.

in·ar·tic·u·late (in″ahr-tik'u-lat) 1. not having joints; disjointed. 2. uttered so as to be unintelligible; incapable of articulate speech.

in ar·tic·u·lo mor·tis (in ahr-tik'u-lo mor'-tis) [L.] at the moment of death.

in·born (in'born″) 1. genetically determined, and present at birth. 2. congenital.

in·breed·ing (-brēd-ing) the mating of closely related individuals or of individuals having closely similar genetic constitutions.

in·car·cer·at·ed (in-kahr'ser-āt″ed) imprisoned; constricted; subjected to incarceration.

in·car·cer·a·tion (in-kahr″ser-a'shun) unnatural retention or confinement of a part.

in·cest (in'sest″) sexual activity between persons so closely related that marriage between them is legally or culturally prohibited.

in·ci·dence (-sid-ins) the rate at which a certain event occurs, as the number of new cases of a specific disease occurring during a certain period in a population at risk.

in·ci·dent (-sid-int) impinging upon, as incident radiation.

in·ci·sal (in-si'z'l) 1. cutting. 2. pertaining to the cutting edge of an anterior tooth.

in·cised (in-sīzd') cut; made by cutting.

in·ci·sion (in-sizh'un) 1. a cut or a wound made by cutting with a sharp instrument. **incis'ional,** adj. 2. the act of cutting.

in·ci·sive (-si'siv) 1. having the power or quality of cutting. 2. pertaining to the incisor teeth.

in·ci·sor (I) (-si'zer) 1. adapted for cutting. 2. incisor tooth.

in·ci·su·ra (in-si-su'rah) pl. *incisu'rae.* [L.] notch.

in·ci·sure (-si'zher) notch. **i's of Lanterman, Lanterman-Schmidt i's,** oblique slashes or lines on the sheath of a myelinated fiber. **Rivinus' i., tympanic i.,** see under *notch.*

in·cli·na·tio (in″klĭ-na'she-o) pl. *inclinatio'nes.* [L.] inclination.

in·cli·na·tion (-klĭ-na'shun) a sloping or leaning; the angle of deviation from a particular line or plane of reference; in dentistry, the deviation of a tooth from the vertical. **pelvic i.,** the angle between the plane of the pelvic inlet and the horizontal plane.

in·clu·sion (in-kloo'zhun) 1. the act of enclosing or the condition of being enclosed. 2. anything that is enclosed; a cell inclusion. **cell i.,** a usually lifeless, often temporary, constituent in the cytoplasm of a cell. **dental i.,** 1. a tooth so surrounded with bony tissue that it is unable to erupt. 2. a cyst of oral soft tissue or bone.

in·com·pat·i·ble (-kom-pat'ĭ-b'l) not suitable for combination, simultaneous administration, or transplantation; mutually repellent.

in·com·pe·tent (-kom'pit-int) 1. unable to function properly. 2. a person who is unable to perform the required functions of daily living. 3. a person determined by the courts to be unable to manage their own affairs.

in·con·ti·nence (-kon'tĭ-nens) 1. inability to control excretory functions. 2. immoderation or excess. **incon'tinent,** adj. **fecal i.,** involuntary passage of feces and flatus. **overflow i.,** urinary incontinence due to pressure of retained urine in the bladder after the bladder has contracted to its limits, with dribbling of urine. **passive i.,** urinary or fecal incontinence in which the bladder or colon is full and cannot be emptied in the usual way but can be induced by pressure. **stress i.,** involuntary escape of urine due to strain on the orifice of the bladder, as in coughing or sneezing. **urge i., urgency i.,** urinary or fecal incontinence preceded by a sudden, uncontrollable impulse to evacuate. **urinary i.,** inability to control the voiding of urine.

in·con·ti·nen·tia (-kon″tĭ-nen′shah) [L.] incontinence. **i. pigmen′ti,** a hereditary disorder in which early vesicular and later verrucous and bizarrely pigmented skin lesions are associated with eye, bone, and central nervous system defects.

in·co·or·di·na·tion (in″ko-or″dĭ-na′shun) ataxia.

in·cor·po·ra·tion (in-kor″por-a′shun) 1. the union of a substance with another, or with others, in a composite mass. 2. a primitive unconscious defense mechanism in which aspects of another person are assimilated into the self.

in·cre·ment (in′krĭ-mint) increase or addition; the amount by which a value or quantity is increased. **incremen′tal,** adj.

in·crus·ta·tion (in″krus-ta′shun) 1. the formation of a crust. 2. a crust, scab, or scale.

in·cu·bate (in′ku-bāt) 1. to subject to or to undergo incubation. 2. material that has undergone incubation.

in·cu·ba·tion (in″ku-ba′shun) 1. the provision of proper conditions for growth and development, as for bacterial or tissue cultures. 2. the development of an infectious disease from time of the entrance of the pathogen to the appearance of clinical symptoms. 3. the development of the embryo in the eggs of oviparous animals. 4. the maintenance of an artificial environment for an infant, especially a premature infant.

in·cu·ba·tor (in′ku-bāt-er) an apparatus for maintaining optimal conditions (temperature, humidity, etc.) for growth and development, as one used in the early care of premature infants, or one used for cultures.

in·cu·dal (-ku-dil) pertaining to the incus.

in·cu·do·mal·le·al (in″ku-do-mal′e-il) pertaining to the incus and malleus.

in·cu·do·sta·pe·di·al (-stah-pe′de-il) pertaining to the incus and stapes.

in·cur·a·ble (in-kūr′ah-b′l) 1. not susceptible of being cured. 2. a person with a disease which cannot be cured.

in·cus (ing′kus) [L.] see *Table of Bones.*

in·cy·clo·pho·ria (in″si-klo-for′e-ah) cyclophoria in which the upper pole of the visual axis deviates toward the nose.

in·cy·clo·tro·pia (-tro′pe-ah) cyclotropia in which the upper pole of the vertical axis deviates toward the nose.

in·dane·di·one (in″dān-di′ōn) any of a group of related synthetic anticoagulants, e.g., anisindione, which impair the hepatic synthesis of the vitamin K–dependent coagulation factors (prothrombin, factors VII, IX, and X).

in·dap·amide (in-dap′ah-mīd) an antihypertensive and diuretic with actions and uses similar to those of chlorothiazide.

in·dex (in′deks) pl. *indexes, in′dices.* [L.] 1. forefinger. 2. a unitless quantity, usually a ratio of two measurable quantities having the same dimensions, or such a ratio multiplied by 100. **body mass i. (BMI),** the weight in kilograms divided by the square of the height in meters, used in the assessment of underweight and obesity. **cardiac i. (CI),** cardiac output per unit time divided by body surface area. **Colour I.,** a publication of the Society of Dyers and Colourists and the American Association of Textile Chemists and Colorists containing an extensive list of dyes and dye intermediates. Each chemically distinct compound is identified by a specific number, the C.I. number, avoiding the confusion of trivial names used for dyes in the dye industry. **I. Medicus,** a monthly publication of the National Library of Medicine in which the world's leading biomedical literature is indexed by author and subject. **mitotic i.,** the ratio of the number of cells in a population undergoing mitosis to the number not undergoing mitosis. **opsonic i.,** a measure of opsonic activity determined by the ratio of the number of microorganisms phagocytized by normal leukocytes in the presence of serum from an individual infected by the microorganism, to the number phagocytized in serum from a normal individual. **phagocytic i.,** the average number of bacteria ingested per leukocyte of the patient's blood. **Quetelet i.,** body mass i. **refractive i.,** the refractive power of a medium compared with that of air (assumed to be 1). Symbol n or *n*. **short increment sensitivity i. (SISI),** a hearing test in which randomly spaced, 0.5-second tone bursts are superimposed at 1- to 5-decibel increments in intensity on a carrier tone having the same frequency and an intensity of 20 decibels above the speech recognition threshold. **therapeutic i.,** originally, the ratio of the maximum tolerated dose to the minimum curative dose; now defined as the ratio of the median lethal dose (LD_{50}) to the median effective dose (ED_{50}). It is used in assessing the safety of a drug. **vital i.,** the ratio of births to deaths within a given time in a population.

in·di·can (in′dĭ-kan) potassium indoxyl sulfate, formed by decomposition of tryptophan in the intestines and excreted in the urine.

in·di·ca·tor (in′dĭ-kāt″er) 1. the index finger, or the extensor muscle of the index finger. 2. any substance that indicates the appearance or disappearance of a chemical by a color change or attainment of a certain pH.

in·dif·fer·ent (in-dif'er-ent) not tending one way or another; neutral; having no preponderating affinity.

in·di·ges·tion (in''dĭ-jes'chun) lack or failure of digestion; commonly used to denote vague abdominal discomfort after meals. **acid i.**, hyperchlorhydria. **fat i.**, steatorrhea. **gastric i.**, that taking place in, or due to a disorder of, the stomach. **intestinal i.**, disorder of the digestive function of the intestine. **sugar i.**, defective ability to digest sugar, resulting in fermental diarrhea.

in·dig·i·ta·tion (in-dij''ĭ-ta'shun) intussusception (1).

in·di·go (in'dĭ-go) 1. a blue dyeing material from various leguminous and other plants, being the aglycone of indican and also made synthetically; sometimes found in the sweat and urine. 2. a color between blue and violet, produced by energy of wavelengths between 420 and 450 nm.

in·dig·o·tin (in''dĭ-go'tin) a neutral, tasteless, insoluble, dark blue powder, the principal ingredient of commercial indigo.

in·di·go·tin·di·sul·fon·ate so·di·um (in''-dĭ-go''tin-di-sul'fon-āt) a dye, occurring as a dusky, purplish blue powder or blue granules, used as a diagnostic aid in cystoscopy.

in·di·na·vir (in-di'nah-vir) an HIV protease inhibitor that causes formation of immature, noninfectious viral particles; used as the sulfate salt in the treatment of HIV infection and AIDS.

in·di·rect (in''di-rekt') 1. not immediate or straight. 2. acting through an intermediary agent.

in·di·um (In) (in'de-um) chemical element (see *Table of Elements*), at. no. 49. **i. 111**, an artificial isotope having a half-life of 2.81 days and emitting gamma rays; it is used to label a variety of compounds for nuclear medicine.

in·di·vid·u·a·tion (in''dĭ-vid''u-a'shun) 1. the process of developing individual characteristics. 2. differential regional activity in the embryo occurring in response to organizer influence.

in·dole (in'dōl) a compound obtained from coal tar and indigo and produced by decomposition of tryptophan in the intestine, where it contributes to the peculiar odor of feces. It is excreted in the urine in the form of indican.

in·do·lent (in'dah-lint) 1. causing little pain. 2. slow growing.

in·do·meth·a·cin (in''do-meth'ah-sin) a nonsteroidal antiinflammatory drug; used in the treatment of various rheumatic and nonrheumatic inflammatory conditions, dysmenorrhea, and vascular headache. The trihydrated sodium salt is used to induce closure in certain cases of patent ductus arteriosus.

in·dox·yl (in-dok'sil) an oxidation product of indole, formed in tryptophan decomposition and excreted in the urine as indican.

in·duced (in-dōost') 1. produced artificially. 2. produced by induction.

in·duc·er (in-dōos'er) a molecule that causes a cell or organism to accelerate synthesis of an enzyme or sequence of enzymes in response to a developmental signal.

in·du·ci·ble (in-doo'sĭ-b'l) produced because of stimulation by an inducer.

in·duc·tance (in-duk'tans) that property of a circuit whereby changing current generates an electromotive force (EMF) in the same or a neighboring circuit; the EMF is proportional to the rate of change of the current and inductance is quantitated as the ratio of these two.

in·duc·tion (in-duk'shun) 1. the act or process of inducing or causing to occur. 2. the production of a specific morphogenetic effect in the embryo through evocators or organizers. 3. the production of anesthesia or unconsciousness by use of appropriate agents. 4. the generation of an electric current or magnetic properties in a body because of its proximity to another electric current or magnetic field.

in·duc·tor (-ter) a tissue elaborating a chemical substance that acts to determine growth and differentiation of embryonic parts.

in·du·ra·tion (in''du-ra'shun) 1. sclerosis or hardening. 2. hardness. 3. an abnormally hard spot or place. **in'durative**, adj. **black i.**, hardening and pigmentation of lung tissue in coal workers' pneumoconiosis. **brown i.**, 1. a deposit of altered blood pigment in the lung. 2. increase of pulmonary connective tissue, dark colored due to anthracosis or chronic congestion from valvular heart disease. **cyanotic i.**, hardening of the kidney from chronic venous congestion. **granular i.**, cirrhosis. **gray i.**, induration of lung tissue in or after pneumonia, without the pigmentation of brown induration. **penile i.**, Peyronie's disease. **red i.**, red, congested lung tissue seen in idiopathic pulmonary fibrosis.

in·du·si·um gris·e·um (in-du'ze-um gris'e-um) [L.] a thin layer of gray matter on the dorsal surface of the corpus callosum.

in·dwell·ing (in'dwel-ing) pertaining to a catheter or other tube left within an organ or body passage for drainage, to maintain patency, or for the administration of drugs or nutrients.

in·e·bri·a·tion (in-e''bre-a'shun) drunkenness; intoxication with, or as if with, alcohol.

in·ert (in-ert') inactive.

in·er·tia (-er'shah) [L.] inactivity; inability to move spontaneously. **colonic i.,** weak muscular activity of the colon, leading to distention of the organ and constipation. **uterine i.,** sluggishness of uterine contractions in labor.

in ex·tre·mis (in ek-stre'mis) [L.] at the point of death.

in·fan·cy (in'fin-se) the early period of life; see *infant*.

in·fant (in'fint) the human young from the time of birth to one year of age. **dysmature i.,** postmature i. **floppy i.,** see under *syndrome*. **immature i.,** one usually weighing less than 2500 grams at birth and not physiologically well developed. **low birth weight (LBW) i.,** one weighing less than 2500 g at birth. **mature i.,** one weighing 2500 g or more at birth, usually at or near full term, physiologically fully developed, and having optimal chance of survival. **moderately low birth weight (MLBW) i.,** one weighing at least 1500 but less than 2500 g at birth. **newborn i.,** the human young during the first four weeks after birth. **postmature i.,** 1. one with postmaturity syndrome. 2. postterm i. **postterm i.,** one born at or after the forty-second completed week (294 days) of gestation. **premature i.,** 1. one usually born after the twentieth completed week and before full term, defined as weighing 500 to 2499 g at birth; the chance of survival depends on the weight. In countries where adults are smaller than in the United States, the upper limit may be lower. 2. preterm i. **preterm i.,** one born before the thirty-seventh completed week (259 days) of gestation. **term i.,** one born in the interval from the thirty-seventh completed week to the forty-second completed week of gestation; 259 days to 293 days, inclusive. **very low birth weight (VLBW) i.,** one weighing less than 1500 g at birth.

in·fan·tile (in'fin-tīl) pertaining to an infant or to infancy.

in·fan·ti·lism (in'fan-til-izm, in-fan'til-izm) persistence of childhood characters into adult life, marked by mental retardation, underdevelopment of sex organs, and often dwarfism. **cachectic i.,** that due to chronic infection or poisoning. **hypophysial i.,** a type of dwarfism with retention of infantile characteristics, due to undersecretion of growth hormone and gonadotropin deficiency. **sexual i.,** continuance of prepubertal sex characters and behavior after the usual age of puberty. **universal i.,** general dwarfishness in stature, with absence of secondary sex characteristics.

in·farct (in'fahrkt) a localized area of ischemic necrosis produced by occlusion of the arterial supply or the venous drainage of the part. **anemic i.,** one due to the sudden arrest of circulation in a vessel, or to decoloration of hemorrhagic blood. **hemorrhagic i.,** one that is red owing to oozing of erythrocytes into the injured area.

in·farc·tion (in-fahrk'shun) 1. the formation of an infarct. 2. infarct. **acute myocardial i. (AMI),** that occurring during the period when circulation to a region of the heart is obstructed and necrosis is occurring. **cardiac i.,** myocardial i. **cerebral i.,** an ischemic condition of the brain, causing a persistent focal neurologic deficit in the area affected. **mesenteric i.,** coagulation necrosis of the intestines due to a decrease in blood flow in the mesenteric vasculature. **migrainous i.,** a focal neurologic defect that constituted part of a migrainous aura but that has persisted for a long period and may be permanent. **myocardial i. (MI),** gross necrosis of the myocardium, due to interruption of the blood supply to the area. **non–Q wave i.,** myocardial infarction not characterized by abnormal Q waves. **pulmonary i.,** localized necrosis of lung tissue, due to obstruction of the arterial blood supply. **Q wave i.,** myocardial infarction characterized by Q waves that are abnormal either in character or number or both. **silent myocardial i.,** myocardial infarction occurring without pain or other symptoms; often detected only by electrographic or postmortem examination. **watershed i.,** cerebral infarction in a watershed area during a time of prolonged systemic hypotension.

in·fect (in-fekt') 1. to invade and produce infection in. 2. to transmit a pathogen or disease to.

in·fec·tion (-fek'shun) 1. invasion and multiplication of microorganisms in body tissues, especially that causing local cellular injury due to competitive metabolism, toxins, intracellular replication, or antigen–antibody response. 2. an infectious disease. **airborne i.,** one that is contracted by inhalation of microorganisms or spores suspended in air on water droplets or dust particles.

droplet i., infection due to inhalation of respiratory pathogens suspended on liquid particles exhaled by someone already infected (*droplet nuclei*). **endogenous i.,** that due to reactivation of organisms present in a dormant focus, as occurs in tuberculosis, etc. **tunnel i.,** subcutaneous infection of an artificial passage into the body that has been kept patent. **opportunistic i.,** infection by an organism that does not ordinarily cause disease but becomes pathogenic under certain circumstances (e.g., impaired immune responses).

in·fec·tious (-fek′shus) 1. caused by or capable of being communicated by infection, as an infectious disease. 2. infective (1).

in·fec·tive (in-fek′tiv) 1. capable of producing infection. 2. infectious (1).

in·fe·ri·or (-fēr′e-er) situated below, or directed downward; in anatomy, used in reference to the lower surface of a structure, or to the lower of two (or more) similar structures.

in·fer·til·i·ty (in″fer-til′ĭ-te) diminution or absence of ability to produce offspring. **infer′tile,** adj. **immunologic i.,** any of several types believed to be caused by presence in the female of antibodies that interfere with functioning of the sperm.

in·fes·ta·tion (-fes-ta′shun) parasitic attack or subsistence on the skin and/or its appendages, as by insects, mites, or ticks; sometimes used to denote parasitic invasion of the organs and tissues, as by helminths.

in·fib·u·la·tion (in-fib″u-la′shun) the act of buckling or fastening as if with buckles, particularly the practice of fastening the prepuce or labia minora together to prevent coitus.

in·fil·trate (in-fil′trāt) 1. to penetrate the interstices of a tissue or substance. 2. the material or solution so deposited.

in·fil·tra·tion (in″fil-tra′shun) 1. the pathological diffusion or accumulation in a tissue or cells of substances not normal to it or in amounts in excess of the normal. 2. infiltrate (2). 3. the deposition of a solution directly into tissue; see under *anesthesia*. **adipose i.,** fatty i. **calcareous i.,** deposit of lime and magnesium salts in the tissues. **cellular i.,** the migration and accumulation of cells within the tissues. **fatty i.,** 1. a deposit of fat in tissues, especially between cells; the term describes an older concept now included in *fatty change*. 2. the presence of fat vacuoles in the cell cytoplasm.

in·fil·tra·tive (in′fil-tra″tiv) pertaining to or characterized by infiltration.

in·firm (in-firm′) weak; feeble, as from disease or old age.

in·fir·ma·ry (-ah-re) a hospital or place where the sick or infirm are maintained or treated.

in·flam·ma·gen (in-flam′ah-jen) an irritant that elicits both edema and the cellular response of inflammation.

in·flam·ma·tion (in″flah-ma′shun) a protective tissue response to injury or destruction of tissues, which serves to destroy, dilute, or wall off both the injurious agent and the injured tissues. The classical signs of acute inflammation are pain (dolor), heat (calor), redness (rubor), swelling (tumor), and loss of function (functio laesa). **inflam′matory,** adj. **acute i.,** inflammation, usually of sudden onset, marked by the classical signs (see *inflammation*), in which vascular and exudative processes predominate. **catarrhal i.,** a form affecting mainly a mucous surface, marked by a copious discharge of mucus and epithelial debris. **chronic i.,** prolonged and persistent inflammation marked chiefly by new connective tissue formation; it may be a continuation of an acute form or a prolonged low-grade form. **exudative i.,** one in which the prominent feature is an exudate. **fibrinous i.,** one marked by an exudate of coagulated fibrin. **granulomatous i.,** a form, usually chronic, marked by granuloma formation. **hyperplastic i.,** one leading to the formation of new connective tissue fibers. **interstitial i.,** one affecting chiefly the stroma of an organ. **parenchymatous i.,** one affecting chiefly the essential tissue elements of an organ. **plastic i., productive i., proliferous i.,** hyperplastic i. **pseudomembranous i.,** an acute inflammatory response to a powerful necrotizing toxin, e.g., diphtheria toxin, with formation, on a mucosal surface, of a false membrane composed of precipitated fibrin, necrotic epithelium, and inflammatory white cells. **purulent i.,** suppurative i. **serous i.,** one producing a serous exudate. **subacute i.,** a condition intermediate between chronic and acute inflammation, exhibiting some of the characteristics of each. **suppurative i.,** one marked by pus formation. **ulcerative i.,** that in which necrosis on or near the surface leads to loss of tissue and creation of a local defect (ulcer).

in·fla·tion (in-fla′shun) distention, or the act of distending, with air, gas, or fluid.

in·flec·tion (-flek′shun) the act of bending inward, or the state of being bent inward.

in·flix·i·mab (-flik'sĭ-mab) an anti–tumor necrosis factor antibody used in treatment of Crohn's disease and rheumatoid arthritis.

in·flu·en·za (in″floo-en'zah) [Ital.] an acute viral infection of the respiratory tract, occurring in isolated cases, epidemics, and pandemics, caused by serologically distinct strains of viruses (influenzaviruses) designated A, B, and C; marked by inflammation of the nasal mucosa, pharynx, and conjunctiva, headache, myalgia; often fever, chills, and prostration; and occasionally involvement of the myocardium or central nervous system **influen′zal**, adj.

In·flu·en·za·vi·rus A (in″floo-en'zah-vi″rus) a genus of viruses of the family Orthomyxoviridae containing the agent of influenza A. See *influenza virus*, under *virus*.

In·flu·en·za·vi·rus B a genus of viruses of the family Orthomyxoviridae containing the agent of influenza B. See *influenza virus*, under *virus*.

In·flu·en·za·vi·rus C a genus of viruses of the family Orthomyxoviridae containing the agent of influenza C. See *influenza virus*, under *virus*.

in·fold·ing (in-fold'ing) 1. the folding inward of a layer of tissue, as in the formation of the neural tube in the embryo. 2. the enclosing of redundant tissue by suturing together the walls of the organ on either side of it.

infra- word element [L.], *beneath*.

in·fra·bulge (in'frah-bulj) the surfaces of a tooth gingival to the height of contour, or sloping cervically.

in·fra·cal·ca·rine (in″frah-kal'kah-rīn) inferior to the calcarine sulcus.

in·fra·cla·vic·u·lar (-klah-vik'u-lar) subclavian.

in·fra·clu·sion (-kloo'zhun) a condition in which the occluding surface of a tooth does not reach the normal occlusal plane and is out of contact with the opposing tooth.

in·frac·tion (in-frak'shun) incomplete bone fracture without displacement.

in·fra·den·ta·le (in″frah-den-ta'le) a cephalometric landmark, being the highest anterior point on the gingiva between the mandibular medial (central) incisors.

in·fra·di·an (-de'in) pertaining to a period longer than 24 hours; applied to the cyclic behavior of certain phenomena in living organisms (infradian rhythm).

in·fra·duc·tion (-duk'shun) downward rotation of an eye around its horizontal axis.

in·fra·no·dal (-no'd'l) below a node.

in·fra·or·bi·tal (-or'bĭ-t'l) suborbital; under, or on the inferior surface of, the orbit.

in·fra·pa·tel·lar (-pah-tel'er) subpatellar; below or beneath the patella.

in·fra·red (-red') denoting electromagnetic radiation of wavelength greater than that of the red end of the spectrum, having wavelengths of 0.75–1000 μm; sometimes subdivided into *long-wave* or *far i.* (about 3.0–1000 μm) and *short-wave* or *near i.* (about 0.75–3.0 μm).

in·fra·son·ic (-son'ik) below the frequency range of sound waves.

in·fra·spi·nous (-spi'nus) beneath the spine of the scapula.

in·fra·tem·po·ral (-tem'pŏ-r'l) inferior to the temple.

in·fra·ver·gence (-ver'jens) rotation of one eye downward while the other one remains still.

in·fra·ver·sion (-ver'zhun) 1. infraclusion. 2. the downward deviation of one eye. 3. conjugate downward rotation of both eyes.

in·fun·dib·u·lar (in″fun-dib'u-lar) 1. pertaining to an infundibulum. 2. funnel-shaped.

in·fun·dib·u·lec·to·my (-dib″u-lek'tah-me) excision of the infundibulum of the heart.

in·fun·dib·u·li·form (-dib'u-lĭ-form) infundibular (2).

in·fun·dib·u·lo·ma (-dib″u-lo'mah) a tumor of the stalk (infundibulum) of the hypophysis.

in·fun·dib·u·lum (-dib'u-lum) pl. *infundib′ula*. [L.] 1. a funnel-shaped structure. 2. conus arteriosus. 3. i. of neurohypophysis. **infundib′ular**, adj. **ethmoidal i.**, 1. a passage connecting the nasal cavity with anterior ethmoidal cells and frontal sinus. 2. a sinuous passage connecting the middle nasal meatus with the anterior ethmoidal cells and often with the frontal sinus. **i. of hypothalamus,** **i. of neurohypophysis,** a hollow, funnel-shaped mass in front of the tuber cinereum, extending to the neurohypophysis. **i. of uterine tube,** the distal, funnel-shaped portion of the uterine tube.

in·fu·sion (in-fu'zhun) 1. the steeping of a substance in water to obtain its soluble principles. 2. the product obtained by this process. 3. the therapeutic introduction of fluid other than blood into a vein.

in·ges·tant (-jes'tant) a substance that is or may be taken into the body by mouth or through the digestive system.

in·ges·tion (-chun) the taking of food, drugs, etc., into the body by mouth.

in·gra·ves·cent (in″grah-ves'ent) gradually becoming more severe.

in·grown (in′grōn) having grown inward, into the flesh.

in·growth (-grōth) an inward growth; something that grows inward or into.

in·guen (ing′gwen) pl. *in′guina*. [L.] groin: the junctional region between the abdomen and thigh. **in′guinal,** adj.

in·gui·nal (in′gwĭ-n′l) pertaining to the groin.

in·hal·ant (in-hāl′ant) 1. something meant to be inhaled; see *inhalation* (def. 3). 2. a class of psychoactive substances whose volatile vapors are subject to abuse. **antifoaming i.,** an agent that is inhaled as a vapor to prevent the formation of foam in the respiratory passages of a patient with pulmonary edema.

in·ha·la·tion (in″hah-la′shun) 1. the drawing of air or other substances into the lungs. **inhala′tional,** adj. 2. the drawing of an aerosolized drug into the lungs with the breath. 3. any drug or solution of drugs administered (as by means of nebulizers or aerosols) by the nasal or oral respiratory route.

in·hal·er (in-hāl′er) 1. an apparatus for administering vapor or volatilized medications by inhalation. 2. ventilator (2).

in·her·ent (in-her′ent) implanted by nature; intrinsic; innate.

in·her·i·tance (in-her′ĭ-tans) 1. the acquisition of characters or qualities by transmission from parent to offspring. 2. that which is transmitted from parent to offspring. **cytoplasmic i.,** mitochondrial i. **dominant i.,** see under *gene*. **extrachromosomal i.,** mitochondrial i. **intermediate i.,** inheritance in which the phenotype of the heterozygote falls between that of either homozygote. **maternal i.,** mitochondrial i. **mitochondrial i.,** the inheritance of traits controlled by genes on the DNA of mitochondria in the ooplasm; thus the genes are inherited entirely from the maternal side, segregate randomly at meiosis or mitosis, and are variably expressed. **recessive i.,** see under *gene*. **sex-linked i.,** see under *gene*.

in·hib·it (in-hib′it) to retard, arrest, or restrain.

in·hi·bi·tion (in″hĭ-bish′un) 1. arrest or restraint of a process. 2. in psychoanalytic theory, the conscious or unconscious restraining of an impulse or desire. **competitive i.,** inhibition of enzyme activity in which the inhibitor (a substrate analogue) competes with the substrate for binding sites on the enzymes. **contact i.,** inhibition of cell division and cell motility in normal animal cells when in close contact with each other. **endproduct i., feedback i.,** inhibition of

the initial steps of a process by an end-product of the reaction. **noncompetitive i.,** inhibition of enzyme activity by substances that combine with the enzyme at a site other than that utilized by the substrate.

in·hib·i·tor (in-hib′ĭ-tor) 1. any substance that interferes with a chemical reaction, growth, or other biologic activity. 2. a chemical substance that inhibits or checks the action of a tissue organizer or the growth of microorganisms. 3. an effector that reduces the catalytic activity of an enzyme. **ACE i's,** angiotensin-converting enzyme i's. **alpha₁-proteinase i.,** alpha₁-antitrypsin. **angiotensin-converting enzyme i's,** competitive inhibitors of angiotensin-converting enzyme; used as antihypertensives, usually in conjunction with a diuretic, and also as vasodilators in the treatment of congestive heart failure. **aromatase i's,** a class of drugs that inhibit aromatase activity and thus block production of estrogens; used to treat breast cancer and endometriosis. **C1 i. (C1 INH),** an inhibitor of activated C1, the initial component of the classic complement pathway. Deficiency of or defect in the protein causes hereditary angioedema. **carbonic anhydrase i.,** any of a class of agents that inhibit carbonic anhydrase activity; used chiefly for the treatment of glaucoma, and for epilepsy, familial periodic paralysis, mountain sickness, and uric acid renal calculi. **cholinesterase i.,** a compound that prevents the hydrolysis of acetylcholine by acetylcholinesterase, so that high levels of acetylcholine accumulate at reactive sites. **COX-2 i's, cyclooxygenase-2 i's,** a group of nonsteroidal antiinflammatory drugs that act by inhibiting cyclooxygenase-2 activity; they have fewer gastrointestinal side effects than other NSAIDs. **gastric acid pump i.,** an agent that inhibits gastric acid secretion by blocking the action of H^+,K^+-ATPase at the secretory surface of gastric parietal cells; called also *proton pump i.* **HIV protease i.,** any of a group of antiretroviral drugs active against the human immunodeficiency virus, preventing protease-mediated cleavage of viral polyproteins and so causing production of immature noninfectious viral particles. **MAO i.,** monoamine oxidase inhibitor. **membrane i. of reactive lysis (MIRL),** protectin. **monoamine oxidase i. (MAOI),** any of a group of antidepressant drugs that act by blocking the action of the enzyme monoamine oxidase; believed to act by thus increasing the level of catecholamines in the central nervous system. **α₂-plasmin i.,** α₂-antiplasmin. **plasminogen activator i.**

(PAI), any of several regulators of the fibrinolytic system that act by binding to and inhibiting free plasminogen activator; the most important are *PAI-1* and *PAI-2.* **platelet i.,** any of a group of agents that inhibit the clotting activity of platelets. **protease i.,** 1. a substance that blocks the activity of an endopeptidase (protease). 2. HIV protease i. **proton pump i.,** gastric acid pump i. **reverse transcriptase i.,** a substance that blocks activity of the reverse transcriptase of a retrovirus and is used as an antiretroviral agent. **selective serotonin reuptake i. (SSRI),** any of a group of drugs that inhibit the inactivation of serotonin by blocking its absorption in the central nervous system; used to treat depressive, obsessive-compulsive, and panic disorders.

in·hib·i·to·ry (-tor″e) restraining or arresting any process; effecting a stay or arrest, partial or complete.

in·i·on (in′e-on) the external occipital protuberance. **in′ial,** adj.

ini·ti·a·tion (ĭ-nĭ″she-a′shun) the creation of a small alteration in the genetic coding of a cell by a low level of exposure to a carcinogen, priming the cell for neoplastic transformation upon later exposure to a carcinogen or a promoter.

in·i·tis (ĭ-ni′tis) myositis.

in·jec·tion (in-jek′shun) 1. the forcing of a liquid into a part, as into the subcutaneous tissues, the vascular tree, or an organ. 2. a substance so forced or administered; in pharmacy, a solution of a medicament suitable for injection. **hypodermic i.,** subcutaneous i. **intracutaneous i.,** intradermal i. **intracytoplasmic sperm i. (ICSI),** a micromanipulation technique used in male factor infertility, with insertion of a spermatocyte directly into an oocyte. **intradermal i.,** one made into the dermis or substance of the skin. **intramuscular i.,** one made into the substance of a muscle. **intrathecal i.,** injection of a substance through the theca of the spinal cord into the subarachnoid space. **intravenous i.,** one made into a vein. **jet i.,** one made through the intact skin by an extremely fine jet of the solution under high pressure. **lactated Ringer's i.,** a sterile solution of calcium chloride, potassium chloride, sodium chloride, and sodium lactate in water for injection, given as a fluid and electrolyte replenisher. **Ringer's i.,** a sterile solution of sodium chloride, potassium chloride, and calcium chloride in water for injection, used as a fluid and electrolyte replenisher. **subcutaneous i.,** one made into the subcutaneous tissues.

in·ju·ry (in′jer-e) wound or trauma; harm or hurt; usually applied to damage inflicted on the body by an external force. **birth i.,** impairment of body function or structure due to adverse influences to which the infant has been subjected at birth. **Goyrand's i.,** pulled elbow. **straddle i.,** injury to the distal urethra from falling astride a blunt object. **whiplash i.,** a popular nonspecific term applied to injury to the spine and spinal cord due to sudden extension of the neck.

in·lay (-la) material laid into a defect in tissue; in dentistry, a filling made outside the tooth to correspond with the cavity form and then cemented into the tooth.

in·let (-let) a means or route of entrance. **pelvic i.,** the upper limit of the pelvic cavity. **thoracic i.,** the elliptical opening at the summit of the thorax.

INN International Nonproprietary Name.

in·nate (ĭ-nāt′) inborn.

in·ner·va·tion (in″er-va′shun) 1. the distribution or supply of nerves to a part. 2. the supply of nervous energy or of nerve stimulation sent to a part. **inner′vatory,** adj.

in·nid·i·a·tion (ĭ-nid″e-a′shun) development of cells in a part to which they have been carried by metastasis.

in·no·cent (in′o-sent) not malignant; benign; not tending of its own nature to a fatal issue.

in·nom·i·nate (ĭ-nom′ĭ-nāt) nameless.

in(o)- word element [Gr.], *fiber.*

ino·chon·dri·tis (in″o-kon-dri′tis) inflammation of a fibrocartilage.

in·oc·u·la·ble (in-ok′u-lah-b′l) 1. susceptible of being inoculated; transmissible by inoculation. 2. not immune against a disease transmissible by inoculation.

in·oc·u·la·tion (-ok″u-la′shun) introduction of microorganisms, infective material, serum, or other substances into tissues of living organisms, or culture media; introduction of a disease agent into a healthy individual to produce a mild form of the disease followed by immunity.

in·oc·u·lum (-ok′u-lum) pl. *inoc′ula.* Material used in inoculation.

ino·di·la·tor (in″o-di-la′ter) an agent with both positive inotropic and vasodilator effects.

in·op·er·a·ble (in-op′er-ah-b′l) not susceptible to treatment by surgery.

in·or·gan·ic (in″or-gan′ik) 1. having no organs. 2. not of organic origin.

in·os·co·py (in-os′kah-pe) the diagnosis of disease by artificial digestion and examination of the fibers or fibrinous matter of sputum, blood, effusions, etc.

in·o·se·mia (in″o-se′me-ah) 1. the presence of inositol in the blood. 2. an excess of fibrin in the blood.

in·o·sine (I) (in′o-sēn) a purine nucleoside containing the base hypoxanthine and the sugar ribose, which occurs in transfer RNAs and as an intermediate in the degradation of purines and purine nucleosides to uric acid and in pathways of purine salvage. **i. monophosphate (IMP),** a nucleotide produced by the deamination of adenosine monophosphate (AMP); it is the precursor of AMP and GMP in purine biosynthesis and an intermediate in purine salvage and in purine degradation.

ino·si·tol (in-o′sĭ-tol) a cyclic sugar alcohol, the fully hydroxylated derivative of cyclohexane; usually referring to the most abundant isomer, *myo*-inositol, which occurs in many plant and animal tissues and microorganisms and is often classified as a member of the vitamin B complex. **i. 1,4,5-triphosphate (InsP₃, IP₃),** a second messenger that causes the release of calcium from certain intracellular organelles.

in·o·tro·pic (in′o-tro″pik) affecting the force of muscular contractions.

in·pa·tient (in′pa-shent) a patient who comes to a hospital or other health care facility for diagnosis or treatment that requires an overnight stay.

in·quest (in′kwest) a legal inquiry before a coroner or medical examiner, and usually a jury, into the manner of death.

in·sa·lu·bri·ous (in″sah-loo′bre-us) injurious to health.

in·san·i·ty (in-san′it-e) a legal term for mental illness of such degree that the individual is not responsible for his or her acts. **insane′,** adj.

in·scrip·tio (-skrip′she-o) pl. *inscriptio′nes.* [L.] inscription. **i. tendi′nea,** see under *intersectio.*

in·scrip·tion (-skrip′shun) 1. a mark, or line. 2. that part of a prescription containing the names and amounts of the ingredients.

In·sec·ta (-sek′tah) a class of arthropods whose members are characterized by division into three parts: head, thorax, and abdomen.

in·sem·i·na·tion (-sem″ĭ-na′shun) the deposit of seminal fluid within the vagina or cervix. **artificial i. (AI),** that done by artificial means. **artificial i. by donor (AID),** donor i. **artificial i. by husband (AIH),** artificial insemination in which the semen used is from the woman's mate. **donor i., heterologous i.,** artificial insemination in which the semen used is not from the woman's mate. **homologous i.,** artificial i. by husband.

in·sen·si·ble (-sen′sĭ-b′l) 1. devoid of sensibility or consciousness. 2. not perceptible to the senses.

in·ser·tion (-ser′shun) 1. the act of implanting, or the condition of being implanted. 2. the site of attachment, as of a muscle to the bone that it moves. 3. in genetics, a rare nonreciprocal type of translocation in which a segment is removed from one chromosome and then inserted into a broken region of a nonhomologous chromosome. **velamentous i.,** attachment of the umbilical cord to the membranes rather than to the placenta.

in·sid·i·ous (-sid′e-us) coming on stealthily; of gradual and subtle development.

in·sight (in′sīt″) 1. in psychiatry, the patient's awareness and understanding of their attitudes, feelings, behavior, and disturbing symptoms; self-understanding. 2. in problem solving, the sudden perception of the appropriate relationships of things that results in a solution.

in si·tu (in si′too) [L.] in its normal place; confined to the site of origin.

in·sol·u·ble (in-sol′u-b′l) not susceptible of being dissolved.

in·som·nia (-som′ne-ah) inability to sleep; abnormal wakefulness. **insom′niac, insom′nic,** adj. **fatal familial i.,** an inherited prion disease affecting primarily the thalamus and characterized by progressive insomnia, hallucinations, stupor, and coma ending in death; autonomic and motor disturbances are also present. **primary i.,** a dyssomnia characterized by persistent difficulty initiating or maintaining sleep or by persistently nonrestorative sleep; not due to any other condition.

in·so·nate (-so′nāt) to expose to ultrasound waves.

in·sorp·tion (-sorp′shun) movement of a substance into the blood, especially from the gastrointestinal tract into the circulating blood.

in·sper·sion (-sper′shun) the act of sprinkling, as with a powder.

in·spi·ra·tion (in″spĭ-ra′shun) inhalation. **inspi′ratory,** adj.

in·spis·sat·ed (in-spis′āt-id) being thickened, dried, or made less fluid by evaporation.

in·sta·bil·i·ty (-stah-bil′ĭ-te) lack of steadiness or stability. **detrusor i.,** involuntary contraction of the detrusor muscle of the bladder caused by nonneurological problems. Cf. *detrusor hyperreflexia.*

in·star (in′stahr) any stage of an arthropod between molts.

in·step (-step) the dorsal part of the arch of the foot.

in·stil·la·tion (in″stĭ-la′shun) administration of a liquid drop by drop.

in·stinct (in′stinkt) a complex of unlearned responses characteristic of a species. **instinc′-tive,** adj. **death i.,** in psychoanalysis, the latent instinctive impulse toward dissolution and death. **herd i.,** the instinct or urge to be one of a group and to conform to its standards of conduct and opinion. **life i.,** in psychoanalysis, all of the constructive tendencies of the organism aimed at maintenance and perpetuation of the individual and species.

in·sti·tu·tion·al·iza·tion (in-stĭ-too″shun-al-ĭ-za′shun) 1. commitment of a patient to a health care facility for treatment, often psychiatric. 2. in patients hospitalized for a long period, the development of excessive dependency on the institution and its routines.

in·stru·ment (in′stroo-ment) any tool, appliance, or apparatus.

in·stru·men·tal (in″stroo-men′t'l) 1. pertaining to or performed by instruments. 2. serving as a means to a particular result.

in·stru·men·ta·tion (in″stroo-men-ta′shun) 1. the use of instruments; work performed with instruments. 2. a group of instruments used for a specific purpose.

in·su·date (in-soo′dāt) the substance accumulated in insudation.

in·su·da·tion (-soo-da′shun) the accumulation, as in the kidney, of substances derived from the blood.

in·suf·fi·cien·cy (-sah-fish′in-se) inability to perform properly an allotted function. **adrenal i.,** 1. hypoadrenalism; abnormally diminished activity of the adrenal gland. 2. adrenocortical i. **adrenocortical i.,** abnormally diminished secretion of corticosteroids by the adrenal cortex, as in Addison's disease. **aortic i.,** defective functioning of the aortic valve, with incomplete closure resulting in aortic regurgitation. **cardiac i.,** heart failure. **coronary i.,** decrease in flow of blood through the coronary blood vessels. **i. of the externi,** deficient power in the externi muscles of the eye, resulting in esophoria. **ileocecal i.,** inability of the ileocecal valve to prevent backflow of contents from the cecum into the ileum. **i. of the interni,** deficient power in the interni muscles of the eye, resulting in exophoria. **mitral i.,** defective functioning of the mitral valve, with incomplete closure causing mitral regurgitation. **pulmonary i.,** defective functioning of the pulmonary valve, with incomplete closure causing pulmonic regurgitation. **thyroid i.,** hypothyroidism. **tricuspid i.,** defective functioning of the tricuspid valve, with incomplete closure causing tricuspid regurgitation; it is usually secondary to systolic overload. **valvular i.,** 1. dysfunction of a cardiac valve, with incomplete closure resulting in valvular regurgitation. 2. venous i. **velopharyngeal i.,** failure of velopharyngeal closure due to cleft palate, muscular dysfunction, etc., resulting in defective speech. **venous i.,** inadequacy of the venous valves with impairment of venous drainage, resulting in edema. **vertebrobasilar i.,** transient ischemia of the brain stem and cerebellum due to stenosis of the vertebral or basilar artery.

in·suf·fla·tion (-sah-fla′shun) 1. the act of blowing a powder, vapor, or gas into a body cavity. 2. finely powdered or liquid drugs carried into the respiratory passages by such devices as aerosols. **perirenal i.,** injection of air around the kidney for radiographic examination of the adrenal glands. **tubal i.,** see *Rubin's test,* under *test.*

in·su·la (in′soo-lah) pl. *in′sulae.* [L.] 1. an islandlike structure. 2. a triangular area of the cerebral cortex forming the floor of the lateral cerebral fossa.

in·su·lar (-soo-ler) pertaining to the insula or to an island, as the islands of Langerhans.

in·su·la·tion (in″soo-la′shun) 1. the surrounding of a space or body with material designed to prevent the entrance or escape of radiant or electrical energy. 2. the material so used.

in·su·lin (in′soo-lin) 1. a protein hormone formed from proinsulin in the beta cells of the pancreatic islets of Langerhans. The major fuel-regulating hormone, it is secreted into the blood in response to a rise in concentration of blood glucose or amino acids. Insulin promotes the storage of glucose and the uptake of amino acids, increases protein and lipid synthesis, and inhibits lipolysis and gluconeogenesis. 2. a preparation of insulin, either of porcine or bovine origin or a recombinant form with sequence the same as or similar to that in humans, used in the treatment of diabetes mellitus; classified as *rapid-acting, intermediate-acting,* or *long-acting* on the basis of speed of onset and duration of activity. 3. regular insulin; a rapid-acting, unmodified form of insulin prepared from crystalline bovine or porcine insulin. **i. aspart,** a rapid-acting analogue of human insulin created by recombinant DNA technology. **buffered i. human,** insulin human buffered with phosphate; used particularly in continuous infusion pumps. **extended i. zinc suspension,**

a long-acting insulin consisting of porcine or human insulin in the form of large zinc-insulin crystals. **i. glargine,** an analogue of human insulin produced by recombinant DNA technology, having a slow, steady release over 24 hours. **i. human,** a protein corresponding to insulin elaborated in the human pancreas, derived from pork insulin by enzymatic action or produced synthetically by recombinant DNA techniques; sometimes used specifically to denote a rapid-acting regular insulin preparation of this protein. **isophane i. suspension,** an intermediate-acting insulin consisting of porcine or human insulin reacted with zinc chloride and protamine sulfate. **Lente i.,** insulin zinc suspension. **i. lispro,** a rapid-acting analogue of human insulin synthesized by means of recombinant DNA technology. **NPH i.,** isophane i. suspension. **prompt i. zinc suspension,** a rapid-acting insulin consisting of porcine insulin with zinc chloride added to produce a suspension of amorphous insulin. **regular i.,** insulin (3). **Semilente i.,** prompt insulin zinc suspension. **Ultralente i.,** extended insulin zinc suspension. **i. zinc suspension,** an intermediate-acting insulin consisting of porcine or human insulin with a zinc salt added such that the solid phase of the suspension contains a 7:3 ratio of crystalline to amorphous insulin.

in·su·lin·o·gen·e·sis (in″soo-lin″o-jen′ĕ-sis) the formation and release of insulin by the islets of Langerhans.

in·su·li·no·ma (in″soo-lin-o′mah) an islet cell tumor of the beta cells, usually benign, that secretes insulin and is one of the chief causes of hypoglycemia.

in·su·lin·o·pe·nic (in″soo-lin″o-pe′nik) diminishing, or pertaining to a decrease in, the level of circulating insulin.

in·su·li·tis (in″soo-li′tis) lymphocytic infiltration of the islets of Langerhans, suggesting an inflammatory or immunologic reaction.

in·sus·cep·ti·bil·i·ty (in″sah-sep″tĭ-bil′it-e) the state of being unaffected; immunity.

in·take (in-tāk′) the substances, or the quantities thereof, taken in and utilized by the body.

in·te·gra·tion (in″tĕ-gra′shun) 1. anabolism. 2. coordination. 3. assimilation. 4. assimilation of genetic material from one bacterium (donor) into the chromosome of another (recipient).

in·te·grin (in′tĕ-grin) any of a family of heterodimeric cell adhesion receptors, each consisting of an α and a β polypetide chain, that mediate cell-to-cell and cell-to-extracellular matrix interactions.

in·teg·u·ment (in-teg′u-ment) a covering or investment. **common i.,** the covering of the body, or skin, including its various layers and their appendages.

in·teg·u·men·ta·ry (in-teg″u-men′tĕ-re) 1. pertaining to or composed of skin. 2. serving as a covering.

in·teg·u·men·tum (-tum) [L.] integument.

in·tel·lect (in′tĭ-lekt) the mind, thinking faculty, or understanding.

in·tel·lec·tu·al·iza·tion (in″tĕ-lek″choo-al-ĭ-za′shun) an unconscious defense mechanism in which reasoning is used to avoid confronting an objectionable impulse, emotional conflict, or other stressor and thus to defend against anxiety.

in·ten·tion (in-ten′shun) 1. a manner of healing; see under *healing.* 2. a goal or desired end.

inter- word element [L.], *between.*

in·ter·ac·tion (in″ter-ak′shun) the quality, state, or process of (two or more things) acting on each other. **drug i.,** the action of one drug upon the effectiveness or toxicity of another (or others).

in·ter·al·ve·o·lar (-al-ve′o-lar) between alveoli.

in·ter·ar·tic·u·lar (-ahr-tik′u-lar) situated between articular surfaces.

in·ter·atri·al (-a′tre-al) situated between the atria of the heart.

in·ter·brain (in′ter-brān″) 1. thalamencephalon. 2. diencephalon.

in·ter·ca·lary, in·ter·ca·lat·ed (in-ter′kah-lar″e, in-ter-kah-la′ted) inserted between; interposed.

in·ter·cap·il·lary (in″ter-kap′ĭ-lar-e) among or between capillaries.

in·ter·car·pal (-kahr′p′l) between the carpal bones.

in·ter·car·ti·lag·i·nous (-kahr″tĭ-laj′ĭ-nus) between, or connecting, cartilages.

in·ter·cav·er·nous (-kav′er-nus) between two cavities.

in·ter·cel·lu·lar (-sel′u-lar) between or among cells.

in·ter·cos·tal (-kos′t′l) between two ribs.

in·ter·course (in′ter-kors) 1. mutual exchange. 2. sexual i. **sexual i.,** 1. coitus. 2. any physical contact between two individuals involving stimulation of the genital organs of at least one.

in·ter·cri·co·thy·rot·o·my (in″ter-kri″ko-thi-rot′ah-me) cricothyrotomy.

in·ter·crit·i·cal (-krit′ĭ-k′l) denoting the period between attacks, as of gout.

in·ter·cur·rent (-kur′ent) occurring during and modifying the course of another disease.

in·ter·cusp·ing (-kusp′ing) the occlusion of the cusps of the teeth of one jaw with the depressions in the teeth of the other jaw.

in·ter·den·tal (-den′t'l) between the proximal surfaces of adjacent teeth in the same arch.

in·ter·den·ti·um (-den′she-um) interproximal space.

in·ter·dig·i·ta·tion (-dij″ĭ-ta′shun) 1. an interlocking of parts by finger-like processes. 2. one of a set of finger-like processes.

in·ter·face (in′ter-fās) the boundary between two systems or phases. **interfa′cial,** adj.

in·ter·fas·cic·u·lar (in″ter-fah-sik′u-ler) between adjacent fascicles.

in·ter·fem·o·ral (-fem′or-al) between the thighs.

in·ter·fer·on (IFN) (-fēr′on) any of a family of glycoproteins, production of which can be stimulated by viral infection, by intracellular parasites, by protozoa, and by bacteria and bacterial endotoxins, that exert antiviral activity and have immunoregulatory functions; they also inhibit the growth of nonviral intracellular parasites. Interferons are designated α, β, γ, and ω on the basis of association with certain producer cells and functions; all animal cells, however, can produce interferons and some cells can produce more than one type. Pharmaceutical preparations of natural or synthetic interferons (e.g., *i. alfa-2a, i. alfa-2b, i. alfa-n1, i. alfa-n3, i. alfacon-1, i. beta-1a, i. beta-1b, i. gamma-1b*) are used as antineoplastics and biological response modifiers.

in·ter·glob·u·lar (-glob′u-lar) between or among globules, as of the dentin.

in·ter·glu·te·al (-gloo′te-al) internatal; between the buttocks.

in·ter·ic·tal (-ik′t'l) occurring between attacks or paroxysms.

in·ter·ki·ne·sis (-kĭ-ne′sis) the period between the first and second divisions in meiosis.

in·ter·leu·kin (-loo′kin) a generic term for a group of multifunctional cytokines that are produced by a variety of lymphoid and nonlymphoid cells and whose effects occur at least partly within the lymphopoietic system. **i.-2 (IL-2),** one produced by T cells in response to antigenic or mitogenic stimulation, acting to regulate the immune response. It stimulates the proliferation of T cells and the synthesis of other T cell–derived cytokines, stimulates the growth and cytolytic function of NK cells to produce lymphokine-activated killer cells, is a growth factor for and stimulates antibody synthesis in B cells, and may promote apoptosis in antigen-activated T cells; it is used pharmaceutically as an antineoplastic.

in·ter·lo·bar (-lo′bar) situated or occurring between lobes.

in·ter·lo·bi·tis (-lo-bi′tis) interlobular pleurisy.

in·ter·lob·u·lar (-lob′u-lar) situated or occurring between lobules.

in·ter·lock·ing (-lok′ing) closely joined, as by hooks or dovetails; locking into one another.

in·ter·me·di·ate (-me′de-at) 1. between; intervening; resembling, in part, each of two extremes. 2. a substance formed in a chemical process that is essential to formation of the end product of the process.

in·ter·me·din (-me′din) melanocyte-stimulating hormone.

in·ter·me·di·us (-me′de-us) [L.] intermediate; in anatomy, denoting a structure lying between a lateral and a medial structure.

in·ter·men·stru·al (-men′stroo-il) occurring between the menstrual periods.

in·ter·mit·tent (-mit′ent) marked by alternating periods of activity and inactivity.

in·ter·mu·ral (-mu′ral) situated between the walls of organs.

in·ter·mus·cu·lar (-mus′ku-lar) situated between muscles.

in·tern (in′tern) a medical graduate serving in a hospital preparatory to being licensed to practice medicine.

in·ter·nal (in-ter′n'l) situated or occurring on the inside; in anatomy, many structures formerly called internal are now termed medial.

in·ter·nal·iza·tion (in-ter″nal-ĭ-za′shun) a mental mechanism whereby certain external attributes, attitudes, or standards of others are unconsciously taken as one's own.

in·ter·na·tal (in″ter-na′t'l) intergluteal.

in·ter·neu·ron (-noor′on) 1. a neuron between the primary sensory neuron and the final motoneuron. 2. any neuron whose processes are entirely confined within a specific area, as within the olfactory lobe.

in·tern·ist (in-ter′nist) a specialist in internal medicine.

in·tern·ship (in′tern-ship) the position or term of service of an intern in a hospital.

in·ter·nu·cle·ar (in″ter-noo′kle-er) situated between nuclei or between nuclear layers of the retina.

in·ter·nun·ci·al (-nun′shil) transmitting impulses between two different parts.

in·ter·nus (in-ter′nus) [L.] internal; in anatomy, denoting a structure nearer to the center of an organ or part.

in·ter·oc·clu·sal (in″ter-ah-kloo′z′l) situated between the occlusal surfaces of opposing teeth in the two dental arches.

in·tero·cep·tor (-sep′ter) a sensory nerve ending that is located in and transmits impulses from the viscera. **interocep′tive,** adj.

in·ter·oc·u·lar (-ok′u-lar) between the eyes.

in·ter·os·se·ous (-os′e-us) between bones.

in·ter·pa·ri·e·tal (-pah-ri′ĕ-t′l) 1. intermural. 2. between the parietal bones.

in·ter·pe·dun·cu·lar (-pĕ-dunk′u-lar) situated between two peduncles, as between two cerebellar peduncles.

in·ter·phase (in′ter-fāz) the interval between two successive cell divisions, during which the chromosomes are not individually distinguishable.

in·ter·pleu·ral (-ploor′al) between two layers of the pleura.

in·ter·po·lat·ed (in-ter′po-la″ted) inserted between other elements or parts.

in·ter·po·la·tion (in-ter″po-la′shun) the determination of intermediate values in a series on the basis of observed values.

in·ter·pre·ta·tion (-prĕ-ta′shun) in psychotherapy, the therapist's explanation to the patient of the latent or hidden meanings of what the patient says, does, or experiences.

in·ter·prox·i·mal (in″ter-prok′sĭ-mal) between two adjoining surfaces.

in·ter·ra·dic·u·lar (-rah-dik′u-lar) between or among roots or radicles.

in·ter·sec·tio (-sek′she-o) pl. *intersectio′nes.* [L.] intersection. **i. tendi′nea,** a fibrous band traversing the belly of a muscle, dividing it into two parts.

in·ter·sec·tion (-sek′shun) a site at which one structure crosses another.

in·ter·sex (in′ter-seks) 1. hermaphrodite. 2. pseudohermaphrodite. 3. intersexuality. **female i.,** a female pseudohermaphrodite. **male i.,** a male pseudohermaphrodite. **true i.,** a true hermaphrodite.

in·ter·sex·u·al·i·ty (in″ter-sek″shoo-al′ĭ-te) 1. hermaphroditism. 2. pseudohermaphroditism. 3. androgyny. **intersex′ual,** adj.

in·ter·space (in′ter-spās) a space between similar structures.

in·ter·stice (in-ter′stis) a small interval, space, or gap in a tissue or structure.

in·ter·sti·tial (in″ter-stish′′l) pertaining to parts or interspaces of a tissue.

in·ter·sti·ti·um (-stish′ĭ-um) 1. interstice. 2. interstitial tissue.

in·ter·tha·lam·ic (-thah-lam′ik) between thalami, particularly the optic thalami.

in·ter·trans·verse (-tranz-vers′) between transverse processes of the vertebrae.

in·ter·tri·go (-tri′go) an erythematous skin eruption occurring on apposed skin surfaces.

in·ter·tro·chan·ter·ic (-tro″kan-ter′ik) situated in or pertaining to the space between the greater and lesser trochanters.

in·ter·ure·ter·al (-u-re′ter-ahl) interureteric.

in·ter·ure·ter·ic (-u-rĕ-ter′ik) between ureters.

in·ter·vag·i·nal (-vaj′ĭ-nil) between sheaths.

in·ter·val (in′ter-val) the space between two objects or parts; the lapse of time between two events. **atrioventricular (AV) i.,** the time between the start of atrial systole and the start of ventricular systole, equivalent to the P–R interval of electrocardiography. **cardioarterial i.,** the time between the apex beat and arterial pulsation. **confidence i.,** an estimated statistical interval for a parameter, giving a range of values that may contain the parameter and the degree of confidence that it is in fact there. **coupling i.,** the length of time between an ectopic beat and the sinus beat preceding it; in an arrhythmia characterized by such beats, the intervals may be constant *(fixed coupling i's)* or inconstant *(variable coupling i's).* **escape i.,** the interval between an escape beat and the normal beat preceding it. **interdischarge i.,** the time between two discharges of the action potential of a single muscle fiber. **interpotential i.,** the time between discharges of action potentials of two different fibers from the same motor unit. **P–R i.,** the portion of the electrocardiogram between the onset of the P wave (atrial depolarization) and the QRS complex (ventricular depolarization). **lucid i.,** 1. a brief period of remission of symptoms in a psychosis. 2. a brief return to consciousness after loss of consciousness in head injury. **pacemaker escape i.,** the period between the last sensed spontaneous cardiac activity and the first beat stimulated by the artificial pacemaker. **P–P i.,** the time from the beginning of one P wave to that of the next P wave, representing the length of the cardiac cycle. **QRS i.,** the interval from the beginning of the Q wave to the termination of the S wave, representing the time for ventricular depolarization. **QRST i., Q–T i.,** the time from the beginning of the Q wave to the end of the T wave, representing the duration of ventricular electrical activity. **systolic time i's (STI),** any of several intervals measured for assessing left ventricular performance, particularly left ventricular ejection time, electromechanical systole, and preejection period. **V–A i.,** the time between a ventricular stimulus and the atrial stimulus following it.

in·ter·ve·nous (in″ter-ve′nus) between veins.

in·ter·ven·tion (-ven′shun) 1. the act or fact of interfering so as to modify. 2. any measure whose purpose is to improve health or alter the course of disease. **crisis i.,** 1. an immediate, short-term, psychotherapeutic approach, the goal of which is to help resolve a personal crisis within the individual's immediate environment. 2. the procedures involved in responding to an emergency. **percutaneous coronary i. (PCI),** the management of coronary artery occlusion by any of various catheter-based techniques, such as percutaneous transluminal coronary angioplasty, atherectomy, excimer laser angioplasty, and implantation of coronary stents and related devices.

in·ter·ven·tric·u·lar (-ven-trik′u-lar) situated between ventricles.

in·ter·ver·te·bral (-ver′tĕ-bral) situated between two contiguous vertebrae; see under *disk.*

in·ter·vil·lous (-vil′us) between or among villi.

in·tes·tine (in-tes′tin) the part of the alimentary canal extending from the pyloric opening of the stomach to the anus. See Plate 27. **intes′tinal,** adj. **large i.,** the distal portion of the intestine, about 5 feet long, extending from its junction with the small intestine to the anus and comprising the cecum, colon, rectum, and anal canal. **small i.,** the proximal portion of the intestine, about 20 feet long, smaller in caliber than the large intestine, extending from the pylorus to the cecum and comprising the duodenum, jejunum, and ileum.

in·tes·ti·num (in″tes-ti′num) pl. *intesti′na.* [L.] intestine.

in·ti·ma (in′tĭ-mah) 1. innermost. 2. tunica intima vasorum. **in′timal,** adj.

in·ti·mi·tis (in″tĭ-mi′tis) endangiitis.

in·tol·er·ance (in-tol′er-ans) inability to withstand or consume; inability to absorb or metabolize nutrients. **congenital lysine i.,** an inherited disorder due to a defect in the degradation of lysine, characterized by vomiting, rigidity, and coma, and high levels of ammonia, lysine, and arginine in the blood. **congenital sucrose i.,** a disaccharide intolerance specific for sucrose, usually due to a congenital defect in the sucrase-isomaltase enzyme complex; see *sucrase-isomaltase deficiency.* **disaccharide i.,** a complex of abdominal symptoms after ingestion of normal quantities of dietary carbohydrates, including diarrhea, flatulence, distention, and pain; it is usually due to deficiency of one or more disaccharidases but may be due to impaired absorption or other causes. **drug i.,** 1. inability to continue taking, or difficulty in continuing to take, a medication because of an adverse side effect that is not immunity-mediated. 2. the state of reacting to the normal pharmacologic doses of a drug with the symptoms of overdosage. **hereditary fructose i.,** an inherited disorder of fructose metabolism due to an enzymatic deficiency, with onset in infancy, characterized by hypoglycemia with variable manifestations of fructosuria, fructosemia, anorexia, vomiting, failure to thrive, jaundice, splenomegaly, and an aversion to fructose-containing foods. **lactose i.,** a disaccharide intolerance specific for lactose, usually due to an inherited deficiency of lactase activity in the intestinal mucosa, which may not be manifest until adulthood. *Congenital lactose i.* may be due to an inherited immediate deficiency of lactase activity or may be a more severe disorder with vomiting, dehydration, failure to thrive, disacchariduria, and cataracts, probably due to abnormal permeability of the gastric mucosa. **lysinuric protein i.,** a hereditary disorder of metabolism involving a defect in dibasic amino acid transport; characterized by growth retardation, episodic hyperammonemia, seizures, mental retardation, hepatomegaly, muscle weakness, and osteopenia; it can be treated with citrulline supplementation.

in·tor·sion (-tor′shun) inward rotation of the upper pole of the vertical meridian of each eye toward the midline of the face.

in·tox·i·ca·tion (-tok″sĭ-ka′shun) 1. stimulation, excitement, or stupefaction caused by a chemical substance, or as if by one. 2. substance i., especially that due to ingestion of alcohol. 3. poisoning; the state of being poisoned. **substance i.,** reversible, substance-specific, maladaptive behavioral or psychological changes directly resulting from the physiologic effects on the central nervous system of recent ingestion of or exposure to a psychoactive substance, particularly alcohol.

intra- word element [L.], *inside; within.*

in·tra·aor·tic (in″trah-a-or′tik) within the aorta.

in·tra·ar·te·ri·al (-ahr-tēr′e-al) within an artery or arteries.

in·tra·ar·tic·u·lar (-ahr-tik′u-lar) within a joint.

in·tra·can·a·lic·u·lar (in″trah-kan″ah-lik′u-ler) within canaliculi.

in·tra·cap·su·lar (-kap′su-lar) within a capsule.

in·tra·car·di·ac (-kahr′de-ak) within the heart.

in·tra·cav·er·no·sal (-kav″er-no′s′l) within the corpus cavernosum.

in·tra·cel·lu·lar (-sel′u-ler) within a cell or cells.

in·tra·cer·vi·cal (-ser′vĭ-k′l) within the canal of the cervix uteri.

in·tra·cra·ni·al (-kra′ne-al) within the cranium.

in·tra·crine (in′trah-krin) denoting a type of hormone function in which a regulatory factor acts within the cell that synthesizes it by binding to intracellular receptors.

in·trac·ta·ble (in-trak′tah-b′l) resistant to cure, relief, or control.

in·tra·cu·ta·ne·ous (in″trah-ku-ta′ne-us) within the skin.

in·tra·cys·tic (-sis′tik) within the bladder or a cyst.

in·tra·cy·to·plas·mic (-si″to-plaz′mik) within the cytoplasm of a cell.

in·tra·der·mal (-der′mal) 1. within the dermis. 2. intracutaneous.

in·tra·duc·tal (-duk′t′l) situated or occurring within the duct of a gland.

in·tra·du·ral (-dūr′′l) within or beneath the dura mater.

in·tra·ep·i·the·li·al (-ep″ĭ-the′le-al) situated among the cells of the epithelium.

in·tra·fal·lo·pi·an (-fah-lo′pe-an) within the uterine (fallopian) tube.

in·tra·fat (-fat′) situated in or introduced into fatty tissue, as the subcutaneous tissue.

in·tra·fu·sal (-fu′z′l) pertaining to the striated fibers within a muscle spindle.

in·tra·lig·a·men·ta·ry (-lig″ah-men′tah-re) intraligamentous.

in·tra·lig·a·men·tous (-lig″ah-men′tus) within a ligament.

in·tra·lob·u·lar (-lob′u-ler) within a lobule.

in·tra·med·ul·lary (-med′u-lar″e) within (1) the spinal cord, (2) the medulla oblongata, or (3) the marrow cavity of a bone.

in·tra·mem·bra·nous (-mem′brah-nus) within a membrane.

in·tra·mu·ral (-mu′r′l) within the wall of an organ.

in·tra·mus·cu·lar (-mus′ku-ler) within the muscular substance.

in·tra·oc·u·lar (-ok′u-lar) within the eye.

in·tra·op·er·a·tive (-op′er-ah-tiv″) occurring during a surgical operation.

in·tra·pa·ri·e·tal (-pah-ri′ĕ-t′l) 1. intramural. 2. within the parietal region of the brain.

in·tra·par·tal (in″trah-pahr′tal) intrapartum.

in·tra·par·tum (-pahr′tum) occurring during childbirth or during delivery.

in·tra·pel·vic (-pel′vik) within the pelvis.

in·tra·peri·to·ne·al (-per″ĭ-to-ne′′l) within the peritoneal cavity.

in·tra·psy·chic (-si′kik) arising, occurring, or situated within the mind.

in·tra·re·nal (-re′n′l) within the kidney.

in·tra·spi·nal (-spīn′′l) within the spinal column.

in·tra·the·cal (-the′k′l) within a sheath; through the theca of the spinal cord into the subarachnoid space.

in·tra·tho·rac·ic (-thah-ras′ik) endothoracic.

in·tra·tra·che·al (-tra′ke-al) endotracheal.

in·tra·tym·pan·ic (-tim-pan′ik) within the tympanic cavity.

in·tra·uter·ine (-u′ter-in) within the uterus.

in·trav·a·sa·tion (in-trav″ah-sa′shun) the entrance of foreign material into vessels.

in·tra·vas·cu·lar (in″trah-vas′ku-lar) within a vessel.

in·tra·ve·nous (-ve′nus) within a vein or veins. **intrave′nously,** adj.

in·tra·ven·tric·u·lar (-ven-trik′u-lar) within a ventricle.

in·tra·ves·i·cal (-ves′ĭ-k′l) within the urinary bladder.

in·tra·vi·tal (-vīt′′l) occurring during life.

in·tra vi·tam (in′trah vīt′am) [L.] during life.

in·trin·sic (in-trin′sik) situated entirely within or pertaining exclusively to a part.

in·troi·tus (-tro′ĭ-tus) pl. *intro′itus.* [L.] the entrance to a cavity or space.

in·tro·jec·tion (in″trah-jek′shun) a mental mechanism in which the standards and values of other persons or groups are unconsciously and symbolically taken within oneself.

in·tro·mis·sion (-mish′un) the entrance of one part into another.

in·tron (in′tron) a noncoding sequence between two coding sequences within a gene, processed out in the formation of mature mRNA.

in·tro·spec·tion (in″trah-spek′shun) contemplation or observation of one's own thoughts and feelings; self-analysis. **introspec′tive,** adj.

in·tro·sus·cep·tion (-sah-sep′shun) intussusception.

in·tro·ver·sion (-ver′zhun) 1. the turning outside in, more or less completely, of an organ, or the resulting condition. 2. preoccupation with oneself, with reduction of interest in the outside world.

in·tro·vert (in′tro-vert) 1. a person whose interest is turned inward to the self. 2. to turn one's interest inward to the self. 3. a structure that can be turned or drawn inwards. 4. to turn a part or organ inward upon itself.

in·tu·ba·tion (in″too-ba′shun) the insertion of a tube into a body canal or hollow organ, as into the trachea. **endotracheal i.**, insertion of a tube into the trachea for purposes of anesthesia, airway maintenance, aspiration of secretions, lung ventilation, or prevention of entrance of foreign material into the airway; the tube goes through the nose (*nasotracheal i.*) or mouth (*orotracheal i.*). **nasal i.**, insertion of a tube into the respiratory or gastrointestinal tract through the nose. **oral i.**, insertion of a tube into the respiratory or gastrointestinal tract through the mouth.

in·tu·mes·cence (in″too-mes′ins) 1. a swelling, normal or abnormal. 2. the process of swelling. **intumes′cent**, adj.

in·tu·mes·cen·tia (in-too-mĕ-sen′shah) pl. *intumescen′tiae*. [L.] intumescence.

in·tus·sus·cep·tion (in″tah-sah-sep′shun) prolapse of one part of the intestine into the lumen of an immediately adjacent part.

in·tus·sus·cep·tum (-sep′tum) the portion of intestine that has prolapsed in intussusception.

in·tus·sus·cip·i·ens (-sip′e-ens) the portion of intestine containing the intussusceptum.

in·u·lin (in′ūl-in) a starch occurring in the rhizome of certain plants, yielding fructose on hydrolysis, and used in tests of renal function.

in·unc·tion (in-unk′shun) the act of anointing or applying an ointment by rubbing.

in utero (in u′ter-o) [L.] within the uterus.

in vac·uo (vak′u-o) [L.] in a vacuum.

in·vag·i·na·tion (in-vaj″ĭ-na′shun) 1. the infolding of one part within another part of a structure, as of the blastula during gastrulation. 2. intussusception. **basilar i.**, a developmental deformity of the occipital bone and upper end of the cervical spine in which the latter appears to have pushed the floor of the occipital bone upward.

in·va·sion (-va′zhun) 1. the attack or onset of a disease. 2. the simple, harmless entrance of bacteria into the body or their deposition in tissue, as opposed to infection. 3. the infiltration and destruction of surrounding tissue, characteristic of malignant tumors.

in·va·sive (-siv) 1. having the quality of invasiveness. 2. involving puncture of the skin or insertion of an instrument or foreign material into the body; said of diagnostic techniques.

in·va·sive·ness (-nis) 1. the ability of microorganisms to enter the body and spread in the tissues. 2. the ability to infiltrate and actively destroy surrounding tissue, a property of malignant tumors.

in·ven·to·ry (in′ven-tor″e) a comprehensive list of personality traits, aptitudes, and interests; some of the most popular include the *California Personality I. (CPI)*, *Millon Clinical Multiaxial I. (MCMI)*, and *Minnesota Multiphasic Personality I. (MMPI)*.

in·verse (in′vers) 1. reversed in order, effect, or nature. 2. the reciprocal of a particular quantity.

in·ver·sion (in-ver′zhun) 1. a turning inward, inside out, or other reversal of the normal relation of a part. 2. a term used by Freud for homosexuality. 3. a chromosomal aberration due to the inverted reunion of the middle segment after breakage of a chromosome at two points, resulting in a change in sequence of genes or nucleotides. **i. of uterus**, a turning of the uterus whereby the fundus is forced through the cervix, protruding into or completely outside of the vagina. **visceral i.**, the more or less complete right and left transposition of the viscera.

in·ver·te·brate (-ver′tĕ-brāt) 1. having no spinal column. 2. any animal having no spinal column.

in·vest·ment (-vest′mint) material in which a denture, tooth, crown, or model for a dental restoration is enclosed for curing, soldering, or casting, or the process of such enclosure.

in·vet·er·ate (-vet′er-āt) confirmed and chronic; long-established and difficult to cure.

in vi·tro (in ve′tro) [L.] within a glass; observable in a test tube; in an artificial environment.

in vi·vo (ve′vo) [L.] within the living body.

in·vo·lu·crum (in″vo-loo′krum) pl. *involu′cra*. [L.] a covering or sheath, as of a sequestrum.

in·vol·un·tary (in-vol′un-tar″e) 1. independent of the will. 2. contrary to the will.

in·vo·lu·tion (in″vo-loo′shun) 1. a rolling or turning inward. 2. a retrograde change of the body or of an organ, as the retrograde changes in size of the female genital organs after delivery. 3. the progressive degeneration occurring naturally with age, resulting in shriveling of organs or tissues. **involu′tional**, adj.

io·ben·guane (i″o-ben′gwān) a norepinephrine analogue that is taken up by the neuroendocrine cells and concentrated in the hormone storage vesicles; labeled with radioactive iodine, it is used for diagnostic imaging of neuroendocrine tumors and disorders of the adrenal medulla.

io·ce·tam·ic ac·id (-se-tam′ik) a water-soluble iodinated radiopaque x-ray contrast medium used for oral cholecystography.

iod·ic ac·id (i-o'dik) a monobasic acid, HIO_3, formed by oxidation of iodine with nitric acid or chlorates, which has strong acid and reducing properties.

io·dide (i'o-dīd) a binary compound of iodine.

io·din·a·tion (i''o-din-a'shun) the incorporation or addition of iodine in a compound.

io·dine (I) (i'ah-dīn) chemical element (see *Table of Elements*), at. no. 53; it is essential in nutrition, being necessary for synthesis of the thyroid hormones thyroxine and triiodothyronine. Iodine solution is used as a topical antiinfective. See also *radioiodine*. **protein-bound i.,** iodine firmly bound to protein in the serum, determination of which constitutes one test of thyroid function. **radioactive i.,** radioiodine.

io·din·oph·i·lous (i''o-din-of'ĭ-lus) easily stainable with iodine.

io·dism (i'ah-dizm) chronic poisoning by iodine or iodides, with coryza, ptyalism, frontal headache, emaciation, weakness, and skin eruptions.

io·do·der·ma (i-o''do-der'mah) any skin lesion resulting from iodism.

io·do·hip·pu·rate so·di·um (i-o''-do-hip'u-rāt) an iodine-containing compound that has been used as a radiopaque medium in pyelography. When labeled with radioactive iodine, it may be used as a diagnostic aid in determination of renal function and in renal imaging.

io·do·phil (i-o'do-fil) 1. any cell or other element readily stainable with iodine. 2. iodinophilous.

io·do·phil·ia (i-o''do-fil'e-ah) a reaction shown by leukocytes in certain pathologic conditions, as in toxemia and severe anemia, in which the polymorphonuclears show diffuse brownish coloration when treated with iodine or iodides.

io·dop·sin (i''ah-dop'sin) a photosensitive violet pigment found in the retinal cones of some animals and important for color vision.

io·do·quin·ol (i-o''dah-kwin'ol) an amebicide used in the treatment of amebic dysentery; also used topically as an antibacterial and antifungal.

io·hex·ol (i''o-hek'sol) a nonionic, water-soluble, low-osmolality radiopaque medium.

ion (i'on) an atom or molecule that has gained or lost one or more electrons and acquired a positive charge (a cation) or negative charge (an anion). **ion'ic,** adj. **dipolar i.,** zwitterion.

ion·iza·tion (i''on-ĭ-za'shun) 1. any process by which a neutral atom or molecule gains or loses electrons, acquiring a net charge. 2. iontophoresis.

ion·o·phore (i'on-ah-for'') any molecule, as of a drug, that increases the permeability of cell membranes to a specific ion.

ion·to·pho·re·sis (i-on''to-fah-re'sis) the introduction of ions of soluble salts into the body by means of electric current. **iontophoret'ic,** adj.

io·pa·no·ic ac·id (i''o-pah-no'ik) a radiopaque medium used in cholecystography.

io·phen·dy·late (-fen'dĭ-lāt) a radiopaque medium used in myelography.

io·pro·mide (-pro'mīd) a nonionic, low-osmolality radiopaque medium used for cardiovascular imaging, excretory urology, and contrast enhancement in computed tomography.

io·thal·a·mate (-thal'ah-māt) a radiopaque medium for a variety of radiographic procedures, including angiography, arthrography, urography, cholangiography, and computed tomographic imaging; used as the meglumine or sodium salt, or a combination.

io·ver·sol (-ver'sol) a nonionic contrast medium used in angiography and urography and for contrast enhancement in computed tomography.

iox·ag·late (i''ok-sag'lāt) a low-osmolality radiopaque medium, used as the meglumine or sodium salt.

iox·i·lan (i-ok'sĭ-lan) a low-viscosity, low-osmolality, nonionic contrast agent used in arteriography, excretory urography, and computed tomography.

IP intraperitoneal; isoelectric point.

IPAA International Psychoanalytical Association.

ip·e·cac (ip'ě-kak) the dried rhizome and roots of *Cephaelis ipecacuanha* or *C. acuminata;* used as an emetic or expectorant.

ipra·tro·pi·um (ip''rah-tro'pe-um) a synthetic congener of atropine that acts as an anticholinergic agent; used as the bromide salt by inhalation as a bronchodilator and intranasally to relieve rhinorrhea.

IPPB intermittent positive pressure breathing.

ipsi- word element [L.], *same; self.*

ip·si·lat·er·al (ip''sĭ-lat'er-al) situated on or affecting the same side.

IPV poliovirus vaccine inactivated.

IQ intelligence quotient.

Ir iridium.

ir·be·sar·tan (ir''bě-sahr'tan) an angiotensin II receptor antagonist used as an antihypertensive.

ir·id·aux·e·sis (ir''id-awk-se'sis) thickening of the iris.

iri·dec·to·me·so·di·al·y·sis (ir''ĭ-dek''to-me''so-di-al'ĭ-sis) excision and separation of adhesions around the inner edge of the iris.

iri·dec·to·my (-me) excision of part of the iris.

iri·dec·tro·pi·um (ir″ĭ-dek-tro′pe-um) eversion of the iris.

iri·de·mia (ir″ĭ-dēm′e-ah) hemorrhage from the iris.

iri·den·clei·sis (ir″ĭ-den-kli′sis) surgical incarceration of a slip of the iris within a corneal or limbal incision to act as a wick for aqueous drainage in glaucoma.

iri·den·tro·pi·um (ir″ĭ-den-tro′pe-um) inversion of the iris.

iri·de·re·mia (ir″ĭ-dĕ-re′me-ah) congenital absence of the iris.

irid·i·al (i-rid′e-al) iridic.

iri·des (ir′ĭ-dēz) [Gr.] plural of *iris*.

iri·des·cence (ir″ĭ-des′ens) the condition of gleaming with bright and changing colors. **irides′cent**, adj.

irid·e·sis (i-rid′ĕ-sis) repositioning of the pupil by fixation of a sector of iris in a corneal or limbal incision.

irid·ic (-ik) pertaining to the iris.

irid·i·um (Ir) (ĭ-rid′e-um) chemical element (see *Table of Elements*), at. no. 77. **i. Ir 192,** an artificial radioactive isotope with a half-life of 75 days, used in radiotherapy.

irid(o)- word element [Gr.], *iris of the eye; a colored circle.*

iri·do·avul·sion (ir″ĭ-do-ah-vul′shun) complete tearing away of the iris from its periphery.

iri·do·cele (i-rid′ah-sēl) hernial protrusion of part of the iris through the cornea.

iri·do·col·o·bo·ma (ir″ĭ-do-kol″ah-bo′mah) congenital fissure or coloboma of the iris.

iri·do·con·stric·tor (-kon-strik′ter) a muscle element or an agent which acts to constrict the pupil of the eye.

iri·do·cor·ne·al (-kor′ne-al) pertaining to the iris and cornea.

iri·do·cy·cli·tis (-sĭ-kli′tis) inflammation of the iris and ciliary body. **heterochromic i.,** a unilateral low-grade form leading to depigmentation of the iris of the affected eye.

iri·do·cys·tec·to·my (-sis-tek′tah-me) excision of part of the iris to form an artificial pupil.

iri·do·dod·e·sis (ir″ĭ-dod′ĭ-sis) iridesis.

iri·do·di·al·y·sis (ir″ĭ-do-di-al′ĭ-sis) the separation or loosening of the iris from its attachments.

iri·do·di·la·tor (-di-la′ter) a muscle element or an agent which acts to dilate the pupil of the eye.

iri·do·do·ne·sis (-do-ne′sis) tremulousness of the iris on movement of the eye, occurring in subluxation of the lens.

iri·do·ker·a·ti·tis (-ker″ah-ti′tis) inflammation of the iris and cornea.

iri·do·ki·ne·sia (-kĭ-ne′zhah) iridokinesis.

iri·do·ki·ne·sis (-kĭ-ne′sis) contraction and expansion of the iris. **iridokinet′ic,** adj.

iri·do·lep·tyn·sis (-lep-tin′sis) thinning or atrophy of the iris.

iri·do·ma·la·cia (-mah-la′shah) softening of the iris.

iri·do·me·so·di·al·y·sis (-me″so-di-al′ĭ-sis) surgical loosening of adhesions around the inner edge of the iris.

iri·do·mo·tor (-mōt′er) pertaining to movements of the iris.

iri·don·cus (ir″id-ong′kus) tumor or swelling of the eye.

iri·do·peri·pha·ki·tis (ir″ĭ-do-per″ĭ-fah-ki′tis) inflammation of the lens capsule.

iri·do·ple·gia (-ple′jah) paralysis of the sphincter of the iris.

iri·dop·to·sis (ir″id-op-to′sis) prolapse of the iris.

iri·do·rhex·is (ir″ĭ-do-rek′sis) 1. rupture of the iris. 2. the tearing away of the iris.

iri·dos·chi·sis (ir″ĭ-dos′kĭ-sis) splitting of the mesodermal stroma of the iris into two layers, with fibrils of the anterior layer floating in the aqueous.

iri·do·ste·re·sis (ir″ĭ-do-stĕ-re′sis) removal of all or part of the iris.

iri·dot·a·sis (ir″ĭ-dot′ah-sis) surgical stretching of the iris for glaucoma.

iri·dot·o·my (-ah-me) incision of the iris.

iri·no·te·can (i″rĭ-no-te′kan) a DNA topoisomerase inhibitor used as the hydrochloride salt as an antineoplastic in the treatment of colorectal carcinoma.

iris (i′ris) pl. *i′rides.* [Gr.] the circular pigmented membrane behind the cornea, perforated by the pupil. See Plate 30.

iri·tis (i-ri′tis) inflammation of the iris. **irit′ic,** adj. **serous i.,** iritis with a serous exudate.

iri·to·ec·to·my (ir″it-o-ek′tah-me) surgical excision of deposits of after-cataract on the iris, together with iridectomy, to form an artificial pupil.

irit·o·my (i-rit′ah-me) iridotomy.

iron (Fe) (i′ern) chemical element (see *Table of Elements*), at. no. 26; it is an essential constituent of hemoglobin, cytochrome, and other components of respiratory enzyme systems. Depletion of iron stores may result in iron-deficiency anemia, and various salts or complexes of iron are used as hematinics, including *i. dextran, i.-polysaccharide, i. sorbitex,* and *i. sucrose.*

irot·o·my (i-rot′ah-me) iridotomy.

ir·ra·di·ate (ĭ-rād′e-āt) to treat with radiant energy.

ir·ra·di·a·tion (ĭ-ra″de-a′shun) 1. radiotherapy. 2. the dispersion of nervous impulse beyond the normal path of conduction. 3. the application of rays, such as ultraviolet rays, to a substance to increase its vitamin efficiency.

ir·re·duc·i·ble (ir″ĭ-doo′sĭ-b'l) not susceptible to reduction, as a fracture, hernia, or chemical substance.

ir·ri·ga·tion (ir″ĭ-ga′shun) 1. washing by a stream of water or other fluid. 2. a liquid used for such washing. **Ringer's i.,** Ringer's injection packaged for irrigation and used as a topical physiologic salt solution.

ir·ri·ta·bil·i·ty (ir″ĭ-tah-bil′ĭ-te) the quality of being irritable. **myotatic i.,** the ability of a muscle to contract in response to stretching.

ir·ri·ta·ble (ir′ĭ-tah-b'l) 1. capable of reacting to a stimulus. 2. abnormally sensitive to stimuli. 3. prone to excessive anger, annoyance, or impatience.

ir·ri·ta·tion (ir″ĭ-ta′shun) 1. the act of stimulating. 2. a state of overexcitation and undue sensitivity. **ir′ritative,** adj.

IRV inspiratory reserve volume.

is·che·mia (is-ke′me-ah) deficiency of blood in a part, usually due to functional constriction or actual obstruction of a blood vessel. **ische′mic,** adj. **silent i.,** cardiac ischemia without pain or other symptoms.

is·chi·al (is′ke-il) ischiatic; pertaining to the ischium.

is·chi·at·ic (is″ke-at′ik) ischial.

ischi(o)- word element [Gr.], *ischium.*

is·chio·anal (is″ke-o-a′n'l) pertaining to the ischium and anus.

is·chio·cap·su·lar (-kap′su-lar) pertaining to the ischium and the capsular ligament of the hip joint.

is·chio·coc·cyg·e·al (-kok-sij′e-il) pertaining to the ischium and coccyx.

is·chio·dyn·ia (-din′e-ah) pain in the ischium.

is·chio·glu·te·al (-gloo′te-al) pertaining to the ischium and the buttocks.

is·chio·pu·bic (-pu′bik) pertaining to the ischium and pubes.

is·chio·rec·tal (-rek′t'l) pertaining to the ischium and rectum.

is·chi·um (is′ke-um) pl. *is′chia.* [L.] see *Table of Bones* and Plate 1.

isch·uria (is-kūr′e-ah) retention of the urine. **ischuret′ic,** adj.

is·ei·ko·nia (i″si-ko′ne-ah) isoiconia. **iseikon′ic,** adj.

is·eth·i·o·nate (i″sĕ-thi′ah-nāt) USAN contraction for 2-hydroxyethanesulfonate.

is·land (i′lind) a cluster of cells or isolated piece of tissue. **blood i's,** aggregations of mesenchymal cells in the angioblast of the early embryo, developing into vascular endothelium and blood cells. **bone i.,** a benign focus of mature cortical bone within trabecular bone on a radiograph. **i's of Langerhans,** see under *islet.* **i's of pancreas,** islets of Langerhans. **i. of Reil,** insula.

is·let (-lit) an island. **i's of Langerhans,** irregular microscopic structures scattered throughout the pancreas and comprising its endocrine portion. They contain the *alpha cells,* which secrete the hyperglycemic factor glucagon; the *beta cells,* which secrete insulin; the *delta cells,* which secrete somatostatin; and the *PP* (or *F*) *cells,* which secrete pancreatic polypeptide. Degeneration of the beta cells is one of the causes of diabetes mellitus.

is(o)- word element [Gr.], *equal; alike; same; uniform.*

iso·ag·glu·ti·nin (i″so-ah-gloot′in-in) an isoantigen that acts as an agglutinin.

iso·al·lele (-ah-lēl′) an allelic gene that is considered as being normal but can be distinguished from another allele by its differing phenotypic expression when in combination with a dominant mutant allele.

iso·an·ti·body (-an′tĭ-bod″e) an antibody produced by one individual that reacts with isoantigens of another individual of the same species.

iso·an·ti·gen (-jen) an antigen existing in alternative (allelic) forms, thus inducing an immune response when one form is transferred to members who lack it; typical isoantigens are the blood group antigens.

iso·bar (i′so-bahr) one of two or more chemical species with the same atomic weight but different atomic numbers.

iso·bar·ic (i″so-bar′ik) having equal or constant pressure or weight across space or time.

iso·car·box·a·zid (i″so-kahr-bok′sah-zid) a monoamine oxidase inhibitor used as an antidepressant and in the prophylaxis of migraine.

iso·cel·lu·lar (-sel′u-ler) made up of identical cells.

iso·chro·mat·ic (-kro-mat′ik) of the same color throughout.

iso·chro·mo·some (-kro′mah-sōm) an abnormal chromosome having a median centromere and two identical arms, formed by transverse, rather than normal longitudinal, splitting of a replicating chromosome.

iso·chron·ic (-kron′ik) isochronous.

isoch·ro·nous (i-sok′rah-nus) performed in equal times; said of motions and vibrations occurring at the same time and being equal in duration.

iso·ci·trate (i″so-sǐ′trāt) a salt of isocitric acid.

iso·cit·ric ac·id (-sit′rik) an intermediate in the tricarboxylic acid cycle, formed from oxaloacetic acid and converted to ketoglutaric acid.

iso·co·ria (-kor′e-ah) equality of size of the pupils of the two eyes.

iso·cor·tex (-kor′teks) the neocortex as opposed to the allocortex.

iso·cy·tol·y·sin (-si-tol′ĭ-sin) an isoantigen that acts as a cytolysin.

iso·cy·to·sis (-si-to′sis) equality of size of cells, especially of erythrocytes.

iso·dac·tyl·ism (-dak′tĭ-lizm) relatively even length of the fingers.

iso·dose (i′so-dōs) a radiation dose of equal intensity to more than one body area.

iso·elec·tric (i″so-e-lek′trik) showing no variation in electric potential.

iso·en·er·get·ic (-en″er-jet′ik) exhibiting equal energy.

iso·en·zyme (-en′zīm) isozyme.

iso·eth·a·rine (-eth′ah-rēn) a β₂-adrenergic receptor agonist, administered by inhalation in the form of the hydrochloride or mesylate salt as a bronchodilator.

iso·flu·rane (-floo′rān) a potent inhalational anesthetic similar to enflurane, used for induction and maintenance of general anesthesia.

isog·a·my (i-sog′ah-me) reproduction resulting from union of two gametes identical in size and structure, as in protozoa. **isog′a·mous,** adj.

iso·ge·ne·ic (i″so-jĭ-ne′ik) syngeneic.

iso·gen·e·sis (-jen′ě-sis) similarity in the processes of development.

iso·gen·ic (-jen′ik) syngeneic.

isog·e·nous (i-soj′ě-nus) developed from the same cell.

iso·graft (i′sah-graft) syngraft.

iso·hem·ag·glu·ti·nin (i″so-hem″ah-gloot′in-in) an isoantigen that agglutinates erythrocytes.

iso·he·mol·y·sin (-he-mol′ĭ-sin) an isoantigen that causes hemolysis.

iso·ico·nia (-i-ko′ne-ah) a condition in which the image of an object is the same in both eyes. **isoicon′ic,** adj.

iso·im·mu·ni·za·tion (-im″u-nǐ-za′shun) development of antibodies in response to isoantigens.

iso·ki·net·ic (-kǐ-net′ik) maintaining constant torque or tension as muscles shorten or lengthen; see *isokinetic exercise,* under *exercise.*

iso·late (i′sah-lāt) 1. to separate from others. 2. a group of individuals prevented by geographic, genetic, ecologic, social, or artificial barriers from interbreeding with others of their kind.

iso·la·tion (i″sah-la′shun) 1. the process of isolating, or the state of being isolated. 2. the physiologic separation of a part, as by tissue culture or by interposition of inert material. 3. the extraction and purification of a chemical substance of unknown structure from a natural source. 4. the separation of infected individuals from those uninfected for the communicable period. 5. the successive propagation of a growth of microorganisms until a pure culture is obtained. 6. a defense mechanism in which emotions are detached from the ideas, impulses, or memories to which they usually connect.

iso·lec·i·thal (-les′ĭ-thal) having small amounts of yolk evenly distributed throughout the cytoplasm, as in the eggs of mammals.

iso·leu·cine (Ile, I) (-loo′sēn) an essential amino acid produced by hydrolysis of fibrin and other proteins; necessary for optimal infant growth and for nitrogen equilibrium in adults.

isol·o·gous (i-sol′ah-gus) characterized by an identical genotype.

isol·y·sin (i-sol′ĭ-sin) a lysin acting on cells of animals of the same species as that from which it is derived.

iso·mal·tase (i″so-mawl′tās) α-dextrinase.

iso·mer (i′sah-mer) any compound exhibiting, or capable of exhibiting, isomerism. **isomer′ic,** adj.

isom·er·ase (i-som′er-ās) a major class of enzymes comprising those that catalyze the process of isomerization.

isom·e·rism (-ah-rizm) the possession by two or more distinct compounds of the same molecular formula, each molecule having the same number of atoms of each element, but in different arrangement. **geometric i.,** stereoisomerism in which isomers differ in the arrangement of substituents of a rigid structure, such as double-bonded carbon atoms or a ring. **optical i.,** stereoisomerism in which isomers differ in the arrangement of substituents at one or more asymmetric carbon atoms; thus some, but not necessarily all, are optically active. **structural i.,** isomerism in which the compounds have the same molecular but different structural formulas, the linkages of the atoms being different.

isom·er·iza·tion (i-som″er-ĭ-za′shun) the process whereby any isomer is converted into another isomer, usually requiring special conditions of temperature, pressure, or catalysts.

iso·meth·ep·tene mu·cate (i″so-mĕ-thep′tēn mu′kāt) an indirect-acting sympathomimetic amine that constricts dilated carotid and cerebral vessels, used in combination with dichloralphenazone and acetaminophen in the treatment of migraine and tension headache.

iso·met·ric (-met′rik) maintaining, or pertaining to, the same measure of length; of equal dimensions.

iso·me·tro·pia (-mĕ-tro′pe-ah) equality in refraction of the two eyes.

iso·mor·phism (-mor′fizm) identity in form; in genetics, referring to genotypes of polyploid organisms which produce similar gametes even though containing genes in different combinations on homologous chromosomes. **isomor′phous,** adj.

iso·ni·a·zid (-ni′ah-zid) an antibacterial used as a tuberculostatic.

iso·pho·ria (-for′e-ah) equality in the tension of the vertical muscles of each eye.

iso·plas·tic (-plas′tik) syngeneic.

iso·pre·cip·i·tin (-pre-sip′it-in) an isoantigen that acts as a precipitin.

iso·prene (i′so-prēn) an unsaturated, branched chain, five-carbon hydrocarbon that is the molecular unit of the isoprenoid compounds.

iso·pre·noid (i″so-pre′noid) any compound biosynthesized from or containing isoprene units, including terpenes, carotenoids, fat-soluble vitamins, ubiquinone, rubber, and some steroids.

iso·pro·pa·nol (-pro′pah-nol) isopropyl alcohol.

iso·pro·te·re·nol (-pro-ter′ĕ-nol) a sympathomimetic used in the form of the hydrochloride and sulfate salts as a bronchodilator, and in the form of the hydrochloride salt as a cardiac stimulant.

isop·ter (i-sop′ter) a curve representing areas of equal visual acuity in the field of vision.

iso·pyk·no·sis (i″so-pik-no′sis) the quality of showing uniform density throughout, especially the uniformity of condensation observed in comparison of different chromosomes or in different areas of the same chromosome. **isopyknot′ic,** adj.

iso·sen·si·ti·za·tion (i″so-sen″sĭ-tĭ-za′shun) allosensitization.

iso·sex·u·al (-sek′shoo-al) pertaining to or characteristic of the same sex.

isos·mot·ic (i″soz-mot′ik) having the same osmotic pressure.

iso·sor·bide (i″so-sor′bīd) an osmotic diuretic used to reduce intraocular pressure; its dinitrate and mononitrate esters are used

as coronary vasodilators to treat coronary insufficiency and angina pectoris.

Isos·po·ra (i-sos′por-ah) a genus of sporozoan parasites (order Coccidia), found in birds, amphibians, reptiles, and various mammals, including humans; *I. bel′li* and *I. hom′inis* cause coccidiosis in humans.

iso·spore (i′so-spor) 1. an isogamete of organisms that reproduce by spores. 2. an asexual spore produced by a homosporous organism.

isos·then·uria (i″sos-thin-ūr′e-ah) excretion of urine that has not been concentrated by the kidneys and has the same osmolality as that of plasma.

iso·tone (i′so-tōn) one of several nuclides having the same number of neutrons, but differing in number of protons in their nuclei.

iso·to·nia (i″so-to′ne-ah) 1. a condition of equal tone, tension, or activity. 2. equality of osmotic pressure between two elements of a solution or between two different solutions.

iso·ton·ic (-ton′ik) 1. denoting a solution in which body cells can be bathed without net flow of water across the semipermeable cell membrane. 2. denoting a solution having the same tonicity as another solution with which it is compared. 3. maintaining uniform tonus.

iso·tope (i′so-tōp) a chemical element having the same atomic number as another (i.e., the same number of nuclear protons), but having a different atomic mass (i.e., a different number of nuclear neutrons).

iso·trans·plan·ta·tion (i″so-trans-plan-ta′-shun) syngeneic transplantation.

iso·tret·i·noin (i″so-tret′in-o-in) a synthetic form of retinoic acid, used orally to clear cystic and conglobate acne.

iso·tro·pic (-tro′pik) 1. having the same value of a property, e.g., refractive index, in all directions. 2. being singly refractive.

iso·va·ler·ic ac·id (i″so-vah-ler′ik) a carboxylic acid occurring in excess in the plasma and urine in isovalericacidemia.

iso·va·ler·ic·ac·i·de·mia (i″so-vah-ler″ik-as″ĭ-de′me-ah) an aminoacidopathy due to a defect in the pathway of leucine catabolism, characterized by elevated levels of isovaleric acid in the plasma and urine, causing a characteristic odor of sweaty feet, severe acidosis and ketosis, lethargy, convulsions, pernicious vomiting, psychomotor retardation, and in severe cases coma and death.

iso·vo·lu·mic (i″so-vah-loo′mik) maintaining the same volume.

isox·su·prine (i-sok′su-prēn) an adrenergic used as a vasodilator in the form of the hydrochloride salt.

iso·zyme (i'so-zīm) one of the multiple forms in which an enzyme may exist in an organism or in different species, the various forms differing chemically, physically, or immunologically, but catalyzing the same reaction.

is·rad·i·pine (is-rad'ĭ-pēn) a calcium channel blocking agent used alone or with a thiazide diuretic for the treatment of hypertension.

is·sue (ish'oo) a discharge of pus, blood, or other matter; a suppurating lesion emitting such a discharge.

isth·mec·to·my (is-mek'tah-me) excision of an isthmus, especially the isthmus of the thyroid.

isth·mo·pa·ral·y·sis (is″mo-pah-ral'ĭ-sis) isthmoplegia.

isth·mo·ple·gia (-ple'jah) paralysis of the isthmus of the fauces.

isth·mus (is'mus) pl. *isth'mi.* A narrow connection between two larger bodies or parts. **isth'mian,** adj. **i. of auditory tube, i. of eustachian tube,** the narrowest part of the auditory tube at the junction of its bony and cartilaginous parts. **i. of fauces,** the constricted aperture between the cavity of the mouth and the pharynx. **i. of rhombencephalon,** the narrow segment of the fetal brain, forming the plane of separation between the rhombencephalon and cerebrum. **i. of thyroid gland,** the band of tissue joining the lobes of the thyroid gland. **i. of uterine tube,** the narrower, thicker-walled portion of the uterine tube closest to the uterus. **i. of uterus,** the constricted part of the uterus between the cervix and the body of the uterus.

itch (ich) a skin disorder attended with itching. **bakers' i.,** any of several inflammatory dermatoses of the hands, especially chronic monilial paronychia, seen with special frequency in bakers. **barbers' i.,** 1. tinea barbae. 2. sycosis vulgaris. **grain i.,** itching dermatitis due to a mite, *Pyemotes ventricosus,* which preys on certain insect larvae which live on straw, grain, and other plants. **grocers' i.,** a vesicular dermatitis caused by certain mites found in stored hides, dried fruits, grain, copra, and cheese. **ground i.,** the itching eruption caused by the entrance into the skin of the larvae of *Ancylostoma duodenale* or *Necator americanus;* see *hookworm disease.* **jock i.,** tinea cruris. **swimmers' i.,** an itching dermatitis due to penetration into the skin of larval forms (cercariae) of schistosomes, occurring in bathers in waters infested with these organisms. **winter i.,** xerotic eczema.

itch·ing (ich'ing) pruritus; an unpleasant cutaneous sensation, provoking the desire to scratch or rub the skin.

iter (i'ter) a tubular passage. **i'teral,** adj. **i. ad infundi'bulum,** the passage from the third ventricle of the brain to the infundibulum (1). **i. chor'dae ante'rius,** the opening through which the chorda tympani nerve exits the tympanic cavity. **i. chor'dae poste'rius,** the opening through which the chorda tympani nerve enters the tympanic cavity. **i. den'tium,** the passage through which a permanent tooth erupts through the gums.

IU International unit.

-itis word element [Gr.], *inflammation.*

it·ra·co·na·zole (it″rah-kon'ah-zōl) a triazole antifungal used in a variety of infections.

IUD intrauterine device.

IUGR intrauterine growth retardation (or restriction).

IV intravenous.

IVF in vitro fertilization.

Ix·o·des (iks-o'dēz) a genus of parasitic ticks (family Ixodidae); some species are disease vectors.

ix·o·di·a·sis (ik″sah-di'ah-sis) any disease or lesion due to tick bites; infestation with ticks.

ix·o·did (ik'so-did) a tick, or pertaining to a tick, of the genus *Ixodes.*

Ix·od·i·dae (iks-od'ĭ-de) a family of ticks (superfamily Ixodoidea), comprising the hard-bodied ticks.

Ix·od·i·des (-dēz) the ticks, a suborder of Acarina, including the superfamily Ixodoidea.

Ix·o·doi·dea (iks″o-doid'e-ah) a superfamily of arthropods (suborder Ixodides), comprising both the hard- and soft-bodied ticks.

J

J joule.

jack·et (jak'it) an enveloping structure or garment for the trunk or upper part of the body. **plaster-of-Paris j.,** a casing of plaster of Paris enveloping the body, to support or correct deformities. **strait j.,** informal name for *camisole.*

jack·screw (-skroo) a screw-turned device to expand the dental arch and move individual teeth.

jac·ti·ta·tion (jak"tĭ-ta'shun) restless tossing to and fro in acute illness.

jaun·dice (jawn'dis) icterus; yellowness of the skin, scleras, mucous membranes, and excretions due to hyperbilirubinemia and deposition of bile pigments. **acholuric j.,** jaundice without bilirubinemia, associated with elevated unconjugated bilirubin that is not excreted by the kidney. **acholuric familial j.,** hereditary spherocytosis. **breast milk j.,** elevated unconjugated bilirubin in some breast-fed infants due to the presence of 5-β-pregnane-3-α-20-β-diol in breast milk, which inhibits glucuronyl transferase conjugating activity, or to dehydration. **cholestatic j.,** that resulting from abnormal bile flow in the liver. **hemolytic j.,** that due to increased production of bilirubin from hemoglobin under conditions causing accelerated degradation of erythrocytes. **hepatocellular j.,** that due to injury to or disease of liver cells. **hepatogenic j., hepatogenous j.,** that due to disease or disorder of the liver. **leptospiral j.,** Weil's syndrome. **mechanical j.,** obstructive j. **neonatal j., j. of the newborn,** icterus neonatorum. **nuclear j.,** kernicterus. **obstructive j.,** that due to blocking of bile flow. **physiologic j.,** mild icterus neonatorum lasting the first few days of life. **retention j.,** that due to inability of the liver to dispose of the bilirubin provided by the circulating blood.

jaw (jaw) either of the two bony tooth-bearing structures (mandible and maxilla) in the head of dentate vertebrates. **cleft j.,** a cleft between the median nasal and maxillary prominences through the alveolus. **Hapsburg j.,** a mandibular prognathous jaw, often accompanied by Hapsburg lip. **phossy j.,** phosphorus necrosis.

JCV JC virus.

je·ju·nal (jĕ-joo'n'l) pertaining to the jejunum.

je·ju·nec·to·my (jĕ"joo-nek'tah-me) excision of the jejunum.

je·ju·no·ce·cos·to·my (jĕ-joo"no-se-kos'-tah-me) anastomosis of the jejunum to the cecum.

je·ju·no·il·e·itis (-il"e-i'tis) inflammation of the jejunum and ileum.

je·ju·no·je·ju·nos·to·my (-jĕ"joo-nos'tah-me) anastomosis between two portions of the jejunum.

je·ju·nos·to·my (jĕ"joo-nos'tah-me) the creation of a permanent opening between the jejunum and the surface of the abdominal wall.

je·ju·not·o·my (-not'ah-me) incision of the jejunum.

je·ju·num (jĕ-joo'num) that part of the small intestine extending from the duodenum to the ileum.

jel·ly (jel'e) a soft substance that is coherent, tremulous, and more or less translucent; generally, a colloidal semisolid mass. **cardiac j.,** a gelatinous substance present between the endothelium and myocardium of the embryonic heart, which transforms into the connective tissue of the endocardium. **contraceptive j.,** a nongreasy jelly used in the vagina for prevention of conception. **petroleum j.,** petrolatum. **Wharton's j.,** the intracellular mucoid connective tissue of the umbilical cord.

jerk (jurk) a sudden reflex or involuntary movement. **jer'ky,** adj. **Achilles j., ankle j.,** triceps surae reflex. **biceps j.,** see under *reflex.* **elbow j.,** triceps reflex. **jaw j.,** see under *reflex.* **knee j., quadriceps j.,** patellar reflex. **tendon j.,** see under *reflex.* **triceps surae j.,** see under *reflex.*

jim·son weed (jim'son wēd) stramonium.

jing (jing) [Chinese] one of the basic substances that according to traditional Chinese medicine pervade the body, usually translated as "essence"; the body reserves or constitutional makeup, replenished by food and rest, that supports life and is associated with developmental changes in the organism.

joint (joint) the site of junction or union between bones, especially one that allows motion of the bones. **amphidiarthrodial j.,**

463

amphidiarthrosis. **arthrodial** j., plane j. **ball-and-socket** j., spheroidal j. **biaxial** j., one with two chief axes of movement, at right angles to each other. **bicondylar** j., a condylar joint with a meniscus between the articular surfaces, such as the temporomandibular joint. **bilocular** j., one with two synovial compartments separated by an interarticular cartilage. **cartilaginous** j., a type of synarthrosis in which the bones are united by cartilage. **Charcot's** j., neuropathic arthropathy. **Chopart's** j., one between the calcaneus and the cuboid bone and the talus and navicular bone. **cochlear** j., a hinge joint that permits some rotation or lateral motion. **composite** j., **compound** j., one in which several bones articulate. **condylar** j., **condyloid** j., ellipsoidal joint; one in which an ovoid head of one bone moves in an elliptical cavity of another, permitting all movements except axial rotation. **diarthrodial** j., synovial j. **elbow** j., the articulation between the humerus, ulna, and radius. **ellipsoidal** j., condylar j. **enarthrodial** j., spheroidal j. **facet j's,** the articulations of the vertebral column. **false** j., pseudarthrosis. **fibrocartilaginous** j., symphysis. **fibrous** j., a type of synarthrosis in which the bones are united by continuous intervening fibrous tissue. **flail** j., an unusually mobile joint. **ginglymoid** j., ginglymus. **gliding** j., plane j. **hinge** j., ginglymus. **hip** j., the spheroidal joint between the head of the femur and the acetabulum of the hip bone. **immovable** j., fibrous j. **intercarpal j's,** the articulations between the carpal bones. **knee** j., the compound joint between the femur, patella, and tibia. **Lisfranc's** j., the articulation between the tarsal and metatarsal bones. **mixed** j., one combining features of different types of joints. **multiaxial** j., spheroidal j. **neurocentral** j., a synchondrosis between the body of a vertebra and either half of the vertebral arch. **peg-and-socket** j., gomphosis. **pivot** j., a uniaxial joint in which one bone pivots within a bony or an osseoligamentous ring. **plane** j., a synovial joint in which the opposed surfaces are flat or only slightly curved. **polyaxial** j., spheroidal j. **rotary** j., pivot j. **saddle** j., one having two saddle-shaped surfaces at right angles to each other. **simple** j., one in which only two bones articulate. **spheroidal** j., ball-and-socket joint; a synovial joint in which a round surface on one bone ("ball") moves within a concavity ("socket") on the other bone. **spiral** j., cochlear j. **synarthrodial** j., fibrous j. **synovial** j., diarthrosis; a joint that permits more or less free motion, the union of the bony elements being surrounded by an articular capsule enclosing a cavity lined by synovial membrane. **temporomandibular** j., a bicondylar joint formed by the head of the mandible and the mandibular fossa, and the articular tubercle of the temporal bone. **trochoid** j., pivot j. **uniaxial** j., one which permits movement in one axis only. **unilocular** j., a synovial joint having only one cavity.

joule (J) (jōol) the SI unit of energy, being the work done by a force of 1 newton acting over a distance of 1 meter.

ju·gal (joo′g'l) pertaining to the cheek.

ju·ga·le (joo-ga′le) jugal point.

jug·u·lar (jug′u-lar) 1. cervical. 2. pertaining to a jugular vein. 3. a jugular vein.

ju·gum (joo′gum) pl. *ju′ga.* [L.] yoke; a depression or ridge connecting two structures.

juice (jōos) any fluid from animal or plant tissue. **gastric** j., the secretion of the gastric glands. **intestinal** j., the secretion of glands in the intestinal lining. **pancreatic** j., the enzyme-containing secretion of the pancreas, conducted through its ducts to the duodenum.

jump·ing (jump′ing) 1. the skipping of several steps in a series. 2. see under *disease.*

junc·tio (junk′she-o) pl. *junctio′nes.* [L.] junction.

junc·tion (-shun) the place of meeting or coming together. **junc′tional,** adj. **adherent** j., a type of intercellular junction that links cell membranes and cytoskeletal elements within and between cells, connecting adjacent cells mechanically. **ameloodentinal** j., dentinoenamel j. **atrioventricular** j., **AV** j., part or all of the region comprising the atrioventricular node and the bundle of His, with the bundle branches sometimes specifically excluded. **cementoenamel** j., the line at which the cementum covering the root of a tooth and the enamel covering its crown meet, designated anatomically as the cervical line. **dentinocemental** j., the line of meeting of the dentin and cementum on the root of a tooth. **dentinoenamel** j., the plane of meeting between dentin and enamel on the crown of a tooth. **esophagogastric** j., the site of transition from the stratified squamous epithelium of the esophagus to the simple columnar epithelium of the cardia of the stomach. **gap** j., a narrowed portion of the intercellular space containing channels linking adjacent cells and through which pass ions, most sugars, amino acids, nucleotides, vitamins, hormones, and cyclic AMP. In electrically excitable tissues, these gap junctions transmit electrical impulses via ionic currents and are known as *electrotonic synapses.*

or eliminating the intercellular passage of molecules. **ureteropelvic j.,** the junction between the ureter and the renal pelvis.

gastroesophageal j., esophagogastric j. **ileocecal j.,** the junction of the ileum and cecum, located at the lower right side of the abdomen and fixed to the posterior abdominal wall. **intercellular j's,** specialized regions on the borders of cells that provide connections between adjacent cells. **mucocutaneous j.,** the site of transition between skin and mucous membrane. **mucogingival j.,** the histologically distinct line marking the separation of the gingival tissue from the oral mucosa. **myoneural j., neuromuscular j.,** the site of apposition between a nerve fiber and the motor end plate of the skeletal muscle which it innervates. **occluding j.,** tight j. **sclerocorneal j.,** corneal limbus. **tight j.,** an intercellular junction at which adjacent plasma membranes are joined tightly together by interlinked rows of integral membrane proteins, limiting

junc·tu·ra (junk-too′rah) pl. *junctu′rae.* [L.] junction; joint.

jur·is·pru·dence (joor″is-proo′dens) the science of the law. **medical j.,** the science of the law as applied to the practice of medicine.

ju·ve·nile (ju′vin-īl) 1. pertaining to youth or childhood. 2. a youth or child; a young animal. 3. a cell or organism intermediate between immature and mature forms.

juxta- word element [L.], *situated near; adjoining.*

jux·ta·ar·tic·u·lar (juks″tah-ahr-tik′u-lar) situated near or in the region of a joint.

jux·ta·glo·mer·u·lar (-glo-mer′u-ler) near or next to a renal glomerulus.

jux·ta·po·si·tion (-pah-zish′un) apposition.

K

K kelvin; lysine; potassium (L. *ka′lium*).

K_M, K_m Michaelis constant.

k kilo-.

κ (kappa, the tenth letter of the Greek alphabet) one of the two types of immunoglobulin light chains.

kak- for words beginning thus, see those beginning *cac-*.

ka·la-azar (kah″lah-ah-zahr′) [Hindi] visceral leishmaniasis.

ka·li·ure·sis (ka″le-u-re′sis) the excretion of potassium in the urine. **kaliuret′ic,** adj.

kal·li·din (kal′ĭ-din) lysyl-bradykinin, a decapeptide kinin produced by the action of tissue and glandular kallikreins on LMW kininogen and having physiologic effects similar to those of bradykinin.

kal·li·kre·in (kal″ĭ-kre′in) any of several serine proteinases that cleave kininogens to form kinins. **plasma k.,** a plasma hydrolase that cleaves HMW kininogen to produce bradykinin and also activates blood coagulation factors XII and VII and plasminogen. **tissue k.,** a hydrolase of tissues and various glandular secretions that cleaves LMW kininogen to form kallidin.

kal·li·kre·in·o·gen (-kre-in′ah-jen) prekallikrein.

kam·po (kahm′po) [Japanese] herbal medicine as practiced in Japan, having its origin in traditional Chinese medicine.

kan·a·my·cin (kan″ah-mi′sin) an aminoglycoside antibiotic derived from *Streptomyces kanamyceticus,* effective against aerobic gramnegative bacilli and some gram-positive bacteria, including mycobacteria; used as the sulfate salt.

kan·po (kahn′po) kampo.

ka·o·lin (ka′o-lin) native hydrated aluminum silicate, powdered and freed from gritty particles by elutriation; used as an adsorbent and, often with pectin, an antidiarrheal.

ka·o·lin·o·sis (ka″o-lin-o′sis) pneumoconiosis from inhaling particles of kaolin.

ka·pha (kah′fah) [Sanskrit] in ayurveda, one of the three doshas, condensed from the elements water and earth. It is the principle of stabilizing energy, governs growth in the body and mind, is concerned with structure, stability, lubrication, and fluid balance, and is eliminated from the body through the urine.

kar·ma (kahr′mah) [Sanskrit] in Indian philosophy, the total effect of a person's actions, both mental and physical, on his or her existence; a person's present state, including health, is determined by actions from previous existence, and present actions determine their destiny for future existence.

kary(o)- word element [Gr.], *nucleus.*

kary·og·a·my (kar″e-og′ah-me) cell conjugation with union of nuclei.

karyo·ki·ne·sis (kar″e-o-kǐ-ne′sis) division of the nucleus, usually an early stage in the process of cell division, or mitosis. **karyokinet′ic,** adj.

karyo·lymph (kar′e-o-limf′) the liquid portion of the nucleus of a cell, in which the other elements are dispersed.

kary·ol·y·sis (kar″e-ol′ǐ-sis) the dissolution of the nucleus of a cell. **karyolyt′ic,** adj.

karyo·mor·phism (kar″e-o-mor′fizm) the shape of a cell nucleus.

karyo·phage (kar′e-o-fāj″) a protozoan that phagocytizes the nucleus of the cell it infects.

karyo·pyk·no·sis (kar″e-o-pik-no′sis) shrinkage of a cell nucleus, with condensation of the chromatin. **karyopyknot′ic,** adj.

kary·or·rhex·is (-rek′sis) rupture of the cell nucleus in which the chromatin disintegrates into formless granules that are extruded from the cell. **karyorrhec′tic,** adj.

karyo·some (kar′e-o-sōm″) any of the condensed irregular clumps of chromatin dispersed in the chromatin network of a cell.

karyo·type (-tīp″) the chromosomal constitution of the cell nucleus; by extension, the photomicrograph of chromosomes arranged according to the Denver classification.

kat katal.

kat(a)- word element [Gr.], *down; against.* See also words beginning *cat(a)-.*

kat·al (kat′al) a unit of measurement proposed to express activities of all catalysts, being that amount of a catalyst that catalyzes a reaction rate of 1 mole of substrate per second. Symbol kat.

ka·tol·y·sis (kah-tol′ǐ-sis) the incomplete or intermediate conversion of complex chemical bodies into simpler compounds; applied especially to digestive processes.

ka·va ka·va a preparation of the rhizome of *Piper methysticum,* (kava plant), having muscle-relaxing, anticonvulsive, anxiolytic, and sedative effects; used for the relief of stress and restlessness, and for sleep induction; also used in homeopathy and folk medicine.

kcal kilocalorie.

kD, kDa kilodalton; 1000 daltons.

ke·loid (ke′loid) a sharply elevated, irregularly shaped, progressively enlarging scar due to excessive collagen formation in the dermis during connective tissue repair. **keloid′al,** adj.

kel·vin (K) (kel′vin) the base SI unit of temperature, equal to 1/273.16 of the absolute temperature of the triple point of water.

Ke·pone (ke′pōn) trademark for a nonbiodegradable polychlorinated ketone, used as an insecticide; workers exposed to it have suffered neurologic symptoms such as tremors and slurred speech.

ker·a·sin (ker′ah-sin) older name for a glucocerebroside in which the fatty acid is lignoceric acid.

ker·a·tan sul·fate (ker′ah-tan) either of two glycosaminoglycans (I and II), consisting of repeating disaccharide units of N-acetylglucosamine and galactose, but differing slightly in carbohydrate content and localization. It occurs in cartilage, the cornea, and in the nucleus pulposus and is also an accumulation product in Morquio's syndrome.

ker·a·tec·ta·sia (ker″ah-tek-ta′zhah) protrusion of a thinned, scarred cornea.

ker·a·tec·to·my (ker″ah-tek′to-me) excision of a portion of the cornea; kerectomy. **photorefractive k.,** the correction of ametropia by using an excimer laser to remove a portion of the anterior corneal stroma in order to create a new radius of curvature.

ker·at·ic (ker-at′ik) 1. keratinous. 2. corneal.

ker·a·tin (ker′ah-tin) any of a family of scleroproteins that are the main constituents of epidermis, hair, nails, and horny tissues. The high-sulfur keratin polypeptides of ectodermally derived structures, e.g., hair and nails, are also called *hard k's.*

ker·a·tin·ase (-ās) a proteolytic enzyme that catalyzes the cleavage of keratin.

ker·a·tin·i·za·tion (ker″ah-tin″ǐ-za′shun) conversion into keratin.

ke·rat·i·no·cyte (ker-at′in-o-sīt) the epidermal cell that synthesizes keratin, known in its successive stages in the layers of the skin as basal cell, prickle cell, and granular cell.

ker·a·tin·oid (ker′ah-tin-oid″) a form of keratin-coated tablet insoluble in the stomach but readily soluble in the intestine.

ke·rat·i·no·some (kě-rat′ǐ-no-sōm) lamellar body; a type of spherical granule in cells of the skin that migrates to the cytoplasm and discharges its contents into the intercellular space, where the granules are believed to function as a barrier against foreign substances.

ker·a·tin·ous pertaining to or containing keratin.

ker·a·ti·tis (ker″ah-ti′tis) inflammation of the cornea. **k. bullo′sa,** presence of blebs upon the cornea. **dendriform k., dendritic k.,** herpetic keratitis which results in a branching ulceration of the cornea. **herpetic k.,** 1. that, commonly with dendritic ulceration (*dendriform* or *dendritic k.*), due to infection with herpes simplex virus. 2. that occurring in herpes zoster ophthalmicus. **interstitial k.,** chronic keratitis with deep deposits in the cornea, which becomes hazy. **lattice k.,** bilateral hereditary corneal dystrophy with formation of interwoven filamentous lesions. **microbial k.,** that resulting from bacterial or fungal infection of the cornea, usually associated with soft contact lens wear. **neuroparalytic k.,** that due to injury to the trifacial nerve which prevents closing of the eyelids, marked by dryness and fissuring of the corneal epithelium. **phlyctenular k.,** see under *keratoconjunctivitis.* **sclerosing k.,** keratitis with scleritis. **trachomatous k.,** pannus trachomatosus. **ulcerative k.,** keratitis with ulceration of the corneal epithelium, frequently a result of bacterial invasion of the cornea.

kerat(o)- word element [Gr.], *horny tissue; cornea.*

ker·a·to·ac·an·tho·ma (ker″ah-to-ak″an-tho′mah) a benign, locally destructive, epithelial tumor closely resembling squamous cell carcinoma, manifested as one or more craters, each filled with a keratin plug and usually resolving spontaneously.

ker·a·to·cele (ker′ah-to-sēl″) hernial protrusion of Descemet's membrane.

ker·a·to·cen·te·sis (ker″ah-to-sen-te′sis) puncture of the cornea.

ker·a·to·con·junc·ti·vi·tis (-kon-junk″tĭ-vi′tis) inflammation of the cornea and conjunctiva. **epidemic k.,** a highly infectious form, commonly with regional lymph node involvement, occurring in epidemics; an adenovirus has been repeatedly isolated from affected patients. **phlyctenular k.,** a form marked by formation of a small, gray, circumscribed lesion at the corneal limbus. **k. sic′ca,** a condition marked by hyperemia of the conjunctiva, thickening and drying of the corneal epithelium, itching and burning of the eye and, often, reduced visual acuity. **viral k.,** epidemic k.

ker·a·to·co·nus (-ko′nus) conical protrusion of the central part of the cornea.

ker·a·to·cyst (ker′ah-to-sist) an odontogenic cyst lined with a layer of keratinized squamous epithelium and commonly associated with a primordial cyst.

ker·a·to·der·ma (ker″ah-to-der′mah) 1. hypertrophy of the stratum corneum of the skin. 2. a horny skin or covering. **k. blennorrha′gicum,** pustular psoriasis associated with gonorrhea. **k. climacte′ricum,** an acquired form on the palms and soles, sometimes with fissuring of the thickened patches, in perimenopausal women. **palmoplantar k.,** congenital, hereditary thickening of the skin of the palms and soles,

sometimes with painful fissuring; often associated with other anomalies.

ker·a·tog·e·nous (ker″ah-toj′ĕ-nus) giving rise to a growth of horny material.

ker·a·to·glo·bus (ker″ah-to-glo′bus) a bilateral anomaly in which the cornea is enlarged and globular in shape.

ker·a·to·hel·co·sis (-hel-ko′sis) ulceration of the cornea.

ker·a·to·hy·a·lin (-hi′ah-lin) 1. a substance in the granules in the stratum granulosum of the epidermis, which may be involved in keratinization. 2. a substance found in granules in Hassall corpuscles of the thymus.

ker·a·to·hy·a·line (-hi′ah-līn) 1. both horny and hyaline. 2. pertaining to keratohyalin or to the keratohyalin granules or the stratum granulosum of the epidermis. 3. keratohyalin.

ker·a·to·i·ri·tis (-i-ri′tis) inflammation of the cornea and iris.

ker·a·to·lep·tyn·sis (-lep-tin′sis) removal of the anterior portion of the cornea and replacement with bulbar conjunctiva.

ker·a·to·leu·ko·ma (-loo-ko′mah) a white opacity of the cornea.

ker·a·tol·y·sis (ker″ah-tol′ĭ-sis) softening and separation of the stratum corneum of the epidermis. **pitted k., k. planta′re sulca′tum,** a tropical disease marked by thickening and deep fissuring of the skin of the soles, occurring during the rainy season.

ker·a·to·lyt·ic (ker″ah-to-lit′ik) pertaining to, characterized by, or producing keratolysis, or an agent that so acts.

ker·a·to·ma (ker″ah-to′mah) pl. *keratomas, kerato′mata.* A callus or callosity.

ker·a·to·ma·la·cia (ker″ah-to-mah-la′shah) softening and necrosis of the cornea associated with vitamin A deficiency.

ker·a·tome (ker′ah-tōm) a knife for incising the cornea.

ker·a·tom·e·try (ker″ah-tom′ĭ-tre) measurement of corneal curves. **keratomet′ric,** adj.

ker·a·to·mi·leu·sis (ker″ah-to-mĭ-loo′sis) keratoplasty in which a slice of the patient's cornea is removed, shaped to the desired curvature, and then sutured back on the remaining cornea to correct optical error. **laser-assisted in-situ k. (LASIK),** keratoplasty in which the excimer laser and microkeratome are combined for vision correction; the microkeratome is used to shave a thin slice and create a hinged flap in the cornea, the exposed cornea is reshaped by the laser, and the flap is replaced, without sutures, to heal back into position.

ker·a·to·my·co·sis (-mi-ko′sis) fungal infection of the cornea.

ker·a·to·nyx·is (-nik´sis) keratocentesis.

ker·a·top·a·thy (ker″ah-top´ah-the) noninflammatory disease of the cornea. **band k.**, a condition characterized by an abnormal gray circumcorneal band.

ker·a·to·pha·kia (ker″ah-to-fa´ke-ah) keratoplasty in which a slice of donor's cornea is shaped to a desired curvature and inserted between layers of the recipient's cornea to change its curvature.

ker·a·to·plas·ty (ker´ah-to-plas″te) plastic surgery of the cornea; corneal transplantation. **optic k.**, transplantation of corneal material to replace scar tissue which interferes with vision. **refractive k.**, removal of a section of cornea from a patient or donor, which is shaped to the desired curvature and inserted either between (keratophakia) layers of or on (keratomileusis) the patient's cornea to change its curvature and correct optical errors. **tectonic k.**, transplantation of corneal material to replace tissue which has been lost.

ker·a·to·rhex·is (ker″ah-to-rek´sis) rupture of the cornea.

ker·a·tor·rhex·is keratorhexis.

ker·a·tos·co·py (ker″ah-tos´kah-pe) inspection of the cornea.

ker·a·to·sis (ker″ah-to´sis) pl. *kerato´ses.* Any horny growth, such as a wart or callosity. **keratot´ic,** adj. **actinic k.**, a sharply outlined verrucous or keratotic growth, which may develop into a cutaneous horn, and may become malignant; it usually occurs in the middle-aged or elderly and is due to excessive exposure to the sun. **k. blennorrha´gica,** keratoderma blennorrhagicum. **k. follicula´ris,** a hereditary form marked by areas of crusting, itching, verrucous papular growths which may fuse to form papillomatous and warty malodorous growths. **inverted follicular k.**, a benign usually solitary epithelial tumor originating in a hair follicle and occurring as a flesh-colored nodule or papule. **k. palma´ris et planta´ris,** palmoplantar keratoderma. **k. pharyn´gea,** that characterized by horny projections from the tonsils and the orifices of the lymph follicles in the pharyngeal walls. **k. pila´ris,** hyperkeratosis limited to the hair follicles. **k. puncta´ta,** a hereditary hyperkeratosis in which the lesions are localized in multiple points on the palms and soles. **seborrheic k., k. seborrhe´ica,** a benign tumor of epidermal origin, marked by soft friable plaques with slight to intense pigmentation, most often on the face, trunk, and limbs. **senile k., solar k.**, actinic k.

ker·a·to·sul·fate (ker″ah-to-sul´fāt) keratan sulfate.

ker·a·tot·o·my (ker″ah-tot´ah-me) incision of the cornea. **radial k.**, a series of incisions made in the cornea from its outer edge toward its center in spokelike fashion; done to flatten the cornea and thus to correct myopia.

ker·a·to·to·rus (ker″ah-to-tor´us) a vaultlike protrusion of the cornea.

ke·ri·on (kēr´e-on) a boggy, exudative tumefaction covered with pustules; associated with tinea infections.

ker·nic·ter·us (ker-nik´ter-us) [Ger.] a condition with severe neural symptoms, associated with high levels of bilirubin in the blood.

keta·mine (ke´tah-mēn) a rapid-acting general anesthetic, used as the hydrochloride salt.

ket(o)- word element, *ketone group.*

ke·to ac·id (ke´to) a carboxylic acid containing a carbonyl group.

ke·to·ac·i·do·sis (ke″to-as″ĭ-do´sis) acidosis accompanied by the accumulation of ketone bodies in the body tissues and fluids. **diabetic k.**, see under *acidosis.*

ke·to·ac·id·uria (-as″ĭ-du´re-ah) the presence of keto acids in the urine. **branched-chain k.**, maple syrup urine disease.

ke·to·a·mi·no·ac·i·de·mia (-ah-me″no-as″ĭ-de´me-ah) maple syrup urine disease.

β-ke·to·bu·tyr·ic ac·id (-bu-tēr´ik) acetoacetic acid.

ke·to·gen·e·sis (-jen´ĕ-sis) the production of ketone bodies. **ketogenet´ic, ketogen´ic,** adj.

ke·to·co·na·zole (ke″to-kon´ah-zōl) a derivative of imidazole used as an antifungal agent.

α-ke·to·glu·ta·rate (-gloo´tah-rāt) a salt or anion of α-ketoglutaric acid.

α-ke·to·glu·tar·ic ac·id (-gloo-tar´ik) a metabolic intermediate involved in the tricarboxylic acid cycle, in amino acid metabolism, and in transamination reactions as an amino group acceptor.

ke·tol·y·sis (ke-tol´ĭ-sis) the splitting up of ketone bodies. **ketolyt´ic,** adj.

ke·tone (ke´tōn) any of a class of organic compounds containing the carbonyl group, $C=O$, whose carbon atom is joined to two other carbon atoms, i.e., with the carbonyl group occurring within the carbon chain.

ketonemia excessive ketone bodies in the blood.

ke·ton·uria (ke″to-nu´re-ah) an excess of ketone bodies in the urine.

ke·to·pro·fen (-pro´fen) a nonsteroidal antiinflammatory drug used in the treatment of various rheumatic and nonrheumatic inflammatory disorders, pain, dysmenorrhea, and vascular headaches.

ke·to·ro·lac (ke″to-ro′lak) a nonsteroidal antiinflammatory drug available as the tromethamine salt; used systemically for short-term management of pain; also applied topically to the conjunctiva in the treatment of allergic conjunctivitis and of ocular inflammation following cataract surgery.

ke·tose (ke′tōs) a subgroup of the monosaccharides, being those having a nonterminal carbonyl (keto) group.

ke·to·sis (ke-to′sis) accumulation of excessive amounts of ketone bodies in body tissues and fluids, occurring when fatty acids are incompletely metabolized. **ketot′ic**, adj.

ke·to·ster·oid (ke″to-ster′oid) a steroid having ketone groups on functional carbon atoms. The *17-ketosteroids*, found in normal urine and in excess in certain tumors and in congenital adrenal hyperplasia, have a ketone group on the 17th carbon atom and include certain androgenic and adrenocortical hormones.

ke·to·ti·fen (-ti′fen) a noncompetitive H_1-receptor antagonist and mast cell stabilizer; used topically as the fumarate salt as an antipruritic in the treatment of allergic conjunctivitis.

keV kiloelectron volt; 1000 electron volts.

key·note (ke′nōt) in homeopathy, the characteristic property of a drug that indicates its use in treating a similar symptom of disease.

kg kilogram.

kHz kilohertz; 1000 hertz.

ki (ke) [Japanese] qi.

kid·ney (kid′ne) either of the two organs in the lumbar region that filter the blood, excreting the end-products of body metabolism in the form of urine, and regulating the concentrations of hydrogen, sodium, potassium, phosphate, and other ions in the extracellular fluid. **abdominal k.,** an ectopic kidney just above the iliac crest. **amyloid k.,** one with renal amyloidosis. **artificial k.,** an extracorporeal device through which blood may be circulated for removal of elements that normally are excreted in the urine; a hemodialyzer. **cake k.,** a solid, irregularly lobed organ of bizarre shape, formed by fusion of the two renal anlagen. **cicatricial k.,** a shriveled, irregular, and scarred kidney due to suppurative pyelonephritis. **fatty k.,** one with fatty degeneration. **flea-bitten k.,** one with scattered petechiae on its surface. **floating k.,** nephroptosis. **fused k.,** a single anomalous organ developed as a result of fusion of the renal anlagen. **head k.,** pronephros. **horseshoe**

k., an anomaly in which the right and left kidneys are linked at one end by tissue. **hypermobile k.,** nephroptosis. **lumbar k.,** an ectopic kidney found opposite the sacral promontory in the iliac fossa, anterior to the iliac vessels. **lump k.,** cake k. **medullary sponge k.,** a usually asymptomatic, congenital condition in which small cystic dilatations of the collecting tubules of the renal medulla give the kidney a spongy feeling and appearance. **middle k.,** mesonephros. **pelvic k.,** an ectopic kidney found opposite the sacrum and below the aortic bifurcation. **polycystic k's,** see *polycystic kidney disease*, under *disease*. **primordial k.,** pronephros. **sigmoid k.,** an anomaly in which the two kidneys are fused in the form of a capital Greek letter sigma. **sponge k.,** medullary sponge k. **thoracic k.,** an ectopic kidney that protrudes above the diaphragm into the posterior mediastinum. **waxy k.,** amyloid k.

kilo- word element [Gr.], *one thousand* (10^3), used in naming units of measurement. Symbol k.

kilo·cal·o·rie (kil′o-kal″o-re) a unit of heat equal to 1000 calories. Abbreviated kcal.

kilo·gram (kil′o-gram) the basic SI unit of mass, being 1000 grams, or one cubic decimeter of water; equivalent to 2.205 pounds avoirdupois.

kin·an·es·the·sia (kin″an-es-the′zhah) akinesthesia.

ki·nase (ki′nās) 1. a subclass of the transferases, comprising the enzymes that catalyze the transfer of a high-energy group from a donor (usually ATP) to an acceptor. 2. a suffix used in the names of some enzymes that convert an inactive or precursor form.

kine- word element [Gr.], *movement*. See also words beginning *cine-*.

kine·plas·ty (kin′ĕ-plas″te) use of the stump of an amputated limb to produce motion of the prosthesis.

kine·scope (-skōp) an instrument for ascertaining ocular refraction.

ki·ne·sia (kĭ-ne′zhah) motion sickness.

ki·ne·si·at·rics (ki-ne′se-at′riks) kinesitherapy.

ki·ne·sics (ki-ne′siks) the study of body movement as a part of the process of communication.

ki·ne·si·gen·ic (kĭ-ne″sĭ-jen′ik) caused by movement.

kine·sim·e·ter (kin″ĕ-sim′ĕ-ter) an instrument for quantitative measurement of movements.

kinesi(o)- word element [Gr.], *movement*.

ki·ne·si·ol·o·gy (ki-ne″se-ol′ah-je) 1. the sum of what is known regarding human motion; the study of motion of the human body. 2. a system of diagnosis based on the theory that muscle dysfunction is secondary to subclinical structural, chemical, or mental dysfunction in other parts of the body; using manual muscle testing to help identify the primary dysfunction and treating by attempting to correct the underlying state.

ki·ne·sio·neu·ro·sis (ki-ne″se-o-noor-o′sis) a functional nervous disorder marked by motor disturbances.

ki·ne·sis (kĭ-ne′sis) [Gr.] 1. movement. 2. stimulus-induced motion responsive only to the intensity of the stimulus, not the direction; cf. *taxis*.

-kinesis word termination, *movement* or *activation*.

ki·ne·si·ther·a·py (kĭ-ne″sĭ-ther′ah-pe) the treatment of disease by movements or exercise.

kin·es·the·sia (kin″es-the′zhah) 1. the awareness of position, weight, tension and movement. 2. movement sense. **kinesthet′ic,** adj.

kin·es·the·sis (-sis) kinesthesia.

ki·net·ic (kĭ-net′ik) pertaining to or producing motion.

ki·net·ics (-iks) the scientific study of the turnover, or rate of change, of a specific factor in the body, commonly expressed as units of amount per unit time. **chemical k.,** the study of the rates and mechanisms of chemical reactions.

ki·ne·to·car·dio·gram (kĭ-ne″to-kahr′de-o-gram″) the graphic record obtained by kinetocardiography.

ki·ne·to·car·di·og·ra·phy (-kahr″de-og′rah-fe) the graphic recording of slow vibrations of the anterior chest wall in the region of the heart, the vibrations representing the absolute motion at a given point on the chest.

ki·ne·to·chore (ki-nēt′ah-kōr) centromere.

ki·ne·to·gen·ic (ki-ne″to-jen′ik) causing or producing movement.

ki·ne·to·plast (ki-nēt′o-plast) a structure associated with the basal body in many protozoa, primarily the Mastigophora; it is rich in DNA and, like the basal body, it replicates independently.

ki·ne·to·sis (kĭ″nĕ-to′sis) pl. *kineto′ses.* Any disorder due to unaccustomed motions; see *motion sickness.*

king·dom (king′dum) 1. in the classification of living organisms, the highest of the categories; there are usually considered to be five: Monera, Protista, Fungi, Planta (the plants), and Animalia (the animals). 2. traditionally, one of three major categories into which natural objects are classified: the animal, plant, and mineral kingdoms.

ki·nin (ki′nin) any of a group of vasoactive straight-chain polypeptides formed by kallikrein-catalyzed cleavage of kininogens; causing vasodilation and also altering vascular permeability.

ki·nin·ase II (-ās) see *peptidyl-dipeptidase A.*

ki·nin·o·gen (ki-nin′o-jen) either of two plasma α_2-globulins that are kinin precursors, *HMW (high-molecular-weight) k.,* precursor to bradykinin, and *LMW (low-molecular-weight) k.,* precursor to kallidin.

ki·no·cil·i·um (ki″no-sil′e-um) pl. *kinocil′ia.* A motile, protoplasmic filament on the free surface of a cell.

kin·ship (kin′ship) a group of individuals of varying degrees of descent from a common ancestor.

Kleb·si·el·la (kleb″se-el′ah) a genus of gram-negative bacteria (family Enterobacteriaceae); *K. pneumo′niae* is the etiologic agent of Friedländer's pneumonia and other respiratory infections.

klee·blatt·schä·del (kla′blaht-sha′d′l) [Ger.] cloverleaf skull; a congenital anomaly in which there is intrauterine synostosis of multiple or all cranial sutures.

klep·to·ma·nia (klep″to-ma′ne-ah) compulsive stealing of objects unnecessary for personal use or monetary value.

knee (ne) 1. genu; the area around the articulation of the femur and tibia. 2. any structure resembling this part of the leg. **housemaid's k.,** inflammation of the bursa of the patella, with fluid accumulating within it. **knock k.,** knock-knee. **trick k.,** a popular term for a knee joint susceptible to locking in position, most often due to longitudinal splitting of the medial meniscus.

knock-knee (nok′ne) genu valgum; a deformity of the thigh or leg, or both, in which the knees are abnormally close together and the space between the ankles is increased.

knot (not) 1. an intertwining of the ends or parts of one or more threads, sutures, or strips of cloth. 2. in anatomy, a knoblike swelling or protuberance. **primitive k.,** see under *node.* **surgeon's k., surgical k.,** a knot in which the thread is passed twice through the first loop.

knuck·le (nuk′′l) the dorsal aspect of any phalangeal joint, or any similarly bent structure.

koil(o)- word element [Gr.], *hollowed; concave.*

koi·lo·cyte (koi′lo-sīt″) a concave or hollow cell.

koi·lo·cy·to·sis (koi″lo-si-to′sis) the presence of abnormal koilocytes that are vacuolated with clear cytoplasm or perinuclear halos and nuclear pyknosis. **koilocytot′ic,** adj.

koil·onych·ia (-nik′e-ah) dystrophy of the fingernails in which they are thinned and concave, with raised edges.

koi·lor·rhach·ic (-rak′ik) having a vertebral column in which the lumbar curvature is anteriorly concave.

koi·lo·ster·nia (-sturn′e-ah) pectus excavatum.

kolp- for words beginning thus, see those beginning *colp-*.

ko·ly·pep·tic (ko″le-pep′tik) hindering or checking digestion.

Kr krypton.

krait (krāt) any member of the genus *Bungarus*, extremely venomous crotalid snakes found from India across Southeast and East Asia.

krau·ro·sis (kraw-ro′sis) a dried, shriveled condition. **k. vul′vae,** lichen sclerosus of the female external genitalia, characterized by atrophy, leukoplakic patches on the mucosa, and intense itching.

krypt(o)- for words beginning thus, see those beginning *crypt(o)-*.

kryp·ton (Kr) (krip′ton) chemical element (see *Table of Elements*), at. no. 36. **k. 81m,** an unstable radioactive isotope of krypton having a half-life of 13 seconds and emitting gamma rays (0.19 MeV); used in pulmonary ventilation studies.

kun·da·li·ni (koon″dah-le′ne) 1. in Hindu tradition, psychospiritual energy that lies dormant in the lowest chakra. 2. see under *yoga*.

ku·ru (koo′roo) an infectious form of prion disease with a long incubation period found only in New Guinea and thought to be associated with ritual cannibalism.

kV kilovolt; 1000 volts.

kVp kilovolts peak.

kwash·i·or·kor (kwahsh″e-or′kor) a form of protein-energy malnutrition produced by severe protein deficiency; caloric intake is usually also deficient. Symptoms include retarded growth, changes in skin and hair pigment, edema, immune deficiency, and pathologic changes in the liver. **marasmic k.,** a condition in which there is a deficiency of both calories and protein, with severe tissue wasting, loss of subcutaneous fat, and usually dehydration.

ky·ma·tism (ki′mah-tizm) myokymia.

kyn·uren·ic ac·id (kin″u-ren′ik) a bicyclic aromatic compound formed from kynurenine in a pathway of tryptophan catabolism and excreted in the urine in several disorders of tryptophan catabolism.

kyn·ure·nine (kin″u-rĕ′nēn) an aromatic amino acid, first isolated from dog urine; it is an intermediate in the catabolism of tryptophan.

ky·phos (ki′fos) the hump in the spine in kyphosis.

ky·pho·sco·li·o·sis (ki″fo-sko″le-o′sis) backward and lateral curvature of the spinal column.

ky·pho·sis (ki-fo′sis) abnormally increased convexity in the curvature of the thoracic spine as viewed from the side. **kyphot′ic,** adj. **k. dorsa′lis juveni′lis, juvenile k., Scheuermann's k.,** osteochondrosis of the vertebrae.

kyr·tor·rhach·ic (kir″to-rak′ik) having a vertebral column in which the lumbar curvature is convex anteriorly.

kyt(o)- for words beginning thus, see those beginning *cyt(o)-*.

L

L left; leucine; liter; lung; lumbar vertebrae (L1–L5).

L- chemical prefix specifiying the relative configuration of an enantiomer, indicating a carbohydrate with the same configuration around a specific carbon atom as L-glyceraldehyde or an amino acid having the same configuration as L-serine. Opposed to D-.

l former symbol for *liter*.

l. [L.] ligamen′tum (ligament).

l length.

l- levo- (left, counterclockwise, levorotatory). Opposed to *d*-.

λ (lambda, the eleventh letter of the Greek alphabet) wavelength; one of the two types of immunoglobulin light chains.

La lanthanum.

la·bel (la′b'l) 1. a mark, tag, or other characteristic that identifies something. 2. to provide something with such a characteristic.

radioactive l., a radioisotope that is incorporated into a compound to mark it.

la·bet·a·lol (lah-bet′ah-lol) a beta-adrenergic blocking agent with some alpha-adrenergic blocking activity; used in the form of the hydrochloride salt as an antihypertensive.

la·bia (la′be-ah) plural of *labium*.

la·bi·al (la′be-al) 1. pertaining to a lip or labium. 2. in dental anatomy, pertaining to the tooth surface that faces the lip.

la·bi·al·ly (la′be-il-e) toward the lips.

la·bile (la′bīl) 1. gliding; moving from point to point over the surface; unstable; fluctuating. 2. chemically unstable.

la·bil·i·ty (lah-bil′ĭ-te) 1. the quality of being labile. 2. in psychiatry, emotional instability.

labio- word element [L.], *lip*.

la·bio·al·ve·o·lar (la″be-o-al-ve′ah-ler) 1. pertaining to the lip and dental alveoli. 2. pertaining to the labial side of a dental alveolus.

la·bio·cho·rea (-ko-re′ah) a choreic affection of the lips in speech, with stammering.

la·bio·cli·na·tion (-klī′na-shun) deviation of an anterior tooth from the vertical, in the direction of the lips.

la·bio·graph (la′be-o-graf″) an instrument for recording lip motions in speaking.

la·bio·men·tal (la″be-o-ment′′l) pertaining to the lip and chin.

la·bio·place·ment (-plās′mint) displacement of a tooth toward the lip.

la·bio·ver·sion (-ver′zhun) labial displacement of a tooth from the line of occlusion.

la·bi·um (la′be-um) pl. *la′bia*. [L.] 1. lip. 2. a fleshy border or edge; a liplike structure. 3. in the plural, often used to denote the *labia majora* and *minora pudendi*. **la′bial,** adj. **la′bia majo′ra puden′di,** elongated folds running downward and backward from the mons pubis in the female, one on either side of the rima pudendi. **la′bia mino′ra puden′di,** small skin folds, one on each side, running backward from the clitoris between the labia majora and the vaginal opening. **la′bia o′ris,** the lips of the mouth.

la·bor (la′ber) [L.] the function of the female by which the infant is expelled through the vagina to the outside world: the *first stage* begins with onset of regular uterine contractions and ends when the os is completely dilated and flush with the vagina; the *second* extends from the end of the first stage until the expulsion of the infant is completed; the *third* extends from expulsion of the infant until the placenta and membranes are expelled; the *fourth* denotes the hour or two after delivery, when uterine tone is established. **artificial l.,** induced l. **dry l.,** that in which the amniotic fluid escapes before the onset of uterine contractions. **false l.,** see under *pain.* **induced l.,** that brought on by mechanical or other extraneous means, usually by the intravenous infusion of oxytocin. **missed l.,** that in which contractions begin and then cease, the fetus being retained for weeks or months. **postmature l., postponed l.,** that occurring two weeks or more after the expected date of confinement. **precipitate l.,** that occurring with undue rapidity. **premature l.,** expulsion of a viable infant before the normal end of gestation; usually applied to interruption of pregnancy between the twenty-eighth and thirty-seventh week.

lab·o·ra·to·ry (lab′rah-tor″e) a place equipped for making tests or doing experimental work. **clinical l.,** one for examination of materials derived from the human body for the purpose of providing information on diagnosis, prognosis, prevention, or treatment of disease.

la·brum (la′brum) pl. *la′bra.* [L.] an edge, rim, or lip.

lab·y·rinth (lab′ĭ-rinth) the internal ear, made up of the vestibule, cochlea, and canals. See Plate 29. **labyrin′thine,** adj. **bony l.,** the bony part of the internal ear. **cochlear l.,** the part of the membranous labyrinth that includes the perilymphatic space and the cochlear duct. **endolymphatic l.,** membranous l. **ethmoidal l.,** either of the paired lateral masses of the ethmoid bone, which contain many thin-walled cellular cavities. **membranous l.,** a system of communicating epithelial sacs and ducts within the bony labyrinth, containing the endolymph. **osseous l.,** bony l. **perilymphatic l.,** perilymphatic space. **vestibular l.,** the part of the membranous labyrinth that includes the utricle and saccule and the semicircular ducts.

lab·y·rin·thi·tis (lab″ĭ-rin-thi′tis) otitis interna; inflammation of the labyrinth. **acute serous l.,** a type caused by chemical or toxic irritants that invade the labyrinth, usually from the middle ear. **acute suppurative l.,** a type in which pus enters the labyrinth, usually either through a fistula after infection of the middle ear or through temporal bone erosion from meningitis. **circumscribed l.,** perilabyrinthitis; acute serous labyrinthitis in a discrete area, due to erosion of the bony wall of a semicircular canal with exposure of the membranous labyrinth.

lab·y·rin·thus (lab″ĭ-rin′thus) pl. *labyrin′thi.* [L.] labyrinth.

lac (lak) [L.] 1. milk. 2. any milklike medicinal preparation.

lac·er·at·ed (las'er-āt″ed) torn; mangled; wounded by a jagged instrument.

lac·er·a·tion (las″er-a'shun) 1. the act of tearing. 2. a torn, ragged, mangled wound.

la·cer·tus (lah-ser'tus) [L.] a name given certain fibrous attachments of muscles.

lac·ri·mal (lak'rĭ-mal) pertaining to the tears.

lac·ri·ma·tion (lak″rĭ-ma'shun) secretion and discharge of tears.

lac·ri·ma·tor (lak'rĭ-māt″er) an agent, as a gas, that induces the flow of tears.

lac·ri·mot·o·my (lak″rĭ-mot'ah-me) incision of the lacrimal gland, duct, or sac.

lac·ta·gogue (lak'tah-gog) galactagogue.

lac·tam (lak'tam) a cyclic amide formed from aminocarboxylic acids by elimination of water; lactams are isomeric with lactims, which are enol forms of lactams. **β-l.,** see under *antibiotic.*

β-lac·ta·mase (lak'tah-mās) any of a group of enzymes, produced by almost all gram-negative bacteria, that hydrolyze the β-lactam ring of penicillins and cephalosporins, destroying their antibiotic activity. Individual enzymes may be called *penicillinases* or *cephalosporinases* based on their specificities.

lac·tase (lak'tās) a β-galactosidase occurring in the brush border membrane of the intestinal mucosa that catalyzes the cleavage of lactose to galactose and glucose; it is part of the β-glycosidase enzyme complex.

lac·tase de·fi·cien·cy reduced or absent lactase activity in the intestinal mucosa; the hereditary adult form is the normal state in most populations other than white Northern Europeans and may be characterized by abdominal pain, flatulence, and diarrhea after milk ingestion (lactose intolerance); the rare congenital form (congenital lactose intolerance) is characterized by diarrhea, vomiting, and failure to thrive.

lac·tate (lak'tāt) 1. any salt or ester of lactic acid. 2. to secrete milk.

L-lac·tate de·hy·dro·gen·ase (LDH) (de-hi'dro-jen-ās) an enzyme that catalyzes the interconversion of lactate and pyruvate. It is widespread in tissues and is abundant in kidney, skeletal muscle, liver, and myocardium, appearing in elevated concentrations in the blood when these tissues are injured.

lac·ta·tion (lak-ta'shun) 1. the secretion of milk. 2. the period of milk secretion.

lac·te·al (lak'te-il) any of the intestinal lymphatics that transport chyle.

lac·tes·cence (lak-tes'ins) resemblance to milk.

lac·tic (lak'tik) pertaining to milk.

lac·tic ac·id (lak'tik) CH₃CHOHCOOH, a compound formed in the body in anaerobic metabolism of carbohydrate and also produced by bacterial action in milk. The sodium salt of racemic or inactive lactic acid (*sodium lactate*) is used as an electrolyte and fluid replenisher.

lac·tic·ac·i·de·mia (lak″tik-as″ĭ-de'me-ah) excess of lactic acid in the blood.

lac·ti·ce·mia (lak″tĭ-se'me-ah) lacticacidemia.

lac·tif·er·ous (lak-tif'er-us) conveying milk.

lac·ti·fuge (lak'tĭ-fūj) antigalactic.

lac·tig·er·ous (lak-tij'er-us) lactiferous.

lac·tim (lak'tim) see *lactam.*

lac·ti·tol (-tĭ-tol) a disaccharide analogue of lactulose used as a bulk sweetener; it is also laxative and is used to treat constipation.

lac·tiv·o·rous (lak-tiv'er-us) feeding or subsisting upon milk.

lact(o)- word element [L.], *milk.*

Lac·to·bac·il·la·ceae (lak″to-bas″il-a'se-e) a family of bacteria (order Eubacteriales).

Lac·to·bac·il·lus (-bah-sil'us) a genus of the family Lactobacillaceae. They are anaerobic or microaerophilic and occur widely in nature and in the human mouth, vagina, and intestinal tract. In the oral cavity, they are found associated with dental caries but have no known etiologic role. Some produce only lactic acid and others produce other end products of fermentation. **L. acid·o'philus,** a lactobacillus producing the fermented product, acidophilus milk; preparations are used as digestive aids, for the production of B-complex vitamins, and to help prevent infections after antibiotic treatment.

lac·to·bac·il·lus (-bah-sil'us) pl. *lactobacil′li.* An organism of the genus *Lactobacillus.*

lac·to·cele (lak'to-sēl) galactocele.

lac·to·gen (lak'to-jen) any substance that enhances lactation. **human placental l.,** a hormone secreted by the placenta; it has lactogenic, luteotropic, and growth-promoting activity, and inhibits maternal insulin activity.

lac·to·gen·ic (lak″to-jen'ik) galactopoietic.

lac·to·glob·u·lin (-glob'u-lin) a globulin occurring in milk.

lac·tone (lak'tōn) a cyclic organic compound in which the chain is closed by ester formation between a carboxyl and a hydroxyl group in the same molecule.

lac·to·ovo·ve·ge·ta·ri·an (lak″to-o″vo-vej″ĕ-ter'e-an) ovolactovegetarian.

lac·tor·rhea (-re'ah) galactorrhea.

lac·tose (lak'tōs) a disaccharide occurring in mammalian milk, which on hydrolysis yields glucose and galactose; used as a tablet and capsule diluent, a powder bulking agent, and as a component of infant feeding formulas.

lac·to·side (lak'to-sīd) glycoside in which the sugar constituent is lactose.

lac·tos·uria (-su're-ah) excessive lactose in the urine.

lac·to·trope (lak'to-trōp) lactotroph.

lac·to·troph (-trōf) an acidophil of the adenohypophysis that secretes prolactin.

lac·to·veg·e·tar·i·an (-vej″ĕ-tar'e-an) 1. one who practices lactovegetarianism. 2. pertaining to lactovegetarianism.

lac·to·veg·e·tar·i·an·ism (-tar'e-ah-nizm″) restriction of the diet to vegetables and dairy products, eschewing other foods of animal origin.

lac·tu·lose (lak'tu-lōs) a synthetic disaccharide used as a laxative and to enhance excretion or formation of ammonia in the treatment of hepatic encephalopathy.

la·cu·na (lah-ku'nah) pl. *lacu'nae*. [L.] 1. a small pit or hollow cavity. 2. a defect or gap, as in the field of vision (scotoma). **lacu'nar**, adj. **absorption l.**, resorption l. **bone l.**, a small cavity within the bone matrix, containing an osteocyte; from it slender canaliculi radiate and penetrate the adjacent lamellae to anastomose with the canaliculi of neighboring lacunae, thus forming a system of cavities interconnected by minute canals. **cartilage l.**, any of the small cavities within the cartilage matrix, containing a chondrocyte. **Howship's l.**, resorption l. **intervillous l.**, one of the blood spaces of the placenta in which the fetal villi are found. **lateral lacunae**, venous meshworks within the dura mater on either side of the superior sagittal sinus. **osseous l.**, bone l. **l. pharyn'gis**, a depression at the pharyngeal end of the eustachian tube. **resorption l.**, a pit or groove in developing bone that is undergoing resorption; frequently found to contain osteoclasts. **trophoblastic l.**, intervillous l.

la·cu·nule (lah-ku'nūl) a minute lacuna.

la·cus (la'kus) pl. *la'cus*. [L.] lake.

lae- for words beginning thus, see those beginning *le*-.

La·e·trile (la'ĕ-tril) trademark for *l*-mandelonitrile-β-glucuronic acid, a semisynthetic derivative of amygdalin; it is alleged to have antineoplastic properties. Cf. *laetrile*.

la·e·trile amygdalin (*l*-mandelonitrile-β-gentiobioside) derived from crushed pits of certain fruits, usually apricots, and alleged to have antineoplastic properties. Cf. *Laetrile*.

lae·ve (le've) [L.] nonvillous.

lag (lag) 1. the time between application of a stimulus and the reaction. 2. the period after inoculation of bacteria into a culture medium, in which growth or cell division is slow. **anaphase l.**, delayed movement during anaphase of one homologous chromosome in mitosis or of one chromatid in meiosis, so that the chromosome is not incorporated into the nucleus of one of the daughter cells; the result is one normal cell and one cell with monosomy.

la·ge·na (lah-je'nah) 1. a part of the upper end of the cochlear duct. 2. the organ of hearing in nonmammalian vertebrates.

la·gen·i·form (lah-jen'ĭ-form) flask-shaped.

lag·oph·thal·mos (lag″of-thal'mos) inability to shut the eyes completely.

lake (lāk) 1. to undergo separation of hemoglobin from erythrocytes. 2. a circumscribed collection of fluid in a hollow or depressed cavity. **lacrimal l.**, the triangular space at the medial angle of the eye, where the tears collect. **marginal l's**, discontinuous venous lacunae, relatively free of villi, near the edge of the placenta, formed by merging of the marginal portions of the intervillous space with the subchorial lake. **subchorial l.**, the portion of the placenta, relatively free of villi, just beneath the chorionic plate; at the edge of the placenta it becomes continuous with irregular channels to form the marginal lakes.

lal·la·tion (lah-la'shun) a babbling, infantile form of speech.

lal(o)- word element [Gr.], *speech; babbling.*

lalo·ple·gia (lal″o-ple'jah) logoplegia.

lal·or·rhea (-re'ah) logorrhea.

lamb·da (lam'dah) point of union of the lambdoid and sagittal sutures.

lamb·doid (lam'doid) shaped like the Greek letter lambda, Λ or λ.

Lam·blia (lam'ble-ah) *Giardia.*

lam·bli·a·sis (lam-bli'ah-sis) giardiasis.

lam·bli·o·sis (lam″ble-o'sis) giardiasis.

lame (lām) incapable of normal locomotion; deviating from normal gait.

la·mel·la (lah-mel'ah) pl. *lamel'lae*. [L.] 1. a thin leaf or plate, as of bone. 2. a medicated disk or wafer to be inserted under the eyelid. **circumferential l.**, one of the layers of bone that underlie the periosteum and endosteum. **concentric l.**, haversian l. **endosteal l.**, one of the bony plates lying beneath the endosteum. **ground l.**, interstitial l. **haversian l.**, one of the concentric bony plates surrounding a haversian canal.

intermediate l., interstitial l., one of the bony plates that fill in between the haversian systems. **vitreous l.,** lamina basalis (1).

la·mel·lar (lah-mel′ar) 1. pertaining to or resembling lamellae. 2. lamellated (1).

lam·el·lat·ed (lam′ĕ-lāt″ed) 1. having, composed of, or arranged in lamellae. 2. lamelliform.

la·mel·li·form (lah-mel′ĭ-form) resembling lamellae.

la·mel·li·po·dia (lah-mel″ĭ-po′de-ah) sing. *lamellipo′dium.* Delicate sheetlike extensions of cytoplasm which form transient adhesions with the cell substrate and wave gently, enabling the cell to move along the substrate.

lam·i·na (lam′ĭ-nah) pl. *la′minae.* [L.] 1. layer; a thin, flat plate of a larger composite structure. 2. l. of vertebra. **basal l.,** 1. the layer of the basement membrane lying next to the basal surface of the adjoining cell layer, comprising two layers, the electron-lucent lamina lucida and the electron-dense lamina densa. 2. sometimes, the entire basement membrane. 3. l. basalis. **l. basa′lis,** 1. one of the pair of longitudinal zones of the embryonic neural tube, from which develop the ventral gray columns of the spinal cord and the motor centers of the brain. 2. basal l. (1). **l. basila′ris,** the posterior wall of the cochlear duct, separating it from the scala tympani. **Bowman's l.,** see under *membrane.* **l. choroidocapilla′ris,** the inner layer of the choroid, composed of a single-layered network of small capillaries. **l. cribro′sa,** 1. fascia cribrosa. 2. *(of ethmoid bone)* the horizontal plate of ethmoid bone forming the roof of the nasal cavity, and perforated by many foramina for passage of olfactory nerves. 3. *(of sclera)* the perforated part of the sclera through which pass the axons of the retinal ganglion cells. **l. den′sa,** see *basal l.* (1). **elastic l.,** 1. Bowman's membrane. 2. Descemet's membrane. **epithelial l.,** the layer of ependymal cells covering the choroid plexus. **l. lu′cida,** see *basal l.* (1). **nuclear l.,** a tightly woven meshwork that lines the nuclear side of the inner nuclear membrane; it is believed to control the shape of the nucleus. **l. pro′pria,** 1. the connective tissue layer of mucous membrane. 2. the middle fibrous layer of the tympanic membrane. **l. ra′ra,** lamina lucida; see *basal l.* (1). In the lung alveoli and renal glomeruli, one may occur on each side of the lamina densa. **reticular l.,** 1. a layer of the basement membrane, adjacent to the connective tissue, seen in some

epithelia. 2. l. reticularis. **l. reticula′ris,** the perforated hyaline membrane covering the organ of Corti. **Rexed's laminae, spinal laminae,** an architectural scheme used to classify the structure of the spinal cord, based on the cytological features of the neurons in different regions of the gray substance. **l. spira′lis,** 1. a double plate of bone winding spirally around the modiolus, dividing the spiral canal of the cochlea into the scala tympani and scala vestibuli. 2. a bony projection on the outer wall of the cochlea in the lower part of the first turn. **terminal l. of hypothalamus,** the thin plate derived from the telencephalon, forming the anterior wall of the third ventricle of the cerebrum. **l. of vertebra, l. of vertebral arch,** either of the pair of broad plates of bone flaring out from the pedicles of the vertebral arches and fusing together at the midline to complete the posterior part of the arch and provide a base for the spinous process.

lam·i·nag·ra·phy (lam″ĭ-nag′rah-fe) tomography.

lam·i·na·plas·ty (lam′in-ah-plas″te) relief of compression of the spinal cord or nerve roots by incision completely through one lamina of a vertebral arch, creation of a trough in the contralateral lamina, and opening of the arch like a door.

lam·i·nar (lam′ĭ-nar) 1. pertaining to a lamina or laminae. 2. laminated. 3. of, pertaining to, or being a streamlined, smooth fluid flow.

lam·i·nat·ed (-nāt″ed) having, composed of, or arranged in layers or laminae.

lam·i·nec·to·my (lam″ĭ-nek′tah-me) excision of the posterior arch of a vertebra.

lam·i·not·o·my (lam″ĭ-not′ah-me) transection of a lamina of a vertebra.

la·miv·u·dine (lah-miv′u-dēn) a nucleoside analogue that inhibits reverse transcriptase, used as an antiviral agent in the treatment of chronic hepatitis B and, in combination with zidovudine, the treatment of HIV infection and AIDS.

la·mo·tri·gine (lah-mo′trī-jēn) an anticonvulsant used in the treatment of certain forms of epilepsy.

lamp (lamp) an apparatus for furnishing heat or light. **mercury arc l., mercury vapor l., quartz l.,** one in which the arc is in mercury vapor, enclosed in a quartz burner; used in light therapy; it may be air- or water-cooled. **xenon arc l.,** one producing light of high intensity in a wide continuum of wavelengths; used with optical filters to simulate solar radiation.

lance (lans) 1. lancet. 2. to cut or incise with a lancet.

lan·cet (lan'set) a small, pointed, two-edged surgical knife.

lan·ci·nat·ing (lan'sĭ-nāt″ing) tearing, darting, or sharply cutting; said of pain.

lan·o·lin (lan'ah-lin) a purified, waxlike substance from the wool of sheep, *Ovis aries*, occurring in an anhydrous form and also a form containing 25 to 30 percent water; used as a water-in-oil ointment or cream base. *Modified l.* has been additionally processed to reduce the amount of free lanolin alcohols and detergent and pesticide residues.

lan·so·pra·zole (lan-so'prah-zōl) a proton pump inhibitor used to inhibit gastric acid secretion for the treatment of duodenal or gastric ulcer, gastroesophageal reflux disease, and hyperchlorhydria.

lan·tha·num (La) (lan'thah-num) .chemical element (see *Table of Elements*), at. no. 57.

la·nu·go (lah-noo'go) the fine hair on the body of the fetus.

lapar(o)- word element [Gr.], *loin* or *flank*; loosely, *abdomen*.

lap·a·ro·hys·ter·ec·to·my (lap″ah-ro-his″-ter-ek'tah-me) abdominal hysterectomy.

lap·a·ro·hys·ter·ot·o·my (-his″ter-ot'ah-me) abdominal hysterotomy.

lap·a·ro·scope (lap'ah-rah-skōp″) an endoscope for examining the peritoneal cavity.

lap·a·ros·co·py (lap″ah-ros'kah-pe) examination or treatment of the interior of the abdomen by means of a laparoscope.

lap·a·rot·o·my (-rot'ah-me) incision through the flank or, more generally, through any part of the abdominal wall.

lap·in·iza·tion (lap″in-ĭ-za'shun) serial passage of a virus or vaccine through rabbits to modify its characteristics.

lard (lahrd) purified internal fat of the abdomen of the hog.

lar·va (lahr'vah) pl. *lar'vae*. [L.] an independent, motile, sometimes feeding, developmental stage in the life history of an animal. **l. cur'rens**, a variant of larva migrans caused by *Strongyloides stercoralis*, in which the progression of the linear lesion is much more rapid. **cutaneous l. migrans, l. mi'grans**, creeping eruption; a convoluted threadlike pruritic, erythematous, papular or vesicular skin eruption that appears to migrate, caused by burrowing beneath the skin of roundworm larvae, particularly *Ancylostoma larvae*. Also applied to similar lesions caused by other parasites. **ocular l. migrans**, infection of the eye with larvae of *Toxocara canis* or *T. cati*, which may lodge in the choroid or retina or migrate to the vitreous; on the death of the larvae, a granulomatous inflammation occurs, the lesion varying from a translucent elevation of the retina to massive retinal detachment and pseudoglioma. **visceral l. migrans**, a condition due to prolonged migration of nematode larvae in human tissue other than skin; commonly caused by the larvae of *Toxocara canis* or *T. cati*, which do not complete their life cycle in humans.

lar·vate (-vāt) masked; concealed; said of a disease or symptom of disease.

lar·yn·ge·al (lah-rin'je-al) pertaining to the larynx.

lar·yn·gec·to·my (lar″in-jek'tah-me) surgical removal of the larynx.

lar·yn·gis·mus (-jiz'mus) spasm of the larynx. **laryngis'mal**, adj. **l. stri'dulus**, pseudocroup; sudden laryngeal spasm with crowing inhalation and cyanosis, usually seen in children at night.

lar·yn·gi·tis (-ji'tis) inflammation of the larynx. **laryngit'ic**, adj. **subglottic l.**, inflammation of the undersurface of the vocal cords.

laryng(o)- word element [Gr.], *larynx*.

la·ryn·go·cele (lah-ring'go-sēl) a congenital anomalous air sac communicating with the cavity of the larynx, which may bulge outward on the neck.

la·ryn·go·fis·sure (-fish″er) median laryngotomy.

lar·yn·gog·ra·phy (lar″ing-gog'rah-fe) radiography of the larynx.

lar·yn·gol·o·gy (-gol'ah-je) the branch of medicine dealing with the throat, pharynx, larynx, nasopharynx, and tracheobronchial tree.

lar·yn·gop·a·thy (-gop'ah-the) any disorder of the larynx.

la·ryn·go·pha·ryn·ge·al (lah-ring″go-fah-rin'je-al) pertaining to the larynx and pharynx or to the laryngopharynx.

la·ryn·go·phar·yn·gec·to·my (lah″ring-go-far″in-jek'tah-me) excision of the larynx and pharynx.

la·ryn·go·phar·ynx (-far'inks) the portion of the pharynx below the upper edge of the epiglottis, opening into the larynx and esophagus. **laryngopharyn'geal**, adj.

lar·yn·goph·o·ny (lar″in-gof'ah-ne) a voice sound heard over the larynx.

la·ryn·go·plas·ty (lah-ring'go-plas″te) plastic repair of the larynx.

la·ryn·go·ple·gia (lah-ring″go-ple'jah) paralysis of the larynx.

la·ryn·go·pto·sis (-to'sis) lowering and mobilization of the larynx as sometimes seen in the aged.

lar·yn·gos·co·py (lar″ing-gos′kah-pe) visual examination of the interior larynx. **laryngoscop′ic,** adj.

la·ryn·gos·te·no·sis (lah-ring″go-stĕ-no′sis) narrowing or stricture of the larynx.

la·ryn·gos·to·my (lar″ing-gos′tah-me) surgical fistulization of the larynx.

lar·yn·got·o·my (-got′ah-me) incision of the larynx. **inferior l.,** laryngotomy through the cricothyroid membrane. **median l.,** laryngotomy through the thyroid cartilage. **subhyoid l., superior l.,** laryngotomy through the thyrohyoid membrane.

la·ryn·go·tra·che·itis (lah-ring″go-tra″ke-i′tis) inflammation of the larynx and trachea.

la·ryn·go·tra·che·ot·o·my (-tra″ke-ot′ah-me) incision of the larynx and trachea.

lar·ynx (lar′inks) pl. *laryn′ges.* [L.] the organ of voice; the air passage between the lower pharynx and the trachea, containing the vocal cords and formed by nine cartilages: the thyroid, cricoid, and epiglottis and the paired arytenoid, corniculate, and cuneiform cartilages. See Plate 25.

la·ser (la′zer) a device that transfers light of various frequencies into an extremely intense, small, and nearly nondivergent beam of monochromatic radiation in the visible region, with all the waves in phase; capable of mobilizing immense heat and power when focused at close range, it is used as a tool in surgery, in diagnosis, and in physiological studies. **argon l.,** a laser with ionized argon as the active medium, whose beam is in the blue and green visible light spectrum; used for photocoagulation. **carbon-dioxide l.,** a laser with carbon dioxide gas as the active medium, which produces infrared radiation at 10,600 nm; used to excise and incise tissue and to vaporize. **dye l.,** a laser with organic dye as the active medium, whose beam is in the visible light spectrum. **excimer l.,** a laser with rare gas halides as the active medium, whose beam is in the ultraviolet spectrum and penetrates tissues only a short distance; used in ophthalmological procedures and laser angioplasty. **helium-neon l.,** a laser with a mixture of ionized helium and neon gases as the active medium, whose beam is in the red visible light spectrum; used as a guiding beam for lasers operating at nonvisible wavelengths. **krypton l.,** a laser with krypton ionized by electric current as the active medium, whose beam is in the yellow-red visible light spectrum; used for photocoagulation. **KTP l.,** one in which a beam generated by a neodymium:YAG laser is directed through a potassium titanyl phosphate crystal to produce a beam in the green visible spectrum; used for photoablation and photocoagulation. **neodymium: yttrium-aluminum-garnet (Nd:YAG) l.,** a laser whose active medium is a crystal of yttrium, aluminum, and garnet doped with neodymium ions, and whose beam is in the near infrared spectrum at 1060 nm; used for photocoagulation and photoablation. **potassium titanyl phosphate l.,** KTP l.

LASIK laser-assisted in-situ keratomileusis.

las·si·tude (las′ĭ-tood) weakness; exhaustion.

la·tan·o·prost (lah-tan′o-prost″) an antiglaucoma agent applied topically to the conjunctiva in the treatment of open-angle glaucoma and ocular hypertension.

la·ten·cy (la′ten-se) 1. a state of seeming inactivity. 2. the time between the instant of stimulation and the beginning of a response. 3. see under *stage.*

la·tent (la′tent) concealed; not manifest; potential; dormant; quiescent.

la·ten·ti·a·tion (la-ten″she-a′shun) the process of making latent; in pharmacology, chemical modification of a biologically active compound to affect its absorption, distribution, etc., the modified compound being transformed after administration to the active compound by biological processes.

lat·er·ad (lat′er-ad) toward the lateral aspect.

lat·er·al (-il) 1. denoting a position farther from the median plane or midline of the body or a structure. 2. pertaining to a side.

lat·er·a·lis (lat″er-a′lis) [L.] lateral.

lat·er·al·i·ty (lat″er-al′ĭ-te) a tendency to use preferentially the organs (hand, foot, ear, eye) of the same side in voluntary motor acts. **crossed l.,** the preferential use of contralateral members of the different pairs of organs in voluntary motor acts, e.g., right eye and left hand. **dominant l.,** lateral dominance.

lat·ero·dor·sal (lat″er-o-dor′s'l) denoting a position farther from the median plane or midline and more toward the back surface.

lat·ero·duc·tion (-duk′shun) movement of an eye to either side.

lat·ero·flex·ion (-flek′shun) flexion to one side.

lat·ero·tor·sion (-tor′shun) twisting of the vertical meridian of the eye to either side.

lat·ero·ver·sion (-ver′zhun) abnormal turning to one side.

la·tex (la′teks) a viscid, milky juice secreted by some seed plants.

lath·y·rism (lath′ĭ-rizm) spastic paraplegia, pain, hyperesthesia, and paresthesia due to excessive ingestion of the seeds of leguminous plants of the genus *Lathyrus,* which includes many kinds of peas. **lathyrit′ic,** adj.

la·tis·si·mus (lah-tis'ĭ-mus) [L.] widest; in anatomy, denoting a broad structure.

lat·ro·dec·tism (lat″ro-dek'tizm) intoxication due to venom of spiders of the genus *Latrodectus.*

Lat·ro·dec·tus (-dek'tus) a genus of poisonous spiders, including *L. mac′tans,* the black widow spider, whose bite may cause severe symptoms or even death.

LATS long-acting thyroid stimulator.

la·tus[1] (la'tus) [L.] broad, wide.

la·tus[2] pl. *la'tera.* [L.] the side or flank.

lau·rate (law'rāt) a salt, ester, or anionic form of lauric acid.

lau·ric ac·id (-rik) a twelve-carbon saturated fatty acid found in many vegetable fats, particularly coconut oil and palm kernel oil.

la·vage (lah-vahzh') 1. the irrigation or washing out of an organ, as of the stomach or bowel. 2. to wash out, or irrigate.

lav·en·der (lav'en-der) 1. any plant of the genus *Lavandula.* 2. a preparation of the flowers of *L. angustifolia* or of the lavender oil extracted from them; used for loss of appetite, dyspepsia, nervousness, and insomnia; also widely used in folk medicine.

law (law) a uniform or constant fact or principle. **Allen's paradoxic l.,** the more sugar a normal person is given the more is utilized; the reverse is true in diabetics. **all-or-none l.,** see *all or none.* **Beer's l., Beer-Lambert l.,** in spectrophotometry, the absorbance of a solution is proportional to the concentration of the absorbing solute and to the path length of the light beam through the solution. **Boyle's l.,** at a constant temperature the volume of a perfect gas varies inversely as the pressure, and the pressure varies inversely as the volume. **Charles' l.,** at a constant pressure the volume of a given mass of a perfect gas varies directly with the absolute temperature. **l. of conservation of energy,** in any given system the amount of energy is constant; energy is neither created nor destroyed, but only transformed from one form to another. **l. of conservation of mass, l. of conservation of matter,** mass (or matter) can be neither created nor destroyed; this law can be violated on the microscopic level. **Dalton's l.,** the pressure exerted by a mixture of nonreacting gases is equal to the sum of the partial pressures of the separate components; it holds true only at very low pressures. **Hellin's l., Hellin-Zeleny l.,** one in about 89 pregnancies ends in the birth of twins; one in 89×89 (7921), of triplets; one in $89 \times 89 \times 89$ (704,969), of quadruplets. **Henry's l.,** the solubility of a gas in a liquid solution at a constant temperature

is proportional to the partial pressure of the gas above the solution. **l. of independent assortment,** genes that are not alleles are distributed to the gametes independently of one another; one of Mendel's laws. **Mendel's l's, mendelian l's,** two laws of inheritance of single-gene traits that form the basis of genetics; the *law of segregation* and the *law of independent assortment.* **Nysten's l.,** rigor mortis affects first the muscles of mastication, next those of the face and neck, then those of the trunk and arms, and last those of the legs and feet. **Ohm's l.,** the strength of an electric current varies directly as the electromotive force and inversely as the resistance. **Raoult's l.,** the vapor pressure of a volatile component of an ideal solution is equal to the mole fraction of that substance in solution times its vapor pressure in the pure state at the temperature of the solution; it is true only for ideal solutions and ideal gases. **l. of segregation,** the members of a pair of allelic genes segregate from one another and pass to different gametes; one of Mendel's laws. **l. of similars,** in homeopathy, the principle that a substance that in large doses will produce symptoms of a specific disease will, in extremely small doses, cure it. **l's of thermodynamics,** *Zeroth law:* two systems in thermal equilibrium with a third are in thermal equilibrium with each other. *First law:* energy is conserved in any process. *Second law:* there is always an increase in entropy in any naturally occurring (spontaneous) process. *Third law:* absolute zero is unattainable.

law·ren·ci·um (Lw) (law-ren'se-um) chemical element (see *Table of Elements*), at. no. 103.

lax·a·tive (lak'sah-tiv) 1. mildly cathartic. 2. a cathartic or purgative. **bulk l., bulk-forming l.,** one promoting bowel evacuation by increasing fecal volume. **contact l.,** one that increases the motor activity of the intestinal tract. **lubricant l.,** one that promotes softening of the stool and facilitates passage of the feces through the intestines by its lubricant effect. **saline l.,** a salt administered in hypertonic solution to draw water into the intestinal lumen by osmosis, distending it and promoting peristalsis and evacuation. **stimulant l.,** contact l.

lax·i·ty (lak'sĭ-te) 1. slackness or looseness; a lack of tautness, firmness, or rigidity. 2. slackness or displacement in the motion of a joint. **lax',** adj.

lay·er (la'er) a stratum or lamina. **bacillary l.,** l. of rods and cones. **basal l.,** stratum basale. **blastodermic l.,** germ l. **l's of cerebral cortex,** six anatomical divisions

(I–VI) of the cerebral cortex (specifically the neocortex), distinguished according to the types of cells and fibers they contain. **clear l.,** stratum lucidum. **columnar l.,** mantle l. **compact l. of endometrium,** stratum compactum. **enamel l.,** either of two walls, the inner concave wall or the outer convex wall, of the enamel organ. **functional l. of endometrium,** stratum functionale. **ganglionic l. of cerebellum,** Purkinje l. **germ l.,** any of the three primary layers of cells of the embryo (ectoderm, endoderm, and mesoderm), from which the tissues and organs develop. **germinative l.,** stratum germinativum. **granular l.,** 1. stratum granulosum. 2. the deep layer of the cortex of the cerebellum. **Henle's l.,** the outermost layer of the inner root sheath of the hair follicle. **horny l.,** stratum corneum. **malpighian l.,** stratum germinativum. **mantle l.,** the middle layer of the wall of the primordial neural tube, containing primordial nerve cells and later forming the gray matter of the central nervous system. **odontoblastic l.,** the epithelioid layer of odontoblasts in contact with the dentin of teeth. **prickle cell l.,** stratum spinosum. **Purkinje l., Purkinje cell l.,** the layer of Purkinje neurons situated between the external molecular layer and the internal granular layer of the cerebellar cortex. **l. of rods and cones,** a layer of the retina immediately beneath the pigment epithelium, between it and the external limiting membrane, containing the rods and cones. **spinous l.,** stratum spinosum. **spongy l. of endometrium,** stratum spongiosum. **subendocardial l.,** the layer of loose fibrous tissue uniting the endocardium and myocardium and containing the vessels and nerves of the conducting system of the heart. **subepicardial l.,** the layer of loose connective tissue uniting the epicardium and myocardium.

lb [L.] pound (L. *libra*).

LBBB left bundle branch block; see *bundle branch block*, under *block*.

LCAT lecithin-cholesterol acyltransferase.

LCIS lobular carcinoma in situ.

LD₅₀ median lethal dose.

LDH L-lactate dehydrogenase.

LDL low-density lipoprotein.

LDL-C low-density-lipoprotein cholesterol

L-dopa levodopa.

LE left eye; lupus erythematosus.

lead¹ (Pb) (led) chemical element (see *Table of Elements*), at. no. 82. Absorption or ingestion causes poisoning, which affects the brain, nervous and digestive systems, and blood.

lead² (lēd) any of the conductors connected to the electrocardiograph, each comprising two or more electrodes that are attached at specific body sites and used to examine electrical activity by monitoring changes in the electrical potential between them. **l. I,** the standard bipolar limb lead attached to the right and left arms. **l. II,** the standard bipolar limb lead attached to the right arm and left leg. **l. III,** the standard bipolar limb lead attached to the left arm and left leg. **augmented unipolar limb l.,** a modified unipolar limb lead; the three standard leads are: aV_F (left leg), aV_L (left arm), and aV_R (right arm). **aV_F l.,** an augmented unipolar limb lead in which the positive electrode is on the left leg. **aV_L l.,** an augmented unipolar limb lead in which the positive electrode is on the left arm. **aV_R l.,** an augmented unipolar limb lead in which the positive electrode is on the right arm. **bipolar l.,** an array involving two electrodes placed at different body sites. **limb l.,** an array in which any registering electrodes are attached to limbs. **pacemaker l., pacing l.,** the connection between the heart and the power source of an artificial cardiac pacemaker. **precordial l's,** leads in which the exploring electrode is placed on the chest and the other is connected to one or more limbs; usually used to denote one of the V leads. **standard l's,** the 12 leads used in a standard electrocardiogram, comprising the standard bipolar limb leads I–III, the augmented unipolar limb leads, and the standard precordial leads. **unipolar l.,** an array of two electrodes, only one of which transmits potential variation. **V l's,** the series of six standard unipolar leads in which the exploring electrode is attached to the chest, designated V₁ to V₆. **XYZ l's,** leads used in one system of spatial vectorcardiography.

learn·ing (lern'ing) a long-lasting adaptive behavioral change due to experience. **latent l.,** that which occurs without reinforcement, becoming apparent only when a reinforcement or reward is introduced.

lec·i·thal (les'ĭ-thal) having a yolk; used especially as a word termination (*isolecithal*, etc.).

lec·i·thin (les'ĭ-thin) phosphatidylcholine.

lec·i·thin–cho·les·ter·ol ac·yl·trans·fer·ase (LCAT) (kah-les'ter-ol a″sil-trans'fer-ās) an enzyme that catalyzes the formation of cholesteryl esters in high-density lipoproteins; deficiency of enzyme activity, an inherited disorder, results in accumulation of cholesterol and phosphatidylcholine in plasma and tissues, which causes corneal opacities, anemia, and often proteinuria.

lec·tin (lek′tin) any of a group of hemagglutinating proteins found primarily in plant seeds, which bind specifically to the branching sugar molecules of glycoproteins and glycolipids on the surface of cells.

leech (lēch) any of the annelids of the class Hirudinea, especially *Hirudo medicinalis*; some species are bloodsuckers. Leeches have been used for drawing blood.

le·flu·no·mide (lĕ-floo′no-mīd) an immunomodulator used in treatment of rheumatoid arthritis.

leg (leg) 1. the part of the lower limb between the knee and ankle. 2. in common usage, the entire lower limb, with the part below the knee being called the *lower leg*. 3. any of the four limbs of a quadruped. **bandy l.,** bowleg. **bayonet l.,** ankylosis of the knee after backward displacement of the tibia and fibula. **bow l.,** see *bowleg*. **milk l.,** phlegmasia alba dolens. **restless l's,** a disagreeable, creeping, irritating sensation in the legs, usually the lower legs, relieved only by walking or keeping the legs moving. **scissor l.,** deformity with crossing of the legs in walking.

Le·gion·el·la (le″jah-nel′ah) a genus of gram-negative, aerobic, rod-shaped bacteria (family Legionellaceae), normal inhabitants of lakes, streams, and moist soil; they have often been isolated from cooling-tower water, evaporative condensers, tap water, shower heads, and treated sewage. *L. micda′dei* is the causative agent of Pittsburgh pneumonia. *L. pneumo′phila* is the causative agent of legionnaires' disease.

le·gion·el·lo·sis (le″jin-el-o′sis) disease caused by infection with *Legionella pneumophila;* see *legionnaires' disease* and *Pontiac fever.*

le·gume (lĕ′gūm) 1. any plant of the large family Leguminosae. 2. the pod or fruit of one of these plants, such as a pea or bean.

leio·der·mia (li″o-derm′e-ah) abnormal smoothness and glossiness of the skin.

leio·myo·fi·bro·ma (-mi″o-fi-bro′mah) epithelioid leiomyoma.

leio·myo·ma (-mi-o′mah) a benign tumor derived from smooth muscle, most often of the uterus. **l. cu′tis,** one or more smooth, firm, painful, often waxy nodules arising from cutaneous or subcutaneous smooth muscle fibers. **epithelioid l.,** leiomyoma, usually of the stomach, in which the cells are polygonal rather than spindle shaped.

leio·my·o·ma·to·sis (-mi″o-mah-to′sis) the occurrence of multiple leiomyomas throughout the body.

leio·myo·sar·co·ma (-sahr-ko′mah) a sarcoma containing spindle cells of smooth muscle.

Leish·ma·nia (lēsh-ma′ne-ah) a genus of parasitic protozoa, including several species pathogenic for humans. In some classifications, organisms are placed in four complexes comprising species and subspecies: *L. donova′ni* (causing visceral leishmaniasis), *L. tro′pica* (causing the Old World form of cutaneous leishmaniasis), *L. mexica′na* (causing the New World form of cutaneous leishmaniasis), and *L. vian′nia* (causing mucocutaneous leishmaniasis).

leish·ma·ni·a·sis (lēsh″mah-ni′ah-sis) infection with *Leishmania.* **American l.,** any of the types of cutaneous or visceral leishmaniasis occurring in South America, Central America, or Mexico. **cutaneous l.,** an endemic granulomatous disease, divided into two forms: an Old World form caused by *Leishmania major, L. tropica* or *L. aethiopica* and a New World form caused by *L. mexicana* or *L. viannia.* **mucocutaneous l.,** chronic, progressive, metastatic spread of the lesions of New World leishmaniasis caused by *Leishmania viannia braziliensis* to the nasal, pharyngeal, and buccal mucosa long after the appearance of the initial cutaneous lesion, causing widespread destruction of tissue with marked deformity. **post-kala-azar dermal l.,** a condition associated with visceral leishmaniasis, characterized by hypopigmented or erythematous macules on the face and sometimes also the trunk and limbs, the facial lesions progressing to papules and nodules resembling those of lepromatous leprosy. **l. reci′divans,** a prolonged, relapsing form of cutaneous leishmaniasis resembling tuberculosis of the skin. **visceral l.,** a chronic, highly fatal if untreated, infectious disease caused by *Leishmania donovani,* characterized by hepatosplenomegaly, fever, chills, vomiting, anemia, leukopenia, hypergammaglobulinemia, and an earth-gray color of the skin.

-lemma word element [Gr.], *sheath.*

lem·mo·blas·tic (lem″o-blas′tik) forming or developing into neurilemma tissue.

lem·nis·cus (lem-nis′kus) pl. *lemnis′ci.* [L.] 1. a ribbon or band. 2. a band or bundle of fibers in the central nervous system.

length (*l*) (length) the longest dimension of an object, or of the measurement between the two ends. **crown-heel l. (CHL),** the distance from the crown of the head to the heel in embryos, fetuses, and infants; the equivalent of standing height in older persons. **crown-rump l. (CRL),** the distance from the crown of the head to the breech in embryos, fetuses, and infants; the equivalent of sitting height in older persons. **focal l.,** the distance between a lens and an object from which all rays of light are brought to a focus.

lens (lenz) 1. a piece of glass or other transparent material so shaped as to converge or scatter light rays; see also *glasses*. 2. crystalline l.; the transparent, biconvex body separating the posterior chamber and vitreous body, and constituting part of the refracting mechanism of the eye; see Plate 30. **achromatic l.,** one corrected for chromatic aberration. **aplanatic l.,** one for correcting spherical aberrations. **bandage l.,** a soft contact lens worn on a diseased or injured cornea to protect or treat it. **biconcave l.,** one concave on both faces. **biconvex l.,** one convex on both faces. **bifocal l.,** one with two parts of different refracting powers, the upper for distant and the lower for near vision. **concavoconvex l.,** one with one concave and one convex face. **contact l.,** a curved shell of glass or plastic applied directly over the globe or cornea to correct refractive errors. It may be a *soft (hydrophilic) contact l.,* flexible and water absorbent, or a *hard (hydrophobic) contact l.,* rigid and not water absorbent; the latter type is subdivided into gas permeable and non–gas permeable, usually polymethylmethacrylate (PMMA), lenses. **convexoconcave l.,** one with one convex and one concave face. **crystalline l.,** lens (2). **cylindrical l.,** one for correcting astigmatism, with one plane surface and one cylindrical, or one spherical surface and one toroidal. Symbol C. **decentered l.,** one whose optical axis does not pass through the center. **honeybee l.,** a magnifying lens resembling the multifaceted eye of the honeybee, consisting of three or six small telescopes mounted in the upper part of the lens and directed toward the center and right and left visual fields. Prisms are included to provide a continuous, unbroken magnified field of view. **omnifocal l.,** one whose power increases continuously and regularly in a downward direction, avoiding the discontinuity of bifocal and trifocal lenses. **planoconvex l.,** a lens with one plane and one convex side. **spherical l. (S, sph),** one that is a segment of a sphere. **trial l.,** one used to test vision. **trifocal l.,** one with three parts of different refracting powers, the upper for distant, the middle for intermediate, and the lower for near vision.

len·ti·co·nus (len″tĭ-ko′nus) a congenital conical bulging, anteriorly or posteriorly, of the lens of the eye.

len·tic·u·lar (len-tik′u-ler) 1. pertaining to or shaped like a lens. 2. pertaining to the lens of the eye. 3. pertaining to the lenticular nucleus.

len·ti·form (len′tĭ-form) lens-shaped.

len·tig·i·nes (len-tij′ĭ-nēz) plural of *lentigo*.

len·tig·i·no·sis (len-tĭj″ĭ-no′sis) a condition marked by multiple lentigines. **progressive cardiomyopathic l.,** multiple symmetrical lentigines, hypertrophic obstructive cardiomyopathy, and retarded growth, sometimes with mental retardation.

len·ti·glo·bus (len″tĭ-glo′bus) exaggerated curvature of the lens of the eye, producing an anterior spherical bulging.

len·ti·go (len-ti′go) pl. *lentig′ines.* [L.] a flat brownish pigmented spot on the skin, due to increased deposition of melanin and an increased number of melanocytes. **l. malig′na,** a circumscribed macular patch of hyperpigmentation, with shades of dark brown, tan, or black, that enlarges slowly and may be a precursor to lentigo maligna melanoma.

Len·ti·vi·rus (len′tĭ-vi″rus) a genus of retroviruses that cause persistent infection that typically results in chronic, progressive, usually fatal disease; it includes the human immunodeficiency viruses.

len·ti·vi·rus (len′tĭ-vi″rus) any virus of the subfamily Lentivirinae.

le·on·ti·a·sis (le″on-ti′ah-sis) the leonine facies of lepromatous leprosy, due to nodular invasion of the subcutaneous tissue. **l. os′sea, l. os′sium,** hypertrophy of the bones of the cranium and face, giving it a vaguely leonine appearance.

lep·er (lep′er) a person with leprosy; a term now in disfavor.

le·pid·ic (lĕ-pid′ik) pertaining to scales.

lep·i·ru·din (lep″ĭ-roo′din) a recombinant form of hirudin used as an anticoagulant in patients with heparin-induced thrombocytopenia.

lep·ra (lep′rah) leprosy.

lep·re·chaun·ism (lep′rĕ-kon″izm) a lethal familial congenital condition in which the infant is small and has elfin facies and severe endocrine disorders, as indicated by enlarged clitoris and breasts.

lep·rid (lep′rid) cutaneous lesion or lesions of tuberculoid leprosy: hypopigmented or erythematous nodules or plaques, lacking bacilli.

lep·ro·ma (lep-ro'mah) a superficial granulomatous nodule rich in leprosy bacilli, the characteristic lesion of lepromatous leprosy.

lep·ro·ma·tous (-tus) pertaining to lepromas; see under *leprosy*.

lep·ro·min (lep'rah-min) a repeatedly boiled, autoclaved, gauze-filtered suspension of finely triturated lepromatous tissue and leprosy bacilli, used in the skin test for tissue resistance to leprosy.

lep·ro·stat·ic (-stat'ik) inhibiting the growth of *Mycobacterium leprae*, or an agent that so acts.

lep·ro·sy (lep'rah-se) a chronic communicable disease caused by *Mycobacterium leprae* and characterized by the production of granulomatous lesions of the skin, mucous membranes, and peripheral nervous system. Two principal, or polar, types are recognized: lepromatous and tuberculoid. **lepromatous l.**, that form marked by the development of lepromas and by an abundance of leprosy bacilli from the onset; nerve damage occurs only slowly, and the skin reaction to lepromin is negative. It is the only form which may regularly serve as a source of infection. **tuberculoid l.**, the form in which leprosy bacilli are few or lacking and nerve damage occurs early, so that all skin lesions are denervated from the onset, often with dissociation of sensation; the skin reaction to lepromin is positive, and the patient is rarely a source of infection to others.

lept(o)- word element [Gr.], *slender; delicate.*

lep·to·ceph·a·lus (lep"to-sef'ah-lus) a person with an abnormally tall, narrow skull.

lep·to·cyte (lep'to-sīt) target cell (1).

lep·to·me·nin·ges (lep"to-mĕ-nin'jēz) sing. *leptome'ninx*. The pia mater and arachnoid taken together; the pia-arachnoid. **leptomenin'geal**, adj.

lep·to·me·nin·gi·tis (-men"in-ji'tis) inflammation of the leptomeninges.

lep·to·men·in·gop·a·thy (-men"ing-gop'ah-the) any disease of the leptomeninges.

lep·to·mo·nad (-mo'nad) 1. of or pertaining to *Leptomonas*. 2. denoting the leptomonad form; see *promastigote*. 3. a protozoan exhibiting the leptomonad (promastigote) form.

Lep·to·mo·nas (-mo'nis) a genus of protozoa of the family Trypanosomatidae, parasitic in the digestive tract of insects.

lep·to·pel·lic (-pel'ik) having a narrow pelvis.

Lep·to·spi·ra (-spi'rah) a genus of aerobic spirochete bacteria (family Leptospiraceae); all pathogenic strains (i.e., those that cause leptospirosis) are contained in the species *L. inter'rogans*, which is divided into several serogroups, which are in turn divided into serotypes.

lep·to·spi·ra an individual organism belonging to the genus *Leptospira*. **leptospi'ral**, adj.

Lep·to·spi·ra·ceae (-spi-ra'se-e) a family of bacteria, spirochetes that are flexible helical cells and are aerobic; it consists of one genus, *Leptospira*.

lep·to·spi·ro·sis (-spi-ro'sis) any infectious disease due to a serotype of *Leptospira*, manifested by lymphocytic meningitis, hepatitis, and nephritis, separately or in combination, and varying in severity from a mild carrier state to fatal disease.

lep·to·tene (lep'to-tēn) the stage of meiosis in which the chromosomes are threadlike in shape.

lep·to·thri·co·sis (lep"to-thrĭ-ko'sis) leptotrichosis.

Lep·to·thrix (lep'tah-thriks) a genus of schizomycetes (family Chlamydobacteriaceae), widely distributed and usually found in fresh water.

lep·to·tri·cho·sis (lep"to-trĭ-ko'sis) any infection with *Leptothrix*. **l. conjuncti'vae**, Parinaud's oculoglandular syndrome caused by *Leptothrix*.

les·bi·an (lez'be-an) 1. pertaining to homosexuality between women. 2. a female homosexual.

les·bi·an·ism (lez'be-in-izm") homosexuality between women.

le·sion (le'zhun) any pathological or traumatic discontinuity of tissue or loss of function of a part. **angiocentric immunoproliferative l.**, a multisystem disease consisting of invasion and destruction of body tissues and structures by atypical lymphocytoid and plasmacytoid cells resembling a lymphoma, often progresssing to lymphoma. **Armanni-Ebstein l.**, vacuolization of the renal tubular epithelium in diabetes. **benign lymphoepithelial l.**, enlargement of the salivary glands with infiltration of the parenchyma by polyclonal B cells and T cells, atrophy of acini, and formation of lymphoepithelial islands. **Blumenthal l.**, a proliferative vascular lesion in the smaller arteries in diabetes. **central l.**, any lesion of the central nervous system. **Ghon's primary l.**, Ghon focus. **Janeway l.**, a small erythematous or hemorrhagic lesion, usually on the palms or soles, in bacterial endocarditis. **primary l.**, the original lesion manifesting a disease, as a chancre.

le·thal (le'th'l) fatal.

leth·ar·gy (leth'ar-je) 1. a lowered level of consciousness, with drowsiness, listlessness, and apathy. 2. a condition of indifference.

let·ro·zole (let'rah-zōl) an antineoplastic used in the treatment of advanced breast cancer in postmenopausal women.

Leu leucine.

leu·cine (Leu, L) (loo'sēn) an essential amino acid necessary for optimal growth in infants and for nitrogen equilibrium in adults.

leuc(o)- for words beginning thus, see also those beginning *leuko-*.

Leu·co·nos·toc (loo″ko-nos'tok) a genus of slime-forming saprophytic bacteria (tribe Streptococcaceae) found in milk and fruit juices, including *L. citro'vorum*, *L. dextran'icum*, and *L. mesenteroi'des*.

leu·co·vo·rin (-vor'in) folinic acid; the calcium salt is used as an antidote for folic acid antagonists, e.g., methotrexate, and in the treatment of megaloblastic anemias due to folic acid deficiency and colorectal carcinoma.

leu·ka·phe·re·sis (loo″kah-fĕ-re'sis) the selective separation and removal of leukocytes from withdrawn blood, the remainder of the blood then being retransfused into the donor.

leu·ke·mia (loo-ke'me-ah) a progressive, malignant disease of the blood-forming organs, marked by distorted proliferation and development of leukocytes and their precursors in the blood and bone marrow. **leuke'mic**, adj. **acute l.**, leukemia in which the involved cell line shows little or no differentiation, usually consisting of blast cells; it comprises two types, acute lymphocytic leukemia and acute myelogenous leukemia. **acute granulocytic l.**, acute myelogenous l. **acute lymphoblastic l. (ALL)**, one of the two major categories of acute leukemia, characterized by anemia, fatigue, weight loss, easy bruising, thrombocytopenia, granulocytopenia with bacterial infections, bone pain, lymphadenopathy, hepatosplenomegaly, and sometimes spread to the central nervous system. It is subclassified on the basis of the surface antigens expressed, e.g., *B-cell type*, *T-cell type*. **acute lymphocytic l.**, acute lymphoblastic l. **acute megakaryoblastic l.**, **acute megakaryocytic l.**, a form of acute myelogenous leukemia in which megakaryocytes are predominant and platelets are increased in the blood. **acute monocytic l.**, an uncommon form of acute myelogenous leukemia in which the predominating cells are monocytes. **acute myeloblastic l.**, 1. a common type of acute myelogenous leukemia in which myeloblasts predominate;

it is divided into two types on the basis of degree of cell differentiation. 2. acute myelogenous l. **acute myelocytic l.**, acute myelogenous l. **acute myelogenous l. (AML)**, one of the two major categories of acute leukemia, with symptoms including anemia, fatigue, weight loss, easy bruising, thrombocytopenia, and granulocytopenia. **acute myeloid l.**, 1. acute myeloblastic l. (1). 2. acute myelogenous l. **acute myelomonocytic l.**, a common type of acute myelogenous leukemia, with both malignant monocytes and monoblasts. **acute non-lymphocytic l.**, acute myelogenous l. **acute promyelocytic l.**, acute myelogenous leukemia in which more than half the cells are malignant promyelocytes. **acute undifferentiated l. (AUL)**, acute myelogenous leukemia in which the predominating cell is so immature it cannot be classified. **adult T-cell l./lymphoma (ATL)**, an adult-onset, subacute or chronic malignancy of mature T lymphocytes, believed to be caused by human T lymphotropic virus type I. **aleukemic l.**, a form in which the total white blood cell count in the peripheral blood is not elevated; it may be lymphocytic, monocytic, or myelogenous. **basophilic l.**, leukemia in which the basophilic leukocytes predominate. **chronic l.**, leukemia in which the involved cell line is well differentiated, usually B lymphocytes, but immunologically incompetent. **chronic granulocytic l.**, chronic leukemia of the myelogenous type, usually associated with a specific chromosomal abnormality and occurring in adulthood. **chronic lymphocytic l. (CLL)**, chronic leukemia of the lymphocytic type, characterized by lymphadenopathy, fatigue, renal involvement, and pulmonary leukemic infiltrates. **chronic myelocytic l.**, **chronic myelogenous l.**, **chronic myeloid l.**, chronic granulocytic l. **chronic myelomonocytic l.**, a chronic, slowly progressing form characterized by malignant monocytes and myeloblasts, splenomegaly, and thrombocytopenia. **l. cu'tis**, a cutaneous manifestation of leukemia resulting from infiltration of the skin by malignant leukocytes. **eosinophilic l.**, a form in which eosinophils are the predominating cells. **granulocytic l.**, myelogenous l. **hairy cell l.**, chronic leukemia marked by splenomegaly and an abundance of large, mononuclear abnormal cells with numerous irregular cytoplasmic projections that give them a flagellated or hairy appearance in the bone marrow, spleen, liver, and peripheral blood. **histiocytic l.**, acute monocytic l. **lymphatic l., lymphoblastic l.**,

lymphocytic l., a form associated with hyperplasia and overactivity of the lymphoid tissue, with increased levels of circulating malignant lymphocytes or lymphoblasts. **lymphogenous l., lymphoid l.,** lymphatic l. **lymphosarcoma cell l.,** (B-cell type) acute lymphoblastic l. **mast cell l.,** a rare form marked by overwhelming numbers of tissue mast cells in the peripheral blood. **megakaryoblastic l.,** acute megakaryocytic l. **megakaryocytic l.,** 1. acute megakaryocytic l. 2. hemorrhagic thrombocythemia. **micromyeloblastic l.,** a form of myelogenous leukemia in which the immature nucleoli-containing cells are small and similar to lymphocytes. **monocytic l.,** acute monocytic l. **myeloblastic l.,** 1. myelogenous l. 2. acute myeloblastic l. **myelocytic l., myelogenous l., myeloid granulocytic l.,** a form arising from myeloid tissue in which the granular polymorphonuclear leukocytes and their precursors predominate. See also *acute myelogenous l.* and *chronic granulocytic l.* **myelomonocytic l.,** acute myelomonocytic l. **plasma cell l., plasmacytic l.,** a form in which the predominating cell in the peripheral blood is the plasma cell. **promyelocytic l.,** acute promyelocytic l. **Rieder cell l.,** a form of acute myelogenous leukemia in which the blood contains asynchronously developed cells with immature cytoplasm and a lobulated, relatively more mature nucleus. **stem cell l.,** acute undifferentiated l.

leu·ke·mid (loo-ke′mid) any of the polymorphic skin eruptions associated with leukemia; clinically, they may be nonspecific, i.e., papular, macular, purpuric, etc., but histopathologically they may represent true leukemic infiltrations.

leu·ke·mo·gen (loo-ke′mo-jen) any substance which produces leukemia. **leukemogen′ic,** adj.

leu·ke·moid (loo-ke′moid) exhibiting blood and sometimes clinical findings resembling those of leukemia, but due to some other cause.

leu·kin (loo′kin) a bactericidal substance from leukocyte extract.

leuk(o)- word element [Gr.], *white; leukocyte.*

leu·ko·ag·glu·ti·nin (loo″ko-ah-gloo′tĭ-nin) an agglutinin which acts upon leukocytes.

leu·ko·blas·to·sis (-blas-to′sis) abnormal proliferation of leukocytes, as seen in leukemia.

leu·ko·ci·din (-si′din) a substance produced by some pathogenic bacteria that is toxic to polymorphonuclear leukocytes (neutrophils).

leu·ko·cyte (loo′ko-sīt) white cell, white blood cell; a colorless blood corpuscle capable of ameboid movement, whose chief function is to protect the body against microorganisms causing disease and which may be classified in two main groups: *granular* and *nongranular.* **leukocyt′ic,** adj. **agranular l.,** nongranular l. **basophilic l.,** basophil (2). **eosinophilic l.,** eosinophil. **granular l.,** granulocyte; a leukocyte containing abundant granules in the cytoplasm, such as a neutrophil, eosinophil, or basophil. **neutrophilic l.,** neutrophil (1). **nongranular l.,** a leukocyte without specific granules in the cytoplasm, such as a lymphocyte or monocyte.

leu·ko·cy·to·gen·e·sis (loo″ko-si″to-jen′ĕ-sis) leukopoiesis.

leu·ko·cy·tol·y·sis (-si-tol′ĭ-sis) leukolysis. **leukocytolyt′ic,** adj.

leu·ko·cy·to·ma (-si-to′mah) a tumor-like mass of leukocytes.

leu·ko·cy·to·pe·nia (-si″to-pe′ne-ah) leukopenia.

leu·ko·cy·to·pla·nia (-si″to-pla′ne-ah) wandering of leukocytes; passage of leukocytes through a membrane.

leu·ko·cy·to·poi·e·sis (-si″to-poi-e′sis) leukopoiesis.

leu·ko·cy·to·sis (-si-to′sis) a transient increase in the number of leukocytes in the blood, due to various causes. **basophilic l.,** basophilia (1). **eosinophilic l.,** eosinophilia. **mononuclear l.,** mononucleosis. **neutrophilic l.,** neutrophilia. **pathologic l.,** that due to some morbid condition, such as infection or trauma. **physiologic l.,** that due to a nonpathologic condition such as strenuous exercise.

leu·ko·cy·to·sper·mia (-si″to-sper′me-ah) excessive leukocytes in the seminal fluid.

leu·ko·cy·to·tax·is (-si″to-tak′sis) leukotaxis.

leu·ko·cy·to·tox·ic·i·ty (-si″to-tok-sis′ĭ-te) lymphocytotoxicity.

leu·ko·der·ma (-der′mah) an acquired condition with localized loss of pigmentation of the skin. **l. acquisi′tum centri′fugum,** halo nevus. **syphilitic l.,** indistinct coarsely mottled hypopigmentation, usually on the sides of the neck, in late secondary syphilis.

leu·ko·dys·tro·phy (-dis′trah-fe) disturbance of the white substance of the brain; see also *leukoencephalopathy.* **globoid cell l.,** Krabbe's disease. **hereditary adult-onset l.,** an inherited leukoencephalopathy characterized by progressive degeneration of the white matter, with motor disturbances, bowel and bladder incontinence, and orthostatic

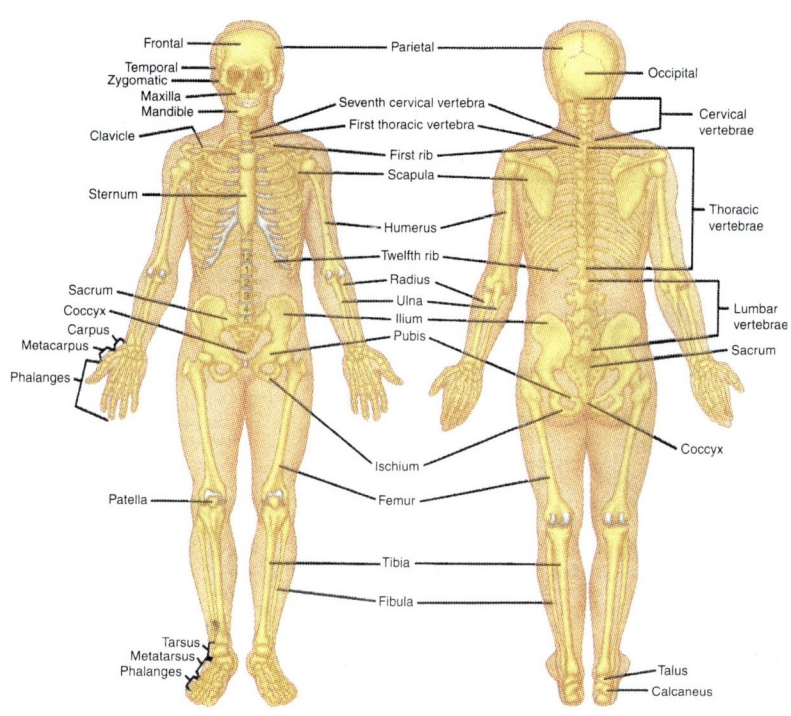

PLATE 1—Anterior and Posterior Views of the Skeleton

Frontal — Parietal
Temporal
Zygomatic
Maxilla
Mandible — Seventh cervical vertebra
Clavicle — First thoracic vertebra
Occipital
Cervical vertebrae
First rib
Sternum — Scapula
Humerus
Thoracic vertebrae
Twelfth rib
Sacrum — Radius
Coccyx — Ulna
Carpus — Ilium
Metacarpus — Pubis
Lumbar vertebrae
Sacrum
Phalanges
Ischium
Coccyx
Patella — Femur
Tibia
Fibula
Tarsus
Metatarsus
Phalanges
Talus
Calcaneus

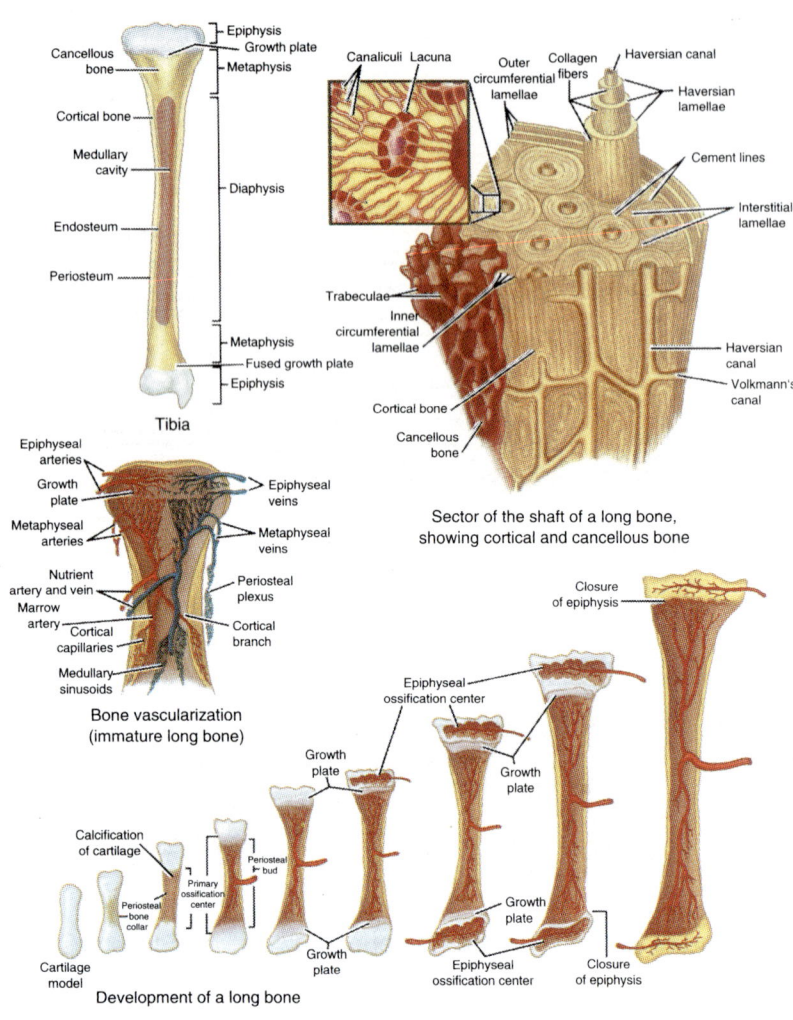

Epiphysis
Growth plate
Metaphysis
Cancellous bone
Cortical bone
Medullary cavity
Endosteum
Periosteum
Diaphysis
Metaphysis
Fused growth plate
Epiphysis

Tibia

Canaliculi
Lacuna
Outer circumferential lamellae
Collagen fibers
Haversian canal
Haversian lamellae
Cement lines
Interstitial lamellae
Trabeculae
Inner circumferential lamellae
Cortical bone
Cancellous bone
Haversian canal
Volkmann's canal

Sector of the shaft of a long bone,
showing cortical and cancellous bone

Epiphyseal arteries
Growth plate
Metaphyseal arteries
Nutrient artery and vein
Marrow artery
Cortical capillaries
Medullary sinusoids
Epiphyseal veins
Metaphyseal veins
Periosteal plexus
Cortical branch

Bone vascularization
(immature long bone)

Closure of epiphysis
Epiphyseal ossification center
Growth plate
Growth plate
Growth plate
Epiphyseal ossification center
Closure of epiphysis

Calcification of cartilage
Periosteal bone collar
Primary ossification center
Periosteal bud
Growth plate

Cartilage model

Development of a long bone

PLATE 2—Structure, Vascularization, and Development of Bone

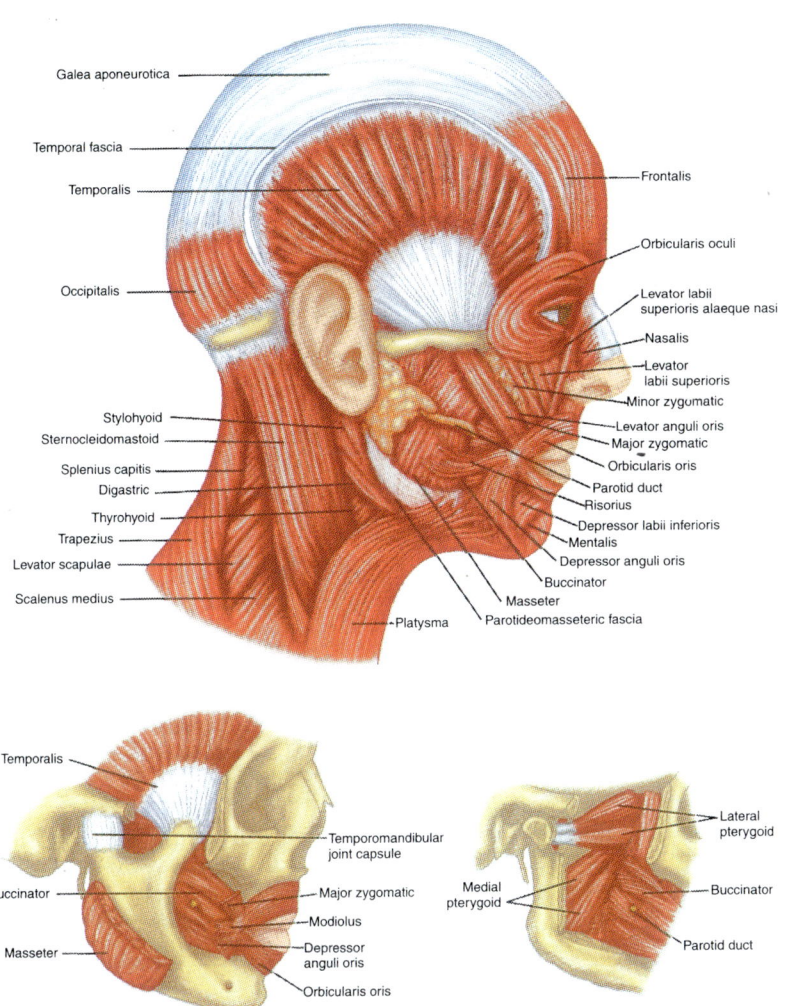

Galea aponeurotica

Temporal fascia

Temporalis

Occipitalis

Stylohyoid

Sternocleidomastoid

Splenius capitis

Digastric

Thyrohyoid

Trapezius

Levator scapulae

Scalenus medius

Frontalis

Orbicularis oculi

Levator labii superioris alaeque nasi

Nasalis

Levator labii superioris

Minor zygomatic

Levator anguli oris

Major zygomatic

Orbicularis oris

Parotid duct

Risorius

Depressor labii inferioris

Mentalis

Depressor anguli oris

Buccinator

Masseter

Parotideomasseteric fascia

Platysma

Temporalis

Buccinator

Masseter

Temporomandibular joint capsule

Major zygomatic

Modiolus

Depressor anguli oris

Orbicularis oris

Medial pterygoid

Lateral pterygoid

Buccinator

Parotid duct

PLATE 3—Muscles of the Head and Neck

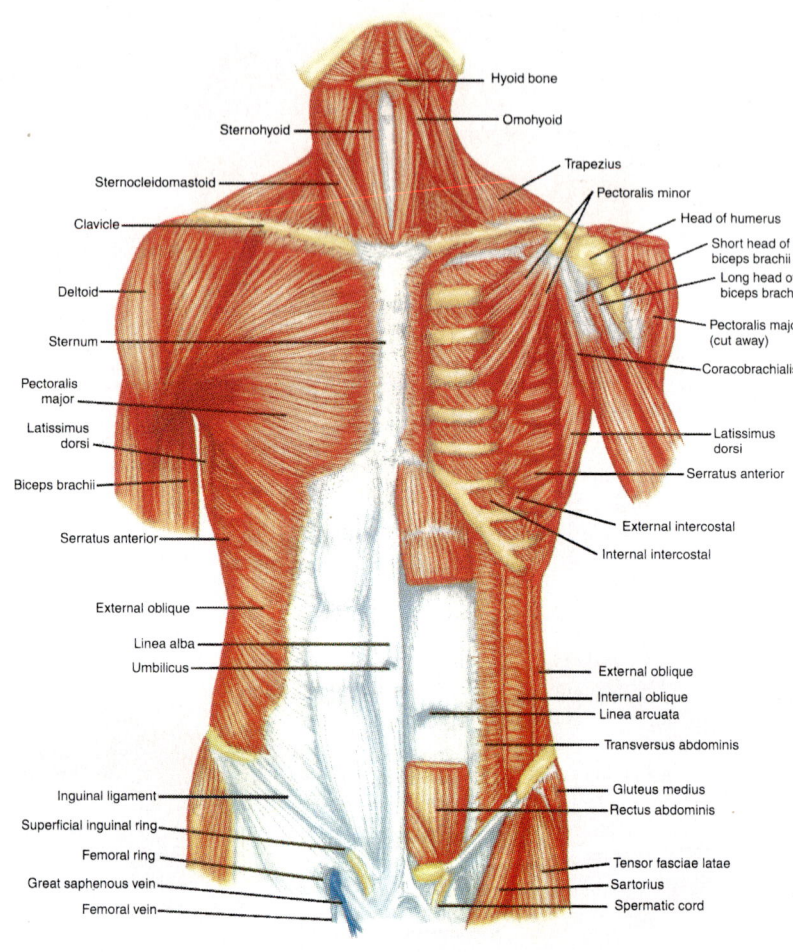

PLATE 4—Muscles of the Trunk, Anterior View

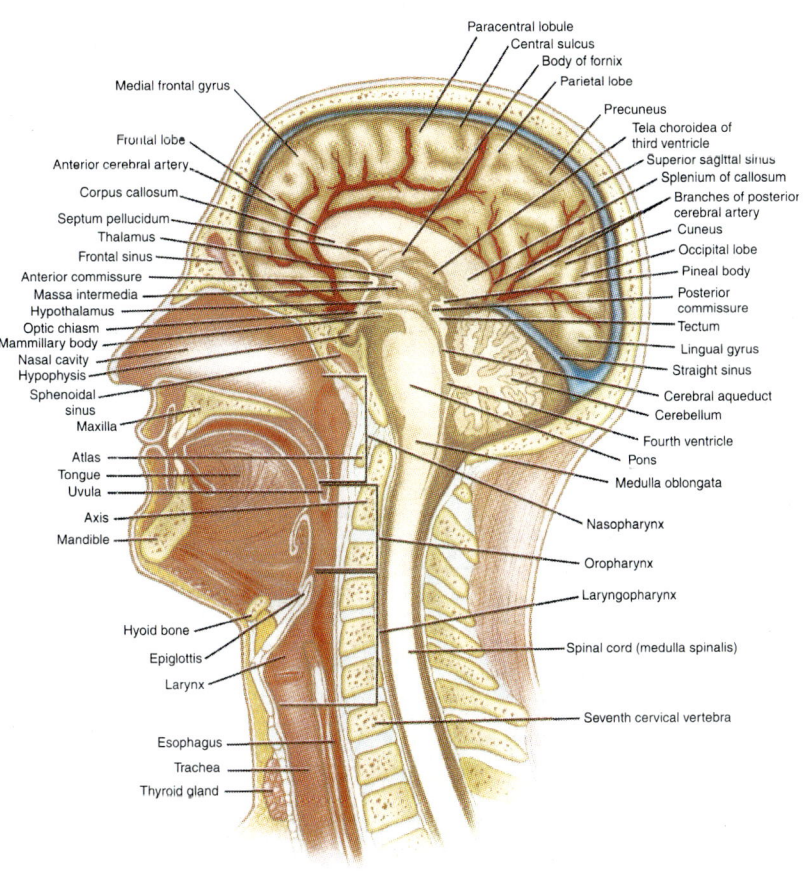

Paracentral lobule
Central sulcus
Body of fornix
Parietal lobe
Precuneus
Tela choroidea of third ventricle
Superior sagittal sinus
Splenium of callosum
Branches of posterior cerebral artery
Cuneus
Occipital lobe
Pineal body
Posterior commissure
Tectum
Lingual gyrus
Straight sinus
Cerebral aqueduct
Cerebellum
Fourth ventricle
Pons
Medulla oblongata
Nasopharynx
Oropharynx
Laryngopharynx
Spinal cord (medulla spinalis)
Seventh cervical vertebra

Medial frontal gyrus
Frontal lobe
Anterior cerebral artery
Corpus callosum
Septum pellucidum
Thalamus
Frontal sinus
Anterior commissure
Massa intermedia
Hypothalamus
Optic chiasm
Mammillary body
Nasal cavity
Hypophysis
Sphenoidal sinus
Maxilla
Atlas
Tongue
Uvula
Axis
Mandible
Hyoid bone
Epiglottis
Larynx
Esophagus
Trachea
Thyroid gland

PLATE 9—Brain in Relation to Other Structures of the Head and Neck

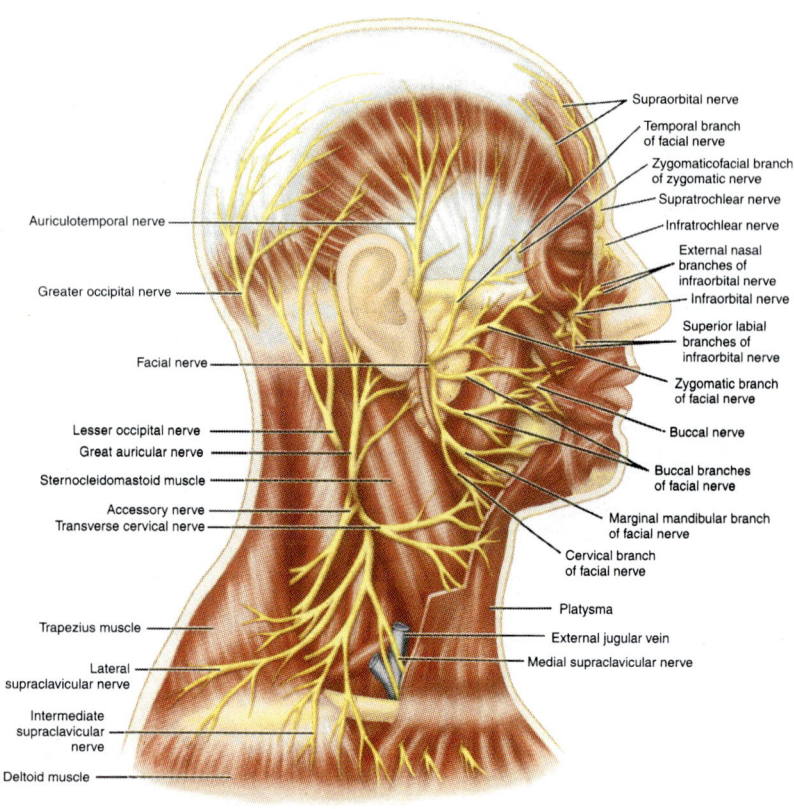

Supraorbital nerve

Temporal branch
of facial nerve

Zygomaticofacial branch
of zygomatic nerve

Supratrochlear nerve

Infratrochlear nerve

External nasal
branches of
infraorbital nerve

Infraorbital nerve

Superior labial
branches of
infraorbital nerve

Zygomatic branch
of facial nerve

Buccal nerve

Buccal branches
of facial nerve

Marginal mandibular branch
of facial nerve

Cervical branch
of facial nerve

Platysma

External jugular vein

Medial supraclavicular nerve

Auriculotemporal nerve

Greater occipital nerve

Facial nerve

Lesser occipital nerve

Great auricular nerve

Sternocleidomastoid muscle

Accessory nerve

Transverse cervical nerve

Trapezius muscle

Lateral
supraclavicular nerve

Intermediate
supraclavicular
nerve

Deltoid muscle

PLATE 10—Superficial Nerves of the Head and Neck

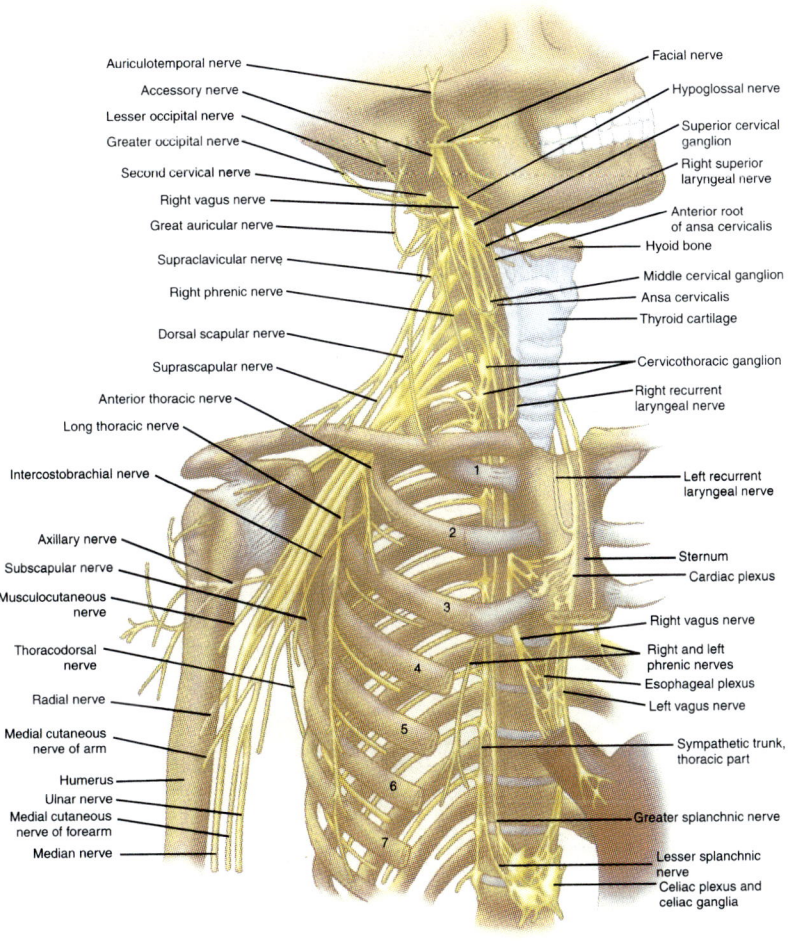

Auriculotemporal nerve
Accessory nerve
Lesser occipital nerve
Greater occipital nerve
Second cervical nerve
Right vagus nerve
Great auricular nerve
Supraclavicular nerve
Right phrenic nerve
Dorsal scapular nerve
Suprascapular nerve
Anterior thoracic nerve
Long thoracic nerve
Intercostobrachial nerve
Axillary nerve
Subscapular nerve
Musculocutaneous nerve
Thoracodorsal nerve
Radial nerve
Medial cutaneous nerve of arm
Humerus
Ulnar nerve
Medial cutaneous nerve of forearm
Median nerve

Facial nerve
Hypoglossal nerve
Superior cervical ganglion
Right superior laryngeal nerve
Anterior root of ansa cervicalis
Hyoid bone
Middle cervical ganglion
Ansa cervicalis
Thyroid cartilage
Cervicothoracic ganglion
Right recurrent laryngeal nerve
Left recurrent laryngeal nerve
Sternum
Cardiac plexus
Right vagus nerve
Right and left phrenic nerves
Esophageal plexus
Left vagus nerve
Sympathetic trunk, thoracic part
Greater splanchnic nerve
Lesser splanchnic nerve
Celiac plexus and celiac ganglia

PLATE 11—Deep Nerves of the Neck, Axilla, and Upper Thorax

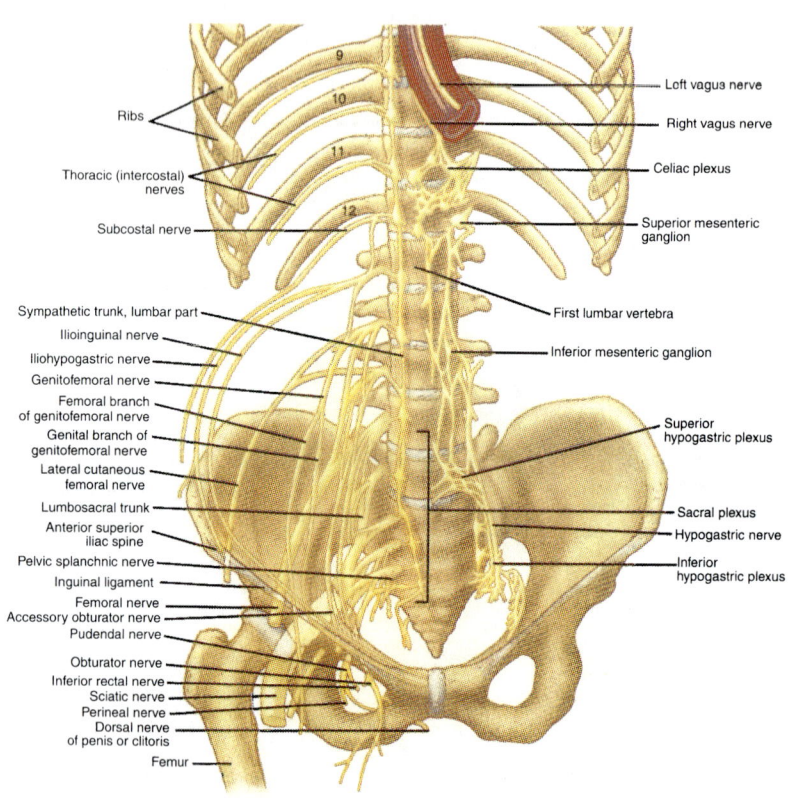

Ribs

Thoracic (intercostal) nerves

Subcostal nerve

Sympathetic trunk, lumbar part
Ilioinguinal nerve
Iliohypogastric nerve
Genitofemoral nerve
Femoral branch of genitofemoral nerve
Genital branch of genitofemoral nerve
Lateral cutaneous femoral nerve
Lumbosacral trunk
Anterior superior iliac spine
Pelvic splanchnic nerve
Inguinal ligament
Femoral nerve
Accessory obturator nerve
Pudendal nerve
Obturator nerve
Inferior rectal nerve
Sciatic nerve
Perineal nerve
Dorsal nerve of penis or clitoris
Femur

Left vagus nerve
Right vagus nerve
Celiac plexus
Superior mesenteric ganglion
First lumbar vertebra
Inferior mesenteric ganglion
Superior hypogastric plexus
Sacral plexus
Hypogastric nerve
Inferior hypogastric plexus

9
10
11
12

PLATE 12—Deep Nerves of the Lower Trunk

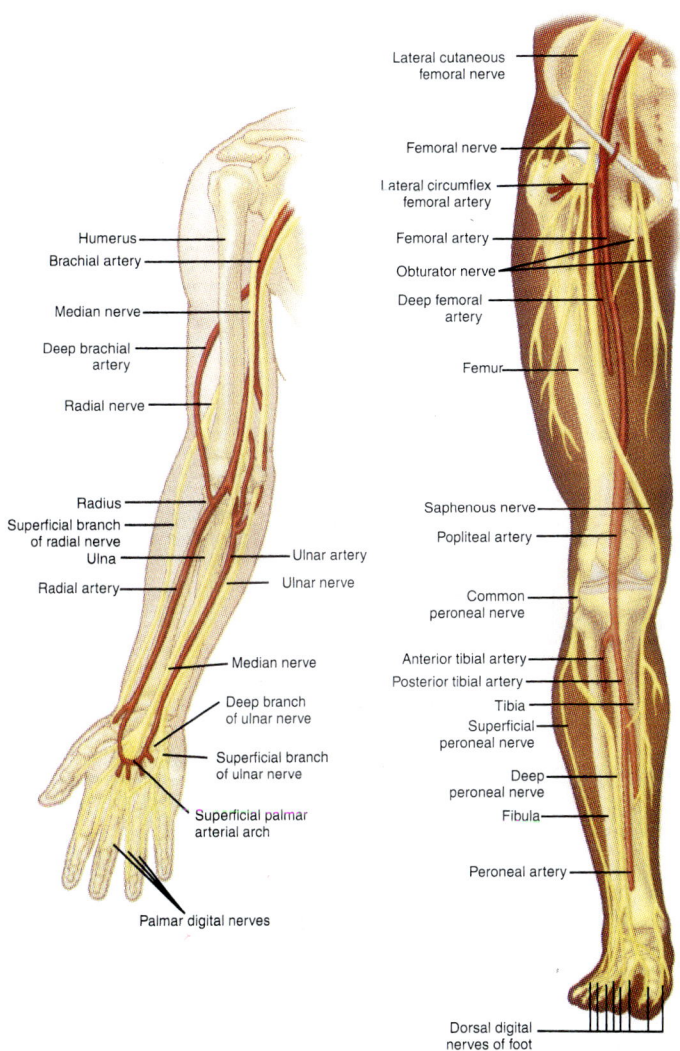

Lateral cutaneous femoral nerve

Femoral nerve

Lateral circumflex femoral artery

Femoral artery

Obturator nerve

Deep femoral artery

Femur

Humerus

Brachial artery

Median nerve

Deep brachial artery

Radial nerve

Radius

Superficial branch of radial nerve

Ulna

Radial artery

Ulnar artery

Ulnar nerve

Median nerve

Deep branch of ulnar nerve

Superficial branch of ulnar nerve

Superficial palmar arterial arch

Palmar digital nerves

Saphenous nerve

Popliteal artery

Common peroneal nerve

Anterior tibial artery

Posterior tibial artery

Tibia

Superficial peroneal nerve

Deep peroneal nerve

Fibula

Peroneal artery

Dorsal digital nerves of foot

PLATE 13—Nerves of the Limbs

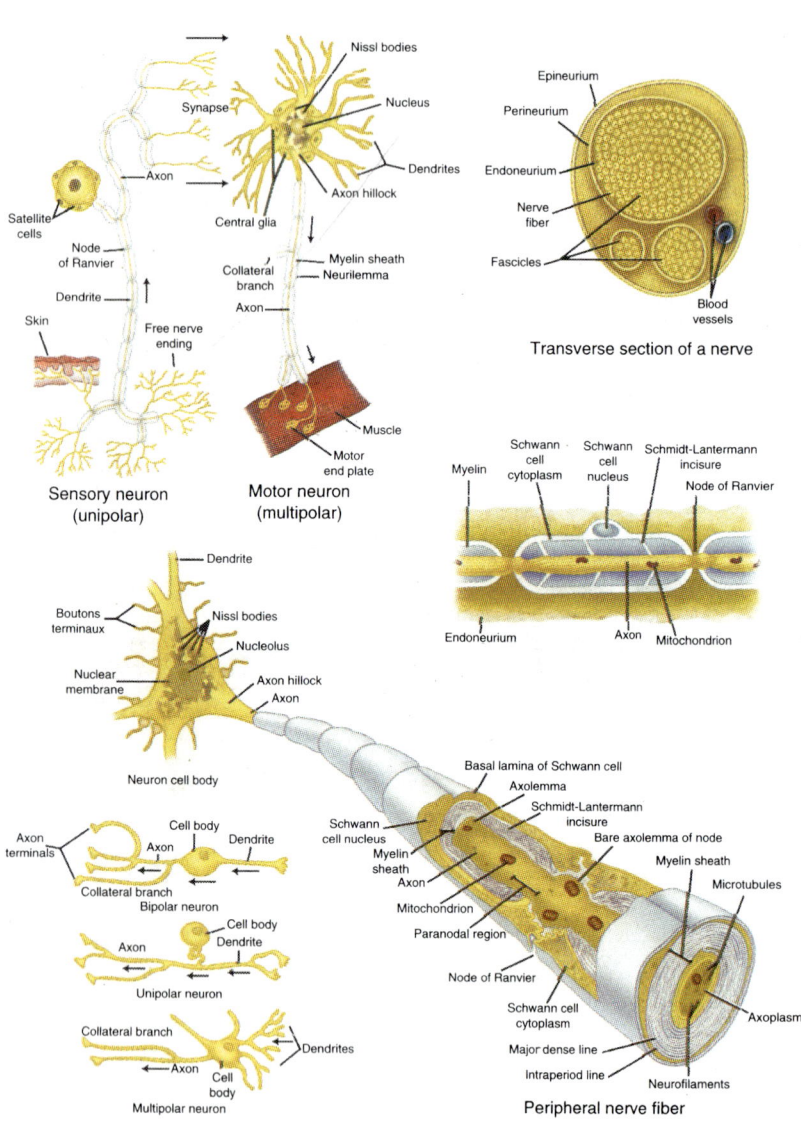

PLATE 14—Structure of Nerve Tissue

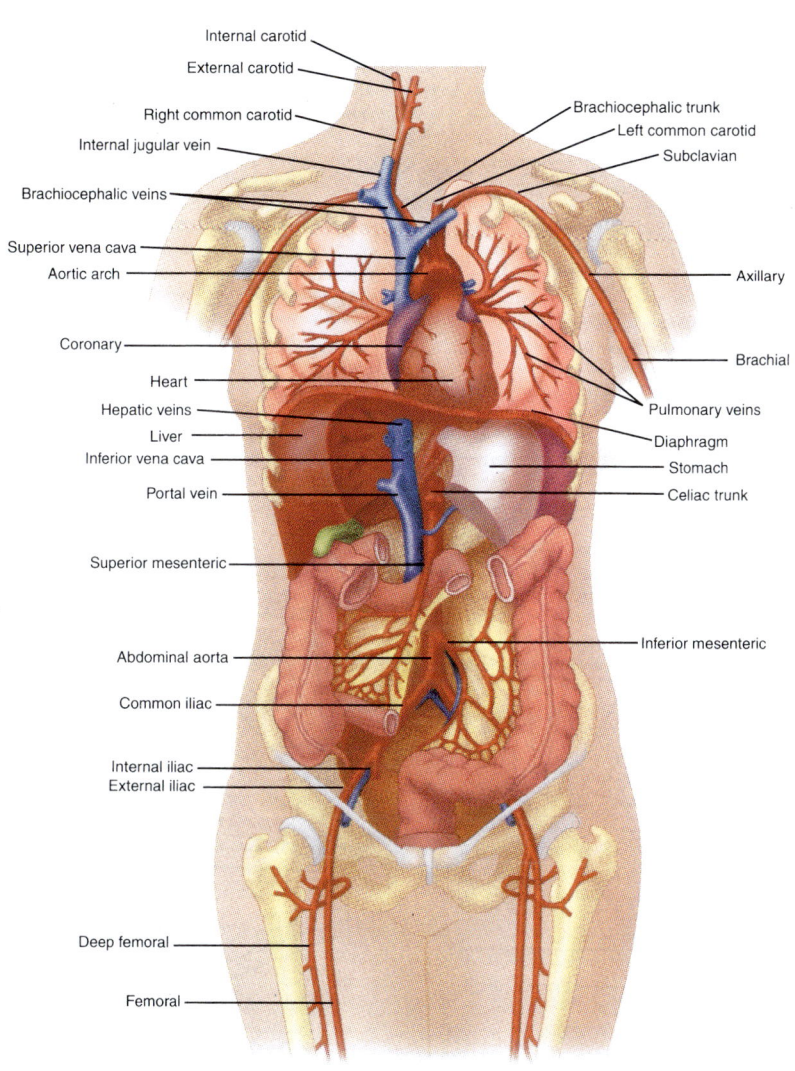

Internal carotid
External carotid
Right common carotid
Internal jugular vein
Brachiocephalic veins
Superior vena cava
Aortic arch
Coronary
Heart
Hepatic veins
Liver
Inferior vena cava
Portal vein
Superior mesenteric
Abdominal aorta
Common iliac
Internal iliac
External iliac
Deep femoral
Femoral

Brachiocephalic trunk
Left common carotid
Subclavian
Axillary
Brachial
Pulmonary veins
Diaphragm
Stomach
Celiac trunk
Inferior mesenteric

PLATE 15—Principal Arteries of the Body and the Pulmonary Veins

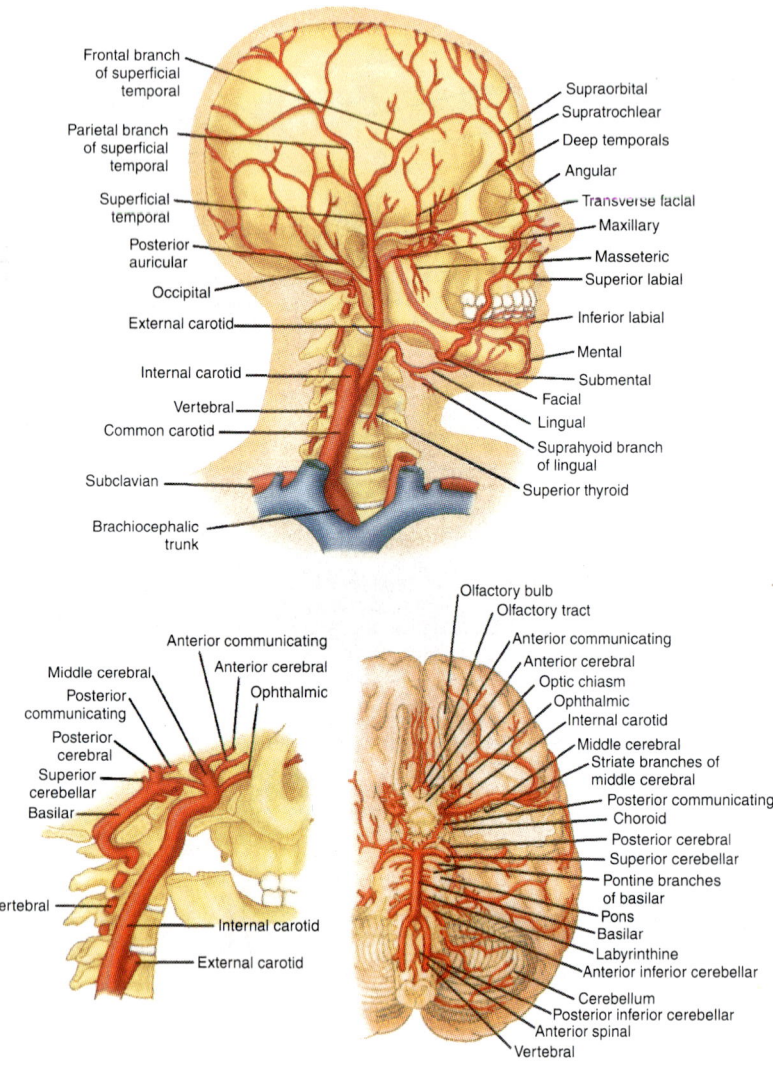

Frontal branch
of superficial
temporal

Parietal branch
of superficial
temporal

Superficial
temporal

Posterior
auricular

Occipital

External carotid

Internal carotid

Vertebral

Common carotid

Subclavian

Brachiocephalic
trunk

Supraorbital

Supratrochlear

Deep temporals

Angular

Transverse facial

Maxillary

Masseteric

Superior labial

Inferior labial

Mental

Submental

Facial

Lingual

Suprahyoid branch
of lingual

Superior thyroid

Anterior communicating

Middle cerebral

Posterior
communicating

Anterior cerebral

Ophthalmic

Posterior
cerebral

Superior
cerebellar

Basilar

Vertebral

Internal carotid

External carotid

Olfactory bulb

Olfactory tract

Anterior communicating

Anterior cerebral

Optic chiasm

Ophthalmic

Internal carotid

Middle cerebral

Striate branches of
middle cerebral

Posterior communicating

Choroid

Posterior cerebral

Superior cerebellar

Pontine branches
of basilar

Pons

Basilar

Labyrinthine

Anterior inferior cerebellar

Cerebellum

Posterior inferior cerebellar

Anterior spinal

Vertebral

PLATE 16—Arteries of the Head, Neck, and Base of the Brain

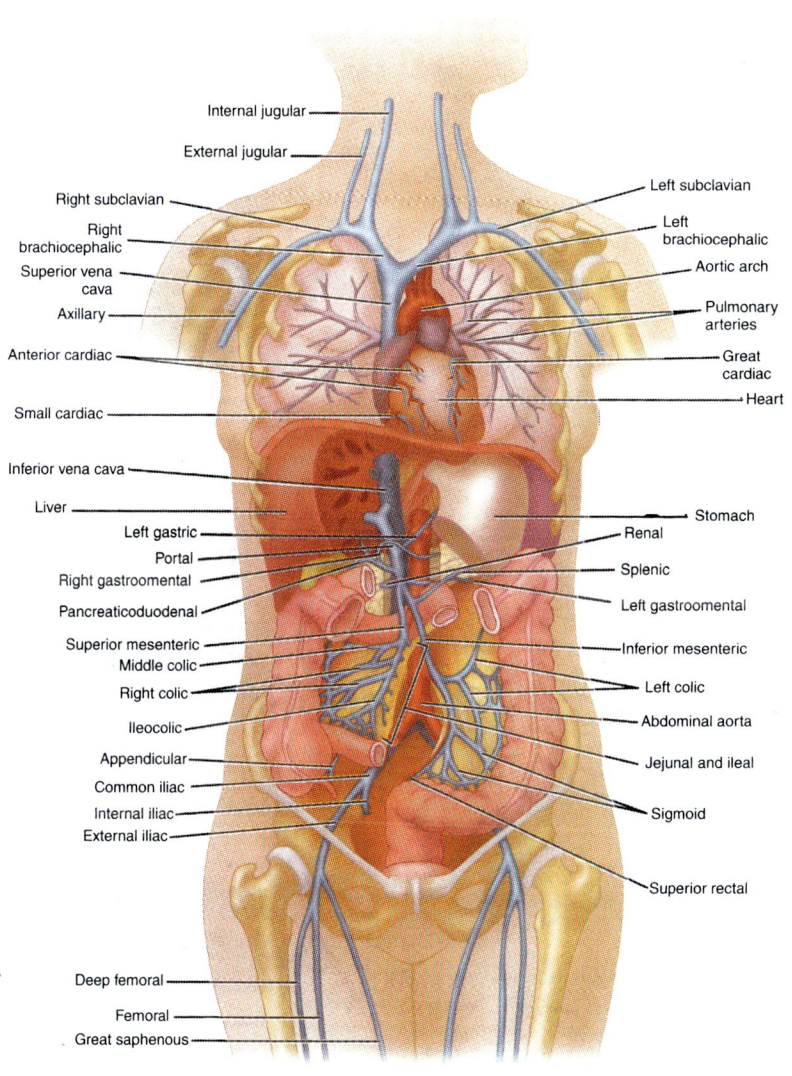

Internal jugular

External jugular

Right subclavian

Right brachiocephalic

Superior vena cava

Axillary

Anterior cardiac

Small cardiac

Inferior vena cava

Liver

Left gastric

Portal

Right gastroomental

Pancreaticoduodenal

Superior mesenteric

Middle colic

Right colic

Ileocolic

Appendicular

Common iliac

Internal iliac

External iliac

Deep femoral

Femoral

Great saphenous

Left subclavian

Left brachiocephalic

Aortic arch

Pulmonary arteries

Great cardiac

Heart

Stomach

Renal

Splenic

Left gastroomental

Inferior mesenteric

Left colic

Abdominal aorta

Jejunal and ileal

Sigmoid

Superior rectal

PLATE 21—Principal Veins of the Body

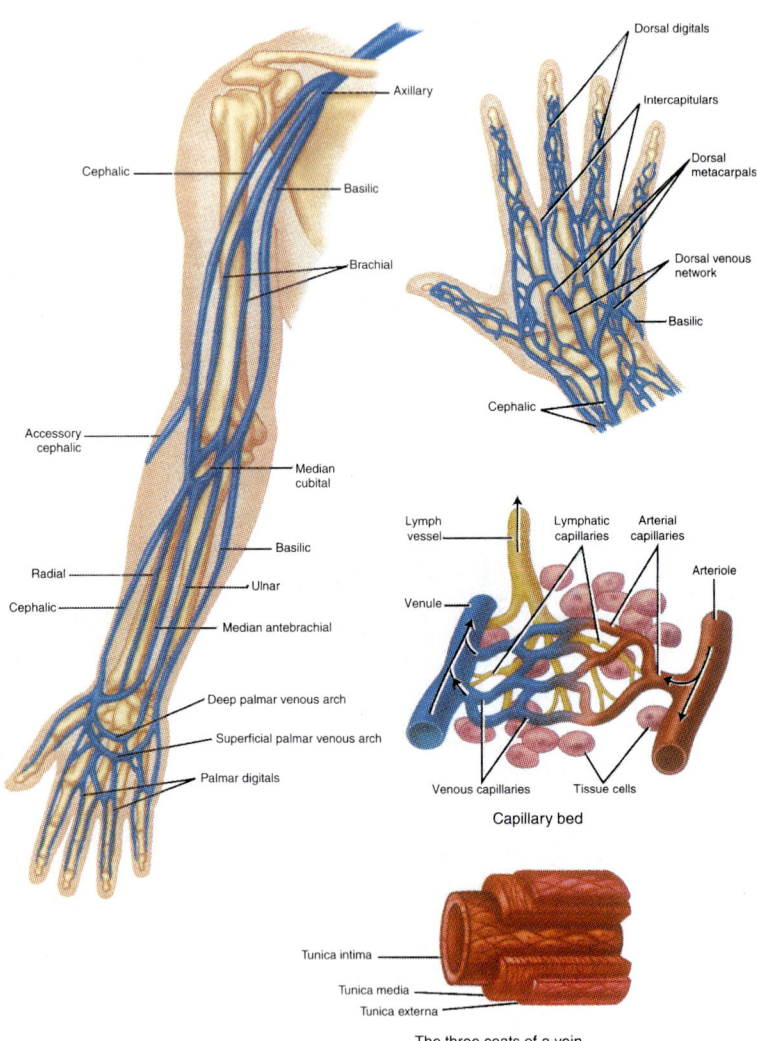

Axillary

Cephalic

Basilic

Brachial

Accessory cephalic

Median cubital

Basilic

Radial

Ulnar

Cephalic

Median antebrachial

Deep palmar venous arch

Superficial palmar venous arch

Palmar digitals

Dorsal digitals

Intercapitulars

Dorsal metacarpals

Dorsal venous network

Basilic

Cephalic

Lymph vessel

Lymphatic capillaries

Arterial capillaries

Arteriole

Venule

Venous capillaries

Tissue cells

Capillary bed

Tunica intima

Tunica media

Tunica externa

The three coats of a vein

PLATE 22—Superficial Veins of the Upper Limb and Venous Structure

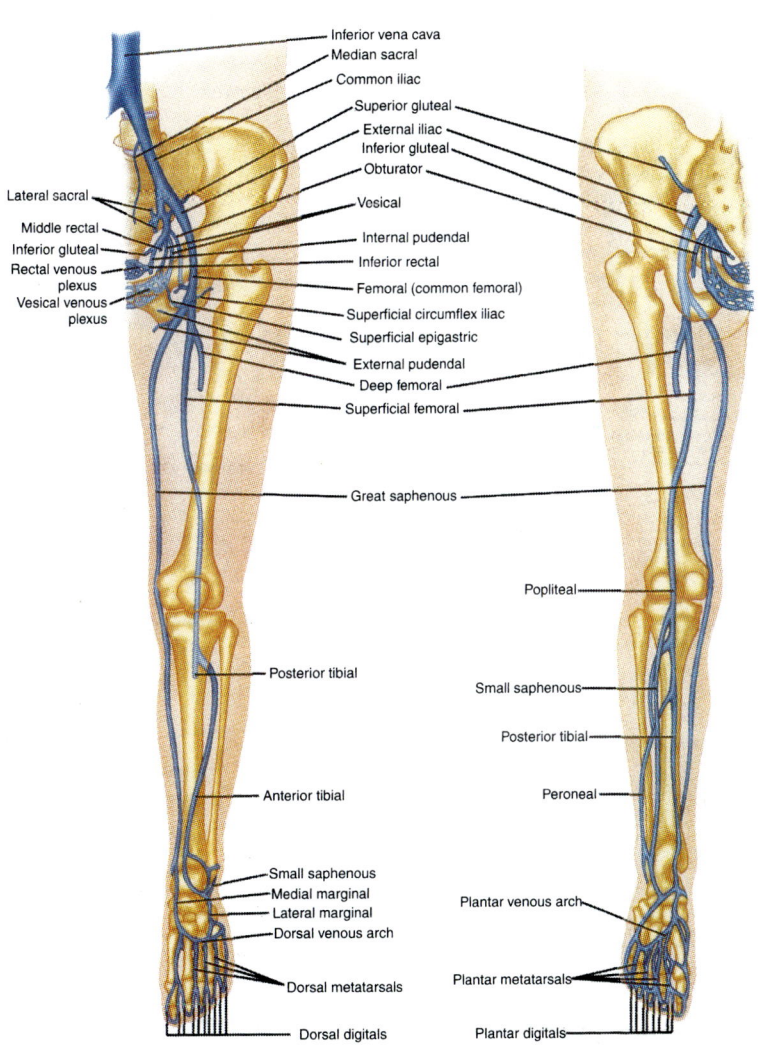

Inferior vena cava
Median sacral
Common iliac
Superior gluteal
External iliac
Inferior gluteal
Obturator
Lateral sacral
Vesical
Middle rectal
Inferior gluteal
Internal pudendal
Rectal venous plexus
Inferior rectal
Vesical venous plexus
Femoral (common femoral)
Superficial circumflex iliac
Superficial epigastric
External pudendal
Deep femoral
Superficial femoral

Great saphenous

Popliteal

Posterior tibial

Small saphenous

Posterior tibial

Anterior tibial

Peroneal

Small saphenous
Medial marginal
Lateral marginal
Dorsal venous arch
Plantar venous arch
Dorsal metatarsals
Plantar metatarsals
Dorsal digitals
Plantar digitals

PLATE 23—Superficial Veins of the Lower Limb

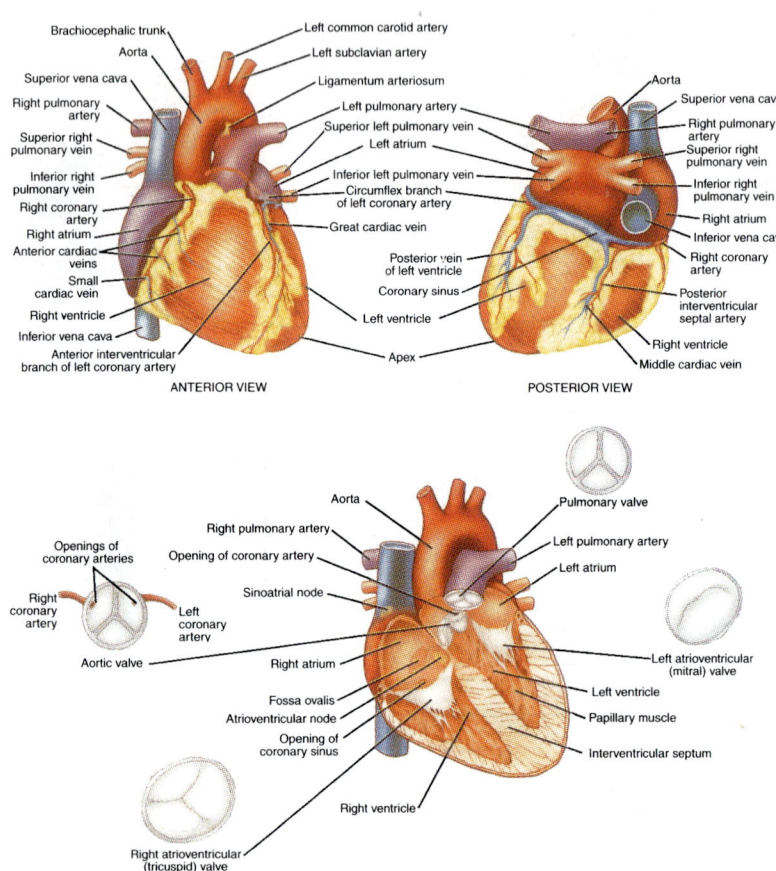

ANTERIOR VIEW

Brachiocephalic trunk
Aorta
Superior vena cava
Right pulmonary artery
Superior right pulmonary vein
Inferior right pulmonary vein
Right coronary artery
Right atrium
Anterior cardiac veins
Small cardiac vein
Right ventricle
Inferior vena cava
Anterior interventricular branch of left coronary artery

Left common carotid artery
Left subclavian artery
Ligamentum arteriosum
Left pulmonary artery
Superior left pulmonary vein
Left atrium
Inferior left pulmonary vein
Circumflex branch of left coronary artery
Great cardiac vein
Posterior vein of left ventricle
Coronary sinus
Left ventricle
Apex

POSTERIOR VIEW

Aorta
Superior vena cava
Right pulmonary artery
Superior right pulmonary vein
Inferior right pulmonary vein
Right atrium
Inferior vena cava
Right coronary artery
Posterior interventricular septal artery
Right ventricle
Middle cardiac vein

Openings of coronary arteries
Right coronary artery
Left coronary artery
Aortic valve

Aorta
Right pulmonary artery
Opening of coronary artery
Sinoatrial node
Right atrium
Fossa ovalis
Atrioventricular node
Opening of coronary sinus
Right ventricle
Right atrioventricular (tricuspid) valve

Pulmonary valve
Left pulmonary artery
Left atrium
Left atrioventricular (mitral) valve
Left ventricle
Papillary muscle
Interventricular septum

PLATE 24—Structures of the Heart

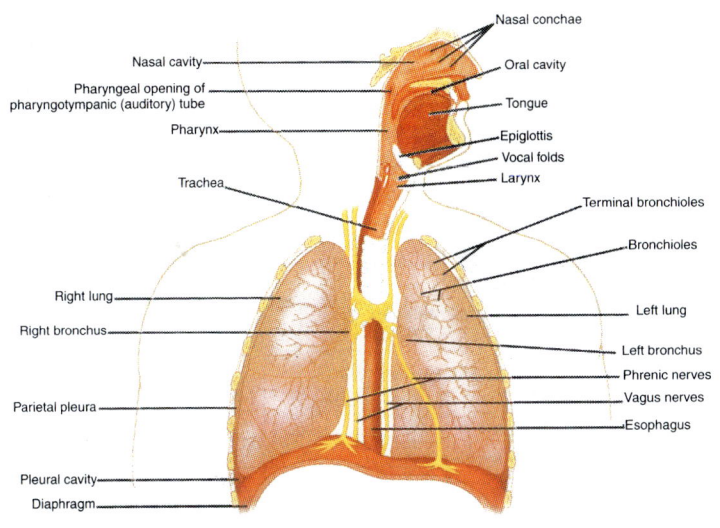

Nasal conchae

Nasal cavity

Pharyngeal opening of pharyngotympanic (auditory) tube

Oral cavity

Pharynx

Tongue

Epiglottis

Vocal folds

Trachea

Larynx

Terminal bronchioles

Bronchioles

Right lung

Left lung

Right bronchus

Left bronchus

Phrenic nerves

Vagus nerves

Parietal pleura

Esophagus

Pleural cavity

Diaphragm

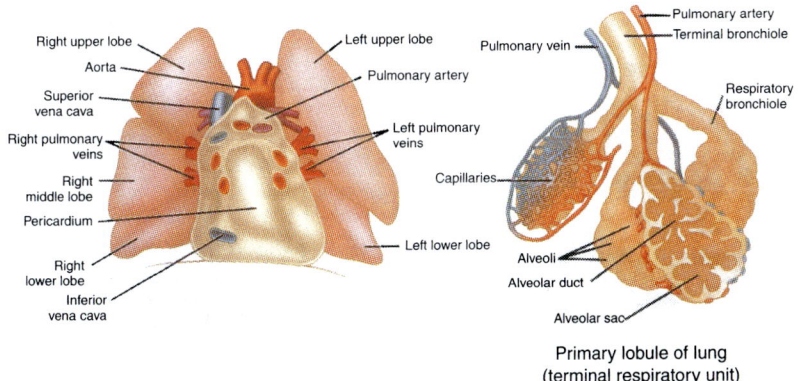

Right upper lobe

Left upper lobe

Aorta

Pulmonary artery

Superior vena cava

Left pulmonary veins

Right pulmonary veins

Right middle lobe

Pericardium

Left lower lobe

Right lower lobe

Inferior vena cava

Pulmonary artery

Terminal bronchiole

Pulmonary vein

Respiratory bronchiole

Capillaries

Alveoli

Alveolar duct

Alveolar sac

Primary lobule of lung
(terminal respiratory unit)

PLATE 25—Organs of the Respiratory System

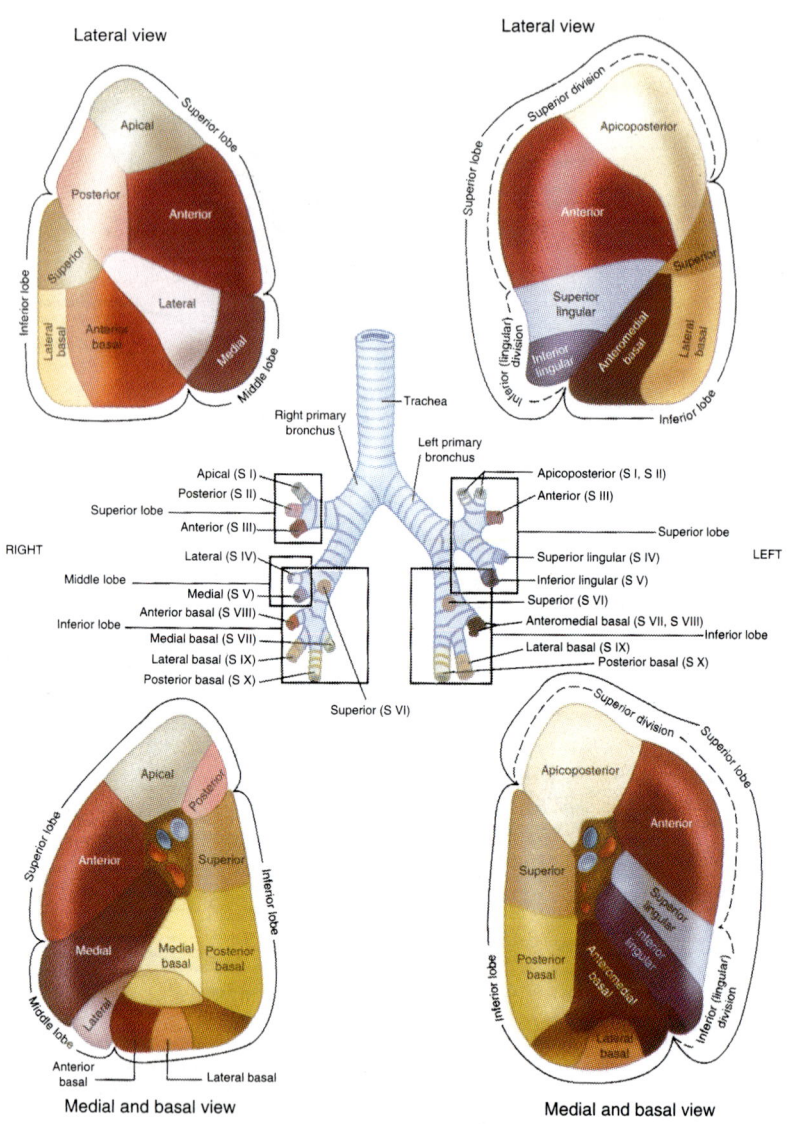

Lateral view

Apical
Posterior
Anterior
Lateral
Medial
Superior lobe
Superior
Anterior basal
Lateral basal
Inferior lobe
Middle lobe

Lateral view

Superior division
Apicoposterior
Anterior
Superior lingular
Inferior lingular
Anteromedial basal
Superior lobe
Superior
Lateral basal
Inferior lobe
Inferior (lingular) division

Trachea
Right primary bronchus
Left primary bronchus

RIGHT

Apical (S I)
Posterior (S II)
Anterior (S III)
Superior lobe

Lateral (S IV)
Middle lobe
Medial (S V)
Anterior basal (S VIII)
Inferior lobe
Medial basal (S VII)
Lateral basal (S IX)
Posterior basal (S X)
Superior (S VI)

LEFT

Apicoposterior (S I, S II)
Anterior (S III)
Superior lobe

Superior lingular (S IV)
Inferior lingular (S V)
Superior (S VI)
Anteromedial basal (S VII, S VIII)
Inferior lobe
Lateral basal (S IX)
Posterior basal (S X)

Apical
Posterior
Anterior
Superior
Medial
Medial basal
Posterior basal
Lateral
Superior lobe
Inferior lobe
Middle lobe
Anterior basal
Lateral basal

Medial and basal view

Apicoposterior
Anterior
Superior
Superior lingular
Inferior lingular
Posterior basal
Anteromedial basal
Lateral basal
Superior division
Superior lobe
Inferior lobe
Inferior (lingular) division

Medial and basal view

**PLATE 26—Pulmonary Segments: Tracheobronchial Branching
Correlated with Subdivision of the Lungs**

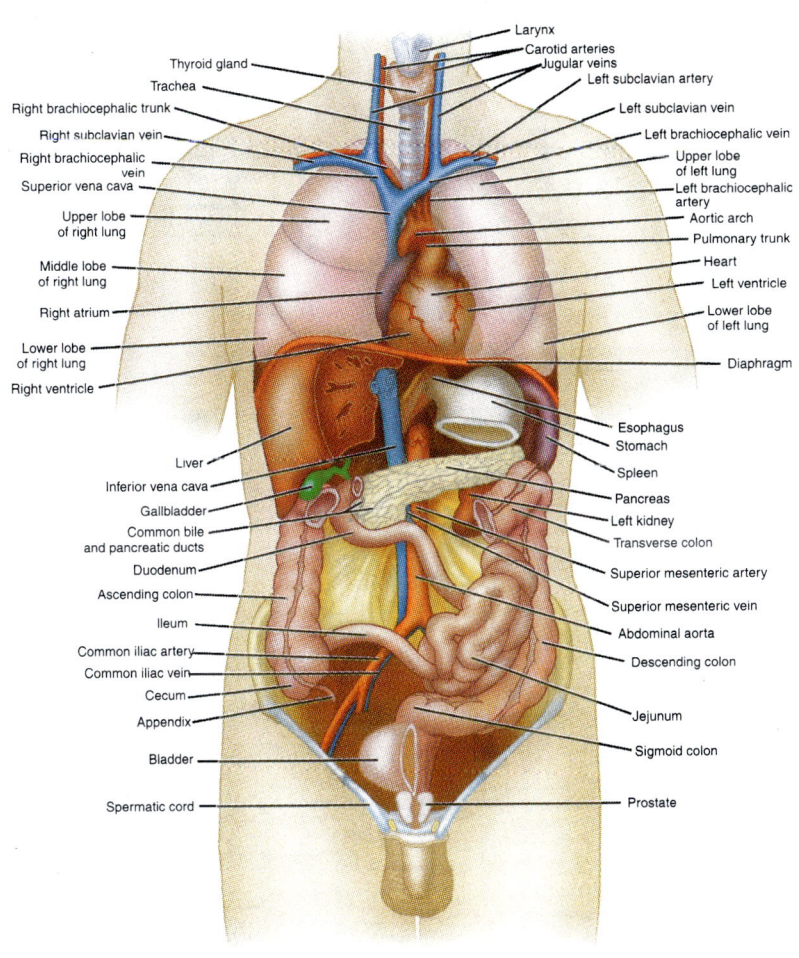

Larynx
Carotid arteries
Jugular veins
Left subclavian artery
Thyroid gland
Trachea
Left subclavian vein
Right brachiocephalic trunk
Right subclavian vein
Left brachiocephalic vein
Right brachiocephalic vein
Upper lobe of left lung
Superior vena cava
Left brachiocephalic artery
Upper lobe of right lung
Aortic arch
Pulmonary trunk
Middle lobe of right lung
Heart
Left ventricle
Right atrium
Lower lobe of left lung
Lower lobe of right lung
Diaphragm
Right ventricle
Esophagus
Stomach
Spleen
Liver
Pancreas
Inferior vena cava
Left kidney
Gallbladder
Transverse colon
Common bile and pancreatic ducts
Duodenum
Superior mesenteric artery
Ascending colon
Superior mesenteric vein
Ileum
Abdominal aorta
Common iliac artery
Descending colon
Common iliac vein
Cecum
Appendix
Jejunum
Bladder
Sigmoid colon
Spermatic cord
Prostate

PLATE 27—Thoracic and Abdominal Viscera

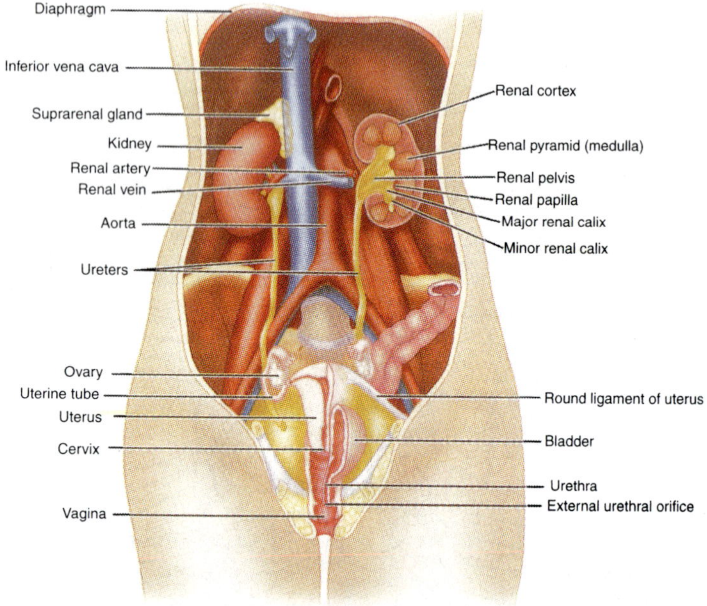

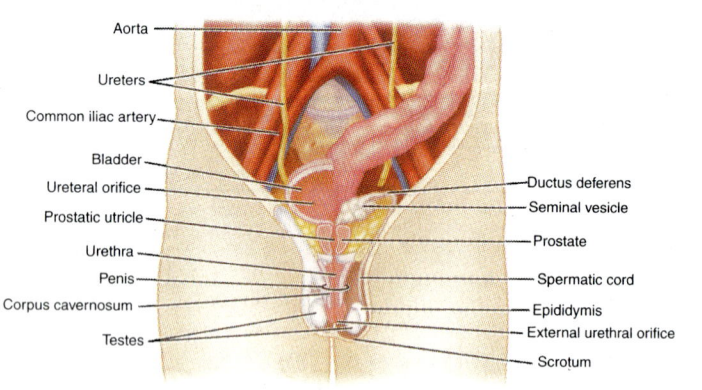

Diaphragm

Inferior vena cava

Suprarenal gland

Kidney

Renal artery

Renal vein

Aorta

Ureters

Ovary

Uterine tube

Uterus

Cervix

Vagina

Renal cortex

Renal pyramid (medulla)

Renal pelvis

Renal papilla

Major renal calix

Minor renal calix

Round ligament of uterus

Bladder

Urethra

External urethral orifice

Aorta

Ureters

Common iliac artery

Bladder

Ureteral orifice

Prostatic utricle

Urethra

Penis

Corpus cavernosum

Testes

Ductus deferens

Seminal vesicle

Prostate

Spermatic cord

Epididymis

External urethral orifice

Scrotum

PLATE 28—Organs of the Urogenital System

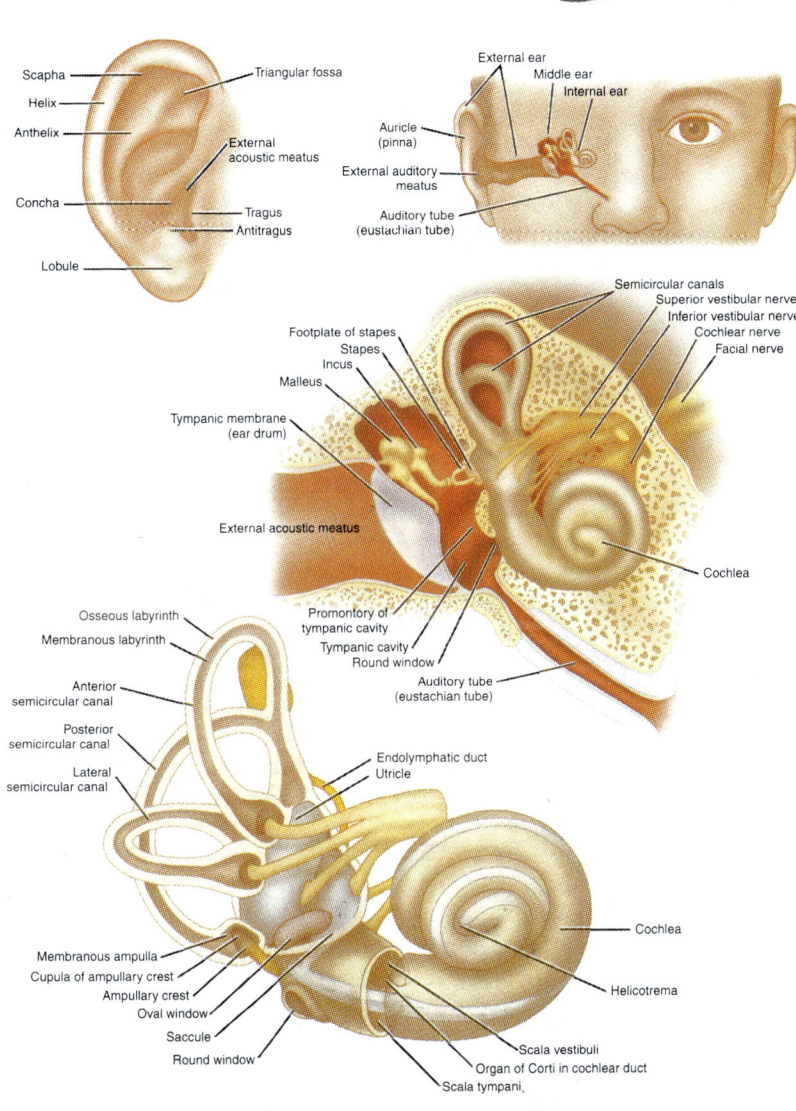

Scapha

Helix

Anthelix

Concha

Lobule

Triangular fossa

External acoustic meatus

Tragus

Antitragus

External ear
Middle ear
Internal ear

Auricle (pinna)

External auditory meatus

Auditory tube (eustachian tube)

Footplate of stapes
Stapes
Incus
Malleus

Tympanic membrane (ear drum)

External acoustic meatus

Semicircular canals
Superior vestibular nerve
Inferior vestibular nerve
Cochlear nerve
Facial nerve

Cochlea

Promontory of tympanic cavity
Tympanic cavity
Round window
Auditory tube (eustachian tube)

Osseous labyrinth

Membranous labyrinth

Anterior semicircular canal

Posterior semicircular canal

Lateral semicircular canal

Endolymphatic duct
Utricle

Membranous ampulla
Cupula of ampullary crest
Ampullary crest
Oval window
Saccule
Round window

Cochlea

Helicotrema

Scala vestibuli
Organ of Corti in cochlear duct
Scala tympani

PLATE 29—Structures of the Ear

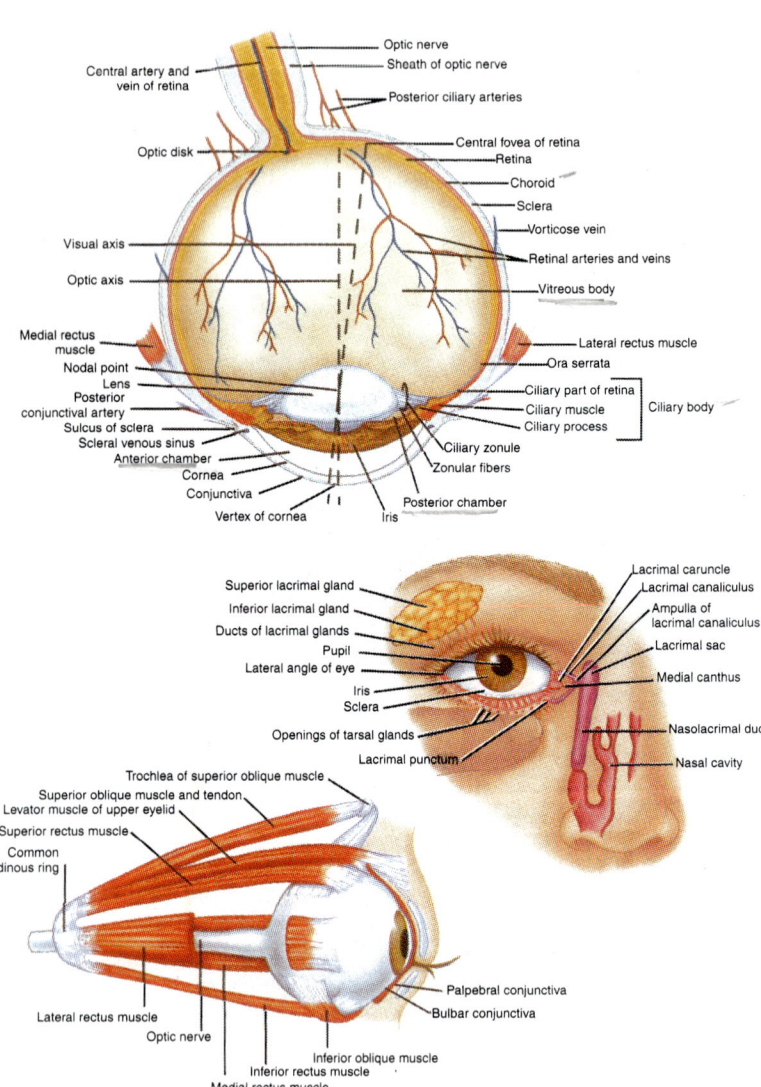

Optic nerve
Sheath of optic nerve
Central artery and vein of retina
Posterior ciliary arteries
Optic disk
Central fovea of retina
Retina
Choroid
Sclera
Vorticose vein
Visual axis
Retinal arteries and veins
Optic axis
Vitreous body
Medial rectus muscle
Lateral rectus muscle
Nodal point
Ora serrata
Lens
Posterior conjunctival artery
Ciliary part of retina
Ciliary muscle
Ciliary process
Ciliary body
Sulcus of sclera
Scleral venous sinus
Ciliary zonule
Anterior chamber
Zonular fibers
Cornea
Conjunctiva
Posterior chamber
Vertex of cornea
Iris

Superior lacrimal gland
Lacrimal caruncle
Lacrimal canaliculus
Inferior lacrimal gland
Ampulla of lacrimal canaliculus
Ducts of lacrimal glands
Pupil
Lacrimal sac
Lateral angle of eye
Iris
Medial canthus
Sclera
Openings of tarsal glands
Nasolacrimal duct
Lacrimal punctum
Nasal cavity

Trochlea of superior oblique muscle
Superior oblique muscle and tendon
Levator muscle of upper eyelid
Superior rectus muscle
Common tendinous ring
Palpebral conjunctiva
Bulbar conjunctiva
Lateral rectus muscle
Optic nerve
Inferior oblique muscle
Inferior rectus muscle
Medial rectus muscle

PLATE 30—The Eye and Related Structures

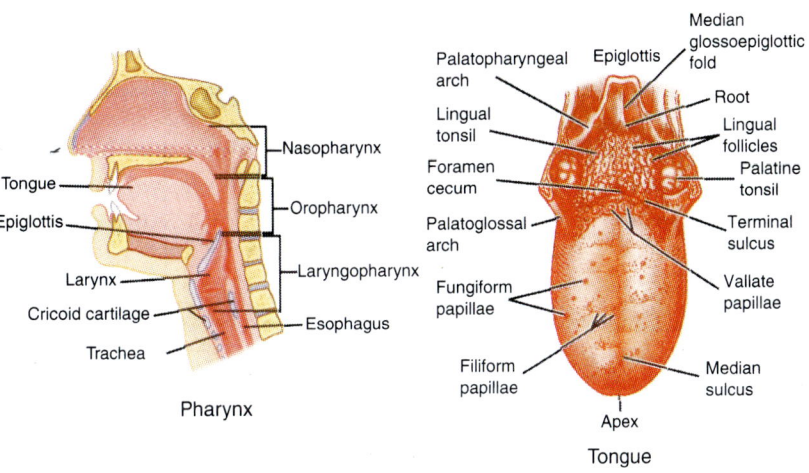

Pharynx

- Nasopharynx
- Oropharynx
- Laryngopharynx
- Esophagus
- Tongue
- Epiglottis
- Larynx
- Cricoid cartilage
- Trachea

Tongue

- Palatopharyngeal arch
- Epiglottis
- Median glossoepiglottic fold
- Lingual tonsil
- Root
- Lingual follicles
- Foramen cecum
- Palatine tonsil
- Palatoglossal arch
- Terminal sulcus
- Fungiform papillae
- Vallate papillae
- Filiform papillae
- Median sulcus
- Apex

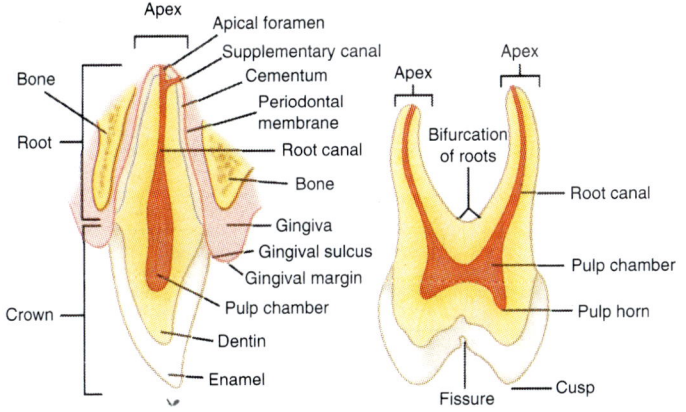

Cross sections of incisor and molar teeth

- Apex
- Apical foramen
- Supplementary canal
- Cementum
- Periodontal membrane
- Root canal
- Bone
- Bone
- Root
- Gingiva
- Gingival sulcus
- Gingival margin
- Pulp chamber
- Crown
- Dentin
- Enamel
- Apex
- Bifurcation of roots
- Apex
- Root canal
- Pulp chamber
- Pulp horn
- Fissure
- Cusp

PLATE 31—Structures of the Pharynx and Oral Cavity

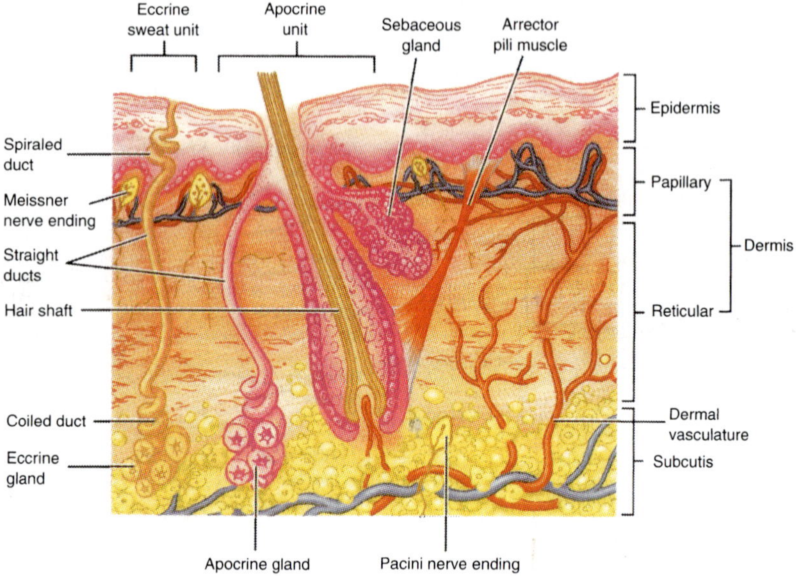

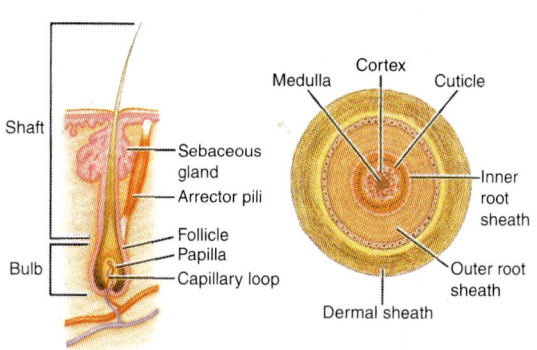

Eccrine sweat unit

Apocrine unit

Sebaceous gland

Arrector pili muscle

Epidermis

Spiraled duct

Meissner nerve ending

Straight ducts

Hair shaft

Papillary

Dermis

Reticular

Coiled duct

Eccrine gland

Dermal vasculature

Subcutis

Apocrine gland

Pacini nerve ending

Skin

Shaft

Sebaceous gland

Arrector pili

Follicle

Papilla

Capillary loop

Bulb

Medulla

Cortex

Cuticle

Inner root sheath

Outer root sheath

Dermal sheath

Hair, in longitudinal and cross-section

PLATE 32—Sections of Skin and Hair

hypotension. **metachromatic l.,** an inherited disorder due to accumulation of sulfatide in tissues with a diffuse loss of myelin in the central nervous system; it occurs in several forms, with increasing age of onset correlated to decreasing severity, all initially presenting as mental regression and motor disturbances.

leu·ko·ede·ma (-ĕ-de′mah) a variant condition of the buccal mucosa, consisting of an increase in thickness of the epithelium and intracellular edema of the stratum spinosum or stratum germinativum.

leu·ko·en·ceph·a·li·tis (-en-sef″ah-li′tis) inflammation of the white substance of the brain.

leu·ko·en·ceph·a·lop·a·thy (-en-sef″ah-lop′ah-the) any of a group of diseases affecting the white substance of the brain. The term *leukodystrophy* is used to denote such disorders due to defective formation and maintenance of myelin in infants and children. **progressive multifocal l.,** a form due to opportunistic infection of the central nervous system by the JC virus, with demyelination occurring usually in the cerebral hemispheres and rarely in the brain stem and cerebellum.

leu·ko·eryth·ro·blas·to·sis (-ĕ-rith″ro-blas-to′sis) anemia associated with space-occupying lesions of the bone marrow that cause bone marrow suppression with a variable number of immature cells of the erythrocytic and granulocytic series in the circulation.

leu·ko·ker·a·to·sis (-ker″ah-to′sis) leukoplakia.

leu·ko·ko·ria (-kor′e-ah) any condition marked by the appearance of a whitish reflex or mass in the pupillary area behind the lens.

leu·ko·krau·ro·sis (-kraw-ro′sis) kraurosis vulvae.

leu·ko·lym·pho·sar·co·ma (-lim″fo-sahr-ko′mah) leukosarcoma.

leu·kol·y·sis (-kol′ĭ-sis) destruction or disintegration of leukocytes. **leukolyt′ic,** adj.

leu·ko·ma (loo-ko′mah) pl. *leuko′mata.* [Gr.] 1. a dense, white corneal opacity. 2. leukoplakia of the buccal mucosa. **leukom′atous,** adj. **adherent l.,** a white tumor of the cornea enclosing a prolapsed adherent iris.

leu·ko·my·eli·tis (loo″ko-mi″ĕ-li′tis) inflammation of the white substance of the spinal cord.

leu·ko·ne·cro·sis (-nĕ-kro′sis) gangrene with formation of a white slough.

leu·ko·nych·ia (-nik′e-ah) abnormal whiteness of the nails, either total or in spots or streaks.

leu·ko·path·ia (-path′e-ah) 1. leukoderma. 2. disease of the leukocytes. **l. un′guium,** leukonychia.

leu·ko·pe·de·sis (-pĕ-de′sis) leukocyte emigration.

leu·ko·pe·nia (-pe′ne-ah) reduction of the number of leukocytes in the blood below about 5000 per cubic mm. **leukope′nic,** adj. **basophilic l.,** basophilopenia. **malignant l., pernicious l.,** agranulocytosis.

leu·ko·pla·kia (-pla′ke-ah) 1. a white patch on a mucous membrane that will not rub off. 2. oral l. **atrophic l.,** lichen sclerosus in females. **oral l.,** white, thick patches on the oral mucosa due to hyperkeratosis of the epithelium, producing favorable conditions for development of epidermoid carcinoma; often occurring on the cheeks (*l. bucca′lis*), gums, or tongue (*l. lingua′lis*). **oral hairy l.,** a white filiform to flat patch on the tongue or the buccal mucosa, caused by infection with Epstein-Barr virus and associated with human immunodeficiency virus infection. **l. vul′vae,** 1. lichen sclerosus in females. 2. any white-appearing lesion of the vulva.

leu·ko·poi·e·sis (-poi-e′sis) production of leukocytes.

leu·kor·rhea (-re′ah) a whitish, viscid discharge from the vagina and uterine cavity.

leu·ko·sar·co·ma (-sahr-ko′mah) the development of leukemia in patients originally having a well-differentiated, lymphocytic type of malignant lymphoma.

leu·ko·sis (loo-ko′sis) pl. *leuko′ses.* Proliferation of leukocyte-forming tissue.

leu·ko·tax·is (loo″ko-tak′sis) cytotaxis of leukocytes; the tendency of leukocytes to collect in regions of injury and inflammation. **leukotac′tic,** adj.

leu·kot·o·me (loo″ko-tōm) a neurosurgical tool in which a wire loop on one end of a rigid shaft is used to cut tissue.

leu·kot·o·my (loo-kot′ah-me) prefrontal lobotomy.

leu·ko·tox·in (loo″ko-tok″sin) a cytoxin destructive to leukocytes.

leu·ko·trich·ia (loo″ko-trik′e-ah) whiteness of the hair in a circumscribed area.

leu·ko·tri·ene (-tri′ēn) any of a group of biologically active compounds derived from arachidonic acid that function as regulators of allergic and inflammatory reactions. They are identified by the letters A, B, C, D, and E, with subscript numerals indicating the number of double bonds in each molecule.

leu·pro·lide (loo-pro′līd) a synthetic analogue of gonadotropin-releasing hormone, used in the form of the acetate ester as an antiendometriotic agent, antineoplastic, and gonadotropin inhibitor.

lev·al·bu·ter·ol (lev″al-bu′ter-ol) *R*-albuterol; a β-adrenergic agent used as the hydrochloride salt as a bronchodilator for the treatment and prophylaxis of reversible bronchospasm.

le·vam·i·sole (le-vam′ĭ-sōl) an immunomodulator used with fluorouracil in the treatment of colon cancer, administered as the hydrochloride salt.

lev·ar·te·re·nol (lev″ar-tĕ-re′nol) the levorotatory isomer of norepinephrine, a much more potent pressor agent than the natural dextrorotatory isomer.

le·va·tor (le-va′tor) pl. *levato′res*. 1. A muscle that elevates an organ or structure. 2. an instrument for raising depressed osseous fragments in fractures.

lev·el (lev′el) relative position, rank, or concentration. confidence l., the probability that a confidence interval does not contain the population parameter. l. of significance, the probability of incorrectly rejecting the null hypothesis.

le·ve·ti·rac·e·tam (le″vĕ-ti-ras′ĕ-tam) an anticonvulsant used in the treatment of partial seizures in adults with epilepsy.

lev·i·ga·tion (lev″ĭ-ga′shun) the grinding to a powder of a moist or hard substance.

lev(o)- word element [L.], *left*.

le·vo·be·tax·o·lol (le″vo-ba-tak′sah-lol) a cardioselective β-adrenergic blocking agent, used topically in the form of the hydrochloride salt in the treatment of glaucoma and ocular hypertension.

le·vo·bu·no·lol (le″vo-bu′no-lol) a nonspecific beta-adrenergic blocking agent used as the hydrochloride salt in the treatment of glaucoma and ocular hypertension.

le·vo·bu·piv·a·caine (le″vo-bu-piv′ah-kān) the *S* enantiomer of bupivacaine; a local anesthetic used as the hydrochloride salt for local infiltration anesthesia, peripheral nerve block, and epidural anesthesia.

le·vo·cab·as·tine (-kab′ah-stēn) an antihistamine applied topically to the conjunctiva as the hydrochloride salt to treat seasonal allergic conjunctivitis.

le·vo·car·dia (-kahr′de-ah) a term denoting normal position of the heart associated with transposition of other viscera (situs inversus).

le·vo·car·ni·tine (-kahr′nĭ-tēn) a preparation of the biologically active L-isomer of carnitine used in the treatment of carnitine deficiency.

le·vo·cli·na·tion (-klĭ-na′shun) rotation of the upper poles of the vertical meridians of the two eyes to the left.

le·vo·do·pa (-do′pah) L-dopa; the levorotatory isomer of dopa, used as an antiparkinsonian agent.

le·vo·flox·a·cin (-flok′sah-sin) a broad-spectrum antibacterial agent for systemic and ophthalmic use.

le·vo·meth·a·dyl (-meth′ah-dil) an opioid analgesic used as an adjunct in the treatment of opioid addiction; administered as the acetate hydrochloride salt.

le·vo·nor·ges·trel (-nor-jes′trel) the levorotatory form of norgestrel; used as an oral or subdermal contraceptive.

le·vo·ro·ta·to·ry (-ro′tah-tor″e) turning the plane of polarization of polarized light to the left (counterclockwise).

le·vor·pha·nol (le-vor′fah-nol) an opioid analgesic with properties and actions similar to those of morphine; used as the bitartrate salt as an analgesic and an anesthesia adjunct.

le·vo·thy·rox·ine (le″vo-thi-rok′sēn) L-thyroxine, obtained from the thyroid gland of domesticated food animals or prepared synthetically; used as the sodium salt in the treatment of hypothyroidism and the treatment and prophylaxis of goiter and thyroid carcinoma.

le·vo·tor·sion (-tor′shun) levoclination.

le·vo·ver·sion (-ver′zhun) a turning toward the left.

LFA left frontoanterior (position of the fetus).

LFP left frontoposterior (position of the fetus).

LFT left frontotransverse (position of the fetus).

LH luteinizing hormone.

LH–RH luteinizing hormone–releasing hormone.

Li lithium.

li·bi·do (lĭ-be′do, lĭ-bi′do) pl. *libid′ines*. [L.] 1. sexual desire. 2. the psychic energy derived from instinctive biological drives; in early freudian theory it was restricted to the sexual drive, then expanded to all expressions of love and pleasure, but has evolved to include also the death instinct. **libid′inal**, adj.

lice (līs) plural of *louse*.

li·cen·ti·ate (li-sen′she-āt) one holding a license from an authorized agency giving the right to practice a particular profession.

li·chen (līk′'n) 1. any of certain plants formed by the mutualistic combination of an alga and a fungus. 2. any of various papular skin diseases in which the lesions are typically small, firm papules set close

together.   **l. amyloido′sus,** a condition characterized by localized cutaneous amyloidosis.
l. fibromucinoido′sus, l. myxedemato′sus, a condition resembling myxedema but unassociated with hypothyroidism, marked by a fibrocystic proliferation, increased deposition of acid mucopolysaccharides in the skin, and the presence of a circulating paraprotein; it may present as lichenoid papules or urticaria-like plaques and nodules.   **l. ni′tidus,** a chronic inflammatory eruption consisting of many, pinhead-sized pale, flat, sharply marginated, glistening, discrete papules, scarcely raised above the skin level.
l. planopila′ris, a variant of lichen planus characterized by formation of acuminate horny papules around the hair follicles, in addition to the typical lesions of ordinary lichen planus.   **l. pla′nus,** an inflammatory skin disease with wide, flat, violaceous, shiny papules in circumscribed patches; it may involve the hair follicles, nails, and buccal mucosa.   **l. ru′ber monilifor′mis,** a variant of lichen simplex chronicus with papules arranged in linear beaded bands.
l. ru′ber pla′nus, l. planus.   **l. sclero′sus,** a chronic atrophic skin disease marked by white papules with an erythematous halo and keratotic plugging, usually around the external genitalia or in the perianal region.
l. scrofuloso′rum, l. scrofulo′sus, any eruption of minute reddish lichenoid follicular papules in children and young adults with tuberculosis.   **l. sim′plex chro′nicus,** a dermatosis of psychogenic origin, marked by a pruritic discrete or, more often, confluent papular eruption, usually confined to a localized area.   **l. spinulo′sus,** a condition in which there is a horn or spine in the center of each hair follicle.   **l. stria′tus,** a self-limited condition characterized by a linear lichenoid eruption, usually in children.

li·chen·i·fi·ca·tion   (li-ken″ĭ-fĭ-ka′shun) thickening and hardening of the skin, with exaggeration of its normal markings.

lic·o·rice   (lik′ah-ris)   glycyrrhiza; the dried rhizome, roots, and stolons of various species of the perennial herb *Glycyrrhiza,* used as an expectorant and for the treatment of gastritis; also used in traditional Chinese medicine, ayurveda, and folk medicine.

li·do·caine   (li′do-kān) an anesthetic with sedative, analgesic, and cardiac depressant properties, applied topically in the form of the base or hydrochloride salt as a local anesthetic; also used in the latter form as a cardiac antiarrhythmic and to produce infiltration anesthesia and various nerve blocks.

lie   (li)   the relation of the long axis of the fetus with respect to that of the mother; cf. *presentation* and *position.*   **oblique l.,** the situation during labor when the long axis of the fetal body crosses the long axis of the maternal body at an angle close to 45 degrees.   **transverse l.,** the situation during labor when the long axis of the fetus crosses the long axis of the mother; see table under *position.*

li·en   (li′en)   [L.]   spleen.   **lie′nal,** adj.   **l. accesso′rius,** accessory spleen.   **l. mo′bilis,** floating spleen.

lien(o)-   word element [L.], *spleen;* see also words beginning *splen(o)-.*

li·eno·cele   (li-e′no-sēl)   hernia of the spleen.

li·en·tery   (li′en-tĕ″re)   diarrhea with passage of undigested food.   **lienter′ic,** adj.

LIF   left iliac fossa; leukocyte inhibitory factor.

life   (līf)   the aggregate of vital phenomena; the quality or principle by which living things are distinguished from inorganic matter, as manifested by such phenomena as metabolism, growth, reproduction, adaptation, etc.

lig·a·ment   (lig′ah-mint)   1. a band of fibrous tissue connecting bones or cartilages, serving to support and strengthen joints.
2. a double layer of peritoneum extending from one visceral organ to another.   3. cord-like remnants of fetal tubular structures that are nonfunctional after birth.   **ligamen′tous,** adj.   **accessory l.,** one that strengthens or supports another.   **alar l′s,** 1. two bands passing from the apex of the dens to the medial side of each occipital condyle.   2. a pair of folds of the synovial membrane of the knee joint.   **annular stapedial l.,** a ring of fibrous tissue that attaches the base of the stapes to the fenestra vestibuli of the inner ear.   **anococcygeal l.,** a fibrous band connecting the posterior fibers of the sphincter of the anus to the coccyx.   **arcuate l′s,** 1. the arched ligaments connecting the diaphragm with the lowest ribs and the first lumbar vertebra.   2. ligamenta flava.
Bérard's l., the suspensory ligament of the pericardium.   **Bertin's l., Bigelow's l.,** iliofemoral l.   **l. of Botallo,** a strong thick fibromuscular cord extending from the pulmonary artery to the aortic arch; it is the remains of the ductus arteriosus.
Bourgery's l., oblique popliteal ligament; a broad band of fibers extending from the medial condyle of the tibia across the back of the knee joint to the lateral epicondyle of the femur.   **broad l.,** 1. a broad fold of peritoneum supporting the uterus, extending from the uterus to the wall of the pelvis

on either side. 2. a sickle-shaped sagittal fold of perineum helping attach the liver to the diaphragm and separating the left and right hepatic lobes. **Brodie's l.**, transverse humeral l. **Burns' l.**, falciform process (1). **Campbell's l.**, suspensory l. (2). **cardinal l.**, part of a thickening of the visceral pelvic fascia beside the cervix and vagina, passing laterally to merge with the upper fascia of the pelvic diaphragm. **carpal l., transverse**, flexor retinaculum of hand. **Colles' l.**, a triangular band of fibers arising from the lacunar ligament and pubic bone and passing to the linea alba. **conoid l.**, the posteromedial portion of the coracoclavicular ligament, extending from the coracoid process to the inferior surface of the clavicle. **conus l.**, a collagenous band connecting the posterior surface of the pulmonary annulus and the muscular infundibulum to the root of the aorta. **Cooper's l.**, pectineal l. **coracoclavicular l.**, a band joining the coracoid process of the scapula and the acromial extremity of the clavicle, consisting of two ligaments, the conoid and trapezoid. **cotyloid l.**, a ring of fibrocartilage connected with the rim of the acetabulum. **cruciate l's of knee**, more or less cross-shaped ligaments, one anterior and one posterior, arising from the femur and passing through the intercondylar space to attach to the tibia. **cystoduodenal l.**, an anomalous fold of peritoneum extending between the gallbladder and the duodenum. **diaphragmatic l.**, the involuting urogenital ridge that becomes the suspensory ligament of the ovary. **falciform l.**, a sickle-shaped sagittal fold of peritoneum that helps attach the liver to the diaphragm. **flaval l's**, ligamenta flava. **glenohumeral l's**, bands, usually three, on the inner surface of the articular capsule of the humerus, extending from the glenoid lip to the anatomical neck of the humerus. **glenoid l.**, 1. (pl.) dense bands on the plantar surfaces of the metatarsophalangeal joints. 2. see under *lip*. **Henle's l.**, falx inguinalis. **Hey's l.**, falciform process (1). **iliofemoral l.**, a very strong triangular or inverted Y-shaped band covering the anterior and superior portions of the hip joint. **iliotrochanteric l.**, a portion of the articular capsule of the hip joint. **inguinal l.**, a fibrous band running from the anterior superior spine of the ilium to the spine of the pubis. **lacunar l.**, a membrane with its base just medial to the femoral ring, one side attached to the inguinal ligament and the other to the pectineal line of the pubis. **Lisfranc's l.**,

a fibrous band extending from the medial cuneiform bone to the second metatarsal. **Lockwood's l.**, a suspensory sheath supporting the eyeball. **medial l.**, 1. a large fan-shaped ligament on the medial side of the ankle. 2. the medial ligament of temporomandibular articulation. **meniscofemoral l's**, two small fibrous bands of the knee joint attached to the lateral meniscus, one (the anterior) extending to the anterior cruciate ligament and the other (the posterior) to the medial femoral condyle. **nephrocolic l.**, fasciculi from the fatty capsule of the kidney passing down on the right side to the posterior wall of the ascending colon and on the left side to the posterior wall of the descending colon. **nuchal l.**, a broad, fibrous, roughly triangular sagittal septum in the back of the neck, separating the right and left sides. **patellar l.**, the continuation of the central portion of the tendon of the quadriceps femoris muscle distal to the patella, extending from the patella to the tuberosity of the tibia. **pectineal l.**, a strong aponeurotic lateral continuation of the lacunar ligament along the pectineal line of the pubis. **periodontal l.**, the fibrous connective tissue that surrounds the root of a tooth, separating it from and attaching it to the alveolar bone, and serving to hold the tooth in its socket. It extends from the base of the gingival mucosa to the fundus of the bony socket. **phrenicocolic l.**, a peritoneal fold passing from the left colic flexure to the adjacent part of the diaphragm. **Poupart's l.**, inguinal l. **pulmonary l.**, a vertical fold extending from the hilus to the base of the lung. **rhomboid l. of clavicle**, a ligament connecting cartilage of the first rib to the undersurface of the clavicle. **Robert's l.**, posterior meniscofemoral l. **round l.**, 1. (*of femur*) a broad ligament arising from the fatty cushion of the acetabulum and inserted on the head of the femur. 2. (*of uterus*) a fibromuscular band attached to the uterus near the uterine tube, passing through the inguinal ring to the labium majus. **Schlemm's l's**, two ligamentous bands of the capsule of the shoulder joint. **subflaval l's**, ligamenta flava. **suspensory l.**, 1. (*of lens*) ciliary zonule. 2. (*of axilla*) a layer ascending from the axillary fascia and ensheathing the pectoralis minor muscle. 3. (*of ovary*) the portion of the broad ligament lateral to and above the ovary. 4. (*of breast*) one of numerous fibrous processes extending from the body of the mammary gland to the dermis. 5. (*of clitoris*) a strong fibrous band attaching the root of the clitoris to the linea alba and pubic symphysis. 6. (*of penis*) a strong fibrous band that attaches the root of the penis to the linea alba and pubic symphysis. **synovial l.,** a large synovial fold. **tendino-trochanteric l.,** a portion of the capsule of the hip joint. **tracheal l's,** circular horizontal ligaments that join the tracheal cartilages together. **transverse l.,** short fibers that connect the posterior surface of the neck of a rib with the anterior surface of the transverse process of the corresponding vertebra. **transverse humeral l.,** a band of fibers bridging the intertubercular groove of the humerus and holding the tendon in the groove. **trapezoid l.,** the anterolateral portion of the coracoclavicular ligament, extending from the upper surface of the coracoid process to the trapezoid line of the clavicle. **umbilical l., median,** a fibrous cord, the remains of the obliterated umbilical artery, running cranialward beside the bladder to the umbilicus. **uteropelvic l's,** expansions of muscular tissue in the broad ligament, radiating from the fascia over the internal obturator to the side of the uterus and the vagina. **ventricular l.,** vestibular l. **vesicoumbilical l.,** median umbilical l. **vesicouterine l.,** a ligament that extends from the anterior aspect of the uterus to the bladder. **vestibular l.,** the membrane extending from the thyroid cartilage in front to the anterolateral surface of the arytenoid cartilage behind. **vocal l.,** the elastic tissue membrane extending from the thyroid cartilage in front to the vocal process of the arytenoid cartilage behind. **Weitbrecht's l.,** a small ligamentous band extending from the ulnar tuberosity to the radius. **Wrisberg's l.,** posterior meniscofemoral l. **Y l.,** iliofemoral l. **yellow l's,** ligamenta flava.

lig·a·men·to·pexy (lig″ah-men′to-pek″se) fixation of the uterus by shortening or suturing the round ligament.

lig·a·men·tum (lig″ah-men′tum) pl. *ligamen′ta*. [L.] ligament. **ligamen′ta fla′va,** yellow ligaments: a series of bands of yellow elastic tissue attached to and extending between the ventral portions of the laminae of two adjacent vertebrae, from the axis to the sacrum. They assist in maintaining or regaining the erect position and serve to close in the spaces between the arches.

li·gand (li′gand, lig′and) an organic molecule that donates the necessary electrons to form coordinate covalent bonds with metallic ions. Also, an ion or molecule that reacts to form a complex with another molecule.

li·gase (li′gās, lig′ās) any of a class of enzymes that catalyze the joining together of two molecules coupled with the breakdown of a pyrophosphate bond in ATP or a similar triphosphate.

li·ga·tion (li-ga′shun) the application of a ligature. **tubal l.,** sterilization of the female by constricting, severing, or crushing the uterine tubes.

lig·a·ture (lig′ah-cher) any material, such as thread or wire, used for tying a vessel or to constrict a part.

light (līt) electromagnetic radiation with a range of wavelength between 3900 (violet) and 7700 (red) angstroms, capable of stimulating the subjective sensation of sight; sometimes considered to include ultraviolet and infrared radiation as well. **idioretinal l.,** the sensation of light in the complete absence of external stimuli. **intrinsic l.,** the dim light always present in the visual field. **polarized l.,** light of which the vibrations are made over one plane or in circles or ellipses. **Wood's l.,** ultraviolet radiation from a mercury vapor source, transmitted through a nickel-oxide filter (Wood's filter, or glass), which holds back all but a few violet rays and passes ultraviolet wavelengths of about 365 nm.

light·en·ing (līt′en-ing) the sensation of decreased abdominal distention produced by the descent of the uterus into the pelvic cavity, two to three weeks before labor begins.

lig·no·cer·ic ac·id (lig″no-sēr′ik) a saturated 24-carbon fatty acid occurring in sphingomyelin and as a minor constituent of many plant fats.

limb (lim) 1. member or extremity; one of the paired appendages of the body used in locomotion or grasping; in humans, an arm or leg with all its parts. 2. a structure or part resembling an arm or leg. **anacrotic l.,** ascending l. (2). **ascending l.,** 1. the distal part of the loop of Henle. 2. anacrotic l.; the ascending portion of an arterial pulse tracing. **catacrotic l.,** descending l. (2). **descending l.,** 1. the proximal part of the loop of Henle. 2. catacrotic l.; the descending portion of an arterial pulse tracing. **lower l.,** the limb of the body extending from the gluteal region to the foot; it is specialized for weight-bearing and locomotion. See also *leg*. **pectoral l.,** thoracic l. **pelvic l.,** 1. the leg, or a homologous part. 2. the limb attached to the pelvic girdle; the lower limb of a human or a homologous structure such as a hind limb on another animal. **phantom l.,** the sensation, after amputation of a limb, that the absent part is still present; there may also be paresthesias, transient aches, and intermittent or continuous pain perceived as originating in the absent limb. **thoracic l.,** the limb attached to the thoracic girdle; the upper limb of a human or a homologous structure (wing, foreleg, etc.) in another animal. **upper l.,** the limb of the body extending from the deltoid region to the hand; it is specialized for functions such as grasping and manipulating. See also *arm.*

lim·bic (lim′bik) pertaining to a limbus, or margin; see also under *system.*

lim·bus (lim′bus) pl. *lim′bi.* [L.] an edge, fringe, or border. **corneal l.,** the edge of the cornea where it joins the sclera. **spiral l.,** the thickened periosteum of the osseous spiral lamina of the cochlea.

lime (līm) 1. calcium oxide, a corrosively alkaline and caustic earth, CaO; having various industrial uses and also a pharmaceutic necessity. 2. the acid fruit of the tropical tree, *Citrus aurantifolia;* its juice contains ascorbic acid. **soda l.,** see under *soda.*

li·men (li′men) pl. *li′mina.* [L.] a threshold or boundary. **l. of insula, l. in′sulae,** the point at which the cortex of the insula is continuous with the cortex of the frontal lobe. **l. na′si,** the ridge marking the boundary between the vestibule of the nose and the nasal cavity proper.

lim·i·nal (lim′ĭ-n′l) barely perceptible; pertaining to a threshold.

lim·i·nom·e·ter (lim″ĭ-nom′it-er) an instrument for measuring the strength of a stimulus that just induces a tendon reflex.

lim·i·tans (lim′ĭ-tanz) [L.] limiting.

lim·it dex·trin·ase (lim′it deks′trin-ās) α-dextrinase.

limp (limp) any gait that avoids weight bearing by one leg.

lin·co·my·cin (lin″ko-mi′sin) an antibiotic, primarily a gram-positive specific antibacterial, produced by a variant of *Streptomyces lincolnensis;* used as the hydrochloride salt.

lin·dane (lin′dān) the gamma isomer of benzene hexachloride, used as a topical pediculicide and scabicide.

line (līn) 1. a stripe, streak, or narrow ridge. 2. an imaginary line connecting different anatomic landmarks. **lin′ear,** adj. **absorption l's,** dark lines in the spectrum due to absorption of light by the substance through which the light has passed. **anocutaneous l.,** pectinate l. **Beau's l's,** transverse furrows on the fingernails, usually a sign of a systemic disease but also due to other causes. **bismuth l.,** a thin

blue-black line along the gingival margin in bismuth poisoning. **blood l.,** a line of direct descent through several generations. **cement l.,** a line visible in microscopic examination of bone in cross section, marking the boundary of an osteon (haversian system). **cervical l.,** anatomical designation for the cementoenamel junction, the dividing line between the crown and root portions of a tooth. **cleavage l's,** linear clefts in the skin indicative of direction of the fibers. **costoclavicular l.,** parasternal l. **l. of Douglas,** a crescentic line marking the termination of the posterior layer of the sheath of the rectus abdominis muscle. **epiphyseal l.,** 1. a plane or plate on a long bone, visible as a line, marking the junction of the epiphysis and diaphysis. 2. a strip of lesser density on the radiograph of a long bone, representing that plane or plate. **l's of expression,** the natural skin lines and creases of the face and neck; the preferred lines of incision in facial and cervical surgery. **gingival l.,** 1. a line determined by the level to which the gingiva extends on a tooth. 2. any linear mark visible on the surface of the gingiva. **gluteal l.,** any of the three rough curved lines (anterior, inferior, and posterior) on the gluteal surface of the ala of the ilium. **Harris l's,** lines of retarded growth seen radiographically at the epiphyses of long bones. **hot l.,** see under *H.* **iliopectineal l.,** a ridge on the ilium and pubes showing the brim of the true pelvis. **intertrochanteric l.,** a line running obliquely from the greater to the lesser trochanter on the anterior surface of the femur. **lead l.,** a gray or bluish black line at the gingival margin in lead poisoning. **mammary l.,** see under *ridge.* **mammillary l.,** an imaginary vertical line passing through the center of the nipple. **median l.,** an imaginary line dividing the body surface equally into right and left sides. **milk l.,** mammary ridge. **mylohyoid l.,** a ridge on the inner surface of the lower jaw from the base of the symphysis to the ascending rami behind the last molar tooth. **nasobasilar l.,** one through the basion and nasion. **Nélaton's l.,** one from the anterior superior spine of the ilium to the most prominent part of the tuberosity of the ischium. **nuchal l's,** three lines (inferior, superior, highest) on the outer surface of the occipital bone; see also *external occipital crest.* **parasternal l.,** an imaginary line midway between the mammillary line and the border of the sternum. **pectinate l.,** one marking the junction of the zone of the anal canal lined with stratified squamous epithelium and the zone lined with columnar epithelium. **pectineal l.,** 1. a line running down the posterior surface of the shaft of the femur, giving attachment to the pectineus muscle. 2. the anterior border of the superior ramus of the pubis. **semilunar l.,** a curved line along the lateral border of each rectus abdominis muscle, marking the meeting of the aponeuroses of the internal oblique and transverse abdominal muscles. **Shenton's l.,** a curved line seen in radiographs of the normal hip, formed by the top of the obturator foramen. **sternal l.,** an imaginary vertical line on the anterior body surface, corresponding to the lateral border of the sternum. **subcostal l.,** a transverse line on the surface of the abdomen at the level of the lower edge of the tenth costal cartilage. **Sydney l.,** a palmar crease correlated with an increased risk for leukemia and other malignancies in childhood. **temporal l.,** 1. either of the curved ridges, inferior and superior, on the outside of the parietal bone, continuous with the temporal line of the frontal bone. 2. a ridge extending superiorly and posteriorly from the zygomatic process of the frontal bone. **terminal l. of pelvis,** one on the inner surface of each pelvic bone, from the sacroiliac joint to the iliopubic eminence anteriorly, separating the false from the true pelvis. **trapezoid l.,** a ridge on the inferior surface of the clavicle for attachment of the trapezoid ligament. **Voigt's l.,** a dorsoventral pigmented line of demarcation on the skin along the lateral edge of the biceps muscle; seen in 20 to 26 per cent of blacks and rarely in whites.

li·nea (lin'e-ah) pl. *li'neae.* [L.] line; in anatomy, a narrow ridge or streak on the surface of a structure. **l. al'ba,** white line; the tendinous median line on the anterior abdominal wall between the two rectus muscles. **l. as'pera,** a rough longitudinal line on the back of the femur for muscle attachments. **li'neae atro'phicae,** striae atrophicae. **l. epiphysia'lis,** epiphyseal line. **l. glu'tea,** gluteal line. **l. ni'gra,** the linea alba when it has become pigmented in pregnancy. **l. splen'dens,** the sheath for the anterior spinal artery formed by the pia mater in the anterior median fissure of the spinal cord.

lin·er (līn'er) material applied to the inside of the walls of a cavity or container for protection or insulation of the surface.

li·nez·o·lid (lī-nez'o-lid) a synthetic oxazolidinone antibacterial, effective against gram-positive organisms.

lin·gua (ling'gwah) pl. *lin'guae.* [L.] tongue. **lin'gual,** adj. **l. geogra'phica,** benign migratory glossitis. **l. ni'gra,** black tongue. **l. plica'ta,** fissured tongue.

lin·gual (ling'gwal) 1. pertaining to or near the tongue. 2. in dental anatomy, facing the tongue or oral cavity.

Lin·guat·u·la (ling-gwat'u-lah) a genus of wormlike arthropods, the adults of which inhabit the respiratory tract of vertebrates; the larvae are found in the lungs and other internal organs. It includes *L. serra'ta (L. rhina'ria),* which parasitizes dogs and cats and sometimes humans.

lin·gu·la (ling'gu-lah) pl. *lin'gulae.* [L.] a small, tonguelike structure, such as the projection from the lower portion of the upper lobe of the left lung *(l. pulmo'nis sinis'tri),* or the bony ridge between the body and great wing of the sphenoid *(l. sphenoida'lis).* **ling'ular,** adj.

lin·gu·lec·to·my (ling″gu-lek'tah-me) excision of the lingula of the left lung.

lingu(o)- word element [L.], *tongue.*

lin·guo·pap·il·li·tis (ling″gwo-pap″ĭ-li'tis) inflammation or ulceration of the papillae of the edges of the tongue.

lin·guo·ver·sion (-ver'zhun) displacement of a tooth lingually from the line of occlusion.

lin·i·ment (lin'ĭ-mint) an oily liquid preparation to be used on the skin.

li·ni·tis (lĭ-ni'tis) inflammation of gastric cellular tissue. **l. plas'tica,** diffuse fibrous proliferation of the submucous connective tissue of the stomach, resulting in thickening and fibrosis so that the organ is constricted, inelastic, and rigid (like a leather bottle).

link·age (lingk'ij) 1. the connection between different atoms in a chemical compound, or the symbol representing it in structural formulas; see also *bond.* 2. in genetics, the association of genes having loci on the same chromosome, which results in the tendency of a group of such nonallelic genes to be associated in inheritance. 3. in psychology, the connection between a stimulus and its response.

li·no·le·ate (lĭ-no'le-āt) a salt (soap), ester, or anionic form of linoleic acid.

lin·o·le·ic ac·id (lin″o-le'ik) a polyunsaturated fatty acid, occurring as a major constituent of many vegetable oils; it is used in the biosynthesis of prostaglandins and cell membranes.

li·no·le·nate (lĭ-no'lĕ-nāt) a salt (soap), ester, or anionic form of linolenic acid.

lin·o·len·ic ac·id (lin″o-len'ik) a polyunsaturated 18-carbon essential fatty acid occurring in some fish oils and many seed-derived oils.

lin·seed (lin'sēd) flaxseed; the dried ripe seed of *Linum usitatissimum*, the common flax plant, used as a laxative and a topic demulcent and emollient, and a source of α-linolenic acid.

lint (lint) an absorbent surgical dressing material.

li·o·thy·ro·nine (li″o-thi'ro-nēn) a synthetic pharmaceutical preparation of the levorotatory isomer of triiodothyronine, used as the sodium salt in the treatment of hypothyroidism and the treatment and prophylaxis of goiter and thyroid carcinoma.

li·o·trix (li'o-triks) a 1:4 mixture of liothyronine sodium and levothyroxine sodium by weight; used as the sodium salt in the treatment of hypothyroidism and the treatment and prophylaxis of goiter and thyroid carcinoma.

lip (lip) 1. the upper or lower fleshy margin of the mouth. 2. any liplike part; labium. **cleft l.,** a congenital cleft or defect in the upper lip. **glenoid l.,** a ring of fibrocartilage joined to the rim of the glenoid cavity. **Hapsburg l.,** a thick, overdeveloped lower lip that often accompanies Hapsburg jaw.

lip·ac·i·du·ria (lip″as-ĭ-du're-ah) fatty acids in the urine.

lip·ase (li'pās, lip'ās) any enzyme that catalyzes the cleavage of a fatty acid anion from a triglyceride or phospholipid.

lip·ec·to·my (lĭ-pek'tah-me) excision of a localized area of subcutaneous adipose tissue. **suction l., suction-assisted l.,** liposuction; surgical removal of localized fat deposits via high pressure vacuum, applied by means of a suction curet or cannula inserted subdermally through small incisions.

lip·ede·ma (lip″ĕ-de'mah) an accumulation of excess fat and fluid in subcutaneous tissues.

lip·emia (lĭ-pe'me-ah) hyperlipidemia. **lipe'mic,** adj. **alimentary l.,** that occurring after ingestion of food. **l. retina'lis,** that manifested by a milky appearance of the veins and arteries of the retina.

lip·id (lip'id) any of a heterogeneous group of fats and fatlike substances, including fatty acids, neutral fats, waxes, and steroids, which are water-insoluble and soluble in nonpolar solvents. Lipids, which are easily stored in the body, serve as a source of fuel, are an important constituent of cell structure, and serve other biological functions. Compound lipids comprise the glycolipids, lipoproteins, and phospholipids.

lip·i·de·mia (lip″ĭ-dēm'e-ah) hyperlipidemia.

lip·i·do·sis (lip″ĭ-do'sis) pl. *lipido'ses.* Any disorder of lipid metabolism involving abnormal accumulation of lipids in the reticuloendothelial cells.

lip·i·du·ria (lip″ĭ-du're-ah) adiposuria; lipids in the urine.

lip(o)- word element [Gr.], *fat; lipid.*

lipo·am·ide (lip″o-am'īd) the functional form of lipoic acid, linked to the lysine side chain of any of several enzyme complexes that catalyze the oxidative decarboxylation of keto acids.

lipo·ar·thri·tis (lip″o-ahr-thri'tis) inflammation of fatty tissue of a joint.

lipo·at·ro·phy (-at'ro-fe) atrophy of subcutaneous fatty tissues of the body.

lipo·blast (lip'o-blast) a connective tissue cell which develops into a fat cell. **lipoblas'tic,** adj.

lipo·blas·to·ma (lip″o-blas-to'mah) a benign fatty tumor composed of a mixture of embryonic lipoblastic cells in a myxoid stroma and mature fat cells, with the cells arranged in lobules.

lipo·blas·to·ma·to·sis (-blas-to″mah-to'sis) the occurrence of multiple lipoblastomas locally diffused but without a tendency to metastasize.

lipo·car·di·ac (-kahr'de-ak) relating to a fatty heart.

lipo·chon·dro·ma (-kon-dro'mah) chondrolipoma.

lipo·chrome (lip'o-krōm) any of a group of fat-soluble hydrocarbon pigments, such as carotene, xanthophyll, lutein, chromophane, and the natural coloring material of butter, egg yolk, and yellow corn.

lipo·cyte (-sīt) 1. a fat cell. 2. a fat-storing cell of the liver.

lipo·dys·tro·phia (lip″o-dis-tro'fe-ah) lipodystrophy. **l. progressi'va,** progressive lipodystrophy.

lipo·dys·tro·phy (-dis'tro-fe) any disturbance of fat metabolism. **congenital generalized l., congenital progressive l.,** total l. **generalized l.,** total l. **partial l., progressive l.,** progressive and symmetrical loss of subcutaneous fat from the parts above the pelvis, beginning with facial emaciation and progressing downward, giving an apparent and possibly real accumulation of fat about the thighs and buttocks. **total l.,** a recessive condition marked by the virtual absence of subcutaneous adipose tissue, macrosomia, visceromegaly, hypertrichosis, acanthosis nigricans, and reduced glucose tolerance in the presence of high insulin levels.

lipo·fi·bro·ma (-fi-bro'mah) fibrolipoma.

li·po·fus·cin (-fu'sin) any of a class of fatty pigments formed by the solution of a pigment in fat.

li·po·fus·cin·o·sis (-fu"sin-o'sis) any disorder due to abnormal storage of lipofuscins. **neuronal ceroid-l.,** any of several genetic lipidoses characterized by progressive neurodegeneration, loss of vision, and a fatal course; included are *Jansky-Bielschowsky disease*, *Vogt-Spielmeyer disease*, and *Kufs' disease*.

li·po·gen·e·sis (-jen'ĕ-sis) the formation of fat; the transformation of nonfat food materials into body fat. **lipogenet'ic,** adj.

lip·o·gen·ic (-jen'ik) forming, producing, or caused by fat.

li·po·gran·u·lo·ma (-gran"u-lo'mah) a foreign body inflammation of adipose tissue containing granulation tissue and oil cysts.

li·po·gran·u·lo·ma·to·sis (-gran"u-lo"mah-to'sis) a condition of faulty lipid metabolism in which yellow nodules of lipoid material are deposited in the skin and mucosae, giving rise to granulomatous reactions.

li·po·hy·per·tro·phy (-hi-per'tro-fe) hypertrophy of subcutaneous fat. **insulin l.,** localized hypertrophy of subcutaneous fat at insulin injection sites caused by the lipogenic effect of insulin.

lipo·ic ac·id (lip-o'ik) a necessary cofactor for several enzyme complexes involved in the oxidative decarboxylation of keto acids, where it occurs in the form lipoamide. It is used as a dietary supplement for its antioxidant properties.

lip·oid (lip'oid) fatlike.

li·pol·y·sis (lĭ-pol'ĭ-sis) the splitting up or decomposition of fat. **lipolyt'ic,** adj.

lip·o·ma (lip-o'mah) a benign, soft, rubbery, encapsulated tumor of adipose tissue, usually composed of mature fat cells.

lip·o·ma·to·sis (lip"o-mah-to'sis) abnormal localized or tumorlike accumulations of fat in the tissues. **renal l.,** fatty masses within the kidney.

lipo·me·nin·go·cele (-mĕ-ning'go-sēl) meningocele associated with an overlying lipoma.

lipo·my·e·lo·me·nin·go·cele (-mi"ĕ-lo-mĕ-ning-go'sĕl) myelomeningocele with an overlying lipoma.

lipo·my·o·ma (-mi-o'mah) myolipoma.

lipo·myx·o·ma (-mik-so'mah) myxolipoma.

li·po·pe·nia (-pe'ne-ah) deficiency of lipids in the body.

lipo·phage (lip'o-fāj) a cell which absorbs or ingests fat.

lipo·pha·gia (lip"o-fa'jah) lipolysis. **lipopha'gic,** adj.

li·poph·a·gy (lĭ-pof'ah-je) lipolysis. **lipopha'gic,** adj.

lipo·phil·ia (lip"o-fil'e-ah) 1. affinity for fat. 2. solubility in lipids. **lipophil'ic,** adj.

lipo·plas·ty (-plas'te) liposuction.

lipo·poly·sac·cha·ride (-pol"e-sak'ah-rīd) 1. a molecule in which lipids and polysaccharides are linked. 2. a major component of the cell wall of gram-negative bacteria; lipopolysaccharides are endotoxins and important antigens.

lipo·pro·tein (-pro'tēn) a complex of lipids and apolipoproteins, the form in which lipids are transported in the blood. **α-l., alpha l.,** one with electrophoretic mobility equivalent to that of the α_1-globulins, e.g., high-density lipoprotein. **β-l., beta l.,** one with electrophoretic mobility equivalent to that of the β-globulins, e.g., low-density lipoprotein. **floating beta l's,** β-VLDL. **high-density l. (HDL),** a class of plasma lipoproteins that promote transport of cholesterol from extrahepatic tissue to the liver for excretion in the bile; serum levels have been negatively correlated with premature coronary heart disease. **intermediate-density l. (IDL),** a class of lipoproteins formed in the degradation of very-low-density lipoproteins; some are cleared rapidly into the liver and some are degraded to low-density lipoproteins. **low-density l. (LDL),** a class of plasma lipoproteins that transport cholesterol to extrahepatic tissues; high serum levels have been correlated with premature coronary heart disease. **Lp(a) l.,** a lipoprotein particle containing apolipoprotein B-100 as well as an antigenically unique apolipoprotein; its occurrence at high levels in plasma has been correlated with increased risk of heart disease. **pre-β-l., pre-beta l.,** very-low-density lipoprotein **sinking pre-β-l.,** Lp(a) l. **very-high-density l. (VHDL),** a class of lipoproteins composed predominantly of proteins and also containing a high concentration of free fatty acids. **very-low-density l. (VLDL),** a class of lipoproteins that transport triglycerides from the intestine and liver to adipose and muscle tissues; they contain primarily triglycerides with some cholesteryl esters.

lipo·pro·tein li·pase (li'pās) an enzyme that catalyzes the hydrolytic cleavage of fatty acids from triglycerides (or di- or monoglycerides) in chylomicrons, very-low-density lipoproteins, and low-density lipoproteins.

lipo·sar·co·ma (lip"o-sahr-ko'mah) a malignant mesenchymal tumor usually occurring in the intermuscular fascia in the upper thigh, characterized by primitive lipoblastic cells with varying degrees of lipoblastic or lipomatous differentiation, sometimes with foci of normal fat cells.

li·po·sis (lĭ-po'sis) lipomatosis.

lipo·sol·u·ble (lip"o-sol'u-b'l) soluble in fats.

lipo·some (lip'o-sōm) a microscopic spherical particle formed by a lipid bilayer enclosing an aqueous compartment.

lipo·suc·tion (lip'o-suk"shun) suction-assisted lipectomy.

li·pot·ro·phy (lĭ-pot'rah-fe) increase of bodily fat. **lipotroph'ic**, adj.

lipo·tro·pic (lip"o-tro'pik) acting on fat metabolism by hastening removal or decreasing the deposit of fat in the liver; also, an agent having such effects.

lip·o·tro·pin (lip'o-tro"pin) any of several prohormones that promote lipolysis; the most important one in humans is *β-lipotropin*. *β-l.*, a prohormone synthesized by cells of the adenohypophysis; it promotes fat mobilization and skin darkening by stimulation of melanocytes and is the precursor of the endorphins.

lipo·vac·cine (-vak'sēn) a vaccine in a vegetable oil vehicle.

li·pox·i·dase (lĭ-pok'sĭ-dās) lipoxygenase.

li·poxy·ge·nase (lĭ-pok'sĭ-jĕ-nās) an enzyme that catalyzes the oxidation of polyunsaturated fatty acids to form a peroxide of the acid.

lip·ping (lip'ing) 1. a wedge-shaped shadow in the radiograph of chondrosarcoma between the cortex and the elevated periosteum. 2. bony overgrowth in osteoarthritis.

liq·ue·fa·cient (lik"wĭ-fa'shint) 1. producing or pertaining to liquefaction. 2. an agent that produces liquefaction.

liq·ue·fac·tion (-fak'shun) conversion into a liquid form. **liquefac'tive**, adj.

liq·ue·fy (lik'wĭ-fi) to become or cause to become liquid.

liq·uid (lik'wid) 1. a substance that flows readily in its natural state. 2. flowing readily; neither solid nor gaseous.

li·quor (lik'er, li'kwor) pl. *liquors, liquo'res*. [L.] 1. a liquid, especially an aqueous solution containing a medicinal substance. 2. a term applied to certain body fluids. **l. am'nii**, amniotic fluid. **l. cerebrospina'lis**, cerebrospinal fluid. **l. folli'culi**, follicular fluid.

li·sin·o·pril (li-sin'o-pril) an angiotensin-converting enzyme inhibitor used in the treatment of hypertension, congestive heart failure, and acute myocardial infarction.

lis·sen·ceph·a·ly (lis"en-sef'ah-le) agyria. **lissencephal'ic**, adj.

Lis·ter·el·la (lis"ter-el'ah) *Listeria*.

Lis·te·ria (lis-tēr'e-ah) a genus of gram-negative bacteria (family Corynebacterium); *L. monocyto'genes* causes listeriosis.

lis·ter·i·o·sis (lis-te"re-o'sis) infection caused by *Listeria monocytogenes*. Infection in utero results in abortion, stillbirth, or prematurity; that during birth causes cardiorespiratory distress, diarrhea, vomiting, and meningitis; and in adults it causes meningitis, endocarditis, and disseminated granulomatous lesions.

lis·ter·ism (lis'ter-izm) the principles and practice of antiseptic and aseptic surgery.

li·ter (L) (lēt'er) a basic unit of volume used for liquids with the SI system, equal to 1000 cubic centimeters, or 1 cubic decimeter, or to 1.0567 quarts liquid measure.

li·thi·a·sis (lĭ-thi'ah-sis) the formation or presence of calculi or other concretions.

lith·i·um (Li) (lith'e-um) chemical element (see *Table of Elements*), at. no. 3. Its salts, especially *l. carbonate* and *l. citrate*, are used to treat and prevent manic states in bipolar disorder.

lith(o)- word element [Gr.], *stone; calculus*.

litho·clast (lith'o-klast) lithotrite.

litho·gen·e·sis (-jen'ĕ-sis) formation of calculi. **lithogen'ic, lithog'enous**, adj.

li·thol·a·paxy (lĭ-thol"ah-pak'se) lithotripsy.

li·thol·y·sis (lĭ-thol'ĭ-sis) dissolution of calculi. **litholyt'ic**, adj.

litho·ne·phri·tis (lith"o-nĕ-fri'tis) inflammation of the kidney due to irritation by calculi.

li·thot·o·my (lĭ-thot'ah-me) 1. incision of a duct or organ for removal of calculi. 2. cystolithotomy.

litho·trip·sy (lith'o-trip"se) the crushing of a calculus within the urinary system or gallbladder, followed at once by the washing out of the fragments; it may be performed surgically or by noninvasive methods, such as by laser or by shock waves. **extracorporeal shock wave l.**, a procedure for treating upper urinary tract stones: the patient is immersed in a large tub of water and a high-energy shock wave generated by a high-voltage spark is focused on the stone by an ellipsoid reflector. The stone disintegrates into particles, which are passed in the urine. **pneumatic l.**, lithotripsy in which a rigid probe is inserted through the ureter and pneumatic pressure is applied directly to the calculus.

litho·trip·ter (lith'o-trip"ter) an instrument for crushing calculi in lithotripsy.

litho·trip·tic (lith"o-trip'tik) dissolving vesical calculi; also, an agent that so acts.

litho·trip·tor (lith'o-trip"tor) lithotripter.

litho·trite (lith′o-trīt) an instrument for crushing a urinary calculus.

li·thot·ri·ty (lĭ-thot′rĭ-te) lithotripsy.

lith·ure·sis (lith″u-re′sis) the passage of gravel in the urine.

lit·mus (lit′mus) a pigment prepared from *Rocella tinctoria* and other lichens; used as an acid-base (pH) indicator.

lit·ter (lit′er) stretcher.

lit·to·ral (lit′ah-r′l) pertaining to the shore of a large body of water.

li·ve·do (lĭ-ve′do) [L.] a discolored patch on the skin. **l. racemo′sa, l. reticula′ris,** a red to blue, netlike mottling of the skin on the limbs and trunk, which becomes more intense on exposure to cold.

liv·e·doid (liv′id-oid) pertaining to livedo.

liv·er (liv′er) 1. the large, dark-red gland in the upper part of the abdomen on the right side, just beneath the diaphragm. See Plate 27. Its functions include storage and filtration of blood, secretion of bile, conversion of sugars into glycogen, and many other metabolic activities. 2. the same gland of certain animals, sometimes used as food or from which pharmaceutical products are prepared. **fatty l.,** one affected with fatty infiltration, the fat in large droplets and the liver enlarged but of normal consistency. **hobnail l.,** a liver whose surface is marked with nail-like points from cirrhosis.

liv·er phos·phor·y·lase (fos-for′ĭ-lās) the liver isozyme of glycogen phosphorylase; deficiency causes glycogen storage disease, type VI.

liv·er phos·phor·y·lase ki·nase (ki′nās) the liver isozyme of phosphorylase kinase; deficiency causes phosphorylase *b* kinase deficiency.

liv·id (liv′id) discolored, as from a contusion or bruise; black and blue.

li·vor (li′vor) pl. *livo′res.* [L.] discoloration. **l. mor′tis,** discoloration of dependent parts of the body after death.

lix·iv·i·a·tion (lik-siv″e-a′shun) separation of soluble from insoluble material by use of an appropriate solvent, and drawing off the solution.

LMA left mentoanterior (position of fetus).

LMF lymphocyte mitogenic factor.

LMP left mentoposterior (position of fetus); last menstrual period.

LMT left mentotransverse (position of fetus).

LNMP last normal menstrual period.

LNPF lymph node permeability factor.

LOA left occipitoanterior (position of fetus).

Loa (lo′ah) a genus of filarial nematodes, including *L. lo′a,* a West African species that migrates freely throughout the subcutaneous

connective tissue, seen especially about the orbit and even under the conjunctiva, and occasionally causing edematous swellings.

load·ing (lōd′ing) 1. administering sufficient quantities of a substance to test a subject's ability to metabolize or absorb it. 2. exertion of lengthening force on a part such as a muscle or ligament.

lo·bate (lo′bāt) divided into lobes.

lo·ba·tion (lo-ba′shun) the formation of lobes; the state of having lobes. **renal l.,** the appearance on x-ray films of small notches along the surface of the kidney, indicating the location of renal lobes.

lobe (lōb) 1. a more or less well-defined portion of an organ or gland. 2. one of the main divisions of a tooth crown. **lo′bar,** adj. **caudate l.,** a small lobe of the liver between the inferior vena cava and the left lobe. **ear l.,** the lower fleshy part of the external ear. **frontal l.,** the rostral (anterior) portion of the cerebral hemisphere. **hepatic l's,** the lobes of the liver, designated the right and left and the caudate and quadrate. **insular l.,** insula. **occipital l.,** the most posterior portion of the cerebral hemisphere, forming a small part of its dorsolateral surface. **parietal l.,** the upper central portion of the cerebral hemisphere, between the frontal and occipital lobes, and above the temporal lobe. **polyalveolar l.,** a congenital disorder characterized in early infancy by far more than the normal number of alveoli in the lung lobes; thereafter, normal multiplication of alveoli does not take place and they become enlarged, i.e., emphysematous. **quadrate l.,** 1. precuneus. 2. a small lobe of the liver, between the gallbladder on the right, and the left lobe. **spigelian l.,** caudate l. of liver. **temporal l.,** the lower lateral lobe of the cerebral hemisphere.

lo·bec·to·my (lo-bek′tah-me) excision of a lobe, as of the lung, brain, or liver.

lo·bot·o·my (lo-bot′ah-me) incision of a lobe; in psychosurgery, incision of all the fibers of a lobe of the brain. **frontal l., prefrontal l.,** incision of the white matter of the frontal lobe with a leukotome passed via a cannula through holes drilled in the skull.

lob·u·lat·ed (lob′ūl-āt-id) made up of lobules.

lob·ule (lob′ūl) a small segment or lobe, especially one of the smaller divisions making up a lobe. **lob′ular,** adj. **l's of epididymis,** the wedge-shaped parts of the head of the epididymis, each comprising an efferent ductule of the testis. **hepatic l's,** the small vascular units composing the substance of the liver. **paracentral l.,** a lobe on the medial surface of the cerebral hemisphere, continuous with the pre- and postcentral gyri, limited below by the cingulate sulcus. **parietal l.,** one of the two divisions, inferior and superior, of the parietal lobe of the cerebrum. **portal l.,** a polygonal mass of liver tissue containing portions of three adjacent hepatic lobules, and having a portal vein at its center and a central vein peripherally at each corner. **primary l. of lung, respiratory l.,** terminal respiratory unit. **l's of testis,** the pyramidal subdivisions of the testicular substance, each with its base against the tunica albuginea of the testis and its apex at the mediastinum, and composed largely of seminiferous tubules.

lob·u·lus (lob'u-lus) pl. *lo'buli.* [L.] lobule.

lo·bus (lo'bus) pl. *lo'bi.* [L.] lobe.

lo·cal (lo'k'l) restricted to or pertaining to one spot or part; not general.

lo·cal·iza·tion (lo"kal-ĭ-za'shun) 1. the determination of the site or place of any process or lesion. 2. restriction to a circumscribed or limited area. 3. the localization in the oocyte or blastomere of materials that will develop into a particular tissue or organ. **cerebral l.,** determination of areas of the cortex involved in performance of certain functions. **germinal l.,** the location on a blastoderm of prospective organs.

lo·ca·tor (lo'kăt-er) a device for determining the site of foreign objects within the body. **electroacoustic l.,** a device which amplifies into an audible click the contact of the probe with a solid object in tissue.

lo·chia (lo'ke-ah) a vaginal discharge occurring during the first week or two after childbirth. **lo'chial,** adj. **l. al'ba,** the final vaginal discharge after childbirth, when the amount of blood is decreased and the leukocytes are increased. **l. cruen'ta,** l. rubra. **l. ru'bra,** that occurring immediately after childbirth, consisting almost entirely of blood. **l. sanguinolen'ta,** l. serosa. **l. sero'sa,** the serous vaginal discharge occurring four or five days after childbirth.

lo·chio·me·tra (lo"ke-o-me'trah) distention of the uterus by retained lochia.

lo·chio·me·tri·tis (-me-tri'tis) puerperal metritis.

lo·chi·or·rha·gia (-ra'jah) lochiorrhea.

lo·chi·or·rhea (-re'ah) an abnormally profuse lochia.

lo·chi·os·che·sis (lo"ke-os'kĕ-sis) retention of the lochia.

lock·jaw (lok'jaw) 1. tetanus. 2. trismus.

lo·co·mo·tion (lo"kah-mo'shun) movement or the ability to move from one place to another. **locomo'tive, locomo'tor,** adj.

lo·co·re·gion·al (lo"ko-re'jun-al) limited to a localized area, as contrasted with systemic or metastatic.

loc·u·lus (lok'u-lus) pl. *lo'culi.* [L.] 1. a small space or cavity. 2. an enlargement in the uterus in some mammals, containing an embryo. **loc'ular,** adj.

lo·cum (lo'kum) [L.] place. **l. te'nens, l. te'nent,** a practitioner who temporarily takes the place of another.

lo·cus (lo'kus) pl. *lo'ci, lo'ca.* [L.] 1. place; site. 2. in genetics, the specific site of a gene on a chromosome. **l. caeru'leus,** a pigmented eminence in the superior angle of the floor of the fourth ventricle of the brain.

lo·dox·a·mide (lo-dok'sah-mīd) a mast cell stabilizer and antiallergic; applied topically to the eye as the tromethamine salt for the treatment of allergen-induced conjunctivitis, keratitis, and keratoconjunctivitis.

log·a·dec·to·my (log"ah-dek'tah-me) excision of a portion of the conjunctiva.

log·am·ne·sia (-am-ne'zhah) receptive aphasia.

log·a·pha·sia (-ah-fa'zhah) motor aphasia.

log(o)- word element [Gr.], *words; speech.*

lo·go·clo·nia (log"o-klo'ne-ah) spasmodic repetition of words or parts of words, particularly the end syllables; often occurring in Alzheimer's disease. Cf. *stuttering.*

log·op·a·thy (log-op'ah-the) speech disorder.

logo·pe·dics (log"o-pe'diks) the study and treatment of speech defects.

logo·ple·gia (-ple'jah) paralysis of the speech organs.

log·or·rhea (-re'ah) pressured speech; excessive and rapid speech, seen in certain mental disorders.

logo·spasm (log'o-spazm) 1. logoclonia. 2. stuttering.

-logy word element [Gr.], *science; treatise; sum of knowledge in a particular subject.*

lo·i·a·sis (lo-i'ah-sis) infection with nematodes of the genus *Loa.*

loin (loin) the part of the back between the thorax and pelvis.

lo·me·flox·a·cin (lo"mě-flok'sah-sin) a broad-spectrum antibiotic effective against a wide range of aerobic gram-negative and gram-positive organisms; used as the hydrochloride salt.

lo·mus·tine (lo-mus'tēn) an alkylating agent of the nitrosourea group, used as an antineoplastic in the treatment of Hodgkin's disease and brain tumors.

lon·gis·si·mus (lon-jis'ĭ-mus) [L.] longest.

lon·gi·tu·di·na·lis (lon″jĭ-tood″in-a′lis) [L.] lengthwise.

lon·gus (long′gus) [L.] long.

loop (loop) a turn or sharp curve in a cord-like structure. **capillary l's,** minute endothelial tubes that carry blood in the papillae of the skin. **closed l.,** a type of feedback in which the input to one or more of the subsystems is affected by its own output. **l. of Henle, Henle's l.,** the long U-shaped part of the renal tubule, extending through the medulla from the end of the proximal convoluted tubule. It begins with a *descending limb* (comprising the *proximal straight tubule* and the *thin tubule*), followed by the *ascending limb* (the *distal straight tubule*), and ending at the *distal convoluted tubule.* **open l.,** a system in which an input alters the output, but the output has no effect on the input.

loo·sen·ing (loo′sen-ing) freeing from restraint or strictness. **l. of associations,** in psychiatry, a disorder of thinking in which associations of ideas become so shortened, fragmented, and disturbed as to lack logical relationship.

LOP left occipitoposterior (position of fetus).

lo·per·amide (lo-per′ah-mīd) an antiperistaltic used as the hydrochloride salt as an antidiarrheal and to reduce the volume of discharge from ileostomies.

lo·phot·ri·chous (lo-fot′rĭ-kus) having two or more flagella at one end (of a bacterial cell).

lo·pin·a·vir (lo-pin′ah-vir) an antiviral HIV protease inhibitor, used with ritonavir in the treatment of HIV infection.

lor·a·car·bef (lor″ah-kahr′bef) a carbacephem antibiotic closely related to cefaclor and having similar antibacterial actions and uses.

lor·at·a·dine (lah-rat′ah-dēn) a nonsedating antihistamine used in the treatment of allergic rhinitis, chronic idiopathic urticaria, and asthma.

lor·a·ze·pam (lor-az′ĕ-pam) a benzodiazepine used as an antianxiety agent, sedative-hypnotic, preanesthetic medication, and anticonvulsant.

lor·do·sis (lor-do′sis) 1. the anterior concavity in the curvature of the lumbar and cervical spine as viewed from the side. 2. abnormal increase in this curvature.

lo·sar·tan (lo-sahr′tan) an angiotensin II receptor antagonist, used as an antihypertensive; used as the potassium salt.

LOT left occipitotransverse (position of fetus).

lo·te·pred·nol (lo″tĕ-pred′nol) a corticosteroid applied topically to the conjunctiva in the treatment of seasonal allergic conjunctivitis, postoperative inflammation, and ocular inflammatory disorders.

lo·tion (lo′shun) a liquid suspension, solution, or emulsion for external application to the body.

loupe (loop) [Fr.] a magnifying lens.

louse (lous) pl. *lice.* Any of various parasitic insects; species parasitic on humans are *Pediculus humanus capitis* (head l.), *P. humanus corporis* (body, or clothes, l.), and *Phthirus pubis* (crab, or pubic, l.). Lice are major vectors of typhus, relapsing fever, and trench fever.

lo·va·stat·in (lo′vah-stat″in) an antihyperlipidemic agent that acts by inhibiting cholesterol synthesis, used in the treatment of hypercholesterolemia and other forms of dyslipidemia and to lower the risks associated with atherosclerosis and coronary heart disease.

low-grade (lo′grād′) occurring near the low end of a range, as of a fever or malignancy.

lox·a·pine (lok′sah-pēn) a tricyclic dibenzoxazepine derivative used as the succinate and hydrochloride salts as an antipsychotic.

lox·os·ce·lism (lok-sos′sil-izm) a morbid condition due to the bite of the spiders *Loxosceles laeta* and *L. reclusa,* beginning with a painful erythematous vesicle and progressing to a gangrenous slough of the affected area.

lox·ot·o·my (lok-sot′ah-me) oval amputation.

loz·enge (loz′enj) [Fr.] 1. troche; a discoid-shaped, solid, medicinal preparation for solution in the mouth, consisting of an active ingredient incorporated in a suitably flavored base. 2. a triangular area of tissue marked for excision in plastic surgery.

Lp(a) see under *lipoprotein.*

LPN licensed practical nurse.

LPV lymphotropic papovavirus.

LSA left sacroanterior (position of fetus).

LScA left scapuloanterior (position of fetus).

LScP left scapuloposterior (position of fetus).

LSD lysergic acid diethylamide.

LSP left sacroposterior (position of fetus).

L-spine lumbar spine.

LST left sacrotransverse (position of fetus).

LTF lymphocyte transforming factor.

Lu lutetium.

lubb-dupp (lub-dup′) syllables used to represent the first and second heart sounds.

lu·bri·cant (loo′brĭ-kant) a substance applied as a surface film to reduce friction between moving parts.

lu·cid·i·ty (loo-sid′it-e) clearness of mind. **lu′cid,** adj.

lu·es (loo′ēz) syphilis. **luet′ic,** adj.

lum·ba·go (lum-ba′go) pain in the lumbar region.

lum·bar (lum′bar) pertaining to the loins.

lum·bar·iza·tion (lum″bar-ĭ-za′shun) non-fusion of the first and second segments of the sacrum so that there is one additional articulated vertebra, the sacrum consisting of only four segments.

lumb(o)- word element [L.], *loin.*

lum·bo·cos·tal (lum″bo-kos′t'l) pertaining to the loin and ribs.

lum·bo·dyn·ia (-din′e-ah) lumbago.

lum·bo·in·gui·nal (-ing′gwĭ-nil) pertaining to the loin and groin.

lum·bo·sa·cral (-sa′kral) pertaining to the loins and sacrum.

lum·bri·cide (lum′brĭ-sīd) ascaricide.

lum·bri·coid (-koid) resembling an earthworm; said particularly of *Ascaris lumbricoides.*

lum·bri·co·sis (lum″brĭ-ko′sis) ascariasis.

lum·bri·cus (lum-bri′kus) pl. *lumbri′ci.* [L.] 1. the earthworm. 2. old term for *ascaris.*

lum·bus (lum′bus) [L.] loin.

lu·men (loo′men) pl. *lu′mina.* [L.] 1. the cavity or channel within a tube or tubular organ. 2. the SI unit of luminous flux; it is the light emitted in a unit solid angle by a uniform point source with luminous intensity of one candela. **lu′minal,** adj. **residual l.,** the remains of Rathke's pouch, between the distal and intermediate parts of the pituitary gland.

lu·mi·nes·cence (loo″mĭ-nes′ens) the property of giving off light without a corresponding degree of heat.

lu·mi·no·phor (loo′mĭ-nah-for″) a chemical group which gives the property of luminescence to organic compounds.

lu·mi·rho·dop·sin (loo″mĭ-rah-dop′sin) an intermediate product of exposure of rhodopsin to light.

lum·pec·to·my (lum-pek′tah-me) 1. surgical excision of only the palpable lesion in carcinoma of the breast. 2. surgical removal of a mass.

lu·nate (loo′nāt) 1. moon-shaped or crescentic. 2. lunate bone; see *Table of Bones.*

lung (lung) the organ of respiration; either of the pair of organs that effect aeration of blood, lying on either side of the heart within the chest cavity. See Plates 25 and 26. **black l.,** pneumoconiosis of coal workers. **brown l.,** byssinosis. **farmer's l.,** hypersensitivity pneumonitis from inhalation of moldy hay dust. **humidifier l.,** hypersensitivity pneumonitis caused by breathing air that has passed through humidifiers, dehumidifiers, or air conditioners contaminated

by certain fungi, amebas, or thermophilic actinomycetes. **iron l.,** popular name for *Drinker respirator.* **pigeon breeder's l.,** hypersensitivity pneumonia from inhalation of particles of bird feces by those who work closely with pigeons or other birds; it may eventually result in pulmonary fibrosis. **white l.,** pneumonia alba.

lung·worm (-wurm″) any parasitic worm that invades the lungs, e.g., *Paragonimus westermani* in humans.

lu·nu·la (loo′nu-lah) pl. *lu′nulae.* [L.] a small, crescentic or moon-shaped area or structure, e.g., the white area at the base of the nail of a finger or toe, or one of the segments of the semilunar valves of the heart.

lu·poid (loo′poid) pertaining to or resembling lupus.

lu·pus (loo′pus) any of a group of skin diseases in which the lesions are characteristically eroded. **chilblain l. erythematosus,** a form due to cold-induced microvascular injury, aggravated by cold; the lesions initially resemble chilblains but eventually assume the form of discoid lupus erythematosus. **cutaneous l. erythematosus,** one of the two main forms of lupus erythematosus, in which the skin may be either the only or the first organ or system involved. It may be chronic (*discoid l. erythematosus*), subacute (*systemic l. erythematosus*), or acute (characterized by an acute, edematous, erythematous eruption). **discoid l. erythematosus (DLE),** a chronic form of cutaneous lupus erythematosus marked by red macules covered with scanty adherent scales that fall off and leave scars; lesions typically form a butterfly pattern over the bridge of the nose and cheeks, but other areas may be involved. **drug-induced l.,** a syndrome closely resembling systemic lupus erythematosus, precipitated by prolonged use of certain drugs, most commonly hydralazine, isoniazid, various anticonvulsants, and procainamide. **l. erythemato′sus (LE),** a group of chronic connective tissue diseases manifested in two main types: *cutaneous l. erythematosus* and *systemic l. erythematosus.* **l. erythemato′sus profun′dus,** a form of cutaneous lupus erythematosus in which deep brawny indurations or subcutaneous nodules occur under normal or, less often, involved skin; the overlying skin may be erythematous, atrophic, and ulcerated and on healing may leave a depressed scar. **l. erythemato′sus tu′midus,** a variant of discoid or systemic lupus erythematosus in which the lesions are raised reddish purple or brown plaques. **hypertrophic l. erythematosus,** a form of discoid lupus erythematosus characterized by verrucous hyperkeratotic lesions. **l. hyper-tro'phicus,** 1. a variant of lupus vulgaris in which the lesions consist of a warty vegetative growth, often crusted or slightly exudative, usually occurring on moist areas near body orifices. 2. hypertrophic l. erythematosus. **l. milia'ris dissemina'tus fa'ciei,** a form marked by multiple, discrete, superficial nodules on the face, particularly on the eyelids, upper lip, chin, and nares. **neonatal l.,** a rash resembling discoid lupus erythematosus, sometimes with systemic abnormalities such as heart block or hepatosplenomegaly, in infants of mothers with systemic lupus erythematosus; it is usually benign and self-limited. **l. per'nio,** 1. a cutaneous manifestation of sarcoidosis consisting of violaceous smooth shiny plaques on the ears, forehead, nose, and digits, frequently associated with bone cysts. 2. chilblain l. erythematosus. **systemic l. erythematosus (SLE),** a chronic generalized connective tissue disorder, ranging from mild to fulminating, marked by skin eruptions, arthralgia, arthritis, leukopenia, anemia, visceral lesions, neurologic manifestations, lymphadenopathy, fever, and other constitutional symptoms. Typically, there are many abnormal immunologic phenomena, including hypergammaglobulinemia and hypocomplementemia, deposition of antigen-antibody complexes, and the presence of antinuclear antibodies and LE cells. **l. vulga'ris,** the most common and severe form of tuberculosis of the skin, most often affecting the face, with formation of red-brown patches of nodules in the dermis that progressively spread peripherally with central atrophy, causing ulceration and scarring and destruction of cartilage in involved sites.

lute (loot) 1. a substance such as cement, wax, or clay that coats a surface or joint area to make a tight seal. 2. to coat or seal with such a substance.

lu·te·al (loo'te-al) pertaining to or having the properties of the corpus luteum or its active principle.

lu·te·in (-in) 1. a lipochrome from the corpus luteum, fat cells, and egg yolk. 2. any lipochrome.

lu·te·in·ic (loo″te-in'ik) 1. pertaining to lutein. 2. luteal. 3. pertaining to luteinization.

lu·te·in·iza·tion (-in″ĭ-za'shun) the process by which a postovulatory ovarian follicle transforms into a corpus luteum through vascularization, follicular cell hypertrophy, and lipid accumulation, the latter in some species giving the yellow color indicated by the term.

lu·te·ol·y·sis (-ol'ĭ-sis) degeneration of the corpus luteum. **luteolyt'ic,** adj.

lu·te·o·ma (loo″te-o'mah) 1. a luteinized granulosa-theca cell tumor. 2. nodular hyperplasia of ovarian lutein cells sometimes occurring in the last trimester of pregnancy.

lu·te·o·tro·pic (-tro'pik) stimulating formation of the corpus luteum.

lu·te·ti·um (Lu) (loo-te'she-um) chemical element (see *Table of Elements*), at. no. 71.

Lut·zo·my·ia (loot″zo-mi'ah) a genus of sandflies of the family Psychodidae, the females of which suck blood.

lux (lx) (luks) the SI unit of illumination, being 1 lumen per square meter.

lux·a·tion (luk-sa'shun) dislocation.

lux·u·ri·ant (lug-zhoor'e-ant) growing freely or excessively.

LVAD left ventricular assist device; see *ventricular assist device*, under *device*.

LVN licensed vocational nurse.

Lw lawrencium.

ly·ase (li'ās) any of a class of enzymes that remove groups from their substrates (other than by hydrolysis or oxidation), leaving double bonds, or that conversely add groups to double bonds.

ly·can·thro·py (li-kan'thrah-pe) delusion in which the patient believes he or she is a wolf or other animal or can change into one.

ly·co·pene (li'ko-pēn) the red carotenoid pigment of tomatoes and various berries and fruits.

ly·co·per·do·no·sis (li″ko-per″do-no'sis) hypersensitivity pneumonitis due to inhalation of spores of the puffball fungus, *Lycoperdon*.

ly·ing-in (li'ing-in) 1. puerperal. 2. puerperium.

lymph (limf) a transparent, usually slightly yellow, often opalescent liquid found within the lymphatic vessels, and collected from tissues in all parts of the body and returned to the blood via the lymphatic system. Its cellular component consists chiefly of lymphocytes. **aplastic l., corpuscular l.,** lymph that contains an excess of leukocytes and does not tend to become organized. **euplastic l., fibrinous l.,** that which tends to coagulate and become organized. **inflammatory l.,** lymph produced by inflammation, as in wounds. **tissue l.,** lymph derived from body tissues and not from the blood.

lym·pha (lim'fah) [L.] lymph.

lym·phad·e·nec·to·my (lim-fad″ĕ-nek′tah-me) surgical excision of a lymph node or nodes.

lym·phad·e·ni·tis (lim-fad″ĕ-ni′tis) inflammation of one or more lymph nodes. **cervical l.,** see under *adenitis*. **mesenteric l.,** a condition clinically resembling acute appendicitis, in which there is inflammation of the mesenteric lymph nodes receiving lymph from the intestine. **tuberculous l.,** tuberculosis of lymph nodes, usually either cervical (*tuberculous cervical l.*) or mediastinal. **tuberculous cervical l.,** tuberculosis of the cervical lymph nodes; formerly called *scrofula*.

lym·phad·e·no·cele (lim-fad′ĕ-no-sēl) a cyst of a lymph node.

lym·phad·e·nog·ra·phy (lim″fad-in-og′rah-fe) radiography of lymph nodes after injection of a contrast medium in a lymphatic vessel.

lym·phad·e·noid (lim-fad′ĕ-noid) resembling the tissue of lymph nodes; see under *tissue*.

lym·phad·e·no·ma (lim-fad″in-o′mah) lymphoma.

lym·phad·e·nop·a·thy (-op′ah-the) disease of the lymph nodes. **angioimmunoblastic l., angioimmunoblastic l. with dysproteinemia (AILD),** a systemic lymphoma-like disorder characterized by malaise, generalized lymphadenopathy, and constitutional symptoms; it is a nonmalignant hyperimmune reaction to chronic antigenic stimulation. **dermatopathic l.,** regional lymph node enlargement associated with melanoderma and other dermatoses marked by chronic erythroderma. **immunoblastic l.,** angioimmunoblastic l.

lym·pha·gogue (lim′fah-gog) an agent promoting the production of lymph.

lym·phan·gi·ec·ta·sia (lim-fan″je-ek-ta′zhah) lymphangiectasis.

lym·phan·gi·ec·ta·sis (-ek′tah-sis) dilatation of the lymphatic vessels. **lymphangiectat′ic,** adj.

lym·phan·gio·en·do·the·li·o·ma (lim-fan″je-o-en″do-the″le-o′mah) endothelioma of the lymphatic vessels.

lym·phan·gi·og·ra·phy (lim-fan″je-og′rah-fe) angiography of lymphatic vessels.

lym·phan·gio·leio·myo·ma·to·sis (lim-fan″je-o-li″o-mi″o-mah-to′sis) lymphangiomyomatosis.

lym·phan·gi·ol·o·gy (lim-fan″je-ol′ah-je) the scientific study of the lymphatic system.

lym·phan·gi·o·ma (-o′mah) a tumor composed of newly formed lymph spaces and channels. **cavernous l.,** 1. a deeply seated lymphangioma composed of cavernous lymphatic spaces and occurring in the head or neck. 2. cystic hygroma. **cystic l.,** cystic hygroma.

lym·phan·gio·my·o·ma·to·sis (lim-fan″je-o-mi″o-mah-to′sis) a progressive disorder of women of child-bearing age, marked by nodular and diffuse interstitial proliferation of smooth muscle in the lungs, lymph nodes, and thoracic duct. Called also *lymphangioleiomyomatosis*.

lym·phan·gio·phle·bi·tis (-flĕ-bi′tis) inflammation of the lymphatic vessels and the veins.

lym·phan·gio·sar·co·ma (-sahr-ko′mah) a malignant tumor of vascular endothelial cells arising from lymphatic vessels, usually in a limb that is the site of chronic lymphedema.

lym·phan·gi·tis (lim″fan-ji′tis) inflammation of a lymphatic vessel or vessels. **lymphangit′ic,** adj.

lym·pha·phe·re·sis (lim″fah-fĕ′rĭ-sis) lymphocytapheresis.

lym·phat·ic (lim-fat′ik) 1. pertaining to lymph or to a lymphatic vessel. 2. a lymphatic vessel.

lym·pha·tism (lim′fah-tizm) status lymphaticus.

lym·pha·ti·tis (lim″fah-ti′tis) inflammation of some part of the lymphatic system.

lym·pha·tol·y·sis (-tol′ĭ-sis) destruction of lymphatic tissue. **lymphatolyt′ic,** adj.

lym·phec·ta·sia (lim″fek-ta′zhah) distention with lymph.

lym·phe·de·ma (lim″fah-de′mah) chronic swelling of a part due to accumulation of interstitial fluid (edema) secondary to obstruction of lymphatic vessels or lymph nodes. **congenital l.,** Milroy's disease.

lymph·no·di·tis (limf″no-di′tis) lymphadenitis.

lymph(o)- word element [L.], *lymph; lymphoid tissue; lymphatics; lymphocytes*.

lym·pho·blast (lim′fo-blast) a morphologically immature lymphocyte, representing an activated lymphocyte that has been transformed in response to antigenic stimulation. **lymphoblas′tic,** adj.

lym·pho·blas·to·ma (lim″fo-blas-to′mah) poorly differentiated lymphocytic malignant lymphoma.

lym·pho·blas·to·sis (-blas-to′sis) an excess of lymphoblasts in the blood.

Lym·pho·cryp·to·vi·rus (lim″fo-krip′to-vi′rus) Epstein-Barr–like viruses; a genus of viruses of the subfamily Gammaherpesvirinae containing both animal and human pathogens, including Epstein-Barr virus and Marek's disease virus.

lym·pho·cy·ta·phe·re·sis (-si″tah-fĕ-re′sis) the selective removal of lymphocytes from withdrawn blood, which is then retransfused into the donor.

lym·pho·cyte (lim′fo-sīt) a mononuclear, nongranular leukocyte having a deeply staining nucleus containing dense chromatin and a pale-blue–staining cytoplasm. Chiefly a product of lymphoid tissue, it participates in immunity. **lymphocyt′ic,** adj. **B l's,** B cells, bursa-dependent lymphocytes; the precursors of antibody-producing cells (plasma cells) and the cells primarily responsible for humoral immunity. **cytotoxic T l's (CTL),** differentiated T lymphocytes that can recognize and lyse target cells bearing specific antigens recognized by their antigen receptors; they are important in graft rejection and killing of tumor cells and virus-infected host cells. **Rieder's l.,** a myeloblast sometimes seen in acute leukemia and chronic lymphocytic leukemia, having a nucleus with several wide and deep indentations suggesting lobulation. **T l's,** T cells, thymus-dependent lymphocytes; those that pass through or are influenced by the thymus before migrating to tissues; they are responsible for cell-mediated immunity and delayed hypersensitivity.

lym·pho·cy·to·blast (lim″fo-si′to-blast) lymphoblast.

lym·pho·cy·to·ma (-si-to′mah) well-differentiated lymphocytic malignant lymphoma. **l. cu′tis,** a manifestation of cutaneous lymphoid hyperplasia, with one or more skin lesions usually on the face, ears, limbs, or areolae of the breasts.

lym·pho·cy·to·pe·nia (-si″to-pe′ne-ah) lymphopenia; reduction of the number of lymphocytes in the blood.

lym·pho·cy·to·phe·re·sis (-si″to-fĕ-re′sis) lymphocytapheresis.

lym·pho·cy·to·sis (-si-to′sis) an excess of normal lymphocytes in the blood or an effusion.

lym·pho·cy·to·tox·ic·i·ty (-si″to-tok-sis′ĭ-te) the quality or capability of lysing lymphocytes, as in procedures in which lymphocytes having a specific cell surface antigen are lysed when incubated with antisera and complement.

lym·pho·duct (lim′fo-dukt) lymphatic vessel.

lym·pho·epi·the·li·o·ma (lim″fo-ep″ĭ-thēl″e-o′mah) a pleomorphic, poorly differentiated carcinoma arising from modified epithelium overlying lymphoid tissue of the nasopharynx.

lym·phog·e·nous (lim-foj′ĕ-nus) 1. producing lymph. 2. produced from lymph or in the lymphatics.

lym·pho·glan·du·la (lim″fo-glan′du-lah) pl. *lymphoglan′dulae.* A lymph node.

lym·pho·gran·u·lo·ma (-gran″u-lo′mah) Hodgkin's disease. **l. inguina′le,** l. vene′reum, a venereal infection due to strains of *Chlamydia trachomatis,* marked by a primary transient ulcerative lesion of the genitals, followed by acute lymphadenopathy. In men, primary infection on the penis usually leads to inguinal lymphadenitis; in women, primary infection of the labia, vagina, or cervix often leads to hemorrhagic proctocolitis, and may progress to ulcerations, rectal strictures, rectovaginal fistulas, and genital elephantiasis.

lym·pho·gran·u·lo·ma·to·sis (-gran″u-lo″mah-to′sis) European synonym for *Hodgkin's disease.*

lym·phog·ra·phy (lim-fog′rah-fe) radiography of the lymphatic channels and lymph nodes after injection of radiopaque material.

lym·phoid (lim′foid) resembling or pertaining to lymph or tissue of the lymphoid system.

lym·pho·kine (lim′fo-kīn) a general term for soluble protein mediators postulated to be released by sensitized lymphocytes on contact with antigen, and believed to play a role in macrophage activation, lymphocyte transformation, and cell-mediated immunity.

lym·pho·ki·ne·sis (lim″fo-kĭ-ne′sis) 1. movement of endolymph in the semicircular canals. 2. the circulation of lymph in the body.

lym·pho·lyt·ic (-lit′ik) causing destruction of lymphocytes.

lym·pho·ma (lim-fo′mah) any neoplastic disorder of lymphoid tissue. Often used to denote *malignant l.,* classifications of which are based on predominant cell type and degree of differentiation; various categories may be subdivided into nodular and diffuse types depending on the predominant pattern of cell arrangement. **adult T-cell l., adult T-cell leukemia/l.,** see under *leukemia.* **B-cell l.,** any in a large group of non-Hodgkin's lymphomas characterized by malignant transformation of the B lymphocytes. **B-cell monocytoid l.,** a low-grade lymphoma in which cells resemble those of hairy cell leukemia. **Burkitt's l.,** a form of small noncleaved-cell lymphoma, usually occurring in Africa, manifested usually as a large osteolytic lesion in the jaw or as an abdominal mass; Epstein-Barr virus has been implicated as a causative agent. **centrocytic**

l., mantle cell l. **convoluted T-cell l.,** lymphoblastic lymphoma with markedly convoluted nuclei. **cutaneous T-cell l.,** a group of lymphomas exhibiting (1) clonal expansion of malignant T lymphocytes arrested at varying stages of differentiation of cells committed to the series of helper T cells, and (2) malignant infiltration of the skin, which may be the chief or only manifestation of disease. **diffuse l.,** in an older classification method, malignant lymphoma in which the neoplastic cells diffusely infiltrate the entire lymph node, without any definite organized pattern. **follicular l.,** any of several types of non-Hodgkin's lymphoma in which the lymphomatous cells are clustered into nodules or follicles. **follicular center cell l.,** B-cell lymphoma classified by the similarity of the cell size and nuclear characteristics to those of normal follicular center cells; the four previous subtypes are scattered among several types of follicular and diffuse lymphomas. **giant follicular l.,** follicular l. **granulomatous l.,** Hodgkin's disease. **histiocytic l.,** a rare type of non-Hodgkin's lymphoma characterized by the presence of large tumor cells resembling histiocytes morphologically but considered to be of lymphoid origin. **Hodgkin's l.,** see under *disease.* **intermediate lymphocytic l., lymphocytic l., intermediately differentiated,** mantle cell l. **large cell l.,** any of several types of lymphoma characterized by the formation of one or more types of malignant large lymphocytes, such as large cleaved or noncleaved follicular center cells, in a diffuse pattern. **large cell, immunoblastic l.,** a highly malignant type of non-Hodgkin's lymphoma characterized by large lymphoblasts (B or T lymphoblasts or a mixture) resembling histiocytes and having a diffuse pattern of infiltration. **Lennert's l.,** a type of non-Hodgkin's lymphoma with a high content of epithelioid histiocytes and frequently with bone marrow involvement. **lymphoblastic l.,** a highly malignant type of non-Hodgkin's lymphoma composed of a diffuse, relatively uniform proliferation of cells with round or convoluted nuclei and scanty cytoplasm. **malignant l.,** a group of malignancies characterized by the proliferation of cells native to the lymphoid tissues, i.e., lymphocytes, histiocytes, and their precursors and derivatives; the group is divided into two major clinicopathologic categories: *Hodgkin's disease* and *non-Hodgkin's lymphoma.* **mantle cell l., mantle zone l.,** a rare form of non-Hodgkin's lymphoma having a usually diffuse pattern with both small lymphocytes and small cleaved cells. **marginal zone l.,** a group of related B-cell neoplasms that involve the lymphoid tissues in the marginal zone, the patchy area outside the follicular mantle zone. **mixed lymphocytic-histiocytic l.,** non-Hodgkin's lymphoma characterized by a mixed population of cells, the smaller cells resembling lymphocytes and the larger ones histiocytes. **nodular l.,** follicular l. **non-Hodgkin's l.,** a heterogeneous group of malignant lymphomas, the only common feature being an absence of the giant Reed-Sternberg cells characteristic of Hodgkin's disease. **plasmacytoid lymphocytic l.,** a rare variety of small lymphocytic lymphoma in which the predominant cell type is the plasma cell. **primary effusion l.,** a B-cell lymphoma associated with human herpesvirus 8 infection, characterized by the occurrence of lymphomatous effusions in body cavities without the presence of a solid tumor. **small B-cell l.,** the usual type of small lymphocytic lymphoma, having predominantly B lymphocytes. **small cleaved cell l.,** a group of non-Hodgkin's lymphomas characterized by the formation of malignant small cleaved follicular center cells, with either a follicular or diffuse pattern. **small lymphocytic l.,** a diffuse form of non-Hodgkin's lymphoma representing the neoplastic proliferation of well-differentiated B lymphocytes, with focal lymph node enlargement or generalized lymphadenopathy and splenomegaly. **small lymphocytic T-cell l.,** small lymphocytic lymphoma that has predominantly T lymphocytes. **small noncleaved cell l.,** a highly malignant type of non-Hodgkin's lymphoma characterized by the formation of small noncleaved follicular center cells, usually in a diffuse pattern. **T-cell l's,** a heterogeneous group of lymphoid neoplasms representing malignant transformation of the T lymphocytes. **U-cell l., undefined l.,** a category of non-Hodgkin's lymphomas that cannot be classified into a definite type by either morphologic or known immunocytochemical markers. **undifferentiated l.,** small noncleaved cell l.

lym·pho·ma·to·sis (lim″fo-mah-to′sis) the formation of multiple lymphomas in the body.

lym·pho·myx·o·ma (-mik-so′mah) any benign growth consisting of adenoid tissue.

lym·pho·no·dus (-no′dus) pl. *lymphono′di.* Lymph node.

lym·phop·a·thy (lim-fop′ah-the) any disease of the lymphatic system.

lym·pho·pe·nia (lim″fo-pēn′e-ah) lymphocytopenia.

lym·pho·plas·ma·phe·re·sis (-plaz-mah-fĕ′ris-is) selective separation and removal of plasma and lymphocytes from withdrawn blood, the remainder of the blood then being retransfused to the donor.

lym·pho·pro·lif·er·a·tive (-pro-lif′er-ah″tiv) pertaining to or characterized by proliferation of the cells of the lymphoreticular system.

lym·pho·re·tic·u·lar (-rĕ-tik′u-ler) pertaining to the cells or tissues of both the lymphoid and reticuloendothelial systems.

lym·pho·re·tic·u·lo·sis (-re-tik″ūl-o′sis) proliferation of the reticuloendothelial cells of the lymph nodes. **benign l.,** cat-scratch fever.

lym·phor·rha·gia (-ra′jah) lymphorrhea.

lym·phor·rhea (-re′ah) flow of lymph from cut or ruptured lymph vessels.

lym·phor·rhoid (lim′fah-roid) a localized dilatation of a perianal lymph channel, resembling a hemorrhoid.

lym·pho·sar·co·ma (lim″fo-sahr-ko′mah) a general term applied to malignant neoplastic disorders of lymphoid tissue, but not including Hodgkin's disease; see *lymphoma.*

lym·pho·scin·tig·ra·phy (-sin-tig′rah-fe) scintigraphic detection of metastatic tumor in radioactively labeled lymph nodes, particularly that using radioactively labeled technetium colloid (*radiocolloid l.*).

lym·phos·ta·sis (lim-fos′tah-sis) stoppage of lymph flow.

lym·pho·tax·is (lim″fo-tak′sis) the property of attracting or repulsing lymphocytes.

lym·pho·tox·in (lim′fo-tok″sin) tumor necrosis factor β; a lymphokine produced by activated T lymphocytes that inhibits growth of tumors and blocks transformation of cells.

lym·pho·tro·pic (lim″fo-trop′ik) having an affinity for lymphatic tissue.

ly·on·iza·tion (li″on-ĭ-za′shun) the process by which or the condition in which all X chromosomes of the cells in excess of one are inactivated on a random basis.

lyo·phil·ic (li″o-fil′ik) having an affinity for, or stable in, solution.

ly·oph·i·li·za·tion (li-of″ĭ-lĭ-za′shun) the creation of a stable preparation of a biological substance by rapid freezing and dehydration of the frozen product under high vacuum.

lyo·pho·bic (li″ah-fo′bik) not having an affinity for, or unstable in, solution.

lyo·tro·pic (-tro′pik) lyophilic.

ly·pres·sin (li-pres′in) a synthetic preparation of lysine vasopressin, used as an antidiuretic and vasoconstrictor in the treatment of central diabetes insipidus.

lyse (līz) 1. to cause or produce disintegration of a compound, substance, or cell. 2. to undergo lysis.

Lys lysine.

ly·ser·gic ac·id di·eth·yl·amide (LSD) (li-ser′jik as′id di-eth′il-ah-mīd) a widely abused psychomimetic derived from lysergic acid, with both sympathomimetic and serotoninergic blocking effects. Side effects can include ataxia, fever, hyperreflexia, mydriasis, piloerection, tremor, nausea and vomiting, visual perception disorders, and varying psychiatric disturbances. Anxiety may develop into acute panic reactions, and a persistent toxic psychotic state may result.

ly·ser·gide (li-ser′jīd) lysergic acid diethylamide.

ly·sin (li′sin) 1. an antibody that causes complement-dependent lysis of cells; often used with a prefix indicating the target cells, e.g., hemolysin. 2. any substance that causes cytolysis.

ly·sine (Lys, K) (li′sēn) a naturally occurring, essential amino acid, necessary for optimal growth in human infants and for maintenance of nitrogen equilibrium in adults. The acetate and hydrochloride salts are used in dietary supplementation and the hydrochloride salt is used in the treatment of severe metabolic alkalosis refractory to treatment.

ly·sin·o·gen (li-sin′ah-jen) an antigenic substance capable of inducing the formation of lysins.

ly·sin·uria (li″sĭ-nu′re-ah) an aminoaciduria consisting of excessive lysine in the urine, as in hyperlysinemia. **lysinu′ric,** adj.

ly·sis (li′sis) 1. destruction or decomposition, as of a cell or other substance, under influence of a specific agent. 2. mobilization of an organ by division of restraining adhesions. 3. gradual abatement of the symptoms of a disease.

-lysis word element [Gr.], *dissolution, reduction, abatement, relief.*

ly·so·gen (li′so-jen) 1. an agent that induces lysis. 2. lysinogen. 3. a lysogenized bacterium.

ly·so·gen·ic (li-so-jen′ik) 1. producing lysins or causing lysis. 2. pertaining to lysogeny.

ly·so·ge·nic·i·ty (li″so-jĕ-nis′ĭ-te) 1. the ability to produce lysins or cause lysis. 2. the potentiality of a bacterium to produce phage. 3. the specific association of the phage genome (prophage) with the bacterial genome in such a way that only a few, if any, phage genes are transcribed.

ly·sog·e·ny (li-soj′ĕ-ne) the phenomenon in which a bacterium is infected by a temperate bacteriophage, the viral DNA is integrated in the chromosome of the host cell and replicated along with the host chromosome for many generations (the lysogenic cycle), and then production of virions and lysis of host cells (the lytic cycle) begins again.

ly·so·so·mal α-glu·co·si·dase (li″so-so′mal gloo-ko′sĭ-dās) acid maltase.

ly·so·some (li′so-sōm) one of the minute bodies occurring in many types of cells, containing various hydrolytic enzymes and normally involved in the process of localized intracellular digestion. **lysoso′mal,** adj. **secondary l.,** one that has fused with a phagosome (or pinosome), bringing hydrolases in contact with the ingested material and resulting in digestion of the material.

ly·so·zyme (-zīm) an enzyme present in saliva, tears, egg white, and many animal fluids, functioning as an antibacterial agent by catalyzing the hydrolysis of specific glycosidic linkages in peptidoglycans and chitin, breaking down some bacterial cell walls.

lys·sa (lis′ah) [Gr.] rabies. **lys′sic,** adj.

Lys·sa·vi·rus (lis′ah-vi″rus) rabies-like viruses; a genus of viruses of the family Rhabdoviridae comprising the rabies virus and other related African viruses infecting mammals and arthropods.

lys·so·pho·bia (lis″o-fo′be-ah) irrational fear of rabies.

lyt·ic (lit′ik) 1. pertaining to lysis or to a lysin. 2. producing lysis.

-lytic a word termination denoting lysis of the substance indicated by the stem to which it is affixed.

lyze (līz) lyse.

M

M mega-; methionine; molar^1; molar^2; myopia.

M. [L.] mis′ce (mix); mistu′ra (a mixture).

M molar^1.

*M*r relative molecular mass; see *molecular weight,* under *weight.*

m median; meter; milli-.

m. [L.] mus′culus (muscle).

m mass; molal.

m- meta- (2).

μ (mu, the twelfth letter of the Greek alphabet) micro-; the heavy chain of IgM (see *immunoglobulin*).

MA Master of Arts; mental age.

mA milliampere; one thousandth (10^{-3}) of an ampere.

MAC membrane attack complex; *Mycobacterium avium* complex (see under *disease*).

mac·er·ate (mas′er-āt) to soften by wetting or soaking.

ma·chine (mah-shēn′) a mechanical contrivance for doing work or generating energy. **heart-lung m.,** a combination blood pump (artificial heart) and blood oxygenator (artificial lung) used in open-heart surgery.

Mac·ra·can·tho·rhyn·chus (mak″rah-kan″thor-ing′kus) a genus of parasitic worms (phylum Acanthocephala), including *M. hirudina′ceus,* found in swine.

mac·ren·ceph·a·ly (mak″ren-sef′ah-le) hypertrophy of the brain.

macr(o)- word element [Gr.], *large; abnormal size.*

mac·ro·ad·e·no·ma (mak″ro-ad″ĕ-no′mah) a pituitary adenoma over 10 mm in diameter.

mac·ro·am·y·lase (-am′ĭ-lās) a complex in which normal serum amylase is bound to a variety of specific binding proteins, forming a complex too large for renal excretion.

mac·ro·bi·o·ta (-bi-ōt′ah) the macroscopic living organisms of a region. **macrobiot′ic,** adj.

mac·ro·blast (mak′ro-blast) an abnormally large immature erythrocyte; a large young erythroblast with megaloblastic features.

mac·ro·ble·pha·ria (mak″ro-blĕ-far′e-ah) abnormal largeness of the eyelid.

mac·ro·ceph·a·ly (-sef′ah-le) megalocephaly; unusually large size of the head. **macrocephal′ic,** adj.

mac·ro·chei·lia (-ki′le-ah) excessive size of the lip.

mac·ro·chei·ria (-ki′re-ah) megalocheiria.

mac·ro·co·lon (-ko′lon) megacolon.

mac·ro·cra·nia (-kra′ne-ah) abnormal increase in the size of the skull, the face appearing small in comparison.

mac·ro·cyte (mak'ro-sīt) an abnormally large erythrocyte.

mac·ro·cy·the·mia (mak"ro-si-thēm'e-ah) the presence of macrocytes in the blood.

mac·ro·cyt·ic (-sit'ik) pertaining to or characterized by macrocytes.

mac·ro·cy·to·sis (-si-to'sis) macrocythemia.

mac·ro·dac·ty·ly (-dak'tĭ-le) megalodactyly.

mac·ro·el·e·ment (-el'ĕ-ment) any of the macronutrients that are chemical elements.

mac·ro·fau·na (-faw'nah) the macroscopic animal organisms of a region.

mac·ro·flo·ra (-flor'ah) the macroscopic vegetable organisms of a region.

mac·ro·fol·lic·u·lar (-fah-lik'u-lar) pertaining to or characterized by large follicles.

mac·ro·gam·ete (-gam'ēt) 1. the larger, less active female anisogamete. 2. the larger of two types of malarial parasites; see *gamete* (2).

mac·ro·ga·me·to·cyte (-gah-mēt'ah-sīt) 1. a cell that produces macrogametes. 2. the female gametocyte of certain Sporozoa, such as malarial plasmodia, which matures into a macrogamete.

mac·ro·gen·i·to·so·mia (-jen"it-ah-so'me-ah) excessive bodily development, with unusual enlargement of the genital organs. **m. prae'cox,** macrogenitosomia occurring at an early age.

mac·rog·lia (mah-krog'le-ah) neuroglial cells of ectodermal origin, i.e., the astrocytes and oligodendrocytes considered together.

mac·ro·glob·u·lin (mak"ro-glob'ŭl-in) a globulin of unusually high molecular weight, in the range of 1,000,000. **α₂-m.,** a plasma protein that inhibits a wide variety of proteolytic enzymes, including trypsin, plasmin, thrombin, kallikrein, and chymotrypsin, by entrapping and reducing the accessibility of their functional sites to large molecules.

mac·ro·glob·u·lin·emia (-glob"ŭl-in-ēm'e-ah) increased levels of macroglobulins in the blood. **Waldenström's m.,** a plasma cell dyscrasia resembling leukemia, with cells of lymphocytic, plasmacytic, or intermediate morphology that secrete an IgM M component, diffuse infiltration of bone marrow, weakness, fatigue, bleeding disorders, and visual disturbances.

mac·ro·gna·thia (-nath'e-ah) enlargement of the jaw. **macrognath'ic,** adj.

mac·ro·gy·ria (-ji're-ah) moderate reduction in the number of sulci of the cerebrum, sometimes with increase in the brain substance, resulting in excessive size of the gyri.

mac·ro·lide (mak'ro-līd) 1. a compound characterized by a large lactone ring with multiple keto and hydroxyl groups. 2. any of a group of antibiotics containing this ring

linked to one or more sugars, produced by certain species of *Streptomyces*.

mac·ro·mas·tia (mak"ro-mas'te-ah) excessive size of the breasts.

mac·ro·me·lia (-mēl'e-ah) abnormal largeness of one or more limbs.

mac·ro·mere (mak'ro-mēr) one of the large blastomeres formed by unequal cleavage of a zygote as a result of asymmetric positioning of the mitotic spindle.

mac·ro·meth·od (-meth"id) a chemical method using customary (not minute) quantities of the substance being analyzed.

mac·ro·min·er·al (mak"ro-min'er-al) macroelement.

mac·ro·mol·e·cule (mak"ro-mol'ĭ-kūl) a very large molecule having a polymeric chain structure, as in proteins, polysaccharides, etc. **macromolec'ular,** adj.

mac·ro·mono·cyte (-mon'ah-sīt) an abnormally large monocyte.

mac·ro·my·elo·blast (-mi'ĭ-lo-blast") an abnormally large myeloblast.

mac·ro·nod·u·lar (-nod'u-lar) characterized by large nodules.

mac·ro·nor·mo·blast (-nor'mo-blast) macroblast.

mac·ro·nu·cle·us (-noo'kle-us) the larger of two types of nuclei when more than one is present in a cell.

mac·ro·nu·tri·ent (-noo'tre-ent) an essential nutrient required in relatively large amounts, such as carbohydrates, fats, proteins, or water; sometimes certain minerals are included, such as calcium, chloride, or sodium.

mac·ro·nych·ia (-nik'e-ah) abnormal length of the fingernails.

mac·ro·ovalo·cyte (mak"ro-o'vah-lo-sīt) an enlarged, oval erythrocyte seen in megaloblastic anemia.

mac·ro·pe·nis (-pe'nis) excessive size of the penis.

mac·ro·phage (mak'ro-fāj) any of the large, mononuclear, highly phagocytic cells derived from monocytes that occur in the walls of blood vessels (adventitial cells) and in loose connective tissue (histiocytes, phagocytic reticular cells). They are components of the reticuloendothelial system. Macrophages are usually immobile but become actively mobile when stimulated by inflammation; they also interact with lymphocytes to facilitate antibody production. **alveolar m.,** one of the rounded granular, mononuclear phagocytes within the alveoli of the lungs that ingest inhaled particulate matter. **armed m's,** those capable of inducing cytotoxicity as a consequence of antigen-binding by cytophilic antibodies on their surfaces or by factors derived from T lymphocytes.

mac·roph·thal·mia (mak″rof-thal′me-ah) megalophthalmos; enlargement of the eyeball.

mac·ro·poly·cyte (mak″ro-pol′ĭ-sīt) a hypersegmented polymorphonuclear leukocyte of greater than normal size.

mac·ro·pro·lac·ti·no·ma (-pro-lak″tĭ-no′mah) a prolactinoma more than 10 mm in diameter, usually associated with serum prolactin levels above 500 ng per mL.

ma·crop·sia (mah-krop′se-ah) a disorder of visual perception in which objects appear larger than their actual size.

mac·ro·scop·ic (mak″ro-skop′ik) gross (2).

mac·ro·shock (mak′ro-shok″) in cardiology, a moderate to high level of electric current passing over two areas of intact skin, which can cause ventricular fibrillation.

mac·ro·so·ma·tia (mak″ro-so-ma′shah) great bodily size.

mac·ro·sto·mia (-sto′me-ah) greatly exaggerated width of the mouth.

mac·ro·tia (mak-ro′shah) abnormal enlargement of the pinna of the ear.

mac·u·la (mak′u-lah) pl. *ma′culae.* [L.] 1. a stain, spot, or thickening; in anatomy, an area distinguishable by color or otherwise from its surroundings. Often used alone to refer to the macula retinae. 2. m. lutea. 3. macule. 4. a corneal scar, appreciated as a gray spot. **mac′ular, mac′ulate,** adj. **acoustic maculae,** maculae acusticae. **ma′culae acus′ticae,** the macula sacculi and macula utriculi considered together. **m. adhe′rens,** desmosome. **ma′culae atro′phicae,** white scarlike patches formed on the skin by atrophy. **ma′culae ceru′leae,** faint grayish blue spots sometimes found peripheral to the axilla or groin in pediculosis. **cerebral m.,** tache cérébrale. **ma′culae cribro′sae,** three perforated areas (inferior, medial, and superior) on the vestibular wall through which branches of the vestibulocochlear nerve pass to the saccule, utricle, and semicircular canals. **m. den′sa,** a zone of heavily nucleated cells in the distal renal tubule. **m. fla′va laryn′gis,** a yellow nodule at one end of a vocal cord. **m. lu′tea, m. lu′tea re′tinae, m. re′tinae,** an irregular yellowish depression on the retina, lateral to and slightly below the optic disk. **m. sac′culi,** a thickening on the wall of the saccule where the epithelium contains hair cells that are stimulated by linear acceleration and deceleration and by gravity. **m. utri′culi,** a thickening in the wall of the utricle where the epithelium contains hair cells that are stimulated by linear acceleration and deceleration and by gravity.

mac·ule (mak′ūl) a discolored spot on the skin that is not raised above the surface.

mac·u·lo·cer·e·bral (mak″ūl-o-ser′ĭ-bril) cerebromacular.

mac·u·lop·a·thy (mak″u-lop′ah-the) any pathological condition of the macula retinae. **bull's eye m.,** increase of pigment of a circular area of the macula retinae accompanying degeneration, occurring in various toxic states and diseases.

mad·a·ro·sis (mad″ah-ro′sis) loss of eyelashes or eyebrows.

Mad·u·rel·la (mad″ūr-el′ah) a genus of imperfect fungi. *M. gris′ea* and *M. myceto′mi* are etiologic agents of maduromycosis.

ma·du·ro·my·co·sis (mah-doo″ro-mi-ko′sis) mycetoma.

maf·en·ide (maf′in-īd) an antibacterial, used topically as the monoacetate salt in superficial infections.

mag·al·drate (mag′al-drāt) a chemical combination of aluminum and magnesium hydroxides and sulfate; an antacid.

ma·gen·ta (mah-jen′tah) fuchsin or other salt of rosaniline.

mag·got (mag′it) the soft-bodied larva of an insect, especially a form living in decaying flesh.

mag·ma (mag′mah) 1. a thick, viscous, aqueous suspension of finely divided, insoluble, inorganic material. 2. a thin, pastelike substance composed of organic material.

mag·ne·si·um (Mg) (mag-ne′ze-um) chemical element (see *Table of Elements*), at. no. 12; its salts are essential in nutrition, being required for the activity of many enzymes, especially those concerned with oxidative phosphorylation. Various salts, including *m. chloride, m. gluceptate, m. gluconate,* and *m. lactate* are used as electrolyte replenishers. **m. carbonate,** an antacid. **m. chloride,** an electrolyte replenisher and a pharmaceutic necessity for hemodialysis and peritoneal dialysis fluids. **m. citrate,** a saline laxative used for bowel evacuation before diagnostic procedures or surgery of the colon. **m. hydroxide,** an antacid and laxative. **m. oxide,** an antacid and laxative; also used as a preventative for hypomagnesemia and as a sorbent in pharmaceutical preparations. **m. salicylate,** see *salicylate.* **m. silicate,** $MgSiO_3$, a silicate salt of magnesium; the most common hydrated forms found in nature are asbestos and talc. **m. sulfate,** Epsom salt; an anticonvulsant and electrolyte replenisher, also used as a laxative and local antiinflammatory. **m. trisilicate,**

a compound of magnesium oxide and silicon dioxide with varying proportions of water; an antacid.

mag·net (mag'nit) an object having polarity and capable of attracting iron. **magnet'ic,** adj.

mag·net·ro·pism (mag-net'ro-pizm) a growth response in a nonmotile organism under the influence of a magnet.

mag·ni·fi·ca·tion (mag″nĭ-fĭ-ka'shun) 1. apparent increase in size, as under the microscope. 2. the process of making something appear larger, as by use of lenses. 3. the ratio of apparent (image) size to real size.

ma huang (mah hwahng') [Chinese] any of various species of *Ephedra* used as herbs in Chinese medicine.

main·te·nance (mān'tĕ-nans) providing a stable state over a long period, or the stable state so produced.

ma·jor (ma'jer) large; significant; great or greatest in scope, effect, number, size, extent, or importance.

mal (mahl) [Fr. and Sp.] disease. **grand m.** (grahn), see under *epilepsy*. **m. de Meleda** (dĕ mel'ĕ-dah), a chronic, inherited, symmetrical hyperkeratosis of the palms and soles with spreading to their dorsal aspects and to other parts of the body; cutaneous lesions are erythematous, scaling, malodorous, and fissured. **petit m.** (pĕ-te'), see under *epilepsy*.

ma·la¹ (ma'lah) [L.] 1. cheek. 2. zygomatic bone; see *Table of Bones*.

ma·la² (mŭ'lah) [Sanskrit] in ayurveda, waste products of the body formed during metabolism, including urine, feces, mucus, and sweat.

mal·ab·sorp·tion (mal″ab-sorp'shun) impaired intestinal absorption of nutrients.

ma·la·cia (mah-la'shah) morbid softening or softness of a part or tissue.

-malacia word element [Gr.], *morbid softness.*

mal·a·co·ma (mal″ah-ko'mah) a morbidly soft part or spot.

mal·a·co·pla·kia (mal″ah-ko-pla'ke-ah) the formation of soft patches of the mucous membrane of a hollow organ. **m. vesi'cae,** a soft, yellowish, fungus-like growth on the mucosa of the bladder and ureters.

mal·a·co·sis (mal″ah-ko'sis) malacia.

mal·a·cos·te·on (mal″ah-kos'te-on) osteomalacia.

mal·ad·just·ment (mal″ah-just'ment) in psychiatry, defective adaptation to the environment.

mal·a·dy (-ah-de) disease.

mal·aise (mal-āz') a vague feeling of discomfort.

mal·align·ment (mal″ah-līn'mint) displacement, especially of teeth from their normal relation to the line of the dental arch.

ma·lar (ma'lar) 1. buccal; pertaining to the cheek. 2. zygomatic.

ma·lar·ia (mah-lar'e-ah) an infectious febrile disease endemic in many warm regions of the world, caused by protozoa of the genus *Plasmodium*, which are parasitic in red blood cells; it is transmitted by *Anopheles* mosquitoes and marked by attacks of chills, fever, and sweating occurring at intervals that depend on the time required for development of a new generation of parasites in the body. **malar'ial,** adj. **falciparum m.,** the most serious form, due to *Plasmodium falciparum*, with severe constitutional symptoms and sometimes causing death. **ovale m.,** a mild form due to *Plasmodium ovale*, with recurring tertian febrile paroxysms and a tendency to end in spontaneous recovery. **quartan m.,** that in which the febrile paroxysms occur every 72 hours, or every fourth day counting the day of occurrence as the first day of each cycle; due to *Plasmodium malariae*. **quotidian m.,** vivax malaria in which the febrile paroxysms occur daily. **tertian m.,** vivax malaria in which the febrile paroxysms occur every 42 to 47 hours, or every third day counting the day of occurrence as the first day of the cycle. **vivax m.,** that due to *Plasmodium vivax*, in which the febrile paroxysms commonly occur every other day (*tertian m.*), but may occur daily (*quotidian m.*), if there are two broods of parasites segmenting on alternate days.

ma·lar·i·a·ci·dal (mah-lar'e-ah-si″dal) plasmodicidal.

Mal·as·se·zia (mal″ah-se'zhah) a genus of fungi of the form-class Hyphomycetes, including *M. fur'fur*, which causes tinea versicolor in susceptible individuals, and *M. pachyder'matis*.

mal·as·sim·i·la·tion (mal″ah-sim″ĭ-la'shun) 1. imperfect, or disordered, assimilation. 2. the inability of the gastrointestinal tract to take up ingested nutrients, due to faulty digestion (maldigestion) or to impaired intestinal mucosal transport (malabsorption).

ma·late (ma'lāt) any salt of malic acid.

mal·a·thi·on (mal-ah-thi'on) an organophosphorus insecticide used as a topical pediculicide.

mal·ax·a·tion (mal″ak-sa'shun) an act of kneading.

mal·de·vel·op·ment (-dĭ-vel'op-mint) abnormal growth or development.

male (māl) 1. the sex that produces spermatozoa. 2. masculine.

mal·e·ate (mal'e-āt) any salt or ester of maleic acid.

ma·le·ic ac·id (mah-le′ik) an unsaturated dibasic acid, the *cis*-isomer of fumaric acid.

mal·erup·tion (mal″e-rup′shun) eruption of a tooth out of its normal position.

mal·for·ma·tion (-for-ma′shun) 1. a type of anomaly. 2. a morphologic defect of an organ or larger region of the body, resulting from an intrinsically abnormal developmental process.

mal·ic ac·id (mal′ik) a crystalline acid from the juices of many fruits and plants and an intermediate in the tricarboxylic acid cycle.

ma·lig·nan·cy (mah-lig′nan-se) 1. a tendency to progress in virulence. 2. the quality of being malignant. 3. a cancer, especially one with the potential to cause death.

ma·lig·nant (-nant) 1. tending to become worse and end in death. 2. having the properties of anaplasia, invasiveness, and metastasis; said of tumors.

ma·lin·ger·ing (mah-ling′ger-ing) willful, fraudulent feigning or exaggeration of the symptoms of illness or injury to attain a consciously desired end.

mal·le·a·ble (mal′e-ah-b′l) susceptible of being beaten out into a thin plate.

mal·leo·in·cu·dal (mal″e-o-ing′kūd′l) pertaining to the malleus and incus.

mal·le·o·lus (mah-le′o-lus) pl. *malle′oli*. [L.] a rounded process, such as the protuberance on either side of the ankle joint at the lower end of the fibula and the tibia. **malle′olar,** adj.

mal·le·ot·o·my (mal″e-ot′ah-me) 1. operative division of the malleus. 2. operative separation of the malleoli.

mal·le·us (mal′e-us) [L.] see *Table of Bones*.

mal·nu·tri·tion (mal″noo-trish′un) any disorder of nutrition.

mal·oc·clu·sion (-ah-kloo′zhun) improper relations of apposing teeth when the jaws are in contact.

mal·po·si·tion (-pah-zish′un) abnormal or anomalous placement.

mal·prac·tice (mal-prak′tis) improper or injurious practice; unskillful and faulty medical or surgical treatment.

mal·pres·en·ta·tion (mal″prez-en-ta′shun) faulty fetal presentation.

mal·ro·ta·tion (-ro-ta′shun) 1. abnormal or pathologic rotation, as of the vertebral column. 2. failure of normal rotation of an organ, as of the gut, during embryonic development.

mal·tase (mawl′tās) 1. α-glucosidase. 2. any enzyme with similar glycolytic activity, cleaving α-1,4 and sometimes α-1,6 linked glucose residues from nonreducing termini; in humans there are considered to be four such enzymes; two are the heat-stable enzymes, usually called maltases, constituting the glucoamylase complex; the other two are the heat-labile enzymes, usually called sucrase and isomaltase.

MALT·oma (mawl-to′mah) a form of extranodal marginal zone lymphoma originating in mucosa-associated lymphoid tissue, particularly that of the gastrointestinal tract.

mal·ti·tol (mawl′tĭ-tol) a hydrogenated, partially hydrolyzed starch used as a bulk sweetener.

mal·tose (mawl′tōs) a disaccharide composed of two glucose residues, the fundamental structural unit of glycogen and starch.

ma·lum (ma′lum) [L.] disease.

mal·un·ion (mal-ūn′yon) faulty union of the fragments of a fractured bone.

mam·ba (mahm′bah) any member of the genus *Dendroaspis*, extremely venomous elapid snakes. Included are the black mamba (*D. polylepis*), a large black African tree snake, and the green mamba (*D. angusticeps*), a large green or black tree snake of eastern and southern Africa.

ma·mil·la (mah-mil′ah) [L.] mammilla.

mam·ma (mam′ah) pl. *mam′mae*. [L.] the breast.

mam·mal (mam′l) an individual of the class Mammalia. **mamma′lian,** adj.

mam·mal·gia (mah-mal′je-ah) mastalgia.

mam·ma·plas·ty (mam′ah-plas″te) mammoplasty; plastic reconstruction of the breast, either to augment or reduce its size.

Mam·ma·lia (mah-māl′e-ah) a class of warm-blooded vertebrate animals, including all that have hair and suckle their young.

mam·ma·ry (mam′ah-re) pertaining to the mammary gland, or breast.

mam·mec·to·my (mah-mek′tah-me) mastectomy.

mam·mil·la (mah-mil′ah) pl. *mammil′lae*. [L.] 1. nipple (1). 2. papilla. **mam′millary,** adj.

mam·mil·li·plas·ty (mah-mil′ĭ-plas″te) theleplasty.

mam·mil·la·tion (mam″ĭ-la′shun) a nipple-like elevation or projection. **mam′millated,** adj.

mam·mil·li·tis (mam″ĭ-li′tis) thelitis.

mam·mi·tis (mam-i′tis) mastitis.

mamm(o)- word element [L.], *breast; mammary gland.*

mam·mo·gram (mam′o-gram) a radiograph of the breast.

mam·mog·ra·phy (mah-mog′rah-fe) radiography of the mammary gland.

mam·mo·pla·sia (mam″ah-pla′zhah) development of breast tissue.

mam·mo·plas·ty (mam′ah-plas″te) mammaplasty.

mam·mose (mam′ōs) 1. having large breasts. 2. mammillated.

mam·mot·o·my (mah-mot′ah-me) mastotomy.

mam·mo·tro·phic (mam″ah-tro′fik) mammotropic.

mam·mo·tro·pic (-tro′pik) having a stimulating effect on the mammary gland.

mam·mo·tro·pin (mam′o-tro″pin) prolactin.

man·di·ble (man′dĭ-b′l) the lower jaw; see *Table of Bones*. **mandib′ular**, adj.

man·dib·u·la (man-dib′u-lah) pl. *mandib′ulae*. [L.] mandible.

man·drel (man′dril) the shaft on which a dental tool is held in the dental handpiece, for rotation by the dental engine.

man·drin (-drin) a metal guide for a flexible catheter.

ma·neu·ver (mah-noo′ver) a skillful or dextrous method or procedure. **Bracht's m.**, a method of extraction of the aftercoming head in breech presentation. **Brandt-Andrews m.**, a method of expressing the placenta from the uterus. **forward-bending m.**, a method of detecting retraction signs in neoplastic changes in the mammae; the patient bends forward from the waist with chin held up and arms extended toward the examiner. If retraction is present, an asymmetry in the breast is seen. **Heimlich m.**, a method of dislodging food or other material from the throat of a choking victim: wrap one's arms around the victim, allowing their upper torso to hang forward; with both hands against the victim's abdomen (slightly above the navel and below the rib cage), make a fist with one hand, grasp it with the other, and forcefully press into the abdomen with a quick upward thrust. Repeat several times if necessary. **Pajot's m.**, a method of forceps delivery with traction along the axis of the superior pelvic aperture. **Pinard's m.**, a method of bringing down the foot in breech extraction. **Prague m.**, a method of extracting the aftercoming head in breech presentation. **Scanzoni m.**, double application of forceps blades for delivery of a fetus in the occiput posterior position. **Toynbee m.**, pinching the nostrils and swallowing; if the auditory tube is patent, the tympanic membrane will retract medially. **Valsalva m.**, 1. increase in intrathoracic pressure by forcible exhalation effort against the closed glottis. 2. increase in the pressure in the eustachian tube and middle ear by forcible exhalation effort against occluded nostrils and closed mouth.

man·ga·fo·di·pir (mang″gah-fo′dĭ-pir) a contrast-enhancing agent used as the trisodium salt in magnetic resonance imaging (MRI) of hepatic lesions.

man·ga·nese (Mn) (man′gah-nēs) chemical element (see *Table of Elements*), at. no. 25; its salts occur in the body tissue in very small amounts and activate liver arginase and other enzymes. Poisoning, usually due to inhalation of manganese dust, is manifested by symptoms including mental disorders accompanying a syndrome resembling parkinsonism, and inflammation of the respiratory system.

ma·nia (ma′ne-ah) [Gr.] a phase of bipolar disorders characterized by expansiveness, elation, agitation, hyperexcitability, hyperactivity, and increased speed of thought and ideas. **man′ic**, adj.

-mania word element [Gr.], *obsessive preoccupation with something*.

man·ic-de·pres·sive (man″ik-de-pres′iv) alternating between attacks of mania and depression, as in bipolar disorders.

man·i·kin (man′ĭ-kin) a model to illustrate anatomy or on which to practice surgical or other manipulations.

ma·nip·u·la·tion (mah-nip″u-la-shun) skillful or dextrous treatment by the hands.

man·ni·tol (man′ĭ-tol) a sugar alcohol formed by reduction of mannose or fructose and widely distributed in plants and fungi; an osmotic diuretic used to prevent and treat acute renal failure, to promote excretion of toxic substances, to reduce cerebral edema or elevated intracranial or intraocular pressure, and to prevent hemolysis during transurethral surgical procedures.

man·nose (man′ōs) a six-carbon sugar epimeric with glucose and occurring in oligosaccharides of many glycoproteins and glycolipids.

man·no·si·do·sis (man″ōs-ĭ-do′sis) a lysosomal storage disease due to a defect in α-mannosidase activity that results in lysosomal accumulation of mannose-rich substrates; it is characterized by coarse facies, upper respiratory problems, mental retardation, hepatosplenomegaly, and cataracts.

ma·nom·e·ter (mah-nom′it-er) an instrument for measuring the pressure of liquids or gases. **manomet′ric**, adj.

ma·nom·e·try (-ĕ-tre) the measurement of pressure by means of a manometer. **anal m.**, the measurement of pressure generated by the anal sphincter; used in the evaluation of fecal incontinence.

Man·son·el·la (man″son-el′ah) a genus of filarial nematodes. *M. ozzar′di* is found in the mesentery and visceral fat of humans in Central and South America.

Man·so·nia (man-so′ne-ah) a genus of mosquitoes, several species of which transmit *Brugia malayi*; some may also transmit viruses, such as those of equine encephalomyelitis.

man·tle (man′t′l) 1. an enveloping cover or layer. 2. cerebral cortex.

man·u·al (man′u-al) 1. of or pertaining to the hand; performed by the hand or hands. 2. a small reference book, particularly one giving instructions or guidelines. **Diagnostic and Statistical M. of Mental Disorders (DSM),** see under *D*.

ma·nu·bri·um (mah-noo′bre-um) pl. *manu′bria.* [L.] a handle-like structure or part, such as the manubrium of the sternum. **m. mal′lei, m. of malleus,** the longest process of the malleus; it is attached to the middle layer of the tympanic membrane and has the tensor tympani muscle attached to it. **m. ster′ni, m. of sternum,** the cranial part of the sternum, articulating with the clavicles and first two pairs of ribs.

ma·nus (ma′nus) pl. *ma′nus.* [L.] hand.

MAO monoamine oxidase; see *monoamine oxidase inhibitor,* under *inhibitor*.

MAOI monoamine oxidase inhibitor.

MAP mean arterial pressure.

map (map) a two-dimensional graphic representation of arrangement in space. **cytogenetic m., cytologic m.,** a gene map giving the position of gene loci relative to chromosome bands. **fate m.,** a plan of a blastula or other early stage of an embryo, showing areas of prospective significance in normal development. **gene m.,** one showing the positions of genetic loci on the chromosomes and usually giving some indication of the distance between loci. **genetic m., linkage m.,** a gene map giving the relative locations of genetic markers, based on recombination frequencies. **physical m.,** a gene map showing the locations of genetic markers along with the physical distances between them. **restriction m.,** a physical map indicating restriction enzyme cleavage sites. **transduction m.,** in bacterial genetics, a gene map giving distances between loci based on relative cotransduction frequencies.

ma·pro·ti·line (mah-pro′tĭ-lēn) a tetracyclic antidepressant with actions similar to those of the tricyclic antidepressants; used as the hydrochloride salt.

ma·ras·mus (mah-raz′mus) a form of protein-energy malnutrition predominantly due to prolonged severe caloric deficit, chiefly occurring in the first year of life, with growth retardation and wasting of subcutaneous fat and muscle. **maran′tic, maras′mic,** adj.

march (mahrch) the progression of electrical activity through the motor cortex. **jacksonian m.,** the spread of abnormal electrical activity from one area of the cerebral cortex to adjacent areas, characteristic of jacksonian epilepsy.

mar·fan·oid (mahr′fan-oid) having the characteristic symptoms of Marfan syndrome.

mar·gin (mahr′jin) an edge or border. **mar′ginal,** adj. **dentate m.,** pectinate line. **gingival m.,** gum m. **gum m.,** the border of the gingiva surrounding, but unattached to, the substance of the teeth.

mar·gi·na·tion (mahr″jĭ-na′shun) accumulation and adhesion of leukocytes to the epithelial cells of blood vessel walls at the site of injury in the early stages of inflammation.

mar·gino·plas·ty (mahr′jin-o-plas″te) surgical restoration of a border, as of the eyelid.

mar·go (mahr′go) pl. *mar′gines.* Margin.

mar·i·hua·na (mar′ĭ-hwah′nah) marijuana.

mar·i·jua·na (mar′ĭ-hwah′nah) a preparation of the leaves and flowering tops of hemp plants (*Cannabis sativa*), usually smoked in cigarettes for its euphoric properties.

mar·i·tal (mar′ĭ-t′l) of or pertaining to marriage.

mark (mahrk) a spot, blemish, or other circumscribed area visible on a surface. **birth m.,** see *birthmark.* **port-wine m.,** nevus flammeus. **strawberry m.,** 1. strawberry hemangioma (1). 2. cavernous hemangioma.

mark·er (mahrk′er) something that identifies or that is used to identify. **tumor m.,** a biochemical substance indicative of neoplasia, ideally specific, sensitive, and proportional to tumor load.

mar·row (mar′o) bone marrow; the soft organic material filling the cavities of bones, made up of a fiber-rich meshwork of connective tissue, the meshes being filled with marrow cells, which consist variously of fat cells, large nucleated cells or myelocytes, and megakaryocytes. *Yellow bone m.* is that in which fat cells predominate; *red bone m.* is the site of production of erythrocytes and granular leukocytes and occurs in developing bone, as of the ribs and vertebrae. **spinal m.,** the spinal cord.

Mar·su·pi·a·lia (mahr-soo″pe-a′le-ah) an order of mammals characterized by the possession of a marsupium, including opossums, kangaroos, wallabies, koala bears, and wombats.

marsh·mal·low (mahrsh′mel″o, -mal″o) a perennial Eurasian herb, *Althaea officinalis*, or preparations of its flowers, leaves, or roots, which are used in the treatment of cough and for irritation of the oral and pharyngeal mucosa; also used in folk medicine.

mar·su·pi·al·iza·tion (mahr-soo″pe-al-ĭ-za′shun) conversion of a closed cavity into an open pouch, by incising it and suturing the edges of its wall to the edges of the wound.

mas·cu·line (mas′kūl-in) pertaining to or having qualities normally associated with the male sex.

mas·cu·lin·i·ty (mas″ku-lin′ĭ-te) virility; the possession of masculine qualities.

mas·cu·lin·iza·tion (-lin-ĭ-za′shun) 1. normal development of male primary or secondary sex characters in a male. 2. development of male secondary sex characters in a female or prepubescent male. 3. the condition of having such sex characters.

ma·ser (ma′zer) a device which produces an extremely intense, small and nearly nondivergent beam of monochromatic radiation in the microwave region, with all the waves in phase.

mask (mask) 1. a covering or appliance for shading, protecting, or medicating the face. 2. to cover or conceal. 3. in audiometry, to obscure or diminish a sound by the presence of another sound of different frequency. 4. in dentistry, to camouflage metal parts of a prosthesis by covering with opaque material.

masked (maskt) 1. concealed from view; hidden. 2. not presenting or producing the usual symptoms. 3. blind (2).

maso·chism (mas′ah-kizm) the act or instance of gaining pleasure from physical or psychological pain; usually used to denote *sexual masochism*. **masochis′tic,** adj. **sexual m.,** a paraphilia in which sexual gratification is derived from being hurt, humiliated, or otherwise made to suffer physically or psychologically.

mass (mas) 1. a lump or collection of cohering particles. 2. a cohesive mixture to be made into pills. 3. the characteristic of matter that gives it inertia. Symbol *m*. **atomic m.,** atomic weight; used particularly when describing a single isotope of a nuclide. **inner cell m.,** embryoblast. **lean body m.,** that part of the body including all its components except neutral storage lipid; in essence, the fat-free mass of the body. **molar m.** (M), the mass of a molecule in grams (or kilograms) per mole. **molecular m.,** the mass of a molecule in daltons, derived by addition of the component atomic masses. Its dimensionless equivalent is molecular weight. **relative molecular m.,** technically preferable term for *molecular weight*. Symbol M_r.

mas·sa (mas′ah) pl. *mas′sae*. [L.] mass (1).

mas·sage (mah-sahzh′) [Fr.] systematic therapeutic friction, stroking, or kneading of the body. **cardiac m.,** intermittent compression of the heart by pressure applied over the sternum *(closed cardiac m.)* or directly to the heart through an opening in the chest wall *(open cardiac m.);* done to reinstate and maintain circulation. **carotid sinus m.,** firm rotatory pressure applied to one side of the neck over the carotid sinus, causing vagal stimulation and used to slow or terminate tachycardia. **electrovibratory m., vibratory m.,** that performed with an electric vibrator.

mas·sa·sau·ga (mas″ah-saw′gah) *Sistrurus catenatus*, a small venomous rattlesnake in the United States and northern Mexico.

mas·se·ter (mas-ēt′er) see *Table of Muscles.* **masseter′ic,** adj.

mas·seur (mah-sur′) [Fr.] 1. a man who performs massage. 2. an instrument for performing massage.

mas·seuse (-sooz′) [Fr.] a woman who performs massage.

MAST acronym for Military Anti-Shock Trousers, inflatable trousers used to induce autotransfusion of blood from the lower to the upper part of the body.

mas·tad·e·ni·tis (mas″tad-ĕ-ni′tis) mastitis.

Mas·tad·e·no·vi·rus (mast-ad′ĕ-no-vi″rus) mammalian adenoviruses; a genus of viruses of the family Adenoviridae that infect mammals, causing disease of the gastrointestinal tract, conjunctiva, central nervous system, and urinary tract; many species induce malignancy.

mas·tal·gia (mas-tal′je-ah) pain in the breast.

mas·tat·ro·phy (mas-tat′rah-fe) atrophy of the breast.

mas·tec·to·my (mast-ek′tah-me) excision of the breast. **modified radical m.,** total mastectomy with axial node dissection, but leaving the pectoral muscles intact. **radical m.,** amputation of the breast with wide excision of the pectoral muscles and axillary lymph nodes. **subcutaneous m.,** excision of breast tissue with preservation of overlying skin, nipple, and areola so that the breast form may be reconstructed.

mas·ti·ca·tion (mas″tĭ-ka′shun) chewing; the biting and grinding of food.

mas·ti·ca·to·ry (mas′tĭ-kah-tor″e) 1. subserving or pertaining to mastication; affecting the muscles of mastication. 2. a remedy to be chewed but not swallowed.

Mas·ti·goph·o·ra (mas″tĭ-gof′o-rah) a subphylum of Protozoa comprising those having one or more flagella throughout most of their life cycle, and a simple, centrally located nucleus; many are parasitic in both invertebrates and vertebrates, including humans.

mas·ti·gote (mas'tĭ-gōt) any member of the subphylum Mastigophora.

mas·ti·tis (mas-ti'tis) inflammation of the breast. **m. neonato'rum,** any abnormal condition of the breast in the newborn. **periductal m.,** inflammation of the tissues about the ducts of the mammary gland. **plasma cell m.,** infiltration of the breast stroma with plasma cells and proliferation of the cells lining the ducts.

mast(o)- word element [Gr.], *breast; mastoid process.*

mas·to·cyte (mas'tah-sīt) mast cell.

mas·to·cy·to·sis (-si-to'sis) an accumulation, local or systemic, of mast cells in the tissues; known as *urticaria pigmentosa* when widespread in the skin.

mas·toid (mas'toid) 1. breast-shaped. 2. mastoid process. 3. pertaining to the mastoid process.

mas·toid·al·gia (mas"toid-al'jah) pain in the mastoid region.

mas·toid·ec·to·my (mas"toi-dek'tah-me) excision of the mastoid cells or the mastoid process.

mas·toi·deo·cen·te·sis (mas-toid"e-o-sen-te'sis) paracentesis of the mastoid cells.

mas·toid·itis (mas"toid-i'tis) inflammation of the mastoid antrum and cells.

mas·top·a·thy (mas-top'ah-the) any disease of the mammary gland.

mas·to·pexy (mas'to-pek"se) surgical fixation of a pendulous breast.

mas·to·plas·ty (mas'to-plas"te) mammaplasty.

mas·to·pto·sis (mas"to-to'sis) pendulous breasts.

mas·to·scir·rhus (-skir'us) hardening of the mammary gland.

mas·to·squa·mous (-skwah'mus) pertaining to the mastoid and squama of the temporal bone.

mas·tot·o·my (mas-tot'ah-me) surgical incision of a breast.

mas·tur·ba·tion (mas"ter-ba'shun) self-stimulation of the genitals for sexual pleasure.

MAT multifocal atrial tachycardia; see *chaotic atrial tachycardia,* under *tachycardia.*

match·ing (mach'ing) 1. comparison and selection of objects having similar or identical characteristics. 2. selection of compatible donors and recipients for transfusion or transplantation. 3. selection of subjects for clinical trials or other studies so that the different groups are similar in selected characteristics. **cross m.,** crossmatching.

ma·te·ria (mah-tēr'e-ah) [L.] matter. **m. al'ba,** whitish deposits on the teeth, composed of mucus and epithelial cells containing bacteria and filamentous organisms. **m. me'dica,** pharmacology.

ma·ter·nal (mah-ter'nal) pertaining to the mother.

ma·ter·ni·ty (mah-ter'nĭ-te) 1. motherhood. 2. a lying-in hospital.

mat·ing (māt'ing) pairing of individuals of opposite sexes, especially for reproduction. **assortative m., assorted m., assortive m.,** the mating of individuals having similar qualities or constitutions. **random m.,** the mating of individuals without regard to any similarity between them.

ma·trix (ma'triks) pl. *ma'trices.* [L.] 1. the intercellular substance of a tissue or the tissue from which a structure develops. 2. groundwork; the base in which or from which a thing develops. 3. a mold or form for casting. 4. a metal or plastic strip used to provide form to a dental restoration. 5. the continuous phase of a composite dental restoration. **bone m.,** the intercellular substance of bone, consisting of collagenous fibers, ground substance, and inorganic salts. **cartilage m.,** the intercellular substance of cartilage, consisting of cells and extracellular fibers embedded in an amorphous ground substance. **extracellular m. (ECM),** any substance produced by cells and excreted to the extracellular space within the tissues, serving as a scaffolding to hold tissues together and helping to determine their characteristics. **interterritorial m.,** a paler staining region among the darker territorial matrices. **nail m.,** m. unguis. **territorial m.,** basophilic matrix around groups of cartilage cells. **m. un'guis,** nail bed; also, the proximal part of the nail bed where growth occurs.

mat·ter (mat'er) 1. substance; anything that occupies space. 2. pus. **gray m. of nervous system,** substantia grisea. **white m. of nervous system,** substantia alba.

mat·u·ra·tion (mach-u-ra'shun) 1. the process of becoming mature. 2. attainment of emotional and intellectual maturity. 3. in biology, a process of cell division during which the number of chromosomes in the germ cells is reduced to one half the number characteristic of the species. 4. suppuration.

ma·ture (mah-chōōr') 1. to develop to maturity; to ripen. 2. fully developed; ripe.

ma·tu·ti·nal (mah-too'tĭ-nal) occurring in the morning.

max·il·la (mak-sil'ah) pl. *maxil'las, maxil'lae.* [L.] the bone of the upper jaw; see *Table of Bones.* **max'illary,** adj.

max·il·lo·eth·moi·dec·to·my (mak″sil-o-eth″moid-ek′tah-me) excision of the portion of the maxilla surrounding the maxillary sinus and of the cribriform plate and anterior ethmoid cells.

max·il·lo·fa·cial (-fa′sh′l) pertaining to the maxilla and the face.

max·il·lo·man·dib·u·lar (-man-dib′u-ler) pertaining to the upper and lower jaws.

max·il·lot·o·my (mak″si-lot′ah-me) surgical sectioning of the maxilla which allows movement of all or part of the maxilla into the desired position.

max·i·mum (mak′sĭ-mum) pl. *max′ima*. [L.] 1. the greatest possible, or actual, effect or quantity. 2. largest; utmost. **max′imal,** adj. **transport m., tubular m. (T_m),** the highest rate (milligrams per minute) at which the renal tubules can transfer a substance either from the tubular luminal fluid to the interstitial fluid or from the interstitial fluid to the tubular luminal fluid, beyond which it may be excreted in the urine.

maze (māz) a complicated system of intersecting paths used in intelligence tests and in demonstrating learning in experimental animals.

ma·zin·dol (ma′zin-dōl) a sympathomimetic amine having amphetamine-like actions; used as an anorectic.

ma·zo·pexy (ma′zo-pek″se) mastopexy.

ma·zo·pla·sia (ma″zo-pla′zhah) degenerative epithelial hyperplasia of the mammary acini.

MB [L.] Medici′nae Baccalau′reus (Bachelor of Medicine).

MC¹ [L.] Magis′ter Chirur′giae (Master of Surgery).

MC² Medical Corps.

mcg microgram.

MCH mean corpuscular hemoglobin.

MCHC mean corpuscular hemoglobin concentration.

mCi millicurie; one thousandth (10^{-3}) of a curie.

μCi microcurie; one millionth (10^{-6}) of a curie.

MCP membrane cofactor protein.

MCV mean corpuscular volume.

MD [L.] Medici′nae Doc′tor (Doctor of Medicine).

Md mendelevium.

MDA methylenedioxyamphetamine.

MDF myocardial depressant factor.

MDMA 3,4-methylenedioxymethamphetamine.

meal (mēl) a portion of food or foods taken at some particular and usually stated or fixed time. **Boyden m.,** a test meal for the study of gallbladder evacuation in cholecystographic studies. **test m.,** a meal containing material given to aid in diagnostic examination of the stomach.

mean (mēn) an average; a numerical value that in some sense represents the central value of a set of numbers. **arithmetic m.,** the sum of *n* numbers divided by *n*. **geometric m.,** the *n*th root of the product of *n* numbers.

mea·sles (mēz″lz) rubeola; a highly contagious viral infection, usually of childhood, involving primarily the respiratory tract and reticuloendothelial tissues, marked by an eruption of discrete, red papules, which become confluent, flatten, turn brown, and desquamate. **atypical m.,** a form of natural measles infection affecting those who previously received killed measles virus vaccine. **black m.,** a severe form in which the eruption is very dark and petechial. **German m.,** rubella. **hemorrhagic m.,** black m.

meas·ure (mezh′er) see tables accompanying *weight*.

me·a·ti·tis (me″ah-ti′tis) inflammation of the urinary meatus.

me·a·to·plas·ty (me-at′o-plas″te) plastic surgery of a meatus.

me·a·tos·co·py (me″ah-tos′kah-pe) inspection of a meatus, especially the urinary meatus.

me·a·tot·o·my (-tot′ah-me) incision of an acoustic or urinary meatus to enlarge it.

me·a·tus (me-a′tus) pl. *mea′tus.* [L.] an opening or passage. **mea′tal,** adj. **acoustic m., auditory m.,** either of two passages in the ear, one leading to the tympanic membrane (*external acoustic m.*), and one for passage of nerves and blood vessels (*internal acoustic m.*). **nasal m.,** one of the four portions (common, inferior, middle, and superior) of the nasal cavity on either side of the septum. **urinary m.,** the opening of the urethra on the body surface through which urine is discharged.

me·ben·da·zole (mĕ-ben′dah-zōl) an anthelmintic used against trichuriasis, enterobiasis, ascariasis, and hookworm disease.

mec·a·myl·amine (mek″ah-mil′ah-min) a ganglionic blocking agent used in the form of the hydrochloride salt as an antihypertensive.

me·chan·ics (mĕ-kan′iks) the science dealing with the motions of bodies. **body m.,** the application of kinesiology to prevent and correct problems related to posture.

mech·a·nism (mek′ah-nizm) 1. a machine or machine-like structure. 2. the manner of combination of parts, processes, etc., which subserve a common function. **defense m.,** a usually unconscious mental mechanism by which psychic tension is diminished, e.g., repression, rationalization, etc. **escape m.**, in the heart, the mechanism of impulse initiation by lower centers in response to lack of impulse propagation by the sinoatrial node. **mental m.**, 1. the organization of mental operations. 2. an unconscious and indirect manner of gratifying a repressed desire.

mech·a·no·re·cep·tor (mek″ah-no-re-sep′-ter) a receptor that is excited by mechanical pressures or distortions, as those responding to touch and muscular contractions.

me·cha·no·sen·so·ry (-scn′sŏ-rc) pertaining to sensory activation in response to mechanical pressures or distortions.

mech·lor·eth·amine (mek″lor-eth′ah-mēn) one of the nitrogen mustards, used in the form of the hydrochloride salt as an antineoplastic, particularly in disseminated Hodgkin's disease.

mec·li·zine (mek′lĭ-zēn) an antihistamine used as the hydrochloride salt as an antinauseant in motion sickness and to manage vertigo associated with disease affecting the vestibular system.

mec·lo·cy·cline (mek″lo-si′klēn) a tetracycline antibiotic used topically as *m. sulfosalicylate* for the treatment of acne vulgaris.

me·clo·fen·am·ate (mek″lo-fen′ah-māt) a nonsteroidal antiinflammatory drug used as the sodium salt in the treatment of rheumatic and nonrheumatic inflammatory disorders, pain, dysmenorrhea, hypermenorrhea, and vascular headaches.

me·co·ni·um (mĭ-ko′ne-um) dark green mucilaginous material in the intestine of the full-term fetus.

me·dia (me′de-ah) 1. plural of *medium*. 2. middle. 3. tunica media vasorum.

me·di·al (me′de-il) 1. situated toward the median plane or midline of the body or a structure. 2. pertaining to the middle layer of structures.

me·di·a·lis (me″de-a′lis) [L.] medial.

me·di·an (me′de-in) 1. situated in the median plane or in the midline of a body or structure. 2. the value of the middle item of a series when the items are arranged in numerical order. Symbol m.

me·di·a·nus (me″de-a′nus) [L.] median.

me·di·as·ti·nal (-as-ti′n'l) of or pertaining to the mediastinum.

me·di·as·ti·ni·tis (-as″tĭ-ni′tis) inflammation of the mediastinum. **fibrosing m.**, **fibrous m.**, mediastinal fibrosis.

me·di·as·ti·nog·ra·phy (me″de-as″tĭ-nog′rah-fe) radiography of the mediastinum.

me·di·as·ti·no·peri·car·di·tis (me″de-as″tĭ-no-per″ĭ-kahr-di′tis) pericarditis with adhesions extending from the pericardium to the mediastinum.

me·di·as·ti·nos·co·py (me″de-as″ti-nos′-kah-pe) examination of the mediastinum by means of an endoscope inserted through an anterior midline incision just above the thoracic inlet.

me·di·as·ti·num (me″de-ah-sti′num) pl. *mediasti′na*. [L.] 1. a median septum or partition. 2. the mass of tissues and organs separating the two pleural sacs, between the sternum in front and the vertebral column behind, containing the heart and its large vessels, trachea, esophagus, thymus, lymph nodes, and other structures and tissues; it is divided into superior and inferior regions, the latter subdivided into anterior, middle, and posterior parts. **m. tes′tis**, the partial septum of the testis, formed near its posterior border by a continuation of the tunica albuginea.

me·di·ate¹ (me′de-it) indirect; accomplished by means of an intervening medium.

me·di·ate² (me′de-āt) to serve as an intermediate agent.

med·i·ca·ble (med′ĭ-kah-b'l) subject to treatment with reasonable expectation of cure.

med·i·cal (med′ĭ-k'l) pertaining to medicine.

Med·i·care (med′ĭ-kār) a program of the Social Security Administration which provides medical care to the aged.

med·i·cat·ed (med′ĭ-kāt″id) imbued with a medicinal substance.

med·i·ca·tion (med″ĭ-ka′shun) 1. medicine (1). 2. impregnation with a medicine. 3. administration of a medicine or other remedy. **ionic m.**, iontophoresis.

me·dic·i·nal (mĭ-dis′in-il) having healing qualities; pertaining to a medicine.

med·i·cine (med′ĭ-sin) 1. any drug or remedy. 2. the diagnosis and treatment of disease and the maintenance of health. 3. the treatment of disease by nonsurgical means. **alternative m.**, see *complementary and alternative medicine.* **aviation m.**, that dealing with the physiologic, medical, psychologic, and epidemiologic problems involved in aviation. **Chinese herbal m.**, a highly complex system of diagnosis and treatment using medicinal herbs, one of the branches of traditional Chinese medicine. Herbs range from the nontoxic and rejuvenating, used to support the body's healing system, to highly toxic ones, used to treat disease. **clinical m.**, 1. the study of disease by direct examination of the living patient. 2. the last two years of the usual curriculum in a medical college. **complementary m., complementary and alternative m. (CAM),** a large and diverse set of systems of diagnosis, treatment, and prevention based on philosophies and techniques other than those used in conventional Western medicine. Such practices may be described as *alternative*, existing as a body separate from and as a replacement for conventional Western medicine, or *complementary*, used in addition to conventional Western practice. CAM is characterized by its focus on the whole person as a unique individual, on the energy of the body and its influence on health and disease, on the healing power of nature and the mobilization of the body's own resources to heal itself, and on the treatment of the underlying causes, not symptoms, of disease. Many of the techniques used are controversial and have not been validated by controlled studies. **emergency m.,** the medical specialty dealing with the acutely ill or injured who require immediate medical treatment. **environmental m.,** that dealing with the effects of the environment on humans, including rapid population growth, water and air pollution, travel, etc. **experimental m.,** the study of diseases based on experimentation in animals. **family m.,** see under *practice.* **folk m.,** the use of home remedies and procedures as handed down by tradition. **forensic m.,** medical jurisprudence. **geographic m.,** 1. geomedicine. 2. tropical m. **group m.,** the practice of medicine by a group of physicians, usually representing various specialties, who are associated together for the cooperative diagnosis, treatment, and prevention of disease. **herbal m.,** herbalism. **holistic m.,** a system of medicine which considers man as an integrated whole, or as a functioning unit. **internal m.,** that dealing especially with diagnosis and medical treatment of diseases and disorders of internal structures of the body. **legal m.,** medical jurisprudence. **mind-body m.,** a holistic approach to medicine that takes into account the effect of the mind on physical processes, including the effects of psychosocial stressors and conditioning, particularly as they affect the immune system. **naturopathic m.,** naturopathy. **nuclear m.,** the branch of medicine concerned with the use of radionuclides in the diagnosis and treatment of disease. **occupational m.,** the branch of medicine dealing with the study, prevention, and treatment of workplace-related injuries and occupational diseases. **orthomolecular m.,** a system for the prevention and treatment of disease based on the theory that each person's biochemical environment is genetically determined and individually specific. Therapy involves supplementation with substances naturally present in the body (e.g., vitamins, minerals, trace elements, amino acids) in individually optimized amounts. **patent m.,** a drug or remedy protected by a trademark, available without a prescription; formerly used for quack remedies sold by peddlers. **physical m.,** physiatry. **preclinical m.,** 1. preventive m. 2. the first two years of the usual curriculum in a medical college. **preventive m.,** science aimed at preventing disease. **proprietary m.,** a remedy whose formula is owned exclusively by the manufacturer and which is marketed usually under a name registered as a trademark. **psychosomatic m.,** the study of the interactions between psychological processes and physiological states. **rehabilitation m.,** the branch of physiatry concerned with the restoration of form and function after injury or illness. **socialized m.,** a system of medical care controlled by the government. **space m.,** the branch of aviation medicine concerned with conditions encountered by humans in space. **sports m.,** the branch of medicine concerned with injuries sustained in athletics, including their prevention, diagnosis, and treatment. **traditional Chinese m. (TCM),** the diverse body of medical theory and practice that has evolved in China, comprising four branches: acupuncture and moxibustion, herbal medicine, qi gong, and tui na. In all of these, the body and mind are considered together as a dynamic system subject to cycles of change and affected by the environment, and emphasis is on supporting the body's self-healing ability. Fundamental to TCM are the yin/yang principle and the concept of basic substances that pervade the body: qi, jing, and shen, collectively known as the three treasures, and the blood (a fluid and material manifestation of qi) and body fluids (which moisten and lubricate the body). **travel m., travelers' m.,** the subspecialty of tropical medicine consisting of the diagnosis and treatment or prevention of diseases of travelers. **tropical m.,** the branch of medicine concerned with diseases of the tropics and subtropics. **veterinary m.,** the diagnosis and treatment of diseases of animals other than humans.

med·i·co·le·gal (med″ĭ-ko-le′g′l) pertaining to medical jurisprudence.

med·i·co·so·cial (-so′shil) having both medical and social aspects.

me·dio·lat·er·al (me″de-o-lat′er-il) pertaining to the midline and one side.

me·dio·ne·cro·sis (-ně-kro′sis) necrosis of the tunica media of a blood vessel.

med·i·ta·tion (med″ĭ-ta′shun) an intentional and self-regulated focusing of attention, whose purpose is to relax and calm the mind and body. **mindfulness m.,** a form in which distracting thoughts and feelings are not ignored but instead acknowledged and observed nonjudgmentally as they arise in order to detach from them and gain insight and awareness. **transcendental m.,** a technique for attaining a state of physical relaxation and psychological calm by the regular practice of a relaxation procedure that entails the repetition of a mantra to block distracting thoughts.

me·di·um (me′de-um) pl. *mediums, me′dia.* [L.] 1. a substance that transmits impulses. 2. culture medium; see under *C.* 3. a preparation used in treating histologic specimens. **active m.,** the aggregated atoms, ions, or molecules contained in a laser's optical cavity, in which stimulated emission will occur under the proper excitation. **clearing m.,** a substance to render histologic specimens transparent. **contrast m.,** a radiopaque substance used in radiography to permit visualization of internal body structures. **culture m.,** see under *C.* **dioptric media,** refracting media. **disperse m., dispersion m., dispersive m.,** the continuous phase of a colloid system; the medium in which the particles of the disperse phase are distributed, analogous to the solvent in a true solution. **nutrient m.,** a culture medium to which nutrient materials have been added. **refracting media,** the transparent tissues and fluid in the eye through which light rays pass and by which they are refracted and focused on the retina.

me·di·us (me′de-us) [L.] situated in the middle.

med·roxy·pro·ges·ter·one (med-rok″se-pro-jes′ter-ōn) a progestin used as the acetate ester in treatment of menstrual disorders, in postmenopause hormone replacement therapy, as a test for endogenous estrogen production, as an antineoplastic in the treatment of metastatic endometrial, breast, and renal carcinoma, and as a long-acting contraceptive.

med·ry·sone (med′rĭ-sōn″) a synthetic glucocorticoid used topically in the treatment of corticosteroid-responsive allergic and inflammatory conditions of the eye.

me·dul·la (mě-dul′ah) pl. *medul′lae.* [L.] the innermost part; marrow. **adrenal m., m.**

of adrenal gland, the inner, reddish brown, soft part of the adrenal gland; it synthesizes, stores, and releases catecholamines. **m. of bone,** bone marrow. **m. oblonga′ta,** that part of the brainstem continuous with the pons above and the spinal cord below. **m. os′sium,** bone marrow. **renal m.,** the inner part of the kidney substance, composed chiefly of collecting elements, Henle's loops, and vasa recta, organized grossly into pyramids. **spinal m., m. spina′lis,** spinal cord. **m. of thymus,** the central portion of each lobule of the thymus; it contains many more reticular cells and far fewer lymphocytes than does the surrounding cortex.

med·ul·lary (med′ah-lar″e) 1. pertaining to a medulla. 2. pertaining to bone marrow. 3. pertaining to the spinal cord.

med·ul·lat·ed (med′ah-lāt″ed) myelinated.

med·ul·li·za·tion (med″ah-lĭ-za′shun) enlargement of marrow spaces, as in rarefying osteitis.

me·dul·lo·blast (mě-dul′o-blast) an undifferentiated cell of the embryonic neural tube that may develop into either a neuroblast or spongioblast.

me·dul·lo·epi·the·li·o·ma (-ep″ĭ-the-le-o′mah) a rare type of neuroepithelial tumor, usually in the brain or retina, composed of primitive neuroepithelial cells lining the tubular spaces.

me·fe·nam·ic ac·id (mef″ah-nam′ik) a nonsteroidal antiinflammatory drug used to treat or prevent pain, inflammation, dysmenorrhea, and vascular headache.

mef·lo·quine (mef′lo-kwin) an antimalarial effective against chloroquine-resistant strains of *Plasmodium falciparum* and *P. vivax;* used as the hydrochloride salt.

mega- word element [Gr.], *large;* also used in naming units of measurement (symbol M) to designate an amount one million (10^6) times the size of the unit to which it is joined.

mega·cal·i·co·sis (meg″ah-kal″ĭ-ko′sis) nonobstructive dilatation of the renal calices due to malformation of the renal papillae.

mega·caryo·cyte (-kar′e-o-sīt) megakaryocyte.

mega·co·lon (meg′ah-ko″lon) dilatation and hypertrophy of the colon. **acquired m.,** colonic enlargement associated with chronic constipation, but with normal ganglion cell innervation. **aganglionic m., congenital m.,** Hirschsprung's disease; that due to congenital lack of myenteric ganglion cells in a segment of the large bowel, with loss of motor function in that segment and massive dilatation of the colon proximally. **idiopathic m.**, acquired m. **toxic m.**, that associated with amebic or ulcerative colitis.

mega·cys·tis (meg″ah-sis′tis) an abnormally enlarged urinary bladder.

mega·esoph·a·gus (-ĕ-sof′ah-gus) see *achalasia.*

mega·karyo·blast (-kar′e-o-blast″) the earliest cytologically identifiable precursor in the thrombocytic series, which matures to form the promegakaryocyte. **megakaryoblas′tic**, adj.

mega·karyo·cyte (-sīt″) the giant cell of bone marrow containing a greatly lobulated nucleus, from which mature blood platelets originate. **megakaryocyt′ic**, adj.

meg·al·gia (meg-al′jah) a severe pain.

megal(o)- word element [Gr.], *large; abnormal enlargement.*

meg·a·lo·blast (meg′ah-lo-blast″) a large, nucleated, immature progenitor of an abnormal erythrocytic series; the abnormal form corresponding to the normoblast. **megaloblas′tic**, adj.

meg·a·lo·ceph·a·ly (meg″ah-lo-sef′ah-le) macrocephaly. **megalocephal′ic**, adj.

meg·a·lo·chei·ria (-ki′re-ah) abnormal largeness of the hands.

meg·a·lo·cyte (meg′ah-lo-sīt″) macrocyte.

meg·a·lo·dac·ty·ly (meg″ah-lo-dak′tĭ-le) excessive size of the fingers or toes. **megalodac′tylous**, adj.

meg·a·lo·gas·tria (-gas′tre-ah) enlargement or abnormally large size of the stomach.

meg·a·lo·kar·y·o·cyte (-kar′e-o-sīt″) megakaryocyte.

meg·a·lo·ma·nia (-ma′ne-ah) unreasonable conviction of one's own extreme greatness, goodness, or power. **megaloma′niac**, adj.

meg·a·lo·pe·nis (-pe′nis) macropenis.

meg·a·loph·thal·mos (meg″ah-lof-thal′mos) macrophthalmia.

meg·a·lo·pia (meg″ah-lo′pe-ah) macropsia.

meg·a·lo·po·dia (-po′de-ah) abnormal largeness of the feet.

meg·a·lop·sia (meg″ah-lop′se-ah) macropsia.

meg·a·lo·syn·dac·ty·ly (meg″ah-lo-sin-dak′tĭ-le) a condition in which the digits are very large and more or less completely grown together.

meg·a·lo·ure·ter (-u-re′ter) megaureter.

meg·a·lo·ure·thra (-u-re′thrah) congenital dilation of the urethra, due usually to abnormal development of the corpus spongiosum but occasionally to some abnormality of the corpus cavernosum.

mega·u·re·ter (meg″ah-u-re′ter) congenital ureteral dilatation, which may be either primary or secondary to something else.

-megaly word element [Gr.], *enlargement.*

mega·vi·ta·min (meg′ah-vi″tah-min) a dose of vitamin(s) vastly exceeding the amount recommended for nutritional balance.

mega·volt (MV) (meg′ah-volt) one million (10^6) volts.

mega·volt·age (-vōl″taj) in radiotherapy, voltage greater than 1 megavolt, in contrast to orthovoltage and supervoltage.

me·ges·trol (mĕ-jes′trol) a synthetic progestational agent, used as the acetate ester in the palliative treatment of some breast, endometrial, and prostate carcinomas and in the treatment of anorexia, cachexia, and weight loss associated with cancer or AIDS.

meg·lu·mine (meg′loo-mēn) a crystalline base used in preparing salts of certain acids for use as a diagnostic radiopaque media, e.g., *diatrizoate m., iothalamate m.*

meg·ohm (meg′ōm) one million (10^6) ohms.

meg·oph·thal·mos (meg″of-thal′mos) hydrophthalmos.

mei·o·sis (mi-o′sis) cell division occurring in maturation of sex cells, wherein, over two successive cell divisions, each daughter nucleus receives half the number of chromosomes typical of the somatic cells of the species, so that the gametes are haploid. **meiot′ic**, adj.

mel·ag·ra (mel-ag′rah) muscular pain in the limbs.

mel·al·gia (mel-al′jah) pain in the limbs.

mel·an·cho·lia (mel″an-ko′le-ah) depression; curently used to denote severe forms of major depressive disorder. **melanchol′ic**, adj.

mel·a·nin (mel′ah-nin) any of several closely related dark pigments of the skin, hair, choroid coat of the eye, substantia nigra, and various tumors, produced by polymerization of oxidation products of tyrosine and dihydroxyphenol compounds.

mel·a·nism (mel′ah-nizm) melanosis.

melan(o)- word element [Gr.], *black; melanin.*

mel·a·no·a·melo·blas·to·ma (mel″ah-no-ah-mel″o-blas-to′mah) melanotic neuroectodermal tumor.

mel·a·no·blast (mel′ah-no-blast″) a cell that originates from the neural crest and develops into a melanocyte.

mel·a·no·blas·to·ma (mel″ah-no-blas-to′mah) malignant melanoma.

mel·a·no·car·ci·no·ma (-kahr″sĭ-no′mah) malignant melanoma.

mel·a·no·cyte (mel′ah-no-sīt, mĕ-lan′o-sīt) any of the dendritic clear cells of the epidermis that synthesize tyrosinase and, within their melanosomes, the pigment melanin; the melanosomes are then transferred from melanocytes to keratinocytes. **melanocyt′ic**, adj.

mel·a·no·cy·to·ma (mel″ah-no-si-to′mah) a neoplasm or hamartoma composed of melanocytes.

mel·a·no·der·ma (-der′mah) abnormally increased melanin in the skin.

mel·a·no·der·ma·ti·tis (-der″mah-ti′tis) dermatitis with deposit of melanin in the skin.

me·lan·o·gen (mĭ-lan′ah-jen) a colorless chromogen, convertible into melanin, which may occur in the urine in certain diseases.

mel·a·no·gen·e·sis (mel″ah-no-jen′ĕ-sis) the production of melanin.

mel·a·no·glos·sia (-glos′e-ah) black tongue.

mel·a·noid (mel′ah-noid) 1. resembling melanin. 2. a substance resembling melanin.

mel·a·no·leu·ko·der·ma (mel″ah-no-loo″kah-der′mah) a mottled appearance of the skin. **m. col′li**, syphilitic leukoderma about the neck.

mel·a·no·ma (mel″ah-no′mah) a tumor arising from the melanocytic system of the skin and other organs; used alone, it refers to *malignant m.*. **acral-lentiginous m.**, an irregular, enlarging black macule with a prolonged noninvasive stage, occurring chiefly on the palms and soles; it is the most common type of melanoma in nonwhite persons. **amelanotic m.**, an unpigmented malignant melanoma. **juvenile m.**, spindle and epithelioid cell nevus. **lenti′go malig′na m.**, a cutaneous malignant melanoma arising in the site of a preexisting lentigo maligna, occurring on sun exposed areas, particularly of the face. **malignant m.**, a malignant tumor usually developing from a nevus or lentigo maligna and consisting of black masses of cells with a marked tendency to metastasis. **nodular m.**, a type of malignant melanoma without a perceptible radial growth phase, usually occurring on the head, neck, or trunk as a uniformly pigmented, elevated, bizarrely colored, rapidly enlarging nodule that ulcerates. **ocular m.**, malignant melanoma arising from the structures of the eye, frequently metastasizing and rapidly causing death. **subungual m.**, acral-lentiginous melanoma in the nail fold or bed. **superficial spreading m.**, malignant melanoma characterized by a period of radial growth atypical of epidermal melanocytes, which may be followed by invasive growth or may regress; it usually occurs as a small pigmented macule or papule with irregular outline on the lower leg or back. **uveal m.**,

ocular melanoma consisting of overgrowth of uveal melanocytes.

mel·a·no·nych·ia (-nik′e-ah) blackening of the nails by melanin pigmentation.

mel·a·no·phage (mel′ah-no-fāj″) a histiocyte laden with phagocytosed melanin.

mel·a·no·phore (-for″) a pigment cell containing melanin, especially such a cell in fishes, amphibians, and reptiles.

mel·a·no·pla·kia (mel″ah-no-pla′ke-ah) the formation of melanotic patches on the oral mucosa.

mel·a·no·sis (mel″ah-no′sis) melanism; disordered production of melanin, with darkening of the skin. **m. co′li**, black or dark brown discoloration of the mucosa of the colon, due to the presence of pigment-laden (not true melanin) macrophages within the lamina propria. **neurocutaneous m.**, giant hairy nevus accompanied by malignant melanomas of the meninges.

mel·a·no·some (mel′ah-no-sōm″) any of the granules within the melanocytes that contain tyrosinase and synthesizes melanin; they are transferred from the melanocytes to keratinocytes.

mel·a·not·ic (mel″ah-not′ik) 1. pertaining to or characterized by the presence of melanin. 2. characterized by melanosis.

mel·an·uria (mel″an-ūr′e-ah) excretion of urine that is darkly stained or turns dark on standing. **melanu′ric**, adj.

me·las·ma (mĕ-laz′mah) sharply demarcated, blotchy, brown macules, usually in a symmetrical distribution on the cheeks and forehead and sometimes the upper lip and neck, often associated with pregnancy or other altered hormonal state.

mel·a·to·nin (mel″ah-to′nin) a catecholamine hormone synthesized and released by the pineal body; in mammals it influences hormone production and in many species regulates seasonal changes such as reproductive pattern and fur color. In humans it is implicated in the regulation of sleep, mood, puberty, and ovarian cycles and it has been tried therapeutically for insomnia, jet lag, and other conditions.

me·le·na (mĕ-le′nah) the passage of dark stools stained with altered blood.

me·li·oi·do·sis (mel″e-oi-do′sis) a glanderslike disease of rodents, transmissible to humans, and caused by *Pseudomonas pseudomallei*.

melo·plas·ty (mel′ah-plas″te) plastic surgery of the cheek.

melo·rhe·os·to·sis (mel″ŏ-re″os-to′sis) a form of osteosclerosis, with linear tracks extending through a long bone; see *rheostosis*.

mel·ox·i·cam (mĕ-lok'sĭ-kam) a nonsteroidal antiinflammatory drug used in the treatment of osteoarthritis.

mel·pha·lan (mel'fah-lan) a cytotoxic alkylating agent derived from mechlorethamine, used as an antineoplastic.

mem·ber (mem'ber) 1. a distinct part of the body. 2. limb.

mem·bra (mem'brah) [L.] plural of *membrum*.

mem·bra·na (mem-bra'nah) pl. *membra'nae*. [L.] membrane.

mem·brane (mem'brān) a thin layer of tissue that covers a surface, lines a cavity, or divides a space or organ. **alveolar-capillary m., alveolocapillary m.,** a thin tissue barrier through which gases are exchanged between the alveolar air and the blood in the pulmonary capillaries. Called also *blood-air barrier* and *blood-gas barrier*. **alveolodental m.,** periodontium. **arachnoid m.,** arachnoid (2). **atlantooccipital m.,** either of two midline ligamentous structures, one (the *anterior*) passing from the anterior arch of the atlas to the anterior margin of the foramen magnum, and the other (the *posterior*) connecting the posterior aspects of the same structures. **basement m.,** a sheet of amorphous extracellular material upon which the basal surfaces of epithelial cells rest; it is also associated with muscle cells, Schwann cells, fat cells, and capillaries, interposed between the cellular elements and the underlying connective layer. **basilar m. of cochlear duct,** lamina basilaris. **Bichat's m.,** fenestrated m. **Bowman's m.,** a thin layer of cornea between the outer layer of stratified epithelium and the substantia propria. **Bruch's m.,** the inner layer of the choroid, separating it from the pigmentary layer of the retina. **Brunn's m.,** the epithelium of the olfactory region of the nose. **cloacal m.,** the thin temporary barrier between the embryonic hindgut and the exterior. **Corti's m.,** a gelatinous mass resting on the organ of Corti, connected with the hairs of the hair cells. **croupous m.,** the false membrane of true croup. **cytoplasmic m.,** plasma m. **decidual m's, deciduous m's,** decidua. **Descemet's m.,** a thin hyaline membrane between the substantia propria and endothelial layer of the cornea. **diphtheritic m.,** a false membrane characteristic of diphtheria, formed by coagulation necrosis. **drum m.,** tympanic m. **elastic m.,** one made up largely of elastic fibers. **enamel m.,** 1. dental cuticle. 2. the inner layer of cells within the enamel organ of the fetal dental germ. **epiretinal m.,** a pathologic membrane partially covering the surface of the retina, probably originating chiefly from the retinal pigment epithelial and glial cells. **extraembryonic m's,** those that protect the embryo or fetus and provide for its nutrition, respiration, and excretion; the yolk sac (umbilical vesicle), allantois, amnion, chorion, decidua, and placenta. **false m.,** neomembrane; a membranous exudate, such as the diphtheritic membrane. **fenestrated m.,** one of the perforated elastic sheets of the tunica intima and tunica media of arteries. **fetal m's,** extraembryonic m's. **fibroelastic m. of larynx,** the fibroelastic layer beneath the mucous coat of the larynx. **germinal m.,** blastoderm. **glomerular m.,** the membrane covering a glomerular capillary. **hemodialyzer m.,** the semipermeable membrane that filters the blood in a hemodialyzer, commonly made of cuprophane, cellulose acetate, polyacrylonitrile, or polymethyl methacrylate. **hyaline m.,** 1. a membrane between the outer root sheath and inner fibrous layer of a hair follicle. 2. a layer of eosinophilic hyaline material lining alveoli, alveolar ducts, and bronchioles, found at autopsy in infants who have died of respiratory distress syndrome of the newborn. **hyaloid m.,** vitreous m. (1). **Jackson's m.,** a web of adhesions sometimes covering the cecum and causing obstruction of the bowel. **keratogenous m.,** matrix unguis. **limiting m.,** one which constitutes the border of some tissue or structure. **medullary m.,** endosteum. **mucous m.,** the membrane lining various canals and cavities of the body. **Nasmyth's m.,** dental cuticle. **nuclear m.,** 1. either of the membranes, inner and outer, comprising the nuclear envelope. 2. nuclear envelope. **olfactory m.,** the olfactory portion of the mucous membrane lining the nasal fossa. **ovular m.,** vitelline m. **peridental m., periodontal m.,** periodontal ligament. **placental m.,** the membrane separating the fetal from the maternal blood in the placenta; sometimes inappropriately called the *placental barrier*. **plasma m.,** the structure, composed of lipids, proteins, and some carbohydrates, that encloses the cytoplasm of a cell, forming a selectively permeable barrier. **pupillary m.,** a mesodermal layer attached to the rim or front of the iris during embryonic development. **Reissner's m.,** the thin anterior wall of the cochlear duct, separating it from the scala vestibuli. **reticular m., reticulated m.,** a netlike membrane over the spiral organ of the ear, through which pass the free ends of the outer hair cells. **m. of round window,** secondary tympanic m. **Ruysch's m., ruyschian m.,**

lamina choroidocapillaris. **Scarpa's m.,** secondary tympanic m. **schneiderian m.,** the mucous membrane lining the nose. **secondary tympanic m.,** the membrane enclosing the fenestra cochlearis. **serous m.,** tunica serosa. **Shrapnell's m.,** the thin upper part of the tympanic membrane. **suprapleural m.,** the strengthened portion of the endothoracic fascia attached to the inner part of the first rib and the transverse process of the seventh cervical vertebra. **synaptic m.,** the part of the plasma membrane of a neuron that is within a synapse. **synovial m.,** 1. the inner of the two layers of the articular capsule of a synovial joint, composed of loose connective tissue and having a free smooth surface that lines the joint cavity. 2. either of two membranes, superior and inferior, lining the articular capsule of the temporomandibular joint. **tectorial m.,** Corti's m. **tympanic m.,** the thin partition between the external acoustic meatus and the middle ear. **undulating m.,** a protoplasmic membrane running like a fin along the bodies of certain protozoa. **unit m.,** the trilaminar structure of the plasma membrane and other cellular membranes (e.g., nuclear m's, mitochondrial m's) revealed by the electron microscope. **vestibular m. of cochlear duct,** the thin anterior wall of the cochlear duct, separating it from the scala tympani. **vitelline m.,** the cytoplasmic, noncellular membrane surrounding an oocyte. **vitreous m.,** 1. a delicate boundary layer investing the vitreous body. 2. Bruch's m. 3. Descemet's m. 4. hyaline m. (1). **yolk m.,** vitelline m. **Zinn's m.,** ciliary zonule.

mem·bra·no·car·ti·lag·i·nous (mem″-brah-no-kahr″tĭ-laj′ĭ-nus) 1. developed in both membrane and cartilage. 2. partly cartilaginous and partly membranous.

mem·bra·noid (mem′brah-noid) resembling a membrane.

mem·bran·ol·y·sis (mem″brān-ol′ĭ-sis) disruption of a cell membrane.

mem·bra·nous (mem′brah-nus) pertaining to or of the nature of a membrane.

mem·brum (mem′brum) pl. *mem′bra.* [L.] 1. member. 2. limb.

mem·o·ry (mem′o-re) that faculty by which sensations, impressions, and ideas are stored and recalled. **immunologic m.,** anamnesis; the capacity of the immune system to respond more rapidly and strongly to subsequent antigenic challenge than to the first exposure. **remote m.,** memory that is serviceable for events long past, but not able to acquire new recollections. **replacement m.,** the replacing of one memory with another.

screen m., a consciously tolerable memory serving to conceal another memory that might be disturbing or emotionally painful if recalled. **short-term m.,** memory that is lost within a brief period (from a few seconds to a maximum of about 30 minutes) unless reinforced.

MEN multiple endocrine neoplasia.

me·nac·me (mĕ-nak′me) the period of a woman's life which is marked by menstrual activity.

men·a·di·ol (men″ah-di′ol) a vitamin K analogue; its sodium diphosphate salt is used as a prothrombinogenic vitamin.

men·a·di·one (men″ah-di′ōn) vitamin K_3. 1. a synthetic fat-soluble vitamin that can be converted in the body to active vitamin K. 2. the basic double ring quinone structure that is the parent structure of the related compounds with vitamin K activity, which can be formed by addition of long side chain substituents.

men·a·quin·one (men″ah-kwin′ōn) vitamin K_2; any of a series of compounds having vitamin K activity and structurally similar to phytonadione (vitamin K_1) but having a different side chain; synthesized by the intestinal flora.

me·nar·che (mĕ-nahr′ke) establishment or beginning of the menstrual function. **menar′cheal,** adj.

men·de·le·vi·um (Md) (men″dĕ-le′ve-um) chemical element (see *Table of Elements*), at. no. 101.

me·nin·ges (mĕn-in′jēz) sing. *meninx.* [Gr.] the three membranes covering the brain and spinal cord: dura mater, arachnoid, and pia mater. **menin′geal,** adj.

me·nin·gi·o·ma (mĕ-nin″je-o′mah) a benign, slow-growing tumor of the meninges, usually next to the dura mater, which may invade the skull or cause hyperostosis, and often causes increased intracranial pressure; it is usually subclassified on the basis of anatomic location. **angioblastic m.,** one containing many blood vessels of various sizes. **convexity m's,** a diverse group of meningiomas located within the sulci of the brain, usually anterior to the rolandic fissure. **psammomatous m.,** one containing many psammoma bodies.

me·nin·gism (men′in-jizm) the symptoms of meningitis with acute febrile illness or dehydration without infection of the meninges.

men·in·gis·mus (men″in-jiz′mus) meningism.

men·in·gi·tis (men″in-ji′tis) pl. *meningi′tides.* [Gr.] inflammation of the meninges. **meningit′ic,** adj. **basilar m.,** that affecting the meninges at the base of the brain. **cerebral m.,** inflammation of the membranes of the brain. **cerebrospinal m.,** inflammation of the membranes of the brain and spinal cord. **chronic m.,** a variable syndrome of prolonged fever, headache, lethargy, stiff neck, confusion, nausea, and vomiting, with pleocytosis; due to a variety of infectious and noninfectious causes. **cryptococcal m.,** cryptococcosis in which the meninges are invaded by *Cryptococcus*. **eosinophilic m.,** meningitis characterized by an increase in lymphocytes and a high percentage of eosinophils in the cerebrospinal fluid, usually due to *Angiostrongylus cantonensis* infection. **epidemic cerebrospinal m.,** meningococcal m. **meningococcal m.,** an acute infectious, usually epidemic, disease attended by a seropurulent meningitis, due to *Neisseria meningitidis*, usually with an erythematous, herpetic, or hemorrhagic skin eruption. **occlusive m.,** leptomeningitis of children, with closure of the lateral and median apertures of the fourth ventricle. **m. ossi'ficans,** ossification of the cerebral meninges. **otitic m.,** that secondary to otitis media. **spinal m.,** inflammation of the membranes of the spinal cord. **tubercular m., tuberculous m.,** severe meningitis due to *Mycobacterium tuberculosis*. **viral m.,** that due to a virus, e.g., coxsackieviruses, mumps virus, or the virus of lymphocytic choriomeningitis, marked by malaise, fever, headache and other aches, nausea, and cerebrospinal fluid pleocytosis (mainly lymphocytic); it usually runs a short uncomplicated course.

mening(o)- word element [Gr.], *meninges; membrane*.

me·nin·go·cele (mě-ning'gah-sēl) hernial protrusion of the meninges through a defect in the cranium *(cranial m.)* or vertebral column *(spinal m.)*.

me·nin·go·coc·ce·mia (-kok-sēm'e-ah) invasion of the blood by meningococci.

me·nin·go·coc·cus (mě-ning''go-kok'us) pl. *meningococ'ci*. An individual organism of *Neisseria meningitidis*. **meningococ'cal, meningococ'cic,** adj.

me·nin·go·cyte (mě-ning'go-sīt) a histiocyte of the meninges.

me·nin·go·en·ceph·a·li·tis (mě-ning''go-en-sef''ah-li'tis) inflammation of the brain and meninges. **toxoplasmic m.,** meningoencephalitis occurring in toxoplasmosis, with seizures and mental confusion followed by coma; often fatal if untreated.

me·nin·go·en·ceph·a·lo·cele (-en-sef'ah-lo-sēl'') encephalocele.

me·nin·go·en·ceph·a·lop·a·thy (-en-sef''ah-lop'ah-the) noninflammatory disease of the cerebral meninges and brain.

me·nin·go·gen·ic (-jen'ik) arising in the meninges.

me·nin·go·ma·la·cia (-mah-la'shah) softening of a membrane.

me·nin·go·my·eli·tis (-mi''ě-li'tis) inflammation of the spinal cord and its membranes.

me·nin·go·my·elo·ra·dic·u·li·tis (-mi''ě-lo-rah-dik''u-li'tis) inflammation of the meninges, spinal cord, and roots of the spinal nerves.

me·nin·go·os·teo·phle·bi·tis (-os''te-o-flě-bi'tis) periostitis with inflammation of the veins of a bone.

men·in·gop·a·thy (men''in-gop'ah-the) any disease of the meninges.

me·nin·go·ra·dic·u·lar (mě-ning''go-rah-dik'u-ler) pertaining to the meninges and the cranial or spinal nerve roots.

me·nin·gor·rha·gia (-ra'jah) hemorrhage from cerebral or spinal membranes.

men·in·go·sis (men''ing-go'sis) attachment of bones by membrane.

me·ninx (me'ninks) pl. *menin'ges*. [Gr.] singular of *meninges*.

men·is·ci·tis (men''ĭ-si'tis) inflammation of a meniscus of the knee joint.

me·nis·co·cyte (mě-nis'ko-sīt) sickle cell.

me·nis·co·fem·o·ral (mě-nis''ko-fem'or-al) pertaining to or connecting the femur and a meniscus.

me·nis·co·syn·o·vi·al (-sin-o've-il) pertaining to a meniscus and the synovial membrane.

me·nis·cus (mě-nis'kus) pl. *menis'ci*. [L.] something of crescent shape, as the concave or convex surface of a column of liquid in a pipet or buret, or a crescent-shaped cartilage in the knee joint. **menis'cal,** adj. **tactile m.,** one of the small, cup-shaped nerve endings found in the deep epidermis, in hair follicles, and in the hard palate; they function as touch receptors.

men(o)- word element [Gr.], *menstruation*.

meno·lip·sis (men''ah-lip'sis) temporary cessation of menstruation.

meno·met·ror·rha·gia (-met''ro-ra'jah) excessive and prolonged uterine bleeding occurring at irregular, frequent intervals.

meno·pause (men'ah-pawz) cessation of menstruation. **menopaus'al,** adj. **premature m.,** cessation of ovulation and menstrual cycles before age 40.

men·or·rha·gia (men''ah-ra'jah) hypermenorrhea.

men·or·rhal·gia (-ral'jah) dysmenorrhea.

men·or·rhea (-re′ah) 1. the normal discharge of the menses. 2. profuse menstruation. **menorrhe′al**, adj.

me·nos·che·sis (mĕ-nos′kĕ-sis) retention of the menses.

meno·stax·is (men″ah-stak′sis) excessively prolonged menstruation.

meno·tro·pins (-tro′pins) a purified preparation of gonadotropins extracted from the urine of postmenopausal women containing follicle-stimulating hormone (FSH) and luteinizing hormone (LH); used to treat male hypogonadism, to induce ovulation and pregnancy in certain infertile, anovulatory women, and to stimulate oocyte development and maturation in patients using assisted reproductive technologies.

men·ses (men′sēz) the monthly flow of blood from the female genital tract.

men·stru·al (men′stroo-al) pertaining to the menses or to menstruation.

men·stru·a·tion (men″stroo-a′shun) the cyclic, physiologic discharge through the vagina of blood and muscosal tissues from the nonpregnant uterus; it is under hormonal control and normally recurs usually at approximately four-week intervals, except during pregnancy and lactation, throughout the reproductive period (puberty through menopause). **anovular m., anovulatory m.,** periodic uterine bleeding without preceding ovulation. **infrequent m.,** oligomenorrhea. **profuse m.,** hypermenorrhea. **retrograde m.,** backflow of menstrual fluid, epithelial cells ,and debris through the uterine tubes and into the peritoneal cavity. **scanty m.,** hypomenorrhea. **vicarious m.,** discharge of blood from an extragenital source at the time menstruation is normally expected.

men·su·ra·tion (men″ser-a′shun) the act or process of measuring.

men·tal (ment′l) 1. pertaining to the mind. 2. pertaining to the chin.

men·thol (men′thol) an alcohol from various mint oils or produced synthetically; used topically to relieve itching and as an inhalation to treat upper respiratory tract disorders.

men·to·la·bi·al (men″to-la′be-al) pertaining to the chin and lip.

men·to·plas·ty (men′to-plas″te) plastic surgery of the chin; surgical correction of deformities and defects of the chin.

men·tum (men′tum) [L.] chin.

MEP maximum expiratory pressure.

me·pen·zo·late (mĕ-pen′zo-lāt) a quaternary ammonium compound with anticholinergic and antimuscarinic effects, used in the form of the bromide salt in the treatment of peptic ulcers and disorders characterized by colon hypermotility.

meperidine (mĕ-per′ĭ-dēn) an opioid analgesic, used as the hydrochloride salt as an analgesic and an anesthesia adjunct.

me·phen·ter·mine (mĕ-fen′ter-mēn) an adrenergic used as the sulfate salt for its vasopressor effects in the treatment of certain hypotensive states.

me·phen·y·to·in (mĕ-fen′ĭ-to″in) an anticonvulsant used for the control of a variety of epileptic seizures.

me·phit·ic (mĕ-fit′ik) emitting a foul odor.

meph·o·bar·bi·tal (mef″o-bahr′bĭ-tal) a long-acting barbiturate used as an anticonvulsant.

me·pi·va·caine (mĕ-pi′vah-kān) a lidocaine analogue used in the form of the hydrochloride salt as a local anesthetic.

me·pro·ba·mate (mĕ-pro′bah-māt, mep″ro-bam′āt) a carbamate derivative with tranquilizing and muscle relaxant actions.

mEq milliequivalent.

mer·ad·i·mate (mer-ad′ĭ-māt) an absorber of ultraviolet A radiation, used topically as a sunscreen.

me·ral·gia (mĕ-ral′jah) pain in the thigh. **m. paresthe′tica,** paresthesia, pain, and numbness in the outer surface of the thigh due to entrapment of the lateral femoral cutaneous nerve at the inguinal ligament.

mer·cap·tan (mer-kap′tan) thiol (2).

mer·cap·to·pur·ine (6-MP) (mer-kap″to-pūr′ēn) a sulfur-containing purine analogue, used as an antineoplastic and as an immunosuppressant.

mer·cu·ri·al (mer-kūr′e-il) 1. pertaining to mercury. 2. a preparation containing mercury.

mer·cur·ic (mer-kūr′ik) pertaining to mercury as a bivalent element.

mer·cu·rous (mer′kūr-us) pertaining to mercury as a monovalent element.

mer·cu·ry (Hg) (mer′kūr-e) chemical element (see *Table of Elements*), at. no. 80. Acute mercury poisoning, due to ingestion, is marked by severe abdominal pain, vomiting, bloody diarrhea with watery stools, oliguria or anuria, and corrosion and ulceration of the digestive tract; in the chronic form, due to absorption through skin and mucous membranes, inhalation, or ingestion, there is stomatitis, blue line along the gum border, sore hypertrophied gums that bleed easily, loosening of teeth, erethism, ptyalism, tremors, and incoordination.

me·rid·i·an (mĕ-rid′e-an) 1. an imaginary line on the surface of a spherical body, marking the intersection with the surface of a plane passing through its axis. 2. in acupuncture, a system of 20 lines connecting acupoints and regarded as channels through which qi flows.

me·rid·i·a·nus (mĕ-rid″e-a′nus) pl. *meridia′ni.* [L.] meridian.

mer(o)- word element [Gr.], 1. *part.* 2. *thigh.*

mero·blas·tic (mer″o-blas′tik) partially dividing; undergoing cleavage in which only part of the zygote participates.

mero·crine (mer′o-krin) discharging only the secretory product and maintaining the secretory cell intact (e.g., salivary glands, pancreas).

mero·gen·e·sis (mer″o-jen′ĕ-sis) cleavage of a zygote. **merogenet′ic,** adj.

mero·me·lia (-me′le-ah) congenital absence of any part of a limb; cf. *amelia.*

mero·myo·sin (-mi′o-sin) a fragment of the myosin molecule isolated by treatment with proteolytic enzyme; there are two types, heavy (H-meromyosin) and light (L-meromyosin).

mer·o·pen·em (-pen′em) a broad-spectrum antibacterial effective against a wide variety of gram-positive and gram-negative organisms; used in the treatment of intra-abdominal infections and bacterial meningitis.

me·ro·pia (mĕ-ro′pe-ah) partial blindness.

mero·ra·chis·chi·sis (mer″o-rah-kis′kĭ-sis) fissure of a part of the vertebral column.

me·rot·o·my (mĕ-rot′ah-me) dissection into segments, especially dissection of a cell.

mero·zo·ite (mer″o-zo′īt) one of the organisms formed by multiple fission (schizogony) of a sporozoite within the body of the host.

MESA microsurgical epididymal sperm aspiration.

me·sal·amine (mĕ-sal′ah-mēn) 5-aminosalicylic acid, an active metabolite of sulfasalazine, used in the prophylaxis and treatment of inflammatory bowel disease.

me·sal·a·zine (mĕ-sal′ah-zēn) mesalamine.

mes·an·gio·cap·il·lary (mes-an″je-o-kap′ĭ-lar″e) pertaining to or affecting the mesangium and the associated capillaries.

mes·an·gi·um (mes-an′je-um) the thin membrane supporting the capillary loops in renal glomeruli. **mesan′gial,** adj.

mes·ax·on (mes-ak′son) a pair of parallel membranes marking the line of edge-to-edge contact of Schwann cells encircling an axon.

mes·ca·line (mes′kah-lēn) a poisonous alkaloid from the flowering heads (mescal buttons) of a Mexican cactus, *Lophophora williamsii;* it produces an intoxication with delusions of color and sound.

mes·ec·to·derm (mez-ek′tah-derm) embryonic migratory cells derived from the neural crest of the head that contribute to the formation of the meninges and become pigment cells.

mes·en·ceph·a·lon (mez″-en-sef′ah-lon) midbrain. 1. the part of the brain developed from the middle of the three primary vesicles of the embryonic neural tube, comprising the tectum and the cerebral peduncles. 2. the middle of the three primary brain vesicles in the embryo, lying between the prosencephalon and the rhombencephalon. **mesencephal′ic,** adj.

mes·en·ceph·a·lot·o·my (-sef″ah-lot′ah-me) surgical production of lesions in the midbrain, especially for relief of intractable pain.

mes·en·chy·ma (mez-eng′kĭ-mah) mesenchyme.

mes·en·chyme (mez′eng-kīm) the meshwork of embryonic connective tissue in the mesoderm from which are formed the connective tissues of the body and the blood and lymphatic vessels. **mesen′chymal,** adj.

mes·en·chy·mo·ma (mez″en-ki-mo′mah) a mixed mesenchymal tumor composed of two or more cellular elements not commonly associated, exclusive of fibrous tissue.

mes·en·ter·ic (-ter′ik) pertaining to the mesentery.

mes·en·ter·io·pexy (-ter′e-o-pek″se) fixation or suspension of a torn mesentery.

mes·en·ter·i·pli·ca·tion (-ter″ĭ-plĭ-ka′shun) shortening of the mesentery by plication.

mes·en·ter·i·um (-ter′e-um) [L.] mesentery (1).

mes·en·ter·on (mez-en′ter-on) the midgut.

mes·en·tery (mez′en-ter″e) 1. the peritoneal fold attaching the small intestine to the posterior body wall. 2. a membranous fold attaching an organ to the body wall.

me·si·ad (me′ze-ad) toward the middle or center.

me·si·al (me′ze-al) nearer the center of the dental arch.

me·si·al·ly (me′ze-al″-e) toward the median line.

me·sio·clu·sion (me″ze-o-kloo′zhun) anteroclusion; malrelation of the dental arches with the mandibular arch anterior to the maxillary arch (prognathism).

me·sio·dens (me′ze-o-dens) pl. *mesioden′tes.* A small supernumerary tooth, occurring singly or paired, generally palatally between the maxillary central incisors.

me·si·on (me′ze-on) the plane dividing the body into right and left symmetrical halves.

me·sio·ver·sion (me″ze-o-ver′zhun) displacement of a tooth along the dental arch toward the midline of the face.

mes·mer·ism (mez′mer-izm) hypnotism.

mes·na (mez′nah) a sulfhydryl compound given with urotoxic antineoplastic agents because it inactivates some of their urotoxic metabolites.

mes(o)- word element [Gr.], *middle*.

meso·ap·pen·dix (mez″o-ah-pen′diks) the peritoneal fold connecting the appendix to the ileum.

meso·bil·i·ru·bin·o·gen (-bil″ĭ-roo-bin′ah-jen) a reduced form of bilirubin, formed in the intestine, which on oxidation forms stercobilin.

meso·blast (mez′o-blast) mesoderm, especially in the early, undifferentiated stages.

meso·blas·te·ma (mez″o-blas-te′mah) the cells composing the mesoblast.

meso·blas·tic (-blas′tik) pertaining to or derived from the mesoblast.

meso·car·dia (-kahr′de-ah) atypical location of the heart, with the apex in the midline of the thorax.

meso·car·di·um (-kahr′de-um) that part of the embryonic mesentery connecting the heart with the body wall in front and the foregut behind.

meso·ce·cum (-se′kum) the occasionally occurring mesentery of the cecum.

meso·co·lon (-ko′lon) the peritoneal process attaching the colon to the posterior abdominal wall, and called ascending, descending, etc., according to the portion of colon to which it attaches. **mesocol′ic,** adj.

meso·co·lo·pexy (-ko′lo-pek″se) suspension or fixation of the mesocolon.

meso·co·lo·pli·ca·tion (-ko″lo-pli-ka′shun) plication of the mesocolon to limit its mobility.

meso·cor·tex (-kor′teks) the cortex of the cingulate gyrus, intermediate in form between the allocortex and the isocortex and having five or six layers.

meso·derm (mez′o-derm) the middle of the three primary germ layers of the embryo, lying between the ectoderm and endoderm; from it are derived the connective tissue, bone, cartilage, muscle, blood and blood vessels, lymphatics, lymphoid organs, notochord, pleura, pericardium, peritoneum, kidneys, and gonads. **mesoder′mal, mesoder′mic,** adj.

meso·du·o·de·num (mez″o-doo″o-de′num) the mesenteric fold enclosing the duodenum of the early fetus. **mesoduode′nal,** adj.

meso·epi·did·y·mis (-ep″ĭ-did′ĭ-mis) a fold of tunica vaginalis testis sometimes connecting the epididymis and testis.

meso·gas·tri·um (-gas′tre-um) the portion of the primitive mesentery which encloses the stomach and from which the greater omentum develops. **mesogas′tric,** adj.

meso·glu·te·us (-gloo′te-us) gluteus medius muscle; see *Table of Muscles*. **mesoglu′teal,** adj.

meso·ile·um (-il′e-um) the mesentery of the ileum.

meso·je·ju·num (-jĕ-joo′num) the mesentery of the jejunum.

meso·mere (mez′o-mēr) 1. a blastomere of size intermediate between a macromere and a micromere. 2. a midzone of the mesoderm between the epimere and hypomere.

meso·me·tri·um (mez″o-me′tre-um) the portion of the broad ligament below the mesovarium.

meso·morph (mez′o-morf) an individual having the type of body build in which mesodermal tissues predominate: relative preponderance of muscle, bone, and connective tissue, usually with heavy, hard physique of rectangular outline.

mes·on (me′zon, mes′on) 1. mesion. 2. a subatomic particle having a rest mass intermediate between the mass of the electron and that of the proton, carrying either a positive, negative, or neutral electric charge.

meso·neph·ric (mez″o-nef′rik) pertaining to the mesonephros.

mes·o·ne·phro·ma (-nĕ-fro′mah) clear cell adenocarcinoma.

meso·neph·ros (-nef′ros) pl. *mesoneph′roi.* [Gr.] the excretory organ of the embryo, arising caudad to the pronephric rudiments or the pronephros and using its ducts.

meso·phile (mez′o-fil) an organism which grows best at 20°–55° C. **mesophil′ic,** adj.

meso·phle·bi·tis (mez″o-flĕ-bi′tis) inflammation of the middle coat of a vein.

me·soph·ry·on (mĕ-sof′re-on) the glabella, or its central point.

meso·pul·mo·num (mez″o-pul-mo′num) the embryonic mesentery enclosing the laterally expanding lung.

me·sor·chi·um (mĕ-sor′ke-um) the portion of the primordial mesentery enclosing the fetal testis, represented in the adult by a fold between the testis and epididymis. **mesor′chial,** adj.

meso·rec·tum (mez″o-rek′tum) the fold of peritoneum connecting the upper portion of the rectum with the sacrum.

meso·rid·a·zine (mes″o-rid′ah-zēn) a phenothiazine antipsychotic, used as the besylate salt.

meso·sal·pinx (mez″o-sal′pinks) the portion of the broad ligament above the mesovarium.

meso·sig·moid (-sig'moid) the peritoneal fold attaching the sigmoid flexure to the posterior abdominal wall.

meso·sig·moido·pexy (-sig-moi'do-pek"se) fixation of the mesosigmoid for prolapse of the rectum.

meso·some (mez'o-sōm) an invagination of the bacterial cell membrane, forming organelles thought to be the site of cytochrome enzymes and the enzymes of oxidative phosphorylation and the citric acid cycle.

meso·ster·num (mez"o-ster'num) body of sternum.

meso·ten·din·e·um (-ten-din'e-um) the connective tissue sheath attaching a tendon to its fibrous sheath.

meso·the·li·o·ma (-the"le-o'mah) a tumor derived from mesothelial tissue (peritoneum, pleura, pericardium), occurring in both benign and malignant forms.

meso·the·li·um (-the'le-um) the layer of cells, derived from mesoderm, lining the body cavity of the embryo; in the adult, it forms the simple squamous epithelium that covers all true serous membranes (peritoneum, pericardium, pleura). **mesothe'lial**, adj.

meso·tym·pa·num (-tim'pah-num) the portion of the middle ear medial to the tympanic membrane.

meso·va·ri·um (-var'e-um) the portion of the broad ligament between the mesometrium and mesosalpinx, which encloses and holds the ovary in place.

mes·sen·ger (mes'en-jer) an information carrier. **second m.**, any of several classes of intracellular signals acting at or situated within the plasma membrane and translating electrical or chemical messages from the environment into cellular responses.

mes·tra·nol (mes'trah-nol) an estrogen related to ethinyl estradiol; used in combination with a progestational agent as an oral contraceptive.

mes·y·late (mes'ĭ-lāt) USAN contraction for methanesulfonate.

Met methionine.

met(a)- word element [Gr.], (1) a prefix indicating (*a*) change; transformation; exchange; (*b*) after; next; (2) symbol *m*-, a prefix indicating a 1,3-substituted position in derivatives of benzene; (3) a prefix indicating a polymeric acid anhydride.

meta-anal·y·sis (met"ah-ah-nal'ĭ-sis) a systematic method that takes data from a number of independent studies and integrates them using statistical analysis.

me·tab·a·sis (mĕ-tab'ah-sis) a change in the manifestations or course of a disease.

meta·bi·o·sis (met"ah-bi-o'sis) dependence of one organism upon another for its existence; commensalism.

me·tab·o·lism (mĕ-tab'ŏ-lizm) 1. the sum of all the physical and chemical processes by which living organized substance is produced and maintained (anabolism), and also the transformation by which energy is made available for the uses of the organism (catabolism). 2. biotransformation. **metabol'ic**, adj. **basal m.**, the minimal energy expended to maintain respiration, circulation, peristalsis, muscle tonus, body temperature, glandular activity, and the other vegetative functions of the body.

meta·bo·lite (-līt) any substance produced by metabolism or by a metabolic process.

meta·car·pal (met"ah-kahr'pal) 1. pertaining to the metacarpus. 2. a bone of the metacarpus.

meta·car·pus (-kahr'pus) the part of the hand between the wrist and fingers, its skeleton being five bones (metacarpals) extending from the carpus to the phalanges.

meta·cen·tric (-sen'trik) having the centromere near the middle, so that the arms of the replicating chromosome are approximately equal in length.

meta·cer·ca·ria (-ser-kar'e-ah) pl. *metacercar'iae*. The encysted resting or maturing stage of a trematode parasite in the tissues of an intermediate host or on vegetation.

meta·chro·ma·sia (-kro-ma'zhah) 1. failure to stain true with a given stain. 2. the different coloration of different tissues produced by the same stain. 3. change of color produced by staining.

meta·chro·mat·ic (-kro-mat'ik) staining differently with the same dye; said of tissues in which a dye gives different colors to different elements.

meta·chro·mo·phil (-kro'mo-fil) not staining in the usual manner with a given stain.

meta·cone (met'ah-kōn) the distobuccal cusp of an upper molar tooth.

meta·con·id (met"ah-kōn'id) the mesiolingual cusp of a lower molar tooth.

meta·gas·ter (-gas'ter) the permanent intestinal canal of the embryo.

meta·gen·e·sis (-jen'ĕ-sis) alternation of generations; alternation in regular sequence of asexual and sexual reproductive methods, as in certain fungi.

Meta·gon·i·mus (met"ah-gon'ĭ-mus) a genus of flukes, including *M. yokoga'wai*, parasitic in the small intestine of humans and other mammals in Japan, China, Indonesia, the Balkans, and Israel.

met·al (met′′l) any element marked by luster, malleability, ductility, and conductivity of electricity and heat and which will ionize positively in solution. **metal′lic**, adj. **alkali m.**, any of a group of monovalent metals, including lithium, sodium, potassium, rubidium, and cesium. **heavy m.**, one with a high specific gravity, usually defined as over 5.0; some cause heavy metal poisoning.

me·tal·lo·en·zyme (mě-tal′′o-en′zīm) any enzyme containing tightly bound metal atoms, e.g., the cytochromes.

me·tal·lo·por·phy·rin (mě-tal′′o-por′fĭ-rin) a combination of a metal with porphyrin, as in heme.

me·tal·lo·pro·tein (-pro′tēn) a protein molecule with a bound metal ion, e.g., hemoglobin.

met·al·lur·gy (met′al-urj-e) the science and art of using metals.

meta·mere (met′ah-mēr) 1. one of a series of homologous segments of the body of an animal. 2. in genetic theory, one of a varying number of common repeating units that make up the repressor segment of a chromosome segment.

meta·mor·pho·sis (met′′ah-mor′fah-sis) change of structure or shape, particularly, transition from one developmental stage to another, as from larva to adult form. **metamor′phic**, adj. **fatty m.**, fatty change.

meta·my·elo·cyte (-mi′il-o-sīt′′) a precursor in the granulocytic series, being a cell intermediate in development between a promyelocyte and the mature, segmented (polymorphonuclear) granular leukocyte, and having a U-shaped nucleus.

meta·neph·ric (-nef′rik) of or pertaining to the metanephros.

meta·neph·rine (-nef′rin) a metabolite of epinephrine excreted in urine and found in certain tissues.

meta·neph·ros (-nef′ros) pl. *metaneph′roi.* [Gr.] the primordium of the permanent kidney, developing later than and caudad to the mesonephros.

meta·phase (met′ah-fāz) the second stage of cell division (mitosis or meiosis), in which the chromosomes, each consisting of two chromatids, are arranged in the equatorial plane of the spindle prior to separation.

meta·phos·phor·ic ac·id (met′′ah-fos-for′ik) a polymer of phosphoric acid, used as a reagent for chemical analysis and as a test for albumin in the urine.

meta·phys·e·al (met′′ah-fiz′e-al) pertaining to or of the nature of a metaphysis.

meta·phys·i·al metaphyseal.

me·taph·y·sis (mě-taf′ĭ-sis) pl. *metaph′yses.* [Gr.] the wider part at the end of a long bone, adjacent to the epiphyseal disk.

meta·pla·sia (met′′ah-pla′zhah) the change in the type of adult cells in a tissue to a form abnormal for that tissue. **metaplas′tic**, adj. **myeloid m.**, a syndrome characterized by myeloid tissue in extramedullary sites with nucleated erythrocytes and immature granulocytes in the circulating blood and extramedullary hematopoiesis in the liver and spleen, as well as anemia and splenomegaly. Both a primary form (*agnogenic myeloid m.*) and forms secondary to carcinoma, leukemia, leukoerythroblastosis, and tuberculosis are known.

meta·pneu·mon·ic (-noo-mon′ik) succeeding or following pneumonia.

meta·pro·ter·e·nol (met′′ah-pro-ter′ě-nol) a β_2-adrenergic receptor agonist with significant β_1-adrenergic activity, used in the form of the sulfate salt as a bronchodilator.

meta·psy·chol·o·gy (-si-kol′ah-je) the branch of speculative psychology that deals with the significance of mental processes that are beyond empirical verification.

meta·ram·i·nol (-ram′ĭ-nol) a sympathomimetic agent acting mainly as an α-adrenergic agonist but also stimulating the β_1-adrenergic receptors of the heart and having potent vasopressor activity; used as the bitartrate salt in the treatment of certain hypotensive states.

meta·ru·bri·cyte (-roo′′bri-sīt) orthochromatic erythroblast.

me·tas·ta·sec·to·my (mě-tas′′tah-sek′tah-me) excision of one or more metastases.

me·tas·ta·sis (mě-tas′tah-sis) pl. *metas′tases.* 1. Transfer of disease from one organ or part of the body to another not directly connected with it, due either to transfer of pathogenic microorganisms or to transfer of cells; all malignant tumors are capable of metastasizing. 2. a growth of pathogenic microorganisms or of abnormal cells distant from the site primarily involved by the morbid process. **metastat′ic**, adj.

meta·tar·sal (met′′ah-tahr′sal) 1. pertaining to the metatarsus. 2. a bone of the metatarsus.

meta·tar·sal·gia (-tahr-sal′jah) pain and tenderness in the metatarsal region.

meta·tar·sus (-tahr′sus) the part of the foot between the ankle and the toes, its skeleton being the five bones (metatarsals) extending from the tarsus to the phalanges.

meta·thal·a·mus (-thal′ah-mus) the part of the diencephalon composed of the medial and lateral geniculate bodies; often considered to be part of the thalamus.

me·tath·e·sis (mĕ-tath′ĕ-sis) 1. artificial transfer of a morbid process. 2. a chemical reaction in which an element or radical in one compound exchanges places with another element or radical in another compound.

meta·tro·phic (met″ah-tro′fik) utilizing organic matter for food.

me·tax·a·lone (mĕ-taks′ah-lōn) a skeletal muscle relaxant used in the treatment of painful musculoskeletal conditions.

Meta·zoa (met″ah-zo′ah) that division of the animal kingdom embracing the multicellular animals whose cells differentiate to form tissues, i.e., all animals except the Protozoa. **metazo′al, metazo′an,** adj.

meta·zo·on (-zo′on) pl. *metazo′a.* An individual organism of the Metazoa.

met·en·ceph·a·lon (met″en-sef′ah-lon) [Gr.] 1. the anterior part of the rhombencephalon, comprising the cerebellum and pons. 2. the anterior of two brain vesicles formed by specialization of the rhombencephalon in the developing embryo.

me·te·or·ism (mĕt′e-ah-rizm″) tympanites.

me·te·orot·ro·pism (me″te-o-rot′rah-pizm) response to influence by meteorologic factors noted in certain biological events. **meteorotrop′ic,** adj.

me·ter (me′ter) 1. the base SI unit of linear measure, approximately equivalent to 39.37 inches. Symbol m. 2. an apparatus to measure the quantity of anything passing through it.

-meter word element [Gr.], *relationship to measurement; instrument for measuring.*

met·for·min (met-for′min) an antihyperglycemic agent that potentiates the action of insulin, used in the treatment of type 2 diabetes mellitus.

meth·ac·ry·late (meth-ak′rĭ-lāt) an ester of methacrylic acid, or the resin derived from polymerization of the ester. See also *acrylic resins,* under *resin.*

meth·a·cryl·ic ac·id (meth″ah-kril′ik) an organic acid that polymerizes easily to form a ceramic-like mass. Its esters, methyl and polymethyl methacrylate, are used in the manufacture of acrylic resins and plastics.

meth·a·done (meth′ah-dōn) a synthetic opioid analgesic with actions similar to those of morphine and heroin, and almost equal in potential for addiction; the hydrochloride salt is used as an analgesic and in the management of heroin addiction.

meth·am·phet·amine (meth″am-fet′ah-mēn) a central nervous system stimulant and pressor substance with actions similar to amphetamine; used as the hydrochloride salt in

the treatment of attention-deficit/hyperactivity disorder. Abuse may lead to dependence.

meth·a·nal (meth′ah-nal) formaldehyde.

meth·ane (meth′ān) an inflammable, explosive gas, CH_4, from decomposition of organic matter.

meth·a·no·gen (meth′ah-nah-jen″) an anaerobic microorganism that grows in the presence of carbon dioxide and produces methane gas. Methanogens are found in the stomach of cows, in swamp mud, and in other environments in which oxygen is not present.

meth·a·nol (meth′ah-nol) methyl alcohol.

meth·a·zo·la·mide (meth″ah-zo′lah-mīd) a carbonic anhydrase inhibitor used as an adjunct to reduce intraocular pressure in the treatment of glaucoma.

meth·di·la·zine (meth-di′lah-zēn) an antihistamine with anticholinergic and sedative effects, used as the base or the hydrochloride salt as an antipruritic.

met·hem·al·bu·min (met″hēm-al-bu′min) a brownish pigment formed in the blood by the binding of albumin with heme; indicative of intravascular hemolysis.

met·he·mo·glo·bin (met-he′mo-glo″bin) a hematogenous pigment formed from hemoglobin by oxidation of the iron atom from the ferrous to the ferric state. A small amount is found in the blood normally, but injury or toxic agents convert a larger proportion of hemoglobin into methemoglobin, which does not function as an oxygen carrier.

meth·en·amine (meth″en-am′in) an antibacterial used in urinary tract infections; administered as the hippurate and mandelate salts.

meth·i·cil·lin (meth″ĭ-sil′in) a semisynthetic penicillin highly resistant to inactivation by penicillinase; used as the sodium salt.

meth·im·a·zole (meth-im′ah-zōl) a thyroid inhibitor used in the treatment of hyperthyroidism.

me·thi·o·nine (Met, M) (mĕ-thi′ŏ-nēn) a naturally occurring, essential amino acid that furnishes both methyl groups and sulfur necessary for normal metabolism. Labeled with carbon 11, it is used in positron emission tomography for detection of neoplasms.

meth·o·car·ba·mol (meth″o-kahr′bah-mol) a skeletal muscle relaxant used in the treatment of painful musculoskeletal conditions.

meth·od (meth′od) the manner of performing any act or operation; a procedure or technique. **dye dilution m.,** a type of indicator dilution method for assessing flow through the circulatory system, using a dye as an indicator. **indicator dilution m.,** any of several methods for assessing flow through the circulatory system by injecting a known quantity of an indicator and monitoring its concentration over time at a specific point in the system. **Lamaze m.,** a method of preparing for delivery, involving education of the prospective mother in the physiology of pregnancy and parturition as well as in techniques such as breathing exercises and bearing down for the easing of delivery. **rhythm m.,** a method of preventing conception by restricting coitus to the so-called safe period, avoiding the days just before and after the expected time of ovulation. **Westergren m.,** the most common method for testing the erythrocyte sedimentation rate, measuring the timed fall of the level of red cells after mixing whole blood and sodium citrate anticoagulant-diluent solution. **Yuzpe m.,** a regimen for postcoital contraception, consisting of a combination of ethinyl estradiol and norgestrel taken twice, 12 hours apart.

meth·od·ol·o·gy (meth″id-ol′ah-je) the science of method; the science dealing with principles of procedure in research and study.

meth·o·hex·i·tal (meth″o-hek′sit-al) an ultrashort-acting barbiturate; its sodium salt is used as a general anesthetic, a general and local anesthesia adjunct, and a sedative for certain diagnostic procedures in children.

meth·o·trex·ate (-trek′sāt) a folic acid antagonist used as the base or the sodium salt as an antineoplastic, antipsoriatic, and antiarthritic.

me·thox·amine (mĕ-thok′sah-mēn) an α_1-adrenergic agonist, used as the hydrochloride salt as a vasopressor.

me·thox·sa·len (mĕ-thok′sah-len) a psoralen that induces melanin production on exposure of the skin to ultraviolet light; used in the treatment of idiopathic vitiligo, mycosis fungoides, and psoriasis.

meth·oxy·flu·rane (mĕ-thok″se-floo′rān) a highly potent inhalational anesthetic agent.

meth·sux·i·mide (meth-suk′sĭ-mīd) an anticonvulsant used in the treatment of seizures in absence epilepsy.

meth·y·clo·thi·a·zide (meth″ĭ-klo-thi′ah-zīd) a thiazide diuretic used for treatment of hypertension and edema.

meth·yl (meth′il) the chemical group or radical CH_3—. **m. methacrylate,** a methyl ester of methacrylic acid, which polymerizes to form polymethyl methacrylate; used in the manufacture of acrylic resins and plastics. **m. salicylate,** a volatile oil with a characteristic wintergreen odor and taste; used as a flavoring agent and as a topical counterirritant for muscle pain.

meth·yl·amine (meth′il-ah-mēn″) a flammable, explosive gas used in tanning and organic synthesis and produced naturally in some decaying fish, certain plants, and crude methanol; it is irritating to the eyes.

meth·yl·ate (meth′ĭ-lāt) 1. a compound of methyl alcohol and a base. 2. to add a methyl group to a substance.

meth·yl·ben·ze·tho·ni·um (meth″il-ben″zĕ-tho′ne-um) a disinfectant quaternary compound; applied topically to skin coming in contact with urine, feces, or perspiration, and used in a rinse for diapers and linens of incontinent patients.

meth·yl·cel·lu·lose (-sel′ūl-ōs) a methyl ester of cellulose; used as a bulk laxative and as a suspending agent for drugs and applied topically to the conjunctiva to protect and lubricate the cornea during certain ophthalmic procedures.

meth·yl·co·bal·a·min (-ko-bal′ah-min) a metabolically active cobalamin derivative synthesized upon ingestion of vitamin B_{12}.

meth·yl·do·pa (-do′pah) a phenylalanine derivative used in the treatment of hypertension.

meth·yl·do·pate (-do′pāt) the ethyl ester of methyldopa; its hydrochloride salt is used as an antihypertensive.

meth·y·lene (meth′ĭ-lēn) the bivalent hydrocarbon radical —CH_2— or CH_2=.

meth·y·lene·di·oxy·am·phet·amine (MDA) (-di-ok″se-am-fet′ah-mēn) a hallucinogenic compound chemically related to amphetamine and mescaline; it is widely abused and causes dependence.

3,4-meth·y·lene·di·oxy·meth·am·phet·amine (-meth″am-fet′ah-mēn) MDMA; a compound chemically related to amphetamine and having hallucinogenic properties; it is widely abused. Popularly called *Ecstasy.*

meth·yl·er·go·no·vine (meth″il-er″go-no′vēn) an oxytocic, used as the maleate salt to prevent or combat postpartum or post-abortion hemorrhage and atony.

meth·yl·glu·ca·mine (-gloo′kah-mēn) meglumine.

meth·yl·ma·lon·ic ac·id (-mah-lon′ik) a carboxylic acid intermediate in fatty acid metabolism.

meth·yl·ma·lon·ic·ac·i·de·mia (-mah-lon″ik-as″ĭ-de′me-ah) 1. an aminoacidopathy characterized by an excess of methylmalonic acid in the blood and urine, with metabolic ketoacidosis, hyperglycinemia, hyperglycinuria, and hyperammonemia, resulting from any of several enzymatic defects. 2. excess of methylmalonic acid in the blood.

meth·yl·ma·lon·ic·ac·id·uria (-as″ĭ-du′re-ah) 1. excess of methylmalonic acid in the urine. 2. methylmalonicacidemia (1).

meth·yl·meth·ac·ry·late (meth″il-meth-ak′rĭ-lāt) see under *methyl.*

meth·yl·phen·i·date (meth″il-fen′ĭ-dāt) a central stimulant, used in the form of the hydrochloride salt in the treatment of attention-deficit/hyperactivity disorder in children and narcolepsy.

meth·yl·pred·nis·o·lone (-pred-nis′ah-lōn) a synthetic glucocorticoid derived from progesterone, used in replacement therapy for adrenocortical insufficiency and as an antiinflammatory and immunosuppressant; also used as *m. acetate* and *m. sodium succinate.*

meth·yl·tes·tos·ter·one (-tes-tos′ter-ōn) a synthetic androgenic hormone with actions and uses similar to those of testosterone.

5-meth·yl·tet·ra·hy·dro·fo·late (-tet″rah-hi″dro-fo′lāt) a derivative of folic acid that is the principal form of folic acid during transport and storage in the body and that also acts as a source of methyl groups for the regeneration of methionine.

meth·yl·trans·fer·ase (-trans′fer-ās) any of a group of enzymes that catalyze the transfer of a methyl group from one compound to another.

meth·y·ser·gide (-sur′jīd) a potent serotonin antagonist with direct vasoconstrictor effects, used as the maleate salt in prophylaxis of migraine and cluster headaches.

met·i·pran·o·lol (met″ĭ-pran′ah-lol) a beta-adrenergic blocking agent, used as the hydrochloride salt in the treatment of glaucoma and ocular hypertension.

met·myo·glo·bin (met-mi″ah-glo′bin) a compound formed from myoglobin by oxidation of the ferrous to the ferric state.

met·o·clo·pra·mide (met″o-klo′prah-mīd) a dopamine receptor antagonist and prokinetic that stimulates gastric motility, used as the hydrochloride salt as an antiemetic, an adjunct in gastrointestinal radiology and intestinal intubation, and in the treatment of gastroparesis and gastroesophageal reflux.

me·to·la·zone (mĕ-to′lah-zōn) a sulfonamide derivative with actions similar to the thiazide diuretics; used in the treatment of hypertension and edema.

me·top·ic (mĕ-top′ik) frontal (1).

me·to·pi·on (mĕ-to′pe-on) glabella.

met·o·pro·lol (met″ah-pro′lol) a cardioselective β_1-adrenergic blocking agent used in the form of the succinate and tartrate salts in the treatment of hypertension, chronic angina pectoris, and myocardial infarction.

me·tox·e·nous (mĕ-tok′sĕ-nus) requiring two hosts for the life cycle; said of parasites.

me·tra (me′trah) the uterus.

me·tra·tro·phia (-tro′fe-ah) atrophy of the uterus.

me·trec·to·pia (me″trek-to′pe-ah) uterine displacement.

me·treu·ryn·ter (me″troo-rin′ter) an inflatable bag for dilating the cervical canal.

met·ric (mĕ′trik) 1. pertaining to measures or measurement. 2. having the meter as a basis.

me·tri·tis (me-tri′tis) inflammation of the uterus.

me·triz·a·mide (mĕ-triz′ah-mīd) a nonionic, water-soluble, iodinated radiographic contrast medium used in myelography and cisternography.

metr(o)- word element [Gr.], *uterus.*

me·tro·col·po·cele (me″tro-kol′pah-sēl) hernia of uterus with prolapse into the vagina.

met·ro·ni·da·zole (-ni′dah-zōl) an antiprotozoal and antibacterial effective against obligate anaerobes; used as the base or the hydrochloride salt. It is also used as a topical treatment for rosacea.

me·trop·a·thy (me-trop′ah-the) hysteropathy.

me·tro·peri·to·ni·tis (me″tro-per″ĭ-to-ni′tis) inflammation of the peritoneum about the uterus.

me·tro·phle·bi·tis (-flĕ-bi′tis) inflammation of the uterine veins.

me·tro·plas·ty (-plas′te) plastic surgery on the uterus.

me·tror·rha·gia (-ra′jah) uterine bleeding occurring at irregular intervals, and sometimes of prolonged duration.

me·tror·rhea (-re′ah) a free or abnormal uterine discharge.

me·tror·rhex·is (-rek′sis) rupture of the uterus.

me·tro·stax·is (me″tro-stak′sis) slight but persistent uterine bleeding.

me·tro·ste·no·sis (-stĕ-no′sis) contraction or stenosis of the uterine cavity.

-metry word element [Gr.], *measurement.*

me·tyr·a·pone (mĕ-tēr′ah-pōn) a synthetic compound that selectively inhibits an enzyme responsible for the biosynthesis of corticosteroids; it is used as a diagnostic aid for determination of hypothalamicopituitary-adrenocortical reserve.

me·ty·ro·sine (mĕ-ti′ro-sēn) an inhibitor of the first step in catecholamine synthesis, used to control hypertensive attacks in pheochromocytoma.

MeV megaelectron volt; one million (10^6) electron volts.

mex·il·e·tine (mek′sĭ-lĕ-tēn) an antiarrhythmic agent used as the hydrochloride salt in the treatment of ventricular arrhythmias.

mez·lo·cil·lin (mez″lo-sil′in) a semisynthetic broad-spectrum penicillin used as the sodium salt, particularly in the treatment of mixed infections.

μF microfarad.

Mg magnesium.

mg milligram.

μg microgram.

MHC major histocompatibility complex.

MHz megahertz; one million (10^6) hertz.

MI myocardial infarction.

mi·ca·tion (mi-ka′shun) a quick motion, such as winking.

mi·con·a·zole (mi-kon′ah-zōl) an imidazole antifungal agent used as the base or the nitrate salt against tinea and cutaneous or vulvovaginal candidiasis.

mi·cren·ceph·a·ly (mi″kren-sef′ah-le) abnormal smallness of the brain. **micrenceph′alous**, adj.

micr(o)- word element [Gr.], *small;* also used in naming units of measurement (symbol μ) to designate an amount one millionth (10^{-6}) the size of the unit to which it is joined, e.g., microgram.

mi·cro·ab·scess (mi″kro-ab′ses) a very small, localized collection of pus. **Pautrier′s m.,** one of the well-defined collections of mycosis cells located within the epidermis in T-cell lymphoma and mycosis fungoides.

mi·cro·ad·e·no·ma (-ad″ĕ-no′mah) a pituitary adenoma less than 10 mm in diameter.

mi·cro·aero·phil·ic (-a″er-o-fil′ik) requiring oxygen for growth but at lower concentration than is present in the atmosphere; said of bacteria.

mi·cro·ag·gre·gate (-ag′rĕ-gat) a microscopic collection of particles, as of platelets, leukocytes, and fibrin, that occurs in stored blood.

mi·cro·al·bu·min·uria (-al-bu-min-u′re-ah) a very small increase in urinary albumin.

mi·cro·anal·y·sis (-ah-nal′ĭ-sis) the chemical analysis of minute quantities of material.

mi·cro·anat·o·my (-ah-nat′ah-me) histology.

mi·cro·an·eu·rysm (-an′ūr-izm) a microscopic aneurysm, a characteristic of thrombotic purpura.

mi·cro·an·gi·op·a·thy (-an″je-op′ah-the) angiopathy involving the small blood vessels. **microangiopath′ic**, adj. **thrombotic m.,** thrombi in arterioles and capillaries, as in thrombotic thrombocytopenic purpura and hemolytic uremic syndrome.

mi·crobe (mi′krōb) a microorganism, especially a pathogenic one such as a bacterium, protozoan, or fungus. **micro′bial, micro′bic**, adj.

mi·cro·bi·cide (mi-kro′bĭ-sīd) 1. a substance that destroys microbes. 2. a substance that destroys infectious agents, including also viruses; sometimes used specifically for that used to prevent transmission of sexually transmitted diseases. **microbici′dal**, adj.

mi·cro·bi·ol·o·gy (mi″kro-bi-ol′ah-je) the science dealing with the study of microorganisms. **microbiolog′ical**, adj.

mi·cro·bio·pho·tom·e·ter (-bi″o-fo-tom′it-er) an instrument for measuring the growth of bacterial cultures by the turbidity of the medium.

mi·cro·bi·o·ta (-bi-ot′ah) the microscopic living organisms of a region. **microbiot′ic**, adj.

mi·cro·blast (mi′kro-blast) an erythroblast of 5 microns or less in diameter.

mi·cro·ble·pha·ria (mi″kro-blĕ-far′e-ah) abnormal shortness of the vertical dimensions of the eyelids.

mi·cro·body (mi′kro-bod″e) 1. any of the membrane-bound, ovoid or spherical, granular cytoplasmic particles containing enzymes and other substances, which originate in the endoplasmic reticulum of vertebrate liver and kidney cells and other cells, and in protozoa, yeast, and many cell types of higher plants. 2. peroxisome (1).

mi·cro·bu·ret (mi″kro-būr-et′) a buret with a capacity of the order of 0.1 to 10 mL, with graduated intervals of 0.001 to 0.02 mL.

mi·cro·ca·lix (mi″kro-ka′liks) a very small renal calix arising by caliceal branching, usually at the side of a calix of normal size.

mi·cro·car·dia (-kahr′de-ah) abnormal smallness of the heart.

mi·cro·ceph·a·ly abnormal smallness of the head. **microcephal′ic**, adj.

mi·cro·chei·lia (-ki′le-ah) abnormal smallness of the lip.

mi·cro·chei·ria (-ki′re-ah) abnormal smallness of the hands.

mi·cro·chem·is·try (-kem′is-tre) chemistry concerned with exceedingly small quantities of chemical substances.

mi·cro·cin·e·ma·tog·ra·phy (-sin″ĭ-mah-tog′rah-fe) moving picture photography of microscopic objects.

mi·cro·cir·cu·la·tion (-sir″ku-la′shun) the flow of blood through the fine vessels (arterioles, capillaries, and venules). **microcirculato′ry**, adj.

Mi·cro·coc·ca·ceae (-kok-a′se-e) a family of gram-positive, aerobic or facultatively anaerobic bacteria of the order Eubacteriales, made up of spherical cells dividing primarily in two or three planes.

Mi·cro·coc·cus (-kok'us) a genus of gram-positive bacteria (family Micrococcaceae) found in soil, water, etc.

mi·cro·coc·cus (-kok'us) pl. *micrococ'ci*. 1. An organism of the genus *Micrococcus*. 2. a very small spherical microorganism.

mi·cro·co·lon (-ko'lon) an abnormally small colon.

mi·cro·co·ria (-kor'e-ah) smallness of the pupil.

mi·cro·crys·tal·line (-kris'tah-lin) made up of minute crystals.

mi·cro·cyte (-sit) 1. an abnormally small erythrocyte, 5 microns or less in diameter. **microcyt'ic**, adj. 2. microglial cell.

mi·cro·cy·to·tox·ic·i·ty (-si″to-tok-sis'it-e) the capability of lysing or damaging cells as detected in procedures (e.g., lymphocytotoxicity procedures) using extremely minute amounts of material.

mi·cro·de·ter·mi·na·tion (-de-ter″mĭ-na'shun) chemical examination of minute quantities of substance.

mi·cro·dis·kec·to·my (mi″kro-dis-kek'tah-me) debulking of a herniated nucleus pulposus using an operating microscope or loupe for magnification.

mi·cro·dis·sec·tion (-di-sek'shun) dissection of tissue or cells under the microscope.

mi·cro·drep·a·no·cyt·ic (-drep″ah-no-sit'ik) containing microcytic and drepanocytic elements.

mi·cro·en·vi·ron·ment (-en-vi'ron-ment) the environment at the microscopic or cellular level.

mi·cro·eryth·ro·cyte (-ĕ-rith'rah-sit) microcryte.

mi·cro·far·ad (μF) (-far'ad) one millionth (10^{-6}) of a farad.

mi·cro·fau·na (-faw'nah) the microscopic animal organisms of a special region.

mi·cro·fil·a·ment (-fil'ah-ment) any of the submicroscopic filaments composed chiefly of actin, found in the cytoplasmic matrix of almost all cells, often with the microtubules.

mi·cro·fi·la·ria (-fĭ-lar'e-ah) [L.] the prelarval stage of Filarioidea in the blood of humans and in the tissues of the vector; sometimes incorrectly used as a genus name.

mi·cro·flo·ra (-flor'ah) the microscopic vegetable organisms of a special region.

mi·cro·fol·lic·u·lar (-fah-lik'u-lar) pertaining to or characterized by small follicles.

mi·cro·frac·ture (-frak'cher) a minute, incomplete break or small area of discontinuity in a bone.

mi·cro·gam·ete (-gam'ēt) 1. the smaller, often flagellated, actively motile male anisogamete. 2. the smaller of two types of malarial parasites; see *gamete* (2).

mi·cro·ga·me·to·cyte (-gah-mēt'ah-sit) 1. a cell that produces microgametes. 2. the male gametocyte of certain Sporozoa, such as malarial plasmodia.

mi·crog·lia (mi-krog'le-ah) small nonneural cells forming part of the supporting structure of the central nervous system. They are migratory and act as phagocytes to waste products of nerve tissue. **microg'lial**, adj.

mi·crog·lio·cyte (mi-krog'le-o-sit) microglial cell.

mi·cro·glob·u·lin (mi″kro-glob'ūl-in) any globulin, or any fragment of a globulin, of low molecular weight.

mi·crog·na·thia (-nath'e-ah) unusual smallness of the jaws, especially the lower jaw. **micrognath'ic**, adj.

mi·cro·go·nio·scope (-go'ne-o-skōp) a gonioscope with a magnifying lens.

mi·cro·gram (μg) (mi'kro-gram) one millionth (10^{-6}) of a gram.

mi·cro·graph (-graf) 1. an instrument used to record very minute movements by making a greatly magnified photograph of the minute motions of a diaphragm. 2. a photograph of a minute object or specimen as seen through a microscope.

mi·cro·graph·ia (mi″kro-graf'e-ah) tiny handwriting, or handwriting that decreases in size from normal to minute, seen in parkinsonism.

mi·cro·gyr·ia (-ji're-ah) polymicrogyria.

mi·cro·gy·rus (-ji'rus) pl. *microgy'ri*. An abnormally small, malformed convolution of the brain.

mi·cro·in·farct (-in'fahrkt) a very small infarct due to obstruction of circulation in capillaries, arterioles, or small arteries.

mi·cro·in·jec·tor (-in-jek'ter) an instrument for infusion of very small amounts of fluids or drugs.

mi·cro·in·va·sion (-in-va'zhun) microscopic extension of malignant cells into adjacent tissue in carcinoma in situ. **microinva'sive**, adj.

mi·cro·ker·a·tome (-ker'ah-tōm) an instrument for removing a thin slice, or creating a thin hinged flap, on the surface of the cornea.

mi·cro·lec·i·thal (-les'ĭ-thal) containing little yolk, as the eggs of mammals.

mi·cro·li·ter (μL) (mi′kro-le″ter) one millionth (10^{-6}) of a liter.

mi·cro·li·thi·a·sis (mi″kro-lǐ-thi′ah-sis) the formation of minute concretions in an organ. **m. alveola′ris pulmo′num, pulmonary alveolar m.,** deposition of minute, sand-like calculi in the pulmonary alveoli.

mi·cro·ma·nip·u·la·tion (mi″kro-mah-nip″u-la′shun) surgery, injection, or other procedures done with a micromanipulator.

mi·cro·ma·nip·u·la·tor (-mah-nip′u-la-ter) an instrument for the moving, dissecting, etc., of minute specimens under the microscope.

mi·cro·mere (mi′kro-mēr) one of the small blastomeres formed by unequal cleavage of a fertilized oocyte as the result of asymmetric positioning of the mitotic spindle.

mi·cro·me·tas·ta·sis (mi″kro-mě-tas′-tah-sis) the spread of cancer cells from the primary tumor to distant sites to form microscopic secondary tumors. **micrometa-stat′ic,** adj.

mi·crom·e·ter¹ (mi-krom′ě-ter) an instrument for measuring objects seen through the microscope.

mi·cro·me·ter² (μm) (mi′kro-me″ter) one millionth (10^{-6}) of a meter.

mi·cro·meth·od (-meth″id) any technique dealing with exceedingly small quantities of material.

mi·cro·my·elia (-mi-e′le-ah) abnormal smallness of the spinal cord.

mi·cro·my·elo·blast (-mi′ě-lo-blast) a small, immature myelocyte. **micromyeloblas′tic,** adj.

mi·cro·nee·dle (mi″kro-ne′d′l) a fine glass needle used in micromanipulation.

mi·cro·neu·ro·sur·gery (-nōōr″o-sur′jě-re) surgery conducted under high magnification with miniaturized instruments on microscopic vessels and structures of the nervous system.

mi·cro·nu·cle·us (-noo′kle-us) 1. in ciliate protozoa, the smaller of two types of nucleus in each cell, which functions in sexual reproduction; cf. *macronucleus.* 2. a small nucleus. 3. nucleolus.

mi·cro·or·gan·ism (-or′gah-nizm) a microscopic organism; those of medical interest include bacteria, fungi, and protozoa. Viruses are often included, but are sometimes excluded because they are not cellular and are unable to replicate without a host cell.

mi·cro·pa·thol·o·gy (-pah-thol′ah-je) 1. the sum of what is known about minute pathologic change. 2. pathology of diseases caused by microorganisms.

mi·cro·pe·nis (-pe′nis) abnormal smallness of the penis.

mi·cro·per·fu·sion (-per-fu′zhun) perfusion of a minute amount of a substance.

mi·cro·phage (mi′kro-fāj) a small phagocyte; an actively motile neutrophil capable of phagocytosis.

mi·cro·pha·kia (mi″kro-fa′ke-ah) abnormal smallness of the crystalline lens.

mi·cro·phone (mi′krah-fōn) a device to pick up sound for amplification or transmission.

mi·cro·phon·ic (mi″kro-fon′ik) 1. serving to amplify sound. 2. cochlear microphonic **cochlear m.,** the electrical potential generated in the hair cells of the organ of Corti in response to acoustic stimulation.

mi·cro·pho·to·graph (-fōt′ah-graf) a photograph of small size.

mi·croph·thal·mos (mi″krof-thal′mus) abnormal smallness in all dimensions of one or both eyes.

mi·cro·pi·no·cy·to·sis (mi″kro-pi″no-si-to′sis) the taking up into a cell of specific macromolecules by invagination of the plasma membrane which is then pinched off, resulting in small vesicles in the cytoplasm.

mi·cro·pi·pet (-pi-pet′) a pipet for handling small quantities of liquids (up to 1 mL).

mi·cro·pleth·ys·mog·ra·phy (-pleth″is-mog′rah-fe) the recording of minute changes in the size of a part as produced by circulation of blood.

mi·cro·probe (mi′kro-prōb″) a minute probe, as one used in microsurgery.

mi·crop·sia (mi-krop′se-ah) a visual disorder in which objects appear smaller than their actual size.

mi·cro·punc·ture (mi′kro-punk″cher) 1. the creation of minute openings by piercing. 2. in renal physiology, the process by which nephron segments are pierced.

mi·cro·ra·di·og·ra·phy (mi″kro-ra″de-og′rah-fe) radiography under conditions which permit subsequent microscopic examination or enlargement of the radiograph up to several hundred linear magnifications.

mi·cro·re·frac·tom·e·ter (-re″frak-tom′it-er) a refractometer for the discernment of variations in minute structures.

mi·cro·res·pi·rom·e·ter (-res″pǐ-rom′it-er) an apparatus to investigate oxygen usage in isolated tissues.

mi·cro·scope (mi′kro-skōp) an instrument used to obtain an enlarged image of small objects and reveal details of structure not otherwise distinguishable. **acoustic m.,** one using very high frequency ultrasound waves, which are focused on the object; the reflected beam is converted to an image by electronic processing. **binocular m.,** one with two eyepieces, permitting use of both eyes. **compound m.,** one consisting of two lens systems. **corneal m.,** one with a lens of high magnifying power, for observing minute changes in the cornea and iris. **dark-field m.,** one designed to permit diversion of light rays and illumination from the side, so that details appear light against a dark background. **electron m.,** one in which an electron beam, instead of light, forms an image for viewing on a fluorescent screen, or for photography. **fluorescence m.,** one used for the examination of specimens stained with fluorochromes or fluorochrome complexes, e.g., a fluorescein-labeled antibody, which fluoresces in ultraviolet light. **infrared m.,** one in which radiation of 800 nm or longer wavelength is used as the image-forming energy. **light m.,** one in which the specimen is viewed under visible light. **phase m., phase-contrast m.,** one altering the phase relationships of the light passing through and that passing around the object, the contrast permitting visualization without the necessity of staining or other special preparation. **scanning m., scanning electron m.,** an electron microscope in which a beam of electrons scans over a specimen point by point and builds up an image on the fluorescent screen of a cathode ray tube. **simple m.,** one consisting of a single lens. **slit lamp m.,** a corneal microscope with a special attachment that permits examination of the endothelium on the posterior surface of the cornea. **stereoscopic m.,** a binocular microscope modified to give a three-dimensional view of the specimen. **ultraviolet m.,** one that utilizes reflecting optics or quartz and other ultraviolet-transmitting lenses. **x-ray m.,** one in which x-rays are used instead of light, the image usually being reproduced on film.

mi·cro·scop·ic (mi″kro-skop′ik) 1. of extremely small size; visible only by the aid of the microscope. 2. pertaining or relating to a microscope or to microscopy.

mi·cros·co·py (mi-kros′kah-pe) examination under or observation by means of the microscope.

mi·cro·shock (-shok″) in cardiology, a low level of electric current applied directly to myocardial tissue; as little as 0.1 mA causes ventricular fibrillation.

mi·cros·mat·ic (mi″kros-mat′ik) having a feebly developed sense of smell, as in humans.

mi·cro·some (mi′krah-sōm) any of the vesicular fragments of endoplasmic reticulum formed after disruption and centrifugation of cells. **microso′mal,** adj.

mi·cro·spec·tro·scope (mi″kro-spek′trah-skōp) a spectroscope and microscope combined.

mi·cro·sphe·ro·cyte (-sfēr′ah-sīt) spherocyte.

mi·cro·sphero·cy·to·sis (-sfēr″o-si-to′sis) spherocytosis.

mi·cro·sphyg·mia (-sfig′me-ah) a pulse that is difficult to perceive by the finger.

mi·cro·sple·nia (-sple′ne-ah) smallness of the spleen.

Mi·cros·po·ron (mi″kro-spor′on) *Microsporum.*

Mi·cros·po·rum (-spor′um) a genus of fungi that cause diseases of skin and hair, including *M. audoui′ni, M. ca′nis, M. ful′vum,* and *M. gyp′seum.*

mi·cro·sto·mia (-sto′me-ah) unusually small size of the mouth.

mi·cro·sur·gery (-sur′jĕ-re) dissection of minute structures under the microscope by means of hand-held instruments. **microsur′gical,** adj.

mi·cro·syr·inge (-sĭ-rinj′) a syringe fitted with a screw-thread micrometer for accurate measurement of minute quantities.

mi·cro·tia (mi-kro′she-ah) gross hypoplasia or aplasia of the auricle of the ear, with a blind or absent external acoustic meatus.

mi·cro·tome (mi′krah-tōm) an instrument for cutting thin sections for microscopic study.

mi·cro·tu·bule (mi″kro-too′būl) any of the slender, tubular structures composed chiefly of tubulin, found in the cytoplasmic ground substance of nearly all cells; they are involved in maintenance of cell shape and in the movements of organelles and inclusions, and form the spindle fibers of mitosis.

mi·cro·vas·cu·la·ture (-vas′kūl-ah-cher) the finer vessels of the body, as the arterioles, capillaries, and venules. **microvas′cular,** adj.

mi·cro·ves·sel (mi′kro-ves″el) any of the finer vessels of the body.

mi·cro·vil·lus (-vil′us) a minute process from the free surface of a cell, especially cells of the proximal convolution in renal tubules and of the intestinal epithelium.

mi·cro·wave (-wāv) a wave of electromagnetic radiation between far infrared and radio waves, regarded as extending from 300,000 to 100 megahertz (wavelength of 1 mm to 30 cm).

mi·cro·zo·on (mi″kro-zo′on) pl. *microzo′a.* A microscopic animal organism.

mi·crur·gy (mi′krur-je) manipulative technique in the field of a microscope. **micrur′gic,** adj.

Mi·cru·roi·des (mi″kroo-roi′dēz) a genus of venomous snakes of the family Elapidae. *M. euryxan′thus* is the Arizona or Sonoran coral snake of Mexico and the southwestern United States.

Mi·cru·rus (mi-kroo′rus) a genus of venomous snakes of the family Elapidae. *M. ful′vius*, the Eastern or Texas coral snake, is found in the southern United States and tropical America; its body is marked with bright red, yellow, and black bands.

mic·tu·rate (mik′cher-āt) urinate.

mic·tu·ri·tion (mik″tu-ri′shun) urination.

mid·azo·lam (mid′a-zo-lam″) a benzodiazepine tranquilizer, used as the maleate ester for sedation and in the induction of anesthesia.

mid·brain (mid′brān) mesencephalon.

midg·et (mij′it) old term for *normal dwarf*.

mid·gut (mid′gut) the region of the embryonic digestive tube into which the yolk sac opens and which gives rise to most of the intestines; ahead of it is the foregut and caudal to it is the hindgut.

mi·do·drine (mi′do-drēn″) a vasopressor used as the hydrochloride salt in the treatment of orthostatic hypotension.

mid·riff (-rif) the diaphragm; the region between the breast and waistline.

mid·wife (-wīf) an individual who practices midwifery; see *nurse-midwife*.

mif·e·pris·tone (mif″ĕ-pris′tōn) RU-486; an antiprogestin used with misoprostol or other prostaglandin to terminate pregnancy in the first trimester.

mig·li·tol (mig′lĭ-tol) an enzyme inhibitor that slows the absorption of glucose into the bloodstream and reduces postprandial hyperglycemia; used in the treatment of type 2 diabetes.

mi·graine (mi′grān) a symptom complex of periodic headaches, usually temporal and unilateral, often with irritability, nausea, vomiting, constipation or diarrhea, and photophobia, preceded by constriction of the cranial arteries, often with resultant prodromal sensory, especially ocular, symptoms (aura), and commencing with the vasodilation that follows. **mi′grainous,** adj. **abdominal m.,** that in which abdominal symptoms are predominant. **basilar m., basilar artery m.,** a type of ophthalmic migraine whose aura fills both visual fields and which may be accompanied by dysarthria and disturbances of equilibrium. **ophthalmic m.,** migraine accompanied by amblyopia, teichopsia, or other visual disturbance. **ophthalmoplegic m.,** periodic migraine accompanied by ophthalmoplegia. **retinal m.,** a type of

ophthalmic migraine with retinal symptoms, probably secondary to constriction of one or more retinal arteries.

mi·gra·tion (mi-gra′shun) 1. an apparently spontaneous change of place, as of symptoms. 2. diapedesis.

mi·gra·to·ry (mi′grah-tor″e) 1. roving or wandering. 2. of, pertaining to, or characterized by migration; undergoing periodic migration.

mil·dew (mil′doo) colloquialism for any superficial fungous growth on plants or any organic material.

mil·i·a·ria (mil″e-ar′e-ah) a cutaneous condition with retention of sweat, which is extravasated at different levels in the skin; when used alone, it refers to *miliaria rubra*. **m. ru′bra,** heat rash; prickly heat; a condition due to obstruction of the ducts of the sweat glands; the sweat escapes into the epidermis, producing pruritic red papulovesicles.

mil·i·ary (mil′e-ar″e) 1. like millet seeds. 2. characterized by lesions resembling millet seeds.

mil·i·um (mil′e-um) pl. *mil′ia.* [L.] a tiny spheroidal epithelial cyst lying superficially within the skin, usually of the face, containing lamellated keratin and often associated with vellus hair follicles.

milk (milk) 1. the fluid secretion of the mammary gland forming the natural food of young mammals. 2. any whitish milklike substance, e.g., coconut milk or plant latex. 3. a liquid (emulsion or suspension) resembling the secretion of the mammary gland. **m. of magnesia,** a suspension of magnesium hydroxide, used as an antacid and laxative. **modified m.,** cow's milk made to correspond to the composition of human milk. **soy m.,** a liquid made from soybeans, used as a milk substitute and a source of calcium. **vitamin D m.,** cow's milk supplemented with 400 IU of vitamin D per quart. **witch's m.,** milk secreted in the breast of the newborn infant.

milk·ing (milk′ing) the pressing out of the contents of a tubular structure by running the finger along it.

milky (mil′ke) 1. having the appearance of milk; whitish, cloudy, fluid. 2. filled with or consisting of milk or a milklike fluid.

milli- word element [L.], *one thousand;* also used in naming units of measurement (symbol m) to designate an amount 10^{-3} the size of the unit to which it is joined, e.g., milligram.

mil·li·equiv·a·lent (mEq) (mil″e-e-kwiv′ah-lint) one thousandth (10^{-3}) of the equivalent weight of an element, radical, or compound.

mil·li·gram (mg) (mil′ĭ-gram) one thousandth (10^{-3}) of a gram.

mil·li·li·ter (mL) (-le″ter) one thousandth (10^{-3}) of a liter.

mil·li·me·ter (mm) (-me″ter) one thousandth (10^{-3}) of a meter.

mil·li·mo·lar (mM) (-mo″ler) denoting a concentration of 1 millimole per liter.

mil·li·mole (mmol) (-mōl) one thousandth (10^{-3}) of a mole.

mil·pho·sis (mil-fo′sis) the falling out of the eyelashes.

mil·ri·none (mil′rĭ-nōn) a cardiotonic used in the treatment of congestive heart failure.

mi·me·sis (mĭ-me′sis) the simulation of one disease by another. **mimet′ic,** adj.

mi·met·ic (mĭ-met′ik) pertaining to or exhibiting imitation or simulation, as of one disease for another.

mim·ic (mim′ik) 1. pertaining to imitation or simulation. 2. one who imitates, or that which imitates.

mind (mīnd) 1. the organ or seat of consciousness; the faculty, or brain function, by which one is aware of surroundings, and by which one experiences feelings, emotions, and desires, and is able to attend, remember, learn, reason, and make decisions. 2. the organized totality of an organism's mental and psychological processes, conscious and unconscious. 3. the characteristic thought process of a person or group.

min·er·al (min′er-al) any nonorganic homogeneous solid substance of the earth's crust. **trace m.,** a mineral trace element.

min·er·alo·cor·ti·coid (min″er-il-o-kor′tĭ-koid) 1. any of the group of corticosteroids, principally aldosterone, primarily involved in the regulation of electrolyte and water balance through their effect on ion transport in epithelial cells of the renal tubules, resulting in retention of sodium and loss of potassium. Cf. *glucocorticoid.* 2. of, pertaining to, or resembling a mineralocorticoid.

min·i·mal (min′ĭ-m′l) smallest or least; the smallest possible.

mini·pill (min′e-pil) an oral contraceptive consisting of a small daily dose of a progestational agent.

mini·plate (-plāt) a small bone plate.

mi·no·cy·cline (mĭ-no-si′klēn) a semisynthetic broad-spectrum tetracycline antibiotic, used as the hydrochloride salt.

mi·nor (mi′ner) insignificant; small or least in scope, effect, number, size, extent, or importance.

mi·nox·i·dil (mĭ-nok′sĭ-dil) a potent, long-acting vasodilator acting primarily on arterioles; used as an antihypertensive, also applied topically in androgenetic alopecia.

mi·nute (mi-nōōt′) extremely small. **double m's,** acentric chromosomal fragments created by gene amplification and newly integrated into the chromosome; they are tumor markers indicative of solid neoplasms with a poor prognosis.

mio·car·dia (mi″ah-kahr′de-ah) systole.

mi·o·sis (mi-o′sis) contraction of the pupil.

mi·ot·ic (mi-ot′ik) 1. pertaining to, characterized by, or producing miosis. 2. an agent that causes contraction of the pupil.

MIP maximum inspiratory pressure.

mi·ra·cid·i·um (mi″rah-sid′e-um) pl. *miraci′dia.* The first stage larva of a trematode, which undergoes further development in the body of a snail.

mire (mēr) [Fr.] one of the figures on the arm of an ophthalmometer whose images are reflected on the cornea; measurement of their variations determines the amount of corneal astigmatism.

MIRL membrane inhibitor of reactive lysis; see *protectin.*

mir·ror (mir′er) a polished surface that reflects sufficient light to yield images of objects in front of it. **dental m.,** mouth m. **frontal m., head m.,** a circular mirror strapped to the head of the examiner, used to reflect light into a cavity, especially the nose, pharynx, or larynx. **mouth m.,** a small mirror attached at an angle to a handle, for use in dentistry.

mir·taz·a·pine (mir″taz-ah-pēn) an antidepressant structurally unrelated to any of the classes of antidepressants.

mis·car·riage (mis′kar-aj) popular term for *spontaneous abortion.*

mis·ci·ble (mis′ĭ-b′l) able to be mixed.

mi·sog·a·my (mĭ-sog′ah-me) hatred of or aversion to marriage.

mi·sog·y·ny (mĭ-soj′ĭ-ne) hatred of women.

mi·so·pro·stol (mi″so-pros′tol) a synthetic prostaglandin E_1 analogue used to treat gastric irritation resulting from long-term therapy with nonsteroidal antiinflammatory drugs; also used in conjunction with mifepristone (q.v.) for termination of pregnancy.

mis·tle·toe (mis′il-to) any of several related parasitic shrubs. *European m. (Viscum album)* contains small amounts of several toxins and is used for rheumatism and as an adjunct in cancer therapy; also used in traditional Chinese medicine and homeopathy.

mite (mīt) any arthropod of the order Acarina except the ticks; they are minute animals, usually transparent or semitransparent, and may be parasitic on humans and domestic animals, causing various skin irritations. **chigger m., harvest m.,** chigger. **itch m., mange m.,** see *Notoedres* and *Sarcoptes*.

mith·ra·my·cin (mith″rah-mi′sin) plicamycin.

mi·ti·cide (mi′tĭ-sīd) an agent destructive to mites.

mi·to·chon·dria (mi″to-kon′dre-ah) sing. *mitochon′drion* [Gr.] small spherical to rod-shaped cytoplasmic organelles, enclosed by two membranes separated by an intermembranous space; the inner membrane is infolded, forming a series of projections (cristae). Mitochondria are the principal sites of ATP synthesis; they contain enzymes of the tricarboxylic acid cycle and for fatty acid oxidation, oxidative phosphorylation, and many other biochemical pathways. They contain their own nucleic acids and ribosomes, replicate independently, and code for the synthesis of some of their own proteins. **mitochon′drial,** adj.

mi·to·gen (mīt″o-jen) a substance that induces mitosis and cell tranformation, especially lymphocyte transformation. **mitogen′ic,** adj.

mi·to·my·cin (mi″to-mi′sin) 1. any of a group of antitumor antibiotics (e.g., mitomycin A, B, C) produced by *Streptomyces caespitosus.* 2. mitomycin C; used as a palliative antineoplastic.

mi·to·sis (mi-to′sis) a method of indirect cell division in which the two daughter nuclei normally receive identical complements of the number of chromosomes characteristic of the somatic cells of the species. **mitot′ic,** adj.

mi·to·tane (mi′to-tān) an antineoplastic similar to the insecticide DDT; used for the treatment of inoperable adrenocortical carcinoma.

mi·to·xan·trone (mi″to-zan′trōn) a DNA-intercalating anthracenedione, used as the hydrochloride salt as an antineoplastic agent in the treatment of acute myelogenous leukemia and advanced, hormone-refractory prostate cancer; also used in the treatment of secondary multiple sclerosis.

mi·tral (mi′tril) shaped like a miter; pertaining to the mitral valve.

mi·tral·iza·tion (mi″tril-ĭ-za′shun) a straightening of the left border of the cardiac shadow, commonly seen radiographically in mitral stenosis.

mit·tel·schmerz (mit′el-shmertz) pain associated with ovulation, usually occurring in the middle of the menstrual cycle.

mi·va·cu·rium (mi″vah-ku′re-um) a nondepolarizing neuromuscular blocking agent

of short duration, used as the chloride salt as an adjunct to anesthesia.

mixed (mikst) affecting various parts at once; showing two or more different characteristics.

mix·ture (miks′cher) a combination of different drugs or ingredients, as a fluid with other fluids or solids, or of a solid with a liquid.

Mi·ya·ga·wa·nel·la (me″yah-gah″wah-nel′ah) *Chlamydia.*

mL, ml milliliter.

μ**L** microliter.

MLD median lethal dose; minimum lethal dose.

mM millimolar.

mm millimeter.

μ**m** micrometer (2).

MMIHS megacystis-microcolon–intestinal hypoperistalsis syndrome.

mmol millimole.

MMR measles-mumps-rubella (vaccine); see *measles, mumps, and rubella vaccine live,* under *vaccine.*

Mn manganese.

mne·mon·ics (ne-mon′iks) improvement of memory by special methods or techniques. **mnemon′ic,** adj.

MO Medical Officer.

Mo molybdenum.

mo·bi·li·za·tion (mo″bĭ-lĭ-za′shun) the rendering of a fixed part movable. **stapes m.,** surgical correction of immobility of the stapes in treatment of deafness.

Mo·bi·lun·cus (mo″bĭ-lung′kus) a genus of gram-negative, anaerobic bacteria, frequently isolated from women with bacterial vaginosis.

mo·daf·i·nil (mo-daf′ĭ-nil″) a central nervous system stimulant used in the treatment of narcolepsy.

mo·dal·i·ty (mo-dal′ĭ-te) 1. a method of application of, or the employment of, any therapeutic agent, especially a physical agent. 2. in homeopathy, a condition that modifies drug action; a condition under which symptoms develop, becoming better or worse. 3. a specific sensory entity, such as taste.

mode (mōd) 1. a manner, way, or method of acting; a particular condition of functioning. 2. in statistics, the most frequently occurring value or item in a distribution.

mod·el (mod′'l) 1. something that represents or simulates something else. 2. a reasonable facsimile of the body or any of its parts. 3. cast (2). 4. to imitate another's behavior. 5. an hypothesis or theory.

mod·i·fi·ca·tion (mod″ĭ-fĭ-ka′shun) the process or result of changing the form or characteristics of an object or substance. **behavior m.**, see under *therapy*.

mod·i·fi·er (mod′ĭ-fi″er) an agent that changes the form or characteristics of an object or substance. **biologic response m. (BRM),** a method or agent that alters host-tumor interaction, usually by amplifying the antitumor mechanisms of the immune system, or by some mechanism directly or indirectly affecting host or tumor cell characteristics.

mo·di·o·lus (mo-di′o-lus) the central pillar or columella of the cochlea.

mod·u·la·tion (mod″u-la′shun) 1. the act of tempering. 2. the normal capacity of cell adaptability to its environment. 3. embryologic induction in a specific region. **antigenic m.**, the alteration of antigenic determinants in a living cell surface membrane following interaction with antibody. **biochemical m.**, in combination chemotherapy, the use of a substance to modulate the negative side effects of the primary agent, increasing its effectiveness or allowing a higher dose to be used.

mod·u·la·tor (mod′u-la″ter) a specific inductor that brings out characteristics peculiar to a definite region.

mo·ex·i·pril (mo-ek′sĭ-pril″) an angiotensin-converting enzyme inhibitor used as the hydrochloride salt as an antihypertensive.

moi·e·ty (moi′it-e) any equal part; a half; also any part or portion, as a portion of a molecule.

mol (mol) mole (1).

mo·lal (*m*) (mo′lal) containing one mole of solute per kilogram of solvent. NOTE: *molal* refers to the weight of the solvent, *molar* to the volume of the solution.

mo·lal·i·ty (mo-lal′it-e) the number of moles of a solute per kilogram of pure solvent. Cf. *molarity*.

mo·lar¹ (mo′lar) 1. pertaining to a mole of a substance. 2. a measure of the concentration of a solute, expressed as the number of moles of solute per liter of solution. Symbol M, *M*, or mol/L.

mo·lar² (M) (mo′lar) 1. see under *tooth* and see Plate 31. 2. pertaining to a molar tooth.

mo·lar·i·ty (mo-lar′ĭ-te) the number of moles of a solute per liter of solution. Cf. *molality*.

mold (mōld) 1. any of a group of parasitic and saprobic fungi causing a cottony growth on organic substances; also the deposit or growth produced by such fungi. 2. a form in which an object is shaped, or cast. 3. in dentistry, the shape of an artificial tooth.

mold·ing (mōld′ing) the adjusting of the shape and size of the fetal head to the birth canal during labor.

mole¹ (mōl) the base SI unit of amount of matter, being that amount of substance that contains as many elementary entities as there are carbon atoms in 0.012 kg of carbon 12 (^{12}C), Avogadro's number (6.023×10^{23}).

mole² a nevocytic nevus; also, a pigmented fleshy growth or, loosely, any blemish of the skin. **pigmented m.**, see under *nevus*.

mole³ a fleshy mass or tumor formed in the uterus by the degeneration or abnormal development of a zygote. **hydatid m., hydatidiform m.**, an abnormal pregnancy characterized by placental abnormality involving swollen chorionic villi, which form a large, grapelike mass of vesicles, by trophoblastic hyperplasia, and by loss of fetal blood vessels in the villi. It is *complete* when all villi are swollen and fetal tissues are absent, and *partial* when only some villi are swollen and fetal tissues are present. Complete moles usually possess only paternal chromosomes; partial moles are usually triploid and possess both maternal and paternal chromosomes.

mol·e·cule (mol′ĕ-kūl) a small mass of matter; the smallest amount of a substance which can exist alone; an aggregation of atoms, specifically a chemical combination of two or more atoms forming a specific chemical substance. **molec′ular,** adj.

mo·li·men (mo-li′men) pl. *moli′mina*. [L.] a laborious effort made for the performance of any normal bodily function, especially that manifested by a variety of unpleasant symptoms preceding or accompanying menstruation.

mo·lin·done hy·dro·chlo·ride (mo-lin′dōn) an antipsychotic agent, used as the hydrochloride salt.

mol·li·ti·es (mo-lish′e-ēz) [L.] softness; abnormal softening. **m. os′sium,** osteomalacia.

mol·lus·cum (mŏ-lus′kum) 1. any of various skin diseases marked by the formation of soft rounded cutaneous tumors. 2. m. contagiosum. **mollus′cous,** adj. **m. contagio′sum,** a viral skin disease caused by a poxvirus, with firm, round, translucent, crateriform papules containing caseous matter and peculiar capsulated bodies.

Mol wt, mol wt molecular weight.

mo·lyb·date (mah-lib′dāt) any salt of molybdic acid.

mo·lyb·den·um (Mo) (mah-lib′dĭ-num) chemical element (see *Table of Elements*), at. no. 42.

mo·lyb·do·pro·tein (mah-lib″do-pro′tēn) an enzyme containing molybdenum.

mo·met·a·sone (mo-met′ah-sōn) a synthetic corticosteroid used in the form of *m. furoate* for the relief of inflammation and pruritus in certain dermatoses and the treatment of allergic rhinitis and other inflammatory nasal conditions..

mon·ad (mon′ad) 1. a single-celled protozoan or coccus. 2. a univalent radical or element. 3. in meiosis, one member of a tetrad.

mon·ar·thri·tis (mon″ahr-thri′tis) inflammation of a single joint.

mon·ar·tic·u·lar (-tik′u-ler) pertaining to a single joint.

mon·as·ter (mon-as′ter) the single star-shaped figure at the end of prophase in mitosis.

mon·ath·e·to·sis (-ath″ĭ-to′sis) athetosis of one limb.

mon·atom·ic (mon″ah-tom′ik) 1. monovalent (1). 2. monobasic. 3. containing one atom.

mon·au·ral (mon-aw′ral) pertaining to one ear.

mo·ne·cious (mo-ne′shus) monoecious.

Mo·ne·ra (mo-ne′rah) a kingdom comprising the prokaryotes, unicellular organisms lacking true nuclei, i.e. the bacteria.

mon·es·thet·ic (mon″es-thet′ik) pertaining to or affecting a single sense or sensation.

mon·go·lism (mong′go-lizm) former (now offensive) name for *Down syndrome*.

mo·nil·e·thrix (mo-nil′ĕ-thriks) a hereditary condition in which the hairs exhibit marked multiple constrictions, giving a beading effect, and are very brittle.

Mo·nil·ia (mo-nil′e-ah) 1. former name for *Candida*. 2. a genus of imperfect fungi of the family Moniliaceae.

mo·nil·i·al (-al) pertaining to or caused by *Monilia* (*Candida*).

mo·nil·i·form (mo-nil′ĭ-form) beaded.

mon·i·tor (mon′it-er) 1. to check constantly on a given condition or phenomenon, e.g., blood pressure or heart or respiratory rate. 2. an apparatus by which such conditions can be constantly observed or recorded. **ambulatory ECG m., Holter m.,** a portable continuous electrocardiographic recorder used to detect the frequency and duration of rhythm disturbances.

mon·key·pox (mung′ke-poks) a mild, epidemic, exanthematous disease occurring in monkeys and other mammals; when transmitted to humans, it causes a disease clinically similar to smallpox.

mon(o)- word element [Gr.], *one; single; limited to one part; combined with one atom.*

mono·am·ide (mon″o-am′ĭd) an amide compound with only one amide group.

mono·amine (mon″o-ah-mēn′) an amine containing one amino group, e.g., serotonin, dopamine, epinephrine, and norepinephrine.

mono·am·in·er·gic (-am″in-er′jik) of or pertaining to neurons that secrete monoamine neurotransmitters (e.g., dopamine, serotonin).

mono·am·ni·ot·ic (-am″ne-ot′ik) having or developing within a single amniotic cavity, such as monozygotic twins.

mono·bac·tam (-bak′tam) 1. a class of synthetic antibiotics with a cyclic beta-lactam nucleus. 2. a class of synthetic antibiotics having a monocyclic β-lactam nucleus.

mono·ba·sic (-ba′sik) having but one atom of replaceable hydrogen.

mono·ben·zone (-ben′zōn) a melanin-inhibiting agent used as a topical depigmenting agent in vitiligo.

mono·blast (mon′o-blast) the earliest precursor in the monocytic series, which matures to develop into the promocyte.

mono·blep·sia (mon″o-blep′se-ah) 1. a condition in which vision is better when only one eye is used. 2. blindness to all colors but one.

mono·cho·rea (-ko-re′ah) chorea affecting only one limb.

mono·cho·ri·on·ic (-kor″e-on′ik) having or developing in a common chorionic sac, such as monozygotic twins.

mono·chro·mat (-kro′mat) a person with monochromatic vision.

mono·chro·mat·ic (-kro-mat′ik) 1. existing in or having only one color. 2. pertaining to or affected by monochromatic vision. 3. staining with only one dye at a time.

mono·chro·ma·tism (-kro′mah-tizm) monochromatic vision. **cone m.,** that in which there is some cone function. **rod m.,** that in which there is complete absence of cone function.

mono·chro·mato·phil (-kro-mat′ah-fil) 1. stainable with only one kind of stain. 2. any cell or other element taking only one stain.

mono·clo·nal (-klōn′al) 1. derived from a single cell. 2. pertaining to a single clone.

mon·oc·u·lar (mon-ok′u-ler) 1. pertaining to or having only one eye. 2. having only one eyepiece, as in a microscope.

mono·cyte (mon′o-sīt) a mononuclear, phagocytic leukocyte, 13μ to 25μ in diameter, with an ovoid or kidney-shaped nucleus, and azurophilic cytoplasmic granules. Formed in the bone marrow from promonocytes, monocytes are transported to tissues, such as the lung and liver, where they develop into macrophages. **monocyt′ic,** adj.

mono·cy·toid (mon″o-si′toid) resembling a monocyte.

mono·cy·to·pe·nia (-si″to-pe′ne-ah) deficiency of monocytes in the blood.

mono·der·mo·ma (-der-mo′mah) a tumor developed from one germ layer.

mo·noe·cious (mo-ne′shus) having reproductive organs typical of both sexes in a single individual.

mono·eth·a·nol·amine (mon″o-eth″ah-nōl′ah-mēn) an amino alcohol used as a pharmaceutical surfactant. The oleate salt is *ethanolamine oleate*.

mono·gen·ic (-jen′ik) pertaining to or influenced by a single gene.

mono·io·do·ty·ro·sine (-i-o″do-ti′ro-sēn) an iodinated amino acid intermediate in the synthesis of thyroxine and triiodothyronine.

mono·kine (mon′o-kīn) a general term for soluble mediators of immune responses that are not antibodies or complement components and that are produced by mononuclear phagocytes (monocytes or macrophages).

mono·loc·u·lar (mon″o-lok′u-lar) unilocular.

mono·ma·nia (-ma′ne-ah) a form of mental disorder characterized by preoccupation with one subject or idea.

mono·mer (mon′o-mer) 1. a simple molecule of relatively low molecular weight, capable of reacting to form by repetition a dimer, trimer, or polymer. 2. some basic unit of a molecule, either the molecule itself or some structural or functional subunit of it.

mono·mer·ic (mon″o-mer′ik) 1. pertaining to, composed of, or affecting a single segment. 2. in genetics, determined by a gene or genes at a single locus.

mono·mi·cro·bi·al (-mi-kro′be-al) marked by the presence of a single species of microorganisms.

mono·mo·lec·u·lar (-mo-lek′u-ler) pertaining to a single molecule or to a layer one molecule thick.

mono·mor·phic (-mor′fik) existing in only one form; maintaining the same form throughout all developmental stages.

mono·neu·ri·tis (-noo-ri′tis) inflammation of a single nerve. **m. mul′tiplex,** see under *mononeuropathy.*

mono·neu·rop·a·thy (-noo-rop′ah-the) disease affecting a single nerve. **multiple m., m. mul′tiplex,** mononeuropathy of several different nerves simultaneously.

mono·nu·cle·ar (-noo′kle-er) 1. having but one nucleus. 2. a cell having a single nucleus, especially a monocyte of the blood or tissues.

mono·nu·cle·o·sis (-noo″kle-o′sis) excess of mononuclear leukocytes (monocytes) in the blood. **chronic m.,** chronic fatigue syndrome. **cytomegalovirus m.,** an infectious disease caused by a cytomegalovirus and resembling infectious mononucleosis. **infectious m.,** an acute infectious disease caused by the Epstein-Barr virus; symptoms include fever, malaise, sore throat, lymphadenopathy, atypical lymphocytes (resembling monocytes) in the peripheral blood, and various immune reactions.

mono·nu·cle·o·tide (-noo′kle-ah-tīd″) nucleotide.

mono·oc·ta·no·in (-ok″tah-no′in) a semisynthetic glycerol derivative used to dissolve cholesterol stones in the common and intrahepatic bile ducts.

mono·pha·sia (-fa′zhah) aphasia with ability to utter only one word or phrase. **mono·pha′sic,** adj.

mono·phe·nol mono·oxy·gen·ase (-fe′nol mon″o-ok′si-jen″ās) any of a group of oxidoreductases that catalyze a step in the formation of melanin pigments from tyrosine.

mon·oph·thal·mus (mon″of-thal′mus) cyclops.

mono·phy·let·ic (mon″o-fi-let′ik) descended from a common ancestor or stem cell.

mono·ple·gia (-ple′jah) paralysis of a single part. **monople′gic,** adj.

mono·pty·chi·al (-ti′ke-al) arranged in a single layer; said of glands whose cells are arranged on the basement membrane in a single layer.

mon·or·chid (mon-or′kid) 1. pertaining to or characterized by monorchism. 2. an individual with monorchism.

mon·or·chid·ism (-or′kid-izm) monorchism.

mon·or·chism (mon′or-kizm) the condition of having only one testis in the scrotum.

mono·sac·cha·ride (mon″o-sak′ah-rīd) a simple sugar, having the general formula $C_nH_{2n}O_n$; a carbohydrate that cannot be decomposed by hydrolysis. The two main types are the aldoses and the ketoses.

mono·so·di·um glu·ta·mate (-so′de-um) the monosodium salt of L-glutamic acid, used as a pharmaceutic necessity and to enhance the flavor of foods.

mono·so·my (mon′o-so″me) existence in a cell of only one instead of the normal diploid pair of a particular chromosome. **monoso′mic,** adj.

mono·spasm (mon′o-spazm) spasm of a single limb or part.

mono·spe·cif·ic (mon″o-spě-sif′ik) having an effect only on a particular kind of cell or tissue or reacting with a single antigen, as a monospecific antiserum.

mono·sper·my (mon'o-sper"me) fertilization in which only one spermatozoon enters the oocyte.

Mono·spo·ri·um (mon"o-spor'e-um) a genus of fungi, including *M. apiosper'mum*, a cause of maduromycosis.

mono·stra·tal (-strāt'al) pertaining to a single layer or stratum.

mono·syn·ap·tic (-sĭ-nap'tik) pertaining to or passing through a single synapse.

mono·ther·a·py (-ther'ah-pe) treatment of a condition by means of a single drug.

mono·ther·mia (-ther'me-ah) maintenance of the same body temperature throughout the day.

mo·not·o·cous (mo-not'ah-kus) giving birth to but one offspring at a time.

mon·ot·ri·chous (mon-ot'rĭ-kus) having a single polar flagellum.

mono·un·sat·u·rat·ed (mon"o-un-sach'er-āt"ed) of a chemical compound, containing one double or triple bond.

mono·va·lent (-va'lent) 1. having a valency of one. 2. capable of combining with only one antigenic specificity or with only one antibody specificity.

mono·ov·u·lar (mon-ov'u-l'r) pertaining to or derived from a single oocyte, as monozygotic twins.

mono·xen·ic (-zen'ik) associated with a single known species of microorganisms; said of otherwise germ-free animals.

mo·nox·e·nous (mon-ok'sĕ-nus) requiring only one host to complete the life cycle.

mon·ox·ide (mon-ok'sīd) an oxide with one oxygen atom in the molecule.

mono·zy·got·ic (mon"o-zi-got'ik) pertaining to or derived from a single zygote; as monozygotic twins.

mons (mons) [L.] an elevation or eminence. **m. pu'bis, m. ve'neris,** the rounded fleshy prominence over the symphysis pubis in the female.

mon·ster (mon'ster) a term formerly used to denote a fetus or infant with such pronounced developmental anomalies as to be grotesque and usually nonviable.

mon·te·lu·kast (mon"tĕ-loo'kast) a leukotriene antagonist used as the sodium salt in prophylaxis and chronic treatment of asthma.

mon·tic·u·lus (mon-tik'u-lus) pl. *monti'culi.* [L.] a small eminence. **m. cerebel'li,** the projecting or central part of the vermis.

mood (mood) the emotional state or state of mind of an individual.

MOPP a cancer chemotherapy regimen consisting of mechlorethamine, Oncovin (vincristine), procarbazine, and prednisone.

Mo·rax·ei·ia (mo-rak-sel'ah) a genus of bacteria (family Neisseriaceae), made up of gram-negative, short, aerobic, nonpigmented organisms found as parasites and pathogens on the mucous membranes of mammals; it includes two subgenera: *M. (Moraxella)* and *M. (Branhamella). M. (Branhamel'la) catarrha'lis* is a normal inhabitant of the human nasal cavity and nasopharynx, occasionally causing otitis media or respiratory disease. *M. (Moraxel'la) lacuna'ta* causes conjunctivitis and corneal infections.

mor·bid (mor'bid) 1. pertaining to, affected with, or inducing disease; diseased. 2. unhealthy or unwholesome. 3. characterized by preoccupation with gloomy or unwholesome feelings or thoughts.

mor·bid·i·ty (mor-bid'it-e) 1. a diseased condition or state. 2. the incidence or prevalence of a disease or of all diseases in a population.

mor·bil·li (mor-bil'i) [L.] measles.

mor·bil·li·form (mor-bil'ĭ-form) measles-like; resembling the eruption of measles.

Mor·bil·li·vi·rus (-vi"rus) measles-like viruses; a genus of viruses of the family Paramyxoviridae, including the agents of measles and canine distemper.

mor·bus (mor'bus) [L.] disease.

mor·cel·la·tion (mor"sel-a'shun) the division of solid tissue (such as a tumor) into pieces, which can then be removed.

mor·dant (mord'int) 1. a substance capable of intensifying or deepening the reaction of a specimen to a stain. 2. to subject to the action of a mordant before staining.

morgue (morg) a place where dead bodies may be kept for identification or until claimed for burial.

mor·i·bund (mor'ĭ-bund) in a dying state.

mor·i·ci·zine (mor-ĭ'sĭ-zēn) a phenothiazine derivative used as the hydrochloride salt as an antiarrhythmic in treatment of ventricular arrhythmias.

-morph word element [Gr.], *shape; form.*

mor·phea (mor-fe'ah) a condition in which there is connective tissue replacement of the skin and sometimes the subcutaneous tissues, with formation of firm ivory white or pinkish patches, bands, or lines.

mor·phine (mor'fēn) an opioid analgesic, the principal and most active alkaloid of opium; used as the sulfate or hydrochloride salt as an analgesic, antitussive, and as an adjunct to anesthesia or to treatment of pulmonary edema secondary to left ventricular failure.

mor·pho·gen (mor'fah-jen) a substance in embryonic tissue that forms a concentration gradient and influences morphogenesis.

mor·pho·gen·e·sis (mor″fo-jen'ĕ-sis) the evolution and development of form, as the development of the shape of a particular organ or part of the body, or the development undergone by individuals who attain the type to which the majority of the individuals of the species approximate.

mor·pho·ge·net·ic (mor″fo-jĕ-net'ik) producing growth; producing form or shape.

mor·phol·o·gy (mor-fol'ah-je) the science of the forms and structure of organisms; the form and structure of a particular organism, organ, or part. **morpholog′ic, morpholog′ical,** adj.

mor·pho·sis (mor-fo'sis) the process of formation of a part or organ. **morphot′ic,** adj.

mor·rhu·ate (mor'u-āt) the fatty acids of cod liver oil; the sodium salt is used as a sclerosing agent, especially for the treatment of varicose veins and hemorrhoids.

mors (mōrs) [L.] death.

mor·sus (mor'sus) [L.] bite.

mor·tal (mor't'l) 1. subject to death, or destined to die. 2. fatal.

mor·tal·i·ty (mor-tal'it-e) 1. the quality of being mortal. 2. see *death rate,* under *rate.* 3. the ratio of actual deaths to expected deaths.

mor·tar (mor'ter) a bell- or urn-shaped vessel in which drugs are beaten, crushed, or ground with a pestle.

mor·ti·fi·ca·tion (mor″tĭ-fĭ-ka'shun) gangrene.

mor·u·la (mor'u-lah) 1. the solid mass of blastomeres formed by cleavage of a zygote. 2. an inclusion body seen in circulating leukocytes in ehrlichiosis.

mor·u·lar (-ler) 1. pertaining to a morula. 2. resembling a mulberry.

mo·sa·ic (mo-za'ik) 1. a pattern made of numerous small pieces fitted together. 2. in genetics, an individual or cell cultures having two or more cell lines that are karyotypically or genotypically distinct but are derived from a single zygote. 3. in embryology, the condition in the fertilized eggs of some species whereby the cells of early stages have developed cytoplasm which determines the parts that are to develop. 4. in plant pathology, a viral disease characterized by mottling of the foliage.

mo·sa·i·cism (mo-za'ĭ-sizm) in genetics, the presence in an individual of two or more cell lines that are karyotypically or genotypically distinct and are derived from a single zygote.

mOsm milliosmole; one thousandth (10^{-3}) of an osmole.

mos·qui·to (mos-ke'to) [Sp.] a bloodsucking and venomous insect of the family Culicidae, including the genera *Aedes, Anopheles, Culex,* and *Mansonia.*

mo·til·in (mo-til'in) a polypeptide hormone secreted by enterochromaffin cells of the gut; it causes increased motility of several portions of the gut and stimulates pepsin secretion. Its release is stimulated by the presence of acid and fat in the duodenum.

mo·til·i·ty (mo-til'ite) the ability to move spontaneously. **mo′tile,** adj.

mo·to·neu·ron (mōt″o-nōōr′on) motor neuron; a neuron having a motor function; an efferent neuron conveying motor impulses. **lower m.,** a peripheral neuron whose cell body lies in the ventral gray columns of the spinal cord and whose termination is in a skeletal muscle. **peripheral m.,** in a reflex arc, a motoneuron that receives impulses from interneurons. **upper m.,** a neuron in the cerebral cortex that conducts impulses from the motor cortex to a motor nucleus of one of the cerebral nerves or to a ventral gray column of the spinal cord.

mo·tor (mōt'er) 1. a muscle, nerve, or center that effects or produces motion. 2. producing or subserving motion.

mot·tled (mot'ld) marked by spots or blotches of different colors or shades.

mot·tling (-ling) a condition of spotting with patches of color.

mou·lage (moo-lahzh′) [Fr.] the making of molds or models in wax or plaster; also, a mold or model so produced.

mound·ing (mound'ing) myoedema (1).

mount (mount) 1. to fix in or on a support. 2. a support on which something may be fixed. 3. to prepare specimens and slides for study. 4. a specimen or slide for study.

mourn·ing (mor'ning) 1. the normal psychological processes that follow the loss of a loved one; grief is the accompanying emotional state. 2. social expressions of grief, such as funeral and burial services, prayers, or other rituals.

mouse (mous) 1. a small rodent, various species of which are used in laboratory experiments. 2. a small weight or movable structure. **joint m.,** a movable fragment of cartilage or other body within a joint. **peritoneal m.,** a free body in the peritoneal cavity, probably a small detached mass of omentum, sometimes visible radiographically.

mouth (mouth) 1. an opening. 2. the anterior opening of the alimentary canal, the cavity containing the tongue and teeth. **trench m.**, necrotizing ulcerative gingivitis.

mouth·wash (mouth′wosh) a solution for rinsing the mouth.

move·ment (mo͞ov′ment) 1. an act of moving; motion. 2. an act of defecation. **ameboid m.**, movement like that of an ameba, accomplished by protrusion of cytoplasm of the cell. **associated m.**, 1. movement of parts which act together, as the eyes. 2. synkinesis. **brownian m.**, the random zigzag or dancing movement of minute solute particles suspended in a solvent, due to bombardment by rapidly moving solvent molecules. **rapid eye m. (REM)**, the rapid conjugate movement of the eyes that occurs during REM sleep (see under *sleep*). **vermicular m's**, the wormlike movements of the intestines in peristalsis.

mov·er (mo͞o′ver) that which produces motion. **prime m.**, a muscle that acts directly to bring about a desired movement.

moxa (mok′sah) [Japanese] the dried leaves of *Artemisia vulgaris*, burned on or near acupoints in moxibustion.

mox·a·lac·tam (mok″sah-lak′tam) a semisynthetic antibiotic chemically related to the third-generation cephalosporins and having a broad spectrum of antibacterial activity; used as the disodium salt.

mox·i·bus·tion (mok″sĭ-bus′chun) the stimulation of an acupoint by the burning of a cone or cylinder of moxa placed at or near the point.

mox·i·flox·a·cin (-flok′sah-sin) a fluoroquinolone antibacterial effective against many gram-positive and gram-negative bacteria; used as the hydrochloride salt.

6-MP mercaptopurine.

MPD maximum permissible dose.

MPH Master of Public Health.

MPO myeloperoxidase.

MR mitral regurgitation.

mR milliroentgen; one thousandth (10^{-3}) of a roentgen.

MRA Medical Record Administrator.

mrad millirad; one thousandth (10^{-3}) of a rad.

MRC Medical Reserve Corps.

MRCP Member of Royal College of Physicians.

MRCS Member of Royal College of Surgeons.

mrem millirem; one thousandth (10^{-3}) of a rem.

MRI magnetic resonance imaging.

MRL Medical Record Librarian; now called Medical Record Administrator.

mRNA messenger RNA.

MS Master of Science; Master of Surgery; mitral stenosis; multiple sclerosis.

ms millisecond; one thousandth (10^{-3}) of a second.

μs microsecond; one millionth (10^{-6}) of a second.

MSG monosodium glutamate.

MSH melanocyte-stimulating hormone.

MSUD maple syrup urine disease.

MT Medical Technologist.

mtDNA mitochondrial DNA.

mu·cif·er·ous (mu-sif′er-us) muciparous.

mu·ci·gen (mu′sĭ-jen) the substance from which mucin is derived.

mu·ci·lage (-lij) an aqueous solution of a gummy substance, used as a vehicle or demulcent. **mucilag′inous**, adj.

mu·cil·loid (-loid) a preparation of a mucilaginous substance. **psyllium hydrophilic m.**, a powdered preparation of the mucilaginous portion of the seeds of blond psyllium (*Plantago ovata*), used as a bulk-forming laxative.

mu·cin (mu′sin) 1. any of a group of protein-containing glycoconjugates with high sialic acid or sulfated polysaccharide content that compose the chief constituent of mucus. 2. any of a wide variety of glycoconjugates, including mucoproteins, glycoproteins, glycosaminoglycans, and glycolipids.

mu·ci·noid (mu′sĭ-noid) resembling or pertaining to mucin.

mu·ci·no·sis (mu″si-no′sis) a state with abnormal deposits of mucins in the skin. **follicular m.**, a disease of the pilosebaceous unit, characterized by plaques of follicular papules and alopecia.

mu·ci·nous (mu′sĭ-nus) resembling, or marked by formation of, mucin.

mu·cin·uria (mu″sin-ūr′e-ah) the presence of mucin in the urine, suggesting vaginal contamination.

mu·cip·a·rous (mu-sip′ah-rus) secreting mucus.

muc(o)- word element [L.], *mucus; pertaining to a mucous membrane.*

mu·co·cele (mu′ko-sēl) 1. dilatation of a cavity with mucous secretion. 2. mucus retention cyst.

mu·co·cil·i·ary (mu″ko-sil′e-ar-e) pertaining to mucus and to the cilia of the epithelial cells in the airways.

mu·co·cu·ta·ne·ous (-ku-ta′ne-us) pertaining to or affecting the mucous membrane and the skin.

mu·co·en·ter·itis (-en″ter-i′tis) mucous colitis.

mu·co·ep·i·der·moid (-ep″ĭ-der′moid) composed of mucus-producing epithelial cells.

mu·co·gin·gi·val (-jin′jĭ-val) pertaining to the oral mucosa and gingiva, or to the line of demarcation between them.

mu·coid (mu′koid) 1. resembling mucus. 2. mucinoid.

mu·co·lip·i·do·sis (mu″ko-lip″ĭ-do′sis) pl. *mucolipido′ses*. Any of a group of lysosomal storage diseases in which both glycosaminoglycans (mucopolysaccharides) and lipids accumulate in tissues but without excess of the former in the urine.

mu·co·lyt·ic (-lit′ik) capable of reducing the viscosity of mucus, or an agent that so acts.

mu·co·peri·chon·dri·um (-pĕ″re-kon′dre-um) perichondrium having a mucosal surface, as that of the nasal septum. **mucoperichon′drial,** adj.

mu·co·peri·os·te·um (-os′te-um) periosteum having a mucous surface. **mucoperios′teal,** adj.

mu·co·poly·sac·cha·ride (-sak′ah-rīd) 1. glycosaminoglycan. 2. any polysaccharide with high hexosamine content, including the glycosaminoglycans and also neutral polysaccharides such as chitin.

mu·co·pol·y·sac·cha·ri·do·sis (-sak″ah-ri-do′sis) pl. *mucopolysaccharido′ses*. Any of a group of lysosomal storage disorders due to defective metabolism of glycosaminoglycans, causing their accumulation and excretion and affecting the bony skeleton, joints, liver, spleen, eye, ear, skin, teeth, and the cardiovascular, respiratory, and central nervous systems.

mu·co·pro·tein (-pro′tēn) a covalently linked conjugate of protein and polysaccharide, the latter containing many hexosamine residues and constituting 4 to 30 per cent of the weight of the compound; they occur mainly in mucus secretions.

mu·co·pu·ru·lent (-pūr′ah-lint) containing both mucus and pus.

mu·co·pus (mu′ko-pus) mucus blended with pus.

Mu·cor (mu′kor) a genus of fungi, some species of which cause mucormycosis.

Mu·co·ra·les (mu″kor-a′lēz) an order of fungi, including bread molds and related fungi, most of which are saprobes. Species of genera *Absidia*, *Mucor*, and *Rhizopus* cause mucormycosis.

mu·cor·my·co·sis (-mi-ko′sis) mycosis due to fungi of the order Mucorales, usually occurring in debilitated or immunocompromised patients, often beginning in the upper respiratory tract or lungs, from which mycelial growths metastasize to other organs.

mu·co·sa (mu-ko′sah) [L.] mucous membrane. **muco′sal,** adj.

mu·cous (mu′kus) 1. pertaining to or resembling mucus. 2. covered with mucus. 3. secreting, producing, or containing mucus.

mu·co·vis·ci·do·sis (mu″ko-vis″ĭ-do′sis) cystic fibrosis.

mu·cus (mu′kus) the free slime of the mucous membranes, composed of secretion of the glands, various salts, desquamated cells, and leukocytes.

mug·wort (mug′wort) 1. any of several plants of the genus *Artemisia*, particularly *A. vulgaris*. 2. a preparation of *A. vulgaris*, used internally for gastrointestinal complaints and as a tonic; also used in homeopathy and traditional Chinese medicine.

mu·li·e·bria (mu″le-eb′re-ah) the female genitalia.

multi- word element [L.], *many*.

mul·ti·cen·tric (mul″te-sen′trik) polycentric.

Mul·ti·ceps (mul′tĭ-seps) a genus of tapeworms, including *M. mul′ticeps*, whose adult stage is parasitic in dogs and whose larval stage (*Coenurus cerebralis*) usually develops in the central nervous system of goats and sheep and occasionally in humans.

mul·ti·fac·to·ri·al (mul″te-fak-tor′e-al) 1. of or pertaining to, or arising through the action of many factors. 2. in genetics, arising as the result of the interaction of several genes and usually, to some extent, of nongenetic factors.

mul·ti·fid (mul′tĭ-fid) cleft into many parts.

mul·ti·fo·cal (mul″te-fo′k′l) arising from or pertaining to many foci.

mul·ti·form (mul′tĭ-form) polymorphic.

mul·ti·grav·i·da (mul″te-grav′ĭ-dah) a woman who is pregnant and has been pregnant at least twice before.

mul·ti·in·fec·tion (-in-fek′shun) infection with several kinds of pathogens.

mul·ti·loc·u·lar (-lok′u-ler) having many cells or compartments.

mul·ti·nod·u·lar (-nod′u-ler) composed of many nodules.

mul·tip·a·ra (mul-tip′ah-rah) a woman who has had two or more pregnancies resulting in viable fetuses, whether or not the offspring were alive at birth. **multip′arous,** adj. **grand m.,** a woman who has had six or more pregnancies resulting in viable fetuses.

mul·ti·par·i·ty (mul″te-par′ĭ-te) 1. the condition of being a multipara. 2. the production of several offspring in one gestation.

mul·ti·ple (mul′tĭ-p′l) manifold; occurring in or affecting various parts of the body at once.

mul·ti·sen·so·ry (mul″te-sen′sah-re) capable of responding to more than one kind of sensory input, as certain neurons in the central nervous system.

mul·ti·va·lent (-vāl′ent) 1. having the power of combining with three or more univalent atoms. 2. active against several strains of an organism.

mum·mi·fi·ca·tion (mum″ĭ-fĭ-ka′shun) the shriveling up of a tissue, as in dry gangrene, or of a dead, retained fetus.

mumps (mumps) an acute contagious paramyxovirus disease seen mainly in childhood, involving chiefly the salivary glands, most often the parotids, but other tissues, e.g., the meninges and testes (in postpubertal males), may be affected.

mu·pir·o·cin (mu-pir′o-sin) an antibacterial derived from *Pseudomonas fluorescens*, effective against staphylococci and nonenteric streptococci; used topically in the treatment of impetigo and, intranasally as the calcium salt, in the treatment of nasal colonization by *Staphylococcus aureus*.

mu·ral (mūr″l) pertaining to or occurring in the wall of a body cavity.

mu·ram·i·dase (mu-ram′ĭ-das) lysozyme.

mu·rex·ine (mu-rek′sin) a neurotoxin from the hypobranchial gland of the snail *Murex*. It is called purpurine when derived from snails of the genus *Purpura*.

mu·rine (mūr′ēn) pertaining to, derived from, or characteristic of mice or rats.

mur·mur (mur′mer) [L.] an auscultatory sound, particularly a periodic sound of short duration of cardiac or vascular origin. **anemic m.**, a cardiac murmur heard in anemia. **aortic m.**, one generated by blood flowing through a diseased aorta or aortic valve. **arterial m.**, one over an artery, sometimes aneurysmal and sometimes constricted. **Austin Flint m.**, a presystolic murmur heard at the apex in aortic regurgitation. **cardiac m.**, one of finite length generated by turbulence of blood flow through the heart. **Carey Coombs m.**, a rumbling mid-diastolic murmur occurring in the active phase of rheumatic fever. **continuous m.**, a humming cardiac murmur heard throughout systole and diastole. **Cruveilhier-Baumgarten m.**, one heard at the abdominal wall over veins connecting the portal and caval systems. **diastolic m's**, cardiac murmurs heard during diastole, usually due to semilunar valve regurgitation or to altered blood flow through atrioventricular valves. **Duroziez's m.**, a double murmur over the femoral or other large peripheral artery; due to aortic insufficiency. **ejection m.**, a type of systolic murmur usually heard in midsystole when ejection volume and velocity of blood flow are maximal, such as in aortic or pulmonary stenosis. **extracardiac m.**, one heard over the heart but originating from another structure. **friction m.**, see *rub*. **functional m.**, a cardiac murmur generated in the absence of organic cardiac disease. **Gibson m.**, a long, rumbling cardiac murmur heard for most of systole and diastole, usually in the second left interspace near the sternum, indicative of patent ductus arteriosus. **Graham Steell's m.**, one due to pulmonary regurgitation in patients with pulmonary hypertension and mitral stenosis. **heart m.**, cardiac m. **innocent m.**, functional m. **machinery m.**, Gibson m. **musical m.**, a cardiac murmur having a periodic harmonic pattern. **organic m.**, one due to a lesion in an organ, e.g., the heart, a vessel, or a lung. **pansystolic m.**, a regurgitant murmur heard throughout systole. **pericardial m.**, see under *rub*. **prediastolic m.**, a cardiac murmur heard just before and with diastole; due to mitral obstruction, or to aortic or pulmonary regurgitation. **presystolic m.**, a cardiac murmur heard just before ventricular ejection, usually associated with atrial contraction and the acceleration of blood flow through a narrowed atrioventricular valve. **pulmonic m.**, one due to disease of the pulmonary valve or artery. **regurgitant m.**, one due to regurgitation of blood through an abnormal valvular orifice. **seagull m.**, a raucous murmur with musical qualities, such as that heard occasionally in aortic insufficiency. **Still's m.**, a low-frequency, vibratory or buzzing, functional cardiac murmur of childhood, heard in midsystole. **systolic m's**, cardiac murmurs heard during systole; usually due to mitral or tricuspid regurgitation or to aortic or pulmonary obstruction. **to-and-fro m.**, a friction rub heard in both systole and diastole. **vascular m.**, one heard over a blood vessel. **vesicular m.**, vesicular breath sounds.

mu·ro·mo·nab-CD3 (mu″ro-mo′nab) a murine monoclonal antibody to the CD3 antigen of human T cells that functions as an immunosuppressant in the treatment of acute allograft rejection of renal, hepatic, and cardiac transplants.

Mus (mus) a genus of rodents, including *M. mus′culus*, the common house mouse.

Mus·ca (mus′kah) [L.] a genus of flies, including the common housefly, *M. domes′tica*, which may serve as a vector of various pathogens; its larvae may cause myiasis.

mus·ca (mus′kah) pl. *mus′cae*. A fly. **mus′cae volitan′tes**, specks seen as floating before the eyes.

mus·ca·rine (-rēn) a deadly alkaloid from various mushrooms, e.g., *Amanita muscaria* (the fly agaric), and also from rotten fish.

mus·ca·rin·ic (mus″kah-rin′ik) denoting the cholinergic effects of muscarine on postganglionic parasympathetic neural impulses.

mus·cle (mus″′l) an organ that by contraction produces movement of an animal organism; see *Table of Muscles*, and see Plates 3–7. **agonistic m.**, one opposed in action by another muscle (the antagonistic m.). **antagonistic m.**, one that counteracts the action of another muscle (the agonistic m.). **antigravity m's**, those muscles, mainly extensors of the knees, hips, and back, that by their tone resist the constant pull of gravity in the maintenance of normal posture. **appendicular m's**, the muscles of a limb. **articular m.**, one that has one end attached to a joint capsule. **m's of auditory ossicles**, the two muscles of the middle ear, the tensor tympani and the stapedius. **auricular m's**, 1. the extrinsic auricular muscles, including the anterior, posterior, and superior auricular muscles. 2. the intrinsic auricular muscles that extend from one part of the auricle to another, including the helicis major, helicis minor, tragicus, antitragicus, transverse auricular, and oblique auricular muscles. See table. **Bell's m.**, the muscular strands between the ureteric orifices and the uvula vesicae, bounding the trigone of the urinary bladder. **bipennate m.**, pennate m. **Brücke's m.**, the longitudinal fibers of the ciliary muscle. **cardiac m.**, the muscle of the heart, composed of striated but involuntary muscle fibers, comprising the chief component of the myocardium and lining the walls of the adjoining large vessels. **cervical m's**, the muscles of the neck, including the sternocleidomastoid, longus colli, suprahyoid, infrahyoid, and scalene muscles. **coccygeal m's**, the muscles acting upon the coccyx, including the coccygeal and the dorsal and ventral sacrococcygeal muscles. **congenerous m's**, muscles having a common action or function. **cruciate m.**, a muscle in which the fiber bundles are arranged in the shape of an X. **cutaneous m.**, striated muscle that inserts into the skin. **dilator m.**, a muscle that dilates. **dorsal m's**, the muscles of the back. **epimeric m.**, one derived from an epimere and innervated by a posterior ramus of a spinal nerve. **m's of expression**, a group of cutaneous muscles of the facial structures, including the muscles of the scalp, ear, eyelids, nose, and mouth, and the platysma. **extraocular m's**, the six voluntary muscles that move the eyeball: superior, inferior, middle, and lateral recti, and superior and inferior oblique muscles. **extrinsic m.**, one not originating in the limb or part in which it is inserted. **m's of eye**, extraocular m's. **facial m's**, m's of expression. **fixation m's, fixator m's**, accessory muscles that serve to steady a part. **fusiform m.**, a spindle-shaped muscle in which the fibers are approximately parallel to the long axis of the muscle but converge upon a tendon at either end. **hamstring m's**, the muscles of the back of the thigh: biceps femoris, semitendinous, and semimembranous muscles. **Horner's m.**, the lacrimal part of the orbicularis oculi muscle. **Houston's m.**, fibers of the bulbocavernosus muscle compressing the dorsal vein of the penis. **m's of hyoid bone**, the infrahyoid and suprahyoid muscles. **hypaxial m's**, the long muscle of head, long muscle of neck, vertebral portion of the diaphragm, and anterior sacrococcygeal muscle. **hypomeric m.**, one derived from a hypomere and innervated by an anterior ramus of a spinal nerve. **hypothenar m's**, the intrinsic muscles of the little finger; flexing, abducting, and opposing it, and comprising the short palmar, abductor of little finger, short flexor of little finger, and opponens of little finger muscles. **infrahyoid m's**, the muscles that anchor the hyoid bone to the sternum, clavicle, and scapula, including the sternohyoid, omohyoid, sternothyroid, and thyrohyoid muscles. **inspiratory m's**, those acting during inhalation, such as the diaphragm and the intercostal and pectoral muscles. **intra-auricular m's**, the stapedius and tensor tympani muscles. **intraocular m's**, the intrinsic muscles of the eyeball. **intrinsic m.**, one that is contained (origin, belly, and insertion) in the same limb or part. **involuntary m.**, one that is not under the control of the will. **iridic m's**, those controlling the iris. **Landström's m.**, minute muscle fibers in the fascia around and behind the eyeball, attached in front to the anterior orbital fascia and eyelids. **m's of larynx**, the intrinsic and extrinsic muscles of the larynx, including the oblique and transverse arytenoid, ceratocricoid, lateral and posterior cricoarytenoid, cricothyroid, thyroarytenoid, and vocal muscles. **lingual m's**, the extrinsic

TABLE OF MUSCLES

Common Name*	TA Term†	Origin*	Insertion*	Innervation*	Action
abductor m. of great toe	m. abductor hallucis	medial tubercle of calcaneus, plantar fascia	medial side of base of proximal phalanx of great toe	medial plantar	abducts, flexes great toe
abductor m. of little finger	m. abductor digiti minimi manus	pisiform bone, tendon of ulnar flexor m. of wrist	medial side of base of proximal phalanx of little finger	ulnar	abducts little finger
abductor m. of little toe	m. abductor digiti minimi pedis	medial and lateral tubercles of calcaneus, plantar fascia	lateral side of base of proximal phalanx of little toe	lateral plantar	abducts little toe
abductor m. of thumb, long	m. abductor pollicis longus	posterior surfaces of radius and ulna	radial side of base of first metacarpal bone	posterior interosseous	abducts, extends thumb
abductor m. of thumb, short	m. abductor pollicis brevis	scaphoid, ridge of trapezium, flexor retinaculum of hand	lateral side of base of proximal phalanx of thumb	median	abducts thumb
adductor m., great	m. adductor magnus	deep part—inferior ramus of pubis, ramus of ischium; superficial part—ischial tuberosity	deep part—linea aspera of femur; superficial part—adductor tubercle of femur	deep part—obturator; superficial part—sciatic	deep part—adducts thigh; superficial part—extends thigh
adductor m. of great toe	m. adductor hallucis	oblique head—bases of metatarsals 2,3,4; sheath of peroneus longus; transverse head—capsules of metatarso-phalangeal joints	lateral side of base of proximal phalanx of great toe	lateral plantar	flexes, adducts great toe
adductor m., long	m. adductor longus	body of pubis	linea aspera of femur	obturator	adducts, rotates, flexes thigh
adductor m., short	m. adductor brevis	body and inferior ramus of pubis	upper part of linea aspera of femur	obturator	adducts, rotates, flexes thigh
adductor m., smallest	m. adductor minimus	a name given to the anterior portion of the great adductor m.	ischium, body, and ramus of pubis	obturator, sciatic	adducts thigh
adductor m. of thumb	m. adductor pollicis	oblique head—second and third metacarpals, capitate, sheath of tendon of flexor carpi radialis, palmar ligaments of carpus; transverse head—front of third metacarpal	medial side of base of proximal phalanx of thumb	ulnar	adducts, opposes thumb
anconeus m.	m. anconeus	back of lateral epicondyle of humerus	olecranon and posterior surface of ulna	radial	extends forearm
anorectoperineal m's	mm. anorectoper-ineales	bands of smooth muscle fibers in male, extending from perineal flexure of rectum to membranous part of urethra			

546

antitragicus m.	m. antitragicus	outer part of antitragus	caudate process of helix and antihelix	temporal, posterior auricular branches of facial
arrector m. of hair	m. arrector pili	dermis	hair follicle	sympathetic	elevate hair of skin
articular m. of elbow	m. articularis cubiti	a few fibers of the deep surface of the triceps m. of arm that insert into the posterior ligament and synovial membrane of the elbow joint			
articular m. of knee	m. articularis genus	front of lower part of femur	upper part of capsule of knee joint	femoral	raises capsule of knee joint
aryepiglottic m.	pars aryepiglottica musculi arytenoidei obliqui	an inconstant fascicle of oblique arytenoid m., from apex of arytenoid cartilage to lateral margin of epiglottis			
arytenoid m., oblique	m. arytenoideus obliquus	muscular process of arytenoid cartilage	apex of opposite arytenoid cartilage	recurrent laryngeal	closes inlet of larynx
arytenoid m., transverse	m. arytenoideus transversus	medial surface of arytenoid cartilage	medial surface of opposite arytenoid cartilage	recurrent laryngeal	approximates arytenoid cartilage
auricular m., anterior	m. auricularis anterior	superficial temporal fascia	cartilage of ear	facial	draws auricle forward
auricular m., oblique	m. obliquus auriculae	cranial surface of concha	cranial surface of auricle above concha	posterior auricular, temporal	
auricular m., posterior	m. auricularis posterior	mastoid process	cartilage of ear	facial	draws auricle backward
auricular m., superior	m. auricularis superior	galea aponeurotica	cartilage of ear	facial	raises auricle
auricular m., transverse. See transverse m. of auricle					
biceps m. of arm (biceps brachii m.)	m. biceps brachii	*long head*—upper border of glenoid cavity; *short head*—apex of coracoid process	tuberosity of radius, fascia of forearm	musculocutaneous	flexes, supinates forearm
biceps m. of thigh (biceps femoris m.)	m. biceps femoris	*long head*—ischial tuberosity; *short head*—linea aspera of femur	head of fibula, lateral condyle of tibia	*long head*—tibial; *short head*—peroneal, popliteal	flexes, rotates leg laterally, extends thigh
brachial m.	m. brachialis	anterior aspect of humerus	coronoid process of ulna	musculocutaneous, radial	flexes forearm
brachioradial m.	m. brachioradialis	lateral supracondylar ridge of humerus	lower end of radius	radial	flexes forearm
bronchoesophageal m.	m. bronchoesophageus	a name applied to muscle fibers arising from wall of left bronchus, reinforcing musculature of esophagus			

*m. = muscle; m's = (pl.) muscles.
†m. = [L.] musculus; mm. = ([L.] pl.) musculi.

TABLE OF MUSCLES *Continued*

Common Name*	TA Term†	Origin*	Insertion*	Innervation*	Action
buccinator m.	m. buccinator	buccinator ridge of mandible, alveolar processes of maxilla, pterygomandibular ligament	orbicularis oris m. at angle of mouth	buccal branch of facial	compresses cheek and retracts angle of mouth
bulbocavernous m., bulbocavernosus m.	m. bulbospongiosus	central point of perineum, median raphe of bulb	fascia of penis or clitoris	pudendal	constricts urethra in male, vaginal orifice in female, contributes to erection of penis or clitoris
ceratocricoid m.	m. ceratocricoideus	a name applied to muscle fibers from cricoid cartilage to inferior horn of thyroid cartilage			
chin m.	m. mentalis	incisive fossa of mandible	skin of chin	facial	wrinkles skin of chin
chondroglossus m.	m. chondroglossus	lesser horn and body of hyoid bone	substance of tongue	hypoglossal	depresses, retracts tongue
ciliary m.	m. ciliaris	scleral spur	outer layers of choroid and ciliary processes	oculomotor, parasympathetic	makes lens more convex in visual accommodation
coccygeal m.	m. ischiococcygeus	ischial spine	lateral border of lower part of sacrum, coccyx	third and fourth sacral	supports and raises coccyx
constrictor m. of pharynx, inferior	m. constrictor pharyngis inferior	undersurfaces of cricoid and thyroid cartilages	median raphe of posterior wall of pharynx	glossopharyngeal, pharyngeal plexus, branches of superior laryngeal and recurrent laryngeal	constricts pharynx
constrictor m. of pharynx, middle	m. constrictor pharyngis medius	horns of hyoid bone, stylohyoid ligament	median raphe of posterior wall of pharynx	pharyngeal plexus of vagus, glossopharyngeal	constricts pharynx
constrictor m. of pharynx, superior	m. constrictor pharyngis superior	pterygoid plate, pterygomandibular raphe, mylohyoid ridge of mandible, mucous membrane of floor of mouth	median raphe of posterior wall of pharynx	pharyngeal plexus of vagus	constricts pharynx
coracobrachial m.	m. coracobrachialis	coracoid process of scapula	medial surface of shaft of humerus	musculocutaneous	flexes, adducts arm
corrugator m., supercilii	m. corrugator supercilii	medial end of superciliary arch	skin of eyebrow	facial	draws eyebrow downward and medially
cremaster	m. cremaster	inferior margin of internal oblique m. of abdomen	pubic tubercle	genital branch of genitofemoral	elevates testis
cricoarytenoid m., lateral	m. cricoarytenoideus lateralis	lateral surface of cricoid cartilage	muscular process of arytenoid cartilage	recurrent laryngeal	approximates vocal folds
cricoarytenoid m., posterior	m. cricoarytenoideus posterior	back of cricoid cartilage	muscular process of arytenoid cartilage	recurrent laryngeal	separates vocal folds

548

English name	Latin name	Origin	Insertion	Nerve	Action
cricothyroid m.	m. cricothyroideus	front and side of cricoid cartilage	lamina of thyroid cartilage	external branch of superior laryngeal	tenses vocal folds
dartos m.	m. dartos	nonstriated muscle fibers of the tunica dartos, the deeper layers of which help to form the scrotal septum			
deltoid m.	m. deltoideus	clavicle, acromion, spine of scapula	deltoid tuberosity of humerus	axillary	abducts, flexes, extends arm
depressor m., superciliary	m. depressor supercilii	a name applied to a few fibers of orbital part of orbicularis oculi m. that are inserted into the eyebrow, which they depress			
depressor m. of angle of mouth	m. depressor anguli oris	lateral border of mandible	angle of mouth	facial	pulls down angle of mouth
depressor m. of lower lip	m. depressor labii inferioris	anterior surface of lower border of mandible	orbicularis oris m. and skin of lower lip	facial	depresses lower lip
depressor m. of nasal septum	m. depressor septi nasi	incisive fossa of maxilla	ala and septum of nose	facial	constricts nostril and depresses ala
detrusor m. of bladder	m. detrusor vesicae	bundles of smooth muscle fibers forming the muscular coat of the urinary bladder, which are arranged in a longitudinal and a circular layer and on contraction serve to expel urine			
detrusor urinae. See detrusor m. of bladder					
diaphragm	diaphragma	back of xiphoid process, inner surfaces of lower 6 costal cartilages and lower 4 ribs, medial and lateral arcuate ligaments, bodies of upper lumbar vertebrae	central tendon of diaphragm	phrenic	increases volume of thorax in inspiration
digastric m.	m. digastricus	*anterior belly*—digastric fossa on lower border of mandible near symphysis; *posterior belly*—mastoid notch of temporal bone	intermediate tendon on hyoid bone	*anterior belly*—mylohyoid; *posterior belly*—digastric branch of facial	elevates hyoid bone, lowers jaw
dilator m. of pupil	m. dilatator pupillae	a name applied to fibers extending radially from sphincter of pupil to ciliary margin		sympathetic	dilates iris
epicranial m.	m. epicranius	a name applied to muscular covering of scalp, including occipitofrontal and temporoparietal m's and galea aponeurotica			
erector m. of spine	m. erector spinae	a name applied to fibers of the more superficial of deep muscles of back, originating from sacrum, spines of lumbar and eleventh and twelfth thoracic vertebrae, and iliac crest, which split and insert as iliocostal, longissimus, and spinal m's			
extensor m. of fingers	m. extensor digitorum	lateral epicondyle of humerus	extensor expansion of each (nonthumb) finger	posterior interosseous	extends wrist joint and phalanges

TABLE OF MUSCLES *Continued*

Common Name*	TA Term†	Origin*	Insertion*	Innervation*	Action
extensor m. of great toe, long	m. extensor hallucis longus	front of fibula, interosseous membrane	base of distal phalanx of great toe	deep peroneal	extends great toe, dorsiflexes ankle joint
extensor m. of great toe, short	m. extensor hallucis brevis	a name applied to portion of short extensor m. of toes that goes to great toe			
extensor m. of index finger	m. extensor indicis	posterior surface of ulna, interosseous membrane	extensor expansion of index finger	posterior interosseous	extends index finger
extensor m. of little finger	m. extensor digiti minimi	common extensor tendon	extensor expansion of little finger	deep branch of radial	extends little finger
extensor m. of thumb, long	m. extensor pollicis longus	posterior surface of ulna, interosseous membrane	base of distal phalanx of thumb	posterior interosseous	extends thumb, adducts and rotates thumb
extensor m. of thumb, short	m. extensor pollicis brevis	posterior surface of radius, interosseous membrane	base of proximal phalanx of thumb	posterior interosseous	extends thumb
extensor m. of toes, long	m. extensor digitorum longus	anterior surface of fibula, lateral condyle of tibia, interosseous membrane	extensor expansion of each of 4 lateral toes	deep peroneal	extends toes
extensor m. of toes, short	m. extensor digitorum brevis	upper surface of calcaneus	tendons of long extensor muscle of first, second, third, fourth toes	deep peroneal	extends toes
extensor m. of wrist, long radial	m. extensor carpi radialis longus	lateral supracondylar ridge of humerus	base of second metacarpal bone	radial	extends, abducts wrist joint
extensor m. of wrist, short radial	m. extensor carpi radialis brevis	lateral epicondyle of humerus	base of third metacarpal bone	deep branch of radial	extends, abducts wrist joint
extensor m. of wrist, ulnar	m. extensor carpi ulnaris	*humeral head*—lateral epicondyle of humerus; *ulnar head*—posterior border of ulna	base of fifth metacarpal bone	deep branch of radial	extends, adducts wrist joint
fibular m's. *See* peroneal m's.					
flexor accessorius m. *See* quadratus plantae m.					
flexor m. of fingers, deep	m. flexor digitorum profundus	shaft of ulna, coronoid process, interosseous membrane	bases of distal phalanges of 4 medial fingers	anterior interosseous, ulnar	flexes distal phalanges
flexor m. of fingers, superficial	m. flexor digitorum superficialis	*humeroulnar head*—medial epicondyle of humerus, coronoid process of ulna; *radial head*—anterior border of radius	sides of middle phalanges of 4 (nonthumb) fingers	median	primarily flexes middle phalanges

550

flexor m. of great toe, long	m. flexor hallucis longus	posterior surface of fibula	base of distal phalanx of great toe	tibial	flexes great toe
flexor m. of great toe, short	m. flexor hallucis brevis	undersurface of cuboid, lateral cuneiform	both sides of base of proximal phalanx of great toe	medial plantar	flexes great toe
flexor m. of little finger, short	m. flexor digiti minimi manus	hook of hamate bone, transverse carpal ligament	medial side of proximal phalanx of little finger	ulnar	flexes little finger
flexor m. of little toe, short	m. flexor digiti minimi pedis	base of fifth metatarsal, sheath of long peroneal muscle	lateral surface of base of proximal phalanx of little toe	lateral plantar	flexes little toe
flexor m. of thumb, long	m. flexor pollicis longus	anterior surface of radius, interosseous membrane, and medial epicondyle of humerus or coronoid process of ulna	base of distal phalanx of thumb	anterior interosseous	flexes thumb
flexor m. of thumb, short	m. flexor pollicis brevis	tubercle of trapezium, flexor retinaculum	radial side of base of proximal phalanx of thumb	median, ulnar	flexes, adducts thumb
flexor m. of toes, long	m. flexor digitorum longus	posterior surface of shaft of tibia	distal phalanges of 4 lateral toes	tibial	flexes toes, plantar flexes foot
flexor m. of toes, short	m. flexor digitorum brevis	medial tuberosity of calcaneus, plantar fascia	middle phalanges of 4 lateral toes	medial plantar	flexes toes
flexor m. of wrist, radial	m. flexor carpi radialis	medial epicondyle of humerus	base of second metacarpal bone	median	flexes, abducts wrist joint
flexor m. of wrist, ulnar	m. flexor carpi ulnaris	*humeral head*—medial epicondyle of humerus; *ulnar head*—olecranon, ulna, intermuscular septum	pisiform, hook of hamate, base of fifth metacarpal	ulnar	flexes, adducts wrist joint
gastrocnemius m.	m. gastrocnemius	*medial head*—popliteal surface of femur, upper part of medial condyle, capsule of knee; *lateral head*—lateral condyle, capsule of knee	aponeurosis unites with tendon of soleus to form Achilles tendon	tibial	plantar flexes foot, flexes knee joint
gemellus m., inferior	m. gemellus inferior	tuberosity of ischium	greater trochanter of femur	nerve to quadratus femoris m.	rotates thigh laterally
gemellus m., superior	m. gemellus superior	spine of ischium	greater trochanter of femur	nerve to internal obturator	rotates thigh laterally
genioglossus m.	m. genioglossus	superior mental spine	hyoid bone, undersurface of tongue	hypoglossal	protrudes, depresses tongue
geniohyoid m.	m. geniohyoideus	inferior mental spine	body of hyoid bone	a branch of first cervical nerve through hypoglossal	elevates and draws hyoid bone forward, or depresses mandible when hyoid fixed
glossopalatine m. *See* palatoglossus m.					

TABLE OF MUSCLES *Continued*

Common Name*	TA Term†	Origin*	Insertion*	Innervation*	Action
gluteus maximus m. (gluteal m., greatest)	m. gluteus maximus	posterior aspect of ilium, posterior surfaces of sacrum, coccyx, sacrotuberous ligament, fascia covering gluteus medius	iliotibial tract of fascia lata, gluteal tuberosity of femur	inferior gluteal	extends, abducts, rotates thigh laterally
gluteus medius m. (gluteal m., middle)	m. gluteus medius	lateral surface of ilium between anterior and posterior gluteal lines	greater trochanter of femur	superior gluteal	abducts, rotates thigh medially
gluteus minimus m. (gluteal m., least)	m. gluteus minimus	lateral surface of ilium between anterior and inferior gluteal lines	greater trochanter of femur	superior gluteal	abducts, rotates thigh medially
gracilis m.	m. gracilis	body and inferior ramus of pubis	medial surface of shaft of tibia	obturator	adducts thigh, flexes knee joint
m. of helix, greater	m. helicis major	spine of helix	anterior border of helix	auriculotemporal, posterior auricular	tenses skin of acoustic meatus
m. of helix, smaller	m. helicis minor	anterior rim of helix	concha	temporal, posterior auricular	
hyoglossus m.	m. hyoglossus	body and greater horn of hyoid bone	side of tongue	hypoglossal	depresses, retracts tongue
iliac m.	m. iliacus	iliac fossa, base of sacrum	greater psoas tendon, lesser trochanter of femur	femoral	flexes thigh, trunk on limb
iliococcygeal m.	m. iliococcygeus	a name applied to posterior portion of levator ani m., including fibers originating as far forward as obturator canal, and inserting on side of coccyx and in anococcygeal ligament		third and fourth sacral	helps support pelvic viscera, resists increases in intraabdominal pressure
iliocostal m.	m. iliocostalis	a name applied to lateral division of erector m. of spine			
iliocostal m., lumbar	m. iliocostalis lumborum	iliac crest	angles of lower 6 or 7 ribs	thoracic and lumbar	extends lumbar spine
iliocostal m. of neck	m. iliocostalis cervicis	angles of third, fourth, fifth, and sixth ribs	transverse processes of fourth, fifth, and sixth cervical vertebrae	cervical	extends cervical spine
iliocostal m. of thorax	m. iliocostalis thoracis	upper borders of angles of 6 lower ribs	angles of 6 upper ribs and transverse process of seventh cervical vertebra	thoracic	keeps thoracic spine erect
iliopsoas m.	m. iliopsoas	a name applied collectively to iliac and greater psoas m's			
incisive m's of inferior lip		incisive fossae of mandible	angle of mouth	facial	apply lower lip to teeth and alveolar arch
incisive m's of superior lip		incisive fossae of maxilla	angle of mouth	facial	apply upper lip to teeth and alveolar arch

Common name	Latin name	Origin	Insertion	Nerve	Action
infraspinous m.	m. infraspinatus	infraspinous fossa of scapula	greater tubercle of humerus	suprascapular	rotates arm laterally
intercostal m's, external	mm. intercostales externi	inferior border of rib	superior border of rib below	intercostal	primarily elevate ribs in inspiration
intercostal m's, innermost	mm. intercostales intimi	the layer of muscle fibers separated from the internal intercostal m's by the intercostal nerves			
intercostal m's, internal	mm. intercostales interni	inferior border of rib and costal cartilage	superior border of rib and costal cartilage below	intercostal	primarily act on ribs in expiration
interosseous m's of foot, dorsal	mm. interossei dorsales pedis	sides of adjacent metatarsal bones	base of proximal phalanges of second, third, and fourth toes and extensor expansions	lateral plantar	flex, abduct toes
interosseous m's of hand, dorsal	mm. interossei dorsales manus	each by two heads from adjacent sides of metacarpal bones	bases of proximal phalanges and corresponding extensor expansions of second, third, and fourth fingers	ulnar	abduct fingers, flex proximal, extend middle and distal phalanges
interosseous m's, palmar	mm. interossei palmares	sides of second, fourth, and fifth metacarpal bones	bases of proximal phalanges and corresponding extensor expansions of second, fourth, and fifth fingers	ulnar	adduct fingers, flex proximal, extend middle and distal phalanges
interosseous m's, plantar	mm. interossei plantares	medial side of third, fourth, and fifth metatarsal bones	medial side of base of proximal phalanges of third, fourth, and fifth toes and extensor expansions	lateral plantar	flex, adduct toes
interspinal m's	mm. interspinales	a name applied to short bands of muscle fibers extending on each side between spinous processes of contiguous vertebrae		spinal	extend vertebral column
interspinal m's, lumbar	mm. interspinales lumborum	extend between contiguous lumbar vertebrae		spinal	extend vertebral column
interspinal m's of neck	mm. interspinales cervicis	extend between contiguous cervical vertebrae		spinal	extend vertebral column
interspinal m's of thorax	mm. interspinales thoracis	extend between contiguous thoracic vertebrae		spinal	extend vertebral column
intertransverse m's	mm. intertransversarii	a name applied to small muscles passing between transverse processes of adjacent vertebrae		anterior branches of spinal	bend vertebral column laterally
intertransverse m's, lateral lumbar	mm. intertransversarii laterales lumborum	extend between transverse processes of adjacent lumbar vertebrae		posterior branches of spinal	bend vertebral column laterally
intertransverse m's, medial lumbar	mm. intertransversarii mediales lumborum	extend between accessory process of one lumbar vertebra to mammillary process of contiguous vertebra		anterior branches of spinal	bend vertebral column laterally
intertransverse m's of neck, anterior	mm. intertransversarii anteriores cervicis	extend between anterior tubercles of adjacent cervical vertebrae		anterior branches of spinal	bend vertebral column laterally

Common Name*	TA Term†	Origin*	Insertion*	Innervation*	Action
intertransverse m's of neck, lateral posterior	mm. intertransversarii posteriores laterales cervicis	extend between posterior tubercles of adjacent cervical vertebrae		anterior branches of spinal	bend vertebral column laterally
intertransverse m's of neck, medial posterior	mm. intertransversarii posteriores mediales cervicis	extend between posterior tubercles of adjacent cervical vertebrae		posterior branches of spinal	bend vertebral column laterally
intertransverse m's of thorax	mm. intertransversarii thoracis	extend between anterior tubercles of adjacent thoracic vertebrae		posterior branches of spinal	bend vertebral column laterally
ischiocavernous m.	m. ischiocavernosus	ramus of ischium	crus of penis or clitoris	perineal	maintains erection of penis or clitoris
ischiococcygeal m. *See* coccygeal m.					
latissimus dorsi m.	m. latissimus dorsi	spines of lower thoracic vertebrae, spines of lumbar and sacral vertebrae through attachment to thoracolumbar fascia, iliac crest, lower ribs, inferior angle of scapula	floor of intertubercular groove of humerus	thoracodorsal	adducts, extends, rotates humerus medially
levator m. of angle of mouth	m. levator anguli oris	canine fossa of maxilla	orbicularis oris m., skin at angle of mouth	facial	raises angle of mouth
levator ani m.	m. levator ani	a name applied collectively to important muscular components of pelvic diaphragm; includes pubococcygeal, puborectal, and iliococcygeal m's		third and fourth sacral	helps support pelvic viscera and resist increases in intra-abdominal pressure
levator m. of prostate. *See* pubo-prostatic m.					
levator m's of ribs	mm. levatores costarum	transverse processes of seventh cervical and first 11 thoracic vertebrae	medial to angle of a lower rib	intercostal	aid elevation of ribs in respiration
levator m's of ribs, long	mm. levatores costarum longi	the lower levator m's of ribs of each side, which have fascicles extending down to the second rib below the vertebra of origin			
levator m's of ribs, short	mm. levatores costarum breves	the levator m's of ribs of each side that insert into the rib next below the vertebra of origin			

levator m. of scapula	m. levator scapulae	transverse processes of 4 upper cervical vertebrae	medial border of scapula	third and fourth cervical	raises scapula
levator m. of thyroid gland	m. levator glandulae thyroideae	isthmus or pyramid of thyroid gland	body of hyoid bone		
levator m. of upper eyelid	m. levator palpebrae superioris	sphenoid bone above optic canal	skin and tarsal plate of upper eyelid	oculomotor	raises upper eyelid
levator m. of upper lip	m. levator labii superioris	lower margin of orbit	musculature of upper lip	facial	raises upper lip
levator m. of upper lip and ala of nose	m. levator labii superioris alaeque nasi	frontal process of maxilla	skin and cartilage of ala nasi, upper lip	infraorbital branch of facial	raises upper lip, dilates nostril
levator veli palatini m.	m. levator veli palatini	apex of petrous part of temporal bone and cartilage of auditory tube	aponeurosis of soft palate	pharyngeal plexus	raises and draws back soft palate
long m. of head	m. longus capitis	transverse processes of third to sixth cervical vertebrae	basilar part of occipital bone	cervical	flexes head
long m. of neck	m. longus colli	*superior oblique portion*—transverse processes of third to fifth cervical vertebrae; *inferior oblique portion*—bodies of first to third thoracic vertebrae; *vertical portion*—bodies of 3 upper thoracic and 3 lower cervical vertebrae	*superior oblique portion*—tubercle of anterior arch of atlas; *inferior oblique portion*—transverse processes of fifth and sixth cervical vertebrae; *vertical portion*—bodies of second to fourth cervical vertebrae	anterior cervical	flexes, supports cervical vertebrae
longissimus m.	m. longissimus	the largest element of the erector spinae m., including the longissimus m's of head, neck, and thorax			
longissimus m. of head	m. longissimus capitis	transverse processes of 4 or 5 upper thoracic vertebrae, articular processes of 3 or 4 lower cervical vertebrae	mastoid process of temporal bone	cervical	draws head backward, rotates head
longissimus m. of neck	m. longissimus cervicis	transverse processes of 4 or 5 upper thoracic vertebrae	transverse processes of second or third to sixth cervical vertebrae	lower cervical and upper thoracic	extends cervical vertebrae
longissimus m. of thorax	m. longissimus thoracis	transverse and articular processes of lumbar vertebrae and thoracolumbar fascia	transverse processes of all thoracic vertebrae, 9 or 10 lower ribs	lumbar and thoracic	extends thoracic vertebrae
longitudinal m. of tongue, inferior	m. longitudinalis inferior linguae	undersurface of tongue at base	tip of tongue	hypoglossal	changes shape of tongue in mastication and deglutition
longitudinal m. of tongue, superior	m. longitudinalis superior linguae	submucosa and septum of tongue	margins of tongue	hypoglossal	changes shape of tongue in mastication and deglutition

Common Name*	TA Term†	Origin*	Insertion*	Innervation*	Action
lumbrical m's of foot	mm. lumbricales pedis	tendons of long flexor m's of toes	extensor expansions of 4 lateral toes	medial and lateral plantar	flex metatarsophalangeal joints, extend distal phalanges
lumbrical m's of hand	mm. lumbricales manus	tendons of deep flexor m's of fingers	extensor expansions of 4 non-thumb fingers	median, ulnar	flex metacarpophalangeal joints, extend middle and distal phalanges
masseter m.	m. masseter	*superficial part*—zygomatic process of maxilla, lower border of zygomatic arch; *deep part*—lower border and medial surface of zygomatic arch	*superficial part*—angle and ramus of mandible; *deep part*—upper half of ramus and lateral surface of coronoid process of mandible	masseteric, from mandibular division of trigeminal	raises mandible, closes jaws
multifidus m's	mm. multifidi	sacrum, sacroiliac ligament, mammillary processes of lumbar, transverse processes of thoracic, and articular processes of cervical vertebrae	spines of contiguous vertebrae above	spinal	extend, rotate vertebral column
mylohyoid m.	m. mylohyoideus	mylohyoid line of mandible	body of hyoid bone, median raphe	mylohyoid branch of inferior alveolar	elevates hyoid bone, supports floor of mouth
nasal m.	m. nasalis	maxilla	*alar part*—ala nasi; *transverse part*—by aponeurotic expansion with fellow of opposite side	facial	*alar part*—aids in widening nostril; *transverse part*—depresses cartilage of nose
oblique m. of abdomen, external	m. obliquus externus abdominus	lower 8 ribs at costal cartilages	crest of ilium, linea alba through rectus sheath	lower intercostal	flexes, rotates vertebral column, compresses abdominal viscera
oblique m. of abdomen, internal	m. obliquus internus abdominis	thoracolumbar fascia, iliac crest, inguinal ligament	lower 3 or 4 costal cartilages, linea alba, conjoined tendon to pubis	lower intercostal, first lumbar	flexes, rotates vertebral column, compresses abdominal viscera
oblique m. of auricle. *See* auricular m., oblique					
oblique m. of eyeball, inferior	m. obliquus inferior bulbi	orbital surface of maxilla	sclera	oculomotor	rotates eyeball upward and outward
oblique m. of eyeball, superior	m. obliquus superior bulbi	lesser wing of sphenoid above optic canal	sclera	trochlear	rotates eyeball downward and outward
oblique m. of head, inferior	m. obliquus capitis inferior	spinous process of axis	transverse process of atlas	spinal	rotates atlas and head
oblique m. of head, superior	m. obliquus capitis superior	transverse process of atlas	occipital bone	spinal	extends and moves head laterally

		Origin	Insertion	Nerve	Action
obturator m., external	m. obturatorius externus	pubis, ischium, external surface of obturator membrane	trochanteric fossa of femur	obturator	rotates thigh laterally
obturator m., internal	m. obturatorius internus	pelvic surface of hip bone and obturator membrane, margin of obturator foramen, ramus of ischium, inferior ramus of pubis	greater trochanter of femur	fifth lumbar, first and second sacral	rotates thigh laterally
occipitofrontal m.	m. occipitofrontalis	*frontal belly*—galea aponeurotica; *occipital belly*—highest nuchal line of occipital bone	*frontal belly*—skin of eyebrow, root of nose; *occipital belly*—galea aponeurotica	*frontal belly*—temporal branch of facial; *occipital belly*—posterior auricular branch of facial	*frontal belly*—raises eyebrow; *occipital belly*—draws scalp backward
omohyoid m.	m. omohyoideus	superior border of scapula	body of hyoid bone	upper cervical through ansa cervicalis	depresses hyoid bone
opposing m. of little finger	m. opponens digiti minimi manus	hook of hamate bone, flexor retinaculum	ulnar margin of fifth metacarpal	eigth cervical through ulnar	abducts, flexes, rotates fifth metacarpal
opposing m. of thumb	m. opponens pollicis	tubercle of trapezium, flexor retinaculum	radial side of first metacarpal	sixth and seventh metacarpal through median	flexes, opposes thumb
orbicularis oculi m.	m. orbicularis oculi	*orbital part*—medial margin of orbit, including frontal process of maxilla; *palpebral part*—medial palpebral ligament; *lacrimal part*—posterior lacrimal crest	*orbital part*—near origin after encircling orbit; *palpebral part*—fibers intertwine into lateral palpebral raphe; *lacrimal part*—lateral palpebral raphe, upper and lower tarsi	facial	closes eyelids, wrinkles forehead, compresses lacrimal sac
orbicularis oris m.	m. orbicularis oris	a name applied to complicated sphincter muscle of mouth, comprising 2 parts: *labial part*—consisting of fibers restricted to lips; *marginal part*—consisting of fibers blending with those of adjacent muscles		facial	closes, protrudes lips
orbital m.	m. orbitalis	bridges inferior orbital fissure	fascia of inferior orbital fissure	sympathetic fibers	
palatoglossus m.	m. palatoglossus	undersurface of soft palate	side of tongue	pharyngeal plexus	elevates tongue, constricts fauces
palatopharyngeal m.	m. palatopharyngeus	soft palate	posterior border of thyroid cartilage, aponeurosis of pharynx	pharyngeal plexus	aids swallowing
palmar m., long	m. palmaris longus	medial epicondyle of humerus	flexor retinaculum, palmar aponeurosis	median	flexes wrist joint, anchors skin and fascia of hand
palmar m., short	m. palmaris brevis	palmar aponeurosis	skin of medial border of hand	ulnar	assists in deepening hollow of palm
papillary m's	mm. papillares cordis	a name applied to conical muscular projections from walls of cardiac ventricles, attached to cusps of atrioventricular valves by chordae tendineae; there are anterior and posterior papillary m's in each ventricle and a group of small papillary m's on the septum in the right ventricle			steady and strengthen atrioventricular valves and prevent eversion of their cusps

TABLE OF MUSCLES *Continued*

Common Name*	TA Term†	Origin*	Insertion*	Innervation*	Action
pectinate m's	mm. pectinati atrii	a name applied to small ridges of muscular fibers projecting from inner walls of auricles of heart, and extending in right atrium from auricle to crista terminalis			
pectineal m.	m. pectineus	pectineal line of pubis	pectineal line of femur	femoral, obturator	flexes, adducts thigh
pectoral m., greater	m. pectoralis major	clavicle, sternum, 6 upper costal cartilages, aponeurosis of external oblique m. of abdomen	crest of greater tubercle of humerus	lateral and medial pectoral	adducts, flexes, rotates arm medially
pectoral m., smaller	m. pectoralis minor	third, fourth, and fifth ribs	coracoid process of scapula	medial and lateral pectoral	draws shoulder forward and downward, raises third, fourth, and fifth ribs in forced inspiration
peroneal n., long	m. peroneus longus	lateral condyle of tibia, head and lateral surface of fibula	medial cuneiform, first metatarsal	superficial peroneal	plantar flexes, everts, abducts foot
peroneal n., short	m. peroneus brevis	lateral surface of fibula	base of fifth metatarsal	superficial peroneal	everts, abducts, plantar flexes foot
peroneal m., third	m. peroneus tertius	anterior surface of fibula, interosseous membrane	base of fifth metatarsal	deep peroneal	everts, dorsiflexes foot
piriform m.	m. piriformis	ilium, second to fourth sacral vertebrae	greater trochanter of femur	first and second sacral	rotates thigh laterally
plantar m.	m. plantaris	ridge at lower end of femur	posterior part of calcaneus	tibial	plantar flexes foot, flexes knee
platysma	platysma	a name applied to a platelike muscle originating from the fascia of cervical region and inserting in mandible and skin around mouth		cervical branch of facial	wrinkles skin of neck, depresses jaw
pleuroesophageal m.	m. pleuroesophageus	a bundle of smooth muscle fibers usually connecting esophagus with left mediastinal pleura			
popliteal m.	m. popliteus	lateral condyle of femur, lateral meniscus	posterior surface of tibia	tibial	flexes leg, rotates leg medially
procerus m.	m. procerus	fascia over nasal bone	skin of forehead	facial	draws medial angle of eyebrows down
pronator m., quadrate	m. pronator quadratus	anterior surface and border of distal third or fourth of shaft of radius	anterior surface and border of distal fourth of shaft of radius	anterior interosseous	pronates forearm
pronator m., round	m. pronator teres	*humeral head*—medial epicondyle of humerus; *ulnar head*—coronoid process of ulna	lateral surface of radius	median	pronates forearm, flexes elbow
psoas m., greater	m. psoas major	lumbar vertebrae	lesser trochanter of femur	second and third lumbar	flexes thigh or trunk

558

Common name	Latin name	Origin	Insertion	Nerve	Action
psoas m., smaller	m. psoas minor	last thoracic and first lumbar vertebrae	pectineal line, iliopectineal eminence, iliac fascia	first lumbar	flexes trunk
pterygoid m., lateral (external)	m. pterygoideus lateralis	*superior head*—infratemporal surface of greater wing of sphenoid, infratemporal crest; *inferior head*—lateral surface of lateral pterygoid plate	neck of condyle of mandible, capsule of temporomandibular joint	mandibular	protrudes mandible, opens jaws, moves mandible from side to side
pterygoid m., medial (internal)	m. pterygoideus medialis	medial surface of lateral pterygoid plate, tuberosity of maxilla	medial surface of ramus and angle of mandible	mandibular	closes jaws
pubococcygeal m.	m. pubococcygeus	a name applied to anterior portion of levator ani m., originating in front of obturator canal and inserting in anococcygeal ligament and side of coccyx		third and fourth sacral	helps support pelvic viscera and resist increases in intra-abdominal pressure
puboprostatic m.	m. puboprostaticus	a name applied to part of anterior portion of pubococcygeal m., which in male is inserted into prostate and tendinous center of perineum		pudendal	supports, compresses prostate, helps control micturition
puborectal m.	m. puborectalis	a name applied to portion of levator ani m., with a more lateral origin from pubic bone, and continuous posteriorly with corresponding muscle of opposite side		third and fourth sacral	helps support pelvic viscera and resist increases in intraabdominal pressure
pubovaginal m.	m. pubovaginalis	a name applied to part of anterior portion of pubococcygeal m., which is inserted into urethra and vagina		pudendal	helps control micturition
pubovesical m.	m. pubovesicalis	smooth muscle fibers extending from neck of urinary bladder to pubis			
pyloric sphincter	m. sphincter pyloricus	a thickening of the circular muscle of the stomach around its opening into the duodenum			
pyramidal m.	m. pyramidalis	anterior aspect of pubis, anterior pubic ligament	linea alba	last thoracic	tenses abdominal wall
pyramidal m. of auricle	m. pyramidalis auriculae	a name applied to inconstant prolongation of fibers of m. of tragus to spine of helix			
quadratus femoris m.	m. quadratus femoris	tuberosity of ischium	intertrochanteric crest and quadrate tubercle of femur	fourth and fifth lumbar, first sacral	adducts, rotates thigh laterally
quadratus lumborum m.	m. quadratus lumborum	iliac crest, thoracolumbar fascia	twelfth rib, transverse processes of 4 upper lumbar vertebrae	first and second lumbar, twelfth thoracic	flexes lumbar vertebrae laterally, fixes last rib
quadratus plantae m.	m. quadratus plantae	calcaneus, plantar fascia	tendons of long flexor m. of toes	lateral plantar	aids in flexing toes
quadriceps m. of thigh	m. quadriceps femoris	a name applied collectively to rectus femoris m. and intermediate, lateral, and medial vastus m's, inserting by a common tendon that surrounds patella and ends on tuberosity of tibia		femoral	extends leg upon thigh

TABLE OF MUSCLES *Continued*

Common Name*	TA Term†	Origin*	Insertion*	Innervation*	Action
rectococcygeal m.	m. rectococcygeus	smooth muscle fibers originating on anterior surface of second and third coccygeal vertebrae and inserting on posterior surface of rectum		autonomic	retracts, elevates rectum
rectourethral m. *See anorectoperineal m's*					
rectouterine m.	m. rectouterinus	a band of fibers in female, running between cervix uteri and rectum, in rectouterine fold		lower thoracic	flexes lumbar vertebrae, supports abdomen
rectovesical m.	m. rectovesicalis	a band of fibers in male, connecting longitudinal musculature of rectum with external muscular coat of bladder		first and second cervical	flexes, supports head
rectus abdominis m.	m. rectus abdominis	pubic crest and symphysis	xiphoid process, fifth, sixth, and seventh costal cartilages	first and second cervical	flexes, supports head
rectus capitis anterior m.	m. rectus capitis anterior	lateral mass of atlas	basilar part of occipital bone	suboccipital, greater occipital	extends head
rectus capitis lateralis m.	m. rectus capitis lateralis	transverse process of atlas	jugular process of occipital bone	suboccipital, greater occipital	extends head
rectus capitis posterior major m.	m. rectus capitis posterior major	spinous process of axis	occipital bone	oculomotor	adducts, rotates eyeball downward and medially
rectus capitis posterior minor m.	m. rectus capitis posterior minor	tubercle on posterior arch of atlas	occipital bone	abducens	abducts eyeball
rectus m. of eyeball, inferior	m. rectus inferior bulbi	common tendinous ring	underside of sclera	oculomotor	adducts eyeball
rectus m. of eyeball, lateral	m. rectus lateralis bulbi	common tendinous ring	lateral side of sclera	oculomotor	adducts, rotates eyeball upward and medially
rectus m. of eyeball, medial	m. rectus medialis bulbi	common tendinous ring	medial side of sclera	femoral	extends knee, flexes thigh at hip
rectus m. of eyeball, superior	m. rectus superior bulbi	common tendinous ring	upper aspect of sclera	dorsal scapular	adducts, elevates scapula
rectus femoris m.	m. rectus femoris	anterior inferior iliac spine, rim of acetabulum	base of patella, tuberosity of tibia	dorsal scapular	adducts, elevates scapula
rhomboid major m.	m. rhomboideus major	spinous processes of second, third, fourth, and fifth thoracic vertebrae	medial margin of scapula		
rhomboid minor m.	m. rhomboideus minor	spinous processes of seventh cervical and first thoracic vertebrae, lower part of nuchal ligament	medial margin of scapula at root of spine		

risorius m.	m. risorius	fascia over masseter	skin at angle of mouth	buccal branch of facial	draws angles of mouth laterally
rotator m's	mm. rotatores	a name applied to a series of small muscles deep in groove between spinous and transverse processes of vertebrae, connecting a vertebra with the vertebra one or two above it		spinal	extend and rotate vertebral column toward opposite side
sacrococcygeal m., dorsal (posterior)		a name applied to muscular slip passing from dorsal surface of sacrum to coccyx			
sacrococcygeal m., ventral (anterior)		a name applied to musculotendinous slip passing from lower sacral vertebrae to coccyx			
sacrospinal m. See erector m. of spine					
salpingopharyngeal m.	m. salpingopharyngeus	cartilage of auditory tube	posterior part of palatopharyngeal m.	pharyngeal plexus	raises pharynx
sartorius m.	m. sartorius	anterior superior iliac spine	upper part of medial surface of tibia	femoral	flexes knee at leg, thigh at pelvis
scalene m., anterior	m. scalenus anterior	transverse processes of third to sixth cervical vertebrae	scalene tubercle of first rib	fourth to sixth cervical	raises first rib, flexes cervical vertebrae laterally and forward and rotates to opposite side
scalene m., middle	m. scalenus medius	transverse processes of second to seventh cervical vertebrae and often atlas	upper surface of first rib	third to eighth cervical	raises first rib, flexes cervical vertebrae laterally and forward and rotates to opposite side
scalene m., posterior	m. scalenus posterior	transverse processes of fourth to sixth cervical vertebrae	second rib	sixth to eighth cervical	raises second rib, flexes cervical vertebrae laterally
scalene m., smallest	m. scalenus minimus	transverse process of seventh cervical vertebra	first rib, suprapleural membrane	seventh cervical	raises first rib, flexes and rotates cervical vertebrae, supports suprapleural membrane
semimembranous m.	m. semimembranosus	tuberosity of ischium	lateral condyle of femur, medial condyle and border of tibia	tibial	flexes and rotates leg medially, extends thigh
semispinal m. of head	m. semispinalis capitis	transverse processes of upper thoracic and lower cervical vertebrae	occipital bone	suboccipital, greater occipital, other branches of cervical	extends, rotates head
semispinal m. of neck	m. semispinalis cervicis	transverse processes of upper thoracic vertebrae	spinous processes of second to fifth cervical vertebrae	branches of cervical	extends, rotates vertebral column
semispinal m. of thorax	m. semispinalis thoracis	transverse processes of lower thoracic vertebrae	spinous processes of lower cervical and upper thoracic vertebrae	spinal	extends, rotates vertebral column
semitendinous m.	m. semitendinosus	tuberosity of ischium	upper part of medial surface of tibia	tibial	flexes and rotates leg medially, extends thigh

TABLE OF MUSCLES *Continued*

Common Name*	TA Term†	Origin*	Insertion*	Innervation*	Action
serratus m., anterior	m. serratus anterior	8 or 9 upper ribs	medial border of scapula	long thoracic	draws scapula forward, rotates scapula to raise shoulder in abduction of arm
serratus m., inferior posterior	m. serratus posterior inferior	spines of lower thoracic and upper lumbar vertebrae	4 lower ribs	ninth to twelfth (or eleventh) thoracic	lowers ribs in expiration
serratus m., superior posterior	m. serratus posterior superior	nuchal ligament, spinous processes of upper thoracic vertebrae	second to fifth ribs	upper 4 thoracic	raises ribs in inspiration
soleus m.	m. soleus	fibula, tibia, tendinous arch between tibia and fibula	calcaneus by Achilles tendon	tibial	plantar flexes foot
sphincter m. of anus, external	m. sphincter ani externus	tip of coccyx, anococcygeal ligament	tendinous center of perineum	inferior rectal, perineal branch of fourth sacral	closes anus
sphincter m. of anus, internal	m. sphincter ani internus	a thickening of circular layer of muscular tunic at caudal end of rectum			
sphincter m. of bile duct	m. sphincter ductus choledochi	an annular sheath of circular layer of muscle fibers investing bile duct within wall of duodenum			
sphincter m. of female urethra, external	m. sphincter urethrae externus urethrae femininae	ramus of pubis	median raphe behind and in front of urethra	perineal	compresses central part of urethra
sphincter m. of hepatopancreatic ampulla	m. sphincter ampullae hepato-pancreaticae	an annular band of muscle fibers investing hepatopancreatic ampulla within wall of duodenum			
sphincter m. of male urethra, external	m. sphincter urethrae externus urethrae masculinae	ramus of pubis	median raphe behind and in front of urethra	perineal	compresses membranous part of urethra
sphincter m. of pupil	m. sphincter pupillae	a name applied to circular fibers of iris		parasympathetic through ciliary	constricts pupil
sphincter m. of urethra, internal	m. sphincter urethrae internus	a name applied to circular layer of fibers surrounding internal urethral orifice in males		vesical	closes internal orifice of urethra
spinal m. of head	m. spinalis capitis	spinous processes of upper thoracic and lower cervical vertebrae	occipital bone	branches of cervical	extends head
spinal m. of neck	m. spinalis cervicis	spinous process of seventh cervical vertebra, nuchal ligament	spinous processes of axis	branches of cervical	extends vertebral column

spinal m. of thorax	m. spinalis thoracis	spinous processes of upper lumbar and lower thoracic vertebrae	spinous processes of upper thoracic vertebrae	branches of thoracic and lumbar	extends vertebral column
splenius m. of head	m. splenius capitis	lower half of nuchal ligament, spinous processes of seventh cervical and upper thoracic vertebra	mastoid part of temporal bone, occipital bone	cervical	extends, rotates head
splenius m. of neck	m. splenius cervicis	spinous processes of third to sixth thoracic vertebrae	transverse processes of upper cervical vertebrae	cervical	extends, rotates head and neck
stapedius m.	m. stapedius	interior of pyramidal eminence of tympanic cavity	posterior of neck of stapes	facial	dampens movement of stapes
sternal m.	m. sternalis	a name applied to muscular band occasionally found parallel to sternum on sternocostal end of greater pectoral m.			
sternocleidomastoid m.	m. sternocleidomastoideus	*sternal head*—manubrium sterni; *clavicular head*—medial third of clavicle	mastoid process, superior nuchal line of occipital bone	accessory, cervical plexus	flexes vertebral column, rotates head to opposite side
sternohyoid m.	m. sternohyoideus	manubrium sterni, clavicle, posterior sternoclavicular ligament	body of hyoid bone	ansa cervicalis	depresses hyoid bone and larynx
sternothyroid m.	m. sternothyroideus	manubrium sterni	lamina of thyroid cartilage	ansa cervicalis	depresses thyroid cartilage
styloglossus m.	m. styloglossus	styloid process	margin of tongue	hypoglossal	raises, retracts tongue
stylohyoid m.	m. stylohyoideus	styloid process	body of hyoid bone	facial	draws hyoid bone and tongue upward and backward
stylopharyngeal m.	m. stylopharyngeus	styloid process	thyroid cartilage, side of pharynx	glossopharyngeal, pharyngeal plexus	raises, dilates pharynx
subclavius m.	m. subclavius	first rib and its cartilage	lower surface of clavicle	fifth and sixth cervical	depresses lateral end of clavicle
subcostal m's	mm. subcostales	inner surface of ribs	inner surface of second or third rib below	intercostal	draw adjacent ribs together, depress ribs
subscapular m.	m. subscapularis	subscapular fossa of scapula	lesser tubercle of humerus	subscapular	rotates arm medially
supinator m.	m. supinator	lateral epicondyle of humerus, ligaments of elbow, ulna	radius	deep branch of radial	supinates forearm
supraspinous m.	m. supraspinatus	supraspinous fossa of scapula	greater tubercle of humerus	suprascapular	abducts arm
suspensory m. of duodenum	m. suspensorius duodeni	a name applied to flat band of smooth muscle fibers originating from left crus of diaphragm and inserting continuous with muscular coat of duodenum at its junction with jejunum			
tarsal m., inferior	m. tarsalis inferior	inferior rectus m. of eyeball	tarsal plate of lower eyelid	sympathetic	widens palpebral fissure
tarsal m., superior	m. tarsalis superior	levator m. of upper eyelid	tarsal plate of upper eyelid	sympathetic	widens palpebral fissure
temporal m.	m. temporalis	temporal fossa and fascia	coronoid process of mandible	mandibular	closes jaws

Common Name*	TA Term†	Origin*	Insertion*	Innervation*	Action
temporoparietal m.	m. temporoparietalis	temporal fascia above ear	galea aponeurotica	temporal branches of facial	tightens scalp
tensor fasciae latae m.	m. tensor fasciae latae	iliac crest	iliotibial tract of fascia lata	superior gluteal	flexes, rotates thigh medially
tensor tympani m.	m. tensor tympani	cartilaginous portion of auditory tube	manubrium of malleus	mandibular	tenses tympanic membrane
tensor veli palatini m.	m. tensor veli palatini	scaphoid fossa of pterygoid process, spine of sphenoid, wall of auditory tube	aponeurosis of soft palate, horizontal part of palatine bone	mandibular	tenses soft palate, opens auditory tube
teres major m.	m. teres major	inferior angle of scapula	lip of intertubercular sulcus of humerus	lower subscapular	adducts, extends, and rotates arm medially
teres minor m.	m. teres minor	lateral margin of scapula	greater tubercle of humerus	axillary	rotates arm laterally
m. of terminal notch	m. incisurae terminalis	an inconstant muscular slip continuing forward from m. of tragus to bridge notch of cartilaginous part of meatus			
thyroarytenoid m.	m. thyroarytenoideus	lamina of thyroid cartilage	muscular process of arytenoid cartilage	recurrent laryngeal	relaxes, shortens vocal folds
thyroepiglottic m.	pars thyroepiglottica musculi thyroarytenoidei	lamina of thyroid cartilage	epiglottis	recurrent laryngeal	closes inlet to larynx
thyrohyoid m.	m. thyrohyoideus	lamina of thyroid cartilage	greater horn of hyoid bone	first cervical	raises and changes form of larynx
tibial m., anterior	m. tibialis anterior	lateral condyle and surface of tibia, interosseous membrane	medial cuneiform, base of first metatarsal	deep peroneal	dorsiflexes, inverts foot
tibial m., posterior	m. tibialis posterior	tibia, fibula, interosseous membrane	bases of second to fourth metatarsal bones and tarsal bones, except talus	tibial	plantar flexes, inverts foot
tracheal m.	m. trachealis	a transverse layer of smooth muscle fibers filling gap at back of each cartilage of trachea		autonomic	lessens caliber of trachea
m. of tragus	m. tragicus	a short, flattened vertical band on lateral surface of tragus, innervated by auriculotemporal and posterior auricular nerves			
transverse m. of auricle	m. transversus auriculae	cranial surface of auricle	circumference of auricle	posterior auricular	retracts helix
transverse perineal m., deep	m. transversus perinei profundus	ramus of ischium	tendinous center of perineum	perineal	fixes tendinous center of perineum
transverse perineal m., superficial	m. transversus perinei superficialis	ramus of ischium	tendinous center of perineum	perineal	fixes tendinous center of perineum

564

transverse m. of tongue	m. transversus linguae	median septum of tongue	dorsum and margins of tongue	hypoglossal	changes shape of tongue in mastication and swallowing
transversospinal m's	mm. transversospinales	a name applied collectively to semispinal, multifidus, and rotator m's			
transversus abdominis m.	m. transversus abdominis	lower 6 costal cartilages, thoracolumbar fascia, iliac crest, inguinal ligament	linea alba through rectus sheath, conjoined tendon to pubis	lower intercostals, iliohypogastric, ilioinguinal	compresses abdominal viscera
transversus menti m.	m. transversus menti	superficial fibers of depressor m. of angle of mouth which turn medially and cross to opposite side			
transversus nuchae m.	m. transversus nuchae	a small muscle often present, passing from occipital protuberance to posterior auricular m.; it may be either superficial or deep to trapezius			
transversus thoracis m.	m. transversus thoracis	posterior surface of body of sternum and of xiphoid process	second to sixth costal cartilages	intercostal	draws ribs downward
trapezius m.	m. trapezius	occipital bone, nuchal ligament, spinous processes of seventh cervical and all thoracic vertebrae	clavicle, acromion, spine of scapula	accessory, cervical plexus	elevates shoulder, rotates scapula to raise shoulder in abduction of arm, draws scapula backward
triceps m. of arm (triceps brachii m.)	m. triceps brachii	*long head*—infraglenoid tubercle of scapula; *lateral head*—posterior surface and lateral border of humerus, lateral intermuscular septum; *medial head*—posterior surface of humerus below groove for radial nerve, medial border of humerus, medial intermuscular septum	olecranon of ulna	radial	extends forearm; *long head* adducts, extends arm
triceps m. of calf (triceps surae m.)	m. triceps surae	a name applied collectively to gastrocnemius and soleus m's			
trigonal m's	mm. trigoni vesicae urinariae	a submucous sheet of smooth muscle at the bladder trigone, continuous with ureteral muscles above and those of the proximal urethra below			
trigonal m., deep	m. trigoni vesicae urinariae profundus	the deep layer of the trigonal muscles, continuous with the detrusor m. of bladder			
trigonal m., superficial	m. trigoni vesicae urinariae superficialis	the superficial layer of the trigonal muscles, continuous proximally with the muscles of the ureteral wall			
m. of uvula	m. uvulae	posterior nasal spine of palatine bone and aponeurosis of soft palate	uvula	pharyngeal plexus	raises uvula

TABLE OF MUSCLES Continued

Common Name*	TA Term†	Origin*	Insertion*	Innervation*	Action
vastus m., intermediate	m. vastus intermedius	anterior and lateral surfaces of femur	patella, common tendon of quadriceps femoris m.	femoral	extends leg
vastus m., lateral	m. vastus lateralis	lateral aspect of femur	patella, common tendon of quadriceps femoris m.	femoral	extends leg
vastus m., medial	m. vastus medialis	medial aspect of femur	patella, common tendon of quadriceps femoris m.	femoral	extends leg
vertical m. of tongue	m. verticalis linguae	dorsal fascia of tongue	sides and base of tongue	hypoglossal	changes shape of tongue in mastication and deglutition
vocal m.	m. vocalis	angle between laminae of thyroid cartilage	vocal process of arytenoid cartilage	recurrent laryngeal	causes local variations in tension of vocal fold
zygomatic m., greater	m. zygomaticus major	zygomatic bone	angle of mouth	facial	draws angle of mouth upward and backward
zygomatic m., smaller	m. zygomaticus minor	zygomatic bone	orbicularis oris m., levator m. of upper lip	facial	draws upper lip upward and laterally

and intrinsic muscles that move the tongue. **m's of lower limb,** the muscles acting on the thigh, leg, and foot. **masticatory m's,** a group of muscles responsible for the movement of the jaws during mastication, including the masseter, temporal, and medial and lateral pterygoid muscles. **Müller's m.,** 1. the circular fibers of the ciliary muscle. 2. orbital muscle; see *Table of Muscles.* **multipennate m.,** one in which the fiber bundles converge to several tendons. **m's of neck,** cervical m's. **nonstriated m.,** a type without transverse striations in its constituent fibers; such muscles are almost always involuntary. **ocular m's,** extraocular m's. **orbicular m.,** one that encircles a body opening, e.g., the eye or mouth. **palatine m's,** the intrinsic and extrinsic muscles that act upon the soft palate and the adjacent pharyngeal wall. **pennate m., penniform m.,** a muscle in which the fibers approach the tendon of insertion from a wide area and are inserted through a large segment of its circumference. **pharyngeal m's,** the muscular coat of the pharynx, comprising the three constrictor muscles and the stylopharyngeal, salpingopharyngeal, and palatopharyngeal muscles. **quadrate m.,** a square-shaped muscle. **Reisseisen's m's,** the smooth muscle fibers of the smallest bronchi. **Ruysch's m.,** the muscular tissue of the fundus uteri. **semipennate m.,** a muscle in which the fiber bundles approach the tendon of insertion from only one direction and are inserted through only a small segment of its circumference. **skeletal m's,** striated muscles attached to bones, typically crossing at least one joint. **smooth m.,** nonstriated m. **sphincter m.,** sphincter. **strap m's,** muscles of the neck, particularly those of the thyroid cartilage and hyoid bone. **striated m., striped m.,** any muscle whose fibers are divided by transverse bands into striations; such muscles are voluntary. **suboccipital m's,** those situated just below the occipital bone, including the rectus capitis muscles and the oblique, splenius, and long muscles of head. **suprahyoid m's,** the muscles that attach the hyoid bone to the skull, including the digastric, stylohyoid, mylohyoid, and geniohyoid muscles. **synergic m's, synergistic m's,** those that assist one another in action. **thenar m's,** the abductor and flexor muscles of the thumb. **m's of tongue,** lingual m's. **triangular m.,** 1. a muscle that is triangular in shape. 2. depressor m. of angle of mouth; see *Table of Muscles.* **unipennate m.,** semipennate m. **unstriated m.,** nonstriated m. **m's of**

upper limb, the muscles acting on the arm, forearm, and hand. **vestigial m.,** a muscle that was once well developed but through evolution has become rudimentary. **visceral m.,** muscle fibers associated chiefly with the hollow viscera; except for the striated fibers in the heart, they are smooth muscle fibers bound together by reticular fibers. **voluntary m.,** any muscle that is normally under the control of the will; usually composed of striated muscle fibers. **yoked m's,** those that normally act simultaneously and equally, as in moving the eyes.

mus·cle phos·pho·fruc·to·ki·nase (mus′l fos″fo-frook″to-ki′nās) the muscle isozyme of 6-phosphofructokinase.

mus·cle phos·phor·y·lase (fos-for′ĭ-lās) the muscle isozyme of glycogen phosphorylase; deficiency causes glycogen storage disease, type V.

mus·cu·lar (mus′ku-lar) 1. pertaining to or composing muscle. 2. having a well-developed musculature.

mus·cu·la·ris (mus″ku-la′ris) [L.] 1. muscular. 2. pertaining to a muscular layer or coat; see *tunica muscularis.*

mus·cu·la·ture (mus′kūl-ah-cher) the muscular apparatus of the body or of a part.

mus·cu·lo·apo·neu·rot·ic (mus″kūl-o-ap″o-nōōr-ot′ik) pertaining to a muscle and its aponeurosis.

mus·cu·lo·cu·ta·ne·ous (-ku-ta′ne-us) myocutaneous; pertaining to, composed of, or supplying both muscles and skin.

mus·cu·lo·phren·ic (-fren′ik) pertaining to or supplying the diaphragm and adjoining muscles.

mus·cu·lo·skel·e·tal (-skel′ĕ-t′l) pertaining to or comprising the skeleton and muscles.

mus·cu·lo·spi·ral (-spi′r′l) pertaining to muscles and having a spiral direction, as the radial nerve.

mus·cu·lo·ten·di·nous (-ten′dĭ-nus) pertaining to or composed of muscle and tendon.

mus·cu·lus (mus′ku-lus) pl. *mus′culi.* [L.] muscle; see *Table of Muscles.*

mush·room (mush′rōōm) the fruiting body of certain fungi; some are edible and some are poisonous. See also *mushroom poisoning.*

mus·tard (mus′terd) 1. a plant of the genus *Brassica.* 2. the ripe seeds of *Brassica alba* (white mustard) and *B. nigra* (black mustard), whose oils have irritant, stimulant, and emetic properties. 3. resembling, or something resembling, mustard in one or more of its properties. **nitrogen m.,** 1. mechlorethamine. 2. any of a group of cytotoxic, blistering alkylating agents homologous to the vesicant war gas dichlorodiethyl sulfide (mustard gas), some of which have been used as antineoplastics and immunosuppressants.

mu·ta·gen (mu″tah-jen) an agent which induces genetic mutation.

mu·ta·gen·e·sis (mu″tah-jen′ĕ-sis) 1. the production of change. 2. the induction of genetic mutation.

mu·ta·ge·nic·i·ty (-jĕ-nis′it-e) the property of being able to induce genetic mutation.

mu·tant (mūt′nt) 1. an organism that has undergone genetic mutation. 2. produced by mutation.

mu·ta·ro·tase (mu″tah-ro′tās) an isomerase that catalyzes the interconversion of the α- and β-forms of D-glucose, L-arabinose, D-galactose, D-xylose, lactose, and maltose.

mu·ta·ro·ta·tion (-ro-ta′shun) a change in optical activity of a freshly prepared solution of a pure compound, occurring because of the formation of diastereoisomers having different optical activity.

mu·tase (mu′tās) a group of enzymes (transferases) that catalyze the intramolecular shifting of a chemical group from one position to another.

mu·ta·tion (mu-ta′shun) a permanent transmissible change in the genetic material. Also, an individual exhibiting such change; a sport. **point m.,** a mutation resulting from a change in a single base pair in the DNA molecule. **somatic m.,** a genetic mutation occurring in a somatic cell, providing the basis for a mosaic condition. **suppressor m.,** a mutation that partially or completely masks phenotypic expression of a mutation but occurs at a different site from it (i.e., causes suppression); it may be intragenic or intergenic. It is used particularly to describe a secondary mutation that suppresses a nonsense codon created by a primary mutation.

mute (mūt) 1. unable to speak. 2. to muffle or soften a sound.

mu·ti·la·tion (mu″tĭ-la′shun) the act of depriving an individual of a limb, member, or other important part. Also, the condition resulting therefrom.

mu·tism (mu′tizm) inability or refusal to speak. **akinetic m.,** a state in which the person can make no spontaneous movement or vocal sound; it often may be caused by a lesion in the third ventricle or be psychogenic. Called also *abulia.* **selective m.,** a mental disorder of childhood characterized by continuous refusal to speak in social situations by a child who is able and willing to speak to selected persons.

mu·tu·al·ism (mu′choo-al-izm″) the biologic association of two individuals or populations of different species, both of which are benefited by the relationship and sometimes unable to exist without it.

MV¹ [L.] Med′icus Veterina′rius (veterinary physician).

MV² megavolt; minute volume.

mV millivolt; one thousandth (10^{-3}) of a volt.

μV microvolt; one millionth (10^{-6}) of a volt.

MVP mitral valve prolapse; see under *syndrome.*

MW molecular weight.

my·al·gia (mi-al′jah) muscular pain. **myal′gic,** adj. **epidemic m.,** see under *pleurodynia.*

my·as·the·nia (mi″as-the′ne-ah) muscular debility or weakness. **myasthen′ic,** adj. **familial infantile m. gravis,** an inherited disorder of infants, characterized by feeding difficulties, episodes of apnea, ophthalmoparesis, and weakness or fatigue, often improving with age. **m. gas′trica,** weakness and loss of tone in the muscular coats of the stomach; atony of the stomach. **m. gra′vis,** an autoimmune disease of neuromuscular function, possibly due to presence of antibodies to acetylcholine receptors at the neuromuscular junction, marked by fatigue and exhaustion of the muscular system, often with fluctuating severity, without sensory disturbance or atrophy. **neonatal m.,** a transient myasthenia affecting offspring of myasthenic women.

my·a·to·nia (mi″ah-to′ne-ah) amyotonia.

my·at·ro·phy (mi-at′ro-fe) atrophy of a muscle.

my·ce·li·um (mi-se′le-um) pl. *myce′lia.* The mass of threadlike processes (hyphae) constituting the fungal thallus. **myce′lial,** adj.

my·cete (mi′sēt) a fungus.

my·ce·tis·mus (mi″sĕ-tiz′mus) mushroom poisoning.

my·ce·to·ma (mi″sĕ-to′mah) a chronic, progressive, destructive infection of the cutaneous and subcutaneous tissues, fascia, and bone caused by traumatic implantation of certain actinomycetes (*actinomycotic m.*), true fungi (*eumycotic m.*), or other organisms; it usually involves the foot (*Madura foot*) or leg.

myc(o)- word element [Gr.], *fungus.*

My·co·bac·te·ri·a·ceae (mi″ko-bak-tēr″e-a′se-e) a family of bacteria (order Actinomycetales) found in soil and dairy products and as parasites in humans and other animals.

My·co·bac·te·ri·um (-bak-tēr′e-um) a genus of gram-positive, acid-fast bacteria (family Mycobacteriaceae), including *M. a′vium-intracellula′re,* a complex that causes opportunistic infections in patients with HIV infection, *M. bal′nei* (*M. mari′num*), the cause of swimming pool granuloma; *M. bo′vis,* the

my·co·bac·te·ri·um (mi″ko-bak-tēr′e-um) pl. *mycobacte′ria*. An individual organism of the genus *Mycobacterium*. **anonymous mycobacteria, atypical mycobacteria,** nontuberculous mycobacteria. **Group I–IV mycobacteria,** see *nontuberculous mycobacteria*. **nontuberculous mycobacteria,** mycobacteria other than *Mycobacterium tuberculosis* or *M. bovis*; they are divided into four groups, I–IV, on the basis of several physical characteristics.

my·co·der·ma·ti·tis (-der″mah-ti′tis) candidiasis.

my·co·lo·gy (mi-kol′ah-je) the science and study of fungi.

my·co·myr·in·gi·tis (mi″ko-mir″in-ji′tis) myringomycosis.

my·co·phe·no·late (-fen′o-lāt) an immunosuppressant used as *m. mofetil* to prevent rejection of allogeneic cardiac, hepatic, and renal transplants.

My·co·plas·ma (mi′ko-plaz″mah) a genus of pleomorphic, gram-negative, aerobic to facultatively anerobic bacteria lacking cell walls, including the pleuropneumonia-like organisms; species include *M. ho′minis*, which is associated with nongonococcal urethritis and mild pharyngitis, and *M. pneumo′niae*, a cause of primary atypical pneumonia.

my·co·plas·mal (mi″ko-plaz′m′l) of, pertaining to, or caused by *Mycoplasma*.

My·co·plas·ma·ta·ceae (mi″ko-plaz″mahta′se-e) a family of schizomycetes, made up of a single genus, *Mycoplasma*.

my·co·sis (mi-ko′sis) any disease caused by fungi. **m. fungoi′des,** a chronic, malignant, lymphoreticular neoplasm of the skin and, in late stages, lymph nodes and viscera, with development of large, painful, ulcerating tumors.

my·cot·ic (mi-kot′ik) 1. pertaining to mycosis. 2. caused by a fungus.

my·co·tox·i·co·sis (mi″ko-tok-sĭ-ko′sis) 1. poisoning due to a fungal or bacterial toxin. 2. poisoning due to ingestion of fungi, especially mushrooms; see also *Amanita*.

my·co·tox·in (mi′ko-tok″sin) a fungal toxin.

my·dri·a·sis (mĭ-dri′ah-sis) [Gr.] dilatation of the pupil.

myd·ri·at·ic (mid″re-at′ik) dilating the pupil, or an agent that so acts.

my·ec·to·my (mi-ek′tah-me) excision of a muscle.

my·ec·to·pia (mi″ek-to′pe-ah) displacement of a muscle.

my·el·ap·o·plexy (mi″il-ap′ah-plek″se) hematomyelia.

my·el·ate·lia (-ah-te′le-ah) myelodysplasia.

my·el·at·ro·phy (-at′rah-fe) atrophy of the spinal cord.

my·el·emia (-ēm′e-ah) myelocytosis.

my·el·en·ceph·a·lon (-en-sef′ah-lon) 1. medulla oblongata. 2. the posterior of two brain vesicles formed by specialization of the rhombencephalon in embryonic development.

my·elin (mi′ĕ-lin) the lipid-rich substance of the cell membrane of Schwann cells that coils to form the myelin sheath surrounding the axon of myelinated nerve fibers. **myelin′ic,** adj.

my·eli·nat·ed (mi′ĕ-lĭ-nāt″ed) having a myelin sheath.

my·elin·a·tion (mi′ĕ-lin-a′shun) myelinization.

my·elin·i·za·tion (mi″ĕ-lin″ĭ-za′shun) the act of adding myelin; formation of a myelin sheath.

my·elin·ol·y·sis (-ol′ĭ-sis) demyelination.

my·eli·no·sis (-o′sis) fatty degeneration, with formation of myelin.

my·elino·tox·ic (mi″ĕ-lin′o-tok″sik) having a deleterious effect on myelin; causing demyelination.

my·eli·tis (mi″ĕ-li′tis) 1. inflammation of the spinal cord; often expanded to include noninflammatory spinal cord lesions. 2. inflammation of the bone marrow (osteomyelitis). **myelit′ic,** adj.

myel(o)- word element [Gr.], *marrow* (often with specific reference to the *spinal cord*).

my·elo·ab·la·tion (mi″ĕ-lo-ab-la′shun) the severe or complete depletion of bone marrow cells; as the administration of high doses of chemotherapy or radiation therapy prior to bone marrow transplantation. **myeloab′la-tive,** adj.

my·elo·blast (mi′ĕ-lo-blast″) an immature cell found in the bone marrow and not normally in the peripheral blood; it is the most primitive precursor in the granulocytic series, which matures to develop into the promyelocyte and eventually the granular leukocyte. **myeloblas′tic,** adj.

my·elo·blas·te·mia (-blas-tēm′ah) the presence of myeloblasts in the blood.

my·elo·blas·to·ma (-blas-to′mah) a focal malignant tumor composed of myeloblasts or early myeloid precursors occurring outside the bone marrow.

my·elo·cele (mi″ĕ-lo-sēl″) protrusion of the spinal cord through a defect in the vertebral arch.

my·elo·cyst (-sist″) a benign cyst developed from rudimentary medullary canals.

my·elo·cys·to·cele (mi″ĕ-lo-sis′to-sēl) myelomeningocele.

my·elo·cys·to·me·nin·go·cele (-mĕ-ning′go-sēl) myelomeningocele.

my·elo·cyte (mi′ĕ-lo-sīt″) a precursor in the granulocyte series, being a cell intermediate in development between a promyelocyte and a metamyelocyte. **myelocyt′ic,** adj.

my·elo·cy·to·ma (-si-to′mah) 1. chronic granulocytic leukemia. 2. myeloma.

my·elo·cy·to·sis (mi″ĕ-lo-si-to′sis) excessive number of myelocytes in the blood.

my·elo·dys·pla·sia (-dis-pla′zhah) 1. a neural tube defect causing defective development of any part of the spinal cord. 2. dysplasia of myelocytes and other elements of the bone marrow. **myelodysplas′tic,** adj.

my·elo·en·ceph·a·li·tis (-en-sef″ah-li′tis) inflammation of the spinal cord and brain.

my·elo·fi·bro·sis (-fi-bro′sis) replacement of bone marrow by fibrous tissue.

my·elo·gen·e·sis (-jen′ĕ-sis) myelinization.

my·elog·e·nous (mi″ĕ-loj′ĕ-nus) produced in bone marrow.

my·elog·ra·phy (mi″ĕ-log′rah-fe) radiography of the spinal cord after injection of a contrast medium into the subarachnoid space.

my·eloid (mi′ĕ-loid) 1. medullary; pertaining to, derived from, or resembling bone marrow or the spinal cord. 2. having the appearance of myelocytes, but not derived from bone marrow.

my·eloi·do·sis (mi″ĕ-loi-do′sis) formation of myeloid tissue, especially hyperplastic development of such tissue.

my·elo·li·po·ma (mi″ĕ-lo-lĭ-po′-mah) a rare benign tumor of the adrenal gland composed of adipose tissue, lymphocytes, and primitive myeloid cells.

my·elo·ma (mi″ĕ-lo′mah) a tumor composed of cells of the type normally found in the bone marrow. **giant cell m.,** see under *tumor* (1). **multiple m.,** a disseminated type of plasma cell dyscrasia characterized by multiple bone marrow tumor foci and secretion of an M component, manifested by skeletal destruction, pathologic fractures, bone pain, the presence of anomalous circulating immunoglobulins, Bence Jones proteinuria, and anemia. **plasma cell m.,** multiple m. **sclerosing m.,** myeloma associated with osteosclerosis, most often manifested by peripheral neuropathy. **solitary m.,** a variant of multiple myeloma in which there is a single localized tumor focus.

my·elo·ma·la·cia (mi″ĕ-lo-mah-la′shah) morbid softening of the spinal cord.

my·elo·ma·to·sis (-mah-to′sis) multiple myeloma.

my·elo·men·in·gi·tis (-men″in-ji′tis) meningomyelitis.

my·elo·me·nin·go·cele (-mĕ-ning′go-sēl) hernial protrusion of the spinal cord and its meninges through a defect in the vertebral arch.

my·elo·mere (mi′ĕ-lo-mēr″) one of the segments of the embryonic brain or spinal cord.

my·elo·mono·cyt·ic (mi″ĕ-lo-mon″o-sit′ik) characterized by both myelocytes and monocytes.

my·elop·a·thy (mi″ĕ-lop′ah-the) 1. any functional disturbance and/or pathological change in the spinal cord; often used to denote nonspecific lesions, as opposed to *myelitis.* 2. pathological bone marrow changes. **myelopath′ic,** adj. **carcinomatous m.,** rapidly progressive degeneration or necrosis of the spinal cord associated with a carcinoma. **chronic progressive m.,** gradually progressive spastic paraparesis associated with infection by human T-lymphotropic virus 1. **HTLV-1–associated m.,** chronic progressive m. **paracarcinomatous m., paraneoplastic m.,** carcinomatous m. **spondylotic cervical m.,** that secondary to encroachment of cervical spondylosis upon a congenitally small cervical spinal canal. **transverse m.,** that extending across the spinal cord. **vacuolar m.,** loss of myelin and spongy degeneration of the spinal cord with microscopic vacuolization, caused by infection with human immunodeficiency virus.

my·elo·per·ox·i·dase (mi″ĕ-lo-per-ok′sĭ-das) a green hemoprotein in neutrophils and monocytes that catalyzes the reaction of hydrogen peroxide and halide ions to form cytotoxic acids and other intermediates; these play a role in the oxygen-dependent killing of tumor cells and microorganisms. Abbreviated MPO.

my·elo·pe·tal (mi″ĕ-lop′ĭ-t′l) moving toward the spinal cord.

my·e·loph·thi·sis (mi″ĕ-lo-thi′sis) 1. wasting of the spinal cord. 2. bone marrow suppression secondary to marrow infiltration by tumor with local production of myelosuppressive cytokines.

my·e·lo·plast (mi′ĕ-lo-plast″) any leukocyte of the bone marrow.

my·e·lo·poi·e·sis (mi″ĕ-lo-poi-e′sis) the formation of marrow or the cells arising from it. **myelopoiet′ic,** adj.

my·e·lo·pro·lif·er·a·tive (-pro-lif′er-ah-tiv) pertaining to or characterized by medullary and extramedullary proliferation of bone marrow constituents; see under *disorder.*

my·e·lo·ra·dic·u·li·tis (-rah-dik″u-li′tis) inflammation of the spinal cord and posterior nerve roots.

my·e·lo·ra·dic·u·lo·dys·pla·sia (-rah-dik″u-lo-dis-pla′zhah) developmental abnormality of the spinal cord and spinal nerve roots.

my·e·lo·ra·dic·u·lop·a·thy (-rah-dik″u-lop′ah-the) disease of the spinal cord and spinal nerve roots.

my·elor·rha·gia (-ra′jah) hematomyelia.

my·e·lo·sar·co·ma (-sahr-ko′mah) a sarcomatous growth made up of myeloid tissue or bone marrow cells.

my·e·los·chi·sis (mi″ĕ-los′kĭ-sis) a developmental anomaly characterized by a cleft spinal cord.

my·e·lo·scle·ro·sis (-sklĕ-ro′sis) 1. sclerosis of the spinal cord. 2. obliteration of the marrow cavity by small spicules of bone. 3. myelofibrosis.

my·e·lo·sis (mi″ĕ-lo′sis) 1. myelocytosis. 2. formation of a tumor of the spinal cord. **erythremic m.,** erythroleukemia.

my·e·lo·spon·gi·um (mi″ĕ-lo-spun′je-um) a network developing into the neuroglia.

my·e·lo·sup·pres·sion (-sŭ-presh′un) bone marrow suppression.

my·e·lo·sup·pres·sive (-sŭ-pres′iv) 1. causing bone marrow suppression. 2. an agent that so acts.

my·e·lo·tox·ic (mi′ĕ-lo-tok″sik) 1. destructive to bone marrow. 2. myelosuppressive. 3. arising from diseased bone marrow.

my·en·ter·on (mi-en′ter-on) the muscular coat of the intestine. **myenter′ic,** adj.

my·es·the·sia (mi″es-the′zhah) muscle sense (1).

my·i·a·sis (mi-i′ah-sis) invasion of the body by the larvae of flies, characterized as cutaneous (subdermal tissue), gastrointestinal, nasopharyngeal, ocular, or urinary, depending on the region invaded.

my·lo·hy·oid (mi″lo-hi′oid) pertaining to molar teeth and the hyoid bone.

my(o)- word element [Gr.], *muscle.*

myo·ar·chi·tec·ton·ic (mi″o-ahr″kĭ-tek-ton′ik) pertaining to structural arrangement of muscle fibers.

myo·at·ro·phy (-at′rah-fe) muscular atrophy.

myo·blast (mi′o-blast) an embryonic cell which becomes a muscle cell or fiber. **myoblas′tic,** adj.

myo·blas·to·ma (mi″o-blas-to′mah) a benign circumscribed tumor-like lesion of soft tissue, possibly composed of myoblasts. **granular cell m.,** see under *tumor.*

myo·car·di·al (-kahr′de-al) pertaining to the muscular tissue of the heart.

myo·car·di·op·a·thy (-kahr″de-op′ah-the) cardiomyopathy.

myo·car·di·tis (-kahr-di′tis) inflammation of the muscular walls of the heart. **acute isolated m.,** a frequently fatal, idiopathic, acute myocarditis affecting chiefly the interstitial fibrous tissue. **Fiedler's m.,** acute isolated myocarditis **giant cell m.,** a subtype of acute isolated myocarditis characterized by the presence of multinucleate giant cells and other inflammatory cells, and by ventricular dilatation, mural thrombi, and wide areas of necrosis. **granulomatous m.,** giant cell myocarditis, including also granuloma formation. **hypersensitivity m.,** that due to allergic reactions caused by hypersensitivity to various agents, particularly sulfonamides, penicillins, and methyldopa. **interstitial m.,** that affecting chiefly the interstitial fibrous tissue.

myo·car·di·um (-kahr′de-um) the middle and thickest layer of the heart wall, composed of cardiac muscle. **hibernating m.,** see *myocardial hibernation,* under *hibernation.* **stunned m.,** see *myocardial stunning,* under *stunning.*

myo·cele (mi′o-sēl) protrusion of a muscle through its ruptured sheath.

my·oc·lo·nus (mi-ok′lo-nus) shocklike contractions of a muscle or a group of muscles. **myoclon′ic,** adj. **essential m.,** myoclonus of unknown etiology, involving one or more muscles and elicited by excitement or an attempt at voluntary movement. **intention m.,** that occurring when voluntary muscle movement is initiated. **nocturnal m.,** nonpathological myoclonic jerks occurring as a person is falling asleep or is asleep. **palatal m.,** rapid rhythmic, up-and-down movement of one or both sides of the palate, often with ipsilateral synchronous clonic movements of the face, tongue, pharynx, and diaphragm muscles.

myo·coele (mi′o-sēl) the cavity within a myotome (2).

myo·cu·ta·ne·ous (mi″o-ku-ta′ne-us) musculocutaneous.

myo·cyte (mi′o-sīt) a muscle cell. **Anichkov m.,** see under *cell.*

myo·cy·tol·y·sis (mi″o-si-tol′ĭ-sis) disintegration of muscle fibers. **coagulative m.,** contraction band necrosis.

myo·dys·to·nia (-dis-to′ne-ah) disorder of muscular tone.

myo·dys·tro·phy (-dis′trah-fe) 1. muscular dystrophy. 2. myotonic dystrophy.

myo·ede·ma (-ĕ-de′mah) 1. the rising in a lump by a wasting muscle when struck. 2. edema of a muscle.

myo·epi·the·li·o·ma (-ep″ĭ-thēl″e-o′mah) a tumor composed of outgrowths of myoepithelial cells from a sweat gland.

myo·epi·the·li·um (-ep″ĭ-the′le-um) tissue made up of contractile epithelial cells. **myoepithe′lial,** adj.

myo·fas·ci·al (-fash′e-al) pertaining to or involving the fascia surrounding and associated with muscle tissue.

myo·fas·ci·tis (-fah-si′tis) inflammation of a muscle and its fascia.

myo·fi·ber (-fi′ber) muscle fiber.

myo·fi·bril (-fi′bril) muscle fibril; one of the slender threads of a muscle fiber, composed of numerous myofilaments. See Plate 7. **myofi′brillar,** adj.

myo·fi·bro·blast (-fi′bro-blast) an atypical fibroblast combining the ultrastructural features of a fibroblast and a smooth muscle cell.

myo·fi·bro·ma (-fi-bro′mah) leiomyoma.

myo·fi·bro·sis (-fi-bro′sis) replacement of muscle tissue by fibrous tissue.

myo·fi·bro·si·tis (-fi″bro-si′tis) perimysiitis.

myo·fila·ment (-fil′ah-ment) any of the ultramicroscopic threadlike structures composing the myofibrils of striated muscle fibers; thick ones contain myosin, thin ones contain actin, and intermediate ones contain desmin and vimentin. See Plate 7.

myo·gen·e·sis (-jen′ĕ-sis) the development of muscle tissue, especially its embryonic development. **myogenet′ic,** adj.

my·o·gen·ic (-jen′ik) 1. pertaining to myogenesis. 2. originating in myocytes or muscle tissue.

my·og·e·nous (mi-oj′ĕ-nus) originating in muscular tissue.

myo·glo·bin (mi″o-glo′bin) the oxygen-transporting pigment of muscle, a hemoprotein that resembles a single subunit of hemoglobin, being composed of one globin polypeptide chain and one heme group.

myo·glob·u·lin (-glob′ūl-in) a globulin from muscle serum.

myo·graph (mi′o-graf) apparatus for recording effects of muscular contraction.

my·og·ra·phy (mi-og′rah-fe) 1. the use of a myograph. 2. description of muscles. 3. radiography of muscle tissue after injection of a radiopaque medium. **myograph′ic,** adj.

my·oid (mi′oid) resembling muscle.

myo·ki·nase (mi″o-ki′nās) adenylate kinase; an enzyme of muscle that catalyzes the phosphorylation of ADP to molecules of ATP and AMP.

myo·ki·ne·sis (-kĭ-ne′sis) movement of muscles, especially displacement of muscle fibers in operation. **myokinet′ic,** adj.

myo·kym·ia (-ki′me-ah) 1. a benign condition marked by brief spontaneous tetanic contractions of motor units or groups of muscle fibers, usually adjacent groups of fibers contracting alternately. 2. myoky′mic

myo·li·po·ma (-lĭ-po′mah) a benign mesenchymoma containing fatty or lipomatous elements.

my·ol·o·gy (mi-ol′ah-je) the scientific study or description of the muscles and accessory structures (bursae and synovial sheath).

my·ol·y·sis (mi-ol′ĭ-sis) disintegration or degeneration of muscle tissue.

my·o·ma (mi-o′mah) pl. *myomas, myo′mata.* A benign tumor formed of muscle elements. **myom′atous,** adj. **uterine m.,** leiomyoma of the uterus.

my·o·ma·to·sis (mi-o″mah-to′sis) the formation of multiple myomas.

my·o·mec·to·my (mi″o-mek′tah-me) 1. surgical removal of a myoma, particularly of the uterus (leiomyoma). 2. myectomy.

myo·mel·a·no·sis (-mel″ah-no′sis) melanosis of muscle tissue.

myo·mere (mi′o-mēr) myotome (2).

my·om·e·ter (mi-om′it-er) an apparatus for measuring muscle contraction.

myo·me·tri·tis (mi″o-me-tri′tis) inflammation of the myometrium.

myo·me·tri·um (-me′tre-um) the tunica muscularis of the uterus. **myome′trial,** adj.

myo·neme (mi′o-nēm) a fine contractile fiber found in the cytoplasm of certain protozoa.

myo·neu·ral (mi″o-nŏōr″al) pertaining to nerve terminations in muscles.

myo·pal·mus (-pal′mus) muscle twitching.

myo·pa·ral·y·sis (-pah-ral′ĭ-sis) paralysis of a muscle.

myo·par·e·sis (-pah-re′sis) slight muscle paralysis.

my·op·a·thy (mi-op′ah-the) any disease of muscle. **myopath′ic,** adj. **centronuclear m.,** myotubular m. **mitochondrial m.,** any of a group of myopathies associated with an increased number of large, often abnormal, mitochondria in muscle fibers and manifested by exercise intolerance, weakness, lactic acidosis, infantile quadriparesis, ophthalmoplegia, and cardiac abnormalities. **myotubular m.,** an often fatal X-linked myopathy marked by myofibers resembling the myotubules of early fetal muscle. **nema-line m.,** a congenital abnormality of myofibrils in which small threadlike fibers are scattered through the muscle fibers; marked by hypotonia and proximal muscle weakness. **ocular m.,** progressive external ophthalmoplegia. **thyrotoxic m.,** weakness and wasting of skeletal muscles, especially of the pelvic and shoulder girdles, accompanying hyperthyroidism.

myo·peri·car·di·tis (mi″o-per″ĭ-kahr-di′tis) myocarditis combined with pericarditis.

myo·phos·phor·y·lase (mi″o-fos-for′ĭ-lās) the muscle isozyme of glycogen phosphorylase; deficiency causes glycogen storage disease, type V.

my·o·pia (M) (mi-o′pe-ah) nearsightedness; ametropia in which parallel rays come to a focus in front of the retina, vision being better for near objects than for far. **myop′ic,** adj. **curvature m.,** myopia due to changes in curvature of the refracting surfaces of the eye. **index m.,** myopia due to abnormal refractivity of the media of the eye. **malignant m., pernicious m.,** progressive myopia with disease of the choroid, leading to retinal detachment and blindness. **progressive m.,** myopia increasing in adult life.

myo·plasm (mi′o-plazm) the contractile part of a muscle cell, or myofibril.

myo·plas·ty (-plas″te) plastic surgery on muscle. **myoplas′tic,** adj.

my·or·rhex·is (-rek′sis) rupture of a muscle.

myo·sar·co·ma (-sahr-ko′mah) a malignant tumor derived from muscle tissue.

myo·scle·ro·sis (-sklĕ-ro′sis) hardening of muscle tissue.

my·o·sin (mi′o-sin) a protein of the myofibril, occurring chiefly in the A band; with actin it forms actomyosin, which is responsible for the contractile properties of muscle.

myo·si·tis (mi″o-si′tis) inflammation of a voluntary muscle. **m. fibro′sa,** a type in which connective tissue forms within the muscle. **inclusion body m.,** a progressive inflammatory myopathy primarily involving muscles of the pelvic region and legs. **multiple m.,** polymyositis. **m. ossi′ficans,** myositis marked by bony deposits or by ossification of muscle. **proliferative m.,** a benign, rapidly growing, reactive, nodular lesion similar to nodular fasciitis, but characterized by fibroblast proliferation within skeletal muscle. **trichinous m.,** that due to the presence of *Trichinella spiralis.*

myo·tac·tic (mi″o-tak′tik) pertaining to the proprioceptive sense of muscles.

my·ot·a·sis (mi-ot′ah-sis) stretching of muscle. **myotat′ic,** adj.

myo·teno·si·tis (mi″o-ten″o-si′tis) inflammation of a muscle and tendon.

myo·tome (mi′o-tōm) 1. an instrument for performing myotomy. 2. the muscle plate or portion of a somite that develops into noncardiac striated muscle. 3. a group of muscles innervated from a single spinal segment. **myotom′ic,** adj.

myo·to·nia (mi″o-to′ne-ah) dystonia involving increased muscular irritability and contractility with decreased power of relaxation. **myoton′ic,** adj. **m. atro′phica,** myotonic dystrophy. **m. conge′nita,** a hereditary disease marked by tonic spasm and rigidity of certain muscles when attempts are made to move them after rest or when they are mechanically stimulated. **m. dystro′phica,** myotonic dystrophy.

myo·to·noid (mi-ot′o-noid) denoting muscle reactions marked by slow contraction or relaxation.

myo·to·nus (-nus) tonic spasm of a muscle or a group of muscles.

myo·tro·phic (mi″o-tro″fik) 1. increasing the weight of muscle. 2. pertaining to myotrophy.

my·ot·ro·phy (mi-ot″rah-fe) nutrition of muscle.

myo·tu·bule (mi″o-too′būl) a developing muscle cell or fiber with a centrally located nucleus. **myotu′bular,** adj.

Myr·i·ap·o·da (mir″e-ap′ah-dah) a superclass of arthropods, including centipedes and millipedes.

my·rin·ga (mĭ-ring′gah) the tympanic membrane.

my·rin·gec·to·my (mir″in-jek′tah-me) tympanectomy.

my·rin·gi·tis (mir″in-ji′tis) inflammation of the tympanic membrane. **m. bullo′sa, bullous m.,** a form of viral otitis media in which serous or hemorrhagic blebs appear on the tympanic membrane and often on the adjacent wall of the auditory meatus.

myring(o)- word element [L.], *tympanic membrane.*

my·rin·go·my·co·sis (-mi-ko′sis) otomycosis of the tympanic membrane.

my·rin·got·o·my (mi-ring-got′ah-me) tympanotomy; creation of a hole in the tympanic membrane, as for tympanocentesis.

my·ris·tic ac·id (mĭ-ris′tik) a saturated 14-carbon fatty acid occurring in most animal and vegetable fats, particularly butterfat and coconut, palm, and nutmeg oils.

myrrh (mur) the oleo-gum-resin obtained from species of *Commiphora;* applied topically in mild inflammations of the oral and pharyngeal mucosa.

myr·ti·form (mir′tĭ-form) shaped like myrtle or myrtle berries.

my·so·pho·bia (-fo′be-ah) irrational fear of dirt and contamination.

myx·ad·e·ni·tis (miks″ad-ĕ-ni′tis) inflammation of a mucous gland.

myx·as·the·nia (as-the′ne-ah) deficient secretion of mucus.

myx·ede·ma (-sĕ-de′mah) a dry, waxy type of swelling (nonpitting edema) with abnormal deposits of mucin in the skin (mucinosis) and other tissues, associated with hypothyroidism; the facial changes are distinctive, with swollen lips and thickened nose. **myxedem′atous,** adj. **congenital m.,** cretinism. **papular m.,** lichen myxedematosus. **pituitary m.,** that due to deficient secretion of the pituitary hormone thyrotropin. **pretibial m.,** localized edema associated with preceding hyperthyroidism and exophthalmos, occurring typically on the anterior (pretibial) surface of the legs, the mucin deposits appearing as both plaques and papules.

myx(o)- word element [Gr.], *mucus; slime.*

myxo·chon·dro·ma (mik″so-kon-dro′mah) chondroma with stroma resembling primitive mesenchymal tissue.

myxo·fi·bro·ma (-fi-bro′mah) a fibroma containing myxomatous tissue.

myxo·fi·bro·sar·co·ma (-fi″bro-sahr-ko′mah) older term for the myxoid subtype of malignant fibrous histiocytoma.

myx·oid (mik′soid) mucoid.

myxo·li·po·ma (mik″so-lĭ-po′mah) lipoma with foci of myxomatous degeneration.

myx·o·ma (mik-so′mah) pl. *myxomas,* *myxo′mata.* A benign tumor composed of primitive connective tissue cells and stroma resembling mesenchyme.

myx·o·ma·to·sis (mik″so-mah-to′sis) 1. the development of multiple myxomas. 2. myxomatous degeneration.

myx·o·ma·tous (mik-so′mah-tus) of the nature of a myxoma.

myxo·sar·co·ma (-sahr-ko′mah) a sarcoma with myxomatous tissue.

myxo·vi·rus (mik′so-vi″rus) any of a group of RNA viruses, including the viruses of influenza, parainfluenza, mumps, and Newcastle disease, characteristically causing agglutination of erythrocytes.

N newton; nitrogen; normal (2a).

N normal (2a); number; Avogadro's number.

N**A** Avogadro's number.

n nano-; refractive index; neutron.

n. [L.] ner′vus (nerve).

n haploid chromosome number; refractive index; sample size (statistics).

n- normal (2b).

ν (nu, the thirteenth letter of the Greek alphabet) frequency (1).

NA *Nomina Anatomica;* a former official body of anatomical nomenclature, superseded by *Terminologia Anatomica* [TA] (1998).

Na sodium (L. *na′trium*).

na·bu·me·tone (nah-bu′mĕ-tōn) a nonsteroidal antiinflammatory drug used in the treatment of osteoarthritis and rheumatoid arthritis.

na·cre·ous (na′kre-us) having a pearl-like luster.

NAD nicotinamide adenine dinucleotide.

NAD+ the oxidized form of NAD.

NADH the reduced form of NAD.

na·di (nah′de) in ayurveda, any of the channels that carry vital energy through the body.

na·do·lol (na-do′lol) a nonselective β-adrenergic blocking agent used for the treatment of angina pectoris and hypertension.

NADP nicotinamide adenine dinucleotide phosphate.

NADP+ the oxidized form of NADP.

NADPH the reduced form of NADP.

naf·a·rel·in (naf′ah-rel″in) a synthetic preparation of gonadotropin-releasing hormone, used as the acetate ester in the treatment of central precocious puberty and endometriosis.

naf·cil·lin (naf-sil′in) a semisynthetic, acid- and penicillinase-resistant penicillin that is effective against staphylococcal infections; used as the sodium salt.

naf·ti·fine (naf′tĭ-fēn) a broad-spectrum antifungal agent, used topically as the hydrochloride salt.

nail (nāl) 1. the horny cutaneous plate on the dorsal surface of the distal end of a finger or toe. 2. a rod of metal, bone, or other material for fixation of fragments of fractured bones. **ingrown n.,** aberrant growth of a toenail, with one or both lateral margins pushing deeply into adjacent soft tissue. **racket n.,** a short broad thumbnail. **spoon n.,** one with a concave surface.

Nai·ro·vi·rus (ni'ro-vi″rus) a genus of viruses of the family Bunyaviridae, including Crimean-Congo hemorrhagic fever virus.

Na·ja (na'jah) the cobras, a genus of venomous snakes (family Elapidae) found in Asia and Africa.

Na⁺,K⁺-ATP·ase (a-te-pe'ās) an enzyme that spans the plasma membrane and hydrolyzes ATP to provide the energy necessary to drive the cellular sodium pump.

nal·bu·phine (nal'bu-fēn) an opioid analgesic, used as the hydrochloride salt in the treatment of moderate to severe pain and as an anesthesia adjunct.

nal·i·dix·ic ac·id (nal-ĭ-dik'sik) a synthetic antibacterial agent used in the treatment of genitourinary infections caused by gram-negative organisms.

nal·me·fene (nal'mě-fēn″) an opioid antagonist, used as the hydrochloride salt in the treatment of opioid overdose and postoperative opioid depression.

nal·or·phine (nal'or-fēn) a semisynthetic congener of morphine; the hydrochloride salt is used as an antagonist to morphine and related narcotics and in the diagnosis of narcotic addiction.

nal·ox·one (nal-ok'sōn) an opioid antagonist, used as the hydrochloride salt in opioid toxicity, opioid-induced respiratory depression, and hypotension associated with septic shock.

nal·trex·one (nal-trek'sōn) an opioid antagonist used as the hydrochloride salt in treatment of opioid or alcohol abuse.

name (nām) a word or words used to designate a unique entity and distinguish it from others. **generic n.,** 1. in chemistry, a name applied to a class of compounds, e.g., alkane. 2. nonproprietary n. 3. in biology, the name applied to a genus. **International Nonproprietary N. (INN),** the nonproprietary designation recommended by the World Health Organization for any pharmaceutical preparation. **nonproprietary n.,** a short name coined for a drug or chemical not subject to proprietary (trademark) rights and recommended or recognized by an official body. **pharmacy equivalent n. (PEN),** a shortened name for a drug or combination of drugs; when used for a combination of drugs, the term usually consists of the prefix *co-* plus an abbreviation for each drug in the combination. **proprietary n.,** a brand name or trademark under which a proprietary product is marketed. See *proprietary.* **systematic n.,** in chemical nomenclature, a name of a substance based on the chemical structure of a compound. **trivial n.,** in chemical nomenclature, a name of a substance that does not reflect its chemical structure; many trivial names are semisystematic, e.g., the *-ol* in glycerol indicates that it is an alcohol. **United States Adopted N. (USAN),** a nonproprietary designation for any compound used as a drug, established by negotiation between their manufacturers and a council sponsored jointly by the American Medical Association, American Pharmaceutical Association, and United States Pharmacopeial Convention.

nan·dro·lone (nan'dro-lōn) an anabolic steroid with lesser androgenic effects; used as *n. decanoate* and *n. phenpropionate* in the treatment of severe growth retardation in children and of metastatic breast cancer and as an adjunct in the treatment of chronic wasting diseases and anemia associated with renal insufficiency.

na·nism (na'nizm) dwarfism.

nan(o)- word element [Gr.], *dwarf; small size;* also used in naming units of measurement (symbol n) to designate an amount one billionth (10^{-9}) the size of the unit to which it is joined, e.g., nanocurie.

nano·ceph·a·ly (nan″o-sef'ah-le) microcephaly. **nanoceph'alous,** adj.

nano·gram (ng) (nan″o-gram) one billionth (10^{-9}) of a gram.

nan·oid (nan'oid) dwarfish.

nano·me·ter (nm) (nan'o-me″ter) one billionth (10^{-9}) of a meter.

nan·oph·thal·mia (nan″of-thal'me-ah) nanophthalmos.

nan·oph·thal·mos (nan″of-thal'mus) abnormal smallness in all dimensions of one or both eyes in the absence of other ocular defects; pure microphthalmos.

nan·ous (nan'us) dwarfed; stunted.

na·nu·ka·ya·mi (nah″noo-kah-yah'me) a leptospirosis marked by fever and jaundice, first reported in Japan, due to *Leptospira hebdomadis.*

nape (nāp) the back of the neck.

naph·az·o·line (naf-az'o-lēn) an adrenergic used in the form of the hydrochloride salt as a vasoconstrictor to decongest nasal and ocular mucosae.

naph·tha (naf'thah) any of various volatile liquid hydrocarbon mixtures from petroleum, natural gas, or coal tar, sometimes specifically petroleum benzin or ligroin; used as solvents, dry cleaning fluids, in synthesis, in varnishes, or as fuels.

NAPNES National Association for Practical Nurse Education and Services.

na·prap·a·thy (nah-prap'ah-the) a system of therapy employing manipulation of connective tissue (ligaments, muscles, and joints) and dietary measures to facilitate the recuperative and regenerative processes of the body.

na·prox·en (nah-prok'sen) a nonsteroidal antiinflammatory drug used as the base or the sodium salt in the treatment of pain, inflammation, arthritis, gout, calcium pyrophosphate deposition disease, fever, and dysmenorrhea and in the prophylaxis and suppression of vascular headache.

nap·sy·late (nap'sĭ-lāt) USAN contraction for 2-naphthalenesulfonate.

NAPT National Association for Poetry Therapy.

nar·a·trip·tan (nar″ah-trip'tan) a selective serotonin receptor agonist used as the hydrochloride salt in the acute treatment of migraine.

nar·cis·sism (nahr'sĭ-sizm) dominant interest in one's self; the state in which the ego is invested in oneself rather than in another person; self-love. **narcissis'tic,** adj.

narc(o)- word element [Gr.], *stupor; stuporous state.*

nar·co·hyp·no·sis (nahr″ko-hip-no'sis) hypnotic suggestions made while the patient is narcotized.

nar·co·lep·sy (nahr'ko-lep″se) recurrent, uncontrollable, brief episodes of sleep, often with hypnagogic or hypnopompic hallucinations, cataplexy, and sleep paralysis. **narcolep'tic,** adj.

nar·co·sis (nahr-ko'sis) reversible depression of the central nervous system produced by drugs, marked by stupor or insensibility.

nar·cot·ic (nahr-kot'ic) 1. pertaining to or producing narcosis. 2. an agent that produces insensibility or stupor, especially an opioid.

nar·co·tize (nahr'ko-tīz) to put under the influence of a narcotic.

na·res (na'rēs) [L.] the nostrils; the external openings of the nasal cavity.

na·sal (na'zil) pertaining to the nose.

na·sa·lis (na-za'lis) [L.] nasal.

nas·cent (nas'ent, na'sent) 1. being born; just coming into existence. 2. just liberated from a chemical combination, and hence more reactive because uncombined.

na·si·on (na'ze-on) the middle point of the frontonasal suture.

nas(o)- word element [L.], *nose.*

na·so·an·tral (na″zo-an'tral) pertaining to the nose and maxillary antrum.

na·so·an·tros·to·my (-an-tros'tah-me) surgical formation of a nasoantral window for drainage of an obstructed maxillary sinus.

na·so·cil·i·ary (-sil'e-ĕ″re) pertaining to the eyes, brow, and root of the nose.

na·so·fron·tal (-frun't'l) pertaining to the nose and forehead or to nasal and frontal bones.

na·so·gas·tric (-gas'trik) pertaining to the nose and stomach.

na·so·la·bi·al (-la'be-il) pertaining to the nose and lip.

na·so·lac·ri·mal (-lak'rĭ-m'l) pertaining to the nose and lacrimal apparatus.

na·so·pal·a·tine (-pal'ah-tīn) pertaining to the nose and palate.

na·so·phar·yn·gi·tis (-far″in-ji'tis) inflammation of the nasopharynx.

na·so·pha·ryn·go·la·ryn·go·scope (-fah-ring″go-lah-ring'gah-skōp) a flexible fiberoptic endoscope for examining the nasopharynx and larynx.

na·so·phar·ynx (-far'inks) the part of the pharynx above the soft palate. **nasopharyn'geal,** adj.

na·so·si·nu·si·tis (-si″ah-si'tis) rhinosinusitis.

na·so·tra·che·al (-tra'ke-al) pertaining to the nose and the trachea.

na·sus (na'sus) nose.

na·tal (nāt'l) 1. pertaining to birth. 2. gluteal.

nat·a·my·cin (nat″ah-mi'sin) a polyene antibiotic used in topical treatment of fungal keratitis, blepharitis, and conjunctivitis.

na·teg·li·nide (nah-teg'lĭ-nīd) an agent that stimulates release of insulin from pancreatic islet beta cells, used in the treatment of type 2 diabetes.

Na·tion·al For·mu·lary (NF) a book of standards for certain pharmaceuticals and preparations that are not included in the USP (*United States Pharmacopeia*).

na·tri·ure·sis (na″tre-ūr-e'sis) excretion of sodium in the urine, particularly in excessive amounts. **pressure n.,** increased urinary excretion of sodium along with water when arterial pressure increases; a compensatory mechanism to maintain blood pressure within the normal range.

na·tri·uret·ic (-ūr-et′ik) 1. pertaining to, characterized by, or promoting natriuresis. 2. an agent that promotes natriuresis.

nat·u·ral (nach′ah-r′l) neither artificial nor pathologic.

na·tur·op·a·thy (na″cher-op′ah-the) a drugless system of health care, using a wide variety of therapies, including hydrotherapy, heat, massage, and herbal medicine, whose purpose is to treat the whole person to stimulate and support the person's own innate healing capacity. **naturopath′ic,** adj.

nau·sea (naw′ze-ah) an unpleasant sensation vaguely referred to the epigastrium and abdomen, with a tendency to vomit. **n. gravida′rum,** the morning sickness of pregnancy.

nau·se·ant (naw′ze-ant) 1. inducing nausea. 2. an agent causing nausea.

nau·se·ate (naw′ze-āt) to affect with nausea.

nau·seous (naw′shus) pertaining to or producing nausea.

na·vel (na′v′l) the umbilicus.

na·vic·u·la (nah-vik′u-lah) frenulum of pudendal labia.

na·vic·u·lar (-ler) scaphoid.

Nb niobium.

NBTE nonbacterial thrombotic endocarditis.

NCI National Cancer Institute.

nCi nanocurie; one billionth (10^{-9}) of a curie.

NCN National Council of Nurses.

ND Doctor of Naturopathy.

Nd neodymium.

NDA National Dental Association.

nDNA nuclear DNA.

Nd:YAG neodymium:yttrium-aluminum-garnet; see under *laser.*

Ne neon.

near·sight·ed·ness (nēr-sīt′ed-nes) myopia.

ne·ar·thro·sis (ne″ahr-thro′sis) a false or artificial joint.

neb·u·la (neb′u-lah) pl. *ne′bulae.* [L.] 1. a slight corneal opacity. 2. a preparation, particularly an oily preparation, for use in a nebulizer.

neb·u·li·za·tion (neb″u-lĭ-za′shun) 1. conversion into an aerosol or spray. 2. treatment by an aerosol.

neb·u·liz·er (neb′u-li″zer) atomizer; a device for throwing a spray.

Ne·ca·tor (ne-kāt′or) a genus of hookworms. *N. america′nus* (American or New World hookworm) causes hookworm disease.

ne·ca·to·ri·a·sis (ne-kāt″or-i′ah-sis) hookworm disease caused by species of *Necator.*

ne·ces·si·ty (nĕ-ses′ĭ-te) something necessary or indispensable. **pharmaceutical n.,** a substance having slight or no value therapeutically, but used in the preparation of various pharmaceuticals, including preservatives, solvents, ointment bases, and flavoring, coloring, diluting, emulsifying, and suspending agents.

neck (nek) 1. cervix or collum; the constricted part connecting the head and trunk. 2. the constricted part of an organ or other structure. **anatomical n. of humerus,** a constriction of the humerus just below its proximal articular surface. **bladder n.,** a constricted portion of the urinary bladder, formed by the meeting of its inferolateral surfaces proximal to the opening of the urethra. **n. of femur,** the heavy column of bone connecting the head of the femur and the shaft. **Madelung's n.,** diffuse symmetrical lipomas of the neck. **surgical n. of humerus,** the constricted part of the humerus just below the tuberosities. **n. of tooth,** the narrowed part of a tooth between the crown and the root. **uterine n., n. of uterus,** cervix uteri. **webbed n.,** pterygium colli. **wry n.,** torticollis.

neck·lace (nek′lis) a structure encircling the neck. **Casal's n.,** an eruption in pellagra, encircling the lower part of the neck.

nec·rec·to·my (nĕ-krek′tah-me) excision of necrotic tissue.

necr(o)- word element [Gr.], *death.*

nec·ro·bac·il·lo·sis (nek″ro-bas″ĭ-lo′sis) infection of animals with *Fusobacterium necrophorum.*

nec·ro·bi·o·sis (-bi-o′sis) swelling, basophilia, and distortion of collagen bundles in the dermis, sometimes with obliteration of normal structure, but short of actual necrosis. **necrobiot′ic,** adj.

nec·ro·cy·to·sis (-si-to′sis) death and decay of cells.

nec·ro·gen·ic (-jen′ik) productive of necrosis or death.

ne·crog·e·nous (nĕ-kroj′ĕ-nus) originating or arising from dead matter.

ne·crol·o·gy (nĕ-krol′ah-je) statistics or records of death. **necrolog′ic,** adj.

ne·crol·y·sis (nĕ-krol′ĭ-sis) separation or exfoliation of necrotic tissue. **toxic epidermal n.,** a severe cutaneous reaction, primarily to drugs, but also due to other causes such as infections or neoplastic disease, characterized by bulla formation, subepidermal separation, and widespread loss of skin, leaving raw denuded areas.

nec·ro·phil·ia (nek″ro-fil′e-ah) sexual attraction to or sexual contact with dead bodies.

nec·ro·phil·ic (-fil′ik) 1. pertaining to necrophilia. 2. showing preference for dead tissue, as necrophilic bacteria.

ne·croph·i·lous (nĕ-krof′ĭ-lus) necrophilic.

nec·ro·pho·bia (nek″ro-fo′be-ah) irrational fear of death or of dead bodies.

nec·rop·sy (nek′rop-se) examination of a body after death; autopsy.

nec·rose (nek-rōs′) to become necrotic or to undergo necrosis.

ne·cro·sis (ně-kro′sis) pl. *necro′ses*. [Gr.] the morphological changes indicative of cell death caused by progressive enzymatic degradation; it may affect groups of cells or part of a structure or an organ. **aseptic n.,** necrosis without infection, usually in the head of the femur after traumatic hip dislocation. **Balser's fatty n.,** gangrenous pancreatitis with omental bursitis and disseminated patches of necrosis of fatty tissues. **caseous n.,** cheesy n. **central n.,** that affecting the central portion of an affected bone, cell, or lobule of the liver. **cheesy n.,** that in which the tissue is soft, dry, and cottage cheese–like; most often seen in tuberculosis and syphilis. **coagulation n.,** necrosis of a portion of some organ or tissue, with formation of fibrous infarcts, the protoplasm of the cells becoming fixed and opaque by coagulation of the protein elements, the cellular outline persisting for a long time. **colliquative n.,** that in which the necrotic material becomes softened and liquefied. **contraction band n.,** a cardiac lesion characterized by hypercontracted myofibrils and contraction bands and mitochondrial damage, caused by calcium influx into dying cells resulting in arrest of the cells in the contracted state. **fat n.,** that in which the neutral fats in adipose tissue are split into fatty acids and glycerol, usually affecting the pancreas and peripancreatic fat in acute hemorrhagic pancreatitis. **liquefaction n.,** colliquative n. **phosphorus n.,** necrosis of the jaw bone due to exposure to phosphorus. **postpartum pituitary n.,** necrosis of the pituitary during the postpartum period, often associated with shock and excessive uterine bleeding during delivery, and leading to variable patterns of hypopituitarism. **subcutaneous fat n.,** induration of the subcutaneous fat in newborn and young infants. **n. ustilagi′nea,** dry gangrene due to ergotism. **Zenker's n.,** see under *degeneration*.

nec·ro·sper·mia (nek″ro-sperm′e-ah) a condition in which the spermatozoa of the semen are either motionless or dead. **necrosper′mic,** adj.

ne·crot·ic (ně-krot′ik) pertaining to or characterized by necrosis.

nec·ro·tiz·ing (nek′ro-tīz″ing) causing necrosis.

ne·crot·o·my (ně-krot′ah-me) 1. dissection of a dead body. 2. excision of a sequestrum.

ned·o·cro·mil (ned″o-kro′mil) a nonsteroidal antiinflammatory drug used by inhalation in the treatment of bronchial asthma and topically as the sodium salt in the treatment of allergic conjunctivitis.

nee·dle (ne′d′l) 1. a sharp instrument for suturing or puncturing. 2. to puncture or separate with a needle. **aneurysm n.,** one with a handle, used in ligating blood vessels. **aspirating n.,** a long, hollow needle for removing fluid from a cavity. **cataract n.,** one used in removing a cataract. **discission n.,** a special form of cataract needle. **hypodermic n.,** a short, slender, hollow needle, used in injecting drugs beneath the skin. **stop n.,** one with a shoulder that prevents too deep penetration. **transseptal n.,** one used to puncture the interatrial septum in transseptal catheterization.

neem (nēm) *Azadirachta indica*, a large evergreen tree having antifungal, antibacterial, antiviral, and antimalarial activity; long used medicinally for a wide variety of indications.

NEFA nonesterified fatty acids.

ne·fa·zo·done (ně-fa′zo-dōn) an antidepressant, used as the hydrochloride salt.

neg·a·tive (neg′ah-tiv) 1. having a value less than zero. 2. indicating absence, as of a condition or organism. 3. characterized by refusal, denial, resistance, or opposition.

neg·a·tiv·ism (neg′ah-tǐ-vizm″) opposition to suggestion or advice; behavior opposite to that appropriate to a specific situation or against the wishes of others, including direct resistance to efforts to be moved.

ne·glect (ně-glekt′) disregard of or failure to perform some task or function. **unilateral n.,** hemiapraxia with failure to pay attention to bodily grooming and stimuli on one side but not the other, usually due to a lesion in the central nervous system.

Neis·se·ria (ni-sēr′e-ah) a genus of gram-negative bacteria (family Neisseriaceae), including *N. gonorrhoe′ae*, the etiologic agent of gonorrhea, *N. meningi′tidis*, a prominent cause of meningitis and the specific etiologic agent of meningococcal meningitis.

Neis·se·ri·a·ceae (ni-sēr′e-a′se-e) a family of parasitic bacteria (order Eubacteriales).

nel·fin·a·vir (nel-fin′ah-vir) an HIV protease inhibitor that causes formation of immature, noninfectious viral particles; used as the mesylate salt in the treatment of HIV infection.

nem·a·line (nem'ah-lēn) threadlike or rod-shaped.

Nem·a·thel·min·thes (nem''ah-thel-min'-thēz) in some classifications, a phylum including the Acanthocephala and Nematoda.

nem·a·to·cide (nem'ah-to-sīd'') 1. destroying nematodes. 2. an agent that so acts.

Nem·a·to·da (nem''ah-to'dah) a class of helminths (phylum Aschelminthes), the roundworms, many of which are parasites; in some classifications, considered to be a phylum, and sometimes known as Nemathelminthes, or a class of that phylum.

nem·a·tode (nem'ah-tōd) a roundworm; any individual of the class Nematoda.

ne(o)- word element [Gr.], new; recent.

neo·ad·ju·vant (ne''o-aj'oo-vant) referring to preliminary cancer therapy, usually chemotherapy or radiation therapy, that precedes a necessary second modality of treatment.

neo·an·ti·gen (-an'tĭ-jen) tumor-associated antigen.

neo·blad·der (-blad'er) a continent urinary reservoir constructed from a detubularized bowel segment or from a segment of the stomach, with implantation of the ureters and urethra; used to replace the bladder following cystectomy.

neo·blas·tic (-blas'tik) originating in or of the nature of new tissue.

neo·cer·e·bel·lum (-sĕ''rĭ-bel'um) phylogenetically, the newer parts of the cerebellum, consisting of those parts predominantly supplied by corticopontocerebellar fibers.

neo·cor·tex (-kor'teks) the newer, six-layered portion of the cerebral cortex, showing the most highly evolved stratification and organization. Cf. archicortex and paleocortex.

neo·dym·i·um (Nd) (-dim'e-um) chemical element (see Table of Elements), at. no. 60.

neo·glot·tis (-glot'is) a glottis created by suturing the pharyngeal mucosa over the superior end of the transected trachea above the primary tracheostoma and making a permanent stoma in the mucosa; done to permit phonation after laryngectomy. **neoglot'tic,** adj.

ne·ol·o·gism (ne-ol'ah-jizm) a newly coined word; in psychiatry, a new word whose meaning may be known only to the patient using it.

neo·mem·brane (ne''o-mem'brān) false membrane.

neo·my·cin (-mi'sin) a broad-spectrum aminoglycoside antibiotic produced by Streptomyces fradiae, effective against a wide range of gram-negative bacilli and some gram-positive bacteria; used as the sulfate salt.

ne·on (Ne) (ne'on) chemical element (see Table of Elements), at. no. 10.

neo·na·tal (ne''o-nāt'l) pertaining to the first four weeks after birth.

neo·nate (ne'o-nāt) newborn infant.

neo·na·tol·o·gy (ne''o-na-tol'ah-je) the diagnosis and treatment of disorders of the newborn.

neo·pal·li·um (-pal'e-um) neocortex.

neo·pla·sia (-pla'zhah) the formation of a neoplasm. **cervical intraepithelial n. (CIN),** dysplasia of the cervical epithelium, often premalignant, characterized by various degrees of hyperplasia, abnormal keratinization, and the presence of condylomata. **gestational trophoblastic n. (GTN),** a group of neoplastic disorders that originate in the placenta, including hydatidiform mole, chorioadenoma destruens, and choriocarcinoma. **multiple endocrine n. (MEN),** a group of rare diseases caused by genetic defects that lead to hyperplasia and hyperfunction of two or more components of the endocrine system; type I is characterized by tumors of the pituitary, parathyroid glands, and pancreatic islet cells, with peptic ulcers and sometimes Zollinger-Ellison syndrome; type II is characterized by thyroid medullary carcinoma, pheochromocytoma, and parathyroid hyperplasia; type III is similar to type II but includes neuromas of the oral region, neurofibromas, ganglioneuromas of the gastrointestinal tract, and café-au-lait spots.

neo·plasm (ne'o-plazm) tumor; any new and abnormal growth, specifically one in which cell multiplication is uncontrolled and progressive. Neoplasms may be benign or malignant.

neo·plas·tic (ne''o-plas'tik) 1. pertaining to a neoplasm. 2. pertaining to neoplasia.

ne·op·ter·in (ne-op'ter-in) 1. a pteridine derivative excreted at elevated levels in the urine in some disorders of tetrahydrobiopterin synthesis, certain malignant diseases, viral infection, and graft rejection. 2. any of a class of related compounds.

Neo·rick·ett·sia (ne''o-rĭ-ket'se-ah) a genus of rickettsiae (tribe Ehrlichieae), including a single species, N. helmin'thoeca. It is found in the salmon fluke (Troglotrema salmincola), a parasite of various fish, especially salmon and trout, and causes hemorrhagic enteritis in those ingesting raw infected fish.

neo·stig·mine (-stig'mēn) a cholinergic (cholinesterase inhibitor), used as the bromide or methylsulfate salt in the treatment of myasthenia gravis, in the prevention and treatment of postoperative stasis and atony of the gastrointestinal tract or urinary bladder, and for postsurgical reversal of the effects of nondepolarizing neuromuscular blocking agents.

neo·thal·a·mus (-thal′ah-mus) the part of the thalamus connected to the neocortex.

neo·u·re·thra (-u-re′thrah) a surgically created urethra.

neph·e·lom·e·ter (nef″il-om′it-er) an instrument for measuring the concentration of substances in suspension by means of light scattering by the suspended particles.

ne·phral·gia (ne-fral′jah) pain in a kidney.

neph·rec·ta·sia (nef″rek-ta′zhah) distention of the kidney.

ne·phrec·to·my (ně-frek′tah-me) excision of a kidney.

neph·ric (nef′rik) renal.

ne·phrit·ic (ně-frit′ik) pertaining to or affected with nephritis.

ne·phri·tis (ně-fri′tis) pl. *nephri′tides.* [Gr.] inflammation of the kidney; a focal or diffuse proliferative or destructive disease that may involve the glomerulus, tubule, or interstitial renal tissue. **glomerular n.,** glomerulonephritis. **interstitial n.,** primary or secondary disease of the renal interstitial tissue. **lupus n.,** glomerulonephritis associated with systemic lupus erythematosus. **potassium-losing n.,** see under *uropathy.* **radiation n.,** kidney damage caused by ionizing radiation; symptoms include glomerular and tubular damage, hypertension, and proteinuria, sometimes leading to renal failure. It may be acute or chronic, and some varieties do not manifest until years after the radiation exposure. **salt-losing n.,** see under *nephropathy.* **transfusion n.,** nephropathy following transfusion from an incompatible donor. **tubulointerstitial n.,** nephritis of the renal tubules and interstitial tissues, usually secondary to drug sensitization, systemic infection, graft rejection, or autoimmune disease. An acute type and a chronic type have been distinguished.

ne·phrit·o·gen·ic (ně-frit″o-jen′ik) causing nephritis.

nephr(o)- word element [Gr.], *kidney.*

neph·ro·blas·to·ma·to·sis (nef″ro-blas-to″mah-to′sis) clusters of microscopic blastema cells, tubules, and stromal cells at the periphery of the renal lobes in an infant; believed to be a precursor of Wilms' tumor.

neph·ro·cal·ci·no·sis (-kal″sĭ-no′sis) precipitation of calcium phosphate in the renal tubules, with resultant renal insufficiency.

neph·ro·cele (nef′ro-sēl) hernia of a kidney.

neph·ro·col·ic (nef″ro-kol′ik) pertaining to or connecting the kidney and colon.

neph·ro·co·lop·to·sis (-ko″lop-to′sis) downward displacement of the kidney and colon.

neph·ro·gen·ic (-jen′ik) producing kidney tissue.

ne·phrog·e·nous (ně-froj′ě-nus) arising in a kidney.

ne·phrog·ra·phy (ně-frog′rah-fe) radiography of the kidney.

neph·ro·lith (nef′ro-lith) renal calculus.

nephrolithiasis (nef″ro-lĭ-thi′ah-sis) presence of renal calculi.

neph·ro·li·thot·o·my (nef″ro-lĭ-thot′ah-me) incision of the kidney for removal of calculi.

ne·phrol·o·gy (ně-frol′ah-je) the branch of medical science that deals with the kidneys.

ne·phrol·y·sis (ně-frol′ĭ-sis) 1. freeing of a kidney from adhesions. 2. destruction of kidney substance. **nephrolyt′ic,** adj.

ne·phro·ma (ně-fro′mah) a tumor of the kidney or of kidney tissue. **congenital mesoblastic n.,** a renal tumor similar to Wilms' tumor but appearing earlier and infiltrating more surrounding tissue.

neph·ro·meg·a·ly (nef″ro-meg′ah-le) enlargement of the kidney.

neph·ron (nef′ron) the structural and functional unit of the kidney, numbering about a million in the renal parenchyma, each being capable of forming urine; see also *renal tubules,* under *tubule.*

neph·ron·oph·thi·sis (nef″ron-of′thĭ-sis) wasting disease of the kidney substance. **familial juvenile n.,** a progressive hereditary kidney disease, marked by anemia, polyuria, and renal loss of sodium, progressing to chronic renal failure, tubular atrophy, interstitial fibrosis, glomerular sclerosis, and medullary cysts.

ne·phrop·a·thy (ně-frop′ah-the) disease of the kidneys. **nephropath′ic,** adj. **analgesic n.,** interstitial nephritis with renal papillary necrosis, seen with abuse of analgesics such as aspirin or acetaminophen. **diabetic n.,** the nephropathy seen in later stages of diabetes mellitus, with first hyperfiltration, renal hypertrophy, microalbuminuria, and hypertension, and later proteinuria and end-stage renal disease. **gouty n.,** any of a group of chronic kidney diseases associated with the abnormal production and excretion of uric acid. **HIV-associated n.,** renal pathology in patients infected with the human immunodeficiency virus, a condition resembling focal segmental glomerulosclerosis. **IgA n.,** see under *glomerulonephritis.* **ischemic n.,** nephropathy resulting from partial or complete obstruction of a renal artery and the accompanying ischemia; there is a significant reduction in the glomerular filtration rate. **membranous n.**, see under *glomerulonephritis*. **minimal change n.**, see under *disease*. **obstructive n.**, nephropathy from obstruction of the urinary tract with hydronephrosis and a slowed glomerular filtration rate. **potassium-losing n.**, persistent urinary potassium losses in the presence of hypokalemia, such as in metabolic alkalosis or intrinsic renal disease. **reflux n.**, childhood pyelonephritis in which the renal scarring results from vesicoureteric reflux, with radiological appearance of intrarenal reflux. **salt-losing n.**, any intrinsic renal disease causing abnormal urinary sodium loss to the point of hypotension. **sickle cell n.**, chronic kidney disease in sickle cell disease, including vascular abnormalities, fibrosis, and an increased glomerular filtration rate. **urate n, uric acid n.**, any of a group of kidney diseases with hyperuricemia, including an acute form, a chronic form (*gouty n.*), and nephrolithiasis with uric acid calculi.

neph·ro·pexy (nef′ro-pek″se) fixation or suspension of a hypermobile kidney.

neph·rop·to·sis (nef″rop-to′sis) floating or hypermobile kidney; downward displacement of a kidney.

neph·ro·py·eli·tis (nef″ro-pi″ĕ-li′tis) pyelonephritis.

neph·ro·py·elog·ra·phy (-pi″il-og′rah-fe) radiography of the kidney and its pelvis.

neph·ro·py·o·sis (-pi-o′sis) pyonephrosis.

neph·ror·rha·gia (-ra′jah) hemorrhage from the kidney.

neph·ror·rha·phy (nef-ror′ah-fe) suture of the kidney.

neph·ro·scle·ro·sis (nef″ro-sklĕ-ro′sis) hardening of the kidney due to renovascular disease. **arteriolar n.**, that involving mainly arterioles, with degeneration of renal tubules and fibrotic thickening of glomeruli; there are both benign and malignant forms.

neph·ro·scope (nef′rah-skōp) an instrument inserted into an incision in the renal pelvis for viewing the inside of the kidney.

ne·phro·sis (nĕ-fro′sis) [Gr.] any kidney disease characterized by purely degenerative lesions of the renal tubules. **amyloid n.**, renal amyloidosis. **lipid n.**, minimal change disease. **lower nephron n.**, renal insufficiency leading to uremia, due to necrosis of the lower nephron cells, blocking the tubular lumens of this region; seen after severe injuries, especially crushing injury to muscles (*crush syndrome*).

neph·ro·so·ne·phri·tis (nĕ-fro″so-nĕ-fri′tis) renal disease with nephrotic and nephritic components.

ne·phros·to·my (nĕ-fros′tah-me) creation of a permanent fistula leading into the renal pelvis.

ne·phrot·ic (nĕ-frot′ik) pertaining to, resembling, or caused by nephrosis.

neph·ro·tome (nef′ro-tōm″) one of the segmented divisions of the mesoderm connecting the somite with the lateral plates of unsegmented mesoderm; the source of much of the urogenital system.

neph·ro·to·mog·ra·phy (nef″ro-tah-mog′-rah-fe) radiologic visualization of the kidney by tomography. **nephrotomograph′ic**, adj.

ne·phrot·o·my (nĕ-frot′ah-me) incision of a kidney.

neph·ro·tox·ic (nef′ro-tok″sik) destructive to kidney cells.

neph·ro·tox·in (-tok″sin) a toxin having a specific destructive effect on kidney cells.

neph·ro·tro·pic (nef″ro-tro′pik) having a special affinity for kidney tissue.

neph·ro·tu·ber·cu·lo·sis (-too-berk″u-lo′sis) renal tuberculosis.

neph·ro·ure·ter·ec·to·my (-u-re″ter-ek′tah-me) excision of a kidney and all or part of the ureter.

nep·tu·ni·um (Np) (nep-toon′e-um) chemical element (see *Table of Elements*), at. no. 93.

nerve (nerv) a cordlike structure comprising a collection of nerve fibers that convey impulses between a part of the central nervous system and some other body region. See *Table of Nerves* and Plates 8–14. **accelerator n′s**, the cardiac sympathetic nerves, which, when stimulated, accelerate action of the heart. **afferent n.**, any nerve that transmits impulses from the periphery toward the central nervous system; see *sensory n.* **articular n.**, any mixed peripheral nerve that supplies a joint and its associated structures. **autonomic n.**, any of the parasympathetic or sympathetic nerves of the autonomic nervous system. **centrifugal n.**, efferent n. **centripetal n.**, afferent n. **cutaneous n.**, any mixed peripheral nerve that supplies a region of the skin. **depressor n.**, 1. a nerve that lessens the activity of an organ. 2. an afferent nerve whose stimulation causes a fall in blood pressure. **efferent n.**, any that carries impulses from the central nervous system to the periphery, e.g., a motor nerve. **excitor n.**, one that transmits impulses resulting in an increase in functional activity. **excitoreflex n.**, a visceral nerve that produces reflex action. **furcal n.**, the fourth lumbar nerve. **fusimotor n′s**, those with

TABLE OF NERVES

Common Name* [Modality]	TA Term†	Origin*	Branches*	Distribution*
abducens n. (6th cranial) [motor]	n. abducens	a nucleus in the pons, beneath floor of fourth ventricle		lateral rectus muscle of eyeball
accessory n. (11th cranial) [parasympathetic, motor]	n. accessorius	by cranial roots from side of medulla oblongata, and by spinal roots from spinal cord	internal and external branches	internal branch to vagus, thereby to palate, pharynx, larynx, and thoracic viscera; external to sternocleidomastoid and trapezius muscles
acoustic n. See vestibulocochlear n.				
alveolar n., inferior [motor, general sensory]	n. alveolaris inferior	mandibular n.	inferior dental plexus, mental and mylohyoid n's	teeth and gums of lower jaw, skin of chin and lower lip, mylohyoid muscle and anterior belly of digastric muscle
alveolar n's, superior	nn. alveolares superiores	collective name for superior alveolar branches (anterior, middle, and posterior) that arise from infraorbital and maxillary n's, innervating teeth and gums of upper jaw and maxillary sinus, and forming superior dental plexus		
ampullar n., anterior	n. ampullaris anterior	branch of vestibular n. that innervates ampulla of anterior semicircular duct, ending around hair cells of ampullary crest		
ampullar n., inferior. See ampullar n., posterior				
ampullar n., lateral	n. ampullaris lateralis	branch of vestibular n. that innervates ampulla of lateral semicircular duct, ending around hair cells of ampullary crest		
ampullar n., posterior	n. ampullaris posterior	branch of vestibular n. that innervates ampulla of posterior semicircular duct, ending around hair cells of ampullary crest		
ampullar n., superior. See ampullar n., anterior				
anal n's, inferior [general sensory, motor]		pudendal n., or independently from sacral plexus		sphincter ani externus muscle, skin around anus, lining of anal canal up to pectinate line
anococcygeal n. [general sensory]	n. anococcygeus	coccygeal plexus		sacrococcygeal joint, coccyx, skin over normal coccyx
antebrachial cutaneous n's. See cutaneous n's of forearm				
auditory n. See vestibulocochlear n.				
auricular n's, anterior [general sensory]	nn. auriculares anteriores	auriculotemporal n.		skin of anterosuperior part of external ear
auricular n., great [general sensory]	n. auricularis magnus	cervical plexus—C2–C3	anterior and posterior branches	skin over parotid gland and mastoid process, and both surfaces of auricle

582

*n.†				
auricular n., posterior [motor, general sensory]	n. auricularis posterior	facial n.	occipital branch	posterior auricular and occipitofrontal muscles, skin of external acoustic meatus
auriculotemporal n. [general sensory]	n. auriculotemporalis	by two roots from mandibular n.	anterior auricular n's, n. of external acoustic meatus, parotid branches, branch to tympanic membrane, branches communicating with facial n.; terminal branches superficial temporal to scalp	parotid gland, scalp in temporal region, tympanic membrane. See also auricular n., anterior and n. of external acoustic meatus
axillary n. [motor, general sensory]	n. axillaris	posterior cord of brachial plexus—C5–C6	lateral superior brachial cutaneous n., muscular branches	deltoid and teres minor muscles, skin over back of arm
brachial cutaneous n's. See cutaneous n's of arm				
buccal n. [general sensory]	n. buccalis	mandibular n.		skin and mucous membrane of cheeks, gums, and perhaps first two molars and the premolars
cardiac n., inferior. See cardiac n., inferior cervical				
cardiac n., inferior cervical [sympathetic (accelerator), visceral afferent (chiefly pain)]	n. cardiacus cervicalis inferior	cervicothoracic ganglion		heart via cardiac plexus
cardiac n., middle, See cardiac n., middle cervical				
cardiac n., middle cervical [sympathetic (accelerator), visceral afferent (chiefly pain)]	n. cardiacus cervicalis medius	middle cervical ganglion		heart
cardiac n., superior. See cardiac n., superior cervical				
cardiac n., superior cervical [sympathetic (accelerator)]	n. cardiacus cervicalis superior	superior cervical ganglion		heart
cardiac n's, thoracic [sympathetic (accelerator), visceral afferent (chiefly pain)]	rami cardiaci thoracici	ganglia T2–T4 or T5 of sympathetic trunk		heart
caroticotympanic n's (inferior and superior) [sympathetic]	nn. caroticotympanici	internal carotid plexus	with tympanic n. form tympanic plexus	tympanic region, parotid gland

*n. = nerve; n's = (pl.) nerves.
†n. = [L.] nervus; nn. = ([L.] pl.) nervi.

Common Name* [Modality]	TA Term†	Origin*	Branches*	Distribution*
carotid n's, external [sympathetic]	nn. carotici externi	superior cervical ganglion		cranial blood vessels and glands via external carotid plexus
carotid n., internal [sympathetic]	n. caroticus internus	superior cervical ganglion		cranial blood vessels and glands via internal carotid plexus
cavernous n's of clitoris [parasympathetic, sympathetic, visceral afferent]	nn. cavernosi clitoridis	uterovaginal plexus		erectile tissue of clitoris
cavernous n's of penis [sympathetic, parasympathetic, visceral afferent]	nn. cavernosi penis	prostatic plexus		erectile tissue of penis
cerebral n's. See cranial n's				
cervical n's	nn. cervicales	the 8 pairs of n's that arise from cervical segments of spinal cord and, except last pair, leave vertebral column above correspondingly numbered vertebra; the anterior branches of upper 4, on either side, unite to form cervical plexus; those of lower 4, together with anterior branch of first thoracic n., form most of brachial plexus		
cervical n., transverse [general sensory]	n. transversus colli	cervical plexus—C2–C3	superior and inferior branches	skin on side and front of neck
cervical cardiac n's. See cardiac n's, cervical				
ciliary n's, long [sympathetic, general sensory]	nn. ciliares longi	nasociliary n., from ophthalmic n.		dilator muscle of pupil, uvea, cornea
ciliary n's, short [parasympathetic, sympathetic, general sensory]	nn. ciliares breves	ciliary ganglion		smooth muscles and tunics of eye
cluneal n's, inferior [general sensory]	nn. clunium inferiores	posterior femoral cutaneous n.		skin of lower part of buttock
cluneal n's, middle [general sensory]	nn. clunium medii	plexus formed by lateral branches of posterior branches of first 4 sacral nerves		ligaments of sacrum and skin over posterior part of buttock
cluneal n's, superior [general sensory]	nn. clunium superiores	lateral branches of posterior branches of upper lumbar n's		skin of upper part of buttock
coccygeal n.	n. coccygeus	either of the pair of nerves arising from coccygeal segment of spinal cord		
cochlear n.	n. cochlearis	the part of the vestibulocochlear n. concerned with hearing, consisting of fibers that arise from the bipolar cells in the spiral ganglion and have their receptors in the spiral organ of the cochlea		

584

cranial n's	nn. craniales	the 12 pairs of n's connected with brain, including olfactory (I), optic (II), oculomotor (III), trochlear (IV), trigeminal (V), abducens (VI), facial (VII), vestibulocochlear (VIII), glossopharyngeal (IX), vagus (X), accessory (XI), and hypoglossal (XII) nerves		
crural interosseous n. See interosseous n. of leg				
cubital n. See ulnar n.				
cutaneous n's, perforating	n. cutaneus perforans	second and third sacral n's		skin over inferomedial gluteus maximus
cutaneous n. of arm, inferior lateral [general sensory]	n. cutaneus brachii lateralis inferior	radial n.		skin of lateral surface of lower arm
cutaneous n. of arm, medial [general sensory]	n. cutaneus brachii medialis	medial cord of brachial plexus (T1)		skin of medial and posterior aspects of arm
cutaneous n. of arm, posterior [general sensory]	n. cutaneus brachii posterior	radial n. in axilla		skin of back of arm
cutaneous n. of arm, superior lateral [general sensory]	n. cutaneus brachii lateralis superior	axillary n.		skin of back of arm
cutaneous n's of calf. See sural cutaneous n's				
cutaneous cervical n. See cervical n., transverse				
cutaneous n. of foot, intermediate dorsal [general sensory]	n. cutaneus dorsalis intermedius	superficial peroneal n.	dorsal digital n's of foot	skin of front of lower third of leg and dorsum of foot; ankle; skin and joints of adjacent sides of third and fourth, and of fourth and fifth toes
cutaneous n. of foot, lateral dorsal [general sensory]	n. cutaneus dorsalis lateralis	continuation of sural n.		skin and joints of lateral side of foot and fifth toe
cutaneous n. of foot, medial dorsal [general sensory]	n. cutaneus dorsalis medialis	superficial peroneal n.		skin and joints of medial side of foot and big toe; adjacent sides of second and third toes
cutaneous n. of forearm, lateral [general sensory]	n. cutaneus antebrachii lateralis	continuation of musculocutaneous n.		skin over radial side of forearm; sometimes an area of skin of back of hand
cutaneous n. of forearm, medial [general sensory]	n. cutaneus antebrachii medialis	medial cord of brachial plexus (C8, T1)	anterior and ulnar	skin of front, medial, and posteromedial aspects of forearm
cutaneous n. of forearm, posterior [general sensory]	n. cutaneus antebrachii posterior	radial n.		skin of dorsal aspect of forearm
cutaneous n. of neck, transverse. See cervical n., transverse				

TABLE OF NERVES *Continued*

Common Name* [Modality]	TA Term†	Origin*	Branches*	Distribution*
cutaneous n. of thigh, lateral [general sensory]	n. cutaneus femoris lateralis	lumbar plexus—L2–L3		skin of lateral aspect and front of thigh
cutaneous n. of thigh, posterior [general sensory] *See digital n's of radial n., dorsal*	n. cutaneus femoris posterior	sacral plexus—S1–S3	inferior cluneal n's, perineal branches	skin of buttock, external genitalia, back of thigh and calf
digital n's, radial dorsal. *See digital n's of ulnar n., dorsal*				
digital n's of foot, dorsal [general sensory]	nn. digitales dorsales pedis	1. intermediate dorsal cutaneous n. 2. deep peroneal n.		1. skin and joint of adjacent sides of third and fourth, and of fourth and fifth toes 2. skin and joints of adjacent sides of great and second toes
digital n's of lateral plantar n., common plantar [general sensory]	nn. digitales plantares communes nervi plantaris lateralis	superficial branch of lateral plantar n.	medial n. gives rise to 2 proper plantar digital n's	lateral one to short flexor muscle of little toe, skin and joints of lateral side of sole and little toe; medial one to adjacent sides of fourth and fifth toes
digital n's of lateral plantar n., proper plantar [general sensory]	nn. digitales plantares proprii nervi plantaris lateralis	common plantar digital n's		short flexor muscle of little toe, skin and joints of lateral side of sole and little toe, and adjacent surfaces of fourth and fifth toes
digital n's of medial plantar n., common plantar [motor, general sensory]	nn. digitales plantares communes nervi plantaris medialis	medial plantar n.	muscular branches, proper plantar digital n's	short flexor muscle of great toe and first lumbrical muscles, skin and joints of medial side of foot and great toe, and adjacent sides of great and second, second and third, and third and fourth toes
digital n's of medial plantar n., proper plantar [general sensory]	nn. digitales plantares proprii nervi plantaris medialis	common plantar digital n's		skin and joints of great toe, and adjacent sides of great and second, second and third, and third and fourth toes; the nerves extend to the dorsum to supply nail beds and tips of toes
digital n's of median n., common palmar [motor, general sensory]	nn. digitales palmares communes nervi mediani	lateral and medial divisions of median n.	proper palmar digital n's	thumb, index, middle, and ring fingers, and first two lumbrical muscles

586

English name [type]	Latin name	Origin	Branches	Distribution
digital n's of median n., proper palmar [motor, general sensory]	nn. digitales palmares proprii nervi mediani	common palmar digital n's		first two lumbrical muscles, skin and joints of both sides and palmar aspect of thumb, index, and middle fingers, radial side of ring finger, back of distal aspect of these digits
digital n's of radial n., dorsal [general sensory]	nn. digitales dorsales nervi radialis	superficial branch of radial n.		skin and joints of back of thumb, index finger, and part of middle fingers, as far distally as digital phalanx
digital n's of ulnar n., common palmar [general sensory]	nn. digitales palmares communes nervi ulnaris	superficial branch of ulnar n.	proper palmar digital n's	little and ring fingers
digital n's of ulnar n., dorsal [general sensory]	nn. digitales dorsales nervi ulnaris	dorsal branch of ulnar n.		skin and joints of medial side of little finger, dorsal aspects of adjacent sides of little and ring fingers and of ring and middle fingers
digital n's of ulnar n., proper palmar [general sensory]	nn. digitales palmares proprii nervi ulnaris	the lateral of the two common palmar digital n's from superficial branch of ulnar n.		skin and joints of adjacent sides of fourth and fifth fingers
dorsal n. of clitoris [general sensory, motor]	n. dorsalis clitoridis	pudendal n.		deep transverse muscle of perineum, sphincter muscle of urethra, corpus cavernosum clitoridis, and skin, prepuce, and glans of clitoris
dorsal n. of penis [general sensory, motor]	n. dorsalis penis	pudendal n.		deep transverse muscle of perineum, sphincter muscle of urethra, corpus cavernosum penis, and skin, prepuce, and glans of penis
dorsal scapular n. [motor]	n. dorsalis scapulae	brachial plexus—anterior branch of C5		rhomboid muscles and occasionally the levator muscle of scapula
ethmoidal n., anterior [general sensory]	n. ethmoidalis anterior	continuation of nasociliary n., from ophthalmic n.	internal, external, lateral, and medial nasal branches	mucosa of upper and anterior nasal septum, lateral wall of nasal cavity, skin of lower bridge and tip of nose
ethmoidal n., posterior [general sensory]	n. ethmoidalis posterior	nasociliary n., from ophthalmic n.		mucosa of posterior ethmoid cells and of sphenoidal sinus
n. of external acoustic meatus [general sensory]	n. meatus acustici externi	auriculotemporal n.		skin lining external acoustic meatus, and tympanic membrane

Common Name† [Modality]	TA Term†	Origin*	Branches*	Distribution*
facial n. (7th cranial) [motor, parasympathetic, general sensory, special sensory]. See also intermediate n.	n. facialis	inferior border of pons, between olive and inferior cerebellar peduncle	stapedius n.; posterior auricular n.; parotid plexus; digastric, stylohyoid, temporal, zygomatic, buccal, lingual, marginal mandibular, and cervical branches, and communicating branch with tympanic plexus	various structures of face, head, and neck (see also individual branches in this table)
femoral n. [general sensory, motor]	n. femoralis	lumbar plexus—L2–L4; descending behind inguinal ligament to femoral triangle	saphenous n., muscular and anterior cutaneous branches	skin of thigh and leg, muscles of front of thigh, and hip and knee joints (see also individual branches in this table)
femoral cutaneous n's. See cutaneous n's of thigh fibular n's. See peroneal n's				
frontal n. [general sensory]	n. frontalis	ophthalmic division of trigeminal n.; enters orbit through superior orbital fissure	supraorbital and supratrochlear n's	chiefly to forehead and scalp (see individual branches listed in this table)
genitofemoral n. [general sensory, motor]	n. genitofemoralis	lumbar plexus—L1–L2	genital and femoral branches	cremaster muscle, skin of scrotum or labium majus and of adjacent area of thigh and femoral triangle
glossopharyngeal n. (9th cranial) [motor, parasympathetic, general sensory, special sensory, visceral sensory]	n. glossopharyngeus	several rootlets from lateral side of upper medulla oblongata, between olive and inferior cerebellar peduncle	tympanic n., pharyngeal, stylopharyngeal, carotid tonsillar, and lingual branches, communicating branches with auricular and meningeal branches of vagus n., with chorda tympani, and with auriculotemporal n.	has two enlargements (superior and inferior ganglia) and supplies tongue, pharynx, and parotid nerve (see also individual branches in this table)
gluteal n., inferior [motor] gluteal n., superior [motor, general sensory]	n. gluteus inferior n. gluteus superior	sacral plexus—L5–S2 sacral plexus—L4–S1		gluteus maximus muscle gluteus medius and minimus muscles, tensor fasciae latae muscle, and hip joint
hemorrhoidal n's, inferior. See anal n's, inferior				
hypogastric n.	n. hypogastricus	a nerve trunk situated on either side (right and left), interconnecting superior and inferior hypogastric plexuses		
hypoglossal n. (12th cranial) [motor]	n. hypoglossus	several rootlets in anterolateral sulcus between olive and pyramid of medulla oblongata; passes through hypoglossal canal to tongue	lingual branches	styloglossus, hyoglossus, and genioglossus muscles, intrinsic muscles of tongue

iliohypogastric n. [motor, general sensory]	n. iliohypogastricus	lumbar plexus—L1 (sometimes T12)	lateral and anterior cutaneous branches	skin above pubis and over lateral side of buttock, and occasionally pyramidal muscle
ilioinguinal n. [general sensory]	n. ilioinguinalis	lumbar plexus—L1 (sometimes T12); accompanies spermatic cord through inguinal canal	anterior scrotal or labial branches	skin of scrotum or labia majora, and adjacent part of thigh
infraorbital n. [general sensory]	n. infraorbitalis	continuation of maxillary n., entering orbit through inferior orbital fissure, occupying in succession infraorbital groove, canal, and foramen	middle and anterior superior alveolar, inferior palpebral, internal and external nasal, and superior labial branches	incisor, cuspid, and premolar teeth of upper jaw, skin and conjunctiva of lower eyelid, mobile septum and skin of side of nose, mucous membrane of mouth, skin of upper lip
infratrochlear n. [general sensory]	n. infratrochlearis	nasociliary n., from ophthalmic n.	palpebral branches	skin of root and upper bridge of nose and lower eyelid, conjunctiva, lacrimal duct
intercostal n's	nn. intercostales	branches of the first 11 thoracic spinal n's, situated between the ribs. The first 3 send branches to the brachial plexus and thoracic wall; 4 through 6 supply only the thoracic wall; and 7 through 11 are thoracoacromial in distribution		
intercostobrachial n's [general sensory]	nn. intercostobrachiales	second and third intercostal n's		skin of axilla and of back and medial aspect of arm
intermediate n. [parasympathetic, special sensory]	n. intermedius	smaller root of facial n., between main root and vestibulocochlear n.	greater petrosal n., chorda tympani	lacrimal, nasal, palatine, submandibular, and sublingual glands, and anterior two-thirds of tongue
interosseous n. of forearm, anterior [motor, general sensory]	n. interosseus antebrachii anterior	median n.		long flexor of thumb, deep flexor of fingers, and pronator quadratus muscles, wrist and intercarpal joints
interosseous n. of forearm, posterior [motor, general sensory]	n. interosseus antebrachii posterior	continuation of deep branch of radial n.		long abductor muscle of thumb, extensor muscles of thumb and index finger, and wrist and intercarpal joints
interosseous n. of leg [general sensory]	n. interosseus cruris	tibial n.		interosseous membrane and tibiofemoral syndesmosis
ischiadic n. See sciatic n.				
jugular n.	n. jugularis	a branch of the superior cervical ganglion that communicates with glossopharyngeal and vagus n's		
labial n's, anterior [general sensory]	nn. labiales anteriores	ilioinguinal n.		skin of anterior labial region of labia majora and adjacent part of thigh

TABLE OF NERVES Continued

Common Name* [Modality]	TA Term†	Origin*	Branches*	Distribution*
labial n's, posterior [general sensory]	nn. labiales posteriores	perineal n's		labium majus
lacrimal n. [general sensory]	n. lacrimalis	ophthalmic division of trigeminal n., entering orbit through superior orbital fissure		lacrimal gland, conjunctiva, lateral commissure of eye, skin of upper eyelid
laryngeal n., external [motor]	ramus externus nervi laryngei superioris	superior laryngeal n.		cricothyroid, inferior constrictor of pharynx
laryngeal n., inferior [motor]		recurrent laryngeal n., especially the terminal portion		intrinsic muscles of larynx, except cricothyroid, communicates with internal laryngeal n.
laryngeal n., internal [general sensory]	ramus internus nervi laryngealis superioris	superior laryngeal n.		mucosa of epiglottis, base of tongue, and larynx
laryngeal n., recurrent [parasympathetic, visceral afferent, motor]	n. laryngeus recurrens	vagus n. (chiefly the cranial part of the accessory n.)	inferior laryngeal n., tracheal, esophageal, pharyngeal, and inferior cardiac branches	tracheal mucosa, esophagus, inferior constrictor muscle of pharynx, cardiac plexus (see also individual branches in this table)
laryngeal n., superior [motor, general sensory, visceral afferent, parasympathetic]	n. laryngeus superior	inferior ganglion of vagus n.	external, internal, and communicating branches	cricothyroid muscle and inferior constrictor muscle of pharynx, mucosa of epiglottis, base of tongue, and larynx
lingual n. [general sensory]	n. lingualis	mandibular n., descending to tongue, first medial to mandible and then under cover of mucosa of mouth	sublingual n, lingual branches, branches to isthmus of fauces, branches communicating with hypoglossal n. and chorda tympani	anterior two-thirds of tongue, adjacent areas of mouth, gums, isthmus of fauces, sublingual gland and overlying mucosa
lumbar n's	nn. lumbales	the 5 pairs of n's that arise from lumbar segments of spinal cord, each pair leaving vertebral column below correspondingly numbered vertebrae; anterior branches of these nerves participate in formation of lumbosacral plexus		
mandibular n. (third division of trigeminal n.) [general sensory, motor]	n. mandibularis	mandibular division of trigeminal n.	meningeal branch, masseteric, deep temporal, lateral and medial pterygoid, buccal, auriculotemporal, lingual, and inferior alveolar n's	extensive distribution to muscles of mastication, skin of face, mucous membrane of mouth, teeth, dura mater, mucous membrane of mastoid air cells (see also individual branches in this table)
masseteric n. [motor, general sensory]	n. massetericus	mandibular division of trigeminal n.		masseter muscle, temporomandibular joint

590

maxillary n. (second division of trigeminal n.) [general sensory]	n. maxillaris	trigeminal ganglion	meningeal branch, zygomatic, superior alveolar, and infraorbital n's, ganglionic branches to pterygopalatine ganglion, and (indirectly) branches of pterygopalatine ganglion	dura mater, extensive distribution to skin of face and scalp, mucous membrane of maxillary sinus and nasal cavity, and teeth (see also individual branches in this table)
median n. [general sensory]	n. medianus	lateral and medial cords of brachial plexus—C6-T1	anterior interosseous n. of forearm, common palmar digital n's, and muscular and palmar branches, a communicating branch with ulnar n.	the elbow, wrist, and intercarpal joints, anterior muscles of the forearm, muscles of the digits, skin of the palm, thenar eminence, and digits (see also individual branches in this table)
mental n. [general sensory]	n. mentalis	inferior alveolar n.	mental, gingival, and inferior labial branches	skin of chin, lower lip
musculocutaneous n. [general sensory, motor]	n. musculocutaneus	lateral cord of brachial plexus—C5-C7	lateral cutaneous n. of forearm, muscular branches	coracobrachial, biceps brachii, and brachial muscles, elbow joint, skin of radial side of forearm
mylohyoid n. [motor]	n. mylohyoideus	inferior alveolar n.		mylohyoid muscle, anterior belly of digastric muscle
nasociliary n. [general sensory]	n. nasociliaris	ophthalmic division of trigeminal n.	long ciliary, posterior ethmoidal, anterior ethmoidal, and infratrochlear n's, and a communicating branch to ciliary ganglion	(see individual branches in this table)
nasopalatine n. [parasympathetic, general sensory]	n. nasopalatinus	pterygopalatine ganglion		mucosa and glands of most of nasal septum and anterior part of hard palate
obturator n. [general sensory, motor]	n. obturatorius	lumbar plexus—L3-L4	anterior, posterior, and muscular branches	gracilis and adductor muscles, skin of medial part of thigh, and hip and knee joints
obturator n., accessory [general sensory, motor]	n. obturatorius accessorius	anterior branches of L3-L4		pectineal muscle, hip joint, communicates with obturator n.
obturator n., internal [general sensory, motor]	n. musculi obturatorii interni	anterior branches of L5, S1-S2		superior gemellus, internal obturator muscles
occipital n., greater [general sensory, motor]	n. occipitalis major	medial branch of posterior branch of C2		semispinal muscle of head and skin of scalp as far forward as vertex
occipital n., lesser [general sensory]	n. occipitalis minor	superficial cervical plexus—C2-C3		ascends behind auricle and supplies some of the skin of side of head and on cranial surface of auricle

TABLE OF NERVES *Continued*

Common Name* [Modality]	TA Term†	Origin*	Branches*	Distribution*
occipital n., third [general sensory]	n. occipitalis tertius	medial branch of posterior branch of C3		skin of upper part of back of neck and head
oculomotor n. (3rd cranial) [motor, parasympathetic]	n. oculomotorius	brainstem, emerging medial to cerebral peduncles, running forward in the cavernous sinus	superior and inferior branches	entering orbit through superior orbital fissure, the branches supply levator muscle of upper lid, all extrinsic muscles except lateral rectus and superior oblique, and carry para-sympathetic fibers for the ciliary muscle and sphincter muscle of pupil
olfactory n. (1st cranial) [special sensory]	n. olfactorius	the nerve of smell, consisting of about 20 bundles (sometimes called olfactory nerves) arising in the olfactory epithelium and passing through the cribriform plate of ethmoid bone to olfactory bulb		
ophthalmic n. (first division of trigeminal n.) [general sensory]	n. ophthalmicus	trigeminal ganglion	tentorial, frontal, lacrimal, nasociliary n's	eyeball and conjunctiva, lacrimal sac and gland, nasal mucosa and frontal sinus, external nose, eyelid, forehead, and scalp (see also individual branches in this table)
optic n. (2nd cranial) [special sensory]	n. opticus	the nerve of sight (actually part of the central nervous system), consisting chiefly of axons and central processes of cells of the ganglionic layer of retina leaving each orbit through the optic canal, joining with the contralateral optic n. to form the optic chiasm (the medial fibers of each nerve crossing over to opposite side), and continuing as the optic tract		
palatine n., anterior. *See* palatine n., greater				
palatine n., greater [parasym-pathetic, sympathetic; general sensory]	n. palatinus major	pterygopalatine ganglion	posterior inferior [lateral] nasal branches	emerges through greater palatine foramen and supplies palate
palatine n's, lesser [parasym-pathetic, sympathetic; general sensory]	nn. palatini minores	pterygopalatine ganglion		emerge through lesser palatine foramen and supply soft palate and tonsil
pectoral n., lateral [motor, general sensory]	n. pectoralis lateralis	lateral cord of brachial plexus or anterior divisions of upper and middle trunks (C5–C7)		usually several nerves supplying the smaller pectoral muscle and acromioclavicular and shoulder joints

592

Common name [modality]	NA term	Origin	Branches	Distribution
pectoral n., medial [motor]	n. pectoralis medialis	medial cord or lower trunk of brachial plexus (C8, T1)		usually several nerves supplying the greater and smaller pectoral muscles
perforating cutaneous n. See cutaneous n., perforating				
perineal n's [motor, general sensory]	nn. perineales	pudendal n. in pudendal canal	muscular branches and posterior scrotal or labial n's	muscular branches supply bulbospongiosus, ischiocavernosus, superficial transverse perineal muscles and bulb of penis and, in part, sphincter ani externi and levator ani; the scrotal (labial) n's supply the scrotum or labium majus
peroneal n., common [general sensory, motor]	n. fibularis communis	sciatic n. in lower part of thigh		supplies short head of biceps femoris muscle; gives off lateral sural cutaneous n. and communicating branch as it descends in popliteal fossa, supplies knee and superior tibiofibular joints and anterior tibial muscle; divides into superficial and deep peroneal n's
peroneal n., deep [general sensory, motor]	n. fibularis profundus	common peroneal n.		winds around neck of fibula and descends on the interosseous membrane to front of ankle; muscular branches given off to anterior tibial, extensor of great toe, long extensor of toes, and third peroneal muscles, and a twig to ankle joint; a lateral terminal division supplies short extensor muscle of toes and tarsal joints; medial terminal division, or digital branch, divides into dorsal digital n's for skin and joints of adjacent sides of first and second toes
peroneal n., superficial common [general sensory, motor]	n. fibularis superficialis	common peroneal n.		descends in front of fibula, supplies long and short peroneal muscles and, in the lower part of the leg, divides into the muscular rami, medial and intermediate dorsal cutaneous n's (see also individual branches listed in this table)
petrosal n., deep [sympathetic]	n. petrosus profundus	internal carotid plexus		joins greater petrosal n. to form n. of pterygoid canal, and supplies lacrimal, nasal, and palatine glands via pterygopalatine ganglion and its branches
petrosal n., greater [parasympathetic, general sensory]	n. petrosus major	intermediate n. via geniculate ganglion		running forward from geniculate ganglion, joins deep petrosal n. of pterygoid canal, and reaches lacrimal, nasal, and palatine glands and nasopharynx, via pterygopalatine ganglion and its branches

TABLE OF NERVES *Continued*

Common Name* [Modality]	TA Term†	Origin*	Branches*	Distribution*
petrosal n., lesser [parasympathetic]	n. petrosus minor	tympanic plexus		parotid gland via otic ganglion and auriculotemporal n.
pharyngeal n.	n. pharyngeus	posterior part of pterygo-palatine ganglion		mucosa of nasopharynx behind auditory tube
phrenic n. [motor, general sensory]	n. phrenicus	cervical plexus—C4-C5	pericardial and phrenicoabdominal branches	pleura, pericardium, diaphragm, peritoneum, sympathetic plexuses
phrenic n's, accessory	nn. phrenici accessorii	inconstant contribution of fifth cervical n. to phrenic n.; when present, they run a separate course to root of neck or into thorax before joining phrenic n.		
piriform n. [general sensory, motor]	n. musculi piriformis	posterior branches of anterior branches of S1-S2		anterior piriform muscle
plantar n., lateral [general sensory, motor]	n. plantaris lateralis	smaller of terminal branches of tibial n.	muscular, superficial, and deep branches; the superficial gives off common plantar digital n.	lying between first and second layers of muscles of sole, supplies quadratus plantae, abductor of little toe, short flexor of little toe, adductor of great toe, interosseous, and second, third, and fourth lumbrical muscles, and gives off cutaneous and articular twigs to lateral side of sole and fourth and fifth toes
plantar n., medial [general sensory, motor]	n. plantaris medialis	larger of terminal branches of tibial n.	common plantar digital n's and muscular branches	abductor of great toe, short flexor of great toe, short flexor of toes, and first lumbrical muscles, and cutaneous and articular twigs to medial side of sole and to the first to fourth toes (see also individual branches in this table)
pneumogastric n. *See* vagus n.				
popliteal n., lateral. *See* peroneal n., common				
popliteal n., medial. *See* tibial n.				
pterygoid n., lateral [motor]	n. pterygoideus lateralis	mandibular n.		lateral pterygoid muscle

English name [type]	Latin name	Origin/course	Distribution
pterygoid n., medial [motor]	n. pterygoideus medialis	mandibular n.	medial pterygoid, tensor tympani, and tensor veli palatini muscles
n. of pterygoid canal [parasympathetic, sympathetic]	n. canalis pterygoidei	union of deep and greater petrosal n's	pterygopalatine ganglion and branches
pudendal n. [general sensory, motor, parasympathetic]	n. pudendus	enters pudendal canal, gives off inferior anal n's, then divides into perineal n's and dorsal n. of penis (clitoris)	muscles, skin, and erectile tissue of perineum (see also individual branches in this table)
		sacral plexus—S2–S4	
n. to quadratus femoris muscle [general sensory, motor]	n. musculi quadrati femoris	anterior branches of L4–L5	inferior gemellus and anterior quadratus femoris muscles, hip joint
radial n. [general sensory, motor]	n. radialis	posterior cord of brachial plexus—C6–C8, and sometimes C5 and T1	descending in back of arm and forearm, ultimately distributed to skin on back of forearm, arm, and hand, extensor muscles on back of arm and forearm, and elbow joint and many joints of hand (see also branches in this table)
		posterior cutaneous and inferior lateral cutaneous n's of arm, posterior cutaneous n. of forearm, muscular, deep, and superficial branches	
rectal n's, inferior. See anal n's, inferior			
recurrent n. See laryngeal n., recurrent			
saccular n.	n. saccularis	the branch of the vestibular n. that innervates macula of saccule	
sacral n's	nn. sacrales	the 5 pairs of n's (S1–S5) that arise from sacral segments of spinal cord; the anterior branches of first 4 pairs participate in formation of sacral plexus	
saphenous n. [general sensory]	n. saphenus	termination of femoral n.	knee joint, subsartorial and patellar plexuses, skin on medial side of leg and foot
			infrapatellar and medial crural cutaneous branches
sciatic n. [general sensory, motor]	n. ischiadicus	divides into common peroneal and tibial n's, usually in lower third of thigh	(see individual branches in this table)
		sacral plexus—L4–S3; leaves pelvis through greater sciatic foramen	
scrotal n's, anterior [general sensory]	nn. scrotales anteriores	ilioinguinal n.	skin of anterior scrotal region
scrotal n's, posterior [general sensory]	nn. scrotales posteriores	perineal n's	skin of scrotum
spinal n's	nn. spinales	the 31 pairs of n's that arise from spinal cord, and pass between the vertebrae, including 8 cervical, 12 thoracic, 5 lumbar, 5 sacral, and 1 coccygeal	
splanchnic n., greater [preganglionic sympathetic, visceral afferent]	n. splanchnicus major	thoracic sympathetic trunk and thoracic ganglia T5–T10 of sympathetic trunk	descending through diaphragm or its aortic opening, ends in celiac ganglia and plexuses, with a splanchnic ganglion commonly near the diaphragm

595

TABLE OF NERVES *Continued*

Common Name* [Modality]	TA Term†	Origin*	Branches*	Distribution*
splanchnic n., lesser [preganglionic sympathetic, visceral afferent]	n. splanchnicus minor	thoracic ganglia T9, T10 of sympathetic trunk	renal branch	pierces diaphragm, joins aorticorenal ganglion and celiac plexus, and communicates with renal and superior mesenteric plexuses
splanchnic n., lowest [sympathetic, visceral afferent]	n. splanchnicus imus	last ganglion of sympathetic trunk or lesser splanchnic n.		aorticorenal ganglion and adjacent plexus
splanchnic n's, lumbar [preganglionic sympathetic, visceral afferent]	nn. splanchnici lumbales	lumbar ganglia or sympathetic trunk		upper nerves join celiac and adjacent plexuses, middle ones go to mesenteric and adjacent plexuses, lower ones descend to superior hypogastric plexus
splanchnic n's, pelvic [preganglionic parasympathetic, visceral afferent]	radix parasympathica ganglionorum pelvicorum	sacral plexus—S3–S4		leaving sacral plexus, they enter inferior hypogastric plexus and supply pelvic organs
splanchnic n's, sacral [preganglionic sympathetic, visceral afferent]	nn. splanchnici sacrales	sacral part of sympathetic trunk		pelvic organs and blood vessels via inferior hypogastric plexus
stapedius n. [motor]	n. stapedius	facial n.		stapedius muscle
subclavian n. [motor, general sensory]	n. subclavius	upper trunk of brachial plexus—C5		subclavius muscle, sternoclavicular joint
subcostal n. [general sensory, motor]	n. subcostalis	anterior branch of thoracic n. T12		skin of lower abdomen and lateral side of gluteal region, parts of transverse, oblique, and rectus muscles, and usually pyramidal muscle, and adjacent peritoneum
sublingual n. [parasympathetic, general sensory]	n. sublingualis	lingual n.		sublingual gland and overlying mucous membrane
suboccipital n. [motor]	n. suboccipitalis	posterior branch of cervical n. C1		emerges above posterior arch of atlas, supplies muscles of suboccipital triangle and semispinal muscle of head
subscapular n's [motor]	nn. subscapulares	posterior cord of brachial plexus—C5		usually two or more nerves, upper and lower, supplying subscapular and teres major muscles

596

supraclavicular n's	nn. supraclaviculares	a term denoting collectively the common trunk, which is a branch of the cervical plexus (C3–C4) and which emerges under cover of the posterior border of the sternocleidomastoid muscle and divides into the intermediate, lateral, and medial supraclavicular n's		
supraclavicular n's, anterior. *See supraclavicular n's, medial*				
supraclavicular n's, intermediate [general sensory]	nn. supraclaviculares intermedii	cervical plexus—C3–C4		descend in posterior triangle, cross clavicle, supplying skin over pectoral and deltoid regions
supraclavicular n's, lateral [general sensory]	nn. supraclaviculares laterales	cervical plexus—C3–C4		descend in posterior triangle, cross clavicle, supplying skin of superior and posterior aspects of shoulder
supraclavicular n's, medial [general sensory]	nn. supraclaviculares mediales	cervical plexus—C3–C4		descend in posterior triangle, cross clavicle, supplying skin of medial infraclavicular region
supraclavicular n's, middle. *See supraclavicular n's, intermediate*				
supraclavicular n's, posterior. *See supraclavicular n's, lateral*				
supraorbital n. [general sensory]	n. supraorbitalis	continuation of frontal n., from ophthalmic n.	lateral and medial branches	leaves orbit through supraorbital notch or foramen, supplying skin of upper eyelid, forehead, anterior part of scalp (to vertex), mucosa of frontal sinus
suprascapular n. [motor, general sensory]	n. suprascapularis	brachial plexus—C5–C6		descends through suprascapular and spinoglenoid notches, supplying acromioclavicular and shoulder joints, and supraspinous and infraspinous muscles
supratrochlear n. [general sensory]	n. supratrochlearis	frontal n., from ophthalmic n.		leaves orbit at medial end of supraorbital margin, supplying forehead and upper eyelid

597

TABLE OF NERVES *Continued*

Common Name* [Modality]	TA Term†	Origin*	Branches*	Distribution*
sural n. [general sensory]	n. suralis	medial sural cutaneous n. and communicating branch of common peroneal n.	lateral dorsal cutaneous n. and lateral calcaneal branches	skin on back of leg, and skin and joints on lateral side of foot and heel
sural cutaneous n., lateral [general sensory]	n. cutaneus surae lateralis	common peroneal n.		skin of lateral side of back of leg, rarely may continue as sural n.
sural cutaneous n., medial [general sensory]	n. cutaneus surae medialis	tibial n.; usually joins peroneal communicating branch of common peroneal n. to form sural n.		may continue as sural n.
temporal n's, deep [motor]	nn. temporales profundi	mandibular n.		temporal muscles
n. to tensor tympani muscle [motor]	n. musculi tensoris tympani	medial pterygoid n.		tensor tympani muscle
n. to tensor veli palatini muscle [motor]	n. musculi tensoris veli palatini	medial pterygoid n.		tensor veli palatini muscle
tentorial n. [general sensory]	ramus meningeus recurrens nervi ophthalmici	ophthalmic n.		dura mater of tentorium cerebelli and falx cerebri
terminal n.	n. terminalis	the collection of nerve filaments in the pia mater between the olfactory bulb and crista galli, and passing through the cribriform plate to the nasal mucosa		
thoracic n's	nn. thoracici	the 12 pairs of spinal n's that arise from thoracic segments of spinal cord, each pair leaving vertebral column below correspondingly numbered vertebra		
thoracic n., long [motor]	n. thoracicus longus	brachial plexus—anterior branches of C5–C7		body wall of thorax and upper part of abdomen
thoracic splanchnic n., greater. *See* splanchnic n., greater				
thoracic splanchnic n., lesser. *See* splanchnic n., lesser				
thoracic splanchnic n., lowest. *See* splanchnic n., lowest				
thoracodorsal n. [motor]	n. thoracodorsalis	posterior cord of brachial plexus—C7–C8		descends behind brachial plexus to anterior serratus muscle latissimus dorsi muscle

598

neu·ro·nop·a·thy (noor″on-op′ah-the) polyneuropathy involving destruction of the cell bodies of neurons.

neu·ro·oph·thal·mol·o·gy (noor″o-of″thal-mol′ah-je) the specialty dealing with the portions of the nervous system related to the eye.

neu·ro·pap·il·li·tis (-pap″ĭ-li′tis) papillitis (2).

neu·ro·par·a·lyt·ic (-par″ah-lit′ik) affected with or pertaining to paralysis of a nerve or nerves.

neu·ro·path·ic (-path′ik) pertaining to or characterized by neuropathy.

neu·ro·patho·ge·nic·i·ty (-path″ah-jin-is′it-e) the quality of producing or the ability to produce pathologic changes in nerve tissue.

neu·ro·pa·thol·o·gy (-pah-thol′ah-je) pathology of diseases of the nervous system.

neu·rop·a·thy (nŏŏ-rop′ah-the) a functional disturbance or pathological change in the peripheral nervous system, sometimes limited to noninflammatory lesions as opposed to those of neuritis. **angiopathic n.,** that caused by arteritis of the blood vessels supplying the nerves, usually a systemic complication of disease. **axonal n.,** axonopathy. **diabetic n.,** any of several clinical types of peripheral neuropathy (sensory, motor, autonomic, and mixed) occurring with diabetes mellitus; the most common is a chronic, symmetrical sensory polyneuropathy affecting first the nerves of the lower limbs and often affecting autonomic nerves. **entrapment n.,** any of a group of neuropathies, e.g., carpal tunnel syndrome, due to mechanical pressure on a peripheral nerve. **hereditary motor and sensory n. (HMSN),** any of a group of hereditary polyneuropathies involving muscle weakness, atrophy, sensory deficits, and vasomotor changes in the lower limbs. **hereditary optic n.,** Leber's hereditary optic n. **hereditary sensory n.,** hereditary sensory radicular n. **hereditary sensory and autonomic n. (HSAN),** any of several inherited neuropathies that involve slow ascendance of lesions of the sensory nerves, resulting in pain, distal trophic ulcers, and autonomic disturbances. **hereditary sensory radicular n.,** an inherited polyneuropathy characterized by signs of radicular sensory loss in the limbs, shooting pains, chronic trophic ulceration of the feet, and sometimes deafness. **ischemic n.,** an injury to a peripheral nerve caused by a reduction in blood supply. **Leber's hereditary optic n.,** an inherited disorder of ATP manufacture, usually in males, usually as bilateral progressive optic atrophy and loss of central vision that may remit spontaneously. **multiple n.,** 1. polyneuropathy. 2. multiple mononeuropathy. **peripheral n.,** polyneuropathy. **pressure n.,** entrapment n. **progressive hypertrophic n.,** a slowly progressive familial disease beginning in early life, marked by hyperplasia of interstitial connective tissue causing thickening of peripheral nerve trunks and posterior roots, and by sclerosis of the posterior columns of the spinal cord. **sarcoid n.,** a polyneuropathy sometimes seen in sarcoidosis, characterized by either cranial polyneuritis or spinal nerve deficits. **tomaculous n.,** an inherited neuropathy characterized by pain, weakness, and pressure palsy in the arms and hands, with swelling of the myelin sheaths. **toxic n.,** that due to ingestion of a toxin. **vasculitic n.,** angiopathic n.

neu·ro·pep·tide (noor″o-pep′tīd) any of the molecules composed of short chains of amino acids (endorphins, enkephalins, vasopressin, etc.) found in brain tissue.

neu·ro·phar·ma·col·o·gy (-fahr″mah-kol′ah-je) the scientific study of the effects of drugs on the nervous system.

neu·ro·phy·sin (-fi′sin) any of a group of soluble proteins secreted in the hypothalamus that serve as binding proteins for vasopressin and oxytocin, playing a role in their transport in the neurohypophyseal tract and their storage in the posterior pituitary.

neu·ro·phys·i·ol·o·gy (-fiz″e-ol′ah-je) physiology of the nervous system.

neu·ro·pil (noor′o-pil) a feltwork of interwoven dendrites and axons and of neuroglial cells in the gray matter of the central nervous system.

neu·ro·plasm (-plazm) the protoplasm of a nerve cell. **neuroplas′mic,** adj.

neu·ro·plas·ty (-plas″te) plastic repair of a nerve.

neu·ro·pore (-por) the open anterior (*rostral n.*) or posterior (*caudal n.*) end of the neural tube of the early embryo, which closes as the embryo develops.

neu·ro·psy·chi·a·try (noor″o-si-ki′ah-tre) the combined specialties of neurology and psychiatry.

neu·ro·psy·chol·o·gy (-si-kol′ah-je) a discipline combining neurology and psychology to study the relationship between the functioning of the brain and cognitive processes or behavior. **neuropsycholog′ical,** adj.

neu·ro·ra·di·ol·o·gy (-ra″de-ol′ah-je) radiology of the nervous system.

neu·ro·ret·i·ni·tis (-ret″ĭ-ni′tis) inflammation of the optic nerve and retina.

neu·ro·ret·i·nop·a·thy (-ret″ĭ-nop′ah-the) pathologic involvement of the optic disk and retina.

neu·ror·rha·phy (nōō-ror′ah-fe) suture of a divided nerve.

neu·ro·sar·co·ma (noor″o-sahr-ko′mah) a sarcoma with neural elements.

neu·ro·se·cre·tion (-sĕ-kre′shun) 1. secretory activities of nerve cells. 2. the product of such activities; a neurosecretory substance. **neurosecre′tory,** adj.

neu·ro·sis (nōō-ro′sis) pl. *neuro′ses.* 1. Former name for a category of mental disorders characterized by anxiety and avoidance behavior, with symptoms distressing to the patient, intact reality testing, no violations of gross social norms, and no apparent organic etiology. 2. in psychoanalytic theory, the process that gives rise to these disorders as well as personality disorders and some psychotic disorders, being triggering of unconscious defense mechanisms by unresolved conflicts. **character n.,** a type of high-level personality disorder with some neurotic characteristics. **hysterical n.,** former name for a group of conditions now divided between *conversion disorder* and *dissociative disorders.*

neu·ro·spasm (noor′o-spazm) a spasm caused by a disorder in the motor nerve supplying the muscle.

neu·ro·splanch·nic (noor″o-splank′nik) pertaining to the cerebrospinal and sympathetic nervous systems.

neu·ro·spon·gi·o·ma (-spun″je-o′mah) glioma.

neu·ro·sur·gery (noor′o-sur″jer-e) surgery of the nervous system.

neu·ro·su·ture (noor″o-soo′cher) neurorrhaphy.

neu·ro·syph·i·lis (-sif′il-is) syphilis of the central nervous system.

neu·ro·ten·di·nous (-ten′dĭ-nus) pertaining to both nerve and tendon.

neu·ro·ten·sin (-ten′sin) a tridecapeptide found in small intestine and brain tissue; it induces vasodilation and hypotension, and in the brain it is a neurotransmitter.

neu·rot·ic (nōō-rot′ik) 1. pertaining to or characterized by a neurosis. 2. a person affected with a neurosis.

neu·rot·iza·tion (nōō-rot″ĭ-za′shun) regeneration of a nerve after its division.

neu·rot·me·sis (noor″ot-me′sis) partial or complete severance of a nerve, with disruption of the axon and its myelin sheath and the connective tissue elements.

neu·ro·tome (noor′o-tōm) 1. a needlelike knife for dissecting nerves. 2. neuromere (1).

neu·ro·to·mog·ra·phy (noor″o-tah-mog′rah-fe) tomography of the central nervous system.

neu·rot·o·my (nōō-rot′ah-me) dissection or cutting of nerves.

neu·rot·o·ny (nōō-rot′ah-ne) stretching of a nerve.

neu·ro·tox·ic·i·ty (noor″o-tok-sis′it-e) the quality of exerting a destructive or poisonous effect upon nerve tissue. **neurotox′ic,** adj.

neu·ro·tox·in (noor′o-tok′sin) a substance that is poisonous or destructive to nerve tissue.

neu·ro·trans·duc·er (noor″o-tranz-doo′ser) a neuron that synthesizes and releases hormones which serve as the functional link between the nervous system and the pituitary gland.

neu·ro·trans·mit·ter (-tranz′mit-er) a substance released from the axon terminal of a presynaptic neuron on excitation, which diffuses across the synaptic cleft to either excite or inhibit the target cell. **false n.,** an amine that can be stored in and released from presynaptic vesicles but that has little effect on postsynaptic receptors.

neu·ro·trau·ma (-traw′mah) mechanical injury to a nerve.

neu·rot·ro·pism (nōō-rot′ro-pizm) 1. the quality of having a special affinity for nervous tissue. 2. the alleged tendency of regenerating nerve fibers to grow toward specific portions of the periphery. **neurotro′pic,** adj.

neu·ro·tu·bule (noor″o-too′bŭl) a microtubule occurring in a neuron.

neu·ro·vac·cine (-vak′sēn) vaccine virus prepared by growing the virus in a rabbit's brain.

neu·ro·vas·cu·lar (-vas′ku-ler) pertaining to both nervous and vascular elements, or to nerves controlling the caliber of blood vessels.

neu·ro·vis·cer·al (-vis′er′l) neurosplanchnic.

neu·ru·la (noor′u-lah) the early embryonic stage following the gastrula, marked by the first appearance of the nervous system.

neu·ru·la·tion (noor″u-la′shun) formation in the early embryo of the neural plate, followed by its closure with development of the neural tube.

neu·tral (noo′tril) neither basic nor acidic.

neu·tro·cyte (noo′tro-sīt) neutrophil (1). **neutrocyt′ic,** adj.

neu·tron (noo′tron) an electrically neutral or uncharged particle of matter existing along with protons in the nucleus of atoms of all elements except the mass 1 isotope of hydrogen. Symbol n.

neu·tro·pe·nia (noo″tro-pe′ne-ah) diminished number of neutrophils in the blood.

neu·tro·phil (noo′tro-fil) 1. a granular leukocyte having a nucleus with three to five lobes connected by threads of chromatin, and cytoplasm containing very fine granules; cf. *heterophil.* 2. any cell, structure, or histologic element readily stainable with neutral dyes. **rod n., stab n.,** one whose nucleus is not divided into segments.

neu·tro·phil·ia (noo″tro-fil′e-ah) increase in the number of neutrophils in the blood.

neu·tro·phil·ic (-fil′ik) 1. pertaining to neutrophils. 2. stainable by neutral dyes.

ne·vir·a·pine (nĕ-vir′ah-pēn) a nonnucleoside inhibitor of HIV-1 reverse transcriptase, used in combination with other antiretroviral agents in the treatment of HIV infection.

ne·vo·cyte (ne′vo-sīt) nevus cell. **nevocyt′ic,** adj.

ne·void (ne′void) resembling a nevus.

ne·vo·li·po·ma (ne″vo-lĭ-po′mah) a nevus containing a large amount of fibrofatty tissue.

ne·vus (ne′vus) pl. *ne′vi.* [L.] 1. any congenital skin lesion; a birthmark. 2. a type of hamartoma representing a circumscribed stable malformation of the skin and occasionally of the oral mucosa, which is not due to external causes; the excess (or deficiency) of tissue may involve epidermal, connective tissue, adnexal, nervous, or vascular elements. **balloon cell n.,** an intradermal nevus consisting of balloon cells with pale cytoplasm that contains large vacuoles formed of altered melanosomes. **blue n.,** a dark blue nodular lesion composed of closely grouped melanocytes and melanophages situated in the mid-dermis. **blue rubber bleb n.,** a hereditary condition marked by multiple bluish cutaneous hemangiomas with soft raised centers, frequently associated with hemangiomas of the gastrointestinal tract. **cellular blue n.,** a large blue to blue-black, multilobulated, well-circumscribed, nodular tumor composed of melanocytes and spindle cells, tending to occur on the buttocks and sacrococcygeal region and having a low incidence of transformation to melanoma. **compound n.,** a nevocytic nevus composed of fully formed nests of nevus cells in the epidermis and newly forming ones in the dermis. **connective tissue n.,** any of a group of hamartomas involving various components of the connective tissue, usually present at birth or soon after. **dysplastic n.,** an acquired atypical nevus with an irregular border, indistinct margin, and mixed coloration, characterized by intraepidermal melanocytic dysplasia and often a precursor of malignant melanoma. **n. flam′meus,** a common congenital vascular malformation involving mature capillaries, ranging from pink (*salmon patch*) to dark bluish red (*portwine stain*) and usually occurring on the face and neck. **giant congenital pigmented n., giant hairy n., giant pigmented n.,** any of a group of large, darkly pigmented, hairy nevi, present at birth; they are associated with other cutaneous and subcutaneous lesions, neurofibromatosis, and leptomeningeal melanocytosis and exhibit a predisposition to the development of malignant melanoma. **halo n.,** a pigmented nevus surrounded by a ring of depigmentation. **intradermal n.,** a nevocytic nevus, clinically indistinguishable from compound nevus, in which the nests of nevus cells lie exclusively within the dermis. **n. of Ito,** a mongolian spot–like lesion similar to nevus of Ota but localized to areas of distribution of the posterior supraclavicular and lateral cutaneous brachial nerves. **junction n.,** a nevocytic nevus in which the nests of nevus cells are confined to the dermoepidermal junction. **n. lipomato′sus,** nevolipoma. **nevocytic n., n. cell n.,** a tumor composed of nests of nevus cells, usually presenting as tan to brown small macules or papules with well-defined, rounded borders; they are subclassified as compound, intradermal, and junction. **n. of Ota, Ota's n.,** a mongolian spot–like lesion usually present at birth, involving the conjunctiva and lids, as well as adjacent facial skin, sclera, ocular muscles, periosteum, and buccal mucosa, usually unilaterally. **pigmented n.,** a nevus containing melanin, usually restricted to nevocytic nevi and moles. **sebaceous n., n. sebaceus of Jadassohn,** a syndrome characterized by single or linear hamartomas of the scalp, face, or neck that may change through life; neurologic symptoms and ophthalmic abnormalities may be present. Over time, some lesions become nodular and tend to develop benign or malignant adnexal tumors or basal cell carcinoma. **n. spi′lus,** a smooth, tan to brown, macular nevus composed of melanocytes, and speckled with smaller, darker macules. **spindle and epithelioid cell n.,** a benign compound nevus, seen usually in children, composed of dermal spindle and epithelioid cells, resembling malignant melanoma histologically and appearing as a smoothish, raised, firm, pink to purplish nodule or papule. **n. spongio′sus al′bus muco′sae,** white sponge n. **n. uni′us la′teris,** a verrucous epidermal nevus occurring as a linear band, patch, or streak, usually along the margin between two neuromeres. **vascular n., n. vascula′ris, n. vasculo′sus,** a reddish swelling or patch on the skin due to hypertrophy of the skin capillaries. **white sponge n.,** a benign, congenital, inherited disorder characterized by extensive spongy whiteness and gray-white, soft, fissured lesions of the mucous membranes, especially of the oral mucosa.

new·born (noo'born″) 1. recently born. 2. newborn infant.

new·ton (N) (noo'ton) the SI unit of force; that when applied in a vacuum to a body having a mass of 1 kilogram accelerates it at the rate of 1 meter per second squared.

nex·us (nek'sus) pl. *nex'us.* [L.] 1. a bond, especially one between members of a series or group. 2. gap junction.

NF *National Formulary.*

NFLPN National Federation for Licensed Practical Nurses.

ng nanogram.

Ni nickel.

ni·a·cin (ni'ah-sin) nicotinic acid; a water-soluble vitamin of the B complex required by the body for the formation of the coenzymes NAD and NADP, important in biochemical oxidations; used to prevent and treat pellagra and to treat hyperlipidemia.

ni·a·cin·amide (ni″ah-sin'ah-mīd) nicotin-amide, a B complex vitamin used in the prophylaxis and treatment of pellagra.

NIAID National Institute of Allergy and Infectious Diseases.

ni·car·di·pine (ni-kahr'dĭ-pēn) a calcium channel blocker that acts as a vasodilator; used as the hydrochloride salt in the treatment of angina pectoris and hypertension.

niche (nich) a defect in an otherwise even surface, especially a depression or recess in the wall of a hollow organ, as seen in a radiograph, or such a depression in an organ visible to the naked eye. **enamel n.,** either of two depressions between the dental lamina and the developing tooth germ, one pointing distally (*distal enamel n.*) and the other mesially (*mesial enamel n.*).

NICHD National Institute of Child Health and Human Development.

nick·el (Ni) (nik'l) chemical element (see *Table of Elements*), at. no. 28. Long-term exposure to metallic nickel, as in jewelry, can cause contact (nickel) dermatitis; nickel fumes can be carcinogenic.

nick·ing (nik'ing) localized constriction of the retinal blood vessels.

nic·o·tin·a·mide (nik″o-tin'ah-mīd) niaci-namide. **n. adenine dinucleotide (NAD),** a coenzyme composed of nicotinamide mono-nucleotide in pyrophosphate linkage with adenosine monophosphate; it is involved in numerous enzymatic reactions, in which it serves as an electron carrier by being alternately oxidized (NAD$^+$) and reduced (NADH). **n. adenine dinucleotide phos-phate (NADP),** a coenzyme composed of nicotinamide mononucleotide coupled by pyrophosphate linkage to adenosine 2',5'-bis-phosphate; it serves as an electron carrier in numerous reactions, being alternately oxi-dized (NADP$^+$) and reduced (NADPH).

nic·o·tine (nik'o-tēn, nik'o-tin) a very poi-sonous alkaloid, obtained from tobacco or produced synthetically; used as an agricultural insecticide, and as an aid to smoking ces-sation. **n. polacrilex,** nicotine bound to a cation exchange resin; used in nicotine chewing gum as an aid to smoking cessation.

nic·o·tin·ic (nik″o-tin'ik) denoting the effect of nicotine and other drugs in initially stimu-lating and subsequently, in high doses, in-hibiting neural impulses at autonomic ganglia and the neuromuscular junction.

nic·o·tin·ic ac·id (nik″o-tin'ik) niacin.

nic·o·tin·ism (nik'ah-tin-izm) nicotine poi-soning.

nic·ti·ta·tion (nik″tĭ-ta'shun) winking.

ni·dal (nīd'l) pertaining to a nidus.

ni·da·tion (ni-da'shun) implantation (1).

NIDCR National Institute of Dental and Craniofacial Research.

NIDD, NIDDM non–insulin-dependent dia-betes mellitus; see *type 2 diabetes mellitus,* under *diabetes.*

ni·dus (ni'dus) pl. *ni'di.* [L.] 1. the point of origin or focus of a morbid process. 2. nucleus (2). **n. a'vis,** a depression in the cerebellum between the posterior velum and uvula.

ni·fed·i·pine (ni-fed'ĭ-pēn) a calcium chan-nel blocking agent used as a coronary vasodilator in the treatment of coronary insufficiency and angina pectoris; also used in the treatment of hypertension.

night·mare (nīt'mār″) a terrifying dream, usually awakening the dreamer.

night·shade (nīt'shād″) a plant of the genus *Solanum.* **deadly n.,** belladonna.

NIGMS National Institute of General Medical Sciences.

ni·gra (ni'grah) [L.] substantia nigra. **ni'gral,** adj.

ni·gro·sin (ni'gro-sin) an aniline dye having a special affinity for ganglion cells.

ni·gro·stri·a·tal (ni″gro-stri-āt'l) projecting from the substantia nigra to the corpus stria-tum; said of a bundle of nerve fibers.

NIH National Institutes of Health.

ni·hil·ism (ni'il-izm) 1. an attitude of skep-ticism regarding traditional values and beliefs or their frank rejection. 2. a delusion of nonexistence of part or all of the self or the world. **nihilis′tic,** adj.

ni·lu·ta·mide (ni-loo′tah-mīd) a nonsteroidal antiandrogen used as an antineoplastic in the treatment of prostatic carcinoma.

NIMH National Institute of Mental Health.

ni·mo·di·pine (ni-mo′dĭ-pēn) a calcium channel blocker used as a vasodilator in the treatment of neurologic deficits associated with subarachnoid hemorrhage from a ruptured intracranial aneurysm.

ni·o·bi·um (Nb) (ni-o′be-um) chemical element (see *Table of Elements*), at. no. 41.

nip·ple (nip′′l) 1. mammary papilla; the pigmented projection on the anterior surface of the breast, surrounded by the areola; in women it gives outlet to the lactiferous ducts. 2. any similarly shaped structure.

ni·sol·di·pine (ni-sol′dĭ-pēn) a calcium channel blocker used in the treatment of hypertension.

nit (nit) the egg of a louse.

ni·trate (ni′trāt) any salt of nitric acid; organic nitrates are used in the treatment of angina pectoris.

ni·tric (ni′trik) pertaining to or containing nitrogen in one of its higher valences. **n. oxide,** endothelium-derived relaxing factor; a naturally occurring gas that in the body is a short-lived dilator substance released from vascular endothelial cells in response to the binding of vasodilators; it inhibits muscular contraction and produces relaxation, and is toxic in the central nervous system. A preparation is used in the treatment of persistent fetal circulation in term and near-term neonates.

ni·tric ac·id (ni′trik) a colorless liquid, HNO_3, which fumes in moist air and has a characteristic choking odor; used as a cauterizing agent. Its potassium salt (*potassium nitrate*) is used in potassium deficiencies and as a diuretic; its sodium salt (*sodium nitrate*) as a reagent.

ni·tri·fi·ca·tion (ni′′trĭ-fĭ-ka′shun) the bacterial oxidation of ammonia to nitrite and then to nitrate in the soil.

ni·trite (ni′trīt) any salt or ester of nitrous acid.

ni·tro·cel·lu·lose (ni′′tro-sel′ūl-ōs) pyroxylin.

ni·tro·fu·ran (-fu′ran) any of a group of antibacterials, including nitrofurantoin, nitrofurazone, etc., that are effective against a wide range of bacteria.

ni·tro·fu·ran·to·in (-fu-ran′to-in) an antibacterial effective against many gram-negative and gram-positive organisms; used in urinary tract infections.

ni·tro·fu·ra·zone (-fūr′ah-zōn) an antibacterial effective against a wide variety of gram-negative and gram-positive organisms; used topically as a local antiinfective.

ni·tro·gen (N) (ni′tro-jen) chemical element (see *Table of Elements*), at. no. 7. It forms about 78 per cent of the atmosphere and is a constituent of all proteins and nucleic acids. **n. 13,** a radioactive isotope of nitrogen having a half-life of 9.97 minutes and decaying by positron emission (1.190 MeV); used as a tracer in positron emission tomography. **n. mustard,** see under *mustard.* **nonprotein n.,** the nitrogenous constituents of the blood exclusive of the protein bodies, consisting of the nitrogen of urea, uric acid, creatine, creatinine, amino acids, polypeptides, and an undetermined part known as *rest nitrogen.*

ni·trog·e·nous (ni-troj′ĕ-nus) containing nitrogen.

ni·tro·glyc·er·in (ni′′tro-glis′er-in) an antianginal, antihypertensive, and vasodilator used for the prophylaxis and treatment of angina pectoris, the treatment of congestive heart failure and myocardial infarction, and blood pressure control or controlled hypotension during surgery.

ni·tro·prus·side (-prus′īd) the anion $[Fe(CN)_5)NO]^{2-}$; see *sodium nitroprusside.*

ni·tro·so·urea (ni-tro′′so-u′re-ah) any of a group of lipid-soluble biological alkylating agents, including carmustine and lomustine, which cross the blood-brain barrier and are used as antineoplastic agents.

ni·trous (ni′trus) pertaining to nitrogen in its lowest valency. **n. oxide,** a gas, N_2O, used as a general anesthetic, usually in combination with another agent.

ni·trous ac·id (ni′trus) a weak acid, HNO_2, existing only in aqueous solution.

ni·za·ti·dine (nĭ-zat′ĭ-dēn) a histamine H_2 receptor antagonist, used to inhibit gastric acid secretion in the treatment of gastric and duodenal ulcer, gastroesophageal reflux disease, and conditions that cause gastric hypersecretion.

NLN National League for Nursing.

nm nanometer.

NMR nuclear magnetic resonance.

nn. [L. pl.] nervi (nerves).

No nobelium.

no·bel·i·um (No) (no-bel′e-um) chemical element (see *Table of Elements*), at. no. 102.

No·car·dia (no-kahr′de-ah) a genus of bacteria (family Nocardiaceae), including *N. asteroï′des,* which produces a tuberculosis-like infection in humans, *N. farci′nica* (probably identical with *N. asteroï′des*), which produces a tuberculosis-like infection in cattle and causes actinomycotic mycetoma, and *N. brasilien'sis*, which causes nocardiosis and actinomycotic mycetoma in humans.

No·car·di·a·ceae (no-kahr″de-a′se-e) a family of bacteria (order Actinomycetales), including the genera *Actinomadura* and *Nocardia*.

no·car·di·al (-de-al) pertaining to or caused by *Nocardia*.

no·car·di·o·sis (-de-o′sis) infection with *Nocardia*.

no·ce·bo (no-se′bo) [L.] an adverse, nonspecific side effect occurring in conjunction with a medication but not directly resulting from the pharmacologic action of the medication.

noci- word element [L.], *harm; injury*.

no·ci·as·so·ci·a·tion (no″se-ah-so″se-a′shun) unconscious discharge of nervous energy under the stimulus of trauma.

no·ci·cep·tion (no″sĭ-sep′shun) pain sense.

no·ci·cep·tor (-sep′ter) a receptor for pain caused by injury, physical or chemical, to body tissues. **nocicep′tive,** adj.

no·ci·per·cep·tion (-per-sep′shun) pain sense.

noc·tu·ria (nok-tūr′e-ah) excessive urination at night.

noc·tur·nal (nok-tur′n'l) pertaining to, occurring at, or active at night.

node (nōd) a small mass of tissue in the form of a swelling, knot, or protuberance, either normal or pathological. **no′dal,** adj. **atrioventricular n., AV n. (AVN),** a collection of Purkinje fibers beneath the endocardium of the right atrium, continuous with the atrial muscle fibers and atrioventricular bundle; it receives the cardiac impulses from the sinoatrial node and passes them on to the ventricles. **Bouchard's n's,** cartilaginous and bony enlargements of the proximal interphalangeal joints of the fingers in degenerative joint disease. **Dürck's n's,** granulomatous perivascular infiltrations in the cerebral cortex in trypanosomiasis. **Flack's n.,** sinoatrial n. **Heberden's n's,** small hard nodules, usually at the distal interphalangeal joints of the fingers, formed by calcific spurs of the articular cartilage and associated with osteoarthritis. **Hensen's n.,** primitive node. **Keith's n., Keith-Flack n.,** sinoatrial n. **lymph n.,** any of the accumulations of lymphoid tissue organized as definite lymphoid organs along the course of lymphatic vessels, consisting of an outer cortical and an inner medullary part; they are the main source of lymphocytes of the peripheral blood and, as part of the reticuloendothelial system, serve as a defense

mechanism by removing noxious agents, e.g., bacteria and toxins, and probably play a role in antibody formation. **Osler's n's,** small, raised, swollen, tender areas, bluish or sometimes pink or red, occurring commonly in the pads of the fingers or toes, in the thenar or hypothenar eminences, or the soles of the feet; they are practically pathognomonic of subacute bacterial endocarditis. **primitive n.,** a mass of cells at the cranial end of the primitive streak in the early embryo. **n's of Ranvier,** constrictions of myelinated nerve fibers at regular intervals at which the myelin sheath is absent and the axon is enclosed only by Schwann cell processes; see Plate 14. **Schmorl's n.,** an irregular or hemispherical bone defect in the upper or lower margin of the body of a vertebra. **sentinel n.,** 1. the first lymph node to receive drainage from a tumor; used to determine whether there is lymphatic metastasis in certain types of cancer. 2. signal n. **signal n.,** an enlarged supraclavicular lymph node; often the first sign of a malignant abdominal tumor. **singer's n's,** vocal cord nodules. **sinoatrial n., sinuatrial n., sinus n.,** a microscopic collection of atypical cardiac muscle fibers (Purkinje fibers) at the junction of the superior vena cava and right atrium, in which the cardiac rhythm normally originates and which is therefore called the cardiac pacemaker. **teacher's n's,** vocal cord nodules. **Troisier's n., Virchow's n.,** signal n.

no·di (no′di) [L.] plural of *nodus*.

no·dose (no′dōs) having nodes or projections.

no·dos·i·ty (no-dos′it-e) 1. a node. 2. the quality of being nodose.

no·do·ven·tric·u·lar (no″do-ven-trik′u-lar) connecting the atrioventricular node to the ventricle.

nod·ule (nod′ūl) a small node or boss which is solid and can be detected by touch. **nod′ular,** adj. **Albini's n's,** gray nodules of the size of small grains, sometimes seen on the free edges of the atrioventricular valves of infants; they are remains of fetal structures. **apple jelly n's,** minute, yellowish or reddish brown, translucent nodules, seen on diascopic examination of the lesions of lupus vulgaris. **n's of Arantius,** see under *body*. **Aschoff's n's,** see under *body*. **Bianchi's n's,** bodies of Arantius. **Brenner n's,** nodular masses of tumor in the cyst wall in cases of Brenner tumor. **Gamna n's, Gandy-Gamna n's,** brown or yellow pigmented nodules sometimes seen in the enlarged spleen, e.g., in Gamna's disease and sidesrotic splenomegaly. **Jeanselme's n's,** juxta-articular n's. **juxtaarticular n's,** gummata of tertiary syphilis and of nonvenereal treponemal diseases, located on joint capsules, bursae, or tendon sheaths. **Lisch n's,** hamartomas of the iris occurring in neurofibromatosis. **lymphatic n.,** 1. lymph node. 2. a small, dense accumulation of lymphocytes within the lymph node cortex, expressing tissue cytogenetic and defense functions. **milker's n's,** paravaccinia. **Morgagni's n's,** bodies of Arantius. **pulp n.,** denticle (2). **rheumatic n's,** small, round or oval, mostly subcutaneous nodules similar to Aschoff bodies; seen in rheumatic fever. **rheumatoid n's,** subcutaneous nodules consisting of central foci of necrosis surrounded by palisade-like coronas of fibroblasts, seen in rheumatoid arthritis. **Schmorl's n.,** an irregular or hemispherical bone defect in the upper or lower margin of the body of the vertebra. **triticeous n.,** see under *cartilage.* **typhus n's,** minute nodules, originally described in typhus, produced by perivascular infiltration of polymorphonuclear leukocytes and mononuclear cells in typhus. **n. of vermis,** the part of the vermis of the cerebellum, on the ventral surface, where the inferior medullary velum attaches. **vocal cord n's,** singer's or teacher's nodes; small white nodule on the vocal cords in those who use their voice excessively.

nod·u·lus (nod'u-lus) pl. *no'duli.* [L.] nodule.

no·dus (no'dus) pl. *no'di.* [L.] node.

no·ma (no'mah) gangrenous processes of the mouth or genitalia. In the mouth (*cancrum oris, gangrenous stomatitis*), it begins as a small gingival ulcer and results in gangrenous necrosis of surrounding facial tissues; on the genitalia, the appearance is similar, affecting the penis in males and the labia majora, one after the other, in females.

no·men·cla·ture (no'men-kla"cher) a classified system of names, as of anatomical structures, organisms, etc. **binomial n.,** the system of designating plants and animals by two latinized words signifying the genus and species.

nom·i·nal (nom'ĭ-n'l) pertaining to a name or names.

nom·o·gram (nom'o-gram) a graph with several scales arranged so that a straightedge laid on the graph intersects the scales at related values of the variables; the values of any two variables can be used to find the values of the others.

non- word element [L.] *not.*

non com·pos men·tis (non kom'pos men'tis) [L.] not of sound mind, and so not legally responsible.

non·con·duc·tor (non"kon-duk'ter) a substance that does not readily transmit electricity, light, or heat.

non·di·a·bet·ic (-di-ah-bet'ik) not caused by or affected with diabetes.

non·dis·junc·tion (-dis-junk'shun) failure either of two homologous chromosomes to pass to separate cells during the first meiotic division, or of the two chromatids of a chromosome to pass to separate cells during mitosis or during the second meiotic division. As a result, one daughter cell has two chromosomes or two chromatids, and the other has none.

non·elec·tro·lyte (-e-lek'tro-līt) a substance that does not dissociate into ions; in solution it is a nonconductor of electricity.

non·heme (non'hēm) not bound within a porphyrin ring; said of iron so contained within a protein.

non·neu·ro·nal (non"noo-ro'n'l) pertaining to or composed of nonconducting cells of the nervous system, e.g., neuroglial cells.

non·ox·y·nol 9 (non-ok'sĭ-nol) a spermaticide used in contraceptive agents.

non·re·spond·er (non-re-spon'der) a person or animal that after vaccination against a given virus does not show any immune response when challenged with the virus.

non·se·cre·tor (non"sĭ-krēt'er) a person with A or B type blood whose body secretions do not contain the particular (A or B) substance.

non·self (non'self) in immunology, pertaining to foreign antigens.

non·spe·cif·ic (non"spĭ-sif'ik) 1. not due to any single known cause. 2. not directed against a particular agent, but rather having a general effect.

non·union (non-ūn'yun) failure of the ends of a fractured bone to unite.

non·vi·a·ble (-vi'ah-b'l) not capable of living.

NOPHN National Organization for Public Health Nursing.

nor- chemical prefix denoting (*a*) a compound of normal structure (having an unbranched chain of carbon atoms) that is isomeric with one having a branched chain, or (*b*) a compound whose chain or ring contains one less methylene (CH_2) group than does that of its homologue.

nor·adren·a·line (nor"ah-dren'ah-lin) norepinephrine.

nor·ad·ren·er·gic (-ah-dren-urj'ik) activated by or secreting norepinephrine.

nor·epi·neph·rine (-ep-ĭ-nef'rin) a catecholamine, which is the principal neurotransmitter of postganglionic adrenergic neurons, having predominant α-adrenergic activity; also secreted by the adrenal medulla in response to splanchnic stimulation, being released predominantly in response to hypotension. It is a powerful vasopressor and is used, in the form of the bitartrate salt, to restore the blood pressure in certain cases of acute hypotension and to improve cardiac function during decompensation associated with congestive heart failure or cardiovascular surgery.

nor·eth·in·drone (nor-eth'in-drōn) a progestational agent having some anabolic, estrogenic, and androgenic properties; used as the base or the acetate ester in the treatment of amenorrhea, dysfunctional uterine bleeding, and endometriosis, and as an oral contraceptive.

nor·ethy·no·drel (nor'ĕ-thi'no-drel) a progestin, used in combination with an estrogen as an oral contraceptive, to control endometriosis, for the treatment of hypermenorrhea, and to produce cyclic withdrawal bleeding.

nor·flox·a·cin (nor-flok'sah-sin) a broad-spectrum antibacterial effective against a wide range of aerobic gram-negative and gram-positive organisms.

nor·ges·ti·mate (-jes'tĭ-māt) a synthetic progestational agent with little androgenic activity, used in combination with an estrogen component as an oral contraceptive.

nor·ges·trel (-jes'trel) a synthetic progestational agent used as an oral contraceptive.

norm (norm) a fixed or ideal standard.

nor·mal (nor'm'l) 1. agreeing with the regular and established type. 2. in chemistry, (a) denoting a solution containing, in each 1000 mL, 1 g equivalent weight of the active substance, symbol N or *N*; (b) denoting aliphatic hydrocarbons in which no carbon atom is combined with more than 2 other carbon atoms, symbol *n*-; (c) denoting salts not containing replaceable hydrogen or hydroxide ions.

nor·meta·neph·rine (nor''met-ah-nef'rin) a metabolite of norepinephrine excreted in the urine and found in certain tissues.

norm(o)- word element [L.], *normal; usual; conforming to the rule.*

nor·mo·blast (nor'mo-blast) 1. orthochromatic erythroblast. 2. term now often used as a synonym of *erythroblast;* sometimes more specifically, a nucleated cell in the normal course of erythrocyte maturation, as opposed to a megaloblast. When used in the latter sense, the four developmental stages of the nucleated cells of the erythrocytic series are usually named pronormoblasts (*proerythroblasts*) and basophilic, polychromatophilic,

and orthochromatic normoblasts (see under *erythroblast*). **normoblas'tic,** adj.

nor·mo·blas·to·sis (nor''mo-blas-to'sis) excessive production of normoblasts by the bone marrow.

nor·mo·cal·ce·mia (-kal-sēm'e-ah) a normal level of calcium in the blood. **normocalce'mic,** adj.

nor·mo·chro·mia (-krōm'e-ah) normal color; indicating the color of erythrocytes having a normal hemoglobin content. **normochro'mic,** adj.

nor·mo·cyte (nor'mo-sīt) an erythrocyte that is normal in size, shape, and color. **normocyt'ic,** adj.

nor·mo·cy·to·sis (nor''mo-si-to'sis) a normal state of the blood in respect to erythrocytes.

nor·mo·gly·ce·mia (-gli-sēm'e-ah) euglycemia. **normoglyce'mic,** adj.

nor·mo·ka·le·mia (-kah-lēm'e-ah) a normal level of potassium in the blood. **normokale'mic,** adj.

nor·mo·sper·mia (-sper'me-ah) production of spermatozoa normal in number and motility. **normosperm'ic,** adj.

nor·mo·ten·sive (-ten'siv) 1. characterized by normal tone, tension, or pressure, as by normal blood pressure. 2. a person with normal blood pressure.

nor·mo·ther·mia (-therm'e-ah) a normal state of temperature. **normother'mic,** adj.

nor·mo·vo·le·mia (-vo-lēm'e-ah) normal blood volume.

nor·trip·ty·line (nor-trip'tĭ-lēn) a tricyclic antidepressant, used as the hydrochloride salt to treat depression and panic disorder and to relieve chronic severe pain.

nose (nōz) the specialized facial structure serving as an organ of the sense of smell and as part of the respiratory apparatus; see Plate 25. **saddle n., swayback n.,** a nose with a sunken bridge.

nose·bleed (nōz'blēd) epistaxis.

No·se·ma (no-se'mah) a genus of intracellular protozoa, including *N. ocula'rum,* which causes corneal infections.

nose·piece (nōz'pēs'') the portion of a microscope nearest to the stage, which bears the objective or objectives.

nos(o)- word element [Gr.], *disease.*

noso·co·mi·al (nos''o-ko'me-il) pertaining to or originating in a hospital.

no·sog·e·ny (no-soj'ĭ-ne) pathogenesis.

no·sol·o·gy (no-sol'ah-je) the science of the classification of diseases. **nosolog'ic,** adj.

noso·para·site (nos''o-par'ah-sīt) an organism found in conjunction with a disease which it is able to modify, but not to produce.

No·so·psyl·lus (nos″o-sil′us) a genus of fleas, including *N. fascia′tus*, the common rat flea of North America and Europe, a vector of murine typhus and probably of plague.

nos·tril (nos′tril) either of the nares.

nos·trum (nos′trum) a quack, patent, or secret remedy.

no·tal·gia (no-tal′jah) pain in the back.

notch (noch) incisure; an indentation on the edge of a bone or other organ. **aortic n.**, dicrotic n. **cardiac n.**, 1. (*of stomach*) a notch at the junction of the esophagus and the greater curvature of the stomach. 2. (*of left lung*) a notch in the anterior border of the left lung. **dicrotic n.**, a small downward deflection in the arterial pulse or pressure contour immediately following the closure of the semilunar valves and preceding the dicrotic wave, sometimes used as a marker for the end of systole or the ejection period. **mastoid n.**, a deep groove on the medial surface of the mastoid process of the temporal bone, giving attachment to the posterior belly of the digastric muscle. **parotid n.**, the notch between the ramus of the mandible and the mastoid process of the temporal bone. **Rivinus' n., tympanic n.**, a defect in the upper tympanic part of the temporal bone, filled by the upper portion of the tympanic membrane.

No·tech·is (no-tek′is) a genus of extremely venomous Australian snakes of the family Elapidae. *N. scuta′tus* is the tiger snake, whose body is brown with dark bands.

no·ti·fi·a·ble (no″tĭ-fi′ah-b'l) necessary to be reported to a government health agency.

not(o)- word element [Gr.], *the back*.

no·to·chord (nōt′o-kord) a rod-shaped cord of cells on the dorsal aspect of an embryo, defining the primitive axis of the body and serving as the center of development of the axial skeleton; it is the common factor of all chordates.

No·to·ed·res (no″to-ed′rēz) a genus of mites, including *N. ca′ti*, an itch mite causing a persistent, often fatal, mange in cats; it also infests domestic animals and sometimes temporarily humans.

No·vo·cain (no′vah-kān) trademark for preparations of procaine.

nox·ious (nok′shus) hurtful; injurious; pernicious.

Np neptunium.

NPN nonprotein nitrogen.

NPO [L.] nil per os (nothing by mouth).

NREM non–rapid eye movement (see under *sleep*).

ns nanosecond; one billionth (10^{-9}) of a second.

NSAIA nonsteroidal antiinflammatory analgesic (or agent); see under *drug*.

NSAID nonsteroidal antiinflammatory drug.

NSCLC non–small cell lung carcinoma (or cancer).

NSNA National Student Nurse Association.

NST nonstress test.

nu·cha (noo′kah) nape. **nu′chal**, adj.

nu·cle·ar (noo′kle-ar) pertaining to a nucleus.

nu·cle·ase (noo′kle-ās) any of a group of enzymes that split nucleic acids into nucleotides and other products.

nu·cle·at·ed (noo′kle-āt″id) having a nucleus or nuclei.

nu·clei (noo′kle-i) [L.] plural of *nucleus*.

nu·cle·ic ac·id (noo-kle′ik) a high-molecular-weight nucleotide polymer. There are two types: *deoxyribonucleic acid* (DNA) and *ribonucleic acid* (RNA).

nu·cleo·cap·sid (noo″kle-o-kap′sid) a unit of viral structure, consisting of a capsid with the enclosed nucleic acid.

nu·cle·of·u·gal (noo″kle-of′u-gil) moving away from a nucleus.

nu·cleo·his·tone (noo″kle-o-his′tōn) the nucleoprotein complex made up of DNA and histones, the principal constituent of chromatin.

nu·cle·oid (noo′kle-oid) 1. resembling a nucleus. 2. a nucleus-like body sometimes seen in the center of an erythrocyte. 3. the genetic material (nucleic acid) of a virus situated in the center of the virion. 4. the nuclear region of a bacterium, which contains the chromosome but is not limited by a nuclear membrane.

nu·cleo·lo·ne·ma (noo″kle-o″lo-ne′mah) a network of strands formed by organization of a finely granular substance, perhaps containing RNA, in the nucleolus of a cell.

nu·cle·o·lus (noo-kle′o-lus) pl. *nucle′oli*. [L.] a rounded refractile body in the nucleus of most cells, which is the site of synthesis of ribosomal RNA.

nu·cle·op·e·tal (noo″kle-op′ĭ-t′l) moving toward a nucleus.

nu·cleo·phago·cy·to·sis (noo″kle-o-fag″o-si-to′sis) the engulfing of the nuclei of other cells by phagocytes.

nu·cleo·phile (noo′kle-o-fĭl) an electron donor in chemical reactions involving covalent catalysis in which the donated electrons bond other chemical groups (electrophiles). **nucleophil′ic**, adj.

nu·cleo·plasm (-plazm″) the protoplasm of the nucleus of a cell.

nu·cleo·pro·tein (noo″kle-o-pro′tēn) a substance composed of a simple basic protein (e.g., a histone) combined with a nucleic acid.

nu·cleo·si·dase (-si′dās) an enzyme that catalyzes the splitting of a nucleoside to form a purine or pyrimidine base and a sugar.

nu·cleo·side (noo′kle-o-sīd″) one of the compounds into which a nucleotide is split by the action of nucleotidase or by chemical means; it consists of a sugar (a pentose) with a purine or pyrimidine base.

nu·cleo·some (-sōm) any of the complexes of histone and DNA in eukaryotic cells, seen under the electron microscope as bead-like bodies on a string of DNA.

nu·cleo·ti·dase (noo″kle-o-ti′dās) an enzyme that catalyzes the cleavage of a nucleotide into a nucleoside and orthophosphate.

nu·cleo·tide (noo′kle-o-tīd″) one of the compounds into which nucleic acid is split by action of nuclease; nucleotides are composed of a base (purine or pyrimidine), a sugar (ribose or deoxyribose), and a phosphate group. **cyclic n's,** those in which the phosphate group bonds to two atoms of the sugar forming a ring, as in cyclic AMP and cyclic GMP, which act as intracellular second messengers.

nu·cleo·tid·yl (noo″kle-o-tīd′il) a nucleotide residue.

nu·cleo·tox·in (noo′kle-o-tok″sin) 1. a toxin from cell nuclei. 2. any toxin affecting cell nuclei.

nu·cle·us (noo′kle-us) pl. *nu′clei.* [L.] 1. the central core of a body or object. 2. cell nucleus; a spheroid body within a cell, consisting of a thin nuclear membrane, organelles, one or more nucleoli, chromatin, linin, and nucleoplasm. 3. a group of nerve cells, usually within the central nervous system, bearing a direct relationship to the fibers of a particular nerve. 4. in organic chemistry, the combination of atoms forming the central element or basic framework of the molecule of a specific compound or class of compounds. 5. see *atomic n.* **nu′clear,** adj. **ambiguous n.,** the nucleus of origin of motor fibers of the vagus, glossopharyngeal, and accessory nerves in the medulla oblongata. **anterior olfactory n.,** scattered groups of neurons intermingled with the olfactory tract that run caudally from the end of the olfactory bulb, some receiving synaptic stimuli from the fibers of the olfactory tract. **arcuate n.,** 1. a nucleus of nerve cells in the posterior hypothalamic region, extending into the median eminence and almost entirely surrounding the base of the infundibulum. 2. one of the small irregular areas of gray substance on the ventromedial aspect of the pyramid of the medulla oblongata. **atomic n.,** the central core of an atom, composed of protons and neutrons, constituting most of its mass but only a small part of its volume. **basal n., n. basa′lis,** specific interconnected groups of masses of gray substance deep in the cerebral hemispheres and in the upper brain stem. **n. caeru′leus,** a compact aggregation of pigmented neurons subjacent to the locus caeruleus, sometimes considered one of the medial reticular nuclei. **n. cauda′tus,** an elongated, arched gray mass closely related to the lateral ventricle throughout its entire extent, which, together with the putamen, forms the neostriatum. **central nuclei of thalamus,** two small intralaminar nuclei, medial and lateral, situated in the internal medullary lamina. **centromedian n. of thalamus,** the largest and most caudal of the intralaminar nuclei of the dorsal thalamus. **cochlear nuclei,** the nuclei, anterior and posterior, of termination of sensory fibers of the cochlear part of the vestibulocochlear nerve, which partly encircle the inferior cerebellar peduncle at the junction of the medulla oblongata and pons. **cuneate n., n. cunea′tus,** a nucleus in the medulla oblongata, in which the fibers of the fasciculus cuneatus synapse. **Deiters' n.,** lateral vestibular nucleus; see *nuclei vestibulares.* **dentate n., n. denta′tus,** the largest of the deep cerebellar nuclei lying in the white matter of the cerebellum. **droplet nuclei,** see under *infection.* **emboliform n., n. embolifor′mis,** a small cerebellar nucleus that lies between the dentate nucleus and globose nucleus and contributes to the superior cerebellar peduncles. **n. endopeduncula′ris,** a small nucleus in the internal capsule of the hypothalamus, adjacent to the medial edge of the globus pallidus. **fastigial n., n. fastigia′tus, n. fasti′gii,** the most medial of the deep cerebellar nuclei, near the midline in the roof of the fourth ventricle. **n. gra′cilis,** a nucleus in the medulla oblongata, in which the fibers of the fasciculus gracilis of the spinal cord synapse. **hypoglossal n., n. of hypoglossal nerve,** the nucleus of origin of the hypoglossal nerve in the medulla oblongata. **interpeduncular n., n. interpeduncula′ris,** a nucleus between the cerebral peduncles immediately dorsal to the interpeduncular fossa. **lenticular n., lentiform n.,** the part of the corpus striatum just lateral to the internal capsule, comprising the putamen and globus pallidus. **Meynert's n.,** a group of neurons in the basal forebrain that has wide projections to the neocortex and is rich in acetylcholine and choline acetyltransferase; it undergoes degeneration in paralysis agitans and Alzheimer's disease. **motor n.,** any collection of cells in the central nervous system giving origin to a motor nerve. **oculomotor n., n. oculomoto′rius,** the origin of the fibers of the oculomotor nerve, situated in the tegmentum of the mesencephalon immediately ventral to the central gray matter, between the medial longitudinal fasciculi. Innervation of the superior rectus of one eye originates in the contralateral oculomotor nerve nucleus; the other elements of the nucleus supply ipsilateral eye muscles via the oculomotor nerve. **olivary n.,** 1. a folded band of gray substance enclosing a white core and producing the elevation (olive) of the medulla oblongata. 2. olive (2). **n. of origin,** any of the groups of nerve cells in the central nervous system from which arise the motor, or efferent, fibers of the cranial nerves. **paraventricular n. of hypothalamus,** a band of cells in the wall of the third ventricle in the anterior hypothalamic region; many of its cells are neurosecretory in function (secreting oxytocin) and project to the neurohypophysis. **pontine nuclei, nu′clei pon′tis,** groups of nerve cell bodies in the part of the pyramidal tract within the ventral part of the pons, upon which the fibers of the corticopontine tract synapse, and whose axons in turn cross to the opposite side and form the middle cerebellar peduncle. **n. pulpo′sus, pulpy n.,** a semifluid mass of fine white and elastic fibers forming the center of an intervertebral disk. **raphe nuclei, nuclei of raphe,** a subgroup of the reticular nuclei of the brainstem, found in narrow longitudinal sheets along the raphae of the medulla oblongata, pons, and mesencephalon; they include many neurons that synthesize serotonin. **red n.,** a distinctive oval nucleus (pink in fresh specimens) centrally placed in the upper mesencephalic reticular formation. **reticular nuclei,** nuclei found in the reticular formation of the brainstem, occurring primarily in longitudinal columns in three groups: medial or intermediate reticular nuclei, lateral reticular nuclei, and reticular nuclei of the raphe. **n. ru′ber,** red n. **salivary nuclei,** two columns of cells in the posterolateral part of the reticular formation of the pons, together comprising the parasympathetic outflow for the supply of the salivary glands. **sensory n.,** the nucleus of termination of the afferent (sensory) fibers of a peripheral nerve. **solitary nuclei,** any of various nuclei of termination of the visceral afferent fibers of the facial, glossopharyngeal, and vagus nerves, which enter the solitary tract. **subthalamic n., n. subthala′micus,** a nucleus on the medial side of the junction of the internal capsule and crus cerebri. **supraoptic n.,** one just above the lateral part of the optic chiasm; many of its cells are neurosecretory in function (secreting antidiuretic hormone) and project to the neurohypophysis; other cells are osmoreceptors which respond to increased osmotic pressure to signal the release of antidiuretic hormone by the neurohypophysis. **tegmental n., laterodorsal,** several nuclear masses of the reticular formations of the pons and midbrain, especially of the latter, where they are in close approximation to the superior cerebellar peduncles. **terminal n.,** groups of nerve cells within the central nervous system on which the axons of primary afferent neurons of various cranial nerves synapse. **thoracic n.,** see under *column.* **nuclei of trapezoid body,** two groups of nerve cell bodies in or next to the trapezoid body. **trigeminal nuclei,** four nuclei located along the trigeminal nerve, chiefly in the pons and medulla oblongata. **nu′clei vestibula′res,** the four (superior, lateral, medial, and inferior) cellular masses in the floor of the fourth ventricle in which the branches of the vestibulocochlear nerve terminate.

nu·clide (noo′klīd) a species of atom characterized by the charge, mass, number, and quantum state of its nucleus, and capable of existing for a measurable lifetime (usually more than 10^{-10} sec.).

null (nul) 1. insignificant; having no consequence or value. 2. absent or nonexistent. 3. zero; nothing.

nul·lip·a·ra (nul-ip′ah-rah) para 0; a woman who has never borne a viable child. See *para.* **nullip′arous,** adj.

nul·li·par·i·ty (nul″ĭ-par′ĭ-te) the state of being a nullipara.

numb (num) anesthetic (1).

num·ber (num′ber) a symbol, as a figure or word, expressive of a certain value or a specified quantity determined by count. **atomic n.** *(Z),* a number expressive of the number of protons in an atomic nucleus. **Avogadro's n.** *(N, N_A),* the number of molecules in one mole of a substance: 6.023×10^{23}. **mass n.** *(A),* the number expressive of the mass of a nucleus, being the total number of protons and neutrons in the nucleus of an atom or nuclide. **oxidation n.,** a number assigned to each atom in a molecule or ion that represents the number of electrons theoretically lost (negative numbers) or gained (positive numbers) in converting the atom to the elemental form (which has an oxidation number of zero). The sum of the oxidation numbers for all atoms in a neutral compound is zero; for polyatomic ions, it is equal to the ionic charge. **tooth n.**, a number assigned for each of the permanent teeth in consecutive order, with 1 for the upper right third molar and 17 for the lower left third molar, and proceeding around each jaw. **turnover n.**, the number of molecules of substrate acted upon by one molecule of enzyme per minute.

numb·ness (num'nes) anesthesia (1).

num·mu·lar (num'u-ler) 1. coin-sized and coin-shaped. 2. made up of round, flat disks. 3. arranged like a stack of coins.

nurse (nurs) 1. one who is especially prepared in the scientific basis of nursing and who meets certain prescribed standards of education and clinical competence. 2. to provide services essential to or helpful in the promotion, maintenance, and restoration of health and well-being. 3. to breast-feed an infant. **clinical n. specialist**, a registered nurse with a high degree of knowledge, skill, and competence in a specialized area of nursing, and usually having a master's degree in nursing. **community n.**, in Great Britain, a public health nurse. **community health n.**, public health n. **district n.**, community n. **general duty n.**, a registered nurse, usually one who has not undergone training beyond the basic nursing program, who sees to the general nursing care of patients in a hospital or other health agency. **graduate n.**, a graduate of a school of nursing; often used to designate one who has not been registered or licensed. **licensed practical n.**, a graduate of a school of practical nursing whose qualifications have been examined by a state board of nursing and who has been legally authorized to practice as a licensed practical or vocational nurse (L.P.N. or L.V.N.), under supervision of a physician or registered nurse. **licensed vocational n.**, see *licensed practical n.* **n. practitioner**, a registered nurse with advanced education and clinical training within a specialty area. **private n., private duty n.**, one who attends an individual patient, usually on a fee-for-service basis, and who may specialize in a specific class of diseases. **probationer n.**, a person who has entered a school of nursing and is under observation to determine fitness for the nursing profession; applied principally to nursing students enrolled in hospital schools of nursing. **public health n.**, an especially prepared registered nurse employed in a community agency to safeguard the health of persons in the community, giving care to the sick in their homes, promoting health and well-being by teaching families how to keep well, and assisting in programs for the prevention of disease. **Queen's n.**, in Great Britain, a district nurse who has been trained at or in accordance with the regulations of the Queen Victoria Jubilee Institute for Nurses. **registered n.**, a graduate nurse who has been legally authorized (registered) to practice after examination by a state board of nurse examiners or similar regulatory authority, and who is legally entitled to use the designation RN. **scrub n.**, one who directly assists the surgeon in the operating room. **n. specialist**, clinical n. specialist. **visiting n.**, public health n. **wet n.**, a woman who breast-feeds the infant of another.

nurse-mid·wife (-mid'wīf) an individual educated in the two disciplines of nursing and midwifery, who possesses evidence of certification according to the requirements of the American College of Nurse-Midwives. Abbreviated C.N.M. (Certified Nurse-Midwife).

nurse-mid·wi·fery (-mid'wi-fer-e) the independent management of care of essentially normal newborns and women, antepartally, intrapartally, postpartally, and/or gynecologically, occurring within a health care system which provides for medical consultation, collaborative management, or referral, and is in accord with the functions, standards, and qualifications as defined by the American College of Nurse-Midwives.

nur·se·ry (nurs'er-e) the department in a hospital where the newborn are cared for.

nurs·ing (nurs'ing) 1. the provision, at various levels of preparation, of services essential to or helpful in the promotion, maintenance, and restoration of health and well-being or in prevention of illness, as of infants, of sick and injured, or of others for any reason unable to provide such services for themselves. 2. breast-feeding.

nu·ta·tion (noo-ta'shun) the act of nodding, especially involuntary nodding.

nu·tri·ent (noo'tre-int) 1. nourishing; providing nutrition. 2. a food or other substance that provides energy or building material for the survival and growth of a living organism.

nu·tri·ment (noo'trĭ-mint) nutrient (2).

nu·tri·tion (noo-trish'un) the taking in and metabolism of nutrients (food and other nourishing material) by an organism so that life is maintained and growth can take place. **nutri'tional**, adj. **enteral n.**, the delivery of nutrients in liquid form directly into the stomach, duodenum, or jejunum. **par·enteral n.**, administration of nutriment intravenously. **total parenteral n. (TPN)**, intravenous administration, via a central venous catheter, of the total nutrient requirements of a patient with gastrointestinal dysfunction.

nu·tri·tious (noo-trish'us) affording nourishment.

nu·tri·tive (noo'trĭ-tiv) nutritional.

nu·tri·ture (-cher) the status of the body in relation to nutrition.

nyc·ta·lo·pia (nik″tah-lo′pe-ah) 1. night blindness. 2. in French (and incorrectly in English), day blindness.

nyct(o)- word element [Gr.], *night; darkness.*

nyc·to·hem·er·al (nik″to-hem′er-il) pertaining to both day and night.

nymph (nimf) a developmental stage in certain arthropods, e.g., ticks, between the larval form and the adult, and resembling the latter in appearance.

nym·pha (nim′fah) pl. *nym′phae.* [Gr.] one of the labia minora pudendi.

nym·phec·to·my (nim-fek′tah-me) excision of the nymphae (labia minora).

nym·phi·tis (nim-fi′tis) inflammation of the nymphae (labia minora).

nymph(o)- word element [Gr.], *nymphae* (labia minora).

nym·pho·ma·nia (nim″fo-ma′ne-ah) excessive sexual desire in a female. **nymphoman′iac,** adj.

nym·phon·cus (nim-fong′kus) swelling of the nymphae (labia minora).

nym·phot·o·my (nim-fot′ah-me) surgical incision of the nymphae (labia minora) or clitoris.

nys·tag·mi·form (nis-tag′mĭ-form) nystagmoid.

nys·tag·mo·graph (nis-tag′mah-graf) an instrument for recording the movements of the eyeball in nystagmus.

nys·tag·moid (nis-tag′moid) resembling nystagmus.

nys·tag·mus (nis-tag′mus) involuntary rapid movement (horizontal, vertical, rotatory, or mixed, i.e., of two types) of the eyeball. **nystag′mic,** adj. **aural n.,** vestibular n. **caloric n.,** rotatory nystagmus induced by irrigating the ears with warm or cold water or air; see *caloric test,* under *test.* **Cheyne's n., Cheyne-Stokes n.,** a peculiar rhythmical eye movement. **dissociated n.,** that in which the movements in the two eyes are dissimilar. **end-position n.,** that occurring in normal individuals only at extremes of gaze. **fixation n.,** that occurring only on gazing fixedly at an object. **gaze n.,** nystagmus made apparent by looking to the right or to the left. **gaze paretic n.,** a form of gaze nystagmus seen in patients recovering from central nervous system lesions; the eyes fail to stay fixed to the affected side with a cerebral or pontine lesion. **labyrinthine n.,** vestibular n. **latent n.,** that occurring only when one eye is covered. **lateral n.,** involuntary horizontal movement of the eyes. **opticokinetic n., optokinetic n.,** the normal nystagmus occurring when looking at objects passing across the field of vision, as in viewing from a moving vehicle. **pendular n.,** that which consists of to-and-fro movements of equal velocity. **positional n.,** that which occurs, or is altered in form or intensity, on assumption of certain positions of the head. **retraction n., n. retracto′rius,** a spasmodic backward movement of the eyeball occurring on attempts to move the eye; a sign of midbrain disease. **rotatory n.,** involuntary rotation of eyes about the visual axis. **spontaneous n.,** that occurring without specific stimulation of the vestibular system. **undulatory n.,** pendular n. **vertical n.,** involuntary up-and-down movement of the eyes. **vestibular n.,** that due to disturbance of the vestibular system; eye movements are rhythmic, with slow and fast components.

ny·sta·tin (ni-stat′in) an antifungal produced by growth of *Streptomyces noursei;* used in treatment of infections caused by *Candida albicans* and other *Candida* species.

nyx·is (nik′sis) puncture, or paracentesis.

O oxygen.

O. [L.] o′culus (eye).

o- ortho- (2).

Ω ohm.

ω- (omega, the twenty-fourth letter of the Greek alphabet) (1) the carbon atom farthest from the principal functional group in a molecule. (2) last in a series of related entities or chemical compounds.

OA ocular albinism.

OAF osteoclast activating factor.

OB obstetrics.

obes·i·ty (o-bēs′ĭ-te) an increase in body weight beyond the limitation of skeletal and physical requirements, as the result of excessive accumulation of body fat. **obese′**, adj. **adult-onset o.**, that beginning in adulthood and characterized by increase in size (hypertrophy) of adipose cells with no increase in number. **lifelong o.**, that beginning in childhood and characterized by an increase both in number (hyperplasia) and in size (hypertrophy) of adipose cells. **morbid o.**, the condition of weighing two or more times the ideal weight; so called because it is associated with many serious and life-threatening disorders.

obex (o′beks) the ependyma-lined junction of the taeniae of the fourth ventricle of the brain at the inferior angle.

ob·jec·tive (ob-jek′tiv) 1. perceptible by the external senses. 2. a result for whose achievement an effort is made. 3. the lens or system of lenses of a microscope (or telescope) nearest the object that is being examined.

ob·li·gate (ob′lĭ-gāt) pertaining to or characterized by the ability to survive only in a particular environment or to assume only a particular role, as an obligate anaerobe.

ob·lig·a·to·ry (ob-lig′ah-tor″e) obligate.

obliq·ui·ty (ob-lik′wit-e) the state of being inclined or slanting. **oblique′**, adj. **Litzmann's o.**, inclination of the fetal head so that the posterior parietal bone presents to the birth canal. **Nägele's o.**, presentation of the anterior parietal bone to the birth canal, the biparietal diameter being oblique to the brim of the pelvis.

oblit·er·a·tion (ob-lit″er-a′shun) complete removal by disease, degeneration, surgical procedure, irradiation, etc.

ob·lon·ga·ta (ob-long-gah′tah) medulla oblongata. **oblonga′tal**, adj.

ob·ses·sion (ob-sesh′un) a persistent unwanted idea or impulse that cannot be eliminated by reasoning. **obses′sive**, adj.

ob·ses·sive-com·pul·sive (ob-ses′iv-kom-pul′siv) pertaining to obsessions and compulsions, to obsessive-compulsive disorder, or to obsessive-compulsive personality disorder.

ob·ste·tri·cian (ob″stĕ-trish′in) one who practices obstetrics.

ob·stet·rics (ob-stet′riks) the branch of medicine dealing with pregnancy, labor, and the puerperium. **obstet′ric, obstet′rical**, adj.

ob·sti·pa·tion (ob″stĭ-pa′shun) intractable constipation.

ob·struc·tion (ob-struk′shun) 1. the act of blocking or clogging. 2. block; occlusion; the state or condition of being clogged. **obstruc′tive**, adj.

ob·tund (ob-tund′) to render dull, blunt, or less acute, or to reduce alertness.

ob·tun·da·tion (ob-tun-da′shun) mental blunting with mild to moderate reduction in alertness and a diminished sensation of pain.

ob·tun·dent (ob-tun′dent) 1. pertaining to or causing obtundation. 2. having the power to soothe pain. 3. an agent that blunts irritation or soothes pain.

ob·tu·ra·tor (ob′tu-rāt″er) a disk or plate, natural or artificial, that closes an opening.

ob·tu·sion (ob-too′zhun) a deadening or blunting of sensitiveness.

OCA oculocutaneous albinism.

oc·cip·i·tal (ok-sip′ĭ-t′l) pertaining to the occiput; located near the occipital bone.

oc·cip·i·tal·iza·tion (ok-sip″ĭ-tal-ĭ-za′shun) synostosis of the atlas with the occipital bone.

oc·cip·i·to·cer·vi·cal (ok-sip″ĭ-to-ser′vĭ-k′l) pertaining to the occiput and neck.

oc·cip·i·to·fron·tal (-frun′t′l) pertaining to the occiput and the forehead.

oc·cip·i·to·mas·toid (-mas′toid) pertaining to the occipital bone and mastoid process.

oc·cip·i·to·men·tal (-men′t′l) pertaining to the occiput and chin.

oc·cip·i·to·pa·ri·e·tal (-pah-ri′ĕ-t′l) pertaining to the occipital and parietal bones or lobes of the brain.

oc·cip·i·to·tem·po·ral (-tem′per-il) pertaining to the occipital and temporal bones.

oc·cip·i·to·tha·lam·ic (-thah-lam′ik) pertaining to the occipital lobe and thalamus.

oc·ci·put (ok′si-put) the back part of the head. **occip′ital,** adj.

oc·clude (ŏ-klood′) to fit close together; to close tight; to obstruct or close off.

oc·clu·sal (ŏ-kloo′z'l) 1. pertaining to the masticating surfaces of the premolar and molar teeth. 2. occlusive.

oc·clu·sion (ŏ-kloo′zhun) 1. obstruction. 2. the trapping of a liquid or gas within cavities in a solid or on its surface. 3. the relation of the teeth of both jaws when in functional contact during activity of the mandible. 4. momentary complete closure of some area in the vocal tract, causing the breath to stop and pressure to accumulate. **abnormal o.,** malocclusion. **balanced o.,** occlusion in which the teeth are in harmonious working relation. **centric o.,** that in the vertical and horizontal position of the mandible in which the cusps of the mandibular and maxillary teeth interdigitate maximally. **coronary o.,** complete obstruction of an artery of the heart. **eccentric o.,** occlusion of the teeth when the lower jaw has moved from the centric position. **habitual o.,** the consistent relationship of the teeth in the maxilla to those of the mandible when the teeth in both jaws are brought into maximum contact. **lateral o.,** occlusion of the teeth when the lower jaw is moved to the right or left of centric occlusion. **lingual o.,** malocclusion in which the tooth is lingual to the line of the normal dental arch. **mesial o.,** the position of a lower tooth when it is mesial to its opposite number in the maxilla. **normal o.,** the contact of the upper and lower teeth in the centric relationship. **protrusive o.,** anteroclusion. **retrusive o.,** distocclusion. **venous o.,** the blocking of venous return.

oc·clu·sive (ŏ-kloo′siv) pertaining to or causing occlusion.

oc·cult (ŏ-kult′) obscure or hidden from view.

OCD obsessive-compulsive disorder.

ochrom·e·ter (ŏ-krom′ĕ-ter) an instrument for measuring capillary blood pressure.

ochro·no·sis (o″kron-o′sis) deposition of dark pigment in the body tissues, usually secondary to alkaptonuria, characterized by urine that darkens on standing and dusky discoloration of the sclerae and ears. **ochronot′ic,** adj.

OCT ornithine carbamoyltransferase; oxytocin challenge test.

oct(a)- word element [Gr., L.], eight.

oc·tin·ox·ate (ok-tin′ok-sāt) an absorber of ultraviolet B radiation, used topically as a sunscreen.

oc·ti·sal·ate (ok″tĭ-sal′āt) a substituted salicylate that absorbs ultraviolet light in the UVB range, used as a sunscreen.

oc·to·cryl·ene (ok′to-kril″ēn) a sunscreen that absorbs ultraviolet light in the UVB range.

oc·to·pam·ine (ok″to-pam′ēn) a sympathomimetic amine thought to result from inability of the diseased liver to metabolize tyrosine; it is called a false neurotransmitter, since it can be stored in presynaptic vesicles, replacing norepinephrine, but has little effect on postsynaptic receptors.

oc·tre·o·tide (ok-tre′o-tīd) a synthetic analogue of somatostatin, used as the acetate ester in the palliative treatment of the symptoms of gastrointestinal endocrine tumors and in the treatment of acromegaly.

oc·tyl meth·oxy·cin·na·mate (ok′til mĕthok″se-sin′ah-māt) octinoxate.

oc·u·lar (ok′u-lar) 1. of, pertaining to, or affecting the eye. 2. eyepiece.

oc·u·list (ok′u-list) ophthalmologist.

ocul(o)- word element [L.], eye.

oc·u·lo·cu·ta·ne·ous (ok″u-lo-ku-ta′ne-us) pertaining to or affecting the eyes and the skin.

oc·u·lo·fa·cial (-fa′shal) pertaining to the eyes and the face.

oc·u·lo·gy·ra·tion (-ji-ra′shun) movement of the eye about the anteroposterior axis. **oculogy′ric,** adj.

oc·u·lo·man·dib·u·lo·dys·ceph·a·ly (-mandib″u-lo-dis-sef′ah-le) malformation of the cranium and facial bones with optic abnormalities.

oc·u·lo·mo·tor (-mōt′er) pertaining to or effecting eye movements.

oc·u·lo·my·co·sis (-mi-ko′sis) any fungal disease of the eye.

oc·u·lo·na·sal (-na′z'l) pertaining to the eye and the nose.

oc·u·lo·pu·pil·lary (-pu′pĭ-lar-e) pertaining to the pupil of the eye.

oc·u·lo·zy·go·mat·ic (-zi″go-mat′ik) pertaining to the eye and the zygoma.

oc·u·lus (ok′u-lus) pl. o′culi. [L.] eye.

OD¹ [L.] o′culus dex′ter (right eye).

OD² Doctor of Optometry; overdose.

odon·tal·gia (o″don-tal′jah) toothache.

odon·tec·to·my (o″don-tek′tah-me) excision of a tooth.

odon·tic (o-don′tik) pertaining to the teeth.

odont(o)- word element [Gr.], tooth.

odon·to·blast (o-don′to-blast) one of the connective tissue cells that deposit dentin and form the outer surface of the dental pulp. **odontoblas′tic,** adj.

odon·to·blas·to·ma (o-don″to-blas-to′mah) a tumor made up of odontoblasts.

odon·to·clast (o-don′to-klast) an osteoclast associated with absorption of the roots of deciduous teeth.

odon·to·gen·e·sis (o-don″to-jen′ĕ-sis) the origin and histogenesis of the teeth. **odontogenet′ic,** adj. **o. imperfec′ta,** dentinogenesis imperfecta.

odon·to·gen·ic (-jen′ik) 1. forming teeth. 2. arising in tissues that give origin to the teeth.

odon·toid (o-don′toid) like a tooth.

odon·tol·o·gy (o″don-tol′ah-je) 1. scientific study of the teeth. 2. dentistry.

odon·tol·y·sis (o″don-tol′ĭ-sis) the resorption of dental tissue.

odon·to·ma (o″don-to′mah) any odontogenic tumor, especially a composite odontoma. **composite o.,** one consisting of both enamel and dentin in an abnormal pattern. **radicular o.,** one associated with a tooth root, or formed when the root was developing.

odon·top·a·thy (o″don-top′ah-the) any disease of the teeth. **odontopath′ic,** adj.

odon·tot·o·my (o″don-tot′ah-me) incision of a tooth.

odor (o′der) a volatile emanation perceived by the sense of smell.

odor·ant (o′der-int) any substance capable of stimulating the sense of smell.

-odynia word element [Gr.], *pain.*

odyn·om·e·ter (o″din-om′ĕ-ter) algesimeter.

od·y·no·pha·gia (o-din″o-fa′jah) a dysphagia in which swallowing causes pain.

oe- for words beginning thus, see also those beginning *e-.*

oesoph·a·go·sto·mi·a·sis (e-sof″ah-go-sto-mi′ah-sis) infection with *Oesophagostomum.*

Oesoph·a·gos·to·mum (e-sof″ah-gos′to-mum) a genus of nematode worms found in the intestines of various animals.

Oes·trus (es′trus) a genus of botflies. *O. o′vis* deposits its larvae in nasal passages of sheep and goats, and may cause ocular myiasis in humans.

of·fi·cial (o-fi′shal) authorized by a current pharmacopeia or recognized formulary.

of·fic·i·nal (o-fis′ĭ-nal) denoting pharmaceutical preparations that are regularly kept at pharmacies.

oflox·a·cin (o-flok′sah-sin) an antibacterial agent effective against a wide variety of gram-negative and gram-positive aerobic organisms.

ohm (Ω) (ōm) the SI unit of electrical resistance, being that of a resistor in which a current of 1 ampere is produced by a potential difference of 1 volt.

ohm·me·ter (ōm′me-ter) an instrument that measures electrical resistance in ohms.

OI osteogenesis imperfecta.

-oid word element [Gr.], *resembling.*

oil (oil) 1. an unctuous, combustible substance that is liquid, or easily liquefiable, on warming, and is soluble in ether but not in water. Oils may be animal, vegetable, or mineral in origin, and volatile or nonvolatile (fixed). A number of oils are used as flavoring or perfuming agents in pharmaceutical preparations. 2. a fat that is liquid at room temperature. **borage o.,** that extracted from the seeds of borage; used for the treatment of neurodermatitis and as a food supplement. **cajeput o.,** a volatile oil from the fresh leaves and twigs of cajeput; used as a stimulant and rubefacient in rheumatism and other muscle and joint pain. **canola o.,** rapeseed oil, specifically that prepared from rapeseed plants bred to be low in erucic acid. **castor o.,** a fixed oil obtained from the seed of *Ricinus communis;* used as a bland topical emollient and also occasionally as a strong cathartic. **clove o.,** a volatile oil from cloves; used externally in the treatment of colds and headache and as a dental antiseptic and analgesic; it also has various uses in Indian medicine. **cod liver o.,** partially destearinated, fixed oil from fresh livers of *Gadus morrhua* and other fish of the family Gadidae; used as a source of vitamins A and D. **corn o.,** a refined fixed oil obtained from the embryo of *Zea mays;* used as a solvent and vehicle for various medicinal agents and as a vehicle for injections. It has also been promoted as a source of polyunsaturated fatty acids in special diets. **cottonseed o.,** a fixed oil from seeds of cultivated varieties of the cotton plant (*Gossypium*); used as a solvent and vehicle for drugs. **essential o.,** volatile o. **ethiodized o.,** an iodine addition product of the ethyl ester of fatty acids of poppyseed oil; used as a diagnostic radiopaque medium. **eucalyptus o.,** a volatile oil from the fresh leaf of species of *Eucalyptus;* used as a pharmaceutical flavoring agent, as an expectorant and local antiseptic, for rheumatism, and in folk medicine. **evening primrose o.,** that produced from the ripe seeds of evening primrose (*Oenothera biennis*); used in the treatment of mastalgia, premenstrual syndrome, and atopic eczema. **expressed o., fatty o., fixed o.,** a nonvolatile oil, i.e., one that does not evaporate on warming; such oils consist of a mixture of fatty acids and their esters, and are classified as solid, semisolid, and liquid, or as drying, semidrying, and nondrying as a function of their tendency to solidify on exposure to air. **fennel o.,** a volatile oil distilled from fennel (the seeds of *Foeniculum vulgare*); used for cough, bronchitis, and dyspepsia and as a pharmaceutical flavoring agent. **iodized o.,** an iodine addition product of vegetable oil; used as a diagnostic radiopaque medium. **lavender o.,** a volatile oil distilled from the flowering tops of lavender or prepared synthetically; used for loss of appetite, dyspepsia, nervousness, and insomnia; also widely used in folk medicine. **mineral o.,** a mixture of liquid hydrocarbons from petroleum; used as a lubricant laxative, drug vehicle, and skin emollient and cleanser. *Light mineral o.,* of lesser density, is used similarly. **olive o.,** a fixed oil obtained from ripe fruit of *Olea europaea;* used as a setting retardant for dental cements, topical emollient, pharmaceutic necessity, and sometimes as a laxative. **peanut o.,** the refined fixed oil from peanuts (*Arachis hypogaea);* used as a solvent and vehicle for drugs. **peppermint o.,** a volatile oil from fresh overground parts of the flowering plant of peppermint (*Mentha piperita);* used as a flavoring agent for drugs, and as a gastric stimulant and carminative. **rapeseed o.,** the oil expressed from the seeds of the rapeseed plant; used in the manufacture of soaps, margarines, and lubricants. See also *canola o.* **safflower o.,** an oily liquid extracted from the seeds of the safflower, *Carthamus tinctorius,* containing predominantly linoleic acid; used as a pharmaceutical aid, a component of total parenteral nutrition solutions, and in the management of hypercholesterolemia. **silicone o.,** any of various long-chain fluid silicone polymers, some of which are injected into the vitreous to serve as a vitreous substitute during or after vitreoretinal surgery. **tea tree o.,** an essential oil from the leaves and branch tips of tea tree, having bacteriostatic and weak antiviral and antimycotic properties, used topically for skin infections and used internally and externally in folk medicine for various indications. **thyme o.,** the volatile oil extracted from fresh, flowering thyme; used as an antitussive and expectorant. **volatile o.,** one that evaporates readily, usually found in aromatic plants; most are a mixture of two or more terpenes. **volatile o. of mustard,** a volatile oil distilled from the seeds of black mustard (*Brassica nigra);* used as a strong counterirritant and rubefacient.

oint·ment (oint′ment) a semisolid preparation for external application to the skin or mucous membranes, usually containing a medicinal substance.

oja (o′jah) in ayurveda, the imprint of self in the physical body, which arises from the strength of the metabolism and balance a body maintains in knowing itself, thus governing the immune system

OL [L.] o′culus lae′vus (left eye).

-ol word termination indicating a hydroxyl derivative of a hydrocarbon, e.g., an alcohol or a phenol.

ol·amine (ol′ah-mēn) USAN contraction for ethanolamine.

olan·za·pine (o-lan′zah-pēn) a monoaminergic antagonist used as an antipsychotic.

ole·ag·i·nous (o″le-aj′ĭ-nus) oily; greasy.

ole·ate (o′le-āt) 1. a salt, ester, or anion of oleic acid. 2. a solution of a substance in oleic acid; used as an ointment.

olec·ran·ar·thri·tis (o-lek″ran-ahr-thri′tis) anconitis.

olec·ran·ar·throp·a·thy (-ahr-throp′ah-the) disease of the elbow joint.

olec·ra·non (o-lek′rah-non) bony projection of the ulna at the elbow. **olec′ranal,** adj.

ole·ic ac·id (o-le′ik) a monounsaturated 18-carbon fatty acid found in most animal fats and vegetable oils; used in pharmacy as an emulsifier and to assist absorption of some drugs by the skin.

ole·in (o′le-in) the triglyceride formed from oleic acid, occurring in most fats and oils.

ole(o)- word element [L.], *oil.*

oleo·res·in (o″le-o-rez′in) 1. a natural combination of a resin and a volatile oil, such as exudes from pines, etc. 2. a compound extracted from a drug, containing both volatile oil and resin, by percolation with a volatile solvent, such as acetone, alcohol, or ether, and removal of the solvent.

oleo·vi·ta·min (-vīt′ah-min) a preparation of fish liver oil or edible vegetable oil containing one or more fat-soluble vitamins or their derivatives.

ole·um (o′le-um) pl. *o′lea.* [L.] oil.

ol·fact (ol′fakt) a unit of odor, the minimum perceptible odor, being the minimum concentration of a substance in solution that can be perceived by a large number of normal individuals; expressed in grams per liter.

ol·fac·tion (ol-fak′shun) 1. smell; the ability to perceive and distinguish odors. 2. the act of perceiving and distinguishing odors.

ol·fac·tol·o·gy (ol″fak-tol′ah-je) the science of the sense of smell.

ol·fac·tom·e·ter (ol″fak-tom′ĕ-ter) an instrument for testing the sense of smell.

ol·fac·to·ry (ol-fak′ter-e) pertaining to the sense of smell.

olig(o)- word element [Gr.], *few; little; scanty.*

ol·i·go·as·then·o·sper·mia (ol″ĭ-go-as″-thĕ-no-sper′me-ah) oligospermia with decreased sperm motility.

ol·i·go·clo·nal (-klo′n′l) pertaining to or derived from only a few clones.

ol·i·go·cys·tic (-sis′tik) containing few cysts.

ol·i·go·dac·ty·ly (-dak′tĭ-le) the presence of less than the usual number of fingers or toes.

ol·i·go·den·dro·cyte (-den′dro-sīt) a cell of the oligodendroglia.

ol·i·go·den·drog·lia (-den-drog′le-ah) 1. the nonneural cells of ectodermal origin forming part of the adventitial structure (neuroglia) of the central nervous system. 2. the tissue composed of such cells.

ol·i·go·den·dro·gli·o·ma (-den″dro-gli-o′mah) a neoplasm derived from and composed of oligodendrocytes in varying stages of differentiation.

ol·i·go·dip·sia (-dip′se-ah) hypodipsia.

ol·i·go·don·tia (-don′shah) presence of fewer than the normal number of teeth.

ol·i·go·ga·lac·tia (-gah-lak′she-ah) hypogalactia.

ol·i·go·hy·dram·ni·os (-hi-dram′ne-os) deficiency in the amount of amniotic fluid.

ol·i·go·meg·a·ne·phro·nia (-meg″ah-nĕ-fro′ne-ah) congenital renal hypoplasia in which there is a reduced number of lobes and nephrons, with hypertrophy of the nephrons. **oligomeganephron′ic**, adj.

ol·i·go·men·or·rhea (-men″o-re′ah) abnormally infrequent menstruation.

ol·i·go·mer (ol′ĭ-go-mer) a polymer formed by the combination of relatively few monomers.

ol·i·go·nu·cle·o·tide (ol″ĭ-go-noo′kle-o-tīd) a polymer made up of a few (2–20) nucleotides.

ol·i·go·sac·cha·ride (-sak′ah-rīd) a carbohydrate which on hydrolysis yields a small number of monosaccharides.

ol·i·go·sper·mia (-sper′me-ah) decreased number of spermatozoa in the semen.

ol·i·go·syn·ap·tic (-sin-ap′tik) involving a few synapses in series and therefore a sequence of only a few neurons.

ol·i·go·zo·o·sper·mia (-zo″o-sper′me-ah) oligospermia.

ol·i·gu·ria (ol″ĭ-gu′re-ah) diminished urine production and excretion in relation to fluid intake. **oligu′ric**, adj.

oli·va (o-li′vah) pl. *oli′vae*. [L.] olive (2).

ol·i·vary (ol′ĭ-var″e) 1. shaped like an olive. 2. pertaining to the olive.

ol·ive (ol′iv) 1. the tree *Olea europaea* and its fruit. 2. olivary body; a rounded elevation lateral to the upper part of each pyramid of the medulla oblongata.

ol·i·vif·u·gal (ol″ĭ-vif′u-g′l) moving or conducting away from the olive.

ol·i·vip·e·tal (ol″ĭ-vip′ĭ-t′l) moving or conducting toward the olive.

ol·i·vo·pon·to·cer·e·bel·lar (ol″ĭ-vo-pon″to-ser″ĕ-bel′er) pertaining to the olive, the middle peduncles, and the cerebellar cortex.

olo·pa·ta·dine (o″-lo-pat′ah-dēn) an antihistamine used as the hydrochloride salt in the topical treatment of allergic conjunctivitis.

ol·sal·a·zine (ol-sal′ah-zēn) a derivative of mesalamine used as the sodium salt as an antiinflammatory in ulcerative colitis.

-oma word element [Gr.], *tumor; neoplasm.*

OMD Doctor of Oriental Medicine.

omen·tal (o-men′t′l) pertaining to the omentum.

omen·tec·to·my (o″men-tek′tah-me) excision of all or part of the omentum.

omen·ti·tis (o″men-ti′tis) inflammation of the omentum.

omen·to·pexy (o-men′to-pek″se) fixation of the omentum, especially to establish collateral circulation in portal obstruction.

omen·tor·rha·phy (o″men-tor′ah-fe) suture or repair of the omentum.

omen·tum (o-men′tum) pl. *omen′ta*. [L.] a fold of peritoneum extending from the stomach to adjacent abdominal organs. **colic o.**, **gastrocolic o.**, greater o. **gastrohepatic o.**, lesser o. **greater o.**, a peritoneal fold suspended from the greater curvature of the stomach and attached to the anterior surface of the transverse colon. **lesser o.**, a peritoneal fold joining the lesser curvature of the stomach and the first part of the duodenum to the porta hepatis. **o. ma′jus**, greater o. **o. mi′nus**, lesser o.

omep·ra·zole (o-mep′ra-zōl) an inhibitor of gastric acid secretion used in the treatment of dyspepsia, gastroesophageal reflux disease, disorders of gastric hypersecretion, and peptic ulcer, including that associated with *Helicobacter pylori* infection.

omo·cla·vic·u·lar (o″mo-klah-vik′u-ler) pertaining to the shoulder and clavicle.

omo·hy·oid (-hi′oid) pertaining to the shoulder and the hyoid bone.

om·pha·lec·to·my (om″fah-lek′tah-me) excision of the umbilicus.

om·phal·ic (om-fal′ik) umbilical.

om·pha·li·tis (om″fah-li′tis) inflammation of the umbilicus.

omphal(o)- word element [Gr.], *umbilicus.*

om·pha·lo·cele (om′fah-lo-sēl″) protrusion, at birth, of part of the intestine through a defect in the abdominal wall at the umbilicus.

om·pha·lo·mes·en·ter·ic (om″fah-lo-mes″en-ter′ik) pertaining to the umbilicus and mesentery.

om·pha·lo·phle·bi·tis (-flĕ-bi′tis) inflammation of the umbilical veins.

om·pha·lor·rha·gia (-ra′jah) hemorrhage from the umbilicus.

om·pha·lor·rhea (-re′ah) effusion of lymph at the umbilicus.

om·pha·lor·rhex·is (-rek′sis) rupture of the umbilicus.

om·pha·lot·o·my (om″fah-lot′ah-me) the cutting of the umbilical cord.

onan·ism (o′nah-nizm) 1. coitus interruptus. 2. masturbation.

On·cho·cer·ca (ong″ko-ser′kah) a genus of nematode parasites of the superfamily Filarioidea, including *O. vol′vulus*, which causes onchocerciasis.

on·cho·cer·ci·a·sis (-ser-ki′ah-sis) infection by nematodes of the genus *Onchocerca*. Parasites invade the skin, subcutaneous tissues, and other parts of the body, producing fibrous nodules; blindness occurs after ocular invasion.

on·cho·cer·co·ma (-ser-ko′mah) one of the dermal or subcutaneous nodules containing *Onchocerca volvulus* in human onchocerciasis.

onc(o)-¹ word element [Gr.], *tumor; swelling; mass.*

onc(o)-² word element [Gr.], *barb; hook.*

on·co·cyte (ong′ko-sīt″) a large epithelial cell with an extremely acidophilic and granular cytoplasm, containing vast numbers of mitochondria; such cells may undergo neoplastic transformation. **oncocyt′ic**, adj.

on·co·cy·to·ma (ong″ko-si-to′mah) 1. a usually benign adenoma composed of oncocytes with granular, eosinophilic cytoplasm. 2. a benign Hürthle cell tumor. renal o., a benign neoplasm of the kidney resembling a renal cell carcinoma but encapsulated and not invasive.

on·co·cy·to·sis (-sis) metaplasia of oncocytes.

on·co·fe·tal (-fe′t′l) carcinoembryonic.

on·co·gen·e·sis (-jen′ĕ-sis) tumorigenesis; the production or causation of tumors. **oncogenet′ic**, adj.

on·co·gen·ic (-jen′ik) giving rise to tumors or causing tumor formation; said especially of tumor-inducing viruses.

on·cog·e·nous (ong-koj′ĕ-nus) arising in or originating from a tumor.

on·col·o·gy (ong-kol′ah-je) the sum of knowledge regarding tumors; the study of tumors.

on·col·y·sate (on-kol′ĭ-sāt) any agent that lyses or destroys tumor cells.

on·col·y·sis (ong-kol′ĭ-sis) destruction or dissolution of a neoplasm. **oncolyt′ic**, adj.

on·co·sis (ong-ko′sis) a morbid condition marked by the development of tumors.

on·co·sphere (ong′ko-sfēr) the larva of the tapeworm contained within the external embryonic envelope and armed with six hooks.

on·cot·ic (ong-kot′ik) 1. pertaining to swelling. 2. see under *pressure.*

on·cot·o·my (ong-kot′ah-me) the incision of a tumor or swelling.

on·co·tro·pic (ong″ko-tro′pik) having special affinity for tumor cells.

On·co·vin (ong′ko-vin) trademark for a preparation of vincristine sulfate.

on·co·vi·rus (ong′ko-vi″rus) any of the tumor-producing RNA viruses of the family Oncovirinae.

on·dan·se·tron (on-dan′sĕ-tron) an antiemetic used as the hydrochloride salt, in conjunction with cancer chemotherapy, radiotherapy, or after surgery.

onei·ric (o-ni′rik) pertaining to or characterized by dreaming or oneirism.

onei·rism (o-ni′rizm) a waking dream state.

oneir(o)- word element [Gr.], *dream.*

on·lay (on′la) 1. a graft applied or laid on the surface of an organ or structure. 2. a cast metal restoration that overlays cusps and lends strength to the restored tooth.

on·o·mato·ma·nia (on″ah-mat″ah-ma′ne-ah) irresistible preoccupation with specific words or names.

on·to·gen·e·sis (on″to-jen′ĕ-sis) ontogeny.

on·tog·e·ny (on-toj′ĭ-ne) the complete developmental history of an individual organism. **ontogenet′ic, ontogen′ic**, adj.

ony·al·ai (o″ne-al′a-e) a form of thrombocytopenic purpura due to a nutritional disorder occurring in blacks in Africa.

on·y·cha·tro·phia (o-nik″ah-tro′fe-ah) atrophy of a nail or the nails.

on·y·chaux·is (on″ĭ-kawk′sis) hypertrophy of the nails.

on·y·chec·to·my (on″ĭ-kek′tah-me) excision of a nail or nail bed.

onych·ia (o-nik′e-ah) inflammation of the nail bed, resulting in loss of the nail.

on·y·chi·tis (on″ĭ-ki′tis) onychia.

onych(o)- word element [Gr.], *the nails.*

on·y·cho·cryp·to·sis (on″ĭ-ko-krip-to′sis) ingrown nail.

on·y·cho·dys·tro·phy (-dis′trah-fe) malformation of a nail.

on·y·cho·gen·ic (-jen′ik) producing nail substance.

on·y·cho·graph (o-nik′o-graf) an instrument for observing and recording the nail pulse and capillary circulation.

on·y·cho·gry·pho·sis (on″ĭ-ko-grĭ-fo′sis) hypertrophy and curving of the nails, giving them a clawlike appearance.

on·y·cho·gry·po·sis (-grĭ-po′sis) onychogryphosis.

on·y·cho·het·ero·to·pia (-het″er-o-to′pe-ah) abnormal location of the nails.

on·y·chol·y·sis (on″ĭ-kol′ĭ-sis) loosening or separation of a nail from its bed.

on·y·cho·ma·de·sis (on″ĭ-ko-mah-de′sis) complete loss of the nails.

on·y·cho·ma·la·cia (-mah-la′shah) softening of the fingernail.

on·y·cho·my·co·sis (-mi-ko′sis) tinea unguium.

on·y·chop·a·thy (on″ĭ-kop′ah-the) any disease of the nails. **onychopath′ic,** adj.

on·y·cho·pha·gia (on″ĭ-ko-fa′jah) biting of the nails.

on·y·choph·a·gy (on″ĭ-kof′ah-je) onychophagia.

on·y·chor·rhex·is (on″ĭ-ko-rek′sis) spontaneous splitting or breaking of the nails.

on·y·cho·schi·zia (-skiz′e-ah) splitting of a nail in layers, usually at the free edge.

on·y·cho·sis (on″ĭ-ko′sis) disease or deformity of a nail or the nails.

on·y·cho·til·lo·ma·nia (on″ĭ-ko-til″o-ma′ne-ah) compulsive picking or tearing at the nails.

on·y·chot·o·my (on″ĭ-kot′ah-me) incision into a fingernail or toenail.

on·yx (on′iks) 1. nail (1). 2. a type of hypopyon.

oo- word element [Gr.], *egg; oocyte.*

oo·blast (o′o-blast) a primordial cell from which an oocyte ultimately develops.

oo·cyst (-sist) the encysted or encapsulated ookinete in the wall of a mosquito's stomach; also, the analogous stage in the development of any sporozoan.

oo·cyte (-sīt) the immature female reproductive cell prior to fertilization; derived from an oogonium. It is a *primary o.* prior to completion of the first maturation division, and a *secondary o.* in the period between the first and second maturation divisions.

oog·a·my (o-og′ah-me) in the most restrictive sense, fertilization of a large nonmotile female gamete by a small motile male gamete, as in certain algae; often used more generally to mean the sexual union of two dissimilar gametes (heterogamy). **oog′amous,** adj.

oo·gen·e·sis (o″o-jen′ĕ-sis) the process of formation of female gametes (oocytes). **oogenet′ic,** adj.

oo·go·ni·um (-go′ne-um) pl. *oogo′nia.* [Gr.] 1. a primordial oocyte during fetal development; it is derived from a primordial germ cell and before birth becomes a primary oocyte. 2. the female reproductive structure in certain fungi and algae.

oo·ki·ne·sis (-kĭ-ne′sis) the mitotic movements of the oocyte during maturation and fertilization.

oo·ki·nete (-ki-nēt′) the fertilized form of the malarial parasite in a mosquito's body, formed by fertilization of a macrogamete by a microgamete and developing into an oocyst.

oo·lem·ma (-lem′ah) zona pellucida.

ooph·o·rec·to·my (o-of″ah-rek′tah-me) excision of one or both ovaries.

ooph·o·ri·tis (-ri′tis) inflammation of an ovary.

oophor(o)- word element [Gr.], *ovary.*

ooph·o·ro·cys·tec·to·my (o-of″ah-ro-sis-tek′tah-me) excision of an ovarian cyst.

ooph·o·ro·cys·to·sis (-sis-to′sis) the formation of ovarian cysts.

ooph·o·ro·hys·ter·ec·to·my (-his″ter-ek′tah-me) excision of the ovaries and uterus.

ooph·o·ron (o-of′ah-ron) ovary.

ooph·o·ro·pexy (o-of′ah-ro-pek″se) ovariopexy.

ooph·o·ro·plas·ty (-plas″te) plastic surgery of an ovary.

ooph·o·ros·to·my (o-of″ah-ros′tah-me) the creation of an opening into an ovarian cyst.

ooph·o·rot·o·my (o-of″ah-rot′ah-me) incision of an ovary.

oo·plasm (o′o-plazm) the cytoplasm of an oocyte.

oo·tid (-tid) a mature oocyte; one of four cells derived from the two consecutive divisions of the primary oocyte. In mammals, the second maturation division is not completed unless fertilization occurs.

opac·i·fi·ca·tion (o-pas″ĭ-fĭ-ka′shun) 1. the development of an opacity. 2. the rendering opaque to x-rays of a tissue or organ by introduction of a contrast medium.

opac·i·ty (o-pas′it-e) 1. the condition of being opaque. 2. an opaque area.

opal·es·cent (o″pah-les′int) showing a milky iridescence, like an opal.

opaque (o-pāk′) impervious to light rays or, by extension, to x-rays or other electromagnetic radiation.

open (o′pen) 1. not obstructed or closed. 2. exposed to the air; not covered by unbroken skin. 3. pertaining to a study in which both subjects and experimenters know which treatment is administered to each subject.

open·ing (o′pin-ing) an aperture or open space; anatomic openings may be called *aditus, foramen, fossa, hiatus, orifice,* or *ostium.* **aortic o.,** 1. the aperture in the diaphragm for passage of the descending aorta. 2. see under *orifice.* **cardiac o.,** the opening from the esophagus into the stomach. **caval o.,** foramen venae cavae. **pyloric o.,** the opening between the stomach and duodenum. **saphenous o.,** see under *hiatus.*

op·er·a·ble (op'er-ah-b'l) subject to being operated upon with a reasonable degree of safety; appropriate for surgical removal.

op·er·ant (op'er-ant) in psychology, any response that is not elicited by specific external stimuli but that recurs at a given rate in a particular set of circumstances.

op·er·a·tion (op″er-a′shun) 1. any action performed with instruments or by the hands of a surgeon; a surgical procedure. 2. any effect produced by a therapeutic agent. **op′erative,** adj. **Albee's o.,** an operation for ankylosis of the hip. **Babcock's o.,** a technique for eradication of varicose veins by extirpation of the saphenous vein. **Bassini's o.,** plastic repair of inguinal hernia. **Beer's o.,** a flap method for cataract. **Belsey Mark IV o.,** an operation for gastroesophageal reflux performed through a thoracic incision; the fundus is wrapped 270 degrees around the circumference of the esophagus, leaving its posterior wall free. **Billroth's o.,** partial resection of the stomach with anastomosis to the duodenum (Billroth I) or to the jejunum (Billroth II). **Blalock-Taussig o.,** side-to-side anastomosis of the left subclavian artery to the left pulmonary artery to shunt some of the systemic circulation into the pulmonary circulation; performed as palliative treatment of tetralogy of Fallot or other congenital anomalies associated with insufficient pulmonary arterial flow. **Browne o.,** a type of urethroplasty for hypospadias repair, in which an intact strip of epithelium is left on the ventral surface of the penis to form the roof of the urethra, and the floor of the urethra is formed by epithelialization from the lateral wound margins. **Brunschwig o.,** pancreatoduodenectomy performed in two stages. **Caldwell-Luc o.,** 1. antrostomy in which an opening is made into the maxillary sinus via an incision into the supradental fossa opposite the premolar teeth. 2. in compound zygomaticomaxillary fractures, a method of packing of the maxillary sinus to allow reduction of displaced fragments of the zygoma by upward and outward pressure. **Cotte's o.,** removal of the presacral nerve. **Daviel's o.,** extraction of a cataract through a corneal incision without cutting the iris. **Denis Browne o.,** Browne o. **Dührssen's o.,** vaginal fixation of the uterus. **Dupuy-Dutemps o.,** blepharoplasty of the lower lid with tissue from the upper lid. **Elliot's o.,** sclerectomy

by trephine. **equilibrating o.,** tenotomy of the direct antagonist of a paralyzed eye muscle. **exploratory o.,** incision into a body area to determine the cause of unexplained symptoms. **flap o.,** 1. any operation involving the raising of a flap of tissue. 2. in periodontics, an operation to secure greater access to granulation tissue and osseous defects, consisting of detachment of the gingivae, the alveolar mucosa, and/or a portion of the alveolar mucosa. **Fothergill o.,** an operation for uterine prolapse by fixation of the cardinal ligaments. **Frazier-Spiller o.,** trigeminal rhizotomy using an approach through the middle cranial fossa. **Fredet-Ramstedt o.,** pyloromyotomy. **Frost-Lang o.,** insertion of a gold ball in place of an enucleated eyeball. **Gonin's o.,** thermocautery of the fissure in the retina, performed through an opening in the sclera, for retinal detachment. **Hartmann's o.,** resection of a diseased portion of the colon, with the proximal end of the colon brought out as a colostomy and the distal stump or rectum being closed by suture. **Kelly's o.,** see under *plication.* **King's o.,** arytenoidopexy. **Kraske's o.,** removal of the coccyx and part of the sacrum for access to a rectal carcinoma. **Lagrange's o.,** sclerectoiridectomy. **Le Fort's o., Le Fort-Neugebauer o.,** uniting the anterior and posterior vaginal walls at the middle line to repair or prevent uterine prolapse. **Lorenz's o.,** an operation for congenital dislocation of the hip. **McBurney o.,** radical surgery for the cure of inguinal hernia. **Macewen's o.,** an operation for the radical cure of hernia by closing the internal ring with a pad made of the hernial sac. **McDonald o.,** an operation for incompetent cervix, in which the cervical os is closed with a purse-string suture. **McGill's o.,** suprapubic transvesical prostatectomy. **McVay o.,** see under *repair.* **Manchester o.,** Fothergill o. **Marshall-Marchetti-Krantz o.,** suture of the anterior portion of the urethra, vesical neck, and bladder to the posterior surface of the pubic bone for correction of stress incontinence. **Motais' o.,** transplantation of a portion of the tendon of the superior rectus muscle of the eyeball into the upper lid, for ptosis. **Partsch's o.,** a technique for marsupialization of a dental cyst. **radical o.,** one involving extensive resection of tissue for complete extirpation of disease. **Ramstedt's o.,** pyloromyotomy. **Saemisch's o.,** transfixion of the cornea and of the base of the ulcer for cure of hypopyon. **Shirodkar's o.,** an operation for incompetent cervix in which the cervical os is closed with a surrounding purse-string suture. **Wertheim's o.,** radical hysterectomy. **Ziegler's o.,** V-shaped iridectomy for forming an artificial pupil.

oper·cu·lum (o-per′ku-lum) pl. *oper′cula*. [L.] 1. a lid or covering. 2. the folds of pallium from the frontal, parietal, and temporal lobes of the cerebrum overlying the insula. **oper′cular,** adj. **dental o.,** the hood of gingival tissue overlying the crown of an erupting tooth. **trophoblastic o.,** the plug of trophoblast that helps close the gap in the endometrium made by the implanting blastocyst.

op·er·on (op′er-on) a segment of a chromosome comprising an operator gene and closely linked structural genes having related functions.

ophi·a·sis (o-fi′ah-sis) a form of alopecia areata involving the temporal and occipital margins of the scalp in a continuous band.

ophi·dism (o′fi-dizm) poisoning by snake venom.

oph·ry·on (of′re-on) the middle point of the transverse supraorbital line.

oph·ry·o·sis (of″re-o′sis) spasm of the eyebrow.

oph·thal·mag·ra (of″thal-mag′rah) sudden pain in the eye.

oph·thal·mal·gia (of″thal-mal′jah) pain in the eye.

oph·thal·mec·to·my (of″thal-mek′tah-me) excision of an eye; enucleation of the eyeball.

oph·thal·men·ceph·a·lon (of″thal-men-sef′ah-lon) the retina, optic nerve, and visual apparatus of the brain.

oph·thal·mia (of-thal′me-ah) severe inflammation of the eye. **Egyptian o.,** trachoma. **gonorrheal o.,** gonorrheal conjunctivitis. **o. neonato′rum,** any hyperacute purulent conjunctivitis occurring during the first 10 days of life, usually contracted during birth from infected vaginal discharge of the mother. **phlyctenular o.,** see under *keratoconjunctivitis.* **purulent o.,** a form with a purulent discharge, commonly due to gonorrheal infection. **sympathetic o.,** granulomatous inflammation of the uveal tract of the uninjured eye following a wound involving the uveal tract of the other eye, resulting in bilateral granulomatous inflammation of the entire uveal tract.

oph·thal·mic (of-thal′mik) ocular (1).

oph·thal·mi·tis (of″thal-mi′tis) inflammation of the eyeball. **ophthalmit′ic,** adj.

ophthalm(o)- word element [Gr.], *eye.*

oph·thal·mo·blen·nor·rhea (of-thal″mo-blen″o-re′ah) gonorrheal conjunctivitis.

oph·thal·mo·cele (of-thal′mo-sēl) exophthalmos.

oph·thal·mo·dy·na·mom·e·try (of-thal″mo-di″nah-mom′ĭ-tre) determination of the blood pressure in the retinal artery.

oph·thal·mo·dyn·ia (-din′e-ah) pain in the eye.

oph·thal·mo·ei·ko·nom·e·ter (-i″ko-nom′ĕ-ter) an instrument for determining both the refraction of the eye and the relative size and shape of the ocular images.

oph·thal·mog·ra·phy (of″thal-mog′rah-fe) description of the eye and its diseases.

oph·thal·mo·gy·ric (of-thal″mo-ji′rik) oculogyric.

oph·thal·mol·o·gist (of″thal-mol′ah-jist) a physician who specializes in ophthalmology.

oph·thal·mol·o·gy (of″thal-mol′ah-je) the branch of medicine dealing with the eye, including its anatomy, physiology, and pathology. **ophthalmolog′ic,** adj.

oph·thal·mo·ma·la·cia (of-thal″mo-mah-la′shah) abnormal softness of the eyeball.

oph·thal·mom·e·try (of″thal-mom′ĭ-tre) determination of the refractive powers and defects of the eye.

oph·thal·mo·my·co·sis (of-thal″mo-mi-ko′sis) any disease of the eye caused by a fungus.

oph·thal·mo·my·ot·o·my (-mi-ot′ah-me) surgical division of the muscles of the eyes.

oph·thal·mo·neu·ri·tis (-noo-ri′tis) optic neuritis.

oph·thal·mop·a·thy (of″thal-mop′ah-the) any disease of the eye.

oph·thal·mo·plas·ty (of-thal′mo-plas″te) plastic surgery of the eye or its appendages.

oph·thal·mo·ple·gia (of-thal″mo-ple′jah) paralysis of the eye muscles. **ophthalmople′gic,** adj. **external o.,** paralysis of the external ocular muscles. **internal o.,** paralysis of the iris and ciliary apparatus. **nuclear o.,** that due to a lesion of nuclei of motor nerves of the eye. **Parinaud's o.,** paralysis of conjugate upward movement of the eyes without paralysis of convergence, associated with midbrain lesions. **partial o.,** that affecting some of the eye muscles. **progressive external o.,** gradual paralysis affecting the extraocular muscles, and sometimes also the orbicularis oculi, leading to ptosis and progressive total ocular paresis. **total o.,** paralysis of all the eye muscles, both intraocular and extraocular.

oph·thal·mor·rha·gia (-ra′jah) hemorrhage from the eye.

oph·thal·mor·rhea (-re′ah) oozing of blood from the eye.

oph·thal·mor·rhex·is (-rek'sis) rupture of an eyeball.

oph·thal·mo·scope (of-thal'mo-skōp) an instrument containing a perforated mirror and lenses used to examine the interior of the eye. **direct o.,** one that produces an upright, or unreversed, image of approximately 15 times magnification. **indirect o.,** one that produces an inverted, or reversed, direct image of two to five times magnification. **scanning laser o.,** an instrument for retinal imaging in which the retina is scanned by a low-power laser and the reflected light is used to create a digital image.

oph·thal·mos·co·py (of″thal-mos'kah-pe) examination of the eye by means of the ophthalmoscope. **medical o.,** that performed for diagnostic purposes. **metric o.,** that performed for measurement of refraction.

oph·thal·mos·ta·sis (of″thal-mos'tah-sis) fixation of the eye with the ophthalmostat.

oph·thal·mo·stat (of-thal'mo-stat) an instrument for holding the eye steady during operation.

oph·thal·mot·o·my (of″thal-mot'ah-me) incision of the eye.

oph·thal·mo·trope (of-thal'mo-trōp) a mechanical eye that moves like a real eye.

opi·ate (o'pe-it) 1. any drug derived from opium. 2. hypnotic (2).

opi·oid (o'pe-oid) 1. any synthetic narcotic that has opiate-like activities but is not derived from opium. 2. any of a group of naturally occurring peptides, e.g., enkephalins, that bind at or otherwise influence opiate receptors, either with opiate-like or opiate antagonist effects.

opis·thi·on (o-pis'the-on) the midpoint of the lower border of the foramen magnum.

opis·thor·chi·a·sis (o″pis-thor-ki'ah-sis) infection of the biliary tract by *Opisthorchis*.

Opis·thor·chis (o″pis-thor'kis) a genus of flukes parasitic in the liver and biliary tract of various birds and mammals; *O. feli'neus* and *O. viver'rini* cause opisthorchiasis and *O. sinen'sis* causes clonorchiasis in humans.

opis·thot·o·nos (o″pis-thot'ŏ-nos) a form of extreme hyperextension of the body in which the head and heels are bent backward and the body bowed forward. **opisthoton'ic,** adj.

opi·um (o'pe-um) [L.] air-dried milky exudation from incised unripe capsules of *Papaver somniferum* or its variety *album*, containing some 20 alkaloids, the more important being morphine, codeine, and thebaine; the alkaloids are used for their narcotic and analgesic effect. Because it is highly addictive, opium production is restricted and cultivation of the plants from which it is obtained is prohibited by most nations under an international agreement.

op·por·tu·nis·tic (op″er-toon-is'tik) 1. denoting a microorganism which does not ordinarily cause disease but becomes pathogenic under certain circumstances. 2. denoting a disease or infection caused by such an organism.

oprel·ve·kin (o-prel'vĕ-kin″) recombinant interleukin-11, used as a hematopoietic stimulator to prevent thrombocytopenia following myelosuppressive chemotherapy.

op·sin (op'sin) a protein of the retinal rods (scotopsin) and cones (photopsin) that combines with 11-*cis*-retinal to form visual pigments.

op·so·clo·nus (op″so-clo'nus) involuntary, nonrhythmic horizontal and vertical oscillations of the eyes.

op·so·nin (op'son-in) an antibody that renders bacteria and other cells susceptible to phagocytosis. **opson'ic,** adj. **immune o.,** an antibody that sensitizes a particulate antigen to phagocytosis, after combination with the homologous antigen in vivo or in vitro.

op·so·ni·za·tion (op″sah-nĭ-za'shun) the rendering of bacteria and other cells subject to phagocytosis.

op·so·no·cy·to·phag·ic (op″son-o-sīt″o-faj'ik) denoting the phagocytic activity of blood in the presence of serum opsonins and homologous leukocytes.

op·tic (op'tik) ocular (1).

op·ti·cal (op'tĭ-k'l) visual.

op·ti·cian (op-tish'in) a specialist in opticianry.

op·ti·cian·ry (-re) the translation, filling, and adapting of ophthalmic prescriptions, products, and accessories.

op·ti·co·chi·as·mat·ic (op″tĭ-ko-ki″az-mat'ik) pertaining to the optic nerves and chiasma.

op·ti·co·cil·i·ary (-sil'e-ar″e) pertaining to the optic and ciliary nerves.

op·ti·co·pu·pil·lary (-pu'pĭ-lar″e) pertaining to the optic nerve and pupil.

op·tics (op'tiks) the science of light and vision.

opt(o)- word element [Gr.], *visible; vision; sight.*

op·to·gram (op'to-gram) the retinal image formed by the bleaching of visual purple under the influence of light.

op·to·ki·net·ic (op″to-kĭ-net'ik) pertaining to movement of the eyes, as in nystagmus.

op·tom·e·ter (op-tom'ĕ-ter) a device for measuring the power and range of vision.

op·tom·e·trist (op-tom'ĕ-trist) a specialist in optometry.

op·tom·e·try (op-tom′ĕ-tre) the professional practice consisting of examination of the eyes to evaluate health and visual abilities, diagnosis of eye diseases and conditions of the eye and visual system, and provision of necessary treatment by the use of eyeglasses, contact lenses, and other functional, optical, surgical, and pharmaceutical means as regulated by state law.

op·to·my·om·e·ter (op″to-mi-om′ĕ-ter) a device for measuring the power of ocular muscles.

OPV poliovirus vaccine live oral.

OR operating room.

ora[1] (o′rah) pl. *o′rae*. [L.] an edge or margin. **o. serra′ta re′tinae,** the zigzag margin of the retina of the eye.

ora[2] plural of *os*[1].

orad (o′rad) toward the mouth.

oral (or′al) 1. pertaining to the mouth; taken through or applied in the mouth. 2. lingual (2).

oral·i·ty (or-al′it-e) the psychic organization of all the sensations, impulses, and personality traits derived from the oral stage of psychosexual development.

or·ange (or′anj) 1. the trees *Citrus aurantium* and *Citrus sinensis* or their fruits; the flowers and peels are used in pharmaceutical preparations. 2. a color between red and yellow, produced by energy of wavelengths between 590 and 630 nm. 3. a dye or stain with this color.

or·bic·u·lar (or-bik′u-ler) circular; rounded.

or·bic·u·la·re (or-bik″u-la′re) a small oval knob on the long limb of the incus, articulating with or ossified to the head of the stapes.

or·bic·u·lus (or-bik′u-lus) pl. *orbi′culi*. [L.] a small disk.

or·bit (or′bit) the bony cavity containing the eyeball and its associated muscles, vessels, and nerves. **or′bital,** adj.

or·bi·ta (or′bĭ-tah) pl. *or′bitae*. [L.] orbit.

or·bi·ta·le (or″bĭ-ta′le) the lowest point on the inferior edge of the orbit.

or·bi·ta·lis (or″bĭ-ta′lis) [L.] pertaining to the orbit.

or·bi·tog·ra·phy (or″bĭ-tog′rah-fe) visualization of the orbit and its contents using radiography or computed tomography.

or·bi·to·na·sal (or″bit-o-na′zal) pertaining to the orbit and nose.

or·bi·to·nom·e·ter (-nom′ĕ-ter) an instrument for measuring backward displacement of the eyeball produced by a given pressure on its anterior aspect.

or·bi·top·a·thy (or″bĭ-top′ah-the) disease affecting the orbit and its contents.

or·bi·tot·o·my (or″bĭ-tot′ah-me) incision into the orbit.

Or·bi·vi·rus (or′bĭ-vi″rus) orbiviruses; a genus of viruses of the family Reoviridae, infecting a variety of vertebrates, including humans; it includes Orungo virus.

or·bi·vi·rus (or′bĭ-vi″rus) any virus of the genus *Orbivirus*.

or·ce·in (or-se′in) a brownish-red coloring substance obtained from orcinol; used as a stain for elastic tissue.

or·chi·al·gia (or″ke-al′jah) pain in a testis.

or·chi·dec·to·my (or″kĭ-dek′tah-me) orchiectomy.

orchid(o)- [Gr. *orchidion*, dim. of *orchis* testis] word element [Gr.], *testis*.

or·chi·ec·to·my (or″ke-ek′tah-me) excision of one or both testes. If bilateral it is called also *castration*.

or·chi·epi·did·y·mi·tis (-ep″ĭ-did″ĭ-mi′tis) epididymo-orchitis.

orchi(o)- word element [Gr.], *testis*.

or·chi·op·a·thy (or″ke-op′ah-the) any disease of the testis.

or·chio·pexy (or′ke-o-pek″se) fixation in the scrotum of an undescended testis.

or·chio·plas·ty (-plas″te) plastic surgery of a testis.

or·chi·ot·o·my (or″kĭ-ot′ah-me) incision into a testis.

or·chi·tis (or-ki′tis) inflammation of a testis. **orchit′ic,** adj.

or·ci·nol (or′sĭ-nol) an antiseptic principle, mainly derived from lichens, used as a reagent in various tests.

or·der (or′der) a taxonomic category subordinate to a class and superior to a family (or suborder).

or·der·ly (or′der-le) an attendant in a hospital who works under the direction of a nurse.

or·di·nate (or′dĭ-nat) the vertical line in a graph along which is plotted one of two sets of factors considered in the study. Symbol *y*.

orex·i·gen·ic (o-rek″sĭ-jen′ik) increasing or stimulating the appetite.

orf (orf) a contagious pustular viral dermatitis of sheep, communicable to humans.

or·gan (or′gan) a somewhat independent body part that performs a special function. **o. of Corti,** the organ lying against the basilar membrane in the cochlear duct, containing special sensory receptors for hearing, and consisting of neuroepithelial hair cells and several types of supporting cells. **effector o.,** effector (2). **end o.,** end-organ. **enamel o.,** a process of epithelium forming a cap over a dental papilla and developing into the enamel. **genital o's,** reproductive o's. **Golgi tendon o.,** any of the mechanoreceptors arranged in series with muscle in the tendons of mammalian muscles, being the receptors for stimuli responsible for the lengthening reaction. **Jacobson's o.,** vomeronasal o. **reproductive o's,** the various internal and external organs that are concerned with reproduction. **rudimentary o.,** 1. a primordium. 2. an imperfectly or incompletely developed organ. **sense o's, sensory o's,** organs that receive stimuli that give rise to sensations, i.e., organs that translate certain forms of energy into nerve impulses that are perceived as special sensations. **spiral o.,** o. of Corti. **vestigial o.,** an undeveloped organ that, in the embryo or in some ancestor, was well developed and functional. **vomeronasal o.,** a small sac just above the vomeronasal cartilage; rudimentary in adult humans but well developed in many other animals. **Weber's o.,** prostatic utricle. **o's of Zuckerkandl,** para-aortic bodies.

or·ga·nelle (or″gah-nel′) a specialized structure of a cell, such as a mitochondrion, Golgi complex, lysosome, endoplasmic reticulum, ribosome, centriole, chloroplast, cilium, or flagellum.

or·gan·ic (or-gan′ik) 1. pertaining to or arising from an organ or organs. 2. having an organized structure. 3. arising from an organism. 4. pertaining to substances derived from living organisms. 5. denoting chemical substances containing covalently bonded carbon atoms, excluding such binary compounds as the carbon oxides, carbides, etc. 6. pertaining to or cultivated by use of animal or vegetable fertilizers, rather than synthetic chemicals.

or·gan·ism (or′gan-izm) an individual living thing, whether animal or plant. **pleuropneumonia-like o's,** any of various bacteria of the genus *Mycoplasma,* originally found causing pleuropneumonia in cattle and later found in other animals, including humans.

or·ga·ni·za·tion (or″gah-nĭ-za′shun) 1. the process of organizing or of becoming organized. 2. the replacement of blood clots by fibrous tissue. 3. an organized body, group, or structure. **Professional Standards Review O. (PSRO),** a regional organization of physicians and in some cases allied health professionals established to monitor health care services paid for by Medicare, Medicaid, and Maternal and Child Health programs.

or·ga·nize (or′gan-īz) 1. to provide with an organic structure. 2. to form into organs.

or·ga·niz·er (or′gah-nīz″er) a region of the embryo that is capable of determining the differentiation of other regions.

organ(o)- word element [Gr.], *organ, organic.*

or·ga·no·gen·e·sis (or″gah-no-jen′ĕ-sis) the origin and development of organs. **organogenet′ic,** adj.

or·ga·nog·e·ny (or″gah-noj′ĕ-ne) organogenesis.

or·ga·noid (or′gah-noid) 1. resembling an organ. 2. a structure that resembles an organ.

or·ga·no·meg·a·ly (or″gan-o-meg′ah-le) visceromegaly.

or·ga·no·mer·cu·ri·al (-mer-ku′re-al) any mercury-containing organic compound.

or·ga·no·me·tal·lic (-mĕ-tal′ik) consisting of a metal combined with an organic radical, used particularly for a compound in which the metal is linked directly to a carbon atom.

or·ga·no·phos·phate (or″gah-no-fos′fāt) an organic ester of phosphoric or thiophosphoric acid; such compounds are powerful acetylcholinesterase inhibitors and are used as insecticides and nerve gases. **organophos′phorous,** adj.

or·ga·no·tro·phic (-tro′fik) heterotrophic.

or·ga·not·ro·pism (or″gah-not′rah-pizm) the special affinity of chemical compounds or pathogenic agents for particular tissues or organs of the body. **organotrop′ic,** adj.

or·gasm (or′gazm) the apex and culmination of sexual excitement. **orgas′mic,** adj.

ori·en·ta·tion (or″e-en-ta′shun) 1. awareness of one's environment with reference to time, place, and people. 2. the relative positions of atoms or groups in a chemical compound.

or·i·fice (or′ĭ-fis) 1. the entrance or outlet of any body cavity. 2. any opening or meatus. **orific′ial,** adj. **aortic o.,** the opening of the left ventricle into the aorta. **cardiac o.,** see under *opening.* **external urethral o.,** urinary meatus. **left atrioventricular o., mitral o.,** the opening between the left atrium and ventricle of the heart. **pulmonary o., o. of pulmonary trunk,** the opening between the pulmonary trunk and the right ventricle. **right atrioventricular o., tricuspid o.,** the opening between the right atrium and ventricle of the heart.

or·i·gin (or′ĭ-jin) the source or beginning of anything, especially the more fixed end or attachment of a muscle (as distinguished from its insertion), or the site of emergence of a peripheral nerve from the central nervous system.

or·li·stat (or′lĭ-stat) an inhibitor of gastrointestinal lipases that prevents the digestion, and therefore absorption, of dietary fat; used in the treatment of obesity.

or·ni·thine (or′nĭ-thēn) an amino acid obtained from arginine by splitting of urea; it is an intermediate in urea biosynthesis.

or·ni·thine car·ba·mo·yl·trans·fer·ase (kahr″bah-mo″il-trans′fer-ās) an enzyme that catalyzes the carbamoylation of ornithine to form citrulline, a step in the urea cycle; deficiency of the enzyme is an X-linked aminoacidopathy causing hyperammonemia, neurologic abnormalities, and oroticaciduria and is usually fatal in the neonatal period in males.

or·ni·thin·emia (or″nĭ-thī-ne′me-ah) hyperornithinemia.

Or·ni·thod·o·ros (or″nĭ-thod′ah-ros) a genus of soft-bodied ticks, many species of which are reservoirs and vectors of the spirochetes (*Borrelia*) of relapsing fevers.

or·ni·tho·sis (or″nĭ-tho′sis) psittacosis.

oro·lin·gual (o″ro-ling′gwal) pertaining to the mouth and tongue.

oro·na·sal (-na′z′l) pertaining to the mouth and nose.

oro·pha·ryn·ge·al (-fah-rin′je-al) 1. pertaining to the mouth and pharynx. 2. pertaining to the oropharynx.

oro·phar·ynx (-far′inks) the part of the pharynx between the soft palate and the upper edge of the epiglottis.

oro·tra·che·al (-tra′ke-al) pertaining to the mouth and trachea.

or·phen·a·drine (or-fen′ah-drēn) an analogue of diphenhydramine having anticholinergic, antihistaminic, and antispasmodic actions; its citrate salt is used as a skeletal muscle relaxant.

ORS oral rehydration salts.

ORT oral rehydration therapy.

ortho- 1. word element [Gr.], *straight; normal; correct.* 2. in organic chemistry, a prefix indicating a cyclic derivative having two substituents in adjacent positions. Symbol *o-*. 3. in organic chemistry, the common form of an acid.

or·tho·cho·rea (or″tho-ko-re′ah) choreic movements in the erect posture.

or·tho·chro·mat·ic (-kro-mat′ik) staining normally.

or·tho·de·ox·ia (-de-ok′se-ah) accentuation of arterial hypoxemia in the erect position.

or·tho·don·tics (-don′tiks) the branch of dentistry concerned with irregularities of teeth and malocclusion, and associated facial abnormalities. **orthodon′tic,** adj.

or·tho·don·tist (-don′tist) a dentist who specializes in orthodontics.

or·tho·drom·ic (-drom′ik) conducting impulses in the normal direction; said of nerve fibers.

or·thog·nath·ia (or″thog-nath′e-ah) the branch of oral medicine dealing with the cause and treatment of malposition of the bones of the jaw.

or·thog·na·thic (or″thog-na′thik) 1. pertaining to orthognathia. 2. orthognathous.

or·thog·na·thous (or-thog′nah-thus) pertaining to or characterized by minimal protrusion of the mandible or minimal prognathism.

or·tho·grade (or′tho-grād) walking with the body upright.

Or·tho·hep·ad·na·vi·rus (or″tho-hep-ad′nah-vi″rus) [ortho- + hepadnavirus] hepatitis B viruses that infect mammals; a genus of the family Hepadnaviridae that includes hepatitis B virus.

or·thom·e·ter (or-thom′ĕ-ter) instrument for determining relative protrusion of the eyeballs.

or·tho·mo·lec·u·lar (or″tho-mo-lek′u-lar) relating to or aimed at restoring the optimal concentrations and functions at the molecular level of the substances (e.g., vitamins) normally present in the body.

or·tho·myxo·vi·rus (-mik″so-vi″rus) a subgroup of myxoviruses that includes the viruses of human and animal influenza.

or·tho·pe·dic (-pe′dik) pertaining to the correction of deformities of the musculoskeletal system; pertaining to orthopedics.

or·tho·pe·dics (-pe′diks) the branch of surgery dealing with the preservation and restoration of the function of the skeletal system, its articulations, and associated structures.

or·tho·pe·dist (-pe′dist) an orthopedic surgeon.

or·tho·per·cus·sion (-per-kush′un) percussion with the distal phalanx of the finger held perpendicularly to the body wall.

or·tho·pho·ria (-for′e-ah) normal equilibrium of the eye muscles, or muscular balance. **orthophor′ic,** adj.

or·tho·phos·phor·ic ac·id (-fos-for′ik) phosphoric acid.

or·thop·nea (or″thop-ne′ah) dyspnea that is relieved in the upright position. **orthopne′ic,** adj.

Or·tho·pox·vi·rus (or′tho-poks-vi″rus) a genus of viruses of the subfamily Chordopoxvirinae (family Poxviridae) that cause generalized infections with a rash in mammals, including cowpox, monkeypox, and variola viruses.

or·tho·prax·is (or″tho-prak′sis) orthopraxy.

or·tho·praxy (or′tho-prak-se) mechanical correction of deformities.

or·thop·tic (or-thop′tik) correcting obliquity of one or both visual axes.

or·thop·tics (-tiks) treatment of strabismus by exercise of the ocular muscles.

Or·tho·reo·vi·rus (or″tho-re′o-vi″rus) a genus of viruses of the family Reoviridae; no causative relationship to any disease has been proved in humans but in other mammals they have been associated with respiratory and enteric disease, and in chickens and turkeys with arthritis.

or·tho·scope (or′tho-skōp) an apparatus which neutralizes corneal refraction by means of a layer of water.

or·tho·scop·ic (or″tho-skop′ik) 1. affording a correct and undistorted view. 2. pertaining to an orthoscope.

or·tho·sis (or-tho′sis) pl. *ortho'ses*. [Gr.] an orthopedic appliance or apparatus used to support, align, prevent, or correct deformities or to improve function of movable parts of the body. **cervical o.,** one that encircles the neck and supports the chin, used in the treatment of injuries of the cervical spine. **dynamic o.,** a support or protective apparatus for the hand or other body part which also aids in initiating, performing, and reacting to motion. **halo o.,** a cervical orthosis consisting of a stiff halo attached to the upper skull and to a rigid jacket on the chest, providing maximal rigidity.

or·tho·stat·ic (or″tho-stat′ik) pertaining to or caused by standing erect.

or·tho·stat·ism (-stat′izm) an erect standing position of the body.

or·thot·ic (or-thot′ik) serving to protect or to restore or improve function; pertaining to the use or application of an orthosis.

or·thot·ics (-iks) the field of knowledge relating to orthoses and their use.

or·thot·ist (or-thot′ist) a person skilled in orthotics and practicing its application in individual cases.

or·thot·o·nos (or-thot′ah-nos) tetanic spasm which fixes the head, body, and limbs in a rigid straight line.

or·thot·o·nus (or-thot′ah-nus) orthotonos.

or·tho·top·ic (or″tho-top′ik) occurring at the normal place.

or·tho·vol·tage (or′tho-vōl″taj) in radiotherapy, voltage in the range of 140 to 400 kilovolts, as contrasted to supervoltage and megavoltage.

OS [L.] *o'culus sinis'ter* (left eye).

Os osmium.

os[1] (os) pl. *o'ra*. [L.] 1. any body orifice. 2. the mouth.

os[2] pl. *os'sa*. [L.] bone; see *Table of Bones*.

os·cil·la·tion (os″ĭ-la′shun) a backward and forward motion, like that of a pendulum.

oscill(o)- word element [L.], *oscillation*.

os·cil·lom·e·ter (os″ĭ-lom′ĕ-ter) an instrument for measuring oscillations.

os·cil·lop·sia (os″ĭ-lop′se-ah) a visual sensation that stationary objects are swaying back and forth.

os·cil·lo·scope (ŏ-sil′o-skōp) an instrument that displays a visual representation of electrical variations on the fluorescent screen of a cathode-ray tube.

os·cu·lum (os′ku-lum) pl. *os'cula*. [L.] a small aperture or minute opening.

-ose a suffix indicating that the substance is a carbohydrate.

osel·tam·i·vir (o″sel-tam′ĭ-vir) an inhibitor of viral neuraminidase, used as the phosphate salt in the treatment of influenza.

-osis word element [Gr.], *disease; morbid state; abnormal increase*.

os·mate (oz′māt) a salt containing the osmium tetroxide anion.

os·mat·ic (oz-mat′ik) olfactory.

os·mic ac·id (oz′mik) osmium tetroxide.

os·mi·um (Os) (oz′me-um) chemical element (see *Table of Elements*), at. no. 76. **o. tetroxide,** a fixative used in preparing histologic specimens, OsO_4.

osm(o)-[1] word element [Gr.], *odor; smell*.

osm(o)-[2] word element [Gr.], *impulse; osmosis*.

os·mo·lal·i·ty (oz″mo-lal′it-e) the concentration of a solution in terms of osmoles of solute per kilogram of solvent.

os·mo·lar (oz-mo′ler) pertaining to the concentration of osmotically active particles in solution.

os·mo·lar·i·ty (oz″mo-lar′ĭ-te) the concentration of a solution in terms of osmoles of solutes per liter of solution.

os·mole (oz′mol) a unit of osmotic pressure equivalent to the amount of solute that dissociates in solution to form one mole (Avogadro's number) of particles (molecules and ions). Symbol Osm.

os·mom·e·ter (oz-mom′ĕ-ter) an instrument for measuring osmotic concentration or pressure.

os·mo·phil·ic (oz″mo-fil′ik) having an affinity for solutions of high osmotic pressure.

os·mo·phore (oz′mo-fōr) the group of atoms responsible for the odor of a compound.

os·mo·re·cep·tor (oz″mo-re-sep′ter) 1. any of a group of specialized neurons in the hypothalamus that are stimulated by increased osmolality (chiefly, increased sodium concentration) of the extracellular fluid; their excitation promotes the release of antidiuretic hormone by the posterior pituitary. 2. olfactory receptor.

os·mo·reg·u·la·tion (-reg″u-la′shun) adjustment of internal osmotic pressure of a simple organism or body cell in relation to that of the surrounding medium. **osmo-reg′ulatory**, adj.

os·mo·sis (oz-mo′sis, os-mo′sis) the diffusion of pure solvent across a membrane in response to a concentration gradient, usually from a solution of lesser to one of greater solute concentration. **osmot′ic**, adj.

os·mo·stat (oz′mo-stat″) the regulatory centers that control the osmolality of the extracellular fluid.

os·sa (os′ah) [L.] plural of *os²*.

os·se·in (os′e-in) the collagen of bone.

osse(o)- word element [L.], *a bone; containing a bony element.*

os·seo·car·ti·lag·i·nous (os″e-o-kahr″tĭ-laj-ĭ-nus) composed of bone and cartilage.

os·seo·fi·brous (-fi′brus) made up of fibrous tissue and bone.

os·seo·mu·cin (-mu′sin) the ground substance that binds together the collagen and elastic fibrils of bone.

os·se·ous (os′e-us) of the nature or quality of bone; bony.

os·si·cle (os′ĭ-k′l) a small bone, especially one of those in the middle ear. **ossic′ular**, adj. **Andernach's o′s**, sutural bones. **auditory o′s**, the small bones of the middle ear: incus, malleus, and stapes. See Plate 29.

os·sic·u·lec·to·my (os″ĭ-kūl-ek′tah-me) excision of one or more ossicles of the middle ear.

os·sic·u·lot·o·my (os″ĭ-kūl-ot′ah-me) incision of the auditory ossicles.

os·sic·u·lum (ŏ-sik′u-lum) pl. *ossi′cula*. [L.] ossicle.

os·sif·er·ous (ŏ-sif′er-us) producing bone.

os·sif·ic (ŏ-sif′ik) forming or becoming bone.

os·si·fi·ca·tion (os″ĭ-fĭ-ka′shun) formation of or conversion into bone or a bony substance. **ectopic o.**, a pathological condition in which bone arises in tissues not in the osseous system and in connective tissues usually not manifesting osteogenic properties. **endochondral o.**, ossification that occurs in and replaces cartilage. **heterotopic o.**, the formation of bone in abnormal locations, secondary to pathology. **intramembranous o.**, ossification that occurs in and replaces connective tissue.

os·si·fy·ing (os′ĭ-fi″ing) changing or developing into bone.

os·te·al·gia (os″te-al′jah) pain in the bones.

os·te·ar·throt·o·my (-ahr-throt′ah-me) excision of an articular end of a bone.

os·tec·to·my (os-tek′tah-me) excision of a bone or part of a bone.

os·te·ec·to·pia (os″te-ek-to′pe-ah) displacement of a bone.

os·te·itis (os″te-i′tis) inflammation of bone. **condensing o.**, osteitis with hard deposits of earthy salts in affected bone. **o. defor′mans**, rarefying osteitis resulting in weakened, deformed bones of increased mass, which may lead to bowing of long bones and deformation of flat bones; when the bones of the skull are affected, deafness may result. Called also *Paget's disease of bone*. **o. fibro′sa cys′tica, o. fibro′sa cys′tica generalisa′ta, o. fibro′sa osteoplas′tica**, rarefying osteitis with fibrous degeneration and formation of cysts and with the presence of fibrous nodules on the affected bones, due to marked osteoclastic activity secondary to hyperparathyroidism. **o. fragi′litans**, osteogenesis imperfecta. **o. fungo′sa**, chronic osteitis in which the haversian canals are dilated and filled with granulation tissue. **parathyroid o.**, o. fibrosa cystica. **sclerosing o.**, 1. sclerosing nonsuppurative osteomyelitis. 2. condensing o.

os·tem·py·e·sis (ost″em-pi-e′sis) suppuration within a bone.

oste(o)- word element [Gr.], *bone*.

os·teo·ana·gen·e·sis (os″te-o-an′ah-jen″ĕ-sis) regeneration of bone.

os·teo·ar·thri·tis (-ahr-thri′tis) noninflammatory degenerative joint disease marked by degeneration of the articular cartilage, hypertrophy of bone at the margins, and changes in the synovial membrane, accompanied by pain and stiffness. **osteoarthrit′ic**, adj.

os·teo·ar·throp·a·thy (-ahr-throp′ah-the) any disease of the joints and bones. **hypertrophic pulmonary o.**, **secondary hypertrophic o.**, symmetrical osteitis of the four limbs, chiefly localized to the phalanges and terminal epiphyses of the long bones of the forearm and leg; it is often secondary to chronic lung and heart conditions.

os·teo·ar·thro·sis (-ahr-thro′sis) osteoarthritis.

os·teo·ar·throt·o·my (-ahr-throt′ah-me) osteoarthrotomy.

os·teo·blast (os′te-o-blast″) a cell arising from a fibroblast, which, as it matures, is associated with bone production.

os·teo·blas·to·ma (os″te-o-blas-to′mah) a benign, painful, rather vascular tumor of bone marked by formation of osteoid tissue and primitive bone.

os·teo·camp·sia (-kamp′se-ah) curvature of a bone.

os·teo·chon·dral (-kon′dril) pertaining to bone and cartilage.

os·teo·chon·dri·tis (-kon-dri′tis) inflammation of bone and cartilage. **o. defor′mans juveni′lis**, osteochondrosis of the capitular epiphysis of the femur. **o. defor′mans**

juveni′lis dor′si, osteochondrosis of vertebrae. **o. dis′secans,** that resulting in splitting of pieces of cartilage into the affected joint.

os·te·o·chon·dro·dys·pla·sia (-kon″dro-dis-pla′zhah) any disorder of cartilage and bone growth.

os·te·o·chon·dro·dys·tro·phy (-dis′trah-fe) Morquio's syndrome.

os·te·o·chon·drol·y·sis (-kon-drol′ĭ-sis) osteochondritis dissecans.

os·te·o·chon·dro·ma (-kon-dro′mah) a benign bone tumor consisting of projecting adult bone capped by cartilage projecting from the lateral contours of endochondral bones.

os·te·o·chon·dro·ma·to·sis (-kon-dro″mah-to′sis) occurrence of multiple osteochondromas, sometimes specifically denoting one of the disorders multiple cartilaginous exostoses or enchondromatosis.

os·te·o·chon·dro·myx·o·ma (-mik-so′mah) osteochondroma containing myxoid elements.

os·te·o·chon·dro·sis (-kon-dro′sis) a disease of the growth ossification centers in children, beginning as a degeneration or necrosis followed by regeneration or recalcification; known by various names, depending on the bone involved.

os·te·o·oc·la·sis (os″te-ok′lah-sis) surgical fracture or refracture of bones.

os·te·o·clast (os′te-o-klast″) 1. a large multinuclear cell associated with absorption and removal of bone. 2. an instrument used for osteoclasis. **osteoclas′tic,** adj.

os·te·o·clas·to·ma (os″te-o-klas-to′mah) giant cell tumor of bone.

os·te·o·cope (os′te-o-kōp″) severe pain in a bone. **osteocop′ic,** adj.

os·te·o·cra·ni·um (os″te-o-kra′ne-um) the fetal skull during its stage of ossification.

os·te·o·cys·to·ma (-sis-to′mah) a bone cyst.

os·te·o·cyte (os′te-o-sīt″) an osteoblast that has become embedded within the bone matrix, occupying a bone lacuna and sending, through the canaliculi, slender cytoplasmic processes that make contact with processes of other osteocytes.

os·te·o·di·as·ta·sis (os″te-o-di-as′tah-sis) the separation of two adjacent bones.

os·te·odyn·ia (-din′e-ah) ostealgia.

os·te·o·dys·tro·phy (-dis′trah-fe) abnormal development of bone. **renal o.,** a condition due to chronic kidney disease and renal failure, with elevated serum phosphorus levels, low or normal serum calcium levels, and stimulation of parathyroid function, resulting in a variable admixture of bone disease.

os·te·o·epiph·y·sis (-e-pif′ĭ-sis) any bony epiphysis.

os·te·o·fi·bro·ma (-fi-bro′mah) a benign tumor combining both osseous and fibrous elements.

os·te·o·flu·o·ro·sis (-floo-ro′sis) skeletal changes, usually consisting of osteomalacia and osteosclerosis, caused by the chronic intake of excessive quantities of fluorides.

os·te·o·gen (os′te-o-jen″) the substance composing the inner layer of the periosteum, from which bone is formed.

os·te·o·gen·e·sis (os″te-o-jen′ĕ-sis) the formation of bone; the development of the bones. **osteogenet′ic,** adj. **o. imperfec′ta (OI),** any of several types of collagen disorders, of variable inheritance, due to defective biosynthesis of type I collagen and characterized by brittle, osteoporotic, easily fractured bones; other defects are blue sclerae, wormian bones, and dentinogenesis imperfecta.

os·te·o·gen·ic (-jen′ik) derived from or composed of any tissue concerned in bone growth or repair.

os·te·o·ha·lis·ter·e·sis (-hah-lis″ter-e′sis) deficiency in mineral elements of bone.

os·te·oid (os′te-oid) 1. resembling bone. 2. the organic matrix of bone; young bone that has not undergone calcification.

os·te·o·in·duc·tion (os″te-o-in-duk′shun) the act or process of stimulating osteogenesis.

os·te·o·lipo·chon·dro·ma (-lip″o-kon-dro′mah) a benign cartilaginous tumor with osseous and fatty elements.

os·te·ol·o·gy (os″te-ol′ah-je) scientific study of the bones.

os·te·ol·y·sis (os″te-ol′ĭ-sis) dissolution of bone; applied especially to the removal or loss of the calcium of bone. **osteolyt′ic,** adj.

os·te·o·ma (os″te-o′mah) a benign, slow-growing tumor composed of well-differentiated, densely sclerotic, compact bone, occurring particularly in the skull and facial bones. **compact o.,** a small, dense, compact tumor of mature lamellar bone with little medullary space, usually in the craniofacial or nasal bones. **o. cu′tis,** 1. formation of bone-containing nodules in the skin. 2. progressive dermal ossification during childhood, with development of islands of heterotopic bone within the dermis or subcutis, coalescence of the lesions into plaques, and invasion of ossification into deep connective tissue. **o. du′rum, o. ebur′neum,** compact o. **ivory o.,** compact o. **o. medulla′re,** one having marrow spaces. **osteoid o.,** a small, benign but painful, circumscribed tumor of spongy bone, usually in the bones of the limbs or vertebrae of young persons. **o. spon·gio′sum, spongy o.,** one having cancellated bone.

os·te·o·ma·la·cia (os″te-o-mah-la′shah) inadequate or delayed mineralization of osteoid in mature cortical and spongy bone; it is the adult equivalent of rickets and accompanies that disorder in children. **osteomala′cic,** adj. **hepatic o.,** osteomalacia as a complication of cholestatic liver disease, which may lead to severe bone pain and multiple fractures. **oncogenic o., tumor-induced o.,** osteomalacia occurring in association with mesenchymal neoplasms, which are usually benign.

os·te·o·mere (os′te-o-mēr″) one of a series of similar bony structures, such as the vertebrae.

os·te·om·e·try (os″te-om′ĭ-tre) measurement of the bones.

os·te·o·my·eli·tis (os″te-o-mi″ĕ-li′tis) inflammation of bone, localized or generalized, due to infection, usually by pyogenic organisms. **osteomyelit′ic,** adj. **Garré′s o.,** sclerosing nonsuppurative o., a chronic form involving the long bones, especially the tibia and femur, marked by a diffuse inflammatory reaction, increased density and spindle-shaped sclerotic thickening of the cortex, and an absence of suppuration.

os·te·o·my·elo·dys·pla·sia (-mi″ĕ-lo-dis-pla′zhah) a condition characterized by thinning of the osseous tissue of bones and increase in size of the marrow cavities, attended by leukopenia and fever.

os·te·o·myxo·chon·dro·ma (-mik″so-kon-dro′mah) osteochondromyxoma.

os·te·on (os′te-on) [Gr.] the basic unit of structure of compact bone, comprising a haversian canal and its concentrically arranged lamellae.

os·te·o·ne·cro·sis (os″te-o-nĕ-kro′sis) necrosis of a bone.

os·te·o·neu·ral·gia (-noo-ral′jah) neuralgia of a bone.

os·te·o·path (os′te-o-path″) a practitioner of osteopathy.

os·te·o·path·ia (os″te-o-path′e-ah) osteopathy (1). **o. conden′sans dissemina′ta,** osteopoikilosis. **o. stria′ta,** an asymptomatic condition characterized radiographically by multiple condensations of cancellous bone tissue, giving a striated appearance.

os·te·op·a·thy (os″te-op′ah-the) 1. any disease of a bone. 2. a system of therapy based on the theory that the body is capable of making its own remedies against disease and other toxic conditions when it is in normal structural relationship and has favorable environmental conditions and adequate nutrition; it utilizes generally accepted physical methods of diagnosis and therapy, while emphasizing the importance of normal body mechanics and manipulative methods of detecting and correcting faulty structure. **osteopath′ic,** adj.

os·te·o·pe·nia (os″te-o-pe′ne-ah) 1. reduced bone mass due to a decrease in the rate of osteoid synthesis to a level insufficient to compensate for normal bone lysis. 2. any decrease in bone mass below the normal. **osteopen′ic,** adj.

os·te·o·peri·os·te·al (-per″e-os′te-il) pertaining to bone and its periosteum.

os·te·o·peri·os·ti·tis (-per″e-os-ti′tis) inflammation of a bone and its periosteum.

os·te·o·pe·tro·sis (-pĭ-tro′sis) a hereditary disease marked by abnormally dense bone, and by the common occurrence of fractures of affected bone.

os·te·o·phle·bi·tis (-flĕ-bi′tis) inflammation of the veins of a bone.

os·te·o·phy·ma (-fi′mah) a tumor or outgrowth of bone.

os·te·o·phyte (os′te-o-fīt″) a bony excrescence or outgrowth of bone.

os·te·o·plas·ty (-plas″te) plastic surgery of the bones.

os·te·o·poi·ki·lo·sis (os″te-o-poi″kĭ-lo′sis) a mottled condition of bones, apparent radiographically, due to the presence of multiple sclerotic foci and scattered stippling. **osteopoikilot′ic,** adj.

os·te·o·po·ro·sis (-por-o′sis) abnormal rarefaction of bone; it may be idiopathic or occur secondary to other diseases. **osteoporot′ic,** adj. **posttraumatic o.,** loss of bone substance following a nerve-damaging injury, sometimes due to an increased blood supply caused by the neurogenic insult, or to disuse secondary to pain; a component of reflex sympathetic dystrophy.

os·te·o·ra·dio·ne·cro·sis (-ra″de-o-nĕ-kro′sis) necrosis of bone as a result of exposure to radiation.

os·te·or·rha·gia (-ra′jah) hemorrhage from bone.

os·te·or·rha·phy (os″te-or′ah-fe) fixation of fragments of bone with sutures or wires.

os·te·o·sar·co·ma (os″te-o-sahr-ko′mah) a malignant primary neoplasm of bone composed of a malignant connective tissue stroma with evidence of malignant osteoid, bone, or cartilage formation; it is subclassified as osteoblastic, chondroblastic, or fibroblastic. **osteosarco′matous,** adj. **parosteal o.,** a variant consisting of a slowly growing tumor resembling cancellous bone but arising from the cortex of the bone and slowly growing outward to surround the bone. **periosteal**

o., a variant of osteochondroma consisting of a soft, lobulated tumor arising from the periosteum of a long bone and growing outward. **small-cell o.**, a variant of osteosarcoma resembling Ewing's sarcoma, with areas of osteoid and sometimes chondroid formation.

os·teo·sar·co·ma·to·sis (os″te-o-sahr-ko″mah-to′sis) the simultaneous occurrence of multiple osteosarcomas; synchronous multicentric osteosarcoma.

os·teo·scle·ro·sis (-sklĕ-ro′sis) the hardening or abnormal density of bone. **osteosclerot′ic**, adj. **o. conge′nita**, achondroplasia. **o. fra′gilis**, osteopetrosis. **o. fra′gilis generalisa′ta**, osteopoikilosis.

os·te·o·sis (os″te-o′sis) the formation of bony tissue. **o. cu′tis**, osteoma cutis.

os·teo·su·ture (os″te-o-soo′cher) osteorrhaphy.

os·teo·syn·o·vi·tis (-sin″o-vi′tis) synovitis with osteitis of neighboring bones.

os·teo·syn·the·sis (-sin′this-is) surgical fastening of the ends of a fractured bone.

os·teo·ta·bes (-ta′bēz) a disease, chiefly of infants, in which bone marrow cells are destroyed and the marrow disappears.

os·teo·throm·bo·sis (-throm-bo′sis) thrombosis of the veins of a bone.

os·teo·tome (os′te-o-tōm″) a chisel-like knife for cutting bone.

os·te·ot·o·my (os″te-ot′ah-me) incision or transection of a bone. **cuneiform o.**, removal of a wedge of bone. **displacement o.**, surgical division of a bone and shifting of the divided ends to change the alignment of the bone or to alter weight-bearing stresses. **Le Fort o.**, transverse sectioning and repositioning of the maxilla; the incision for each of the three types (*Le Fort I, II,* and *III o's*) is placed along the line defined by the corresponding Le Fort fracture. **linear o.**, the sawing or linear cutting of a bone. **sandwich o.**, a surgical procedure for augmenting an atrophic mandible, resembling a visor osteotomy but having a horizontal split confined between the mental foramina. **visor o.**, a surgical technique for augmenting an atrophic mandible, in which the mandible is split sagitally and the cranial fragment is slid upward and supported with grafts.

os·ti·tis (os-ti′tis) osteitis.

os·ti·um (os′te-um) pl. *os′tia.* [L.] an opening or orifice. **os′tial**, adj. **o. abdomina′le tu′bae uteri′nae**, the funnel-shaped opening where the uterine tube meets the abdominal cavity. **coronary o.**, either of the two openings in the aortic sinus that mark the origin of the (left and right) coronary arteries.

o. inter′num u′teri, o. uterinum tubae uterinae. **o. pharyn′geum tu′bae auditi′vae**, the pharyngeal opening of the auditory tube. **o. pri′mum**, an opening in the lower portion of the membrane dividing the embryonic heart into right and left sides. **o. secun′dum**, an opening high in the septum of the embryonic heart, approximately where the foramen ovale will later appear. **tympanic o., o. tympa′nicum tu′bae auditi′vae**, the opening of the auditory tube on the carotid wall of the tympanic cavity. **o. u′teri**, the external opening of the uterine cervix into the vagina. **o. uteri′num tu′bae uteri′nae**, the point where the cavity of the uterine tube becomes continuous with that of the uterus. **o. vagi′nae**, the external orifice of the vagina.

os·to·mate (os′tah-māt) one who has undergone enterostomy or ureterostomy.

os·to·my (os′tah-me) general term for an operation in which an artificial opening is formed.

-ostomy word element [Gr.], *surgical creation of an artificial opening.*

OT Old tuberculin.

otal·gia (o-tal′jah) pain in the ear; earache.

OTC over the counter; said of drugs not required by law to be sold on prescription only.

otic (ōt′ik) auditory (1).

oti·tis (o-ti′tis) inflammation of the ear. **otit′ic**, adj. **aviation o.**, barotitis media. **o. exter′na**, inflammation of the external ear, usually caused by a bacterial or fungal infection; it may be either *circumscribed*, with formation of a furuncle, or *diffuse*. **furuncular o.**, otitis externa with formation of a furuncle. **o. inter′na**, labyrinthitis. **o. me′dia**, inflammation of the middle ear, classified as either *serous (secretory)*, due to obstruction of the eustachian tube, or *suppurative (purulent)*, due to bacterial infection. Both types may involve hearing loss.

ot(o)- word element [Gr.], *ear.*

Oto·bi·us (o-to′be-us) a genus of soft-bodied ticks parasitic in the ears of various animals, including humans.

oto·ceph·a·ly (o″to-sef′ah-le) a congenital anomaly characterized by lack of a lower jaw and by ears that are united below the face.

oto·cra·ni·um (-kra′ne-um) the area of the petrous part of the temporal bone surrounding the osseous labyrinth. **otocra′nial**, adj.

oto·cyst (o′to-sist) the auditory vesicle of the embryo.

Oto·dec·tes (o″to-dek′tēz) a genus of mites.

oto·en·ceph·a·li·tis (-en-sef″ah-li′tis) inflammation of the brain due to extension from an inflamed middle ear.

oto·gen·ic (-jen′ik) otogenous.

otog·e·nous (o-toj′ĕ-nus) originating within the ear.

oto·lar·yn·gol·o·gy (o″to-lar″ing-gol′ah-je) the branch of medicine dealing with disease of the ear, nose, and throat.

oto·lith (o′to-lith) statolith.

otol·o·gy (o-tol′ah-je) the branch of medicine dealing with the ear, its anatomy, physiology, and pathology. **otolog′ic,** adj.

oto·mu·cor·my·co·sis (o″to-mu″kor-mi-ko′sis) mucormycosis of the ear.

oto·my·co·sis (-mi-ko′sis) otitis externa caused by a fungal infection.

oto·neu·rol·o·gy (-noo-rol′ah-je) the branch of otology dealing especially with those portions of the nervous system related to the ear. **otoneurolog′ic,** adj.

oto·pha·ryn·ge·al (o″to-fah-rin′je-al) pertaining to the ear and pharynx.

oto·plas·ty (o′to-plas″te) plastic surgery of the ear.

oto·py·or·rhea (o″to-pi″o-re′ah) otorrhea that is purulent.

oto·rhi·no·lar·yn·gol·o·gy (-ri″no-lar″ing-gol′ah-je) the branch of medicine dealing with the ear, nose, and throat.

oto·rhi·nol·o·gy (-ri-nol′ah-je) the branch of medicine dealing with the ear and nose.

otor·rhea (-re′ah) a discharge from the ear.

oto·scle·ro·sis (-sklĕ-ro′sis) a condition in which otospongiosis may cause bony ankylosis of the stapes, resulting in conductive hearing loss. **otosclerot′ic,** adj.

oto·scope (o′to-skōp) an instrument for inspecting or auscultating the ear.

oto·spon·gi·o·sis (o″to-spon″je-o′sis) the formation of spongy bone in the bony labyrinth of the ear.

oto·tox·ic (o′to-tok″sik) having a deleterious effect upon the eighth nerve or on the organs of hearing and balance.

OU [L.] o′culus uter′que (each eye).

ounce (oz) (ouns) a measure of weight. In the avoirdupois system, $\frac{1}{16}$ lb, 28.3495 g, or 437.5 grains; in the apothecaries' system, $\frac{1}{12}$ lb, 31.03 g, or 480 grains. **fluid o. (fl oz),** a unit of liquid measure of the apothecaries' system; in the United States it is one-sixteenth of a pint, or 29.57 mL. In Great Britain, *(imperial ounce)*, it is one-twentieth of an (imperial) pint, or 28.41 mL.

out·breed·ing (out′brēd″ing) the mating of unrelated individuals, which often produces more vigorous offspring than the parents are in terms of growth, survival, and fertility.

out·let (-let) a means or route of exit or egress. **pelvic o.,** the inferior opening of the pelvis. **thoracic o.,** the irregular opening at the inferior part of the thorax, bounded by the twelfth thoracic vertebra, the twelfth ribs, and the lower edge of the costal cartilages.

out·li·er (out′li-er) an observation so distant from the central mass of the data that it noticeably influences results.

out·pa·tient (-pa-shent) a patient who comes to the hospital, clinic, or dispensary for diagnosis and/or treatment but does not occupy a bed.

out·pock·et·ing (out-pok′et-ing) evagination.

out·pouch·ing (-pouch-ing) evagination.

out·put (-poot) the yield or total of anything produced by any functional system of the body. **cardiac o. (CO),** the effective volume of blood expelled by either ventricle of the heart per unit of time (usually per minute). **stroke o.,** see under *volume.* **urinary o.,** the amount of urine excreted by the kidneys.

ova (o′vah) plural of *ovum.*

ovar·i·an (o-var′e-an) pertaining to an ovary or ovaries.

ovar·i·ec·to·my (o-var″e-ek′tah-me) oophorectomy.

ovari(o)- word element [L.], *ovary.*

ovar·io·cele (o-var′e-o-sēl″) hernial protrusion of an ovary.

ovar·io·cen·te·sis (o-var″e-o-sen-te′sis) surgical puncture of an ovary.

ovar·io·pexy (-pek′se) the operation of elevating and fixing an ovary to the abdominal wall.

ovar·i·or·rhex·is (-rek′sis) rupture of an ovary.

ovar·i·os·to·my (o-var″e-os′tah-me) oophorostomy.

ovar·i·ot·o·my (-ot′ah-me) 1. oophorectomy. 2. removal of an ovarian tumor.

ovar·io·tu·bal (o-var″e-o-too′b′l) tuboovarian.

ova·ri·tis (o″vah-ri′tis) oophoritis.

ova·ri·um (o-var′e-um) pl. *ova′ria.* [L.] ovary.

ova·ry (o′vah-re) the female gonad: either of the paired female sexual glands in which oocytes are formed. **ova′rian,** adj. **polycystic o's,** ovaries containing multiple small follicular cysts filled with yellow or blood-stained thin serous fluid, as in polycystic ovary syndrome.

over·bite (o′ver-bīt″) the extension of the upper incisor teeth over the lower ones vertically when the opposing posterior teeth are in contact.

over·com·pen·sa·tion (o″ver-kom″pen-sa′shun) exaggerated correction of a real or imagined physical or psychologic defect.

over·den·ture (-den′cher) a complete denture supported both by mucosa and by a few remaining natural teeth that have been altered to permit the denture to fit over them.

over·de·ter·mi·na·tion (-de-ter″mĭ-na′-shun) the concept that every dream, disorder, aspect of behavior, or other emotional reaction or symptom has multiple causative factors.

over·do·sage (o″ver-do′sij) 1. the administration of an excessive dose. 2. the condition resulting from an excessive dose.

over·dose (o′ver-dōs″) 1. to administer an excessive dose. 2. an excessive dose.

over·drive (o′ver-drīv) a more rapid heart rate produced in the correction of an underlying pathologic rhythm; see also under *pacing*.

over·hy·dra·tion (-hi-dra′shun) hyperhydration.

over·jet (o′ver-jet) extension of the incisal or buccal cusp ridges of the upper teeth labially or buccally to the incisal margins and ridges of the lower teeth when the jaws are closed normally.

over·rid·ing (o″ver-rīd′ing) 1. the slipping of either part of a fractured bone past the other. 2. extending beyond the usual position.

over·ven·ti·la·tion (-ven″tĭ-la′shun) hyperventilation.

ovi- see *ov(o)-*.

ovi·cide (o′vĭ-sīd) an agent destructive to the eggs of certain organisms.

ovi·duct (-dukt) 1. uterine tube. 2. in nonmammals, a passage through which ova leave the female or pass to an organ that communicates with the exterior of the body. **ovidu′cal, oviduct′al,** adj.

ovif·er·ous (o-vif′er-us) producing ova.

ovi·gen·e·sis (o″vĭ-jen′ĕ-sis) oogenesis.

ovip·a·rous (o-vip′ah-rus) producing eggs in which the embryo develops outside the maternal body, as in birds.

ovi·pos·i·tor (o″vĭ-pos′it-er) a specialized organ by which many female insects deposit their eggs.

ov(o)- word element [L.], *egg; ovum.* Also, *ovi-.*

ovo·lac·to·veg·e·tar·i·an (o″vo-lak″to-vej″ĕ-tar′e-an) 1. one whose diet is restricted to vegetables, dairy products, and eggs, eschewing other foods of animal origin. 2. pertaining to ovolactovegetarianism. 3. one who practices ovolactovegetarianism.

ovo·lac·to·veg·e·tar·i·an·ism (-tar′e-ah-nizm″) restriction of the diet to vegetables, dairy products, and eggs, eschewing other foods of animal origin.

ovo·plasm (o′vo-plazm) ooplasm.

ovo·tes·tis (o″vo-tes′tis) a gonad containing both testicular and ovarian tissue.

ovo·veg·e·tar·i·an (-vej″ĕ-tar′e-an) 1. pertaining to ovovegetarianism. 2. one who practices ovovegetarianism.

ovo·veg·e·tar·i·an·ism (-tar′e-ah-nizm″) restriction of the diet to vegetables and eggs, eschewing other foods of animal origin.

ovu·lar (ov′u-lar) 1. pertaining to an ovule. 2. pertaining to an oocyte.

ovu·la·tion (ov″u-la′shun) the discharge of a secondary oocyte from a graafian follicle. **ov′ulatory,** adj.

ovule (o′vūl) 1. the oocyte within the graafian follicle. 2. any small, egglike structure.

ovum (o′vum) pl. *o′va.* [L.] 1. the female reproductive cell which, after fertilization, becomes a zygote that develops into a new member of the same species. 2. imprecise term for *oocyte.* 3. formerly, any of various stages from the primary oocyte to the implanting blastocyst. 4. in some species, any stage from the unfertilized female reproductive cell, through the developing embryo surrounded by nutrient material and protective covering, up to the point when the young emerge.

ox·a·cil·lin (ok″sah-sil′in) a semisynthetic penicillinase-resistant penicillin used as the sodium salt in infections due to penicillin-resistant, gram-positive organisms.

ox·a·late (ok′sah-lāt) any salt of oxalic acid.

ox·a·le·mia (ok″sah-le′me-ah) excess of oxalates in the blood.

ox·al·ic ac·id (ok-sal′ik) a dicarboxylic acid occurring in various fruits and vegetables and as a metabolic product of glyoxylic or ascorbic acid; it is not metabolized but is excreted in the urine. Excess may lead to formation of calcium oxalate calculi in the kidney.

ox·al·ism (ok′sal-izm) poisoning by oxalic acid or by an oxalate.

ox·a·lo·ac·e·tate (ok″sal-o-as′ĕ-tāt) a salt or ester of oxaloacetic acid.

ox·a·lo·ace·tic ac·id (ok″sah-lo-ah-sēt′ik) a metabolic intermediate in the tricarboxylic acid cycle; it is convertible to aspartic acid by aspartate transaminase.

ox·a·lo·sis (ok″sah-lo′sis) generalized deposition of calcium oxalate in renal and extrarenal tissues, as may occur in primary hyperoxaluria.

ox·al·uria (ok″sal-u′re-ah) hyperoxaluria.

ox·an·dro·lone (ok-san′dro-lōn) an androgenic and anabolic steroid that is used in the treatment of catabolic or tissue-wasting diseases or states.

ox·a·pro·zin (ok″sah-pro′zin) a nonsteroidal antiinflammatory drug, used in the treatment of rheumatoid arthritis and osteoarthritis.

ox·az·e·pam (ok-saz′ĕ-pam) a benzodiazepine tranquilizer, used as an antianxiety agent and as an adjunct in the treatment of acute alcohol withdrawal symptoms.

oxa·zo·li·din·one (ok″sah-zo-lid′ĭ-nōn) any of a class of synthetic antibacterial agents effective against gram-positive organisms.

ox·car·baz·e·pine (oks″kahr-baz′ĕ-pēn) an anticonvulsant used in the treatment of partial seizures.

ox·i·con·a·zole (ok″sĭ-kon′ah-zōl) an imidazole antifungal used topically as the nitrate salt in the treatment of various forms of tinea.

ox·i·dant (ok′sĭ-dant) the electron acceptor in an oxidation-reduction (redox) reaction.

ox·i·dase (ok′sĭ-dās) any enzyme of the class of oxidoreductases in which molecular oxygen is the hydrogen acceptor.

ox·i·da·tion (ok″sĭ-da′shun) the act of oxidizing or state of being oxidized. **ox·i·da·tive**, adj.

ox·i·da·tion-re·duc·tion (-re-duk′shun) the chemical reaction whereby electrons are removed (oxidation) from atoms of the substance being oxidized and transferred to those being reduced (reduction).

ox·ide (ok′sīd) a compound of oxygen with an element or radical.

ox·i·dize (ok′sĭ-dīz) to cause to combine with oxygen or to remove hydrogen.

ox·i·do·re·duc·tase (ok″sĭ-do-re-duk′tās) any of a class of enzymes that catalyze the reversible transfer of electrons from a substrate that becomes oxidized to one that becomes reduced (oxidation-reduction, or redox reaction).

ox·im (ok′sim) oxime.

ox·ime (ok′sēm) any of a series of compounds containing the CH(=NOH) group, formed by the action of hydroxylamine upon an aldehyde or a ketone.

ox·im·e·ter (ok-sim′ĕ-ter) a photoelectric device for determining the oxygen saturation of the blood.

ox·im·e·try (ok-sim′ĕ-tre) determination of the oxygen saturation of arterial blood using an oximeter.

5-oxo·pro·line (-pro′lēn) an acidic lactam of glutamic acid occurring at the N-terminus of several peptides and proteins.

5-oxo·pro·lin·u·ria (-pro″lin-u′re-ah) 1. excess of 5-oxoproline in the urine. 2. generalized deficiency of glutathione synthetase.

ox·triph·yl·line (oks-trif′ĭ-lēn) the choline salt of theophylline, used chiefly as a bronchodilator.

oxy- word element [Gr.], *sharp; quick; sour; the presence of oxygen in a compound.*

oxy·ben·zone (ok″se-ben′zōn) a topical sunscreen that absorbs UVB and some UVA rays.

oxy·bu·ty·nin (-bu′tĭ-nin) an anticholinergic having direct antispasmodic effect on smooth muscle; used as the chloride salt in the treatment of uninhibited or reflex neurogenic bladder.

oxy·ceph·a·ly (-sef′ah-le) a condition in which the top of the skull is pointed or conical owing to premature closure of the coronal and lambdoid sutures. **oxycephal′ic**, adj.

oxy·co·done (-ko′dōn) an opioid analgesic derived from morphine; used in the form of the hydrochloride and terephthalate salts.

ox·y·gen (O) (ok′sĭ-jen) chemical element (see *Table of Elements*), at. no. 8. It constitutes about 20 per cent of atmospheric air, is the essential agent in the respiration of plants and animals, and is necessary to support combustion. **o. 15**, an artificial radioactive isotope of oxygen having a half-life of 2.04 minutes and decaying by positron emission; used as a tracer in positron emission tomography. **hyperbaric o.**, oxygen under greater than atmospheric pressure.

ox·y·gen·ase (-jen-ās) any oxidoreductase that catalyzes the incorporation of both atoms of molecular oxygen into a single substrate.

ox·y·gen·ate (-jĕ-nāt) to saturate with oxygen.

ox·y·gen·a·tion (ok″sĭ-jĕ-na′shun) 1. the act or process of adding oxygen. 2. the result of having oxygen added. **extracorporeal membrane o. (ECMO)**, a technique for providing respiratory support for newborns, in which the blood is circulated through an artificial lung consisting of two compartments separated by a gas-permeable membrane, with the blood on one side and the ventilating gas on the other.

oxy·hem·a·to·por·phy·rin (-hem″ah-to-por′fĭ-rin) a pigment sometimes found in the urine, closely allied to hematoporphyrin.

oxy·he·mo·glo·bin (-he″mo-glo′bin) hemoglobin that contains bound O_2, a compound formed from hemoglobin on exposure to alveolar gas in the lungs.

oxy·met·az·o·line (-met-az′o-lēn) an adrenergic used as the hydrochloride salt as a vasoconstrictor to reduce nasal or conjunctival congestion.

oxy·meth·o·lone (-meth′o-lōn) an anabolic steroid used in the treatment of anemia and for the prophylaxis and treatment of hereditary angioedema.

oxy·mor·phone (-mor′fōn) an opioid analgesic, used as the hydrochloride salt as an analgesic and anesthesia adjunct.

oxy·myo·glo·bin (-mi'o-glo"bin) myoglobin charged with oxygen.

ox·yn·tic (ok-sint'ik) secreting acid, as the parietal (oxyntic) cells.

oxy·phil (ok'se-fil) 1. (*in pl.*) Askanazy cells. 2. (*in pl.*) oxyphil cells. 3. oxyphilic.

oxy·phil·ic (ok"se-fil'ik) stainable with an acid dye.

oxy·quin·o·line (ok"sĭ-kwin'o-lēn) a dicyclic aromatic compound used as a chelating agent; also used in the form of the base or the sulfate salt as a bacteriostatic, fungistatic, antiseptic, and disinfectant.

oxy·tet·ra·cy·cline (ok"se-tet"rah-si'klēn) a broad-spectrum tetracycline antibiotic produced by *Streptomyces rimosus*, used as the base or the hydrochloride salt.

oxy·to·cia (-to'se-ah) rapid labor.

oxy·to·cic (-to'sik) 1. pertaining to, marked by, or promoting oxytocia. 2. an agent that promotes rapid labor by stimulating contractions of the myometrium.

oxy·to·cin (-to'sin) a hypothalamic hormone stored in the posterior pituitary, which has uterine-contracting and milk-releasing actions; it may also be prepared synthetically or obtained from the posterior pituitary of domestic animals; used to induce active labor,

increase the force of contractions in labor, contract uterine muscle after delivery of the placenta, control postpartum hemorrhage, and stimulate milk ejection.

oxy·uri·a·sis (-ūr-i'ah-sis) 1. infection with an oxyurid such as *Enterobius vermicularis*. 2. enterobiasis.

oxy·uri·cide (-ūr'ĭ-sīd) an agent that destroys oxyurids.

oxy·urid (-ūr'id) a pinworm, seatworm, or threadworm; any individual of the superfamily Oxyuroidea.

Oxy·uris (-ūr'is) a genus of intestinal nematodes (superfamily Oxyuroidea).

Oxy·uroi·dea (-ūr"oi-de'ah) a superfamily of small nematodes—the pinworms, seatworms, or threadworms—parasitic in the cecum and colon of vertebrates and sometimes infecting invertebrates.

oz ounce.

oze·na (o-ze'nah) an atrophic rhinitis marked by a thick mucopurulent discharge, mucosal crusting, and fetor.

ozone (o'zōn) a bluish explosive gas or blue liquid, being an allotropic form of oxygen, O_3; it is antiseptic and disinfectant, and irritating and toxic to the pulmonary system.

P

P para; peta-; phosphate (group); phosphorus; posterior; premolar; proline; pupil.

P power; pressure.

P₁ parental generation.

P₂ pulmonic second sound.

p pico-; proton; the short arm of a chromosome.

p- para- (2).

PA physician assistant; posteroanterior; pulmonary artery.

Pa pascal; protactinium.

PAB, PABA *p*-aminobenzoic acid.

pace·mak·er (pās'māk"er) 1. that which sets the pace at which a phenomenon occurs. 2. the natural cardiac pacemaker or an artificial cardiac pacemaker. 3. in biochemistry, a substance whose rate of reaction sets the pace for a series of related reactions. **artificial cardiac p.,** a device designed to reproduce or regulate the rhythm of the heart. It is worn by or implanted in the body of the patient, is battery-driven, is usually triggered or

inhibited to modify output by sensing the intracardiac potential in one or more cardiac chambers, and may also have antitachycardia functions. Many are designated by a three to five letter code used to categorize them functionally. **cardiac p.,** a group of cells rhythmically initiating the heartbeat, characterized physiologically by a slow loss of membrane potential during diastole; usually it is the sinoatrial node. **demand p.,** an implanted cardiac pacemaker in which the generator stimulus is inhibited by a signal derived from the heart's electrical activation (depolarization), thus minimizing the risk of pacemaker-induced fibrillation. **dual chamber p.,** an artificial pacemaker with two leads, one in the atrium and one in the ventricle, so that electromechanical synchrony can be approximated. **ectopic p.,** any biological cardiac pacemaker other than the sinoatrial node; it is normally inactive. **escape p.,** an ectopic pacemaker that assumes control of cardiac impulse propagation because of failure of the sinoatrial node to initiate one or more impulses. **fixed-rate p.**, an artificial cardiac pacemaker set to pace at only a single rate. **rate responsive p.**, an artificial cardiac pacemaker that can deliver stimuli at a rate adjustable to some parameter independent of atrial activity. **runaway p.**, a malfunctioning artificial cardiac pacemaker that abruptly accelerates its pacing rate, inducing tachycardia. **secondary p.**, ectopic p. **single chamber p.**, an implanted cardiac pacemaker with only one lead, placed in either the atrium or the ventricle. **wandering atrial p.**, a condition in which the site of origin of the impulses controlling the heart rate shifts from one point to another within the atria, almost with every beat.

pachy- word element [Gr.], *thick*.

pachy·bleph·a·ron (pak″e-blef′ah-ron) thickening of the eyelids.

pachy·ceph·a·ly (-sef′ah-le) abnormal thickness of the bones of the skull. **pachycephal′ic**, adj.

pachy·chei·lia (-ki′le-ah) thickening of the lips.

pachy·chro·mat·ic (-kro-mat′ik) having the chromatin in thick strands.

pachy·dac·ty·ly (-dak′tĭ-le) megalodactyly.

pachy·der·ma (-der′mah) abnormal thickening of the skin. **pachyder′matous**, adj.

pachy·der·ma·to·cele (-der-mat′ah-sēl) plexiform neuroma attaining large size, producing an elephantiasis-like condition.

pachy·der·mo·peri·os·to·sis (-der″moper″e-os-to′sis) pachyderma affecting the face and scalp, thickening of the bones of the distal limbs, and acropachy.

pachy·glos·sia (-glos′e-ah) abnormal thickness of the tongue.

pachy·gy·ria (-ji′re-ah) macrogyria.

pachy·lep·to·men·in·gi·tis (-lep″to-men″in-ji′tis) inflammation of the dura mater and pia mater.

pachy·men·in·gi·tis (-men″in-ji′tis) inflammation of the dura mater.

pachy·men·in·gop·a·thy (-men″ing-gop′ah-the) noninflammatory disease of the dura mater.

pachy·me·ninx (-me′ninks) pl. *pachymenin′ges*. Dura mater.

pa·chyn·sis (pah-kin′sis) an abnormal thickening. **pachyn′tic**, adj.

pachy·onych·ia (pak″e-o-nik′e-ah) abnormal thickening of the nails. **p. conge′nita**, a rare, congenital, dominantly inherited disorder marked by great thickening of the nails, hyperkeratosis of palms and soles, and leukoplakia.

pachy·peri·os·ti·tis (-per″e-os-ti′tis) periostitis of the long bones resulting in abnormal thickness of affected bones.

pachy·peri·to·ni·tis (-per″ĭ-to-ni′tis) inflammation and thickening of the peritoneum.

pachy·pleu·ri·tis (-ploo-ri′tis) 1. fibrothorax. 2. pleural fibrosis.

pachy·sal·pin·gi·tis (-sal″pin-ji′tis) chronic salpingitis with thickening.

pachy·sal·pin·go·ova·ri·tis (-sal-ping″go-o″vah-ri′tis) chronic inflammation of the ovary and uterine tube, with thickening.

pachy·tene (pak′ĭ-tēn) in the prophase of meiosis, the stage following zygotene during which the chromosomes shorten, thicken, and separate into two sister chromatids joined at their centromeres. Paired homologous chromosomes, which were joined by synapsis, now form a tetrad of four chromatids. Where crossing over has occurred between nonsister chromatids, they are joined by X-shaped chiasmata.

pach·y·vag·i·ni·tis (-vaj″ĭ-ni′tis) chronic vaginitis with thickening of the vaginal walls.

pac·ing (pās′ing) setting of the pace. **asynchronous p.**, cardiac pacing in which impulse generation by the pacemaker occurs at a fixed rate, independent of underlying cardiac activity. **burst p.**, overdrive p. **cardiac p.**, regulation of the rate of contraction of the heart muscle by an artificial cardiac pacemaker. **coupled p.**, a variation of paired pacing in which the patient's natural depolarization serves as the first of the two stimuli, with the second induced by an artificial cardiac pacemaker. **diaphragm p.**, **diaphragmatic p.**, electrophrenic respiration. **overdrive p.**, the process of increasing the heart rate by means of an artificial cardiac pacemaker in order to suppress certain arrhythmias. **paired p.**, cardiac pacing in which two impulses are delivered to the heart in close succession, to slow tachyarrhythmias and to improve cardiac performance. **ramp p.**, cardiac pacing in which stimuli are delivered at a rapid but continually altering rate, either from faster to slower (*rate decremental* or *tune down*), from fast to faster (*cycle length decremental* or *ramp up*), or in some cyclic combination of increasing and decreasing rates; used to control tachyarrhythmias. **synchronous p.**, cardiac pacing in which information about sensed activity in one or more cardiac chambers is used to determine the timing of impulse generation by the pacemaker. **underdrive p.**, a method for terminating certain tachycardias by means of slow asynchronous pacing at a rate not an even fraction of the tachycardia rate.

pack (pak) 1. treatment by wrapping a patient in blankets or sheets or a limb in towels, either wet or dry and hot or cold; also, the blankets or towels used for this purpose. 2. a tampon.

pack·er (pak′er) an instrument for introducing a dressing into a cavity or a wound.

pack·ing (-ing) the filling of a wound or cavity with gauze, sponges, pads, or other material; also, the material used for this purpose.

pac·li·tax·el (pak″lĭ-tak′sel) an antineoplastic that promotes and stabilizes polymerization of microtubules, isolated from the Pacific yew tree *(Taxus brevifolia);* used in the treatment of advanced ovarian or breast carcinoma, non–small cell lung carcinoma, and AIDS-related Kaposi's sarcoma.

pad (pad) a cushionlike mass of soft material. **abdominal p.,** a pad for the absorption of discharges from abdominal wounds or for packing off abdominal viscera to improve exposure during surgery. **buccal fat p.,** sucking p. **dinner p.,** a pad placed over the stomach before a plaster jacket is applied; the pad is then removed, leaving space under the jacket to accommodate expansion of the stomach after eating. **infrapatellar fat p.,** a large pad of fat lying behind and below the patella. **knuckle p's,** nodular thickenings of the skin on the dorsal surface of the interphalangeal joints. **retromolar p.,** a cushionlike mass of tissue situated at the distal termination of the mandibular residual ridge. **sucking p., suctorial p.,** a lobulated mass of fat that occupies the space between the masseter and the external surface of the buccinator; it is well developed in infants.

pad·i·mate O (pad′ĭ-māt) a substituted aminobenzoate used as a sunscreen, absorbing UVB rays.

pae- for words beginning thus, see those beginning with *pe-*.

PAF platelet activating factor.

-pagus word element [Gr.], *conjoined twins.*

PAH, PAHA *p*-aminohippuric acid.

PAI plasminogen activator inhibitor.

pain (pān) a feeling of distress, suffering, or agony, caused by stimulation of specialized nerve endings. **bearing-down p.,** pain accompanying uterine contractions during the second stage of labor. **false p's,** ineffective pains resembling labor pains, not accompanied by cervical dilatation. **growing p's,** recurrent quasirheumatic limb pains peculiar to early youth. **hunger p.,** pain coming on at the time for feeling hunger for a meal; a symptom of gastric disorder. **intermenstrual p.,** pain accompanying ovulation, occurring during the period between the menses, usually about midway. **labor p's,** the rhythmic pains of increasing severity and frequency due to contraction of the uterus at childbirth. **phantom limb p.,** pain felt as though arising in an absent (amputated) limb. **psychogenic p.,** symptoms of physical pain having psychological origin. **referred p.,** pain felt in a part other than that in which the cause that produced it is situated. **rest p.,** a continuous burning pain due to ischemia of the lower leg, which begins or is aggravated after reclining and is relieved by sitting or standing.

paint (pānt) 1. a liquid designed for application to a surface, as of the body or a tooth. 2. to apply a liquid to a specific area as a remedial or protective measure.

pair (par) 1. a combination of two related, similar, or identical entities or objects. 2. in cardiology, two successive premature beats, particularly two ventricular premature complexes. **base p.,** either of the two pairs—guanine and cytosine, adenine and thymine—of purine-pyrimidine bases joined by hydrogen bonds that make up DNA.

palae(o)- see *pale(o)-.*

pal·ate (pal′it) roof of the mouth; the partition separating the nasal and oral cavities. **pal′atal, pal′atine,** adj. **cleft p.,** congenital fissure of median line of palate. **hard p.,** the anterior portion of the palate, separating the oral and nasal cavities, consisting of the bony framework and covering membranes. **soft p.,** the fleshy part of the palate, extending from the posterior edge of the hard palate; the uvula projects from its free inferior border.

pal·a·ti·tis (pal″ah-ti′tis) inflammation of the palate.

palat(o)- word element [L.], *palate.*

pal·a·to·glos·sal (pal″ah-to-glos′al) pertaining to the palate and tongue.

pal·a·tog·na·thous (pal″ah-tog′nah-thus) having a cleft palate.

pal·a·to·pha·ryn·ge·al (pal″ah-to-fah-rin′je-al) pertaining to the palate and pharynx.

pal·a·to·plas·ty (pal′ah-to-plas″te) plastic reconstruction of the palate.

pal·a·to·ple·gia (pal″ah-to-ple′jah) paralysis of the palate.

pal·a·tor·rha·phy (pal″ah-tor′ah-fe) surgical correction of a cleft palate.

pa·la·tum (pah-la′tum) pl. *pala′ta.* [L.]. palate.

pale(o)- word element [Gr.], *old.* Also *palae(o)-.*

pa·leo·cer·e·bel·lum (pa″le-o-ser″ĕ-bel′um) the phylogenetically second oldest part of the cerebellum, namely the vermis of the anterior lobe and the pyramis, uvula, and paraflocculus of the posterior lobe. Because this corresponds roughly to the primary site of termination of the major spinocerebellar afferents, the term is sometimes equated with *spinocerebellum*.. Spelled also *palaeocerebellum*. **paleocerebel′lar**, adj.

pa·leo·cor·tex (-kor′teks) [*paleo-* + *cortex*] that portion of the cerebral cortex that, with the archicortex, develops in association with the olfactory system and is phylogenetically older and less stratified than the neocortex. It is composed chiefly of the piriform cortex and the parahippocampal gyrus. Spelled also *palaeocortex*. **paleocor′tical**, adj.

pa·leo·pa·thol·o·gy (-pah-thol′ah-je) study of disease in bodies which have been preserved from ancient times.

pa·leo·stri·a·tum (-stri-a′tum) the phylogenetically older portion of the corpus striatum, represented by the globus pallidus. **paleostria′tal**, adj.

pa·leo·thal·a·mus (-thal′ah-mus) the phylogenetically older part of the thalamus, i.e., the medial portion that lacks reciprocal connections with the neopallium.

pali- word element [Gr.], *again; pathologic repetition*. Also *palin-*.

palin- see *pali-*.

pal·in·dro·mia (pal″in-dro′me-ah) [Gr.] a recurrence or relapse. **palindro′mic**, adj.

pal·i·nop·sia (-op′se-ah) visual perseveration; the continuance of a visual sensation after the stimulus is gone.

pal·i·viz·u·mab (pal″ĭ-viz′u-mab) a monoclonal antibody against respiratory syncytial virus (RSV); used as a passive immunizing agent in susceptible infants and children.

pal·la·di·um (Pd) (pah-la′de-um) chemical element (see *Table of Elements*), at. no. 46; used in alloys for dental and orthodontic appliances.

pall·an·es·the·sia (pal″an-es-the′zhah) loss or absence of pallesthesia.

pall·es·the·sia (pal″es-the′zhah) the ability to feel mechanical vibrations on or near the body, such as when a vibrating tuning fork is placed over a bony prominence. **pallesthet′ic**, adj.

pal·li·a·tive (pal′e-a″tiv) affording relief; also, a drug that so acts.

pal·li·dec·to·my (pal″ĭ-dek′tah-me) extirpation of the globus pallidus.

pal·li·do·an·sot·o·my (pal″ĭ-do-an-sot′ah-me) production of lesions in the globus pallidus and ansa lenticularis.

pal·li·dot·o·my (pal″ĭ-dot′ah-me) a stereotaxic surgical technique for the production of lesions in the globus pallidus for treatment of extrapyramidal disorders.

pal·li·dum (pal′ĭ-dum) globus pallidus. **pal′lidal**, adj.

pal·li·um (pal′e-um) [L.] 1. cerebral cortex. 2. the cerebral cortex during its period of development. **pal′lial**, adj.

pal·lor (pal′er) paleness, as of the skin.

palm (pahm) the hollow or flexor surface of the hand. **pal′mar**, adj.

pal·ma (pahl′mah) pl. *pal′mae*. [L.] palm.

pal·mar·is (pahl-mar′is) palmar.

pal·mate (pahl′māt) having a shape resembling that of a hand with the fingers spread.

pal·mit·ic ac·id (pal-mit′ik) a 16-carbon saturated fatty acid found in most fats and oils, particularly associated with stearic acid; one of the most prevalent saturated fatty acids in body lipids.

pal·mi·tin (pal′mĭ-tin) glyceryl tripalmitate; a crystallizable and saponifiable fat from various fats and oils.

pal·mi·to·le·ate (pal″mĭ-to′le-āt) a salt (soap), ester, or anionic form of palmitoleic acid.

pal·mi·to·le·ic ac·id (pal-mit-o-le′ik) a monounsaturated 16-carbon fatty acid occurring in many oils, particularly those derived from marine animals.

pal·pa·tion (pal-pa′shun) the act of feeling with the hand; the application of the fingers with light pressure to the surface of the body for the purpose of determining the condition of the parts beneath in physical diagnosis. **pal′patory**, adj.

pal·pe·bra (pal′pĕ-brah) pl. *pal′pebrae*. [L.] eyelid. **pal′pebral**, adj.

pal·pe·bri·tis (pal″peb-bri′tis) blepharitis.

pal·pi·ta·tion (pal″pĭ-ta′shun) a subjective sensation of an unduly rapid or irregular heartbeat.

pal·sy (pawl′ze) paralysis. **Bell's p.**, unilateral facial paralysis of sudden onset due to a lesion of the facial nerve, resulting in characteristic facial distortion. **cerebral p.**, any of a group of persisting qualitative motor disorders appearing in young children, resulting from brain damage caused by birth trauma or intrauterine pathology. **Erb's p.**, **Erb-Duchenne p.**, Erb-Duchenne paralysis. **facial p.**, Bell's p. **progressive bulbar p.**, chronic, progressive, generally fatal paralysis and atrophy of the muscles of the lips, tongue, mouth, pharynx, and larynx due to lesions of the motor nuclei of the lower brain stem, usually occurring in late adult years. **wasting p.**, spinal muscular atrophy.

pam·a·brom (pam′ah-brom) a mild diuretic used in preparations for the relief of premenstrual symptoms.

pam·i·dro·nate (pam″ĭ-dro′nāt) an inhibitor of bone resorption used to treat malignancy-associated hypercalcemia, osteitis deformans, and osteolytic metastasis secondary to breast cancer or myeloma; used as the disodium salt. Complexed with technetium 99m, it is used in bone imaging.

pam·pin·i·form (pam-pin′ĭ-form) shaped like a tendril.

PAN polyarteritis nodosa.

pan- word element [Gr.], *all.*

pan·ag·glu·ti·nin (-ah-gloo′tĭ-nin) an agglutinin which agglutinates the erythrocytes of all human blood groups.

pan·ar·ter·i·tis (-ahr-ter-i′tis) polyarteritis.

pan·at·ro·phy (pan-at′rah-fe) atrophy of several parts; diffuse atrophy.

pan·au·to·nom·ic (pan″aw-tah-nom′ik) pertaining to or affecting the entire autonomic (sympathetic and parasympathetic) nervous system.

pan·car·di·tis (-kahr-di′tis) diffuse inflammation of the heart.

pan·cha·kar·ma (pahn″chah-kahr′mah) [Sanskrit] a fivefold purification treatment used in ayurveda, usually including a purgative to eliminate kapha, a laxative to eliminate pitta, an enema to eliminate vata, inhalation treatment to clear doshas from the head, and bloodletting to purify the blood.

pan·co·lec·to·my (pan″ko-lek′tah-me) excision of the entire colon, with creation of an ileostomy.

pan·cre·as (pan′kre-as) pl. *pancre′ata.* [Gr.] a large, elongated, racemose gland lying transversely behind the stomach, between the spleen and duodenum. Its external secretion contains digestive enzymes. One internal secretion, insulin, is produced by the beta cells, and another, glucagon, is produced by the alpha cells. The alpha, beta, and delta cells form aggregates, called *islands of Langerhans.* See Plate 27. **endocrine p.,** that part of the pancreas that acts as an endocrine gland, consisting of the islets of Langerhans, which secrete insulin and other hormones. **exocrine p.,** that part of the pancreas that acts as an exocrine gland, consisting of the pancreatic acini, which produce pancreatic juice and secrete it into the duodenum to aid in protein digestion.

pan·cre·a·tec·to·my (pan″kre-ah-tek′tah-me) excision of the pancreas.

pan·cre·at·ic (pan″kre-at′ik) pertaining to the pancreas.

pan·cre·at·ic elas·tase (e-las′tās) an endopeptidase catalyzing the cleavage of specific peptide bonds in protein digestion; it is activated in the duodenum by trypsin-induced cleavage of its inactive precursor proelastase. In humans the form expressed is *p. e. II.*

pancreatic(o)- word element [Gr.], *pancreas; pancreatic duct.*

pan·cre·at·i·co·du·o·de·nal (pan″kre-at″ĭ-ko-doo″ah-de′n′l) pertaining to the pancreas and duodenum.

pan·cre·at·i·co·du·o·de·nos·to·my (-doo″ah-dĕ-nos′tah-me) anastomosis of the pancreatic duct to a different site on the duodenum.

pan·cre·at·i·co·en·ter·os·to·my (-en″ter-os′tah-me) anastomosis of the pancreatic duct to the intestine.

pan·cre·at·i·co·gas·tros·to·my (-gas-tros′tah-me) anastomosis of the pancreatic duct to the stomach.

pan·cre·at·i·co·je·ju·nos·to·my (-jĕ″joo-nos′tah-me) anastomosis of the pancreatic duct to the jejunum.

pan·cre·a·tin (pan′kre-ah-tin) a substance from the pancreas of the hog or ox containing enzymes, principally amylase, protease, and lipase; used as a digestive aid.

pan·cre·a·ti·tis (pan″kre-ah-ti′tis) inflammation of the pancreas. **acute hemorrhagic p.,** a condition due to autolysis of pancreatic tissue caused by escape of enzymes into the substance, resulting in hemorrhage into the parenchyma and surrounding tissues.

pancreat(o)- word element [Gr.], *pancreas.*

pan·cre·a·to·du·o·de·nec·to·my (pan″-kre-ah-to-doo″o-dĕ-nek′tah-me) excision of the head of the pancreas along with the encircling loop of the duodenum.

pan·cre·a·to·gen·ic (-to-jen′ik) arising in the pancreas.

pan·cre·a·tog·ra·phy (-tog′rah-fe) radiography of the pancreas.

pan·cre·a·to·li·thec·to·my (-to-lĭ-thek′tah-me) excision of a calculus from the pancreas.

pan·cre·a·to·li·thi·a·sis (-to-lĭ-thi′ah-sis) presence of calculi in the ductal system or parenchyma of the pancreas.

pan·cre·a·to·li·thot·o·my (-to-lĭ-thot′ah-me) incision of the pancreas for the removal of calculi.

pan·cre·a·tol·y·sis (-tol′ĭ-sis) destruction of pancreatic tissue. **pancreatolyt′ic,** adj.

pan·cre·a·tot·o·my (-tot′ah-me) incision of the pancreas.

pan·cre·a·to·tro·pic (-to-tro′pik) having an affinity for the pancreas.

pan·cre·li·pase (pan″kre-li′pās) a preparation of hog pancreas containing enzymes, principally lipase with amylase and protease;

used as a digestive aid in pancreatic insufficiency.

pan·creo·priv·ic (pan″kre-o-priv′ik) lacking a pancreas.

pan·creo·zy·min (-zi′min) cholecystokinin.

pan·cu·ro·ni·um (pan″ku-ro′ne-um) a neuromuscular blocking agent used as the bromide salt as an adjunct to anesthesia.

pan·cys·ti·tis (-sis-ti′tis) cystitis involving the entire thickness of the wall of the urinary bladder, as occurs in interstitial cystitis.

pan·cy·to·pe·nia (-sit-ah-pe′ne-ah) abnormal depression of all the cellular elements of the blood.

pan·dem·ic (pan-dem′ik) 1. a widespread epidemic of a disease. 2. widely epidemic.

pan·en·ceph·a·li·tis (pan″en-sef″ah-li′tis) encephalitis, probably of viral origin, which produces intranuclear or intracytoplasmic inclusion bodies that result in parenchymatous lesions of both the gray and white matter of the brain.

pan·en·do·scope (pan-en′dah-skōp) 1. an endoscope that permits wide-angle viewing. 2. a cystoscope that permits wide-angle viewing of the bladder and urethra.

pan·hy·po·pi·tu·i·ta·rism (pan-hi″po-pĭ-too′ĭ-tah-rizm) generalized hypopituitarism due to absence or damage of the pituitary gland, which, in its complete form, leads to absence of gonadal function and insufficiency of thyroid and adrenal function. When cachexia is a prominent feature, it is called *Simmonds' disease* or *pituitary cachexia.*

pan·hys·tero·sal·pin·gec·to·my (-his-ter-o-sal″pin-jek′tah-me) excision of the body of the uterus, cervix, and uterine tubes.

pan·hys·ter·o·sal·pin·go·ooph·o·rec·to·my (-sal-ping″go-o″of-ah-rek′tah-me) excision of the uterus, cervix, uterine tubes, and ovaries.

pan·ic (pan′ik) acute, extreme, and unreasoning fear and anxiety. **homosexual p.**, an acute, extreme anxiety reaction brought on by circumstances that induce the unconscious fear of being homosexual or of succumbing to homosexual impulses.

pan·my·eloph·thi·sis (pan-mi″ĕ-lof′thĭ-sis) aplastic anemia.

pan·nic·u·lec·to·my (pah-nik″u-lek′tah-me) surgical excision of the abdominal apron of superficial fat in the obese.

pan·nic·u·li·tis (-li′tis) inflammation of the panniculus adiposus, especially of the abdomen. **nodular nonsuppurative p.**, **relapsing febrile nodular nonsuppurative p.**, a disease marked by fever and the formation of crops of tender nodules in subcutaneous fatty tissues.

pan·nic·u·lus (pah-nik′u-lus) pl. *panni′culi.* [L.] a layer of membrane. **p. adipo′sus**, the subcutaneous fat: a layer of fat underlying the dermis.

pan·nus (pan′us) [L.]. 1. superficial vascularization of the cornea with infiltration of granulation tissue. 2. an inflammatory exudate overlying the synovial cells on the inside of a joint. 3. panniculus adiposus. **p. trachomato′sus**, pannus of the cornea secondary to trachoma.

pan·oph·thal·mi·tis (pan″of-thal-mi′tis) inflammation of all the eye structures or tissues.

pan·oti·tis (-o-ti′tis) inflammation of all the parts or structures of the ear.

pan·pho·bia (pan-fo′be-ah) fear of everything; vague and persistent dread of an unknown evil.

pan·ret·i·nal (-ret′ĭ-nal) pertaining to or encompassing the entire retina.

Pan·stron·gy·lus (-stron′jĭ-lus) a genus of hemipterous insects, species of which transmit trypanosomes.

pan·sys·tol·ic (pan″sis-tol′ik) pertaining to or affecting all of, or occurring throughout, systole.

pan·te·the·ine (pan″tĭ-the′in) an amide of pantothenic acid, an intermediate in the biosynthesis of CoA, a growth factor for *Lactobacillus bulgaricus*, and a cofactor in certain enzyme complexes.

pant(o)- word element [Gr.], *all; the whole.*

pan·to·pra·zole (pan-to′prah-zōl) a gastric acid pump inhibitor similar to omeprazole, used as the sodium salt in the treatment of erosive esophagitis associated with gastroesophageal reflux disease and of pathological hypersecretion associated with Zollinger-Ellison syndrome or other neoplastic cindition.

pan·to·then·ate (pan″to-then′āt) any salt of pantothenic acid; *calcium p.* is used as a dietary source of pantothenic acid.

pan·to·the·nic ac·id (-ik) a component of coenzyme A and a member of the vitamin B complex; necessary for nutrition in some animal species, but of uncertain importance for humans.

pan·tro·pic (pan-tro′pik) having an affinity for or affecting many tissues or cells.

pa·pa·in (pah-pa′in, pah-pi′in) a proteolytic enzyme from the latex of papaw, *Carica papaya*, which catalyzes the hydrolysis of proteins and polypeptides to amino acids; used as a protein digestant and as a topical application for enzymatic débridement.

pa·pav·er·ine (pah-pav′er-in) a smooth muscle relaxant and vasodilator used as the hydrochloride salt to relieve arterial spasms causing cerebral, peripheral, or myocardial ischemia and also injected into the penis in the diagnosis and treatment of erectile dysfunction.

pa·per (pa′per) a material manufactured in thin sheets from fibrous substances that have first been reduced to a pulp. **litmus p.,** moisture-absorbing paper impregnated with a solution of litmus: if slightly acid, it is red, and alkalis turn it blue; if slightly alkaline, it is blue and acid turns it red. **test p.,** paper stained with a compound that changes visibly on occurrence of a chemical reaction.

pa·pil·la (pah-pil′ah) pl. *papil′lae.* [L.] a small nipple-shaped projection or elevation. **circumvallate papillae,** vallate papillae. **conical papillae,** sparsely scattered elevations on the tongue, often considered to be modified filiform papillae. **p. of corium,** dermal p. **dental p., dentinal p.,** a small mass of condensed mesenchyme in the enamel organ; it differentiates into the dentin and dental pulp. **dermal p.,** any of the conical extensions of the fibers, capillary blood vessels, and sometimes nerves of the dermis into corresponding spaces among downward- or inward-projecting rete ridges on the undersurface of the epidermis. **duodenal p.,** either of two small elevations on the mucosa of the duodenum, the *major* at the entrance of the conjoined pancreatic and common bile ducts and the *minor* at the entrance of the accessory pancreatic duct. **filiform papillae,** threadlike elevations covering most of the tongue surface. **foliate papillae,** parallel mucosal folds on the tongue margin at the junction of its body and root. **fungiform papillae,** knoblike projections of the tongue scattered among the filiform papillae. **gingival p.,** the cone-shaped pad of gingiva filling the space between the teeth up to the contact area. **hair p.,** the fibrovascular mesodermal papilla enclosed within the hair bulb. **incisive p.,** an elevation at the anterior end of the raphe of the palate. **interdental p.,** gingival p. **lacrimal p.,** one in the conjunctiva near the medial angle of the eye. **p., conical, filiform, foliate, fungiform,** and *vallate papillae.* **mammary p.,** nipple (1). **optic p.,** optic disk. **palatine p.,** incisive p. **p. pi′li,** hair p. **renal papillae,** the blunted apices of the renal pyramids. **tactile p.,** see under *corpuscle.* **urethral p.,** a slight elevation in the vestibule of the vagina at the external orifice of the urethra. **vallate papillae,** eight

to twelve large papillae arranged in a V near the base of the tongue.

pap·il·lary (pap′ĭ-lar″e) pertaining to or resembling a papilla, or nipple.

pa·pil·le·de·ma (pap″il-ĕ-de′mah) edema of the optic disk.

pa·pil·li·tis (pap″ĭ-li′tis) 1. inflammation of a papilla. 2. a form of optic neuritis involving the optic papilla (disk).

pa·pil·lo·ad·e·no·cys·to·ma (pap″il-o-ad″ĭ-no-sis-to′mah) papillary cystadenoma.

pap·il·lo·ma (pap″il-o′mah) a benign tumor derived from epithelium. **papillo′matous,** adj. **fibroepithelial p.,** a type containing extensive fibrous tissue. **intracanalicular p.,** an arborizing nonmalignant growth within the ducts of certain glands, particularly of the breast. **intraductal p.,** a tumor in a lactiferous duct, usually attached to the wall by a stalk; it may be solitary, often with a serous or bloody nipple discharge, or multiple. **inverted p.,** one in which the proliferating epithelial cells invaginate into the underlying stroma.

pap·il·lo·ma·to·sis (pap″il-o′mah-to′sis) development of multiple papillomas.

Pa·pil·lo·ma·vi·ri·nae (pap″ĭ-lo″mah-vir-i′ne) the papillomaviruses; a subfamily of viruses (family Papovaviridae) that induce papillomas in susceptible hosts; the single genus is *Papillomavirus.*

Pa·pil·lo·ma·vi·rus (pap″ĭ-lo″mah-vi″rus) papillomaviruses; a genus of viruses (subfamily Papillomavirinae) that induce papillomas in humans and other animals; some have been associated with malignancy.

pap·il·lo·ma·vi·rus (pap″ĭ-lo″mah-vi″rus) any virus of the subfamily Papillomavirinae. **human p. (HPV),** any of a number of species that cause warts, particularly plantar warts and genital warts, on the skin and mucous membranes in humans; some are associated with malignancies of the genital tract.

pap·il·lo·ret·i·ni·tis (pap″ĭ-lo-ret″ĭ-ni′tis) inflammation of the optic disk and retina.

pap·il·lot·o·my (pap″il-ot′ah-me) incision of a papilla, as of a duodenal papilla.

Pa·po·va·vi·ri·dae (pah-po″vah-vir′ĭ-de) the papovaviruses: a family of DNA viruses, many of which are oncogenic or potentially oncogenic; it includes two subfamilies, Papillomavirinae and Polyomavirinae.

pa·po·va·vi·rus (pah-po′vah-vi″rus) any virus of the family Papovaviridae. **lympho·tropic p. (LPV),** a polyomavirus originally isolated from a B-lymphoblastic cell line of an African green monkey; antigenically related viruses are widespread in primates and may infect humans.

pap·u·la·tion (pap″u-la′shun) the formation of papules.

pap·ule (pap′ūl) a small, circumscribed, solid, elevated lesion of the skin. **pap′ular**, adj.

pap·u·lo·ne·crot·ic (pap″u-lo-nĕ-krot′ik) characterized by both papules and necrosis.

pap·u·lo·sis (pap″ūl-o′sis) the presence of multiple papules. **bowenoid p.**, benign reddish brown papules occurring primarily on the genitalia, particularly the penis, in young adults; believed to have a viral etiology.

pap·y·ra·ceous (pap″ĭ-ra′shus) like paper.

para (par′ah) a woman who has produced one or more viable offspring, regardless of whether the child or children were living at birth. Used with Roman numerals to designate the number of such pregnancies, as *para 0* (none—nullipara), *para I* (one—primipara), *para II* (two—secundipara), etc. Symbol P.

para- 1. word element [Gr.], *beside; near; resembling; accessory to; beyond; apart from; abnormal.* 2. symbol *p-.* In organic chemistry, indicating a substituted benzene ring whose substituents are on opposite carbon atoms in the ring.

para-ami·no·ben·zo·ic ac·id (par″ah-ah-me″no-ben-zo′ik) *p-*aminobenzoic acid.

para-ami·no·hip·pu·ric ac·id (-ah-me″no-hĭ-pūr′ik) *p-*aminohippuric acid.

para-ami·no·sal·i·cyl·ic ac·id (-ah-me″no-sal-ĭ-sil′ik) *p-*aminosalicylic acid.

para-an·es·the·sia (-an″es-the′zhah) anesthesia of the lower part of the body.

para-aor·tic (-a-or′tik) near or next to the aorta.

para·bio·sis (-bi-o′sis) the union of two individuals, as conjoined twins, or of experimental animals by surgical operation. **parabiot′ic**, adj.

para·ca·sein (-ka′se-in) the chemical product of the action of rennin on casein.

para·cen·te·sis (-sen-te′sis) surgical puncture of a cavity for the aspiration of fluid. **paracentet′ic**, adj.

para·cen·tral (-sen′tr'l) near a center.

para·cer·vi·cal (-ser′vĭ-k'l) near a neck or cervix, particularly the uterine cervix.

para·chol·era (-kol′er-ah) a disease resembling Asiatic cholera but not caused by *Vibrio cholerae.*

para·chor·dal (-kor′d'l) situated beside the notochord.

para·clin·i·cal (-klin′ĭ-k'l) pertaining to abnormalities (e.g., morphological or biochemical) underlying clinical manifestations (e.g., chest pain or fever).

para·coc·cid·i·oi·dal (-kok-sid″e-oi′d'l) pertaining to or caused by fungi of the genus *Paracoccidioides.*

Para·coc·cid·i·oi·des (-kok-sid″e-oi′dēz) a genus of Fungi Imperfecti of the family Moniliaceae; they proliferate by multiple budding yeast cells in the tissues. *P. brasilien′sis* is the etiologic agent of paracoccidioidomycosis.

para·coc·cid·i·oi·do·my·co·sis (-kok-sid″e-oi″do-mi-ko′sis) an often fatal, chronic granulomatous disease caused by *Paracoccidioides brasiliensis*, primarily involving the lungs, but spreading to the skin, mucous membranes, lymph nodes, and internal organs.

para·co·li·tis (-ko-li′tis) inflammation of the outer coat of the colon.

para·crine (par′ah-krin) 1. denoting a type of hormone function in which hormone synthesized in and released from endocrine cells binds to its receptor in nearby cells and affects their function. 2. denoting the secretion of a hormone by an organ other than an endocrine gland.

par·acu·sia (par″ah-ku′se-ah) 1. any deficiency in the sense of hearing. 2. auditory hallucination.

par·acu·sis (-ku′sis) paracusia.

para·did·y·mis (-did′ĭ-mis) a group of several convoluted tubules in the anterior part of the spermatic cord; probably a remnant of the mesonephros.

para·dox (par′ah-doks) a seemingly contradictory occurrence. **paradox′ic**, **paradox′ical**, adj. **Weber's p.**, elongation of a muscle that has been so stretched that it cannot contract.

para·du·o·de·nal (par″ah-doo″o-de′n'l, -doo-od′ah-n'l) alongside, near, or around the duodenum.

para·esoph·a·ge·al (-e-sof″ah-je′al) near or beside the esophagus.

par·af·fin (par′ah-fin) 1. a purified hydrocarbon wax used for embedding histological specimens and as a stiffening agent in pharmaceutical preparations. 2. alkane. **liquid p.**, mineral oil.

par·af·fin·o·ma (par″ah-fin-o′mah) a chronic granuloma produced by prolonged exposure to paraffin.

para·floc·cu·lus (-flok′u-lus) a small lobe of the cerebellar hemisphere, immediately cranial to the flocculus.

para·gan·gli·o·ma (-gang″gle-o′mah) a tumor of the tissue composing the paraganglia. **nonchromaffin p.**, chemodectoma.

para·gan·gli·on (-gang′gle-on) pl. *paragan′glia.* A collection of chromaffin cells derived from neural ectoderm, occurring outside the adrenal medulla, usually near the sympathetic ganglia and in relation to the aorta and its branches.

para·geu·sia (-goo′zhah) 1. perversion of the sense of taste. 2. a bad taste in the mouth.

par·a·gon·i·mi·a·sis (-gon′ĭ-mi′ah-sis) infection with flukes of the genus *Paragonimus*.

Par·a·gon·i·mus (-gon-ĭ-mus) a genus of parasitic flukes that have two invertebrate hosts, the first a snail, the second a crab or crayfish. *P. westerma′ni* is the lung fluke, seen especially in Asia, found in cysts in the lungs and sometimes elsewhere in humans and other animals that have eaten infected freshwater crayfish and crabs.

para·gran·u·lo·ma (-gran″u-lo′mah) the most benign form of Hodgkin's disease, largely confined to the lymph nodes.

para·he·mo·phil·ia (-he″mo-fil′e-ah) a hereditary hemorrhagic tendency due to deficiency of coagulation factor V.

para·hip·po·cam·pal (-hip″o-kam′p′l) near or next to the hippocampus.

para·hor·mone (-hor′mōn) a substance, not a true hormone, which has a hormone-like action in controlling the functioning of some distant organ.

para·in·fec·tious (-in-fek′shus) pertaining to manifestations of infectious disease that are caused by the immune response to the infectious agent.

para·ker·a·to·sis (-ker″ah-to′sis) persistence of the nuclei of keratinocytes as they rise into the stratum corneum of the epidermis. It is normal in the epithelium of the true mucous membrane of the mouth and vagina.

para·ki·ne·sia (-kĭ-ne′zhah) perversion of motor function; in ophthalmology, irregular action of an individual ocular muscle.

para·la·lia (-la′le-ah) a disorder of speech, especially the production of a vocal sound different from the one desired.

par·al·lag·ma (-lag′mah) displacement of a bone or of the fragments of a broken bone.

par·al·ler·gy (par-al′er-je) a condition in which an allergic state, produced by specific sensitization, predisposes the body to react to other allergens with clinical manifestations that differ from the original reaction. **paraller′gic**, adj.

pa·ral·y·sis (pah-ral′ĭ-sis) pl. *paral′yses*. Loss or impairment of motor function in a part due to lesion of the neural or muscular mechanism; also, by analogy, impairment of sensory function (*sensory p.*). **p. a′gitans**, Parkinson's disease. **ascending p.**, spinal paralysis that progresses cephalad. **bulbar p.**, progressive bulbar palsy. **compression p.**, that caused by pressure on a nerve. **conjugate p.**, loss of ability to perform some parallel ocular movements. **crossed p.**, **cruciate p.**, that affecting one side of the face and the other side of the body. **decubitus p.**, that due to pressure on a nerve from lying for a long time in one position. **divers′ p.**, decompression sickness. **Duchenne's p.**, 1. Erb-Duchenne p. 2. progressive bulbar palsy. **Erb-Duchenne p.**, paralysis of the upper roots of the brachial plexus, caused by birth injury. **facial p.**, weakening or paralysis of the facial nerve, as in Bell's palsy. **familial periodic p.**, a rare inherited disorder with recurring attacks of rapidly progressive flaccid paralysis associated with serum potassium levels that are decreased (type I or hypokalemic type), increased (type II or hyperkalemic type), or normal (type III or normokalemic type). **hyperkalemic periodic p.**, see *familial periodic p.* **hypokalemic periodic p.**, see *familial periodic p.* **immune p.**, **immunologic p.**, older name for *immunologic tolerance*. **juvenile p. agitans (of Hunt)**, increased muscle tonus with the characteristic attitude and facies of paralysis agitans, occurring in early life and due to progressive degeneration of the globus pallidus. **Klumpke's p.**, **Klumpke-Dejerine p.**, lower brachial plexus paralysis caused by birth injury, particularly during a breech delivery. **Landry's p.**, acute idiopathic polyneuritis. **mixed p.**, combined motor and sensory paralysis. **motor p.**, paralysis of voluntary muscles. **musculospiral p.**, paralysis of the extensor muscles of the wrist and fingers. **normokalemic periodic p.**, see *familial periodic p.* **periodic p.**, 1. any of various diseases characterized by episodic flaccid paralysis or muscular weakness. 2. familial periodic p. **postepileptic p.**, Todd's p. **progressive bulbar p.**, see under *palsy*. **pseudobulbar p.**, spastic weakness of the muscles innervated by the cranial nerves, i.e., the facial muscles, pharynx, and tongue, due to bilateral lesions of the corticospinal tract, often accompanied by uncontrolled weeping or laughing. **pseudohypertrophic muscular p.**, see under *dystrophy*. **sensory p.**, loss of sensation due to a morbid process. **thyrotoxic periodic p.**, recurrent episodes of generalized or local paralysis accompanied by hypokalemia, occurring in association with Graves' disease, especially after exercise or a high carbohydrate or high sodium meal. **Todd's p.**, transient hemiplegia or monoplegia after an epileptic seizure. **vasomotor p.**, cessation of vasomotor control.

par·a·lyt·ic (par″ah-lit′ik) 1. affected with or pertaining to paralysis. 2. a person affected with paralysis.

par·a·lyz·ant (par'ah-līz"ant) 1. causing paralysis. 2. a drug that causes paralysis.

para·mas·ti·gote (par"ah-mas'tĭ-gōt) having an accessory flagellum by the side of a larger one.

para·mas·ti·tis (-mas-ti'tis) inflammation of tissues around the mammary gland.

Par·a·me·ci·um (-me'se-um) a genus of ciliate protozoa.

par·a·me·ci·um (-me'se-um) pl. *parame'cia*. An organism of the genus *Paramecium*.

pa·ram·e·ter (pah-ram'ĕ-ter) 1. a constant that distinguishes specific cases, having a definite fixed value in one case but different values in other cases. 2. in statistics, a value that specifies one of the members of a family of probability distributions, such as the mean or standard deviation. 3. a variable whose measure is indicative of a quantity or function that cannot itself be directly determined precisely.

para·me·tric¹ (par"ah-me'trik) situated near the uterus; parametrial.

para·met·ric² (-met'rik) pertaining to or defined in terms of a parameter.

para·me·tri·tis (-me-tri'tis) inflammation of the parametrium.

para·me·tri·um (-me'tre-um) the extension of the subserous coat of the supracervical portion of the uterus laterally between the layers of the broad ligament. **parame'trial**, adj.

par·am·ne·sia (par"am-ne'zhah) a disturbance of memory in which reality and fantasy are confused.

Par·amoe·ba (par"ah-me'bah) a genus of parasitic or free-living ameboid protozoa.

para·mu·cin (-mu'sin) a colloid substance from ovarian cysts, differing from mucin and pseudomucin in that it reduces Fehling's solution before boiling with acid.

par·am·y·loi·do·sis (par-am"ĭ-loi-do'sis) accumulation of an atypical form of amyloid in tissues.

para·my·oc·lo·nus (par"ah-mi-ok'lo-nus) myoclonus in several unrelated muscles. **p. mul'tiplex,** a form of myoclonus of unknown etiology starting in the muscles of the upper arms and shoulders and spreading to other parts of the upper body.

para·myo·to·nia (-mi"o-to'ne-ah) a disease marked by tonic spasms due to disorder of muscular tonicity, especially a hereditary and congenital affection. **p. conge'nita,** an inherited disorder similar to myotonia congenita, except that the precipitating factor is cold exposure, the myotonia is aggravated by activity, and only the proximal muscles of the limbs, eyelids, and tongue are affected.

Para·myxo·vi·ri·dae (-mik"so-vir'ĭ-de) the paramyxoviruses; a family of RNA viruses with a single-stranded, negative-sense RNA genome, including two subfamilies, Paramyxovirinae and Pneumovirinae.

Para·myxo·vi·ri·nae (-mik"so-vir-i'ne) a subfamily of the family Paramyxoviridae, containing three genera: *Morbillivirus, Paramyxovirus,* and *Rubulavirus.*

Para·myxo·vi·rus (-mik'so-vi"rus) 1. a genus of viruses (family Paramyxoviridae) that cause chiefly respiratory infections in a variety of vertebrate hosts; included are mumps and parainfluenza viruses. 2. paramyxovirus; a genus of viruses of the subfamily Paramyxovirinae (family Paramyxoviridae) that cause chiefly respiratory infections in a variety of vertebrate hosts.

para·myxo·vi·rus (-mik'so-vi"rus) any virus of the family Paramyxoviridae.

para·na·sal (-na'z'l) alongside or near the nose.

para·neo·plas·tic (-ne"o-plas'tik) pertaining to changes produced in tissue remote from a tumor or its metastases.

para·neph·ric (-nef'rik) near the kidney.

para·ne·phri·tis (-nĕ-fri'tis) 1. inflammation of the adrenal gland. 2. inflammation of the connective tissue around the kidney.

par·an·es·the·sia (par"an-es-the'zhah) para-anesthesia.

par·a·noia (par"ah-noi'ah) 1. behavior characterized by well-systematized delusions of grandeur or persecution or a combination. 2. former name for *delusional disorder.* **paranoi'ac, par'anoid,** adj.

par·a·no·mia (-no'me-ah) amnestic aphasia.

para·nu·cle·us (-noo'kle-us) a body sometimes seen in cell protoplasm near the nucleus. **paranu'clear,** adj.

para·oral (-or'al) 1. near or adjacent to the mouth. 2. administered by some route other than by the mouth; said of medication.

para·pa·re·sis (-pah-re'sis) partial paralysis of the lower limbs. **tropical spastic p.,** chronic progressive myelopathy.

para·per·tus·sis (-per-tus'is) an acute respiratory disease clinically indistinguishable from mild or moderate pertussis, caused by *Bordetella parapertussis.*

para·pha·sia (-fa'zhah) partial aphasia in which the patient employs wrong words, or uses words in wrong and senseless combinations (*choreic p.*).

para·phe·mia (-fe'me-ah) paraphasia.

pa·ra·phia (pah-ra'fe-ah) perversion of the sense of touch.

para·phil·ia (par"ah-fil'e-ah) a psychosexual disorder marked by sexual urges, fantasies, and behavior involving objects, suffering or humiliation, or children or other nonconsenting partners. **paraphil′iac,** adj.

para·phi·mo·sis (-fi-mo′sis) retraction of phimotic foreskin, causing a painful swelling of the glans, sometimes progressing to dry gangrene.

para·phra·sia (-fra′zhah) paraphasia.

para·plasm (par′ah-plazm) 1. any abnormal growth. 2. hyaloplasm (1). **paraplas′tic,** adj.

para·plec·tic (par″ah-plek′tik) paraplegic.

para·ple·gia (-ple′jah) paralysis of the lower part of the body, including the legs.

para·ple·gic (-ple′jik) 1. pertaining to or of the nature of paraplegia. 2. an individual with paraplegia.

Para·pox·vi·rus (-poks′vi-rus) parapoxviruses; a genus of viruses comprising viruses of ungulates, including those causing orf and paravaccinia.

para·prax·is (-prak′sis) pl. *paraprax′es.* A faulty action, as a slip of the tongue or misplacement of an object, which in psychoanalytic theory is due to unconscious associations and motives.

para·pro·tein (-pro′tēn) a normal or abnormal plasma protein appearing in large quantities as a result of a pathological condition; term now largely replaced by *M component.*

para·pro·tein·emia (-pro″tēn-e′me-ah) plasma cell dyscrasia.

par·ap·sis (par-ap′sis) paraphia.

para·pso·ri·a·sis (par″ah-sah-ri′ah-sis) any of a group of slowly developing, persistent, maculopapular scaly erythrodermas, devoid of subjective symptoms and resistant to treatment.

para·quat (par′ah-kwaht) a poisonous compound, some of whose salts are used as contact herbicides. Contact with concentrated solutions causes irritation of the skin, cracking and shedding of the nails, and delayed healing of cuts and wounds. After ingestion of large doses, renal and hepatic failure may develop, followed by pulmonary insufficiency.

para·ro·san·i·line (par″ah-ro-zan′ĭ-lin) a basic dye; a triphenylmethane derivative, one of the components of basic fuchsin.

par·ar·rhyth·mia (-rith′me-ah) parasystole.

para·sa·cral (-sa′kr′l) beside or near the sacrum.

para·sex·u·al (-sek′shoo-al) accomplished by other than sexual means, as by genetic study of in vitro somatic cell hybrids.

para·si·noi·dal (-si-noi′d′l) situated along the course of a sinus.

par·a·site (par′ah-sīt) 1. a plant or animal that lives upon or within another living organism at whose expense it obtains some advantage; see *symbiosis.* 2. the smaller, less complete member of asymmetrical conjoined twins, attached to and dependent upon the autosite. **parasit′ic,** adj. **malarial p.,** *Plasmodium.* **obligatory p.,** one that is entirely dependent on a host for its survival.

par·a·si·te·mia (par″ah-si-te′me-ah) the presence of parasites, especially malarial forms, in the blood.

par·a·sit·ism (par″ah-si″tizm) 1. symbiosis in which one population (or individual) adversely affects another, but cannot live without it. 2. infection or infestation with parasites.

par·a·si·to·gen·ic (par″ah-si″to-jen′ik) due to parasites.

par·a·si·tol·o·gy (-si-tol′ah-je) the scientific study of parasites and parasitism.

par·a·si·to·tro·pic (-si″to-tro′pik) having an affinity for parasites.

para·som·nia (-som′ne-ah) a category of sleep disorders in which abnormal events occur during sleep, such as sleepwalking or talking; due to inappropriately timed activation of physiological systems.

para·spa·di·as (-spa′de-as) a congenital condition in which the urethra opens on one side of the penis.

para·ster·nal (-ster′n′l) situated beside the sternum.

para·sui·cide (-soo′ĭ-sīd) attempted suicide, emphasizing that in most such attempts death is not the desired outcome.

para·sym·pa·thet·ic (-sim″pah-thet′ik) see under *system.*

para·sym·pa·tho·lyt·ic (-sim″pah-tho-lit′ik) anticholinergic.

para·sym·pa·tho·mi·met·ic (-sim″pah-tho-mi-met′ik) cholinergic.

para·syn·ap·sis (-sĭ-nap′sis) the union of chromosomes side by side during meiosis.

para·sys·to·le (-sis′tah-le) a cardiac irregularity attributed to the interaction of two foci independently initiating cardiac impulses at different rates.

para·ten·on (-ten′on) the fatty areolar tissue filling the interstices of the fascial compartment in which a tendon is situated.

para·thi·on (-thi′on) a highly toxic agricultural insecticide.

para·thor·mone (-thor′mōn) parathyroid hormone.

para·thy·mia (-thi′me-ah) a perverted, contrary, or inappropriate mood.

par·a·thy·roid (-thi′roid) 1. situated beside the thyroid gland. 2. see under *gland.*

para·thy·ro·pri·val (-thi″ro-pri′v′l) hypoparathyroid.

para·thy·ro·tro·pic (-thi″ro-tro′pik) having an affinity for the parathyroid glands.

para·tope (par′ah-tōp) the site on the antibody molecule that attaches to an antigen.

pa·rat·ro·phy (pah-rat′rah-fe) dystrophy.

para·tu·ber·cu·lo·sis (par″ah-too-ber″ku-lo′sis) a tuberculosis-like disease not due to *Mycobacterium tuberculosis*.

para·ty·phoid (-ti′foid) infection due to *Salmonella* of all groups except *S. typhi*.

para·ure·thral (-u-re′thr'l) near the urethra.

para·vac·cin·ia (-vak-sin′e-ah) an infection due to the paravaccinia virus, producing papular, and later vesicular, pustular, and scabular, lesions on the udders and teats of milk cows, the oral mucosa of suckling calves, and the hands of humans milking infected cows.

para·vag·i·ni·tis (-vaj″ĭ-ni′tis) inflammation of the tissues alongside the vagina.

para·ver·te·bral (-ver′tĕ-br'l) beside the vertebral column.

para·ves·i·cal (-ves′ĭ-k'l) perivesical.

para·zone (par′ah-zōn) one of the white bands alternating with dark bands (diazones) seen in cross section of a tooth.

pa·ren·chy·ma (pah-reng′kĭ-mah) [Gr.] the essential or functional elements of an organ, as distinguished from its stroma or framework. **paren′chymal, parenchym′atous,** adj. **renal p.,** the functional tissue of the kidney, consisting of the nephrons.

pa·ren·ter·al (pah-ren′ter-al) not through the alimentary canal, but rather by injection through some other route, as subcutaneous, intramuscular, etc.

pa·re·sis (pah-re′sis) slight or incomplete paralysis. **general p.,** paralytic dementia; a form of neurosyphilis in which chronic meningoencephalitis causes gradual loss of cortical function, progressive dementia, and generalized paralysis.

par·es·the·sia (par″es-the′zhah) morbid or perverted sensation; an abnormal sensation, as burning, prickling, formication, etc.

pa·ret·ic (pah-ret′ik) pertaining to or affected with paresis.

par·i·cal·ci·tol (par″ĭ-kal′sĭ-tol) a synthetic vitamin D analogue, used for the prevention and treatment of hyperparathyroidism secondary to chronic renal failure.

par·i·es (par′e-ēz) pl. *pari′etes.* [L.] a wall, as of an organ or cavity.

pa·ri·e·tal (pah-ri′ĕ-t'l) 1. of or pertaining to the walls of a cavity. 2. pertaining to or located near the parietal bone.

pa·ri·e·to·fron·tal (pah-ri″ĕ-to-frun′t'l) pertaining to the parietal and frontal bones, gyri, or fissures.

pa·ri·e·to·oc·cip·i·tal (-ok-sip′ĭ-t'l) pertaining to the parietal and occipital bones or lobes.

par·i·ty (par′ĭ-te) 1. para; the condition of a woman with respect to having borne viable offspring. 2. equality; close correspondence or similarity.

par·kin·son·ism (pahr′kin-son-izm″) a group of neurological disorders marked by hypokinesia, tremor, and muscular rigidity; see *parkinsonian syndrome,* under *syndrome,* and *Parkinson's disease,* under *disease.* **parkinson′ian,** adj.

par·oc·cip·i·tal (par″ok-sip′ĭ-t'l) near the occipital bone.

par·o·mo·my·cin (par′ah-mo-mi″sin) a broad-spectrum antibiotic derived from *Streptomyces rimosus* var. *paromomycinus;* the sulfate salt is used as an antiamebic.

par·onych·ia (par″-ah-nik′e-ah) inflammation involving the folds of tissue around the fingernail.

par·o·nych·i·al (-nik′e-al) pertaining to paronychia or to the nail folds.

par·oöph·o·ron (par″o-of′ŏ-ron) an inconstantly present small group of coiled tubules between the layers of the mesosalpinx, being a remnant of the excretory part of the mesonephros.

par·oph·thal·mia (par″-of-thal′me-ah) inflammation of the connective tissue around the eye.

par·os·te·al (par-os′te-al) pertaining to the outer surface of the periosteum.

par·os·to·sis (par″os-to′sis) ossification of tissues outside the periosteum.

pa·rot·id (pah-rot′id) near the ear.

pa·rot·i·di·tis (pah-rot″ĭ-di′tis) parotitis.

par·oti·tis (par″o-ti′tis) inflammation of the parotid gland. **epidemic p.,** mumps.

par·ovar·i·an (par″o-var′e-an) 1. beside the ovary. 2. pertaining to the epoöphoron.

par·ox·e·tine (pah-rok′sĕ-tēn) a selective serotonin uptake inhibitor used as the hydrochloride salt to treat depression and obsessive-compulsive, panic, and social anxiety disorders.

par·ox·ysm (par′ok-sizm) 1. a sudden recurrence or intensification of symptoms. 2. a spasm or seizure. **paroxys′mal,** adj.

pars (pahrz) pl. *par′tes.* [L.] part.

pars pla·ni·tis (pahrz pla-ni′tis) granulomatous uveitis of the pars plana of the ciliary body.

part (pahrt) a division of a larger structure. **mastoid p. of temporal bone,** mastoid bone; the irregular, posterior part of the temporal bone. **petromastoid p. of temporal bone,** see *petrous p. of temporal bone.* **petrous p. of**

temporal bone, petrous bone; the part of the temporal bone at the base of the cranium, containing the inner ear. Some divide it into two subparts, calling the posterior section the *mastoid part,* reserving the term *petrous part* for the anterior section only, and calling the entire area the *petromastoid part.* **squamous p. of temporal bone,** squamous bone; the flat, scalelike, anterior superior portion of the temporal bone. **tympanic p. of temporal bone,** tympanic bone; the part of the temporal bone forming the anterior and inferior walls and part of the posterior wall of the external acoustic meatus.

par·ti·cle (pahr′tĭ-k′l) a tiny mass of material. **Dane p.,** an intact hepatitis B viral particle. **elementary p's of mitochondria,** numerous minute, club-shaped granules with spherical heads attached to the inner membrane of a mitochondrion. **viral p., virus p.,** virion.

par·ti·tion·ing (pahr-tish′un-ing) dividing into parts. **gastric p.,** a form of gastroplasty in which a small stomach pouch is formed whose filling signals satiety; used in the treatment of morbid obesity.

par·tu·ri·ent (pahr-tu′re-ent) giving birth or pertaining to birth; by extension, a woman in labor.

par·tu·ri·om·e·ter (pahr″tu-re-om′ĕ-ter) device used in measuring the expulsive power of the uterus.

par·tu·ri·tion (pahr″tu-ri′shun) childbirth.

pa·ru·lis (pah-roo′lis) a subperiosteal abscess of the gum.

par·vi·cel·lu·lar (pahr″vĭ-sel′u-ler) composed of small cells.

Par·vo·vi·ri·dae (pahr″vo-vir′ĭ-de) the parvoviruses: a family of DNA viruses with a linear single-stranded DNA genome, including the genera *Parvovirus* and *Dependovirus.*

Par·vo·vi·rus (pahr′vo-vi″rus) parvoviruses; a genus of viruses (family Parvoviridae) infecting mammals and birds; human parvoviruses cause aplastic crisis, erythema infectiosum, hydrops fetalis, spontaneous abortion, and fetal death.

par·vo·vi·rus (pahr′vo-vi″rus) any virus belonging to the family Parvoviridae.

PAS, PASA *p*-aminosalicylic acid.

pas·cal (Pa) (pas-kal′, pas′kal) the SI unit of pressure, which corresponds to a force of one newton per square meter.

pas·sive (pas′iv) neither spontaneous nor active; not produced by active efforts.

paste (pāst) a semisolid preparation containing one or more drug substances, for topical application.

Pas·teur·el·la (pas″ter-el′ah) a genus of gram-negative bacteria (family Pasteurellaceae), including *P. multo′cida,* the etiologic agent of the hemorrhagic septicemias.

pas·teur·el·lo·sis (pas″ter-ĕ-lo′sis) infection with organisms of the genus *Pasteurella.*

pas·teur·iza·tion (pas″cher-ĭ-za′shun) heating of milk or other liquids to moderate temperature for a definite time, often 60°C. for 30 min., which kills most pathogenic bacteria and considerably delays other bacterial development.

patch (pach) 1. a small area differing from the rest of a surface. 2. a macule more than 3 or 4 cm in diameter. **Peyer's p's,** oval elevated patches of closely packed lymph follicles on the mucosa of the small intestines. **salmon p.,** see *nevus flammeus.*

pa·tel·la (pah-tel′ah) [L.] see *Table of Bones.* **patel′lar,** adj.

pat·el·lec·to·my (pat″il-ek′tah-me) excision of the patella.

pat·ent (pāt′nt) 1. open, unobstructed, or not closed. 2. apparent, evident.

path·er·gy (path′er-je) 1. a condition in which the application of a stimulus leaves the organism unduly susceptible to subsequent stimuli of a different kind. 2. a condition of being allergic to numerous antigens. **pather′gic,** adj.

path·find·er (path′find″er) 1. an instrument for locating urethral strictures. 2. a dental instrument for tracing the course of root canals.

path(o)- word element [Gr.], *disease.*

patho·an·a·tom·i·cal (path″o-an″ah-tom′ik′l) pertaining to anatomic pathology.

patho·bi·ol·o·gy (-bi-ol′ah-je) pathology.

patho·cli·sis (-klis′is) a specific sensitivity to specific toxins, or a specific affinity of certain toxins for certain systems or organs.

patho·gen (path′ah-jen) any disease-producing agent or microorganism. **pathogen′ic,** adj.

patho·gen·e·sis (path″ah-jen′ĕ-sis) the development of morbid conditions or of disease; more specifically the cellular events and reactions and other pathologic mechanisms occurring in the development of disease. **pathogenet′ic,** adj.

pa·thog·no·mon·ic (path″ug-no-mon′ik) specifically distinctive or characteristic of a disease or pathologic condition; denoting a sign or symptom on which a diagnosis can be made.

patho·log·ic (path″ah-loj′ik) 1. indicative of or caused by some morbid condition. 2. pertaining to pathology.

patho·log·i·cal (-loj′ĭ-k′l) pathologic.

pa·thol·o·gy (pah-thol'ah-je) 1. the branch of medicine dealing with the essential nature of disease, especially changes in body tissues and organs that cause or are caused by disease. 2. the structural and functional manifestations of disease. **anatomic p.,** the anatomical study of changes in the function, structure, or appearance of organs or tissues, including postmortem examinations and the study of biopsy specimens. **cellular p.,** cytopathology. **clinical p.,** pathology applied to the solution of clinical problems, especially the use of laboratory methods in clinical diagnosis. **comparative p.,** that which considers human disease processes in comparison with those of other animals. **oral p.,** that treating of conditions causing or resulting from morbid anatomic or functional changes in the structures of the mouth. **surgical p.,** the pathology of disease processes that are surgically accessible for diagnosis or treatment.

patho·mi·me·sis (path″o-mi-me'sis) mimicry of a disease or disorder, particularly malingering.

patho·mor·phism (-mor'fizm) perverted or abnormal morphology.

patho·phys·i·ol·o·gy (-fiz″e-ol'ah-je) the physiology of disordered function.

patho·psy·chol·o·gy (-si-kol'ah-je) the psychology of mental disease.

path·way (path'wa) 1. a course usually followed. 2. the nerve structures through which an impulse passes between groups of nerve cells or between the central nervous system and an organ or muscle. 3. metabolic p. **accessory conducting p.,** myocardial fibers that propagate the atrial contraction impulse to the ventricles but are not a part of the normal atrioventricular conducting system. **afferent p.,** the nerve structures through which an impulse, especially a sensory impression, is conducted to the cerebral cortex. **alternative complement p.,** a pathway of complement activation initiated by a variety of factors other than those initiating the classical pathway, including IgA immune complexes, bacterial endotoxins, microbial polysaccharides, and cell walls. It does not include factors C1, C2, and C4 of the classical complement pathway but does include factors B and D and properdin. **amphibolic p.,** a group of metabolic reactions providing small metabolites for further metabolism to end products or for use as precursors in synthetic, anabolic reactions. **circus p.,** a ring or circuit traversed by an abnormal excitatory waveform, as in reentry. **classical complement p.,** a pathway of complement

activation, comprising nine components (C1 to C9), initiated by antigen-antibody complexes containing immunoglobulins IgG or IgM. **common p. of coagulation,** the steps in the mechanism of coagulation from the activation of factor X through the conversion of fibrinogen to fibrin. **efferent p.,** the nerve structures through which an impulse passes away from the brain, especially for the innervation of muscles, effector organs, or glands. **Embden-Meyerhof p.,** the series of enzymatic reactions in the anaerobic conversion of glucose to lactic acid, resulting in energy in the form of adenosine triphosphate (ATP). **extrinsic p. of coagulation,** the mechanism that produces fibrin following tissue injury, beginning with formation of an activated complex between tissue factor and factor VII and leading to activation of factor X, inducing the reactions of the common pathway of coagulation. **final common p.,** a motor pathway consisting of the motor neurons by which nerve impulses from many central sources pass to a muscle or gland in the periphery. **intrinsic p. of coagulation,** a sequence of reactions leading to fibrin formation, beginning with the contact activation of factor XII, and resulting in the activation of factor X to initiate the common pathway of coagulation. **lipoxygenase p.,** a pathway for the formation of leukotrienes and hydroxyeicosatetraenoic acid from arachidonic acid. **metabolic p.,** a series of enzymatic reactions that converts one biological material to another. **motor p.,** an efferent pathway conducting impulses from the central nervous system to a muscle. **pentose phosphate p.,** a major branching of the Embden-Meyerhof pathway of carbohydrate metabolism, successively oxidizing hexoses to form pentose phosphates. **reentrant p.,** that over which the impulse is conducted in reentry.

-pathy word element [Gr.], *morbid condition* or *disease;* generally used to designate a noninflammatory condition.

pa·tri·lin·e·al (pat″ri-lin'e-il) descended through the male line.

pat·u·lous (pat'u-lus) spread widely apart; open; distended.

pauci- word element [L.], *few.* Cf. *olig(o)-.*

pau·ci·syn·ap·tic (paw″se-sin-ap'tik) oligosynaptic.

pause (pawz) an interruption or rest. **compensatory p.,** the pause in impulse generation after an extrasystole, either *full* if the sinus node is not reset or *incomplete* or *noncompensatory* if the node is reset and the cycle length is disrupted. **sinus p.,** a transient interruption in the sinus rhythm, of a duration that is not an exact multiple of the normal cardiac cycle.

pa·vor (pa'vor) [L.] terror. **p. noctur'nus** [L. "night terrors"], a sleep disturbance of children causing them to cry out in fright and awake in panic, with poor recall of a nightmare. Repeated occurrences are called *sleep terror disorder.*

PAWP pulmonary artery wedge pressure.

Pb lead[1] (L. *plum'bum*).

PBI protein-bound iodine.

PC phosphocreatine.

p.c. [L.] post ci'bum (after meals).

PCB polychlorinated biphenyl.

PCC prothrombin complex concentrate.

PCE pseudocholinesterase; see *cholinesterase.*

PCI percutaneous coronary intervention.

Pco₂ carbon dioxide partial pressure; also written P_{CO_2}, pCO_2, or pCO_2.

PCOS polycystic ovary syndrome.

PCR polymerase chain reaction.

PCT porphyria cutanea tarda.

PCV packed-cell volume.

PCWP pulmonary capillary wedge pressure.

Pd palladium.

PDA patent ductus arteriosus.

peak (pēk) the top or upper limit of a graphic tracing or of any variable. **kilovolts p. (kVp),** the highest kilovoltage used in producing a radiograph.

pearl (perl) 1. a small rounded mass or body. 2. a rounded mass of tough sputum as seen in the early stages of an attack of bronchial asthma. **epidermic p's, epithelial p's,** rounded concentric masses of epithelial cells found in squamous cell carcinomas. **Laënnec's p's,** soft casts of the smaller bronchial tubes expectorated in bronchial asthma.

pec·ten (pek'ten) pl. *pec'tines.* [L.] 1. a comb; in anatomy, any of certain comblike structures. 2. p. analis. **p. of anal canal, p. ana'lis,** the zone in the lower half of the anal canal between the pectinate line and the anal verge. **p. os'sis pu'bis,** pectineal line (2).

pec·te·no·sis (pek"tĕ-no'sis) stenosis of the anal canal due to an inelastic ring of tissue between the anal groove and anal crypts.

pec·tin (pek'tin) a polymer of sugar acids of fruit that forms gels with sugar at the proper pH; a purified form obtained from the acid extract of the rind of citrus fruits or from apple pomace is used as an antidiarrheal and as a pharmaceutic aid. **pec'tic,** adj.

pec·ti·nate (pek'tĭ-nāt) comb-shaped.

pec·tin·e·al (pek-tin'e-il) pertaining to the os pubis.

pec·tin·i·form (pek-tin'ĭ-form) comb-shaped.

pec·to·ral (pek'ter-il) thoracic.

pec·to·ra·lis (pek"tah-ra'lis) [L.] thoracic.

pec·to·ril·o·quy (pek-tah-ril'ah-kwe) voice sounds of increased resonance heard through the chest wall.

pec·tus (pek'tus) pl. *pec'tora.* [L.] thorax. **p. carina'tum,** pigeon breast or chest; a condition of the chest in which the sternum is prominent, due to obstruction of infantile respiration or to rickets. **p. excava'tum,** funnel breast or chest; a congenital deformity in which the sternum is depressed.

ped·al (ped'l) pertaining to the foot or feet.

ped·er·as·ty (ped"er-as'te) anal intercourse between a man and a boy.

pe·di·at·ric (pe"de-at'rik) pertaining to the health of children.

pe·di·at·rics (-riks) the branch of medicine dealing with children, their development and care, and with the nature and treatment of diseases of children.

ped·i·cel (ped'ĭ-sel) a footlike part, especially any of the secondary processes of a podocyte.

ped·i·cel·la·tion (ped"ĭ-sel-a'shun) the development of a pedicle.

ped·i·cle (ped'ĭ-k'l) a footlike, stemlike, or narrow basal part or structure.

pe·dic·u·lar (pĕ-dik'u-lar) pertaining to or caused by lice.

pe·dic·u·la·tion (pĕ-dik"u-la'shun) 1. the process of forming a pedicle. 2. infestation with lice.

pe·dic·u·li·cide (pĕ-dik'u-lĭ-sīd) 1. destroying lice. 2. an agent that destroys lice.

pe·dic·u·lo·sis (pĕ-dik"u-lo'sis) infestation with lice of the family Pediculidae, especially *Pediculus humanus.*

pe·dic·u·lous (pĕ-dik'u-lus) infested with lice.

Pe·dic·u·lus (pĕ-dik'u-lus) a genus of lice. *P. huma'nus,* a species feeding on human blood, is a major vector of typhus, trench fever, and relapsing fever; it has two subspecies: *P. huma'nus cap'itis* (head louse) found on the scalp hair, and *P. huma'nus cor'poris* (body, or clothes, louse) found on the body.

pe·dic·u·lus (pĕ-dik'u-lus) pl. *pedic'uli.* [L.] 1. louse. 2. pedicle.

ped·i·gree (ped'ĭ-gre) a table, chart, diagram, or list of an individual's ancestors, used in genetics in the analysis of mendelian inheritance.

ped(o)-[1] word element [Gr.], *child.*

ped(o)-[2] word element [L.], *foot.*

pe·do·don·tics (pe-do-don'tiks) the branch of dentistry dealing with the teeth and mouth conditions of children.

pe·do·phil·ia (-fĭl'e-ah) a paraphilia in which an adult has recurrent, intense sexual urges or sexually arousing fantasies of engaging or repeatedly engages in sexual activity with a prepubertal child. **pedophil'ic**, adj.

pe·dor·thics (pe-dor'thiks) the design, manufacture, fitting, and modification of shoes and related foot appliances as prescribed for the amelioration of painful or disabling conditions of the foot and leg. **pedor'thic**, adj.

pe·dun·cle (pĕ-dung'k'l) a stemlike connecting part, especially (a) a collection of nerve fibers coursing between different areas in the central nervous system, or (b) the stalk by which a nonsessile tumor is attached to normal tissue. **pedun'cular**, adj. **cerebellar p's**, three sets of paired bundles of the hindbrain (superior, middle, and inferior), connecting the cerebellum to the midbrain, pons, and medulla oblongata, respectively. **cerebral p.**, the anterior half of the midbrain, divisible into an anterior part (crus cerebri) and a posterior part (tegmentum), which are separated by the substantia nigra. **pineal p.**, habenula (2). **p's of thalamus**, thalamic radiations.

pe·dun·cu·lus (pĕ-dung'ku-lus) pl. **pedun'culi**. [L.] peduncle.

PEEP positive end-expiratory pressure; see under pressure.

PEF peak expiratory flow.

PEG pneumoencephalography; polyethylene glycol.

peg (peg) a projecting structure. **rete p's**, see under ridge.

peg·ad·e·mase (peg-ad'ĕ-mās) adenosine deaminase derived from bovine intestine and attached covalently to polyethylene glycol, used in replacement therapy for adenosine deaminase deficiency in immunocompromised patients.

peg·as·par·gase (-as'pahr-jās) L-asparaginase covalently linked to polyethylene glycol, used as an antineoplastic in the treatment of acute lymphoblastic leukemia.

peg·in·ter·fer·on (peg"in"ter-fēr'on) a covalent conjugate of recombinant interferon and polyethylene glycol (PEG), with the former moiety responsible for the biological activity; conjugates of interferon alfa-2a and interferon alfa-2b are administered subcutaneously in the treatment of chronic hepatitis C infection.

pel·age (pel'ahj) [Fr.] 1. the hairy coat of mammals. 2. hairs of the body, limbs, and head collectively.

pel·i·o·sis (pel"e-o'sis) purpura. **p. hepatis**, a mottled blue liver, due to blood-filled lacunae in the parenchyma.

pel·lag·ra (pĕ-lag'rah) a syndrome due to niacin deficiency (or failure to convert tryptophan to niacin), marked by dermatitis on parts of the body exposed to light or trauma, inflammation of the mucous membranes, diarrhea, and psychic disturbances. **pellag'rous**, adj.

pel·la·groid (pah-lag'roid) resembling pellagra.

pel·li·cle (pel'ik'l) a thin scum forming on the surface of liquids.

pel·lu·cid (pel-oo'sid) translucent.

pel·vic (pel'vik) pertaining to the pelvis.

pel·vi·cal·i·ce·al (pel"vĭ-kal"ĭ-se'il) pertaining to the renal pelves and calices.

pel·vi·ceph·a·lom·e·try (-sef"ah-lom'ĭ-tre) measurement of the fetal head in relation to the maternal pelvis.

pel·vi·fix·a·tion (-fik-sa'shun) surgical fixation of a displaced pelvic organ.

pel·vim·e·try (pel-vim'ĭ-tre) measurement of the capacity and diameter of the pelvis.

pel·vi·ot·o·my (pel"ve-ot'ah-me) 1. incision or transection of a pelvic bone. 2. pyelotomy.

pel·vis (pel'vis) pl. **pel'ves**. [L.] the lower (caudal) portion of the trunk, bounded anteriorly and laterally by the two hip bones and posteriorly by the sacrum and coccyx. Also applied to any basinlike structure, e.g., the renal pelvis. **pel'vic**, adj. **android p.**, one with a wedge-shaped inlet and narrow anterior segment; used to describe a female pelvis with characteristics usually found in the male. **anthropoid p.**, a female pelvis in which the anteroposterior diameter of the inlet equals or exceeds the transverse diameter. **assimilation p.**, one in which the ilia articulate with the vertebral column higher (high assimilation p.) or lower (low assimilation p.) than normal, the number of lumbar vertebrae being correspondingly decreased or increased. **beaked p.**, one with the pelvic bones laterally compressed and their anterior junction pushed forward. **brachypellic p.**, one in which the transverse diameter exceeds the anteroposterior diameter by 1 to 3 cm. **contracted p.**, one showing a decrease of 1.5 to 2 cm in any important diameter; when all dimensions are proportionately diminished it is a generally contracted p. (p. justo minor). **dolichopellic p.**, an elongated pelvis, the anteroposterior diameter being greater than the transverse diameter. **extrarenal p.**, see renal p. **false p.**, the part of the pelvis superior to a plane passing through the iliopectineal lines. **flat p.**, one in which the anteroposterior dimension is abnormally reduced. **funnel-shaped p.,** one with a normal inlet but a greatly narrowed outlet. **gynecoid p.,** the normal female pelvis: a rounded oval pelvis with well-rounded anterior and posterior segments. **infantile p.,** a generally contracted pelvis with an oval shape, high sacrum, and marked inclination of the walls. **p. jus′to ma′jor,** an unusually large gynecoid pelvis, with all dimensions increased. **p. jus′to mi′nor,** a small gynecoid pelvis, with all dimensions symmetrically reduced; see also *contracted p.* **juvenile p.,** infantile p. **p. ma′jor,** false p. **mesatipellic p.,** one in which the transverse diameter is equal to the anteroposterior diameter or exceeds it by no more than 1 cm. **p. mi′nor,** true p. **platypellic p., platypelloid p.,** one shortened in the anteroposterior aspect, with a flattened transverse oval shape. **rachitic p.,** one distorted as a result of rickets. **renal p.,** the funnel-shaped expansion of the upper end of the ureter into which the renal calices open; it is usually within the renal sinus, but under certain conditions a large part of it may be outside the kidney *(extrarenal p.)*. **scoliotic p.,** one deformed as a result of scoliosis. **split p.,** one with a congenital separation at the pubic symphysis. **spondylolisthetic p.,** one in which the last, or rarely the fourth or third, lumbar vertebra is dislocated in front of the sacrum, more or less occluding the pelvic brim. **true p.,** the part of the pelvis inferior to a plane passing through the iliopectineal lines.

pel·vo·spon·dy·li·tis (pel″vo-spon″dĭ-li′tis) inflammation of the pelvic portion of the spine. **p. ossi′ficans,** ankylosing spondylitis.

pe·mir·o·last (pĕ-mir′o-last″) a mast cell stabilizer that inhibits type I hypersensitivity reactions; administered topically as the potassium salt to prevent pruritus associated with allergic conjunctivitis.

pem·o·line (pem′ah-lēn) a central nervous system stimulant used in the treatment of attention-deficit/hyperactivity disorder.

pem·phi·goid (pem′fĭ-goid) 1. resembling pemphigus. 2. any of a group of dermatological syndromes similar to but clearly distinguishable from the pemphigus group.

pem·phi·gus (-gus) 1. a distinctive group of diseases marked by successive crops of bullae. 2. pemphigus vulgaris. **benign familial p.,** a hereditary, recurrent vesiculobullous dermatitis, usually involving the axillae, groin, and neck, with crops of lesions that regress over several weeks or months. **p. erythemato′sus,** a chronic form in which the lesions, limited to the face and chest,

resemble those of disseminated lupus erythematosus. **p. folia′ceus,** a chronic, generalized, vesicular and scaling eruption somewhat resembling dermatitis herpetiformis or, later in its course, exfoliative dermatitis. **p. ve′getans,** a variant of pemphigus vulgaris in which the bullae are replaced by verrucoid hypertrophic vegetative masses. **p. vulga′ris,** a rare relapsing disease with suprabasal, intraepidermal bullae of the skin and mucous membranes; invariably fatal if untreated.

pen·bu·to·lol (pen-bu′tah-lol) a beta-adrenergic blocking agent with intrinsic sympathomimetic activity; used as the sulfate salt in the treatment of hypertension.

pen·ci·clo·vir (-si′klo-vir) a compound that inhibits viral DNA synthesis in herpesviruses 1 and 2, used in the treatment of recurrent herpes labialis.

pen·del·luft (pen′del-looft) the movement of air back and forth between the lungs, resulting in increased dead space ventilation.

pen·du·lar (pen′du-lar) having a pendulum-like movement.

pen·du·lous (-lus) hanging loosely; dependent.

pe·nec·to·my (pe-nek′tah-me) surgical removal of the penis.

pen·e·trance (pen′ĭ-trins) the frequency with which a heritable trait is manifested by individuals carrying the principal gene or genes conditioning it.

pen·e·trom·e·ter (pen″ĕ-trom′ĕ-ter) an instrument for measuring the penetrating power of x-rays.

-penia word element [Gr.], *deficiency.*

pen·i·cil·la·mine (pen″ĭ-sil′ah-mēn) a degradation product of penicillin that chelates certain heavy metals and also binds cystine and promotes its excretion; used in the treatment of Wilson's disease, cystinuria, recurrent cystine renal calculi, and rheumatoid arthritis.

pen·i·cil·lin (pen″ĭ-sil′in) any of a large group of natural *(p. G, p.V)* or semisynthetic antibacterial antibiotics derived directly or indirectly from strains of fungi of the genus *Penicillium* and other soil-inhabiting fungi, which exert a bactericidal as well as a bacteriostatic effect on susceptible bacteria by interfering with the final stages of the synthesis of peptidoglycan, a substance in the bacterial cell wall. The penicillins, despite their relatively low toxicity for the host, are active against many bacteria, especially grampositive pathogens (streptococci, staphylococci, pneumococci); clostridia; some gram-negative forms (gonococci, meningococci); some spirochetes *(Treponema pallidum* and *T.*

pertenue); and some fungi. Certain strains of some target species, e.g., staphylococci, secrete the enzyme penicillinase, which inactivates penicillin and confers resistance to the antibiotic.

pen·i·cil·lin·ase (pen″ĭ-sil′ĭ-nās) a β-lactamase preferentially cleaving penicillin.

Pen·i·cil·li·um (-sil′e-um) a genus of fungi.

pen·i·cil·lo·yl pol·y·ly·sine (pen″ĭ-sil′o-il pol″e-li′sēn) benzylpenicilloyl polylysine.

pen·i·cil·lus (pen″ĭ-sil′us) pl. *penicil′li.* [L.] a brushlike structure, particularly any of the brushlike groups of arterial branches in the lobules of the spleen.

pe·nile (pe′nīl) of or pertaining to the penis.

pe·nis (pe′nis) the male organ of urination and copulation. **concealed p.,** a small penis hidden by a skin abnormality or the suprapubic fat pad. **webbed p.,** a penis that is enclosed by the skin of the scrotum, which extends onto its shaft.

pe·ni·tis (pe-ni′tis) inflammation of the penis.

pen·ni·form (pen′ĭ-form) shaped like a feather.

pe·no·plas·ty (pe′no-plas″te) phalloplasty.

pent(a)- word element [Gr.], *five.*

pen·ta·gas·trin (-gas′trin) a synthetic pentapeptide consisting of β-alanine and the C-terminal tetrapeptide of gastrin; used as a test of gastric secretory function.

pen·tam·i·dine (pen-tam′ĭ-dēn) an antiinfective used as the isethionate salt in the treatment of *Pneumocystis carinii* pneumonia, leishmaniasis, and early African trypanosomiasis.

pen·ta·starch (pen′tah-stahrch″) an artificial colloid derived from a waxy starch and used as an adjunct in leukapheresis to increase the erythrocyte sedimentation rate.

pen·taz·o·cine (pen-taz′o-sēn) a synthetic opioid analgesic, used in the form of the hydrochloride and lactate salts as an analgesic and anesthesia adjunct.

pen·te·tate (pen′tĕ-tāt) a salt, anion, ester, or complex of pentetic acid.

pen·te·tic ac·id (pen-tet′ik) diethylenetriamine pentaacetic acid, DTPA; a chelating agent (iron) with the general properties of the edetates; used in preparing radiopharmaceuticals.

pen·to·bar·bi·tal (pen″to-bahr′bĭ-tal) a short- to intermediate-acting barbiturate; the sodium salt is used as a hypnotic and sedative, usually presurgery, and as an anticonvulsant.

pen·to·san (pen′to-san″) a carbohydrate derivative used in the form of *p. polysulfate sodium* as an antiinflammatory in the treatment of interstitial cystitis.

pen·tose (pen′tōs) a monosaccharide containing five carbon atoms in a molecule.

pen·to·stat·in (pen″to-stat′in) an antineoplastic used in the treatment of hairy cell leukemia.

pen·tos·uria (pen″to-su′re-ah) excretion of pentoses in the urine. **alimentary p.,** that occurring as a normal consequence of excessive ingestion of some fruits or their juices. **essential p.,** a benign autosomal recessive deficiency of the enzyme L-xylulose reductase resulting in excessive urinary excretion of L-xylulose.

pen·tox·i·fyl·line (pen″tok-sif′ah-lin) a xanthine derivative that reduces blood viscosity; used for the symptomatic relief of intermittent claudication.

pep·lo·mer (pep′lo-mer) a subunit of a peplos.

pep·los (pep′lohs) envelope (2).

pep·per (pep′er) 1. any of various plants of the genus *Piper*, or their fruits, particularly the black pepper (*P. nigrum*), the common spice. 2. any of various plants of the genus *Capsicum*, or their fruits. **cayenne p., red p.,** capsicum.

pep·per·mint (-mint) the perennial herb *Mentha piperita*, or a preparation of its dried leaves and flowering tops, which have carminative, gastric stimulant, and counterirritant properties; used for gastrointestinal, liver, and gallbladder disturbances; also used in folk medicine and in homeopathy.

pep·sin (pep′sin) the proteolytic enzyme of gastric juice which catalyzes the hydrolysis of native or denatured proteins to form a mixture of polypeptides; it is formed from pepsinogen in the presence of acid or, autocatalytically, in the presence of pepsin.

pep·sin·o·gen (pep-sin′ah-jin) a zymogen secreted by the chief cells of the gastric glands and converted into pepsin in the presence of gastric acid or of pepsin itself.

pep·tic (pep′tik) pertaining to pepsin or to digestion or to the action of gastric juices.

pep·ti·dase (pep′tĭ-dās) any of a subclass of proteolytic enzymes that catalyze the hydrolysis of peptide linkages; it comprises the exopeptidases and endopeptidases.

pep·tide (pep′tīd, pep′tid) any of a class of compounds of low molecular weight that yield two or more amino acids on hydrolysis; known as di-, tri-, tetra-, etc.) peptides, depending on the number of amino acids in the molecule. Peptides form the constituent parts of proteins. **atrial natriuretic p. (ANP),** a hormone involved in natriuresis and the regulation of renal and cardiovascular homeostasis. **opioid p.,** opioid (2).

pep·ti·der·gic (pep″tĭ-der′jik) of or pertaining to neurons that secrete peptide hormones.

pep·ti·do·gly·can (pep″tĭ-do-gli′kan) a glycan (polysaccharide) attached to short cross-linked peptides; found in bacterial cell walls.

pep·ti·dyl·di·pep·ti·dase A (pep′tĭ-dil di-pep′tĭ-dās) an enzyme that catalyzes the cleavage of a dipeptide from the C-terminal end of oligopeptides; when catalyzing the cleavage of angiotensin I to form the activated angiotensin II, it is also called *angiotensin-converting enzyme;* when catalyzing the cleavage and inactivation of kinins, it is also called *kininase II.*

pep·to·gen·ic (pep″tah-jen′ik) 1. producing pepsin or peptones. 2. promoting digestion.

pep·tol·y·sis (pep-tol′ĭ-sis) the splitting up of peptones. **peptolyt′ic,** adj.

pep·tone (pep′tōn) a derived protein, or a mixture of cleavage products produced by partial hydrolysis of native protein. **pepton′ic,** adj.

per- word element [L.], (1) *throughout; completely; extremely;* (2) in chemistry, *a large amount; combination of an element in its highest valence.*

per·ac·id (per-as′id) an acid containing more than the usual quantity of oxygen.

per·acute (per″ah-kūt′) excessively acute or sharp.

per anum (per a′num) [L.] through the anus.

per·cept (per′sept″) the object perceived; the mental image of an object in space perceived by the senses.

per·cep·tion (per-sep′shun) the conscious mental registration of a sensory stimulus. **percep′tive,** adj.

per·cep·tiv·i·ty (per″sep-tiv′ĭ-te) ability to receive sense impressions.

per·chlor·ic ac·id (per-klor′ik) a colorless volatile liquid, $HClO_4$, which can cause powerful explosions in the presence of organic matter or anything reducible.

per·co·late (per′kah-lāt) 1. to strain; to submit to percolation. 2. to trickle slowly through a substance. 3. a liquid that has been submitted to percolation.

per·co·la·tion (per″kah-la′shun) the extraction of soluble parts of a drug by passing a solvent liquid through it.

per·cus·sion (per-kush′un) the act of striking a part with short, sharp blows as an aid in diagnosing the condition of the underlying parts by the sound obtained. **auscultatory p.,** auscultation of the sound produced by percussion. **immediate p.,** that in which the blow is struck directly against the body surface. **mediate p.,** that in which a pleximeter is used. **palpatory p.,** a combination of palpation and percussion, affording tactile rather than auditory impressions.

per·cus·sor (per-kus′or) a vibrator that produces relatively coarse movements.

per·cu·ta·ne·ous (per″ku-ta′ne-us) performed through the skin.

per·en·ceph·a·ly (per″en-sef′ah-le) porencephaly.

per·en·ni·al (pah-ren′e-al) lasting through the year or for several years.

per·fect (per′fekt) of a fungus, capable of reproducing sexually (with sexual spores).

per·fo·rans (per′fo-ranz) pl. *perforan′tes.* [L.] penetrating; applied to various muscles, nerves, arteries, and veins.

per·fu·sate (per-fu′zāt) a liquid that has been subjected to perfusion.

per·fu·sion (-zhun) 1. the act of pouring over or through, especially the passage of a fluid through the vessels of a specific organ. 2. a liquid poured over or through an organ or tissue. **luxury p.,** abnormally increased flow of blood to an area of the brain, leading to swelling.

per·go·lide (per′go-līd) a long-acting ergot derivative with dopaminergic properties; used as the mesylate salt in the treatment of parkinsonism.

peri- word element [Gr.], *around; near.* See also words beginning *para-.*

peri·ac·i·nal (per″e-as′ĭ-nal) around an acinus.

peri·ac·i·nous (-as′ĭ-nus) periacinal.

peri·ad·e·ni·tis (-ad″ĕ-ni′tis) inflammation of tissues around a gland. **p. muco′sa necro′tica recur′rens,** the more severe form of aphthous stomatitis, marked by recurrent attacks of aphtha-like lesions that begin as small firm nodules and enlarge, ulcerate, and heal to leave numerous atrophied scars on the oral mucosa.

peri·am·pul·lary (-am′pu-lar″e) around an ampulla.

peri·ap·i·cal (-ap′ĭ-k′l) around the apex of the root of a tooth.

peri·ap·pen·di·ci·tis (-ah-pen″dĭ-si′tis) inflammation of the tissues around the vermiform appendix.

peri·ar·ter·i·tis (-ahr-ter-i′tis) inflammation of the external coats of an artery and of the tissues around the artery. **p. nodo′sa,** 1. polyarteritis nodosa. 2. a group comprising polyarteritis nodosa, allergic granulomatous angiitis, and many systemic necrotizing vasculitides with clinicopathologic characteristics overlapping these two.

peri·ar·thri·tis (-ahr-thri′tis) inflammation of tissues around a joint.

peri·ar·tic·u·lar (-ahr-tik′u-lar) around a joint.

peri·ax·i·al (-ak′se-al) near or around an axis.

peri·bron·chio·li·tis (per″ĭ-brong″ke-o-li′tis) inflammation of tissues around the bronchioles.

peri·bron·chi·tis (-brong-ki′tis) bronchitis with inflammation and thickening of tissues around the bronchi.

peri·cal·i·ce·al (-kal″ĭ-se′al) near a renal calix.

peri·cal·lo·sal (-kah-lo′s′l) around the corpus callosum.

peri·car·di·al (-kahr′de-al) 1. pertaining to the pericardium. 2. surrounding the heart.

peri·car·di·ec·to·my (-kahr″de-ek′tah-me) excision of a portion of the pericardium.

peri·car·dio·cen·te·sis (-kahr″de-o-sen-te′sis) surgical puncture of the pericardial cavity for the aspiration of fluid.

peri·car·di·ol·y·sis (-kahr″de-ol′ĭ-sis) the operative freeing of adhesions between the visceral and parietal pericardium.

peri·car·dio·phren·ic (-kahr″de-o-fren′ik) pertaining to the pericardium and diaphragm.

peri·car·di·or·rha·phy (-kahr″de-or′ah-fe) suture of the pericardium.

peri·car·di·os·to·my (-kahr″de-os′tah-me) creation of an opening into the pericardium, usually for the drainage of effusions.

peri·car·di·ot·o·my (-kahr″de-ot′ah-me) incision of the pericardium.

peri·car·di·tis (-kahr-di′tis) inflammation of the pericardium. **pericardit′ic**, adj. **adhesive p.**, a condition due to the presence of dense fibrous tissue between the parietal and visceral layers of the pericardium. **constrictive p.**, a chronic form in which a fibrotic, thickened, adherent pericardium restricts diastolic filling and cardiac output, usually resulting from a series of events beginning with fibrin deposition on the pericardial surface followed by fibrotic thickening and scarring and obliteration of the pericardial space. **fibrinous p., fibrous p.**, that characterized by a fibrinous exudate, sometimes accompanied by a serous effusion; usually manifested as a pericardial friction rub. **p. obli′terans, obliterating p.**, adhesive pericarditis that leads to obliteration of the pericardial cavity.

peri·car·di·um (-kahr′de-um) the fibroserous sac enclosing the heart and the roots of the great vessels. **pericar′dial**, adj. **adherent p.**, one abnormally connected with the heart by dense fibrous tissue.

peri·ce·ci·tis (-se-si′tis) inflammation of the tissues around the cecum.

peri·ce·men·ti·tis (-se″men-ti′tis) periodontitis.

peri·cho·lan·gi·tis (-ko″lan-ji′tis) inflammation of the tissues around the bile ducts.

peri·cho·le·cys·ti·tis (-ko″lĕ-sis-ti′tis) inflammation of tissues around the gallbladder.

peri·chon·dri·um (-kon′dre-um) the layer of fibrous connective tissue investing all cartilage except the articular cartilage of synovial joints. **perichon′dral**, adj.

peri·chor·dal (-kor′d′l) around the notochord.

peri·cho·roi·dal (-ko-roid″l) surrounding the choroid coat.

peri·co·li·tis (-ko-li′tis) inflammation around the colon, especially of its peritoneal coat.

peri·co·lon·itis (-ko″lon-i′tis) pericolitis.

peri·col·pi·tis (-kol-pi′tis) inflammation of tissues around the vagina.

peri·cor·o·nal (-kor′o-n′l) around the crown of a tooth.

peri·cra·ni·tis (-kra-ni′tis) inflammation of the pericranium.

peri·cra·ni·um (-kra′ne-um) the periosteum of the skull. **pericra′nial**, adj.

peri·cyte (per′ĭ-sīt) one of the peculiar elongated, contractile cells found wrapped about precapillary arterioles outside the basement membrane.

peri·cy·ti·al (per″ĭ-si′shal) around a cell.

peri·den·tal (-den′t′l) periodontal.

peri·derm (per′ĭ-derm) 1. the outer layer of the bilaminar fetal epidermis, generally disappearing before birth. 2. the cuticle (eponychium and hyponychium), the only part of the periderm persisting after birth. **periderm′al**, adj.

peri·des·mi·um (per″ĭ-dez′me-um) the areolar membrane that covers the ligaments.

peri·di·ver·tic·u·li·tis (-di″ver-tik″u-li′tis) inflammation of the structures around a diverticulum of the intestine.

peri·duc·tal (-duk′t′l) surrounding a duct, particularly of the mammary gland.

peri·du·o·de·ni·tis (-doo-od″ĕ-ni′tis) inflammation around the duodenum.

peri·en·ceph·a·li·tis (per″e-en-sef″ah-li′tis) meningoencephalitis.

peri·en·ter·itis (-en″ter-i′tis) inflammation of the peritoneal coat of the intestines.

peri·esoph·a·gi·tis (-e-sof″ah-ji′tis) inflammation of tissues around the esophagus.

peri·fol·lic·u·lar (per″ĭ-fah-lik′u-lar) surrounding a follicle, particularly a hair follicle.

peri·fol·lic·u·li·tis (-fah-lik″u-li′tis) inflammation around the hair follicles.

peri·gan·gli·itis (-gang″gle-i′tis) inflammation of tissues around a ganglion.

peri·gas·tri·tis (-gas-tri′tis) inflammation of the peritoneal coat of the stomach.

peri·hep·a·ti·tis (-hep″ah-ti′tis) inflammation of the peritoneal capsule of the liver and the surrounding tissue.

peri·is·let (per″e-i′let) situated around the islets of Langerhans.

peri·je·ju·ni·tis (per″ĭ-je″joo-ni′tis) inflammation around the jejunum.

peri·kary·on (-kar′e-on) the cell body as distinguished from the nucleus and the processes; applied particularly to neurons.

peri·lab·y·rin·thi·tis (-lab″ĭ-rin-thi′tis) circumscribed labyrinthitis.

peri·lymph (per′ĭ-limf) the fluid within the space separating the membranous and osseous labyrinths of the ear.

peri·lym·pha (per″ĭ-lim′fah) perilymph.

peri·lym·phan·gi·tis (-lim″fan-ji′tis) inflammation around a lymphatic vessel.

peri·lym·phat·ic (-lim-fat′ik) 1. pertaining to the perilymph. 2. around a lymphatic vessel.

peri·men·in·gi·tis (-men″in-ji′tis) pachymeningitis.

peri·meno·pause (-men′o-pawz) the time just before and after menopause. **perimenopau′sal,** adj.

peri·me·tri·um (-me′tre-um) the tunica serosa surrounding the uterus.

peri·my·eli·tis (-mi″ĕ-li′tis) inflammation of (a) the pia of the spinal cord, or (b) the endosteum.

peri·myo·si·tis (-mi″ah-si′tis) inflammation of connective tissue around a muscle.

peri·mys·i·i·tis (-mis″e-i′tis) inflammation of the perimysium; myofibrositis.

peri·mys·i·um (-mis′e-um) pl. *perimys′ia.* The connective tissue demarcating a fascicle of skeletal muscle fibers. See Plate 7. **perimys′ial,** adj.

peri·na·tal (-na′t'l) relating to the period shortly before and after birth; from the twentieth to twenty-ninth week of gestation to one to four weeks after birth.

peri·na·tol·o·gy (-na-tol′ah-je) the branch of medicine (obstetrics and pediatrics) dealing with the fetus and infant during the perinatal period.

peri·ne·al (-ne′al) pertaining to the perineum.

peri·neo·cele (-ne′ah-sēl) a hernia between the rectum and the prostate or between the rectum and the vagina.

peri·neo·plas·ty (-ne′ah-plas″te) plastic repair of the perineum.

peri·ne·or·rha·phy (-ne-or′ah-fe) suture of the perineum.

peri·ne·ot·o·my (-ne-ot′ah-me) incision of the perineum.

peri·neo·vag·i·nal (-ne″ah-vaj′ĭ-nal) pertaining to or communicating with the perineum and vagina.

peri·neph·ric (-nef′rik) perirenal; surrounding the kidney.

peri·ne·phri·tis (-nĕ-fri′tis) inflammation of the perinephrium.

peri·neph·ri·um (-nef′re-um) the peritoneal envelope and other tissues around the kidney. **perineph′rial,** adj.

peri·ne·um (-ne′um) 1. the pelvic floor and associated structures occupying the pelvic outlet, bounded anteriorly by the pubic symphysis, laterally by the ischial tuberosities, and posteriorly by the coccyx. 2. the region between the thighs, bounded in the male by the scrotum and anus and in the female by the vulva and anus.

peri·neu·ri·tis (-noŏ-ri′tis) inflammation of the perineurium.

peri·neu·ri·um (-noor′e-um) an intermediate layer of connective tissue in a peripheral nerve, surrounding each bundle of nerve fibers. See Plate 14. **perineu′rial,** adj.

peri·nu·cle·ar (-noo′kle-ar) near or around a nucleus.

pe·ri·od (pēr′e-od) an interval or division of time. **ejection p.,** the second phase of ventricular systole, being the interval between the opening and closing of the semilunar valves, during which the blood is discharged into the aortic and pulmonary arteries; it is divided into a *p. of rapid ejection* followed by a *p. of reduced ejection.* **gestation p.,** the duration of pregnancy, in humans being about 266 days (38 weeks) from the time of fertilization until birth. In obstetrics, it is instead considered to begin on the first day of the woman's last normal menstrual period prior to fertilization, thus being about 280 days (40 weeks). **incubation p.,** 1. the interval of time required for development. 2. the interval between the receipt of infection and the onset of the consequent illness or the first symptoms of the illness. 3. the interval between the entrance into a vector of an infectious agent and the time at which the vector is capable of transmitting the infection. **latency p.,** 1. latent p. 2. see under *stage.* **latent p.,** a seemingly inactive period, as that between exposure to an infection and subsequent illness, or that between the instant of stimulation and the beginning of response. **menstrual p., monthly p.,** the time of menstruation. **pacemaker refractory p.,** the period immediately following either pacemaker sensing or pacing, during which improper inhibition of the pacemaker by inappropriate signals is prevented by inactivation of pacemaker sensing. **refractory p.,** the period of depolarization and repolarization of the cell membrane after excitation; during the first portion (*absolute refractory p.*), the nerve or muscle fiber cannot respond to a second stimulus, whereas during the *relative refractory period*, it can respond only to a strong stimulus. **safe p.,** the period during the menstrual cycle when conception is considered least likely to occur; it is approximately the ten days after menstruation begins and the ten days preceding menstruation. **sphygmic p.,** ejection p. **Wenckebach p.,** the steadily lengthening P–R interval occurring in successive cardiac cycles in Wenckebach block.

pe·ri·od·ic (pēr′e-od′ik) 1. recurring at regular intervals of time. 2. recurring intermittently or occasionally.

pe·ri·o·dic·i·ty (pēr″e-ah-dis′ĭ-te) recurrence at regular intervals of time.

peri·odon·tal (per″e-o-don′t′l) 1. pertaining to the periodontal ligament or periodontium. 2. near or around a tooth.

peri·odon·tics (-don′tiks) the branch of dentistry dealing with the study and treatment of diseases of the periodontium.

peri·odon·ti·tis (-don-ti′tis) inflammatory reaction of the periodontium.

peri·odon·ti·um (-don′she-um) pl. *periodon′tia.* The tissues investing and supporting the teeth, including the cementum, periodontal ligament, alveolar bone, and gingiva. In official nomenclature, restricted to the periodontal ligament.

peri·odon·to·sis (-don-to′sis) a degenerative disorder of the periodontal structures, marked by tissue destruction.

peri·onych·i·um (-o-nik′e-um) eponychium (1).

peri·ooph·o·ri·tis (-o-of″o-ri′tis) inflammation of tissues around the ovary.

peri·ooph·o·ro·sal·pin·gi·tis (-o-of″o-ro-sal″pin-ji′tis) inflammation of tissues around an ovary and uterine tube.

peri·op·er·a·tive (-op′er-ah-tiv) pertaining to the period extending from the time of hospitalization for surgery to the time of discharge.

peri·oph·thal·mic (-of-thal′mik) around the eye.

peri·op·tom·e·try (per″e-op-tom′ĕ-tre) measurement of acuity of peripheral vision or of limits of the visual field.

peri·or·bi·ta (-or′bĭ-tah) periosteum of the bones of the orbit, or eye socket. **perior′bital,** adj.

peri·or·bi·ti·tis (-or″bĭ-ti′tis) inflammation of the periorbita.

peri·or·chi·tis (-or-ki′tis) inflammation of the tunica vaginalis testis.

peri·os·te·al (-os′te-al) pertaining to the periosteum.

peri·os·te·itis (-os″te-i′tis) periostitis.

peri·os·te·o·ma (-os-te-o′mah) a morbid bony growth surrounding a bone.

peri·os·teo·my·eli·tis (-os″te-o-mi″ĕ-li′tis) inflammation of the entire bone, including periosteum and marrow.

peri·os·teo·phyte (-os′te-ah-fīt″) a bony growth on the periosteum.

peri·os·te·ot·o·my (-os″te-ot′ah-me) incision of the periosteum.

peri·os·te·um (-os′te-um) a specialized connective tissue covering all bones and having bone-forming potentialities.

peri·os·ti·tis (-os-ti′tis) inflammation of the periosteum.

peri·os·to·sis (-os-to′sis) abnormal deposition of periosteal bone; the condition manifested by development of periosteomas.

peri·otic (-o′tik) 1. situated about the ear, especially the internal ear. 2. the petrous and mastoid portions of the temporal bone, at one stage a distinct bone.

peri·ovu·lar (-ov′u-lar) 1. surrounding an ovum. 2. around the time of ovulation.

peri·pap·il·lary (per″ĭ-pap′ĭ-lar″e) around the optic papilla.

peri·par·tum (-pahr′tum) occurring during the last month of gestation or the first few months after delivery, with reference to the mother.

peri·pha·ci·tis (-fah-si′tis) inflammation of the capsule of the eye lens.

pe·riph·er·ad (pĕ-rif′er-ad) toward the periphery.

pe·riph·ery (pĕ-rif′er-e) an outward surface or structure; the portion of a system outside the central region. **periph′eral,** adj.

peri·phle·bi·tis (per″ĭ-flĕ-bi′tis) inflammation of tissues around a vein, or of the external coat of a vein.

Per·i·pla·ne·ta (-plah-ne′tah) a genus of roaches, including *P. america′na,* the American cockroach, and *P. austra′lasiae,* the Australian cockroach.

peri·plas·mic (-plas′mik) around the plasma membrane; between the plasma membrane and the cell wall of a bacterium.

peri·proc·ti·tis (-prok-ti′tis) inflammation of tissues around the rectum and anus.

peri·pros·ta·ti·tis (-pros″tah-ti′tis) inflammation of tissues around the prostate.

peri·py·le·phle·bi·tis (-pi″le-flĕ-bi′tis) inflammation of tissues around the portal vein.

peri·rec·ti·tis (-rek-ti′tis) periproctitis.

peri·re·nal (-re′n'l) perinephric.

peri·sal·pin·gi·tis (-sal″pin-ji′tis) inflammation of the tissues and peritoneum around a uterine tube.

peri·sig·moid·itis (-sig″moid-i′tis) inflammation of the peritoneum of the sigmoid flexure.

peri·sin·u·si·tis (-si″nah-si′tis) inflammation of tissues about a sinus.

peri·splanch·ni·tis (-splank-ni′tis) inflammation of tissues around the viscera.

peri·sple·ni·tis (-splĕ-ni′tis) inflammation of the peritoneal surface of the spleen.

peri·spon·dy·li·tis (-spon″di-li′tis) inflammation of tissues around a vertebra.

peri·stal·sis (-stahl′sis) the wormlike movement by which the alimentary canal or other tubular organs having both longitudinal and circular muscle fibers propel their contents, consisting of a wave of contraction passing along the tube for variable distances. **peri·stal′tic**, adj.

peri·staph·y·line (-staf′ĭ-lēn) around the uvula.

peri·tec·to·my (-tek′tah-me) excision of a ring of conjunctiva around the cornea in treatment of pannus.

peri·ten·din·e·um (-ten-din′e-um) connective tissue investing larger tendons and extending between the fibers composing them.

peri·ten·di·ni·tis (-ten″dĭ-ni′tis) tenosynovitis.

peri·ten·o·ni·tis (-ten″o-ni′tis) tenosynovitis.

peri·the·li·o·ma (-the″le-o′mah) hemangiopericytoma.

peri·the·li·um (-the′le-um) the connective tissue layer surrounding the capillaries and smaller vessels.

peri·thy·roi·di·tis (-thi″roi-di′tis) inflammation of the capsule of the thyroid gland.

pe·rit·o·my (pĕ-rit′ah-me) incision of the conjunctiva and subconjunctival tissue about the entire circumference of the cornea.

peri·to·ne·al (per″ĭ-to-ne′al) pertaining to the peritoneum.

peri·to·ne·al·gia (-to″ne-al′jah) pain in the peritoneum.

peri·to·neo·cen·te·sis (-to-ne″o-sen-te′sis) paracentesis of the abdominal cavity.

peri·to·ne·oc·ly·sis (-to″ne-ok′lĭ-sis) injection of fluid into the peritoneal cavity.

peri·to·ne·os·co·py (-to″ne-os′kah-pe) laparoscopy.

peri·to·ne·ot·o·my (-to″ne-ot′ah-me) incision into the peritoneum.

peri·to·neo·ve·nous (-to-ne″o-ve′nus) communicating with the peritoneal cavity and the venous system.

peri·to·ne·um (-to-ne′um) the serous membrane lining the walls of the abdominal and pelvic cavities (*parietal p.*) and investing the contained viscera (*visceral p.*), the two layers enclosing a potential space, the peritoneal cavity. **perito·ne′al**, adj.

peri·to·ni·tis (-to-ni′tis) inflammation of the peritoneum, which may be due to chemical irritation or bacterial invasion.

peri·ton·sil·lar (-ton′sĭ-ler) around a tonsil.

peri·ton·sil·li·tis (-ton″sĭ-li′tis) inflammation of peritonsillar tissues.

pe·rit·ri·chous (pĕ-rit′rĭ-kus) 1. having flagella around the entire surface; said of bacteria; sometimes used to describe the flagella themselves. 2. having flagella around the cytostome only; said of Ciliophora.

peri·tu·bu·lar (per″ĭ-too′bu-lar) situated around or near tubules.

peri·um·bil·i·cal (per″e-um-bil′ĭ-k'l) around the umbilicus.

peri·un·gual (-ung′gw'l) around the nail.

peri·ure·ter·itis (-u-re″ter-i′tis) inflammation of tissues around a ureter.

peri·ure·thri·tis (-u-rĕ-thri′tis) inflammation of the tissues around the urethra.

peri·vag·i·ni·tis (per″ĭ-vaj″ĭ-ni′tis) pericolpitis.

peri·vas·cu·lar (-vas′ku-lar) near or around a vessel.

peri·vas·cu·li·tis (-vas″ku-li′tis) inflammation of a perivascular sheath and surrounding tissue.

peri·ves·i·cal (-ves′ĭ-k'l) near the urinary bladder.

peri·ve·sic·u·li·tis (-vĕ-sik″u-li′tis) inflammation of tissue around the seminal vesicle.

per·lèche (per-lesh′) inflammation with exudation, maceration, and fissuring at the labial commissures.

per·man·ga·nate (per-mang′gah-nāt) a salt containing the MnO_4^- ion.

per·me·a·ble (per′me-ah-b'l) not impassable; pervious; permitting passage of a substance.

per·me·a·bil·i·ty (per″me-ah-bil′ĭ-te) the property or state of being permeable.

per·me·ase (per′me-ās) former name for *transport protein*.

per·me·ate (-āt″) 1. to penetrate or pass through, as through a filter. 2. the constituents of a solution or suspension that pass through a filter.

per·meth·rin (per-meth′rin) a topical insecticide used in the treatment of infestations by *Pediculus humanus capitis*, *Sarcoptes scabiei*, or any of various ticks; also applied to objects such as furniture and bedding.

perm·se·lec·tiv·i·ty (perm″sĕ-lek-tiv′ĭ-te) restriction of permeation of macromolecules across a glomerular capillary wall on the basis of molecular size, charge, and physical configuration.

per·ni·cious (per-nish′us) tending toward a fatal issue.

per·nio (per′ne-o) pl. *pernio′nes*. [L.] chilblain.

pero- word element [Gr.], *deformity; maimed*.

pe·ro·me·lia (pe″ro-me′le-ah) severe dysmelia.

per·o·ne·al (-ne′al) pertaining to the fibula or to the lateral aspect of the leg; fibular.

per·oral (per-or′al) performed or administered through the mouth.

per os (per os) [L.] by mouth.

per·ox·i·dase (per-ok′sĭ-dās) any of a group of iron-porphyrin enzymes that catalyze the oxidation of some organic substrates in the presence of hydrogen peroxide.

per·ox·ide (-ok′sīd) that oxide of any element containing more oxygen than any other; more correctly applied to compounds having such linkage as —O—O—.

per·ox·i·some (-ok′sĭ-sōm) 1. any of the microbodies present in vertebrate animal cells, especially liver and kidney cells, which are rich in the enzymes peroxidase, catalase, D-amino acid oxidase, and, to a lesser extent, urate oxidase. 2. microbody (1).

per·phen·a·zine (-fen′ah-zēn) a phenothiazine used as an antipsychotic and as an antiemetic.

per pri·mam in·ten·ti·o·nem (per pri′mam in-ten″she-o′nem) [L.] by first intention; see under *healing*. Written also *per primam*.

per rec·tum (per rek′tum) [L.] by way of the rectum.

per se·cun·dam in·ten·ti·o·nem (per se-kun′dam in-ten″she-o′nem) [L.] by second intention; see under *healing*. Written also *per secundam*.

per·sev·er·a·tion (per-sev″er-a′shun) persistent repetition of the same verbal or motor response to varied stimuli; continuance of activity after cessation of the causative stimulus.

per·so·na (per-so′nah) [L.] in jungian psychology, the personality mask or facade presented by a person to the outside world, as opposed to the anima, the inner being.

per·so·nal·i·ty (per″sah-nal′ĭ-te) the characteristic, relatively stable, and predictable way a person thinks, feels, and behaves, including conscious attitudes, values, and styles, and also unconscious conflicts and defense mechanisms. **antisocial p. (disorder),** a personality disorder characterized

by continuous and chronic antisocial behavior in which the rights of others or generally accepted social norms are violated. **avoidant p. (disorder),** a personality disorder characterized by social discomfort, hypersensitivity to criticism, low self-esteem, and an aversion to activities that involve significant interpersonal contact. **borderline p. (disorder),** a personality disorder marked by a pervasive instability of mood, self-image, and interpersonal relationships, with fears of abandonment, chronic feelings of emptiness, threats, anger, and self-damaging behavior. **cyclothymic p.,** a temperament characterized by rapid, frequent swings between sad and cheerful moods. **dependent p. (disorder),** a personality disorder marked by an excessive need to be taken care of, with submissiveness and clinging, feelings of helplessness when alone, and preoccupation with fears of being abandoned. **depressive p. (disorder),** a persistent and pervasive pattern of depressive cognitions and behaviors, such as unhappiness, low self-esteem, pessimism, critical and derogatory attitudes, guilt or remorse, and an inability to relax or feel enjoyment. **histrionic p. (disorder),** a personality disorder marked by excessive emotionality and attention-seeking behavior. **multiple p. (disorder),** dissociative identity disorder. **narcissistic p. (disorder),** a personality disorder characterized by grandiosity (in fantasy or behavior), lack of social empathy combined with hypersensitivity to the judgments of others, interpersonal exploitativeness, a sense of entitlement, and a need for constant signs of admiration. **obsessive-compulsive p. (disorder),** a personality disorder characterized by an emotionally constricted manner that is unduly rigid, stubborn, perfectionistic, and stingy, with preoccupation with trivial details, overconcern with having everything done one's own way, excessive devotion to work and productivity, and overconscientiousness. **paranoid p. (disorder),** a personality disorder marked by a view of other people as hostile, devious, and untrustworthy and a combative response to disappointments or to events experienced as rebuffs or humiliations. **passive-aggressive p. (disorder),** a personality disorder characterized by indirect resistance to demands for adequate social or occupational performance and by negative, defeatist attitudes. **sadistic p. (disorder),** a pervasive pattern of cruel, demeaning, and aggressive behavior; satisfaction is gained from intimidating, coercing, hurting, and humiliating others. **schizoid p. (disorder),** a personality disorder marked by indifference to social relationships and restricted range of emotional experience and expression. **schizotypal p. (disorder),** a personality disorder characterized by marked deficits in interpersonal competence and eccentricities in ideation, appearance, or behavior. **self-defeating p. (disorder),** a persistent pattern of behavior detrimental to the self, including being drawn to problematic situations or relationships and failing to accomplish tasks crucial to life objectives. **split p.,** an obsolete term formerly used colloquially for either schizophrenia or dissociative identity disorder.

per·spi·ra·tion (per″spĭ-ra′shun) 1. sweating. 2. sweat.

per·sul·fate (per-sul′fāt) a salt of persulfuric acid.

per tu·bam (per too′bam) [L.] through a tube.

per·tus·sis (per-tus′is) whooping cough; an infectious disease caused by *Bordetella pertussis*, marked by catarrh of the respiratory tract and peculiar paroxysms of cough, ending in a prolonged crowing or whooping respiration.

per·tus·soid (-oid) 1. resembling whooping cough. 2. an influenzal cough resembling that of whooping cough.

per va·gi·nam (per vah-ji′nam) [L.] through the vagina.

per·ver·sion (per-ver′zhun) 1. deviation from the normal course. 2. sexual perversion; see under *deviation*.

pes (pes) pl. *pe′des*. [L.] 1. foot. 2. any footlike part.

pes·sa·ry (pes′ah-re) 1. an instrument placed in the vagina to support the uterus or rectum or as a contraceptive device. 2. a medicated vaginal suppository.

pes·ti·lence (pes′tĭ-lins) a virulent contagious epidemic or infectious epidemic disease. **pestilen′tial,** adj.

pes·tle (pes′′l) an implement for pounding drugs in a mortar.

PET positron emission tomography.

peta- (P), a word element used in naming units of measurement to designate a quantity 10^{15} (a quadrillion) times the unit to which it is joined.

-petal word element [L.], *directed* or *moving toward*.

pe·te·chia (pĕ-te′ke-ah) pl. *pete′chiae*. [L.] a minute red spot due to escape of a small amount of blood. **pete′chial,** adj.

pet·i·ole (pet′e-ōl) a stalk or pedicle. **epi-glottic p.,** the pointed lower end of the epiglottic cartilage, attached to the thyroid cartilage.

pe·ti·o·lus (pah-ti′-o-lus) petiole.

pe·tit mal (pĕ-te′ mahl′) [Fr.] see under *epilepsy*.

pé·tris·sage (pa″tre-sahzh′) [Fr.] massage in which the muscles are kneaded and pressed.

pet·ro·la·tum (pet″rah-la′tum) a purified mixture of semisolid hydrocarbons obtained from petroleum; used as an ointment base, protective dressing, and soothing application to the skin. **liquid p.,** mineral oil.

pe·tro·le·um (pĕ-tro′le-um) a thick natural mixture of gaseous, liquid, and solid hydrocarbons obtained from beneath the surface of the earth. **p. benzin,** a colorless, volatile, flammable fraction from petroleum distillation, containing largely hydrocarbons of the methane series; it has been variously described as a special grade of ligroin or as a separate but similar fraction with a lower boiling range. It is used chiefly as an extractive solvent.

pet·ro·mas·toid (-mas′toid) 1. pertaining to the petrous portion of the temporal bone and its mastoid process. 2. otocranium (2).

pet·ro·oc·cip·i·tal (-ok-sip′it′l) pertaining to the petrous portion of the temporal bone and to the occipital bone.

pe·tro·sal (pĕ-tro′sil) pertaining to the petrous portion of the temporal bone.

pet·ro·si·tis (pet″ro-si′tis) inflammation of the petrous portion of the temporal bone.

pet·ro·sphe·noid (-sfe′noid) pertaining to the petrous portion of the temporal bone and to the sphenoid bone.

pet·ro·squa·mous (-skwah′mus) pertaining to the petrous and squamous portions of the temporal bone.

pet·rous (pet′rus) resembling a rock; hard; stony.

pex·is (pek′sis) 1. the fixation of matter by a tissue. 2. surgical fixation. **pex′ic,** adj.

-pexy word element [Gr.], *surgical fixation*. **-pec′tic,** adj.

pey·o·te (pa-ōt′e) a stimulant drug from mescal buttons, whose active principle is mescaline; used by North American Indians in certain ceremonies to produce an intoxication marked by feelings of ecstasy.

pg picogram.

pH the symbol relating the hydrogen ion (H^+) concentration or activity of a solution to that of a given standard solution. Numerically the pH is approximately equal to the negative logarithm of H^+ concentration expressed in molarity. pH 7 is neutral; above it alkalinity increases and below it acidity increases.

phac(o)- word element [Gr.], *lens*. See also words beginning *phak(o)-*.

pha·co·ana·phy·lax·is (fak″o-an″ah-fi-lak′sis) hypersensitivity to the protein of the crystalline lens of the eye, induced by escape of material from the lens capsule.

phaco·cele (fak′ah-sēl) hernia of the eye lens.

phaco·cys·tec·to·my (fak″o-sis-tek′tah-me) excision of part of the lens capsule for cataract.

phaco·cys·ti·tis (-sis-ti′tis) inflammation of the capsule of the eye lens.

phaco·emul·si·fi·ca·tion (-ĕ-mul″sĭ-fi-ka′shun) a method of cataract extraction in which the lens is fragmented by ultrasonic vibrations and simultaneously irrigated and aspirated.

phaco·ery·sis (-ĕ-re′sis) removal of the eye lens in cataract by suction.

phac·oid (fak′oid) shaped like a lens.

phac·oid·itis (fak″oi-di′tis) phakitis.

pha·coido·scope (fah-koid′-ah-skōp) phacoscope.

pha·col·y·sis (fah-kol′ĭ-sis) dissolution or discission of the eye lens. **phacolyt′ic,** adj.

phaco·ma·la·cia (fak″o-mah-la′shah) softening of the lens; a soft cataract.

phaco·meta·cho·re·sis (-met″ah-kor-e′sis) displacement of the eye lens.

phaco·scle·ro·sis (-sklĕ-ro′sis) hardening of the crystalline lens; a hard cataract.

phaco·scope (fak′ah-skōp″) instrument for viewing accommodative changes of the eye lens.

phaco·tox·ic (fak′o-tok″sik) exerting a deleterious effect upon the crystalline lens.

phaeo·hy·pho·my·co·sis (fe″o-hi″fo-mi-ko′sis) any opportunistic infection caused by dematiaceous fungi.

phage (fāj) bacteriophage.

-phage word element [Gr.], *one that eats or destroys.*

phag·e·den·ic (faj″ĕ-den′ik) pertaining to or characterized by a progressive, rapidly spreading, sloughing ulceration.

-phagia word element [Gr.], *eating; swallowing.*

phag(o)- word element [Gr.], *eating; ingestion.*

phago·cyte (fag′o-sīt) any cell that ingests microorganisms or other cells and foreign particles, such as a microphage, macrophage, or monocyte. **phagocyt′ic,** adj.

phago·cy·tin (fag″o-sī′tin) a bactericidal substance from neutrophilic leukocytes.

phago·cy·tol·y·sis (-si-tol′ĭ-sis) destruction of phagocytes. **phagocytolyt′ic,** adj.

phago·cy·to·sis (-si-to′sis) the engulfing of microorganisms or other cells and foreign particles by phagocytes. **phagocytot′ic,** adj.

phago·some (fag′o-sōm) a membrane-bound vesicle in a phagocyte containing the phagocytized material.

phago·type (-tīp) phage type; see under *type.*

-phagy see *-phagia.*

pha·ki·tis (fa-ki′tis) inflammation of the crystalline lens.

phak(o)- see *phac(o)-.*

pha·ko·ma (fah-ko′mah) any of the hamartomas found in the phakomatoses, such as the herald lesions of tuberous sclerosis. See also *tuber* (2).

phak·o·ma·to·sis (fak″o-mah-to′sis) pl. *phakomato′ses.* Any of a group of congenital hereditary developmental anomalies having selective involvement of tissues of ectodermal origin, which develop disseminated glial hamartomas; examples are neurofibromatosis, tuberous sclerosis, Sturge-Weber syndrome, and von Hippel-Lindau disease.

pha·lan·ge·al (fah-lan′je-al) pertaining to a phalanx.

phal·an·gec·to·my (fal″an-jek′tah-me) excision of a phalanx.

phal·an·gi·tis (-ji′tis) inflammation of one or more phalanges.

phalang(o)- word element [Gr.], *phalanx* or *phalanges.*

pha·lanx (fa′langks) pl. *phalan′ges.* [Gr.] 1. any bone of a finger or toe; see *phalanges,* in *Table of Bones.* 2. any one of a set of plates that are disposed in rows and make up the reticular membrane of the organ of Corti. **phalan′geal,** adj.

phal·lec·to·my (fal-ek′tah-me) penectomy.

phal·li (fal′i) plural of *phallus.*

phal·lic (-ik) pertaining to or resembling a phallus.

phal·li·tis (fah-li′tis) penitis.

phal·loi·din (fah-loid′in) a hexapeptide poison from the mushroom *Amanita phalloides,* which causes asthenia, vomiting, diarrhea, convulsions, and death.

phal·lo·plas·ty (fal′o-plas″te) plastic surgery of the penis.

phal·lus (fal′us) pl. *phal′li.* 1. Penis. 2. a representation of the penis. 3. the primordium of the penis or clitoris that develops from the genital tubercle.

phan·er·o·sis (fan″er-o′sis) the process of becoming visible.

phan·tasm (fan′tazm) an impression or image not evoked by actual stimuli, and usually recognized as false by the observer.

phan·tom (fant′um) 1. phantasm. 2. a model of the body or of a part thereof. 3. a device for simulating the in vivo effect of radiation on tissues.

phan·tos·mia (fan-toz'me-ah) a parosmia consisting of a sensation of smell in the absence of any external stimulus.

phar, pharm pharmacy; pharmaceutical; pharmacopeia.

phar·ma·ceu·tic (fahr″mah-soo'tik) pharmaceutical (1).

phar·ma·ceu·ti·cal (-soo'tĭ-k'l) 1. pertaining to pharmacy or drugs. 2. a medicinal drug.

phar·ma·cist (fahr'mah-sist) one who is licensed to prepare and sell or dispense drugs and compounds, and to make up prescriptions.

pharmaco- word element [Gr.], *drug; medicine.*

phar·ma·co·an·gi·og·ra·phy (fahr″mah-ko-an-je-og'rah-fe) angiography in which visualization is enhanced by manipulating the flow of blood by the administration of vasodilating and vasoconstricting agents.

phar·ma·co·dy·nam·ics (-di-nam'iks) the study of the biochemical and physiological effects of drugs and the mechanisms of their actions, including the correlation of their actions and effects with their chemical structure. **pharmacodynam'ic,** adj.

phar·ma·co·ge·net·ics (-jĭ-net'iks) the study of the relationship between genetic factors and the nature of responses to drugs.

phar·ma·cog·no·sy (fahr″mah-kog'nah-se) the branch of pharmacology dealing with natural drugs and their constituents.

phar·ma·co·ki·net·ics (fahr″mah-ko-kĭ-net'iks) the action of drugs in the body over a period of time, including the processes of absorption, distribution, localization in tissues, biotransformation, and excretion. **pharmacokinet'ic,** adj.

phar·ma·co·log·ic (-kah-loj'ik) pertaining to pharmacology or to the properties and reactions of drugs.

phar·ma·col·o·gist (-kol'ah-jist) one who makes a study of the actions of drugs.

phar·ma·col·o·gy (-kol'ah-je) the science that deals with the origin, nature, chemistry, effects, and uses of drugs; it includes pharmacognosy, pharmocokinetics, pharmacodynamics, pharmacotherapeutics, and toxicology.

phar·ma·co·pe·ia (-ko-pe'ah) an authoritative treatise on drugs and their preparations. See also *USP*. **pharmacopei'al,** adj. **United States P.,** see under *U.*

phar·ma·co·ther·a·py (-ther'ah-pe) treatment of disease with medicines.

phar·ma·cy (fahr'mah-se) 1. the branch of the health sciences dealing with the preparation, dispensing, and proper utilization of drugs. 2. a place where drugs are compounded or dispensed.

Pharm D [L.] Pharma'ciae Doc'tor (Doctor of Pharmacy).

phar·yn·gal·gia (far″ing-gal'jah) pharyngodynia.

pha·ryn·ge·al (fah-rin'je-al) pertaining to the pharynx.

phar·yn·gec·to·my (far″in-jek'tah-me) excision of part of the pharynx.

phar·yn·gis·mus (-jiz'mus) muscular spasm of the pharynx.

phar·yn·gi·tis (-ji'tis) sore throat; inflammation of the pharynx. **pharyngit'ic,** adj.

pharyng(o)- word element [Gr.], *pharynx.*

pha·ryn·go·cele (fah-ring'go-sēl″) herniation or cystic deformity of the pharynx.

pha·ryn·go·dyn·ia (fah-ring″go-din'e-ah) pain in the pharynx.

pha·ryn·go·esoph·a·ge·al (-ĕ-sof'ah-je″al) pertaining to the pharynx and esophagus.

pha·ryn·go·my·co·sis (-mi-ko'sis) any fungal infection of the pharynx.

pha·ryn·go·pa·ral·y·sis (-pah-ral'ĭ-sis) paralysis of the pharyngeal muscles.

pha·ryn·go·ple·gia (-ple'jah) pharyngoparalysis.

phar·yn·gos·co·py (far″ing-gos'kah-pe) direct visual examination of the pharynx.

pha·ryn·go·ste·no·sis (fah-ring″go-stĕ-no'sis) narrowing of the pharynx.

phar·yn·got·o·my (far″ing-got'ah-me) incision of the pharynx.

phar·ynx (far'inks) the throat; the musculomembranous cavity behind the nasal cavities, mouth, and larynx, communicating with them and with the esophagus.

phase (fāz) 1. one of the aspects or stages through which a varying entity may pass. 2. in physical chemistry, any physically or chemically distinct, homogeneous, and mechanically separable part of a system. **pha'sic,** adj. **erythrocytic p.,** that phase in the life cycle of a malarial plasmodium in which the parasites multiply in the red blood cells. **five p's,** in traditional Chinese medicine, a set of dynamic relations (designated earth, metal, water, wood, and fire) that can be used to categorize relationships among phenomena. **follicular p.,** the first half of the human menstrual cycle, lasting from cessation of menstrual flow to the surge of luteinizing and follicle-stimulating hormones at the start of the ovulatory phase. **G₁ p.,** a part of the cell cycle during interphase, lasting from the end of cell division (the M phase) until the start of DNA synthesis (the S phase). **G₂ p.,** a relatively quiescent part of the cell cycle during interphase, lasting from the end of DNA synthesis (the S phase) until the start of cell division (the M phase). **luteal p.,** the third phase of the human menstrual cycle, beginning with ovulation and ending, in the absence of fertilization, with the menstrual phase. **M p.,** the part of the cell cycle during which mitosis occurs; subdivided into prophase, metaphase, anaphase, and telophase. **menstrual p.,** the fourth phase of the human menstrual cycle, following the luteal phase in the absence of fertilization. The corpus luteum regresses and is shed through menstruation and growth begins for the ovarian follicle, leading to the next follicular phase. **ovulatory p.,** the second phase of the human menstrual cycle, encompassing the surges of luteinizing and follicle-stimulating hormones, and ovulation; it is followed by the luteal phase. **S p.,** a part of the cell cycle, near the end of interphase, during which DNA is synthesized; between the G_1 and G_2 phases.

phas·mid (faz'mid) 1. either of the two caudal chemoreceptors occurring in certain nematodes (Phasmidia). 2. any nematode containing phasmids.

phe·nac·e·tin (fĕ-nas'ĕ-tin) an analgesic and antipyretic, whose major metabolite is acetaminophen, now little used because of its toxicity.

phe·nan·threne (fĕ-nan'thrēn) a tricyclic aromatic hydrocarbon occurring in coal tar; toxic and carcinogenic.

phen·ar·sa·zine chlor·ide (fen-ahr'sah-zēn) diphenylamine chlorarsine.

phen·a·zone (fen'ah-zōn) antipyrine.

phen·a·zo·pyr·i·dine (fen″ah-zo-pir'ĭ-dēn) a urinary tract analgesic, used as the hydrochloride salt.

phen·cy·cli·dine (PCP) (fen-si'klĭ-dēn) a potent veterinary analgesic and anesthetic, used as a drug of abuse in the form of the hydrochloride salt; its abuse by humans may lead to serious psychological disturbances.

phen·di·met·ra·zine (fen″di-met'rah-zēn) a sympathomimetic amine used as an anorectic in the form of the tartrate salt.

phen·el·zine (fen'el-zēn) a monoamine oxidase inhibitor used as the sulfate salt as an antidepressant and in the prophylaxis of migraine.

phe·nin·da·mine (fĕ-nin'dah-mēn) an antihistamine with anticholinergic and sedative effects, used as the tartrate salt.

phen·ir·amine (fen-ir'ah-mēn) an antihistamine with anticholinergic and sedative effects, used as the maleate salt.

phen·met·ra·zine (-met'rah-zēn) a central nervous system stimulant used as an anorectic in the form of the hydrochloride salt; abuse may lead to habituation.

phen(o)- word element [Gr.], 1. *showing; displaying.* 2. *a compound derived from benzene.*

phe·no·bar·bi·tal (fe″no-bahr'bĭ-tal) a long-acting barbiturate, used as the base or sodium salt as a sedative, hypnotic, and anticonvulsant.

phe·no·copy (fe'no-kop″e) an environmentally induced phenotype mimicking one usually produced by a specific genotype.

phe·no·de·vi·ant (fe″no-de've-ant) an individual whose phenotype differs significantly from that of the typical phenotype in the population.

phe·nol (fe'nol) 1. an extremely poisonous compound, C_6H_5OH, which is caustic and disinfectant; used as a pharmaceutic preservative and in dilution as an antimicrobial and topical anesthetic and antipruritic. Poisoning, due to ingestion or transdermal absorption, causes symptoms including colic, local irritation, corrosion, seizures, cardiac arrhythmias, shock, and respiratory arrest. 2. any organic compound containing one or more hydroxyl groups attached to an aromatic carbon ring.

phe·no·late (fe'no-lāt) 1. to treat with phenol for purposes of sterilization. 2. a salt formed by union of a base with phenol, in which a monovalent metal, such as sodium or potassium, replaces the hydrogen of the hydroxyl group.

phe·nol·phthal·ein (fe″nol-thal'ēn) a cathartic and pH indicator, with a range of 8.5 to 9.0.

phe·nom·e·non (fĕ-nom'ĕ-non) pl. *phenom'ena.* Any sign or objective symptom; an observable occurrence or fact. **booster p.,** on a tuberculin test, an initial false-negative result due to a diminished amnestic response, becoming positive on subsequent testing. **dawn p.,** the early morning increase in plasma glucose concentration and thus insulin requirement in patients with type 1 diabetes mellitus. **Koebner's p.,** a cutaneous response seen in certain dermatoses, manifested by the appearance on uninvolved skin of lesions typical of the skin disease at the site of trauma, on scars, or at points where articles of clothing produce pressure. **Marcus Gunn's pupillary p.,** with unilateral optic nerve or retinal disease, a difference between the pupillary reflexes of the two eyes; on the affected side there is abnormally slight contraction or even dilatation of the pupil when a light is shone in the eye. **no-reflow p.,** when cerebral blood flow is restored following prolonged global cerebral ischemia, there is initial hyperemia followed by a gradual decline in perfusion until there is almost no blood flow. **Somogyi p.,** a rebound phenomenon occurring in diabetes: overtreatment with insulin induces hypoglycemia, thus initiating hormone release; this stimulates lipolysis, gluconeogenesis, and glycogenolysis, which in turn cause rebound hyperglycemia and ketosis.

phe·no·thi·a·zine (fe″no-thi′ah-zēn) any of a group of antipsychotic agents having a similar tricyclic structure and acting as potent alpha-adrenergic and dopaminergic blocking agents, as well as having hypotensive, antispasmodic, antihistaminic, analgesic, sedative, and antiemetic activity..

phe·no·type (fe′nah-tīp) the entire physical, biochemical, and physiological makeup of an individual as determined both genetically and environmentally. Also, any one or any group of such traits. **phenotyp′ic,** adj.

phe·noxy·benz·amine (fĕ-nok″se-ben′zah-mēn) an irreversible α-adrenergic blocking agent; the hydrochloride salt is used to control hypertension in pheochromocytoma and to treat urinary symptoms in benign prostatic hyperplasia.

phen·pro·pi·o·nate (-pro′pe-ah-nāt″) USAN contraction for 3-phenylpropionate.

phen·ter·mine (fen′ter-mēn) a sympathomimetic amine related to amphetamine, used as an anorectic either as the hydrochloride salt or as the base complexed with an ion exchange resin.

phen·yl (fen′il, fe′nil) the monovalent radical C_6H_5—, derived from benzene by removal of a hydrogen. **phenyl′ic,** adj.

phen·yl·a·ce·tic ac·id (fen″il-ah-se′tik) a catabolite of phenylalanine, excessively formed and excreted in the urine in phenylketonuria.

phen·yl·al·a·nine (Phe, F) (-al′ah-nēn) an aromatic essential amino acid necessary for optimal growth in infants and for nitrogen equilibrium in human adults.

phen·yl·bu·ta·zone (-bu′tah-zōn) a nonsteroidal antiinflammatory drug used in the short-term treatment of severe rheumatoid disorders unresponsive to less toxic agents.

***p*-phen·yl·ene·di·amine** (fen″il-ēn-di′ah-mēn) a derivative of benzene used as a dye for hair, garments, and other textiles, as a photographic developing agent, and in a variety of other processes; it is a strong allergen, causing contact dermatitis and bronchial asthma.

phen·yl·eph·rine (-ef′rin) an adrenergic used as the hydrochloride salt for its potent vasoconstrictor properties.

phen·yl·ke·ton·uria (-ke″to-nu′re-ah) PKU or PKU1, an inborn error of metabolism marked by inability to convert phenylalanine into tyrosine, so that phenylalanine and its metabolic products accumulate in body fluids; it results in mental retardation, neurologic manifestations, light pigmentation, eczema, and a mousy odor, all preventable by early restriction of dietary phenylalanine. **phenylketonu′ric,** adj.

phen·yl·mer·cu·ric (-mer-ku′rik) denoting a compound containing the radical C_6H_5Hg—, forming various antiseptic, antibacterial, and fungicidal salts; compounds of the acetate and nitrate salts are used as bacteriostatic pharmaceutical preservatives, and the former is used as a herbicide.

phen·yl·pro·pa·nol·amine (-pro″pah-nol′ah-mēn) an adrenergic, used in the form of the hydrochloride salt as a nasal and sinus decongestant, as an appetite suppressant, and in the treatment of stress incontinence.

phen·yl·py·ru·vic ac·id (-pi-roo′vik) an intermediary product produced when the normal pathway of phenylalanine catabolism is blocked and excreted in the urine in phenylketonuria.

phen·yl·thio·urea (-thi″o-u-re′ah) a compound used in genetics research; the ability to taste it is inherited as a dominant trait. It is intensely bitter to about 70 per cent of the population and nearly tasteless to the rest.

phen·yl·tol·ox·amine (-tol-ok′sah-mēn) a sedating antihistamine, used as the citrate salt.

phen·y·to·in (fen′ĭ-toin′) an anticonvulsant used in the control of various kinds of epilepsy and of seizures associated with neurosurgery.

pheo·chrome (fe′ah-krōm) chromaffin.

pheo·chro·mo·blast (fe″o-kro′mah-blast) any of the embryonic structures that develop into chromaffin (pheochrome) cells.

pheo·chro·mo·cyte (-kro′mah-sīt) chromaffin cell.

pheo·chro·mo·cy·to·ma (-kro″mah-si-to′mah) a tumor of chromaffin tissue of the adrenal medulla or sympathetic paraganglia; symptoms, notably hypertension, reflect the increased secretion of epinephrine and norepinephrine.

phe·re·sis (fĕ-re′sis) apheresis.

pher·o·mone (fer′ah-mōn) a substance secreted to the outside of the body and perceived (as by smell) by other individuals of the same species, releasing specific behavior in the percipient.

PhG Graduate in Pharmacy.

Phi·a·loph·o·ra (fi″ah-lof′ah-rah) a genus of imperfect fungi. *P. verruco′sa* is a cause of chromoblastomycosis; *P. jeansel'mi* is a cause of maduromycosis.

-phil word element [Gr.], *one having an affinity for something.* Also *-phile.* **-phil′ic,** adj.

-phile see *phil.*

-philia word element [Gr.], *affinity for; morbid fondness of.* **-phil′ic,** adj.

phil·trum (fil′trum) the vertical groove in the median portion of the upper lip.

phi·mo·sis (fi-mo′sis) constriction of the orifice of the prepuce so that it cannot be drawn back over the glans. **phimot′ic,** adj.

phleb·an·gi·o·ma (fleb″an-je-o′mah) a venous aneurysm.

phleb·ar·te·ri·ec·ta·sia (-ahr-tēr″e-ek-ta′zhah) general dilatation of veins and arteries.

phleb·ec·ta·sia (-ek-ta′zhah) varicosity (1).

phle·bec·to·my (flĕ-bek′tah-me) excision of a vein, or a segment of a vein.

phleb·em·phrax·is (fleb″em-frak′sis) stoppage of a vein by a plug or clot.

phle·bis·mus (flĕ-biz′mus) obstruction and consequent dilation of veins.

phle·bi·tis (flĕ-bi′tis) inflammation of a vein. **phlebit′ic,** adj. **sinus p.,** inflammation of a cerebral sinus.

phleb(o)- word element [Gr.], *vein.*

phle·boc·ly·sis (flĕ-bok′lĭ-sis) injection of fluid into a vein.

phle·bog·ra·phy (flĕ-bog′rah-fe) 1. venography; angiography of a vein. 2. the graphic recording of the venous pulse.

phle·bo·li·thi·a·sis (fleb″o-lĭ-thi′ah-sis) the development of calculi in veins.

phle·bo·ma·nom·e·ter (-mah-nom′ĕ-ter) an instrument for the direct measurement of venous blood pressure.

phle·bo·phle·bos·to·my (-flĕ-bos′tah-me) operative anastomosis of vein to vein.

phle·bo·rhe·og·ra·phy (-re-og′rah-fe) a technique employing a plethysphygmograph with cuffs applied to the abdomen, thigh, calf, and foot, for measuring venous volume changes in response to respiration and to compression of the foot or calf.

phle·bor·rha·phy (flĕ-bor′ah-fe) suture of a vein.

phle·bo·scle·ro·sis (fleb″o-sklĕ-ro′sis) fibrous thickening of the walls of veins.

phle·bos·ta·sis (flĕ-bos′tah-sis) 1. venous stasis. 2. temporary sequestration of a portion of blood from the general circulation by compressing the veins of a limb.

phle·bo·throm·bo·sis (fleb″o-throm-bo′sis) the development of venous thrombi in the absence of associated inflammation.

Phle·bot·o·mus (flĕ-bot′ah-mus) a genus of biting sandflies, the females of which suck blood. They are vectors of various diseases, including visceral leishmaniasis (*P. argen′tipes, P. chinen′sis, P. ma′jor, P. marti′ni, P. orienta′lis, P. pernicio′sus*), Carrión's disease (*P. nogu′chi, P. verruca′rum*), cutaneous leishmaniasis (*P. lon′gipes, P. sergen′ti*), and phlebotomus fever (*P. papata′sii*).

phle·bot·o·my (flĕ-bot′ah-me) venotomy; incision of a vein.

Phlebovirus (fleb′o-vi″rus) sandfly fever viruses; a genus of the family Bunyaviridae including sandfly fever and Rift Valley fever viruses.

phlegm (flem) viscid mucus excreted in abnormally large quantities from the respiratory tract.

phleg·ma·sia (fleg-ma′zhah) [Gr.] old term for *inflammation.* **p. al′ba do′lens,** milk leg; phlebitis of the femoral vein with swelling of the leg, occasionally following parturition or an acute febrile illness. **p. ceru′lea do′lens,** an acute fulminating form of deep venous thrombosis, with pronounced edema and severe cyanosis of the limb.

phleg·mat·ic (fleg-mat′ik) of dull and sluggish temperament.

phleg·mon (fleg′mon) diffuse inflammation of the soft or connective tissue due to infection. **phleg′monous,** adj.

phlog(o)- word element [Gr.], *inflammation.*

phlo·go·gen·ic (flog″ah-jen′ik) producing inflammation.

phlo·rhi·zin hy·dro·lase (flo-ri′zin hi′dro-lās) glycosylceramidase.

phlyc·te·na (flik-te′nah) pl. *phlycte′nae.* [Gr.] 1. a small blister made by a burn. 2. a small vesicle containing lymph seen on the conjunctiva in certain conditions. **phlyc′tenar,** adj.

phlyc·ten·u·lar (flik-ten′u-lar) associated with the formation of phlyctenules, or of vesicle-like prominences.

phlyc·ten·ule (flik′tin-ūl) a minute vesicle; an ulcerated nodule of cornea or conjunctiva.

pho·bia (fo′be-ah) a persistent, irrational, intense fear of a specific object, activity, or situation (the phobic stimulus), fear that is recognized as being excessive or unreasonable by the individual himself. When a phobia is a significant source of distress or interferes with social functioning, it is considered a mental disorder (sometimes called a *phobic disorder*); in DSM-IV phobias are classified with the anxiety disorders and are subclassified as agoraphobia, specific phobias, and social phobias. **pho′bic,** adj. **simple p.,** specific p. **social p.,** an anxiety disorder characterized by fear and avoidance of social or performance situations in which the individual fears possible embarrassment and humiliation. **specific p.,** persistent and excessive or unreasonable fear of a circumscribed, well-defined object or situation.

-phobia word element [Gr.], *fear of; aversion to.*

pho·co·me·lia (fo″kah-me′le-ah) congenital absence of the proximal portion of a limb or limbs, the hands or feet being attached to the trunk by a small, irregularly shaped bone. **phocome′lic,** adj.

pho·com·e·lus (fo-kom′ĕ-lus) an individual exhibiting phocomelia.

phon·as·the·nia (fo″nas-the′ne-ah) weakness of the voice; difficult phonation from fatigue.

phon·en·do·scope (fo-nen′dah-skōp) a stethoscopic device that intensifies auscultatory sounds.

phon(o)- word element [Gr.], *sound; voice; speech.*

pho·no·car·di·og·ra·phy (fo″no-kahr″de-og′rah-fe) the graphic representation of heart sounds or murmurs; by extension, the term also includes pulse tracings (carotid, apex, and jugular pulses). **phonocardiograph′ic,** adj.

pho·no·cath·e·ter (-kath′ĕ-ter) a device similar to a conventional catheter, with a microphone at the tip.

pho·nol·o·gy (fah-nol′ah-je) the science of vocal sounds. **phonolog′ical,** adj.

pho·no·my·oc·lo·nus (fo″no-mi-ok′lah-nus) myoclonus in which a sound is heard on auscultation of an affected muscle, indicating fibrillar contractions.

pho·no·my·og·ra·phy (-mi-og′rah-fe) the recording of sounds produced by muscle contraction.

pho·no·stetho·graph (-steth′o-graf) an instrument by which chest sounds are amplified, filtered, and recorded.

pho·no·sur·gery (-sur″jer-e) a group of surgical procedures whose purpose is to restore, maintain, or enhance the voice.

phor·bol (for′bol) a polycyclic alcohol occurring in croton oil; it is the parent compound of the phorbol esters. **p. ester,** any of several esters of phorbol that are potent cocarcinogens, activating a cellular protein kinase; used in research to enhance the induction of mutagenesis or tumors by carcinogens.

-phore word element [Gr.], *a carrier.*

-phoresis word element [Gr.], *transmission.*

pho·ria (fo′re-ah) heterophoria.

phose (fōz) any subjective visual sensation, as of light or color.

phos·gene (fos′jēn) a suffocating and highly poisonous gas, carbonyl chloride, $COCl_2$, which causes rapidly fatal pulmonary edema or pneumonia on inhalation; used in the synthesis of organic compounds and formerly as a war gas.

phos·pha·gen (fos′fah-jen) any of a group of high-energy compounds, including phosphocreatine, that act as reservoirs of phosphate bond energy, donating phosphoryl groups for ATP synthesis when supplies are low.

phos·pha·tase (-tās) any of a group of enzymes that catalyze the hydrolytic cleavage of inorganic phosphate from esters.

phos·phate (fos′fāt) any salt or ester of phosphoric acid. **phosphat′ic,** adj.

phos·pha·te·mia (fos″fah-tēm′e-ah) an excess of phosphates in the blood.

phos·pha·ti·dic ac·id (-tid′ik) any of a group of compounds formed by esterification of three hydroxyl groups of glycerol with two fatty acid groups and one phosphoric acid group; from it are derived the phosphoglycerides.

phos·pha·ti·dyl·cho·line (-ti″dil-ko′lēn) a phospholipid comprising choline linked to phosphatidic acid; it is a major component of cell membranes and is localized preferentially in the outer surface of the plasma membrane.

phos·pha·tu·ria (-tūr′e-ah) 1. excretion of phosphates in the urine. 2. hyperphosphaturia.

phos·phene (fos′fēn) a sensation of light due to a stimulus other than light rays, e.g., a mechanical stimulus.

phos·pho·cre·a·tine (PC) (fos″fo-kre′ah-tin) the phosphagen of vertebrates, a creatine–phosphoric acid compound occurring in muscle, being an important storage form of high-energy phosphate, the energy source in muscle contraction.

phos·pho·di·es·ter·ase (-di-es′ter-ās) any of a group of enzymes that catalyze the hydrolytic cleavage of an ester linkage in a phosphoric acid compound containing two such ester linkages.

phos·pho·enol·py·ru·vate (-e″nol-pi′roo-vāt) a high energy derivative of pyruvate occurring as an intermediate in the Embden-Meyerhof pathway of glucose metabolism, in gluconeogenesis, and in the biosynthesis of some amino acids.

6-phos·pho·fruc·to·ki·nase (-frook″to-ki′nās) an enzyme catalyzing the phosphorylation of fructose 6-phosphate, a site of regulation in the Embden-Meyerhof pathway of glucose metabolism; deficiency of the muscle isozyme causes glycogen storage disease, type VII.

phos·pho·glyc·er·ate (-glis′er-āt) an anionic form of phosphoglyceric acid; 2-p. and 3-p. are interconvertible intermediates in the

Embden-Meyerhof pathway of glucose metabolism.

phos·pho·glyc·er·ide (-glis′er-īd) a class of phospholipids, whose parent compound is phosphatidic acid; they consist of a glycerol backbone, two fatty acids, and a phosphorylated alcohol (e.g., choline, ethanolamine, serine, or inositol) and are a major component of cell membranes.

phos·pho·ino·si·tide (-in-o′sĭ-tīd) any of a number of phosphorylated inositol-containing compounds that play roles in cell activation and calcium mobilization in response to hormones.

phos·pho·lip·ase (-lip′ās) any of four enzymes (phospholipase A to D), that catalyze the hydrolysis of specific ester bonds in phospholipids.

phos·pho·lip·id (-lip′id) any lipid that contains phosphorus, including those with a glycerol backbone (phosphoglycerides and plasmalogens) or a backbone of sphingosine or a related substance (sphingomyelins). They are the major lipids in cell membranes.

phos·pho·ne·cro·sis (-nĕ-kro′sis) phosphorus necrosis.

phos·pho·pro·tein (-pro′tēn) a conjugated protein in which phosphoric acid is esterified with a hydroxy amino acid.

phos·phor·ic ac·id (fos-for′ik) 1. orthophosphoric acid, the monomeric form H_3PO_4. 2. a general term encompassing the monomeric (orthophosphoric acid), dimeric (pyrophosphoric acid), and polymeric (metaphosphoric acid) forms of the acid. *Diluted p.a.* is used as a pharmaceutical solvent and a gastric acidifier.

phos·pho·rism (fos′fah-rizm) chronic phosphorus poisoning; see *phosphorus*.

phos·pho·rol·y·sis (fos″fah-rol′ĭ-sis) cleavage of a chemical bond with simultaneous addition of the elements of phosphoric acid to the residues.

phos·pho·rous ac·id (fos-for′us) H_3PO_3; its salts are the phosphites.

phos·pho·rus (P) (fos′fah-rus) chemical element (see *Table of Elements*), at. no. 15. Ingestion or inhalation produces toothache, phosphonecrosis (phossy jaw), anorexia, weakness, and anemia. Phosphorus is an essential element in the diet; in the form of phosphates, it is a major component of the mineral phase of bone and occurs in all tissues, being involved in almost all metabolic processes. **phos′phorous, phosphor′ic,** adj. **p. 32,** a radioisotope of phosphorus having a halflife of 14.28 days and emitting beta particles (1.71 MeV); therapeutic uses include treatment of polycythemia vera, chronic myelocytic leukemia, chronic lymphocytic leukemia, and certain ovarian and prostate carcinomas, palliation of metastatic skeletal disease, and treatment of intraperitoneal and intrapleural malignant effusions.

phos·phor·y·lase (fos-for′ĭ-lās) 1. any of a group of enzymes that catalyze the phosphorolysis of glycosides, transferring the cleaved glycosyl group to inorganic phosphate. When not qualified with the substrate name, the term usually denotes *glycogen phosphorylase* (animals) or *starch phosphorylase* (plants). 2. any of a group of enzymes that catalyze the transfer of a phosphate group to an organic acceptor.

phos·phor·y·lase ki·nase (fos-for′ĭ-lās ki′nās) phosphorylase *b* kinase; an enzyme that catalyzes the phosphorylation and activation of glycogen phosphorylase, a step in the cascade of reactions regulating glycogenolysis.

phos·phor·y·lase b ki·nase de·fi·cien·cy an X-linked disorder of glycogen storage due to deficiency of the enzyme in the liver, characterized in affected males by hepatomegaly, occasional fasting hypoglycemia, and some growth retardation.

phos·phor·y·la·tion (fos-for″ĭ-la′shun) the metabolic process of introducing a phosphate group into an organic molecule. **oxidative p.,** the formation of high-energy phosphate bonds by phosphorylation of ADP to ATP coupled to the transfer of electrons from reduced coenzymes to molecular oxygen via the electron transport chain; it occurs in the mitochondria. **substrate-level p.,** the formation of high-energy phosphate bonds by phosphorylation of ADP to ATP (or GDP to GTP) coupled to cleavage of a high-energy metabolic intermediate.

phos·pho·trans·fer·ase (fos″fo-trans′fer-ās) any of a subclass of enzymes that catalyze the transfer of a phosphate group.

pho·tal·gia (fo-tal′jah) pain, as in the eye, caused by light.

pho·tic (fo′tik) pertaining to light.

phot(o)- word element [Gr.], *light.*

pho·to·abla·tion (fo″to-ab-la′shun) volatilization of tissue by ultraviolet radiation emitted by a laser.

pho·to·ac·tive (-ak′tiv) reacting chemically to sunlight or ultraviolet radiation.

pho·to·al·ler·gen (-al′er-jen) an agent that elicits an allergic response to light.

pho·to·al·ler·gy (-al′er-je) a delayed immunologic type of photosensitivity involving a chemical substance to which the individual has previously become sensitized, combined with radiant energy. **photoaller′gic,** adj.

pho·to·bi·ol·o·gy (-bi-ol'ah-je) the branch of biology dealing with the effect of light on organisms. **photobiolog'ic, photobiolog'ical,** adj.

pho·to·bi·ot·ic (-bi-ot'ik) living only in the light.

pho·to·ca·tal·y·sis (-kah-tal'ĭ-sis) promotion or stimulation of a chemical reaction by light. **photocatalyt'ic,** adj.

pho·to·cat·a·lyst (-kat'ah-list) a substance, e.g., chlorophyll, that brings about a chemical reaction to light.

pho·to·chem·is·try (-kem'is-tre) the branch of chemistry dealing with the chemical properties or effects of light rays or other radiation. **photochem'ical,** adj.

pho·to·che·mo·ther·a·py (-ke"mo-ther'ah-pe) treatment by means of drugs (e.g., methoxsalen) that react to ultraviolet radiation or sunlight.

pho·to·co·ag·u·la·tion (-ko-ag"u-la'shun) condensation of protein material by the controlled use of an intense beam of light (e.g., argon laser) used especially in the treatment of retinal detachment and destruction of abnormal retinal vessels or intraocular tumor masses.

pho·to·der·ma·ti·tis (-der"mah-ti'tis) an abnormal state of the skin in which light is an important causative factor.

pho·to·dy·nam·ic (-di-nam'ik) powerful in the light; used particularly for the action exerted by fluorescent substances in the light.

pho·to·flu·o·rog·ra·phy (-floor"og'rah-fe) the photographic recording of fluoroscopic images on small films, using a fast lens.

pho·to·gen·ic (-jen'ik) 1. produced by light, as photogenic epilepsy. 2. producing or emitting light.

pho·to·lu·min·es·cence (-loo"min-es'ins) the quality of being luminescent after exposure to light or other electromagnetic radiation.

pho·tol·y·sis (fo-tol'ĭ-sis) chemical decomposition or change by the action of light or other radiant energy. **photolyt'ic,** adj.

pho·tom·e·try (fo-tom'ĕ-tre) measurement of the intensity of light.

pho·to·mi·cro·graph (fo"to-mi'kro-graf) a photograph of an object as seen through an ordinary light microscope.

pho·ton (fo'ton) a particle (quantum) of radiant energy.

pho·to·par·ox·ys·mal (fo"to-par"ok-siz'mil) photoconvulsive; denoting an abnormal electroencephalographic response to photic stimulation (brief flashes of light), marked by diffuse paroxysmal discharge recorded as spike-wave complexes; the response may be accompanied by minor seizures.

pho·to·pe·ri·od (fo'to-pēr"e-od) the period of time per day that an organism is exposed to daylight (or to artificial light). **photoperiod'ic,** adj.

pho·to·pe·ri·od·ism (fo"to-pēr'e-ah-dizm) the physiologic and behavioral reactions brought about in organisms by changes in the duration of daylight and darkness.

pho·to·phe·re·sis (-fĕ-re'sis) a technique for treating cutaneous T-cell lymphoma, in which a photoactive chemical is administered, the blood is removed and circulated through a source of ultraviolet radiation, then returned to the patient; it is believed to stimulate the immune system.

pho·to·phil·ic (-fil'ik) thriving in light.

pho·to·pho·bia (-fo'be-ah) abnormal visual intolerance to light. **photopho'bic,** adj.

pho·toph·thal·mia (fōt"of-thal'me-ah) ophthalmia due to exposure to intense light, as in snow blindness.

pho·to·pia (fo-to'pe-ah) day vision. **photop'ic,** adj.

pho·to·pig·ment (fo"to-pig'ment) a pigment that is unstable in the presence of light.

pho·top·sia (fo-top'se-ah) appearance as of sparks or flashes in retinal irritation.

pho·top·sin (fo-top'sin) the protein moiety of the cones of the retina that combines with retinal to form photochemical pigments.

pho·to·ptar·mo·sis (fo"to-tahr-mo'sis) sneezing caused by the influence of light.

pho·top·tom·e·ter (fo"top-tom'ĕ-ter) an instrument for measuring visual acuity by determining the smallest amount of light that will render an object just visible.

pho·to·re·ac·ti·va·tion (fo"to-re-ak"tĭ-va'shun) reversal of the biological effects of ultraviolet radiation on cells by subsequent exposure to visible light.

pho·to·re·cep·tor (-re-sep'ter) a nerve end-organ or receptor sensitive to light.

pho·to·re·frac·tive (-re-frak'tiv) pertaining to the refraction of light.

pho·to·ret·i·ni·tis (-ret"ĭ-ni'tis) retinitis due to exposure to intense light.

pho·to·scan (-skan) a two-dimensional representation of gamma rays emitted by a radioactive isotope in body tissue, produced by a printout mechanism utilizing a light source to expose a photographic film.

pho·to·sen·si·tive (-sen'sĭ-tiv) 1. reacting to light; said of a cell or organism. 2. having abnormally heightened sensitivity of the skin or eyes to sunlight.

pho·to·sen·si·ti·za·tion (-sen″sĭ-tĭ-za′shun) development of abnormally heightened reactivity of the skin or eyes to sunlight.

pho·to·sta·ble (fōt′o-sta″b'l) unchanged by the influence of light.

pho·to·syn·the·sis (fo″to-sin′thĭ-sis) a chemical combination caused by the action of light; specifically, the formation of carbohydrates from carbon dioxide and water in the chlorophyll tissue of plants under the influence of light. **photosynthet′ic,** adj.

pho·to·tax·is (-tak′sis) the movement of cells and microorganisms in response to light. **phototac′tic,** adj.

pho·to·ther·a·py (-ther′ah-pe) 1. treatment of disease by exposure to light. 2. photodynamic therapy.

pho·to·tox·ic (fo′to-tok″sik) having a toxic effect triggered by exposure to light.

pho·to·tro·phic (fo″to-tro′fik) capable of deriving energy from light.

pho·tot·ro·pism (fo-tot′rah-pizm) 1. the tendency of an organism to turn or move toward or away from light. 2. color change produced in a substance by the action of light. **phototrop′ic,** adj.

phren·ic (fren′ik) 1. diaphragmatic. 2. mental (1).

phren·i·co·col·ic (fren″ĭ-ko-kol′ik) pertaining to or connecting the diaphragm and colon.

phre·ni·tis (frĕ-ni′tis) diaphragmitis; inflammation of the diaphragm.

phren(o)- word element [Gr.], (1) *diaphragm;* (2) *mind;* (3) *phrenic nerve.*

phreno·gas·tric (fren″o-gas′trik) pertaining to the diaphragm and stomach.

phreno·he·pat·ic (-hĕ-pat′ik) pertaining to the diaphragm and liver.

phreno·ple·gia (-ple′jah) paralysis of the diaphragm.

phren·o·tro·pic (fren″o-tro′pik) exerting its principal effect upon the mind.

phryno·der·ma (frin″o-der′mah) a follicular hyperkeratosis probably due to deficiency of vitamin A or of essential fatty acids.

phthal·ein (thal′ēn) any one of a series of coloring matters formed by the condensation of phthalic anhydride with the phenols.

phthir·i·a·sis (thi-ri′ah-sis) infestation with *Phthirus pubis.*

Phthir·us (thir′us) a genus of lice, including *P. pu′bis* (the pubic, or crab, louse), which infests the hair of the pubic region, and sometimes the eyebrows and eyelashes.

phthi·sis (thi′sis, ti′sis) a wasting of the body.

Phy·co·my·ce·tes (fi″ko-mi-sēt′ēz) a group of fungi comprising common water, leaf, and bread molds; they can cause phycomycosis in humans.

phy·co·my·co·sis (-mi-ko′sis) 1. any of a group of acute fungal diseases caused by members of Phycomycetes. 2. mucormycosis.

phy·log·e·ny (fi-loj′ĭ-ne) the complete developmental history of a group of organisms. **phylogen′ic,** adj.

phy·lum (fi′lum) pl. *phy′la.* [L.] a primary division of a kingdom, composed of a group of related classes; in the taxonomy of plants and fungi, the term *division* is used instead. Mycologists sometimes use the word to denote any important group of organisms.

phy·ma (fi′mah) pl. *phy′mata.* [Gr.] a skin swelling or tumor larger than a tubercle.

phys·iat·rics (fiz″e-a′triks) physiatry.

phys·iat·rist (-trist) a physician who specializes in physiatry.

phys·iat·ry (-tre) the branch of medicine that deals with the prevention, diagnosis, and treatment of disease or injury, and the rehabilitation from resultant impairments and disabilities, using physical and sometimes pharmaceutical agents.

phys·i·cal (fiz′ik-il) pertaining to the body, to material things, or to physics.

phy·si·cian (fi-zish′in) 1. an authorized practitioner of medicine, as one graduated from a college of medicine or osteopathy and licensed by the appropriate board; see also *doctor.* 2. one who practices medicine as distinct from surgery. **p. assistant,** one who has been trained in an accredited program and certified by an appropriate board to perform certain of a physician's duties, including history taking, physical examination, diagnostic tests, treatment, and certain minor surgical procedures, all under the responsible supervision of a licensed physician. Abbreviated P.A. **attending p.,** 1. a physician who has admitting privileges at a hospital. 2. the physician with primary responsibility for the care of a patient in a particular case. **emergency p.,** a specialist in emergency medicine. **family p.,** a medical specialist who plans and provides the comprehensive primary health care of all members of a family, regardless of age or sex, on a continuous basis. **resident p.,** a graduate and licensed physician receiving training in a specialty, usually in a hospital.

phys·i·co·chem·i·cal (fiz″ĭ-ko-kem′ik-il) pertaining to both physics and chemistry.

phys·ics (fiz′iks) the study of the laws and phenomena of nature, especially of forces and general properties of matter and energy.

physi(o)- word element [Gr.], *nature; physiology; physical.*

phys·io·chem·i·cal (fiz″e-o-kem′ik-il) pertaining to both physiology and chemistry.

phys·i·og·no·my (fiz″e-og′nah-me) 1. determination of mental or moral character and qualities by the face.   2. the countenance, or face.   3. the facial expression and appearance as a means of diagnosis.

phys·i·o·log·ic (fiz″e-o-loj′ik) physiological.

phys·i·o·log·i·cal (-loj′ĭ-kal) pertaining to physiology; normal; not pathologic.

phys·i·ol·o·gist (fiz″e-ol′ah-jist) a specialist in physiology.

phys·i·ol·o·gy (-je) 1. the science which treats of the functions of the living organism and its parts, and of the physical and chemical factors and processes involved.   2. the basic processes underlying the functioning of a species or class of organism, or any of its parts or processes.   **morbid p., pathologic p.,** the study of disordered function or of function in diseased tissues.

phys·io·patho·log·ic (fiz″e-o-path″o-loj′ik) pertaining to pathologic physiology.

phys·io·ther·a·pist (-ther′ah-pist) physical therapist.

phys·io·ther·a·py (-ther′ah-pe) physical therapy.

phy·sique (fĭ-zēk′) the body organization, development, and structure.

phys(o)- word element [Gr.], *air; gas.*

phy·so·hem·a·to·me·tra (fi″so-hem″ah-to-me′trah) gas and blood in the uterine cavity.

phy·so·hy·dro·me·tra (-hi″dro-me′trah) gas and serum in the uterine cavity.

phy·so·me·tra (-me′trah) gas in the uterine cavity.

phy·so·stig·mine (-stig′mēn) a cholinergic alkaloid usually obtained from dried ripe seed of *Physostigma venenosum* (Calabar bean), used as a topical miotic and to reverse the central nervous system effects of an overdosage of anticholinergic drugs; used in the form of the salicylate and sulfate salts.

phy·tan·ic ac·id (fi-tan′ik) a 20-carbon branched-chain fatty acid occurring at high levels in dairy products and the fat of ruminants and accumulated in the tissues in Refsum's disease.

phy·tic ac·id (fi′tik) the hexaphosphoric acid ester of inositol, found in many plants and microorganisms and in animal tissues.

phyt(o)- word element [Gr.], *plant; an organism of the vegetable kingdom.*

phy·to·be·zoar (fi″to-be′zor) a bezoar composed of vegetable fibers.

phy·to·es·tro·gen (-es′tro-jen) any of a group of weakly estrogenic, nonsteroidal compounds widely occurring in plants.

phy·to·hem·ag·glu·ti·nin (-hem″ah-glōōt′in-in) a hemagglutinin of plant origin.

phy·to·hor·mone (-hor′mōn) plant hormone; any of the hormones produced in plants; they are active in controlling growth and other functions at a site remote from their place of production.

phy·to·med·i·cine (-med′ĭ-sin) 1. a preparation of a medicinal herb.   2. herbalism.

phy·to·na·di·one (fi-to″nah-di′ōn) vitamin K₁: a vitamin found in green plants or prepared synthetically, used as a prothrombinogenic agent.

phy·to·par·a·site (fi″to-par″ah-sīt) any parasitic vegetable organism or species.

phy·to·path·o·gen·ic (-path″ah-jen′ik) producing disease in plants.

phy·to·pa·thol·o·gy (-pah-thol′ah-je) the pathology of plants.

phy·to·pho·to·der·ma·ti·tis (-fo″to-der″mah-ti′tis) phototoxic dermatitis induced by exposure to certain plants and then to sunlight.

phy·to·pre·cip·i·tin (-pre-sip′ĭ-tin) a precipitin formed in response to vegetable antigen.

phy·to·sis (fi-to′sis) any disease caused by a phytoparasite.

phy·to·ther·a·py (fi″to-ther′ah-pe) treatment by use of plants.

phy·to·tox·ic (fi′to-tok″sik) 1. pertaining to phytotoxin.   2. poisonous to plants.

phy·to·tox·in (-tok″sin) an exotoxin produced by certain species of higher plants; any toxin of plant origin.

pia-ar·ach·ni·tis (pi″ah-ar″ak-ni′tis) leptomeningitis.

pia-arach·noid (-ah-rak′noid) the pia mater and arachnoid considered together as one functional unit; the leptomeninges.

pia-glia (pi″ah-gli′ah) a membrane constituting one of the layers of the pia-arachnoid.

pi·al (pi′il) pertaining to the pia mater.

pia ma·ter (pi′ah ma′ter) [L.] the innermost of the three meninges covering the brain and spinal cord.

pi·arach·noid (pi″ah-rak′noid) pia-arachnoid.

pi·ca (pi′kah) [L.] compulsive eating of nonnutritive substances, such as ice, dirt, flaking paint, clay, hair, or laundry starch.

pico- word element [It.] designating one trillionth (10^{-12}) part of the unit to which it is joined. Symbol p.

pi·co·gram (pg) (pi′ko-gram) one-trillionth (10^{-12}) of a gram.

pi·cor·na·vi·rus (pi-kor″nah-vi′rus) an extremely small, ether-resistant RNA virus, one of the group comprising the enteroviruses and the rhinoviruses.

pic·rate (pik'rāt) any salt of picric acid.

pic·ric ac·id (-rik) trinitrophenol.

picr(o)- word element [Gr.], 1. *bitter.* 2. *related to picric acid.*

pic·ro·car·mine (pik″ro-kahr'min) a histological stain consisting of a mixture of carmine, ammonia, distilled water, and aqueous solution of picric acid.

PID pelvic inflammatory disease.

pie·bald·ism (pi-bawld'izm) a condition in which the skin is partly brown and partly white, as in partial albinism and vitiligo.

pi·e·dra (pe-a'drah) a fungal disease of the hair in which white or black nodules of fungi form on the shafts.

pi·eses·the·sia (pi-e″zes-the'zhah) the sense by which pressure stimuli are felt.

pi·esim·e·ter (pi″ĕ-sim'ĕ-ter) instrument for testing the sensitiveness of the skin to pressure.

-piesis word element [Gr.], *pressure.* **-pies'ic,** adj.

pig·ment (pig'mint) 1. any coloring matter of the body. 2. a stain or dyestuff. 3. a paintlike medicinal preparation to be applied to the skin. **pig'mentary,** adj. **bile p.,** any of the coloring matters of the bile, including bilirubin, biliverdin, etc. **blood p., hematogenous p.,** any of the pigments derived from hemoglobin. **respiratory p's,** substances, e.g., hemoglobin, myoglobin, or cytochromes, which take part in the oxidative processes of the animal body. **retinal p's, visual p's,** the photopigments in retinal rods and cones that respond to certain colors of light and initiate the process of vision.

pig·men·ta·tion (pig″men-ta'shun) the deposition of coloring matter; the coloration or discoloration of a part by a pigment.

pig·ment·ed (pig-ment'id) colored by deposit of pigment.

pig·men·to·phage (pig-men'tah-fāj) any pigment-destroying cell, especially such a cell of the hair.

pi·lar (pi'lar) pertaining to the hair.

pile (pīl) 1. hemorrhoid. 2. an aggregation of similar elements for generating electricity. **sentinel p.,** a hemorrhoid-like thickening of the mucous membrane at the lower end of an anal fissure.

pi·le·us (pil'e-us) caul.

pi·li (pi'li) [L.] plural of *pilus.*

pi·lif·er·ous (pi-lif'er-us) bearing or producing hair.

pill (pil) tablet.

pil·lar (pil'er) a supporting column, usually occurring in pairs. **articular p's,** columnlike structures formed by the articulation of the superior and inferior articular processes of the vertebrae. **p's of fauces,** folds of mucous membrane at the sides of the fauces.

pil(o)- word element [L.], *hair; composed of hair.*

pi·lo·car·pine (pi″lo-kahr'pēn) a cholinergic alkaloid, used as the base or the hydrochloride or nitrate salt as an antiglaucoma agent and miotic and as the hydrochloride salt in the treatment of xerostomia associated with radiotherapy or Sjögren's syndrome.

pi·lo·cys·tic (-sis'tik) hollow or cystlike, and containing hair; said of dermoid tumors.

pi·lo·erec·tion (-e-rek'shun) erection of the hair.

pi·lo·leio·myo·ma (-li″o-mi-o'mah) cutaneous leiomyoma arising from the arrectores pilorum muscles.

pi·lo·ma·trix·o·ma (-ma-trik'so-mah) a benign, circumscribed, calcifying epithelial neoplasm derived from hair matrix cells, manifested as a small, firm, intracutaneous spheroid mass, usually on the face, neck, or arms.

pi·lo·mo·tor (-mōt'er) pertaining to the arrector muscles, the contraction of which produces cutis anserina (goose flesh) and piloerection.

pi·lo·ni·dal (-nīd'l) having a nidus of hairs.

pi·lose (pi'lōs) hairy; covered with hair.

pi·lo·se·ba·ceous (pi″lo-sĕ-ba'shus) pertaining to the hair follicles and the sebaceous glands.

pi·lus (pi'lus) pl. *pi'li.* [L.] 1. a hair. **pi'lial,** adj. 2. one of the minute filamentous appendages of certain bacteria, associated with antigenic properties of the cell surface. **pi'liate,** adj. **pi'li cunicula'ti,** a condition characterized by burrowing hairs. **pi'li incarna'ti,** a condition characterized by ingrown hairs. **pi'li tor'ti,** a condition characterized by twisted hairs.

pim·e·li·tis (pim″ĕ-li'tis) inflammation of the adipose tissue.

pim·e·lop·ter·yg·i·um (pim″ĕ-lo-ter-ij'e-um) a fatty outgrowth on the conjunctiva.

pi·mo·zide an antipsychotic and antidyskinetic agent used in the treatment of Gilles de la Tourette's syndrome.

pim·ple (pim'p'l) a papule or pustule.

pin (pin) a slender, elongated piece of metal used for securing fixation of parts. **Steinmann p.,** a metal rod for the internal fixation of fractures.

pin·do·lol (pin'dah-lol) a nonselective betaadrenergic blocking agent with intrinsic sympathomimetic activity; used in the treatment of hypertension.

pin·e·al (pin'e-il) 1. pertaining to the pineal body. 2. shaped like a pine cone.

pin·e·al·ec·to·my (pin"e-ah-lek'tah-me) excision of the pineal body.

pin·e·al·ism (pin'e-ah-lizm) the condition due to deranged secretion of the pineal body.

pin·e·a·lo·blas·to·ma (pin"e-ah-lo-blas-to'mah) pinealoma in which the pineal cells are not well differentiated.

pin·e·a·lo·cyte (pin'e-ah-lo-sīt") an epithelioid cell of the pineal body.

pin·e·a·lo·ma (pin"e-ah-lo'mah) a tumor of the pineal body composed of neoplastic nests of large epithelial cells; it may cause hydrocephalus, precocious puberty, and gait disturbances.

pin·gue·cu·la (ping-gwek'u-lah) pl. *pin-gue'culae*. [L.] a benign yellowish spot on the bulbar conjunctiva.

pin·i·form (pin'ĭ-form) conical or cone shaped.

pink·eye (pink'i") acute contagious conjunctivitis.

pin·na (pin'ah) auricle (1). **pin'nal**, adj.

pino·cyte (pi'nah-sīt) a cell that exhibits pinocytosis. **pinocyt'ic**, adj.

pino·cy·to·sis (pi"nah-si-to'sis) a mechanism by which cells ingest extracellular fluid and its contents; it involves the formation of invaginations by the cell membrane, which close and break off to form fluid-filled vacuoles in the cytoplasm. **pinocytot'ic**, adj.

pino·some (pi'no-sōm) the intracellular vacuole formed by pinocytosis.

pint (pīnt) a unit of liquid measure; in the United States it is 16 fluid ounces (0.473 liter). In Great Britain, it is the *imperial pint*, equal to 20 fluid ounces (0.568 liter).

pin·ta (pin'tah) a treponemal infection of tropical America, characterized by bizarre pigmentary changes in the skin.

pin·worm (pin'wurm) oxyurid.

pi·o·glit·a·zone (pi"o-glit'ah-zōn) an antidiabetic agent that decreases insulin resistance in the peripheral tissues and liver; used as the hydrochloride salt in the treatment of type 2 diabetes mellitus.

pip·ecol·ic ac·id (pip"ĕ-kol'ik) a cyclic amino acid occurring as an intermediate in a minor pathway of lysine degradation and at elevated levels in the blood in cerebrohepatorenal syndrome and in hyperlysinemia.

pip·e·cu·ro·ni·um (-ku-ro'ne-um) a nondepolarizing neuromuscular blocking agent used as the bromide salt as an adjunct to anesthesia, inducing skeletal muscle relaxation.

pi·per·a·cil·lin (pi-per'ah-sil"in) a semisynthetic broad-spectrum penicillin effective against a wide variety of gram-positive and gram-negative bacteria; used as the sodium salt.

pi·per·a·zine (-zēn) an anthelmintic used against *Ascaris lumbricoides* and *Enterobius vermicularis*; used as the citrate salt.

pi·pet (pi-pet') pipette.

pi·pette (pi-pet') [Fr.] 1. a glass or transparent plastic tube used in measuring or transferring small quantities of liquid or gas. 2. to dispense by means of a pipette.

pir·bu·ter·ol (pir-bu'ter-ol) a β_2-adrenergic receptor agonist, used in the form of the acetate ester as a bronchodilator.

pir·i·form (pir'ĭ-form) pear-shaped.

Pi·ro·plas·ma (pi"ro-plaz'mah) *Babesia*.

pi·ro·plas·mo·sis (-plaz-mo'sis) babesiasis.

pir·ox·i·cam (pir-ok'sĭ-kam) a nonsteroidal antiinflammatory drug used in the treatment of various rheumatic disorders and dysmenorrhea.

pi·si·form (pi'sĭ-form) resembling a pea in shape and size.

PIT plasma iron turnover.

pit (pit) 1. a hollow fovea or indentation. 2. a pockmark. 3. a small depression or fault in the dental enamel. 4. to indent, or to become and remain for a few minutes indented, by pressure. 5. a small depression in the nail plate. **anal p.**, proctodeum. **arm p.**, the axilla or axillary fossa. **coated p's**, small clathrin-coated pits occurring in the plasma membrane of many cells and involved in receptor-mediated endocytosis. **ear p.**, preauricular p. **lens p.**, a pitlike depression in the ectoderm of the lens placode where the primordial lens is developing. **olfactory p.**, the primordium of a nasal cavity. **otic p.**, a depression appearing in each otic placode, marking the beginning of embryonic development of the internal ear. **preauricular p.**, a small depression anterior to the helix of the ear, sometimes leading to a fistula or congenital preauricular cyst.

pitch (pich) 1. a dark viscous residue from distillation of tar and other substances. 2. any of various bituminous substances such as natural asphalt. 3. a resin from the sap of some coniferous trees. 4. the quality of sound dependent principally on its frequency.

pith·e·coid (pith'ĭ-koid) apelike.

pit·ta (pit'ah) [Sanskrit] in ayurveda, one of the three doshas, condensed from the elements fire and water. It is the principle of transformation energy and governs heat and metabolism in the body, is concerned with the digestive, enzymatic, and endocrine systems, and is eliminated from the body through sweat.

pit·ting (pit′ing) 1. the formation, usually by scarring, of a small depression. 2. the removal from erythrocytes, by the spleen, of such structures as iron granules, without destruction of the cells. 3. remaining indented for a few minutes after removal of firm finger pressure, distinguishing fluid edema from myxedema.

pi·tu·i·cyte (pĭ-tu′ĭ-sīt) the distinctive fusiform cell composing most of the neurohypophysis.

pi·tu·i·ta·rism (pĭ-too′ĭ-tah-rizm″) disorder of pituitary function; see *hyper-* and *hypopituitarism.*

pi·tu·i·tary (pĭ-too′ĭ-tar″e) 1. hypophysial. 2. pituitary gland; see under *gland.* **anterior p.,** adenohypophysis. **posterior p.,** neurohypophysis.

pit·y·ri·a·sis (pit″ĭ-ri′ah-sis) any of various skin diseases characterized by the formation of fine, branny scales. **p. al′ba,** a chronic condition with patchy scaling and hypopigmentation of the skin of the face. **p. ro′sea,** a dermatosis marked by scaling, pink, oval macules arranged with the long axes parallel to the cleavage lines of the skin. **p. ru′bra pila′ris,** a chronic inflammatory skin disease marked by pink scaling macules and horny follicular papules, beginning usually with seborrhea of the scalp and face, with keratoderma of palms and soles. **p. versi′color,** tinea versicolor.

pit·y·roid (pit′ĭ-roid) furfuraceous; branny.

Pit·y·ros·po·rum (pit″ĭ-ros′pĕ-rum) former name for *Malassezia.*

piv·a·late (piv′ah-lāt) USAN contraction for trimethylacetate.

pKₐ the negative logarithm of the ionization constant (K) of an acid, the pH of a solution in which half of the acid molecules are ionized.

PKU, PKU1 phenylketonuria.

pla·ce·bo (plah-se′bo) [L.] any dummy medical treatment; originally, a medicinal preparation having no specific pharmacological activity against the patient's illness or complaint given solely for the psychophysiological effects of the treatment; more recently, a dummy treatment administered to the control group in a controlled clinical trial in order that the specific and nonspecific effects of the experimental treatment can be distinguished.

pla·cen·ta (plah-sen′tah) pl. *placentas, placen′tae.* [L.] an organ characteristic of true mammals during pregnancy, joining mother and fetus, providing endocrine secretion and selective exchange of soluble bloodborne substances through apposition of uterine and trophoblastic vascularized parts. **placen′tal,** adj. **p. accre′ta,** one abnormally adherent to the myometrium, with partial or complete absence of the decidua basalis. **circumvallate p.,** one in which a dense peripheral ring is raised from the surface and the attached membranes are doubled back over the placental edge. **deciduate p., deciduous p.,** a placenta or type of placentation in which the decidua or maternal parts of the placenta separate from the uterus and are cast off together with the trophoblastic parts. **fetal p.,** the part of the placenta derived from the chorionic sac that encloses the embryo, consisting of a chorionic plate and villi. **hemochorial p.,** one in which maternal blood comes in direct contact with the chorion, as in humans. **p. incre′ta,** placenta accreta with penetration of the myometrium. **maternal p.,** the maternally contributed part of the placenta, derived from the decidua basalis. **p. membrana′cea,** one that is abnormally thin and spread out over an unusually large area of the uterine wall. **p. percre′ta,** placenta accreta with invasion of the myometrium to its peritoneal covering, sometimes causing rupture of the uterus. **p. pre′via,** one located in the lower uterine segment, so that it partially or completely covers or adjoins the internal os. **p. spu′ria,** an accessory portion having no blood vessel attachment to the main placenta. **p. succenturia′ta, succenturiate p.,** an accessory portion attached to the main placenta by an artery or vein. **villous p.,** one characterized by the presence of villi that are outgrowths of the chorion.

pla·cen·ta·tion (pla″sen-ta′shun) the series of events following implantation of the embryo and leading to development of the placenta.

pla·cen·ti·tis (-ti′tis) inflammation of the placenta.

pla·cen·tog·ra·phy (-tog′rah-fe) radiological visualization of the placenta after injection of a contrast medium.

pla·cen·toid (plah-sen′toid) resembling the placenta.

plac·ode (plak′ōd) a platelike structure, especially a thickened plate of ectoderm in the early embryo, from which a sense organ develops, e.g., *otic p.* (ear), *lens p.* (eye), and *nasal p.* (nose).

pla·gio·ceph·a·ly (pla″je-o-sef′ah-le) an asymmetric condition of the head, due to irregular closure of the cranial sutures. **plagiocephal′ic,** adj.

plague (plāg) a severe acute or chronic infectious disease due to *Yersinia pestis,* beginning with chills and fever, quickly followed by prostration, often with delirium, headache, vomiting, and diarrhea; primarily a disease of rats and other rodents, it is transmitted to humans by flea bites, or communicated from patient to patient. **bubonic p.,** plague with swelling of the lymph nodes, which form buboes in the femoral, inguinal, axillary, and cervical regions; in the severe form, septicemia occurs, producing petechial hemorrhages. **pneumonic p., pulmonic p.,** a rapidly progressive, highly contagious pneumonia with extensive involvement of the lungs and productive cough with mucoid, bloody, foamy, plague bacilli-laden sputum. **sylvatic p.,** plague in wild rodents, such as the ground squirrel, which serve as a reservoir from which humans may be infected.

pla·nar (pla′nar) 1. flat. 2. of or pertaining to a plane.

plane (plān) 1. a flat surface determined by the position of three points in space. 2. a specified level, as the plane of anesthesia. 3. to rub away or abrade; see *planing.* 4. a superficial incision in the wall of a cavity or between tissue layers, especially in plastic surgery, made so that the precise point of entry into the cavity or between the layers can be determined. **axial p.,** one parallel with the long axis of a structure. **base p.,** an imaginary plane upon which is estimated the retention of an artificial denture. **coronal p's,** frontal p's. **Frankfort horizontal p.,** a horizontal plane represented in profile by a line between the lowest point on the margin of the orbit and the highest point on the margin of the auditory meatus. **frontal p's,** those passing longitudinally through the body from side to side, at right angles to the median plane, dividing the body into front and back parts. **horizontal p.,** 1. one passing through the body, at right angles to both the frontal and median planes, dividing the body into upper and lower parts. 2. one passing through a tooth at right angles to its long axis. **median p.,** one passing longitudinally through the middle of the body from front to back, dividing it into right and left halves. **nuchal p.,** the outer surface of the occipital bone between the foramen magnum and the superior nuchal line. **occipital p.,** the outer surface of the occipital bone above the superior nuchal line. **orbital p.,** 1. the orbital surface of the maxilla. 2. visual p. **sagittal p's,** vertical planes passing through the body parallel to the median plane (or to the sagittal suture), dividing the body into left and right portions. **temporal p.,** the depressed area on the side of the skull below the inferior

temporal line. **transverse p.,** one passing horizontally through the body, at right angles to the sagittal and frontal planes, and dividing the body into upper and lower portions. **vertical p.,** one perpendicular to a horizontal plane, dividing the body into left and right, or front and back portions. **visual p.,** one passing through the visual axes of the two eyes.

pla·nig·ra·phy (plah-nig′rah-fe) tomography. **planigraph′ic,** adj.

plan·ing (pla′ning) abrasion of disfigured skin to promote reepithelialization with minimal scarring; done by mechanical means (dermabrasion) or by application of a caustic (chemabrasion).

plan·ning (plan′ing) consciously setting forth a scheme to achieve a desired end or goal. **natural family p.,** rhythm method.

pla·no·cel·lu·lar (pla″no-sel′u-lar) composed of flat cells.

pla·no·con·cave (-kon′kāv) flat on one side and concave on the other.

pla·no·con·vex (-kon′veks) flat on one side and convex on the other.

plan·ta (plan′tah) the sole of the foot.

plant (plant) any multicellular eukaryotic organism that performs photosynthesis to obtain its nutrition; plants comprise one of the five kingdoms in the most widely used classification of living organisms.

Plan·ta·go (plan-ta′go) a genus of herbs, including *P. in′dica, P. psyl′lium* (Spanish psyllium), and *P. ova′ta* (blond psyllium); see also *psyllium.*

plan·tal·gia (plan-tal′jah) pain in the sole of the foot.

plan·tar (plan′tar) pertaining to the sole of the foot.

plan·ta·ris (plan-ta′ris) [L.] plantar.

plan·ti·grade (plan′tĭ-grād) walking on the full sole of the foot.

plan·u·la (plan′ūl-ah) 1. a larval coelenterate. 2. something resembling such an animal.

pla·num (pla′num) pl. *pla′na.* [L.] plane.

plaque (plak) 1. any patch or flat area. 2. a superficial, solid, elevated skin lesion. **attachment p's,** small regions of increased density along the sarcolemma of skeletal muscles to which myofilaments seem to attach. **bacterial p., dental p.,** a soft thin film of food debris, mucin, and dead epithelial cells on the teeth, providing the medium for bacterial growth. It contains calcium, phosphorus, and other salts, polysaccharides, proteins, carbohydrates, and lipids, and plays a role in the development of caries, dental calculus, and periodontal and gingival diseases. **fibrous p.,** the lesion of atherosclerosis, a pearly white area within an artery that causes the intimal surface to bulge into the lumen; it is composed of lipid, cell debris, smooth muscle cells, collagen, and, in older persons, calcium. **Hollenhorst p's,** atheromatous emboli containing cholesterol crystals in the retinal arterioles, a sign of impending serious cardiovascular disease. **senile p's,** microscopic argyrophilic masses composed of fragmented axon terminals and dendrites surrounding a core of amyloid, seen in small amounts in the cerebral cortex of healthy elderly people and in larger amounts in those with Alzheimer's disease.

-plasia word element [Gr.], *development; formation.*

plasm (plazm) 1. plasma. 2. formative substance (cytoplasm, hyaloplasm, etc.).

plas·ma (plaz'mah) 1. blood plasma; the fluid portion of the blood in which the particulate components are suspended. 2. the fluid portion of the lymph. **plasmat'ic,** adj. **antihemophilic human p.,** human plasma which has been processed promptly to preserve the antihemophilic properties of the original blood; used for temporary correction of bleeding tendency in hemophilia. **blood p.,** plasma (1). **citrated p.,** blood plasma treated with sodium citrate, which prevents clotting. **seminal p.,** the fluid portion of the semen, in which the spermatozoa are suspended.

plas·ma·blast (-blast) the immature precursor of a plasma cell.

plas·ma·cyte (-sīt) plasma cell. **plasmacyt'ic,** adj.

plas·ma·cy·to·ma (plaz″mah-si-to'mah) 1. plasma cell dyscrasias. 2. solitary myeloma.

plas·ma·cy·to·sis (-si-to'sis) an excess of plasma cells in the blood.

plas·ma·lem·ma (-lem'ah) 1. plasma membrane. 2. a thin peripheral layer of the ectoplasm in a fertilized egg.

plas·ma·lo·gen (plaz-mal'ŏ-jen) any of various phospholipids in which the group at one C1 of glycerol is an ether-linked alcohol in place of an ester-linked fatty acid, found in myelin sheaths of nerve fibers, cell membranes of muscle, and platelets.

plas·ma·phe·re·sis (plaz″mah-fĕ-re'sis) the removal of plasma from withdrawn blood, with retransfusion of the formed elements into the donor; generally, type-specific fresh frozen plasma or albumin is used to replace the withdrawn plasma. The procedure may be done for purposes of collecting plasma components or for therapeutic purposes.

plas·mid (plaz'mid) an extrachromosomal self-replicating structure of bacterial cells that carries genes for a variety of functions not essential for cell growth and that can be transferred to other cells by conjugation or transduction. See also *episome.* **F p.,** a conjugative plasmid found in F⁺ (male) bacterial cells that leads with high frequency to its transfer, and much less often to transfer of the bacterial chromosome, to an F⁻ (female) cell lacking such a plasmid. **R p., resistance p.,** a conjugative factor in bacterial cells that promotes resistance to agents such as antibiotics, metal ions, ultraviolet radiation, and bacteriophages.

plas·min (plaz'min) an endopeptidase occurring in plasma as plasminogen, which is activated via cleavage by plasminogen activators; it solubilizes fibrin clots, degrades other coagulation-related proteins, and can be activated for use in therapeutic thrombolysis.

plas·min·o·gen (plaz-min'ah-jen) the inactive precursor of plasmin, occurring in plasma and converted to plasmin by the action of urokinase.

plas·min·o·gen ac·ti·va·tor (ak'tĭ-va″tor) see under *activator.*

plas·mo·cyte (plaz'mo-sīt) plasma cell.

plas·mo·di·ci·dal (plaz-mōd'ĭ-si'd'l) malariacidal; destructive to plasmodia.

Plas·mo·di·um (plaz-mo'de-um) a genus of sporozoa parasitic in the red blood cells of animals and humans. Four species, *P. falci'parum, P. mala'riae, P. ova'le,* and *P. vi'vax,* cause the four specific types of malaria in humans.

plas·mo·di·um (plaz-mo'de-um) pl. *plasmo'-dia.* 1. A parasite of the genus *Plasmodium.* 2. a multinucleate continuous mass of protoplasm formed by aggregation and fusion of myxamebae. **plasmo'dial,** adj.

plas·mol·y·sis (plaz-mol'ĭ-sis) contraction of cell protoplasm due to loss of water by osmosis. **plasmolyt'ic,** adj.

plas·mon (plaz'mon) the hereditary factors of the egg cytoplasm.

plas·mor·rhex·is (plaz″mo-rek'sis) erythrocytorrhexis.

plas·mos·chi·sis (plaz-mos'kĭ-sis) the splitting up of cell protoplasm.

plas·ter (plas'ter) 1. a gypsum material that hardens when mixed with water, used for immobilizing or making impressions of body parts. 2. a pastelike mixture that can be spread over the skin and that is adhesive at body temperature; varied uses include skin protectant and counterirritant. **p. of Paris,** calcined calcium sulfate; on addition of water it forms a porous mass that is used in making casts and bandages to support or immobilize body parts, and in dentistry for making study models.

plas·tic (-tik) 1. tending to build up tissues to restore a lost part. 2. capable of being molded. 3. a high-molecular-weight polymeric material, usually organic, capable of being molded, extruded, drawn, or otherwise shaped and hardened into a form. 4. material that can be molded.

-plasty word element [Gr.], *formation* or *plastic repair of.*

plate (plāt) 1. a flat structure or layer, as a thin layer of bone. 2. dental p. 3. to apply a culture medium to a Petri dish. 4. to inoculate such a plate with bacteria. **bite p.,** biteplate. **bone p.,** a metal bar with perforations for the insertion of screws, used to immobilize fractured segments. **cribriform p.,** fascia cribrosa. **dental p.,** a plate of acrylic resin, metal, or other material, which is fitted to the shape of the mouth and serves to support artificial teeth. **dorsal p.,** roof p. **epiphyseal p.,** the thin plate of cartilage between the epiphysis and the metaphysis of a growing long bone. **equatorial p.,** the collection of chromosomes at the equator of the spindle in mitosis. **floor p.,** the unpaired ventral longitudinal zone of the neural tube. **foot p.,** 1. see *footplate.* 2. the embryonic precursor of a foot. **growth p.,** epiphyseal p. **hand p.,** a flattened expansion at the end of the embryonic limb; the precursor of the hand. **medullary p.,** neural p. **motor end p.,** end plate. **muscle p.,** myotome (2). **nail p.,** nail (1). **neural p.,** the thickened plate of ectoderm in the embryo that develops into the neural tube. **roof p.,** the unpaired dorsal longitudinal zone of the neural tube. **tarsal p.,** tarsus (2). **tympanic p.,** the bony plate forming the floor and sides of the meatus auditorius. **ventral p.,** floor p.

plate·let (plāt′let) thrombocyte; a disk-shaped structure, 2 to 4 μm in diameter, found in the blood of mammals and important for its role in blood coagulation; platelets, which are formed by detachment of part of the cytoplasm of a megakaryocyte, lack a nucleus and DNA but contain active enzymes and mitochondria.

plate·let·phe·re·sis (plāt″let-fĭ-re′sis) thrombocytapheresis.

plat·i·num (Pt) (plat′ĭ-num) chemical element (see *Table of Elements*), at. no. 78.

platy- word element [Gr.], *flat.*

platy·ba·sia (plat″ĭ-ba′zhah) 1. basilar impression. 2. malformation of the base of the skull due to softening of skull bones or a developmental anomaly, with bulging upwards of the floor of the posterior cranial fossa, upward displacement of the upper cervical vertebrae, and bony impingement on the brainstem.

platy·co·ria (-kor′e-ah) a dilated condition of the pupil of the eye.

platy·hel·minth (-hel′minth) one of the Platyhelminthes; a flatworm.

Platy·hel·min·thes (-hel-min′thēz) a phylum of acoelomate, dorsoventrally flattened, bilaterally symmetrical animals, commonly known as flatworms; it includes the classes Cestoidea (tapeworms) and Trematoda (flukes).

platy·hi·er·ic (-hi-er′ik) having a sacral index above 100.

platy·pel·lic (-pel′ik) having a wide, flat pelvis.

platy·pel·loid (-pel′oid) platypellic.

platy·po·dia (-po′de-ah) flatfoot.

pla·tys·ma (plah-tiz′mah) see *Table of Muscles.*

pledge (plej) a solemn statement of intention. **Nightingale p.,** a statement of principles for the nursing profession, formulated by a committee in 1893 and subscribed to by student nurses at the time of the capping ceremonies.

pled·get (plej′it) a small compress or tuft.

-plegia word element [Gr.], *paralysis; a stroke.*

plei·ot·ro·pism (pli-ot′rah-pizm) pleiotropy.

plei·ot·ro·py (-pe) the production by a single gene of multiple phenotypic effects. **pleiotrop′ic,** adj.

pleo- word element [Gr.], *more.*

pleo·cy·to·sis (ple″o-si-to′sis) presence of a greater than normal number of cells in cerebrospinal fluid.

pleo·mor·phism (-mor′fizm) the occurrence of various distinct forms by a single organism or within a species. **pleomor′phic, pleomor′phous,** adj.

ple·on·os·te·o·sis (ple″on-os″te-o′sis) abnormally increased ossification. **Léri's p.,** a hereditary syndrome of premature and excessive ossification, with short stature, limitation of movement, broadening and deformity of digits, and mongolian facies.

ples·ses·the·sia (ples″es-the′ze-ah) palpatory percussion.

pleth·o·ra (pleth′ah-rah) 1. an excess of blood. 2. by extension, a red florid complexion. **pletho′ric,** adj.

ple·thys·mo·graph (plĕ-thiz′mo-grah) an instrument for recording variations in volume of an organ, part, or limb.

ple·thys·mog·ra·phy (plĕ″thiz-mog′rah-fe) the determination of changes in volume by means of a plethysmograph.

pleu·ra (ploor'ah) pl. *pleu'rae*. [Gr.] the serous membrane investing the lungs (*visceral p.*) and lining the walls of the thoracic cavity (*parietal p.*); the two layers enclose a potential space, the *pleural cavity*. The two pleurae, right and left, are entirely distinct from each other. **pleu'ral**, adj.

pleu·ra·cot·o·my (ploor"ah-kot'ah-me) thoracotomy.

pleu·ral·gia (ploor-al'jah) 1. pleurodynia (1). 2. costalgia (2). **pleural'gic**, adj.

pleu·rec·to·my (ploor-ek'tah-me) excision of part of the pleura.

pleu·ri·sy (ploor'ĭ-se) inflammation of the pleura. **pleurit'ic**, adj. **adhesive p.**, fibrinous p. **dry p.**, fibrinous p. **p. with effusion**, that marked by serous exudation. **fibrinous p.**, a type with fibrinous adhesions between the visceral and parietal pleurae, obliterating part or all of the pleural space. **interlobular p.**, a form enclosed between the lobes of the lung. **plastic p.**, fibrinous p. **purulent p.**, empyema (2). **serous p.**, that marked by free exudation of fluid. **suppurative p.**, empyema (2). **wet p.**, p. with effusion.

pleu·ri·tis (ploo-ri'tis) pleurisy. **pleurit'ic**, adj.

pleur(o)- word element [Gr.], *pleura; rib; side.*

pleu·ro·cele (ploor'o-sēl) pneumonocele (1).

pleu·ro·cen·te·sis (ploor"o-sen-te'sis) thoracentesis.

pleu·ro·dyn·ia (-din'e-ah) 1. pain in the pleural cavity. 2. costalgia (2). **epidemic p.**, an epidemic disease due to coxsackievirus B, marked by sudden violent pain in the chest, fever, and a tendency toward recrudescence on the third day.

pleu·ro·gen·ic (-jen'ik) pleurogenous.

pleu·rog·e·nous (ploo-roj'ĕ-nus) originating in the pleura.

pleu·rog·ra·phy (ploor-og'rah-fe) radiography of the pleural cavity.

pleu·ro·hep·a·ti·tis (ploor"o-hep"ah-ti'tis) hepatitis with inflammation of a portion of the pleura near the liver.

pleu·rol·y·sis (ploo-rol'ĭ-sis) surgical separation of pleural adhesions.

pleu·ro·pa·ri·e·to·pexy (ploor"o-pah-ri'ĕ-to-pek"se) fixation of the lung to the chest wall by adhesion of the visceral and parietal pleura.

pleu·ro·peri·car·di·tis (-per"ĭ-kahr-di'tis) inflammation of the pleura and pericardium.

pleu·ro·peri·to·ne·al (-per"ĭ-to-ne'al) pertaining to the pleura and peritoneum.

pleu·ro·pneu·mo·nia (-noo-mo'ne-ah) pleurisy complicated by pneumonia.

pleu·ro·thot·o·nos (-thot'ah-nos) tetanic bending of the body to one side.

pleu·rot·o·my (ploo-rot'ah-me) thoracotomy.

plex·ec·to·my (plek-sek'tah-me) surgical excision of a plexus.

plex·i·form (plek'sĭ-form) resembling a plexus or network.

plex·im·e·ter (plek-sim'ĕ-ter) 1. a plate to be struck in mediate percussion. 2. diascope.

plex·i·tis (plek-si'tis) inflammation of a nerve plexus.

plex·o·gen·ic (plek'sah-jen"ik) giving rise to a plexus or plexiform structure.

plex·op·a·thy (pleks-op'ah-the) any disorder of a plexus, especially of nerves. **lumbar p.**, neuropathy of the lumbar plexus.

plex·or (plek'ser) a hammer used in diagnostic percussion.

plex·us (plek'sus) pl. *plex'us, plexuses*. [L.] a network or tangle, chiefly of vessels or nerves. **plex'al**, adj. **aortic p., abdominal**, one composed of fibers that arise from the celiac and superior mesenteric plexuses and descend along the aorta. Receiving branches from the lumbar splanchnic nerves, it becomes the superior hypogastric plexus below the bifurcation of the aorta. Branches are distributed along the adjacent branches of the aorta. **aortic p., thoracic**, one around the thoracic aorta formed by filaments from the sympathetic trunks and vagus nerves, and from which fine twigs accompany branches of the aorta; continuous below with the celiac plexus and the abdominal aortic plexus. **autonomic p.**, any of the extensive networks of nerve fibers and cell bodies associated with the autonomic nervous system; found particularly in the thorax, abdomen, and pelvis, and containing sympathetic, parasympathetic, and visceral afferent fibers. **Batson's p.**, the vertebral plexus (1) considered as a whole system. **brachial p.**, a nerve plexus originating from the anterior branches of the last four cervical and the first thoracic spinal nerves, giving off many of the principal nerves of the shoulder, chest, and arms. **cardiac p.**, the plexus around the base of the heart, chiefly in the epicardium, formed by cardiac branches from the vagus nerves and the sympathetic trunks and ganglia. **carotid p.**, any of three nerve plexuses surrounding the common, external, and internal carotid arteries, particularly the last. **cavernous p.**, a plexus of sympathetic nerve fibers related to the cavernous sinus of the dura mater. **celiac p.**, 1. a network of ganglia and nerves lying in front of the aorta behind the stomach, supplying the abdominal viscera. 2. a network of lymphatic vessels, the superior mesenteric lymph nodes, and the celiac lymph nodes. **cervical p.,** a nerve plexus formed by the anterior branches of the first four cervical nerves, supplying structures in the neck region. **choroid p's,** infoldings of blood vessels of the pia mater covered by a thin coat of ependymal cells that form tufted projections into the third, fourth, and lateral ventricles of the brain; they secrete the cerebrospinal fluid. **coccygeal p.,** a nerve plexus formed by the anterior branches of the coccygeal and fifth sacral nerves and by a communication from the fourth sacral nerve, giving off the anococcygeal nerve. **cystic p.,** a nerve plexus near the gallbladder. **dental p.,** either of two plexuses (inferior and superior) of nerve fibers, one from the inferior alveolar nerve situated around the roots of the lower teeth, and the other from the superior alveolar nerve situated around the roots of the upper teeth. **enteric p.,** a plexus of autonomic nerve fibers within the wall of the digestive tube, made up of the submucosal, myenteric, and subserosal plexuses. **esophageal p.,** a plexus surrounding the esophagus, formed by branches of the left and right vagi and sympathetic trunks and containing also visceral afferent fibers from the esophagus. **Exner's p.,** superficial tangential fibers in the molecular layer of the cerebral cortex. **gastric p's,** subdivisions of the celiac portions of the prevertebral plexuses, accompanying the gastric arteries and branches and supplying nerve fibers to the stomach. **Heller's p.,** an arterial network in the submucosa of the intestine. **hemorrhoidal p.,** rectal p. **hypogastric p., inferior,** the plexus formed on each side anterior to the lower part of the sacrum, formed by the junction of the hypogastric and pelvic splanchnic nerves; branches are given off to the pelvic organs. **hypogastric p., superior,** the downward continuation of the abdominal aortic plexus; it lies in front of the upper part of the sacrum, just below the bifurcation of the aorta, receives fibers from the lower lumbar splanchnic nerves, and divides into right and left hypogastric nerves. **lumbar p., 1.** one formed by the anterior branches of the second to fifth lumbar nerves in the psoas major muscle (the branches of the first lumbar nerve often are included). **2.** a lymphatic plexus in the lumbar region. **lumbosacral p.,** the lumbar and sacral plexuses considered together, because of their continuous nature. **Meissner's p.,** submucosal p. **mesenteric p., inferior,** a subdivision of the abdominal aortic plexus accompanying the inferior mesenteric artery. **mesenteric p., superior,** a subdivision of the celiac plexus accompanying the superior mesenteric artery. **myenteric p.,** that part of the enteric plexus within the tunica muscularis. **pampiniform p., 1.** a plexus of veins from the testicle and epididymis, constituting part of the spermatic cord. **2.** a plexus of ovarian veins in the broad ligament. **pelvic p.,** inferior hypogastric p. **pharyngeal p., 1.** a venous plexus posterolateral to the pharynx, formed by the pharyngeal veins, communicating with the pterygoid venous plexus, and draining into the internal jugular vein. **2.** one formed chiefly by fibers from branches of the vagus nerves, but also by fibers from the glossopharyngeal nerves and sympathetic trunks, and supplying most of the muscles and mucosa of the pharynx and soft palate. **phrenic p.,** a nerve plexus accompanying the inferior phrenic artery to the diaphragm and adrenal glands. **prevertebral p's,** autonomic nerve plexuses situated in the thorax, abdomen, and pelvis, anterior to the vertebral column; they consist of visceral afferent fibers, preganglionic parasympathetic fibers, preganglionic and postganglionic sympathetic fibers, and ganglia containing sympathetic ganglion cells, and they give rise to postganglionic fibers. **prostatic p., 1.** a subdivision of the inferior hypogastric plexus that supplies nerve fibers to the prostate and adjacent organs. **2.** a venous plexus around the prostate gland, receiving the deep dorsal vein of the penis and draining through the vesical plexus and the prostatic veins. **pterygoid p.,** a network of veins corresponding to the second and third parts of the maxillary artery; situated on the medial and lateral pterygoid muscles and draining into the facial vein. **pulmonary p.,** one formed by several strong trunks of the vagus nerve that are joined at the root of the lung by branches from the sympathetic trunk and cardiac plexus; it is often divided into anterior and posterior parts. **rectal p., 1.** a venous plexus that surrounds the lower part of the rectum and drains into the rectal veins. **2.** any of the rectal nerve plexuses (inferior, middle, or superior). **rectal p., external,** inferior rectal p. (1). **rectal p., inferior, 1.** the subcutaneous portion of the rectal venous plexus, below the pectinate line. **2.** a nerve plexus accompanying the inferior rectal artery, derived chiefly from the inferior rectal nerve. **rectal p., internal,** superior rectal p. (1). **rectal p., middle,** a subdivision of the inferior hypogastric plexus, in proximity with and supplying nerve fibers to the rectum. **rectal p., superior, 1.** the submucosal portion of the rectal venous plexus, above the pectinate line. 2. a nerve plexus accompanying the superior rectal artery to the rectum, derived from the inferior mesenteric and hypogastric plexuses. **sacral p.,** 1. one arising from the anterior branches of the last two lumbar and the first four sacral nerves. 2. a venous plexus on the pelvic surface of the sacrum, receiving the sacral intervertebral veins. **solar p.,** celiac p. (1). **submucosal p.,** the part of the enteric plexus that is situated in the submucosa. **subserosal p.,** the part of the enteric plexus situated deep to the serosal surface of the tunica serosa. **tympanic p.,** a network of nerve fibers supplying the mucous lining of the tympanum, mastoid air cells, and pharyngotympanic tube. **uterine p.,** 1. the part of the uterovaginal plexus that supplies nerve fibers to the cervix and lower part of the uterus. 2. the venous plexus around the uterus, draining into the internal iliac veins by way of the uterine veins. **uterovaginal p.,** 1. the subdivision of the inferior hypogastric plexus that supplies nerve fibers to the uterus, ovary, vagina, urethra, and erectile tissue of the vestibule. 2. the uterine and vaginal venous plexuses considered together. **vaginal p.,** 1. the part of the uterovaginal plexus that supplies nerve fibers to the walls of the vagina. 2. a venous plexus in the walls of the vagina, which drains into the internal iliac veins by way of the internal pudendal veins. **vascular p.,** 1. a network of intercommunicating blood vessels. 2. a plexus of peripheral nerves through which blood vessels receive innervation. **venous p.,** a network of interconnecting veins. **vertebral p.,** 1. a plexus of veins related to the vertebral column. 2. a nerve plexus accompanying the vertebral artery, carrying sympathetic fibers to the posterior cranial fossa via cranial nerves. **vesical p.,** 1. the subdivision of the inferior hypogastric plexus that supplies sympathetic nerve fibers to the urinary bladder and parts of the ureter, ductus deferens, and seminal vesicle. 2. a venous plexus surrounding the upper part of the urethra and the neck of the bladder, communicating with the vaginal plexus in the female and with the prostatic plexus in the male.

-plexy word element [Gr.], *stroke; seizure.* **-plectic,** adj.

pli·ca (pli′kah) pl. *pli′cae.* [L.] a fold.

pli·ca·my·cin (pli″kah-mi′sin) an antineoplastic antibiotic produced by *Streptomyces plicatus;* used in the treatment of advanced testicular carcinoma. It also has an inhibiting effect on osteoclasts and is used to treat hypercalcemia and hypercalciuria associated with malignancy.

pli·cate (pli′kāt) plaited or folded.

pli·ca·tion (pli-ka′shun) the operation of taking tucks in a structure to shorten it. **Kelly p.,** suture of the connective tissue between the vagina and the urethra and the floor of the bladder for correction of stress incontinence in women.

pli·cot·o·my (pli-kot′ah-me) surgical division of the posterior fold of the tympanic membrane.

PLT psittacosis-lymphogranuloma venereum-trachoma (group); see *Chlamydia.*

plug (plug) an obstructing mass. **closing p.,** a fibrinous coagulum of blood that fills the defect in the endometrial epithelium created by implantation of the blastocyst. **Dittrich's p's,** masses of fat globules, fatty acid crystals, and bacteria sometimes seen in the bronchi in bronchitis and bronchiectasis. **epithelial p.,** 1. a mass of ectodermal cells that temporarily closes an opening in the fetus, particularly in the external nares. 2. a mass of epithelium clogging or obstructing an opening. **mucous p.,** 1. a plug formed by secretions of the mucous glands of the cervix uteri and closing the cervical canal during pregnancy. 2. abnormally thick mucus occluding the bronchi and bronchioles.

plug·ger (plug′er) an instrument for compacting filling material in a tooth cavity.

plum·bic (plum′bik) pertaining to lead.

plum·bism (plum′bizm) chronic lead poisoning; see *lead*[1].

pluri- word element [L.], *more.*

plu·ri·glan·du·lar (ploor″ĭ-glan′du-ler) pertaining to or affecting several glands.

plu·ri·hor·mo·nal (-hor-mo′n'l) of or pertaining to several hormones.

plu·rip·o·ten·cy (-po′ten-se) 1. the ability to develop or act in any one of several possible ways. 2. the ability to affect more than one organ or tissue. **plurip′otent, pluripoten′tial,** adj.

plu·ri·po·ten·ti·al·i·ty (-po-ten″she-al′ĭ-te) pluripotency.

plu·to·ni·um (Pu) (ploo-to′ne-um) chemical element (see *Table of Elements*), at. no. 94.

Pm promethium.

PMI point of maximal impulse (of the heart).

PMMA polymethyl methacrylate.

-pnea word element [Gr.], *respiration; breathing.* **-pneic,** adj.

PNET primitive neuroectodermal tumor.

pneu·mar·throg·ra·phy (noo″mahr-throg′rah-fe) radiography of a joint after injection of air or gas as a contrast medium.

pneu·mar·thro·sis (-thro′sis) 1. gas or air in a joint. 2. inflation of a joint with air or gas for radiographic examination.

pneu·mat·ic (noo-mat′ik) 1. pertaining to air. 2. respiratory.

pneu·ma·ti·za·tion (noo″mah-tĭ-za′shun) the formation of air cells or cavities in tissue, especially in the temporal bone.

pneumat(o)- word element [Gr.], *air; gas; lung.*

pneu·ma·to·cele (noo-mat′o-sēl) 1. aerocele; a tumor or cyst formed by air or other gas filling an adventitious pouch, such as a laryngocele, tracheocele, or gaseous swelling of the scrotum. 2. a usually benign, thin-walled, air-containing cyst of the lung, as in staphylococcal pneumonia.

pneu·ma·to·graph (-graf) spirograph.

pneu·ma·to·sis (-to′sis) [Gr.] air or gas in an abnormal location in the body. **p. cystoi′des intestina′lis,** presence of thin-walled, gas-containing cysts in the wall of the intestines.

pneu·ma·tu·ria (-tu′re-ah) gas or air in the urine.

pneum(o)- word element [Gr.], *air or gas; lung.*

pneu·mo·ar·throg·ra·phy (noo″mo-ahr-throg′rah-fe) pneumarthrography.

pneu·mo·bil·ia (-bil′e-ah) gas in the biliary system.

pneu·mo·cele (noo′mo-sēl) 1. pneumonocele (1). 2. pneumatocele (1). 3. pneumatocele (2).

pneu·mo·ceph·a·lus (-sef′ah-lus) air in the intracranial cavity.

pneu·mo·coc·cal (-kok′al) pertaining to or caused by pneumococci.

pneu·mo·coc·ce·mia (-kok-sēm′e-ah) pneumococci in the blood.

pneu·mo·coc·ci·dal (-kok-si′d′l) destroying pneumococci.

pneu·mo·coc·co·sis (-kok-o′sis) infection with pneumococci.

pneu·mo·coc·co·su·ria (-kok″o-su′re-ah) pneumococci in the urine.

pneu·mo·coc·cus (-kok′us) pl. *pneumococ′ci.* An individual organism of the species *Streptococcus pneumoniae.*

pneu·mo·co·ni·o·sis (-ko″ne-o′sis) deposition of large amounts of dust or other particulate matter in the lungs, causing a tissue reaction, usually in workers in certain occupations and in residents of areas with excessive particulates in the air; there are many types, including anthracosis, asbestosis, bituminosis, and silicosis. **coal workers' p.,** black lung; a form caused by deposition of coal dust in the lungs, usually characterized by centrilobular emphysema. Different varieties of coal have

different risks; bituminosis is usually more severe than anthracosis. **talc p.,** talcosis; a type of silicatosis caused by the inhalation of talc; prolonged exposure may result in pulmonary fibrosis.

pneu·mo·cra·ni·um (-kra′ne-um) pneumocephalus.

pneu·mo·cys·ti·a·sis (-sis-ti′ah-sis) interstitial plasma cell pneumonia.

Pneu·mo·cys·tis (-sis′tis) a genus of yeast-like fungi. *P. cari′nii* is the causative agent of interstitial plasma cell pneumonia.

pneu·mo·cys·tog·ra·phy (-sis-tog′rah-fe) cystography after injection of air or gas into the bladder.

pneu·mo·der·ma (-der′mah) subcutaneous emphysema.

pneu·mo·en·ceph·a·lo·cele (-en-sef′ah-lo-sēl) pneumocephalus.

pneu·mo·en·ceph·a·log·ra·phy (PEG) (-en-sef″ah-log′rah-fe) radiography of fluid-containing structures of the brain after cerebrospinal fluid is intermittently withdrawn by lumbar puncture and replaced by a gas.

pneu·mo·en·ter·itis (-en″ter-i′tis) inflammation of the lungs and intestine.

pneu·mog·ra·phy (noo-mog′rah-fe) 1. spirography. 2. radiography of a part after injection of a gas.

pneu·mo·he·mo·peri·car·di·um (noo″-mo-he″mo-pě″re-kahr′de-um) air or gas and blood in the pericardium.

pneu·mo·he·mo·tho·rax (-hemo-thor′aks) hemopneumothorax.

pneu·mo·hy·dro·me·tra (-hi″dro-me′trah) gas and fluid in the uterus.

pneu·mo·hy·dro·peri·car·di·um (-hydro-per″e-kahr′de-um) air or gas and fluid in the pericardium.

pneu·mo·hy·dro·tho·rax (-hydro-thor′aks) hydropneumothorax.

pneu·mo·li·thi·a·sis (-lĭ-thi′ah-sis) the presence of concretions in the lungs.

pneu·mo·me·di·as·ti·num (-me″de-as-ti′num) air or gas in the mediastinum, which may be pathological or introduced intentionally.

pneu·mo·my·co·sis (-mi ko′sis) any fungal disease of the lungs.

pneu·mo·my·elog·ra·phy (-mi″ě-log″rah-fe) radiography of the spinal canal after withdrawal of cerebrospinal fluid and injection of air or gas.

pneu·mo·nec·to·my (-nek′tah-me) excision of lung tissue; it may be total, partial, or of a single lobe (*lobectomy*).

pneu·mo·nia (noo-mo′ne-ah) inflammation of the lungs with exudation and consolidation. **p. al′ba,** a fatal desquamative pneumonia of the newborn due to congenital syphilis, with fatty degeneration of the lungs. **aspiration p.**, that due to aspiration of foreign material into the lungs. **atypical p.**, primary atypical p. **bacterial p.**, that due to bacteria, usually species of *Streptococcus*, *Staphylococcus*, *Klebsiella*, and *Mycoplasma*. **bronchial p.**, bronchopneumonia. **desquamative interstitial p.**, chronic pneumonia with desquamation of large alveolar cells and thickening of the walls of distal air passages; marked by dyspnea and nonproductive cough. **double p.**, that affecting both lungs. **Friedländer's p.**, **Friedländer's bacillus p.**, *Klebsiella* p. **hypostatic p.**, a type seen in the weak or elderly, due to excessive lying on the back. **influenzal p.**, **influenza virus p.**, an acute, usually fatal type due to influenza virus, with high fever, prostration, sore throat, aching pains, dyspnea, massive edema, and consolidation. It may be complicated by bacterial pneumonia. **inhalation p.**, 1. aspiration p. 2. bronchopneumonia due to inhalation of irritating vapors. **interstitial p.**, 1. any of various types of pneumonia characterized by thickening of the interstitial tissue. 2. idiopathic pulmonary fibrosis. **interstitial plasma cell p.**, *Pneumocystis carinii* pneumonia; a form caused by *Pneumocystis carinii*, seen in infants and debilitated or immunocompromised persons; cellular detritus containing plasma cells appears in lung tissue. *Klebsiella* **p.**, Friedländer's pneumonia; a form with massive mucoid inflammatory exudates in a lobe of the lung, due to *Klebsiella pneumoniae*. **lipid p.**, **lipoid p.**, aspiration pneumonia due to aspiration of oil. **lobar p.**, 1. acute bacterial pneumonia with edema, usually in one lung; the most common type is pneumococcal p. 2. pneumococcal p. **lobular p.**, bronchopneumonia. **mycoplasmal p.**, primary atypical pneumonia caused by *Mycoplasma pneumoniae*. **Pittsburgh p.**, a type resembling legionnaires' disease, caused by *Legionella micdadei*, seen in immunocompromised patients. **pneumococcal p.**, the most common type of lobar pneumonia, caused by *Streptococcus pneumoniae*. **pneumocystis p.**, *Pneumocystis carinii* p., interstitial plasma cell p. **primary atypical p.**, any of numerous types of acute pneumonia, caused by bacteria such as species of *Mycoplasma*, *Rickettsia*, or *Chlamydia*, or viruses such as adenoviruses or parainfluenza virus. **rheumatic p.**, a rare, usually fatal complication of acute rheumatic fever, with extensive pulmonary consolidation and rapidly progressive functional deterioration, alveolar exudate, interstitial infiltrates, and necrotizing arteritis. **varicella p.**, that developing after the skin eruption in varicella (chickenpox), apparently due to the same virus; symptoms may be severe, with violent cough, hemoptysis, and severe chest pain. **viral p.**, that due to a virus, e.g., adenovirus, influenza virus, parainfluenza virus, or varicella virus. **white p.**, p. alba.

pneu·mon·ic (noo-mon′ik) 1. pulmonary (1). 2. pertaining to pneumonia.

pneu·mo·ni·tis (noo″mo-ni′tis) inflammation of the lung; see also *pneumonia*. **hypersensitivity p.**, extrinsic allergic alveolitis; a hypersensitivity reaction to repeated inhalation of organic particles, usually on the job, with onset a few hours after exposure to the allergen.

pneumon(o)- word element [Gr.], *lung*.

pneu·mo·no·cele (noo-mon′o-sēl) 1. pleurocele; pneumocele; hernial protrusion of lung tissue, as through a fissure in the chest wall. 2. pneumatocele (2).

pneu·mo·no·cen·te·sis (noo-mo″no-sen-te′sis) paracentesis of a lung.

pneu·mo·no·cyte (noo-mon′ah-sīt) alveolar cell.

pneu·mo·nop·a·thy (-nop′ah-the) pneumonosis; any lung disease.

pneu·mo·no·pexy (noo-mo′nah-pek″se) surgical fixation of the lung to the thoracic wall.

pneu·mo·nor·rha·phy (noo″mo-nor′ah-fe) suture of the lung.

pneu·mo·no·sis (-no′sis) pneumonopathy.

pneu·mo·not·o·my (-not′ah-me) incision of the lung.

pneu·mo·peri·car·di·um (-per′ĭ-kahr′de-um) air or gas in the pericardial cavity.

pneu·mo·peri·to·ne·um (-per″ĭ-to-ne′um) air or gas in the peritoneal cavity.

pneu·mo·peri·to·ni·tis (-per″ĭ-to-ni′tis) peritonitis with air or gas in the peritoneal cavity.

pneu·mo·pleu·ri·tis (-plŏo-ri′tis) pleuropneumonia (1).

pneu·mo·py·elog·ra·phy (-pi″ĕ-log′rah-fe) radiography after injection of oxygen or air into the renal pelvis.

pneu·mo·pyo·peri·car·di·um (-pi″o-per″ĭ-kahr′de-um) pyopneumopericardium.

pneu·mo·pyo·tho·rax (-pi″o-thor′aks) pyopneumothorax.

pneu·mo·ra·di·og·ra·phy (-ra″de-og′rah-fe) radiography after injection of air or oxygen.

pneu·mo·ret·ro·peri·to·ne·um (-ret″ro-per″ĭ-to-ne′um) air in the retroperitoneal space.

pneu·mo·ta·chom·e·ter (-tah-kom′ĕ-ter) a transducer for measuring exhaled air flow.

pneu·mo·tach·y·graph (-tak′e-graf) an instrument for recording the velocity of respired air.

pneu·mo·tax·ic (-tak′sik) regulating the respiratory rate.

pneu·mo·tho·rax (-thor′aks) air or gas in the pleural space, usually as a result of trauma (traumatic or open p.) or some pathological process.

pneu·mot·o·my (noo-mot′ah-me) pneumonotomy.

pneu·mo·ven·tric·u·log·ra·phy (noo″mo-ven-trik″u-log′rah-fe) radiography of the cerebral ventricles after injection of air or gas.

Pneu·mo·vi·rus (noo′mo-vi″rus) respiratory syncytial viruses; a genus of viruses of the family Paramyxoviridae that includes human and bovine respiratory syncytial viruses and pneumonia virus of mice.

PNH paroxysmal nocturnal hemoglobinuria.

PO [L.] per os (by mouth, orally).

Po₂ oxygen partial pressure (tension); also written P_{O_2}, pO_2, and pO_2.

Po polonium.

pock (pok) a pustule, especially of smallpox.

pock·et (pok′et) a bag or pouch. **endocardial p's,** sclerotic thickenings of the mural endocardium, occurring most often on the left ventricular septum below an insufficient aortic valve. **gingival p.,** a gingival sulcus deepened by pathological conditions, caused by gingival enlargement without destruction of the periodontal tissue. **pacemaker p.,** the subcutaneous area in which the pulse generator and pacing leads of an internal pacemaker are implanted, usually developed in the prepectoralis fascia or the retromammary area. **periodontal p.,** a gingival sulcus deepened into the periodontal ligament apically to the original level of the resorbed alveolar crest.

pock·mark (pok′mahrk) a depressed scar left by a pustule.

po·dag·ra (pah-dag′rah) gouty pain in the great toe.

po·dal·gia (po-dal′jah) pain in the foot.

po·dal·ic (po-dal′ik) accomplished by means of the feet; see under version.

pod·ar·thri·tis (pod″ahr-thri′tis) inflammation of the joints of the feet.

po·di·a·try (pah-di′ah-tre) chiropody; the specialized field dealing with the study and care of the foot, including its anatomy, pathology, medicinal and surgical treatment, etc. **podiat′ric,** adj.

pod(o)- word element [Gr.], foot.

podo·cyte (pod′ah-sīt) an epithelial cell of the visceral layer of a renal glomerulus, having a number of footlike radiating processes (pedicels).

podo·dy·na·mom·e·ter (pod″o-di″nah-mom′ĕ-ter) a device for determining the strength of leg muscles.

podo·dyn·ia (-din′e-ah) podalgia.

po·dof·i·lox (po-dof′ĭ-loks) an agent that inhibits cell mitosis and is used for topical treatment of condyloma acuminatum.

po·dol·o·gy (pah-dol′ah-je) podiatry.

podo·phyl·lin (pod″ah-fil′in) podophyllum resin.

podo·phyl·lum (-fil′um) the dried rhizome and roots of Podophyllum peltatum; see under resin.

poe- for words beginning thus, see those beginning pe-.

po·go·ni·a·sis (po″go-ni′ah-sis) excessive growth of the beard, or growth of a beard on a woman.

po·go·ni·on (po-go′ne-on) the anterior midpoint of the chin.

-poiesis word element [Gr.], formation. **-poiet′ic,** adj.

-poietin word element [Gr.], hormone involved in regulation of the numbers of various cell types in the peripheral blood. **-poiet′ic,** adj.

poikil(o)- word element [Gr.], varied; irregular.

poi·ki·lo·blast (poi′kĭ-lo-blast″) an abnormally shaped erythroblast.

poi·ki·lo·cyte (-sīt) an abnormally shaped erythrocyte, such as a burr cell, sickle cell, target cell, acanthocyte, elliptocyte, schistocyte, spherocyte, or stomatocyte.

poi·ki·lo·cy·to·sis (-si-to′sis) presence in the blood of erythrocytes showing abnormal variation in shape.

poi·ki·lo·der·ma (-der′mah) a condition characterized by pigmentary and atrophic changes in the skin, giving it a mottled appearance.

point (point) 1. a small area or spot; the sharp end of an object. 2. to approach the surface, like the pus of an abscess, at a definite spot or place. **p. A,** a radiographic, cephalometric landmark, determined on the lateral head film; it is the most retruded part of the curved bony outline from the anterior nasal spine to the crest of the maxillary alveolar process. **acupuncture p.,** acupoint. **p. B,** a radiographic cephalometric landmark, determined on the lateral head film; it is the most posterior midline point in the concavity between the infradentale and pogonium. **boiling p.,** the temperature at which a liquid will boil; at sea level, water boils at 100°C

(212°F). **cardinal p's,** 1. the points on the different refracting media of the eye that determine the direction of the entering or emerging light rays. 2. four points within the pelvic inlet—the two sacroiliac articulations and the two iliopectineal eminences. **craniometric p.,** one of the established points of reference for measurement of the skull. **far p.,** the remotest point at which an object is clearly seen when the eye is at rest. **p. of fixation,** 1. the point on which the vision is fixed. 2. the point on the retina on which are focused the rays coming from an object directly regarded. **freezing p.,** the temperature at which a liquid begins to freeze; for water, 0°C, or 32°F. **isoelectric p.,** the pH of a solution at which a charged molecule does not migrate in an electric field. **jugal p.,** the point at the angle formed by the masseteric and maxillary edges of the zygomatic bone. **lacrimal p.,** the opening on the lacrimal papilla of an eyelid, near the medial angle of the eye, into which tears from the lacrimal lake drain to enter the lacrimal canaliculi. **McBurney p.,** a point of special tenderness in appendicitis, about one-third the distance between the right anterior superior iliac spine and the umbilicus. **p. of maximal impulse,** the point on the chest where the impulse of the left ventricle is felt most strongly, normally in the fifth costal interspace inside the mammillary line. Abbreviated PMI. **melting p. (mp),** the minimum temperature at which a solid begins to liquefy. **near p.,** the nearest point of clear vision, the *absolute near p.* being that for either eye alone with accommodation relaxed, and the *relative near p.* that for both eyes with the employment of accommodation. **nodal p's,** two points on the axis of an optical system situated so that a ray falling on one will produce a parallel ray emerging through the other. **pressure p.,** 1. a point that is particularly sensitive to pressure. 2. one of various locations on the body at which digital pressure may be applied for the control of hemorrhage. **subnasal p.,** the central point at the base of the nasal spine. **trigger p.,** a spot on the body at which pressure or other stimulus gives rise to specific sensations or symptoms. **triple p.,** the temperature and pressure at which the solid, liquid, and gas phases of a substance are in equilibrium.

point·er (point'er) contusion at a bony eminence. **hip p.,** a contusion of the bone of the iliac crest, or avulsion of muscle attachments at the iliac crest.

poi·son (poiz'n) a substance that, on ingestion, inhalation, absorption, application, injection, or development within the body, in relatively small amounts, may cause structural damage or functional disturbance. **poi'-sonous,** adj.

poi·son·ing (poiz'ning) the morbid condition produced by a poison. **blood p.,** septicemia. **food p.,** a group of acute illnesses due to ingestion of contaminated food. It may result from allergy; toxemia from foods, such as those inherently poisonous or those contaminated by poisons; foods containing poisons formed by bacteria; or foodborne infections. **heavy metal p.,** poisoning with any of the heavy metals, particularly antimony, arsenic, cadmium, lead, mercury, thallium, or zinc. **mushroom p.,** that due to ingestion of poisonous mushrooms; see *Amanita.* **nicotine p.,** poisoning by nicotine, such as in tobacco workers or children who eat cigarettes, marked by stimulation and then depression of the central and autonomic nervous systems, and sometimes death from respiratory paralysis. **salmon p.,** see *Neorickettsia.* **sausage p.,** allantiasis. **scombroid p.,** epigastric pain, nausea, vomiting, headache, dysphagia, thirst, urticaria, and pruritus, usually lasting for less than 24 hours, caused by the ingestion of a toxic histamine-like substance produced by bacterial action on histidine in fish flesh; occurring when inadequately preserved scombroid fish (tuna, bonito, mackerel, etc.) are eaten. **shellfish p.,** poisoning from eating bivalve mollusks contaminated with a neurotoxin secreted by protozoa.

poi·son ivy (poiz'n i've) *Rhus radicans.*

poi·son oak (ōk) *Rhus diversiloba* or *R. toxicodendron.*

poi·son su·mac (soo'mak) *Rhus vernix.*

po·lar (po'lar) 1. of or pertaining to a pole. 2. being at opposite ends of a spectrum of manifestations.

po·la·rim·e·try (po"lah-rim'ĕ-tre) measurement of the rotation of plane polarized light.

po·lar·i·ty (pah-lar'ĭ-te) the condition of having poles or of exhibiting opposite effects at the two extremities.

po·lar·iza·tion (po"lar-ĭ-za'shun) 1. the presence or establishment of polarity. 2. the production of that condition in light in which its vibrations take place all in one plane, or in circles and ellipses. 3. the process of producing a relative separation of positive and negative charges, such as in a body, cell, molecule, or atom.

po·lar·og·ra·phy (po″lar-og′rah-fe) an electrochemical technique for identifying and estimating the concentration of reducible elements in an electrochemical cell by means of the dual measurement of the current flowing through the cell and the electrical potential at which each element is reduced. **polarograph′ic,** adj.

pole (pōl) 1. either extremity of any axis, as of the fetal ellipse or a body organ. 2. either one of two points which have opposite physical qualities. **po′lar,** adj. **animal p.,** 1. the site of an oocyte to which the nucleus is approximated, and from which the polar bodies pinch off. 2. in nonmammalian species, the pole of an egg less heavily laden with yolk than the vegetal pole and exhibiting faster cell division. **cephalic p.,** the end of the fetal ellipse at which the head of the fetus is situated. **frontal p. of cerebral hemisphere,** the most prominent part of the anterior end of each hemisphere. **germinal p.,** animal p. **occipital p. of cerebral hemisphere,** the posterior end of the occipital lobe. **pelvic p.,** the end of the fetal ellipse at which the breech of the fetus is situated. **temporal p. of cerebral hemisphere,** the prominent anterior end of the temporal lobe. **vegetal p.,** that pole of an oocyte at which the greater amount of food yolk is deposited.

po·lice·man (pah-lēs′min) a glass rod with a piece of rubber tubing on one end, used as a stirring rod and transfer tool in chemical analysis.

poli·clin·ic (pol″ĭ-klin′ik) a city hospital, infirmary, or clinic; cf. *polyclinic.*

po·lio (pōl′e-o) poliomyelitis.

poli(o)- word element [Gr.], *gray matter.*

po·lio·clas·tic (po″le-o-klas′tik) destroying the gray matter of the nervous system.

po·lio·dys·tro·phia (-dis-tro′fe-ah) poliodystrophy.

po·lio·dys·tro·phy (-dis′trah-fe) atrophy of the cerebral gray matter. **progressive cerebral p., progressive infantile p.,** Alpers' disease.

po·lio·en·ceph·a·li·tis (-en-sef″ah-li′tis) inflammatory disease of the gray matter of the brain. **inferior p.,** progressive bulbar palsy.

po·lio·en·ceph·a·lo·me·nin·go·my·eli·tis (-en-sef″ah-lo-mĕ-ning″go-mi″ĕ-li′tis) inflammation of the gray matter of the brain and spinal cord and of the meninges.

po·lio·en·ceph·a·lo·my·eli·tis (-en-sef″ah-lo-mi″ĕ-li′tis) cerebral poliomyelitis.

po·lio·en·ceph·a·lop·a·thy (-en-sef″ah-lop′ah-the) disease of the gray matter of the brain.

po·lio·my·eli·tis (-mi″ĕ-li′tis) an acute viral disease usually caused by a poliovirus and marked clinically by fever, sore throat, headache, vomiting, and often stiffness of the neck and back; these may be the only symptoms of the minor illness. In the major illness, which may or may not be preceded by the minor illness, there is central nervous system involvement, stiff neck, pleocytosis in spinal fluid, and perhaps paralysis; there may be subsequent atrophy of muscle groups, ending in contraction and permanent deformity. **abortive p.,** the minor illness of poliomyelitis. **acute anterior p.,** the major illness of poliomyelitis. **ascending p.,** poliomyelitis with a cephalad progression. **bulbar p.,** a severe form affecting the medulla oblongata, which may result in dysfunction of the swallowing mechanism, respiratory embarrassment, and circulatory distress. **cerebral p.,** poliomyelitis that extends into the brain. **spinal paralytic p.,** the classic form of acute anterior poliomyelitis, with the appearance of flaccid paralysis of one or more limbs.

po·lio·my·elop·a·thy (-mi″ĕ-lop′ah-the) any disease of the gray matter of the spinal cord.

po·li·o·sis (pōl-e-o′sis) circumscribed loss of pigment of the hair, especially following some pathological process.

po·lio·vi·rus (pōl′-e-o-vi″rus) the causative agent of poliomyelitis, separable, on the basis of specificity of neutralizing antibody, into three serotypes designated types 1, 2, and 3. **po′lioviral,** adj.

pol·len (pol′in) the male fertilizing element of flowering plants.

pol·lex (pol′eks) pl. *pol′lices.* [L.] the thumb. **p. val′gus,** deviation of the thumb toward the ulnar side. **p. va′rus,** deviation of the thumb toward the radial side.

pol·lic·i·za·tion (pol′is-ĭ-za′shun) surgical construction of a thumb from a finger.

pol·li·no·sis (pol″ĭ-no′sis) an allergic reaction to pollen; hay fever.

po·lo·cytes (po′lo-sīts) polar bodies (1).

po·lo·ni·um (Po) (pah-lo′ne-um) chemical element (see *Table of Elements*), at. no. 84.

pol·ox·a·mer (pol-ok′sah-mer) any of a series of nonionic surfactants of the polyoxypropylene-polyoxyethylene copolymer type, used as surfactants, emulsifiers, stabilizers, and food additives.

po·lus (po′lus) pl. *po′li.* [L.] pole.

poly- word element [Gr.], *many; much.*

poly·ad·e·ni·tis (pol″e-ad″ĕ-ni′tis) inflammation of several glands.

poly·ad·e·no·sis (-ad″in-o′sis) disorder of several glands, particularly endocrine glands.

pol·y·al·ve·o·lar (-al-ve′o-lar) having more than the usual number of alveoli, as a polyalveolar pulmonary lobe.

pol·y·am·ine (-am′ēn) any compound, e.g., spermine or spermidine, containing two or more amino groups.

pol·y·an·dry (-an′dre) 1. polygamy in which a woman is concurrently married to multiple men. 2. animal mating in which the female mates with more than one male. 3. union of two or more male pronuclei with one female pronucleus, resulting in polyploidy of the zygote.

pol·y·an·gi·itis (-an″je-i′tis) inflammation involving multiple blood or lymph vessels.

pol·y·ar·cu·ate (-ahr″ku-at) characterized by multiple arch-shaped curves.

pol·y·ar·ter·i·tis (-ahr″ter-i′tis) 1. multiple inflammatory and destructive arterial lesions. 2. polyarteritis nodosa. **p. nodo′sa (PAN)**, classically, a form of systemic necrotizing vasculitis involving small to medium-sized arteries with signs and symptoms resulting from infarction and scarring of the affected organ system.

pol·y·ar·thric (-ahr′thrik) polyarticular.

pol·y·ar·thri·tis (-ahr-thri′tis) inflammation of several joints. **chronic villous p.**, chronic inflammation of the synovial membrane of several joints. **p. rheuma′tica acu′ta**, rheumatic fever.

pol·y·ar·tic·u·lar (-ahr-tik′u-lar) affecting many joints.

pol·y·atom·ic (-ah-tom′ik) made up of several atoms.

pol·y·ba·sic (-ba′sik) having several replaceable hydrogen atoms.

pol·y·car·bo·phil (-kahr′bo-fil) a hydrophilic resin that is a bulk-forming laxative and also a gastrointestinal absorbent in the treatment of diarrhea; usually used as *calcium p.*

pol·y·cen·tric (-sen′trik) having many centers.

pol·y·cho·lia (-kōl′e-ah) excessive flow or secretion of bile.

pol·y·chon·dri·tis (-kon-dri′tis) inflammation of many cartilages of the body. **chronic atrophic p., p. chro′nica atro′phicans**, relapsing p. **relapsing p.**, an acquired idiopathic chronic disease with a tendency to recurrence, marked by inflammatory and degenerative lesions of various cartilaginous structures.

pol·y·chro·ma·sia (-krōm-a′zhah) 1. variation in the hemoglobin content of erythrocytes. 2. polychromatophilia.

pol·y·chro·mat·ic (-krom-at′ik) manycolored.

pol·y·chro·mato·cyte (-krom-at′ah-sīt) a cell stainable with various kinds of stain.

pol·y·chro·mato·phil (-krom-at″ah-fil) a structure stainable with many kinds of stain.

pol·y·chro·ma·to·phil·ia (-krom-at″ah-fil′e-ah) 1. the property of being stainable with various stains; affinity for all sorts of stains. 2. a condition in which the erythrocytes, on staining, show various shades of blue combined with tinges of pink. **polychromatophil′ic**, adj.

pol·y·clin·ic (-klin′ik) a hospital and school where diseases and injuries of all kinds are studied and treated.

pol·y·clo·nal (-klōn″l) 1. derived from different cells. 2. pertaining to several clones.

pol·y·co·ria (-kor′e-ah) 1. more than one pupil in an eye. 2. the deposit of reserve material in an organ or tissue so as to produce enlargement.

pol·yc·ro·tism (pah-lik′rah-tizm) the quality of having several secondary waves to each beat of the pulse. **polycrot′ic**, adj.

pol·y·cy·e·sis (pol″e-si-e′sis) multiple pregnancy.

pol·y·cys·tic (-sis′tik) containing many cysts.

pol·y·cy·the·mia (-si-thēm′e-ah) an increase in the total cell mass of the blood. **absolute p.**, an increase in red cell mass caused by increased erythropoiesis, which may occur as a compensatory physiologic response to tissue hypoxia or as the principal manifestation of polycythemia vera. **hypertonic p.**, stress p. **relative p.**, a decrease in plasma volume without change in red blood cell mass so that the erythrocytes become more concentrated (elevated hematocrit), which may be an acute transient or a chronic condition. **p. ru′bra, p. vera. secondary p.**, any absolute increase in the total red cell mass other than polycythemia vera, occurring as a physiologic response to tissue hypoxia. **stress p.**, chronic relative polycythemia usually affecting white, middle-aged, mildly obese males who are active, anxiety-prone, and hypertensive. **p. ve′ra**, a myeloproliferative disorder of unknown etiology, characterized by abnormal proliferation of all hematopoietic bone marrow elements and an absolute increase in red cell mass and total blood volume, associated frequently with splenomegaly, leukocytosis, and thrombocythemia.

pol·y·dac·tyl·ism (-dak′til-izm) polydactyly.

pol·y·dac·ty·ly (-dak′tĭ-le) the presence of supernumerary digits on the hands or feet.

pol·y·di·meth·yl·si·lox·ane (-di-meth″il-si-lok′sān) a polymeric siloxane in which the substituents are methyl groups; it is the most common form of silicone.

pol·y·dip·sia (-dip′se-ah) chronic excessive thirst and fluid intake.

pol·y·dys·pla·sia (-dis-pla′zhah) faulty development in several types of tissue or several organs or systems.

pol·y·em·bry·o·ny (-em-bri′o-ne) the production of two or more embryos from the same oocyte or seed.

pol·y·ene (pol′e-ēn) 1. a chemical compound with a carbon chain of four or more atoms and several conjugated double bonds. 2. any of a group of antifungal antibiotics with such a structure (e.g., amphotericin and nystatin) produced by species of *Streptomyces* that damage cell membranes by forming complexes with sterols.

pol·y·es·the·sia (-es-the′zhah) a sensation as if several points were touched on application of a stimulus to a single point.

pol·y·es·tra·di·ol phos·phate (-es″trah-di′ol) a polymer of estradiol phosphate having estrogenic activity similar to that of estradiol; used in the palliative therapy of prostatic carcinoma.

pol·y·eth·y·lene (-eth′ĭ-lēn) polymerized ethylene, (—CH₂—CH₂—)ₙ, a synthetic plastic material, forms of which have been used in reparative surgery. **p. glycol (PEG),** a generic name for mixtures of condensation polymers of ethylene oxide and water, available in liquid form (polymers with average molecular weights between 200 and 700) or as waxy solids (average molecular weights above 1000); some are used as pharmaceutic aids, and *p. glycol 3350* is used as a laxative.

pol·y·ga·lac·tia (-gah-lak′she-ah) excessive secretion of milk.

po·lyg·a·my (pah-lig′ah-me) 1. the concurrent marriage of a woman or man to more than one spouse. 2. animal mating in which the individual mates with more than one partner.

pol·y·gene (pol′e-jēn) a group of nonallelic genes that interact to influence the same character with additive effect.

pol·y·gen·ic (pol″e-jēn′ik) pertaining to or determined by several different genes.

pol·y·glac·tin 910 (-glak′tin) a filamentous material that is braided and used for absorbable sutures.

pol·y·glan·du·lar (-glan′du-lar) pluriglandular.

pol·y·graph (pol′e-graf) an apparatus for simultaneously recording blood pressure, pulse, and respiration, and variations in electrical resistance of the skin; popularly known as a lie detector.

po·lyg·y·ny (pah-lij′ĭ-ne) 1. polygamy in which a man is married concurrently to more than one woman. 2. animal mating in which the male mates with more than one

female. 3. union of two or more female pronuclei with one male pronucleus, resulting in polyploidy of the zygote.

pol·y·gy·ria (pol″e-ji′re-ah) polymicrogyria.

pol·y·he·dral (-he′dril) having many sides or surfaces.

pol·y·hi·dro·sis (-hi-dro′sis) hyperhidrosis.

pol·y·hy·dram·ni·os (-hi-dram′ne-os) excess of amniotic fluid, usually exceeding 2000 mL.

pol·y·hy·dric (-hi′drik) containing more than two hydroxyl groups.

pol·y·in·fec·tion (-in-fek′shun) infection with more than one organism.

pol·y·ion·ic (-i-on′ik) containing several different ions (e.g., potassium, sodium, etc.), as a polyionic solution.

pol·y·iso·pre·noid (-i′so-pre-noid″) any isoprenoid that contains multiple isoprene units, such as rubber.

pol·y·lac·tic ac·id (-lak′tik) a hydrophobic hydroxy acid polymer that is formed into granules and used as a surgical dressing for dental extraction sites.

pol·y·lep·tic (-lep′tik) having many remissions and exacerbations.

pol·y·mas·tia (-mas′te-ah) the presence of supernumerary mammary glands.

pol·y·mas·ti·gote (-mas′tĭ-gōt) 1. having several flagella. 2. a mastigote having several flagella.

pol·y·me·lia (-me′le-ah) a developmental anomaly characterized by the presence of supernumerary limbs.

pol·y·men·or·rhea (-men″ah-re′ah) abnormally frequent menstruation.

pol·y·mer (pol′ĭ-mer) a compound, usually of high molecular weight, formed by the combination of simpler molecules (monomers); it may be formed without formation of any other product (*addition p.*) or with simultaneous elimination of water or other simple compound (*condensation p.*).

po·lym·er·ase (pah-lim′er-ās) an enzyme that catalyzes polymerization.

pol·y·mer·ic (pol″ĭ-mer′ik) exhibiting the characteristics of a polymer.

po·lym·er·iza·tion (pah-lim″er-ĭ-za′shun) the combining of several simpler molecules (monomers) to form a polymer.

po·lym·er·ize (pah-lim′er-īz) to subject to or to undergo polymerization.

pol·y·meth·yl meth·ac·ryl·ate (pol″e-meth′il meth-ak′ril-āt) a thermoplastic acrylic resin formed by polymerization of methyl methacrylate. Abbreviated PMMA. Written also *polymethylmethacrylate.*

pol·y·mi·cro·bi·al (-mi-kro′be-al) marked by the presence of several species of microorganisms.

poly·mi·cro·bic (-mi-kro'bik) polymicrobial.

poly·mi·cro·gy·ria (-mi″kro-ji're-ah) a developmental anomaly of the brain marked by development of numerous small convolutions (microgyri), causing mental retardation.

poly·morph (pol'ĭ-morf) colloquial term for polymorphonuclear leukocyte.

poly·mor·phic (pol″e-mor'fik) occurring in several or many forms; appearing in different forms in different developmental stages.

poly·mor·phism (-mor'fizm) the quality of existing in several different forms. **balanced p.,** an equilibrium mixture of homozygotes and heterozygotes maintained by natural selection against both homozygotes.

poly·mor·pho·cel·lu·lar (-mor″fah-sel'u-lar) having cells of many forms.

poly·mor·pho·nu·cle·ar (-noo'kle-er) having a nucleus so deeply lobed or so divided as to appear to be multiple.

poly·mor·phous (-mor'fus) polymorphic.

poly·my·al·gia (-mi-al'jah) pain involving many muscles.

poly·my·oc·lo·nus (-mi-ok'lŏ-nus) myoclonus in several muscles or groups simultaneously or in rapid succession.

poly·my·op·a·thy (-mi-op'ah-the) disease affecting several muscles simultaneously.

poly·myo·si·tis (-mi″ah-si'tis) inflammation of several or many muscles at once, along with degenerative and regenerative changes marked by muscle weakness out of proportion to the loss of muscle bulk.

poly·myx·in (-mik'sin) generic term for antibiotics derived from *Bacillus polymyxa*; they are differentiated by affixing different letters of the alphabet. **p. B,** the least toxic of the polymyxins; its sulfate is used in the treatment of various gram-negative infections.

poly·ne·sic (-ne'sik) occurring in many foci.

poly·neu·ral (-noor'il) pertaining to or supplied by many nerves.

poly·neu·ral·gia (-noor-al'jah) neuralgia of several nerves.

poly·neu·ri·tis (-noo-ri'tis) inflammation of several peripheral nerves simultaneously. **acute febrile p., acute idiopathic p.,** an acute, rapidly progressive, ascending motor neuron paralysis, beginning in the feet and ascending to the other muscles, often occurring after an enteric or respiratory infection.

poly·neu·ro·myo·si·tis (-noor″o-mi″o-si'tis) polyneuritis with polymyositis.

poly·neu·rop·a·thy (-noo-rop'ah-the) neuropathy of several peripheral nerves simultaneously. **amyloid p.,** polyneuropathy caused by amyloidosis; symptoms may include dysfunction of the autonomic nervous system, carpal tunnel syndrome, and sensory disturbances in the limbs. **erythredema p.,** acrodynia. **familial amyloid p.,** autosomal dominant amyloid polyneuropathy occurring in hereditary amyloidosis; subtypes include *Portuguese type, Indiana type, Finnish type,* and *Iowa type.*

poly·neu·ro·ra·dic·u·li·tis (-noor″o-rah-dik″u-li'tis) acute idiopathic polyneuritis.

poly·nu·cle·ar (-noo″kle-er) having several nuclei; said of cells.

poly·nu·cle·ate (-noo'kle-āt) polynuclear.

poly·nu·cleo·tide (-noo'kle-o-tīd) any polymer of mononucleotides.

Poly·o·ma·vi·ri·nae (pol″e-o″mah-vir-i'-ne) the polyomaviruses: a subfamily of viruses of the family Papovaviridae, many members of which induce tumors in experimental animals; the single genus is *Polyomavirus.*

Poly·o·ma·vi·rus (-vi″rus) polyomaviruses; a genus of viruses of the subfamily Polyomavirinae (family Papovaviridae) that induce tumors in experimental animals; two, BK virus and JC virus, infect humans, and others, including simian virus 40 (SV40), infect other mammals.

poly·o·ma·vi·rus any member of the subfamily Polyomavirinae.

poly·opia (pol″e-o'pe-ah) visual perception of several images of a single object.

poly·or·chi·dism (-or'kid-izm) the presence of more than two testes.

poly·os·tot·ic (-os-tot'ik) affecting several bones.

poly·ov·u·lar (-ov'u-lar) pertaining to or produced from more than one oocyte, as in dizygotic twins.

poly·ov·u·la·to·ry (-ov'u-lah-tor″e) discharging several oocytes in one ovarian cycle.

poly·ox·yl (-ok'sil) a group of surfactants consisting of a mixture of mono- and diesters of stearate and polyoxyethylene diols; they are numbered according to the average polymer length of oxyethylene units, e.g., polyoxyl 40 stearate, and many are used in pharmaceutical preparations.

pol·yp (pol'ip) any growth or mass protruding from a mucous membrane. **adenomatous p.,** a benign neoplastic growth with variable malignant potential, representing proliferation of epithelial tissue in the lumen of the sigmoid colon, rectum, or stomach. **juvenile p's,** small, benign hemispheric hamartomas of the large intestine occurring sporadically in children. **retention p's,** juvenile p's.

pol·yp·ec·to·my (pol″ĭ-pek'tah-me) excision of a polyp.

poly·pep·tide (-pep'tīd) a peptide containing more than two amino acids linked by peptide bonds. **vasoactive intestinal p.,**

a hormone that has vasoactive properties, stimulates intestinal secretion of water and electrolytes, inhibits gastric secretion, promotes glycogenolysis, causes hyperglycemia, and stimulates production of pancreatic juice.

poly·pep·ti·de·mia (-pep″tĭ-dēm′e-ah) the presence of polypeptides in the blood.

poly·pha·gia (-fa′jah) excessive eating; see also *bulimia.*

poly·pha·lan·gia (-fah-lan′jah) side-by-side duplication of one or more phalanges in a digit.

poly·pha·lan·gism (-fah-lan′jizm) polyphalangia.

poly·phar·ma·cy (-fahr′mah-se) 1. administration of many drugs together. 2. administration of excessive medication.

poly·pho·bia (-fo′be-ah) irrational fear of many things.

poly·plas·tic (-plas′tik) 1. containing many structural or constituent elements. 2. undergoing many changes of form.

poly·ploi·dy (-ploi″de) possession of more than two sets of homologous chromosomes.

pol·yp·nea (pol″ip-ne′ah) hyperpnea.

pol·yp·oid (pol′ĭ-poid) resembling a polyp.

poly·po·rous (pol′e-por″us) having many pores.

pol·yp·osis (pol″ĭ-po′sis) the formation of numerous polyps. **familial p., familial adenomatous p.,** multiple adenomatous polyps with high malignant potential, lining the intestinal mucosa, especially that of the colon, beginning at about puberty. It occurs in several hereditary conditions, including *Gardner's, Peutz-Jeghers,* and *Turcot's syndromes.*

pol·yp·ous (pol′ĭ-pus) polyp-like.

poly·pro·py·lene (pol″e-pro′pĭ-lēn) a synthetic, crystalline, thermoplastic polymer with a molecular weight of 40,000 or more and the general formula $(C_3H_5)_n$; uses include nonabsorbable sutures, surgical casts, and the membranes for membrane oxygenators.

poly·pty·chi·al (-ti′ke-al) arranged in several layers.

poly·pus (pol′ĭ-pus) pl. *pol′ypi.* [L.] polyp.

poly·ra·dic·u·li·tis (pol″e-rah-dik″u-li′tis) inflammation of the nerve roots.

poly·ra·dic·u·lo·neu·ri·tis (-rah-dik″u-lo-noŏ-ri′tis) acute idiopathic polyneuritis.

poly·ra·dic·u·lo·neu·rop·a·thy (-rah-dik″u-lo-noŏ-rop′ah-the) 1. any disease of the peripheral nerves and spinal nerve roots. 2. acute idiopathic polyneuritis.

poly·ri·bo·some (-ri′bo-sōm) a cluster of ribosomes connected with messenger RNA; they play a role in peptide synthesis.

poly·sac·cha·ride (-sak′ah-rīd) a carbohydrate that on hydrolysis yields many monosaccharides.

poly·se·ro·si·tis (-sēr″ah-si′tis) general inflammation of serous membranes, with effusion.

poly·si·lox·ane (-si′lok-sān) any of various polymeric siloxanes, particularly the silicones.

poly·some (pol′e-sōm) polyribosome.

poly·som·nog·ra·phy (pol″e-som-nog′rah-fe) the polygraphic recording during sleep of multiple physiologic variables related to the state and stages of sleep to assess possible biological causes of sleep disorders.

poly·so·my (pol′e-so″me) an excess of a particular chromosome.

poly·sor·bate (pol″e-sor′bāt) any of various oleate esters of sorbitol and its anhydrides condensed with polymers of ethylene oxide, numbered to indicate chemical composition and used as surfactant agents.

poly·sper·mia (-sper′me-ah) polyspermy.

poly·sper·my (-sper′me) fertilization of an oocyte by more than one spermatozoon; occurring normally in certain species (*physiologic p.*) and sometimes abnormally in others (*pathologic p.*).

poly·sty·rene (-sti′rēn) the resin produced by polymerization of styrol, a clear resin of the thermoplastic type, used in the construction of denture bases.

poly·sy·nap·tic (-sĭ-nap′tik) pertaining to or relayed through two or more synapses.

poly·syn·dac·ty·ly (-sin-dak′tĭ-le) an association of polydactyly and syndactyly of varying degrees of both the hand and foot.

poly·tef (pol′ĭ-tef) a polymer of tetrafluoroethylene, used as a surgical implant material for many prostheses, such as artificial vessels and orbital floor implants and for many applications in skeletal augmentation and skeletal fixation.

poly·tene (pol′ĭ-tēn) composed of or containing many strands of chromatin (chromonemata).

poly·teno·syn·o·vi·tis (pol″e-ten″o-sin″o-vi′tis) inflammation of several or many tendon sheaths at the same time.

poly·the·lia (-thēl′e-ah) the presence of supernumerary nipples.

poly·thi·a·zide (-thi′ah-zīd) a thiazide diuretic used in the treatment of hypertension and edema.

poly·to·mo·gram (-tom′ah-gram) the record produced by polytomography.

poly·to·mog·ra·phy (-to-mog′rah-fe) tomography of tissue at several predetermined planes.

poly·trau·ma (-traw'mah) the occurrence of injuries to more than one body system.

poly·trich·ia (-trik'e-ah) hypertrichosis.

poly·un·sat·u·rat·ed (-un-sach'er-āt-ed) denoting a chemical compound, particularly a fatty acid, having two or more double or triple bonds in its hydrocarbon chain.

poly·uria (-ūr'e-ah) excessive secretion of urine.

poly·va·lent (-va'lent) multivalent.

poly·vi·nyl (-vi'nil) a polymerization product of a monomeric vinyl compound. **p. alco·hol,** see under *alcohol.* **p. chloride,** a taste-less, odorless, clear, hard resin formed by the polymerization of vinyl chloride; its uses include packaging, clothing, and insulating pipes and wires. Workers in its manufacture are at risk because of the toxicity of vinyl chloride.

poly·vi·nyl·pyr·rol·i·done (-vi"nil-pĭ-ro'lĭ-dōn) povidone.

poly·zo·o·sper·mia (-zo"o-sper'me-ah) ex-cessive numbers of highly motile sperm in the semen.

pom·pho·lyx (pom'fo-liks) [Gr.] an intensely pruritic skin eruption on the sides of the digits or on the palms and soles, consisting of small, discrete, round vesicles, typically occurring in repeated self-limited attacks.

pons (ponz) pl. *pon'tes.* [L.] 1. any slip of tissue connecting two parts of an organ. 2. that part of the central nervous system lying between the medulla oblongata and the midbrain, ventral to the cerebellum; see *brainstem.* **p. he'patis,** an occasional pro-jection partially bridging the longitudinal fissure of the liver.

pon·tic (pon'tik) the portion of a dental bridge that substitutes for an absent tooth.

pon·tic·u·lus (pon-tik'u-lus) pl. *ponti'culi.* [L.] a small ridge or bridgelike structure. **pontic'-ular,** adj.

pon·tine (pon'tīn, pon'tēn) pertaining to the pons.

pont(o)- word element [L.], *the pons.*

pon·to·bul·bar (pon"to-bul'ber) pertaining to the pons and the region of the medulla oblongata dorsad to it.

pon·to·cer·e·bel·lar (-ser"ě-bel'ar) per-taining to the pons and cerebellum.

pon·to·mes·en·ce·phal·ic (-mes"en-sef'al-ik) pertaining to or involving the pons and the mesencephalon.

pool (pool) 1. a common reservoir on which to draw; a supply available to be used by a group. 2. to create such a reservoir or supply, as the mixing of plasma from several donors. 3. an accumulation, as of blood in a part of the body due to retardation of the venous circulation.

pop·lit·e·al (pop"lit'e-il) pertaining to the area behind the knee.

POR problem-oriented record.

por·ac·tant al·fa (por-ak'tant al'fah) an extract of porcine lung surfactant used in the treatment of respiratory distress syndrome of the newborn.

por·ad·e·ni·tis (por"ad-ě-ni'tis) inflamma-tion of iliac lymph nodes with formation of small abscesses.

por·cine (por'sīn) pertaining to swine.

pore (por) a small opening or empty space. **alveolar p's,** openings between adjacent pulmonary alveoli that permit passage of air from one to another. **nuclear p's,** small octagonal openings in the nuclear envelope at sites where the two nuclear membranes are in contact, which together with the annuli form the pore complex. **slit p's,** small slitlike spaces between the pedicels of the podocytes of the renal glomerulus.

por·en·ceph·a·li·tis (por"en-sef"ah-li'tis) porencephaly associated with an inflammatory process.

por·en·ceph·a·ly (-en-sef'ah-le) develop-ment or presence of abnormal cysts or cavities in the brain tissue, usually communicating with a lateral ventricle. **porencephal'ic, por-enceph'alous,** adj.

por·fi·mer (por'fi-mer") a light-activated antineoplastic related to porphyrin; used as the sodium salt in the treatment of eso-phageal and non–small cell lung carcinomas.

por(o)-[1] word element [Gr.], *duct; passage-way; opening; pore.*

por(o)-[2] word element [Gr.], *callus; calculus.*

po·ro·ker·a·to·sis (por"o-ker"ah-to'sis) a hereditary dermatosis marked by a centri-fugally spreading hypertrophy of the stratum corneum around the sweat pores followed by atrophy. Called also *p. of Mibelli.* **poro-keratot'ic,** adj.

po·ro·ma (por-o'mah) a tumor arising in a pore. **eccrine p.,** a benign tumor arising from the intradermal portion of an eccrine sweat duct, usually on the sole.

po·ro·sis (por-o'sis) 1. the formation of the callus in repair of a fractured bone. 2. cavity formation.

po·ros·i·ty (por-os'it-e) the condition of being porous; a pore.

por·ous (por'us) penetrated by pores and open spaces.

por·phin (por'fin) the fundamental ring structure of four linked pyrrole nuclei around which porphyrins, hemin, cytochromes, and chlorophyll are built.

condyloid processes of the rami, the base of the skull and its foramina, the petrous pyramids, the sphenoidal, posterior ethmoid, and maxillary sinuses, and the nasal septum. **Waters' p.,** a radiographic position that gives a posteroanterior view of the maxillary sinus, maxilla, orbits, and zygomatic arches.

pos·i·tive (poz'it-iv) 1. having a value greater than zero. 2. indicating existence or presence, as chromatin-positive. 3. characterized by affirmation or cooperation.

pos·i·tron (poz'ĭ-tron) the antiparticle of an electron; a positively charged electron.

po·sol·o·gy (pah-sol'ah-je) the science or a system of dosage. **posolog'ic,** adj.

post- word element [L.], *after; behind.*

post·anal (pōst-a'n'l) behind or beyond the anus.

post·au·ric·u·lar (pōst″aw-rik'u-lar) located or performed behind the auricle of the ear.

post·ax·i·al (pōst-ak'se-il) behind an axis; in anatomy, referring to the medial (ulnar) aspect of the upper arm, and the lateral (fibular) aspect of the lower leg.

post·bra·chi·al (-bra'ke-il) on the posterior part of the upper arm.

post·cap·il·lary (-kap'ĭ-lar'e) 1. located just to the venous side of a capillary. 2. venous capillary.

post·ca·va (-ka'vah) the inferior vena cava. **postca'val,** adj.

post·cen·tral (-sen'tral) posterior to a center, as the postcentral gyrus.

post·ci·bal (-si'bil) postprandial.

post·coi·tal (-koi't'l) after coitus.

post·di·as·tol·ic (-di″as-tol'ik) after diastole.

post·di·crot·ic (pōst″di-krot'ik) after the dicrotic elevation of the sphygmogram.

pos·ter·i·or (pos-tēr'e-er) directed toward or situated at the back; opposite of anterior.

poster(o)- word element [L.], *the back; posterior to.*

pos·tero·an·te·ri·or (pos″ter-o-an-tēr'e-er) directed from the back toward the front.

pos·tero·clu·sion (-kloo'zhun) distoclusion.

pos·tero·ex·ter·nal (-ek-ster'nal) situated on the outside of a posterior aspect.

pos·tero·in·fe·ri·or (-in-fēr'e-er) posterior and inferior.

pos·tero·lat·er·al (-lat'er-al) situated on the side and toward the posterior aspect.

pos·tero·me·di·an (-me'de-an) situated on the middle of a posterior aspect.

pos·tero·su·pe·ri·or (-soo-pēr'e-er) posterior and superior.

post·gan·gli·on·ic (pōst″gang-gle-on'ik) distal to a ganglion.

post·glo·mer·u·lar (-glo-mer'u-ler) located or occurring distal to a renal glomerulus.

pos·thi·tis (pos-thi'tis) inflammation of the prepuce.

post·hyp·not·ic (pōst″hip-not'ik) following the hypnotic state.

post·ic·tal (pōst-ik'tal) following a seizure.

post·in·fec·tious (pōst″in-fek'shus) occurring after infection.

post·in·flam·ma·to·ry (-in-flam'ah-tor″e) occurring after or secondary to inflammation.

post·ma·tur·i·ty (-mah-choōr'it-e) the condition of an infant after a prolonged gestation period. **postmature',** adj.

post mor·tem (pōst mort'im) [L.] after death.

post·mor·tem (pōst-mort'im) performed or occurring after death.

post·na·sal (-na'z'l) posterior to the nose.

post·na·tal (-na't'l) occurring after birth, with reference to the newborn.

post par·tum (pōst pahr'tum) [L.] after parturition.

post·par·tum (pōst-pahr'tum) occurring after childbirth, with reference to the mother.

post·pran·di·al (-pran'de-al) occurring after a meal.

post·pu·ber·al (-pu'ber-al) postpubertal.

post·pu·ber·tal (-pu'ber-tal) after puberty.

post·pu·bes·cent (pōst″pu-bes'ent) postpubertal.

post·re·nal (pōst-re'nal) 1. located behind a kidney. 2. occurring after leaving a kidney.

post·si·nu·soi·dal (pōst″sĭ-nŭ-soi'dal) located behind a sinusoid or affecting the circulation beyond a sinusoid.

post·sphe·noid (pōst-sfe'noid) pertaining to the posterior portion of the body of the sphenoid bone.

post·ste·not·ic (pōst″stĕ-not'ik) located or occurring distal to or beyond a stenosed segment.

post·sy·nap·tic (-sĭ-nap'tik) distal to or occurring beyond a synapse.

post·term (-term') extending beyond term; said of a pregnancy or of an infant.

post·trau·mat·ic (pōst″traw-mat'ik) occurring as a result of or after injury.

pos·tu·late (pos'choo-lāt) anything assumed or taken for granted.

pos·ture (pos'choor) the attitude of the body. **pos'tural,** adj.

post·vac·ci·nal (pōst-vak'sĭ-nil) occurring after vaccination for smallpox.

pot·a·ble (po'tah-b'l) fit to drink.

pot·as·se·mia (pot″ah-se'me-ah) hyperkalemia.

po·tas·si·um (K) (pah-tas'e-um) chemical element (see *Table of Elements*), at. no. 19. Potassium is the chief cation of intracellular fluid, and many of its salts are used as electrolyte replenishers and antihypokalemics, including *p. acetate*, *p. bicarbonate*, *p. chloride*, and *p. gluconate*. For potassium salts not listed here, see under the active ingredient. **p. bitartrate,** a compound administered rectally with sodium bicarbonate to produce carbon dioxide; used for relief of constipation, evacuation of the colon before surgical or diagnostic procedures, and pre- and postpartum bowel emptying. **p. chloride,** an electrolyte replenisher, KCl. **p. citrate,** a systemic and urinary alkalizer, replenisher, and diuretic. **dibasic p. phosphate,** the dipotassium salt, K_2HPO_4; used alone or in combination with other phosphate compounds as an electrolyte replenisher. **p. hydroxide,** an alkalizer used in pharmaceutical preparations. **p. iodide,** a thyroid inhibitor used in the treatment of hyperthyroidism, as a radiation protectant to the thyroid, as an iodine replenisher, and as an antifungal. **monobasic p. phosphate,** the monopotassium salt, KH_2PO_4; used as a buffering agent in pharmaceutical preparations and, alone or in combination with other phosphate compounds, as an electrolyte replenisher, urinary acidifier, and antiurolithic. **p. permanganate,** the potassium salt of permanganic acid, used as a topical anti-infective, oxidizing agent, and as an antidote for certain poisons. **p. phosphate,** a compound combining potassium and phosphoric acid, usually dibasic potassium phosphate.

po·ten·cy (po′ten-se) 1. the ability of the male to perform coitus. 2. the relationship between the therapeutic effect of a drug and the dose necessary to achieve that effect. 3. the ability of an embryonic part to develop and complete its destiny. **po′tent,** adj.

po·ten·tial (po-ten′shal) 1. existing and ready for action, but not active. 2. the work per unit charge necessary to move a charged body in an electric field from a reference point to another point, measured in volts. **action p. (AP),** the electrical activity developed in a muscle or nerve cell during activity. **after-p.,** afterpotential. **electric p., electrical p.,** potential (2). **evoked p. (EP),** the electrical signal recorded from a sensory receptor, nerve, muscle, or area of the central nervous system that has been stimulated, usually by electricity. **membrane p.,** the electric potential existing on the two sides of a membrane or across the cell wall. **resting p.,** the potential difference across the membrane of a normal cell at rest. **spike p.,** the initial, very large change in potential of an excitable cell membrane during excitation.

po·ten·tial·iza·tion (po-ten″shal-ĭ-za′shun) potentiation (1).

po·ten·ti·a·tion (po-ten″she-a′shun) 1. enhancement of one agent by another so that the combined effect is greater than the sum of the effects of each one alone. 2. posttetanic p. **posttetanic p.,** an incrementing response without change of action potential amplitude, occurring with repetitive nerve stimulation.

po·ten·ti·za·tion (po-ten″tĭ-za′shun) in homeopathy, the process of making a remedy more potent by serial dilution (even to extent that it is unlikely to contain a single molecule of the original substance) and succussion.

pouch (pouch) a pocket or sac. **abdominovesical p.,** one formed by reflection of the peritoneum from the abdominal wall to the anterior surface of the bladder. **branchial p.,** pharyngeal p. **p. of Douglas,** rectouterine p. **ileoanal p.,** see under *reservoir*. **Kock p.,** 1. a continent ileal reservoir with a capacity of 500 to 1000 mL and a valve made by intussusception of the terminal ileum. 2. a modification of this pouch, used as a neobladder. **pharyngeal p.,** a lateral endodermal diverticulum of the pharynx that meets a corresponding pharyngeal groove in the embryonic ectoderm, forming a closing membrane. **Prussak's p.,** a recess in the tympanic membrane between the flaccid part of the membrane and the neck of the malleus. **Rathke's p.,** a diverticulum from the embryonic buccal cavity from which the adenohypophysis is developed. **rectouterine p., rectovaginal p.,** the space between the bladder and uterus in the female peritoneal cavity. **rectovesical p.,** the space between the rectum and the bladder in the male peritoneal cavity. **Seessel's p.,** an outpouching of the embryonic pharynx rostrad of the pharyngeal membrane and caudal to Rathke's pouch. **vesicouterine p.,** the space between the bladder and the uterus in the female peritoneal cavity.

pouch·itis (pouch-i′tis) inflammation of the mucosa, or of the full thickness, of the intestinal wall of an ileal or ileoanal reservoir.

poul·tice (pōl′tis) a soft, moist mass about the consistency of cooked cereal, spread between layers of muslin, linen, gauze, or towels and applied hot to a given area in order to create moist local heat or counterirritation.

pound (lb) (pound) a unit of weight in the avoirdupois (453.6 grams, or 16 ounces) or apothecaries' (373.2 grams, or 12 ounces) system.

po·vi·done (po′vĭ-dōn) a synthetic polymer used as a dispersing and suspending agent. **p.-iodine,** a complex produced by reacting iodine with povidone; used as a topical antiinfective.

pow·er (pou′er) 1. capability; potency; the ability to act. 2. a measure of magnification, as of a microscope. 3. the rate at which work is done; symbol *P*. 4. of a statistical test: the probability of correctly rejecting the null hypothesis when a specified alternative holds true. **defining p.,** the ability of a lens to make an object clearly visible. **resolving p.,** the ability of the eye or of a lens to make small objects that are close together separately visible, thus revealing the structure of an object.

pox (poks) any eruptive or pustular disease, especially one caused by a virus, e.g., chickenpox, cowpox, smallpox.

Pox·vi·ri·dae (poks″vir′ĭ-de) the poxviruses: a family of DNA viruses with a double-stranded DNA genome, including viruses causing smallpox and the pox diseases of other animals; the two subfamilies are Chordopoxvirinae (poxviruses of vertebrates) and Entomopoxvirinae (poxviruses of insects).

pox·vi·rus (poks′-vi-rus) any virus of the family Poxviridae.

PPD purified protein derivative; see under *tuberculin*.

ppm parts per million.

PR prosthion; pulmonic regurgitation.

Pr praseodymium; presbyopia; prism.

PRA panel-reactive antibody.

prac·tice (prak′tis) the use of one's knowledge in a particular profession; the practice of medicine is the exercise of one's knowledge for recognition and treatment of disease. **family p.,** the medical specialty concerned with the planning and provision of the comprehensive primary health care of all members of a family on a continuing basis. **general p.,** old term for the provision of comprehensive medical care regardless of age of the patient or presence of a condition that may temporarily require the services of a specialist; the term has largely been replaced by the term *family practice.* **group p.,** see under *medicine*.

prac·ti·tion·er (prak-tish′un-er) one who has met the requirements of and is engaged in the practice of medicine, dentistry, or nursing. **nurse p.,** see under *nurse*.

prae- for words beginning thus, see those beginning *pre-*.

prag·mat·ag·no·sia (prag″mat-ag-no′zhah) agnosia.

prag·mat·am·ne·sia (-am-ne′zhah) visual agnosia.

praj·na·pa·ra·dha (pruj″nah-pah-rah-thah′) [Sanskrit] in ayurveda, deliberate, willful indulgence in unhealthy practices that leads to unbalanced body functions and disease.

pra·kri·ti (prŭ′kre-the) [Sanskrit] according to ayurveda, a person's underlying characteristic physical and mental constitution and tendencies of expression.

pral·i·dox·ime (pral″ĭ-doks′ēm) a cholinesterase reactivator, used as the chloride salt as an antidote in the treatment of organophosphate poisoning and to counteract the effects of overdosage by anticholinesterases used in treating myasthenia gravis.

pram·i·pex·ole (pram″ĭ-pek′sōl) a dopamine agonist used in the form of the dihydrochloride salt as an antidyskinetic in the treatment of Parkinson's disease.

pra·mox·ine (pră-mok′sēn) a local anesthetic applied topically as the hydrochloride salt for temporary relief of pain and pruritus associated with skin and anorectal disorders.

pra·na (prah′nah) [Sanskrit] in ayurvedic tradition, the life force or vital energy, which permeates the body and is especially concentrated along the midline in the chakras.

pra·na·ya·ma (prah″nah-yah′mah) according to ayurveda, breath control, occurring as one of the eight limbs of yoga; used for controlling the energy within the body and the mind and acting as a vitalizing and regenerating force to increase oxygen exchange that can be used for physical healing.

pran·di·al (pran′de-il) pertaining to a meal.

pra·seo·dym·i·um (Pr) (pra″ze-o-dim′e-um) chemical element (see *Table of Elements*), at. no. 59.

prav·a·stat·in (prav′ah-stat″in) an antihyperlipidemic agent that acts by inhibiting cholesterol synthesis, used as the sodium salt in the treatment of hypercholesterolemia and other forms of dyslipidemia and to lower the risks associated with atherosclerosis and coronary heart disease.

prax·i·ol·o·gy (prak″se-ol′ah-je) the science or study of conduct.

pra·zi·quan·tel (pra″zĭ-kwahn′t′l) a broad-spectrum anthelmintic used for the treatment of a wide variety of fluke and tapeworm infections.

pra·zo·sin (pra′zah-sin) an alpha-adrenergic blocking agent with vasodilator properties, used as the hydrochloride salt in the treatment of hypertension.

pre- word element [L.], *before* (in time or space).

pre·ag·o·nal (pre-ag′in′l) immediately before the death agony.

pre·an·es·thet·ic (pre″an-es-thet′ik) occurring before administration of an anesthetic.

pre·au·ric·u·lar (-aw-rik′u-lar) in front of the auricle of the ear.

pre·ax·i·al (pre-ak′se-il) situated before an axis; in anatomy, referring to the lateral (radial) aspect of the upper arm, and the medial (tibial) aspect of the lower leg.

pre·be·ta·lipo·pro·tein·emia (-ba″tah-lip″o-pro″te-ne′me-ah) hyperprebetalipo-proteinemia.

pre·can·cer·ous (-kan′ser-us) pertaining to a pathologic process that tends to become malignant.

pre·cap·il·lary (-kap′ĭ-lar″e) 1. located just to the arterial side of a capillary. 2. arterial capillary.

pre·car·di·ac (-kahr′de-ak) situated anterior to the heart.

pre·ca·va (-ka′vah) the superior vena cava. **preca′val,** adj.

pre·cen·tral (-sen′tral) anterior to a center, as the precentral gyrus.

pre·chor·dal (-kord″l) situated cranial to the notochord.

pre·cip·i·tant (-sip′it-int) a substance that causes precipitation.

pre·cip·i·tate (-sip′ĭ-tāt) 1. to cause settling in solid particles of substance in solution. 2. a deposit of solid particles settled out of a solution. 3. occurring with undue rapidity.

pre·cip·i·tin (-sip′it-in) an antibody to soluble antigen that specifically aggregates the macromolecular antigen in vivo and in vitro to give a visible precipitate.

pre·cip·i·tin·o·gen (-sip″ĭ-tin′ah-jen) a soluble antigen that stimulates the formation of and reacts with a precipitin.

pre·clin·i·cal (-klin′ĭ-k′l) before a disease becomes clinically recognizable.

pre·clot·ting (-klot′ing) the forcing of a patient's blood through the interstices of a knitted vascular prosthesis prior to implantation to render the graft temporarily impervious to blood by short-term deposition of fibrin and platelets in the interstices.

pre·coc·i·ty (-kos′it-e) unusually early development of mental or physical traits. **pre·co′cious,** adj. **sexual p.,** precocious puberty.

pre·cog·ni·tion (pre″kog-nish′un) extrasensory perception of a future event.

pre·co·ma (pre-ko′mah) the neuropsychiatric state preceding coma, as in hepatic encephalopathy. **precom′atose,** adj.

pre·con·scious (-kon′shus) the part of the mind not present in consciousness, but readily recalled into it.

pre·cor·di·um (-kor′de-um) pl. *precor′dia.* The region of the anterior surface of the body covering the heart and lower thorax. **precor′dial,** adj.

pre·cos·tal (-kos′til) in front of the ribs.

pre·cu·ne·us (-ku′ne-us) [L.] a small convolution on the medial surface of the parietal lobe of the cerebrum.

pre·cur·sor (pre′kur-ser) something that precedes. In biological processes, a substance from which another, usually more active or mature, substance is formed. In clinical medicine, a sign or symptom that heralds another. **precur′sory,** adj.

pre·di·a·be·tes (pre-di″ah-bēt′ēz) a state of latent impairment of carbohydrate metabolism in which the criteria for diabetes mellitus are not all satisfied.

pre·di·as·to·le (pre″di-as′tah-le) the interval immediately preceding diastole. **prediastol′ic,** adj.

pre·di·crot·ic (-di-krot′ik) occurring before the dicrotic wave of the sphygmogram.

pre·di·ges·tion (-di-jes′chun) partial artificial digestion of food before its ingestion.

pre·dis·po·si·tion (-dis-po-zish′un) a latent susceptibility to disease that may be activated under certain conditions.

pre·di·ver·tic·u·lar (pre-di″ver-tik′u-lar) denoting a condition of thickening of the muscular wall of the colon and increased intraluminal pressure without evidence of diverticulosis.

pred·ni·car·bate (pred″nĭ-kahr′bāt) a synthetic corticosteroid used topically for the relief of inflammation and pruritus in certain dermatoses.

pred·nis·o·lone (pred-nis′ah-lōn) a synthetic glucocorticoid derived from cortisol, used in the form of the base or the acetate, sodium phosphate, or tebutate ester in replacement therapy for adrenocortical insufficiency, as an antiinflammatory, and as an immunosuppressant.

pred·ni·sone (pred′nĭ-sōn) a synthetic glucocorticoid derived from cortisone, used as an antiinflammatory and immunosuppressant.

pre·eclamp·sia (pre″e-klamp′se-ah) a toxemia of late pregnancy, characterized by hypertension, proteinuria, and edema.

pre·ejec·tion (-e-jek′shun) occurring prior to ejection.

pre·ex·ci·ta·tion (pre-ek″si-ta′shun) premature activation of a portion of the ventricles due to transmission of cardiac impulses along an accessory pathway not subject to the physiologic delay of the atrioventricular node; sometimes used as a synonym of Wolff-Parkinson-White syndrome.

pre·fron·tal (-front′l) situated in the anterior part of the frontal lobe or region.

pre·gan·gli·on·ic (pre″gang-gle-on′ik) proximal to a ganglion.

pre·glo·mer·u·lar (-glo-mer′u-lar) located or occurring proximal to a renal glomerulus.

pre·gen·i·tal (pre-jen′ĭ-t′l) antedating the emergence of genital interests.

preg·nan·cy (preg′nan-se) 1. the condition of having a developing embryo or fetus in the body, after union of an oocyte and spermatozoon. **preg′nant,** adj. 2. the period during which one is pregnant; see *gestation period*, under *period*. **abdominal p.,** ectopic pregnancy within the abdominal cavity. **ampullar p.,** ectopic pregnancy in the ampulla of the uterine tube. **cervical p.,** ectopic pregnancy within the cervical canal. **combined p.,** simultaneous intrauterine and extrauterine pregnancies. **cornual p.,** pregnancy in one of the horns of a bicornuate uterus. **ectopic p., extrauterine p.,** development of the embryo outside of the uterine cavity. **false p.,** development of the signs of pregnancy without the presence of an embryo. **heterotopic p.,** combined p. **interstitial p.,** ectopic pregnancy in the part of the uterine tube within the uterine wall. **intraligamentary p., intraligamentous p.,** ectopic pregnancy within the broad ligament. **molar p.,** conversion of the early embryo into a mole. **multiple p.,** presence of more than one fetus in the uterus at the same time. **mural p.,** interstitial p. **ovarian p.,** ectopic pregnancy occurring in an ovary. **phantom p.,** false pregnancy due to psychogenic factors. **postterm p.,** one that has extended beyond 42 weeks from the onset of the last menstrual period or 40 completed weeks from conception. **tubal p.,** ectopic pregnancy within a uterine tube. **tuboabdominal p.,** ectopic pregnancy partly in the fimbriated end of a uterine tube and partly in the abdominal cavity. **tubo-ovarian p.,** ectopic pregnancy occurring partly in the ovary and partly in a uterine tube.

preg·nane (preg′nān) a crystalline saturated steroid hydrocarbon, $C_{21}H_{36}$; β-*pregnane* is the form from which several hormones, including progesterone, are derived; α-*pregnane* is the form excreted in the urine.

preg·nane·di·ol (preg″nān-di′ol) a crystalline, biologically inactive dihydroxy derivative of pregnane, formed by reduction of progesterone and found especially in urine of pregnant women.

preg·nane·tri·ol (-tri′ol) a metabolite of 17-hydroxyprogesterone; its excretion in the urine is greatly increased in certain disorders of the adrenal cortex.

preg·ne·no·lone (preg-nēn′ŏ-lōn) an intermediate in steroid hormone synthesis.

pre·hal·lux (pre-hal′uks) a supernumerary bone of the foot growing from the medial border of the scaphoid.

pre·hen·sile (-hen′sil) adapted for grasping or seizing.

pre·hen·sion (-hen′shun) the act of grasping.

pre·hor·mone (-hor′mōn) prohormone.

pre·hy·oid (-hi′oid) in front of the hyoid bone.

pre·ic·tal (-ik′tal) occurring before a stroke, seizure, or attack.

pre·in·va·sive (pre″in-va′siv) not yet invading tissues outside the site of origin.

pre·kal·li·kre·in (-kal-ĭ-kre′in) the proenzyme of plasma kallikrein; it is cleaved and activated by coagulation factor XII.

pre·leu·ke·mia (pre″loo-ke′me-ah) myelodysplastic syndrome. **preleuke′mic,** adj.

pre·lim·bic (pre-lim′bik) in front of a limbus.

pre-β-lipo·pro·tein (pre″ba-tah-lip″o-pro′tēn) very-low-density lipoprotein.

pre·load (pre′lōd) the mechanical state of the heart at the end of diastole, the magnitude of the maximal (end-diastolic) ventricular volume or the end-diastolic pressure stretching the ventricles.

pre·ma·lig·nant (pre″mah-lig′nant) precancerous.

pre·ma·tur·i·ty (-mah-chŏŏr′ĭ-te) underdevelopment; the condition of a premature infant. **premature′,** adj.

pre·max·il·la (-mak-sil′ah) 1. incisive bone. 2. the embryonic bone that later fuses with the maxilla to form the incisive bone.

pre·max·il·lary (pre-mak′sĭ-lar-e) 1. in front of the maxilla. 2. pertaining to the premaxilla (incisive bone).

pre·med·i·ca·tion (pre″med-ĭ-ka′shun) 1. preliminary administration of a drug preceding a diagnostic, therapeutic, or surgical procedure, as an antibiotic or antianxiety agent. 2. a drug administered for such a purpose.

pre·me·nar·che·al (-mĕ-nahr′ke-al) pertaining to the period before menarche.

pre·men·stru·al (pre-men′stroo-al) occurring before menstruation.

pre·men·stru·um (-men′stroo-um) pl. *premen′strua.* [L.] the interval immediately preceding a menstrual period.

pre·mo·lar (P) (-mo′ler) 1. see under *tooth.* 2. situated in front of the molar teeth.

pre·mor·bid (-mor′bid) occurring before development of disease.

pre·mu·ni·tion (pre″mu-nish′un) resistance to infection by the same or closely related pathogen established after an acute infection has become chronic, and lasting as long as the infecting organisms are in the body. **premu′nitive,** adj.

pre·my·elo·blast (pre-mi′ě-lo-blast″) precursor of a myeloblast.

pre·na·tal (-na′tal) preceding birth.

pre·neo·plas·tic (pre″ne-o-plas′tik) preceding the development of a tumor.

pre·op·tic (pre-op′tik) in front of the optic chiasm.

pre·pa·tel·lar (pre″pah-tel′ar) in front of the patella.

pre·peri·to·ne·al (-per-ĭ-to-ne′al) 1. situated between the parietal peritoneum and the abdominal wall. 2. occurring anterior to the peritoneum.

pre·pro·in·su·lin (-pro-in′su-lin) the precursor of proinsulin, containing an additional polypeptide sequence at the N-terminal.

pre·pro·pro·tein (-pro-pro′tēn) any precursor of a proprotein.

pre·pros·thet·ic (-pros-thet′ik) performed or occurring before insertion of a prosthesis.

pre·pu·ber·al (pre-pu′ber-al) prepubertal.

pre·pu·ber·tal (-pu′ber-tal) before puberty; pertaining to the period of accelerated growth preceding gonadal maturity.

pre·pu·bes·cent (pre″pu-bes′ent) prepubertal.

pre·puce (pre′pūs) 1. a covering fold of skin. 2. pt. of penis. **prepu′tial,** adj. **p. of clitoris,** a fold capping the clitoris, formed by union of the labia minora and the clitoris. **p. of penis,** foreskin; the fold of skin covering the glans penis.

pre·pu·ti·o·plas·ty (pre-pu′she-o-plas″te) plastic surgery of the prepuce.

pre·pu·ti·ot·o·my (-pu″she-ot′ah-me) incision of the prepuce to relieve phimosis.

pre·pu·ti·um (-pu′she-um) prepuce.

pre·py·lor·ic (pre″pi-lor′ik) just proximal to the pylorus.

pre·re·nal (pre-re′nal) 1. located in front of a kidney. 2. occurring before the kidney is reached.

pre·sa·cral (-sa′kral) anterior to or preceding the sacrum.

presby- word element [Gr.], *old age.*

pres·by·car·dia (prez″bĭ-kahr′de-ah) impaired cardiac function attributed to aging, with senescent changes in the body and no evidence of other cause of heart disease.

pres·by·cu·sis (-ku′sis) progressive, bilaterally symmetrical sensorineural hearing loss occurring with age.

pres·by·opia (Pr) (-o′pe-ah) diminution of accommodation of the lens of the eye occurring normally with aging. **presbyop′ic,** adj.

pre·scrip·tion (prě-skrip′shun) a written directive for the preparation and administration of a remedy; see also *inscription, signature, subscription,* and *superscription.*

pre·se·nile (pre-se′nīl) pertaining to a condition resembling senility, but occurring in early or middle life.

pre·sen·ta·tion (pre″zen-ta′shun) that part of the fetus lying over the pelvic inlet; the presenting body part of the fetus. Cf. *position* and *lie.* **antigen p.,** the hypothesis that macrophages not only ingest and process antigen, refining and complexing it with SRNA, but also present it in concentrated form at their surfaces to lymphocytes, thus inducing an immune response by the lymphocytes. **breech p.,** presentation of the fetal buttocks or feet in labor; the feet may be alongside the buttocks *(complete breech p.);* the legs may be extended against the trunk and the feet lying against the face *(frank breech p.);* or one or both feet or knees may be prolapsed into the maternal vagina *(incomplete breech p.).* **brow p.,** presentation of the fetal brow in labor. **cephalic p.,** presentation of any part of the fetal head in labor, whether the vertex, face, or brow. **compound p.,** prolapse of a limb of the fetus alongside the head in a cephalic presentation or of one or both arms in a breech presentation. **footling p.,** presentation of the fetus with one (single footling) or both (double footling) feet prolapsed into the maternal vagina. **funis p.,** presentation of the umbilical cord in labor. **placental p.,** placenta previa. **shoulder p.,** presentation of the fetal shoulder in labor; see *oblique lie* and *transverse lie.* **transverse p.,** see under *lie.* **vertex p.,** that in which the vertex of the fetal head is the presenting part.

pre·ser·va·tive (pre-zer′vah-tiv) a substance or preparation added to a product to destroy or inhibit the multiplication of microorganisms.

pre·si·nu·soi·dal (pre″si-nŭ-soi′dal) located in front of a sinusoid or affecting the circulation before the sinusoids.

pre·so·mite (pre-so′mīt) referring to embryos before the appearance of somites.

pre·sphe·noid (-sfe′noid) pertaining to the anterior portion of the body of the sphenoid bone.

pres·sor (pres′or) tending to increase blood pressure.

pres·so·re·cep·tive (pres″o-re-sep′tiv) sensitive to stimuli due to vasomotor activity.

pres·so·re·cep·tor (-re-sep′tor) baroreceptor.

pres·so·sen·si·tive (-sen′sĭ-tiv) pressoreceptive.

pres·sure (P) (presh′er) force per unit area. **arterial p.,** blood p. (2). **blood p.,** 1. the pressure of blood against the walls of any blood vessel. 2. the pressure of blood on the walls of the arteries, dependent on the energy of the heart action, elasticity of the arterial walls, and volume and viscosity of the blood; the *maximum* or *systolic* pressure occurs near the end of the stroke output of the left ventricle, and the *minimum* or *diastolic* late in ventricular diastole. **central venous p. (CVP),** the venous pressure as measured at the right atrium, done by means of a catheter introduced through the median cubital vein to the superior vena cava. **cerebrospinal p.,** the pressure or tension of the cerebrospinal fluid, normally 100–150 mm. as measured by the manometer. **detrusor p.,** the pressure exerted inwards by the detrusor urinae muscles of the bladder wall. **diastolic p., diastolic blood p.,** see *blood p.* **end-diastolic p.,** the pressure in the ventricles at the end of diastole, usually measured in the left ventricle as an approximation of the end-diastolic volume, or preload. **intracranial p. (ICP),** pressure of the subarachnoidal fluid. **intraocular p.,** the pressure exerted against the outer coats by the contents of the eyeball. **intravesical p.,** the pressure exerted on the contents of the urinary bladder; the sum of the intra-abdominal pressure from outside the bladder and the detrusor pressure. **maximum expiratory p. (MEP),** a measure of the strength of respiratory muscles, obtained by having the patient exhale as strongly as possible against a mouthpiece; the maximum value is near total lung capacity. **maximum inspiratory p. (MIP),** a measure of the strength of respiratory muscles, obtained by having the patient inhale as strongly as possible with the mouth against a mouthpiece; the maximum value is near the residual volume. **mean arterial p. (MAP),** the average pressure within an artery over a complete cycle of one heartbeat. **mean circulatory filling p.,** a measure of the average (arterial and venous) pressure necessary to cause filling of the circulation with blood; it varies with blood volume and is directly proportional to the rate of venous return and thus to cardiac output. **negative p.,** pressure less than that of the atmosphere. **oncotic p.,** the osmotic pressure due to the presence of colloids in solution. **osmotic p.,** the pressure required to prevent osmosis through a semipermeable membrane between a solution and pure solvent; it is proportional to the osmolality of the solution. Symbol π. **partial p.,** the pressure exerted by each of the constituents of a mixture of gases. **positive p.,** pressure greater than that of the atmosphere. **positive end-expiratory p. (PEEP),** a method of mechanical ventilation in which pressure is maintained to increase the volume of gas left in the lungs at the end of exhalation, reducing shunting of blood through the lungs and improving gas exchange. **pulmonary artery wedge p. (PAWP), pulmonary capillary wedge p. (PCWP),** intravascular pressure as measured by a catheter wedged into the distal pulmonary artery; used to measure indirectly the mean left atrial pressure. **pulse p.,** the difference between systolic and diastolic pressures. **systolic p., systolic blood p.,** see *blood p.* **Valsalva leak point p.,** the amount of pressure on the bladder by a Valsalva maneuver at which leakage of urine occurs; a measure of strength of the urethral sphincters. **venous p.,** the pressure of blood in the veins. **wedge p.,** blood pressure measured by a small catheter wedged into a vessel, occluding it, e.g., pulmonary capillary wedge p. **wedged hepatic vein p.,** the venous pressure measured with a catheter wedged into the hepatic vein; used to locate the site of obstruction in portal hypertension.

pre·su·bic·u·lum (pre″soo-bik′u-lum) a modified six-layered cortex between the subiculum and the main part of the parahippocampal gyrus.

pre·syn·ap·tic (-sĭ-nap′tik) situated or occurring proximal to a synapse.

pre·sys·to·le (pre-sis′tah-le) the interval just before systole.

pre·sys·tol·ic (pre″sis-tol′ik) 1. pertaining to the beginning of systole. 2. occurring just before systole.

pre·tec·tal (pre-tek′tal) located anterior to the tectum mesencephali.

pre·term (-term′) before completion of the full term; said of pregnancy or of an infant.

pre·thy·roid (-thi′roid) anterior to the thyroid gland or thyroid cartilage.

pre·tib·i·al (-tib′e-al) in front of the tibia.

prev·a·lence (prev′ah-lins) the number of cases of a specific disease present in a given population at a certain time.

pre·ven·tive (pre-vent′iv) prophylactic.

pre·ver·te·bral (-ver′tě-bral) anterior to a vertebra or vertebrae.

pre·ves·i·cal (-ves′ĭ-k′l) anterior to the bladder.

pre·zy·got·ic (pre″zi-got′ik) occurring before completion of fertilization.

pri·a·pism (pri′ah-pizm) persistent abnormal erection of penis, accompanied by pain and tenderness.

prick·le (prik′il) 1. a small, sharp spine or point. 2. a tingling or smarting sensation. **prick′ly,** adj.

pril·o·caine (pril′o-kān) a local anesthetic, used parenterally as the hydrochloride salt or topically, together with lidocaine, as the base.

prim·a·quine (prim′ah-kwēn) an 8-amino-quinoline compound used as an antimalarial in the form of the phosphate salt.

pri·mary (pri′mar-e) first in order or in time of development; principal.

Pri·ma·tes (pri-ma′tēz) the highest order of mammals, including humans, apes, monkeys, and lemurs.

prim·i·done (prim′ĭ-dōn) an anticonvulsant used in the treatment of generalized tonic-clonic, nocturnal myoclonic, and partial seizures.

pri·mi·grav·i·da (pri″mĭ-grav′ĭ-dah) a woman pregnant for the first time; gravida I.

pri·mip·a·ra (pri-mip′ah-rah) pl. *primip′arae*. Para I; a woman who has had one pregnancy that resulted in one or more viable young. See *para*. **primip′arous**, adj.

prim·i·tive (prim′ĭ-tiv) first in point of time; existing in a simple or early form that shows little complexity.

pri·mor·di·al (pri-mor′de-al) primitive.

pri·mor·di·um (-um) pl. *primor′dia*. [L.] the earliest indication of an organ or part during embryonic development.

prim·rose (prim′rōz) 1. a plant of the genus *Primula; P. obco′nica* (the cultivated primrose plant) is a common cause of allergic contact dermatitis. 2. evening p. **evening p.,** the herb *Oenothera biennis*, or a preparation of oil from its seeds; see under *oil*.

prin·ceps (prin′seps) [L.] principal; chief.

prin·ci·ple (prin′sip'l) 1. a chemical component. 2. a substance on which certain of the properties of a drug depend. 3. a law of conduct. **p. of infinitesimal dose,** a fundamental principle of homeopathy: the more a remedy is diluted (even to the point that none of the medicinal substance is likely to be present), the more powerful and longer lasting will be its effect. **yin/yang p.,** in Chinese philosophy, the concept of polar complements existing in dynamic equilibrium and always present simultaneously. In traditional Chinese medicine, a disturbance of the proper balance of yin and yang causes disease, and the goal is to maintain or to restore this balance.

pri·on (pri′on) any of several transmissible forms of the core of prion protein that cause a group of neurodegenerative diseases. Prions differ in structure from normal prion protein, lack detectable nucleic acid, and do not elicit an immune response.

prism (prizm) a solid with a triangular or polygonal cross section; used to correct deviations of the eyes. **adamantine p's, enamel p's,** the structural units of the tooth enamel, consisting of parallel rods or prisms composed mainly of hydroxyapatite crystals and organic substance.

pris·mo·sphere (priz′mo-sfēr) a prism combined with a spherical lens.

PRK photorefractive keratectomy.

PRL, Prl prolactin.

p.r.n. [L.] pro re na′ta (according to circumstances).

Pro proline.

pro- word element [L., Gr.], *before; in front of; favoring.*

pro·ac·cel·er·in (pro″ak-sel′er-in) coagulation factor V.

pro·ac·ti·va·tor (pro-akt′ĭ-vāt-er) a precursor of an activator; a factor that reacts with an enzyme to form an activator.

pro·ar·rhyth·mia (pro″ah-rith′me-ah) cardiac arrhythmia that is either drug-induced or drug-aggravated. **proarrhyth′mic**, adj.

pro·at·las (pro-at′lis) a rudimentary vertebra which in some animals lies in front of the atlas; sometimes seen in humans as an anomaly.

prob·a·bil·i·ty the likelihood of occurrence of a specified event, often represented as a number between 0 (never) and 1 (always) corresponding to the long-run frequency at which an event occurs in a sequence of random independent trials as the number of trials approaches infinity.

pro·band (pro′band) an affected person ascertained independently of relatives in a genetic study.

pro·bang (-bang) a flexible rod with a ball, tuft, or sponge at one end; used to apply medications to or remove matter from the esophagus or larynx.

probe (prōb) 1. a long, slender instrument for exploring wounds or body cavities or passages. 2. a radioactive or chemiluminescent DNA or RNA sequence used to detect the presence of a complementary sequence. DNA probes are used clinically to detect and identify infectious disease agents.

pro·ben·e·cid (pro-ben′ĕ-sid) a uricosuric agent used in the treatment of gout; also used to increase serum concentration of certain antibiotics and other drugs.

pro·cain·amide (pro-kān′ah-mīd) a cardiac depressant used as the hydrochloride salt in the treatment of arrhythmias.

pro·caine (pro′kān) a local anesthetic; the hydrochloride salt is used for infiltration and spinal anesthesia and peripheral nerve block.

pro·car·ba·zine (pro-kahr′bah-zēn) an alkylating agent used as the hydrochloride salt as an antineoplastic, primarily in the treatment of Hodgkin's disease.

pro·car·boxy·pep·ti·dase (pro″kahr-bok″se-pep′ti-dās) the inactive precursor of carboxypeptidase, which is converted to the active enzyme by the action of trypsin.

pro·car·cin·o·gen (-kahr-sin″ah-jen) a chemical substance that becomes carcinogenic only after it is altered by metabolic processes.

Pro·caryo·tae (pro-kar″e-o′te) former name for *Monera.*

pro·ce·dure (pro-se′jer) the manner of performing something; a method or technique. **arterial switch p.,** a one-step method for correction of transposition of the great arteries. **Burch p.,** a type of bladder neck suspension. **endocardial resection p. (ERP),** surgical removal of a portion of left ventricular endocardium and underlying myocardium containing an arrhythmogenic area from the base of an aneurysm or infarction in order to relieve ventricular tachycardia associated with ischemic heart disease. **Fontan p.,** functional correction of tricuspid atresia by anastomosis of, or insertion of a nonvalved prosthesis between, the right atrium and pulmonary artery with closure of the interatrial communication. **Pereyra p.,** a type of bladder neck suspension.

pro·cen·tri·ole (-sen′tre-ōl) the immediate precursor of centrioles and ciliary basal bodies.

pro·ce·phal·ic (pro″sĕ-fal′ik) pertaining to the anterior part of the head.

pro·cer·coid (pro-ser′koid) a larval stage of fish tapeworms.

proc·ess (pros′es) 1. a prominence or projection, as from a bone. 2. a series of operations, events, or steps leading to achievement of a specific result; also, to subject to such a series to produce desired changes. **acromial p.,** acromion. **alveolar p.,** the part of the bone in either the maxilla or mandible surrounding and supporting the teeth. **basilar p.,** a quadrilateral plate of the occipital bone projecting superiorly and anteriorly from the foramen magnum. **caudate p.,** the right of the two processes on the caudate lobe of the liver. **ciliary p's,** meridionally arranged ridges or folds projecting from the crown of the ciliary body. **clinoid p.,** any of the three (anterior, medial, and posterior) processes of the sphenoid bone. **coracoid p.,** a curved process arising from the upper neck of the scapula and overhanging the shoulder joint. **coronoid p.,** 1. the anterior part of the upper end of the ramus of the mandible. 2. a projection at the proximal end of the

ulna. **ensiform p. of sternum,** xiphoid p. **ethmoid p.,** a bony projection above and behind the maxillary process of the inferior nasal concha. **falciform p.,** 1. (of fascia lata) the lateral margin of the saphenous hiatus. 2. (of pelvic fascia) thickening of the superior fascia, from the ischial spine to the pubis. 3. Henle's ligament. **frontonasal p.,** see under *prominence.* **funicular p.,** the portion of the tunica vaginalis surrounding the spermatic cord. **lacrimal p.,** a process of the inferior nasal concha that articulates with the lacrimal bone. **malar p.,** zygomatic p. of maxilla. **mammillary p.,** a tubercle on the superior articular process of each lumbar vertebra. **mandibular p.,** see under *prominence.* **mastoid p.,** the conical projection at the base of the mastoid portion of the temporal bone. **maxillary p.,** 1. see under *prominence.* 2. (of inferior nasal concha): a bony process descending from the ethmoid process of the inferior nasal concha. **nasal p., lateral,** see under *prominence.* **nasal p., medial,** see under *prominence.* **odontoid p. of axis,** a toothlike projection of the axis that articulates with the atlas. **pterygoid p.,** one of the wing-shaped processes of the sphenoid. **spinous p.,** spine (1). **spinous p. of vertebrae,** a part of the vertebrae projecting backward from the arches, giving attachment to the back muscles. **styloid p.,** a long, pointed projection, especially a long spine projecting downward from the inferior surface of the temporal bone. **uncinate p.,** any hooklike process, as of a vertebra, the lacrimal bone, or the pancreas. **xiphoid p.,** the pointed process of cartilage, supported by a core of bone, connected with the lower end of the sternum. **zygomatic p.,** a projection in three parts, from the frontal bone, temporal bone, and maxilla, by which each articulates with the zygomatic bone.

pro·ces·sus (pro-ses′us) pl. *proces′sus.* [L.] process; used in official names of various anatomic structures.

pro·chlor·per·a·zine (pro″klor-per′ah-zēn) a phenothiazine derivative, used as the base or the edisylate or maleate salts as an antiemetic and antipsychotic.

pro·chon·dral (pro-kon′dril) occurring before the formation of cartilage.

pro·ci·den·tia (pro″si-den′shah) prolapse (1).

pro·co·ag·u·lant (-ko-ag′ūl-int) 1. tending to promote coagulation. 2. a precursor of a natural substance necessary to coagulation of the blood.

pro·col·la·gen (-kol′ah-jen) the precursor molecule of collagen, synthesized in the fibroblast, osteoblast, etc., and cleaved to form collagen extracellularly.

pro·con·ver·tin (-kon-ver′tin) coagulation factor VII.

pro·cre·a·tion (-kre-a′shun) reproduction (def. 1). **pro′creative,** adj.

proc·tal·gia (prok-tal′jah) pain in the rectum.

proc·tec·ta·sia (prokt″ek-ta′zhah) dilatation of the rectum or anus.

proc·tec·to·my (prok-tek′tah-me) excision of the rectum.

proc·teu·ryn·ter (prok″tu-rin′ter) a baglike device used to dilate the rectum.

proc·ti·tis (prok-ti′tis) inflammation of the rectum.

proct(o)- word element [Gr.], *rectum*; see also words beginning *rect(o)-*.

proc·to·cele (prok′to-sēl) rectocele.

proc·to·co·li·tis (prok″to-ko-li′tis) inflammation of the colon and rectum.

proc·to·col·po·plas·ty (-kol′po-plas″te) repair of a rectovaginal fistula.

proc·to·de·um (-de′um) the ectodermal depression of the caudal end of the embryo, where later the anus is formed.

proc·tol·o·gy (prok-tol′ah-je) the branch of medicine concerned with disorders of the rectum and anus. **proctolog′ic,** adj.

proc·to·pa·ral·y·sis (prok″to-pah-ral′ĭ-sis) paralysis of the anal and rectal muscles.

proc·to·pexy (prok′to-pek″se) surgical fixation of the rectum.

proc·to·plas·ty (-plas″te) plastic repair of the rectum.

proc·to·ple·gia (prok″to-ple′jah) proctoparalysis.

proc·top·to·sis (prok″top-to′sis) prolapse of the rectum.

proc·tor·rha·phy (prok-tor′ah-fe) surgical repair of the rectum.

proc·tor·rhea (prok″to-re′ah) a mucous discharge from the anus.

proc·to·scope (prok′to-skōp) a speculum or tubular instrument with illumination for inspecting the rectum.

proc·to·sig·moi·di·tis (prok″to-sig″moi-di′tis) inflammation of the rectum and sigmoid colon.

proc·to·sig·moi·dos·co·py (-sig″moi-dos′ko-pe) examination of the rectum and sigmoid colon with the sigmoidoscope.

proc·to·ste·no·sis (-stĕ-no′sis) stricture of the rectum.

proc·tos·to·my (prok-tos′tah-me) creation of a permanent artificial opening from the body surface into the rectum.

proc·tot·o·my (prok-tot′ah-me) incision of the rectum.

pro·cum·bent (pro-kum′bint) prone; lying on the face.

pro·cur·sive (-ker′siv) tending to run forward.

pro·cy·cli·dine (-si′klĭ-dēn) an antidyskinetic used as the hydrochloride salt in the treatment of parkinsonism and for the control of drug-induced extrapyramidal reactions.

pro·drome (pro′drōm) a premonitory symptom; a symptom indicating the onset of a disease. **prodro′mal, prodro′mic,** adj.

pro·drug (-drug) a compound that, on administration, must undergo chemical conversion by metabolic processes before becoming an active pharmacological agent; a precursor of a drug.

prod·uct (prod′ukt) something produced. **cleavage p.,** a substance formed by splitting of a compound molecule into a simpler one. **fibrin degradation p's, fibrinogen degradation p's, fibrin split p's,** the protein fragments produced after digestion of fibrinogen or fibrin by plasmin. **fission p.,** an isotope, usually radioactive, of an element in the middle of the periodic table, produced by fission of a heavy element under bombardment with high-energy particles. **spallation p's,** the isotopes of many different chemical elements produced in small amounts in nuclear fission. **substitution p.,** a substance formed by substitution of one atom or radical in a molecule by another atom or radical.

pro·duc·tive (pro-duk′tiv) producing or forming; said especially of an inflammation that produces new tissue or of a cough that brings forth sputum or mucus.

pro·en·zyme (pro-en′zīm) an inactive precursor that can be converted to active enzyme.

pro·eryth·ro·blast (pro″ĕ-rith′ro-blast) the earliest erythrocyte precursor in the *erythrocytic series*, having a large nucleus containing several nucleoli, surrounded by a small amount of cytoplasm.

pro·es·tro·gen (-es′trah-jen) a substance without estrogenic activity but able to be metabolized in the body to active estrogen.

pro·fes·sion·al (pro-fesh′un-al) 1. pertaining to one's profession or occupation. 2. one who is a specialist in a particular field or occupation. **allied health p.,** a person with special training and licensed when necessary, who works under the supervision of a health professional with responsibilities bearing on patient care.

pro·file (pro′fil) 1. a simple outline, as of the side view of the head or face. 2. a graph, table, or other summary representing quantitatively a set of characteristics determined by tests.

pro·fun·dus (pro-fun'dus) [L.] deep.

pro·gas·trin (-gas'trin) an inactive precursor of gastrin.

pro·ge·ria (-jēr'e-ah) premature old age, a condition occurring in childhood marked by small stature, absence of facial and pubic hair, wrinkled skin, gray hair, and eventual development of atherosclerosis.

pro·ges·ta·tion·al (pro″jes-ta'shun-al) 1. referring to that phase of the menstrual cycle just before menstruation, when the corpus luteum is active and the endometrium secreting. 2. having effects similar to those of progesterone; see also under *agent.*

pro·ges·te·rone (pro-jes'ter-ōn) the principal progestational hormone liberated by the corpus luteum, adrenal cortex, and placenta, whose function is to prepare the uterus for the reception and development of the fertilized oocyte by inducing transformation of the endometrium from the proliferative to the secretory stage; used as a progestational agent in the treatment of dysfunctional uterine bleeding and abnormalities of the menstrual cycle, as part of postmenopausal hormone replacement therapy, as a test for endogenous estrogen production, and as an adjunct in infertility therapy.

pro·ges·tin (-jes'tin) progestational agent.

pro·ges·to·gen (-jes'tah-jen) progestational agent.

pro·glos·sis (-glos'is) the tip of the tongue.

pro·glot·tid (-glot'id) one of the segments making up the body of a tapeworm; see *strobila.*

pro·glot·tis (-glot'is) pl. *proglot'tides.* Proglottid.

prog·na·thism (prog'nah-thizm) abnormal protrusion of the mandible. **prognath'ic, prog'nathous,** adj.

prog·no·sis (prog-no'sis) a forecast of the probable course and outcome of a disorder. **prognos'tic,** adj.

pro·grav·id (pro-grav'id) denoting the phase of the endometrium in which it is prepared for pregnancy.

pro·gres·sion (-gresh'un) 1. the act of moving or walking forward. 2. the process of spreading or becoming more severe. **progres'sive,** adj.

pro·hor·mone (-hor'mōn) a hormone preprotein; a biosynthetic, usually intraglandular, hormone precursor, such as proinsulin.

pro·in·su·lin (-in'sūl-in) a precursor of insulin, having low biologic activity.

pro·jec·tion (-jek'shun) 1. a throwing forward, especially the reference of impressions made on the sense organs to their proper source, so as to locate correctly the objects producing them. 2. a connection between the cerebral cortex and other parts of the nervous system or organs of special sense. 3. the act of extending or jutting out, or a part that juts out. 4. an unconscious defense mechanism by which a person attributes to someone else unacknowledged ideas, thoughts, feelings, and impulses that they cannot accept as their own. 5. the orientation of a radiographic machine in relation to the body or a body part.

pro·kary·on (-kar'e-on) 1. nuclear material scattered in the cytoplasm of the cell, rather than bounded by a nuclear membrane; found in some unicellular organisms, such as bacteria. 2. prokaryote.

pro·kary·ote (-kar'e-ōt) a unicellular organism lacking a true nucleus and nuclear membrane, having genetic material composed of a single loop of naked double-stranded DNA. Prokaryotes, with the exception of mycoplasmas, have a rigid cell wall. **prokary-ot'ic,** adj.

pro·ki·net·ic (pro″kĭ-net'ik) stimulating movement or motility.

pro·la·bi·um (pro-la'be-um) the prominent central part of the upper lip.

pro·lac·tin (-lak'tin) a hormone of the anterior pituitary that stimulates and sustains lactation in postpartum mammals, and shows luteotropic activity in certain mammals.

pro·lac·ti·no·ma (-lak″tĭ-no'mah) a pituitary adenoma that secretes prolactin.

pro·lapse (pro'laps) 1. ptosis; the falling down, or downward displacement, of a part or viscus. 2. to undergo such displacement. **p. of the cord,** protrusion of the umbilical cord ahead of the presenting part of the fetus in labor. **p. of the iris,** protrusion of the iris through a wound in the cornea. **Morgagni's p.,** chronic inflammatory hyperplasia of the mucosa and submucosa of the sacculus laryngis. **rectal p., p. of rectum,** protrusion of the rectal mucous membrane through the anus. **p. of uterus,** downward displacement of the uterus so that the cervix is within the vaginal orifice *(first-degree p.),* the cervix is outside the orifice *(second-degree p.),* or the entire uterus is outside the orifice *(third-degree p.).*

pro·lap·sus (pro-lap'sus) [L.] prolapse.

pro·lep·sis (-lep'sis) recurrence of a paroxysm before the expected time. **prolep'tic,** adj.

pro·li·dase (pro'lĭ-dās) an enzyme that catalyzes the hydrolysis of the imide bond between an α-carboxyl group and proline or hydroxyproline.

pro·lif·er·a·tion (pro-lif″er-a'shun) the reproduction or multiplication of similar forms, especially of cells. **prolif′erative, prolif′-erous,** adj.

pro·lig·er·ous (-lij′er-us) producing offspring.

pro·lin·ase (pro′lĭ-nās) an enzyme that catalyzes the hydrolysis of dipeptides containing proline or hydroxyproline as N-terminal groups.

pro·line (Pro, P) (pro′lēn) a cyclic, non-essential amino acid occurring in proteins; it is a major constituent of collagen.

pro·lym·pho·cyte (pro-lim′fo-sīt) a developmental form in the lymphocytic series, intermediate between the lymphoblast and lymphocyte.

pro·mas·ti·gote (-mas′tĭ-gōt) the morphologic stage in the development of certain protozoa, characterized by a free anterior flagellum and resembling the typical adult form of *Leptomonas.*

pro·mega·karyo·cyte (-meg″ah-kar′e-o-sīt) a precursor in the thrombocytic series, being a cell intermediate between the megakaryoblast and the megakaryocyte.

pro·meg·a·lo·blast (-meg′ah-lo-blast″) the earliest form in the abnormal erythrocyte maturation sequence occurring in vitamin B_{12} and folic acid deficiencies; it corresponds to the pronormoblast, and develops into a megaloblast.

pro·meth·a·zine (-meth′ah-zēn) a phenothiazine derivative, used in the form of the hydrochloride salt as an antihistaminic, antiemetic, antivertigo agent, and sedative, and in the prevention and treatment of motion sickness.

pro·me·thi·um (Pm) (-me′the-um) chemical element (see *Table of Elements*), at. no. 61.

prom·i·nence (prom′ĭ-nins) a protrusion or projection. **frontonasal p.,** frontonasal process; an expansive facial process in the embryo that develops into the forehead and bridge of the nose. **laryngeal p.,** Adam's apple; a subcutaneous prominence on the front of the neck produced by the thyroid cartilage of the larynx. **mandibular p.,** mandibular process; the ventral prominence formed by bifurcation of the mandibular (first pharyngeal) arch in the embryo, which unites ventrally with its fellow to form the lower jaw. **maxillary p.,** maxillary process; the dorsal prominence formed by bifurcation of the mandibular (first pharyngeal) arch in the embryo, which joins with the ipsilateral medial nasal prominence in the formation of the upper jaw. **nasal p., lateral,** the more lateral of the two limbs of a horseshoe-shaped elevation in the future nasal region of the embryo; it participates in formation of the side and wing of the nose. **nasal p., medial,** the more central of the two limbs of a horseshoe-shaped elevation in the future nasal region of the embryo; it joins with the ipsilateral maxillary prominence in the formation of half of the upper jaw.

pro·mono·cyte (pro-mon′ah-sīt) a cell of the monocytic series intermediate between the monoblast and monocyte, with coarse chromatin structure and one or two nucleoli.

prom·on·to·ry (prom′on-tor″e) a projecting process or eminence.

pro·mo·ter (pro-mo′ter) 1. a segment of DNA usually occurring upstream from a gene coding region and acting as a controlling element in the expression of that gene. 2. a substance in a catalyst that increases its rate of activity. 3. a type of epigenetic carcinogen that promotes neoplastic growth only after initiation by another substance.

pro·my·elo·cyte (-mi′il-o-sīt″) a precursor in the granulocytic series, intermediate between myeloblast and myelocyte, containing a few, as yet undifferentiated, cytoplasmic granules. **promyelocyt′ic,** adj.

pro·na·tion (-na′shun) the act of assuming the prone position, or the state of being prone. Applied to the hand, the act of turning the palm backward (posteriorly) or downward, performed by medial rotation of the forearm. Applied to the foot, a combination of eversion and abduction movements taking place in the tarsal and metatarsal joints and resulting in lowering of the medial margin of the foot, hence of the longitudinal arch.

prone (prōn) lying face downward.

pro·neph·ros (pro-nef′ros) pl. *proneph′roi.* 1. a vestigial excretory structure developing in the embryo before the mesonephros; its duct is later used by the mesonephros, which arises caudal to it. 2. the definitive excretory organ of primitive fishes. **proneph′ric,** adj.

pro·nor·mo·blast (-nor′mo-blast) term often considered a synonym of *proerythroblast,* but sometimes limited to one in a normal course of erythrocyte maturation, as opposed to a promegaloblast.

pro·nu·cle·us (-noo′kle-us) 1. the precursor of a nucleus. 2. the haploid nucleus occurring after meiosis in a germ cell.

pro·ot·ic (-ot′ik) preauricular.

pro·pa·fe·none (pro″pah-fe′nōn) a sodium channel blocking agent acting on the Purkinje fibers and the myocardium; used as the hydrochloride salt as an antiarrhythmic.

prop·a·ga·tion (prop″ah-ga′shun) reproduction (def. 1). **prop′agative,** adj.

pro·pa·no·ic ac·id (pro″pah-no′ik) systematic name for propionic acid.

pro·pan·the·line (pro-pan'thĕ-lēn) an anticholinergic, used as the bromide salt in the treatment of peptic ulcer and other gastrointestinal disorders.

pro·par·a·caine (-par'ah-kān) a topical ophthalmic anesthetic; used as the hydrochloride salt.

pro·per·din (pro'per-din) factor P; a nonimmunoglobulin gamma globulin component of the alternative pathway of complement activation.

pro·peri·to·ne·al (pro"per-ĭ-to-ne'al) preperitoneal.

pro·phage (pro'fāj) the latent stage of a phage in a lysogenic bacterium, in which the viral genome becomes inserted into a specific portion of the host chromosome and is duplicated in each cell generation.

pro·phase (-fāz) the first stage in cell reduplication in either meiosis or mitosis.

pro·phy·lac·tic (pro"-fī-lak'tik) 1. tending to ward off disease; pertaining to prophylaxis. 2. an agent that tends to ward off disease.

pro·phy·lax·is (-fī-lak'sis) prevention of disease; preventive treatment.

pro·pi·o·nate (pro'pe-o-nāt) any salt of propionic acid.

Pro·pi·on·i·bac·te·ri·um (pro"pe-on"e-bak-tēr'e-um) a genus of gram-positive bacteria found as saprophytes in humans, animals, and dairy products.

pro·pi·on·ic ac·id (pro"pe-on'ik) a three-carbon saturated fatty acid produced as a fermentation product by several species of bacteria; its salts, calcium and sodium propionate, are used as preservatives for food and pharmaceuticals.

pro·pi·on·ic·ac·i·de·mia (pro"pe-on"ik-as"ĭ-de'me-ah) 1. an aminoacidopathy characterized by excess of propionic acid and glycine in the blood and urine, ketosis, acidosis, and often neurologic complications, due to deficiency of an enzyme involved in amino acid and fatty acid catabolism. 2. excess of propionic acid in the blood.

pro·po·fol (pro'pah-fol) a short acting sedative and hypnotic used as a general anesthetic and adjunct to anesthesia.

pro·pos·i·tus (pro-poz'ĭ-tus) pl. *propo'siti.* [L.] proband; often specifically the first proband to be ascertained.

pro·poxy·phene (-pok'sĭ-fēn) an opioid analgesic structurally related to methadone, used as the hydrochloride and napsylate salts.

pro·pran·o·lol (-pran'o-lol) a β-adrenergic blocking agent, used as the hydrochloride salt in the treatment and prophylaxis of certain cardiac disorders, the treatment of tremors

and of inoperable pheochromocytoma, and the prophylaxis of migraine.

pro·pri·e·tary (-pri'ĕ-tar"e) 1. protected against free competition as to name, composition, or manufacturing process by patent, trademark, copyright, or other means. 2. a medicine so protected.

pro·prio·cep·tion (pro"pre-o-sep'shun) perception mediated by proprioceptors or proprioceptive tissues.

pro·prio·cep·tor (-sep'ter) any of the sensory nerve endings that give information concerning movements and position of the body; they occur chiefly in muscles, tendons, and joint capsules; receptors in the labyrinth may be included. **propriocep'tive,** adj.

pro·pro·tein (pro-pro'tēn) a protein that is cleaved to form a smaller protein, e.g., proinsulin, the precursor of insulin.

prop·tom·e·ter (prop-tom'ĕ-ter) an instrument for measuring the degree of exophthalmos.

prop·to·sis (prop-to'sis) forward displacement or bulging, especially of the eye.

pro·pul·sion (pro-pul'shun) 1. a tendency to fall forward in walking. 2. festination.

pro·pyl (pro'pil) the univalent radical $CH_3CH_2CH_2$—, from propane.

pro·pyl·ene (pro'pĭ-lēn) a gaseous hydrocarbon, $CH_3CH=CH_2$. **p. glycol,** a colorless viscous liquid used as a humectant and solvent in pharmaceutical preparations.

pro·pyl·thio·ura·cil (pro"pil-thi"o-u'rah-sil) a thyroid inhibitor used in the treatment of hyperthyroidism.

pro re na·ta (p.r.n.) (pro re na'tah) [L.] according to circumstances.

pro·ren·nin (pro-ren'in) the zymogen (proenzyme) in the gastric glands that is converted to rennin.

pro·ru·bri·cyte (-roo'brĭ-sīt) basophilic erythroblast.

pro·se·cre·tin (-se-krēt'in) the precursor of secretin.

pro·sec·tion (-sek'shun) carefully programmed dissection for demonstration of anatomic structure.

pro·sec·tor (-sek'tor) [L.] one who dissects anatomical subjects for demonstration.

pros·en·ceph·a·lon (pros"en-sef'ah-lon) forebrain 1. the part of the brain developed from the anterior of the three primary brain vesicles, comprising the diencephalon and telencephalon. 2. the most anterior of the primary brain vesicles, later dividing into the telencephalon and diencephalon.

pros(o)- word element [Gr.], *forward; anterior.*

pros·o·de·mic (pros″o-dem′ik) passing directly from one person to another; said of disease.

pros·o·pag·no·sia (-pag-no′se-ah) inability to recognize faces due to damage to the underside of both occipital lobes.

pros·o·pla·sia (-pla′zhah) 1. abnormal differentiation of tissue. 2. development into a higher level of organization or function.

prosop(o)- word element [Gr.], *face*.

pros·o·po·ple·gia (pros″o-po-ple′jah) facial paralysis. **prosopople′gic,** adj.

pros·o·pos·chi·sis (-pos′kĭ-sis) facial cleft (2).

pros·ta·cy·clin (pros″tah-si′klin) a prostaglandin, PGI$_2$, synthesized by endothelial cells lining the cardiovascular system; it is a potent vasodilator and inhibitor of platelet aggregation. It is used pharmaceutically as *epoprostenol.*

pros·ta·glan·din (-glan′din) any of a group of naturally occurring, chemically related fatty acids that stimulate contractility of the uterine and other smooth muscle and have the ability to lower blood pressure, regulate acid secretion of the stomach, regulate body temperature and platelet aggregation, and control inflammation and vascular permeability; they also affect the action of certain hormones. Nine primary types are labeled A through I, the degree of saturation of the side chain of each being designated by subscripts 1, 2, and 3. The types of prostaglandins are abbreviated PGE$_2$, PGF$_{2\alpha}$, and so on.

pros·ta·glan·din syn·thase (sin′thās) an enzyme catalyzing the initial steps in the synthesis of prostaglandins from arachidonic acid; it comprises the component activities cyclooxygenase, catalyzing cyclization and oxidation reactions, and peroxidase, catalyzing a reduction reaction.

pros·ta·noid (pros′tah-noid) any of a group of complex fatty acids derived from arachidonic acid, including the prostaglandins, prostanoic acid, and the thromboxanes.

pros·tate (pros′tāt) a gland surrounding the bladder neck and urethra in the male; it contributes a secretion to the semen. **pros·tat′ic,** adj.

pros·ta·tec·to·my (pros″tah-tek′tah-me) excision of all or part of the prostate. radical p., removal of the prostate with its capsule, seminal vesicles, ductus deferens, some pelvic fasciae, and sometimes pelvic lymph nodes; performed via either the retropubic or the perineal route. radical retropubic p., radical prostatectomy through the retropubic space via a suprapubic incision. suprapubic transvesical p., removal of the prostate

through a suprapubic incision and an incision in the urinary bladder.

pros·ta·tism (pros′tah-tizm) a symptom complex resulting from compression or obstruction of the urethra, due most commonly to nodular hyperplasia of the prostate.

pros·ta·ti·tis (pros″tah-ti′tis) inflammation of the prostate. **prostatit′ic,** adj. allergic p., eosinophilic p., a condition seen in certain allergies, characterized by diffuse infiltration of the prostate by eosinophils, with small foci of fibrinoid necrosis. nonspecific granulomatous p., prostatitis characterized by focal or diffuse tissue infiltration by peculiar, large, pale macrophages.

pros·ta·to·cys·ti·tis (pros″tah-to-sis-ti′tis) inflammation of the bladder, bladder neck, and prostatic urethra.

pros·ta·to·cys·tot·o·my (-sis-tot′ah-me) incision of the bladder and prostate.

pros·ta·to·dyn·ia (-din′e-ah) pain in the prostate.

pros·ta·to·li·thot·o·my (-lĭ-thot′ah-me) incision of the prostate for removal of a calculus.

pros·ta·to·meg·a·ly (-meg′ah-le) enlargement of the prostate.

pros·ta·tor·rhea (-re′ah) a discharge from the prostate.

pros·ta·tot·o·my (pros″tah-tot′ah-me) surgical incision of the prostate.

pros·ta·to·ve·sic·u·lec·to·my (pros″tah-to-vě-sik″ūl-ek′tah-me) excision of the prostate and seminal vesicles.

pros·ta·to·ve·sic·u·li·tis (-vě-sik″u-li′tis) inflammation of the prostate and seminal vesicles.

pros·the·sis (pros-the′sis) pl. *prosthe′ses.* [Gr.] an artificial substitute for a missing body part, such as an arm, leg, eye, or tooth; used for functional or cosmetic reasons or both. **prosthet′ic,** adj. penile p., a semirigid rod or inflatable device implanted in the penis to provide an erection for men with organic impotence.

pros·thi·on (PR) (pros′the-on) the point on the maxillary alveolar process that projects most anteriorly in the midline.

pros·tho·don·tics (pros″thah-don′tiks) the branch of dentistry dealing with construction of artificial appliances designed to restore and maintain oral function by replacing missing teeth and sometimes other oral structures or parts of the face.

pros·tra·tion (pros-tra′shun) extreme exhaustion or lack of energy or power. heat p., see under *exhaustion.*

pro·tac·tin·i·um (Pa) (pro″tak-tin′e-um) chemical element (see *Table of Elements*), at. no. 91.

pro·ta·mine (prōt'ah-min) one of a class of basic proteins occurring in the sperm of certain fish, having the property of neutralizing heparin; the sulfate salt is used as an antidote to heparin overdosage.

pro·ta·nom·a·ly (pro″tah-nom'ah-le) anomalous trichromatic vision with defective perception of red.

pro·ta·no·pia (pro″tah-no'pe-ah) dichromatic vision with perception of two hues only (blue and yellow) of the normal four primaries, lacking that for red and green and their derivatives. **protanop'ic**, adj.

pro·te·ase (pro'te-ās) endopeptidase.

pro·tec·tant (pro-tek'tant) protective.

pro·tec·tin (-tek'tin) a membrane-bound protein that prevents insertion of the membrane attack complex into the membrane, thereby protecting normal bystander cells from complement-induced lysis.

pro·tec·tive (-tek'tiv) 1. affording defense or immunity. 2. an agent affording defense or immunity.

pro·tec·tor (-tek'ter) a substance in a catalyst that prolongs the rate of activity in the latter.

pro·tein (pro'tēn) any of a group of complex organic compounds containing carbon, hydrogen, oxygen, nitrogen, and sulfur. Proteins, the principal constituents of the protoplasm of all cells, are of high molecular weight and consist of α-amino acids joined by peptide linkages. Twenty different amino acids are commonly found in proteins, each protein having a unique, genetically defined amino acid sequence that determines its specific shape and function. Their roles include enzymatic catalysis, transport and storage, coordinated motion, nerve impulse generation and transmission, control of growth and differentiation, immunity, and mechanical support. **acute phase p.,** any of the non-antibody proteins found in increased amounts in serum during the acute phase response, including C-reactive protein and fibrinogen. **Bence Jones p.,** a low-molecular-weight, heat-sensitive urinary protein found in multiple myeloma, which coagulates when heated to 45°–55°C and redissolves partially or wholly on boiling. **binding p.,** 1. any protein able to specifically and reversibly bind other substances, such as ions, sugars, nucleic acids, or amino acids; they are believed to function in transport. 2. transport p. **p. C,** a vitamin K–dependent plasma protein that, when activated by thrombin, inhibits the clotting cascade by enzymatic cleavage of factors V and VIII and also enhances fibrinolysis. Deficiency results in recurrent venous thrombosis. **C4 binding p.,** a complement system regulatory protein that inhibits activation of the classical pathway. **complete p.,** one containing the essential amino acids in the proportion required in the human diet. **compound p., conjugated p.,** any of those in which the protein is combined with nonprotein molecules or prosthetic groups other than as a salt; e.g., nucleoproteins, glycoproteins, lipoproteins, and metalloproteins. **C-reactive p.,** a globulin that forms a precipitate with the C-polysaccharide of the pneumonococcus; the most predominant of the acute phase proteins. **cystic fibrosis transmembrane regulator p.,** a transmembrane protein produced by the cystic fibrosis gene, primarily functioning as a chloride channel. Numerous mutated forms of the gene have been associated with clinical cystic fibrosis. **fibrillar p.,** any of the generally insoluble proteins that comprise the principal structural proteins of the body, e.g., collagens, elastins, keratin, actin, and myosin. **G p.,** any of a family of proteins of the intracellular portion of the plasma membrane that bind activated receptor complexes and, through conformational changes and cyclic binding and hydrolysis of GTP, effect alterations in channel gating and so couple cell surface receptors to intracellular responses. **glial fibrillary acidic p. (GFAP),** the protein forming the glial filaments of the astrocytes and used as an immunohistochemical marker of these cells. **globular p.,** any of the water-soluble proteins yielding only α-amino acids on hydrolysis, including most of the proteins of the body, e.g., albumins and globulins. **guanyl-nucleotide-binding p.,** G p. **heat shock p.,** any of a group of proteins first identified as synthesized in response to hyperthermia, hypoxia, or other stresses and believed to enable cells to recover from these stresses. Many have been found to be molecular chaperones and are synthesized abundantly regardless of stress. **HIV p's,** proteins specific to the human immunodeficiency virus; presence of certain specific HIV proteins together with certain HIV glycoproteins constitutes a serological diagnosis of HIV infection. **incomplete p.,** one having a ratio of essential amino acids different from that of the average body protein. **membrane cofactor p. (MCP),** an inhibitor of complement activation found in most blood cells, endothelial and epithelial cells, and fibroblasts. **myeloma p.,** any of the abnormal immunoglobulins or fragments, such as Bence-Jones proteins, secreted by myeloma cells. **partial p.,** incomplete p. **plasma p's,** all the proteins present in the blood plasma, including the immunoglobulins. **prion p. (PrP),** a protein of uncertain function, in humans coded for by a gene on the short arm of chromosome 20. The protease-resistant core is the functional, and perhaps only, component of prions; several abnormal forms have been identified and are responsible for prion disease. **p. S,** a vitamin K–dependent plasma protein that inhibits blood clotting by serving as a cofactor for activated protein C. **S p.,** see *vitronectin.* **serum p's,** proteins in the blood serum, including immunoglobulins, albumin, complement, coagulation factors, and enzymes. **sphingolipid activator p. (SAP),** any of a group of non-enzymatic lyso-somal proteins that stimulate the actions of specific lysosomal hydrolases by binding and solubilizing their sphingolipid substrates. **transport p.,** a protein that binds to a substance and provides a transport system for it, either in the plasma or across a plasma membrane.

pro·tein·a·ceous (pro″tēn-a′shus) pertaining to or of the nature of protein.

pro·tein·ase (pro′tēn-ās″) endopeptidase.

pro·tein·emia (pro″tēn-e′me-ah) excess of protein in the blood.

pro·tein ki·nase (pro′tēn ki′nās) an enzyme that catalyzes the phosphorylation of serine, threonine, or tyrosine groups in enzymes or other proteins, using ATP as a phosphate donor.

pro·tein·o·sis (pro″tēn-o′sis) the accumulation of excess protein in the tissues. **lipid p.,** a hereditary defect of lipid metabolism marked by yellowish deposits of hyaline lipid-carbohydrate mixture on the inner surface of the lips, under the tongue, on the oropharynx, and on the larynx, and by skin lesions. **pulmonary alveolar p.,** a chronic lung disease in which the distal alveoli become filled with eosinophilic, probably endogenous proteinaceous material that prevents ventilation of affected areas.

pro·tein·uria (-ūr′e-ah) an excess of serum proteins in the urine, as in renal disease or after strenuous exercise. **proteinu′ric,** adj.

pro·teo·gly·can (pro″te-o-gli′kan) any of a group of polysaccharide-protein conjugates present in connective tissue and cartilage, consisting of a polypeptide backbone to which many glycosaminoglycan chains are covalently linked; they form the ground substance in the extracellular matrix of connective tissue and also have lubricant and support functions.

pro·te·ol·y·sis (-ol′ĭ-sis) the splitting of proteins by hydrolysis of the peptide bonds with formation of smaller polypeptides. **proteolyt′ic,** adj.

pro·teo·me·tab·o·lism (pro″te-o-mĕ-tab′ah-lizm) the metabolism of protein.

pro·teo·pep·tic (-pep′tik) digesting protein.

Pro·te·us (pro′te-us) a genus of gram-negative, motile bacteria usually found in fecal and other putrefying matter, including *P. morga′nii,* found in the intestines and associated with summer diarrhea of infants, and *P. vulga′ris,* often found as a secondary invader in various localized suppurative pathologic processes; it is a cause of cystitis.

pro·throm·bin (pro-throm′bin) coagulation factor II.

pro·throm·bin·ase (-throm′bin-ās) 1. the complex of activated coagulation factor X and calcium, phospholipid, and modified factor V; it can cleave and activate prothrombin to thrombin. 2. sometimes specifically the active enzyme center of the complex, activated factor X.

pro·throm·bi·no·gen·ic (-throm″bĭ-no-jen′ik) promoting the production of prothrombin.

pro·ti·re·lin (-ti′rah-lin) a synthetic preparation of thyrotropin-releasing hormone (q.v.), used diagnostically.

pro·tist (prōt′ist) any member of the kingdom Protista.

Pro·tis·ta (pro-tis′tah) 1. a kingdom comprising the unicellular bacteria, algae, slime molds, fungi, and protozoa; it includes all single-celled organisms. 2. a kingdom comprising unicellular organisms with distinct nuclei (the eukaryotes), including protozoa, algae, and certain intermediate forms.

pro·ti·um (pro′te-um) see *hydrogen.*

prot(o)- 1. word element [Gr.], *first.* 2. in chemistry, a prefix denoting the member of a series of compounds with the lowest proportion of the element or radical to which it is affixed.

pro·to·col (pro′to-kol) 1. an explicit, detailed plan of an experiment, procedure, or test. 2. the original notes made on a necropsy, an experiment, or on a case of disease.

pro·to·di·a·stol·ic (prōt″o-di″ah-stol′ik) pertaining to early diastole, i.e., immediately following the second heart sound.

pro·to·du·o·de·num (-doo″o-de′num) the first or proximal portion of the duodenum, extending from the pylorus to the duodenal papilla.

pro·ton (pro′ton) an elementary particle that is the core or nucleus of an ordinary hydrogen atom of mass 1; the unit of positive electricity, being equivalent to the electron in charge and approximately to the hydrogen ion in mass. Symbol p.

pro·to·on·co·gene (pro″to-ong′ko-jēn) a normal gene that with slight alteration by mutation or other mechanism becomes an oncogene; most are believed to normally function in cell growth and differentiation.

pro·to·path·ic (-path′ik) affected first; pertaining to sensing of stimuli in a nonspecific, usually nonlocalized, manner.

pro·to·plasm (pro′to-plazm) the viscid, translucent colloid material, the essential constituent of the living cell, including cytoplasm and nucleoplasm. **protoplas′mic,** adj.

pro·to·plast (-plast) a bacterial or plant cell deprived of its rigid wall but with its plasma membrane intact; the cell is dependent for its integrity on an isotonic or hypertonic medium.

pro·to·por·phyr·ia (prōt″o-por-fēr′e-ah) erythropoietic p. **erythropoietic p. (EPP),** a form of erythropoietic porphyria marked by excessive protoporphyrin in erythrocytes, plasma, liver, and feces, and by widely varying photosensitive skin changes ranging from a burning or pruritic sensation to erythema, plaquelike edema, and wheals.

pro·to·por·phy·rin (-por′fĭ-rin) any of several porphyrin isomers, one of which is an intermediate in heme biosynthesis; it is accumulated and excreted excessively in feces in erythropoietic protoporphyria and variegate porphyria.

pro·to·por·phy·rin·o·gen (-por″fĭ-rin′ŏ-jen) any of fifteen isomers of a porphyrinogen derivative, one of which is an intermediate produced from coproporphyrinogen in heme synthesis.

Pro·to·the·ca (-the′kah) a genus of ubiquitous yeastlike organisms generally considered to be algae; *P. wickerha′mii* and *P. zop′fii* are pathogenic.

pro·to·the·co·sis (-the-ko′sis) infection caused by organisms of the genus *Prototheca,* varying from cutaneous lesions to systemic invasion, occurring as an opportunistic infection or as a result of traumatic implantation of organisms into the tissues.

pro·to·troph (pro′to-trōf) an organism with the same growth factor requirements as the ancestral strain; said of microbial mutants. **prototroph′ic,** adj.

pro·to·ver·te·bra (pro″to-ver′tah-brah) 1. somite. 2. the caudal half of a somite that forms most of a vertebra.

Pro·to·zoa (-zo′ah) a subkingdom comprising the simplest organisms of the animal kingdom, consisting of unicellular organisms ranging in size from submicroscopic to macroscopic. It comprises the Sarcomastigophora, Labyrinthomorpha, Apicomplexa, Microspora, Acetospora, Myxozoa, and Ciliophora.

pro·to·zo·a·cide (-zo′ah-sīd) destructive to protozoa, or an agent that so acts.

pro·to·zo·an (-zo′an) 1. any member of the Protozoa. 2. of or pertaining to the Protozoa.

pro·to·zo·ia·sis (-zo-i′ah-sis) any disease caused by protozoa.

pro·to·zo·ol·o·gy (-zo-ol′ah-je) the study of protozoa.

pro·to·zo·o·phage (-zo′ah-fāj) a cell having a phagocytic action on protozoa.

pro·trac·tion (pro-trak′shun) 1. drawing out or lengthening. 2. extension or protrusion. 3. a condition in which the teeth or other maxillary or mandibular structures are situated anterior to their normal position. **mandibular p.,** 1. the protrusive movement of the mandible initiated by the lateral and medial pterygoid muscles acting simultaneously. 2. a facial anomaly in which the gnathion lies anterior to the orbital plane. **maxillary p.,** a facial anomaly in which the subnasion is anterior to the orbital plane.

pro·trac·tor (-trak′ter) an instrument for extracting foreign bodies from wounds.

pro·trans·glu·tam·i·nase (-tranz″gloo-tam′ĭ-nās) the inactive precursor of transglutaminase; it is the inactive form of coagulation factor XIII.

pro·trip·ty·line (-trip′tĭ-lēn) a tricyclic antidepressant, also used in the treatment of attention-deficit/hyperactivity disorder, and narcolepsy; used as the hydrochloride salt.

pro·tru·sion (-troo′zhun) 1. extension beyond the usual limits, or above a plane surface. 2. the state of being thrust forward or laterally, as in masticatory movements of the mandible. **protrus′ive,** adj.

pro·tu·ber·ance (-too′ber-ans) a projecting part, or prominence. **mental p.,** a triangular prominence on the anterior surface of the body of the mandible, on or near the median line.

pro·tu·ber·an·tia (-too″ber-an′shah) [L.] protuberance.

pro·uro·ki·nase (pro-UK) (pro″u-ro-ki′nās) the single chain proenzyme cleaved by plasmin to form u-plasminogen activator (urokinase); it is slowly activated in the presence of fibrin clots and is used for therapeutic thrombolysis.

pro·ver·te·bra (pro-ver′tah-brah) protovertebra.

prov·ing (proov′ing) in homeopathy, the administration of a medicinal substance to

pro·vi·rus (pro-vi′rus) the genome of an animal virus integrated (by crossing over) into the chromosome of the host cell, and thus replicated in all of its daughter cells. It can be activated to produce a complete virus; it can also cause transformation of the host cell.

pro·vi·sion·al (-vizh′un-al) formed or performed for temporary purposes; temporary.

pro·vi·ta·min (-vi′tah-min) a precursor of a vitamin. **p. A**, usually β-carotene, sometimes including any of the provitamin A carotenoids. **p. D₂**, ergosterol. **p. D₃**, 7-dehydrocholesterol.

prox·i·mad (prok′sĭ-mad) in a proximal direction.

prox·i·mal (-mil) nearest to a point of reference, as to a center or median line or to the point of attachment or origin.

prox·i·ma·lis (prok″sĭ-ma′lis) [L.] proximal.

prox·i·mate (prok′sĭ-mit) immediate or nearest.

prox·i·mo·buc·cal (prok″sĭ-mo-buk′′l) pertaining to the proximal and buccal surfaces of a posterior tooth.

pro·zone (pro′zōn) the phenomenon exhibited by some sera, in which agglutination or precipitation occurs at higher dilution ranges, but is not visible at lower dilutions or when undiluted.

pru·ri·go (proo-ri′go) [L.] any of several itchy skin eruptions in which the characteristic lesion is dome-shaped with a small transient vesicle on top, followed by crusting or lichenification. **prurig′inous**, adj. **p. mi′tis**, a mild type of prurigo that begins in childhood, is intensely pruritic, and is progressive. **nodular p.**, a form of neurodermatitis, usually on the limbs of middle-aged women, marked by discrete, firm, rough-surfaced, dark brownish-gray, intensely itchy nodules. **p. sim′plex**, papular urticaria.

pru·rit·o·gen·ic (prōōr″it-o-jen′ik) causing pruritus, or itching.

pru·ri·tus (proo-ri′tus) itching. **prurit′ic**, adj. **p. a′ni**, intense chronic itching in the anal region. **p. hiema′lis**, xerotic eczema. **senile p.**, **p. seni′lis**, itching in the aged, possibly due to dryness of the skin. **uremic p.**, generalized itching associated with chronic renal failure and not attributable to other internal or skin disease. **p. vul′vae**, intense itching of the female external genitals.

prus·sic ac·id (prus′ik) hydrogen cyanide; see under *hydrogen*.

PS pulmonary stenosis.

PSA prostate-specific antigen.

psal·te·ri·um (sal-tēr′e-um) commissure of the fornix.

psam·mo·ma (sam-o′mah) 1. any tumor containing psammoma bodies. 2. psammomatous meningioma.

psam·mo·ma·tous (-tus) characterized by the presence of or containing psammoma bodies.

Pseu·dal·les·che·ria (sōōd-al-es-kēr′e-ah) a genus of ascomycetous fungi of the family Microascaceae; *P. boy′dii* is frequently isolated from mycetoma and other fungal infections.

pseu·dal·les·che·ri·a·sis (sōōd″al-es-kĕ-ri′ah-sis) infection with *Pseudallescheria boydii*, usually manifest as mycetoma and pulmonary infection.

pseud·ar·thro·sis (soo″dahr-thro′sis) a pathologic condition in which failure of callus formation following pathologic fracture through an area of deossification in a weight-bearing long bone results in formation of a false joint.

Pseud·ech·is (soo-dek′is) a genus of venomous Australian snakes of the family Elapidae. *P. porphyria′cus* is the Australian blacksnake.

pseud·es·the·sia (soo″des-the′zhah) 1. synesthesia. 2. a sensation felt in the absence of any external stimulus.

pseud(o)- word element [Gr.], *false*.

pseu·do·ac·an·tho·sis (soo″do-ak″an-tho′sis) a condition clinically resembling acanthosis. **p. ni′gricans**, a benign form of acanthosis nigricans associated with obesity; the obesity is sometimes associated with endocrine disturbance.

pseu·do·agraph·ia (-ah-graf′e-ah) echographia.

pseu·do·ain·hum (-īn′yoom) annular constrictions around the digits, limbs, or trunk, occurring congenitally (sometimes causing intrauterine autoamputation) and also associated with a wide variety of disorders.

pseu·do·al·leles (-ah-lēlz′) genes that are seemingly allelic but can be shown to have distinctive, closely linked loci. **pseudoallel′ic**, adj.

pseu·do·ane·mia (-ah-nēm′e-ah) marked pallor with no evidence of anemia.

pseu·do·an·eu·rysm (-an′ūr-izm) false aneurysm; dilatation or tortuosity of a vessel, giving the appearance of an aneurysm.

pseu·do·an·gi·na (-an-ji′nah) a nervous disorder resembling angina.

pseu·do·ap·o·plexy (-ap′ah-plek″se) a condition resembling apoplexy, but without hemorrhage.

pseu·do·bul·bar (-bul'bar) apparently, but not really, due to a bulbar lesion.

pseu·do·cast (soo'do-kast) an accidental formation of urinary sediment resembling a true cast.

pseu·do·cele (-sēl) fifth ventricle.

pseu·do·cho·lin·es·ter·ase (PCE) (soo"do-ko"lin-es'ter-ās) cholinesterase.

pseu·do·chro·mid·ro·sis (-kro"mid-ro'sis) discoloration of sweat by surface contaminants.

pseu·do·co·arc·ta·tion (-ko"ahrk-ta'shun) a condition radiographically resembling coarctation but without compromise of the lumen, as occurs in a congenital anomaly of the aortic arch.

pseu·do·col·loid (-kol'oid) a mucoid substance sometimes found in ovarian cysts.

pseu·do·cow·pox (-kou'poks) paravaccinia.

pseu·do·cox·al·gia (-kok-sal'jah) osteochondrosis of the capitular epiphysis of the femur.

pseu·do·cri·sis (-kri'sis) sudden but temporary abatement of febrile symptoms.

pseu·do·croup (soo'do-kroop) laryngismus stridulus.

pseu·do·cy·e·sis (soo"do-si-e'sis) false pregnancy.

pseu·do·cy·lin·droid (-sǐ-lin'droid) a shred of mucin in the urine resembling a cylindroid.

pseu·do·cyst (soo'do-sist) 1. an abnormal or dilated space resembling a cyst but not lined with epithelium. 2. a complication of acute pancreatitis, characterized by a cystic collection of fluid and necrotic debris whose walls are formed by the pancreas and surrounding organs. 3. a cluster of small, comma-shaped forms of *Toxoplasma gondii* found particularly in muscle and brain tissue in toxoplasmosis.

pseu·do·de·men·tia (soo"do-dě-men'shah) a state of general apathy resembling dementia, but due to a psychiatric disorder rather than organic brain disease and potentially reversible.

pseu·do·diph·the·ria (-dif-thēr'e-ah) diphtheroid; any of a group of infections resembling diphtheria but not caused by *Corynebacterium diphtheriae*.

pseu·do·dom·i·nant (-dom'ǐ-nint) giving the appearance of being dominant; said of a recessive genetic trait appearing in the offspring of a homozygous and a heterozygous parent.

pseu·do·ephed·rine (-ě-fed'rin) one of the optical isomers of ephedrine; used as the hydrochloride or sulfate salt as a nasal decongestant.

pseu·do·epi·lepsy (-ep'ǐ-lep-se) pseudoseizure.

pseu·do·ex·stro·phy (-ek'strah-fe) a developmental anomaly marked by the characteristic musculoskeletal defects of exstrophy of the bladder but with no major defect of the urinary tract.

pseu·do·fol·lic·u·li·tis (-fŏ-lik"u-li'tis) a chronic disorder occurring chiefly in black men, most often in the submandibular region of the neck, the characteristic lesions of which are erythematous papules containing buried hairs.

pseu·do·frac·ture (-frak'cher) a condition seen in the radiograph of a bone as a thickening of the periosteum and formation of new bone over what looks like an incomplete fracture.

pseu·do·gli·o·ma (-gli-o'mah) any condition mimicking retinoblastoma, e.g., retrolental fibroplasia or exudative retinopathy.

pseu·do·glot·tis (-glot'is) 1. the aperture between the false vocal cords. 2. neoglottis. **pseudoglot'tic,** adj.

pseu·do·gout (soo'do-gout) see *calcium pyrophosphate deposition disease,* under *disease.*

pseu·do·he·ma·tu·ria (soo"do-hēm"ah-toor'e-a) presence in urine of pigments that make it pink or red with no detectable hemoglobin or blood cells.

pseu·do·he·mo·phil·ia (-hēm"o-fil'e-ah) von Willebrand's disease.

pseu·do·her·maph·ro·dite (-her-maf'ro-dīt) an individual with pseudohermaphroditism.

pseu·do·her·maph·ro·dit·ism (-her-maf'ro-dīt-izm") a state in which the gonads are of one sex, but one or more contradictions exist in the morphologic criteria of sex. In *female p.,* the individual is genetically female and has female gonads (ovaries) but has significant male secondary sex characters. In *male p.,* the individual is genetically male and has male gonads (testes) but has significant female secondary sex characters.

pseu·do·her·nia (-her'ne-ah) an inflamed sac or gland simulating strangulated hernia.

pseu·do·hy·per·ten·sion (-hi"per-ten'-shun) falsely elevated blood pressure reading by sphygmomanometry, caused by loss of compliance of arterial walls.

pseu·do·hy·per·tro·phy (-hi-per'trah-fe) increase in size without true hypertrophy. **pseudohypertro'phic,** adj.

pseu·do·hy·po·al·dos·ter·on·ism (-hi"po-al-dos'ter-ōn-izm) 1. a hereditary disorder of infancy characterized by severe salt and water depletion and other signs of aldosterone deficiency, although aldosterone secretion is

pseu·do·hy·po·para·thy·roi·dism (-hi″po-par″ah-thi′roi-dizm) a hereditary condition resembling hypoparathyroidism, but caused by failure of response to parathyroid hormone, marked by hypocalcemia and hyperphosphatemia.

pseu·do·iso·chro·mat·ic (-i″so-krom-at′ik) seemingly of the same color throughout; applied to a solution for testing color vision deficiency, having two pigments that can be distinguished by the normal eye.

pseu·do·jaun·dice (-jawn′dis) skin discoloration due to blood changes and not to liver disease.

pseu·do·mel·a·no·sis (-mel″ah-no′sis) discoloration of tissue after death by blood pigments.

pseu·do·mem·brane (-mem′brān) false membrane. **pseudomem′branous,** adj.

Pseu·do·mo·nas (-mo′nas) a genus of gram-negative, aerobic bacteria, some species of which are pathogenic for plants and vertebrates. *P. aerugino′sa* produces the blue-green pigment pyocyanin, which gives the color to "blue pus" and causes various human diseases; *P. acido′vorans, P. alcali′genes, P. fluores′cens, P. picket′tii, P. pseudoalcali′genes, P. pu′tida, P. putrefa′ciens, P. stut′zeri,* and *P. vesicula′ris* are opportunistic pathogens.

pseu·do·mu·cin (-mu′sin) a mucin-like substance found in ovarian cysts. **pseudomu′-cinous,** adj.

pseu·do·myx·o·ma (-mik-so′mah) 1. a mass of epithelial mucus resembling a myxoma. 2. p. peritonei. **p. peritone′i,** the presence in the peritoneal cavity of mucoid matter from a ruptured ovarian cyst or a ruptured mucocele of the appendix.

pseu·do·neu·ri·tis (-noo-ri′tis) a congenital hyperemic condition of the optic papilla.

pseu·do·pap·il·le·de·ma (-pap″ĭ-lĕ-de′mah) anomalous elevation of the optic disk.

pseu·do·pa·ral·y·sis (-pah-ral′ĭ-sis) apparent loss of muscular power without real paralysis. **Parrot's p., syphilitic p.,** pseudoparalysis of one or more limbs in infants, due to syphilitic osteochondritis of an epiphysis.

pseu·do·para·ple·gia (-par″ah-ple′jah) spurious paralysis of the lower limbs, as in hysteria or conversion disorder.

pseu·do·pa·re·sis (-pah-re′sis) a hysterical or nonorganic condition simulating paresis.

pseu·do·pe·lade (-pe′lād) patchy alopecia roughly simulating alopecia areata; it may be due to various diseases of the hair follicles, some of which are associated with scarring.

pseu·do·ple·gia (-ple′jah) paralysis due to a conversion disorder.

pseu·do·po·di·um (-po′de-um) pl. *pseudopo′dia.* A temporary protrusion of the cytoplasm of an ameba, serving for locomotion or the engulfment of food.

pseu·do·poly·me·lia (-pol″e-me′le-ah) an illusory sensation that may be referred to many extreme portions of the body, including the hands, feet, nose, nipples, and glans penis.

pseu·do·pol·yp (-pol′ip) a hypertrophied tab of mucous membrane resembling a polyp.

pseu·do·pol·y·po·sis (-pol″ĭ-po′sis) numerous pseudopolyps in the colon and rectum, due to long-standing inflammation.

pseu·do·preg·nan·cy (-preg′nan-se) 1. false pregnancy. 2. the premenstrual stage of the endometrium; so called because it resembles the endometrium just before implantation of the blastocyst.

pseu·do·pseu·do·hy·po·para·thy·roid·ism (-soo″do-hi″po-par″ah-thi′roi-dizm) an incomplete form of pseudohypoparathyroidism marked by the same constitutional features but by normal levels of calcium and phosphorus in the blood serum.

pseu·do·pter·yg·i·um (-ter-ij′e-um) an adhesion of the conjunctiva to the cornea following a burn or other injury.

pseu·do·pto·sis (-to′sis) decrease in the size of the palpebral aperture.

pseu·do·pu·ber·ty (-pu′ber-te) development of secondary sex characters and reproductive organs that is not associated with pubertal levels of gonadotropins and gonadotropin-releasing hormone; it may be either heterosexual or isosexual. **precocious p.,** the appearance of some of the secondary sex characters without maturation of the gonads, before the normal age of onset of puberty.

pseu·do·re·ac·tion (-re-ak′shun) a false or deceptive reaction; a skin reaction in intradermal tests that is not due to the specific test substance but to protein in the medium employed in producing the toxin.

pseu·do·rick·ets (-rik′its) renal osteodystrophy.

pseu·do·sar·co·ma·tous (-sahr-ko′mah-tus) mimicking sarcoma; used of both benign and malignant lesions that histologically resemble sarcoma.

pseu·do·scar·la·ti·na (-skahr″lah-te′nah) a septic condition with fever and eruption resembling scarlet fever.

pseu·do·scle·ro·sis (-sklĕ-ro′sis) a condition with the symptoms but without the lesions of multiple sclerosis. **Strümpell-Westphal p., Westphal-Strümpell p.,** Wilson's disease.

pseu·do·sei·zure (-se′zhur) an attack resembling an epileptic seizure but having purely psychological causes, lacking the electroencephalographic changes of epilepsy, and sometimes able to be stopped by an act of will.

pseu·do·sto·ma (-sto′mah) an apparent communication between silver-stained epithelial cells.

pseu·do·ta·bes (-ta′bēz) any neuropathy with symptoms like those of tabes dorsalis.

pseu·do·tet·a·nus (-tet′ah-nus) persistent muscular contractions resembling tetanus but unassociated with *Clostridium tetani.*

pseu·do·trun·cus ar·te·ri·o·sus (-trunk′us ahr-tēr″e-o′sus) the most severe form of tetralogy of Fallot.

pseu·do·tu·mor (-too′mer) an enlargement that resembles a tumor, resulting from inflammation, fluid accumulation, or other causes. **p. ce′rebri,** cerebral edema and raised intracranial pressure without neurological signs except occasional sixth nerve palsy. **inflammatory p.,** a tumorlike mass representing an inflammatory reaction.

pseu·do·uri·dine (-ūr′ĭ-dēn) a nucleotide derived from uridine by isomerization and occurring in transfer RNA. Symbol ψ.

pseu·do·ver·ti·go (-ver′tĭ-go) any dizziness or other form of lightheadedness that resembles vertigo but does not involve a sense of rotation.

pseu·do·xan·tho·ma elas·ti·cum (-zan-tho′mah e-las′tĭ-kum) a progressive, inherited disorder with skin, eye, and cardiovascular manifestations, most resulting from basophilic degeneration of elastic tissues, including small yellowish macules and papules, lax, inelastic, and redundant skin, premature arterial calcification, symptoms of coronary insufficiency, hypertension, mitral valve prolapse, angioid streaks in the retina, and gastrointestinal and other hemorrhages.

psi pounds per square inch.

psi·lo·cin (si′lah-sin) a hallucinogenic substance closely related to psilocybin.

psi·lo·cy·bin (si″lah-si′bin) a hallucinogen having indole characteristics, isolated from the mushroom *Psilocybe mexicana.*

psit·ta·co·sis (sit″ah-ko′sis) a disease due to a strain of *Chlamydia psittaci,* first seen in parrots and later in other birds and domestic fowl; it is transmissible to humans, usually taking the form of a pneumonia accompanied by fever, cough, and often splenomegaly. See also *ornithosis.*

psor·a·len (sor′ah-len) any of the constituents of certain plants (e.g., *Psoralea corylifolia*) that have the ability to produce phototoxic dermatitis on subsequent exposure of the individual to sunlight; certain perfumes and drugs (e.g., methoxsalen) contain psoralens.

pso·ri·a·sis (sor-i′ah-sis) a chronic, hereditary, recurrent dermatosis marked by discrete vivid red macules, papules, or plaques covered with silvery lamellated scales. **psoriat′ic,** adj. **erythrodermic p.,** a severe, generalized erythrodermic condition developing usually in chronic forms of psoriasis and characterized by massive exfoliation of skin with serious systemic illness.

PSRO Professional Standards Review Organization.

PSVT paroxysmal supraventricular tachycardia.

psy·chal·gia (si-kal′jah) 1. pain, usually in the head and perceived as being of emotional origin, that may accompany intolerable ideas, obsessions, or hallucinations. 2. psychogenic pain. **psychal′gic,** adj.

psy·cha·tax·ia (si″kah-tak′se-ah) a disordered mental condition marked by confusion and inability to concentrate.

psy·che (si′ke) 1. the human faculty for thought, judgment, and emotion; the mental life, including both conscious and unconscious processes; the mind in its totality, as distinguished from the body. 2. the soul or self. **psy′chic,** adj.

psy·che·del·ic (si″kĭ-del′ik) 1. pertaining to or characterized by hallucinations, distortions of perception and awareness, and sometimes psychotic-like behavior. 2. a drug that produces such effects.

psy·chi·a·trist (si-ki′ah-trist) a physician who specializes in psychiatry.

psy·chi·a·try (si-ki′ah-tre) the branch of medicine dealing with the study, treatment, and prevention of mental disorders. **psychiat′ric,** adj. **biological p.,** that which emphasizes physical, chemical, and neurological causes and treatment approaches. **community p.,** that concerned with the detection, prevention, and treatment of mental disorders as they develop within designated psychosocial, cultural, or geographical areas. **descriptive p.,** that based on the study of observable symptoms and behavioral phenomena, rather than underlying psychodynamic processes. **dynamic p.,** that based on the study of emotional processes, their origins, and the mental mechanisms underlying them, rather than observable behavioral phenomena. **forensic p.**, that dealing with the legal aspects of mental disorders. **geriatric p.**, geropsychiatry. **preventive p.**, that broadly concerned with the amelioration, control, and limitation of psychiatric disability. **social p.**, that concerned with the cultural and social factors that engender, precipitate, intensify, or prolong maladaptive patterns of behavior and complicate treatment.

psy·chic (si′kik) 1. pertaining to the psyche. 2. mental (1).

psych(o)- word element [Gr.], *mind.*

psy·cho·acous·tics (si″ko-ah-koos′tiks) a branch of psychophysics studying the relationship between acoustic stimuli and behavior.

psy·cho·ac·tive (-ak′tiv) psychotropic.

psy·cho·an·a·lep·tic (-an″ah-lep′tik) exerting a stimulating effect upon the mind.

psy·cho·anal·y·sis (-ah-nal′ĭ-sis) 1. a theory of human mental phenomena and behavior focusing on the influence of unconscious forces on the mental state (Freud). 2. a method of investigation into the contents of the mind. 3. a therapeutic technique based on Freud's theory, diagnosing and treating mental and emotional disorders through ascertaining and analyzing the facts of the patient's present and past mental life and emotional experiences. **psychoanalyt′ic**, adj.

psy·cho·bi·ol·o·gy (-bi-ol′ŏ-je) 1. biopsychology; a field of study examining the relationship between brain and mind, studying the effect of biological influences on psychological functioning or mental processes. 2. a psychiatric theory in which the human being is viewed as an integrated unit, incorporating psychological, social, and biological functions, with behavior a function of the total organism. **psychobiolog′ical**, adj.

psy·cho·dra·ma (-drah′mah) a form of group psychotherapy in which patients dramatize emotional problems and life situations in order to achieve insight and to alter faulty behavior patterns.

psy·cho·dy·nam·ics (-di-nam′iks) the interplay of motivational forces that gives rise to the expression of mental processes, as in attitudes, behavior, or symptoms.

psy·cho·gen·e·sis (-jen′ĭ-sis) 1. mental development. 2. production of a symptom or illness by psychic factors.

psy·cho·gen·ic (-jen′ik) having an emotional or psychologic origin.

psy·cho·graph (si′ko-graf) 1. a chart for recording graphically a person's personality traits. 2. a written description of a person's mental functioning.

psy·chol·o·gy (si-kol′ah-je) the science dealing with the mind and mental processes, especially in relation to human and animal behavior. **psycholog′ic, psycholog′ical**, adj. **analytic p.**, psychology based on the concept of the collective unconscious and the complex. **child p.**, the study of the development of the mind of the child. **clinical p.**, the use of psychologic knowledge and techniques in the treatment of persons with emotional difficulties. **community p.**, a broad term referring to the organization of community resources for the prevention of mental disorders. **criminal p.**, the study of the mentality, motivation, and social behavior of criminals. **depth p.**, psychoanalysis. **developmental p.**, the study of behavioral change through the life span. **dynamic p.**, that stressing the element of energy in mental processes. **environmental p.**, the study of the effects of the physical and social environment on behavior. **experimental p.**, the study of the mind and mental operations by the use of experimental methods. **gestalt p.**, gestaltism. **physiologic p., physiological p.**, the branch of psychology that studies the relationship between physiologic and psychologic processes. **social p.**, that treating of the social aspects of mental life.

psy·chom·e·try (si-kom′ĕ-tre) the testing and measuring of mental and psychologic ability, efficiency, potentials, and functioning. **psychomet′ric**, adj.

psy·cho·mo·tor (si″ko-mo′ter) pertaining to motor effects of cerebral or psychic activity.

psy·cho·neu·ral (-noor′al) relating to the totality of neural events initiated by a sensory input and leading to storage, to discrimination, or an output of any kind.

psy·cho·neu·ro·im·mu·nol·o·gy (-noor″-o-im″u-nol′ah;-je) the study of the interactions between psychological factors, the central nervous system, and immune function as modulated by the neuroendocrine system.

psy·cho·neu·ro·sis (-noo-ro′sis) neurosis. **psychoneurot′ic**, adj.

psy·cho·pa·thol·o·gy (-pah-thol′ah-je) 1. the branch of medicine dealing with the causes and processes of mental disorders. 2. abnormal, maladaptive behavior or mental activity.

psy·cho·phar·ma·col·o·gy (-fahr″mah-kol′ah-je) 1. the study of the action of drugs on psychological functions and mental states. 2. the use of drugs to modify psychological functions and mental states. **psychopharmacolog′ic**, adj.

psy·cho·phys·i·cal (-fiz′ĭ-k′l) pertaining to the mind and its relation to physical manifestations.

psy·cho·phys·ics (-fiz′iks) scientific study of quantitative relations between characteristics or patterns of physical stimuli and the sensations induced by them.

psy·cho·phys·i·ol·o·gy (-fiz″e-ol′ah-je) physiologic psychology.

psy·cho·ple·gic (-ple′jik) an agent lessening cerebral activity or excitability.

psy·cho·sen·so·ry (-sen′ser-e) perceiving and interpreting sensory stimuli.

psy·cho·sex·u·al (-sek′shoo-al) pertaining to the mental or emotional aspects of sex.

psy·cho·sis (si-ko′sis) pl. *psycho′ses*. Any major mental disorder of organic or emotional origin marked by derangement of personality and loss of contact with reality, with delusions and hallucinations and often with incoherent speech, disorganized and agitated behavior, or illusions. Cf. *neurosis*. **alcoholic p′s,** those associated with excessive use of alcohol and involving organic brain damage. **bipolar p.,** see under *disorder*. **brief reactive p.,** an episode of brief psychotic disorder that is a reaction to a recognizable, distressing life event. **Korsakoff's p.,** see under *syndrome*. **senile p.,** depressive or paranoid delusions or hallucinations or other mental disorders associated with degeneration of the brain in old age, as in senile dementia. **symbiotic p., symbiotic infantile p.,** a condition seen in two- to four-year-old children having an abnormal relationship to the mothering figure, characterized by intense separation anxiety, severe regression, giving up of useful speech, and autism. **toxic p.,** one due to the ingestion of toxic agents or to the presence of toxins within the body.

psy·cho·so·cial (si″ko-so′shul) pertaining to or involving both psychic and social aspects.

psy·cho·so·mat·ic (-sah-mat′ik) pertaining to the mind-body relationship; having bodily symptoms of psychic, emotional, or mental origin.

psy·cho·stim·u·lant (-stim′ūl-int) 1. producing a transient increase in psychomotor activity. 2. a drug that produces such effects.

psy·cho·sur·gery (-ser′jer-e) brain surgery performed for treatment of psychiatric disorders. **psychosur′gical,** adj.

psy·cho·ther·a·py (-ther′ah-pe) treatment of mental disorders and behavioral disturbances using verbal and nonverbal communication, as opposed to agents such as drugs or electric shock, to alter maladaptive patterns of coping, relieve emotional disturbance, and encourage personality growth. **psychoanalytic p.,** psychoanalysis (3).

psy·chot·ic (si-kot′ik) 1. pertaining to, characterized by, or caused by psychosis. 2. a person exhibiting psychosis.

psy·chot·o·gen·ic (si-kot″ah-jen′ik) psychotomimetic.

psy·choto·mi·met·ic (-mi-met′ik) pertaining to, characterized by, or producing symptoms similar to those of a psychosis.

psy·cho·tro·pic (si″ko-tro′pik) exerting an effect on the mind; capable of modifying mental activity; said especially of drugs.

psychr(o)- word element [Gr.], *cold*.

psy·chro·al·gia (si″kro-al′jah) a painful sensation of cold.

psy·chro·phil·ic (-fil′ik) fond of cold; said of bacteria growing best in the cold (15°–20°C).

psyl·li·um (sil′e-um) 1. a plant of the genus *Plantago*. 2. the husk (*psyllium husk*) or seed (*plantago* or *psyllium seed*) of various species of *Plantago*; used as a bulk-forming laxative.

PT prothrombin time.

Pt platinum.

PTA plasma thromboplastin antecedent (coagulation factor XI).

ptar·mic (tahr′mik) causing sneezing.

ptar·mus (tahr′mus) spasmodic sneezing.

PTC plasma thromboplastin component (coagulation factor IX).

pte·ri·on (tēr′e-on) a point of junction of frontal, parietal, temporal, and sphenoid bones.

pter·o·yl·glu·tam·ic ac·id (ter″o-il-glootam′ik) folic acid.

pte·ryg·i·um (tĕ-rij′e-um) pl. *ptery′gia*. [Gr.] a winglike structure, especially an abnormal triangular fold of membrane in the interpalpebral fissure, extending from the conjunctiva to the cornea. **p. col′li,** webbed neck; a thick skin fold on the side of the neck from the mastoid region to the acromion.

pter·y·goid (ter′ĭ-goid) shaped like a wing.

pter·y·go·man·dib·u·lar (ter″ĭ-go-mandib′u-lar) pertaining to the pterygoid process and the mandible.

pter·y·go·max·il·lary (-mak′sĭ-lar″e) pertaining to the pterygoid process and the maxilla.

pter·y·go·pal·a·tine (-pal′ah-tīn) pertaining to the pterygoid process and the palate bone.

pto·maine (to′mān, to-mān′) any of an indefinite class of toxic bases, usually considered to be formed by the action of bacterial metabolism or proteins.

ptosed (tōst) affected with ptosis.

pto·sis (to′sis) 1. prolapse (1). 2. paralytic drooping of the upper eyelid. **ptot′ic**, adj.

-ptosis word element [Gr.], *downward displacement*. **-ptot′ic**, adj.

PTSD posttraumatic stress disorder.

PTT activated partial thromboplastin time.

pty·al·a·gogue (ti-al′ah-gog) sialagogue.

pty·a·lec·ta·sis (ti″ah-lek′tah-sis) 1. a state of dilatation of a salivary duct. 2. surgical dilation of a salivary duct.

pty·a·lin (ti′ah-lin) α-amylase occurring in saliva.

pty·a·lism (ti′ah-lizm) excessive secretion of saliva.

ptyal(o)- word element [Gr.], *saliva*. See also *sial(o)-*.

pty·a·lo·cele (ti-al′o-sēl) a cystic tumor containing saliva.

pty·a·lo·gen·ic (ti″ah-lo-jen′ik) formed from or by the action of saliva.

pty·a·lor·rhea (-re′ah) ptyalism.

Pu plutonium.

pu·bar·che (pu-bahr′ke) the first appearance of pubic hair.

pu·ber·tas (pu-ber′tas) puberty. **p. prae′-cox**, precocious puberty.

pu·ber·ty (pu′ber-te) the period during which the secondary sex characters begin to develop and the capability of sexual reproduction is attained. **pu′beral, pu′bertal**, adj.

central precocious p., precocious puberty due to premature hypothalamic-pituitary-gonadal maturation; it is always isosexual and involves not only development of secondary sex characters but also development of the gonads. Increases in height and weight and osseous maturation are accelerated, and early closing of the epiphyses leads to short stature. **precocious p.**, the onset of puberty at an earlier age than normal, defined as before age 8 in girls and 9 in boys; it is usually hormonal, but occasionally occurs in otherwise normal children.

pu·bes (pu′bez) [L.] 1. the hairs growing over the pubic region. 2. the pubic region. **pu′bic**, adj.

pu·bes·cent (pu-bes′int) 1. arriving at the age of puberty. 2. covered with down or lanugo.

pu·bic (pu′bik) pertaining to or situated near the pubes, the pubic bone, or the pubic region.

pu·bi·ot·o·my (pu″be-ot′ah-me) surgical separation of the pubic bone lateral to the symphysis.

pu·bis (pu′bis) [L.] pubic bone; see *Table of Bones*.

pu·bo·ves·i·cal (pu″bo-ves′ĭ-kil) vesicopubic.

PUBS percutaneous umbilical blood sampling; see *cordocentesis*.

pu·den·dum (pu-den′dum) pl. *puden′da*. [L.] the external genitalia of humans, especially of the female; see *vulva*. **puden′dal, pu′dic**, adj. **p. femini′num, p. mulie′bre**, the female pudendum.

pu·er·ile (pu′er-il) pertaining to childhood or to children; childish.

pu·er·pera (pu-er′per-ah) a woman who has just given birth to a child.

pu·er·per·al (-al) pertaining to a puerpera or to the puerperium.

pu·er·per·al·ism (-al-izm) morbid condition incident to childbirth.

pu·er·pe·ri·um (pu″er-pēr′e-um) the period or state of confinement after childbirth.

PUFA polyunsaturated fatty acid.

Pu·lex (pu′leks) a genus of fleas, including *P. ir′ritans*, the common flea or human flea, which attacks humans and domestic animals, and may act as an intermediate host of certain helminths.

pu·lic·i·cide (pu-lis′ĭ-sīd) an agent destructive to fleas.

pull (pŏŏl) 1. to strain a muscle. 2. the injury sustained in a muscle strain.

pul·lu·la·tion (pul″u-la′shun) development by sprouting or budding.

pul·mo (pul′mo) pl. *pulmo′nes*. [L.] lung.

pul·mo·nary (pŏŏl′mo-nar″e) 1. pertaining to the lungs. 2. pertaining to the pulmonary artery.

pul·mon·ic (pul-mon′ik) pulmonary.

pul·mo·ni·tis (pul″mah-ni′tis) pneumonitis.

pulp (pulp) any soft, juicy animal or vegetable tissue. **pul′pal**, adj. **coronal p.**, the part of the dental pulp contained in the crown portion of the pulp cavity. **dental p.**, richly vascularized and innervated connective tissue inside the pulp cavity of a tooth. **digital p.**, a cushion of soft tissue on the palmar or plantar surface of the distal phalanx of a finger or toe. **red p., splenic p.**, the dark, reddish brown substance filling the interspaces of the splenic sinuses. **white p.**, sheaths of lymphatic tissue surrounding the arteries of the spleen.

pul·pa (pul′pah) pl. *pul′pae*. [L.] pulp.

pul·pec·to·my (pul-pek′tah-me) removal of dental pulp.

pul·pi·tis (pul-pi′tis) pl. *pulpi′tides*. Inflammation of dental pulp.

pul·pot·o·my (pul-pot′ah-me) excision of the coronal pulp.

pul·py (pul′pe) soft or pultaceous.

pul·sa·tile (pul′sah-tīl) characterized by a rhythmic pulsation.

pul·sa·tion (pul-sa′shun) a throb, or rhythmic beat, as of the heart.

pulse (puls) the rhythmic expansion of an artery that may be felt with the finger. **alternating p.,** one with regular alternation of weak and strong beats without changes in cycle length. **anacrotic p.,** one in which the ascending limb of the tracing shows a transient drop in amplitude. **bigeminal p.,** one in which two beats occur in rapid succession, the groups of two being separated by a longer interval. **cannonball p.,** Corrigan's p. **capillary p.,** Quincke's p. **catadicrotic p.,** one in which the descending limb of the tracing shows two small notches. **Corrigan's p.,** jerky pulse with full expansion and sudden collapse. **dicrotic p.,** a pulse characterized by two peaks, the second peak occurring in diastole and being an exaggeration of the dicrotic wave. **entoptic p.,** a phose occurring with each pulse beat. **hard p.,** one characterized by high tension. **jerky p.,** one in which the artery is suddenly and markedly distended. **paradoxical p.,** one that markedly decreases in size during inhalation, as often occurs in constrictive pericarditis. **pistol-shot p.,** Corrigan's p. **plateau p.,** one that is slowly rising and sustained. **quadrigeminal p.,** one with a pause after every fourth beat. **Quincke's p.,** alternate blanching and flushing of the nail bed due to pulsation of subpapillary arteriolar and venous plexuses; seen in aortic insufficiency and other conditions and occasionally in normal persons. **Riegel's p.,** one that is smaller during respiration. **thready p.,** one that is very fine and scarcely perceptible. **tricrotic p.,** one in which the tracing shows three marked expansions in one beat of the artery. **trigeminal p.,** one with a pause after every third beat. **vagus p.,** a slow pulse. **venous p.,** the pulsation over a vein, especially over the right jugular vein. **water-hammer p.,** Corrigan's p. **wiry p.,** a small, tense pulse.

pulse·less (puls'les) lacking a pulse.

pul·sion (pul'shun) a pushing forward or outward.

pul·sus (-sus) pl. *pul'sus.* [L.] pulse. **p. alter'nans,** alternating pulse. **p. bisfe'riens,** a pulse characterized by two strong systolic peaks separated by a midsystolic dip, most commonly occurring in pure aortic regurgitation and in aortic regurgitation with stenosis. **p. dif'ferens,** inequality of the pulse observable at corresponding sites on the two sides of the body.

pul·ta·ceous (pul-ta'shus) like a poultice; pulpy.

pul·vi·nar (pul-vi'nar) the prominent medial part of the posterior end of the thalamus.

pum·ice (pum'is) a very light, hard, rough, porous substance consisting of silicates of aluminum, potassium, and sodium; used in dentistry as an abrasive.

pump (pump) 1. an apparatus for drawing or forcing liquids or gases. 2. to draw or force liquids or gases. **breast p.,** a manual or electric pump for abstracting breast milk. **calcium p.,** the mechanism of active transport of calcium (Ca^{2+}) across a membrane, as of the sarcoplasmic reticulum of muscle cells, against a concentration gradient; the mechanism is driven by enzymatic hydrolysis of ATP. **intra-aortic balloon p. (IABP),** a pump used in intra-aortic balloon counterpulsation. **proton p.,** a system for transporting protons across cell membranes, often exchanging them for other positively charged ions. **sodium p., sodium-potassium p.,** the mechanism of active transport, driven by hydrolysis of ATP, by which sodium (Na^+) is extruded from a cell and potassium (K^+) is brought in, so as to maintain gradients of these ions across the cell membrane.

pump-oxy·gen·a·tor (pump'ok'si-jin-āt"er) an apparatus consisting of a blood pump and oxygenator, plus filters and traps, for saturating the blood with oxygen during heart surgery.

punch·drunk (punch'drunk) boxer's dementia.

punc·tate (punk'tāt) spotted; marked with points or punctures.

punc·ti·form (-ti-form) like a point.

punc·tum (pungk'tum) pl. *punc'ta.* [L.] a point or small spot. **p. cae'cum,** blind spot. **p. lacrima'le,** lacrimal point. **p. prox'imum,** near point. **p. remo'tum,** far point.

punc·ture (-cher) the act of piercing or penetrating with a pointed object or instrument; a wound so made. **cisternal p.,** puncture of the cisterna cerebellomedullaris through the posterior atlanto-occipital membrane to obtain cerebrospinal fluid. **lumbar p., spinal p.,** the withdrawal of fluid from the subarachnoid space in the lumbar region, usually between the third and fourth lumbar vertebrae. **sternal p.,** removal of bone marrow from the manubrium of the sternum through an appropriate needle. **ventricular p.,** puncture of a cerebral ventricle for the withdrawal of fluid.

pu·pa (pu'pah) [L.] the second stage in the development of an insect, between the larva and the imago. **pu'pal,** adj.

pu·pil (P) (pu'pil) the opening in the center of the iris through which light enters the eye. See Plate 30. **pu'pillary,** adj. **Adie's p.,** tonic p. **Argyll Robertson p.,** one that is miotic and responds to accommodative effort, but not to light. **fixed p.,** one that does not react either to light or on convergence, or in accommodation. **Hutchinson's p.,** one that is dilated while the other is not. **tonic p.,** a usually unilateral condition of the eye in which the affected pupil is larger than the other; responds to accommodation and convergence in a slow, delayed fashion; and reacts to light only after prolonged exposure to dark or light.

pu·pil·la (pu-pil'ah) [L.] pupil.

pu·pil·lom·e·try (pu″pĭ-lom'ĭ-tre) measurement of the diameter or width of the pupil of the eye.

pu·pil·lo·ple·gia (pu″pĭ-lo-ple'jah) tonic pupil.

pu·pil·los·co·py (pu″pĭ-los'kah-pe) retinoscopy.

pu·pil·lo·sta·tom·e·ter (pu″pĭ-lo-stah-tom'ĕ-ter) an instrument for measuring the distance between the pupils.

pure (pūr) free from mixture with or contamination by other materials.

pur·ga·tion (pur-ga'shun) evacuation (2).

pur·ga·tive (purg'it-iv) cathartic (1, 2).

purge (purj) 1. to cleanse or purify, to remove undesirable substances from something. 2. to cause evacuation of feces.

pu·ri·fi·ca·tion (pūr″ĭ-fĭ-ka'shun) the separating of foreign or contaminating elements from a substance of interest.

pu·rine (pūr'ēn) a compound, $C_5H_4N_4$, not found in nature, but variously substituted to produce a group of compounds, *purines* or *purine bases*, which include adenine and guanine found in nucleic acids and xanthine and hypoxanthine.

pur·ple (pur'p'l) 1. a color between blue and red. 2. a substance of this color used as a dye or indicator. **visual p.,** rhodopsin.

pur·pu·ra (pur'pu-rah) 1. a small hemorrhage in the skin, mucous membrane, or serosal surface. 2. a group of disorders characterized by the presence of purpuric lesions, ecchymoses, and a tendency to bruise easily. **purpu'ric,** adj. **allergic p., anaphylactoid p.,** Henoch-Schönlein p. **p. annula'ris tel-angiecto'des,** a rare form in which punctate erythematous lesions coalesce to form an annular or serpiginous pattern. **fibrinolytic p.,** purpura associated with increased fibrinolytic activity of the blood. **p. ful'minans,** nonthrombocytopenic purpura seen mainly in children, usually after an infectious disease, marked by fever, shock, anemia, and sudden, rapidly spreading symmetrical skin hemorrhages of the lower limbs, often associated with extensive intravascular thromboses

and gangrene. **p. hemorrha'gica,** idiopathic thrombocytopenic p. **Henoch's p.,** Henoch-Schönlein purpura in which abdominal symptoms predominate. **Henoch-Schönlein p.,** nonthrombocytopenic purpura of unknown cause, usually in children; associated with symptoms such as urticaria, erythema, arthropathy and arthritis, gastrointestinal disorder, and renal involvement. **idiopathic thrombocytopenic p.,** thrombocytopenic purpura not directly associated with a systemic disease, although often following a systemic infection; believed to be due to an IgG immunoglobulin that acts as an antibody against platelets. **malignant p.,** meningococcal meningitis. **nonthrombocytopenic p.,** purpura without any decrease in the platelet count of the blood. **Schönlein p.,** Henoch-Schönlein purpura with articular symptoms and without gastrointestinal symptoms. **Schönlein-Henoch p.,** Henoch-Schönlein p. **p. seni'lis,** dark purplish red ecchymoses occurring on the forearms and backs of the hands in the elderly. **thrombocytopenic p.,** any form in which the platelet count is decreased, occurring as a primary disease (*idiopathic thrombocytopenic p.*) or as a consequence of a primary hematologic disorder (*secondary thrombocytopenic p.*). **thrombotic thrombocytopenic p.,** a form of thrombotic microangiopathy marked by thrombocytopenia, hemolytic anemia, neurological manifestations, azotemia, fever, and thromboses in terminal arterioles and capillaries.

pu·ru·lence (pūr'ah-lins) suppuration. **pur'ulent,** adj.

pu·ru·loid (pūr'ah-loid) pyoid.

pus (pus) a protein-rich liquid inflammation product made up of leukocytes, cellular debris, and a thin fluid (liquor puris).

pus·tu·la (pus'tu-lah) pl. *pus'tulae.* [L.] pustule.

pus·tule (pus'tūl) a small, elevated, circumscribed, pus-containing lesion of the skin. **pus'tular,** adj.

pus·tu·lo·sis (pus″tu-lo'sis) a condition marked by an eruption of pustules.

pu·ta·men (pu-ta'men) the larger and more lateral part of the lentiform nucleus.

pu·tre·fac·tion (pu″tre-fak'shun) enzymatic decomposition, especially of proteins, with the production of foul-smelling compounds, such as hydrogen sulfide, ammonia, and mercaptans. **putrefac'tive,** adj.

pu·tres·cence (pu-tres'ens) the condition of undergoing putrefaction. **putres'cent,** adj.

pu·tres·cine (pu-tres'in) a polyamine precursor of spermidine, first found in decaying meat but now known to occur in almost all tissues and in some bacterial cultures.

pu·trid (pu'trid) rotten; putrefied.

PVC polyvinyl chloride.

PVP polyvinylpyrrolidone (see *povidone*).

PVP-I povidone-iodine.

py·ar·thro·sis (pi″ahr-thro'sis) suppuration within a joint cavity; acute suppurative arthritis.

pycn(o)- see words beginning *pykn(o)-*.

py·elec·ta·sis (pi″ĕ-lek'tah-sis) dilatation of the renal pelvis.

py·eli·tis (-li'tis) inflammation of the renal pelvis. **pyelit'ic**, adj.

pyel(o)- word element [Gr.], *renal pelvis.*

py·elo·cali·ec·ta·sis (pi″ĕ-lo-kal″e-ek'tah-sis) hydronephrosis.

py·elo·cys·ti·tis (-sis-ti'tis) inflammation of the renal pelvis and bladder.

py·elog·ra·phy (pi″ĕ-log'rah-fe) radiography of the renal pelvis and ureter after injection of contrast material. **antegrade p.**, that in which the contrast medium is introduced by percutaneous needle puncture into the renal pelvis. **retrograde p.**, pyelography after introduction of contrast material through the ureter.

py·elo·in·ter·sti·tial (pi″ĕ-lo-in″ter-stish'al) pertaining to the interstitial tissue of the renal pelvis.

py·elo·li·thot·o·my (-lĭ-thot'ah-me) incision of the renal pelvis for removal of calculi.

py·elo·ne·phri·tis (-nĕ-fri'tis) inflammation of the kidney and its pelvis due to bacterial infection.

py·elo·ne·phro·sis (-nĕ-fro'sis) any disease of the kidney and its pelvis.

py·e·lo·plas·ty (pi'ĕ-lo-plas″te) plastic operation on the renal pelvis.

py·elos·to·my (pi″ĕ-los'tah-me) surgical formation of an opening into the renal pelvis.

py·elot·o·my (-lot'ah-me) incision of the renal pelvis.

py·elo·ure·ter·i·tis (pi″ĕ-lo-u-re″ter-i'tis) inflammation of a ureter and the renal pelvis.

py·elo·ve·nous (-ve'nus) pertaining to the renal pelvis and renal veins.

py·em·e·sis (pi-em'ĭ-sis) the vomiting of pus.

py·e·mia (-ēm'e-ah) septicemia in which secondary foci of suppuration occur and multiple abscesses are formed. **pye'mic**, adj. **arterial p.**, that due to dissemination of septic emboli from the heart. **cryptogenic p.**, that in which the source of infection is in an unidentified tissue.

Py·e·mo·tes (pi″ĭ-mōt'ēz) a genus of parasitic mites. *P. ventrico'sus* attacks certain insect larvae found on straw, grain, and other plants, and causes grain itch in humans.

py·en·ceph·a·lus (pi″en-sef'ah-lus) brain abscess.

py·e·sis (pi-e'sis) suppuration.

py·gal (pi'gil) gluteal.

py·gal·gia (pi-gal'jah) pain in the buttocks.

pyk·nic (pik'nik) having a short, thick, stocky build.

pykn(o)- word element [Gr.], *thick; compact; frequent.*

pyk·no·cyte (pik'no-sīt) a distorted and contracted, occasionally spiculed erythrocyte.

pyk·no·dys·os·to·sis (pik″no-dis″os-to'sis) a hereditary syndrome of dwarfism, osteopetrosis, and skeletal anomalies of the cranium, digits, and mandible.

pyk·nom·e·ter (pik-nom'ĕ-ter) an instrument for determining the specific gravity of fluids.

pyk·no·mor·phous (pik″no-mor'fus) having the stained portions of the cell body compactly arranged.

pyk·no·sis (pik-no'sis) a thickening, especially degeneration of a cell in which the nucleus shrinks in size and the chromatin condenses to a solid, structureless mass or masses. **pyknot'ic**, adj.

pyle- word element [Gr.], *portal vein.*

py·le·phle·bec·ta·sis (pi″lĭ-flĕ-bek'tah-sis) dilatation of the portal vein.

py·le·phle·bi·tis (-flĕ-bi'tis) inflammation of the portal vein.

py·lo·ral·gia (pi″lor-al'jah) pain in the region of the pylorus.

py·lo·rec·to·my (pi″lor-ek'tah-me) excision of the pylorus.

py·lo·ric (pi-lor'ik) pertaining to the pylorus or to the pyloric part of the stomach.

py·lo·ri·ste·no·sis (pi-lor″e-stĕ-no'sis) pyloric stenosis.

pylor(o)- word element [Gr.], *pylorus.*

py·lo·ro·di·o·sis (pi-lor″o-di-o'sis) dilation of a pyloric stricture with the finger during operation.

py·lo·ro·du·o·de·ni·tis (-doo-od″ĕ-ni'tis) inflammation of the pyloric and duodenal mucosa.

py·lo·ro·gas·tre·to·my (-gas-trek'tah-me) excision of the pylorus and adjacent portion of the stomach.

py·lo·ro·my·ot·o·my (-mi-ot'ah-me) incision of the longitudinal and circular muscles of the pylorus.

py·lo·ro·plas·ty (pi-lor'ah-plas″te) plastic surgery of the pylorus. **double p.**, posterior pyloromyotomy combined with the Heineke-Mikulicz pyloroplasty. **Finney p.**, enlargement of the pyloric canal by establishment of an inverted U-shaped anastomosis between the stomach and duodenum after longitudinal incision. **Heineke-Mikulicz p.,** enlargement of a pyloric stricture by incising the pylorus longitudinally and suturing the incision transversely.

py·lo·ros·co·py (pi″lor-os′kah-pe) endoscopic inspection of the pylorus.

py·lo·ros·to·my (-os′tah-me) surgical formation of an opening through the abdominal wall into the stomach near the pylorus.

py·lo·rot·o·my (-ot′ah-me) incision of the pylorus.

py·lo·rus (pi-lor′us) the distal aperture of the stomach, opening into the duodenum; variously used to mean pyloric part of the stomach, and pyloric antrum, canal, opening, or sphincter. **pylor′ic,** adj.

py(o)- word element [Gr.], *pus.*

pyo·cele (pi′o-sēl) a collection of pus, as in the scrotum.

pyo·che·zia (pi″o-ke′zhah) pus in the feces.

pyo·coc·cus (-kok′us) any pus-forming coccus.

pyo·col·po·cele (-kol′po-sēl) a vaginal tumor containing pus.

pyo·cyst (pi′o-sist) a cyst containing pus.

pyo·der·ma (pi″o-der′mah) any purulent skin disease. **p. gangreno′sum,** a rapidly evolving cutaneous ulcer or ulcers, with marked undermining of the border.

pyo·gen·e·sis (-jen′ĭ-sis) suppuration; the formation of pus.

pyo·gen·ic (-jen′ik) suppurative.

pyo·he·mo·tho·rax (-he″mo-thor′aks) pus and blood in the pleural space.

pyo·hy·dro·ne·phro·sis (-hi″dro-nĕ-fro′sis) accumulation of pus and urine in the kidney.

py·oid (pi′oid) resembling or like pus.

pyo·me·tri·tis (pi″o-me-tri′tis) purulent inflammation of the uterus.

pyo·myo·si·tis (-mi″o-si′tis) an acute bacterial infection of skeletal muscle, usually seen in the tropics, most commonly caused by *Staphylococcus aureus.*

pyo·ne·phri·tis (-nĕ-fri′tis) purulent inflammation of the kidney.

pyo·neph·ro·sis (-nĕ-fro′sis) suppurative destruction of the renal parenchyma, with total or almost complete loss of kidney function.

pyo·ova·ri·um (-o-var′e-um) abscess of an ovary.

pyo·peri·car·di·um (-per″ĭ-kahr′de-um) pus in the pericardium.

pyo·peri·to·ne·um (-per″ĭ-tah-ne′um) pus in the peritoneal cavity.

py·oph·thal·mi·tis (pi″of-thal-mi′tis) purulent inflammation of the eye.

pyo·phy·so·me·tra (pi″o-fi″so-me′trah) pus and gas in the uterus.

pyo·pneu·mo·cho·le·cys·ti·tis (-noo″mo-ko″lĕ-sis-ti′tis) distention of the gallbladder, with pus and gas.

pyo·pneu·mo·hep·a·ti·tis (-hep″ah-ti′tis) abscess of the liver with pus and gas.

pyo·pneu·mo·peri·car·di·um (-per″ĭ-kahr′de-um) pus and gas or air in the pericardium.

pyo·pneu·mo·peri·to·ni·tis (-per″ĭ-to-ni′tis) peritonitis with pus and gas.

pyo·pneu·mo·tho·rax (-thor′aks) pus and air or gas in the pleural cavity.

pyo·poi·e·sis (pi″o-poi-e′sis) pyogenesis.

py·op·ty·sis (pi-op′tĭ-sis) expectoration of purulent matter.

pyo·py·elec·ta·sis (pi″o-pi″il-ek′tah-sis) dilatation of the renal pelvis with pus.

py·or·rhea (-re′ah) a copious discharge of pus. **pyorrhe′al,** adj. **p. alveola′ris,** compound periodontitis.

pyo·sal·pin·gi·tis (-sal″pin-ji′tis) uterine salpingitis with suppuration.

pyo·sal·pin·go·ooph·o·ri·tis (-sal-ping″go-o″of-ah-ri′tis) purulent inflammation of a uterine tube and ovary.

pyo·sal·pinx (-sal′pinks) a collection of pus in a uterine tube.

pyo·sper·mia (-sper′me-ah) pus in the semen.

pyo·stat·ic (-stat′ik) stopping or hindering pus formation; an agent that does this.

pyo·tho·rax (-thor′aks) empyema (2).

pyo·ure·ter (-u-re′ter) pus in a ureter.

pyr·a·mid (pir′ah-mid) a pointed or cone-shaped structure or part; often used to indicate the pyramid of the medulla oblongata. **p. of cerebellum,** p. of vermis. **Lalouette's p.,** p. of thyroid. **p. of light,** see under *cone.* **p. of medulla oblongata,** either of two rounded masses, one on either side of the median fissure of the medulla oblongata. **renal p's,** the conical masses composing the medullary substance of the kidney. **p. of thyroid,** an occasional third lobe of the thyroid gland, extending upward from the isthmus. **p. of tympanum,** the hollow elevation in the inner wall of the middle ear containing the stapedius muscle. **p. of vermis,** the part of the vermis cerebelli between the tuber vermis and the uvula.

pyr·a·mi·dal (pĭ-ram′ĭ-d′l) 1. shaped like a pyramid. 2. pertaining to the pyramidal tract.

pyr·a·mis (pir′ah-mis) pl. *pyra′mides.* [Gr.] pyramid.

py·ran (pi′ran) a cyclic compound in which the ring consists of five carbon atoms and one oxygen atom.

pyr·a·nose (pir′ah-nōs) any sugar containing the five-carbon pyran ring structure; it is a cyclic form that ketoses and aldoses may take in solution.

py·ran·tel (pĭ-ran′tel) a broad-spectrum anthelmintic effective against roundworms and pinworms, used as the pamoate and tartrate salts.

pyr·a·zin·amide (pir″ah-zin′ah-mīd) an antibacterial derived from nicotinic acid, used as a tuberculostatic.

py·reth·rin (pi-reth′rin) either of two esters, *p. I* and *p. II*, found in the flowers of certain species of *Chrysanthemum;* used as an insecticide and as a topical pediculicide.

py·ret·ic (pi-ret′ik) 1. febrile. 2. pyrogenic. 3. pyrogen.

py·re·to·gen·e·sis (pi-rēt″o-jen′ĕ-sis) the origin and causation of fever.

py·rex·ia (pi-rek′se-ah) pl. *pyrex′iae.* Fever. **pyrex′ial,** adj.

pyr·i·dine (pir′ĭ-din) 1. a coal tar derivative, C_5H_5N, derived also from tobacco and various organic matter. 2. any of a group of substances homologous with normal pyridine.

pyr·i·do·stig·mine (pir″ĭ-do-stig′mēn) a cholinesterase inhibitor, used as the bromide salt in the treatment of myasthenia gravis and as an antidote to nondepolarizing neuromuscular blocking agents.

pyr·i·dox·al (pir″ĭ-dok′sal) a form of vitamin B_6. **p. phosphate,** the prosthetic group of many enzymes involved in amino acid transformations.

pyr·i·dox·amine (pir″ĭ-doks′ah-mēn) one of the three active forms of vitamin B_6.

pyr·i·dox·ine (pir″ĭ-dok′sēn) one of the forms of vitamin B_6, used as the hydrochloride salt in the prophylaxis and treatment of vitamin B_6 deficiency and as an antidote in cycloserine and isoniazid poisoning.

py·ril·amine (pĭ-ril′ah-mēn) an antihistamine with anticholinergic and sedative effects, used as the maleate and tannate salts.

pyr·i·meth·amine (pir″ĭ-meth′ah-mēn) a folic acid antagonist, used in the treatment of malaria and of toxoplasmosis.

py·rim·i·dine (pĭ-rim′ĭ-dēn) an organic compound, $C_4H_4N_2$, the fundamental form of the pyrimidine bases, including uracil, cytosine, and thymine.

pyr(o)- word element [Gr.], *fire; heat;* (in chemistry) *produced by heating.*

py·ro·cat·e·chol (pi″ro-kat′ĕ-kol) a compound comprising the aromatic portion in the synthesis of endogenous catecholamines;

it has been used as a topical antiseptic and as a reagent.

py·ro·gen (pi′ro-jen) a fever-producing substance.

py·ro·gen·ic (pi″ro-jen′ik) febrifacient; causing fever.

py·ro·glob·u·lin·emia (-glob″u-lin-e′me-ah) presence in the blood of an abnormal globulin constituent that is precipitated by heat.

py·ro·ma·nia (-ma′ne-ah) the compulsion to set or watch fires in the absence of monetary or other gain, the act being preceded by tension or arousal and resulting in pleasure or relief.

py·ro·nin (pi′rah-nin) a red aniline histologic stain.

py·ro·pho·bia (pi″ro-fo′be-ah) irrational fear of fire.

py·ro·phos·pha·tase (-fos′fah-tās) any enzyme that catalyzes the hydrolysis of a pyrophosphate bond, cleaving between the two phosphate groups.

py·ro·phos·phate (-fos′fāt) a salt of pyrophosphoric acid.

py·ro·phos·pho·ric ac·id (-fos-for′ik) a dimer of phosphoric acid, $H_4P_2O_7$; its esters are important in energy metabolism and biosynthesis, e.g., ATP.

py·ro·sis (pi-ro′sis) heartburn.

py·rot·ic (pi-rot′ik) 1. caustic; burning. 2. pertaining to heartburn (pyrosis).

py·roxy·lin (pi-rok′sĭ-lin) a product of the action of a mixture of nitric and sulfuric acids on cotton; used to make collodion.

pyr·role (pir′ōl) 1. a toxic, basic, heterocyclic compound; obtained by destructive distillation of various animal substances and used in the manufacture of pharmaceuticals. 2. a substituted derivative of this structure.

pyr·rol·i·dine (pĭ-rol′ĭ-din) a simple base, $(CH_2)_4NH$, obtained from tobacco or prepared from pyrrole.

py·ru·vate (pi′roo-vāt) a salt, ester, or anion of pyruvic acid. Pyruvate is the end product of glycolysis and may be metabolized to lactate or to acetyl CoA.

py·ru·vic ac·id (pi-roo′vik) $CH_3COCOOH$, an intermediate in carbohydrate, lipid, and protein metabolism.

pyth·i·o·sis (pith″i-e-o′sis) a disease, primarily of horses and mules, caused by *Pythium insidiosum* and characterized by enlarging subcutaneous abscesses that destroy the overlying skin.

py·u·ria (pi-ūr′e-ah) pus in the urine.

Q ubiquinone.

Q₁₀ ubiquinone.

q the long arm of a chromosome.

q.d. [L.] qua′que di′e (every day).

q.h. [L.] qua′que ho′ra (every hour).

qi (che) [Chinese] chi or ch′i; one of the basic substances that according to traditional Chinese medicine pervade the body; a subtle influence or vital energy that is the cause of most physiologic processes and whose proper balance is necessary for maintaining health.

q.i.d. [L.] qua′ter in di′e (four times a day).

qi gong (che′ kung′) [Chinese] qi cultivation, a broad range of practices, incorporating meditation, movement exercises, and breath control, whose purpose is to manipulate and develop qi, and ranging in application from the meditative systems of spiritual practitioners to medical practice to the martial arts.

q.s. [L.] quan′tum sa′tis (sufficient quantity).

q-sort (ku′sort) a technique of personality assessment in which the subject (or an observer) indicates the degree to which a standardized set of descriptive statements applies to the subject.

quack (kwak) one who misrepresents their ability and experience in diagnosis and treatment of disease or effects to be achieved by their treatment.

quack·ery (kwak′er-e) the practice or methods of a quack.

quad·rant (kwod′rant) 1. one fourth of the circumference of a circle. 2. one of four corresponding parts, or quarters, as of the surface of the abdomen or of the field of vision.

quad·rant·an·o·pia (kwod″ran-tah-no′pe-ah) defective vision or blindness in one fourth of the visual field.

quad·ran·tec·to·my (-ran-tek′tah-me) a form of partial mastectomy involving en bloc excision of tumor in one quadrant of breast tissue, as well as the pectoralis major muscle fascia and overlying skin.

quad·rate (kwod′rāt) square or squared.

quadri- word element [L.], *four.*

quad·ri·ceps (kwod′rĭ-seps) having four heads.

quad·ri·gem·i·nal (-jem′ĭ-n′l) 1. fourfold; in four parts; forming a group of four. 2. pertaining to the corpora quadrigemina.

quad·ri·gem·i·ny (-jem′ĭ-ne) 1. occurrence in fours. 2. the occurrence of four beats of the pulse followed by a pause.

quad·rip·a·ra (kwod-rip′ah-rah) a woman who has had four pregnancies that resulted in viable offspring; para IV.

quad·ri·ple·gia (kwod″rĭ-ple′jah) paralysis of all four limbs.

quad·ri·ple·gic (-ple′jik) 1. of, pertaining to, or characterized by quadriplegia. 2. an individual with quadriplegia.

quad·ri·tu·ber·cu·lar (-too-ber′ku-ler) having four tubercles or cusps.

quad·ru·ped (kwod′rah-ped) 1. four-footed. 2. an animal having four feet. **quad·ru′pedal,** adj.

quad·rup·let (kwod-roop′let) one of four offspring produced at one birth.

qual·i·ta·tive (kwahl′ĭ-ta″tiv) pertaining to quality. Cf. *quantitative.*

quan·ti·ta·tive (kwahn′tĭ-ta″tiv) 1. denoting or expressing a quantity. 2. relating to the proportionate quantities or to the amount of the constituents of a compound.

quan·tum (kwon′tum) pl. *quan′ta.* [L.] a unit of measure under the quantum theory (q.v.).

quar·an·tine (kwor′an-tēn, kwahr′an-tēn) 1. restriction of freedom of movement of apparently well individuals who have been exposed to infectious disease, which is imposed for the maximal incubation period of the disease. 2. a period of detention for vessels, vehicles, or travelers coming from infected or suspected ports or places. 3. the place where persons are detained for inspection. 4. to detain or isolate on account of suspected contagion.

quart (kwort) one fourth of a gallon; in the United States it is 0.946 liter and in Great Britain (*imperial quart*) it is 1.14 liters.

quar·tan (kwor′tan) recurring in four-day cycles.

quartz (kworts) a crystalline form of silica (silicon dioxide).

qua·ter·nary (kwah′ter-nar″e) 1. fourth in order. 2. containing four elements or groups.

qua·ze·pam (kwah′zĕ-pam) a benzodiazepine used as a sedative and hypnotic in the treatment of insomnia.

quench·ing (kwench′ing) 1. suppressing or diminishing a physical property, as of heat

724

radical that carries an unpaired electron; such radicals are extremely reactive, with a very short half-life.

rad·i·cle (rad′ĭ-k′l) ramulus; one of the smallest branches of a vessel or nerve.

rad·i·cot·o·my (rad″ĭ-kot′ah-me) rhizotomy.

ra·dic·u·lal·gia (rah-dik″u-lal′jah) pain due to disorder of the spinal nerve roots.

ra·dic·u·lar (rah-dik′u-lar) of or pertaining to a root or radicle.

ra·dic·u·li·tis (rah-dik″u-li′tis) inflammation of the spinal nerve roots.

ra·dic·u·lo·gan·gli·o·ni·tis (rah-dik″u-lo-gang″gle o-ni′tis) inflammation of the posterior spinal nerve roots and their ganglia.

ra·dic·u·lo·me·nin·go·my·eli·tis (-mĕ-ning″go-mi″ĕ-li′tis) meningomyeloradiculitis.

ra·dic·u·lo·neu·ri·tis (-noo-ri′tis) acute idiopathic polyneuritis.

ra·dic·u·lo·neu·rop·a·thy (-noo-rop′ah-the) disease of the nerve roots and spinal nerves.

ra·dic·u·lop·a·thy (rah-dik″u-lop′ah-the) disease of the nerve roots. **spondylotic cau·dal r.**, compression of the cauda equina due to encroachment upon a congenitally small spinal canal by spondylosis, resulting in neural disorders of the lower limbs.

radi(o)- word element [L.], *ray; radiation; emission of radiant energy; radium; radius* (bone of the forearm); affixed to the name of a chemical element to designate a radioactive isotope of that element.

ra·dio·ac·tiv·i·ty (ra″de-o-ak-tiv′ĭ-te) emission of corpuscular or electromagnetic radiations consequent to nuclear disintegration; it is a natural property of all chemical elements of atomic number above 83 and can be induced in all other known elements. **radio·ac′tive**, adj. **artificial r.**, **induced r.**, that produced by bombarding an element with high-velocity particles.

ra·dio·al·ler·go·sor·bent (-al″er-go-sor′bent) denoting a radioimmunoassay technique for the measurement of specific IgE antibody to a variety of allergens.

ra·dio·bi·cip·i·tal (-bi-sip′ĭ-tal) pertaining to the radius and the biceps muscle.

ra·dio·bi·ol·o·gy (-bi-ol′ah-je) the branch of science concerned with effects of light and of ultraviolet and ionizing radiations on living tissue or organisms. **radiobiolog′ical**, adj.

ra·dio·car·di·og·ra·phy (-kahr″de-og′rah-fe) graphic recording of variation with time of the concentration, in a selected chamber of the heart, of a radioactive isotope, usually injected intravenously.

ra·dio·car·pal (-kahr′p′l) pertaining to the radius and carpus.

ra·dio·chem·is·try (-kem′is-tre) the branch of chemistry dealing with radioactive materials.

ra·dio·col·loids (ra″de-o-kol′oidz) radioisotopes in pure form in solution; they often behave more like colloids than solutes.

ra·dio·cys·ti·tis (-sis-ti′tis) radiation cystitis.

ra·dio·den·si·ty (-den′sĭ-te) radiopacity.

ra·dio·der·ma·ti·tis (-der″mah-ti′tis) a cutaneous inflammatory reaction to exposure to biologically effective levels of ionizing radiation.

ra·dio·di·ag·no·sis (-di″ag-no′sis) diagnosis by means of x-rays and radiographs.

ra·di·odon·tics (-don′tiks) dental radiology.

ra·di·odon·tist (-don′tist) a dentist who specializes in dental radiology.

ra·dio·gold (ra′de-o-gold″) one of the radioactive isotopes of gold, particularly [198]Au; see *gold 198*.

ra·dio·gram (-gram″) radiograph.

ra·dio·graph (-graf″) the film produced by radiography.

ra·di·og·ra·phy (ra″de-og′rah-fe) the making of film records (radiographs) of internal structures of the body by passing x-rays or gamma rays through the body to act on specially sensitized film. **radiograph′ic**, adj. **body section r.**, tomography. **digital r.**, a technique in which x-ray absorption is quantified by assignment of a number to the amount of x-rays reaching the detector; the information is manipulated by a computer to produce an optimal image. **electron r.**, a technique in which a latent electron image is produced on clear plastic by passing x-ray photons through a gas with a high atomic number; this image is then developed into a black-and-white picture. **mucosal relief r.**, radiography of the mucosa of the gastrointestinal tract in a double-contrast examination. **neutron r.**, that in which a narrow beam of neutrons from a nuclear reactor is passed through tissues, especially useful in visualizing bony tissues. **serial r.**, the making of several exposures of a particular area at arbitrary intervals. **spot-film r.**, the making of localized instantaneous radiographic exposures during fluoroscopy.

ra·dio·hu·mer·al (ra″de-o-hu′mer-al) pertaining to the radius and humerus.

ra·dio·im·mu·ni·ty (-ĭ-mu′nĭ-te) diminished sensitivity to radiation.

ra·dio·im·mu·no·as·say (-im″u-no-as′a) a highly sensitive and specific assay method that uses the competition between radiolabeled and unlabeled substances in an antigen-antibody reaction to determine the concentration of the unlabeled substance, which may be an antibody or a substance against which specific antibodies can be produced.

ra·dio·im·mu·no·dif·fu·sion (-dĭ-fu′zhun) immunodiffusion conducted with radioisotope-labeled antibodies or antigens.

ra·dio·im·mu·no·scin·tig·ra·phy (-sin-tig′rah-fe) immunoscintigraphy.

ra·dio·im·mu·no·sor·bent (-sor′bent) denoting a radioimmunoassay technique for measuring IgE in samples of serum.

ra·dio·io·dine (-i′o-dīn) any radioactive isotope of iodine, particularly ^{123}I, ^{125}I, and ^{131}I; used in diagnosis and treatment of thyroid disease and in scintiscanning.

ra·dio·iso·tope (-i′so-tōp) a radioactive isotope; one having an unstable nucleus and emitting characteristic radiation during its decay to a stable form.

ra·dio·la·bel (ra′de-o-la″b′l) 1. radioactive label. 2. to incorporate such a radioactive label into a compound.

ra·dio·li·gand (-li′gand) a radioisotope-labeled substance, e.g., an antigen, used in the quantitative measurement of an unlabeled substance by its binding reaction to a specific antibody or other receptor site.

ra·di·ol·o·gist (ra″de-ol′ah-jist) a physician specializing in radiology.

ra·di·ol·o·gy (ra″de-ol′ah-je) that branch of the health sciences dealing with radioactive substances and radiant energy and with the diagnosis and treatment of disease by means of both ionizing (e.g., x-rays) and nonionizing (e.g., ultrasound) radiation. **radiolog′ic, radiolog′ical,** adj.

ra·dio·lu·cent (ra″de-o-loo′sent) permitting the passage of radiant energy, such as x-rays, with little attenuation, the representative areas appearing dark on the exposed film.

ra·di·om·e·ter (ra″de-om′ĕ-ter) an instrument for detecting and measuring radiant energy.

ra·dio·ne·cro·sis (ra″de-o-nĕ-kro′sis) tissue destruction due to radiant energy.

ra·dio·neu·ri·tis (-noo-ri′tis) neuritis from exposure to radiant energy.

ra·dio·nu·clide (-noo′klīd) a nuclide that disintegrates with the emission of corpuscular or electromagnetic radiations.

ra·di·opac·i·ty (-pas′ĭ-te) the quality or property of obstructing the passage of radiant energy, such as x-rays, the representative areas appearing light or white on the exposed film. **radiopaque′,** adj.

ra·dio·pa·thol·o·gy (-pah-thol′ah-je) the pathology of the effects of radiation on tissues.

ra·dio·phar·ma·ceu·ti·cal (-fahr″mah-soo′tĭ-k′l) a radioactive pharmaceutical, nuclide, or other chemical used for diagnostic or therapeutic purposes.

ra·dio·pro·tec·tor (-pro-tek′ter) an agent that provides protection against the toxic effects of ionizing radiation.

ra·dio·re·cep·tor (-re-sep′ter) 1. a receptor for the stimuli that are excited by radiant energy, such as light or heat. 2. a receptor to which a radioligand can bind.

ra·dio·re·sis·tance (-re-zis′tins) resistance, as of tissue or cells, to irradiation. **radio-resist′ant,** adj.

ra·di·os·co·py (ra″de-os′kah-pe) fluoroscopy.

ra·dio·sen·si·tiv·i·ty (ra″de-o-sen″sĭ-tiv′ĭ-te) sensitivity, as of the skin, tumor tissue, etc., to radiant energy, such as x-rays or other radiation. **radiosen′sitive,** adj.

ra·dio·sur·gery (-ser′jer-e) surgery in which tissue destruction is performed by means of ionizing radiation rather than by surgical incision. **stereotactic r., stereotaxic r.,** stereotactic surgery in which lesions are produced by ionizing radiation.

ra·dio·ther·a·py (-ther′ah-pe) treatment of disease by means of ionizing radiation; tissue may be exposed to a beam of radiation, or a radioactive element may be contained in devices (e.g., needles or wire) and inserted directly into the tissues *(interstitial r.)*, or it may be introduced into a natural body cavity *(intracavitary r.)*.

ra·dio·tox·emia (-tok-se′me-ah) toxemia produced by radiant energy.

ra·dio·tra·cer (-tra′ser) radioactive tracer.

ra·dio·trans·par·ent (-trans-par′ent) radiolucent.

ra·di·o·trop·ic (-tro′pik) influenced by radiation.

ra·dio·ul·nar (-ul′ner) pertaining to the radius and ulna.

ra·di·um (ra′de-um) a radioactive element (see *Table of Elements*), at. no. 88, symbol Ra; it has a half-life of 1622 years, emitting alpha, beta, and gamma radiation. It decays to radon.

ra·di·us (ra′de-us) pl. *ra′dii*. [L.] 1. a line from the center of a circle to a point on its circumference. 2. see *Table of Bones*. **r. fix′us,** a straight line from the hormion to the inion.

ra·dix (ra′diks) pl. *ra′dices*. [L.] root.

ra·don (ra′don) a gaseous radioactive element (see *Table of Elements*), at. no. 86, symbol Rn, resulting from decay of radium.

rage (rāj) a state of violent anger. **sham r.,** a state resembling rage occurring in decorticated animals or in certain pathologic conditions in humans.

rag·o·cyte (rag′o-sīt) a polymorphonuclear phagocyte, found in the joints in rheumatoid arthritis, with cytoplasmic inclusions of aggregated IgG, rheumatoid factor, fibrin, and complement.

ra·jas (rah-jus′) [Sanskrit] according to ayurveda, one of the three gunas, characterized by activity, stimulation, and movement.

rale (rahl) crackle; a discontinuous sound consisting of a series of short sounds, heard during inhalation. **amphoric r.,** a coarse musical rale due to splashing of fluid in a cavity connected with a bronchus. **clicking r.,** a small sound heard when inhaled air passes through secretions in smaller bronchi. **crackling r.,** subcrepitant r. **crepitant r.,** a sound like that made by rubbing hairs between the fingers, heard at the end of inhalation. **dry r.,** a fine sound heard in interstitial lung diseases such as idiopathic pulmonary fibrosis. **moist r.,** a sound heard over fluid in the bronchial tubes. **subcrepitant r.,** a fine moist rale heard over liquid in the smaller tubes.

ral·ox·i·fene (ral-ok′sĭ-fēn) a selective activator of estrogen receptors that increases bone mineral density and decreases total and LDL cholesterol without affecting breast and uterine tissue; used as the hydrochloride salt for the prevention of postmenopausal osteoporosis.

ra·mal (ra′m′l) pertaining to a ramus.

ram·i·fi·ca·tion (ram″ĭ-fĭ-ka′shun) 1. distribution in branches. 2. a branching.

ram·i·fy (ram′ĭ-fī) 1. to branch; to diverge in different directions. 2. to traverse in branches.

ra·mi·pril (rah-mi′pril) an angiotensin-converting enzyme inhibitor used in treatment of hypertension and congestive heart failure and the prevention of a major cardiovascular event in high-risk patients.

rami·sec·tion (ram″ĭ-sek′shun) section of one or more rami communicantes of the sympathetic nervous system.

ram·itis (ram-i′tis) inflammation of a ramus.

ra·mose (ra′mos) branching; having many branches.

ra·mu·lus (ram′u-lus) pl. *ra′muli.* [L.] radicle.

ra·mus (ra′mus) pl. *ra′mi.* [L.] a branch, as of a nerve, vein, or artery. **r. articula′ris,** a branch of a mixed (afferent or efferent) peripheral nerve supplying a joint and its associated structures. **r. autono′micus,** any of the branches of the parasympathetic or sympathetic nerves of the autonomic nervous system. **r. commu′nicans,** a branch connecting two nerves or two arteries. **r. cuta′neus,** a branch of a mixed (afferent or efferent) peripheral nerve innervating a region of the skin.

ran·dom (ran′dom) pertaining to a chance-dependent process, particularly one that occurs according to a known probability distribution.

range (rānj) 1. the difference between the upper and lower limits of a variable or of a series of values. 2. an interval in which values sampled from a population, or the values in the population itself, are known to lie. **r. of motion,** the range, measured in degrees of a circle, through which a joint can be extended and flexed.

ra·nine (ra′nīn) 1. pertaining to a frog. 2. ranular. 3. sublingual.

ra·ni·ti·dine (rah-nĭ′tĭ-dēn) a histamine H_2 receptor antagonist, used as the hydrochloride salt to inhibit gastric acid secretion in the treatment of gastric and duodenal ulcer, gastroesophageal reflux disease, and conditions that cause gastric hypersecretion.

ran·u·la (ran′u-lah) a cystic tumor beneath the tongue. **ran′ular,** adj. **pancreatic r.,** a retention cyst of the pancreatic duct.

rape (rāp) nonconsensual sexual penetration of an individual, obtained by force or threat, or in cases in which the victim is not capable of consent.

ra·phe (ra′fe) pl. *ra′phae.* A seam; the line of union of the halves of various symmetrical parts. **r. of penis,** a narrow dark streak or ridge continuous posteriorly with the raphe of scrotum and extending forward along the midline on the underside of the penis. **perineal r.,** a ridge along the median line of the perineum that runs forward from the anus; in the male, it is continuous with the raphe of scrotum. **r. of scrotum,** a ridge along the surface of the scrotum in the median line, continuous with the perineal raphe and the raphe of penis.

rap·port (rah-por′) a relation of harmony and accord, as between patient and physician.

rar·e·fac·tion (rar″ĭ-fak′shun) condition of being or becoming less dense.

ra·sa·ya·na (rah″sah-yah′nah) any of a group of herbal remedies with antioxidant properties used in ayurveda to promote health, provide defense against disease, and promote longevity.

rash (rash) a temporary eruption on the skin. **butterfly r.,** a skin eruption across the nose and adjacent areas of the cheeks in the pattern of a butterfly, as in lupus erythematosus and seborrheic dermatitis. **diaper r.**, irritant dermatitis in infants on the areas covered by the diaper, usually due to soiling or fungal contamination. **drug r.**, see under *eruption*. **heat r.**, miliaria rubra.

rasp (rasp) 1. raspatory; a coarse file used in surgery.   2. to file with a rasp.

ras·pa·to·ry (ras'pah-tor-e) rasp (1).

RAST radioallergosorbent test.

rate (rāt) the speed or frequency with which an event or circumstance occurs per unit of time, population, or other standard of comparison. **basal metabolic r.**, an expression of the rate at which oxygen is used by body cells, or the calculated equivalent heat production by the body, in a fasting subject at complete rest. Abbreviated BMR. **birth r.**, the number of births in a specified area during a defined period for the total population, often further qualified as to which portion of the population is being examined. **case fatality r.**, the ratio of the number of deaths caused by a specified disease to the number of diagnosed cases of that disease. **circulation r.**, the amount of blood pumped through the body by the heart per unit time. **death r.**, an expression of the number of deaths in a population at risk during one year. The *crude death r.* is the ratio of the number of deaths to the total population of an area; the *age-specific death r.* is the ratio of the number of deaths in a specific age group to the number of persons in that age group; the *cause-specific death r.* is the ratio of the number of deaths due to a specified cause to the total population. **dose r.**, the amount of any agent administered per unit of time. **erythrocyte sedimentation r. (ESR)**, the rate at which erythrocytes sediment from a well-mixed specimen of venous blood, as measured by the distance that the top of a column of erythrocytes falls in a specified time interval under specified conditions. **fatality r.**, case fatality r. **fertility r.**, a measure of fertility in a specified population over a specified period of time, particularly the *general fertility r.*, the number of live births in a geographic area in a year per 1000 women of childbearing age. **fetal death r.**, the ratio of the number of fetal deaths in one year to the total number of both live births and fetal deaths in that year. **five-year survival r.**, an expression of the number of survivors with no trace of disease five years after each has been diagnosed or treated for the same disease. **glomerular filtration r. (GFR)**, an expression of the quantity of glomerular filtrate formed each minute in the nephrons of both kidneys, usually measured by the rate of clearance of creatinine. **growth r.**, an expression of the increase in size of an organic object per unit of time. **heart r.**, the number of contractions of the cardiac ventricles per unit of time. **incidence r.**, the probability of developing a particular disease during a given period of time; the numerator is the number of new cases during the specified time period and the denominator is the population at risk during the period. **morbidity r.**, an inexact term that can mean either the *incidence rate* or the *prevalence rate*. **mortality r.**, death r. **prevalence r.**, the number of people in a population who have a disease at a given time: the numerator is the number of existing cases of disease at a specified time and the denominator is the total population. **pulse r.**, the number of pulsations noted in a peripheral artery per unit of time. **respiration r.**, the number of movements of the chest wall per unit of time, indicative of inhalation and exhalation. **sedimentation r.**, the rate at which a sediment is deposited in a given volume of solution, especially when subjected to the action of a centrifuge. **stillbirth r.**, fetal death r.

ra·tio (ra'she-o) [L.] an expression of the quantity of one substance or entity in relation to that of another; the relationship between two quantities expressed as the quotient of one divided by the other. **A-G r., albuminglobulin r.**, the ratio of albumin to globulin in blood serum, plasma, or urine in various renal diseases. **cardiothoracic r.**, on a radiograph, the ratio of the transverse diameter of the heart to the internal diameter of the chest at its widest point just above the dome of the diaphragm. **lecithin/sphingomyelin r., L/S r.**, the ratio of lecithin to sphingomyelin concentration in the amniotic fluid, used to predict the degree of pulmonary maturity of the fetus and thus the risk of respiratory distress syndrome (RDS) if the fetus is delivered prematurely. **sex r.**, the proportion of one sex to another, traditionally the number of males in a population per number of females. **ventilation-perfusion r.**, the ratio of oxygen received in the pulmonary alveoli to the flow of blood through the alveolar capillaries.

ra·tion·al (ra'shun-al) based upon reason; characterized by possession of one's reason.

ra·tion·al·iza·tion (ra"shun-al-ĭ-za'shun) an unconscious defense mechanism by which one justifies attitudes and behavior that would otherwise be unacceptable.

rat·tle·snake (rat''l-snāk) any of the New World pit vipers of the genera *Crotalus* and *Sistrurus,* having a series of cornified interlocking segments at the tip of the tail; when disturbed they vibrate the tail to produce the characteristic rattling or buzzing sound. Included are the massasauga, the *eastern diamondback r.* (*C. adamanteus*), the *Mojave r.* (*C. scutulatus scutulatus*), the *prairie r.* (*C. viridis viridis*), the *pygmy r.* (*S. miliarius*), the *timber r.* (*C. horridus*), and the *western diamondback r.* (*C. atrox*).

Rau·wol·fia (rou-wool′fe-ah) a genus of tropical trees and shrubs, including *R. serpentina* and over 100 other species, that provide numerous alkaloids, notably reserpine, of medical interest.

rau·wol·fia 1. any member of the genus *Rauwolfia.* 2. the dried root of *Rauwolfia,* or an extract of it. **r. serpenti′na,** the dried root of *Rauwolfia serpentina;* used as an antihypertensive; also used in folk medicine and Indian medicine.

RAV Rous-associated virus.

ray (ra) 1. a line emanating from a center. 2. a more or less distinct portion of radiant energy (light or heat), proceeding in a specific direction. **α-r's, alpha r's,** high-speed helium nuclei ejected from radioactive substances; they have less penetrating power than beta rays. **β-r's, beta r's,** electrons ejected from radioactive substances with velocities as high as 0.98 of the velocity of light; they have more penetrating power than alpha rays, but less than gamma rays. **digital r.,** 1. a digit of the hand or foot and the corresponding portion of the metacarpus or metatarsus, considered as a continuous structural unit. 2. in the embryo, a mesenchymal condensation of the hand or foot plate that outlines the pattern of a future digit. **γ-r's, gamma r's,** electromagnetic radiation of short wavelengths emitted by an atomic nucleus during a nuclear reaction, consisting of high-energy photons, having no mass and no electric charge, and traveling with the speed of light and with great penetrating power. **grenz r's,** very soft x-rays having wavelengths about 20 nm, lying between x-rays and ultraviolet rays. **medullary r's,** the intracortical prolongations of the renal pyramids. **roentgen r's,** x-r's. **x-r's,** electromagnetic vibrations of short wavelengths (approximately 0.01 to 10 nm) or corresponding quanta that are produced when electrons moving at high velocity impinge on various substances; they are commonly generated by passing high-voltage current (approximately 10,000 volts) through a Coolidge tube. They are able to penetrate most substances to some extent, to affect a photographic plate, to cause certain substances to fluoresce, and to strongly ionize tissue.

Rb rubidium.

RBBB right bundle branch block; see *bundle branch block,* under *block.*

RBC red blood cell.

RBE relative biological effectiveness.

Re rhenium.

re- word element [L.], *back; again; contrary,* etc.

re·ab·sorp·tion (re″ab-sorp′shun) 1. the act or process of absorbing again, as the absorption by the kidneys of substances (glucose, proteins, sodium, etc.) already secreted into the renal tubules. 2. resorption.

re·ac·tant (re-ak′tant) a substance entering into a chemical reaction.

re·ac·tion (-ak′shun) 1. opposite action, or counterreaction; the response to stimuli. 2. a phenomenon caused by the action of chemical agents; a chemical process in which one substance is transformed into another substance or other substances. 3. the mental and/or emotional state that develops in any particular situation. **acrosome r.,** structural changes and liberation of acrosomal enzymes occurring in spermatozoa in the vicinity of an oocyte, facilitating entry into the oocyte. **alarm r.,** the physiologic effects (increase in blood pressure, cardiac output, blood flow to skeletal muscles, rate of glycolysis, and blood glucose concentration; decrease in blood flow to viscera) mediated by sympathetic nervous system discharge and release of adrenal medullary hormones in response to stress, fright, or rage. **allergic r.,** hypersensitivity r., sometimes specifically a type I hypersensitivity reaction. **anaphylactic r.,** anaphylaxis. **anaphylactoid r.,** one resembling generalized anaphylaxis but not caused by IgE-mediated allergic reaction. **antibody-mediated hypersensitivity r.,** 1. type II hypersensitivity r.; see *Gell and Coombs classification,* under *classification.* 2. occasionally, any hypersensitivity reaction in which antibodies are the primary mediators, i.e., types I–III. **antigen-antibody r.,** the reversible binding of antigen to homologous antibody by the formation of weak bonds between antigenic determinants on antigen molecules and antigen binding sites on immunoglobulin molecules. **anxiety r.,** a reaction characterized by abnormal apprehension or uneasiness; see also *anxiety disorders,* under *disorder.* **Arias-Stella r.,** nuclear and cellular hypertrophy of the endometrial epithelium, associated with ectopic pregnancy.

cell-mediated hypersensitivity r., type IV hypersensitivity r.; see *Gell and Coombs classification,* under *classification.* **conversion r.,** see under *disorder.* **cross r.,** the interaction of an antigen with an antibody formed against a different antigen with which the first antigen shares identical or closely related antigenic determinants. **cytotoxic hypersensitivity r.,** type II hypersensitivity r.; see *Gell and Coombs classification,* under *classification.* **defense r.,** see under *mechanism.* **delayed hypersensitivity r., delayed-type hypersensitivity r.,** that taking 24 to 72 hours to develop and mediated by T lymphocytes rather than by antibodies; usually denoting the subset of type IV hypersensitivity reactions involving cytokine release and macrophage activation, as opposed to direct cytolysis, but sometimes used more broadly, even as a synonym of *type IV hypersensitivity r.* (see *Gell and Coombs classification,* under *classification*). **r. of degeneration,** the reaction to electrical stimulation of muscles whose nerves have degenerated, consisting of loss of response to a faradic stimulation in a muscle, and to galvanic and faradic stimulation in the nerve. **foreign body r.,** a granulomatous inflammatory reaction evoked by the presence of exogenous material in the tissues, characterized by the formation of foreign body giant cells. **hemiopic pupillary r.,** in certain cases of hemianopia, light thrown upon one side of the retina causes the iris to contract, while light thrown upon the other side arouses no response. **Herxheimer's r.,** Jarisch-Herxheimer r. **hypersensitivity r.,** one in which the body mounts an exaggerated or inappropriate immune response to a substance perceived as foreign, resulting in local or general tissue damage. Such reactions are usually classified as *types I–IV* on the basis of the Gell and Coombs classification (q.v.). **id r.,** a secondary skin eruption occurring in sensitized patients as a result of circulation of allergenic products from a primary site of infection. **immediate hypersensitivity r.,** 1. type I hypersensitivity r.; see *Gell and Coombs classification,* under *classification.* 2. occasionally, any hypersensitivity reaction mediated by antibodies and developing rapidly, generally in minutes to hours (i.e., *types I–III*), as distinguished from those mediated by T lymphocytes and macrophages and requiring days to develop (*type IV,* or *delayed hypersensitivity r.*). **immune r.,** see under *response.* **immune complex–mediated hypersensitivity r.,** type III hypersensitivity r.; see *Gell and Coombs classification,* under *classification.*

Jarisch-Herxheimer r., a transient immunologic reaction following antibiotic treatment of early and later stages of syphilis and certain other diseases, marked by fever, chills, headache, myalgia, and exacerbation of cutaneous lesions; due to release of toxic or antigenic substances by the infecting microorganisms. **Jones-Mote r.,** a mild skin reaction of the delayed (type IV) hypersensitivity type occurring after challenge with protein antigens. **late phase r.,** an IgE-mediated immune reaction occurring 5 to 8 hours after exposure to antigen, after the wheal and flare reactions of immediate hypersensitivity have diminished, with inflammation peaking around 24 hours, and then subsiding. **lengthening r.,** reflex elongation of the extensor muscles which permits flexion of a limb. **leukemoid r.,** a peripheral blood picture resembling that of leukemia or indistinguishable from it on the basis of morphologic appearance alone; seen in certain infectious diseases, inflammatory conditions, and intoxications. **Neufeld's r.,** swelling of the capsules of pneumococci, seen under the microscope, on mixture with specific immune serum, owing to the binding of antibody with the capsular polysaccharide. **oxidation-reduction r.,** redox r. **Pirquet r.,** appearance of a papule with a red areola 24 to 48 hours after introduction of two small drops of Old tuberculin by slight scarification of the skin; a positive test indicates previous infection. **polymerase chain r. (PCR),** a rapid technique for in vitro amplification of specific DNA or RNA sequences, allowing small quantities of short sequences to be analyzed without cloning. **precipitin r.,** the formation of an insoluble precipitate by reaction of antigen and antibody. **redox r.,** a reaction oxidizing one substrate while reducing another. **Schultz-Charlton r.,** disappearance of scarlet fever rash around the site of an injection of scarlet fever antitoxin. **serum r.,** seroreaction. **startle r.,** the various psychophysiological phenomena, including involuntary motor and autonomic reactions, evidenced by an individual in reaction to a sudden, unexpected stimulus, as a loud noise. **stress r.,** any physiological or psychological reaction to physical, mental, or emotional stress that disturbs the organism's homeostasis. **T cell–mediated hypersensitivity r.,** type IV hypersensitivity r.; see *Gell and Coombs classification,* under *classification.* **Weil-Felix r.,** agglutination by blood serum of typhus patients of a bacillus of the proteus group from the urine and feces. **Wernicke's r.,** hemiopic pupillary r. **wheal**

and erythema r., wheal and flare r., a cutaneous sensitivity reaction to skin injury or administration of antigen, due to histamine production and marked by edematous elevation and erythematous flare.

re·ac·tion-for·ma·tion (-for-ma'shun) an unconscious defense mechanism in which a person assumes an attitude that is the reverse of the wish or impulse actually harbored.

re·ac·tive (re-ak'tiv) characterized by reaction; readily responsive to a stimulus.

read·ing (rēd'ing) understanding of written or printed symbols representing words. **lip r., speech r.,** understanding of speech through observation of the speaker's lip movements.

re·a·gent (re-a'jent) a substance used to produce a chemical reaction so as to detect, measure, produce, etc., other substances.

re·a·gin (re'ah-jin) the antibody that mediates immediate hypersensitivity reactions; in humans, IgE. **reagin'ic,** adj.

ream·er (rēm'er) an instrument used in dentistry for enlarging root canals.

re·can·a·li·za·tion (re-kan″ah-lĭ-za'shun) formation of new canals or paths, especially blood vessels, through an obstruction such as a clot.

re·cep·tac·u·lum (re″sep-tak'u-lum) pl. *receptac'ula.* [L.] a vessel or receptacle. **r. chy'li,** cisterna chyli.

re·cep·tive (re-cep'tiv) capable of receiving or of responding to a stimulus.

re·cep·tor (-ter) 1. a molecule on the surface or within a cell that recognizes and binds with specific molecules, producing a specific effect in the cell; e.g., the cell-surface receptors for antigens or cytoplasmic receptors for steroid hormones. 2. a sensory nerve ending that responds to various stimuli. **α-adrenergic r's,** adrenergic receptors that respond to norepinephrine and to such blocking agents as phenoxybenzamine. They are subdivided into two types: α_1, found in smooth muscle, heart, and liver, with effects including vasoconstriction, intestinal relaxation, uterine contraction and pupillary dilation, and α_2, found in platelets, vascular smooth muscle, nerve termini, and pancreatic islets, with effects including platelet aggregation, vasoconstriction, and inhibition of norepinephrine release and of insulin secretion. **adrenergic r's,** receptors for epinephrine or norepinephrine, such as those on effector organs innervated by postganglionic adrenergic fibers of the sympathetic nervous system. Classified as *α-adrenergic r's* and *β-adrenergic r's.* **alpha-adrenergic r's,** α-adrenergic r's. **β-adrenergic r's,**

beta-adrenergic r's, adrenergic receptors that respond particularly to epinephrine and to such blocking agents as propranolol. They are subdivided into two basic types: β_1, in myocardium and causing lipolysis and cardiac stimulation, and β_2, in smooth and skeletal muscle and liver and causing bronchodilation and vasodilation. The atypical type β_3 may be involved in lipolysis regulation in adipose tissue. **cholinergic r's,** cell-surface receptor molecules that bind the neurotransmitter acetylcholine and mediate its action on postjunctional cells. **complement r's,** cell-surface receptors for products of complement reactions, playing roles including recognition of pathogens, phagocytosis, adhesion, and clearance of immune complexes. The best characterized are C1–C4, which bind C3 fragments already bound to a surface. **cutaneous r.,** any of the various types of sense organs found in the dermis or epidermis, usually a mechanoreceptor, thermoreceptor, or nociceptor. **cytokine r's,** membrane-spanning proteins that bind cytokines via extracellular domains, acting to convert an extracellular signal to an intracellular one. **H_1 r's, H_2 r's,** see *histamine.* **joint r.,** any of several mechanoreceptors that occur in joint capsules and respond to deep pressure and to other stimuli such as stress or change in position. **muscarinic r's,** cholinergic receptors that are stimulated by the alkaloid muscarine and blocked by atropine; they are found on automatic effector cells and on central neurons in the thalamus and cerebral cortex. **muscle r.,** a mechanoreceptor found in a muscle or tendon. **nicotinic r's,** cholinergic receptors that are stimulated initially and blocked at high doses by the alkaloid nicotine and blocked by tubocurarine; they are found on automatic ganglion cells, on striated muscle cells, and on spinal central neurons. **nonadapting r.,** a mechanoreceptor, such as a nociceptor, that responds to stimulation with a continual steady discharge and little or no accommodation over time. **olfactory r.,** a chemoreceptor in the nasal epithelium that is sensitive to stimulation, giving rise to the sensation of odors. **opiate r., opioid r.,** any of a number of receptors for opiates and opioids, grouped into at least seven types on the basis of their substrates and physiological effects. **orphan r.,** a protein identified as a putative receptor on the basis of its structure but without identification of possible ligands or evidence of function. **pain r.,** nociceptor. **rapidly adapting r.,** a mechanoreceptor that responds quickly to stimulation but that rapidly accommodates and stops firing if the stimulus remains constant. **sensory r.,** receptor (2). **slowly adapting r.,** a mechanoreceptor that responds slowly to stimulation and continues firing as long as the stimulus continues. **stretch r.,** a sense organ in a muscle or tendon that responds to elongation. **tactile r.,** a mechanoreceptor for the sense of touch. **thermal r.,** thermoreceptor.

re·cess (re'ses) a small empty space, hollow, or cavity. **epitympanic r.,** attic or epitympanum; the upper part of the tympanic cavity, above the level of the tympanic membrane, containing part of the incus and malleus. **infundibuliform r.,** pharyngeal r. **laryngopharyngeal r.,** piriform r. **pharyngeal r.,** a wide, slitlike lateral extension in the wall of the nasopharynx, cranial and dorsal to the pharyngeal orifice of the auditory tube. **piriform r.,** a pear-shaped fossa in the wall of the laryngeal pharynx. **pleural r's,** the spaces where the different portions of the pleura join at an angle and which are never completely filled by lung tissue. **r. of Rosenmüller,** pharyngeal r. **sphenoethmoidal r.,** the most superior and posterior part of the nasal cavity, above the superior nasal concha, into which the sphenoidal sinus opens. **subpopliteal r.,** a prolongation of the synovial tendon sheath of the popliteus muscle outside the knee joint into the popliteal space. **superior r. of tympanic membrane,** Prussak's pouch. **utricular r.,** utricle (2).

re·ces·sive (re-ses'iv) 1. tending to recede; in genetics, incapable of expression unless the responsible allele is carried by both members of a pair of homologous chromosomes. 2. a recessive allele or trait.

re·ces·sus (re-ses'us) pl. *reces'sus.* [L.] a recess.

re·cid·i·va·tion (re-sid″ĭ-va'shun) relapse, recurrence, or repetition, as of a disease or condition or of a pattern of behavior, particularly a criminal act.

re·cid·i·vism (re-sid'ĭ-vizm) a tendency to relapse, particularly a return to criminal behavior.

rec·i·pe (res'ĭ-pe) [L.] 1. take; used at the head of a prescription, indicated by the symbol ℞. 2. a formula for the preparation of a specific combination of ingredients.

re·cip·i·ent (re-sip'e-ent) one who receives, as a blood transfusion, or a tissue or organ graft. **universal r.,** a person thought to be able to receive blood of any "type" without agglutination of the donor cells.

re·cip·ro·cal (re-sip'ro-k'l″) 1. being equivalent or complementary. 2. inversely related; opposing.

re·cip·ro·ca·tion (re-sip″ro-ka'shun) 1. the act of giving and receiving in exchange; the complementary interaction of two distinct entities. 2. an alternating back-and-forth movement.

re·cog·ni·tion (rek″og-ni'shun) in immunology, the interaction of immunologically competent cells with antigen, involving antigen binding to a specific receptor on the cell surface and resulting in an immune response.

re·coil (re'koil) a quick pulling back. **elastic r.,** the ability of a stretched object or organ, such as the bladder, to return to its resting position.

re·com·bi·nant (re-kom'bĭ-nant) 1. the new entity (e.g., gene, protein, cell, individual) that results from genetic recombination. 2. pertaining or relating to such an entity. See also under *DNA.*

re·com·bi·na·tion (re″kom-bĭ-na'shun) 1. the reunion, in the same or different arrangement, of formerly united elements that have been separated. 2. in genetics, the process that creates new combinations of genes by shuffling the linear order of the DNA.

re·com·pres·sion (-kom-presh'un) return to normal environmental pressure after exposure to greatly diminished pressure.

re·con·struc·tion (-kon-struk'shun) 1. the reassembling or re-forming of something from constituent parts. 2. surgical restoration of function of a body part.

rec·ord (rek'erd) 1. a permanent or long-lasting account of something (as on film, in writing, etc.). 2. in dentistry, a registration. **problem-oriented r. (POR),** a method of patient care record keeping that focuses on specific health care problems and a cooperative health care plan designed to cope with the identified problems. The components of the POR are: *data base,* which contains information required for each patient regardless of diagnosis or presenting problems; *problem list,* which contains the major problems currently needing attention; *plan,* which specifies what is to be done with regard to each problem; *progress notes,* which document the observations, assessments, nursing care plans, physician's orders, etc., of all health care personnel directly involved in the care of the patient. See also *SOAP.*

rec·re·ment (rek'rĭ-ment) saliva, or other secretion, which is reabsorbed into the blood. **recrementi'tious,** adj.

re·cru·des·cence (re″kroo-des′ens) recurrence of symptoms after temporary abatement. **recrudes′cent**, adj.

re·cruit·ment (re-kroot′ment) 1. the gradual increase to a maximum in a reflex when a stimulus of unaltered intensity is prolonged. 2. in audiology, an abnormally rapid increase in the loudness of a sound caused by a slight increase in its intensity. 3. the orderly increase in number of activated motor units with increasing strength of voluntary muscle contractions. 4. the process by which certain primordial ovarian follicles begin growing in a particular menstrual cycle.

rec·tal (rek′tal) pertaining to the rectum.

rec·tal·gia (rek-tal′jah) proctalgia.

rec·tec·to·my (rek-tek′tah-me) proctectomy.

rec·ti·fi·ca·tion (rek″tǐ-fǐ-ka′shun) 1. the act of making straight, pure, or correct. 2. redistillation of a liquid to purify it.

rec·ti·tis (rek-ti′tis) proctitis.

rect(o)- word element [L.], *rectum*. See also words beginning *proct(o)-*.

rec·to·ab·dom·i·nal (rek″to-ab-dom′ǐ-n′l) pertaining to the rectum and abdomen.

rec·to·cele (rek′to-sēl) hernial protrusion of part of the rectum into the vagina.

rec·to·co·li·tis (rek″to-co-li′tis) proctocolitis.

rec·to·cu·ta·ne·ous (-ku-ta′ne-us) pertaining to the rectum and the skin.

rec·to·la·bi·al (-la′be-al) relating to the rectum and a labium majus.

rec·to·pexy (rek′to-pek″se) proctopexy.

rec·to·plas·ty (-plas′te) proctoplasty.

rec·to·scope (-skōp) proctoscope.

rec·to·sig·moid (rek″to-sig′moid) the terminal portion of the sigmoid colon and the proximal portion of the rectum.

rec·to·sig·moi·dec·to·my (-sig″moi-dek′-tah-me) excision of the rectosigmoid.

rec·tos·to·my (rek-tos′tah-me) proctostomy.

rec·to·ure·thral (rek″to-u-re′thral) pertaining to or communicating with the rectum and urethra.

rec·to·uter·ine (-u′ter-in) pertaining to the rectum and uterus.

rec·to·vag·i·nal (-vaj′ǐ-n′l) pertaining to or communicating with the rectum and vagina.

rec·to·ves·i·cal (-ves′ǐ-k′l) pertaining to or communicating with the rectum and bladder.

rec·tum (rek′tum) the distal portion of the large intestine.

rec·tus (rek′tus) [L.] straight.

re·cum·bent (re-kum′bent) lying down.

re·cu·per·a·tion (-koo″per-a′shun) recovery of health and strength.

re·cur·rence (-ker′ens) the return of symptoms after a remission. **recur′rent**, adj.

re·cur·rent (re-kur′ent) [L. *recurrens* returning] 1. running back, or toward the source. 2. returning after remissions.

re·cur·va·tion (re″kur-va′shun) a backward bending or curvature.

red (red) 1. the color produced by the longest waves of the visible spectrum, approximately 630 to 750 nm. 2. a dye or stain with this color. **scarlet r.,** an azo dye used as a biological stain for fats.

re·dia (re′de-ah) pl. *re′diae*. A larval stage of certain trematode parasites, which develops in the body of a snail host and gives rise to daughter rediae, or to the cercariae.

red·in·te·gra·tion (red-in″tě-gra′shun) 1. the restoration or repair of a lost or damaged part. 2. a psychic process in which part of a complex stimulus provokes the complete reaction that was previously made only to the complex stimulus as a whole. 3. reintegration (2).

re·dox (re′doks) oxidation-reduction.

re·duce (re-doos′) 1. to restore to the normal place or relation of parts, as to reduce a fracture. 2. to undergo reduction. 3. to decrease in weight or size.

re·du·ci·ble (re-doo′sǐ-b′l) capable of being reduced.

re·duc·tant (re-duk′tant) the electron donor in an oxidation-reduction (redox) reaction.

re·duc·tase (-tās) a term used in the names of some of the oxidoreductases, usually specifically those catalyzing reactions important solely for reduction of a metabolite. **5α-r.,** an enzyme that catalyzes the irreversible reduction of testosterone to dihydrotestosterone; enzyme deficiency leads to a form of male pseudohermaphroditism.

re·duc·tion (-shun) 1. the correction of a fracture, luxation, or hernia. 2. the addition of hydrogen to a substance, or more generally, the gain of electrons. **closed r.,** the manipulative reduction of a fracture without incision. **open r.,** reduction of a fracture after incision into the fracture site.

re·du·pli·ca·tion (re″doo-plǐ-ka′shun) 1. a doubling back. 2. the recurrence of paroxysms of a double type. 3. duplication (3).

re·en·try (re-en′tre) reexcitation of a region of cardiac tissue by a single impulse, continuing for one or more cycles and sometimes resulting in ectopic beats or tachyarrhythmias; it also requires refractoriness of the tissue to stimulation and an area of unidirectional block to conduction. **re·en′trant,** adj.

re·feed·ing (re-fēd'ing) restoration of normal nutrition after a period of fasting or starvation.

re·fer·red (re-ferd') of sensory phenomena, perceived at a site other than the one being stimulated.

re·flec·tion (-flek'shun) 1. a turning or bending back upon a course. 2. an image produced by reflection. 3. in physics, the turning back of a ray of light, sound, or heat when it strikes against a surface that it does not penetrate. 4. a special form of reentry in which an impulse crosses an area of diminished responsiveness to excite distal tissue then returns, retracing its path rather than traversing a circuit, to seesaw back and forth.

re·flex (re'fleks) a reflected action or movement; the sum total of any particular automatic response mediated by the nervous system. **abdominal r's,** contractions of the abdominal muscles on stimulation of the abdominal skin. **accommodation r.,** the coordinated changes that occur when the eye adapts itself to near vision; constriction of the pupil, convergence of the eyes, and increased convexity of the lens. **Achilles tendon r.,** triceps surae r. **acoustic r.,** contraction of the stapedius muscle in response to intense sound. **anal r.,** contraction of the anal sphincter on irritation of the anal skin. **ankle r.,** triceps surae r. **auditory r.,** any reflex caused by stimulation of the vestibulocochlear nerve, especially momentary closure of both eyes produced by a sudden sound. **Babinski's r.,** dorsiflexion of the big toe on stimulation of the sole, occurring in lesions of the pyramidal tract, although a normal reflex in infants. **Babkin r.,** pressure by the examiner's thumbs on the palms of both hands of the infant results in opening of the infant's mouth. **baroreceptor r.,** the reflex response to stimulation of baroreceptors of the carotid sinus and aortic arch, regulating blood pressure by controlling heart rate, strength of heart contractions, and diameter of blood vessels. **Bezold r., Bezold-Jarisch r.,** reflex bradycardia and hypotension resulting from stimulation of cardiac chemoreceptors by antihypertensive alkaloids and similar substances. **biceps r.,** contraction of the biceps muscle when its tendon is tapped. **Brain's r.,** extension of a hemiplegic flexed arm on assumption of a quadrupedal posture. **brain stem r's,** those regulated at the level of the brain stem, such as pupillary, pharyngeal, and cough reflexes, and the control of respiration; their absence is one criterion for brain death. **bulbospongiosus r.,** contraction of the bulbospongiosus muscle in response to a tap on the dorsum of the penis. **carotid sinus r.,** slowing of the heart beat on pressure on the carotid artery at the level of the cricoid cartilage. **Chaddock's r.,** in lesions of the pyramidal tract, stimulation below the external malleolus causes extension of the great toe. **chain r.,** a series of reflexes, each serving as a stimulus to the next one, representing a complete activity. **ciliary r.,** the movement of the pupil in accommodation. **ciliospinal r.,** dilation of the ipsilateral pupil on painful stimulation of the skin at the side of the neck. **closed loop r.,** a reflex, such as a stretch reflex, in which the stimulus decreases when it receives feedback from the response mechanism. **conditioned r.,** see under *response*. **conjunctival r.,** closure of the eyelid when the conjunctiva is touched. **corneal r.,** closure of the lids on irritation of the cornea. **cough r.,** the events initiated by the sensitivity of the lining of the airways and mediated by the medulla as a consequence of impulses transmitted by the vagus nerve, resulting in coughing. **cremasteric r.,** stimulation of the skin on the front and inner thigh retracts the testis on the same side. **deep r.,** tendon r. **digital r.,** Hoffmann's sign (2). **diving r.,** a reflex involving cardiovascular and metabolic adaptations to conserve oxygen occurring in animals during diving into water; observed in reptiles, birds, and mammals, including humans. **elbow r.,** triceps r. **embrace r.,** Moro's r. **finger-thumb r.,** opposition and adduction of the thumb combined with flexion at the metacarpophalangeal joint and extension at the interphalangeal joint on downward pressure of the index finger. **gag r.,** pharyngeal r. **gastrocolic r.,** increase in intestinal peristalsis after food enters the empty stomach. **gastroileal r.,** increase in ileal motility and opening of the ileocecal valve when food enters the empty stomach. **grasp r.,** flexion or clenching of the fingers or toes on stimulation of the palm or sole, normal only in infancy. **Hering-Breuer r.,** the reflex that limits excessive expansion and contraction of the chest during respiration prior to sending impulses to the brain via the vagus nerve. **Hoffmann's r.,** see under *sign* (2). **hypogastric r.,** contraction of the muscles of the lower abdomen on stroking the skin on the inner surface of the thigh. **jaw r., jaw jerk r.,** closure of the mouth caused by a downward blow on the passively hanging chin; rarely seen in health but very noticeable in corticospinal tract lesions. **knee jerk r.,** patellar r. **light r.,** 1. cone of light.

2. contraction of the pupil when light falls on the eye. 3. a spot of light seen reflected from the retina with the retinoscopic mirror. **Magnus and de Kleijn neck r's,** extension of both ipsilateral limbs, or one, or part of a limb, increase of tonus on the side to which the chin is turned when the head is rotated to the side, and flexion with loss of tonus on the side to which the occiput points; sign of decerebrate rigidity except in infants. **Mayer's r.,** finger-thumb r. **Mendel-Bekhterev r.,** dorsal flexion of the second to fifth toes on percussion of the dorsum of the foot; in certain organic nervous disorders, plantar flexion occurs. **micturition r.,** any of the reflexes necessary for effortless urination and subconscious maintenance of continence. **Moro's r.,** flexion of an infant's thighs and knees, fanning and then clenching of fingers, with arms first thrown outward and then brought together as though embracing something; produced by a sudden stimulus and seen normally in the newborn. **myotatic r.,** stretch r. **neck r's,** reflex adjustments in trunk posture and limb position caused by stimulation of proprioceptors in the neck joints and muscles when the head is turned, tending to maintain a constant orientation between the head and body. **neck righting r.,** rotation of the trunk in the direction in which the head of the supine infant is turned; this reflex is absent or decreased in infants with spasticity. **nociceptive r's,** reflexes initiated by painful stimuli. **oculocardiac r.,** a slowing of the rhythm of the heart following compression of the eyes; slowing of from 5 to 13 beats per minute is normal. **open loop r.,** a reflex in which the stimulus causes activity that it does not further control and from which it does not receive feedback. **Oppenheim r.,** dorsiflexion of the big toe on stroking downward along the medial side of the tibia, seen in pyramidal tract disease. **orbicularis oculi r.,** normal contraction of the orbicularis oculi muscle, with resultant closing of the eye, on percussion at the outer aspect of the supraorbital ridge, over the glabella, or around the margin of the orbit. **orbicularis pupillary r.,** unilateral contraction of the pupil followed by dilatation after closure or attempted closure of eyelids that are forcibly held apart. **palatal r., palatine r.,** stimulation of the palate causes swallowing. **patellar r.,** contraction of the quadriceps and extension of the leg when the patellar ligament is tapped. **peristaltic r.,** when a portion of the intestine is distended or irritated, the area just proximal contracts and the area just distal relaxes. **pharyngeal r.,** contraction of the pharyngeal constrictor muscle elicited by touching the back of the pharynx. **pilomotor r.,** the production of goose flesh on stroking the skin. **placing r.,** flexion followed by extension of the leg when the infant is held erect and the dorsum of the foot is drawn along the under edge of a table top; it is obtainable in the normal infant up to the age of six weeks. **plantar r.,** irritation of the sole contracts the toes. **proprioceptive r.,** one initiated by a stimulus to a proprioceptor. **pupillary r.,** 1. contraction of the pupil on exposure of the retina to light. 2. any reflex involving the iris, resulting in change in the size of the pupil, occurring in response to various stimuli, e.g., change in illumination or point of fixation, sudden loud noise, or emotional stimulation. **quadriceps r.,** patellar r. **quadrupedal extensor r.,** Brain's r. **red r.,** a luminous red appearance seen upon the retina in retinoscopy. **righting r.,** the ability to assume an optimal position when there has been a departure from it. **Rossolimo's r.,** in pyramidal tract lesions, plantar flexion of the toes on taping their plantar surface. **scratch r.,** a spinal reflex by which an itch or other irritation of the skin causes a nearby body part to move over and briskly rub the affected area. **spinal r.,** any reflex action mediated through a center of the spinal cord. **startle r.,** Moro's r. **stepping r.,** movements of progression elicited when the infant is held upright and inclined forward with the soles of the feet touching a flat surface. **stretch r.,** reflex contraction of a muscle in response to passive longitudinal stretching. **sucking r.,** sucking movements of the lips of an infant elicited by touching the lips or the skin near the mouth. **superficial r.,** any withdrawal reflex elicited by noxious or tactile stimulation of the skin, cornea, or mucous membrane, including the corneal reflex, pharyngeal reflex, cremasteric reflex, etc. **swallowing r.,** palatal r. **tendon r.,** one elicited by a sharp tap on the appropriate tendon or muscle to induce brief stretch of the muscle, followed by contraction. **tonic neck r.,** extensions of the arm and sometimes of the leg on the side to which the head is forcibly turned, with flexion of the contralateral limbs; seen normally in the newborn. **triceps r.,** contraction of the belly of the triceps muscle and slight extension of the arm when the tendon of the muscle is tapped directly, with the arm flexed and fully supported and relaxed. **triceps surae r.,** plantar flexion caused by a twitchlike contraction of the triceps surae

muscle, elicited by a tap on the Achilles tendon, preferably while the patient kneels on a bed or chair, the feet hanging free over the edge. **vestibular r's,** the reflexes for maintaining the position of the eyes and body in relation to changes in orientation of the head. **vestibuloocular r.,** nystagmus or deviation of the eyes in response to stimulation of the vestibular system by angular acceleration or deceleration or when the caloric test is performed. **withdrawal r.,** a nociceptive reflex in which a body part is quickly moved away from a painful stimulus.

re·flex·o·gen·ic (re-flek″so-jen′ik) producing or increasing reflex action.

re·flex·og·e·nous (re″flek-soj′ĕ-nus) reflexogenic.

re·flex·o·graph (re-flek′so-graf) an instrument for recording a reflex.

re·flex·ol·o·gy (re″flek-sol′ah-je) 1. the science or study of reflexes. 2. a therapeutic technique based on the premise that areas in the hands or feet correspond to the organs and systems of the body and stimulation of these areas by pressure can affect the corresponding organ or system.

re·flex·om·e·ter (re″flek-som′ĕ-ter) an instrument for measuring the force required to produce myotatic contraction.

re·flux (re′fluks) a backward or return flow. **duodenogastric r.,** reflux of the contents of the duodenum into the stomach; it may occur normally, especially during fasting. **gastroesophageal r.,** reflux of the stomach and duodenal contents into the esophagus. **hepatojugular r.,** distention of the jugular vein induced by applying manual pressure over the liver; it suggests insufficiency of the right heart. **intrarenal r.,** reflux of urine into the renal parenchymal tissue. **valvular r.,** backflow of blood past a venous valve in the lower limb due to venous insufficiency. **vesicoureteral r., vesicoureteric r.,** backward flow of urine from the bladder into a ureter.

re·fract (re-frakt′) 1. to cause to deviate. 2. to ascertain errors of ocular refraction.

re·frac·tion (re-frak′shun) 1. the act or process of refracting; specifically, the determination of the refractive errors of the eye and their correction with lenses. 2. the deviation of light in passing obliquely from one medium to another of different density. **refrac′tive,** adj. **double r.,** refraction in which incident rays are divided into two refracted rays, so as to produce a double image. **dynamic r.,** the normal accommodation of the eye which is continually exerted without conscious effort.

re·frac·tion·ist (-ist) one skilled in determining the refracting power of the eyes and correcting refracting defects.

re·frac·tom·e·ter (re″frak-tom′ĕ-ter) 1. an instrument for measuring the refractive power of the eye. 2. an instrument for determining the indexes of refraction of various substances, particularly for determining the strength of lenses for spectacles.

re·frac·to·ry (re-frak′tor-e) 1. resistant to treatment. 2. not responding to a stimulus.

re·fran·gi·ble (re-fran′jĭ-b'l) susceptible to being refracted.

re·fresh (re-fresh′) to denude an epithelial wound to enhance tissue repair.

re·frig·er·a·tion (re-frij″er-a′shun) therapeutic application of low temperature.

re·fu·sion (re-fu′zhun) the return of blood to the circulation after temporary removal or stoppage of flow.

re·gen·er·a·tion (re-jen″er-a′shun) the natural renewal of a structure, as of a lost tissue or part. **guided tissue r.,** treatment of wound tissue using microporous membranes as barriers, so that only specific, desired types of cells can enter the wound and regenerate.

reg·i·men (rej′ĭ-men) a strictly regulated scheme of diet, exercise, or other activity designed to achieve certain ends.

re·gio (re′je-o) pl. *regio′nes.* [L.] region.

re·gion (re′jun) a plane area with more or less definite boundaries. **re′gional,** adj. **r's of back,** the areas into which the back is divided, including the *vertebral, sacral, scapular, infrascapular,* and *lumbar.* **facial r.,** that comprising the various anatomical regions of the face: *buccal* (side of oral cavity), *infraorbital* (below eye), *mental* (chin), *nasal* (nose), *oral* (lips), *orbital* (eye), *parotid* (angle of jaw), and *zygomatic* (cheek bone) regions. **homogeneously staining r's (HSR),** long unbanded regions of chromosomes created by gene amplification; they are tumor markers indicative of solid neoplasms with poor prognosis. **pectoral r.,** the aspect of the chest bounded by the pectoralis major muscle, and including the lateral pectoral, mammary, and inframammary regions. **perineal r.,** the region overlying the pelvic outlet, including the *anal* and *genitourinary* regions. **precordial r.,** the part of the anterior surface of the body covering the heart and the pit of the stomach.

reg·is·trant (rej′is-trant) a nurse listed on the books of a registry as available for duty.

reg·is·trar (-trahr) 1. an official keeper of records. 2. in British hospitals, a resident specialist who acts as assistant to the chief or attending specialist.

reg·is·tra·tion (rej″is-tra′shun) in dentistry, the making of a record of the jaw relations present or desired, in order to transfer them to an articulator to facilitate proper construction of a dental prosthesis.

reg·is·try (rej′is-tre) 1. an office where a nurse's name may be listed as being available for duty. 2. a central agency for the collection of pathologic material and related data in a specified field of pathology.

re·gres·sion (re-gresh′un) 1. return to a former or earlier state. 2. subsidence of symptoms or of a disease process. 3. in biology, the tendency in successive generations toward the mean. 4. defensive retreat to an earlier, often infantile, pattern of behavior or thought. 5. a functional relationship between a random variable and the corresponding values of one or more independent variables. **regres′sive,** adj.

reg·u·lar (reg′u-ler) [L. *regularis; regula* rule] normal or conforming to rule; occurring at proper or fixed intervals.

reg·u·la·tion (reg″u-la′shun) 1. the act of adjusting or state of being adjusted to a certain standard. 2. in biology, the adaptation of form or behavior of an organism to changed conditions. 3. the power to form a whole embryo from stages before the gastrula. **reg′ulatory,** adj.

re·gur·gi·tant (re-ger′jĭ-tint) flowing backward.

re·gur·gi·ta·tion (re-ger″jĭ-ta′shun) 1. flow in the opposite direction from normal. 2. vomiting. **aortic r. (AR),** backflow of blood from the aorta into the left ventricle due to insufficiency of the aortic semilunar valve. **mitral r. (MR),** backflow of blood from the left ventricle into the left atrium due to insufficiency of the mitral valve. **pulmonic r. (PR),** backflow of blood from the pulmonary artery into the right ventricle due to insufficiency of the pulmonic semilunar valve. **tricuspid r. (TR),** the backflow of blood from the right ventricle into the right atrium due to insufficiency of the tricuspid valve. **valvular r.,** backflow of blood through the orifices of the heart valves due to imperfect closing of the valves.

re·ha·bil·i·ta·tion (re″hah-bil″ĭ-ta′shun) 1. the restoration of normal form and function after illness or injury. 2. the restoration of the ill or injured patient to optimal functional level in all areas of activity.

re·hy·dra·tion (-hi-dra′shun) the restoration of water or fluid content to a patient or to a substance that has become dehydrated.

rei·ki (ra′ke) [Japanese] a healing tradition of Eastern origin whose purpose is to rebalance the complex energy systems that compose the body when they have become out of balance, using channeling of energy from an unlimited universal energy source through the hands of the practitioner.

re·im·plan·ta·tion (-im-plan-ta′shun) replacement of tissue or a structure in the site from which it was previously lost or removed. **ureteral r.,** ureteroneocystostomy.

re·in·fec·tion (-in-fek′shun) a second infection by the same agent or a second infection of an organ with a different agent.

re·in·force·ment (-in-fors′ment) in behavioral science, the presentation of a stimulus following a response that increases the frequency of subsequent responses, whether *positive* to desirable events, or *negative* to undesirable events which are reinforced in their removal.

re·in·forc·er (-in-for′ser) any stimulus that produces reinforcement, a *positive r.* being a desirable event strengthening responses preceding its occurrence and a *negative r.* being an undesirable event strengthening responses leading to its termination.

re·in·fu·sate (-in-fu′zāt) fluid for reinfusion into the body, usually after being subjected to a treatment process.

re·in·fu·sion (-in-fu′zhun) infusion of body fluid that has previously been withdrawn from the same individual, e.g., reinfusion of ascitic fluid after ultrafiltration.

re·in·ner·va·tion (-in-er-va′shun) restoration of nerve supply to a part from which it has been lost; it may occur spontaneously or by nerve grafting.

re·in·te·gra·tion (-in-tĕ-gra′shun) 1. biological integration after a state of disruption. 2. restoration of harmonious mental function after disintegration of the personality in mental illness.

re·jec·tion (re-jek′shun) an immune reaction against grafted tissue that results in failure of the graft to survive.

re·lapse (rĕ-laps′, re′laps) 1. the return of a disease after its apparent cessation. 2. to fall back into an illness after a period of remission.

re·laps·ing (rĕ-lap′sing, re′lap-sing) recurrent; denoting an illness that is characterized by periods of remission alternating with attacks of symptomatic disease.

re·la·tion (re-la′shun) the condition or state of one object or entity when considered in connection with another. **rel′ative,** adj. **object r's,** the emotional bonds formed between one person and another, as contrasted with love for and interest in oneself.

re·lax·ant (re-lak′sant) 1. lessening or reducing tension. 2. an agent that so acts. **muscle r.,** an agent that specifically aids in reducing muscle tension.

re·line (re-līn′) to resurface the tissue side of a denture with new base material in order to achieve a more accurate fit.

REM rapid eye movements (see under *sleep*).

rem (rem) *r*oentgen–*e*quivalent–*m*an: the amount of any ionizing radiation that has the same biological effectiveness as 1 rad of x-rays; 1 rem = 1 rad × RBE (relative biological effectiveness).

rem·e·dy (rem′ah-de) anything that cures, palliates, or prevents disease. **reme′dial,** adj. **concordant r's,** in homeopathy, remedies of similar action but of dissimilar origin. **inimic r's,** in homeopathy, remedies whose actions are antagonistic. **tissue r's,** the twelve remedies which, according to the biochemical school of homeopathy, form the mineral bases of the body.

rem·i·fen·ta·nil (rem″ĭ-fen′tah-nil) an opioid analgesic used as the hydrochloride salt as an anesthesia adjunct.

re·min·er·al·i·za·tion (re-min″er-al-ĭ-za′shun) restoration of mineral elements, as of calcium salts to bone.

re·mis·sion (re-mish′un) diminution or abatement of the symptoms of a disease; the period during which such diminution occurs.

re·mit·tent (re-mit′ent) having periods of abatement and of exacerbation.

re·mod·el·ing (re-mod′el-ing) reorganization or renovation of an old structure. **bone r.,** absorption of bone tissue and simultaneous deposition of new bone; in normal bone the two processes are in dynamic equilibrium.

re·mo·ti·va·tion (re-mo″tĭ-va′shun) any of various group therapy techniques used with long-term, withdrawn patients in mental hospitals to stimulate their communication, vocational, and social skills and interest in their environment.

ren (ren) pl. *re′nes.* [L.] kidney.

re·nal (re′n'l) pertaining to the kidney.

ren·i·form (ren′ĭ-form) kidney-shaped.

re·nin (re′nin) a proteolytic enzyme synthesized, stored, and secreted by the juxtaglomerular cells of the kidney; it plays a role in regulation of blood pressure by catalyzing the conversion of angiotensinogen to angiotensin I.

re·nin·ism (-izm) a condition marked by overproduction of renin. **primary r.,** a syndrome of hypertension, hypokalemia, hyperaldosteronism, and elevated plasma renin activity, due to proliferation of juxtaglomerular cells.

reni·pel·vic (ren″ĭ-pel′vik) pertaining to the pelvis of the kidney.

ren·nin (ren′in) chymosin.

re·no·gas·tric (re″no-gas′trik) pertaining to the kidney and stomach.

re·nog·ra·phy (re-nog′rah-fe) radiography of the kidney.

re·no·in·tes·ti·nal (re″no-in-tes′tĭ-n'l) pertaining to the kidney and intestine.

re·nop·a·thy (re-nop′ah-the) nephropathy.

re·no·pri·val (re″no-pri′val) pertaining to or caused by lack of kidney function.

re·no·vas·cu·lar (-vas′ku-ler) pertaining to or affecting the blood vessels of the kidney.

ren·ule (ren′ūl) an area of kidney supplied by a branch of the renal artery, usually consisting of three or four medullary pyramids and their corresponding cortical substance.

Reo·vi·ri·dae (re″o-vir′ĭ-de) the reoviruses: a family of RNA viruses with a linear double-stranded RNA genome; it includes the genera *Orbivirus, Orthoreovirus, Rotavirus,* and *Coltivirus.*

reo·vi·rus (re′o-vi″rus) 1. any virus belonging to the family Reoviridae. 2. any virus belonging to the genus *Orthoreovirus.*

re·oxy·gen·a·tion (re-ok″sĭ-jen-a′shun) in radiobiology, the phenomenon in which hypoxic (and thus radioresistant) tumor cells become more exposed to oxygen (and thus more radiosensitive) by coming into closer proximity to capillaries after death and loss of other tumor cells due to previous irradiation.

re·pag·li·nide (rĕ-pag′lĭ-nīd) an oral hypoglycemic agent used in the treatment of type 2 diabetes mellitus.

re·pair (re-pār′) the physical or mechanical restoration of damaged or diseased tissues by the growth of healthy new cells or by surgical apposition. **repar′ative,** adj. **Cooper's ligament r., McVay r.,** repair of an inguinal hernia by suturing the inguinal falx to the pectineal (Cooper's) and inguinal ligaments.

re·place·ment (re-plās′ment) 1. substitution; see also *replacement therapy,* under *therapy.* 2. arthroplasty. **joint r.,** arthroplasty.

re·plan·ta·tion (re″plan-ta′shun) reimplantation.

rep·li·case (rep′lĭ-kās) 1. a polymerase synthesizing RNA from an RNA template. 2. more generically, any enzyme that replicates nucleic acids, i.e., a DNA or RNA polymerase.

rep·li·ca·tion (rep″lĭ-ka′shun) 1. a turning back of a part so as to form a duplication. 2. repetition of an experiment to ensure accuracy. 3. the process of duplicating or reproducing, as replication of an exact copy of a polynucleotide strand of DNA or RNA. **rep′lica·tive,** adj.

re·po·lar·iza·tion (re-po″ler-ĭ-za′shun) the reestablishment of polarity, especially the return of cell membrane potential to resting potential after depolarization.

re·pos·i·tor (-poz′ĭ-ter) an instrument used in returning displaced organs to the normal position.

re·pos·i·to·ry (-poz′ĭ-tor-e) a place where something is stored, in pharmacology referring to the injection, usually intramuscularly, of a long-acting drug, which is slowly absorbed and is therefore prolonged in its action.

re·pres·si·ble (re-pres′ĭ-b′l) capable of undergoing repression.

re·pres·sion (-presh′un) 1. the act of restraining, inhibiting, or suppressing. 2. in psychiatry, an unconscious defense mechanism in which unacceptable ideas, fears, and impulses are thrust out or kept out of consciousness. 3. gene r. **enzyme r.,** interference, usually by the endproduct of a pathway, with synthesis of the enzymes of that pathway. **gene r.,** the inhibition of gene transcription of an operon; in prokaryotes repressor binding to the operon is involved.

re·pres·sor (-pres′er) in genetics, a substance produced by a regulator gene that acts to prevent initiation by the operator gene of protein synthesis in the operon.

re·pro·duc·tion (re″pro-duk′shun) 1. the production of offspring by organized bodies. 2. the creation of a similar object or situation; duplication; replication. **reproduc′tive,** adj. **asexual r.,** reproduction without the fusion of sexual cells. **cytogenic r.,** production of a new individual from a single germ cell or zygote. **sexual r.,** reproduction by the fusion of a female gamete and a male gamete (*bisexual r.*) or by development of an unfertilized egg (*unisexual r.*). **somatic r.,** production of a new individual from a multicellular fragment by fission or budding.

rep·til·ase (rep′til-ās) an enzyme from Russell's viper venom used in determining blood clotting time.

re·pul·sion (re-pul′shun) 1. the act of driving apart or away; a force that tends to drive two bodies apart. 2. in genetics, the occurrence on opposite chromosomes in a double heterozygote of the two mutant alleles of interest.

RES reticuloendothelial system.

re·scin·na·mine (re-sin′ah-min) an alkaloid from various species of *Rauwolfia;* used as an antihypertensive.

re·sect (-sekt′) to excise part or all of an organ or other structure.

re·sec·tion (-sek′shun) excision. **root r.,** apicoectomy. **transurethral r. of the prostate (TURP), transurethral prostatic r.,** resection of the prostate by means of an instrument passed through the urethra. **wedge r.,** removal of a triangular mass of tissue.

re·sec·to·scope (-sek′to-skōp) an instrument with a wide-angle telescope and an electrically activated wire loop for transurethral removal or biopsy of lesions of the bladder, prostate, or urethra.

re·ser·pine (rĕ-ser′pēn) an alkaloid from various species of *Rauwolfia;* used as an antihypertensive.

re·serve (re-zerv′) 1. to hold back for future use. 2. a supply, beyond that ordinarily used, which may be utilized in emergency. **alkali r., alkaline r.,** the amount of conjugate base components of the blood buffers, the most important being bicarbonate. **cardiac r.,** potential ability of the heart to perform work beyond that necessary under basal conditions. **ovarian r.,** the number and quality of oocytes in the ovaries of a woman of childbearing age.

re·ser·voir (rez′er-vwahr) 1. a storage place or cavity. 2. cistern. 3. an alternate host or passive carrier of a pathogenic organism. **continent ileal r.,** 1. a valved intra-abdominal pouch that maintains continence of the feces and is emptied by a catheter when full. 2. a neobladder made from a section of ileum. **continent urinary r.,** neobladder. **ileoanal r.,** a pouch for the retention of feces, formed by suturing together multiple limbs of ileum and connected to the anus by an ileal conduit; used with colectomy to maintain continence in the treatment of ulcerative colitis. **Pecquet's r.,** cisterna chyli.

res·i·dent (rez′ĭ-dent) 1. resident physician. 2. being or pertaining to such a physician.

res·i·due (rez′ĭ-doo) 1. a remainder; that remaining after removal of other substances. 2. in biochemistry, that portion of a monomer that is incorporated in a polymer. **resid′ual,** adj.

res·in (rez′in) 1. a solid or semisolid organic substance exuded by plants or by insects feeding on plants, or produced synthetically; they are insoluble in water but mostly soluble in alcohol or ether. 2. a compound made by condensation or polymerization of low-molecular-weight organic compounds. **res′inous,** adj. **acrylic r's,** a class of thermoplastic resins produced by polymerization of acrylic or methacrylic acid or their derivatives; used in the fabrication of medical prostheses and dental restorations and appliances. **anion exchange r.**, see *ion exchange r.* **cation exchange r.**, see *ion exchange r.* **cholestyramine r.**, a synthetic, strongly basic anion exchange resin in the chloride form which chelates bile acids in the intestine, thus preventing their reabsorption; used as an adjunctive therapy to diet in management of certain hypercholesterolemias and in the symptomatic relief of pruritus associated with bile stasis. **composite r.**, a synthetic resin, usually acrylic based, to which a high percentage of inert filler has been added, e.g., coated glass or silica; used chiefly in dental restorations. **epoxy r.**, a heat-set resin with toughness, adhesibility, chemical resistance, dielectric properties, and dimensional stability; several modified types are used as denture base material. **ion exchange r.**, a high-molecular-weight insoluble polymer of simple organic compounds capable of exchanging its attached ions for other ions in the surrounding medium; classified as *(a)* cation or *anion exchange r's*, depending on which ions the resin exchanges; and *(b)* carboxylic, sulfonic, etc., depending on the nature of the active groups. **podophyllum r.**, podophyllin; a mixture of resins from podophyllum, used as a topical caustic in the treatment of certain papillomas, condylomata acuminata, keratoses, and other epitheliomas.

re·sis·tance (re-zis′tans) 1. opposition, or counteracting force. 2. the natural ability of an organism to resist microorganisms or toxins produced in disease. 3. the opposition to the flow of electrical current between two points of a circuit. Symbol R or *R.* 4. in psychiatry, conscious or unconscious defenses that prevent material in the unconscious from coming into awareness. **airway r.**, the opposition of the tracheobronchial tree to air flow. Symbols R_A, R_{AW}. **androgen r.**, resistance of target organs to the action of androgens; the result is any of a spectrum of defects. In mild to incomplete types the person may have a definite male phenotype but infertility, or may have ambiguous genitalia. In the complete type the person has a female phenotype but XY chromosomes. **drug r.**, the ability of a microorganism to withstand the effects of a drug that are lethal to most members of its species. **electrical r.**, resistance (3). **multidrug r., multiple drug r.**, in some malignant cell lines, resistance to many structurally unrelated chemotherapy agents in cells that have developed natural

resistance to a single cytotoxic compound. **vascular r.**, the opposition to blood flow in a vascular bed.

re·sis·tive (re-zis′tiv) pertaining to or characterized by resistance.

res·o·lu·tion (rez″o-loo′shun) 1. subsidence of a pathologic state. 2. perception as separate of two adjacent points; in microscopy, the smallest distance at which two adjacent objects can be distinguished as separate. 3. a measure of the fineness of detail that can be discerned in an image.

re·sol·vent (re-zol′vent) 1. promoting resolution or the dissipation of a pathologic growth. 2. an agent that promotes resolution.

res·o·nance (rez′o-nins) 1. the prolongation and intensification of sound produced by transmission of its vibrations to a cavity, especially such a sound elicited by percussion. 2. a vocal sound heard on auscultation. 3. the existence of organic chemical structures that can not be accurately represented by a single structural formula, the actual formula lying intermediate between several possible representations differing only in electron position. **amphoric r.**, an auscultatory sound like that produced by blowing over the mouth of an empty bottle. **nuclear magnetic r.**, a measure, by means of applying an external magnetic field to a solution in a constant radiofrequency field, of the magnetic moment of atomic nuclei to determine the structure of organic compounds; the technique is used in magnetic resonance imaging. **skodaic r.**, increased percussion resonance at the upper part of the chest, with flatness below it. **tympanitic r.**, 1. the percussion sound heard on an abdomen with tympanites. 2. the drumlike reverberation of a cavity full of air. **vocal r. (VR)**, the sound of ordinary speech as heard through the chest wall.

res·o·na·tor (rez′o-na″ter) 1. an instrument used to intensify sounds. 2. an electric circuit in which oscillations of a certain frequency are set up by oscillations of the same frequency in another circuit.

re·sorb (re-sorb′) to take up or absorb again.

re·sor·ci·nol (re-zor′si-nol) a bactericidal, fungicidal, keratolytic, exfoliative, and anti-pruritic agent, used especially as a topical keratolytic in the treatment of acne and other dermatoses.

re·sorp·tion (re-sorp′shun) 1. the lysis and assimilation of a substance, as of bone. 2. reabsorption.

res·pir·a·ble (re-spīr′ah-b'l) 1. suitable for respiration. 2. small enough to be inhaled.

res·pi·ra·tion (res″pĭ-ra′shun) 1. the exchange of oxygen and carbon dioxide between the atmosphere and the body cells, including ventilation (inhalation and exhalation); diffusion of oxygen from alveoli to blood and of carbon dioxide from blood to alveoli; and transport of oxygen to and carbon dioxide from body cells. 2. ventilation (1). 3. cellular respiration; the exergonic metabolic processes in living cells by which molecular oxygen is taken in, organic substances are oxidized, free energy is released, and carbon dioxide, water, and other oxidized products are given off by the cell. **abdominal r.,** breathing accomplished mainly by the abdominal muscles and diaphragm. **aerobic r.,** the oxidative transformation of certain substrates into secretory products, the released energy being used in the process of assimilation. **anaerobic r.,** respiration in which energy is released from chemical reactions in which free oxygen takes no part. **artificial r.,** that which is maintained by force applied to the body, by stimulation of the phrenic nerve by an electric current, or by *mouth-to-mouth method* (resuscitation of an apneic victim by direct application of the mouth to his, regularly taking a deep breath and blowing into the victim's lungs). **Biot's r.,** rapid, short breathing with pauses of several seconds, indicating increased intracranial pressure. **Cheyne-Stokes r.,** breathing with rhythmic waxing and waning of depth of breaths and regularly recurring apneic periods. **cogwheel r.,** breathing with jerky inhalation. **electrophrenic r.,** diaphragmatic pacing; induction of respiration by electric stimulation of the phrenic nerve. **external r.,** exchange of gases between the lungs and blood. **internal r.,** exchange of gases between the body cells and blood. **Kussmaul's r., Kussmaul-Kien r.,** air hunger; deep rapid breathing as seen in respiratory acidosis. **paradoxical r.,** that in which all or part of a lung is deflated during inhalation and inflated during exhalation, such as in flail chest or paralysis of the diaphragm. **tissue r.,** internal r.

res·pi·ra·tor (res′pĭ-ra″ter) ventilator (2). **cuirass r.,** see under *ventilator*. **Drinker r.,** popularly, "iron lung": an apparatus formerly in wide use for producing artificial respiration over long periods of time, consisting of a metal tank, enclosing the patient's body, with the head outside, and within which artificial respiration is maintained by alternating negative and positive pressure.

res·pi·ra·to·ry (res′pĭ-rah-tor″e) pertaining to respiration.

res·pi·rom·e·ter (res″pĭ-rom′ĕ-ter) an instrument for determining the nature of respiration.

re·sponse (re-spons′) any action or change of condition evoked by a stimulus. **respon′sive,** adj. **acute phase r.,** a group of physiological processes occurring soon after the onset of infection, trauma, inflammatory processes, and some malignant conditions; it includes increase in acute phase proteins in serum, fever, increased vascular permeability, and metabolic and pathologic changes. **anamnestic r.,** secondary immune r. **autoimmune r.,** the immune response against an autoantigen. **conditioned r.,** a response evoked by a conditioned stimulus; a response to a stimulus that was incapable of evoking it before conditioning. **galvanic skin r.,** the alteration in the electrical resistance of the skin associated with sympathetic nerve discharge. **immune r.,** any response of the immune system to an antigenic stimulus, including antibody production, cell-mediated immunity, and immunological tolerance. **primary immune r.,** the immune response occurring on the first exposure to an antigen, with specific antibodies appearing in the blood after a multiple day latent period. **relaxation r.,** a group of physiologic changes that cause decreased activity of the sympathetic nervous system and consequent relaxation after stimulation of certain regions of the hypothalamus. They may be self-induced through techniques such as meditation and biofeedback. **secondary immune r.,** the immune response occurring on second and subsequent exposures to an antigen, with a stronger response to a lesser amount of antigen, and a shorter lag time compared to the primary immune response. **triple r. (of Lewis),** a triphasic skin reaction to being stroked with a blunt instrument: first a red line develops at the site due to histamine release, then a flare develops around the red line, and lastly a wheal is formed as a result of local edema. **unconditioned r.,** an unlearned response, i.e., one that occurs naturally to an unconditioned stimulus.

rest (rest) 1. repose after exertion. 2. a fragment of embryonic tissue retained within the adult organism. 3. an extension that helps support a removable partial denture. **adrenal r's,** accessory adrenal glands. **incisal r., lingual r., occlusal r.,** a metallic part or extension from a removable partial denture to aid in supporting the prosthesis. **suprarenal r's,** accessory adrenal glands.

re·ste·no·sis (re″stĕ-no′sis) recurrent stenosis, especially of a cardiac valve after surgical correction of the primary condition. **reste-not'ic,** adj.

res·ti·form (res'tĭ-form) shaped like a rope.

res·ti·tu·tion (res″tĭ-too'shun) the spontaneous realignment of the fetal head with the fetal body, after delivery of the head.

res·to·ra·tion (res″to-ra'shun) 1. induction of a return to a previous state, as a return to health or replacement of a part to normal position. 2. partial or complete reconstruction of a body part, or the device used in its place. **restor'ative,** adj.

re·straint (re-strānt') the forcible confinement or control of a subject.

re·stric·tion (re-strik'shun) anything that limits; also, a limitation. **restric'tive,** adj. **intrauterine growth r. (IUGR),** see under *restriction.*

re·sus·ci·ta·tion (-sus″ĭ-ta'shun) restoration to life of one apparently dead. **cardiopulmonary r. (CPR),** the reestablishing of heart and lung action after cardiac arrest or apparent sudden death resulting from electric shock, drowning, respiratory arrest, and other causes. The two major components of CPR are artificial ventilation and closed chest cardiac massage.

re·sus·ci·ta·tor (-sus″ĭ-ta″tor) an apparatus for initiating respiration in persons whose breathing has stopped.

re·tain·er (-tān'er) an appliance or device that keeps a tooth or partial denture in proper position.

re·tar·da·tion (re″tahr-da'shun) delay; hindrance; delayed development. **fetal growth r., intrauterine growth r. (IUGR),** birth weight below the tenth percentile for gestational age for infants born in a given population, defined as *symmetric* (both weight and length below normal) or *asymmetric* (weight below normal, length normal). **mental r.,** a mental disorder characterized by significantly subaverage general intellectual functioning associated with impairment in adaptive behavior and manifested in the developmental period; classified according to IQ as *mild* (50–70), *moderate* (35–50), *severe* (20–35), and *profound* (less than 20). **psychomotor r.,** generalized slowing of mental and physical activity.

retch·ing (rech'ing) strong involuntary effort to vomit.

re·te (re'te) pl. *re'tia.* [L.] a network or meshwork, especially of blood vessels. **r. arterio'sum,** an anastomotic network of minute arteries, just before they become arterioles or capillaries. **articular r.,** a network of anastomosing blood vessels in or around a joint. **malpighian r.,** stratum germinativum. **r. mira'bile,** 1. a vascular network formed by division of an artery or vein into many smaller vessels that reunite into a single vessel. 2. arterial anastomosis of the brain occurring between the external and internal carotid arteries due to longstanding thrombosis of the latter. **r. ova'rii,** a homologue of the rete testis, developed in the early female fetus but vestigial in the adult. **r. subpapilla're,** the network of arteries at the boundary between the papillary and reticular layers of the dermis. **r. tes'tis,** a network formed in the mediastinum testis by the seminiferous tubules. **r. veno'sum,** an anastomotic network of small veins.

re·ten·tion (re-ten'shun) the process of holding back or keeping in position, as persistence in the body of material normally excreted, or maintenance of a dental prosthesis in proper position in the mouth.

ret·e·plase (ret'ĕ-plās) a recombinant form of tissue plasminogen activator; used as a thrombolytic agent in the treatment of myocardial infarction.

re·tic·u·la (rĕ-tik'u-lah) [L.] plural of *reticulum.*

re·tic·u·lar (-lar) resembling a net.

re·tic·u·lat·ed (-lāt″ed) reticular.

re·tic·u·la·tion (rĕ-tik″u-la'shun) the formation or presence of a network.

re·tic·u·lin (rĕ-tik'u-lin) a scleroprotein from the connective fibers of reticular tissue.

re·tic·u·lo·cyte (rĕ-tik'u-lo-sīt) a young erythrocyte showing a basophilic reticulum under vital staining.

re·tic·u·lo·cy·to·pe·nia (rĕ-tik″u-lo-si″to-pe'ne-ah) deficiency of reticulocytes in the blood.

re·tic·u·lo·cy·to·sis (-si-to'sis) an excess of reticulocytes in the peripheral blood.

re·tic·u·lo·en·do·the·li·al (-en″do-the'le-al) pertaining to the reticuloendothelium or to the reticuloendothelial system.

re·tic·u·lo·en·do·the·li·o·sis (-en″do-the″le-o'sis) hyperplasia of reticuloendothelial tissue. **leukemic r.,** hairy cell leukemia.

re·tic·u·lo·en·do·the·li·um (-en″do-the'le-um) the tissue of the reticuloendothelial system.

re·tic·u·lo·his·tio·cyt·ic (-his″te-o-sit'ik) pertaining to or of the nature of a reticulohistiocytoma; see under *granuloma.*

re·tic·u·lo·his·ti·o·cy·to·ma (-his″te-o-si-to'mah) a granulomatous aggregation of lipid-laden histiocytes and multinucleated giant cells with pale eosinophilic cytoplasm having a ground glass appearance. It occurs in two forms, *reticulohistiocytic granuloma* and *multicentric reticulohistiocytosis.*

re·tic·u·lo·his·ti·o·cy·to·sis (-si-to'sis) the formation of multiple reticulohistiocytomas. **multicentric r.,** a systemic disease of polyarthritis of the hands and large joints and development of nodular reticulohistiocytomas in the skin, bone, and mucous and synovial membranes, which may progress to polyvisceral involvement and death.

re·tic·u·lo·pe·nia (-pe'ne-ah) reticulocytopenia.

re·tic·u·lo·sis (rĕ-tik″u-lo'sis) an abnormal increase in cells derived from or related to the reticuloendothelial cells. **familial histiocytic r., histiocytic medullary r.,** a fatal hereditary disorder marked by anemia, granulocytopenia, thrombocytopenia, phagocytosis of blood cells, diffuse proliferation of histiocytes, and enlargement of the liver, spleen, and lymph nodes. **malignant midline r., polymorphic r.,** a form of angiocentric immunoproliferative lesion involving midline structures of the nose and face.

re·tic·u·lo·spi·nal (-spi'n'l) pertaining to a reticular formation and the spinal cord.

re·tic·u·lum (rĕ-tik'u-lum) pl. *retic'ula.* [L.] 1. a small network, especially a protoplasmic network in cells. 2. reticular tissue. **endoplasmic r.,** an ultramicroscopic organelle of nearly all higher plant and animal cells, consisting of a system of membrane-bound cavities in the cytoplasm; occurring in two types, rough-surfaced (*granular r.*), bearing large numbers of ribosomes on its outer surface, and smooth-surfaced (*agranular r.*). **sarcoplasmic r.,** a form of agranular reticulum in the sarcoplasm of striated muscle, comprising a system of smooth-surfaced tubules surrounding each myofibril. **stellate r.,** the soft, middle part of the enamel organ of a developing tooth.

re·ti·form (re'tĭ-form, ret'ĭ-form) reticular.

re·ti·na (ret'ĭ-nah) [L.] the innermost tunic of the eyeball, containing the neural elements for reception and transmission of visual stimuli.

re·ti·nac·u·lum (ret″ĭ-nak'u-lum) pl. *retina'cula.* [L.] 1. a structure that retains an organ or tissue in place. 2. an instrument for retracting tissues during surgery. **extensor r. of foot, inferior,** a thickened band of the crural fascia passing from each malleolus across the front of the ankle joint, there crossing the other and passing onto the dorsum of the foot. **extensor r. of foot, superior,** the thickened lower portion of the fascia on the front of the leg, attached to the tibia on one side and the fibula on the other, and holding in place the extensor tendons that pass beneath it. **extensor r. of**

hand, the distal part of the antebrachial fascia, overlying the extensor tendons. **fibular r., inferior,** inferior peroneal r. **fibular r., superior,** superior peroneal r. **flexor r. of foot,** a strong band of fascia that extends from the medial malleolus down onto the calcaneus, holding in place the tendons of the posterior tibial and flexor muscles as they pass to the sole of the foot, and protecting the posterior tibial vessels and tibial nerve. **flexor r. of hand,** a fibrous band forming the carpal canal through which pass the tendons of the flexor muscles of the hand and fingers. **peroneal r., inferior,** a fibrous band that arches over the tendons of the peroneal muscles and holds them in position on the lateral side of the calcaneus. **peroneal r., superior,** a fibrous band that arches over the tendons of the peroneal muscles and helps to hold them in place below and behind the lateral malleolus. **r. ten'dinum,** a tendinous restraining structure, such as an annular ligament.

ret·i·nal (ret'ĭ-n'l) 1. pertaining to the retina. 2. the aldehyde of retinol, derived from absorbed dietary carotenoids or esters of retinol and having vitamin A activity. In the retina, retinal combines with opsins to form visual pigments. The two isomers 11-*cis* retinal and all-*trans* retinal are interconverted in the visual cycle.

ret·i·ni·tis (ret″ĭ-ni'tis) inflammation of the retina. **r. circina'ta, circinate r.,** circinate retinopathy. **exudative r.,** see under *retinopathy.* **r. pigmento'sa,** a group of diseases, often hereditary, marked by progressive loss of retinal response, retinal atrophy, attenuation of retinal vessels, clumping of pigment, and contraction of the visual field. **r. proli'ferans, proliferating r.,** a condition sometimes due to intraocular hemorrhage, with neovascularization and the formation of fibrous tissue extending into the vitreous from the retinal surface; retinal detachment may be a sequel. **suppurative r.,** that due to pyemic infection.

ret·i·no·blas·to·ma (ret″ĭ-no-blas-to'mah) a malignant congenital blastoma, hereditary or sporadic, composed of tumor cells arising from the retinoblasts. **endophytic r., r. endo'phytum,** a retinoblastoma that begins in the inner layers of the retina and spreads toward the center of the globe. **exophytic r., r. exo'phytum,** a retinoblastoma that begins in the outer layers of the retina and spreads away from the center of the globe.

ret·i·no·cer·e·bral (-sĕ-re'bral, -ser'ĕ-bral) affecting both the retina and cerebrum.

ret·i·no·cho·roi·di·tis (-kor″oi-di′tis) in-flammation of the retina and choroid. **r. juxtapapilla′ris**, a small area of inflammation on the fundus near the papilla; seen in young healthy individuals.

ret·i·no·ic ac·id (ret″ĭ-no′ik) an oxidized derivative of retinol, believed to be the form of vitamin A that plays a role in the development and growth of bone and in the maintenance of normal epithelial structures. In pharmacology, it often denotes the all-*trans* isomer (tretinoin); the 13-*cis* isomer is usually called *isotretinoin*.

ret·i·noid (ret′ĭ-noid) 1. resembling the retina. 2. retinal, retinol, or any structurally similar natural derivative or synthetic compound, with or without vitamin A activity.

ret·i·nol (ret′ĭ-nol) vitamin A_1; a 20-carbon primary alcohol in several isomers that is the form of vitamin A found in mammals and that can be converted to the metabolically active forms retinal and retinoic acid.

ret·i·no·ma·la·cia (ret″ĭ-no-mah-la′shah) softening of the retina.

ret·i·no·pap·il·li·tis (-pap″ĭ-li′tis) inflammation of the retina and optic papilla.

ret·i·nop·a·thy (ret″ĭ-nop′ah-the) any noninflammatory disease of the retina. **circinate r.**, a condition in which a circle of white spots encloses the macula, leading to complete foveal blindness. **diabetic r.**, retinopathy associated with diabetes mellitus, which may be of the background type, progressively characterized by microaneurysms, intraretinal punctate hemorrhages, yellow, waxy exudates, cotton-wool patches, and macular edema, or of the proliferative type, characterized by neovascularization of the retina and optic disk, which may project into the vitreous, proliferation of fibrous tissue, vitreous hemorrhage, and retinal detachment. **exudative r.**, that marked by masses of white or yellowish exudate in the posterior part of the fundus oculi, with deposit of cholesterin and blood debris from retinal hemorrhage, and leading to destruction of the macula and blindness. **hypertensive r.**, that associated with essential or malignant hypertension; changes may include irregular narrowing of the retinal arterioles, hemorrhages in the nerve fiber layers and the outer plexiform layer, exudates and cotton-wool patches, arteriosclerotic changes, and, in malignant hypertension, papilledema. **r. of prematurity**, a bilateral retinopathy typically occurring in premature infants treated with high concentrations of oxygen, characterized by vascular dilatation, proliferation, tortuosity, edema, retinal detachment, and fibrous tissue behind the lens.

proliferative r., the proliferative type of diabetic retinopathy. **renal r.**, a retinopathy associated with renal and hypertensive disorders and presenting the same symptoms as hypertensive retinopathy. **stellate r.**, a retinopathy not associated with hypertensive, renal, or arteriosclerotic disorders, but presenting the same symptoms as hypertensive retinopathy.

ret·i·nos·chi·sis (ret″ĭ-nos′kĭ-sis) splitting of the retina, occurring in the nerve fiber layer (*juvenile form*), or in the external plexiform layer (*adult form*).

ret·i·no·scope (ret′ĭ-no-skōp″) an instrument for performing retinoscopy.

ret·i·nos·co·py (ret″ĭ-nos′kah-pe) observation of the pupil under a beam of light projected into the eye, as a means of determining refractive errors.

ret·i·no·sis (ret″ĭ-no′sis) any degenerative, noninflammatory condition of the retina.

ret·i·no·top·ic (ret″ĭ-no-top′ik) relating to the organization of the visual pathways and visual area of the brain.

re·to·the·li·um (re″to-the′le-um) reticuloendothelium.

re·trac·tile (re-trak′til) able to be drawn back.

re·trac·tion (-trak′shun) the act of drawing back, or condition of being drawn back. **clot r.**, the drawing away of a blood clot from the wall of a vessel, a stage of wound healing caused by contraction of platelets.

re·trac·tor (-trak′ter) 1. an instrument for holding open the lips of a wound. 2. a muscle that retracts.

re·triev·al (-tre′v′l) in psychology, the process of obtaining memory information from wherever it has been stored.

retr(o)- word element [L.], *behind; backward.*

ret·ro·ac·tion (ret″ro-ak′shun) action in a reversed direction.

ret·ro·bul·bar (-bul′bar) 1. behind the medulla oblongata. 2. behind the eyeball.

ret·ro·cer·vi·cal (-ser′vĭ-k′l) behind the cervix uteri.

ret·ro·ces·sion (-sesh′un) a going backward; backward displacement.

ret·ro·coch·le·ar (-kok′le-ar) 1. behind the cochlea. 2. denoting the eighth cranial nerve and cerebellopontine angle as opposed to the cochlea.

ret·ro·col·lic (-kol′ik) nuchal.

ret·ro·col·lis (-kol′is) spasmodic torticollis in which the head is drawn back.

ret·ro·cur·sive (-ker′siv) marked by stepping backward.

ret·ro·de·vi·a·tion (-de″ve-a′shun) retrodisplacement; any displacement backwards, such as retroversion or retroflexion.

ret·ro·dis·place·ment (-dis-plās′ment) retrodeviation.

ret·ro·flex·ion (-flek′shun) the bending of an organ or part so that its top is thrust backward.

ret·ro·gas·se·ri·an (-gas-ēr′e-an) pertaining to the sensory (posterior) root of the trigeminal (gasserian) ganglion.

ret·ro·gnath·ism (-nath′izm) retrusion of the mandible. **retrognath′ic**, adj.

ret·ro·grade (ret′ro-grād) going backward; retracing a former course; catabolic.

ret·ro·gres·sion (ret′ro-gresh′un) degeneration; deterioration; regression; return to an earlier, less complex condition.

ret·ro·lab·y·rin·thine (-lab″ĭ-rin′thēn) posterior to the labyrinth.

ret·ro·len·tal (-len′t′l) behind the lens of the eye.

ret·ro·mo·lar (-mo′lar) behind a molar.

ret·ro·peri·to·ne·al (-per″ĭ-to-ne′al) posterior to the peritoneum.

ret·ro·peri·to·ne·um (-per″ĭ-to-ne′um) retroperitoneal space.

ret·ro·peri·to·ni·tis (-per″ĭ-to-ni′tis) inflammation of the retroperitoneal space.

ret·ro·pha·ryn·ge·al (-fah-rin′je-al) 1. pertaining to the posterior part of the pharynx. 2. posterior to the pharynx.

ret·ro·phar·yn·gi·tis (-far″in-ji′tis) inflammation of the posterior part of the pharynx.

ret·ro·pla·sia (-pla′zhah) retrograde metaplasia; degeneration of a tissue or cell into a more primitive type.

ret·ro·posed (-pōzd′) displaced backward.

ret·ro·po·si·tion (pah-zĭ′shun) retrodeviation.

ret·ro·pu·bic (ret″ro-pu′bik) posterior to the pubic arch.

ret·ro·pul·sion (-pul′shun) 1. a driving back, as of the fetal head in labor. 2. tendency to walk backward, as in some cases of tabes dorsalis. 3. an abnormal gait in which the body is bent backward.

ret·ro·sig·moid·al (-sig-moi′dal) posterior to the sigmoid sinus.

ret·ro·spec·tive (-spek′tiv) looking backward, or directed toward the past.

ret·ro·uter·ine (-u′ter-in) behind the uterus.

ret·ro·ver·sion (-ver′zhun) the tipping backward of an entire organ or part.

ret·ro·ves·i·cal (-ves′ĭ-k′l) posterior to the urinary bladder.

ret·ro·vi·rus (ret′ro-vi″rus) a large group of RNA viruses that includes the leukoviruses and lentiviruses; so called because they carry reverse transcriptase.

re·tru·sion (re-troo′zhun) the state of being located posterior to the normal position, such as the mandible or a tooth displaced in the line of occlusion. **retru′sive**, adj.

re·up·take (re-up′tāk) reabsorption of a previously secreted substance.

re·vas·cu·lar·iza·tion (re-vas′ku-lar-ĭ-za′shun) 1. the restoration of blood supply, as after a wound. 2. the restoration of an adequate blood supply to a part by means of a blood vessel graft, as in aortocoronary bypass.

re·ver·ber·a·tion (-ver″bĕ-ra′shun) duration of neuronal activity well beyond an initial stimulus due to transmission of impulses along branches of nerves arranged in a circle, permitting positive feedback.

re·verse tran·scrip·tase (re-vers′ tran-skrip′tās) an enzyme that catalyzes the template-directed, step-by-step addition of deoxyribonucleotides to the end of a DNA or RNA primer or growing DNA chain, using a single-stranded RNA template; it occurs in retroviruses and the DNA formed is an intermediate in the formation of progeny RNA.

re·ver·sion (-ver′zhun) 1. regression (3). 2. in genetics, the mutation of a mutant phenotype so that the original function is restored; it includes mutation of the DNA such that the parental base sequence is regained (*reverse mutation*).

RF rheumatoid factor.

RFA right frontoanterior (position of the fetus).

RFP right frontoposterior (position of the fetus).

RFT right frontotransverse (position of the fetus).

Rh rhodium.

Rh_null symbol for a rare blood type in which all Rh factors are lacking.

Rhab·di·tis (rab-di′tis) a genus of minute nematodes found mostly in damp earth, and as an accidental parasite in humans.

rhabd(o)- word element [Gr.], *rod; rod-shaped*.

rhab·doid (rab′doid) resembling a rod; rod-shaped.

rhab·do·myo·blast (rab″do-mi′o-blast″) a pathologic racket-shaped or spindle-shaped myoblast occurring in rhabdomyosarcoma. **rhabdomyoblas′tic**, adj.

rhab·do·myo·blas·to·ma (mi″o-blas-to′-mah) rhabdomyosarcoma.

rhab·do·my·ol·y·sis (-mi-ol′ĭ-sis) disintegration of striated muscle fibers with excretion of myoglobin in the urine.

rhab·do·my·o·ma (-mi-o'mah) a benign tumor derived from striated muscle; the cardiac form is considered to be a hamartoma and is often associated with tuberous sclerosis.

rhab·do·myo·sar·co·ma (mi″o-sahr-ko'mah) a highly malignant tumor of striated muscle derived from primitive mesenchymal cells. **alveolar r.,** a type having dense proliferations of small round cells among fibrous septa that form alveoli, seen mainly in adolescents and young adults. **embryonal r.,** a type having alternating loosely cellular areas with myxoid stroma and densely cellular areas with spindle cells, seen mainly in infants and small children. **pleomorphic r.,** a type having large cells with bizarre hyperchromatic nuclei, seen in the skeletal muscles, usually in the limbs of adults.

rhab·do·sar·co·ma (-sahr-ko'mah) rhabdomyosarcoma.

rhab·do·sphinc·ter (-sfingk'ter) a sphincter consisting of striated muscle fibers.

Rhab·do·vi·ri·dae (-vir′ĭ-de) the rhabdoviruses: a family of RNA viruses with a negative-sense single-stranded RNA genome, including the genera *Vesiculovirus* and *Lyssavirus.*

rhab·do·vi·rus (rab'do-vi″rus) any virus of the family Rhabdoviridae.

rhachi- for words beginning thus, see those beginning *rachi-.*

rhag·a·des (rag'ah-dēz) fissures, cracks, or fine linear scars in the skin, especially such lesions around the mouth or other regions subjected to frequent movement.

Rham·nus (ram'nus) [L.] a genus of trees and shrubs often having a cathartic bark and fruit. *R. purshia′na* D.C. is the source of cascara sagrada.

rha·phe (ra'fe) raphe.

rheg·ma (reg'mah) a rupture, rent, or fracture.

rheg·ma·tog·e·nous (reg″mah-toj′ĕ-nus) arising from a rhegma, as rhegmatogenous detachment of the retina.

rhe·ni·um (re'ne-um) chemical element (see *Table of Elements*), at. no. 75, symbol Re.

rhe(o)- word element [Gr.], *electric current; flow* (as of fluids).

rhe·ol·o·gy (re-ol'ah-je) the science of the deformation and flow of matter, such as the flow of blood through the heart and blood vessels.

rhe·os·to·sis (re″os-to'sis) a condition of hyperostosis marked by the presence of streaks in the bones; see also *melorheostosis.*

rheo·tax·is (re″o-tak'sis) the orientation of an organism in a stream of liquid, with its long axis parallel with the direction of flow, designated *negative* (moving in the same direction) or *positive* (moving in the opposite direction).

rheum (rōōm) any watery or catarrhal discharge.

rheu·ma·tal·gia (roo″mah-tal′jah) chronic rheumatic pain.

rheu·ma·tid (roo'mah-tid) any skin lesion etiologically associated with rheumatism.

rheu·ma·tism (roo'mah-tizm) any of a variety of disorders marked by inflammation, degeneration, or metabolic derangement of the connective tissue structures, especially the joints and related structures, and attended by pain, stiffness, or limitation of motion. **rheumat′ic,** adj. **muscular r.,** fibrositis. **palindromic r.,** repeated attacks of arthritis and periarthritis without fever and without causing irreversible joint changes.

rheu·ma·toid (roo'mah-toid) 1. resembling rheumatism. 2. associated with rheumatoid arthritis.

rheu·ma·tol·o·gist (roo″mah-tol'ah-jist) a specialist in rheumatology.

rheu·ma·tol·o·gy (-tol'ah-je) the branch of medicine dealing with rheumatic disorders, their causes, pathology, diagnosis, treatment, etc.

rhex·is (rek'sis) the rupture of a blood vessel or of an organ.

rhi·go·sis (rĭ-go'sis) [Gr.] the ability to feel cold.

rhi·nal·gia (ri-nal′jah) rhinodynia; pain in the nose.

rhin·en·ceph·a·lon (ri″nen-sef′ah-lon) 1. the part of the brain once thought to be concerned entirely with olfactory mechanisms, including olfactory nerves, bulbs, tracts, and subsequent connections (all olfactory in function) and the limbic system (not primarily olfactory in function); homologous with olfactory portions of the brain in certain other animals. 2. formerly, the area of the brain comprising the anterior perforated substance, band of Broca, subcallosal area, and paraterminal gyrus. 3. one of the portions of the embryonic telencephalon.

rhin·i·on (rin'e-on) [Gr.] the lower end of the suture between the nasal bones.

rhi·ni·tis (ri-ni'tis) inflammation of the nasal mucous membrane. **allergic r.,** any allergic reaction of the nasal mucosa, occurring perennially (*nonseasonal allergic r.*) or seasonally (*hay fever*). **atrophic r.,** chronic rhinitis with wasting of the mucous membrane and glands. **r. caseo′sa,** that with a caseous, gelatinous, and fetid discharge. **fibrinous r.,** membranous r. **hypertrophic r.,** that with thickening and swelling of the mucous membrane. **membranous r.,** fibrinous r.; chronic rhinitis with the formation of a false membrane, as in nasal diphtheria. **nonseasonal allergic r., perennial r.,** allergic rhinitis occurring continuously or intermittently all year round, due to exposure to a more or less ever-present allergen, marked by sudden attacks of sneezing, swelling of the nasal mucosa with profuse watery discharge, itching of the eyes, and lacrimation. **seasonal allergic r.,** hay fever. **vasomotor r.,** 1. nonallergic rhinitis in which symptoms like those of allergic rhinitis are brought on by such stimuli as chilling, fatigue, anger, or anxiety. 2. any condition of allergic or nonallergic rhinitis, as opposed to infectious rhinitis.

rhin(o)- word element [Gr.], *nose; nose-like structure.*

rhi·no·an·tri·tis (ri″no-an-tri′tis) inflammation of the nasal cavity and maxillary sinus.

rhi·no·can·thec·to·my (-kan-thek′tah-me) rhinommectomy.

rhi·no·cele (ri′no-sēl) rhinocoele.

rhi·no·ceph·a·ly (rhi″no-sef′ah-le) a developmental anomaly characterized by the presence of a proboscis-like nose above eyes partially or completely fused into one.

rhi·no·chei·lo·plas·ty (-ki′lo-plas″te) plastic surgery of the lip and nose.

rhi·no·coele (ri′no-sēl) the ventricle of the olfactory lobe of the brain.

rhi·no·dyn·ia (-din′e-ah) rhinalgia.

rhi·nog·e·nous (ri-noj′ĕ-nus) arising in the nose.

rhi·no·ky·pho·sis (ri″no-ki-fo′sis) an abnormal hump on the ridge of the nose.

rhi·no·la·lia (-la′le-ah) rhinophonia; a nasal quality of the voice from some disease or defect of the nasal passages, such as undue patency (*r. aper′ta*) or undue closure (*r. clau′sa*) of the posterior nares.

rhi·no·lar·yn·gi·tis (-lar″in-ji′tis) inflammation of the mucosa of the nose and larynx.

rhi·no·lith (ri′no-lith) a nasal stone or concretion.

rhi·no·li·thi·a·sis (ri″no-lĭ-thi′ah-sis) a condition associated with formation of rhinoliths.

rhi·nol·o·gist (ri-nol′ah-jist) a specialist in rhinology.

rhi·nol·o·gy (ri-nol′ah-je) the medical specialty that deals with the nose and its diseases.

rhi·no·ma·nom·e·try (ri″no-mah-nom′ĕ-tre) measurement of the airflow and pressure within the nose during respiration; nasal resistance or obstruction can be calculated from the figures obtained.

rhi·nom·mec·to·my (-mek′tah-me) excision of the inner canthus of the eye.

rhi·no·my·co·sis (-mi-ko′sis) fungal infection of the nasal mucosa.

rhi·no·ne·cro·sis (-nĕ-kro′sis) necrosis of the nasal bones.

rhi·nop·a·thy (ri-nop′ah-the) any disease of the nose.

rhi·no·phar·yn·gi·tis (ri″no-far″in-ji′tis) nasopharyngitis.

rhi·no·pho·nia (-fo′ne-ah) rhinolalia.

rhi·no·phy·co·my·co·sis (-fi″ko-mi-ko′sis) a fungal disease caused by *Entomophthora coronata,* marked by formation of large polyps in the subcutaneous tissues of the nose and paranasal sinuses; orbital involvement and unilateral blindness may follow. Cerebral involvement is common.

rhi·no·phy·ma (-fi′mah) a form of rosacea marked by redness, sebaceous hyperplasia, and nodular swelling and congestion of the skin of the nose.

rhi·no·plas·ty (ri′no-plas″te) plastic surgery of the nose.

rhi·nor·rha·gia (ri″no-ra′jah) epistaxis.

rhi·nor·rhea (-re′ah) the free discharge of a thin nasal mucus. **cerebrospinal fluid r.,** discharge of cerebrospinal fluid through the nose.

rhi·no·sal·pin·gi·tis (-sal″pin-ji′tis) inflammation of the mucosa of the nose and eustachian tube.

rhi·no·scle·ro·ma (-sklĕ-ro′mah) a granulomatous disease, ascribed to *Klebsiella rhinoscleromatis,* involving the nose and nasopharynx; the growth forms hard patches or nodules, which tend to enlarge and are painful to the touch.

rhi·no·scope (ri′no-skōp) a speculum for use in nasal examination.

rhi·nos·co·py (ri-nos′kah-pe) examination of the nose with a speculum, either through the anterior nares (*anterior r.)* or the nasopharynx (*posterior r.).*

rhi·no·si·nu·si·tis (ri″no-si″nŭ-si′tis) inflammation of the paranasal sinuses.

rhi·no·spo·rid·i·o·sis (-spor-id″e-o′sis) a fungal disease caused by *Rhinosporidium seeberi,* marked by large polyps on the mucosa of the nose, eyes, ears, and sometimes the penis and vagina.

rhi·not·o·my (ri-not′ah-me) incision into the nose.

Rhi·no·vi·rus (ri′no-vi″rus) a genus of viruses of the family Picornaviridae that infect the upper respiratory tract and cause the common cold. Over 100 antigenically distinct varieties infect humans.

rhi·no·vi·rus (ri′no-vi″rus) any virus belonging to the genus *Rhinovirus.*

Rhi·pi·ceph·a·lus (ri″pĭ-sef′ah-lus) a genus of cattle ticks, many species of which transmit disease-producing organisms, such as

Babesia ovis, B. canis, Rickettsia rickettsii, and *R. conorii.*

rhiz(o)- word element [Gr.], *root.*

rhi·zoid (ri'zoid) 1. resembling a root. 2. a filamentous structure of fungi and some algae that extends into the substrate.

rhi·zol·y·sis (ri-zol'ĭ-sis) percutaneous radiofrequency rhizotomy; percutaneous rhizotomy performed using radio waves.

rhi·zo·mel·ic (ri"zo-mel'ik) pertaining to the hips and shoulders (the roots of the limbs).

Rhi·zop·o·da (ri-zop'ah-dah) a superclass of protozoa of the subphylum Sarcodina, comprising the amebae.

Rhi·zo·pus (ri'zo-pus) a genus of fungi (order Mucorales); some species, including *R. arrhi'zus* and *R. rhizopodofor'mis,* cause mucormycosis.

rhi·zot·o·my (ri-zot'ah-me) interruption of a cranial or spinal nerve root, such as by chemicals or radio waves. **percutaneous r.,** that performed without brain surgery, such as by means of glycerol or radio waves.

rho·da·mine (ro'dah-mēn) any of a group of red fluorescent dyes used to label proteins in various immunofluorescence techniques.

rho·di·um (ro'de-um) chemical element (see *Table of Elements*), at. no. 45, symbol Rh.

Rhod·ni·us (rod'ne-us) a genus of winged hemipterous insects of South America. *R. prolix'us* transmits *Trypanosoma cruzi,* the cause of Chagas' disease.

rhod(o)- word element [Gr.], *red.*

Rho·do·coc·cus (ro"do-kok'us) a genus of nocardioform actinomycetes; *R. bronchia'lis* is associated with pulmonary disease in humans, and *R. e'qui* causes bronchopneumonia in foals and can infect immunocompromised humans.

rho·do·gen·e·sis (-jen'ĕ-sis) regeneration of rhodopsin after its bleaching by light.

rho·do·phy·lax·is (-fĭ-lak'sis) the ability of the retinal epithelium to regenerate rhodopsin. **rhodophylac'tic,** adj.

rho·dop·sin (ro-dop'sin) visual purple; a photosensitive purple-red chromoprotein in the retinal rods that is bleached to visual yellow (all-*trans* retinal) by light, thereby stimulating retinal sensory endings.

rhomb·en·ceph·a·lon (romb"en-sef'ah-lon) hindbrain. 1. the part of the brain developed from the posterior of the three primary brain vesicles of the embryonic neural tube; it comprises the metencephalon (cerebellum and pons) and myelencephalon (medulla oblongata). 2. the most caudal of the three primary brain vesicles in the embryo, later dividing into the metencephalon and myelencephalon.

rhom·bo·coele (rom'bo-sēl) the terminal expansion of the canal of the spinal cord.

rhom·boid (rom'boid) [Gr. *rhombos* rhomb + *-oid*] having a shape similar to a rectangle that has been skewed to one side so that the angles are oblique.

rhon·chus (rong'kus) pl. *rhon'chi.* [L.] a continuous snorelike sound in the throat or bronchial tubes, due to a partial obstruction. **rhon'chal, rhon'chial,** adj.

r-HuEPO epoetin (recombinant human erythropoietin).

Rhus (rus) a genus of trees and shrubs; contact with certain species produces a severe dermatitis in sensitive persons. The most important toxic species are: *R. diversilo'ba* and *R. toxicoden'dron,* or poison oak; *R. ra'dicans,* or poison ivy; and *R. ver'nix,* or poison sumac.

rhythm (rithm) a measured movement; the recurrence of an action or function at regular intervals. **rhyth'mic, rhyth'mical,** adj. **alpha r.,** electroencephalographic waves having a uniform rhythm and average frequency of 10 per second, typical of a normal person awake in a quiet resting state. **atrial escape r.,** a cardiac dysrhythmia occurring when sustained suppression of sinus impulse formation causes other atrial foci to act as cardiac pacemakers. **atrioventricular (AV) junctional r.,** the heart rhythm that results when the atrioventricular junction acts as pacemaker. **atrioventricular (AV) junctional escape r.,** a cardiac rhythm of four or more AV junctional escape beats at a rate below 60 beats per minute. **beta r.,** electroencephalographic waves having a frequency of 18 to 30 per second, typical during periods of intense activity of the nervous system. **circadian r.,** the regular recurrence in cycles of approximately 24 hours from one stated point to another, e.g., certain biological activities that occur at that interval regardless of constant darkness or other conditions of illumination. **coupled r.,** heart beats occurring in pairs, the second beat usually being a ventricular premature beat; see also *bigeminal pulse.* **delta r.,** rhythm on the electroencephalogram consisting of delta waves. **ectopic r.,** a heart rhythm initiated by a focus outside the sinoatrial node. **escape r.,** a heart rhythm initiated by lower centers when the sinoatrial node fails to initiate impulses, when its rhythmicity is depressed, or when its impulses are completely blocked. **gallop r.,** an auscultatory finding of three (*triple r.*) or four (*quadruple r.*) heart sounds; the extra sounds occur in diastole and are related either to atrial contraction (S_4 *gallop*), to early rapid filling of a ventricle (S_3 *gallop*), or to concurrence of both events *(summation gallop)*. **idioventricular r.,** a sustained series of impulses propagated by an independent pacemaker within the ventricles, with a rate of 20 to 50 beats per minute. **infradian r.,** the regular recurrence in cycles of more than 24 hours, as certain biological activities which occur at such intervals, regardless of conditions of illumination. **nodal r.,** atrioventricular junctional r. **pendulum r.,** alternation in the rhythm of the heart sounds in which the diastolic and systolic sounds are nearly identical and the heartbeat resembles the tick of a watch. **quadruple r.,** the gallop rhythm cadence produced when all four heart sounds recur in successive cardiac cycles. **reciprocal r.,** a cardiac dysrhythmia established by a sustained reentrant mechanism in which impulses traveling back toward the atria also travel forward to reexcite the ventricles, so that each cycle contains a reciprocal beat, with two ventricular contractions. **reciprocating r.,** a cardiac dysrhythmia in which an impulse initiated in the atrioventricular node travels toward both the atria and ventricles, followed by cycles of bidirectional propagation of the impulse alternately initiating from those impulses traveling up and those traveling down. **reentrant r.,** an abnormal cardiac rhythm resulting from reentry. **sinoatrial r., sinus r.,** the normal heart rhythm originating in the sinoatrial node. **supraventricular r.,** any cardiac rhythm originating above the ventricles. **theta r.,** rhythm on the electroencephalogram consisting of theta waves. **triple r.,** the cadence produced when three heart sounds recur in successive cardiac cycles; see also *gallop r.* **ultradian r.,** the regular recurrence in cycles of less than 24 hours, as certain biological activities which occur at such intervals, regardless of conditions of illumination. **ventricular r.,** 1. idioventricular r. 2. any cardiac rhythm controlled by a focus within the ventricles.

rhyth·mic·i·ty (rith-mis′ĭ-te) 1. the state of having rhythm. 2. automaticity (2).

rhy·tid (ri′tid) pl. *rhy′tides.* Skin wrinkle.

rhyt·i·dec·to·my (rit″ĭ-dek′tah-me) excision of skin for elimination of wrinkles.

rhyt·i·do·plas·ty (rit′ĭ-do-plas″te) rhytidectomy.

rhyt·i·do·sis (rit″ĭ-do′sis) a wrinkling, as of the cornea.

rib (rib) any one of the paired bones, 12 on either side, extending from the thoracic vertebrae toward the median line on the ventral aspect of the trunk, forming the major part of the thoracic skeleton; see also *Table*

of Bones. **abdominal r′s, asternal r′s,** false r′s. **cervical r.,** a supernumerary rib arising from a cervical vertebra. **false r′s,** the five lower ribs on either side, not attached directly to the sternum. **floating r′s,** the two lower false ribs on either side, usually without ventral attachment. **slipping r.,** one whose attaching cartilage is repeatedly dislocated. **true r′s,** the seven upper ribs on either side, connected to the sternum by their costal cartilages.

ri·ba·vi·rin (ri″bah-vi′rin) a broad-spectrum antiviral used in the treatment of severe viral pneumonia caused by respiratory syncytial virus, particularly in high-risk infants; also used in conjunction with interferon alfa-2b in the treatment of chronic hepatitis C.

ri·bo·fla·vin (ri′bo-fla″vin) vitamin B₂; a heat-stable, water-soluble flavin of the vitamin B complex, found in milk, organ meats, eggs, leafy green vegetables, whole grains and enriched cereals and breads, and various algae; it is an essential nutrient for humans and is a component of two coenzymes, FAD and FMN, of flavoproteins, which function as electron carriers in oxidation-reduction reactions. Deficiency of the vitamin is known as ariboflavinosis.

ri·bo·nu·cle·ase (ri″bo-noo′kle-ās) an enzyme which catalyzes the depolymerization of ribonucleic acid.

ri·bo·nu·cle·ic ac·id (-noo-kle′ik) RNA, a nucleic acid found in all living cells, constituting the genetic material in the RNA viruses, and playing a role in the flow of genetic information; it is a linear polymer which on hydrolysis yields adenine, guanine, cytosine, uracil, ribose, and phosphoric acid and which may contain extensive secondary structure. For specific types of RNA, see under *RNA.*

ri·bo·nu·cleo·pro·tein (-noo″kle-o-pro′tēn) a substance composed of both protein and ribonucleic acid. Abbreviated RNP.

ri·bo·nu·cleo·side (-noo′kle-o-sīd) a nucleoside in which the purine or pyrimidine base is combined with ribose.

ri·bo·nu·cleo·tide (-tīd) a nucleotide in which the purine or pyrimidine base is combined with ribose.

ri·bose (ri′bōs) an aldopentose present in ribonucleic acid (RNA).

ri·bo·some (ri′bo-sōm) any of the intracellular ribonucleoprotein particles concerned with protein synthesis; they consist of reversibly dissociable units and are found either bound to cell membranes or free in the cytoplasm. They may occur singly or occur in clusters (polyribosomes). **riboso′mal,** adj.

ri·bo·syl (-sil) a glycosyl radical formed from ribose.

ri·cin (ri'sin) a phytotoxin in the seeds of the castor oil plant (*Ricinus communis*), used in the synthesis of immunotoxins.

Ric·i·nus (ris'ĭ-nus) a genus of plants, including *R. commu'nis*, or castor oil plant, the seeds of which afford castor oil. See also *ricin*.

rick·ets (rik'ets) a condition due to vitamin D deficiency, especially in infancy and childhood, with disturbance of normal ossification, marked by bending and distortion of the bones, nodular enlargements on the ends and sides of the bones, delayed closure of the fontanelles, muscle pain, and sweating of the head. **adult r.**, osteomalacia. **familial hypophosphatemic r.**, any of several inherited disorders of proximal renal tubule function causing phosphate loss, hypophosphatemia, and skeletal deformities, including rickets and osteomalacia. **fetal r.**, achondroplasia. **hereditary hypophosphatemic r. with hypercalciuria**, a form of familial hypophosphatemic rickets; hypophosphatemia is accompanied by elevated serum 1,25-dihydroxyvitamin D, increased intestinal absorption of calcium and phosphate, and hypercalciuria. **hypophosphatemic r.**, any of a group of disorders characterized by rickets associated with hypophosphatemia, resulting from dietary phosphorus deficiency or due to defects in renal tubular function; skeletal deformities are present but hypocalcemia, myopathy, and tetany are absent and serum parathyroid hormone is normal. **oncogenous r.**, oncogenous osteomalacia occurring in children. **pseudovitamin D–deficiency r.**, vitamin D–dependent r., sometimes specifically the type I form. **refractory r.**, vitamin D–resistant r. **vitamin D–dependent r.**, either of two (types I and II) inherited disorders characterized by myopathy, hypocalcemia, moderate hypophosphatemia, secondary hyperparathyroidism, and subnormal serum concentrations of 1,25-dihydroxyvitamin D; type I can be overcome by high doses of vitamin D, but type II cannot. **vitamin D–resistant r.**, 1. X-linked hypophosphatemia. 2. any of a group of disorders characterized by rickets but not responding to high doses of vitamin D; most are forms of familial hypophosphatemic rickets.

Rick·ett·sia (rĭ-ket'se-ah) a genus of the tribe Rickettsieae, transmitted by lice, fleas, ticks, and mites to humans and other animals, causing various diseases. **R. a'kari**, the etiologic agent of rickettsialpox, transmitted by the mite *Allodermanyssus sanguineus* from the reservoir of infection in house mice. **R.**

austra'lis, the etiologic agent of North Queensland tick typhus, possibly transmitted by *Ixodes* ticks. **R. cono'rii**, the etiologic agent of boutonneuse fever (Marseilles fever, Mediterranean fever) and possibly of Indian tick typhus, Kenya typhus, and South American tick-bite fever; transmitted by *Rhipicephalus* and *Haemaphysalis* ticks. **R. prowaze'kii**, the etiologic agent of epidemic typhus and the latent infection Brill's disease, which are transmitted between humans via *Pediculus humanus*. **R. rickett'sii**, the etiologic agent of Rocky Mountain spotted fever, transmitted by *Dermacentor*, *Rhipicephalus*, *Haemaphysalis*, *Amblyomma*, and *Ixodes* ticks. **R. tsutsugamu'shi**, the etiologic agent of scrub typhus, transmitted by larval mites of the genus *Trombicula*, including *T. akamushi* and *T. deliensis*, from rodent reservoirs of infection.

rick·ett·sia (rĭ-ket'se-ah) pl. *rickett'siae*. An individual organism of the Rickettsiaceae. **rickett'sial**, adj.

Rick·ett·si·a·ceae (rĭ-ket″se-a'se-e) a family of the order Rickettsiales.

rick·ett·si·al (rĭ-ket'se-al) pertaining to or caused by rickettsiae.

Rick·ett·si·a·les (rĭ-ket″se-a'lēz) an order of gram-negative bacteria occurring as elementary bodies that typically multiply only inside cells of the host. Parasitic for vertebrates and invertebrates, which serve as vectors, they may be pathogenic for humans and other animals.

rick·ett·si·al·pox (rĭ-ket'se-al-poks″) a febrile disease with a vesiculopapular eruption, resembling chickenpox clinically, caused by *Rickettsia akari*.

rick·ett·si·ci·dal (rĭ-ket″sĭ-si'd'l) destructive to rickettsiae.

Rick·ett·si·eae (rik″et-si'e-e) a tribe of the family Rickettsiaceae.

rick·ett·si·o·sis (rĭ-ket″se-o'sis) infection with rickettsiae.

ridge (rij) a linear projection or projecting structure; a crest. **dental r.**, any linear elevation on the crown of a tooth. **dermal r's**, cristae cutis. **genital r., gonadal r.**, a bulge on the medial side of the embryonic mesonephros; the primordial germ cells become embedded in it, forming the primordium of the testis or ovary. **healing r.**, an indurated ridge that normally forms deep to the skin along the length of a healing wound. **interureteric r.**, a fold of mucous membrane extending across the bladder between the ureteric orifices. **mammary r.**, a ridge of thickened epithelium from axilla to groin on each side in the mammalian embryo, along which nipples and mammary glands develop, all but one pair usually disappearing in the human. **mesonephric r.,** the more lateral portion of the urogenital ridge, giving rise to the mesonephros. **rete r's,** inward projections of the epidermis into the dermis, as seen histologically in vertical sections. **synaptic r.,** a wedge-shaped projection of a cone pedicle or of a rod spherule, on either side of which lie the horizontal cells whose dendrites are inserted into the ridge. **urogenital r.,** a longitudinal ridge in the embryo, lateral to the mesentery, which later divides into the mesonephric and gonadal ridges.

rif·a·bu·tin (rif″ah-bu′tin) an antibacterial used for the prevention of disseminated *Mycobacterium avium* complex (MAC) disease in patients with advanced HIV infection.

rif·am·pi·cin (rif′am-pĭ-sin) rifampin.

rif·am·pin (rif-am′pin) a semisynthetic derivative of rifamycin, with the antibacterial actions and uses of the rifamycin group.

rif·a·my·cin (rif″ah-mi′sin) any of a family of antibiotics biosynthesized by a strain of *Streptomyces mediterranei,* effective against a broad spectrum of bacteria, including gram-positive cocci, some gram-negative bacilli, and *Mycobacterium tuberculosis* and certain other mycobacteria; used for the treatment of tuberculosis and the prophylaxis of meningococcal infections.

rif·a·pen·tine (-pen′tēn) a synthetic rifamycin antibiotic used in the treatment of pulmonary tuberculosis.

ri·gid·i·ty (rĭ-jid′ĭ-te) inflexibility or stiffness. **clasp-knife r.,** increased tension in the extensors of a joint when it is passively flexed, giving way suddenly on exertion of further pressure. **cogwheel r.,** tension in a muscle which gives way in little jerks when the muscle is passively stretched. **decerebrate r.,** rigid extension of an animal's legs as a result of decerebration; occurring in humans as a result of lesions in the upper brainstem.

rig·or (rig′er) [L.] chill; rigidity. **r. mor′tis,** the stiffening of a dead body accompanying depletion of adenosine triphosphate in the muscle fibers.

ril·u·zole (ril′u-zōl) a compound used to prolong survival time in the treatment of amyotrophic lateral sclerosis.

rim (rim) a border or edge. **bite r., occlusion r., record r.,** a border constructed on temporary or permanent denture bases in order to record the maxillomandibular relation and for positioning of the teeth.

ri·ma (ri′mah) pl. *ri′mae.* [L.] a cleft or crack. **r. glot′tidis,** the elongated opening between the true vocal cords and between the

arytenoid cartilages. **r. o′ris,** the opening of the mouth. **r. palpebra′rum,** palpebral fissure. **r. puden′di,** the cleft between the labia majora.

ri·man·ta·dine (ri-man′tah-dēn) an antiviral agent used in the prophylaxis and treatment of influenza A.

ri·mex·o·lone (rĭ-mek′sah-lōn″) a corticosteroid used as a topical antiinflammatory in the treatment of inflammation following eye surgery and of uveitis affecting the anterior structures of the eye.

rim·u·la (rim′u-lah) pl. *ri′mulae.* [L.] a minute fissure, especially of the spinal cord or brain.

ring (ring) 1. any annular or circular organ or area. 2. in chemistry, a collection of atoms united in a continuous or closed chain. **Albl's r.,** a ring-shaped shadow in radiographs of the skull, caused by aneurysm of a cerebral artery. **Bandl's r.,** pathologic retraction r.; see *retraction r.* **benzene r.,** the closed hexagon of carbon atoms in benzene, from which different benzene compounds are derived by replacement of hydrogen atoms. **Cannon's r.,** a focal contraction seen radiographically at the mid-third of the transverse colon, marking an area of overlap between the superior and inferior nerve plexuses. **common tendinous r.,** the annular ligament of origin common to the recti muscles of the eye, marking the edge of the optic canal and the inner part of the superior orbital fissure. **conjunctival r.,** a ring at the junction of the conjunctiva and cornea. **constriction r.,** a contracted area of the uterus, where the resistance of the uterine contents is slight, as over a depression in the contour of the fetus, or below the presenting part. **femoral r.,** the abdominal opening of the femoral canal, normally closed by the crural septum and peritoneum. **fibrous r's of heart,** see *anulus fibrosus* (1). **greater r. of iris,** the less coarsely striated outer concentric circle on the anterior surface of the iris. **inguinal r., deep,** an aperture in the transverse fascia for the spermatic cord or the round ligament. **inguinal r., superficial,** an opening in the aponeurosis of the external oblique muscle for the spermatic cord or the round ligament. **Kayser-Fleischer r.,** a gray-green to red-gold pigmented ring at the outer margin of the cornea, seen in progressive lenticular degeneration and pseudosclerosis. **Landolt's r's,** broken rings used in testing visual acuity. **lesser r. of iris,** the more coarsely striated inner concentric circle on the anterior surface of the iris. **mitral r.,** see *anulus fibrosus.* **retraction r.,** a ring-like thickening and indentation occurring in normal labor at the junction of the isthmus and corpus uteri, delineating the upper contracting portion and the lower dilating portion (*physiologic retraction r.*), or a persistent retraction ring in abnormal or prolonged labor that obstructs expulsion of the fetus (*pathologic retraction r.*). **Schwalbe's r.**, a circular ridge composed of collagenous fibers surrounding the outer margin of Descemet's membrane. **scleral r.**, a white ring seen adjacent to the optic disk in ophthalmoscopy when the retinal pigment epithelium and choroid do not extend to the disk. **tracheal r's**, tracheal cartilages: the 16 to 20 incomplete rings which, held together and enclosed by a strong, elastic, fibrous membrane, constitute the wall of the trachea. **tricuspid r.**, see *anulus fibrosus*. **tympanic r.**, the bony ring forming part of the temporal bone at birth and developing into the tympanic plate. **umbilical r.**, the aperture in the fetal abdominal wall through which the umbilical cord communicates with the fetus. **vascular r.**, a developmental anomaly of the aortic arch wherein the trachea and esophagus are encircled by vascular structures, many variations being possible.

ring·worm (ring'-werm) tinea.

ris·ed·ro·nate (ris-ed'ro-nāt'') an inhibitor of bone resorption used as the sodium salt in the treatment of osteitis deformans and for the prevention and treatment of osteoporosis.

ris·per·i·done (-per'ĭ-dōn) an antipsychotic agent, which may act by a combination of dopamine and serotonin antagonism.

RIST radioimmunosorbent test.

ri·sus (ri'sus) [L.] laughter. **r. sardo'nicus**, a grinning expression produced by spasm of facial muscles.

rit·o·drine (rit'o-drēn) a beta$_2$-adrenergic agonist used as the hydrochloride salt as a smooth muscle (uterine muscle) relaxant to delay uncomplicated premature labor.

ri·to·na·vir (rĭ-to'nah-vir) an HIV protease inhibitor used in treatment of HIV infection and AIDS.

ri·tux·i·mab (rĭ-tuk'sĭ-mab) a monoclonal antibody that binds the antigen CD20; used as an antineoplastic in the treatment of CD20-positive, B-cell non-Hodgkin's lymphoma.

ri·val·ry (ri'vul-re) a state of competition or antagonism. **sibling r.**, competition between siblings for the love, affection, and attention of one or both parents or for other recognition or gain.

riv·a·stig·mine (riv''ah-stig'mēn) a cholinesterase inhibitor used as the tartrate salt as an adjunct in the treatment of dementia of the Alzheimer type.

ri·za·trip·tan (ri''zah-trip'tan) a selective serotonin receptor agonist used as the benzoate salt in the acute treatment of migraine.

riz·i·form (riz'ĭ-form) resembling grains of rice.

RLF retinopathy of prematurity (retrolental fibroplasia).

RLL right lower lobe (of lungs).

RMA right mentoanterior (position of the fetus).

RML right middle lobe (of lungs).

RMP right mentoposterior (position of the fetus).

RMT right mentotransverse (position of the fetus).

RN registered nurse.

Rn radon.

RNA ribonucleic acid. **complementary RNA (cRNA)**, viral RNA that is transcribed from negative-sense RNA and serves as a template for protein synthesis. **heterogeneous nuclear RNA (hnRNA)**, a diverse group of long primary transcripts formed in the eukaryotic nucleus, many of which will be processed to mRNA molecules by splicing. **messenger RNA (mRNA)**, RNA molecules, usually 400 to 10,000 bases long, that serve as templates for protein synthesis (translation). **negative-sense RNA**, viral RNA with a base sequence complementary to that of mRNA; during replication it serves as a template for the transcription of viral complementary RNA. **positive-sense RNA**, viral RNA with the same base sequence as mRNA; during replication it functions as mRNA, serving as a template for protein synthesis. **ribosomal RNA (rRNA)**, that which together with proteins forms the ribosomes, playing a structural role and also a role in ribosomal binding of mRNA and tRNAs. **small nuclear RNA (snRNA)**, a class of eukaryotic small RNA molecules found in the nucleus, usually as ribonucleoproteins, and apparently involved in processing heterogeneous nuclear RNA. **transfer RNA (tRNA)**, 20 or more varieties of small RNA molecules functioning in translation; each variety carries a specific amino acid to a site specified by an RNA codon, binding to amino acid, ribosome, and to the codon via an anticodon region.

RNase ribonuclease.

ROA right occipitoanterior (position of the fetus).

Ro·cha·li·maea (ro''kah-li-me'ah) see *Bartonella*.

ro·cu·ro·ni·um (ro''ku-ro'ne-um) a nondepolarizing neuromuscular blocking agent, used as the bromide salt as an adjunct in

general anesthesia to facilitate endotracheal intubation and as a skeletal muscle relaxant during surgery or mechanical ventilation.

rod (rod) 1. a straight, slim mass of substance. 2. retinal rod. **Corti's r's**, pillar cells. **enamel r's**, the approximately parallel rods or prisms forming the enamel of the teeth. **olfactory r.**, the slender apical portion of an olfactory bipolar neuron, a modified dendrite extending to the surface of the epithelium. **retinal r.**, a specialized cylindrical segment of the visual cells containing rhodopsin; the rods serve night vision and detection of motion, and together with the retinal cones form the light-sensitive elements of the retina.

ro·dent (ro'dent) 1. an order of mammals characterized by large chisel-shaped incisors, including the rats, mice, and squirrels, many of which are reservoirs for infectious diseases. 2. gnawing; corroding.

ro·den·ti·cide (ro-den'tĭ-sīd) 1. destructive to rodents. 2. an agent destructive to rodents.

roent·gen (rent'gen) the international unit of x- or γ-radiation; it is the quantity of x- or γ-radiation such that the associated corpuscular emission per 0.001293 g of dry air produces in air ions carrying 1 electrostatic unit of electrical charge of either sign. Symbol R.

roent·gen·og·ra·phy (rent"gen-og'rah-fe) radiography. **roentgenograph'ic**, adj.

roent·gen·ol·o·gist (-ol'ah-jist) radiologist.

roent·gen·ol·o·gy (-ol'-ah-je) radiology.

roent·geno·scope (rent'gen-o-skōp") fluoroscope.

roent·gen·os·co·py (rent"gen-os'kah-pe) fluoroscopy.

ro·fe·cox·ib (ro"fĕ-cok'sib) a nonsteroidal anti-inflammatory drug used in the treatment of osteoarthritis, acute pain, and dysmenorrhea.

role (rōl) the behavior pattern that an individual presents to others. **gender r.**, the public expression of gender; the image projected by a person that identifies their maleness or femaleness, which need not correspond to their gender identity.

Rol·fing (rawl'fing) service mark for a bodywork technique consisting of systematic manipulation of the connective tissue in order to improve posture and to relieve chronic musculoskeletal pain and stress.

rom·berg·ism (rom'berg-izm) Romberg's sign.

ron·geur (raw-zhur') [Fr.] a forceps-like instrument for cutting tough tissue, particularly bone.

room (room) a place in a building, enclosed and set apart for occupancy or for performance of certain procedures. **operating r.**, one especially equipped for the performance of surgical operations. **recovery r.**, a hospital unit adjoining operating or delivery rooms, with special equipment and personnel for the care of patients immediately after operation or childbirth.

room·ing-in (room'ing-in") the practice of keeping a newborn infant in a crib near the mother's bed instead of in a nursery during the hospital stay.

root (root) that portion of an organ, such as a tooth, hair, or nail, that is buried in the tissues, or by which it arises from another structure. **anterior r. of spinal nerve**, the anterior, or motor, division of each spinal nerve, attached centrally to the spinal cord and joining peripherally with the posterior root to form the nerve before it emerges from the intervertebral foramen. **dorsal r. of spinal nerve**, posterior r. of spinal nerve. **motor r. of spinal nerve**, anterior r. of spinal nerve. **nerve r's**, the series of paired bundles of nerve fibers that emerge at each side of the spinal cord, termed posterior (or dorsal) or anterior (or ventral) according to their position. There are 31 pairs (8 cervical, 12 thoracic, 5 lumbar, 5 sacral, and 1 coccygeal), each corresponding posterior and anterior root joining to form a spinal nerve. Certain cranial nerves, e.g., the trigeminal, also have nerve roots. **posterior r. of spinal nerve**, the posterior, or sensory, division of each spinal nerve, attached centrally to the spinal cord and joining peripherally with the anterior root to form the nerve before it emerges from the intervertebral foramen. **sensory r.**, posterior r. of spinal nerve. **ventral r. of spinal nerve**, anterior r. of spinal nerve.

ROP right occipitoposterior (position of the fetus).

ro·pin·i·role (ro-pin'ĭ-rōl") a dopamine agonist used as the hydrochloride salt as an antidyskinetic in the treatment of Parkinson's disease.

ro·pi·va·caine (-piv'ah-kān) a local anesthetic of the amide type, used as the hydrochloride salt for percutaneous infiltration anesthesia, peripheral nerve block, and epidural block.

ro·sa·cea (ro-za'she-ah) a chronic disease of the skin of the nose, forehead, and cheeks, marked by flushing, followed by red coloration due to dilatation of the capillaries, with the appearance of papules and acne-like pustules.

ro·san·i·line (ro-zan′ĭ-lin) a triphenyl-methane derivative, the basis of various dyes and a component of basic fuchsin.

ro·sa·ry (ro′zah-re) a structure resembling a string of beads. **rachitic r.**, see under *bead*.

ro·se·o·la (ro-ze′o-lah, ro″ze-o′lah) [L.] 1. any rose-colored rash. 2. exanthema subitum. **r. infan′tum**, exanthema subitum. **syphilitic r.**, eruption of rose-colored spots in early secondary syphilis.

ro·sette (ro-zet′) [Fr.] any structure or formation resembling a rose, such as *(a)* the clusters of polymorphonuclear leukocytes around a globule of lipid nuclear material, as observed in the test for disseminated lupus erythematosus, or *(b)* a figure formed by the chromosomes in an early stage of mitosis. **Flexner-Wintersteiner r.**, a spoke- and wheel-shaped cell formation seen in retino-blastoma and certain other ophthalmic tumors. **Homer Wright r.**, a circular or spherical grouping of dark tumor cells around a pale, eosinophilic, central area that contains neurofibrils but lacks a lumen; seen in some medulloblastomas, neuroblastomas, and retinoblastomas or other ophthalmic tumors.

ro·sig·lit·a·zone (ro-sig-lit′ah-zōn) an anti-diabetic agent that increases insulin sensitivity, used as the maleate salt in the treatment of type 2 diabetes mellitus.

ro·sin (roz′in) a solid resin obtained from species of *Pinus*; it is used in preparation of ointments and plasters and in many products such as chewing gum, polishes, and varnishes, but is a common cause of contact allergy.

ros·tel·lum (ros-tel′um) pl. *rostel′la*. [L.] a small protuberance of beak, especially the fleshy protuberance of the scolex of a tape-worm, which may or may not bear hooks.

ros·trad (ros′trad) 1. toward a rostrum; nearer the rostrum in relation to a specific point of reference. 2. cephalad.

ros·tral (ros′tral) 1. pertaining to or resembling a rostrum; having a rostrum or beak. 2. situated toward a rostrum or toward the beak (oral and nasal region), which may mean superior (in relationships of areas of the spinal cord) or anterior or ventral (in relationships of brain areas).

ros·trate (ros′trāt) having a beaklike process.

ros·trum (ros′trum) pl. *ros′tra, rostrums*. [L.] a beak-shaped process.

rot (rot) 1. decay. 2. a disease of sheep, and sometimes of humans, due to *Fasciola hepatica*.

ro·tab·la·tion (ro″tab-la′shun) an atherec-tomy technique in which a rotating bur is inserted through a catheter into an artery; the burr rotates and debulks atherosclerotic plaque.

ro·ta·tion (ro-ta′shun) the process of turning around an axis. In obstetrics, the turning of the fetal head (or presenting part) for proper orientation to the pelvic axis. **ro′tary, ro′ta-tatory**, adj. **optical r.**, the quality of certain optically active substances whereby the plane of polarized light is changed, so that it is rotated in an arc the length of which is characteristic of the substance. **van Ness r.**, fusion of the knee joint and rotation of the ankle to function as the knee; done to correct a congenitally missing femur.

Ro·ta·vi·rus (ro′tah-vi″rus) rotaviruses; a genus of viruses of the family Reoviridae, having a wheel-like appearance, that cause acute infantile gastroenteritis and cause diarrhea in young children and many animal species.

ro·ta·vi·rus (ro′tah-vi″rus) any member of the genus *Rotavirus*. **ro′taviral**, adj.

ro·te·none (ro′tĕ-nōn) a poisonous compound from derris root and other roots; used as an insecticide.

rough·age (ruf′aj) indigestible material such as fibers or cellulose in the diet.

rou·leau (roo-lo′) pl. *rouleaux′*. [Fr.] an abnormal group of red blood cells adhering together like a roll of coins.

round·worm (round′werm) any worm of the class Nematoda; a nematode.

RPF renal plasma flow.

R Ph Registered Pharmacist.

rpm revolutions per minute.

RQ respiratory quotient.

RRA Registered Record Administrator.

-rrhage, -rrhagia word element [Gr.], *excessive flow*. **-rrha′gic**, adj.

-rrhea word element [Gr.], *profuse flow*. **-rrheic**, adj.

-rrhexis word element [Gr.], *breaking; rupturing; splitting*.

rRNA ribosomal RNA.

RSA right sacroanterior (position of the fetus).

RScA right scapuloposterior (position of the fetus).

RScP right scapuloposterior (position of the fetus).

RSP right sacroposterior (position of the fetus).

RST right sacrotransverse (position of the fetus).

RSV respiratory syncytial virus; Rous sarcoma virus.

RTF resistance transfer factor.

Ru ruthenium.

RU-486 mifepristone.

rub (rub) 1. to move something over a surface with friction. 2. the action of such movement. 3. friction rub **friction r.**, an auscultatory sound caused by the rubbing together of two serous surfaces, as in pericardial rub. **pericardial r., pericardial friction r.,** a scraping or grating friction rub heard with the heart beat, usually a to-and-fro sound, associated with pericarditis or other pathological condition of the pericardium. **pleural r., pleuritic r.,** a friction rub caused by friction between the visceral and costal pleurae.

ru·be·fa·cient (roo″bĕ-fa′shunt) 1. reddening the skin by producing hyperemia. 2. an agent that so acts.

ru·bel·la (roo-bel′ah) German measles: a mild viral infection marked by a pink macular rash, fever, and lymph node enlargement most often affecting children and nonimmune young adults; transplacental infection of the fetus in the first trimester may produce death of the conceptus or severe developmental anomalies. See also *congenital rubella syndrome*, under *syndrome*.

ru·be·o·la (roo-be′o-lah, roo″be-o′lah) a synonym of measles in English and of German measles in French and Spanish.

ru·be·o·sis (roo″be-o′sis) redness. **r. i′ridis,** a condition characterized by a new formation of vessels and connective tissue on the surface of the iris, frequently seen in diabetics.

ru·ber (roo′ber) [L.] red.

ru·bes·cent (roo-bes′int) growing red; reddish.

ru·bid·i·um (roo-bid′e-um) chemical element (see *Table of Elements*), at. no. 37, symbol Rb. **r. 82,** a radioactive isotope of rubidium having a half-life of 1.273 minutes and decaying by positron emission; used as a tracer in positron emission tomography.

Ru·bi·vi·rus (roo′bĭ-vi″rus) rubella virus; a genus of viruses of the family Togaviridae containing the causative agent of rubella.

ru·bor (roo′bor) [L.] redness, one of the cardinal signs of inflammation.

ru·bra (roo′brah) [L.] red.

ru·bri·blast (roo′brĭ-blast) proerythroblast.

ru·bric (roo′brik) red; specifically, pertaining to the red nucleus.

ru·bri·cyte (roo′brĭ-sīt) polychromatophilic erythroblast.

ru·bro·spi·nal (roo″bro-spi′n′l) pertaining to the red nucleus and the spinal cord.

ru·bro·tha·lam·ic (-thah-lam′ik) pertaining to the red nucleus and the thalamus.

Ru·bu·la·vi·rus (roo′bu-lah-vi″rus) a genus of viruses of the subfamily Paramyxovirinae (family Paramyxoviridae) containing a number of species that cause disease in humans and other animals.

ru·di·ment (roo′dĭ-ment) 1. a structure that has remained undeveloped, or one with little or no function at present but which was functionally developed earlier. 2. primordium.

ru·di·men·ta·ry (roo″dĭ-men′tah-re) 1. imperfectly developed. 2. vestigial.

ru·di·men·tum (roo″dĭ-men′tum) pl. *rudimen′ta.* [L.] rudiment.

ru·ga (roo′gah) pl. *ru′gae.* [L.] a ridge or fold. **ru′gose,** adj.

ru·gos·i·ty (roo-gos′ĭ-te) 1. a condition of being rugose. 2. a fold, wrinkle, or ruga.

RUL right upper lobe (of lung).

rule (rool) a statement of conditions commonly observed in a given situation, or of a prescribed procedure to obtain a given result. **Durham r.,** a definition of criminal responsibility from a federal appeals court case, Durham vs. United States, holding that "an accused is not criminally responsible if his unlawful act was the product of mental disease or mental defect." In 1972 the same court reversed itself and adopted the American Law Institute Formulation. **M'Naghten r.,** a definition of criminal responsibility formulated in 1843 by English judges questioned by the House of Lords as a result of the acquittal of Daniel M'Naghten on grounds of insanity. It holds that "to establish a defense on the ground of insanity, it must be clearly proved that at the time of committing the act the party accused was laboring under such a defect of reason from disease of the mind as not to know the nature and quality of the act he was doing, or, if he did know it, that he did not know that what he was doing was wrong." **Nägele's r.,** (for predicting day of labor) subtract three months from the first day of the last menstruation and add seven days. **r. of nines,** a method of estimating the extent of body surface that has been burned in an adult, dividing the body into sections of 9 per cent or multiples of 9 per cent. **van't Hoff's r.,** the velocity of chemical reactions is increased twofold or more for each rise of 10°C in temperature; generally true only when temperatures approximate those normal for the reaction.

ru·mi·nant (roo′mĭ-nant) 1. chewing the cud. 2. one of the order of animals, including cattle, sheep, goats, deer, and antelopes, which have a stomach with four complete cavities (rumen, reticulum, omasum, abomasum), through which the food passes in digestion.

ru·mi·na·tion (roo″mĭ-na′shun) 1. the casting up of the food to be chewed thoroughly a second time, as in cattle. 2. in humans, the regurgitation of food after almost every meal, part of it being vomited and the rest swallowed: a condition sometimes seen in infants (*rumination disorder*) or in mentally retarded individuals. 3. meditation.

rump (rump) the buttock or gluteal region.

ru·pia (roo'pe-ah) thick, dark, raised, lamellated, adherent crusts on the skin, somewhat resembling oyster shells, as in late recurrent secondary syphilis. **ru'pial,** adj.

rup·ture (rup'chur) 1. tearing or disruption of tissue. 2. to forcibly disrupt tissue. 3. hernia.

rush (rush) peristaltic rush; a powerful wave of contractile activity that travels very long distances down the small intestine, caused by intense irritation or unusual distention.

ru·the·ni·um (roo-the'ne-um) chemical element (see *Table of Elements*), at. no. 44, symbol Ru.

ruth·er·ford (ruth'er-ferd) a unit of radioactive disintegration, representing one million disintegrations per second.

RV residual volume.

RVA rabies vaccine adsorbed; see *rabies vaccine*, *under vaccine*.

RVAD right ventricular assist device; see *ventricular assist device*, under *device*.

S

S spherical lens; serine; siemens; substrate; sulfur; Svedberg unit; sacral vertebrae (S1–S5); heart sound (S₁–S₄).

S. [L.] sig'na (mark).

S entropy.

S- a stereodescriptor used to specify the absolute configuration of compounds having asymmetric carbon atoms; opposed to *R-*.

s second.

s. [L.] se'mis (half); sinis'ter (left).

[L.] si'ne (without).

SA sinoatrial.

sab·u·lous (sab'u-lus) gritty or sandy.

sa·bur·ra (sah-bur'ah) foulness of the mouth or stomach. **sabur'ral,** adj.

sac (sak) a pouch or bag. **air s's,** alveolar s's. **allantoic s.,** the dilated portion of the allantois, becoming a part of the placenta in many mammals; it becomes the urachus in humans. **alveolar s's,** the spaces into which the alveolar ducts open distally, and with which the alveoli communicate. **amniotic s.,** that formed by the amnion, containing the amniotic fluid. **chorionic s.,** that formed by the vertebrate chorion, surrounding the embryo, amniotic cavity, and amniotic sac and contributing to the fetal part of the placenta. **conjunctival s.,** the potential space, lined by conjunctiva, between the eyelids and eyeball. **dental s.,** the dense fibrous layer of mesenchyme surrounding the enamel organ and dental papilla. **endolymphatic s.,** the blind, flattened cerebral end of the endolymphatic duct. **gestational s.,** that comprising the extraembryonic membranes that envelop the embryo or fetus; in humans, that formed by the fused amnion and chorion. **heart s.,** pericardium. **hernial s.,** the peritoneal pouch enclosing a hernia. **Hilton's s.,** laryngeal saccule. **lacrimal s.,** the dilated upper end of the nasolacrimal duct. **yolk s.,** the extraembryonic membrane that connects with the midgut; at the end of the fourth week of development it expands into a pear-shaped vesicle (*umbilical vesicle*) connected to the body of the embryo by a long narrow tube (*yolk stalk*). In mammals, it produces a complete vitelline circulation in the early embryo and then undergoes regression.

sac·cade (sah-kād') [Fr.] the series of involuntary, abrupt, rapid, small movements or jerks of both eyes simultaneously in changing the point of fixation. **saccad'ic,** adj.

sac·cate (sak'āt) 1. saccular. 2. contained in a sac.

sac·cha·ride (sak'ah-rīd) one of a series of carbohydrates, including the sugars.

sac·cha·rin (sak'ah-rin) a white, crystalline compound several hundred times sweeter than sucrose; used as the base or the calcium or sodium salt as a flavor and nonnutritive sweetener.

sacchar(o)- word element [L.], *sugar*.

sac·cha·ro·lyt·ic (sak″ah-ro-lit'ik) capable of breaking the glycosidic bonds in saccharides.

sac·cha·ro·me·tab·o·lism (-mĕ-tab'o-lizm) metabolism of sugar. **saccharometabol'ic,** adj.

Sac·cha·ro·my·ces (-mi'sēz) a genus of yeasts, including *S. cerevis'iae*, or brewers' yeast. **saccharomycet'ic,** adj.

sac·cha·ro·pine (sak′ah-ro-pēn) an intermediate in the metabolism of lysine, accumulating abnormally in some disorders of lysine degradation.

sac·cha·ro·pin·emia (sak″ah-ro-pĭ-ne′me-ah) an excess of saccharopine in the blood.

sac·cha·ro·pin·uria (-pĭ-nu′re-ah) 1. excretion of saccharopine in the urine. 2. a variant form of hyperlysinemia, clinically similar but having higher urinary saccharopine and lower lysine levels.

sac·ci·form (sak′sĭ-form) saccular.

sac·cu·lar (sak′u-ler) pertaining to or resembling a sac.

sac·cu·lat·ed (sak′u-lāt″ed) containing saccules.

sac·cu·la·tion (sak″u-la′shun) 1. a saccule or pouch. 2. the quality of being sacculated.

sac·cule (sak′ūl) 1. a little bag or sac. 2. the smaller of the two divisions of the membranous labyrinth of the ear. **alveolar s′s,** see under *sac.* **laryngeal s.,** a diverticulum extending upward from the front of the laryngeal ventricle.

sac·cu·lo·coch·le·ar (sak″u-lo-kok′le-er) pertaining to the saccule and cochlea.

sac·cu·lus (sak′u-lus) pl. *sac′culi.* [L.] saccule.

sac·cus (sak′us) pl. *sac′ci.* [L.] sac.

sa·crad (sa′krad) toward the sacrum.

sa·cral (sa′kral) pertaining to the sacrum.

sa·cral·gia (sa-kral′jah) pain in the sacrum.

sa·cral·iza·tion (sa″kral-ĭ-za′shun) anomalous fusion of the fifth lumbar vertebra with the first segment of the sacrum.

sa·crec·to·my (sa-krek′tah-me) excision or resection of the sacrum.

sacr(o)- word element [L.], *sacrum.*

sa·cro·coc·cy·ge·al (sa″kro-kok-sij′e-al) pertaining to the sacrum and coccyx.

sa·cro·dyn·ia (-din′e-ah) sacralgia.

sa·cro·il·i·ac (-il′e-ak) pertaining to the sacrum and ilium, or to their articulation.

sa·cro·lum·bar (-lum′bar) pertaining to the sacrum and loins.

sa·cro·sci·at·ic (-si-at′ik) pertaining to the sacrum and ischium.

sac·ro·sid·ase (sak-ro′sĭ-dās) an enzyme used as a substitute to replace the sucrase activity lacking in sucrase-isomaltase deficiency.

sa·cro·spi·nal (sa″kro-spi′n′l) pertaining to the sacrum and the spinal column.

sa·cro·ver·te·bral (-ver′tĕ-bral) pertaining to the sacrum and vertebrae.

sa·crum (sa′krum) [L.] see *Table of Bones.* **scimitar s.,** a congenitally deformed sacrum resembling a scimitar, usually accompanied by other defects such as anorectal or neural anomalies.

SAD seasonal affective disorder.

sa·dism (sa′dizm, sad′izm) the act or instance of gaining pleasure from inflicting physical or psychological pain on another; the term is usually used to denote *sexual s.* **sadis′tic,** adj.

sexual s., a paraphilia in which sexual gratification is derived from inflicting physical or psychological pain on another.

sa·do·ma·so·chism (sa″do-mas′o-kizm) a state characterized by both sadistic and masochistic tendencies. **sadomasochis′tic,** adj.

sage (sāj) *Salvia officinalis,* an herb whose leaves contain a volatile oil and are sudorific, carminative, and astringent; they are used as an antisecretory agent in hyperhidrosis, sialorrhea, pharyngitis, and bronchitis.

sag·it·tal (saj′ĭ-t′l) 1. shaped like an arrow. 2. situated in the direction of the sagittal suture; said of an anteroposterior plane or section parallel to the median plane of the body.

sag·it·ta·lis (saj″ĭ-ta′lis) [L.] sagittal.

St. John's wort (sānt jonz wort) any of various species of the genus *Hypericum; H. perforatum* is used as a mild antidepressant, sedative, and anxiolytic, and is also used topically for inflammation of the skin, contusions, myalgia, and first-degree burns.

Sak·se·naea (sak″sĕ-ne′ah) a genus of fungi of the order Mucorales, characterized by flask-shaped sporangia; *S. vasifor′mis* can cause severe opportunistic mucormycosis in debilitated or immunocompromised patients.

sal·bu·ta·mol (sal-bu′tah-mol) albuterol.

sal·i·cin (sal′ĭ-sin) a precursor of salicylic acid, contained in the bark of the willow and poplar, that is responsible for the antiinflammatory and antipyretic effects of willow bark.

sal·i·cyl·amide (sal″ĭ-sil-am′īd) an amide of salicylic acid used as an analgesic and antipyretic.

sal·i·cyl·ate (sal′ĭ-sil″āt, sah-lis′ĭ-lāt) 1. a salt, anion, or ester of salicylic acid. 2. any of a group of related compounds derived from salicylic acid, which inhibit prostaglandin synthesis and have analgesic, antipyretic, and antiinflammatory activity; included are *acetylsalicylic acid, choline s., magnesium s.,* and *sodium s.* **methyl s.,** see under *methyl.*

sal·i·cyl·ic ac·id (sal″ĭ-sil′ik) a topical keratolytic and caustic; see also *salicylate.*

sal·i·cyl·ism (sal′ĭ-sil″izm) toxic effects of overdosage with salicylic acid or its salts, usually marked by tinnitus, nausea, and vomiting.

sal·i·cyl·ur·ic ac·id (sal″ĭ-sil-ūr′ik) the glycine conjugate of salicylic acid, a form in which salicylates are excreted in the urine.

sal·i·fi·a·ble (sal″ĭ-fi′ah-b'l) capable of combining with an acid to form a salt.

sa·line (sa′lēn, sa′līn) salty; of the nature of a salt; containing a salt or salts. **normal s., physiological s.,** physiologic saline solution.

sal·i·va (sah-li′vah) the enzyme-containing secretion of the salivary glands. **sal′ivary,** adj.

sal·i·vant (sal′ĭ-vant) provoking a flow of saliva.

sal·i·va·tion (sal″ĭ-va′shun) 1. the secretion of saliva. 2. ptyalism.

sal·met·er·ol (sal-met′er-ol) a β_2-adrenergic receptor agonist, used as *s. xinafoate* as a bronchodilator.

Sal·mo·nel·la (sal″mo-nel′ah) a genus of gram-negative bacteria. The genus *Salmonella* is very complex and has been described by several different systems of nomenclature. Clinical laboratories frequently report salmonellae as one of three species, differentiated on the basis of serologic and biochemical reactions: *S. ty′phi, S. choleraesu′is,* and *S. enter′i′tidis;* the last contains all serotypes except the first two. In this system many strains familiarly named as species are designated as serotypes of *S. enteritidis.* Salmonellae may also be grouped into five subgenera (I–V) on the basis of biochemical reactions and further into species on the basis of antigenic reactions; subgenus I contains most of the species. Pathogenic species include *S. arizo′nae* (salmonellosis), *S. choleraesuis* (a strain pathogenic for pigs that may infect humans), *S. enteritidis* (gastroenteritis), *S. enteritidis* serotype *para-ty′phi A* (paratyphoid fever), *S. typhi* (typhoid fever), and *S. enteritidis* serotype *typhimu′rium* (food poisoning and paratyphoid fever).

sal·mo·nel·la (sal″mo-nel′ah) pl. *salmonel′lae.* Any organism of the genus *Salmonella.* **salmonel′lal,** adj.

sal·mo·nel·lo·sis (sal″mo-nel-o′sis) infection with *Salmonella.*

sal·pin·gec·to·my (sal″pin-jek′tah-me) tubectomy; excision of a uterine tube.

sal·pin·gem·phrax·is (sal″pin-jem-frak′sis) obstruction of an auditory tube.

sal·pin·gi·an (sal-pin′je-an) tubal.

sal·pin·gi·tis (sal″pin-ji′tis) inflammation of an auditory or a uterine tube. **salpingit′ic,** adj.

salping(o)- word element [Gr.], *tube (eustachian tube* or *uterine tube).*

sal·pin·go·cele (sal-ping′go-sēl) hernial protrusion of a uterine tube.

sal·pin·gog·ra·phy (sal″ping-gog′rah-fe) radiography of the uterine tubes after injection of a radiopaque medium.

sal·pin·gol·y·sis (sal″ping-gol′ĭ-sis) surgical separation of adhesions involving the uterine tubes.

sal·pin·go-ooph·o·rec·to·my (sal-ping″go-o-of″ah-rek′tah-me) excision of a uterine tube and ovary.

sal·pin·go-ooph·o·ri·tis (-o-of″ah-ri′tis) inflammation of a uterine tube and ovary.

sal·pin·go-ooph·oro·cele (-o-of′ah-ro-sēl″) hernia of a uterine tube and ovary.

sal·pin·go·pexy (sal-ping′go-pek″se) fixation of a uterine tube.

sal·pin·go·pha·ryn·ge·al (sal-ping″go-fah-rin′je-al) pertaining to the auditory tube and the pharynx.

sal·pin·go·plas·ty (sal-ping′go-plas″te) plastic repair of a uterine tube.

sal·pin·gos·co·py (sal″ping-gos′kah-pe) endoscopic visualization of the uterine tubes via the fimbrial ends of the tubes.

sal·pin·gos·to·my (sal″ping-gos′tah-me) 1. formation of an opening or fistula into a uterine tube. 2. surgical restoration of the patency of a uterine tube.

sal·pin·got·o·my (sal″ping-got′ah-me) surgical incision of a uterine tube.

sal·pinx (sal′pinks) [Gr.] a tube, particularly an auditory tube or a uterine tube.

sal·sa·late (sal′sah-lāt) a salicylate with analgesic, antipyretic, and anti-inflammatory actions; used in the treatment of osteoarthritis and rheumatoid arthritis.

salt (sawlt) 1. sodium chloride, or common salt. 2. any compound of a base and an acid; any compound of an acid some of whose replaceable atoms have been substituted. 3. in the plural, a saline cathartic. **bile s's,** glycine or taurine conjugates of bile acids, which are formed in the liver and secreted in the bile. They are powerful detergents which break down fat globules, enabling them to be digested. **Epsom s.,** magnesium sulfate. **Glauber's s.,** sodium sulfate. **oral rehydration s's (ORS),** a dry mixture of sodium chloride, potassium chloride, dextrose, and either sodium citrate or sodium bicarbonate; dissolved in water for use in treatment of dehydration. **smelling s's,** aromatized ammonium carbonate; stimulant and restorative.

sal·ta·tion (sal-ta′shun) 1. the action of leaping. 2. the jerky dancing or leaping that sometimes occurs in chorea. 3. saltatory conduction. 4. in genetics, an abrupt variation in species; a mutation. 5. sudden increases or changes in the course of an illness. **sal′tatory,** adj.

salt·ing out (sawl′ting out) the precipitation of proteins by raising the salt concentration.

sa·lu·bri·ous (sah-loo′bre-us) conducive to health; wholesome.

sal·ure·sis (sal″u-re′sis) urinary excretion of sodium and chloride ions.

sal·uret·ic (-u-ret′ik) 1. pertaining to, characterized by, or promoting saluresis. 2. an agent that so acts.

salve (sav) ointment.

sa·mar·i·um (sah-mar′e-um) chemical element (see *Table of Elements*), at. no. 62, symbol Sm. The complex *s. Sm 153 lexidronam* is used in the palliative treatment of bone pain associated with osteoblastic metastatic bone lesions.

sam·pling (sam′pling) the selection or making of a sample. **chorionic villus s. (CVS),** any of several procedures for obtaining fetal tissue to use in prenatal diagnosis, performed at 9 to 12 weeks' gestation, usually by means of a catheter passed through the cervix or by a needle inserted through the abdominal and uterine walls. **percutaneous umbilical blood s. (PUBS),** cordocentesis.

san·a·tive (san′ah-tiv) curative; healing.

san·a·to·ri·um (san″ah-tor′e-um) an institution for treatment of sick persons, especially a private hospital for convalescents or patients with chronic diseases or mental disorders.

san·a·to·ry (san′ah-tor″e) conducive to health.

sanc·tu·ary (sangk′choo-ar″e) an area in the body where a drug tends to collect and to escape metabolic breakdown.

sand (sand) material occurring in small, gritty particles. **brain s.,** sand bodies.

sand·fly (sand′fli) any of various two-winged flies, especially of the genus *Phlebotomus.*

sane (sān) sound in mind.

sangui- word element [L.], *blood.*

san·gui·fa·cient (sang″gwĭ-fa′shent) hematopoietic.

san·guine (sang′gwin) 1. plethoric. 2. ardent or hopeful.

san·guin·e·ous (sang-gwin′e-us) 1. plethoric. 2. hemic.

san·guin·o·lent (-ah-lent) of a bloody tinge.

san·gui·no·pu·ru·lent (sang″gwĭ-no-pu′roo-lent) containing both blood and pus.

san·guis (sang′gwis) [L.] blood.

sa·ni·es (sa′ne-ēz) a fetid ichorous discharge containing serum, pus, and blood. **sa′nious,** adj.

sa·nio·pu·ru·lent (sa″ne-o-pu′roo-lent) partly sanious and partly purulent.

sa·nio·se·rous (-sēr′us) partly sanious and partly serous.

san·i·tar·i·an (san″ĭ-tar′e-an) one skilled in sanitation and public health science.

san·i·tar·i·um (-tar′e-um) an institution for the promotion of health.

san·i·tary (san′ĭ-tar″e) promoting or pertaining to health.

san·i·ta·tion (san″ĭ-ta′shun) the establishment of conditions favorable to health.

san·i·ti·za·tion (-tĭ-za′shun) the process of making or the quality of being made sanitary.

san·i·ty (san″ĭ-te) soundness, especially of mind.

SAP sphingolipid activator protein.

sa·phe·na (sah-fe′nah) [L.] the small saphenous or the great saphenous vein; see *Table of Veins.*

sa·phe·nous (sah-fe′nus) pertaining to or associated with a saphena; applied to certain arteries, nerves, veins, etc.

sa·po·na·ceous (sa″po-na′shus) soapy; of soaplike feel or quality.

sa·pon·i·fi·ca·tion (sah-pon″ĭ-fĭ-ka′shun) conversion of an oil or fat into a soap by combination with an alkali. In chemistry, the term now denotes hydrolysis of an ester by an alkali, producing a free alcohol and an alkali salt of the ester acid.

sap·o·nin (sap′o-nin) any of a group of glycosides widely distributed in plants, which form a durable foam when their watery solutions are shaken, and which even in high dilutions dissolve erythrocytes.

sapr(o)- word element [Gr.], *decay; decayed matter.*

sa·probe (sa′prōb) an organism, usually referring to a fungus, that feeds on dead or decaying organic matter. **sapro′bic,** adj.

sap·ro·phyte (sap′ro-fīt) any organism living upon dead or decaying organic matter. For fungi, the preferred term is *saprobe.* **saprophyt′ic,** adj.

sap·ro·zo·ic (sap″ro-zo′ik) living on decayed organic matter; said of animals, especially protozoa.

sa·quin·a·vir (sah-kwin′ah-vir) an HIV protease inhibitor that causes formation of immature, noninfectious viral particles; used as the base or the mesylate salt in treatment of HIV infection and AIDS.

sar·al·a·sin (sar-al′ah-sin) an angiotensin II antagonist, used in the form of the acetate ester as an antihypertensive in the treatment of severe hypertension and in the diagnosis of renin-dependent hypertension.

Sar·ci·na (sahr′sĭ-nah) a genus of bacteria (family Micrococcaceae) found in soil and water as saprophytes.

sarc(o)- word element [Gr.], *flesh.*

sar·co·blast (sahr′ko-blast) myoblast.

sar·co·cyst (-sist) 1. a protozoon of the genus *Sarcocystis.* 2. a cylindrical cyst containing parasitic spores, found in muscles of those infected with *Sarcocystis.*

Sar·co·cys·tis (sahr″ko-sis′tis) a genus of parasitic protozoa that occur as sporocysts in the muscle tissue of mammals, birds, and reptiles.

sar·co·cys·to·sis (-sis-to′sis) infection with protozoa of the genus *Sarcocystis*, which in humans is usually asymptomatic or manifested by muscle cysts associated with myositis or myocarditis or by intestinal infection. It is usually transmitted by eating undercooked beef or pork containing sporocysts or by ingestion of sporocysts from the feces of an infected animal.

Sar·co·di·na (-di′nah) a subphylum of protozoa consisting of organisms that alter their body shape and that move about and acquire food either by means of pseudopodia or by protoplasmic flow without producing discrete pseudopodia.

sar·coid (sahr′koid) 1. sarcoidosis. 2. a sarcoma-like tumor. 3. fleshlike.

sar·coi·do·sis (sahr″koi-do′sis) a chronic, progressive, generalized granulomatous reticulosis involving almost any organ or tissue, characterized by the presence in all affected tissues of noncaseating epithelioid cell tubercles.

sar·co·lem·ma (sahr″ko-lem′ah) the membrane covering a striated muscle fiber. **sarcolem′mic, sarcolem′mous,** adj.

sar·co·ma (sahr-ko′mah) pl. *sarcomas, sarco′mata.* Any of a group of tumors usually arising from connective tissue, although the term now includes some of epithelial origin; most are malignant. **alveolar soft part s.,** a well-circumscribed, painless, highly metastatic neoplasm with a distinctive alveolar pattern, usually in the limbs, head, and neck of young adults. **ameloblastic s.,** see under *fibrosarcoma.* **botryoid s., s. botryoi′des,** an embryonal rhabdomyosarcoma arising in submucosal tissue, usually in the upper vagina, cervix uteri, or neck of urinary bladder in young children and infants, presenting grossly as a polypoid grapelike structure. **clear cell s. of kidney,** a malignant kidney tumor similar to Wilms' tumor but with poorer prognosis, often metastasizing to bone. **endometrial stromal s.,** a pale, polypoid, fleshy, malignant tumor of the endometrial stroma. **Ewing's s.,** a highly malignant, metastatic, primitive small round cell tumor of bone, usually in the diaphyses of long bones, ribs, and flat bones of children and adolescents. **giant cell s.,** 1. a form of giant cell tumor of bone arising malignant de novo rather than transforming to malignancy. 2. sarcoma characterized by large anaplastic (giant) cells. **hemangioendothelial s.,** hemangiosarcoma. **immunoblastic s. of B cells,** large cell immunoblastic lymphoma composed predominantly of B cells. **immunoblastic s. of T cells,** large cell immunoblastic lymphoma composed predominantly of T cells. **Kaposi s.,** a multicentric, malignant neoplastic vascular proliferation, characterized by the development of bluish-red nodules on the skin, sometimes with widespread visceral involvement; a particularly virulent, disseminated form occurs in immunocompromised patients. **Kupffer cell s.,** hepatic angiosarcoma. **osteogenic s.,** osteosarcoma. **pseudo–Kaposi s.,** unilateral subacute to chronic dermatitis occurring in association with an underlying arteriovenous fistula and closely resembling Kaposi's sarcoma clinically and histologically. **reticulum cell s.,** histiocytic lymphoma. **Rous s.,** a virus-induced sarcoma-like growth of fowls. **soft tissue s.,** a general term for a malignant tumor derived from extraskeletal connective tissue, including fibrous, fat, smooth muscle, nerve, vascular, histiocytic, and synovial tissue, with almost all lesions arising from primitive mesoderm. **spindle cell s.,** 1. any sarcoma composed of spindle-shaped cells. 2. a type of soft tissue sarcoma whose cells are spindle-shaped and which is usually resistant to radiation therapy.

sar·co·ma·toid (-toid) resembling a sarcoma.

sar·co·ma·to·sis (sahr-ko″mah-to′sis) a condition characterized by development of many sarcomas at various sites.

sar·co·ma·tous (sahr-ko′mah-tus) pertaining to or of the nature of a sarcoma.

sar·co·mere (sahr′ko-mēr) the contractile unit of a myofibril; sarcomeres are repeating units, delimited by the Z bands, along the length of the myofibril.

sar·co·pe·nia (sahr″ko-pe′ne-ah) age-related reduction in skeletal muscle mass in the elderly.

sar·co·plasm (sahr′ko-plazm) the interfibrillary matter of striated muscle. **sarcoplas′mic,** adj.

sar·co·plast (-plast) an interstitial cell of muscle, itself capable of being transformed into muscle.

sar·co·poi·et·ic (sahr″ko-poi-et′ik) producing flesh or muscle.

Sar·cop·tes (sahr-kop′tēz) a genus of mites, including *S. scabie′i,* the cause of scabies in humans.

sar·co·si·ne·mia (sahr″ko-sĭ-ne′me-ah) 1. an aminoacidopathy characterized by accumulation and excretion of sarcosine, sometimes associated with neurologic abnormalities. 2. accumulation of sarcosine in the blood.

sar·co·sis (sahr-ko'sis) abnormal increase of flesh.

sar·co·spo·rid·i·an (sahr″ko-spor-id'e-an) similar to or caused by organisms of the genus *Sarcocystis*.

sar·co·spo·rid·i·o·sis (-spor-id″e-o'sis) sarcocystosis.

sar·cos·to·sis (sahr″kos-to'sis) ossification of fleshy tissue.

sar·co·tu·bules (sahr″ko-too'būlz) the membrane-limited structures of the sarcoplasm, forming a canalicular network around each myofibril.

sar·cous (sahr'kus) pertaining to flesh or muscle tissue.

sar·gram·os·tim (sahr-gram'o-stim) granulocyte-macrophage colony-stimulating factor developed by recombinant technology; used to enhance neutrophil function, stimulating hematopoiesis and decreasing neutropenia.

SARS severe acute respiratory syndrome.

sat·el·lite (sat'ĕ-līt″) 1. a vein that closely accompanies an artery, such as the brachial. 2. a minor, or attendant, lesion situated near a larger one. 3. a globoid mass of chromatin attached at the secondary constriction to the ends of the short arms of acrocentric autosomes. 4. exhibiting satellitism.

sat·el·li·tism (sat'el-i-tizm) the phenomenon in which certain bacterial species grow more vigorously in the immediate vicinity of colonies of other unrelated species, owing to the production of an essential metabolite by the latter species.

sat·el·li·to·sis (sat″el-i-to'sis) accumulation of neuroglial cells about neurons; seen whenever neurons are damaged.

sattva (sahtt'vah) [Sanskrit] according to ayurveda, the purest aspect of the three gunas, characterized by equilibrium; responsible for health and contentment of mind and body and associated with the mind, consciousness, or intelligence that maintains health.

sat·u·rat·ed (sach'ah-rāt″ed) 1. denoting a chemical compound that has only single bonds and no double or triple bonds between atoms. 2. unable to hold in solution any more of a given substance.

sat·u·ra·tion (sach″ah-ra'shun) 1. the state of being saturated, or the act of saturating. 2. in radiotherapy, the delivery of a maximum tolerable tissue dose within a short period, then maintenance of the dose by additional smaller fractional doses over a prolonged period. **oxygen s.**, the amount of oxygen bound to hemoglobin in the blood expressed as a percentage of the maximal binding capacity.

sat·y·ri·a·sis (sat″ĭ-ri'ah-sis) abnormal, excessive, insatiable sexual desire in the male.

sau·cer·iza·tion (saw″ser-ĭ-za'shun) 1. the excavation of tissue to form a shallow shelving depression, usually performed to facilitate drainage from infected areas of bone. 2. the shallow saucer-like depression on the upper surface of a vertebra which has suffered a compression fracture.

saw (saw) a cutting instrument with a serrated edge. **Gigli's wire s.**, a flexible wire with saw teeth.

saw pal·met·to (pal-met'to) a small creeping palm of the southeastern United States, *Serenoa repens*, or its fruit, which is used for urination problems associated with benign prostatic hyperplasia.

saxi·tox·in (sak″sĭ-tok″sin) a powerful neurotoxin synthesized and secreted by certain dinoflagellates, which accumulates in the tissues of shellfish feeding on the dinoflagellates and may cause a severe toxic reaction in persons consuming contaminated shellfish.

Sb antimony (L. *sti'bium*).

Sc scandium.

scab (skab) 1. the crust of a superficial sore. 2. to become covered with a crust or scab.

sca·bi·cide (ska'bĭ-sīd) 1. lethal to *Sarcoptes scabiei*. 2. an agent lethal to *Sarcoptes scabiei*.

sca·bies (ska'bēz) a contagious skin disease due to the itch mite, *Sarcoptes scabiei*; the female bores into the stratum corneum, forming burrows (cuniculi), attended by intense itching and eczema caused by scratching. **scabiet'ic**, adj. **Norwegian s.**, a rare, severe form associated with an immense number of mites, with marked scales and crusts, usually accompanied by lymphadenopathy and eosinophilia.

sca·la (ska'lah) pl. *sca'lae*. [L.] a stairlike structure. **s. me'dia**, cochlear duct. **s. tym'pani**, the part of the cochlea below the lamina spiralis. **s. vesti'buli**, the part of the cochlea above the lamina spiralis.

sca·lar (ska'ler) 1. a quantity that has magnitude only (as opposed to also having direction), such as mass or temperature. Cf. *vector*. 2. pertaining to such a quantity.

scald (skawld) to burn with hot liquid or steam; a burn so produced.

scale (skāl) 1. a thin flake or compacted platelike structure, as of cornified epithelial cells on the body surface. 2. a thin fragment of tartar or other concretion on the surface of the teeth. 3. to remove material from a body surface, as encrustations from a tooth surface. 4. a scheme or device by which some property may be measured (as hardness, weight, linear dimension). **absolute temperature s.,** one with its zero at absolute zero (−273.15°C, −459.67°F). **Brazelton behavioral s.,** a method for assessing infant behavior by responses to environmental stimuli. **Celsius s. (C),** a temperature scale on which 0° is officially 273.15 kelvins and 100° is 373.15 kelvins. Formerly (and still, unofficially), the degree Celsius was called the degree centigrade, with 0° at the freezing point of fresh water and 100° at the boiling point under normal atmospheric pressure; see table accompanying *temperature*. **centigrade s.,** one in which the interval between two fixed points is divided into 100 equal units, as the Celsius scale. **Fahrenheit s. (F),** a temperature scale with the ice point at 32 degrees and the normal boiling point of water at 212 degrees (212°F); see table accompanying *temperature*. **French s.,** a scale used for denoting the size of catheters, sounds, etc., each unit (symbol F) being roughly equivalent to 0.33 mm in diameter. **gray s.,** a representation of intensities in shades of gray, as in gray scale ultrasonography. **Kelvin s.,** an absolute temperature scale whose unit of measurement, the kelvin, is equivalent to the degree Celsius, the ice point therefore being at 273.15 kelvins. **temperature s.,** one for expressing degree of heat, based on absolute zero as a reference point, or with a certain value arbitrarily assigned to such temperatures as the ice point and boiling point of water. See table accompanying *temperature*.

sca·lene (ska′lēn) 1. uneven; unequally three-sided. 2. pertaining to one of the scalenus muscles; see *Table of Muscles.*

sca·le·nec·to·my (ska″lĕ-nek′tah-me) resection of the scalenus muscle.

sca·le·not·o·my (ska″lĕ-not′ah-me) division of the scalenus muscle.

sca·ler (skāl′er) a dental instrument for removal of calculus from teeth.

scalp (skalp) the skin covering the cranium.

scal·pel (skal′p'l) a small surgical knife usually having a convex edge.

scan (skan) 1. to examine or map the body, or one or more organs or regions of it, by gathering information with a sensing device. 2. the data or image so obtained. 3. shortened form of *scintiscan*. **A-s.,** display on a cathode ray tube of ultrasonic echoes, in which one axis represents the time required for return of the echo and the other corresponds to the strength of the echo. **B-s.,** display on a cathode ray tube of ultrasonic echoes, depicting time elapsed and echo strength and producing two-dimensional cross-sectional displays by movement of the transducer. **CAT s., CT s.,** computed tomography, or the image obtained from it. **M-mode s.,** the image obtained using M-mode echocardiography, showing the motion (M) over time of a monodimensional ("ice-pick") section of the heart. **PET s.,** positron emission tomography, or the image obtained from it. **ventilation-perfusion s., V/Q s.,** a scintigraphic technique for demonstrating perfusion defects in normally ventilated areas of the lung in the diagnosis of pulmonary embolism.

scan·di·um (skan′de-um) chemical element (see *Table of Elements*), at. no. 21, symbol Sc.

scan·ning (skan′ing) 1. the act of examining by passing over an area or organ with a sensing device. 2. scanning speech. **MUGA s., multiple gated acquisition s.,** equilibrium radionuclide angiocardiography.

sca·pha (ska′fah) [L.] the curved depression separating the helix and antihelix.

scapho·ceph·a·ly (skaf″o-sef′ah-le) abnormal length and narrowness of the skull as a result of premature closure of the sagittal suture. **scaphocephal′ic, scaphoceph′alous,** adj.

scaph·oid (skaf′oid) 1. boat-shaped. 2. see *Table of Bones.*

scaph·oid·itis (skaf″oi-di′tis) inflammation of the scaphoid bone.

scap·u·la (skap′u-lah) pl. *scap′ulae.* [L.] see *Table of Bones.* **scap′ular,** adj.

scap·u·lal·gia (skap″u-lal′jah) pain in the scapular region.

scap·u·lec·to·my (skap″u-lek′tah-me) excision or resection of the scapula.

scap·u·lo·cla·vic·u·lar (skap″u-lo-klah-vik′u-ler) pertaining to the scapula and clavicle.

scap·u·lo·hu·mer·al (-hu′mer-al) pertaining to the scapula and humerus.

scap·u·lo·pexy (skap′u-lo-pek″se) surgical fixation of the scapula.

sca·pus (ska′pus) pl. *sca′pi.* [L.] shaft.

scar (skahr) cicatrix; a mark remaining after the healing of a wound or other morbid process. By extension, any visible manifestation of an earlier event.

scar·i·fi·ca·tion (skar″ĭ-fĭ-ka′shun) production in the skin of many small superficial scratches or punctures, as for introduction of vaccine.

scar·i·fi·ca·tor (skar′ĭ-fĭ-ka″ter) scarifier.

scar·i·fi·er (skar′ĭ-fi″er) an instrument with many sharp points, used in scarification.

scar·la·ti·na (skahr″lah-te′nah) scarlet fever. **scarlat′inal**, adj. **s. angino′sa**, a form with severe throat symptoms.

scar·la·ti·nel·la (skahr-lat″ĭ-nel′ah) Dukes' disease.

scar·la·tin·i·form (skahr″lah-tin′ĭ-form) resembling scarlet fever.

SCAT sheep cell agglutination test.

scat(o)- word element [Gr.], *dung; fecal matter*.

sca·tol·o·gy (skah-tol′ah-je) 1. study and analysis of feces, as for diagnosis. 2. a preoccupation with feces, filth, and obscenities. **scatolog′ical, scatolog′ic**, adj.

sca·tos·co·py (skah-tos′ko-pe) examination of the feces.

ScD [L.] Scien′tiae Doc′tor (Doctor of Science).

Sce·do·spo·ri·um (se″do-spor′e-um) an imperfect fungus of the form-class Hyphomycetes; it is the anamorph of *Pseudallescheria*. *S. angiosper′mum* is the anamorph of *Pseudallescheria boydii* and is an agent of mycetoma.

schin·dy·le·sis (skin″dĭ-le′sis) an articulation in which one bone is received into a cleft in another.

schist(o)- word element [Gr.], *split, cleft, divided*.

schis·to·ceph·a·lus (shis″-, skis″to-sef′ah-lus) a fetus with cranium bifidum.

schis·to·cor·mus (-kor′mus) a fetus with a cleft lower trunk.

schis·to·cyte (shis′-, skis′to-sīt) burr cell; a fragment of an erythrocyte, commonly observed in the blood in hemolytic anemia.

schis·to·cy·to·sis (shis″-, skis″to-si-to′sis) an accumulation of schistocytes in the blood.

Schis·to·so·ma (-so′mah) a genus of blood flukes, including *S. haemato′bium* of Africa, *S. japon′icum* of East Asia, *S. manso′ni* of Africa, South America, and the West Indies, and *S. intercala′tum* of Central Africa, which cause infection in humans by penetrating the skin of those coming in contact with infected waters; the invertebrate hosts are snails. See *schistosomiasis*. **schistoso′mal**, adj.

schis·to·some (shis′-, skis′to-sōm) an individual of the genus *Schistosoma*.

schis·to·so·mi·a·sis (shis″-, skis″to-so-mi′ah-sis) infection with *Schistosoma*. **s. haemato′bia**, urinary s. **s. intercala′tum**, an endemic intestinal disease of Central Africa due to infection with *Schistosoma intercalatum*, with abdominal pain, diarrhea, and other intestinal symptoms. **intestinal s.**, the chronic form of schistosomiasis mansoni and japonica in which the intestinal tract is involved; usually asymptomatic. **s. japo′nica**, infection with *Schistosoma japonica*. The acute form is marked by fever, allergic symptoms,

and diarrhea; chronic effects, which may be severe, are due to fibrosis around eggs deposited in the liver, lungs, and central nervous system. **s. manso′ni**, infection with *Schistosoma mansoni*, living chiefly in the mesenteric veins but migrating to deposit eggs in venules, primarily of the large intestine; eggs lodging in the liver may lead to peripheral fibrosis, hepatosplenomegaly, and ascites. **urinary s., vesical s.**, infection with *Schistosoma haematobium* involving the urinary tract and causing cystitis and hematuria.

schis·to·so·mi·cide (-so′mĭ-sīd) an agent lethal to schistosomes.

schiz·am·ni·on (skiz-am′ne-on) an amnion formed by cavitation over or in the embryoblast, as in human development.

schiz(o)- word element [Gr.], *split, cleft, divided*.

schizo·af·fec·tive (skiz″o-uh-fek′tiv) pertaining to or exhibiting features of both schizophrenic and mood disorders.

schizo·gen·e·sis (-jen′ĕ-sis) reproduction by fission. **schizog′enous**, adj.

schi·zog·o·ny (skĭ-zog′ah-ne) the asexual reproduction of a sporozoan parasite (sporozoite) by multiple fission of the nucleus of the parasite followed by segmentation of the cytoplasm, giving rise to merozoites. **schizogon′ic**, adj.

schizo·gy·ria (skiz″o-ji′re-ah) a condition in which there are wedge-shaped cracks in the cerebral convolutions.

schiz·oid (skit′soid) 1. denoting the traits that characterize the schizoid personality. 2. denoting any of a variety of schizophrenia-related characteristics, including traits said to indicate a predisposition to schizophrenia as well as disorders other than schizophrenia either occurring in a relative of a schizophrenic or occurring more commonly than average in families of schizophrenics.

schiz·ont (skiz′ont) the multinucleate stage in the development of some members of the Sarcodina and some sporozoans during schizogony.

schizo·nych·ia (skiz″o-nik′e-ah) splitting of the nails.

schizo·pha·sia (skit″so-fa′zhah) word salad; see under *W*.

schizo·phre·nia (skit″so-fren′e-ah, -fre′ne-ah) a mental disorder or group of disorders characterized by disturbances in the form and content of thought (e.g., delusions, hallucinations), in mood (e.g., inappropriate affect), in sense of self and relationship to the external world (e.g., loss of ego boundaries, withdrawal), and in behavior (e.g., bizarre or apparently purposeless behavior); it must cause marked decrease in functioning and be present for at least six months. **schizo-phren′ic,** adj. **catatonic s.,** a form characterized by psychomotor disturbance, which may be manifested by a marked decrease in reactivity to the environment and in spontaneous activity, by excited, uncontrollable, and apparently purposeless motor activity, by resistance to instructions or attempts to be moved, or by maintenance of a rigid posture or of fixed bizarre postures. **childhood s.,** former name for schizophrenia-like symptoms with onset before puberty, marked by autistic, withdrawn behavior, failure to develop an identity separate from the mother′s, and gross developmental immaturity, now classified as pervasive developmental disorders. **disorganized s., hebephrenic s.,** a form marked by disorganized and incoherent thought and speech, shallow, inappropriate, and silly affect, and regressive behavior without systematized delusions. **paranoid s.,** a form characterized by delusions, often with auditory hallucinations, with relative preservation of affect and cognitive functioning. **residual s.,** a condition manifested by individuals with symptoms of schizophrenia who, after a psychotic schizophrenic episode, are no longer psychotic. **undifferentiated s.,** a type characterized by the presence of prominent psychotic symptoms but not classifiable as catatonic, disorganized, or paranoid.

schizo·phren·i·form (-fren′ĭ-form) resembling schizophrenia.

schizo·trich·ia (skiz″o-trik′e-ah) splitting of the hairs at the ends.

schizo·ty·pal (skit″so-ti′p′l) exhibiting abnormalities in behavior and communication style similar to those of schizophrenia, but less severe. See under *personality.*

schizo·zo·ite (skiz″o-zo′īt) merozoite.

schwan·no·ma (shwahn-o′mah) a neoplasm originating from Schwann cells (of the myelin sheath) of neurons; schwannomas include neurofibromas and neurilemomas. **granular cell s.,** see under *tumor.*

sci·at·ic (si-at′ik) 1. near or related to the sciatic nerve or vein. 2. ischial.

sci·at·i·ca (si-at′ĭ-kah) neuralgia along the course of the sciatic nerve, most often with pain radiating into the buttock and lower limb, most commonly due to herniation of a lumbar disk.

SCID severe combined immunodeficiency (disease); see under *immunodeficiency.*

sci·ence (si′ens) 1. the systematic observation of natural phenomena for the purpose of discovering laws governing those phenomena.

2. the body of knowledge accumulated by such means. **scientif′ic,** adj.

sci·er·opia (si″er-o′pe-ah) defect of vision in which objects appear in a shadow.

scin·ti·gram (sin′tĭ-gram) the graphic record obtained by scintigraphy.

scin·tig·ra·phy (sin-tig′rah-fe) the production of two-dimensional images of the distribution of radioactivity in tissues after the internal administration of a radiopharmaceutical imaging agent, the images being obtained by a scintillation camera. **scinti-graph′ic,** adj. **exercise thallium s.,** myocardial perfusion using thallium 201 as a tracer and performed in conjunction with an exercise stress test. **gated blood pool s.,** equilibrium radionuclide angiocardiography. **infarct avid s.,** that performed following myocardial infarction to confirm infarction as well as detect, localize, and quantify areas of myocardial necrosis by means of a radiotracer that concentrates in necrotic regions. **myocardial perfusion s.,** that performed using a radiotracer that traverses the myocardial capillary system; immediate and delayed images are obtained to assess regional blood flow and cell viability.

scin·til·la·tion (sin″tĭ-la′shun) 1. an emission of sparks. 2. a subjective visual sensation, as of seeing sparks. 3. a particle emitted in disintegration of a radioactive element; see also under *counter.*

scin·ti·scan (sin′tĭ-skan) a two-dimensional representation of the radiation emitted by a radioisotope, revealing its concentration in specific organs or tissues.

scir·rhoid (skir′oid) resembling scirrhous carcinoma.

scir·rhous (skir′us) hard or indurated; see under *carcinoma.*

scle·ra (sklēr′ah) pl. *scle′rae.* [L.] the tough white outer coat of the eyeball, covering approximately the posterior five-sixths of its surface, continuous anteriorly with the cornea and posteriorly with the external sheath of the optic nerve. **scler′al,** adj.

scle·rad·e·ni·tis (sklēr″ad-ĕ-ni′tis) inflammation and hardening of a gland.

scle·rec·ta·sia (-ek-ta′zhah) a bulging state of the sclera.

scle·rec·to·iri·dec·to·my (sklĕ-rek″to-ir″ĭ-dek′tah-me) excision of part of the sclera and of the iris.

scle·rec·to·iri·do·di·al·y·sis (-ir″ĭ-do-di-al′ĭ-sis) sclerectomy and iridodialysis.

scle·rec·to·my (sklĕ-rek′tah-me) excision of part of the sclera.

scle·re·de·ma (sklēr″ĕ-de′mah) diffuse, symmetrical, woodlike, nonpitting induration of the skin of unknown etiology, typically beginning on the head, face, or neck and spreading to involve the shoulders, arms, and thorax and sometimes extracutaneous sites. **s. neonato′rum,** sclerema.

scle·re·ma (sklĕ-re′mah) a severe, sometimes fatal disorder of adipose tissue occurring chiefly in preterm, sick, debilitated infants, manifested by induration of the involved tissue, causing the skin to become cold, yellowish white, mottled, boardlike, and inflexible.

scle·ri·rit·o·my (sklĕr″ĭ-rit′ah-me) incision of the sclera and iris in anterior staphyloma.

scle·ri·tis (sklĕ-ri′tis) inflammation of the sclera; it may involve the part adjoining the limbus of the cornea *(anterior s.)* or the underlying retina and choroid *(posterior s.).*

scler(o)- word element [Gr.], *hard; sclera.*

scle·ro·blas·te·ma (sklĕr″o-blas-te′mah) the embryonic tissue from which bone is formed. **scleroblaste′mic,** adj.

scle·ro·cho·roi·di·tis (-kor″oi-di′tis) inflammation of the sclera and choroid.

scle·ro·cor·nea (-kor′ne-ah) the sclera and choroid regarded as forming a single layer.

scle·ro·cor·ne·al (-al) pertaining to the sclera and the cornea.

scle·ro·dac·ty·ly (-dak′tĭ-le) localized scleroderma of the digits.

scle·ro·der·ma (-der′mah) hardening and thickening of the skin, a finding in various different diseases, occurring in localized and general forms. **circumscribed s.,** morphea. **systemic s.,** a systemic disorder of connective tissue with skin hardening and thickening, blood vessel abnormalities, and fibrotic degenerative changes in various body organs.

scle·rog·e·nous (sklĕ-roj′ĕ-nus) producing sclerosis or sclerous tissue.

scle·ro·iri·tis (sklĕr″o-i-ri′tis) inflammation of the sclera and iris.

scle·ro·ker·a·ti·tis (-ker″ah-ti′tis) inflammation of the sclera and cornea.

scle·ro·ma (sklĕ-ro′mah) a hardened patch or induration, especially of the nasal or laryngeal tissues. **respiratory s.,** rhinoscleroma.

scle·ro·ma·la·cia (sklĕr″o-mah-la′shah) degeneration and thinning (softening) of the sclera, occurring in rheumatoid arthritis.

scle·ro·mere (sklĕr′o-mēr) 1. any segment or metamere of the skeletal system. 2. the caudal half of a sclerotome (3).

scle·ro·myx·ede·ma (sklĕr″o-mik″sĕ-de′-mah) 1. lichen myxedematosus. 2. a term sometimes used to refer to lichen myxedematosus associated with scleroderma.

scle·ro·nyx·is (-nik′sis) surgical puncture of the sclera.

scle·ro·ooph·o·ri·tis (-o″of-ah-ri′tis) sclerosing inflammation of the ovary.

scle·roph·thal·mia (sklĕr″of-thal′me-ah) a condition, resulting from imperfect differentiation of the sclera and cornea, in which only the central part of the cornea remains clear.

scle·ro·pro·tein (sklĕr″o-pro′tēn) a simple protein characterized by its insolubility and fibrous structure and usually serving a supportive or protective function in the body.

scle·ro·sant (sklĕ-ro′sant) sclerosing agent.

scle·rose (sklĕ-rōs′) to become, or cause to become, hardened or sclerotic.

scle·ros·ing (-rōs′ing) causing or undergoing sclerosis.

scle·ro·sis (-ro′sis) an induration or hardening, especially from inflammation and in diseases of the interstitial substance; applied chiefly to such hardening of the nervous system or to hardening of the blood vessels. **amyotrophic lateral s.,** Lou Gehrig disease: progressive degeneration of the neurons that give rise to the corticospinal tract and of the motor cells of the brain stem and spinal cord, resulting in a deficit of upper and lower motor neurons; it usually has a fatal outcome within 2 to 3 years. **arterial s.,** arteriosclerosis. **arteriolar s.,** arteriolosclerosis. **diffuse cerebral s.,** the infantile form of metachromatic leukodystrophy. **disseminated s.,** multiple s. **familial centrolobar s.,** Pelizaeus-Merzbacher disease. **glomerular s.,** glomerulosclerosis. **hippocampal s.,** loss of neurons in the region of the hippocampus, with gliosis; sometimes seen in epilepsy. **lateral s.,** degeneration of the lateral columns of the spinal cord, leading to spastic paraplegia. See *amyotrophic lateral sclerosis* and *primary lateral sclerosis* **Mönckeberg's s.,** see under *arteriosclerosis.* **multiple s. (MS),** demyelination occurring in patches throughout the white matter of the central nervous system, sometimes extending into the gray matter; symptoms of lesions of the white matter are weakness, incoordination, paresthesias, speech disturbances, and visual complaints. **primary lateral s.,** a form of motor neuron disease in which the degenerative process is limited to the corticospinal pathways. **progressive systemic s.,** systemic scleroderma. **tuberous s.,** an autosomal dominant disease characterized by hamartomas of the brain (tubers), retina, and viscera; mental retardation; seizures; and adenoma sebaceum.

scle·ro·ste·no·sis (sklĕr″o-stĕ-no′sis) induration or hardening combined with contraction.

scle·ros·to·my (sklĕ-ros'tah-me) surgical creation of an opening in the sclera; usually performed in treatment of glaucoma.

scle·ro·ther·a·py (sklĕr"o-ther'ah-pe) injection of a chemical irritant into a vein to produce inflammation and eventual fibrosis and obliteration of the lumen, as for treatment of hemorrhoids.

scle·rot·ic (sklĕ-rot'ik) 1. hard or hardening; affected with sclerosis. 2. scleral.

scle·ro·ti·tis (sklĕr"o-ti'tis) scleritis.

scle·ro·ti·um (sklĕ-ro'she-um) a structure formed by fungi and certain protozoa in response to adverse environmental conditions, which will germinate under favorable conditions; in fungi, it is a hard mass of intertwined mycelia, usually with pigmented walls, and in protozoa it is a multinucleated hard cyst into which the plasmodium divides.

scle·ro·tome (sklĕr'o-tōm) 1. an instrument used in the incision of the sclera. 2. the area of a bone innervated from a single spinal segment. 3. one of the paired masses of mesenchymal tissue, separated from the ventromedial part of a somite, which develop into vertebrae and ribs.

scle·rot·o·my (sklĕ-rot'ah-me) incision of the sclera.

scle·rous (sklĕr'us) hard; indurated.

sco·lex (sko'leks) pl. *sco'leces, sco'lices.* [Gr.] the attachment organ of a tapeworm, generally considered the anterior, or cephalic, end.

scoli(o)- word element [Gr.], *crooked; twisted.*

sco·lio·ky·pho·sis (sko"le-o-ki-fo'sis) combined lateral (scoliosis) and posterior (kyphosis) curvature of the spine.

sco·li·o·si·om·e·try (-se-om'ĕ-tre) measurement of spinal curvature.

sco·li·o·sis (sko"le-o'sis) lateral curvature of vertebral column. **scoliot'ic,** adj.

scom·broid (skom'broid) 1. of or pertaining to the suborder Scombroidea. 2. a fish of the suborder Scombroidea. See also under *poisoning.*

Scom·broi·dea (skom-broi'de-ah) a suborder of larger, bony, marine fish having oily flesh, including tunas, bonitos, mackerels, albacores, and skipjacks; their flesh may contain a toxic histamine-like substance and, if ingested, can cause scombroid poisoning.

sco·pol·a·mine (sko-pol'ah-mēn) an anticholinergic alkaloid obtained from various solanaceous plants; used as the base or the hydrobromide salt as an antiemetic and as the hydrobromide salt as a preanesthetic antisialagogue, adjunct to general anesthesia, and topical mydriatic and cycloplegic.

sco·po·phil·ia (sko"po-fil'e-ah) usually, voyeurism, but it is sometimes divided into active and passive forms, *active s.* being *voyeurism* and *passive s.* being exhibitionism.

sco·po·pho·bia (-fo'be-ah) irrational fear of being seen.

-scopy word element [Gr.], *examination of.*

scor·bu·tic (skor-bu'tik) pertaining to or affected with scurvy.

scor·bu·ti·gen·ic (skor-bu"ti-jen'ik) causing scurvy.

scor·di·ne·ma (skor"di-ne'mah) yawning and stretching with a feeling of lassitude, occurring as a preliminary symptom of some infectious disease.

score (skor) a rating, usually expressed numerically, based on specific achievement or the degree to which certain qualities or conditions are present. **APACHE s.** [*a*cute *p*hysiological *a*ssessment and *c*hronic *h*ealth *e*valuation], a widely-used method for assessing severity of illness in acutely ill patients in intensive care units, taking into account a variety of routine physiological parameters. **Apgar s.,** a numerical expression of an infant's condition, usually determined at 60 seconds after birth, based on heart rate, respiratory effort, muscle tone, reflex irritability, and color. **Bishop s.,** a score for estimating the prospects of induction of labor, arrived at by evaluating the extent of cervical dilatation, effacement, the station of the fetal head, consistency of the cervix, and the cervical position in relation to the vaginal axis.

scot(o)- word element [Gr.], *darkness.*

sco·to·chro·mo·gen (sko"to-kro'mo-jen) a microorganism whose pigmentation develops in the dark as well as in the light. **scotochromogen'ic,** adj.

sco·to·din·ia (-din'e-ah) dizziness with blurring of vision and headache.

sco·to·ma (sko-to'mah) pl. *scoto'mata.* 1. An area of depressed vision in the visual field, surrounded by an area of less depressed or of normal vision. 2. mental s. **scotom'atous,** adj. **annular s.,** circular area of depressed vision surrounding the point of fixation. **central s.,** an area of depressed vision corresponding with the point of fixation and interfering with central vision. **centrocecal s.,** a horizontal oval defect in the field of vision situated between and embracing both the point of fixation and the blind spot. **color s.,** an isolated area of depressed or defective vision for color. **hemianopic s.,** depressed or lost vision affecting half of the central visual field. **mental s.,** a figurative blind spot in a person's psychological awareness, the person being unable to gain insight into and to understand their mental problems; lack of insight. **negative s.,** one which appears as a blank spot or hiatus in the visual field, the patient being unaware of it. **peripheral s.,** an area of depressed vision toward the periphery of the visual field, distant from the point of fixation. **physiologic s.,** that area of the visual field corresponding with the optic disk, in which the photosensitive receptors are absent. **positive s.,** one which appears as a dark spot in the visual field, the patient being aware of it. **relative s.,** an area of the visual field in which perception of light is only diminished, or loss is restricted to light of certain wavelengths. **ring s.,** annular s. **scintillating s.,** teichopsia.

sco·to·ma·graph (-graf) an instrument for recording a scotoma.

sco·tom·e·try (sko-tom′ĕ-tre) the measurement of scotomas.

sco·to·pho·bia (-fo′be-ah) irrational fear of darkness.

sco·to·pia (sko-to′pe-ah) 1. night vision. 2. dark adaptation. **scotop′ic,** adj.

sco·top·sin (sko-top′sin) the opsin of the retinal rods that combines with 11-*cis* retinal to form rhodopsin; see *retinal* (2).

scra·pie (skra′pe) a prion disease occurring in sheep and goats, characterized by severe pruritus, debility, and muscular incoordination, ending in death.

scratch (skrach) 1. to scrape or rub a surface lightly with the nails or with a sharp or jagged instrument, particularly to relieve itching. 2. a slight wound. 3. to make shallow cuts on a surface. 4. to make a thin grating sound.

screen (skrēn) 1. a structure resembling a curtain or partition, used as a protection or shield, e.g., against excessive radiation exposure. 2. a large flat surface upon which light rays are projected. 3. protective (2). 4. to examine by fluoroscopy (Great Britain). 5. to separate well individuals in a population from those with an undiagnosed pathologic condition by means of tests, examinations, or other procedures. **skin s.,** a substance applied to the skin to protect it from the sun's rays or other noxious agents. **solar s., sun s.,** sunscreen.

screen·ing (skrēn′ing) 1. examination of a group to separate well persons from those who have an undiagnosed pathologic condition or who are at high risk. 2. fluoroscopy (Great Britain). **antibody s.,** a method of determining the presence and amount of anti-HLA antibodies in the serum of a potential allograft recipient: aliquots of the recipient's serum are mixed with a panel of leukocytes from well-characterized cell donors, complement is added, and the percentage of cells that lyse (referred to as the *panel-reactive antibody*) indicates the degree of sensitization of the recipient.

screw·worm (skroo′werm) the larva of *Cochliomyia hominivorax.*

scro·bic·u·late (skro-bik′u-lāt) marked with pits.

scrof·u·la (skrof′u-lah) old name for tuberculous cervical lymphadenitis.

scrof·u·lo·der·ma (skrof″u-lo-der′mah) a tuberculous or nontuberculous mycobacterial infection of the skin caused by direct extension of tuberculosis into the skin from underlying structures or by contact exposure to tuberculosis.

scro·tal (skro′t′l) pertaining to the scrotum.

scro·tec·to·my (skro-tek′tah-me) partial or complete excision of the scrotum.

scro·to·cele (skro′to-sēl) scrotal hernia.

scro·to·plasty (-plas″te) plastic reconstruction of the scrotum.

scro·tum (skro′tum) the pouch containing the testes and their accessory organs. **lymph s.,** elephantiasis scroti.

scu-PA single chain urokinase-type plasminogen activator; see *prourokinase.*

scur·vy (sker′ve) a disease due to deficiency of ascorbic acid (vitamin C), marked by anemia, spongy gums, a tendency to mucocutaneous hemorrhages, and brawny induration of calf and leg muscles.

scute (skūt) any squama or scalelike structure, especially the bony plate separating the upper tympanic cavity and mastoid cells (*tympanic s.*).

scu·ti·form (sku′tĭ-form) shaped like a shield.

scu·tu·lum (sku′tu-lum) pl. *scu′tula.* [L.] one of the disklike or saucerlike crusts characteristic of favus.

scu·tum (sku′tum) 1. scute. 2. a hard chitinous plate on the anterior dorsal surface of hard-bodied ticks.

scy·ba·lum (sib′ah-lum) pl. *scy′bala.* [Gr.] a hard mass of fecal matter in the intestines. **scy′balous,** adj.

scy·phoid (si′foid) shaped like a cup.

SD skin dose; standard deviation.

SDS sodium dodecyl sulfate.

SE standard error.

Se selenium.

seam (sēm) a line of union. **osteoid s.,** on the surface of a bone, the narrow region of newly formed organic matrix not yet mineralized.

sea·sick·ness (se′sik-nes) motion sickness malaise caused by the motion of a ship.

sea·son·al (se′zun-al) of, depending on, or occurring in a particular season of the year.

seat·worm (sēt′werm) oxyurid.

se·ba·ceous (sĕ-ba′shus) pertaining to or secreting sebum.

se·bif·er·ous (sĕ-bif′er-us) sebiparous.

se·bip·a·rous (sĕ-bip′ah-rus) producing fatty secretion.

sebo·lith (seb′o-lith) calculus in a sebaceous gland.

seb·or·rhea (seb″o-re′ah) 1. excessive secretion of sebum. 2. seborrheic dermatitis. **seborrhe′al, seborrhe′ic,** adj. **s. sic′ca,** dry, scaly seborrheic dermatitis.

sebo·tro·pic (seb″o-tro′pik) having an affinity for or a stimulating effect on sebaceous glands; promoting the excretion of sebum.

se·bum (se′bum) the oily secretion of the sebaceous glands, composed of fat and epithelial debris.

se·co·bar·bi·tal (se″ko-bahr′bĭ-tal) a short-acting barbiturate used as the sodium salt as a hypnotic and sedative and as an anticonvulsant in tetanus.

sec·on·dary (sek′un-dar″e) second or inferior in order of time, place, or importance; derived from or consequent to a primary event or thing.

se·cre·ta (se-kre′tah) [L., pl.] secretion (2).

se·cret·a·gogue (se-krĕt′ah-gog) stimulating secretion, or an agent that so acts.

se·crete (se-krēt′) to elaborate and release a secretion.

se·cre·tin (se-kre′tin) a hormone secreted by the duodenal and jejunal mucosa when acid chyme enters the intestine; it stimulates secretion of pancreatic juice and, to a lesser extent, bile and intestinal secretion.

se·cre·tion (-shun) 1. the cellular process of elaborating and releasing a specific product; this activity may range from separating a specific substance of the blood to the elaboration of a new chemical substance. 2. material that is secreted.

se·cre·to·in·hib·i·to·ry (se-kre″to-in-hib′ĭ-tor″e) antisecretory.

se·cre·to·mo·tor (-mo′tor) stimulating secretion; said of nerves.

se·cre·to·mo·tory (-mo′tor-e) secretomotor.

se·cre·tor (se-kre′ter) 1. in genetics, one who secretes the ABH antigens of the ABO blood group in the saliva and other body fluids. 2. the gene determining this trait.

se·cre·to·ry (se-kre′tah-re, se′krĕ-tor″e) pertaining to secretion or affecting the secretions.

sec·tio (sek′she-o) pl. *sectio′nes.* [L.] section.

sec·tion (sek′shun) 1. an act of cutting. 2. a cut surface. 3. a segment or subdivision of an organ. 4. a supplemental taxonomic category subordinate to a subgenus but superior to a species or series. **abdominal s.,** laparotomy. **cesarean s.,** delivery of a fetus by incision through the abdominal wall and uterus. **frozen s.,** a specimen cut by microtome from tissue that has been frozen. **perineal s.,** external urethrotomy. **Saemisch's s.,** see under *operation.* **serial s.,** histologic sections made in consecutive order and so arranged for the purpose of microscopic examination.

se·cun·di·grav·i·da (sĕ-kun″dĭ-grav′ĭ-dah) a woman pregnant the second time; gravida II.

se·cun·dines (sĕ-kun′dīnz, -dēnz) afterbirth.

se·cun·dip·a·ra (sē″kun-dip′ah-rah) a woman who has had two pregnancies which resulted in viable offspring; para II.

SED skin erythema dose; see *erythema dose,* under *dose.*

se·da·tion (sĕ-da′shun) 1. the allaying of irritability or excitement, especially by administration of a sedative. 2. the state so induced. **conscious s.,** a state of anesthesia in which the patient is conscious but is rendered free of fear and anxiety.

sed·a·tive (sed′ah-tiv) 1. allaying irritability and excitement. 2. a drug that so acts.

sed·en·tary (sed′en-tar″e) 1. sitting habitually; of inactive habits. 2. pertaining to a sitting posture.

sed·i·ment (sed′ĭ-ment) a precipitate, especially that formed spontaneously.

sed·i·men·ta·tion (sed″ĭ-men-ta′shun) the settling out of sediment.

seed (sēd) 1. the mature ovule of a flowering plant. 2. a small cylindrical shell of gold or other suitable material, used in application of radiation therapy. 3. to inoculate a culture medium with microorganisms. **grape s.,** a preparation of the seeds of grapes, having antioxidant, antimutagenic, and antiinflammatory properties; used for the prevention of atherosclerosis and cancer and in folk medicine for the treatment of circulatory disorders. **plantago s., psyllium s.,** cleaned, dried ripe seed of species of *Plantago;* used as a bulk-forming laxative.

seg·ment (seg′ment) a demarcated portion of a whole. **anterior s. of eye, anterior s. of eyeball,** the sclera, conjunctiva, cornea, anterior chamber, iris, and lens. **bronchopulmonary s's,** one of the smaller subdivisions of the lobes of the lungs, separated by connective tissue septa and supplied by branches of the respective lobar bronchi. See Plate 26. **hepatic s's,** subdivisions of the hepatic lobes based on arterial and biliary supply and venous drainage. **posterior s. of eye, posterior s. of eyeball,** the vitreous, retina, and optic nerve. **renal s's,** subdivisions of the kidney that have independent blood supply from branches of the renal artery, including the *superior, anterior superior, inferior, anterior inferior,* and *posterior* segments. **spinal s's, s's of spinal cord,** the regions of the spinal cord to each of which is attached anterior and posterior roots of the 31 pairs of spinal nerves: eight *cervical,* twelve *thoracic,* five *lumbar,* five *sacral,* and three *coccygeal.* See Plate 8. **ST s.,** the interval from the end of ventricular depolarization to the onset of the T wave. **uterine s.,** either of the portions into which the uterus differentiates in early labor; the upper contractile portion (corpus uteri) becomes thicker as labor advances, and the lower noncontractile portion (the isthmus) is expanded and thin-walled.

seg·men·tal (seg-men't'l) 1. pertaining to or forming a segment or a product of division, especially into serially arranged or nearly equal parts. 2. undergoing segmentation.

seg·men·ta·tion (seg″men-ta'shun) 1. division into similar parts. 2. cleavage.

seg·men·tum (seg-men'tum) pl. *segmen'ta.* [L.] segment.

seg·re·ga·tion (seg″rĕ-ga'shun) 1. the separation of allelic genes during meiosis as homologous chromosomes begin to migrate toward opposite poles of the cell, so that eventually the members of each pair of allelic genes go to separate gametes. 2. the separation of different elements of a population. 3. the progressive restriction of potencies in the zygote to the various regions of the forming embryo.

sei·zure (se'zhur) 1. the sudden attack or recurrence of a disease. 2. a single episode of epilepsy, often named for the type it represents. **absence s.,** the seizure of absence epilepsy, marked by a momentary break in consciousness of thought or activity and accompanied by a symmetrical 3-cps spike and wave activity on the electroencephalogram. **adversive s.,** a type of focal motor seizure in which there is forceful, sustained turning to one side by the eyes, head, or body. **atonic s.,** an absence seizure characterized by sudden loss of muscle tone. **automatic s.,** a type of complex partial seizure characterized by automatisms, often ambulatory and involving quasipurposeful acts. **clonic s.,** one in which there are generalized clonic contractions without a preceding tonic phase. **complex partial s.,** a type of partial seizure associated with disease of the temporal lobe and characterized by varying degrees of impairment of consciousness and automa-

tisms, for which the patient is later amnestic. **febrile s's,** see under *convulsion.* **generalized tonic-clonic s.,** the seizure of grand mal epilepsy, consisting of a loss of consciousness and generalized tonic convulsions followed by clonic convulsions. **myoclonic s.,** one characterized by a brief episode of myoclonus. **partial s.,** any seizure due to a lesion in a specific, known area of the cerebral cortex. **reflex s.,** an episode of reflex epilepsy. **sensory s.,** 1. a simple partial seizure manifested by paresthesias or other hallucinations, including several types of aura. 2. a reflex seizure in response to a sensory stimulus. **simple partial s.,** a localized type of partial seizure, without loss of consciousness; if it progresses to another type of seizure it is called an *aura.* **tonic s.,** one characterized by tonic but not clonic contractions.

se·lec·tion (sĕ-lek'shun) the play of forces that determines the relative reproductive performance of the various genotypes in a population. **directional s.,** selection favoring individuals at one extreme of the distribution. **disruptive s., diversifying s.,** selection favoring the two extremes rather than the intermediate. **natural s.,** the survival in nature of those individuals and their progeny best equipped to adapt to environmental conditions. **sexual s.,** natural selection in which certain characteristics attract male or female members of a species, thus ensuring survival of those characteristics. **stabilizing s.,** selection favoring intermediate phenotypes rather than those at one or both extremes.

se·lec·tive (sĕ-lek'tiv) 1. having a high degree of selectivity. 2. discriminating; making a choice from multiple alternatives; singling out in preference.

se·lec·tiv·i·ty (sĕ-lek-tiv'ĭ-te) in pharmacology, the degree to which a dose of a drug produces the desired effect in relation to adverse effects.

se·le·gil·ine (sĕ-lej'ĭ-lēn) an antiparkinsonian agent used as the hydrochloride salt in conjunction with levodopa and carbidopa.

se·le·ni·ous ac·id (sĕ-le'ne-us) monohydrated selenium dioxide, a source of elemental selenium.

se·le·ni·um (sĕ-le'ne-um) chemical element (see *Table of Elements*), at. no. 34, symbol Se; it is an essential mineral nutrient, being a constituent of the enzyme glutathione peroxidase. **s. sulfide,** a topical antiseborrheic and antifungal, used in the treatment of seborrheic dermatitis and dandruff of the scalp and of tinea versicolor.

self-an·ti·gen (self-an'tĭ-jen) autoantigen.

self·lim·it·ed (-lim'it-ed) limited by its own peculiarities, and not by outside influence; said of a disease that runs a definite limited course.

self·tol·er·ance (-tol'er-ans) immunological tolerance to self-antigens.

sel·la (sel'ah) pl. *sel'lae.* [L.]. 1. a saddle-shaped depression. **sel'lar,** adj. 2. s. turcica. **s. tur'cica,** a depression on the upper surface of the sphenoid bone, lodging the pituitary gland.

sem·el·in·ci·dent (sem"el-in'sĭ-dent) attacking only once, as an infectious disease which induces immunity thereafter.

se·men (se'men) [L.] fluid discharged at ejaculation in the male, consisting of secretions of glands associated with the urogenital tract and containing spermatozoa. **sem'inal,** adj.

semi- word element [L.], *half.*

semi·ca·nal (sem"e-kah-nal') a channel open at one side.

semi·co·ma (-ko'mah) a stupor from which the patient may be aroused. **semico'matose,** adj.

semi·dom·i·nance (-dom'ĭ-nans) incomplete dominance.

semi·flex·ion (-flek'shun) position of a limb midway between flexion and extension; the act of bringing to such a position.

semi·lu·nar (-loo'nahr) resembling a crescent or half-moon.

semi·i·nal (sem'ĭ-n'l) pertaining to semen or to a seed.

sem·i·nif·er·ous (sem"ĭ-nif'er-us) producing or conveying semen.

sem·i·no·ma (-no'mah) a radiosensitive, malignant neoplasm of the testis, thought to be derived from primordial germ cells of the sexually undifferentiated embryonic gonad. Cf. *germinoma.* **classical s.,** the most common type, composed of well-differentiated sheets or cords of polygonal or round cells (seminoma cells). **ovarian s.,** dysgerminoma. **spermatocytic s.,** a less malignant form characterized by cells resembling maturing spermatogonia with filamentous chromatin.

se·mi·nu·ria (se"mĭ-nu're-ah) the presence of semen in the urine.

se·mi·ot·ic (se"me-ot'ik) 1. pertaining to signs or symptoms. 2. pathognomonic.

se·mi·ot·ics (-iks) symptomatology.

semi·per·me·a·ble (sem"e-per'me-ah-b'l) permitting passage only of certain molecules.

semi·quan·ti·ta·tive (-kwon'tĭ-ta"tiv) yielding an approximation of the quantity or amount of a substance; between a qualitative and a quantitative result.

se·mis (ss.) (se'mis) [L.] half.

semi·sul·cus (sem"e-sul'kus) a depression which, with an adjoining one, forms a sulcus.

semi·su·pi·na·tion (-soo"pĭ-na'shun) a position of partial supination.

semi·syn·thet·ic (-sin-thet'ik) produced by chemical manipulation of naturally occurring substances.

se·nes·cence (sĕ-nes'ens) the process of growing old, especially the condition resulting from the transitions and accumulations of the deleterious aging processes.

se·nile (se'nil) pertaining to old age; manifesting senility.

se·nil·ism (se'nil-izm) premature old age.

se·nil·i·ty (sĕ-nil'ĭ-te) the physical and mental deterioration associated with old age.

sen·na (sen'ah) the dried leaflets of *Cassia acutifolia* or *C. angustifolia;* used chiefly as a cathartic.

sen·no·side (sen'o-sīd) either of two anthraquinone glucosides, sennoside A and B, found in senna as the calcium salts; a mixture of the two is used as a cathartic.

se·no·pia (se-no'pe-ah) an apparent decrease in presbyopia in the elderly, which is related to the development of nuclear sclerosis and resultant myopia.

sen·sa·tion (sen-sa'shun) an impression produced by impulses conveyed by an afferent nerve to the sensorium. **girdle s.,** zonesthesia. **referred s., reflex s.,** one felt elsewhere than at the site of application of a stimulus. **subjective s.,** one perceptible only to the subject, and not connected with any object external to the body.

sense (sens) 1. any of the physical processes by which stimuli are received, transduced, and conducted as impulses to be interpreted to the brain. 2. in molecular genetics, referring to the strand of a nucleic acid that directly specifies the product. **body s.,** somatognosis. **color s.,** the faculty by which colors are perceived and distinguished. **s. of equilibrium,** the sense that maintains awareness of being or not being in an upright position, controlled by receptors in the vestibule of the ear. **joint s.,** arthresthesia. **kinesthetic s.,** 1. kinesthesia. 2. muscle s. **light s.,** the sense by which degrees of brilliancy are distinguished. **motion s., movement s.,** the awareness of motion by the head or body. **muscle s., muscular s.,** 1. sensory impressions, such as movement and stretch, that come from the muscles. 2. movement s. **pain s.,** the ability to feel pain, caused by stimulation of a nociceptor. **position s., posture s.,** the awareness of the position of the body or its parts in space, a combination of the sense of equilibrium and kinesthesia.

pressure s., the sense by which pressure upon the surface of the body is perceived. **sixth s.,** somatognosis. **somatic s's,** senses other than the special senses, including touch, pressure, pain, and temperature, kinesthesia, muscle sense, visceral sense, and sometimes sense of equilibrium. **space s.,** the sense by which relative positions and relations of objects in space are perceived. **special s's,** those of seeing, hearing, taste, smell, and sometimes sense of equilibrium. **stereognostic s.,** the sense by which form and solidity are perceived. **temperature s.,** the sense by which differences of temperature are distinguished by the thermoreceptors. **vestibular s.,** s. of equilibrium. **vibration s.,** pallesthesia. **visceral s.,** the awareness of sensations that arise from the viscera and stimulate the interoceptors; sensations include pain, pressure or fullness, and organ movement.

sen·si·bil·i·ty (sen″sĭ-bil′ĭ-te) susceptibility of feeling; ability to feel or perceive. **deep s.,** sensibility to stimuli such as pain, pressure, and movement that activate receptors below the body surface but not in the viscera. **epicritic s.,** the sensibility of the skin to gentle stimulations permitting fine discriminations of touch and temperature. **proprioceptive s.,** proprioception. **protopathic s.,** sensibility to pain and temperature which is low in degree and poorly localized. **splanchnesthetic s.,** visceral sense.

sen·si·ble (sen′sĭ-b′l) 1. capable of sensation. 2. perceptible to the senses.

sen·si·tive (sen′sĭ-tiv) 1. able to receive or respond to stimuli. 2. unusually responsive to stimulation, or responding quickly and acutely.

sen·si·tiv·i·ty (sen″sĭ-tiv′ĭ-te) 1. the state or quality of being sensitive. 2. the smallest concentration of a substance that can be reliably measured by a given analytical method. 3. the probability that a person having a disease will be correctly identified by a clinical test.

sen·si·ti·za·tion (sen″sĭ-tĭ-za′shun) 1. administration of an antigen to induce a primary immune response. 2. exposure to allergen that results in the development of hypersensitivity. **autoerythrocyte s.,** see *painful bruising syndrome,* under *syndrome.*

sen·si·tized (sen′sĭ-tīzd) rendered sensitive.

sen·so·mo·bile (sen″so-mo′b′l) moving in response to a stimulus.

sen·so·mo·tor (-mo′ter) sensorimotor.

sen·so·ri·al (sen-sor′e-al) pertaining to the sensorium.

sen·so·ri·mo·tor (sen″sor-e-mo′ter) both sensory and motor.

sen·so·ri·neu·ral (-noor′al) of or pertaining to a sensory nerve or mechanism; see also under *deafness.*

sen·so·ri·um (sen-sor′e-um) 1. a sensory nerve center. 2. the state of an individual as regards consciousness or mental awareness.

sen·so·ry (sen′sor-e) pertaining to sensation.

sen·ti·ent (sen′she-ent) able to feel; sensitive.

sen·ti·nel (sen′tĭ-n′l) one who gives a warning or indicates danger.

Seph·a·dex (sef′ah-deks) trademark for cross-linked dextran beads. Various forms are used in chromatography.

sep·sis (sep′sis) 1. presence in the blood or other tissues of pathogenic microorganisms or their toxins. 2. septicemia. **catheter s.,** sepsis occurring as a complication of intravenous catheterization. **puerperal s.,** that occurring after childbirth.

sep·ta (sep′tah) [L.] plural of *septum.*

sep·tal (sep′tal) pertaining to a septum.

sep·tate (sep′tāt) divided by a septum.

sep·tec·to·my (sep-tek′tah-me) excision of part of the nasal septum.

sep·tic (sep′tik) pertaining to sepsis.

sep·ti·ce·mia (sep″tĭ-se′me-ah) blood poisoning; systemic disease associated with the presence and persistence of pathogenic microorganisms or their toxins in the blood. **septice′mic,** adj. **cryptogenic s.,** septicemia in which the focus of infection is not evident during life. **puerperal s.,** see under *fever.*

sep·ti·co·py·emia (-ko-pi-e′me-ah) septicemia and pyemia combined. **septicopye′mic,** adj.

sep·to·mar·gi·nal (sep″to-mahr′jĭ-n′l) pertaining to the margin of a septum.

sep·to·na·sal (-na′z′l) pertaining to the nasal septum.

sep·to·plas·ty (sep′to-plas″te) surgical reconstruction of the nasal septum.

sep·tos·to·my (sep-tos′tah-me) surgical creation of an opening in a septum.

sep·tot·o·my (sep-tot′ah-me) incision of the nasal septum.

sep·tu·lum (sep′tu-lum) pl. *sep′tula.* [L.] a small separating wall or partition.

sep·tum (sep′tum) pl. *sep′ta.* [L.] a dividing wall or partition. **alveolar s.,** interalveolar s. **atrioventricular s. of heart,** the part of the membranous portion of the interventricular septum between the left ventricle and the right atrium. **Bigelow's s.,** a layer of hard, bony tissue in the neck of the femur. **s. of Cloquet, crural s., femoral s.,** the thin fibrous membrane that helps close the femoral ring. **gingival s.,** the part of the gingiva interposed between adjoining teeth. **inter-alveolar s.,** 1. one of the thin plates of bone separating the alveoli of the different teeth in the mandible and maxilla. 2. one of the thin septa separating adjacent pulmonary alveoli. **interatrial s. of heart,** the partition separating the right and left atria of the heart. **interdental s.,** interalveolar s. **interradicular s.,** interalveolar s. (1). **interventricular s. of heart,** the partition separating the right and left ventricles of the heart. **lingual s.,** the median vertical fibrous part of the tongue. **nasal s.,** the partition between the two nasal cavities. **s. pectinifor´me,** s. penis. **pellucid s., s. pellu´cidum,** the triangular double membrane separating the anterior horns of the lateral ventricles of the brain. **s. pe´nis,** the fibrous sheet between the corpora cavernosa of the penis. **s. pri´mum,** the first septum in the embryonic heart, dividing the primordial atrium into right and left chambers. **rectovaginal s.,** the membranous partition between the rectum and vagina. **rectovesical s.,** a membranous partition separating the rectum from the prostate and urinary bladder. **scrotal s.,** the partition between the two chambers of the scrotum. **s. secun´dum,** the second septum in the embryonic heart, to the right of the septum primum; after birth it fuses with the septum primum to close the foramen ovale and form the interatrial septum.

sep·tup·let (sep-tup´let) one of seven offspring produced at one birth.

se·quel (se´kwel) sequela.

se·que·la (sĕ-kwel´ah) pl. *seque´lae.* [L.] a morbid condition following or occurring as a consequence of another condition or event.

se·quence (se´kwens) 1. a connected series of events or things. 2. in dysmorphology, a pattern of multiple anomalies derived from a single prior anomaly or mechanical factor. 3. in molecular biology, DNA having a particular nucleotide pattern or occurring in a particular region of the genome. **amniotic band s.,** early rupture of the amnion with formation of strands of amnion that may adhere to or compress parts of the fetus, resulting in a wide variety of deformities. **gene s.,** the ordered arrangement of nucleotides into codons along the stretch of DNA to be transcribed. **oligohydramnios s.,** a group of anomalies, usually fatal shortly after birth, caused by compression of the fetus secondary to oligohydramnios, which may result from renal agenesis or other urinary tract defects or from leakage of amniotic fluid; infants have characteristic flattened facies (*Potter facies*),

skeletal abnormalities, and often hypoplasia of the lungs.

se·ques·ter (se-kwes´ter) 1. to detach or separate abnormally a small portion from the whole. See *sequestration* and *sequestrum.* 2. to isolate a constituent of a chemical system by chelation or other means.

se·ques·trant (se-kwes´trant) a sequestering agent, as, for example, cholestyramine resin, which binds bile acids in the intestine, thus preventing their absorption.

se·ques·tra·tion (se″kwes-tra´shun) 1. the formation of a sequestrum. 2. the isolation of a patient. 3. a net increase in the quantity of blood within a limited vascular area, occurring physiologically, with forward flow persisting or not, or produced artificially by the application of tourniquets. **pulmonary s.,** loss of connection of lung tissue with the bronchial tree and the pulmonary veins.

se·ques·trec·to·my (-trek´tah-me) excision of a sequestrum.

se·ques·trum (se-kwes´trum) pl. *seques´tra.* [L.] 1. any sequestered tissue. 2. a piece of dead bone separated from the sound bone in necrosis.

se·quoi·o·sis (se″kwoi-o´sis) hypersensitivity pneumonitis due to inhalation of and tissue reaction to dust from moldy redwood bark.

Ser serine.

se·ra (se´rah) [L.] plural of *serum.*

se·ries (se´rēz) a group or succession of events, objects, or substances arranged in regular order or forming a kind of chain; in electricity, parts of a circuit connected successively end to end to form a single path for the current. **se´rial,** adj. **erythrocytic s.,** the succession of morphologically distinguishable cells that are stages in erythrocyte development: proerythroblast, basophilic erythroblast, polychromatophilic erythroblast, orthochromatic erythroblast, reticulocyte, and erythrocyte. **granulocytic s.,** the succession of morphologically distinguishable cells that are stages in granulocyte development; there are distinct basophil, eosinophil, and neutrophil series but the morphological stages are the same. **lymphocytic s.,** a series of morphologically distinguishable cells once thought to represent stages in lymphocyte development; now known to represent various forms of mature lymphocytes. **monocytic s.,** the succession of developing cells that ultimately culminates in the monocyte. **thrombocytic s.,** the succession of developing cells that ultimately culminates in the blood platelets (thrombocytes).

ser·ine (Ser, S) (sēr'ēn) a naturally occurring nonessential amino acid present in many proteins.

ser·mo·rel·in (ser"mo-rel'in) a synthetic peptide corresponding to a portion of growth hormone–releasing hormone; used as the acetate salt in the treatment of growth hormone deficiency.

se·ro·co·li·tis (sēr"o-ko-li'tis) inflammation of the serous coat of the colon.

se·ro·con·ver·sion (-con-ver'zhun) the change of a seronegative test from negative to positive, indicating the development of antibodies in response to immunization or infection.

se·ro·di·ag·no·sis (-di"ag-no'sis) diagnosis of disease based on serologic tests. **serodiagnos'tic,** adj.

se·ro·en·te·ri·tis (-en"tĕ-ri'tis) inflammation of the serous coat of the intestine.

se·ro·fib·rin·ous (-fi'bri-nus) composed of serum and fibrin, as a serofibrinous exudate.

se·ro·group (sēr'o-grōōp") an unofficial designation denoting a group of bacteria containing a common antigen, possibly including more than one serotype, species, or genus.

se·rol·o·gy (sēr-ol'ah-je) the study of antigen-antibody reactions in vitro. **serolog'ic,** adj.

se·ro·ma (sēr-o'mah) a tumorlike collection of serum in the tissues.

se·ro·mem·bra·nous (sēr"o-mem'brah-nus) pertaining to or composed of serous membrane.

se·ro·mu·cous (-mu'kus) both serous and mucous.

se·ro·mus·cu·lar (-mus'ku-ler) pertaining to the serous and muscular coats of the intestine.

se·ro·neg·a·tive (-neg'ah-tiv) showing negative results on serological examination; showing a lack of antibody.

se·ro·pos·i·tive (-poz'ĭ-tiv) showing positive results on serological examination; showing a high level of antibody.

se·ro·pu·ru·lent (-pu'roo-lent) both serous and purulent.

se·ro·pus (sēr'o-pus) serum mingled with pus.

se·ro·re·ac·tion (sēr"o-re-ak'shun) a reaction occurring in serum or as a result of the action of a serum.

se·ro·re·ver·sion (-re-ver'zhun) spontaneous or induced conversion from a seropositive to a seronegative state.

se·ro·sa (se-ro'sah, se-ro'zah) 1. tunica serosa. 2. chorion. **sero'sal,** adj.

se·ro·san·guin·e·ous (sēr"o-sang-gwin'e-us) composed of serum and blood.

se·ro·se·rous (-sēr'us) pertaining to two or more serous membranes.

se·ro·si·tis (-si'tis) pl. *serosi'tides.* Inflammation of a serous membrane.

se·ro·sur·vey (-sur'va) a screening test of the serum of persons at risk to determine susceptibility to a particular disease.

se·ro·syn·o·vi·tis (-sin"o-vi'tis) synovitis with effusion of serum.

se·ro·ther·a·py (-ther'ah-pe) treatment of infectious disease by injection of immune serum or antitoxin.

sero·to·nin (ser"o-to'nin) a hormone and neurotransmitter, 5-hydroxytryptamine (5-HT), found in many tissues, including blood platelets, intestinal mucosa, the pineal body, and the central nervous system; it has many physiologic properties including inhibition of gastric secretion, stimulation of smooth muscles, and production of vasoconstriction.

sero·to·nin·er·gic (ser"o-to"nin-er'jik) 1. containing or activated by serotonin. 2. pertaining to neurons that secrete serotonin.

se·ro·type (sēr'o-tīp) the type of a microorganism determined by its constituent antigens; a taxonomic subdivision based thereon.

se·rous (sēr'us) 1. pertaining to or resembling serum. 2. producing or containing serum.

se·ro·vac·ci·na·tion (sēr"o-vak"sĭ-na'shun) injection of serum combined with bacterial vaccination to produce passive immunity by the former and active immunity by the latter.

ser·pig·i·nous (ser-pij'ĭ-nus) creeping; having a wavy or much indented border.

ser·pin (ser'pin) any of a superfamily of inhibitors of serine proteinase, found in plasma and tissues; all are homologous single-chain glycoproteins targeting specific serine proteinases involved in coagulation, complement activation, fibrinolysis, inflammation, and tissue remodeling.

ser·rat·ed (ser'āt-ed) having a sawlike edge.

Ser·ra·tia (sĕ-ra'she-ah) a genus of bacteria (tribe Serraticae) made up of gram-negative rods which produce a red pigment. For the most part, they are free-living saprophytes, but they cause a variety of infections in immunocompromised patients.

ser·ra·tion (se-ra'shun) 1. the state of being serrated. 2. a serrated structure or formation.

ser·tra·line (ser'trah-lēn) a selective serotonin reuptake inhibitor used as the hydrochloride salt in the treatment of depression, obsessive-compulsive disorder, and panic disorder.

se·rum (sēr'um) pl. *serums, se'ra.* [L.] 1. the clear portion of any liquid separated from its more solid elements. 2. blood s. 3. antiserum. **antilymphocyte s. (ALS),** antiserum derived from animals immunized against human lymphocytes; a powerful non-specific immunosuppressive agent that causes destruction of circulating lymphocytes. **an-tirabies s.,** antiserum obtained from the blood serum or plasma of animals immunized with rabies vaccine; used for postexposure prophylaxis against rabies if rabies immune globulin is unavailable. **blood s.,** the clear liquid that separates from blood when it is allowed to clot completely, and is therefore blood plasma from which fibrogen has been removed during clotting. **foreign s.,** hetero-logous s. **heterologous s.,** 1. that obtained from an animal belonging to species different from that of the recipient. 2. that prepared from an animal immunized by an organism differing from that against which it is to be used. **homologous s.,** 1. that obtained from an animal belonging to the same species as the recipient. 2. that prepared from an animal immunized by the same organism against which it is to be used. **immune s.,** anti-serum. **polyvalent s.,** antiserum containing antibody to more than one kind of antigen. **pooled s.,** the mixed serum from a number of individuals.

se·ru·mal (se-roo'mal) pertaining to or formed from serum.

se·rum-fast (sēr'um-fast) resistant to the effects of serum.

ses·a·moid (ses'ah-moid) 1. denoting a small nodular bone embedded in a tendon or joint capsule. 2. a sesamoid bone.

ses·sile (ses'il) attached by a broad base, as opposed to being pedunculated or stalked.

se·ta·ceous (se-ta'shus) bristlelike.

Se·ta·ria (se-tar'e-ah) a genus of filarial nematodes.

set-point (set'point) the target value of a controlled variable that is maintained physio-logically by bodily control mechanisms for homeostasis.

se·vel·a·mer (sĕ-vel'ah-mer) a phosphate-binding substance used as the hydrochloride salt to reduce serum phosphorus concentra-tions in hyperphosphatemia associated with end-stage renal disease.

sex (seks) 1. a distinctive character of most animals and plants, based on the type of gametes produced by the gonads, ova (macro-gametes) being typical of the female, and spermatozoa (microgametes) of the male, or the category in which the individual is placed on such basis. 2. see *gender identity,* under

identity. 3. sexual intercourse. 4. to deter-mine whether an organism is male or fe-male. **chromosomal s., genetic s.,** sex as determined by the presence of the XX (female) or the XY (male) genotype in somatic cells, without regard to phenotypic mani-festations. **gonadal s.,** that part of the phenotypic sex that is determined by the gonadal tissue present (ovarian or testicular). **morphological s.,** that part of the phenotypic sex that is determined by the morphology of the external genitals. **phenotypic s.,** the phenotypic manifestations of sex determined by endocrine influences.

sex-con·di·tioned (-kon-dish'und) sex-influenced.

sex-duc·tion (-duk'shun) the process where-by part of the bacterial chromosome is attached to the autonomous F (sex) factor and thus is transferred from donor (male) bacterium to recipient (female).

sex-in·flu·enced (-in'floo-enst) denoting an autosomal trait that is expressed differently, in either frequency or degree, in males and females, as for example, male-pattern bald-ness.

sex-lim·it·ed (-lim'ĭ-ted) denoting a genetic trait exhibited by one sex only, although not determined by an X-linked gene.

sex-linked (seks'linkt) transmitted by a gene located on the X chromosome.

sex·ol·o·gy (sek-sol'ah-je) the scientific study of sex and sexual relations.

sex·tup·let (seks-tup'let) any one of six offspring produced at the same birth.

sex·u·al (sek'shoo-al) 1. pertaining to, characterized by, involving, or endowed with sex, sexuality, the sexes, or the sex organs and their functions. 2. characterized by the property of maleness or femaleness. 3. per-taining to reproduction involving both male and female gametes. 4. implying or symbol-izing erotic desires or activity.

sex·u·al·i·ty (sek″shoo-al'ĭ-te) 1. the char-acteristic of the male and female reproductive elements. 2. the constitution of an individual in relation to sexual attitudes and behavior. **infantile s.,** in freudian theory, the erotic life of infants and children, encompassing the oral, anal, and phallic stages of psychosexual development.

SGOT serum glutamic-oxaloacetic transami-nase; see *aspartate transaminase.*

SGPT serum glutamic-pyruvic transaminase; see *alanine transaminase.*

shad·ow-cast·ing (shad'o-kast″ing) applica-tion of a coating of gold, chromium, or other metal to ultramicroscopic structures to increase their visibility under the microscope.

shaft (shaft) a long slender part, such as the diaphysis of a long bone.

shag·gy (shag'e) 1. covered with, having, or resembling rough long hair or wool. 2. having a rough texture or surface or hairlike processes.

sham (sham) 1. a hoax; a fraudulent imitation. 2. not genuine; fraudulent; marked by falseness.

sha·man·ism (shah'-, sha'mah-nizm″) a traditional system, occurring in tribal societies, in which certain individuals (shamans) are believed to be gifted with access to an invisible spiritual world and are able to mediate between it and the physical world to heal, divine, and affect events in the latter.

shank (shangk) 1. leg (1). 2. crus (2).

shap·ing (shāp'ing) a technique in behavior therapy in which new behavior is produced by providing reinforcement for progressively closer approximations of the final desired behavior.

shave (shāv) 1. to cut at or parallel to the surface of the skin. 2. to remove the beard or other body hair by such a process. 3. to cut thin slices from or to cut into thin slices.

SHBG sex hormone–binding globulin.

sheath (shēth) a tubular case or envelope. **arachnoid s.,** the continuation of the arachnoidea mater around the optic nerve, forming part of its internal sheath. **carotid s.,** a portion of the cervical fascia enclosing the carotid artery, the internal jugular vein, and the vagus nerve. **crural s.,** femoral s. **dentinal s.,** the layer of tissue forming the wall of a dentinal tubule. **dural s.,** the external investment of the optic nerve. **femoral s.,** the investing fascia of the proximal portion of the femoral vessels. **s. of Henle,** endoneurium. **Hertwig s.,** root s. (1). **s. of Key and Retzius,** endoneurium. **lamellar s.,** the perineurium. **Mauthner's s.,** axolemma. **medullary s., myelin s.,** the sheath surrounding the axon of myelinated nerve cells, consisting of concentric layers of myelin formed in the peripheral nervous system by the plasma membrane of Schwann cells, and in the central nervous system by oligodendrocytes. It is interrupted at intervals along the length of the axon by gaps known as *nodes of Ranvier.* Myelin is an electrical insulator that serves to speed the conduction of nerve impulses. **pial s.,** the continuation of the pia mater around the optic nerve, forming part of its internal sheath. **root s.,** 1. an investment of epithelial cells around the unerupted tooth and inside the dental follicle. 2. the epithelial portion of a hair follicle. **s. of Schwann,** neurilemma. **synovial s.,** synovial membrane lining the cavity of a bone through which a tendon moves. **tendon s.,** epitendineum.

sheet (shēt) 1. an oblong piece of cotton, linen, etc., for a bed covering. 2. any structure resembling such a covering. **draw s.,** one folded and placed under a patient's body so it may be removed with minimal disturbance of the patient.

shen (shen) one of the basic substances that according to traditional Chinese medicine pervade the body, usually translated "spirit," encompassing both the mind of the individual and healthy mental and physical function.

shi·at·su (she-ot'soo) [Japanese] a Japanese form of acupressure, in which pressure is applied using the thumb, elbow, or knee, perpendicularly to the skin at acupoints, combined with passive stretching and rotation of the joints.

shield (shēld) any protecting structure. • **Buller's s.,** a watch glass fitted over the eye to guard it from infection. **nipple s.,** a device to protect the nipple of a nursing woman.

shift (shift) a change or deviation. **chloride s.,** the exchange of chloride (Cl^-) and bicarbonate (HCO_3^-) between plasma and the erythrocytes occurring whenever HCO_3^- is generated or decomposed within the erythrocytes. **Doppler s.,** the magnitude of frequency change due to the Doppler effect. **s. to the left,** an increase in the percentage of neutrophils having only one or a few lobes. **s. to the right,** an increase in the percentage of multilobed neutrophils.

Shi·gel·la (shĭ-gel'ah) a genus of gram-negative bacteria (family Enterobacteriaceae) which cause dysentery. They are separated into four species on the basis of biochemical reactions: *S. dysente′riae, S. flexne′ri, S. boy′dii,* and *S. son′nei.*

shi·gel·la (shĭ-gel'ah) pl. *shigel′lae.* An individual organism of the genus *Shigella.*

shi·gel·lo·sis (shĭ″gel-lo′sis) infection with *Shigella;* bacillary dysentery.

shin (shin) the prominent anterior edge of the tibia or the leg. **saber s.,** marked anterior convexity of the tibia, seen in congenital syphilis and in yaws.

shin·gles (shing′g′lz) herpes zoster.

shiv·er·ing (shiv′er-ing) 1. involuntary shaking of the body, as with cold. 2. a disease of horses, with trembling or quivering of various muscles.

shock (shok) 1. a sudden disturbance of mental equilibrium. 2. a profound hemodynamic and metabolic disturbance due to failure of the circulatory system to maintain adequate perfusion of vital organs. **anaphylactic s.,** see *anaphylaxis.* **cardiogenic s.,** shock resulting from inadequate cardiac function, as from myocardial infarction or mechanical obstruction; characteristics include hypovolemia, hypotension, cold skin, weak pulse, and confusion. **endotoxin s.,** septic shock due to release of endotoxins by gram-negative bacteria. **hypovolemic s.,** shock due to insufficient blood volume, either from hemorrhage or other loss of fluid or from widespread vasodilation so that normal blood volume cannot maintain tissue perfusion; symptoms are like those of cardiogenic shock. **insulin s.,** a hypoglycemic reaction to overdosage of insulin, a skipped meal, or strenuous exercise in an insulin-dependent diabetic, with tremor, dizziness, cool moist skin, hunger, and tachycardia, sometimes progressing to coma and convulsions. **septic s.,** shock associated with overwhelming infection, most commonly infection with gram-negative bacteria, thought to result from the actions of endotoxins and other products of the infectious agent that cause sequestration of blood in the capillaries and veins. **serum s.,** see *anaphylaxis* and see under *sickness.*

shot·ty (shot′e) like shot; resembling the pellets used in shotgun cartridges.

shoul·der (shōl′der) the area where the arm joins the trunk and the clavicle meets the scapula. **frozen s.,** adhesive capsulitis.

shoul·der-blade (-blād) scapula; see *Table of Bones.*

show (sho) appearance of blood forerunning labor or menstruation.

shunt (shunt) 1. to turn to one side; to bypass. 2. a passage or anastomosis between two natural channels, especially between blood vessels, formed physiologically or anomalously. 3. a surgically created anastomosis; also, the operation of forming a shunt. **arteriovenous s.,** 1. the diversion of blood from an artery directly to a vein. 2. a U-shaped plastic tube inserted between an artery and a vein; usually to allow repeated access to the arterial system for hemodialysis. **Blalock-Taussig s.,** see under *operation.* **cardiovascular s.,** diversion of the blood flow through an anomalous opening from the left side of the heart to the right side or from the systemic to the pulmonary circulation (*left-to-right s.*), or from the right side to the left side or from the pulmonary to the systemic circulation (*right-to-left s.*). **left-to-right s.,** see *cardiovascular s.* **LeVeen peritoneovenous s.,** continuous shunting of

ascites fluid from the peritoneal cavity to the jugular vein by means of a surgically implanted subcutaneous plastic tube. **portacaval s.,** surgical anastomosis of the portal vein and the vena cava. **right-to-left s.,** see *cardiovascular s.* **splenorenal s.,** removal of the spleen with anastomosis of the splenic vein to the left renal vein. **ventriculoatrial s.,** the surgical creation of a communication between a cerebral ventricle and a cardiac atrium by means of a plastic tube, to permit drainage of cerebrospinal fluid for relief of hydrocephalus. **ventriculoperitoneal s.,** a communication between a cerebral ventricle and the peritoneum by means of plastic tubing; done for the relief of hydrocephalus.

SI Système International d'Unités, or International System of Units. See *SI unit,* under *unit.*

Si silicon.

SIADH syndrome of inappropriate antidiuretic hormone.

si·al·ad·e·ni·tis (si″al-ad″ĕ-ni′tis) inflammation of a salivary gland.

si·al·ad·e·no·ma (-ad″ĕ-no′mah) a benign tumor of the salivary glands.

si·al·ad·e·nop·a·thy (-ad″ĕ-nop′ah-the) sialadenosis.

si·al·ad·e·no·sis (-ad″en-o′sis) sialadenopathy; a disease of a salivary gland.

si·al·a·gogue (si-al′ah-gog) an agent which stimulates the flow of saliva. **sialagog′ic,** adj.

si·al·ec·ta·sia (si″al-ek-ta′zhah) dilatation of a salivary duct.

si·al·ic ac·id (si-al′ik) any of a group of acetylated derivatives of neuraminic acid; they occur in many polysaccharides, glycoproteins, and glycolipids in animals and bacteria.

si·a·li·tis (si″ah-li′tis) inflammation of a salivary gland or duct.

sial(o)- word element [Gr.], *saliva; salivary glands.*

si·a·lo·ad·e·nec·to·my (si″ah-lo-ad″ĕ-nek′tah-me) excision of a salivary gland.

si·a·lo·ad·e·ni·tis (-ad″ĕ-ni′tis) sialadenitis.

si·a·lo·ad·e·not·o·my (-ad′en-ot′ah-me) incision and drainage of a salivary gland.

si·a·lo·aer·oph·a·gy (-ār-of′ah-je) the swallowing of saliva and air.

si·a·lo·an·gi·ec·ta·sis (-an″je-ek′tah-sis) sialectasia.

si·a·lo·an·gi·itis (-an″je-i′tis) sialoductitis; inflammation of a salivary duct.

si·a·lo·an·gi·og·ra·phy (-an″je-og′rah-fe) radiography of the ducts of the salivary glands after injection of radiopaque material.

si·a·lo·cele (si′ah-lo-sēl″) a salivary cyst.

si·a·lo·do·chi·tis (si″ah-lo-do-ki′tis) sialoangiitis.

si·a·lo·do·cho·plas·ty (-do'ko-plas"te) plastic repair of a salivary duct.

si·a·lo·duc·ti·tis (-duk-ti'tis) sialoangiitis.

si·a·log·e·nous (si"ah-loj'ĕ-nus) producing saliva.

si·a·log·ra·phy (si"ah-log'rah-fe) sialoangiography.

si·a·lo·lith (si-al'o-lith) a calcareous concretion or calculus in the salivary ducts or glands, usually the submaxillary gland and its duct.

si·a·lo·li·thi·a·sis (si"ah-lo-li-thi'ah-sis) the formation of salivary calculi.

si·a·lo·li·thot·o·my (-li-thot'ah-me) excision of a salivary calculus.

si·a·lo·meta·pla·sia (-met"ah-pla'zhah) metaplasia of the salivary glands. **necrotizing s.,** a benign inflammatory condition of the salivary glands, simulating mucoepidermoid and squamous cell carcinoma.

si·a·lo·mu·cin (-mu'sin) a mucin whose carbohydrate groups contain sialic acid.

si·a·lor·rhea (-re'ah) ptyalism.

si·a·los·che·sis (si"ah-los'kĕ-sis) suppression of secretion of saliva.

si·a·lo·ste·no·sis (si"ah-lo-stĕ-no'sis) stenosis of a salivary duct.

si·a·lo·sy·rinx (-sēr'inks) 1. salivary fistula. 2. a syringe for washing out the salivary ducts, or a drainage tube for the salivary ducts.

sib (sib) 1. a blood relative; one of a group of persons all descended from a common ancestor. 2. sibling.

sib·i·lant (sib'i-lant) whistling or hissing.

sib·ling (sib'ling) any of two or more offspring of the same parents; a brother or sister.

sib·ship (-ship) 1. relationship by blood. 2. a group of persons all descended from a common ancestor. 3. a group of siblings.

si·bu·tra·mine (si-bu'trah-mēn") an anorectic used as the hydrochloride salt in the management of obesity.

sic·cus (sik'us) [L.] dry.

sick (sik) 1. not in good health; afflicted by disease; ill. 2. nauseated.

sick·le·mia (sik-le'me-ah) sickle cell anemia.

sick·ling (sik'ling) the development of sickle cells in the blood.

sick·ness (sik'nes) disease. **African sleeping s.,** African trypanosomiasis. **air s.,** airsickness. **altitude s.,** a condition due to difficulty adjusting to lowered oxygen pressure at high altitudes; it may take the form of mountain sickness, high-altitude pulmonary edema, or cerebral edema. **car s.,** carsickness. **decompression s.,** divers' paralysis; joint pain, respiratory problems, skin lesions, and neurologic signs, due to rapid reduction of air pressure in a person's environment.

green tobacco s., transient, recurring nicotine poisoning in tobacco harvesters. **high-altitude s.,** altitude s. **milk s.,** an acute, often fatal disease in humans after they ingest milk, milk products, or flesh of cattle or sheep who have eaten certain toxic plants; human disease is marked by weakness, anorexia, vomiting, and sometimes muscular tremors. **morning s.,** nausea of early pregnancy. **motion s.,** nausea and malaise due to unaccustomed motion, such as in travel by airplane, automobile, ship, or train. **mountain s.,** a type of high altitude sickness with oliguria, dyspnea, blood pressure and pulse rate changes, and neurological disorders. **radiation s.,** a condition resulting from exposure to a whole-body dose of over 1 gray of ionizing radiation and characterized by the symptoms of the acute radiation syndrome. **sea s.,** seasickness. **serum s.,** a hypersensitivity reaction after administration of foreign serum or serum proteins, marked by urticaria, arthralgia, edema, and lymphadenopathy. **sleeping s.,** increasing lethargy and drowsiness due to a disease process such as African trypanosomiasis or types of encephalomyelitis.

s.i.d. [L.] sem'el in di'e (once a day).

sider(o)- word element [Gr.], *iron.*

sid·ero·blast (sid'er-o-blast") a nucleated erythrocyte containing iron granules in its cytoplasm. **sideroblas'tic,** adj. **ringed s.,** an abnormal sideroblast with many iron granules in its mitochondria, found in a ring around the nucleus; seen in sideroblastic anemia.

sid·ero·cyte (-sīt") an erythrocyte containing nonhemoglobin iron.

sid·ero·der·ma (sid"er-o-der'mah) bronzed coloration of the skin due to disordered iron metabolism.

sid·ero·fi·bro·sis (-fi-bro'sis) fibrosis of the spleen with deposits of iron. **siderofibrot'ic,** adj.

sid·ero·my·cin (-mi'sin) any of a class of antibiotics, synthesized by certain actinomycetes, that inhibit bacterial growth by interfering with iron uptake.

sid·ero·pe·nia (-pe'ne-ah) iron deficiency. **siderope'nic,** adj.

sid·ero·phil (sid'er-o-fil) 1. siderophilous. 2. a siderophilous cell or tissue.

sid·er·oph·i·lous (sid"er-of'i-lus) tending to absorb iron.

sid·ero·phore (sid'er-o-for") a macrophage containing hemosiderin.

sid·er·o·sil·i·co·sis (sid"er-o-sil"i-ko'sis) pneumoconiosis from inhalation of dust containing particles of iron ore and silica.

sid·er·o·sis (sid″er-o′sis) 1. pneumoconiosis due to inhalation of iron particles. 2. hyperferremia. 3. hemosiderosis. **hepatic s.,** the deposit of an abnormal quantity of iron in the liver. **urinary s.,** hemosiderinuria.

SIDS sudden infant death syndrome.

sie·mens (S) (se′menz) the SI unit of conductance; the conductance of one ampere per volt in a body with one ohm resistance.

sig. [L.] sig′na (mark).

sight (sīt) vision (1, 2). **far s.,** hyperopia. **near s.,** myopia. **night s.,** hemeralopia. **second s.,** senopia.

sig·ma·tism (sig′mah-tizm) faulty enunciation or too frequent use of the *s* sound.

sig·moid (sig′moid) 1. shaped like the letter C or S. 2. sigmoid colon.

sig·moid·ec·to·my (sig″moi-dek′tah-me) excision of part or all of the sigmoid colon.

sig·moid·itis (sig″moi-di′tis) inflammation of the sigmoid colon.

sig·moido·pexy (sig-moid′o-pek″se) fixation of the sigmoid colon, as for rectal prolapse.

sig·moido·proc·tos·to·my (sig-moid″o-prok-tos′tah-me) surgical anastomosis of the sigmoid colon to the rectum.

sig·moid·os·co·py (sig″moi-dos′kah-pe) direct examination of the interior of the sigmoid colon.

sig·moido·sig·moi·dos·to·my (sig-moid″-o-sig″moi-dos′tah-me) surgical anastomosis of two portions of the sigmoid colon; the opening so created.

sig·moid·os·to·my (sig″moi-dos′tah-me) creation of an artificial opening from the sigmoid colon to the body surface; the opening so created.

sig·moid·ot·o·my (sig″moi-dot′ah-me) incision of the sigmoid colon.

sig·moido·ves·i·cal (sig-moid″o-ves′ĭ-k'l) pertaining to or communicating with the sigmoid colon and the urinary bladder.

sign (sīn) an indication of the existence of something; any objective evidence of a disease, i.e., such evidence as is perceptible to the examining physician, as opposed to the subjective sensations (symptoms) of the patient. **Abadie's s.,** insensibility of the Achilles tendon to pressure in tabes dorsalis. **Babinski's s.,** 1. loss or lessening of the triceps surae reflex in organic sciatica. 2. see under *reflex.* 3. in organic hemiplegia, failure of the platysma muscle to contract on the affected side in opening the mouth, whistling, etc. 4. in organic hemiplegia, flexion of the thigh and lifting of the heel from the ground when the patient tries to sit up from a supine position with arms crossed upon chest. 5. in organic paralysis, when the affected forearm is placed in supination, it turns over to pronation. **Beevor's s.,** 1. in functional paralysis, inability to inhibit the antagonistic muscles. 2. in paralysis of the lower abdominal muscles due to a spinal cord lesion in the region of the lower thoracic vertebrae, there is upward excursion of the umbilicus on attempting to lift the head. **Bergman's s.,** in urologic radiography, *(a)* the ureter is dilated immediately below a neoplasm, rather than collapsed as below an obstructing stone, and *(b)* the ureteral catheter tends to coil in this dilated portion of the ureter. **Biernacki's s.,** analgesia of the ulnar nerve in general paresis and tabes dorsalis. **Blumberg's s.,** pain on abrupt release of steady pressure (rebound tenderness) over the site of a suspected abdominal lesion, indicative of peritonitis. **Branham's s.,** bradycardia produced by digital closure of an artery proximal to an arteriovenous fistula. **Braxton Hicks' s.,** see under *contraction.* **Broadbent's s.,** retraction on the left side of the back, near the eleventh and twelfth ribs, related to pericardial adhesion. **Brudzinski's s.,** 1. in meningitis, flexion of the neck usually causes flexion of the hip and knee. 2. in meningitis, on passive flexion of one lower limb, the contralateral limb shows a similar movement. **Chaddock's s.,** see under *reflex.* **Chadwick's s.,** a dark blue to purplish-red congested appearance of the vaginal mucosa, an indication of pregnancy. **Chvostek's s., Chvostek-Weiss s.,** spasm of the facial muscles elicited by tapping the facial nerve in the region of the parotid gland; seen in tetany. **Cullen's s.,** bluish discoloration around the umbilicus sometimes associated with intraperitoneal hemorrhage, especially after rupture of the uterine tube in ectopic pregnancy; similar discoloration occurs in acute hemorrhagic pancreatitis. **Dalrymple's s.,** abnormal wideness of the palpebral opening in Graves' disease. **Delbet's s.,** in aneurysm of a limb's main artery, if nutrition of the part distal to the aneurysm is maintained despite absence of the pulse, collateral circulation is sufficient. **de Musset's s.,** Musset's s. **Ewart's s.,** bronchial breathing and dullness on percussion at the lower angle of the left scapula in pericardial effusion. **fabere s.,** see *Patrick's test.* **Friedreich's s.,** diastolic collapse of the cervical veins due to adhesion of the pericardium. **Goodell's s.,** softening of the cervix; a sign of pregnancy. **Gorlin's s.,** the ability to touch the tip of the nose with the tongue, often a sign of Ehlers-Danlos syndrome. **Graefe's s.,** tardy or jerky downward movement of the upper eyelids when the gaze is directed downward; noted in thyrotoxicosis. **halo s.,** a halo effect produced in the radiograph of the fetal head between the subcutaneous fat and the cranium; said to be indicative of intrauterine death of the fetus. **harlequin s.,** reddening of the lower half of the laterally recumbent body and blanching of the upper half, due to temporary vasomotor disturbance in newborn infants. **Hegar's s.,** softening of the lower uterine segment; indicative of pregnancy. **Hoffmann's s.,** 1. increased mechanical irritability of the sensory nerves in tetany; the ulnar nerve is usually tested. 2. a sudden nipping of the nail of the index, middle, or ring finger produces flexion of the terminal phalanx of the thumb and of the second and third phalanges of some other finger. **Homans' s.,** discomfort behind the knee on forced dorsiflexion of the foot, due to thrombosis in the calf veins. **Hoover's s.,** 1. in the normal state or in true paralysis, when the supine patient presses the leg against the surface on which he is lying, the other leg will lift. 2. movement of the costal margins toward the midline in inhalation, bilaterally in pulmonary emphysema and unilaterally in conditions causing flattening of the diaphragm. **Joffroy's s.,** in Graves' disease, absence of forehead wrinkling when the gaze is suddenly directed upward. **Kernig's s.,** in meningitis, inability to completely extend the leg when sitting or lying with the thigh flexed upon the abdomen; when in dorsal decubitus position, the leg can be easily and completely extended. **Klippel-Weil s.,** in pyramidal tract disease, flexion and adduction of the thumb when the flexed fingers are quickly extended by the examiner. **Lasègue's s.,** in sciatica, flexion of the hip is painful when the knee is extended, but painless when the knee is flexed. **Léri's s.,** absence of normal flexion of the elbow on passive flexion of the hand at the wrist of the affected side in hemiplegia. **Lhermitte's s.,** electric-like shocks spreading down the body on flexing the head forward; seen mainly in multiple sclerosis but also in compression and other cervical cord disorders. **Macewen's s.,** a more than normal resonant note on percussion of the skull behind the junction of the frontal, temporal, and parietal bones in internal hydrocephalus and cerebral abscess. **McMurray s.,** occurrence of a cartilage click on manipulation of the knee; indicative of meniscal injury. **Möbius' s.,** in Graves' disease, inability to keep the eyes converged due to insufficiency of the internal rectus muscles. **Musset's s.,** rhythmical jerking of the head in aortic aneurysm and aortic insufficiency. **Nikolsky's s.,** in pemphigus vulgaris and some other bullous diseases, the outer epidermis separates easily from the basal layer on exertion of firm sliding manual pressure. **Oliver s.,** tracheal tugging; see *tugging.* **Oppenheim s.,** see under *reflex.* **Queckenstedt's s.,** when the veins in the neck are compressed on one or both sides in healthy persons, there is a rapid rise in the pressure of the cerebrospinal fluid, which then returns quickly to normal when compression ceases. In obstruction of the vertebral canal, the pressure of the cerebrospinal fluid is little or not at all affected. **Romberg's s.,** swaying of the body or falling when the eyes are closed while standing with the feet close together; observed in tabes dorsalis. **Rossolimo's s.,** see under *reflex.* **setting-sun s.,** downward deviation of the eyes so that each iris appears to "set" beneath the lower lid, with white sclera exposed between it and the upper lid; indicative of increased intracranial pressure or irritation of the brain stem. **Stellwag's s.,** infrequent or incomplete blinking, a sign of Graves' disease. **string of beads s.,** a series of rounded shapes resembling a string of beads on a radiograph of the small intestine, indicating bubbles of trapped gas within the fluid of an obstructed and distended bowel. **Tinel's s.,** a tingling sensation in the distal end of a limb when percussion is made over the site of a divided nerve. It indicates a partial lesion or the beginning regeneration of the nerve. **Trousseau's s.,** tache cérébrale. **vital s's,** the pulse, respiration, and temperature.

sig·na (sig′nah) [L.] write or make a mark; abbreviated S. or sig. in prescriptions.

sig·na·ture (-chur) the part of a prescription that gives directions as to the taking of the medicine.

sig·nif·i·cant (sig-nif′ĭ-kant) in statistics, probably resulting from something other than chance.

sign·ing (sīn′ing) dactylology; use of a system of hand movements for communication.

Si·las·tic (sĭ-las′tik) trademark for polymeric silicone substances that have the properties of rubber but are biologically inert; used in surgical prostheses.

sil·den·a·fil (sil-den′ah-fil″) a phosphodiesterase inhibitor that relaxes the smooth muscle of the penis, facilitating blood flow to the corpus cavernosum; used as the citrate salt to treat erectile dysfunction.

si·lent (si′lent) 1. noiseless. 2. producing no detectable signs or symptoms.

sil·i·ca (sil´ĭ-kah) silicon dioxide, SiO_2, occurring in various allotropic forms, some of which are used in dental materials. See also *silicosis*.

sil·i·ca·to·sis (sil˝ĭ-kah-to´sis) pneumoconiosis caused by inhalation of the dust of silicates such as those in asbestos, kaolin, mica, or talc.

sil·i·co·an·thra·co·sis (sil˝ĭ-ko-an˝thrah-ko´sis) anthracosilicosis.

sil·i·con (sil´ĭ-kon) chemical element (see *Table of Elements*), at. no. 14, symbol Si. **s. carbide,** a compound of silicon and carbon used in dentistry as an abrasive agent. **s. dioxide,** silica.

sil·i·cone (sil´ĭ-kōn) any of a large group of organic compounds comprising alternating silicon and oxygen atoms linked to organic radicals, particularly methyl groups; uses have included wetting agents and surfactants, sealants, coolants, contact lenses, and surgical membranes and implants.

sil·i·co·sid·er·o·sis (sil˝ĭ-ko-sid˝er-o´sis) siderosilicosis.

sil·i·co·sis (sil˝ĭ-ko´sis) pneumoconiosis due to inhalation of the dust of stone, sand, or flint containing silica, with generalized nodular fibrotic changes in the lungs. **sili·cot´ic,** adj.

sil·i·quose (sil´ĭ-kwōs) pertaining to or resembling a pod or husk.

silk (silk) the protein filament produced by the larvae of various insects; braided, degummed silk obtained from the cocoons of the silkworm *Bombyx mori* is used as a nonabsorbable suture material.

si·lox·ane (si-lok´sān) any of various compounds based on a substituted backbone of alternating silica and oxygen molecules; in polymeric form they are polysiloxanes, and when the side chain substituents are organic radicals, they are silicones.

sil·ver (sil´ver) chemical element (see *Table of Elements*), at. no. 47, symbol Ag. **s. nitrate,** used as a local anti-infective, as in the prophylaxis of ophthalmia neonatorum. **s. protein,** silver made colloidal by the presence of, or combination with, protein; it may be *mild*, used as a topical anti-infective, or *strong*, used as an active germicide with a local irritant and astringent effect. **s. sulfadiazine,** the silver derivative of sulfadiazine, having bactericidal activity against many gram-positive and gram-negative organisms, as well as being effective against yeasts; used as a topical antiinfective for the prevention and treatment of wound sepsis in patients with second and third degree burns. **toughened s. nitrate,** a compound of silver nitrate,

hydrochloric acid, sodium chloride, or potassium nitrate; used as a caustic, applied topically after being dipped in water.

si·meth·i·cone (sĭ-meth´ĭ-kōn) an antifoaming and antiflatulent agent consisting of a mixture of dimethicones and silicon dioxide.

sim·i·an (sim´e-an) of, pertaining to, or resembling an ape or a monkey.

si·mi·lia si·mi·li·bus cu·ran·tur (sĭ-mĭ´le-ah sĭ-mĭ´lĭ-bus ku-ran´tur) [L. "likes are cured by likes"] the doctrine, which lies at the foundation of homeopathy, that a disease is cured by those remedies which produce effects resembling the disease itself.

si·mil·li·mum (sĭ-mil´ĭ-mum) [L.] the homeopathic remedy that most exactly reproduces the symptoms of any disease.

sim·ple (sim´p'l) neither compound nor complex; single.

Sim·plex·vi·rus (sim´pleks-vi˝rus) herpes simplex–like viruses; a genus of ubiquitous viruses of the subfamily Alphaherpesvirinae (family Herpesviridae) that infect humans and other animals.

sim·ul (sim´ul) [L.] at the same time as.

sim·u·la·tor (sim´u-la˝tor) something that simulates, such as an apparatus that simulates conditions that will be encountered in real life.

Si·mu·li·um (sĭ-mu´le-um) a genus of biting gnats; some species are intermediate hosts of *Onchocerca volvulus.*

si·mul·tan·ag·no·sia (si˝mul-tăn˝ag-no´zhah) partial visual agnosia, consisting of the inability to comprehend more than one element of a visual scene at the same time or to integrate the parts as a whole.

sim·va·stat·in (sim´vah-stat˝in) an antihyperlipidemic agent that acts by inhibiting cholesterol synthesis, used in the treatment of hypercholesterolemia and other forms of dyslipidemia and to lower the risks associated with atherosclerosis and coronary heart disease.

sin·ci·put (sin´sĭ-put) the upper and front part of the head. **sincip´ital,** adj.

sin·ew (sin´u) a tendon of a muscle. **weeping s.,** an encysted ganglion, chiefly on the back of the hand, containing synovial fluid.

sin·gle blind (sing´g'l blīnd) pertaining to an experiment in which subjects do not know which treatment they are receiving.

sin·gul·tus (sing-gul´tus) [L.] hiccup.

si·nis·ter (sin´is-ter) [L.] left; on the left side.

si·nis·trad (sin´is-trad) to or toward the left.

sin·is·tral (-tral) 1. pertaining to the left side. 2. a left-handed person.

sin·is·tral·i·ty (sin˝is-tral´ĭ-te) lateral dominance on the left side.

sin·is·trau·ral (sin″is-traw′ral) hearing better with the left ear.

sinistr(o)- word element [L.], *left; left side.*

sin·is·tro·cer·e·bral (sin″is-tro-ser′ĕ-bral) pertaining to or situated in the left cerebral hemisphere.

sin·is·troc·u·lar (sin″is-trok′u-ler) having the left eye dominant.

sin·is·tro·gy·ra·tion (sin″is-tro-ji-ra′shun) a turning to the left.

sin·is·tro·man·u·al (-man′u-al) left-handed.

sin·is·trop·e·dal (sin″is-trop′ĕ-dal) using the left foot in preference to the right.

sin·is·tro·tor·sion (sin″is-tro-tor′shun) a twisting toward the left, as of the eye.

si·no·atri·al (si″no-a′tre-al) pertaining to the sinus venosus and the atrium of the heart.

si·no·bron·chi·tis (-brong-ki′tis) chronic paranasal sinusitis with recurrent bronchitis.

si·no·pul·mo·nary (-pool′mah-nar″e) involving the paranasal sinuses and the lungs.

sinu·at·ri·al (sin″u-a′tre-al) sinoatrial.

sin·u·ous (sin′u-us) bending in and out; winding.

si·nus (si′nus) pl. *si′nus, sinuses.* [L.]. 1. a recess, cavity, or channel, as (*a*) one in bone or (*b*) a dilated channel for venous blood. 2. an abnormal channel or fistula permitting escape of pus. **si′nusal,** adj. **air s.,** an air-containing space within a bone. **anal s's,** furrows, with pouchlike openings at the distal end, separating the rectal columns. **aortic s.,** a dilatation between the aortic wall and each of the semilunar cusps of the aortic valve; from two of these sinuses the coronary arteries originate. **branchial s.,** an abnormal cavity or space opening externally on the inferior third of the neck; usually a result of persistence of the second pharyngeal groove and cervical sinus. **carotid s.,** a dilatation of the proximal portion of the internal carotid or distal portion of the common carotid artery, containing in its wall pressoreceptors which are stimulated by changes in blood pressure. **cavernous s.,** either of two irregularly shaped sinuses of the dura mater, located at either side of the body of the sphenoid bone and communicating across the midline; it contains the internal carotid artery and abducent nerve. **cervical s.,** a temporary depression caudal to the second pharyngeal arch, containing the succeeding pharyngeal arches; it is overgrown by the second pharyngeal arch and closes off as the cervical vesicle. **circular s.,** the venous channel encircling the hypophysis, formed by the two cavernous sinuses and the anterior and posterior intercavernous sinuses. **coccygeal s.,** a sinus or fistula just over or close to the tip of the coccyx.

coronary s., the terminal portion of the great cardiac vein, lying in the coronary sulcus between the left atrium and ventricle, and emptying into the right atrium. **cortical s's,** lymph sinuses in the cortex of a lymph node, which arise from the marginal sinuses and continue into the medullary sinuses. **dermal s.,** a congenital sinus tract extending from the surface of the body, between the bodies of two adjacent lumbar vertebrae, to the spinal canal. **dural s's,** large venous channels forming an anastomosing system between the layers of the dura mater, draining the cerebral veins and some diploic and meningeal veins into the veins of the neck. **s. of epididymis,** a long, slitlike serous pocket between the upper part of the testis and the overlying epididymis. **ethmoid s's, ethmoidal s's,** see under *cell.* **frontal s.,** one of the paired paranasal sinuses in the frontal bone, each communicating with the middle meatus of the ipsilateral nasal cavity. **intercavernous s's,** two sinuses of the dura mater connecting the two cavernous sinuses, one passing anterior and the other posterior to the infundibulum of the hypophysis. **lacteal s's, lactiferous s's,** enlargements of the lactiferous ducts just before they open on the mammary papilla. **lymphatic s's,** irregular, tortuous spaces within lymphoid tissue (nodes) through which lymph passes, to enter efferent lymphatic vessels. **marginal s's,** 1. see under *lake.* 2. bowl-shaped lymph sinuses separating the capsule from the cortical parenchyma, and from which lymph flows into the cortical sinuses. **maxillary s.,** one of the paired paranasal sinuses in the body of the maxilla on either side, and opening into the middle meatus of the ipsilateral nasal cavity. **medullary s's,** lymph sinuses in the medulla of a lymph node, which divide the lymphoid tissue into a number of medullary cords. **occipital s.,** one of the sinuses of the dura mater, passing upward along the midline of the cerebellum. **oral s.,** stomodeum. **paranasal s's,** mucosa-lined air cavities in bones of the skull, communicating with the nasal cavity and including ethmoidal, frontal, maxillary, and sphenoidal sinuses. **petrosal s.,** either of two sinuses of the dura mater, arising from the cavernous sinus and draining into the internal jugular vein (*inferior petrosal s.*) or into the transverse sinus (*superior petrosal s.*). **pilonidal s.,** a suppurating sinus containing hair, occurring chiefly in the coccygeal region. **prostatic s.,** the posterolateral recess between the seminal colliculus and the wall of the urethra. **s. of pulmonary trunk,** a slight dilatation between the wall of the pulmonary trunk and each of the semilunar cusps of the pulmonary trunk valve. **renal s.,** a recess in the substance of the kidney, occupied by the renal pelvis, calices, vessels, nerves, and fat. **sagittal s., inferior,** a small venous sinus of the dura mater, opening into the straight sinus. **sagittal s., superior,** a venous sinus of the dura mater which ends in the confluence of sinuses. **sigmoid s.,** a venous sinus of the dura mater on either side, continuous with the transverse sinus and draining into the internal jugular vein of the same side. **sphenoid s., sphenoidal s.,** one of the paired paranasal sinuses in the body of the sphenoid bone and opening into the highest meatus of the ipsilateral nasal cavity. **sphenoparietal s.,** either of two sinuses of the dura mater, draining into the anterior part of the cavernous sinus. **s. of spleen,** a dilated venous sinus in the substance of the spleen. **straight s.,** one of the sinuses of the dura mater formed by junction of the great cerebral vein and inferior sagittal sinus, commonly ending in the confluence of the sinuses. **tarsal s.,** a space between the calcaneus and talus. **tentorial s.,** straight s. **terminal s.,** a vein that encircles the vascular area in the blastoderm. **transverse s.,** 1. either of two large sinuses of the dura mater. 2. a passage behind the aorta and pulmonary trunk and in front of the atria. **tympanic s.,** a deep recess in the posterior part of the tympanic cavity. **urogenital s.,** an elongated sac formed by division of the cloaca in the early embryo, forming most of the bladder, the female vestibule, urethra, and vagina, and most of the male urethra. **uterine s's,** venous channels in the wall of the uterus in pregnancy. **s. of venae cavae,** the portion of the right atrium into which the inferior and the superior venae cavae open. **s. veno′sus,** 1. the common venous receptacle in the embryonic midheart, attached to the posterior wall of the primordial atrium. 2. venous s. (1). 3. s. of venae cavae. **venous s.,** 1. a large vein or channel for the circulation of venous blood. 2. s. venosus (1). **venous s's of dura mater,** large channels for venous blood forming an anastomosing system between the layers of the dura mater of the brain, receiving blood from the brain and draining into the veins of the scalp or deep veins at the base of the skull. **venous s. of sclera,** a branching, circumferential vessel in the internal scleral sulcus, a major component of the drainage pathway for aqueous humor.

si·nus·itis (si″nŭ-si′tis) inflammation of a sinus.

si·nus·oid (si′nŭ-soid) 1. resembling a sinus. 2. a form of terminal blood channel consisting of a large, irregular anastomosing vessel having a lining of reticuloendothelium and found in the liver, heart, spleen, pancreas, and the adrenal, parathyroid, carotid, and hemolymph glands.

si·nus·oi·dal (si″nŭ-soi′dal) 1. located in a sinusoid or affecting the circulation in the region of a sinusoid. 2. shaped like or pertaining to a sine wave.

si·nus·ot·o·my (si″nŭ-sot′ah-me) incision of a sinus.

si·phon (si′fun) a bent tube with two arms of unequal length, used to transfer liquids from a higher to a lower level by the force of atmospheric pressure.

si·phon·age (si′fun-ij) the use of the siphon, as in gastric lavage or in draining the bladder.

si·reno·me·lia (si″ren-o-me′le-ah) apodal symmelia.

si·ren·om·e·lus (si″ren-om′ĕ-lus) a fetus with sirenomelia.

si·ro·li·mus (sĭ-ro′lĭ-mus) a macrolide antibiotic having immunosuppressant properties; used to prevent rejection of kidney transplants.

-sis word element [Gr.], *state; condition.*

SISI short increment sensitivity index.

sis·ter (sis′ter) the nurse in charge of a hospital ward (Great Britain).

Sis·tru·rus (sis-troo′rus) a genus of small rattlesnakes of the family Crotalidae; they occur throughout the United States and have symmetrical plates covering their heads. *S. catena′tus* is the massasauga and *S. milia′rius* is the *pygmy rattlesnake.*

site (sīt) a place, position, or locus. **allosteric s.,** a site on a multi-subunit enzyme that is not the substrate binding site but that when reversibly bound by an effector induces a conformational change in the enzyme, altering its catalytic properties. **antigen-binding s., antigen-combining s.,** the region of the antibody molecule that binds to antigens. **binding s.,** in an enzyme or other protein, the three-dimensional configuration of specific groups on specific amino acids that binds specific compounds, such as substrates or effectors, with high affinity and specificity. **operator s.,** a site adjacent to the structural genes in the operon, where repressor molecules are bound, thereby inhibiting the transcription of the genes in the adjacent operon. **restriction s.,** a base sequence in a DNA segment recognized by a particular restriction endonuclease.

sit(o)- word element [Gr.], *food.*

si·tos·ter·ol (si-tos′ter-ol) any of a group of closely related plant sterols, having anti-cholesterolemic activity.

si·tos·ter·ol·emia (si-tos″ter-ol-e′me-ah) the presence of excessive sitosterols in the blood, especially β-sitosterol, from dietary vegetables. Written also β-*sitosterolemia*.

si·tot·ro·pism (si-tot′ro-pizm) response of living cells to the presence of nutritive elements.

si·tus (si′tus) pl. *si′tus*. [L.] site or position. **s. inver′sus vis′cerum,** lateral transposition of the viscera of the thorax and abdomen. **s. transver′sus,** s. inversus viscerum.

SIV simian immunodeficiency virus.

skat·ole (skat′ōl) a strong-smelling crystalline amine from human feces, produced by protein decomposition in the intestine and directly from tryptophan by decarboxylation.

skel·e·tal (skel′ĕ-t′l) pertaining to the skeleton.

skel·e·ti·za·tion (skel″ĕ-tĭ-za′shun) 1. extreme emaciation. 2. removal of soft parts from the skeleton.

skel·e·tog·e·nous (skel″ĕ-toj′ĕ-nus) producing skeletal or bony structures.

skel·e·ton (skel′ĕ-ton) [Gr.] the hard framework of the animal body, especially that of higher vertebrates; the bones of the body collectively. See Plate 1. **appendicular s.,** the bones of the limbs and supporting thoracic (pectoral) and pelvic girdles. **axial s.,** the bones of the body axis, including the skull, vertebral column, ribs, and sternum. **cardiac s.,** the fibrous or fibrocartilaginous framework that supports and gives attachment to the cardiac muscle fibers and valves, and the roots of the aorta and pulmonary trunk.

ske·ni·tis (ske-ni′tis) inflammation of the paraurethral (Skene's) glands.

skin (skin) the outer protective covering of the body, consisting of the dermis (or corium) and the epidermis. **elastic s.,** Ehlers-Danlos syndrome. **farmers' s.,** actinic elastosis. **lax s., loose s.,** cutis laxa. **sailors' s.,** actinic elastosis.

skin·fold (skin′fōld) the layer of skin and subcutaneous fat raised by pinching the skin and letting the underlying muscle fall back to the bone; used to estimate the percentage of body fat.

SKSD streptokinase-streptodornase.

skull (skul) the cranium; the bony framework of the head, composed of the cranial and facial bones. See *Table of Bones.*

slant (slant) 1. a sloping surface of agar in a test tube. 2. slant culture.

SLE systemic lupus erythematosus.

sleep (slēp) a period of rest for the body and mind, during which volition and consciousness are in abeyance and bodily functions are partially suspended; also described as a behavioral state, with characteristic immobile posture and diminished but readily reversible sensitivity to external stimuli. **NREM s.,** non-rapid eye movement sleep; the deep, dreamless period of sleep during which the brain waves are slow and of high voltage, and autonomic activities, such as heart rate and blood pressure, are low and regular. **REM s.,** the period of sleep during which the brain waves are fast and of low voltage, and autonomic activities, such as heart rate and respiration, are irregular. This type of sleep is associated with dreaming, mild involuntary muscle jerks, and rapid eye movements (REM). It usually occurs three to four times each night at intervals of 80 to 120 minutes, each occurrence lasting from 5 minutes to more than an hour.

sleep·walk·ing (slēp′wawk″ing) somnambulism.

slide (slīd) a glass plate on which objects are placed for microscopic examination.

sling (sling) a bandage or suspensory for supporting a part. **mandibular s.,** a structure suspending the mandible, formed by the medial pterygoid and masseter muscles and aiding in mandibulomaxillary articulation. **pubovaginal s.,** a support constructed of rectoabdominal fascia to stabilize the bladder from underneath in treatment of stress incontinence. **suburethral s.,** a support constructed surgically from muscle, ligament, or synthetic material that elevates the bladder from underneath in the treatment of stress incontinence.

slough (sluf) 1. necrotic tissue in the process of separating from viable portions of the body. 2. to shed or cast off.

sludge (sluj) a suspension of solid or semisolid particles in a fluid which itself may or may not be a truly viscous fluid.

sludg·ing (sluj′ing) settling out of solid particles from solution. **s. of blood,** intravascular agglutination.

Sm samarium.

small·pox (smawl′poks) variola; an acute, highly contagious, often fatal infectious disease, now eradicated worldwide by vaccination programs, caused by an orthopoxvirus and marked by fever and distinctive progressive skin eruptions.

smear (smēr) a specimen for microscopic study prepared by spreading the material across the slide. **Pap s., Papanicolaou s.,** see under *test.*

smeg·ma (smeg′mah) the secretion of sebaceous glands, especially the cheesy secretion, consisting principally of desquamated epithelial cells, found chiefly beneath the prepuce. **smegmat′ic**, adj.

smell (smel) olfaction.

Sn tin (L. *stan′num*).

snake (snāk) 1. a limbless reptile of the suborder Ophidia, some of which are poisonous. 2. any of various worms that resemble members of Ophidia. **black s.**, blacksnake. **brown s.**, a venomous elapid snake of Australia and New Guinea belonging to the genus *Demansia*. **coral s.**, any of various venomous snakes of the genera *Micrurus* and *Micruroides*. **crotalid s.**, crotalid (1). **elapid s.**, elapid (1). **harlequin s.**, coral s. **poisonous s′s**, 1. venomous s′s. 2. snakes that contain poison, either in venom glands or in other organs or tissues. **sea s.**, a snake of the family Hydrophiidae. **tiger s.**, *Notechis scutatus*. **venomous s′s**, snakes that secrete venoms capable of producing a deleterious effect on either the blood (hemotoxin) or the nervous system (neurotoxin), with the venom injected into the body of the victim by the snake's bite. **viperine s.**, true viper.

snap (snap) a short, sharp sound. **opening s.**, a short, sharp sound in early diastole caused by abrupt halting at its maximal opening of an abnormal atrioventricular valve.

snare (snār) a wire loop for removing polyps and tumors by encircling them at the base and closing the loop.

sneeze (snēz) 1. to expel air forcibly and spasmodically through the nose and mouth. 2. an involuntary, sudden, violent, and audible expulsion of air through the mouth and nose.

snore (snor) 1. rough, noisy breathing during sleep, due to vibration of the uvula and soft palate. 2. to produce such sounds during sleep.

snow (sno) a freezing or frozen mixture consisting of discrete particles or crystals. **carbon dioxide s.**, solid carbon dioxide, formed by rapid evaporation of liquid carbon dioxide; it gives a temperature of about −79°C (−110°F). It is used in cryotherapy to freeze and anesthetize the skin and, in the form of a slush (carbon dioxide slush), as an escharotic to destroy skin lesions and as a peeling agent for chemabrasion.

snow·blind·ness (sno′blīnd-nes) see under *blindness*.

SNS sympathetic nervous system.

snuf·fles (snuf′′lz) catarrhal discharge from the nasal mucous membrane in infants, generally in congenital syphilis.

SOAP a device for conceptualizing the process of recording the progress notes in the *problem-oriented record* (see under *record*): *S* indicates subjective data obtained from the patient and others close to him; *O* designates objective data obtained by observation, physical examination, diagnostic studies, etc.; *A* refers to assessment of the patient's status through analysis of the problem, possible interaction of the problems, and changes in the status of the problems; *P* designates the plan for patient care.

soap (sōp) any compound of one or more fatty acids, or their equivalents, with an alkali; it is detergent and is used as a cleanser.

SOB shortness of breath.

so·cial·iza·tion (so′′shal-ĭ-za′shun) the process by which society integrates the individual and the individual learns to behave in socially acceptable ways.

so·cio·bi·ol·o·gy (so′′se-o-bi-ol′ah-je) the branch of theoretical biology that proposes that animal (including human) behavior has a biological basis controlled by the genes. **sociobiolog′ic, sociobiolog′ical**, adj.

so·ci·ol·o·gy (so′′se-ol′ah-je) the scientific study of social relationships and phenomena.

so·ci·om·e·try (so′′se-om′ĕ-tre) the branch of sociology concerned with the measurement of human social behavior.

so·cio·ther·a·py (so′′se-o-ther′ah-pe) any treatment emphasizing modification of the environment and improvement in interpersonal relationships rather than intrapsychic factors.

sock·et (sok′it) a hollow into which a corresponding part fits. **dry s.**, a condition sometimes occurring after tooth extraction, with exposure of bone, inflammation of an alveolar crypt, and severe pain. **eye s.**, orbit. **tooth s.**, dental alveolus.

so·da (so′dah) a term loosely applied to sodium bicarbonate, sodium hydroxide, or sodium carbonate. **baking s., bicarbonate of s.**, sodium bicarbonate. **s. lime**, calcium hydroxide with sodium or potassium hydroxide, or both; used as adsorbent of carbon dioxide in equipment for metabolism tests, inhalant anesthesia, or oxygen therapy.

so·di·um (so′de-um) chemical element (see *Table of Elements*), at. no. 11, symbol Na; the chief cation of extracellular body fluids. For sodium salts not listed here, see under the acid or the active ingredient. **s. acetate**, a source of sodium ions for hemodialysis and peritoneal dialysis, also a systemic and urinary alkalizer. **s. ascorbate,** an antiscorbutic vitamin and nutritional supplement; also used as an aid to deferoxamine therapy in the treatment of chronic iron toxicity. **s. benzoate,** an antifungal agent also used in a test of liver function. **s. bicarbonate,** the monosodium salt of carbonic acid, used as a gastric and systemic anatacid and to alkalize urine; also used, in solution, for washing the nose, mouth, and vagina, as a cleansing enema, and as a dressing for minor burns. **s. biphosphate,** monobasic s. phosphate. **s. borate,** the sodium salt of boric acid, used as an alkalizing agent in pharmaceuticals. **s. carbonate,** the disodium salt of carbonic acid, used as an alkalizing agent in pharmaceuticals. **s. chloride,** common table salt, a necessary constituent of the body and therefore of the diet, involved in maintaining osmotic tension of blood and tissues; uses include replenishment of electrolytes in the body, irrigation of wounds and body cavities, enema, inhaled mucolytic, topical osmotic ophthalmic agent, and preparation of pharmaceuticals. **s. chromate Cr 51,** the disodium salt of chromic acid prepared using the radioactive isotope chromium 51; used to tag erythrocytes or platelets for studies of red cell disease, gastrointestinal bleeding, and platelet survival. **s. citrate,** the trisodium salt of citric acid, used as an anticoagulant for blood or plasma for transfusion; also used as a urinary alkalizer. **dibasic s. phosphate,** an electrolyte replenisher, laxative, urinary acidifier, and antiurolithic, often used in combination with other phosphate compounds. Labeled with radiophosphorus (*s. phosphate P 32*), it is used as an antineoplastic in the treatment of polycythemia vera, chronic lymphocytic or myelocytic leukemia, and metastatic bone lesions. **s. dodecyl sulfate (SDS),** the more usual name for sodium lauryl sulfate when used as an anionic detergent to solubilize proteins. **s. fluoride,** a dental caries prophylactic, NaF; used in the fluoridation of water and applied topically to the teeth. **s. glutamate,** monosodium glutamate. **s. hydroxide,** NaOH, a strongly alkaline and caustic compound; used as an alkalizing agent in pharmaceuticals. **s. hypochlorite,** the sodium salt of hypochlorous acid, NaClO, having germicidal and disinfectant properties. **s. hyposulfite,** s. thiosulfate. **s. iodide,** a binary haloid, used as a source of iodine. Labeled with radioactive iodine, it is used in thyroid function tests and thyroid imaging and to treat hyperthyroidism and thyroid carcinoma. **s. lactate,** the sodium salt of racemic or inactive lactic acid,

used as a fluid and electrolyte replenisher to combat acidosis. **monobasic s. phosphate,** the monohydrate, dihydrate, or anhydrous monosodium salt of phosphoric acid; used in buffer solutions. Used alone or in combination with other phosphate compounds, given intravenously as an electrolyte replenisher, orally or rectally as a laxative, and orally as a urinary acidifier and as an antiurolithic. **s. monofluorophosphate,** a dental caries prophylactic applied topically to the teeth. **s. nitrite,** an antidote for cyanide poisoning; also used as a preservative in cured meats and other foods. **s. nitroprusside,** an antihypertensive used in the treatment of acute congestive heart failure and of hypertensive crisis and to produce controlled hypotension during surgery; also used as a reagent. **s. phenylbutyrate,** an antihyperammonemic agent used as adjunctive treatment to control the hyperammonemia of urea cycle enzyme disorders. **s. phosphate,** any of various compounds of sodium and phosphoric acid; usually specifically *dibasic s. phosphate.* **s. polystyrene sulfonate,** a cation exchange resin used as an antihyperkalemic. **s. propionate,** the sodium salt of propionic acid, having antifungal properties; used as a topical antifungal; also used as a preservative. **s. salicylate,** see *salicylate.* **s. sulfate,** an osmotic laxative. **s. tetradecyl sulfate,** an anionic surfactant with sclerosing properties; used as a wetting agent and in the treatment of varicose veins. **s. thiosulfate,** a compound used as an antidote (with s. nitrite) to cyanide poisoning, in the prophylaxis of ringworm (added to foot baths), topically in tinea versicolor, and in some tests of renal function.

so·do·ku (so'do-koo) the spirillary form of rat-bite fever, caused by *Spirillum minus.*

sod·o·my (sod'ah-me) 1. anal intercourse. 2. old term for any form of homosexuality, or sometimes any of numerous paraphilias.

sof·ten·ing (sof'en-ing) malacia.

Sol. [L.] solutio (solution).

sol (sol) a colloid system in which the dispersion medium is liquid or gas; the latter is usually called an *aerosol.*

so·lar (so'ler) denoting the great sympathetic plexus and its principal ganglia (especially the celiac); so called because of their radiating nerves.

sol·a·tion (so-la'shun) the conversion of a gel into a sol.

sole (sōl) the bottom of the foot.

sol·i·tary (sol'ĭ-tar″e) 1. alone; separated from others. 2. living alone or in pairs only.

sol·u·bil·i·ty (sol″u-bil'ĭ-te) quality of being soluble; susceptibility of being dissolved.

sol·u·ble (sol'u-b'l) susceptible of being dissolved.

so·lute (sol'ūt) the substance dissolved in solvent to form a solution.

so·lu·tion (sŏ-loo'shun) 1. a homogeneous mixture of one or more substances (solutes) dispersed molecularly in a sufficient quantity of dissolving medium (solvent). 2. in pharmacology, a liquid preparation of one or more soluble chemical substances usually dissolved in water. 3. the process of dissolving. 4. a loosening or separation. **acetic acid otic s.,** a solution of glacial acetic acid in a nonaqueous solvent, used to treat otitis externa caused by various fungi. **aluminum acetate topical s.,** a preparation of aluminum subacetate solution, glacial acetic acid, and water; an astringent applied topically to the skin as a wet dressing and used as a gargle or mouthwash. **aluminum subacetate topical s.,** a solution of aluminum sulfate, acetic acid, precipitated calcium carbonate, and water; applied topically as an astringent, and also as an antiseptic and a wet dressing. **anisotonic s.,** one having tonicity differing from that of the standard of reference. **anticoagulant citrate dextrose s.,** a solution of citric acid, sodium citrate, and dextrose in water for injection, used for preservation of whole blood. **anticoagulant citrate phosphate dextrose s.,** a solution containing citric acid, sodium citrate, monobasic sodium phosphate, and dextrose in water for injection; used for preservation of whole blood. **anticoagulant citrate phosphate dextrose adenine s.,** a solution consisting of anticoagulant citrate phosphate dextrose solution and adenine; used for the preservation of whole blood. **anticoagulant heparin s.,** a sterile solution of heparin sodium in sodium chloride, used as an anticoagulant in the preservation of whole blood. **anticoagulant sodium citrate s.,** a solution of sodium citrate in water for injection, used for the storage of whole blood, preparation of blood for fractionation, and preparation of citrated human plasma. **APF s.,** sodium fluoride and acidulated phosphate topical s. **aqueous s.,** one in which water is the solvent. **Benedict's s.,** a sodium citrate, sodium carbonate, and cupric sulfate aqueous solution; used to determine presence of glucose in urine. **buffer s.,** one that resists appreciable change in its hydrogen ion concentration upon addition of acid or alkali. **cardioplegic s.,** a cold solution injected into the aortic root or the coronary ostia to induce cardiac arrest and protect the heart during open heart surgery, usually potassium in an electrolyte solution or in blood. **colloid s.,**

colloidal s., imprecise term for a *colloidal system;* see *colloid* (2). **Dakin's s.,** a diluted sodium hypochlorite solution, which has been used as a topical anti-infective for skin and wounds. **formaldehyde s.,** an aqueous solution containing not less than 37 per cent formaldehyde; used as a disinfectant and as a preservative and fixative for pathologic specimens. **hyperbaric s.,** one having a greater specific gravity than a standard of reference. **hypobaric s.,** one having a specific gravity less than that of a standard of reference. **iodine topical s.,** a solution prepared with purified water, each 100 ml containing 1.8 to 2.2 g of iodine and 2.1 to 2.6 g of sodium iodide; a local anti-infective. **isobaric s.,** a solution having the same specific gravity as a standard of reference. **lactated Ringer's s.,** see under *injection.* **Lugol's s.,** strong iodine s. **molar s.,** a solution each liter of which contains 1 mole of the dissolved substance; designated 1 M. The concentration of other solutions may be expressed in relation to that of molar solutions as tenth-molar (0.1 M), etc. **Monsel's s.,** a reddish-brown aqueous solution of basic ferric sulfate; astringent and hemostatic. **normal s.,** a solution each liter of which contains 1 equivalent weight of the dissolved substance: designated 1 N. **normal saline s., normal salt s.,** physiologic salt s. **ophthalmic s.,** a sterile solution, free from foreign particles, for instillation into the eye. **physiologic saline s., physiologic salt s., physiologic sodium chloride s.,** a 0.9 per cent aqueous solution of sodium chloride, which is isotonic with blood serum. **Ringer's s.,** see under *injection* and *irrigation.* **saline s., salt s.,** a solution of sodium chloride in purified water. **saturated s.,** one containing all of the solute which can be held in solution by the solvent. **sclerosing s.,** a solution of a sclerosing agent, for use in sclerotherapy. **Shohl's s.,** an aqueous solution of citric acid and sodium citrate; used to correct electrolyte imbalance in renal tubular acidosis. **sodium fluoride and acidulated phosphate topical s.,** a solution of sodium fluoride, acidulated with phosphoric acid, pH of 3.0 to 3.5; applied topically to the teeth as a dental caries prophylactic. **sodium hypochlorite s.,** a solution containing 4 to 6 per cent by weight of sodium hypochlorite; used to disinfect utensils. In dilution, usually containing approximately 0.5 per cent free chlorine, it is used for skin disinfection and wound irrigation. **standard s.,** one that contains in each liter a definitely stated amount of reagent; usually expressed in terms of normality (equivalent weights of solute per liter of solution) or molarity (moles of solute per liter of solution). **strong iodine s.,** a solution containing, in each 100 ml, 5 g of iodine and 10 g of potassium iodide; a source of iodine. **supersaturated s.,** an unstable solution containing more of the solute than it can permanently hold. **TAC s.,** a solution of tetracaine, epinephrine, and cocaine, used as a local anesthetic in the emergency treatment of uncomplicated lacerations. **volumetric s.,** one that contains a specific quantity of solvent per stated unit of volume.

sol·vent (sol'vent) 1. dissolving; effecting a solution. 2. a substance, usually a liquid, that dissolves or is capable of dissolving; the component of a solution present in greater amount.

so·ma (so'mah) 1. the body as distinguished from the mind. 2. the body tissue as distinguished from the germ cells. 3. the cell body.

som·as·the·nia (so"mas-the'ne-ah) bodily weakness with poor appetite and poor sleep.

so·ma·tal·gia (so"mah-tal'jah) bodily pain.

so·mat·es·the·sia (so"mat-es-the'zhah) somatognosis.

so·mat·ic (so-mat'ik) 1. pertaining to or characteristic of the soma or body. 2. pertaining to the body wall in contrast to the viscera.

so·ma·ti·za·tion (so"mah-tĭ-za'shun) the conversion of mental experiences or states into bodily symptoms.

somat(o)- word element [Gr.], *body.*

so·mato·chrome (so-mat'o-krōm) any neuron that has cytoplasm completely surrounding the nucleus and easily stainable Nissl bodies.

so·mato·form (so-mat'o-form) denoting physical symptoms that cannot be attributed to organic disease and appear to be psychogenic.

so·ma·to·gen·ic (so"mah-to-jen'ik) originating in the cells of the body, as opposed to *psychogenic.*

so·ma·tog·no·sis (so"mah-tog-no'sis) the general feeling of the existence of one's body and of the functioning of the organs.

so·ma·tol·o·gy (so"mah-tol'ah-je) the sum of what is known about the body; the study of anatomy and physiology.

so·ma·to·me·din (so"mah-to-me'din) any of a group of peptides found in plasma, complexed with binding proteins; they stimulate cellular growth and replication as second messengers in the somatotropic actions of growth hormone and also have insulin-like activities. Two such peptides have been isolated, insulin-like growth factors I and II.

so·ma·tom·e·try (so"mah-tom'ĕ-tre) measurement of the body.

so·ma·to·mo·tor (so"mah-to-mo'ter) pertaining to movements of the body.

so·ma·top·a·thy (so"mah-top'ah-the) a bodily disorder as distinguished from a mental one. **somatopath'ic,** adj.

so·mato·plasm (so-mat'o-plazm) the protoplasm of the body cells exclusive of the germ cells.

so·mato·pleure (-ploor) the embryonic body wall, formed by ectoderm and somatic mesoderm. **somatopleur'al,** adj.

so·ma·to·psy·chic (so"mah-to-si'kik) pertaining to both mind and body; relating to the effects of the body on the mind.

so·ma·tos·co·py (so"mah-tos'kah-pe) examination of the body.

so·ma·to·sen·so·ry (so"mah-to-sen'so-re) pertaining to sensations received in the skin and deep tissues.

so·ma·to·sex·u·al (-sek'shoo-al) pertaining to both physical and sex characteristics, or to physical manifestations of sexual development.

so·ma·to·stat·in (SS) (-stat'in) a polypeptide elaborated primarily by the median eminence of the hypothalamus and by the delta cells of the islets of Langerhans; it inhibits release of thyrotropin, somatotropin, and corticotropin by the adenohypophysis, of insulin and glucagon by the pancreas, of gastrin by the gastric mucosa, of secretin by the intestinal mucosa, and of renin by the kidney.

so·ma·to·stat·in·oma (-stat"in-o'mah) an islet cell tumor that secretes somatostatin.

so·ma·to·ther·a·py (-ther'ah-pe) biological treatment of mental disorders, as electric shock or drug therapy.

so·ma·to·top·ic (-top'ik) related to particular areas of the body; describing organization of motor area of the brain, control of the movement of different parts of the body being centered in specific regions of the cortex.

so·mato·trope (so-mat'o-trōp) somatotroph.

so·mato·troph (-trōf") a type of acidophil of the adenohypophysis that secretes growth hormone.

so·ma·to·tro·phic (so"mah-to-tro'fik) somatotropic.

so·ma·to·tro·phin (-tro"fin) growth hormone.

so·ma·to·tro·pic (-tro'pik) 1. having an affinity for or attacking the body cells. 2. having a stimulating effect on nutrition and growth. 3. having the properties of somatotrophin.

so·ma·to·tro·pin (-tro″pin) growth hormone.

so·mato·type (so-mat′o-tīp) a particular type of body build.

so·ma·trem (so′mah-trem) biosynthetic human growth hormone, prepared by recombinant technology and differing from the natural human hormone in containing an additional methionine residue at the terminus; used to treat growth failure and AIDS-associated cachexia or weight loss.

so·mat·ro·pin (so″mah-tro′pin) biosynthetic human growth hormone, prepared by recombinant means and having the same amino acid sequence as the natural hormone; used to treat growth failure and AIDS-associated cachexia or weight loss.

so·mes·the·sia (so″mes-the′zhah) somatognosis.

so·mite (so′mīt) one of the paired, blocklike masses of mesoderm, arranged segmentally alongside the neural tube of the embryo, forming the vertebral column and segmental musculature.

som·nam·bu·lism (som-nam′bu-lizm) sleepwalking; rising out of bed and walking about or performing other complex motor behavior during an apparent state of sleep.

som·ni·fa·cient (som″nĭ-fa′shint) hypnotic (1, 2).

som·nif·er·ous (som-nif′er-us) hypnotic (1).

som·nil·o·quism (som-nil′o-kwizm) talking in one's sleep.

som·no·lence (som′no-lens) drowsiness or sleepiness, particularly in excess.

som·no·len·tia (som″no-len′shah) [L.] 1. drowsiness, or somnolence. 2. sleep drunkenness.

son·i·ca·tion (son″ĭ-ka′shun) exposure to sound waves; disruption of bacteria by exposure to high-frequency sound waves.

so·nog·ra·phy (sŏ-nog′rah-fe) ultrasonography. **sonograph′ic,** adj.

sono·lu·cent (-loo″sent) anechoic; in ultrasonography, permitting the passage of ultrasound waves without reflecting them back to their source (without giving off echoes).

so·por (so′por) [L.] unnaturally deep or profound sleep.

sop·o·rif·ic (sop″ŏ-rif′ik, so″pŏ-rif′ik) 1. producing deep sleep. 2. hypnotic (2).

so·por·ous (so′por-us) associated with coma or profound sleep.

sorb (sorb) to attract and retain substances by absorption or adsorption.

sor·be·fa·cient (sor″bĕ-fa′shint) absorbefacient.

sor·bent (sor′bent) an agent that sorbs; see *absorbent* and *adsorbent.*

sor·bic ac·id (sor′bik) a fungistat used as an antimicrobial inhibitor in pharmaceuticals.

sor·bi·tan (sor′bĭ-tan) any of the anhydrides of sorbitol, the fatty acids of which are surfactants used as emulsifiers in pharmaceutical preparations; see also *polysorbate 80.*

sor·bi·tol (sor′bĭ-tol) a six-carbon sugar alcohol from a variety of fruits, found in lens deposits in diabetes mellitus. A pharmaceutical preparation is used as a sweetening agent and osmotic laxative, and in drugs as a tablet excipient, humectant, and stabilizer.

sor·des (sor′dēz) debris, especially the encrustations of food, epithelial matter, and bacteria that collect on the lips and teeth during a prolonged fever. **s. gas′tricae,** undigested food, mucus, etc., in the stomach.

sore (sor) 1. popularly, almost any lesion of the skin or mucous membranes. 2. painful. **bed s.,** decubitus ulcer. **canker s.,** recurrent aphthous stomatitis. **cold s.,** see *herpes simplex.* **desert s.,** a form of tropical ulcer occurring in desert areas of Africa, Australia, and the Near East.

sorp·tion (sorp′shun) the process or state of being sorbed; absorption or adsorption.

S.O.S. [L.] si o′pus sit (if it is necessary).

so·ta·lol (so′tah-lol) a non-cardioselective beta-adrenergic blocking agent used as the hydrochloride salt in the treatment of life-threatening cardiac arrhythmias.

souf·fle (soo′f'l) a soft, blowing auscultatory sound. **cardiac s.,** any cardiac or vascular murmur of a blowing quality. **funic s., funicular s.,** hissing souffle synchronous with fetal heart sounds, probably from the umbilical cord. **mammary s.,** a functional cardiac murmur with a blowing sound, heard over the breasts in late pregnancy and during lactation. **placental s.,** the sound supposed to be produced by the blood current in the placenta. **uterine s.,** a sound made by the blood within the arteries of the gravid uterus.

sound (sound) 1. a pressure wave propagating through an elastic medium; waves with a frequency of 20–20,000 Hz cause the sensation of hearing. 2. the effect produced on the organ of hearing by vibrations of the air or other medium. 3. a noise, normal or abnormal, heard within the body. 4. an instrument to be introduced into a cavity to detect a foreign body or to dilate a stricture. **adventitious s's,** abnormal auscultatory sounds heard over the lung, such as rales, rhonchi, or abnormal resonance. **aortic second s.,** the audible vibrations related to the closure of the aortic valve; symbol A_2. **auscultatory s's,** those heard on auscultation, such as breath sounds, heart sounds, and adventitious sounds. **breath s's**, respiratory s's; sounds heard on auscultation over the respiratory tract; bronchial and ventricular ones are heard normally at certain places, whereas a cavernous one indicates a lung cavity. **continuous s's**, adventitious sounds lasting longer than 0.2 sec, such as wheezes and rhonchi. **discontinuous s's**, adventitious sounds lasting less than 0.2 sec and coming in a series; the most common are rales. **ejection s's**, high-pitched clicking sounds heard just after the first heart sound, at maximal opening of the semilunar valves; seen in patients with valvular abnormalities or dilatations of aortic or pulmonary arteries. **friction s.**, see under *rub*. **heart s's**, sounds heard over the cardiac region, produced by the functioning of the heart. The *first*, at the beginning of ventricular systole, is dull, firm, and prolonged, and heard as a "lubb" sound; the *second*, produced mainly by closure of the semilunar valves, is shorter and sharper than the first and is heard as a "dupp" sound; the *third* is usually audible only in youth; and the *fourth* is normally inaudible. **hippocratic s's**, succussion s's. **Korotkoff s's**, sounds heard during auscultatory determination of blood pressure. **percussion s.**, any sound obtained by percussion. **pulmonic second s.**, the audible vibrations related to the closure of the pulmonary valve; symbol P_2. **respiratory s's**, breath s's. **succussion s's**, splashing sounds heard on succussion over a distended stomach or in hydropneumothorax. **to-and-fro s.**, see under *murmur*. **urethral s.**, a long, slender instrument for exploring and dilating the urethra. **valvular ejection s.**, an ejection sound resulting from abnormality of one or both semilunar valves. **vascular ejection s.**, an ejection sound resulting from abnormality of the pulmonary artery or aorta without abnormality of either semilunar valve. **voice s's**, auscultatory sounds heard over the lungs or airways when the patient speaks; increased resonance indicates consolidation or effusion. **white s.**, that produced by a mixture of all frequencies of mechanical vibration perceptible as sound.

soy (soi) soybean.

soy·bean (soi'bēn) the bean of the leguminous plant, *Glycine max*, which contains little starch but is rich in protein and phytoestrogens.

space (spās) 1. a delimited area. 2. an actual or potential cavity of the body. **spa'tial**, adj. **apical s.**, the region between the wall of the alveolus and the apex of the root of a tooth. **axillary s.**, axilla. **Bowman's s.**,

capsular s. **bregmatic s.**, the anterior fontanelle, situated at the junction of the frontal, coronal, and sagittal sutures. **capsular s.**, a narrow chalice-shaped cavity between the glomerular and capsular epithelium of the glomerular capsule of the kidney. **cartilage s's**, the spaces in hyaline cartilage containing the cartilage cells. **corneal s's**, the spaces between the lamellae of the substantia propria of the cornea containing corneal cells and interstitial fluid. **cupular s.**, the part of the attic above the malleus. **danger s.**, a subdivision of the retropharyngeal space, extending from the base of the skull to the level of the diaphragm; it provides a route for the spread of infection from the pharynx to the mediastinum. **dead s's**, 1. the space remaining after incomplete closure of surgical or other wounds, permitting accumulation of blood or serum and resultant delay in healing. 2. in the respiratory tract: (1) *anatomical dead s.*, those portions, from the nose and mouth to the terminal bronchioles, not participating in oxygen–carbon dioxide exchange, and (2) *physiologic dead s.*, which reflects nonuniformity of ventilation and perfusion in the lung, is the anatomical dead space plus the space in the alveoli occupied by air that does not participate in oxygen–carbon dioxide exchange. **epidural s.**, the space between the dura mater and the lining of the vertebral canal. **episcleral s.**, the space between the bulbar fascia and the eyeball. **haversian s.**, see under *canal*. **iliocostal s.**, the area between the twelfth rib and the crest of the ilium. **intercostal s.**, the space between two adjacent ribs. **interglobular s's**, small irregular spaces on the outer surface of the dentin in the tooth root. **interpleural s.**, mediastinum. **interproximal s.**, the space between the proximal surfaces of adjoining teeth. **intervillous s.**, the space of the placenta into which the chorionic villi project and through which the maternal blood circulates. **Kiernan's s's**, the triangular spaces bounded by invaginated Glisson's capsule between the liver lobules, containing the larger interlobular branches of the portal vein, hepatic artery, and hepatic duct. **lymph s.**, any space in tissue occupied by lymph. **Meckel's s.**, a recess in the dura mater which lodges the gasserian ganglion. **mediastinal s.**, mediastinum. **medullary s.**, the central cavity and the intervals between the trabeculae of bone which contain the marrow. **palmar s.**, a large fascial space in the hand, divided by a fibrous septum into a midpalmar and a thenar space. **parasinoidal**

s's, lateral lacunae. **perforated s.**, see under *substance*. **periaxial s.**, a fluid-filled cavity surrounding the nuclear bag and myotubule regions of a muscle spindle. **perilymphatic s.**, the fluid-filled space separating the membranous from the osseous labyrinth. **perineal s's**, spaces on either side of the inferior fascia of the urogenital diaphragm, the *deep* between it and the superior fascia, the *superficial* between it and the superficial perineal fascia. **periplasmic s.**, a zone between the plasma membrane and the outer membrane of the cell wall of gram-negative bacteria. **perivascular s's**, spaces, often only potential, that surround blood vessels for a short distance as they enter the brain. **perivitelline s.**, a space between the oocyte and the zona pellucida. **pneumatic s.**, a portion of bone occupied by air-containing cells, especially the spaces constituting the paranasal sinuses. **Poiseuille's s.**, that part of the lumen of a tube, at its periphery, where no flow of liquid occurs. **Reinke's s.**, a potential space between the vocal ligament and the overlying mucosa. **retroperitoneal s.**, the space between the peritoneum and the posterior abdominal wall. **retropharyngeal s.**, the space behind the pharynx, containing areolar tissue. **retropubic s.**, the areolar space bounded by the reflection of peritoneum, symphysis pubis, and bladder. **Retzius s.**, 1. retropubic s. 2. perilymphatic s. **subarachnoid s.**, the space between the arachnoid and the pia mater. **subdural s.**, the space between the dura mater and the arachnoid. **subgingival s.**, gingival crevice. **subphrenic s.**, the space between the diaphragm and subjacent organs. **subumbilical s.**, a somewhat triangular space in the body cavity beneath the umbilicus. **Tenon's s.**, episcleral s. **thenar s.**, the palmar space lying between the middle metacarpal bone and the tendon of the flexor pollicis longus. **zonular s's**, the lymph-filled spaces between the fibers of the ciliary zonule.

spar·flox·a·cin (spahr-flok'sah-sin) a synthetic, broad-spectrum antimicrobial agent.

spar·ga·no·sis (spahr″gah-no'sis) infection with the larvae (spargana) of any of several species of tapeworms, which invade the subcutaneous tissues, causing inflammation and fibrosis.

spar·ga·num (spahr'gah-num) pl. *spar'gana*. [Gr.] the larval stage of certain tapeworms, especially of the genera *Diphyllobothrium* and *Spirometra*; see also *sparganosis*. Also, a genus name applied to such larvae, usually when the adult stage is unknown.

spasm (spazm) 1. a sudden, violent, involuntary muscular contraction. 2. a sudden transitory constriction of a passage, canal, or orifice. **bronchial s.**, bronchospasm. **carpopedal s.**, spasm of the hand or foot, or of the thumbs and great toes, seen in tetany. **clonic s.**, a spasm consisting of clonic contractions. **facial s.**, tonic spasm of the muscles supplied by the facial nerve, involving the entire side of the face or confined to a limited area about the eye. **habit s.**, see under *tic*. **infantile s's**, a syndrome of severe myoclonus appearing in infancy and associated with general cerebral deterioration. **intention s.**, muscular spasm on attempting voluntary movement. **myopathic s.**, spasm accompanying disease of the muscles. **nodding s.**, a nodding motion of the head accompanied by nystagmus, seen in infants and young children. **saltatory s.**, clonic spasm of the muscles of the legs, producing a peculiar jumping or springing motion when standing. **tetanic s., tonic s.**, tetanus (2). **toxic s.**, spasm caused by a toxin.

spas·mod·ic (spaz-mod'ik) of the nature of a spasm; occurring in spasms.

spas·mol·y·sis (spaz-mol'ĭ-sis) the arrest of spasm. **spasmolyt'ic**, adj.

spas·mus (spaz'mus) [L.] spasm. **s. nu'tans**, nodding spasm.

spas·tic (spas'tik) 1. of the nature of or characterized by spasms. 2. hypertonic, so that the muscles are stiff and movements awkward.

spas·tic·i·ty (spas-tis'ĭ-te) the state of being spastic; see *spastic* (2).

spa·tial (spa'shul) pertaining to space.

spa·ti·um (spa'she-um) pl. *spa'tia*. [L.] space.

spat·u·la (spach'u-lah) [L.] 1. a wide, flat, blunt, usually flexible instrument of little thickness, used for spreading material on a smooth surface. 2. a spatulate structure.

spat·u·late (spach'u-lāt) 1. having a flat blunt end. 2. to mix or manipulate with a spatula. 3. to make an enlarged opening in a tubular structure by means of a longitudinal incision which is then spread open.

SPCA serum prothrombin conversion accelerator (coagulation factor VII).

spe·cial·ist (spesh'ah-list) a physician whose practice is limited to a particular branch of medicine or surgery, especially one who, by virtue of advanced training, is certified by a specialty board as being qualified to so limit it. **clinical nurse s., nurse s.**, see under *nurse*.

spe·cial·ty (spesh'ul-te) the field of practice of a specialist.

spe·ci·a·tion (spe″se-a′shun) the evolutionary formation of new species.

spe·cies (spe′shēz) a taxonomic category subordinate to a genus (or subgenus) and superior to a subspecies or variety. **type s.,** the original species from which the description of the genus is formulated.

spe·cies-spe·cif·ic (-spē-sif′ik) 1. characteristic of a particular species. 2. having a characteristic effect on, or interaction with, cells or tissues of members of a particular species; said of an antigen, drug, or infective agent.

spe·cif·ic (spē-sif′ik) 1. pertaining to a species. 2. produced by a single kind of microorganism. 3. restricted in application, effect, etc., to a particular structure, function, etc. 4. a remedy specially indicated for a particular disease. 5. in immunology, pertaining to the special affinity of antigen for the corresponding antibody.

spec·i·fic·i·ty (spes″ĭ-fis′ĭ-te) 1. the quality or state of being specific. 2. the probability that a person who does not have a disease will be correctly identified by a clinical test.

spec·i·men (spes′ĭ-men) a small sample or part taken to show the nature of the whole, as a small quantity of urine for analysis, or a small fragment of tissue for microscopic study.

SPECT single-photon emission computed tomography.

spec·ta·cles (spek′tah-k′ls) glasses.

spec·ti·no·my·cin (spek″tĭ-no-mi′sin) an antibiotic derived from *Streptomyces spectabilis*, used as the hydrochloride salt in the treatment of gonorrhea.

spec·tral (spek′tral) pertaining to a spectrum; performed by means of a spectrum.

spec·trin (spek′trin) a contractile protein attached to glycophorin at the cytoplasmic surface of the cell membrane of erythrocytes, important in maintaining cell shape.

spectr(o)- word element [L.], *spectrum, image.*

spec·trom·e·try (spek-trom′ĕ-tre) determination of the wavelengths or frequencies of the lines in a spectrum.

spec·tro·pho·tom·e·ter (spek″tro-fotom′ĕ-ter) 1. an apparatus for measuring light sense by means of a spectrum. 2. an apparatus for determining quantity of coloring matter in solution by measurement of transmitted light.

spec·tro·scope (spek′trah-skōp) an instrument for developing and analyzing spectra. **spectroscop′ic,** adj.

spec·trum (spek′trum) pl. *spec′tra.* [L.] 1. a charted band of wavelengths of electromagnetic radiation obtained by refraction or diffraction. 2. by extension, a measurable range of activity, as the range of bacteria affected by an antibiotic *(antibacterial s.)* or the complete range of manifestations of a disease. **absorption s.,** that afforded by light which has passed through various gaseous media, each gas absorbing those rays of which its own spectrum is composed. **broad-s.,** effective against a wide range of microorganisms; said of an antibiotic. **electromagnetic s.,** the range of electromagnetic energy from cosmic rays to electric waves, including gamma, x- and ultraviolet rays, visible light, infrared waves, and radio waves. **fortification s.,** a form of migraine aura characterized by scintillating or zigzag bands of colored light forming the edge of an area of teichopsia. **visible s.,** that portion of the range of wavelengths of electromagnetic vibrations (from 770 to 390 nm) which is capable of stimulating specialized sense organs and is perceptible as light.

spec·u·lum (spek′u-lum) pl. *spec′ula.* [L.] an instrument for opening or distending a body orifice or cavity to permit visual inspection.

speech (spēch) the expression of thoughts and ideas by vocal sounds. **esophageal s.,** that produced by vibration of the column of air in the esophagus against the contracting cricopharyngeal sphincter; used after laryngectomy. **explosive s.,** speech uttered with more force than necessary. **mirror s.,** a speech abnormality in which the order of syllables in a sentence is reversed. **pressured s.,** logorrhea. **scanning s.,** that in which syllables of words are separated by noticeable pauses. **staccato s.,** that in which each syllable is uttered separately. **telegraphic s.,** that consisting of only certain prominent words and lacking articles, modifiers, and other ancillary words, a form of agrammaticism in other than young children.

sperm (sperm) 1. spermatozoon. 2. semen.

sper·mat·ic (sper-mat′ik) 1. seminal. 2. pertaining to spermatozoa.

sper·ma·tid (sper′mah-tid) a cell derived from a secondary spermatocyte by fission, and developing into a spermatozoon.

spermat(o)- word element [Gr.], *seed;* specifically, the male germinative element.

sper·ma·to·blast (sper-mat′o-blast) spermatid.

sper·ma·to·cele (-sēl) cystic distention of the epididymis or rete testis, containing spermatozoa.

sper·ma·to·ce·lec·to·my (sper″mah-to-se-lek′tah-me) excision of a spermatocele.

sper·ma·to·ci·dal (-si′d'l) spermicidal; see *spermicide*.

sper·ma·to·cyst (sper-mat′o-sist) spermatocele.

sper·ma·to·cyte (sper-mat′o-sīt) a cell developed from a spermatogonium in spermatogenesis. **spermatocy′tal, spermatocyt′ic,** adj. **primary s.,** a diploid cell that has derived from a spermatogonium and can subsequently begin meiosis and divide into two haploid secondary spermatocytes. **secondary s.,** one of the two haploid cells into which a primary spermatocyte divides, and which in turn gives origin to spermatids.

sper·ma·to·cy·to·gen·e·sis (sper″mah-to-si″to-jen′ĕ-sis) the first stage of formation of spermatozoa, in which the spermatogonia develop into spermatocytes and then into spermatids.

sper·ma·to·gen·e·sis (-jen′ĕ-sis) the process of formation of spermatozoa, including both spermatocytogenesis and spermiogenesis.

sper·ma·to·ge·net·ic (-jĕ-net′ik) 1. pertaining to spermatogenesis. 2. spermatogenic.

sper·ma·to·gen·ic (-jen′ik) producing semen or spermatozoa.

sper·ma·to·go·ni·um (-go′ne-um) pl. *spermatogo′nia.* An undifferentiated male germ cell, originating in a seminiferous tubule and dividing into two primary spermatocytes.

sper·ma·tol·y·sis (sper″mah-tol′ĭ-sis) destruction or dissolution of spermatozoa. **spermatolyt′ic,** adj.

sper·ma·to·tox·ic (sper″mah-to-tok″sik) 1. spermicidal; see *spermicide*. 2. having a destructive or toxic effect on spermatozoa.

sper·ma·to·zo·on (-zo′on) pl. *spermatozo′a.* A mature male germ cell, which fertilizes the oocyte in sexual reproduction and contains the genetic information for the zygote from the male. Spermatozoa, formed in the seminiferous tubules, are derived from spermatogonia, which first develop into spermatocytes; these in turn produce spermatids by meiosis, which then differentiate into spermatozoa. **spermatozo′al,** adj.

sper·ma·tu·ria (sper″mah-tu′re-ah) seminuria.

sper·mi·a·tion (sper″me-a′shun) the release of mature spermatozoa from the Sertoli cells.

sper·mi·cide (sper′mĭ-sīd) an agent destructive to spermatozoa. **spermici′dal,** adj.

sper·mi·duct (-dukt) the ejaculatory duct and ductus deferens together.

sper·mio·gen·e·sis (sper″me-o-jen′ĕ-sis) the second stage in the formation of spermatozoa, when spermatids transform into spermatozoa.

sperm(o)- see spermat(o)-.

sp gr specific gravity.

sphe·ni·on (sfe′ne-on) pl. *sphe′nia.* The point at the sphenoid angle of the parietal bone.

sphen(o)- word element [Gr.], *wedge-shaped; sphenoid bone.*

sphe·no·eth·moi·dal (sfe″no-eth-moi′d'l) pertaining to the sphenoid and ethmoid bones.

sphe·noid (sfe′noid) 1. wedge-shaped. 2. see *Table of Bones.* **sphenoi′dal,** adj.

sphe·noi·di·tis (sfe″noi-di′tis) inflammation of the sphenoid sinus.

sphe·noi·dot·o·my (sfe″noi-dot′ah-me) incision of a sphenoid sinus.

sphe·no·max·il·lary (sfe″no-mak′sĭ-lar″e) pertaining to the sphenoid bone and the maxilla.

sphe·no·oc·cip·i·tal (-ok-sip′ĭ-t'l) pertaining to the sphenoid and occipital bones.

sphe·no·pal·a·tine (-pal′ah-tīn) pertaining to the sphenoid and palatine bones.

sphe·no·pa·ri·e·tal (-pah-ri′ĕ-t'l) pertaining to the sphenoid and parietal bones.

sphere (sfēr) ball or globe; a three-dimensional round body. **spher′ical,** adj.

spher(o)- word element [Gr.], *round; a sphere.*

sphe·ro·cyte (sfēr′o-sīt) a small, globular, completely hemoglobinated erythrocyte without the usual central pallor characteristically found in hereditary spherocytosis but also in acquired hemolytic anemia. **spherocyt′ic,** adj.

sphe·ro·cy·to·sis (sfēr″o-si-to′sis) the presence of spherocytes in the blood. **hereditary s.,** a congenital hereditary form of hemolytic anemia characterized by spherocytosis, abnormal fragility of erythrocytes, jaundice, and splenomegaly.

sphe·roid (sfēr′oid) a spherelike body.

sphe·roi·dal (sfēr-oi′d'l) resembling a sphere.

sphinc·ter (sfingk′ter) [L.] a ringlike muscle which closes a natural orifice or passage. **sphinc′teral, sphincter′ic,** adj. **anal s., s. a′ni,** see *sphincter muscle of anus* (external and internal) in *Table of Muscles.* **cardiac s., cardioesophageal s.,** muscle fibers about the opening of the esophagus into the stomach. **external s. of female urethra,** external sphincter muscle of female urethra; see *Table of Muscles.* **external s. of male urethra,** external sphincter muscle of male urethra; see *Table of Muscles.* **gastroesophageal s.,** the terminal few centimeters of the esophagus, which prevents reflux of gastric contents into the esophagus. **hepatic s.,** a thickened portion of the muscular coat of the hepatic veins near their entrance into the inferior vena cava. **internal s. of urethra,** internal sphincter muscle of urethra; see *Table of Muscles.* **O'Beirne's s.,** a band of muscle at the junction of the sigmoid colon and rectum. **s. of Oddi,** the sheath of muscle fibers investing the associated bile and pancreatic passages as they traverse the wall of the duodenum. **pharyngoesophageal s.,** a region of higher muscular tone at the junction of the pharynx and esophagus, which is involved in movements of swallowing. **precapillary s.,** a smooth muscle fiber encircling a true capillary where it originates from the arterial capillary, which can open and close the capillary entrance. **pyloric s.,** see *Table of Muscles.* **rectal s.,** an incomplete band or thickening of the muscle fibers in the rectum a few inches above the anus in the upper part of the rectal ampulla. **tubal s.,** an encircling band of muscle fibers at the junction of the uterine tube and the uterus. **vesical s.,** internal sphincter muscle of urethra; see *Table of Muscles.*

sphinc·ter·al·gia (sfingk″ter-al′jah) pain in a sphincter muscle.

sphinc·ter·ec·to·my (-ek′tah-me) excision of a sphincter.

sphinc·ter·is·mus (-iz′mus) spasm of a sphincter.

sphinc·ter·itis (-i′tis) inflammation of a sphincter.

sphinc·ter·ol·y·sis (-ol′ĭ-sis) surgical separation of the iris from the cornea in anterior synechia.

sphinc·tero·plas·ty (sfingk′ter-o-plas″te) plastic reconstruction of a sphincter.

sphinc·ter·ot·o·my (sfingk″ter-ot′ah-me) incision of a sphincter.

sphin·ga·nine (sfing′gah-nēn) a dihydroxy derivative of sphingosine, commonly occurring in sphingolipids.

sphin·go·lip·id (sfing″go-lip′id) a lipid in which the backbone is sphingosine or a related base, the basic unit being a ceramide attached to a polar head group; it includes sphingomyelins, cerebrosides, and gangliosides.

sphin·go·lip·i·do·sis (-lip″ĭ-do′sis) any of various lysosomal storage diseases characterized by abnormal storage of sphingolipids.

sphin·go·my·elin (-mi′ĕ-lin) any of the sphingolipids in which the head group is phosphorylated choline; they occur in membranes, primarily in nervous tissue, and accumulate abnormally in Niemann-Pick disease.

sphin·go·sine (sfing′go-sēn) a long-chain, monounsaturated, aliphatic amino alcohol found in sphingolipids.

sphyg·mic (sfig′mik) pertaining to the pulse.

sphygm(o)- word element [Gr.], *the pulse.*

sphyg·mo·dy·na·mom·e·ter (sfig″mo-di″nah-mom′ĕ-ter) an instrument for measuring the force of the pulse.

sphyg·mo·gram (sfig′mo-gram) a record or tracing made by a sphygmograph.

sphyg·mo·graph (-graf) apparatus for registering the movements, form, and force of the arterial pulse. **sphygmograph′ic,** adj.

sphyg·moid (sfig′moid) resembling the pulse.

sphyg·mo·ma·nom·e·ter (sfig″mo-mah-nom′ĕ-ter) an instrument for measuring arterial blood pressure.

sphyg·mom·e·ter (sfig-mom′ĕ-ter) an instrument for measuring the pulse.

sphyg·mo·scope (sfig′mo-skōp) a device for rendering the pulse beat visible.

sphyg·mo·to·nom·e·ter (sfig″mo-to-nom′ĕ-ter) an instrument for measuring elasticity of arterial walls.

spi·ca (spi′kah) [L.] a figure-of-8 bandage, with turns crossing each other.

spic·ule (spik′ūl) a sharp, needle-like body.

spic·u·lum (spik′u-lum) pl. *spic′ula.* [L.] spicule.

spi·der (spi′der) 1. an arthropod of the class Arachnida. 2. vascular s. **arterial s.,** vascular s. **black widow s.,** a spider, *Latrodectus mactans,* whose bite causes severe poisoning. **vascular s.,** a telangiectasis caused by dilatation and ramification of superficial cutaneous arteries, appearing as a bright red central area with branching rays somewhat resembling a spider; commonly associated with pregnancy and liver disease.

spike (spīk) a sharp upward deflection in a curve or tracing, as on the encephalogram.

spi·na (spi′nah) pl. *spi′nae.* [L.] spine. **s. bi′fida,** a developmental anomaly marked by defective closure of the vertebral arch, through which the meninges may (*s. bi′fida cys′tica*) or may not (*s. bi′fida occul′ta*) protrude. **s. vento′sa,** dactylitis, usually in infants and young children, with enlargement of digits, caseation, sequestration, and sinus formation.

spi·nal (spi′n'l) 1. pertaining to a spine or to the vertebral column. 2. pertaining to the spinal cord's functioning independently from the brain.

spi·nate (spi′nāt) having thorns; thorn-shaped.

spin·dle (spin′d'l) 1. a pin tapered at both ends. 2. the fusiform figure occurring during metaphase of cell division, composed of microtubules radiating from the centrioles and connecting to the chromosomes at their centromeres. 3. a type of brain wave occurring on the electroencephalogram in groups at a frequency of about 14 per second, usually while the patient is falling asleep. 4. muscle s. **Krukenberg's s.,** a spindle-shaped, brownish-red opacity of the cornea. **mitotic s.,** spindle (2). **muscle s.,** a fusiform end organ arranged in parallel between the fibers of skeletal muscle and acting as a mechanoreceptor, being the receptor of impulses responsible for the stretch reflex. **nuclear s.,** spindle (2). **tendon s.,** Golgi tendon organ.

spine (spīn) 1. a slender, thornlike process or projection. 2. vertebral column. **alar s., angular s.,** s. of sphenoid bone. **bamboo s.,** the rigid spine produced by ankylosing spondylitis, so called from its radiographic appearance. **cervical s.,** that portion of the spine comprising the cervical vertebrae. **cleft s.,** spina bifida. **ischial s.,** a bony process projecting backward and medialward from the posterior border of the ischium. **lumbar s.,** that portion of the spine comprising the lumbar vertebrae. **mental s., inferior,** the lower part of a small bony projection on the internal surface of the mandible, near the lower end of the midline, serving for attachment of the geniohyoid muscle. **mental s., superior,** the upper part of a small bony projection on the internal surface of the mandible, near the lower end of the midline, serving for attachment of the genioglossus muscle. **nasal s., anterior,** the sharp anterosuperior projection at the anterior extremity of the nasal crest of the maxilla. **nasal s., posterior,** a sharp, backward-projecting bony spine forming the medial posterior angle of the horizontal part of the palatine bone. **neural s.,** the spinous process of a vertebra. **palatine s's,** laterally placed ridges on the lower surface of the maxillary part of the hard palate, separating the palatine sulci. **poker s., rigid s.,** the anky-losed spine produced by rheumatoid spondylitis. **s. of scapula,** a triangular bony plate attached by one end to the back of the scapula. **sciatic s.,** ischial s. **s. of sphenoid bone,** the posterior and downward projection from the lower aspect of the great wing of the sphenoid bone. **thoracic s.,** that part of the spine comprising the thoracic vertebrae. **s. of tibia,** a longitudinally elongated, raised and roughened area on the anterior crest of the tibia. **trochlear s.,** a bony spicule on the anteromedial part of the orbital surface of the frontal bone for attachment of the trochlea of the superior oblique muscle.

spi·nip·e·tal (spi-nip′ĭ-t′l) conducting or moving toward the spinal cord.

spinn·bar·keit (spin′bahr-kīt) [Ger.] the formation of an elastic thread by mucus of the uterine cervix when it is drawn out; the time of maximum elasticity usually precedes or coincides with ovulation.

spi·no·bul·bar (spi″no-bul′ber) pertaining to the spinal cord and medulla oblongata.

spi·no·cer·e·bel·lar (-ser″ĕ-bel′er) pertaining to the spinal cord and cerebellum.

spi·no·cer·e·bel·lum (-ser″ĕ-bel′um) the portion of the cerebellum serving as the primary site of termination of the major spinocerebellar afferents, roughly corresponding to the vermis; therefore, the term is sometimes equated with paleocerebellum.

spi·no·tha·lam·ic (-thah-lam′ik) pertaining to or extending between the spinal cord and the thalamus.

spi·nous (spi′nus) pertaining to or like a spine.

spir·ad·e·no·ma (spīr″ad-ĕ-no′mah) a benign tumor of the sweat glands, particularly of the coil portion.

spi·ral (spi′ral) 1. helical; winding like the thread of a screw. 2. helix; a winding structure. **Curschmann's s's,** coiled mucinous fibrils sometimes found in the sputum in bronchial asthma.

spi·reme (spi′rēm) the threadlike continuous or segmented figure formed by the chromosome material during prophase.

spi·ril·la (spi-ril′ah) [L.] plural of *spirillum*.

spi·ril·li·cide (spi-ril′ĭ-sīd) an agent that destroys spirilla. **spirilli′dal,** adj.

spi·ril·lo·sis (spi″rĭ-lo′sis) a disease caused by presence of spirilla.

Spi·ril·lum (spi-ril′um) a genus of gram-negative bacteria. The species *S. mi′nus* is pathogenic for guinea pigs, rats, mice, and monkeys and is the cause of rat-bite fever (sodoku) in humans.

spi·ril·lum (spi-ril′um) pl. *spiril′la.* [L.] an organism of the genus *Spirillum*.

spir·it (spir′it) 1. any volatile or distilled liquid. 2. an alcoholic or hydroalcoholic solution of a volatile material. 3. in traditional Chinese medicine, shen (q.v.). **aromatic ammonia s.,** an ammonia-containing preparation used as a respiratory stimulant in syncope, weakness, or threatened faint. **camphor s.,** a solution of camphor and alcohol, used topically as a local counter-irritant.

spir(o)-¹ word element [Gr.], *coil; spiral.*

spir(o)-² word element [L.], *breath; breathing.*

Spi·ro·chae·ta (spi″ro-ke′tah) a genus of bacteria (family Spirochaetaceae), found in slime of fresh and salt water; most species formerly assigned to this genus have been assigned to other genera.

Spi·ro·chae·ta·ce·ae (spi″ro-ke-ta′se-e) a family of bacteria that are slender, coiled, undulating, and motile; it includes the pathogenic genera *Borrelia*, *Spirochaeta*, and *Treponema*.

Spi·ro·chae·ta·les (spi″ro-ke-ta′lēz) the spirochetes, an order of bacteria in which some species are free-living and some parasitic; it includes the families Spirochaetaceae and Leptospiraceae.

spi·ro·chete (spi′ro-kēt) 1. any microorganism of the order Spirochaetales. 2. an organism of the genus *Spirochaeta*.

spi·ro·che·ti·cide (spi″ro-ke′tǐ-sīd) 1. destruction of spirochetes. 2. an agent that destroys spirochetes.

spi·ro·che·tol·y·sis (-ke-tol′ǐ-sis) the destruction of spirochetes by lysis. **spirocheto·lyt′ic**, adj.

spi·ro·che·to·sis (-ke-to′sis) infection with spirochetes.

spi·ro·gram (spi′ro-gram) a tracing or graph of respiratory movements.

spi·ro·graph (-graf) an instrument for registering respiratory movements.

spi·rog·ra·phy (spi-rog′rah-fe) pneumography; the graphic measurement of breathing, including breathing movements and breathing capacity.

spi·roid (spi′roid) resembling a spiral.

spi·ro·lac·tone (spi″ro-lak′tōn) any of a group of compounds capable of opposing the action of sodium-retaining steroids on renal transport of sodium and potassium.

spi·rom·e·ter (spi-rom′ĕ-ter) an instrument for measuring the air taken into and exhaled by the lungs.

Spi·ro·me·tra (spi″ro-me′trah) a genus of tapeworms parasitic in fish-eating cats, dogs, and birds; larval infection (sparganosis) in humans is caused by ingestion of inadequately cooked fish.

spi·rom·e·try (spi-rom′ĕ-tre) the measurement of the breathing capacity of the lungs, such as in pulmonary function tests. See also *spirography*. **spiromet′ric**, adj.

spir·o·no·lac·tone (spi″rah-no-lak′tōn) one of the spirolactones, an aldosterone inhibitor that blocks the aldosterone-dependent exchange of sodium and potassium in the distal tubule, thus increasing excretion of sodium and water and decreasing excretion of potassium; used in the treatment of edema, hypokalemia, primary aldosteronism, and hypertension.

spis·sat·ed (spis′ăt-ed) inspissated.

splanch·nec·to·pia (splangk″nek-to′pe-ah) displacement of one or more viscera.

splanch·nes·the·sia (splangk″nes-the′zhah) visceral sense. **splanchnesthet′ic**, adj.

splanch·nic (splangk′nik) pertaining to the viscera.

splanch·ni·cec·to·my (splangk″nǐ-sek′tah-me) resection of one or more of the splanchnic nerves for the treatment of hypertension or intractable pain.

splanch·ni·cot·o·my (-kot′ah-me) splanchnicectomy.

splanchn(o)- word element [Gr.], *viscus (viscera); splanchnic nerve.*

splanch·no·cele (splangk′no-sēl) hernial protrusion of a viscus.

splanch·no·coele (splangk′no-sēl) that portion of the coelom from which the visceral cavities are formed.

splanch·no·di·as·ta·sis (splangk″no-di-as′tah-sis) displacement of a viscus or viscera.

splanch·nog·ra·phy (splangk-nog′rah-fe) descriptive anatomy of the viscera.

splanch·no·lith (splangk′no-lith) enterolith.

splanch·nol·o·gy (splangk-nol′ah-je) the scientific study of the viscera of the body; applied also to the body of knowledge relating thereto.

splanch·no·meg·a·ly (splangk″no-meg′ah-le) visceromegaly.

splanch·nop·a·thy (splangk-nop′ah-the) any disease of the viscera.

splanch·no·pleure (splangk′no-ploor) the layer formed by union of the splanchnic mesoderm with endoderm; from it are developed the muscles and the connective tissue of the digestive tube. **splanchnopleu′ral**, adj.

splanch·no·scle·ro·sis (splangk″no-sklĕ-ro′sis) hardening of the viscera.

splanch·no·skel·e·ton (-skel′ǐ-tǐn) skeletal structures connected with the viscera.

splanch·not·o·my (splangk-not′ah-me) anatomy or dissection of the viscera.

splanch·no·tribe (splangk′no-trīb) an instrument for crushing the intestine to obliterate its lumen.

splay·foot (spla′foot) flatfoot.

spleen (splēn) a large, glandlike organ situated in the upper left part of the abdominal cavity, lateral to the cardiac end of the stomach. Among its functions are the disintegration of erythrocytes and the setting free of hemoglobin, which the liver converts into bilirubin; the genesis of new erythrocytes during fetal life and in the newborn; serving as a blood reservoir; and production of lymphocytes and plasma cells. **accessory s.,** a connected or detached outlying portion, or exclave, of the spleen. **diffuse waxy s.,**

amyloid degeneration of the spleen involving especially the coats of the venous sinuses and the reticulum of the organ. **floating s., movable s.,** one displaced and abnormally movable. **sago s.,** one with amyloid infiltration, the malpighian corpuscles looking like grains of sand. **wandering s.,** floating s. **waxy s.,** a spleen affected with amyloid degeneration.

splen (splen) [Gr.] spleen.

sple·nal·gia (sple-nal′jah) pain in the spleen.

sple·nec·to·my (sple-nek′tah-me) excision of the spleen.

sple·nec·to·pia (sple″nek-to′pe-ah) displacement of the spleen; floating spleen.

sple·nec·to·py (sple-nek′to-pe) splenectopia.

splen·ic (splen′ik) pertaining to the spleen.

sple·ni·tis (sple-ni′tis) inflammation of the spleen.

sple·ni·um (sple′ne-um) [L.] 1. a bandlike structure. 2. a bandage or compress. 3. splenium corporis callosi. **s. cor′poris cal·lo′si,** the posterior, rounded end of the corpus callosum.

splen(o)- word element [Gr.], *spleen.*

sple·no·cele (sple′no-sēl) hernia of the spleen.

sple·no·col·ic (sple″no-kol′ik) pertaining to the spleen and colon.

sple·no·cyte (sple′no-sīt) the monocyte characteristic of splenic tissue.

sple·nog·ra·phy (sple-nog′rah-fe) 1. radiography of the spleen. 2. a description of the spleen.

sple·no·hep·a·to·meg·a·ly (sple″no-hep″-ah-to-meg′ah-le) hepatosplenomegaly.

sple·noid (sple′noid) resembling the spleen.

sple·nol·y·sin (sple-nol′ĭ-sin) a lysin which destroys spleen tissue.

sple·nol·y·sis (sple-nol′ĭ-sis) destruction of splenic tissue.

sple·no·ma (sple-no′mah) pl. *splenomas, spleno′mata.* A splenic tumor.

sple·no·ma·la·cia (sple″no-mah-la′shah) abnormal softness of the spleen.

sple·no·med·ul·lary (-med′u-lar″e) of or pertaining to the spleen and bone marrow.

sple·no·meg·a·ly (-meg′ah-le) enlargement of the spleen. **congestive s.,** Banti's disease; splenomegaly secondary to portal hypertension. **hemolytic s.,** that associated with any disorder causing increased erythrocyte degradation.

sple·no·my·elog·e·nous (-mi″ĕ-loj′ĕ-nus) formed in the spleen and bone marrow.

sple·no·pan·cre·at·ic (-pan″kre-at′ik) pertaining to the spleen and pancreas.

sple·nop·a·thy (sple-nop′ah-the) any disease of the spleen.

sple·no·pexy (sple′no-pek″se) surgical fixation of the spleen.

sple·nop·to·sis (sple″nop-to′sis) downward displacement of the spleen.

sple·no·re·nal (sple″no-re′n′l) pertaining to the spleen and kidney, or to splenic and renal veins.

sple·nor·rha·gia (-ra′jah) hemorrhage from the spleen.

sple·nor·rha·phy (sple-nor′ah-fe) surgical repair of the spleen.

sple·not·o·my (sple-not′ah-me) incision of the spleen.

sple·no·tox·in (sple′no-tok″sin) a toxin produced by or acting on the spleen.

splic·ing (spli′sing) 1. the attachment of individual DNA molecules to each other, as in the production of chimeric genes. 2. RNA s., **RNA s.,** the removal (splicing out) of introns from a primary transcript and the subsequent joining (splicing together) of exons in the production of a mature RNA molecule.

splint (splint) 1. a rigid or flexible appliance for fixation of displaced or movable parts. 2. the act of fastening or confining with such an appliance. **airplane s.,** one which holds the splinted limb suspended in the air. **anchor s.,** one for fracture of the jaw, with metal loops fitting over the teeth and held together by a rod. **Angle's s.,** one for fracture of the mandible. **Balkan s.,** see under *frame.* **coaptation s's,** small splints adjusted about a fractured limb for the purpose of producing coaptation of fragments. **Denis Browne s.,** a splint consisting of a pair of metal foot splints joined by a cross bar; used in talipes equinovarus. **dynamic s.,** a supportive or protective apparatus which aids in initiation and performance of motion by the supported or adjacent parts. **functional s.,** dynamic s. **shin s's,** strain of the flexor digitorum longus muscle occurring in athletes, marked by pain along the shin bone. **Thomas s.,** a leg splint consisting of two rigid rods attached to an ovoid ring that fits around the thigh; it can be combined with other apparatus to provide traction.

splin·ter (splin′ter) 1. a small slender fragment. 2. to break into small fragments.

splint·ing (splin′ting) 1. application of a splint, or treatment by use of a splint. 2. in dentistry, the application of a fixed restoration to join two or more teeth into a single rigid unit. 3. rigidity of muscles occurring as a means of avoiding pain caused by movement of the part.

split·ting (split'ing) 1. the division of a single object into two or more objects or parts. 2. in psychoanalytic theory, a primitive defense mechanism, in which "objects" (persons) are perceived as "all good" or "all bad" rather than as an intermediate or mixture. **s. of heart sounds,** the presence of two components in the first or second heart sound complexes; particularly denoting separation of the elements of the second sound into two, representing aortic valve closure and pulmonic valve closure.

spo·dog·e·nous (spo-doj'ĕ-nus) caused by accumulation of waste material in an organ.

spon·dy·lal·gia (spon″dĭ-lal'jah) spondylodynia.

spon·dyl·ar·thri·tis (spon″dil-ahr-thri'tis) arthritis of the spine.

spon·dy·lit·ic (spon″dĭ-lit'ik) pertaining to or marked by spondylitis.

spon·dy·li·tis (spon″dĭ-li'tis) inflammation of vertebrae. **s. ankylopoie′tica, ankylosing s.,** rheumatoid arthritis of the spine, affecting young persons predominantly, with pain and stiffness as a result of inflammation of the sacroiliac, intervertebral, and costovertebral joints; it may progress to cause complete spinal and thoracic rigidity. **Kümmell's s.,** see under *disease.* **Marie-Strümpell s.,** ankylosing s. **s. tuberculo′sa,** tuberculosis of the spine. **s. typho′sa,** that following typhoid fever.

spon·dy·li·ze·ma (spon″dil-ĭ-ze'mah) downward displacement of a vertebra because of destruction or softening of the one below it.

spondyl(o)- word element [Gr.], *vertebra; vertebral column.*

spon·dy·loc·a·ce (spon″dil-ok'ah-se) tuberculosis of the vertebrae.

spon·dy·lo·dyn·ia (spon″dĭ-lo-din'e-ah) pain in a vertebra.

spon·dy·lo·lis·the·sis (-lis'the-sis) forward displacement of a vertebra over a lower segment, usually of the fourth or fifth lumbar vertebra due to a developmental defect in the pars interarticularis. **spondylolisthet′ic,** adj.

spon·dy·lol·y·sis (spon″dil-ol'ĭ-sis) the breaking down of a vertebra.

spon·dy·lop·a·thy (spon″dil-op'ah-the) any disease of the vertebrae.

spon·dy·lo·py·o·sis (spon″dil-o-pi-o'sis) suppuration of a vertebra.

spon·dy·los·chi·sis (spon″dĭ-los'kĭ-sis) rachischisis.

spon·dy·lo·sis (spon″dĭ-lo'sis) 1. ankylosis of a vertebral joint. 2. degenerative spinal changes due to osteoarthritis. **rhizomelic s.,** ankylosing spondylitis.

spon·dy·lo·syn·de·sis (spon″dĭ-lo-sin-de'sis) spinal fusion.

spon·dy·lot·ic (spon″dĭ-lot'ik) pertaining to or due to spondylosis.

sponge (spunj) 1. a porous, absorbent mass, as a pad of gauze or cotton surrounded by gauze. 2. the elastic fibrous skeleton of certain species of marine animals. **absorbable gelatin s.,** a sterile, absorbable, water-insoluble, gelatin-base material, used as a local hemostatic.

spon·gi·form (spun'jĭ-form) resembling a sponge.

spongi(o)- word element [Gr.], *sponge; spongelike.*

spon·gio·blast (spun'je-o-blast″) 1. any of the embryonic epithelial cells that develop near the neural tube and later become transformed, some into neuroglial and some into ependymal cells. 2. amacrine cell.

spon·gio·blas·to·ma (spun″je-o-blas-to'mah) a tumor containing spongioblasts; considered to be one of the neuroepithelial tumors.

spon·gio·cyte (spun'je-o-sīt″) 1. neuroglial cell. 2. one of the cells with spongy vacuolated protoplasm in the adrenal cortex.

spon·gi·oid (spun'je-oid) resembling a sponge.

spon·gi·o·plasm (spun'je-o-plazm″) a network of fibrils pervading the cell substance; seen in histological specimens following the use of certain fixatives.

spon·gio·sa (spun″je-o'sah) spongy; sometimes used alone to mean the spongy substance of bone (substantia spongiosa ossium).

spon·gio·sa·plas·ty (-plas″te) autoplasty of the substantia spongiosa ossium to potentiate formation of new bone or to cover bone defects.

spon·gi·o·sis (spun″je-o'sis) intercellular edema within the epidermis.

spon·gy (spun'je) of a spongelike appearance or texture.

spon·ta·ne·ous (spon-ta'ne-us) 1. voluntary; instinctive. 2. occurring without external influence.

spo·rad·ic (spo-rad'ik) occurring singly; widely scattered; not epidemic or endemic.

spo·ran·gi·um (spah-ran'je-um) pl. *sporan′gia.* Any encystment containing spores or sporelike bodies, as in certain fungi.

spore (spor) 1. a refractile, oval body formed within bacteria, especially *Bacillus* and *Clostridium,* which is regarded as a resting stage during the life history of the cell, and is characterized by its resistance to environmental changes. 2. the reproductive element, produced sexually or asexually, of one of the lower organisms, such as protozoa, fungi, algae, etc.

spo·ri·cide (spor'ĭ-sīd) an agent that destroys spores. **sporici'dal**, adj.

spo·ro·ag·glu·ti·na·tion (spor"o-ah-gloo"-tĭ-na'shun) agglutination of spores in the diagnosis of sporotrichosis.

spo·ro·blast (spor'o-blast) one of the bodies formed in the oocyst of the malarial parasite in the mosquito and from which the sporozoite later develops; also, similar stages in certain other sporozoa.

spo·ro·cyst (-sist) 1. any cyst or sac containing spores or reproductive cells. 2. a germinal saclike stage in the life cycle of digenetic trematodes, produced by metamorphosis of a miracidium and giving rise to rediae. 3. a stage in the life cycle of certain coccidian protozoa, contained within the oocyst, produced by a sporoblast, and giving rise to sporozoites.

spo·ro·gen·ic (spor"o-jen'ik) producing spores.

spo·rog·o·ny (spo-rog'ah-ne) sporulation involving multiple fission of a sporont, resulting in the formation of sporocysts and sporozoites. **sporogon'ic**, adj.

spo·ront (spor'ont) a zygote of coccidian protozoa enclosed in an oocyst, which undergoes sporogony to produce sporoblasts.

spo·ro·plasm (spor'o-plazm") 1. the protoplasm of spores. 2. in certain protozoa, the central mass of cytoplasm that leaves the spores as an amebula to infect the host.

Spo·ro·thrix (-thriks) a genus of fungi, including *S. schen'ckii* (see *sporotrichosis*) and *S. car'nis*, which causes formation of white mold on meat in cold storage.

spo·ro·tri·cho·sis (spor"o-trĭ-ko'sis) a chronic fungal disease caused by *Sporothrix schenckii*, most commonly characterized by nodular lesions of the cutaneous and subcutaneous tissues and adjacent lymphatics that suppurate, ulcerate, and drain; it may remain localized or be disseminated by the bloodstream.

spo·ro·zo·an (-zo'an) 1. any protozoan of the phyla Apicomplexa, Ascetospora, Microspora, and Myxozoa. 2. pertaining or relating to protozoa of these phyla.

spo·ro·zo·ite (-zo'īt) the motile, infective stage of certain protozoa that results from sporogony.

spo·ro·zo·on (-zo'on) pl. *sporozo'a*. Sporozoan (1).

sport (sport) a mutation.

spor·u·la·tion (spor"u-la'shun) formation of spores.

spor·ule (spor'ūl) a small spore.

spot (spot) a circumscribed area; a small blemish; a macula. **Bitot's s's,** foamy gray, triangular spots of keratinized epithelium on the conjunctiva, associated with vitamin A deficiency. **blind s.,** 1. optic disk. 2. mental scotoma. **café au lait s's,** macules of a distinctive light brown color, such as occur in neurofibromatosis and Albright's syndrome. **cherry-red s.,** the choroid appearing as a red circular area surrounded by gray-white retina, as viewed through the fovea centralis in Tay-Sachs disease. **cold s.,** see *temperature s's.* **cotton-wool s's,** white or gray soft-edged opacities in the retina, seen in hypertensive retinopathy, lupus erythematosus, and other conditions. **Forschheimer s's,** a fleeting exanthem consisting of discrete rose spots on the soft palate sometimes seen in rubella just prior to the onset of the skin rash. **germinal s.,** the nucleolus of an oocyte. **hot s.,** 1. see *temperature s's.* 2. the sensitive area of a neuroma. 3. an area of increased density on an x-ray or thermographic film. **Koplik's s's,** irregular, bright red spots on the buccal and lingual mucosa, with tiny bluish-white specks in the center of each; seen in the prodromal stage of measles. **liver s.,** 1. a lay term for any of the brownish spots on the face, neck, or backs of the hands in many older people. 2. (pl.) tinea versicolor. **Mariotte's s.,** optic disk. **milky s's,** aggregations of macrophages in the subserous connective tissue of the pleura and peritoneum. **mongolian s.,** a smooth, brown to grayish blue nevus, consisting of an excess of melanocytes, typically found at birth in the sacral region in Asians and dark-skinned races; it usually disappears during childhood. **pain s's,** spots on the skin where alone the sense of pain can be produced by a stimulus. **rose s's,** an eruption of rose-colored spots on the abdomen and thighs during the first seven days of typhoid fever. **Roth's s's,** round or oval white spots sometimes seen in the retina early in the course of subacute bacterial endocarditis. **Soemmering's s.,** macula lutea. **Tardieu's s's,** spots of ecchymosis under the pleura after death by suffocation. **temperature s's,** spots on the skin normally anesthetic to pain and pressure but sensitive respectively to heat and cold. **yellow s.,** macula retinae.

sprain (sprān) a joint injury in which some of the fibers of a supporting ligament are ruptured but the continuity of the ligament remains intact.

sprue (sproo) 1. a chronic form of malabsorption syndrome, occurring in both tropical and nontropical forms. 2. in dentistry, the hole through which metal or other material is poured or forced into a mold. **celiac s.,** see under *disease*. **collagenous s.,** an often fatal condition resembling celiac sprue but unresponsive to withdrawal of dietary gluten, characterized by extensive deposition of collagen in the lamina propria of the colon. **nontropical s.,** celiac disease. **refractory s.,** 1. malabsorption and flat jejunal mucosa unresponsive to withdrawal of dietary gluten. 2. celiac disease in which initial responsiveness to gluten withdrawal deteriorates with time. **tropical s.,** a malabsorption syndrome occurring in the tropics and subtropics, marked by stomatitis, diarrhea, and anemia. **unclassified s.,** refractory s.

Spu·ma·vi·rus (spu'mah-vi″rus) foamy viruses; a genus of nonpathogenic viruses of the subfamily Spumavirinae (family Retroviridae) that induce persistent infection in humans, primates, cats, cattle, and hamsters.

spur (spur) 1. calcar; a spiked projecting body, as from a bone. 2. in dentistry, a piece of metal projecting from a plate, band, or other appliance. **calcaneal s.,** a bone excrescence on the lower surface of the calcaneus which frequently causes pain on walking. **scleral s.,** the posterior lip of the venous sinus of the sclera to which most of the fibers of the trabecular reticulum of the iridocorneal angle and the meridional fibers of the ciliary muscle are attached.

spu·tum (spu'tum) [L.] expectoration; matter ejected from the trachea, bronchi, and lungs through the mouth. **s. cruen'tum,** bloody sputum. **nummular s.,** sputum in rounded coinlike disks. **rusty s.,** sputum stained with blood or blood pigments.

SQ subcutaneous.

squa·ma (skwah'mah) pl. *squa'mae*. [L.] a scale or thin, platelike structure. **squa'mate,** adj.

squame (skwām) a scale or scalelike mass.

squa·mo·oc·cip·i·tal (skwah″mo-ok-sip'ĭ-t'l) pertaining to the squamous portion of the occipital bone.

squa·mo·pa·ri·e·tal (-pah-ri'ĕ-t'l) pertaining to the squamous portion of the temporal bone and the parietal bone.

squa·mo·so·pa·ri·e·tal (skwah-mo″so-pah-ri'ĕ-t'l) squamoparietal.

squa·mous (skwah'mus) scaly or platelike.

squat·ting (skwaht'ing) a position with hips and knees flexed, the buttocks resting on the heels; sometimes adopted by the parturient at delivery or by children with certain types of cardiac defects.

squill (skwil) any of various plants of the genus *Urginea*, particularly *U. maritima* or *U. indica*, or the fleshy inner scales of their bulbs. **red s.,** a variety of *Urginea maritima* with red bulbs, or the fleshy inner scales of its bulb, a source of the cardiac glycoside scilliroside; it can cause convulsions or cardiac arrest and is used as a rodenticide. **white s.,** a variety of *Urginea maritima* with white bulbs, or the fleshy inner scales of its bulb, a source of several cardiac glycosides; used as a cardiotonic; also used in folk medicine.

squint (skwint) strabismus.

Sr strontium.

SRH somatotropin-releasing hormone; see *growth hormone–releasing hormone*, under *hormone*.

sro·ta (sro'tah) [Sanskrit] in ayurveda, channels in the body through which nutrients and waste flow for body function, ranging from the gross to the imperceptible and classified by their origin and by the substances that they carry.

SRS-A slow-reacting substance of anaphylaxis; see under *substance*.

SS somatostatin.

ss. [L.] se'mis (half).

SSRI selective serotonin reuptake inhibitor.

ST sinus tachycardia.

stab¹ (stab) 1. to pierce or wound with a pointed instrument. 2. to thrust a pointed instrument into something. 3. stab culture.

stab² shaped like or resembling a staff or rod.

sta·bile (sta'bil) stable; stationary; resistant to change; opposed to *labile*.

sta·ble (sta'b'l) 1. not moving, fixed, firm. 2. constant (def. 1).

stac·ca·to (stah-kah'to) delivered in quick, jerky bursts.

sta·di·um (sta'de-um) pl. *sta'dia*. [L.] stage. **s. decremen'ti,** the period of decrease of severity in a disease; the defervescence of fever. **s. incremen'ti,** the period of increase in the intensity of a disease; the stage of development of fever.

staff (staf) 1. a wooden rod or rodlike structure. 2. a grooved director used as a guide for the knife in surgery. 3. the professional personnel of a hospital. **s. of Aesculapius,** the rod or staff with entwining snake, symbolic of the god of healing, official insignia of the American Medical Association. See also *caduceus*. **attending s.,** the corps of attending physicians and surgeons of a hospital. **consulting s.,** specialists associated with a hospital and acting in an advisory capacity to the attending staff. **house s.,** the resident physicians and surgeons of a hospital.

stage (stāj) 1. a definite period or distinct phase, as of development of a disease or of an organism. 2. the platform of a microscope on which the slide containing the object to be studied is placed. **algid s.,** a period marked by flickering pulse, subnormal temperature, and varied nervous symptoms. **amphibolic s.,** the stage of an infectious disease between the acme and decline in which the diagnosis is uncertain. **anal s.,** in psychoanalytic theory, the second stage of psychosexual development, occurring between the ages of 1 and 3 years, during which the infant's activities, interests, and concerns are on the anal zone. **cold s.,** the period of chill or rigor in a malarial paroxysm. **first s. of labor,** see *labor.* **fourth s. of labor,** see *labor.* **genital s.,** in psychoanalytic theory, the final stage in psychosexual development, occurring during puberty, during which the person can receive sexual gratification from genital-to-genital contact and is capable of a mature relationship with a member of the opposite sex. **hot s.,** period of pyrexia in a malarial paroxysm. **latency s.,** 1. the incubation period of any infectious disorder. 2. the quiescent period following an active period in certain infectious diseases, during which the pathogen lies dormant before again initiating signs of active disease. 3. in psychoanalytic theory, the period of relative quiescence in psychosexual development, lasting from age 5 to 6 years to adolescence, during which interest in persons of the opposite sex ceases and association is mainly with other children of the same sex. **oral s.,** in psychoanalytic theory, the earliest stage of psychosexual development, from birth to about 18 months, during which the infant's needs, expression, and pleasurable experiences center on the oral zone. **phallic s.,** in psychoanalytic theory, the third stage of psychosexual development, lasting from age 2 or 3 years to 5 or 6 years, during which sexual interest, curiosity, and pleasurable experiences center on the penis in boys and the clitoris in girls. **second s. of labor,** see *labor.* **third s. of labor,** see *labor.*

stag·gers (stag′erz) a form of vertigo occurring in decompression sickness.

stag·ing (stāj′ing) 1. the determination of distinct phases or periods in the course of a disease, the life history of an organism, or any biological process. 2. the classification of neoplasms according to the extent of the tumor. **TNM s.,** staging of tumors according to three basic components: primary tumor (T), regional nodes (N), and metastasis (M). Adscripts are used to denote size and degree of involvement; for example, 0 indicates undetectable, and 1, 2, 3, and 4 a progressive increase in size or involvement. Thus, a tumor may be described as T1, N2, M0.

stag·nant (stag′nant) 1. motionless; not flowing or moving. 2. inactive; not developing or progressing.

stain (stān) 1. a substance used to impart color to tissues or cells, to facilitate microscopic study and identification. 2. an area of discoloration of the skin. **differential s.,** one which facilitates differentiation of various elements in a specimen. **Giemsa s.,** a solution containing azure II-eosin, azure II, glycerin, and methanol; used for staining protozoan parasites, such as *Plasmodium* and *Trypanosoma,* for *Chlamydia,* for differential staining of blood smears, and for viral inclusion bodies. **Gram s.,** a staining procedure in which microorganisms are stained with crystal violet, treated with strong iodine solution, decolorized with ethanol or ethanol-acetone, and counterstained with a contrasting dye; those retaining the stain are *gram-positive,* and those losing the stain but staining with the counterstain are *gram-negative.* **hematoxylin-eosin s.,** a mixture of hematoxylin in distilled water and aqueous eosin solution, employed universally for routine tissue examination. **metachromatic s.,** one which produces in certain elements colors different from that of the stain itself. **port-wine s.,** see *nevus flammeus.* **supravital s.,** a stain introduced in living tissue that has been removed from the body, but before cessation of the chemical life of the cells. **tumor s.,** an area of increased density in a radiograph, due to collection of contrast material in distorted and abnormal vessels, prominent in the capillary and venous phase of arteriography, and presumed to indicate neoplasm. **vital s.,** a stain introduced into the living organism, and taken up selectively by various tissues or cellular elements. **Wright's s.,** a mixture of eosin and methylene blue, used for demonstrating blood cells and malarial parasites.

stain·ing (stān′ing) 1. artificial coloration of a substance to facilitate examination of tissues, microorganisms, or other cells under the microscope. For various techniques, see under *stain.* 2. in dentistry, the modification of the color of a tooth or denture base.

stal·ag·mom·e·ter (stal″ag-mom′ĕ-ter) an instrument for measuring surface tension by determining the exact number of drops in a given quantity of a liquid.

stalk (stawk) an elongated anatomical structure resembling the stem of a plant. **allantoic s.,** the slender tube interposed between the urogenital sinus and allantoic sac; it is the precursor of the urachus. **body s., connecting s.,** a bridge of mesoderm connecting the caudal end of the young embryo with the trophoblastic tissues; the precursor of part of the umbilical cord. **pineal s.,** habenula (2). **yolk s.,** a narrow duct connecting the yolk sac (umbilical vesicle) with the midgut of the early embryo.

stam·mer·ing (stam′er-ing) a disorder of speech behavior marked by involuntary pauses in speech; sometimes used synonymously with stuttering, especially in Great Britain.

stan·dard (stan′dard) something established as a measure or model to which other similar things should conform.

stand·still (stand′stil″) cessation of activity, as of the heart (*cardiac s.*) or chest (*respiratory s.*).

stan·nous (stan′us) containing tin as a bivalent element. **s. fluoride,** a dental caries prophylactic, SnF$_2$, applied topically to the teeth.

stan·o·lone (stan′o-lōn) a semisynthetic form of dihydrotestosterone, which has been used as an androgenic and anabolic steroid.

stan·o·zo·lol (-zo-lol″) an androgenic anabolic steroid, used to prevent attacks of hereditary angioedema.

sta·pe·dec·to·my (sta″pĭ-dek′tah-me) excision of the stapes.

sta·pe·di·al (stah-pe′de-al) pertaining to the stapes.

sta·pe·dio·te·not·o·my (stah-pe″de-o-tĕ-not′ah-me) cutting of the tendon of the stapedius muscle.

sta·pe·dio·ves·tib·u·lar (-ves-tib′u-ler) pertaining to the stapes and vestibule.

sta·pe·dot·o·my (sta″pĕ-dot′ah-me) the surgical creation of a small opening in the footplate of the stapes.

sta·pes (sta′pēz) [L.] see *Table of Bones* and Plate 29.

staph·yl·ede·ma (staf″il-ĕ-de′mah) edema of the uvula.

staph·y·line (staf′ĭ-līn) 1. uvular. 2. botryoid.

staph·y·li·tis (staf″ĭ-li′tis) uvulitis.

staphyl(o)- word element [Gr.], *uvula; resembling a bunch of grapes; staphylococci.*

staph·y·lo·coc·ce·mia (staf″ĭ-lo-kok-se′me-ah) staphylococci in the blood.

Staph·y·lo·coc·cus (-kok′us) a genus of gram-positive bacteria that are potential pathogens, causing local lesions and serious opportunistic infections; it includes *S. au′reus,* which causes serious suppurative infections and systemic disease and whose toxins cause food poisoning and toxic shock, *S. epider′midis,* which is commonly found on normal skin and includes many pathogenic strains, and *S. saprophy′ticus,* a usually nonpathogenic form that sometimes causes urinary tract infections.

staph·y·lo·coc·cus (-kok′us) pl. *staphylococ′ci.* Any organism of the genus *Staphylococcus.* **staphylococ′cal, staphylococ′cic,** adj.

staph·y·lo·der·ma (-der′mah) pyogenic skin infection by staphylococci.

staph·y·lol·y·sin (staf″ĭ-lol′ĭ-sin) a hemolysin produced by staphylococci.

staph·y·lo·ma (staf″ĭ-lo′mah) protrusion of the sclera or cornea, usually lined with uveal tissue, due to inflammation. **staphylom′atous,** adj. **anterior s.,** staphyloma in the anterior part of the eye. **corneal s.,** 1. bulging of the cornea with adherent uveal tissue. 2. one formed by protrusion of the iris through a corneal wound. **posterior s.,** backward bulging of the sclera at the posterior pole of the eye. **scleral s.,** protrusion of the contents of the eyeball where the sclera has become thinned.

staph·y·lon·cus (staf″ĭ-long′kus) a tumor or swelling of the uvula.

staph·y·lo·plas·ty (staf′ĭ-lo-plas″te) plastic repair of the soft palate and uvula.

staph·y·lor·rha·phy (staf″ĭ-lor′ah-fe) palatorrhaphy.

staph·y·lot·o·my (staf″ĭ-lot′ah-me) 1. uvulotomy. 2. excision of a staphyloma.

starch (stahrch) 1. any of a group of polysaccharides of the general formula, $(C_6H_{10}O_5)_n$; it is the chief storage form of carbohydrates in plants. 2. granules separated from mature corn, wheat, or potatoes; used as a dusting powder and pharmaceutic aid.

star·tle (stahr′tl) 1. to make a quick involuntary movement as in alarm, surprise, or fright. 2. to become alarmed, surprised, or frightened.

star·va·tion (stahr-va′shun) long-continued and extreme deprivation of food and resulting morbid effects.

sta·sis (sta′sis) 1. a stoppage or diminution of flow, as of blood or other body fluid. 2. a state of equilibrium among opposing forces. **stat′ic,** adj. **intestinal s.,** impairment of the normal passage of intestinal contents, due to mechanical obstruction or to impaired intestinal motility. **urinary s.,** stoppage of the flow or discharge of urine, at any level of the urinary tract. **venous s.,** impairment or cessation of venous flow.

-stasis word element [Gr.], *maintenance* of (or maintaining) a constant level; preventing increase or multiplication. **-stat′ic,** adj.

stat. [L.] sta′tim (at once, immediately).

state (stāt) condition or situation. **alpha s.,** the state of relaxation and peaceful awakefulness, associated with prominent alpha brain wave activity. **persistent vegetative s.,** a condition of profound nonresponsiveness in the wakeful state caused by brain damage at any level and characterized by a nonfunctioning cerebral cortex, absence of response to the external environment, akinesia, mutism, and inability to signal. **refractory s.,** a condition of subnormal excitability of muscle and nerve following excitation. **resting s.,** the physiologic condition achieved by complete bed rest for at least one hour. **steady s.,** dynamic equilibrium.

-static word element [Gr.], *inhibition; maintenance of a constant level.*

sta·tim (sta'tim) [L.] at once.

sta·tion (sta'shun) 1. a position or location. 2. the location of the presenting part of the fetus in the birth canal, designated as −5 to −1 according to the number of centimeters the part is above an imaginary plane passing through the ischial spines, 0 when at the plane, and +1 to +5 according to the number of centimeters the part is below the plane.

sta·tis·tics (stah-tis'tiks) 1. a collection of numerical data. 2. a discipline devoted to the collection, analysis, and interpretation of numerical data using the theory of probability. **vital s.,** data detailing the rates of birth, death, disease, marriage, and divorce in a population.

stato·acous·tic (stat″o-ah-koo'stik) pertaining to balance and hearing.

stato·co·nia (-ko'ne-ah) sing. *stato-co'nium.* Minute calciferous granules within the gelatinous membrane surrounding the acoustic maculae.

stato·lith (stat'o-lith) a granule of the statoconia.

sta·tom·e·ter (stah-tom'ĕ-ter) an apparatus for measuring the degree of exophthalmos.

sta·ture (stach'ur) the height or tallness of a person standing. **stat'ural,** adj.

sta·tus (sta'tus) [L.] state; particularly used in reference to a morbid condition. **s. asthma'ticus,** a particularly severe asthmatic attack that does not respond adequately to usual therapy and may require hospitalization. **complex partial s.,** status epilepticus consisting of a series of complex partial seizures without return to full consciousness in between. **s. epilep'ticus,** a continuous series of generalized tonic-clonic seizures, or similar seizures, without return to consciousness between them. **s. lympha'ticus, s. thymicolympha'ticus,** hyperplasia of lymphoid tissue and the thymus. **s. verru-co'sus,** a wartlike appearance of the cerebral cortex, produced by disorderly arrangement of the neuroblasts so that the formation of fissures and sulci is irregular and unpredictable.

stav·u·dine (stav'u-dēn) a nucleoside analogue of thymidine that inhibits human immunodeficiency virus (HIV) replication, used in the treatment of HIV infection.

stax·is (stak'sis) [Gr.] hemorrhage.

steal (stēl) diversion, as of blood flow, of something from its normal course, as in occlusive arterial disease. **subclavian s.,** in occlusive disease of the subclavian artery, a reversal of blood flow in the ipsilateral vertebral artery from the basilar artery to the subclavian artery beyond the point of occlusion.

ste·a·rate (ste'ah-rāt) any salt (soap), ester, or anionic form of stearic acid.

ste·a·ric ac·id (ste-ar'ik) a saturated 18-carbon fatty acid occurring in most fats and oils, particularly of tropical plants and land animals; used pharmaceutically as a tablet and capsule lubricant and as an emulsifying and solubilizing agent.

stear(o)- word element [Gr.], *fat.*

ste·a·ti·tis (ste″ah-ti'tis) inflammation of adipose tissue.

steat(o)- stear(o)-.

ste·a·to·cys·to·ma (ste″ah-to-sis-to'mah) an epidermal cyst having an intricately infolded thin epidermal lining, without a granular layer, containing an oily liquid and often abortive hair follicles, lanugo hair, and sebaceous apocrine, or eccrine, glands. **s. mul'tiplex,** development of numerous steatocystomas; often an autosomal dominant disorder chiefly affecting males at birth or presenting about the time of puberty.

ste·a·tog·e·nous (ste″ah-toj'ĕ-nus) lipogenic.

ste·a·tol·y·sis (ste″ah-tol'ĭ-sis) the emulsification of fats preparatory to absorption. **steatolyt'ic,** adj.

ste·a·to·ma (ste″ah-to'mah) pl. *steato'mata, steatomas.* 1. Lipoma. 2. a fatty mass retained within a sebaceous gland.

ste·a·to·ma·to·sis (ste″ah-to″mah-to'sis) 1. lipomatosis. 2. steatocystoma multiplex.

ste·a·to·ne·cro·sis (-nĕ-kro'sis) fat necrosis.

ste·a·to·pyg·ia (ste″ah-to-pij'e-ah) excessive fatness of the buttocks. **steatop'ygous,** adj.

ste·a·tor·rhea (-re'ah) excess fat in feces.

ste·a·to·sis (ste″ah-to'sis) fatty change.

steg·no·sis (steg-no'sis) constriction; stenosis. **stegnot'ic,** adj.

stel·late (stel'āt) star-shaped; arranged in rosettes.

stel·lec·to·my (stě-lek'tah-me) excision of a portion of the stellate ganglion.

stem (stem) a supporting structure comparable to the stalk of a plant. **brain s.,** brainstem; see under *B.*

sten(o)- word element [Gr.], *narrow; contracted; constriction.*

steno·cho·ria (sten"o-kor'e-ah) stenosis.

steno·co·ri·a·sis (-kah-ri'ah-sis) contraction of the pupil.

steno·pe·ic (-pe'ik) having a narrow opening or slit.

ste·nosed (stě-nōzd') narrowed; constricted.

ste·no·sis (stě-no'sis) pl. *steno'ses.* [Gr.] stricture; an abnormal narrowing or contraction of a duct or canal. **aortic s. (AS),** a narrowing of the aortic orifice of the heart or of the aorta near the valve. **hypertrophic pyloric s.,** narrowing of the pyloric canal due to muscular hypertrophy and mucosal edema, usually in infants. **hypertrophic subaortic s., idiopathic hypertrophic subaortic s. (IHSS),** a form of hypertrophic cardiomyopathy in which the left ventricle is hypertrophied and the cavity is small; it is marked by obstruction to left ventricular outflow. **infantile hypertrophic gastric s.,** congenital hypertrophy and hyperplasia of the musculature of the pyloric sphincter, leading to partial obstruction of the gastric outlet. **mitral s.,** a narrowing of the left atrioventricular orifice. **pulmonary s. (PS),** narrowing of the opening between the pulmonary artery and the right ventricle, usually at the level of the valve leaflets. **pyloric s.,** obstruction of the pyloric orifice of the stomach; it may be congenital or acquired. **renal artery s.,** narrowing of one or both renal arteries, so that renal function is impaired, resulting in renal hypertension and, if stenosis is bilateral, chronic renal failure. **subaortic s.,** aortic stenosis due to an obstructive lesion in the left ventricle below the aortic valve, causing a pressure gradient across the obstruction within the ventricle. **tricuspid s. (TS),** narrowing or stricture of the tricuspid orifice of the heart.

steno·ther·mal (sten"o-ther'mal) stenothermic.

steno·ther·mic (-ther'mik) developing only within a narrow range of temperature; said of bacteria.

steno·tho·rax (-thor'aks) abnormal narrowness of the chest.

ste·not·ic (stě-not'ik) marked by stenosis; abnormally narrowed.

stent (stent) 1. a device or mold of a suitable material, used to hold a skin graft in place. 2. a slender rodlike or threadlike device used to provide support for tubular structures that are being anastomosed, or to induce or maintain their patency. **Palmaz s.,** an intravascular stent made of rigid wire mesh; it is introduced by a guidewire and expanded into place by a balloon. **pigtail s.,** one with a curl near the end like that of a pig's tail to maintain it in place.

ste·pha·ni·on (stě-fa'ne-on) [Gr.] intersection of the superior temporal line and the coronal suture. **stepha'nial,** adj.

sterc(o)- word element [L.], *feces.*

ster·co·bi·lin (ster"ko-bi'lin) a bile pigment derivative formed by air oxidation of stercobilinogen; it is a brown-orange-red pigmentation contributing to the color of feces and urine.

ster·co·bi·lin·o·gen (-bi-lin'o-jen) a bilirubin metabolite and precursor of stercobilin, formed by reduction of urobilinogen.

ster·co·lith (ster'ko-lith) fecalith.

ster·co·ra·ceous (ster"kah-ra'shus) fecal.

ster·co·ral (ster'kah-r'l) fecal.

ster·co·ro·ma (ster"kah-ro'mah) a tumorlike mass of fecal matter in the rectum.

ster·cus (ster'kus) pl. *ster'cora.* [L.] feces. **ster'coral, ster'corous,** adj.

stereo- word element [Gr.], *solid; three dimensional; firmly established.*

ster·eo·ar·throl·y·sis (ster"e-o-ahr-throl'ĭ-sis) operative formation of a movable new joint in cases of bony ankylosis.

ster·eo·aus·cul·ta·tion (-aus"kul-ta'shun) auscultation with two stethoscopes, on different parts of the chest.

ster·eo·cam·pim·e·ter (-kam-pim'ĕ-ter) an instrument for studying unilateral central scotomas and central retinal defects.

ster·eo·chem·is·try (-kem'is-tre) the branch of chemistry treating of the space relations of atoms in molecules. **stereochem'ical,** adj.

ster·eo·cine·flu·o·rog·ra·phy (-sin"ĕ-floo-rog'rah-fe) recording by motion picture camera of images observed by stereoscopic fluoroscopy.

ster·eo·en·ceph·a·lo·tome (-en-sef'ah-lah-tōm") a guiding instrument used in stereoencephalotomy.

ster·eo·en·ceph·a·lot·o·my (-en-sef"ah-lot'ah-me) stereotaxic surgery.

ster·e·og·no·sis (ster"e-og-no'sis) 1. the faculty of perceiving and understanding the form and nature of objects by the sense of touch. 2. perception by the senses of the solidity of objects. **stereognos'tic,** adj.

ster·eo·iso·mer (ster″e-o-i′so-mer) one of a group of compounds showing stereo-isomerism.

ster·eo·isom·er·ism (-i-som′er-izm) isomerism in which the isomers have the same structure (same linkages between atoms) but different spatial arrangements of the atoms. **stereoisomer′ic**, adj.

Ster·eo·or·thop·ter (-or-thop′ter) trademark for a mirror-reflecting instrument for correcting strabismus.

ster·eo·scope (ster′e-o-skōp″) an instrument for producing the appearance of solidity and relief by combining the images of two similar pictures of an object.

ster·eo·scop·ic (ster″e-o-skop′ik) having the effect of a stereoscope; giving objects a solid or three-dimensional appearance.

ster·eo·spe·cif·ic (ster″e-o-spĕ-sif′ik) exhibiting marked specificity for one of several stereoisomers of a substrate or reactant; said of enzymes or of synthetic organic reactions.

ster·eo·tac·tic (-tak′tik) 1. characterized by precise positioning in space; said especially of discrete areas of the brain that control specific functions. 2. pertaining to stereotactic surgery. 3. pertaining to thigmotaxis (thigmotactic).

ster·eo·tax·ic (-tak′sik) 1. stereotactic. 2. pertaining to or exhibiting thigmotaxis (thigmotactic).

ster·eo·tax·is (-tak′sis) 1. stereotactic surgery. 2. thigmotaxis.

ster·e·ot·ro·pism (ster″e-ot′rah-pizm) tropism in response to contact with a solid or rigid surface. **stereotrop′ic**, adj.

ster·eo·typ·ic (ster″e-o-tip′ik) having a fixed, unvarying form.

ster·eo·ty·py (ster′e-o-ti″pe) persistent repetition or sameness of acts, ideas, or words.

ste·ric (ster′ik) pertaining to the arrangement of atoms in space; pertaining to stereochemistry.

ster·ile (ster′il) 1. unable to produce offspring. 2. aseptic.

ste·ril·i·ty (stĕ-ril′ĭ-te) 1. inability to produce offspring, i.e., either to conceive (*female s.*) or to induce conception (*male s.*) 2. asepsis.

ster·i·li·za·tion (ster″ĭ-lĭ-za′shun) 1. the complete elimination or destruction of all living microorganisms. 2. any procedure by which an individual is made incapable of reproduction.

ster·i·lize (ster′ĭ-līz) 1. to render sterile; to free from microorganisms. 2. to render incapable of reproduction.

ster·i·liz·er (ster′ĭ-līz″er) an apparatus for the destruction of microorganisms.

ster·nal (ster′n′l) of or relating to the sternum.

ster·nal·gia (ster-nal′jah) pain in the sternum.

ster·ne·bra (ster′ne-brah) pl. *ster′nebrae.* Any of the segments of the sternum in early life, which later fuse to form the body of the sternum.

stern(o)- word element [L.], *sternum.*

ster·no·cla·vic·u·lar (ster″no-klah-vik′u-ler) pertaining to the sternum and clavicle.

ster·no·clei·do·mas·toid (-kli″do-mas′-toid) pertaining to the sternum, clavicle, and mastoid process.

ster·no·cos·tal (-kos′t′l) pertaining to the sternum and ribs.

ster·no·hy·oid (-hi′oid) pertaining to the sternum and hyoid bone.

ster·noid (ster′noid) resembling the sternum.

ster·no·mas·toid (ster″no-mas′toid) pertaining to the sternum and mastoid process.

ster·no·peri·car·di·al (-per″ĭ-kahr′de-al) pertaining to the sternum and pericardium.

ster·nos·chi·sis (ster-nos′kĭ-sis) congenital fissure of the sternum.

ster·no·thy·roid (ster″no-thi′roid) pertaining to the sternum and thyroid cartilage or gland.

ster·not·o·my (ster-not′ah-me) the operation of cutting through the sternum.

ster·num (ster′num) [L.] see *Table of Bones.*

ster·nu·ta·to·ry (ster-nu′tah-tor″e) 1. causing sneezing. 2. an agent that causes sneezing.

ster·oid (ster′oid) any of a group of lipids with a specific 7-carbon-atom ring system as a nucleus, such as progesterone, adrenocortical and gonadal hormones, bile acids, sterols, toad poisons, and some carcinogenic hydrocarbons. **steroi′dal**, adj. **anabolic s.,** any of a group of synthetic derivatives of testosterone having pronounced anabolic properties and relatively weak androgenic properties; they are used clinically mainly to promote growth and repair of body tissues in diseases or states promoting catabolism or tissue wasting.

ste·roi·do·gen·e·sis (stĕ-roi″do-jen′ĕ-sis) production of steroids, as by the adrenal glands. **steroidogen′ic**, adj.

ster·ol (ster′ol) any of a group of steroids with a long (8 to 10 carbons) aliphatic side-chain at position 17 and at least one alcoholic group; they have lipidlike solubility.

ster·tor (ster′tor) snore (1). **ster′torous,** adj.

steth(o)- word element [Gr.], *chest.*

stetho·go·ni·om·e·ter (steth″o-go″ne-om′ĕ-ter) apparatus for measuring curvature of the chest.

steth·om·e·ter (steth-om′ĕ-ter) an instrument for measuring the circular dimension or expansion of the chest.

stetho·scope (steth′o-skōp) an instrument for performing mediate auscultation. **stethoscop′ic**, adj.

steth·os·co·py (steth-os′kah-pe) examination with the stethoscope.

stetho·spasm (steth′o-spazm) spasm of the chest muscles.

sthe·nia (sthe′ne-ah) a condition of strength and activity.

sthen·ic (sthen′ik) active; strong.

STI systolic time intervals.

stib·i·al·ism (stib′e-ah-lizm″) antimony poisoning; see *heavy metal poisoning*, under *poisoning.*

stig·ma (stig′mah) pl. *stigmas, stig′mata.* [Gr.] 1. any mental or physical mark or peculiarity that aids in identification or diagnosis of a condition. 2. a mark, spot, or pore on the surface of an organ or organism. 3. follicular s. 4. a distinguishing personal trait that is perceived as or actually is physically, socially, or psychologically disadvantageous. 5. in the plural, purpuric or hemorrhagic lesions of the hands and/or feet, resembling crucifixion wounds. **stig′mal, stigmat′ic**, adj. **follicular s.,** a spot on the surface of an ovary where the vesicular follicle will rupture and permit passage of the secondary oocyte during ovulation. **malpighian s′s,** the points where the smaller veins enter into the larger veins of the spleen.

stig·ma·ti·za·tion (stig″mah-tĭ-za′shun) 1. the developing of or being identified as possessing one or more stigmata. 2. the act or process of negatively labelling or characterizing another. 3. the condition due to or marked by stigmata.

sti·let (sti′let) stylet.

still·birth (stil′berth) delivery of a dead child.

still·born (-born) born dead.

stim·u·lant (stim′u-lant) 1. producing stimulation. 2. an agent which stimulates. **central s.,** a stimulant of the central nervous system. **diffusible s.,** one that acts quickly and strongly, but transiently. **general s.,** one that acts upon the whole body. **local s.,** one that affects only, or mainly, the part to which it is applied.

stim·u·late (stim′u-lāt) to excite functional activity.

stim·u·la·tion (stim″u-la′shun) the act or process of stimulating; the condition of being stimulated. **deep brain s. (DBS),** patient-controlled, continuous, high-frequency electrical stimulation of a specific area of the thalamus, globus pallidus, or subthalamic nucleus by means of an electrode implanted in the brain. **functional electrical s. (FES),** the application of an electric current by means of a prosthesis to stimulate and restore partial function to a muscle disabled by neurologic lesions. **transcutaneous electrical nerve s. (TENS), transcutaneous nerve s. (TNS),** electrical stimulation of nerves for relief of pain by delivering a current through the skin.

stim·u·la·tor (stim′u-la″tor) 1. any agent that excites functional activity. 2. in electrodiagnosis, an instrument that applies pulses of current to stimulate a nerve, muscle, or area of the central nervous system. **long-acting thyroid s. (LATS),** thyroid-stimulating antibody associated with Graves disease; it is an autoantibody reactive against thyroid cell receptors for thyroid stimulating hormone and thus mimics the effects of the hormone.

stim·u·la·to·ry (-lah-tor″e) capable of stimulating or causing stimulation.

stim·u·lus (stim′u-lus) pl. *stim′uli.* [L.] any agent, act, or influence which produces functional or trophic reaction in a receptor or an irritable tissue. **adequate s.,** a stimulus of the specific form of energy to which a given receptor is sensitive. **aversive s.,** one which, when applied following the occurrence of a response, decreases the strength of that response on later occurrences. **conditioned s.,** a stimulus that acquires the capacity to evoke a particular response on repeated pairing with another stimulus naturally capable of eliciting the response. **discriminative s.,** a stimulus, associated with reinforcement, that exerts control over a particular form of behavior; the subject discriminates between closely related stimuli and responds positively only in the presence of that stimulus. **eliciting s.,** any stimulus, conditioned or unconditioned, that elicits a response. **heterologous s.,** one that produces an effect or sensation when applied to any part of a nerve tract. **homologous s.,** adequate s. **threshold s.,** a stimulus that is just strong enough to elicit a response. **unconditioned s.,** any stimulus naturally capable of eliciting a specific response.

sting (sting) 1. injury due to a biotoxin introduced into an individual or with which he comes in contact, together with the mechanical trauma incident to its introduction. 2. the organ used to inflict such injury.

stip·pled (stip″ld) marked by small spots or flecks.

stip·pling (stip′ling) a spotted condition or appearance, as an appearance of the retina as if dotted with light and dark points, or the appearance of red blood cells in basophilia.

stir·rup (stir′up) 1. a structure or device resembling the stirrup of a saddle, or the portion of an apparatus on which to rest the feet. 2. stapes; see *Table of Bones*.

stitch (stich) 1. a sudden, transient cutting pain. 2. a suture.

sto·chas·tic (sto-kas′tik) pertaining to a random process, particularly a time series of random variables.

stoi·chi·ol·o·gy (stoi″ke-ol′ah-je) the science of elements, especially the physiology of the cellular elements of tissues. **stoichiolog′ic**, adj.

stoi·chi·om·e·try (-om′ĕ-tre) the determination of the relative proportions of the compounds involved in a chemical reaction. **stoichiomet′ric**, adj.

sto·ma (sto′mah) pl. *sto′mas, sto′mata.* [Gr.] a mouthlike opening, particularly an incised opening which is kept open for drainage or other purposes. **sto′mal**, adj.

stom·ach (stum′ak) the musculomembranous expansion of the alimentary canal between the esophagus and duodenum, consisting of a cardiac part, a fundus, a body, and a pyloric part. Its (gastric) glands secrete the gastric juice which, when mixed with food, forms chyme, a semifluid substance suitable for further digestion by the intestine. See Plate 27. **stom′achal, stomach′ic**, adj. **cascade s.**, an atypical form of hourglass stomach, characterized radiographically by a drawing up of the posterior wall; an opaque medium first fills the upper sac and then cascades into the lower sac. **hourglass s.**, one more or less completely divided into two parts, resembling an hourglass in shape, due to scarring which complicates chronic gastric ulcer. **leather bottle s.**, linitis plastica.

stom·a·chal·gia (stum″ah-kal′jah) gastrodynia.

sto·ma·tal·gia (sto″mah-tal′jah) pain in the mouth.

sto·ma·ti·tis (sto″mah-ti′tis) pl. *stomati′- tides.* Generalized inflammation of the oral mucosa. **angular s.**, perlèche. **aphthous s.**, recurrent aphthous s. **gangrenous s.**, see *noma*. **herpetic s.**, an acute infection of the oral mucosa with vesicle formation, due to the herpes simplex virus. **mycotic s.**, thrush. **recurrent aphthous s.**, a recurrent stomatitis of unknown etiology characterized by the appearance of small ulcers on the oral mucosa, covered by a grayish exudate and surrounded by a bright red halo; they heal without scarring in 7 to 14 days. **ulcerative s.**, stomatitis with shallow ulcers on the cheeks, tongue, and lips. **Vincent's s.**, necrotizing ulcerative gingivitis.

stomat(o)- word element [Gr.], *mouth*.

sto·ma·to·dyn·ia (sto″mah-to-din′e-ah) stomatalgia.

sto·ma·tog·nath·ic (sto″mah-tog-nath′ik) denoting the mouth and jaws collectively.

sto·ma·tol·o·gy (sto″mah-tol′ah-je) the branch of medicine that deals with the mouth and its diseases. **stomatolog′ic**, adj.

sto·ma·to·ma·la·cia (sto″mah-to-mah-la′shah) softening of the structures of the mouth.

sto·ma·to·me·nia (-me′ne-ah) bleeding from the mouth at the time of menstruation.

sto·ma·to·my·co·sis (-mi-ko′sis) any fungal disease of the mouth.

sto·ma·top·a·thy (sto″mah-top′ah-the) any disorder of the mouth.

sto·ma·to·plas·ty (sto′mah-to-plas″te) plastic reconstruction of the mouth.

sto·ma·tor·rha·gia (sto″mah-to-ra′jah) hemorrhage from the mouth.

sto·mo·de·um (sto″mo-de′um) an invagination of the surface ectoderm of the embryo, at the point where later the mouth is formed. **stomode′al**, adj.

-stomy word element [Gr.], *creation of an opening into* or *a communication between*.

stone (stōn) 1. calculus. 2. a unit of weight in Great Britain, the equivalent of 14 pounds (avoirdupois), or about 6.34 kg.

stool (stōol) feces. **rice-water s's**, the watery diarrhea of cholera. **silver s.**, feces with a silver color due to a mixture of melena and white fatty stools; it occurs in tropical sprue, in children with diarrhea who are given sulfonamides, and with carcinoma of the ampulla of Vater.

stor·i·form (stor′ĭ-form) having an irregularly whorled pattern somewhat like that of a straw mat; said of the microscopic appearance of dermatofibrosarcomas.

storm (storm) a sudden and temporary increase in symptoms. **thyroid s., thyrotoxic s.**, see under *crisis*.

stra·bis·mom·e·ter (strah-biz-mom′ĕ-ter) an apparatus for measuring strabismus.

stra·bis·mus (strah-biz′mus) squint; deviation of the eye which the patient cannot overcome; the visual axes assume a position relative to each other different from that required by the physiological conditions. **strabis′mic**, adj. **concomitant s.**, that due to faulty insertion of the eye muscles, resulting in the same amount of deviation regardless of the direction of the gaze. **convergent s.**, esotropia. **divergent s.**, exotropia. **nonconcomitant s.**, that in which the amount of deviation of the squinting eye varies according to the direction of gaze. **vertical s.,** that in which the visual axis of the squinting eye deviates in the vertical plane (hypertropia or hypotropia).

stra·bot·o·my (strah-bot′ah-me) section of an ocular tendon in treatment of strabismus.

strad·dle (strad″l) 1. to extend over or across, to be on both sides. 2. to have one leg on each opposite side of something.

strain (strān) 1. to overexercise. 2. excessive effort or exercise. 3. an overstretching or overexertion of some part of the musculature. 4. to filter. 5. change in the size or shape of a body as the result of an externally applied force. 6. a group of organisms within a species or variety, characterized by some particular quality. **wild-type s.,** that used as a standard for a given species or variety of organism, usually assumed to be the one found in nature.

strait (strāt) a narrow passage. **s's of pelvis,** the pelvic inlet (*superior pelvic s.*) and pelvic outlet (*inferior pelvic s.*).

strait·jack·et (strāt′jak″et) informal name for *camisole.*

stra·mo·ni·um (strah-mo′ne-um) the flowering plant *Datura stramonium* or a preparation of its dried leaf and flowering or fruiting tops; it is a source of hyoscyamine and scopolamine and has anticholinergic and parasympatholytic effects. It is used in folk medicine, Chinese medicine, and homeopathy.

stran·gle (strang′g′l) choke (1).

stran·gu·lat·ed (strang′gu-lāt″ed) congested by reason of constriction or hernial stricture.

stran·gu·la·tion (strang″gu-la′shun) 1. choke (2). 2. arrest of circulation in a part due to compression. See *hemostasis* (2).

stran·gu·ry (strang′gu-re) slow and painful discharge of the urine, due to spasm of the urethra and bladder.

strap (strap) 1. a band or slip, as of adhesive plaster, used in attaching parts to each other. 2. to bind down tightly. **Montgomery s's,** straps of adhesive tape used to secure dressings that must be changed frequently.

strat·i·fied (strat′ĭ-fīd) formed or arranged in layers.

strat·i·form (-form) having a layered structure.

stra·tig·ra·phy (strah-tig′rah-fe) tomography. **stratigraph′ic,** adj.

stra·tum (strat′um, stra′tum) pl. *stra′ta.* [L.] a layer or lamina. **s. basa′le,** basal layer: the deepest layer, as of the endometrium or epidermis. **s. compac′tum,** compact layer of endometrium: the sublayer of the stratum functionale facing the interior of the uterus and containing the necks of the uterine glands. **s. cor′neum,** horny layer: the outermost layer of the epidermis, consisting of dead and desquamating cells. **s. functiona′le,** functional layer of endometrium: the layer of endometrium facing the uterine lumen, overlying the stratum basale; subdivided into the stratum compactum and stratum spongiosum. Its cells are cast off at menstruation and parturition. It is called the *decidua* during pregnancy. **s. germinati′vum,** germinative layer: the stratum basale and stratum spinosum of the epidermis considered as a single layer; the term is sometimes used to denote only the stratum basale. **s. granulo′sum,** granular layer. 1. the layer of epidermis between the stratum lucidum and stratum spinosum. 2. the layer of follicle cells lining the theca of the vesicular ovarian follicles. **s. lu′cidum,** clear layer: in the epidermis, the clear translucent layer just beneath the stratum corneum. **s. spino′sum,** spinous or prickle cell layer: in the epidermis, the layer between the stratum granulosum and stratum basale, characterized by the presence of prickle cells. **s. spongio′sum,** spongy layer of endometrium: the sublayer of the stratum functionale underlying the stratum compactum; it contains the tortuous portions of the uterine glands.

streak (strēk) a line, stria, or stripe. **angioid s's,** red to black irregular bands in the ocular fundus running outward from the optic disk. **fatty s.,** a small, flat, yellow-gray area, composed mainly of cholesterol, in an artery; possibly an early stage of atherosclerosis. **meningitic s.,** tache cérébrale. **Moore's lightning s's,** vertical flashes of light sometimes seen on the peripheral side of the field of vision when the eyes are moved, a benign condition. **primitive s.,** a faint white trace at the caudal end of the embryonic disc, formed by movement of cells at the onset of mesoderm formation and providing the first evidence of the embryonic axis.

strepho·sym·bo·lia (stref″o-sim-bo′le-ah) 1. a perceptual disorder in which objects seem reversed as in a mirror. 2. a type of dyslexia in which letters are perceived as if in a mirror; it begins with confusion between similar but oppositely oriented letters (b-d, q-p) and there may be a tendency to read backward.

strept(o)- word element [Gr.], *twisted.*

Strep·to·bac·il·lus (strep″to-bah-sil′lus) a genus of gram-negative bacteria of uncertain affiliation; organisms are highly pleomorphic. *S. monilifor′mis* is a cause of rat-bite fever.

strep·to·bac·il·lus (strep″to-bah-sil′us) pl. *streptobacil′li.* An organism of the genus *Streptobacillus.*

strep·to·cer·ci·a·sis (-ser-ki′ah-sis) infection with *Mansonella streptocerca,* whose microfilariae produce a pruritic rash resembling that in onchocerciasis; transmitted by midges of the genus *Culicoides,* it occurs in Central Africa.

Strep·to·coc·ca·ceae (-kok-a′se-e) a family of gram-positive, facultative anaerobic cocci, which are usually nonmotile, and occur in pairs, chains, or tetrads.

strep·to·coc·cal (-kok′al) pertaining to or caused by a streptococcus.

strep·to·coc·ce·mia (-kok-se′me-ah) occurrence of streptococci in the blood.

Strep·to·coc·cus (-kok′us) a genus of gram-positive, facultatively anaerobic cocci occurring in pairs or chains; it is separable into the *pyogenic group,* the *viridans group,* the *enterococcus group,* and the *lactic group.* The first group includes the β-hemolytic human and animal pathogens, the second and third include α-hemolytic parasitic forms that are normal flora in the upper respiratory tract and the intestinal tract, respectively, and the fourth is made up of saprophytic forms associated with the souring of milk. Species include *S. mu′tans,* which may cause dental caries; *S. pneumo′niae,* an α-hemolytic species that is the most common cause of lobar pneumonia and also causes other serious, acute pyogenic disorders; *S. pyo′genes,* a β-hemolytic species that causes septic sore throat, scarlet fever, and rheumatic fever; and *S. san′guinis,* found in dental plaque, blood, and subacute bacterial endocarditis.

strep·to·coc·cus (strep″to-kok′us) pl. *streptococ′ci.* An organism of the genus *Streptococcus.* **streptococ′cal, streptococ′cic,** adj. **hemolytic s.,** any streptococcus capable of hemolyzing erythrocytes, classified as *α-hemolytic type,* producing a zone of greenish discoloration much smaller than the clear zone produced by the β-hemolytic type about the colony on blood agar; and the *β-hemolytic type,* producing a clear zone of hemolysis immediately around the colony on blood agar. The most virulent streptococci belong to the latter group. On immunological grounds, the β-hemolytic streptococci may be divided into groups A through T; most human pathogens belong to groups A through G. **nonhemolytic s.,** any streptococcus that does not cause a change in the medium when cultured on blood agar. **viridans s.,** any of a group of streptococci with no defined Lancefield group antigens but not *Streptococcus pneumoniae,*

usually α-hemolytic; part of the normal flora of the respiratory tract but also causing dental caries, bacterial endocarditis, and other disorders in immunocompromised hosts.

strep·to·dor·nase (-dor′nās) a deoxyribonuclease produced by hemolytic streptococci.

strep·to·ki·nase (-ki′nās) a protein produced by β-hemolytic streptococci, which produces fibrinolysis by binding to plasminogen and causing its conversion to plasmin; used as a thrombolytic agent. **s.-streptodornase (SKSD),** a mixture of enzymes elaborated by hemolytic streptococci; used as a proteolytic and fibrinolytic agent.

strep·tol·y·sin (strep-tol′ĭ-sin) the hemolysin of hemolytic streptococci.

Strep·to·my·ces (strep″to-mi′sēz) a genus of bacteria (order Actinomycetales), usually soil forms, but occasionally parasitic on plants and animals, and notable as the source of various antibiotics, e.g., the tetracyclines. *S. somalien′sis* is a cause of mycetoma.

strep·to·my·cin (-mi′sin) an aminoglycoside antibiotic produced by *Streptomyces griseus* and effective against a wide variety of aerobic gram-negative bacilli and some gram-positive bacteria, including mycobacteria, but to which many of the former have developed resistance; used as the sulfate salt in the treatment of tuberculosis, tularemia, plague, and brucellosis.

strep·to·sep·ti·ce·mia (-sep″tĭ-se′me-ah) septicemia due to streptococci.

strep·to·zo·cin (-zo′sin) an antineoplastic antibiotic derived from *Streptomyces achromogenes;* used principally in the treatment of islet cell and other tumors of the pancreas.

stress (stres) 1. forcibly exerted influence; pressure. 2. force per unit area. 3. in dentistry, the pressure of the upper teeth against the lower in mastication. 4. a state of physiological or psychological strain caused by adverse stimuli, physical, mental, or emotional, internal or external, that tend to disturb the functioning of an organism and which the organism naturally desires to avoid; see also *stress reaction,* under *reaction.* 5. the stimuli that elicit such a state or stress reactions.

stretch·er (strech′er) a contrivance for carrying the sick or wounded.

stria (stri′ah) pl. *stri′ae.* [L.] 1. a band, line, streak, or stripe. 2. in anatomy, a longitudinal collection of nerve fibers in the brain. **stri′ae atro′phicae, stri′ae disten′sae,** atrophic, pinkish or purplish, scarlike lesions, later becoming white, on the breasts, thighs, abdomen, and buttocks, due to weakening of elastic tissues, associated with pregnancy *(striae gravidarum)*, overweight, rapid growth during puberty and adolescence, Cushing's syndrome, and topical or prolonged treatment with corticosteroids. **stri´ae gravida´rum,** see *striae atrophicae.*

stri·ate (stri´āt) striated.

stri·at·ed (stri´āt-ed) having stripes or striae.

stri·a·tion (stri-a´shun) 1. the quality of being marked by stripes or striae. 2. a streak or scratch, or a series of streaks.

stri·a·to·ni·gral (stri´ah-to-ni´gr'l) projecting from the corpus striatum to the substantia nigra.

stri·a·tum (stri-a´tum) corpus striatum. **stria´tal,** adj.

stric·ture (strik´chur) stenosis.

stric·ture·plas·ty (strik´cher-plas″te) surgical enlargement of the caliber of a constricted bowel segment by means of longitudinal incision and transverse suturing of the stricture.

stric·tur·iza·tion (strik″chur-ĭ-za´shun) the process of decreasing in caliber or of becoming constricted.

stri·dor (stri´dor) [L.] a harsh, high-pitched breath sound. **strid´ulous,** adj. **laryngeal s.,** that due to laryngeal obstruction. A *congenital* form with dyspnea is due to infolding of a congenitally flabby epiglottis and aryepiglottic folds during inhalation; it is usually outgrown by two years of age.

strio·cer·e·bel·lar (stri″o-ser″ĕ-bel´er) pertaining to the corpus striatum and cerebellum.

strip (strip) 1. to press the contents from a canal, such as the urethra or a blood vessel, by running the finger along it. 2. to excise lengths of large veins and incompetent tributaries after subcutaneous dissection. 3. to remove tooth structure or restorative material from the mesial or distal surfaces of teeth utilizing abrasive strips; usually done to alleviate crowding.

stro·bi·la (stro-bi´lah) pl. *strobi´lae.* [L.] the chain of proglottids constituting the bulk of the body of adult tapeworms.

stroke (strōk) 1. a sudden and severe attack. 2. stroke syndrome. 3. a pulsation. **completed s.,** stroke syndrome reflecting the infarction of the vascular territory that is put at risk by a stenosis or occlusion of a feeding vessel. **embolic s.,** stroke syndrome due to cerebral embolism. **s. in evolution,** a preliminary, unstable stage in stroke syndrome in which the blockage is present but the syndrome has not progressed to the stage of completed stroke. **heat s.,** a condition due to excessive exposure to heat, with dry skin, vertigo, headache, thirst, nausea, and muscular cramps; the body temperature may

be dangerously elevated. **thrombotic s.,** stroke syndrome due to cerebral thrombosis, most often superimposed on a plaque of atherosclerosis.

stro·ma (stro´mah) pl. *stro´mata.* [Gr.] the matrix or supporting tissue of an organ. **stro´mal, stromat´ic,** adj.

stro·muhr (strōm´oor) [Ger.] an instrument for measuring the velocity of blood flow.

Stron·gy·loi·des (stron″jĭ-loi´dēz) a genus of widely distributed nematodes parasitic in the intestine of humans and other mammals. *S. stercora´lis* is found in the tropics and subtropics and causes strongyloidiasis.

stron·gy·loi·di·a·sis (stron″jĭ-loi-di´ah-sis) infection with *Strongyloides stercoralis.* In the small intestine it causes mucosal ulceration and diarrhea. In the lungs it causes hemorrhaging.

stron·gy·loi·do·sis (-do´sis) strongyloidiasis.

stron·gy·lo·sis (stron″jĭ-lo´sis) infection with *Strongylus.*

Stron·gy·lus (stron´jĭ-lus) a genus of nematode parasites.

stron·ti·um (stron´she-um) chemical element (see *Table of Elements*), at. no. 38, symbol Sr. **s. 89,** a radioactive isotope of strontium having a half-life of 50.55 days and decaying by beta emission; used in the form of the chloride as a radiation source in palliation of bone pain caused by metastatic lesions.

stroph·u·lus (strof´u-lus) papular urticaria.

stru·ma (stroo´mah) [L.] goiter. **stru´mous,** adj. **Hashimoto's s., s. lymphomato´sa,** Hashimoto's disease. **s. malig´na,** carcinoma of the thyroid gland. **s. ova´rii,** a teratoid ovarian tumor composed of thyroid tissue. **Riedel's s.,** Riedel's thyroiditis.

stru·mec·to·my (stroo-mek´tah-me) excision of a goiter.

stru·mi·tis (stroo-mi´tis) thyroiditis.

strych·nine (strik´nīn) a very poisonous alkaloid, obtained chiefly from *Strychnos nux-vomica* and other species of *Strychnos,* which causes excitation of all portions of the central nervous system by blocking postsynaptic inhibition of neural impulses.

stump (stump) the distal end of a limb left after amputation.

stun (stun) to knock senseless; to render unconscious by a blow or other force.

stun·ning (stun´ing) loss of function, analogous to unconsciousness. **myocardial s.,** temporarily impaired myocardial function, resulting from a brief episode of ischemia and persisting for some period afterward.

stupe (stoop) a hot, wet cloth or sponge, charged with a medication for external application.

stu·pe·fa·cient (stoo″pĕ-fa′shent) 1. inducing stupor. 2. an agent that induces stupor.

stu·por (stoo′per) [L.] 1. a lowered level of consciousness. 2. in psychiatry, a disorder marked by reduced responsiveness. **stu′porous**, adj.

stut·ter·ing (stut′er-ing) a speech problem characterized chiefly by spasmodic repetition of sounds, especially of initial consonants, by prolongation of sounds and hesitation, and by anxiety and tension on the part of the speaker about perceived speech difficulties. Cf. *stammering*.

stye (sti) hordeolum.

sty·let (sti′lit) 1. a wire run through a catheter or cannula to render it stiff or to remove debris from its lumen. 2. a slender probe.

styl(o)- word element [L.], *stake; pole; styloid process of the temporal bone.*

sty·lo·hy·oid (sti″lo-hi′oid) pertaining to the styloid process and hyoid bone.

sty·loid (sti′loid) resembling a pillar; long and pointed; relating to the styloid process.

sty·loid·itis (sti″loi-di′tis) inflammation of tissues around the styloid process of the temporal bone.

sty·lo·mas·toid (sti″lo-mas′toid) pertaining to the styloid and mastoid processes of the temporal bone.

sty·lo·max·il·lary (-mak′sĭ-lar″e) pertaining to the styloid process of the temporal bone and the maxilla.

sty·lus (sti′lus) 1. stylet. 2. a pencil-shaped medicinal preparation, as of caustic.

styp·sis (stip′sis) [Gr.] the action or application of a styptic.

styp·tic (stip′tik) 1. contracting the tissues or blood vessels; used particularly to denote that arresting hemorrhage or resulting in hemostasis. 2. an agent that so acts.

sub- word element [L.], *under; near; almost; moderately.*

sub·ab·dom·i·nal (sub″ab-dom′ĭ-n′l) below the abdomen.

sub·acro·mi·al (-ah-kro′me-al) below the acromion.

sub·acute (-ah-kūt′) somewhat acute; between acute and chronic.

sub·al·i·men·ta·tion (sub-al″ĭ-men-ta′shun) hypoalimentation.

sub·aor·tic (sub″a-or′tik) below the aorta or the aortic valve.

sub·apo·neu·rot·ic (-ap″o-noŏ-rot′ik) below an aponeurosis.

sub·arach·noid (sub″ah-rak′noid) between the arachnoid and the pia mater.

sub·ar·cu·ate (sub-ahr′ku-āt) somewhat arched or bent.

sub·are·o·lar (sub″ah-re′o-ler) beneath the areola.

sub·as·trag·a·lar (-as-trag′ah-ler) below the astragalus.

sub·atom·ic (-ah-tom′ik) of or pertaining to the constituent parts of an atom.

sub·au·ral (sub-aw′ral) below the ear.

sub·au·ra·le (sub″aw-ra′le) the lowest point on the inferior border of the ear lobule when the subject is looking straight ahead.

sub·cal·lo·sal (-kah-lo′s′l) inferior to the corpus callosum.

sub·cap·su·lar (sub-kap′su-ler) below a capsule, especially the capsule of the cerebrum.

sub·car·ti·lag·i·nous (-kahr″tĭ-laj′ĭ-nus) 1. beneath a cartilage. 2. partly cartilaginous.

sub·chon·dral (-kon′dr′l) subcartilaginous (1).

sub·cho·ri·al (-kor′e-al) beneath the chorion or some part of the chorion.

sub·class (sub′klas) a taxonomic category subordinate to a class and superior to an order.

sub·cla·vi·an (sub-kla′ve-an) below the clavicle.

sub·cla·vic·u·lar (sub″klah-vik′u-ler) subclavian.

sub·clin·i·cal (sub-klin′ĭ-k′l) without clinical manifestations.

sub·clone (sub′klōn) 1. the progeny of a mutant cell arising in a clone. 2. each new DNA population produced by cleaving DNA from a clonal population into fragments and cloning them.

sub·con·junc·ti·val (sub″kon-jungk-ti′val) beneath the conjunctiva.

sub·con·scious (sub-kon′shus) 1. imperfectly or partially conscious. 2. formerly, the preconscious and unconscious considered together.

sub·con·scious·ness (-nes) the state of being partially conscious.

sub·cor·a·coid (-kor′ah-koid) situated under the coracoid process.

sub·cor·ne·al (-kor′ne-al) 1. beneath the cornea. 2. beneath the stratum corneum of the skin.

sub·cor·tex (-kor′teks) the brain substance underlying the cortex.

sub·cor·ti·cal (-kor′tĭ-k′l) beneath a cortex, such as the cerebral cortex.

sub·cos·tal (-kos′t′l) below a rib or ribs.

sub·cra·ni·al (-kra′ne-al) below the cranium.

sub·crep·i·tant (-krep′ĭ-tant) pertaining to a rale that is slightly more coarse than a crepitant rale.

sub·cul·ture (sub′kul-chur) a culture of bacteria derived from another culture.

sub·cu·ta·ne·ous (sub″ku-ta′ne-us) beneath the skin.

sub·cu·tic·u·lar (-ku-tik′u-ler) subepidermal.

sub·de·lir·i·um (-dĕ-lēr′e-um) mild delirium.

sub·del·toid (sub-del′toid) beneath the deltoid muscle.

sub·di·a·phrag·mat·ic (-di″ah-frag-mat′ik) subphrenic.

sub·duct (-dukt′) to draw down.

sub·du·ral (-door′al) between the dura mater and the arachnoid.

sub·en·do·car·di·al (sub″en-do-kahr′de-al) beneath the endocardium.

sub·en·do·car·di·um (-kahr′de-um) subendocardial layer.

sub·en·do·the·li·al (-the′le-al) beneath the endothelium.

sub·epi·car·di·al (sub″-ep-ĭ-kahr′de-al) situated below the epicardium.

sub·epi·car·di·um (-kahr′de-um) subepicardial layer.

sub·epi·der·mal (-der′mal) beneath the epidermis.

sub·epi·the·li·al (-the′le-al) beneath the epithelium.

sub·fam·i·ly (sub′fam-ĭ-le) a taxonomic division between a family and a tribe.

sub·fas·cial (sub-fash′ul) beneath a fascia.

sub·fer·til·i·ty (sub″fur-til′ĭ-te) hypofertility; diminished reproductive capacity. **subfer′tile,** adj.

sub·fron·tal (sub-frun′tal) situated or extending underneath the frontal lobe.

sub·ge·nus (sub′je-nus) a taxonomic category between a genus and a species.

sub·gin·gi·val (sub-jin′jĭ-v′l) beneath the gingiva.

sub·gle·noid (sub-gle′noid) beneath the glenoid fossa.

sub·glos·sal (-glos′al) sublingual.

sub·glot·tic (-glot′ik) inferior to the glottis.

sub·gron·da·tion (sub″gron-da′shun) [Fr.] a type of depressed skull fracture, with depression of one fragment of bone beneath another.

sub·he·pat·ic (-hĕ-pat′ik) below the liver.

sub·hy·oid (sub-hi′oid) below the hyoid bone.

su·bic·u·lum (sŭ-bik′u-lum) an underlying or supporting structure.

sub·il·i·ac (sub-il′e-ak) below the ilium.

sub·il·i·um (-il′e-um) the lowest portion of the ilium.

sub·in·vo·lu·tion (sub″in-vo-loo′shun) incomplete involution.

sub·ja·cent (sub-ja′sent) located beneath.

sub·ject¹ (sub-jekt′) to cause to undergo or submit to; to render subservient.

sub·ject² (sub′jekt) 1. a person or animal subjected to treatment, observation, or experiment. 2. a body for dissection.

sub·jec·tive (sub-jek′tiv) pertaining to or perceived only by the affected individual; not perceptible to the senses of another person.

sub·ju·gal (-joo′gal) below the zygomatic bone.

sub·la·tio (sub-la′she-o) [L.] a lifting up, or elevation. **s. re′tinae,** detachment of the retina.

sub·le·thal (-le′thal) insufficient to cause death.

sub·li·mate (sub′lĭ-māt) 1. a substance obtained by sublimation. 2. to accomplish sublimation.

sub·li·ma·tion (sub″lĭ-ma′shun) 1. the conversion of a solid directly into the gaseous state. 2. an unconscious defense mechanism by which consciously unacceptable instinctual drives are expressed in personally and socially acceptable channels.

sub·lime (sub-līm′) to volatilize a solid body by heat and then to collect it in a purified form as a solid or powder.

sub·lim·i·nal (-lim′ĭ-n′l) below the threshold of sensation or conscious awareness.

sub·lin·gual (-ling′gwal) hypoglossal; beneath the tongue.

sub·lin·gui·tis (sub″ling-gwi′tis) inflammation of the sublingual gland.

sub·lob·u·lar (sub-lob′u-lar) beneath a lobule.

sub·lux·a·tion (sub″luk-sa′shun) 1. incomplete or partial dislocation. 2. in chiropractic, any mechanical impediment to nerve function; originally, a vertebral displacement believed to impair nerve function.

sub·mam·ma·ry (sub-mam′ah-re) below the mammary gland.

sub·man·dib·u·lar (sub″man-dib′u-ler) below the mandible.

sub·max·il·lar·i·tis (sub-mak″sĭ-ler-i′tis) inflammation of the submaxillary gland.

sub·max·il·lary (-mak′sĭ-lar″e) below the maxilla.

sub·men·tal (-men′t′l) beneath the chin.

sub·meta·cen·tric (-met″ah-sen′trik) having the centromere almost, but not quite, at the metacentric position.

sub·mi·cro·scop·ic (-mi″kro-skop′ik) too small to be visible with the light microscope.

sub·mor·phous (-mor′fus) neither amorphous nor perfectly crystalline.

sub·mu·co·sa (sub″mu-ko′sah) areolar tissue situated beneath a mucous membrane.

sub·mu·co·sal (-mu-ko′sal) 1. pertaining to the submucosa. 2. beneath a mucous membrane.

sub·mu·cous (sub-mu′kus) beneath a mucous membrane.

sub·nar·cot·ic (sub″nahr-kot′ik) moderately narcotic.

sub·na·sal (sub-na′z′l) inferior to the nose.

sub·na·sa·le (sub″na-sa′le) the point at which the nasal septum merges, in the midsagittal plane, with the upper lip.

sub·neu·ral (sub-noor′al) beneath a nerve.

sub·nor·mal (-nor′m′l) below normal.

sub·nu·cle·us (-noo′kle-us) a partial or secondary nucleus.

sub·oc·cip·i·tal (sub″ok-sip′ĭ-t′l) below the occiput.

sub·or·bi·tal (sub-or′bĭ-t′l) infraorbital.

sub·or·der (sub′or-der) a taxonomic category between an order and a family.

sub·pap·u·lar (sub-pap′u-ler) indistinctly papular.

sub·pa·tel·lar (sub″pah-tel′er) infrapatellar.

sub·peri·car·di·al (-per-ĭ-kahr′de-al) beneath the pericardium.

sub·peri·os·te·al (-per-e-os′te-al) beneath the periosteum.

sub·peri·to·ne·al (-per-ĭ-to-ne′al) beneath or deep to the peritoneum.

sub·pha·ryn·ge·al (-fah-rin′je-al) beneath the pharynx.

sub·phren·ic (sub-fren′ik) beneath the diaphragm.

sub·phy·lum (sub′fi-lum) pl. *subphy′la.* A taxonomic category between a phylum and a class.

sub·pla·cen·ta (sub″plah-sen′tah) decidua basalis.

sub·pleu·ral (sub-ploor′al) beneath the pleura.

sub·pre·pu·tial (sub″pre-pu′shal) beneath the prepuce.

sub·pu·bic (sub-pu′bik) beneath the pubic bone.

sub·pul·mo·nary (-pool′mo-nar″e) beneath the lung.

sub·ret·i·nal (-ret′ĭ-n′l) beneath the retina.

sub·scap·u·lar (-skap′u-ler) below the scapula.

sub·scrip·tion (-skrip′shun) that part of a prescription giving directions for compounding the ingredients.

sub·se·ro·sa (sub″sēr-o′sah) a layer of tissue beneath a serous membrane.

sub·se·ro·sal (-sēr-o′s′l) 1. pertaining to the subserosa. 2. subserous.

sub·se·rous (sub-sēr′us) beneath a serous membrane.

sub·spe·cies (sub′spe-sēz) a taxonomic category subordinate to a species, differing morphologically from others of the species but capable of interbreeding with them; a variety or race.

sub·spi·na·le (sub″spi-na′le) point A.

sub·spi·nous (sub-spi′nus) inferior to a spinous process.

sub·stance (sub′stans) 1. matter with a particular set of characteristics. 2. material constituting an organ or body. 3. psychoactive s. **black s.,** substantia nigra. **controlled s.,** any drug regulated under the Controlled Substances Act. **gelatinous s.,** substantia gelatinosa. **gray s.,** substantia grisea. **ground s.,** the gel-like material in which connective tissue cells and fibers are embedded. **H s.,** H antigen (2). **medullary s.,** 1. substantia alba. 2. the soft marrowlike substance of the interior of an organ. **s. P,** an 11–amino acid peptide, present in nerve cells scattered throughout the body and in special endocrine cells in the gut. It increases the contraction of gastrointestinal smooth muscle and causes vasodilatation; it also seems to be a sensory neurotransmitter. **perforated s.,** 1. *anterior perforated s.,* an area anterolateral to each optic tract, pierced by branches of the anterior and middle cerebral arteries. 2. *posterior perforated s.,* an area between the cerebral peduncles, pierced by branches of the posterior cerebral arteries. **psychoactive s.,** any chemical compound that affects the mind or mental processes; used particularly for drugs used therapeutically in psychiatry, the major classes being the antipsychotic, antidepressant, anxiolytic-sedative, and mood-stabilizing drugs. **reticular s.,** 1. see under *formation.* 2. the netlike mass seen in red blood cells after vital staining. **Rolando's gelatinous s.,** substantia gelatinosa. **slow-reacting s. of anaphylaxis (SRS-A),** an inflammatory agent released by mast cells in the anaphylactic reaction, inducing a slow, prolonged contraction of certain smooth muscles and acting as an important mediator of allergic bronchial asthma. **transmitter s.,** neurotransmitter. **white s.,** substantia alba.

sub·stan·tia (sub-stan′shah) pl. *substan′tiae.* [L.] substance. **s. al′ba,** the white nervous tissue, constituting the conducting portion of the brain and spinal cord, composed mostly of myelinated nerve fibers. **s. ferrugi′nea,** locus caeruleus. **s. gelatino′sa,** the gelatinous-appearing cap forming the dorsal part of the posterior horn of the spinal cord. **s. gri′sea,** gray substance; the gray nervous tissue composed of nerve cell bodies, unmyelinated nerve fibers, and supportive tissue. **s. ni′gra,** the layer of gray substance separating the tegmentum of the midbrain from the crus cerebri. **s. pro′pria,** 1. the tough, fibrous, transparent main part of the cornea, between Bowman's membrane and Descemet's membrane. 2. the main part of the sclera, between the episcleral lamina and the lamina fusca.

sub·ster·nal (sub-ster′n′l) below the sternum.

sub·stit·u·ent (-stich′u-ent) 1. a substitute; especially an atom, radical, or group substituted for another in a compound. 2. of or pertaining to such an atom, radical, or group.

sub·sti·tu·tion (sub″stĭ-too′shun) 1. the act of putting one thing in place of another, especially the chemical replacement of one atom or radical by another. 2. a defense mechanism, operating unconsciously, in which an unattainable or unacceptable goal, emotion, or object is replaced by one that is attainable or acceptable.

sub·strate (sub′strāt) 1. a substance upon which an enzyme acts. 2. a neutral substance containing a nutrient solution. 3. a surface upon which a different material is deposited or adhered, usually in a coating or layer.

sub·struc·ture (-struk-chur) the underlying or supporting portion of an organ or appliance; that portion of an implant denture embedded in the tissues of the jaw.

sub·syl·vi·an (sub-sil′ve-an) situated deep in the lateral sulcus (sylvian fissure).

sub·tar·sal (-tahr′sal) below the tarsus.

sub·ten·to·ri·al (sub″ten-to′re-al) beneath the tentorium of the cerebellum.

sub·tha·lam·ic (-thah-lam′ik) 1. inferior to the thalamus. 2. pertaining to the subthalamus.

sub·thal·a·mus (sub-thal′ah-mus) the ventral thalamus or subthalamic tegmental region: a transitional region of the diencephalon interposed between the (dorsal) thalamus, the hypothalamus, and the tegmentum of the mesencephalon (midbrain); it includes the subthalamic nucleus, Forel's fields, and the zona incerta. **subthalam′ic,** adj.

sub·to·tal (sub-to′t′l) less than, but often almost, complete.

sub·tribe (sub′trīb) a taxonomic category between a tribe and a genus.

sub·tro·chan·ter·ic (sub″tro-kan-ter′ik) below the trochanter.

sub·um·bil·i·cal (-um-bil′ĭ-k′l) inferior to the umbilicus.

sub·un·gual (sub-ung′gwal) beneath a nail.

sub·ure·thral (sub″u-re′thral) inferior to the urethra.

sub·vag·i·nal (sub-vaj′ĭ-n′l) under a sheath, or below the vagina.

sub·ver·te·bral (-ver′tĕ-bral) on the ventral side of the vertebrae.

sub·vo·lu·tion (sub″vo-loo′shun) the operation of turning over a flap to prevent adhesions.

suc·cen·tu·ri·ate (suk″sen-tu′re-āt) accessory; serving as a substitute.

suc·ces·sion·al (suk-sesh′un′l) pertaining to that which follows in order or sequence.

suc·ci·mer (suk′sĭ-mer) a heavy metal–chelating agent that is an analogue of dimercaprol, used in the treatment of lead poisoning; also complexed with technetium Tc 99m and used in renal function testing.

suc·ci·nate (suk′sĭ-nāt) any salt or ester of succinic acid. **s. semialdehyde,** γ-hydroxybutyric acid.

suc·ci·nate-semi·al·de·hyde de·hy·dro·gen·ase (sem″e-al′dĕ-hīd de-hi′dro-jen-ās″) an oxidoreductase catalyzing the final step in γ-aminobutyric acid (GABA) inactivation; deficiency (succinic semialdehyde dehydrogenase deficiency) causes increased levels of GABA and γ-hydroxybutyric acid in urine, plasma, and cerebrospinal fluid, mental retardation, hypotonia, and ataxia.

suc·cin·ic ac·id (suk-sin′ik) an intermediate in the tricarboxylic acid cycle.

suc·cin·i·mide (suk-sin′ĭ-mīd) 1. an organic compound comprising a pyrrole ring with two carbonyl substitutions. 2. any of a class of anticonvulsants with such a basic structure.

suc·ci·nyl·cho·line (suk″sĭ-nil-ko′lēn) a depolarizing neuromuscular blocking agent used as the chloride salt as an anesthesia adjunct and in convulsive therapy.

suc·ci·nyl CoA (suk′sĭ-nil ko-a′) a high-energy intermediate formed in the tricarboxylic acid cycle from α-ketoglutaric acid; it is also a precursor in the synthesis of porphyrins.

suc·cor·rhea (suk″o-re′ah) excessive flow of a natural secretion.

suc·cus·sion (sŭ-kush′un) 1. the shaking of the body during an examination, a splashing sound indicating the presence of fluid and air in a body cavity. 2. the vigorous shaking of a diluted homeopathic preparation in order to activate the medicinal substance.

su·cral·fate (soo-kral′fāt) a complex of aluminum and a sulfated polysaccharide, used as a gastrointestinal antiulcerative.

su·crase (soo′krās) a hydrolase that catalyzes the cleavage of the disaccharides sucrose and maltose to their component monosaccharides; it occurs complexed with α-dextrinase in the brush border of the intestinal mucosa and deficiency of the complex causes the disaccharide intolerance sucrase-isomaltase deficiency.

suc·rase-iso·mal·tase de·fi·cien·cy (-i-so-mawl'tās) a disaccharidase deficiency in which deficiency of the sucrase-isomaltase enzyme complex causes malabsorption of sucrose and starch dextrins, with watery, osmotic-fermentative diarrhea, sometimes leading to dehydration and malnutrition, manifest in infancy (congenital sucrose intolerance).

su·crose (soo'krōs) a disaccharide of glucose and fructose from sugar cane, sugar beet, or other sources; used as a food and sweetening agent and pharmaceutical aid.

su·cros·uria (soo″kro-su're-ah) excessive sucrose in the urine.

suc·tion (suk'shun) aspiration of gas or fluid by mechanical means. **post-tussive s.,** a sucking sound heard over a lung cavity just after a cough.

suc·to·ri·al (suk-tor'e-al) adapted for sucking.

su·da·men (soo-da'men) pl. *suda'mina.* [L.] a whitish vesicle caused by retention of sweat in the stratum corneum of the skin.

Su·dan (soo-dan') a group of azo compounds used as biological stains for fats. **S. black B,** a black, fat-soluble diazo dye, used as a stain for fats.

su·dano·phil·ia (soo-dan″o-fil'e-ah) affinity for Sudan stain. **sudanophil'ic,** adj.

su·do·mo·tor (soo″do-mo'ter) stimulating the sweat glands.

su·do·re·sis (soo″do-re'sis) diaphoresis.

su·do·rif·er·ous (soo″do-rif'er-us) 1. conveying sweat. 2. sudoriparous.

su·do·rif·ic (soo″do-rif'ik) diaphoretic.

su·do·rip·a·rous (soo″do-rip'ah-rus) secreting or producing sweat.

su·et (soo'et) the fat from the abdominal cavity of ruminants, especially the sheep, used in preparing cerates and ointments and as an emollient.

su·fen·ta·nil (soo-fen'tah-nil) an opioid analgesic derived from fentanyl, used as the citrate salt as an anesthetic or anesthesia adjunct; also used for the treatment of obstetric pain.

suf·fo·ca·tion (suf″ah-ka'shun) 1. asphyxiation. 2. the asphyxia that results from stoppage of respiration. **suf'focative,** adj.

suf·fu·sion (sŭ-fu'zhun) 1. the process of overspreading, or diffusion. 2. the condition of being moistened or of being permeated through, as by blood.

sug·ar (shoog'er) any of a class of sweet water-soluble carbohydrates, the monosaccharides and smaller oligosaccharides; often specifically sucrose. **blood s.,** glucose occurring in the blood, or the amount of glucose in the blood. **invert s.,** a mixture of equal amounts of dextrose and fructose, obtained by hydrolyzing sucrose; used in solution as a parenteral nutrient.

sug·ges·tion (sug-jes'chun) 1. the act of offering an idea for action or for consideration of action. 2. an idea so offered. 3. in psychiatry, the process of causing uncritical acceptance of an idea. **hypnotic s.,** one imparted to a person in the hypnotic state, by which he is induced to alter perceptions or memory or to perform actions. **post-hypnotic s.,** implantation in the mind of a subject during hypnosis of a suggestion to be acted upon after recovery from the hypnotic state.

sug·gil·la·tion (sug″jĭ-la'shun) 1. ecchymosis. 2. contusion.

su·i·cide (soo'ĭ-sīd) the taking of one's own life.

su·i·ci·dol·o·gy (soo″ĭ-sīd-ol'ŏ-je) the study of the causes and prevention of suicide.

sul·bac·tam (sul-bak'tam) a β-lactamase inhibitor used as the sodium salt to increase the antibacterial activity of penicillins and cephalosporins against β-lactamase–producing organisms.

sul·cate (sul'kāt) furrowed; marked with sulci.

sul·con·a·zole (sul-kon'ah-zōl) a broad-spectrum imidazole antifungal, used as the nitrate salt in the treatment of various forms of tinea and cutaneous candidiasis.

sul·cus (sul'kus) pl. *sul'ci.* [L.] a groove, trench, or furrow; in anatomy, a general term for such a depression, especially one on the brain surface, separating the gyri. **arterial sulci,** grooves on the internal surfaces of the cranial bones for the meningeal arteries. **calcarine s.,** a sulcus of the medial surface of the occipital lobe, separating the cuneus from the lingual gyrus. **central cerebral s.,** one between the frontal and parietal lobes of the cerebral hemisphere. **cerebral sulci,** the furrows between the cerebral gyri. **cerebral s., lateral,** fissure of Sylvius. **cingulate s.,** one on the median surface of the hemisphere midway between the corpus callosum and the margin of the surface. **collateral s.,** one on the inferior surface of the cerebral hemisphere between the fusiform and parahippocampal gyri. **sul'ci cu'tis,** the fine depressions on the surface of the skin between the dermal ridges. **gingival s.,** the groove between the surface of the tooth and the epithelium lining the free gingiva. **hippocampal s.,** one extending from the splenium of the corpus callosum almost to the tip of the temporal lobe. **interlobar sulci,** the sulci that separate the lobes of the brain from each other. **intraparietal s.,** one separating the parietal gyri. **s. of matrix of nail,** the skin fold in which the proximal part of the nail is embedded. **parietooccipital s.,** one marking the boundary between the cuneus and precuneus, and also between the parietal and occipital lobes of the cerebral hemisphere. **posterior median s.,** 1. a shallow vertical groove in the closed part of the medulla oblongata, continuous with the posterior median sulcus of the spinal cord. 2. a shallow vertical groove dividing the spinal cord throughout its whole length in the midline posteriorly. **precentral s.,** one separating the precentral gyrus from the remainder of the frontal lobe. **scleral s.,** a slight groove at the junction of the sclera and cornea. **venous sulci,** grooves on the internal surfaces of the cranial bones for the meningeal veins.

sul·fa·cet·a·mide (sul″fah-set′ah-mīd) a sulfonamide used topically as the sodium salt to treat ophthalmic infections and acne vulgaris.

sul·fa·di·a·zine (-di′ah-zēn) a sulfonamide antibacterial, used as the base or the sodium salt in the treatment of infections including nocardiosis, toxoplasmosis, otitis media, and chloroquine-resistant falciparum malaria. See also under *silver.*

sul·fa·dox·ine (-dok′sēn) a long-acting sulfonamide used in combination with pyrimethamine in the prophylaxis and treatment of chloroquine-resistant falciparum malaria.

sul·fa·meth·i·zole (-meth′ĭ-zōl) a sulfonamide used in urinary tract infections.

sul·fa·meth·ox·a·zole (-meth-ok′sah-zōl) a sulfonamide antibacterial and antiprotozoal, particularly used in acute urinary tract infections.

sul·fa·pyr·i·dine (-pir′ĭ-dēn) a sulfonamide used as an oral suppressant for dermatitis herpetiformis.

sul·fa·sal·a·zine (-sal′ah-zēn) a sulfonamide used in the treatment and prophylaxis of inflammatory bowel disease and the treatment of rheumatoid arthritis.

sul·fa·tase (sul′fah-tās) an enzyme that catalyzes the hydrolytic cleavage of inorganic sulfate from sulfate esters.

sul·fate (sul′fāt) a salt of sulfuric acid.

sul·fa·tide (sul′fah-tīd) any of a class of cerebroside sulfuric esters; they are found largely in the medullated nerve fibers and may accumulate in metachromatic leukodystrophy.

sulf·he·mo·glo·bin (sulf″he′mo-glo″bin) sulfmethemoglobin.

sulf·he·mo·glo·bin·emia (-he″mo-glo″bin-e′me-ah) sulfmethemoglobin in the blood.

sulf·hy·dryl (sulf-hi′dril) the univalent radical, —SH.

sul·fide (sul′fīd) any binary compound of sulfur; a compound of sulfur with another element or radical or base.

sul·fin·py·ra·zone (sul″fin-pi′rah-zōn) a uricosuric agent used in the treatment of gout.

sul·fi·sox·a·zole (sul″fĭ-sok′sah-zōl) a short-acting sulfonamide antibacterial, used particularly as the base or *s. acetyl* for infections of the urinary tract and as *s. diolamine* as a topical ophthalmic antibacterial.

sul·fite (sul′fīt) any salt of sulfurous acid.

sul·fite ox·i·dase (ok′sĭ-dās) an oxidoreductase that catalyzes the oxidation of sulfite to sulfate as well as the detoxification of sulfite and sulfur dioxide from exogenous sources. It is a mitochondrial hemoprotein containing molybdenum; deficiency results in progressive neurologic abnormalities, lens dislocation, and mental retardation.

sulf·met·he·mo·glo·bin (sulf″met-he′mo-glo″bin) a greenish substance formed by treating the blood with hydrogen sulfide or by absorption of this gas from the intestinal tract.

sul·fon·amide (sul-fon′ah-mīd) a compound containing the —SO₂NH₂ group. The sulfonamides, or sulfa drugs, are derivatives of sulfanilamide, competitively inhibit folic acid synthesis in microorganisms, and formerly were bacteriostatic against a wide variety of bacteria and some protozoa. Because many microbes are now resistant, sulfonamides have largely been supplanted by more effective and less toxic antibiotics.

sul·fone (sul′fōn) 1. the radical SO₂. 2. a compound containing two hydrocarbon radicals attached to the —SO₂— group, especially dapsone and its derivatives, which are potent antibacterials effective against many gram-positive and gram-negative organisms and are widely used as leprostatics.

sul·fo·nyl·urea (sul″fo-nil-u-re′ah) any of a class of compounds that exert hypoglycemic activity by stimulating the islet tissue to secrete insulin, used to control hyperglycemia in patients with type 2 diabetes mellitus who cannot be treated solely by diet and exercise.

sul·fur (sul′fer) [L.] chemical element (see *Table of Elements*), at. no. 16, symbol S; it is a laxative and diaphoretic and is used in diseases of the skin. **s. dioxide,** a colorless, nonflammable gas used as a pharmaceutical antioxidant; also an important air pollutant, irritating the eyes and respiratory tract. **precipitated s.,** a topical scabicide, antiparasitic, antibacterial, antifungal, and keratolytic. **sublimed s.,** a topical scabicide and antiparasitic.

sul·fu·rat·ed, sul·fu·ret·ed (sul′fu-rāt″ed) combined with or charged with sulfur.

sul·fur·ic ac·id (sul-fūr′ik) an oily, highly caustic, poisonous acid, H_2SO_4, widely used in chemistry, industry, and the arts.

sul·fur·ous ac·id (sul′fūr-us) 1. a solution of sulfur dioxide in water, H_2SO_3; used as a reagent. 2. sulfur dioxide.

sul·in·dac (sul-in′dak) 1. a nonsteroidal antiinflammatory drug, analgesic, and antipyretic, used in treatment of rheumatic disorders. 2. a nonsteroidal antiinflammatory drug used in the treatment of various rheumatic and nonrheumatic inflammatory disorders.

sulph- for words beginning thus, see those beginning *sulf-*.

su·mac (soo′mak) name of various trees and shrubs of the genus *Rhus*. **poison s.,** a species, *Rhus vernix*, which causes an itching rash on contact with the skin.

su·ma·trip·tan (soo″mah-trip′tan) a selective serotonin receptor agonist used as the succinate salt in the acute treatment of migraine and cluster headaches.

sum·ma·tion (sŭ-ma′shun) the cumulative effect of a number of stimuli applied to a muscle, nerve, or reflex arc.

sun·burn (sun′bern) injury to the skin, with erythema, tenderness, and sometimes blistering, after excessive exposure to sunlight, produced by unfiltered ultraviolet rays.

sun·screen (-skrēn) a substance applied to the skin to protect it from the effects of the sun's rays.

sun·stroke (-strōk) a condition caused by excessive exposure to the sun, marked by high skin temperature, convulsions, and coma.

super- word element [L.], *above; excessive.*

su·per·al·i·men·ta·tion (soo″per-al″ĭ-men-ta′shun) treatment of wasting diseases by feeding beyond appetite requirements.

su·per·al·ka·lin·i·ty (-al″kah-lin′ĭ-te) excessive alkalinity.

su·per·an·ti·gen (-an′tĭ-jen) any of a group of powerful antigens occurring in various bacteria and viruses that binds outside of the normal T cell receptor site, reacting with multiple T cell receptor molecules and activating T cells nonspecifically.

su·per·cil·ia (-sil′e-ah) [pl., L.] the hairs on the arching protrusion over either eye.

su·per·cil·i·um (-sil′e-um) pl. *supercil′lia.* [L.] eyebrow; the transverse elevation at the junction of the forehead and upper eyelid. **supercil′iary,** adj.

su·per·class (soo′per-klas″) a taxonomic category between a phylum and a class.

su·per·ego (soo″per-e′go) in psychoanalysis, the aspect of the personality that acts as a monitor and evaluator of ego functioning, comparing it with an ideal standard.

su·per·fam·i·ly (soo′per-fam″ĭ-le) 1. a taxonomic category between an order and a family. 2. any of a group of proteins having similarities such as areas of structural homology and believed to descend from the same ancestral gene.

su·per·fe·cun·da·tion (soo″per-fe″kun-da′shun) fertilization of two or more oocytes during the same ovulatory cycle by separate coital acts.

su·per·fi·cial (-fish′al) pertaining to or situated near the surface.

su·per·fi·ci·a·lis (-fish″e-a′lis) [L.] superficial.

su·per·fi·ci·es (-fish′e-ēz) [L.] an outer surface.

su·per·in·duce (-in-doos′) to bring on in addition to an already existing condition.

su·per·in·fec·tion (-in-fek′shun) a new infection occurring in a patient having a preexisting infection, such as bacterial superinfection in viral respiratory disease or infection of a chronic hepatitis B carrier with hepatitis D virus.

su·per·in·vo·lu·tion (-in″vo-loo′shun) prolonged involution of the uterus, after delivery, to a size much smaller than the normal, occurring in nursing mothers.

su·pe·ri·or (soo-pēr′e-or) situated above, or directed upward.

su·per·ja·cent (soo″per-ja′sent) located just above.

su·per·lac·ta·tion (-lak-ta′shun) hyperlactation.

su·per·mo·til·i·ty (-mo-til′ĭ-te) excess of motility.

su·per·na·tant (-na′tant) the liquid lying above a layer of precipitated insoluble material.

su·per·nu·mer·ary (-noo′mer-ar″e) in excess of the regular or normal number.

su·per·nu·tri·tion (-noo-trish′un) excessive nutrition.

su·pero·lat·er·al (-o-lat′er-al) above and to the side.

10

su·per·ov·u·la·tion (ov″u-la′shun) extraordinary acceleration of ovulation, producing a greater than normal number of oocytes.

su·per·ox·ide (-ok′sīd) any compound containing the highly reactive and extremely toxic oxygen radical O_2^-, a common intermediate in numerous biological oxidations.

su·per·sat·u·rate (-sach′er-āt) to add more of an ingredient than can be held in solution permanently.

su·per·scrip·tion (-skrip′shun) the heading of a prescription, i.e., the symbol ℞ or the word Recipe, meaning "take."

su·per·struc·ture (soo′per-struk″chur) the overlying or visible portion of a structure.

su·per·vas·cu·lar·iza·tion (soo″per-vas″kular-ĭ-za′shun) in radiotherapy, the relative increase in vascularity that occurs when tumor cells are destroyed so that the remaining tumor cells are better supplied by the (uninjured) capillary stroma.

su·per·vol·tage (soo′per-vol″tij) in radiotherapy, voltage between 500 kilovolts and 1 megavolt, in contrast to orthovoltage and megavoltage.

su·pi·nate (soo′pĭ-nāt) to assume or place in a supine position.

su·pi·na·tion (soo″pĭ-na′shun) [L. *supinatio*] the act of assuming the supine position, or the state of being supine. Applied to the hand, the act of turning the palm forward (anteriorly) or upward, performed by lateral rotation of the forearm. Applied to the foot, it generally implies movements resulting in raising of the medial margin of the foot, hence of the longitudinal arch.

su·pine (soo′pīn) lying with the face upward, or on the dorsal surface.

sup·port (sŭ-port′) 1. to prevent weakening or failing. 2. a structure that bears the weight of something else. 3. a mechanism or arrangement that helps keep something else functioning. **suppor′tive**, adj.

sup·pos·i·to·ry (sŭ-poz′ĭ-tor″e) an easily fusible medicated mass to be introduced into a body orifice, as the rectum, urethra, or vagina.

sup·pres·sant (sŭ-pres′ant) 1. inducing suppression. 2. an agent that stops secretion, excretion, or normal discharge.

sup·pres·sion (sŭ-presh′un) 1. the act of holding back or checking. 2. sudden stoppage of a secretion, excretion, or normal discharge. 3. in psychiatry, conscious inhibition of an unacceptable impulse or idea as contrasted with repression, which is unconscious. 4. in genetics, masking of the phenotypic expression of a mutation by the occurrence of a second (suppressor) mutation at a different site from the first; the organism appears to be reverted but is in fact doubly mutated. 5. inhibition of the erythrocytic stage of *plasmodium* as prophylaxis for clinical attacks of malaria. 6. cortical inhibition of perception of objects in all or part of the visual field of one eye during binocular vision. **bone marrow s.**, suppression of bone marrow activity, resulting in reduction in the number of platelets, red cells, and white cells. **overdrive s.**, transient suppression of automaticity in a cardiac pacemaker following a period of stimulation by a more rapidly discharging pacemaker.

sup·pu·rant (sup′u-rant) 1. suppurative. 2. an agent that causes suppuration.

sup·pu·ra·tion (sup″u-ra′shun) pyogenesis. **sup′purative**, adj.

supra- word element [L.], *above; over*.

su·pra·acro·mi·al (soo″prah-ah-kro′me-al) above the acromion.

su·pra·au·ric·u·lar (-aw-rik′u-ler) above the auricle of the ear.

su·pra·bulge (soo′prah-bulj″) the surface of the crown of a tooth sloping toward the occlusal surface from the height of contour.

su·pra·cer·e·bel·lar (soo″prah-ser-ĕ-bel′ar) superior to the cerebellum.

su·pra·cho·roid (-kor′oid) above or upon the choroid.

su·pra·cho·roi·dea (-ko-roi′de-ah) the outermost layer of the choroid.

su·pra·cla·vic·u·lar (-klah-vik′u-ler) above the clavicle.

su·pra·clu·sion (-kloo′zhun) projection of a tooth beyond the normal occlusal plane.

su·pra·con·dy·lar (-kon′dĭ-ler) above a condyle.

su·pra·cos·tal (-kos′t'l) above or upon the ribs.

su·pra·cot·y·loid (-kot′ĭ-loid) above the acetabulum.

su·pra·di·a·phrag·mat·ic (-di″ah-fragmat′ik) above the diaphragm.

su·pra·duc·tion (-duk′shun) upward rotation of an eye around its horizontal axis.

su·pra·epi·con·dy·lar (-ep″ĭ-kon′dĭ-ler) above an epicondyle.

su·pra·gin·gi·val (-jin′jĭ-v'l) superior to the gingiva or to the gingival margin.

su·pra·gle·noid (soo″prah-gle′noid) superior to the glenoid cavity.

su·pra·glot·tis (-glot′is) the area of the pharynx above the glottis as far as the epiglottis.

su·pra·glot·ti·tis (soo″prah-glŏ-ti′tis) inflammation of the supraglottis, which can lead to life-threatening upper airway obstruction.

su·pra·hy·oid (-hi′oid) above the hyoid bone.

su·pra·lim·i·nal (-lim′ĭ-n′l) above the threshold of sensation.

su·pra·lum·bar (-lum′bahr) above the loin.

su·pra·mal·le·o·lar (-mah-le′o-ler) above a malleolus.

su·pra·mar·gi·nal (-mahr′jĭ-n′l) superior to a margin or border.

su·pra·mas·toid (-mas′toid) superior to the mastoid process.

su·pra·max·il·lary (-mak′sĭ-lar″e) above the maxilla.

su·pra·me·a·tal (-me-a′t′l) above a meatus.

su·pra·men·ta·le (-men-ta′le) point B.

su·pra·oc·clu·sion (-ŏ-kloo′zhun) supraclusion.

su·pra·op·tic (-op′tik) superior to the optic chiasm.

su·pra·or·bi·tal (-or′bĭ-t′l) above the orbit.

su·pra·pel·vic (-pel′vik) above the pelvis.

su·pra·phar·ma·co·log·ic (-fahr″mah-ko-loj′ik) much greater than the usual therapeutic dose or pharmacologic concentration of a drug.

su·pra·pon·tine (-pon′tīn) above or in the upper part of the pons.

su·pra·pu·bic (-pu′bik) superior to the pubic arch.

su·pra·re·nal (-re′nal) 1. above a kidney. 2. adrenal.

su·pra·scap·u·lar (-skap′u-ler) above the scapula.

su·pra·scle·ral (-skler′al) on the outer surface of the sclera.

su·pra·sel·lar (-sel′er) above the sella turcica.

su·pra·spi·nal (-spi′n′l) above the spine.

su·pra·spi·nous (-spi′nus) 1. supraspinal. 2. superior to a spinous process.

su·pra·ster·nal (-ster′n′l) above the sternum.

su·pra·troch·le·ar (-trok′le-ar) situated above a trochlea.

su·pra·vag·i·nal (-vaj′ĭ-n′l) outside or above a sheath; specifically, above the vagina.

su·pra·val·var (-val′ver) situated above a valve, particularly the aortic or pulmonary valve.

su·pra·ven·tric·u·lar (-ven-trik′u-ler) situated or occurring above the ventricles, especially in an atrium or atrioventricular node.

su·pra·ver·gence (-ver′jens) disjunctive reciprocal movement of the eyes in which one eye rotates upward while the other one stays still.

su·pra·ver·sion (-ver′zhun) 1. abnormal elongation of a tooth from its socket. 2. sursumversion.

su·pra·vi·tal (-vi′t′l) beyond living, as in supravital staining.

su·pra·zy·go·mat·ic (-zi″go-mat′ik) situated above the zygomatic bone.

su·preme (soo-prēm′) ultimate, greatest; highest; used in anatomy for the one in a group having the most superior location.

su·pro·fen (soo-pro′fen) a nonsteroidal antiinflammatory drug applied topically to the conjunctiva to inhibit miosis during ophthalmic surgery.

su·ra (soo′rah) [L.] calf. **su′ral,** adj.

sur·face (ser′fas) facies.

sur·fac·tant (ser-fak′tant) 1. surface-active agent. 2. in pulmonary physiology, a mixture of phospholipids that reduces the surface tension of pulmonary fluids and thus contributes to the elastic properties of pulmonary tissue.

sur·geon (ser′jun) 1. a physician who specializes in surgery. 2. the senior medical officer of a military unit.

sur·gery (ser′jer-e) 1. the branch of medicine that treats diseases, injuries, and deformities by manual or operative methods. 2. the place in a hospital, or doctor's or dentist's office, where surgery is performed. 3. in Great Britain, a room or office where a doctor sees and treats patients. 4. the work performed by a surgeon. **antiseptic s.,** surgery using antiseptic methods. **aseptic s.,** that performed in an environment so free from microorganisms that significant infection or suppuration does not supervene. **bench s.,** surgery performed on an organ that has been removed from the body, after which it is reimplanted. **conservative s.,** surgery designed to preserve, or to remove with minimal risk, diseased or injured organs, tissues, or limbs. **cytoreductive s.,** debulking. **dental s.,** oral and maxillofacial s. **general s.,** that which deals with surgical problems of all kinds, rather than those in a restricted area, as in a surgical specialty such as neurosurgery. **major s.,** surgery involving the more important, difficult, and hazardous operations. **minimally invasive s.,** surgery done with only a small incision or no incision at all, such as through a cannula with a laparoscope or endoscope. **minor s.,** surgery restricted to management of minor problems and injuries. **Mohs' s.,** see under *technique.* **oral and maxillofacial s.,** the branch of dentistry that deals with the diagnosis and surgical and adjunct treatment of diseases and defects of the mouth and dental structures. **plastic s.,** surgery concerned with restoration, reconstruction, correction, or improvement in shape and appearance of body structures that are defective, damaged, or misshapen by injury, disease, or growth and development. **radical s.,** surgery designed to extirpate all areas of locally extensive disease and adjacent zones of lymphatic drainage. **stereotactic s., stereotaxic s.,** any of several techniques for the production of sharply circumscribed lesions in specific tiny areas of pathologic tissue in deep-seated brain structures after locating the discrete structure by means of three-dimensional coordinates.

sur·gi·cal (ser′jĭ-k′l) of, pertaining to, or correctable by surgery.

Sur·gi·cel (ser′jĭ-sel) trademark for an absorbable knitted fabric prepared by controlled oxidation of cellulose, used to control intraoperative hemorrhage when other conventional methods are impractical or ineffective.

sur·ro·gate (sur′o-git) a substitute; a thing or person that takes the place of something or someone else, as a drug used in place of another, or a person who takes the place of another in someone's affective existence.

sur·sum·duc·tion (sur″sum-duk′shun) supraduction.

sur·sum·ver·gence (-ver′jens) supravergence.

sur·sum·ver·sion (-ver′zhun) the simultaneous and equal upward turning of the eyes.

sus·cep·ti·ble (sŭ-sep′tĭ-b′l) 1. readily affected or acted upon. 2. lacking immunity or resistance and thus at risk of infection.

sus·pen·sion (sus-pen′shun) 1. a condition of temporary cessation, as of animation, of pain, or of any vital process. 2. attachment of an organ or other body part to a supporting structure, as of the uterus or bladder in the correction of a hernia or prolapse. 3. a liquid preparation consisting of solid particles dispersed throughout a liquid phase in which they are not soluble. **bladder neck s.,** any of various methods of surgical fixation of the urethrovesical junction area and bladder neck to restore the neck to a high retropubic position for relief of stress incontinence. **colloid s.,** a colloid system; see *colloid* (2). Sometimes used specifically for a sol in which the dispersed phase is solid and the particles are large enough to settle out of solution.

sus·pen·soid (sus-pen′soid) lyophobic colloid.

sus·pen·so·ry (sus-pen′sor-e) 1. serving to hold up a part. 2. a ligament, bone, muscle, sling, or bandage that serves to hold up a part.

sus·ten·tac·u·lum (sus″ten-tak′u-lum) pl. *sustentac′ula*. [L.] a support. **sustentac′ular,** adj.

su·tu·ra (soo-tu′rah) pl. *sutu′rae*. [L.] suture; in anatomy, a type of joint in which the apposed bony surfaces are united by fibrous tissue, permitting no movement; found only between bones of the skull. **s. denta′ta,** s. serrata. **s. pla′na,** a type in which there is simple apposition of the contiguous surfaces, with no interlocking of the edges of the participating bones. **s. serra′ta,** a type in which the participating bones are united by interlocking processes resembling the teeth of a saw. **s. squamo′sa,** a type formed by overlapping of the broad beveled edges of the participating bones. **s. ve′ra,** sutura.

su·ture (soo′cher) 1. sutura. 2. a stitch or series of stitches made to secure apposition of the edges of a surgical or traumatic wound. 3. to apply such stitches. 4. material used in closing a wound with stitches. **su′tural,** adj. **absorbable s.,** a strand of material used for closing wounds which is subsequently dissolved by the tissue fluids. **apposition s.,** a superficial suture used for exact approximation of the cutaneous edges of a wound. **approximation s.,** a deep suture for securing apposition of the deep tissue of a wound. **buried s.,** one placed deep in the tissues and concealed by the skin. **catgut s.,** see *surgical gut*, under *gut*. **coaptation s.,** apposition s. **cobblers' s.,** one made with suture material threaded through a needle at each end. **continuous s.,** one in which a continuous, uninterrupted length of material is used. **coronal s.,** the line of junction of the frontal bone with the two parietal bones. **cranial s's,** the lines of junction between the bones of the skull. **Czerny's s.,** 1. an intestinal suture in which the thread is passed through the mucous membrane only. 2. union of a ruptured tendon by splitting one of the ends and suturing the other end into the slit. **false s.,** a line of junction between apposed surfaces without fibrous union of the bones. **figure-of-eight s.,** one in which the threads follow the contours of the figure 8. **Gély's s.,** a continuous stitch for wounds of the intestine, made with a thread having a needle at each end. **glover's s.,** lockstitch s. **Halsted s.,** a modification of the Lembert suture. **interrupted s.,** one in which each stitch is made with a separate piece of material. **Lembert s.,** an inverting suture used in gastrointestinal surgery. **lock-stitch s.,** a continuous hemostatic suture used in intestinal surgery, in which the needle is, after each stitch, passed through the loop of the preceding stitch. **loop s.,** interrupted s. **mattress s.,** a method in which the stitches are parallel with (*horizontal mattress s.*) or at right angles to (*vertical mattress s.*) the wound edges. **nonabsorbable s.**, suture material which is not absorbed in the body. **purse-string s.**, a continuous, circular inverting suture, such as is used to bury the stump of the appendix. **relaxation s.**, any suture so formed that it may be loosened to relieve tension as necessary. **subcuticular s.**, a method of skin closure involving placement of stitches in the subcuticular tissues parallel with the line of the wound. **uninterrupted s.**, continuous s.

SV stroke volume; sinus venosus.

svas·tha (swus′thyah) [Sanskrit] the term for health used in ayurveda.

sved·berg (sfed′berg) Svedberg unit.

SVT supraventricular tachycardia.

swab (swahb) a wad of cotton or other absorbent material attached to the end of a wire or stick, used for applying medication, removing material, collecting bacteriological material, etc.

swage (swāj) 1. to shape metal by hammering or by adapting it to a die. 2. to fuse, as suture material to the end of a suture needle.

swal·low·ing (swahl′o-ing) the taking in of a substance through the mouth and pharynx, past the cricopharyngeal constriction through the esophagus and into the stomach.

sway·back (swa′bak) lordosis (2).

sweat (swet) perspiration; the clear liquid secreted by the sweat glands.

sweat·ing perspiration; the functional secretion of sweat.

swell·ing (swel′ing) 1. transient abnormal enlargement of a body part or area not due to cell proliferation. 2. an eminence, or elevation. **cloudy s.**, an early stage of toxic degenerative changes, especially in protein constituents of organs in infectious diseases, in which the tissues appear swollen, parboiled, and opaque but revert to normal when the cause is removed.

sy·co·si·form (si-ko′sĭ-form) resembling sycosis.

sy·co·sis (si-ko′sis) papulopustular inflammation of hair follicles, especially of the beard. **s. bar′bae**, bacterial folliculitis of the bearded region, usually caused by *Staphylococcus aureus*. **lupoid s.**, a chronic, scarring form of deep sycosis barbae. **s. vulga′ris**, sycosis barbae.

syl·vat·ic (sil-vat′ik) sylvan; pertaining to, located in, or living in the woods.

sym·bal·lo·phone (sim-bal′o-fōn) a stethoscope with two chest pieces, making possible the comparison and localization of sounds.

sym·bi·ont (sim′bi-ont, sim′be-ont) an organism living in a state of symbiosis.

sym·bi·o·sis (sim″bi-o′sis) pl. *symbio′ses*. [Gr.] 1. in parasitology, the close association of two dissimilar organisms, classified as mutualism, commensalism, parasitism, amensalism, or synnecrosis, depending on the advantage or disadvantage derived from the relationship. 2. in psychiatry, a mutually reinforcing relationship between persons who are dependent on each other; a normal characteristic of the relationship between mother and infant.

sym·bi·ote (sim′bi-ōt) symbiont.

sym·bi·ot·ic (sim″bi-ot′ik) associated in symbiosis; living together.

sym·bleph·a·ron (sim-blef′ah-ron) adhesion of the eyelid(s) to the eyeball.

sym·bleph·a·rop·ter·yg·i·um (-blef″ah-ro-ter-ij′e-um) symblepharon in which the adhesion is a cicatricial band resembling a pterygium.

sym·bol (sim′bol) 1. something, particularly an object, that represents something else. 2. in psychoanalytic theory, a representation or perception that replaces unconscious mental content. **phallic s.**, in psychoanalytic theory, any pointed or upright object which may represent the phallus or penis.

sym·bo·lia (sim-bo′le-ah) ability to recognize the nature of objects by the sense of touch.

sym·bol·ism (sim′bo-lizm) 1. the act or process of representing something by a symbol. 2. in psychoanalytic theory, a mechanism of unconscious thinking characterized by substitution of a symbol for a repressed or threatening impulse or object so as to avoid censorship by the superego.

sym·bol·iza·tion (sim″bol-ĭ-za′shun) an unconscious defense mechanism in which one idea or object comes to represent another because of similarity or association between them.

sym·brachy·dac·ty·ly (sim-brak″e-dak′tĭ-le) a condition in which the fingers or toes are short and webbed.

sym·me·lia (sĭ-me′le-ah) a developmental anomaly characterized by an apparent fusion of the lower limbs, having three feet (*tripodial s.*), two feet (*dipodial s.*), one foot (*monopodial s.*), or no feet (*apodal s.* or *sirenomelia*).

sym·me·lus (sim′ĕ-lus) a fetus exhibiting symmelia.

sym·me·try (sim′ĕ-tre) correspondence in size, form, and arrangement of parts on opposite sides of a plane or around an axis. **symmet′ric, symmet′rical**, adj. **bilateral s.**, the configuration of an irregularly shaped body (as the human body or that of higher animals) which can be divided by a longitudinal plane into halves that are mirror images of each other. **inverse s.,** correspondence as between a part and its mirror image, wherein the right (or left) side of one part corresponds with the left (or right) side of the other. **radial s.,** that in which the body parts are arranged regularly around a central axis.

sym·pa·thec·to·my (sim″pah-thek′tah-me) transection, resection, or other interruption of some portion of the sympathetic nervous pathway. **chemical s.,** that accomplished by means of a chemical agent.

sym·pa·thet·ic (sim″pah-thet′ik) 1. pertaining to, exhibiting, or caused by sympathy. 2. pertaining to the sympathetic nervous system or one of its nerves.

sym·path·i·co·blast (sim-path′ĭ-ko-blast″) sympathoblast.

sym·path·i·co·blas·to·ma (sim-path″ĭ-ko-blas-to′mah) a neuroblastoma arising in one of the ganglia of the sympathetic nervous system.

sym·path·i·co·to·nia (-to′ne-ah) a stimulated condition of the sympathetic nervous system, marked by vascular spasm, heightened blood pressure, and gooseflesh. **sympathicoton′ic,** adj.

sym·path·i·co·trip·sy (-trip′se) the surgical crushing of a nerve, ganglion, or plexus of the sympathetic nervous system.

sym·path·i·co·tro·pic (-tro′pik) 1. having an affinity for the sympathetic nervous system. 2. an agent having an affinity for or exerting its principal effect on the sympathetic nervous system.

sym·patho·ad·re·nal (sim″pah-tho-ah-dre′n'l) 1. pertaining to the sympathetic nervous system and the adrenal medulla. 2. involving the sympathetic nervous system and the adrenal glands, especially increased sympathetic activity that causes increased secretion of epinephrine and norepinephrine.

sym·patho·blast (sim-path′o-blast″) a pluripotential cell in the embryo that will develop into a sympathetic nerve cell or a chromaffin cell.

sym·pa·tho·go·nia (sim″pah-tho-go′ne-ah) sing. *sympathogo′nium* [Gr.] undifferentiated embryonic cells that develop into sympathetic neurons.

sym·pa·tho·go·ni·o·ma (-go″ne-o′mah) sympathicoblastoma.

sym·pa·tho·lyt·ic (-lit′ik) 1. antiadrenergic; opposing the effects of impulses conveyed by adrenergic postganglionic fibers of the sympathetic nervous system. 2. an agent that so acts.

sym·pa·tho·mi·met·ic (-mi-met′ik) 1. mimicking the effects of impulses conveyed by adrenergic postganglionic fibers of the sympathetic nervous system. 2. an agent that produces such an effect.

sym·pa·thy (sim′pah-the) 1. compassion for another person's thoughts, feelings, and experiences. 2. an influence produced in any organ by disease, disorder, or other change in another part. 3. a relation which exists between people or things such that change in the state of one is reflected in the other.

sym·pha·lan·gia (sim″fah-lan′jah) congenital end-to-end fusion of contiguous phalanges of a digit.

sym·phys·e·al (sim-fiz′e-al) pertaining to a symphysis.

sym·phys·i·al (sim-fiz′e-al) symphyseal.

sym·phys·i·or·rha·phy (sim-fiz″e-or′ah-fe) suture of a divided symphysis.

sym·phys·i·ot·o·my (sim-fiz″e-ot′ah-me) division of the symphysis pubis to facilitate delivery.

sym·phy·sis (sim′fĭ-sis) pl. *sym′physes*. [Gr.] fibrocartilaginous joint; a type of joint in which the apposed bony surfaces are firmly united by a plate of fibrocartilage. **pubic s.,** the line of union of the bodies of the pubic bones in the median plane.

sym·po·dia (sim-po′de-ah) symmelia.

sym·port (sim′port) a mechanism of transporting two compounds simultaneously across a cell membrane in the same direction, one compound being transported down a concentration gradient, the other against a gradient.

symp·tom (simp′tom) any subjective evidence of disease or of a patient's condition, i.e., such evidence as perceived by the patient; a change in a patient's condition indicative of some bodily or mental state. **objective s.,** one that is evident to the observer; see *sign*. **presenting s.,** the symptom or group of symptoms about which the patient complains or from which he seeks relief. **subjective s.,** one perceptible only to the patient. **withdrawal s's,** substance withdrawal.

symp·to·mat·ic (simp″to-mat′ik) 1. pertaining to or of the nature of a symptom. 2. indicative (of a particular disease or disorder). 3. exhibiting the symptoms of a particular disease but having a different cause. 4. directed at the allaying of symptoms, as symptomatic treatment.

symp·to·ma·tol·o·gy (simp″to-mah-tol′ah-je) 1. the branch of medicine dealing with symptoms. 2. the combined symptoms of a disease.

symp·to·ma·to·lyt·ic (simp″to-mat-o-lit′ik) causing the disappearance of symptoms.

sym·pus (sim'pus) symmelus.

syn- word element [Gr.], *union; association; together with.*

syn·apse (sin'aps) the site of functional apposition between neurons, where an impulse is transmitted from one to another, usually by a chemical neurotransmitter released by the axon terminal of the presynaptic neuron. The neurotransmitter diffuses across the gap to bind with receptors on the postsynaptic cell membrane and cause electrical changes in that neuron (depolarization/excitation or hyperpolarization/inhibition).

syn·ap·sis (sĭ-nap'sis) the point-for-point pairing off of homologous chromosomes from male and female pronuclei during prophase of meiosis.

syn·ap·tic (sĭ-nap'tik) 1. pertaining to or affecting a synapse. 2. pertaining to synapsis.

syn·ap·to·some (sin-ap'to-sōm″) any of the membrane-bound sacs that break away from axon terminals at a synapse after brain tissue has been homogenized in sugar solution; it contains synaptic vessels and mitochondria.

syn·ar·thro·dia (sin″ahr-thro'de-ah) a fibrous joint. **synarthro'dial,** adj.

syn·ar·thro·phy·sis (sin-ahr″thro-fi'sis) any ankylosing process.

syn·ar·thro·sis (sin″ahr-thro'sis) pl. *synarthro'ses.* A bony junction that is immovable and is connected by solid connective tissue, comprising the fibrous joints and the cartilaginous joints.

syn·can·thus (sin-kan'thus) adhesion of the eyeball to the orbital structures.

syn·ceph·a·lus (-sef'ah-lus) conjoined twins with one head and a single face with four ears, two on the back of the head.

syn·chi·ria (-ki're-ah) dyschiria in which a stimulus applied to one side of the body is felt on both sides.

syn·chon·dro·sis (sin″kon-dro'sis) pl. *synchondro'ses.* [Gr.] a type of cartilaginous joint in which the cartilage is usually converted into bone before adult life.

syn·chon·drot·o·my (-kon-drot'ah-me) division of a synchondrosis.

syn·chro·nism (sing'krah-nizm) synchrony. **synchron'ic, syn'chronous,** adj.

syn·chro·ny (-krah-ne) the occurrence of two events simultaneously or with a fixed time interval between them. **atrioventricular (AV) s.,** in the heart, the physiological condition of atrial electrical activity followed by ventricular electrical activity. **bilateral s.,** the occurrence of a secondary synchronous discharge at a location in the brain exactly contralateral to a discharge caused by a lesion.

syn·chy·sis (sin'kĭ-sis) [Gr.] a softening or fluid condition of the vitreous body of the eye. **s. scintil'lans,** floating cholesterol crystals in the vitreous, developing as a secondary degenerative change.

syn·clit·ism (sin'klit-izm) 1. parallelism between the planes of the fetal head and those of the maternal pelvis. 2. normal synchronous maturation of the nucleus and cytoplasm of blood cells. **synclit'ic,** adj.

syn·clo·nus (-klo-nus) muscular tremor or successive clonic contraction of various muscles together.

syn·co·pe (-ko-pe) a faint; temporary loss of consciousness due to generalized cerebral ischemia. **syn'copal, syncop'ic,** adj. **cardiac s.,** sudden loss of consciousness, with momentary premonitory symptoms or without warning, due to cerebral anemia caused by obstructions to cardiac output or arrhythmias such as ventricular asystole, extreme bradycardia, or ventricular fibrillation. **carotid sinus s.,** see under *syndrome.* **convulsive s.,** syncope with convulsive movements that are milder than those seen in epilepsy. **laryngeal s.,** tussive syncope. **stretching s.,** syncope associated with stretching the arms upward with the spine extended. **swallow s.,** syncope associated with swallowing, a disorder of atrioventricular conduction mediated by the vagus nerve. **tussive s.,** brief loss of consciousness associated with paroxysms of coughing. **vasovagal s.,** see under *attack.*

syn·cy·tial (sin-sish'al) of or pertaining to a syncytium.

syn·cyt·i·o·ma (-sit″e-o'mah) syncytial endometritis. **s. malig'num,** choriocarcinoma.

syn·cyt·io·tro·pho·blast (sin-sit″e-o-tro'fo-blast) the outer syncytial layer of the trophoblast. **syncytiotrophoblas'tic,** adj.

syn·cy·ti·um (sin-sish'e-um) a multinucleate mass of protoplasm produced by the merging of cells.

syn·dac·ty·ly (-dak'tĭ-le) persistence of webbing between adjacent digits of the hand or foot, so that they are more or less completely fused together. **syndac'tylous,** adj.

syn·dec·to·my (-dek'tah-me) peritectomy.

syn·de·sis (sin'dĕ-sis) 1. arthrodesis. 2. synapsis.

syn·des·mec·to·my (sin″dez-mek'tah-me) excision of a portion of ligament.

syn·des·mec·to·pia (-mek-to'pe-ah) unusual situation of a ligament.

syn·des·mi·tis (-mi'tis) 1. inflammation of a ligament. 2. conjunctivitis.

syndesm(o)- word element [Gr.], *connective tissue; ligament.*

syn·des·mog·ra·phy (sin″dez-mog′rah-fe) a description of the ligaments.

syn·des·mol·o·gy (-mol′ah-je) arthrology.

syn·des·mo·plas·ty (sin-dez′mo-plas″te) plastic repair of a ligament.

syn·des·mo·sis (sin″dez-mo′sis) pl. *syndesmo′ses*. [Gr.] a joint in which the bones are united by fibrous connective tissue forming an interosseous membrane or ligament.

syn·des·mot·o·my (-mot′ah-me) incision of a ligament.

syn·drome (sin′drōm) a set of symptoms occurring together; the sum of signs of any morbid state; a symptom complex. See also entries under *disease*. **Aarskog s., Aarskog-Scott s.,** a hereditary X-linked condition characterized by ocular hypertelorism, anteverted nostrils, broad upper lip, peculiar scrotal "shawl" above the penis, and small hands. **acquired immune deficiency s., acquired immunodeficiency s.,** an epidemic, transmissible retroviral disease caused by infection with the human immunodeficiency virus, manifested in severe cases as profound depression of cell-mediated immunity, and affecting certain recognized risk groups. Diagnosis is by the presence of a disease indicative of a defect in cell-mediated immunity (e.g., life-threatening opportunistic infection) in the absence of any known causes of underlying immunodeficiency or of any other host defense defects reported to be associated with that disease (e.g., iatrogenic immunosuppression). **acute coronary s.,** a classification encompassing clinical presentations ranging from unstable angina through non–Q wave infarction, sometimes also including Q wave infarction. **acute radiation s.,** a syndrome caused by exposure to a whole body dose of over 1 gray of ionizing radiation; symptoms, whose severity and time of onset depend on the size of the dose, include erythema, nausea and vomiting, fatigue, diarrhea, petechiae, bleeding from the mucous membranes, hematologic changes, gastrointestinal hemorrhage, epilation, hypotension, tachycardia, and dehydration; death may occur within hours or weeks of exposure. **acute respiratory distress s. (ARDS),** fulminant pulmonary interstitial and alveolar edema, which usually develops within a few days after the initiating trauma, thought to result from alveolar injury that has led to increased capillary permeability. **acute retinal necrosis s.,** necrotizing retinitis with uveitis and other retinal pathology, severe loss of vision, and often retinal detachment; of viral etiology. **Adams-Stokes s.,** episodic cardiac arrest and syncope due to failure of normal and escape pacemakers, with or without ventricular fibrillation; the principal manifestation of severe heart attack. **addisonian s.,** the complex of symptoms resulting from adrenocortical insufficiency; see *Addison's disease*, under *disease*. **Adie's s.,** tonic pupil associated with absence or diminution of certain tendon reflexes. **adrenogenital s.,** a group of syndromes in which inappropriate virilism or feminization results from disorders of adrenal function that also affect gonadal steroidogenesis. **adult respiratory distress s. (ARDS),** acute respiratory distress s. **AEC s.,** Hay-Wells s. **afferent loop s.,** chronic partial obstruction of the proximal loop (duodenum and jejunum) after gastrojejunostomy, resulting in duodenal distention, pain, and nausea following ingestion of food. **Ahumada-del Castillo s.,** galactorrhea-amenorrhea syndrome with low gonadotropin secretion. **akinetic-rigid s.,** muscular rigidity with varying degrees of slowness of movement; seen in parkinsonism and disorders of the basal ganglia. **Alagille s.,** inherited neonatal jaundice, cholestasis with peripheral pulmonic stenosis, unusual facies, and ocular, vertebral, and nervous system abnormalities, due to paucity or absence of intrahepatic bile ducts. **Albright's s., Albright-McCune-Sternberg s.,** polyostotic fibrous dysplasia, patchy dermal pigmentation, and endocrine dysfunction. **Aldrich's s.,** Wiskott-Aldrich s. **Allgrove's s.,** inherited glucocorticoid deficiency with achalasia and alacrima. **Alport's s.,** a hereditary disorder marked by progressive nerve deafness, progressive pyelonephritis or glomerulonephritis, and occasionally ocular defects. **Alström s.,** a hereditary syndrome of retinitis pigmentosa with nystagmus and early loss of central vision, deafness, obesity, and diabetes mellitus. **amnestic s.,** a mental disorder characterized by impairment of memory occurring in a normal state of consciousness; the most common cause is thiamine deficiency associated with alcohol abuse. **amniotic band s.,** see under *sequence*. **Angelman's s.,** happy puppet s. **angular gyrus s.,** a syndrome resulting from an infarction or other lesion of the angular gyrus on the dominant side, often characterized by alexia or agraphia. **ankyloblepharon–ectodermal dysplasia–clefting s.,** Hay-Wells s. **anorexia-cachexia s.,** a systemic response to cancer occurring as a result of a poorly understood relationship between anorexia and cachexia, manifested by malnutrition, weight loss, muscular weakness, acidosis, and toxemia. **anterior cord s.,** anterior spinal artery s.

anterior interosseous s., a complex of symptoms caused by a lesion of the anterior interosseous nerve, usually resulting from a fracture or laceration. anterior spinal artery s., localized injury to the anterior portion of the spinal cord, characterized by complete paralysis and hypalgesia and hypesthesia to the level of the lesion, but with relative preservation of posterior column sensations of touch, position, and vibration. Apert's s., acrocephalosyndactyly, type I; an autosomal dominant disorder characterized by acrocephaly and syndactyly, often with other skeletal deformities and mental retardation. Asherman's s., persistent amenorrhea and secondary sterility due to intrauterine adhesions and synechiae, usually as a result of uterine curettage. Asperger's s., a pervasive developmental disorder resembling autistic disorder, being characterized by severe impairment of social interactions and by restricted interests and behaviors; however, patients are not delayed in development of language, cognitive function, and self-help skills. Barrett's s., peptic ulcer of the lower esophagus, often with stricture, due to the presence of columnar-lined epithelium, which may contain functional mucous cells, parietal cells, or chief cells, in the esophagus instead of normal squamous cell epithelium. Bartter s., a hereditary form of hyperaldosteronism secondary to hypertrophy and hyperplasia of the juxtaglomerular cells, with normal blood pressure and hypokalemic alkalosis in the absence of edema, increased concentration of renin, angiotensin II, and bradykinin; usually occurring in children. basal cell nevus s., an autosomal dominant syndrome characterized by the development in early life of numerous basal cell carcinomas, in association with abnormalities of the skin, bone, nervous system, eyes, and reproductive tract. Bassen-Kornzweig s., abetalipoproteinemia. battered-child s., multiple traumatic lesions of the bones and soft tissues of children, often accompanied by subdural hematomas, willfully inflicted by an adult. Beckwith-Wiedemann s., an inherited disorder characterized by exomphalos, macroglossia, and gigantism, often associated with visceromegaly, adrenocortical cytomegaly, and dysplasia of the renal medulla. Behçet's s., severe uveitis and retinal vasculitis, optic atrophy, and aphthalike lesions of the mouth and genitalia, often with other signs and symptoms suggesting a diffuse vasculitis; it most often affects young males. Bernard-Soulier s., a hereditary coagulation disorder marked by mild

thrombocytopenia, giant and morphologically abnormal platelets, hemorrhagic tendency, prolonged bleeding time, and purpura. Bing-Neel s., the central nervous system manifestations of Waldenström's macroglobulinemia, possibly including encephalopathy, hemorrhage, stroke, convulsions, delirium, and coma. Birt-Hogg-Dubé s., an inherited disorder of proliferation of ectodermal and mesodermal components of the pilar system, occurring as multiple trichodiscomas, acrochordons, and fibrofolliculomas on the head, chest, back, and upper limbs. Blackfan-Diamond s., congenital hypoplastic anemia. blue toe s., skin necrosis and ischemic gangrene manifest as a blue color of the toes, resulting from arterial occlusion, usually caused by emboli, thrombi, or injury. Boerhaave's s., spontaneous rupture of the esophagus. Börjeson's s., Börjeson-Forssman-Lehmann s., a hereditary syndrome, transmitted as an X-linked recessive trait, characterized by severe mental retardation, epilepsy, hypogonadism, hypometabolism, marked obesity, swelling of the subcutaneous tissues of the face, and large ears. bowel bypass s., a syndrome of dermatosis and arthritis occurring some time after jejunoileal bypass, probably caused by immune reponse to bacterial overgrowth in the bypassed bowel. Bradbury-Eggleston s., a progressive syndrome of postural hypotension without tachycardia but with visual disturbances, impotence, hypohidrosis, lowered metabolic rate, dizziness, syncope, and slow pulse; due to impaired peripheral vasoconstriction. bradycardia-tachycardia s., brady-tachy s., a clinical manifestation of the sick sinus syndrome characterized by alternating periods of bradycardia and tachycardia. Brown-Séquard s., ipsilateral paralysis and loss of discriminatory and joint sensation, and contralateral loss of pain and temperature sensation; due to damage to one half of the spinal cord. Brown-Vialetto-van Laere s., an inherited syndrome of progressive bulbar palsy with any of several cranial nerve disorders. Budd-Chiari s., symptomatic obstruction or occlusion of the hepatic veins, causing hepatomegaly, abdominal pain and tenderness, intractable ascites, mild jaundice, and eventually portal hypertension and liver failure. Caffey's s., Caffey-Silverman s., infantile cortical hyperostosis. Canada-Cronkhite s., Cronkhite-Canada s. capillary leak s., extravasation of plasma fluid and proteins into the extravascular space, resulting in sometimes fatal hypotension and reduced organ perfusion; an adverse effect of interleukin-2 therapy. **carcinoid s.,** a symptom complex associated with carcinoid tumors, marked by attacks of cyanotic flushing of the skin and watery diarrhea, bronchoconstrictive attacks, sudden drops in blood pressure, edema, and ascites. Symptoms are caused by tumor secretion of serotonin, prostaglandins, and other biologically active substances. **carotid sinus s.,** syncope sometimes associated with convulsions due to overactivity of the carotid sinus reflex when pressure is applied to one or both carotid sinuses. **carpal tunnel s.,** pain and burning or tingling paresthesias in the fingers and hand, sometimes extending to the elbow, due to compression of the median nerve in the carpal tunnel. **Carpenter's s.,** acrocephalopolysyndactyly, type II; an autosomal recessive disorder characterized by acrocephaly, polysyndactyly, brachydactyly, mild obesity, mental retardation, hypogonadism, and other anomalies. **central cord s.,** injury to the central part of the cervical spinal cord resulting in disproportionately more weakness or paralysis in the upper limbs than in the lower; pathological change is caused by hemorrhage or edema. **cerebrocostomandibular s.,** an inherited syndrome of severe micrognathia and costovertebral abnormalities, with palatal defects, prenatal and postnatal growth deficiencies, and mental retardation. **cerebrohepatorenal s.,** a hereditary disorder, transmitted as an autosomal recessive trait, characterized by craniofacial abnormalities, hypotonia, hepatomegaly, polycystic kidneys, jaundice, and death in early infancy. **cervical rib s.,** thoracic outlet syndrome caused by a cervical rib. **Cestan's s., Cestan-Chenais s.,** an association of contralateral hemiplegia, contralateral hemianesthesia, ipsilateral lateropulsion and hemiasynergia, Horner's syndrome, and ipsilateral laryngoplegia, due to scattered lesions of the pyramid, sensory tract, inferior cerebellar peduncle, nucleus ambiguus, and oculopupillary center. **Charcot's s.,** 1. amyotrophic lateral sclerosis. 2. intermittent claudication. **Charcot-Marie s.,** Charcot-Marie-Tooth disease. **CHARGE s.,** see under *association.* **Chédiak-Higashi s.,** a lethal, progressive, autosomal recessive, systemic disorder associated with oculocutaneous albinism, massive leukocyte inclusions (giant lysosomes), histiocytic infiltration of multiple body organs, development of pancytopenia, hepatosplenomegaly, recurrent or persistent bacterial infections, and a possible predisposition to development of malignant lymphoma. **Chinese restaurant s.,** transient arterial dilatation due to ingestion of monosodium glutamate, which is sometimes used liberally in seasoning Chinese food, marked by throbbing head, lightheadedness, tightness of the jaw, neck, and shoulders, and backache. **Chotzen's s.,** acrocephalosyndactyly, type III; an autosomal dominant disorder characterized by acrocephaly and syndactyly in which the latter is mild and by hypertelorism, ptosis, and sometimes mental retardation. **Christ-Siemens-Touraine s.,** anhidrotic ectodermal dysplasia. **chronic fatigue s.,** persistent debilitating fatigue of recent onset, with greatly reduced physical activity and some combination of muscle weakness, sore throat, mild fever, tender lymph nodes, headaches, and depression, not attributable to any other known causes; it is of controversial etiology. **Churg-Strauss s.,** allergic granulomatous angiitis; a systemic form of necrotizing vasculitis in which there is prominent lung involvement. **chylomicronemia s.,** familial hyperchylomicronemia. **Coffin-Lowry s.,** an X-linked syndrome of incapability of speech, severe mental deficiency, and muscle, ligament, and skeletal abnormalities. **Coffin-Siris s.,** hypoplasia of the fifth fingers and toenails associated with growth and mental deficiencies, coarse facies, mild microcephaly, hypotonia, lax joints, and mild hirsutism. **compartmental s.,** a condition in which increased tissue pressure in a confined anatomic space causes decreased blood flow leading to ischemia and dysfunction of contained myoneural elements, marked by pain, muscle weakness, sensory loss, and palpable tenseness in the involved compartment; ischemia can lead to necrosis resulting in permanent impairment of function. **congenital rubella s.,** transplacental infection of the fetus with rubella, usually in the first trimester of pregnancy, as a consequence of maternal infection, resulting in various developmental anomalies in the newborn infant. **Conn's s.,** primary aldosteronism. **cri du chat s.,** a hereditary congenital syndrome characterized by hypertelorism, microcephaly, severe mental deficiency, and a plaintive catlike cry, due to deletion of the short arm of chromosome 5. **Crigler-Najjar s.,** an autosomal recessive form of nonhemolytic jaundice due to absence of the hepatic enzyme glucuronide transferase, marked by excessive amounts of unconjugated bilirubin in the blood, kernicterus, and severe central nervous system disorders. **s. of crocodile tears,** spontaneous lacrimation occurring parallel with the normal salivation of eating, and associated with facial paralysis; it seems to be due to straying of regenerating nerve fibers, some of those destined for the salivary glands going to the lacrimal glands. **Cronkhite-Canada s.,** familial polyposis of the gastrointestinal tract associated with ectodermal defects such as alopecia and onychodystrophy. **Crow-Fukase s.,** POEMS s. **crush s.,** the edema, oliguria, and other symptoms of renal failure that follow crushing of a part, especially a large muscle mass; see *lower nephron nephrosis,* under *nephrosis.* **Cruveilhier-Baumgarten s.,** cirrhosis with portal hypertension associated with congenital patency of the umbilical and paraumbilical veins. **Cushing's s.,** a condition, more commonly seen in females, due to hyperadrenocorticism resulting from neoplasms of the adrenal cortex or anterior lobe of the pituitary; or to prolonged excessive intake of glucocorticoids for therapeutic purposes (*iatrogenic Cushing's s.* or *Cushing's s. medicamentosus*). The symptoms may include adiposity of the face, neck, and trunk, kyphosis caused by softening of the spine, amenorrhea, hypertrichosis (in females), impotence (in males), dusky complexion with purple markings, hypertension, polycythemia, pain in the abdomen and back, and muscular weakness. **Da Costa s.,** neurocirculatory asthenia. **Dandy-Walker s.,** congenital hydrocephalus due to obstruction of the foramina of Magendie and Luschka. **Dejean's s.,** orbital floor s. **de Lange's s.,** a congenital syndrome of mental retardation, short stature (Amsterdam dwarf), flat spadelike hands, and other anomalies. **dialysis dysequilibrium s.,** symptoms such as headache, nausea, muscle cramps, nervous irritability, drowsiness, and convulsions during or after overly rapid hemodialysis or peritoneal dialysis, resulting from an osmotic shift of water into the brain. **disconnection s.,** any neurologic disorder caused by an interruption in impulse transmission along cerebral fiber pathways. **Down s.,** mongoloid features, short phalanges, widened space between the first and second toes and fingers, and moderate to severe mental retardation; associated with a chromosomal abnormality, usually trisomy of chromosome 21. **Drash s.,** an inherited syndrome of Wilms' tumor with glomerulopathy and male pseudohermaphroditism. **Dubin-Johnson s.,** hereditary chronic nonhemolytic jaundice thought to be due to defective excretion of conjugated bilirubin and certain other organic anions by the liver; a brown, coarsely granular pigment in hepatic cells is pathognomonic. **dumping s.,** nausea, weakness, sweating, palpitation, syncope, often a sensation of warmth, and sometimes diarrhea, occurring after ingestion of food in patients who have undergone partial gastrectomy. **dyscontrol s.,** a pattern of episodic abnormal and often violent and uncontrollable social behavior with little or no provocation; it may have an organic cause or be associated with abuse of a psychoactive substance. **dysmaturity s.,** postmaturity s. **Eaton-Lambert s.,** a myasthenia-like syndrome in which the weakness usually affects the limbs and ocular and bulbar muscles are spared; often associated with oat-cell carcinoma of the lung. **EEC s.,** ectrodactyly–ectodermal dysplasia–clefting s.; an inherited congenital syndrome involving both ectodermal and mesodermal tissues, characterized by ectodermal dysplasia with hypopigmentation of skin and hair, and other hair, nail, tooth, lip, and palate abnormalities. **Ehlers-Danlos s.,** a group of inherited disorders of connective tissue, varying in clinical and biochemical evidence, in mode of inheritance, and in severity from mild to lethal; major manifestations include hyperextensible skin and joints, easy bruisability, friability of tissues, bleeding, poor wound healing, subcutaneous nodules, and cardiovascular, orthopedic, intestinal, and ocular defects. **Eisenmenger's s.,** ventricular septal defect with pulmonary hypertension and cyanosis due to right-to-left (reversed) shunt of blood. Sometimes defined as pulmonary hypertension (pulmonary vascular disease) and cyanosis with the shunt being at the atrial, ventricular, or great vessel area. **EMG s.,** Beckwith-Wiedemann s. **Escobar s.,** multiple pterygium s. **excited skin s.,** nonspecific cutaneous hyperirritability of the back, sometimes occurring when multiple positive reactions are elicited in patch test screening of a battery of substances. **exomphalos-macroglossia-gigantism s.,** Beckwith-Wiedemann s. **extrapyramidal s.,** any of a group of clinical disorders considered to be due to malfunction in the extrapyramidal system and marked by abnormal involuntary movements; included are parkinsonism, athetosis, and chorea. **Faber's s.,** hypochromic anemia. **Fanconi s.,** 1. a rare hereditary disorder, transmitted as an autosomal recessive trait, characterized by pancytopenia, hypoplasia of the bone marrow, and patchy brown discoloration of the skin due to the deposition of melanin, and associated with multiple congenital anomalies of the musculoskeletal and genitourinary systems. 2. a general term for a group of diseases marked by dysfunction of the proximal renal tubules, with generalized hyperaminoaciduria, renal glycosuria, hyperphosphaturia, and bicarbonate and water loss; the most common cause is cystinosis, but it is also associated with other genetic diseases and occurs in idiopathic and acquired forms. **Farber s.**, **Farber-Uzman s.**, Farber's disease. **Felty's s.**, a syndrome of splenomegaly with chronic rheumatoid arthritis and leukopenia; there are usually pigmented spots on the skin of the lower extremities, and sometimes there is other evidence of hypersplenism such as anemia or thrombocytopenia. **fetal alcohol s.**, a syndrome of altered prenatal growth and morphogenesis, occurring in infants born of women who were chronically alcoholic during pregnancy; it includes maxillary hypoplasia, prominence of the forehead and mandible, short palpebral fissures, microophthalmia, epicanthal folds, severe growth retardation, mental retardation, and microcephaly. **fetal hydantoin s.**, poor growth and development with craniofacial and skeletal abnormalities, produced by prenatal exposure to hydantoin analogues, including phenytoin. **floppy infant s.**, abnormal posture in an infant suspended prone, the limbs and head hanging down; due to any of numerous conditions, particularly perinatal injury to the brain or spinal cord, spinal muscular atrophy, and various genetic disorders. **Foix-Alajouanine s.**, a fatal necrotizing myelopathy characterized by necrosis of the gray matter of the spinal cord, thickening of the walls of the spinal vessels, and abnormal spinal fluid. **Franceschetti s.**, the complete form of mandibulofacial dysostosis. **galactorrhea-amenorrhea s.**, amenorrhea and galactorrhea, sometimes associated with increased levels of prolactin. **Ganser s.**, the giving of approximate answers to questions, commonly associated with amnesia, disorientation, perceptual disturbances, fugue, and conversion symptoms. **Garcin's s.**, unilateral paralysis of most or all of the cranial nerves due to a tumor at the base of the skull or in the nasopharynx. **Gardner's s.**, familial polyposis of the colon associated with osseous and soft tissue tumors. **gay bowel s.**, an assortment of sexually transmitted bowel and rectal diseases affecting homosexual males and others who engage in anal intercourse, caused by a wide variety of infectious agents. **general adaptation s.**, the total of all nonspecific reactions of the body to prolonged systemic stress, comprising alarm, resistance, and exhaustion. **Gerstmann-Sträussler s.**, **Gerstmann-Sträussler-Scheinker s.**, a

group of rare prion diseases of autosomal dominant inheritance, having the common characteristics of cognitive and motor disturbances, ending in death, and the presence of multicentric amyloid plaques in the brain. **Gianotti-Crosti s.**, monomorphous, usually nonpruritic, dusky or coppery red, flat-topped, firm papules forming a symmetrical eruption on the face, buttocks, and limbs, including the palms and soles, with malaise and low-grade fever; seen in young children and associated with viral infection. **Gilles de la Tourette's s.**, a childhood-onset syndrome comprising both multiple motor and one or more vocal tics, often associated with obsessions, compulsions, hyperactivity, distractibility, and impulsivity; it may diminish or even remit in adolescence or adulthood. **Goodpasture's s.**, glomerulonephritis with pulmonary hemorrhage and circulating antibodies against basement membranes, usually seen in young men and with a course of rapidly progressing renal failure, with hemoptysis, pulmonary infiltrates, and dyspnea. **Gradenigo's s.**, sixth nerve palsy and unilateral headache in suppurative disease of the middle ear, due to involvement of the abducens and trigeminal nerves by direct spread of the infection. **gray s.**, a potentially fatal condition seen in neonates, particularly premature infants, due to a reaction to chloramphenicol, characterized by an ashen gray cyanosis, listlessness, weakness, and hypotension. **Guillain-Barré s.**, acute idiopathic polyneuritis. **Gunn's s.**, unilateral ptosis of the eyelid, with movements of the affected eyelid associated with those of the jaw. **Hamman-Rich s.**, the acute form of idiopathic pulmonary fibrosis. **Hand-Schüller-Christian s.**, see under *disease*. **hantavirus pulmonary s.**, a sometimes fatal febrile illness caused by a hantavirus, characterized by variable respiratory symptoms followed by acute respiratory distress, sometimes progressing to respiratory failure. **happy puppet s.**, an inherited syndrome of jerky puppetlike movements, frequent laughter, mental and motor retardation, peculiar open-mouthed facies, and seizures. **Harada s.**, Vogt-Koyanagi-Harada s. **Hay-Wells s.**, an inherited syndrome of ectodermal dysplasia, cleft lip and palate, and adhesions of the margins of the eyelids, accompanied by tooth, skin, and hair abnormalities. **HELLP s.**, *h*emolysis, *e*levated *l*iver enzymes, and *l*ow *p*latelet count occurring in association with pre-eclampsia. **Helweg-Larsen's s.**, an inherited syndrome of anhidrosis present from birth and labyrinthitis occurring late in life. **hemolytic uremic s.,** a form of thrombotic microangiopathy with renal failure, hemolytic anemia, and severe thrombocytopenia and purpura. **Herrmann's s.,** an inherited syndrome initially characterized by photomyogenic seizures and progressive deafness, with later development of diabetes mellitus, nephropathy, and mental deterioration. **HHH s.,** hyperornithinemia-hyperammonemia-homocitrullinuria s. **Hinman s.,** a psychogenic disorder seen in children, imitating a neurogenic bladder, consisting of detrusor-sphincter dyssynergia without evidence of neural lesion. **Horner s., Horner-Bernard s.,** sinking in of the eyeball, ptosis of the upper lid, slight elevation of the lower lid, miosis, narrowing of the palpebral fissure, and anhidrosis and flushing of the affected side of the face; due to a brain stem lesion on the ipsilateral side that interrupts descending sympathetic nerves. **Hughes-Stovin s.,** thrombosis of the pulmonary arteries and peripheral veins, characterized by headache, fever, cough, papilledema, and hemoptysis. **Hurler's s.,** an inherited mucopolysaccharidosis due to deficiency of the enzyme α-L-iduronidase, characterized by gargoyle-like facies, dwarfism, severe somatic and skeletal changes, severe mental retardation, cloudy corneas, deafness, cardiovascular defects, hepatosplenomegaly, joint contractures, and death in childhood. **Hutchinson-Gilford s.,** progeria. **hypereosinophilic s.,** any of several diseases characterized by a massive increase in the number of eosinophils in the blood and bone marrow, with infiltration of other organs. Symptoms vary from mild to the often fatal outcome of eosinophilic leukemia. **hyperkinetic s.,** former name for *attention-deficit/hyperactivity disorder.* **hyperornithinemia-hyperammonemia-homocitrullinuria s.,** an inherited disorder characterized by elevated levels of ornithine, postprandial hyperammonemia and homocitrullinuria, and aversion to protein ingestion; believed to result from a defect in the transport of ornithine into the mitochondria, which disturbs the cycle of ureagenesis. **hyperventilation s.,** a complex of symptoms that accompany hypocapnia caused by hyperventilation, including palpitations, shortness of breath, lightheadedness or giddiness, profuse perspiration, tingling sensations in the fingertips, face, or toes, and vasomotor collapse and loss of consciousness if prolonged. **hypoplastic left heart s.,** congenital hypoplasia or atresia of the left ventricle, aortic or mitral valve, and ascending aorta, with respiratory distress, cardiac failure, and death in infancy. **impingement s.,** progressive pathologic changes resulting from the impingement of the acromion, coracoacromial ligament, coracoid process, or acromioclavicular joint on the rotator cuff. **s. of inappropriate antidiuretic hormone (SIADH),** persistent hyponatremia, inappropriately elevated urine osmolality, caused by release of vasopressin (antidiuretic hormone) without discernible stimulus. **irritable bowel s., irritable colon s.,** a chronic noninflammatory disease with a psychophysiologic basis, characterized by abdominal pain, diarrhea or constipation or both, and no detectable pathologic change. **Isaacs' s., Isaacs-Mertens s.,** progressive muscle stiffness and spasms, with continuous muscle fiber activity similar to that seen with neuromyotonia. **Jacod's s.,** chronic arthritis after rheumatic fever, with fibrous changes in the joint capsules leading to deformities that may resemble rheumatoid arthritis but lack bone erosion. **Jarcho-Levin s.,** an inherited disorder of multiple vertebral defects, short thorax, rib abnormalities, camptodactyly, syndactyly, and sometimes urogenital abnormalities, usually fatal in infancy. **Joubert's s.,** inherited, usually fatal, partial to complete agenesis of the cerebellar vermis, with hypotonia, episodic hyperpnea, mental retardation, and abnormal eye movements. **Kartagener's s.,** a hereditary syndrome consisting of dextrocardia, bronchiectasis, and sinusitis. **Kimmelstiel-Wilson s.,** intercapillary glomerulosclerosis in which the lesions are nodular. **King s.,** a form of malignant hyperthermia accompanied by characteristic physical abnormalities. **Klinefelter's s.,** smallness of testes with fibrosis and hyalinization of seminiferous tubules, variable degrees of masculinization, azoospermia, and infertility, and increased urinary gonadotropins. It is associated typically with an XXY chromosome complement although variants include XXYY, XXXY, XXXXY, and various mosaic patterns. **Klippel-Feil s.,** shortness of the neck due to reduction in the number of cervical vertebrae or the fusion of multiple hemivertebrae into one osseous mass, with limitation of neck motion and low hairline. **Korsakoff's s.,** a syndrome of anterograde and retrograde amnesia with confabulation associated with alcoholic or nonalcoholic polyneuritis, currently used synonymously with the term amnestic syndrome or, more narrowly, to refer to the amnestic component of the Wernicke-Korsakoff syndrome. **Kugelberg-Welander s.,** an inherited juvenile form of muscular atrophy due to lesions on the anterior horns of the spinal cord, beginning with the proximal muscles of the lower limbs and pelvic girdle and progressing to the distal muscles. **LAMB s.,** a syndrome of familial myomas with cutaneous, cardiac, and endocrine involvement, manifested as *l*entigines, *a*trial *my*xoma, and *b*lue nevi. **Landau-Kleffner s.,** an epileptic syndrome of childhood with partial or generalized seizures, psychomotor abnormalities, and aphasia progressing to mutism. **Launois' s.,** pituitary gigantism. **Laurence-Moon s.,** an autosomal recessive disorder characterized by mental retardation, pigmentary retinopathy, hypogonadism, and spastic paraplegia. **lazy leukocyte s.,** a syndrome in children, marked by recurrent low-grade infections with a defect in neutrophil chemotaxis and deficient random mobility of neutrophils. **Lemieux-Neemeh s.,** an inherited syndrome of Charcot-Marie-Tooth disease with progressive deafness. **Leriche s.,** lower limb fatigue on exercising, lack of femoral pulse, impotence, and often pale, cold lower limbs, usually seen in males due to obstruction of the terminal aorta. **Lesch-Nyhan s.,** an X-linked disorder of purine metabolism with physical and mental retardation, compulsive self-mutilation of fingers and lips by biting, choreoathetosis, spastic cerebral palsy, and impaired renal function, and by extremely excessive purine synthesis and consequently hyperuricemia and excessive urinary secretion of uric acid. **Li-Fraumeni s.,** a familial syndrome of early breast carcinoma associated with soft tissue sarcomas and other tumors. **locked-in s.,** quadriplegia and mutism with intact consciousness and preservation of some eye movements; usually due to a vascular lesion of the anterior pons. **long QT s.,** prolongation of the Q–T interval combined with torsades de pointes and manifest in several forms, either acquired or congenital, the latter with or without deafness; it may lead to serious arrhythmia and sudden death. **Lowe s., Lowe-Terrey-MacLachlan s.,** oculocerebrorenal s. **Lown-Ganong-Levine s.,** a pre-excitation syndrome of electrocardiographic abnormality characterized by a short P–R interval with a normal QRS complex, accompanied by atrial tachycardia. **Lutembacher's s.,** atrial septal defect with mitral stenosis (usually rheumatic). **lymphadenopathy s.,** unexplained lymphadenopathy for 3 or more months at extrainguinal sites, revealing on biopsy nonspecific lymphoid hyperplasia, possibly a prodrome of acquired immunodeficiency syndrome. **Maffucci's s.,**

enchondromatosis with multiple cutaneous or visceral hemangiomas. **malabsorption s.,** a group of disorders marked by subnormal absorption of dietary constituents, and thus excessive loss of nutrients in the stool, which may be due to a digestive defect, a mucosal abnormality, or lymphatic obstruction. **male Turner's s.,** Noonan's s. **Marfan s.,** a hereditary syndrome of abnormal length of limbs, especially fingers and toes, with subluxation of the lens, cardiovascular abnormalities, and other defects. **Marie-Bamberger s.,** hypertrophic pulmonary osteoarthropathy. **maternal deprivation s.,** failure to thrive with severe growth retardation, unresponsiveness to the environment, depression, retarded mental and emotional development, and behavioral problems resulting from loss, absence, or neglect of the mother or other primary caregiver. **Meckel's s.,** an autosomal recessive syndrome, with sloping forehead, posterior meningoencephalocele, polydactyly, polycystic kidneys, and death in the perinatal period. **meconium aspiration s.,** the respiratory complications resulting from the passage and aspiration of meconium prior to or during delivery. **median cleft facial s.,** a hereditary form of defective midline development of the head and face, including ocular hypertelorism, occult cleft nose and maxilla, and sometimes mental retardation or other defects. **megacystis-megaureter s.,** chronic ureteral dilatation (megaureter) associated with hypotonia and dilatation of the bladder (megacystis) and gaping of ureteral orifices, permitting vesicoureteral reflux of urine, and resulting in chronic pyelonephritis. **megacystis-microcolon-intestinal hypoperistalsis s. (MMIHS),** enlarged bladder (megacystis), small colon with decreased or absent peristalsis (microcolon and intestinal hypoperistalsis), and the same abdominal muscle defect as occurs in prune-belly syndrome. **Meige s.,** 1. Milroy's disease. 2. dystonia of facial and oromandibular muscles with blepharospasm, grimacing mouth movements, and protrusion of the tongue. **MELAS s.,** a maternally-inherited syndrome of *m*itochondrial encephalopathy, *l*actic *a*cidosis, and *s*troke-like episodes. **Menkes' s.,** an X-linked recessive disorder of copper absorption marked by severe cerebral degeneration and arterial changes resulting in death in infancy and by sparse, brittle scalp hair. **Meretoja's s.,** a type of familial amyloid polyneuropathy. **MERRF s.,** a maternally-inherited syndrome of *m*yoclonus with *e*pilepsy and with *r*agged *r*ed *f*ibers. **metabolic s.,** a combination including at least three of the following: abdominal obesity, hypertriglyceridemia, low level of high-density lipoproteins, hypertension, and high fasting glucose level. **methionine malabsorption s.,** an inborn aminoacidopathy marked by white hair, mental retardation, convulsions, attacks of hyperpnea, and urine with an odor like an oasthouse (for drying hops) due to alphahydroxybutyric acid formed by bacterial action on the unabsorbed methionine. **middle lobe s.,** lobar atelectasis in the right middle lobe of the lung, with chronic pneumonitis. **Mikulicz's s.,** chronic bilateral hypertrophy of the lacrimal, parotid, and salivary glands, associated with chronic lymphocytic infiltration; it may be associated with other diseases. **milk-alkali s.,** hypercalcemia without hypercalciuria or hypophosphatemia and with only mild alkalosis and other symptoms attributed to ingestion of milk and absorbable alkali for long periods. **Milkman s.,** a generalized bone disease marked by multiple transparent stripes of absorption in the long and flat bones. **Miller s.,** an inherited syndrome of extensive facial and limb defects, sometimes accompanied by heart defects and hearing loss. **mitral valve prolapse s.,** prolapse of the mitral valve, often with regurgitation; a common, usually benign, often asymptomatic condition characterized by midsystolic clicks and late systolic murmurs on auscultation. **Möbius' s.,** agenesis or aplasia of cranial nerve motor nuclei in congenital bilateral facial palsy, with unilateral or bilateral paralysis of abductors of the eye and sometimes cranial nerve involvement and limb anomalies. **Mohr s.,** an autosomal recessive disorder characterized by brachydactyly, clinodactyly, polydactyly, syndactyly, and bilateral hallucal polysyndactyly; by cranial, facial, lingual, palatal, and mandibular anomalies; and by episodic neuromuscular disturbances. **Morquio's s.,** two biochemically distinct but clinically nearly indistinguishable forms of mucopolysaccharidosis, marked by genu valgum, pigeon breast, progressive flattening of the vertebral bodies, short neck and trunk, progressive deafness, mild corneal clouding, and excretion of keratan sulfate in the urine. **mucocutaneous lymph node s.,** Kawasaki disease. **multiple endocrine deficiency s., multiple glandular deficiency s.,** failure of any combination of endocrine glands, often accompanied by nonendocrine autoimmune abnormalities. **multiple pterygium s.,** an inherited syndrome characterized by pterygia of the neck, axillae, and popliteal, antecubital,

and intercrural areas, accompanied by facial, skeletal, and genital abnormalites. **Munchausen s.,** a subtype of factitious disorder; habitual seeking of hospital treatment for apparent acute illness, the patient giving a plausible and dramatic history, all of which is false. **Munchausen s. by proxy,** see *factitious disorder by proxy,* under *disorder.* **MVP s.,** mitral valve prolapse s. **myelodysplastic s.,** any of a group of related bone marrow disorders of varying duration preceding the development of overt acute myelogenous leukemia; characterized by abnormal hematopoietic stem cells, anemia, neutropenia, and thrombocytopenia. **myeloproliferative s's,** see under *disorder.* **NAME s.,** a syndrome of familial myxomas with cutaneous, cardiac, and endocrine involvement, manifested as *n*evi, *a*trial *m*yxoma, and neurofibroma *e*phelides. **Negri-Jacod s.,** Jacod's s. **Nelson's s.,** the development of an ACTH-producing pituitary tumor after bilateral adrenalectomy in Cushing's syndrome; it is characterized by aggressive growth of the tumor and hyperpigmentation of the skin. **nephrotic s.,** any of a group of diseases involving defective kidney glomeruli, with massive proteinuria, lipiduria with edema, hypoalbuminemia, and hyperlipidemia. **nerve compression s.,** entrapment neuropathy. **Noack s.,** Pfeiffer's s. **nonstaphylococcal scalded skin s.,** toxic epidermal necrolysis. **Noonan's s.,** webbed neck, ptosis, hypogonadism, and short stature, i.e., the phenotype of Turner's syndrome without the gonadal dysgenesis. **obesity-hypoventilation s.,** pickwickian syndrome; a syndrome of obesity, somnolence, hypoventilation, and erythrocytosis. **occipital horn s.,** the X-linked recessive form of cutis laxa. **oculocerebrorenal s.,** an X-linked disorder marked by vitamin D–refractory rickets, hydrophthalmia, congenital glaucoma and cataracts, mental retardation, and renal tubule dysfunction as evidenced by hypophosphatemia, acidosis, and aminoaciduria. **oculodentodigital s., ODD s.,** oculodentodigital dysplasia. **OFD s.,** oral-facial-digital s. **Ömenn's s.,** histiocytic medullary reticulosis. **Opitz s., Opitz-Frias s.,** a familial syndrome consisting of hypertelorism and hernias, and in males also characterized by hypospadias, cryptorchidism, and bifid scrotum. Cardiac, laryngotracheal, pulmonary, anal, and renal abnormalities may also be present. **oral-facial-digital s.,** any of a group of congenital syndromes characterized by oral, facial, and digital anomalies. *Type I,* a male-lethal X-linked dominant disorder, is characterized by camptodactyly, polydactyly, and syndactyly; by cranial, facial, lingual, and dental anomalies; and by mental retardation, familial trembling, alopecia, and seborrhea of the face and milia; *type II* is *Mohr s.*; *type III*, an autosomal recessive disorder, characterized by postaxial hexadactyly, by ocular, lingual, and dental anomalies, and by profound mental retardation. **orbital floor s.**, exophthalmos, diplopia, and anesthesia in the areas innervated by the trigeminal nerve, occurring with a lesion in the floor of the orbit. **organic anxiety s.**, a term used in a former system of classification, denoting an organic mental syndrome marked by prominent, recurrent panic attacks or generalized anxiety caused by a specific organic factor and not associated with delirium. **organic brain s.**, organic mental s. **organic delusional s.**, a term used in a former system of classification, denoting an organic mental syndrome marked by delusions caused by a specific organic factor and not associated with delirium. **organic mental s.**, former term for a constellation of psychological or behavioral signs and symptoms associated with brain dysfunction of unknown or unspecified etiology and grouped according to symptoms rather than etiology. See also under *disorder*. **organic mood s.**, a term used in a former system of classification, denoting an organic mental syndrome marked by manic or depressive mood disturbance caused by a specific organic factor and not associated with delirium. **organic personality s.**, a term used in a former system of classification, denoting an organic mental syndrome characterized by a marked change in behavior or personality, caused by a specific organic factor and not associated with delirium or dementia. **orofaciodigital s.**, oral-facial-digital s. **Ortner s.**, laryngeal paralysis associated with heart disease, due to compression of the recurrent laryngeal nerve between the aorta and a dilated pulmonary artery. **ovarian hyperstimulation s.**, mild to severe ovarian enlargement with exudation of fluid and protein, leading to ascites, pleural or pericardial effusion, azotemia, oliguria, and thromboembolism in women undergoing ovulation induction. **ovarian vein s.**, obstruction of the ureter due to compression by an enlarged or varicose ovarian vein; typically the vein becomes enlarged during pregnancy. **overlap s.**, any of a group of connective tissue disorders that either combine scleroderma with polymyositis or systemic lupus erythematosus or combine systemic lupus erythematosus with rheumatoid arthritis or

polymyositis. **overwear s.**, extreme photophobia, pain, and lacrimation associated with contact lenses, particularly non–gas permeable hard lenses, usually caused by wearing them excessively. **pacemaker s.**, vertigo, syncope, and hypotension, often accompanied by dyspnea, cough, nausea, peripheral edema, and palpitations, all exacerbated or caused by pacemakers that stimulate the ventricle and therefore do not maintain normal atrioventricular synchrony. **pacemaker twiddler's s.**, twiddler's syndrome in a patient with an artificial cardiac pacemaker. **painful bruising s.**, occurrence of one or more spontaneous, chronic recurring painful ecchymoses without antecedent trauma or after insufficient trauma; sometimes precipitated by emotional stress. Because certain patients exhibit autoerythrocyte sensitization in which intradermal injection of their own erythrocytes produces a painful ecchymosis, some consider the condition to be an autosensitivity to a component of the erythrocyte membrane; others consider it to be of psychosomatic or factitious origin. **Pancoast's s.**, 1. neuritic pain and muscle atrophy in the upper limb, and Horner's syndrome, seen with a tumor near the apex of the lung when it involves the brachial plexus. 2. osteolysis in the posterior part of a rib or ribs, sometimes spreading to adjacent vertebrae. **paraneoplastic s.**, a symptom complex arising in a cancer-bearing patient that cannot be explained by local or distant spread of the tumor. **Parinaud's s.**, paralysis of conjugate upward movement of the eyes without paralysis of convergence; associated with tumors of the midbrain. **Parinaud's oculoglandular s.**, a general term applied to conjunctivitis, usually unilateral and of the follicular type, followed by tenderness and enlargement of the preauricular lymph nodes; often due to leptotrichosis but may be associated with other infections. **parkinsonian s.**, a form of parkinsonism due to idiopathic degeneration of the corpus striatum or substantia nigra; frequently a sequela of lethargic encephalitis. **PEP s.**, POEMS s. **Pepper s.**, neuroblastoma with metastases to the liver. **persistent müllerian duct s.**, a hereditary syndrome in males of persistence of müllerian structures in addition to male genital ducts. There may be cryptorchidism on just one side with a contralateral inguinal hernia that contains a testis, uterus, and uterine tube (*hernia uteri inguinalis*). **Peutz-Jeghers s.**, familial gastrointestinal polyposis, especially in the small bowel, associated with mucocutaneous pigmentation. **Pfeiffer s.**, acrocephalosyndactyly, type V; an autosomal dominant disorder characterized by acrocephalosyndactyly associated with broad short thumbs and big toes. **pickwickian s.**, obesity-hypoventilation s. **Pierre Robin s.**, micrognathia with cleft palate, glossoptosis, and absent gag reflex. **plica s.**, pain, tenderness, swelling, and crepitus of the knee joint, sometimes with weakness or locking of the joint, caused by fibrosis and calcification of the synovial plicae. **Plummer-Vinson s.**, dysphagia with glossitis, hypochromic anemia, splenomegaly, and atrophy in the mouth, pharynx, and upper end of the esophagus. **POEMS s.**, polyneuropathy, *organomegaly, endocrinopathy, M* component, and *s*kin changes, sometimes linked to a dysproteinemia such as the presence of unusual monoclonal proteins and light chains. **polyangiitis overlap s.**, a form of systemic necrotizing vasculitis resembling polyarteritis nodosa and allergic angiitis but also showing features of hypersensitivity vasculitis. **polycystic ovary s. (PCOS)**, a clinical symptom complex associated with polycystic ovaries and characterized by oligomenorrhea or amenorrhea, anovulation (hence infertility), and hirsutism; both hyperestrogenism and hyperandrogenism are present. **polysplenia s.**, a congenital syndrome of multiple splenic masses, abnormal position and development of visceral organs, complex cardiovascular defects, and abnormal, usually bilobate, lungs. **post–cardiac injury s.**, fever, chest pain, pleuritis, and pericarditis weeks after injury to the heart, including that due to surgery (*postpericardiotomy s.*) and that due to myocardial infarction (*post–myocardial infarction s.*). **postcardiotomy s.**, postpericardiotomy s. **postcardiotomy psychosis s.**, anxiety, confusion, and perception disturbances occurring three or more days after open heart surgery. **postcommissurotomy s.**, postpericardiotomy s. **postconcussional s.**, physical and personality changes that may occur after concussion of the brain, including amnesia, headache, dizziness, tinnitus, irritability, fatigability, sweating, heart palpitations, insomnia, and difficulty concentrating. **postgastrectomy s.**, dumping s. **post–lumbar puncture s.**, headache in the erect posture, sometimes with nuchal pain, vomiting, diaphoresis, and malaise, all relieved by recumbency, occurring several hours after lumbar puncture; it is due to lowering of intracranial pressure by leakage of cerebrospinal fluid through the needle tract. **postmaturity s.**, a syndrome due to placental insufficiency that causes chronic stress and hypoxia, seen in fetuses and neonates in postterm pregnancies, characterized by decreased subcutaneous fat, skin desquamation, and long fingernails, often with yellow meconium staining of the nails, skin, and vernix. **post–myocardial infarction s.**, post–cardiac injury s. after myocardial infarction. **postpericardiotomy s.**, post–cardiac injury s. after surgery with opening of the pericardium. **Potter's s.**, oligohydramnios sequence. **preexcitation s.**, any syndrome with electrocardiographic signs of preexcitation, such as Wolff-Parkinson-White syndrome; sometimes used synonymously with it. **premenstrual s.**, some or all of the symptoms of depressed, anxious, angry, or irritable mood, emotional lability, bloating, edema, headache, increased fatigue or lethargy, altered appetite or food cravings, breast swelling and tenderness, constipation, and decreased ability to concentrate occurring in the period between ovulation and the onset of menstruation. **prune-belly s.**, a congenital syndrome of deficient or absent anterior abdominal wall musculature, urinary tract anomalies, and undescended testicles. The abdomen is protruding and thin-walled, with wrinkled skin. **Putnam-Dana s.**, subacute combined degeneration of the spinal cord. **Raeder s., Raeder paratrigeminal s.**, unilateral paroxysmal neuralgic pain in the face associated with Horner's syndrome. **Ramsay Hunt s.**, 1. geniculate neuralgia; facial paralysis with otalgia and a vesicular eruption in the external canal of the ear, sometimes extending to the auricle, due to herpes zoster virus infection of the geniculate ganglion. 2. juvenile paralysis agitans (of Hunt). 3. dyssynergia cerebellaris progressiva. **Reiter s.**, the triad of nongonococcal urethritis, conjunctivitis, and arthritis, frequently with mucocutaneous lesions. **respiratory distress s. of the newborn,** a condition seen in infants born prematurely, by cesarean section, or to diabetic mothers, marked by dyspnea and cyanosis; a common, usually fatal subtype is hyaline membrane disease. **Reye's s.**, a rare often fatal encephalopathy of childhood, marked by acute brain swelling with hypoglycemia, fatty infiltration of the liver, hepatomegaly, and disturbed consciousness and seizures, usually seen as a sequel of varicella or an upper airway viral infection. **Rh-null s.**, chronic hemolytic anemia affecting individuals who lack all Rh factors (Rh$_{null}$); it is marked by spherocytosis, stomatocytosis, and increased osmotic fragility. **Riley-Day s.**, familial dysautonomia. **Rosenberg-Bergstrom s.**, an inherited syndrome of hyperuricemia, renal insufficiency, ataxia, and deafness. **Rukavina's s.,** a type of familial amyloid polyneuropathy. **Rundles-Falls s.,** hereditary sideroblastic anemia. **Ruvalcaba's s.,** abnormal shortness of the metacarpal or metatarsal bones, hypoplastic genitalia, and mental and physical retardation of unkown etiology, present from birth in males. **Saethre-Chotzen s.,** Chotzen's s. **salt-depletion s., salt-losing s.,** vomiting, dehydration, hypotension, and sudden death due to very large sodium losses from the body. It may be seen in abnormal losses of sodium into the urine (as in congenital adrenal hyperplasia, adrenocortical insufficiency, or one of the forms of salt-losing nephritis) or in large extrarenal sodium losses, usually from the gastrointestinal tract. **Sanfilippo's s.,** four biochemically distinct but clinically indistinguishable forms of mucopolysaccharidosis, characterized by urinary excretion of heparan sulfate, rapid mental deterioration, and mild Hurler-like symptoms, with death usually occurring before 20 years of age. **scalenus s., scalenus anticus s.,** a type of thoracic outlet syndrome due to compression of the nerves and vessels between a cervical rib and the scalenus anticus muscle, with pain over the shoulder, often extending down the arm or radiating up the back. **Schaumann's s.,** sarcoidosis. **Scheie's s.,** a mild allelic variant of Hurler's syndrome, marked by corneal clouding, clawhand, aortic valve involvement, wide-mouthed facies, genu valgus, and pes cavus; stature, intelligence, and life span are normal. **second impact s.,** acute, usually fatal, brain swelling and increased cranial pressure, caused by repeated head trauma in a short space of time, so that a second concussion occurs before recovery from a previous concussion is complete. **Sertoli-cell–only s.,** congenital absence of the germinal epithelium of the testes, the seminiferous tubules containing only Sertoli cells, marked by testes slightly smaller than normal, azoospermia, and elevated titers of follicle-stimulating hormone and sometimes of luteinizing hormone. **severe acute respiratory s. (SARS),** an infectious respiratory illness characterized by fever, dry cough, and breathing difficulties, often accompanied by headache and body aches; believed to be caused by a coronavirus. **Sézary s.,** a form of cutaneous T-cell lymphoma manifested by exfoliative erythroderma, intense pruritus, peripheral lymphadenopathy, and abnormal hyperchromatic mononuclear cells in the skin, lymph nodes, and peripheral blood. **Sheehan's s.,** postpartum pituitary necrosis.

short-bowel s., short-gut s., any of the malabsorption conditions resulting from massive resection of the small bowel, the degree and kind of malabsorption depending on the site and extent of the resection; it is characterized by diarrhea, steatorrhea, and malnutrition. **shoulder-hand s.,** reflex sympathetic dystrophy limited to the upper limb. **Shprintzen's s.,** velocardiofacial s. **Shwachman, Shwachman-Diamond s.,** primary pancreatic insufficiency and bone marrow failure, characterized by normal sweat chloride values, pancreatic insufficiency, and neutropenia; it may be associated with dwarfism and metaphyseal dysostosis of the hips. **sick sinus s.,** intermittent bradycardia, sometimes with episodes of atrial tachyarrhythmias or periods of sinus arrest, due to malfunction originating in the supraventricular portion of the cardiac conducting system. **Silver-Russell s.,** a syndrome of low birth weight despite normal gestation duration, and short stature, lateral asymmetry, and some increase in gonadotropin secretion. **Sipple's s.,** multiple endocrine neoplasia, type II. **Sjögren's s.,** a symptom complex usually in middle-aged or older women, marked by keratoconjunctivitis sicca, xerostomia, and enlargement of the parotid glands; it is often associated with rheumatoid arthritis and sometimes with systemic lupus erythematosus, scleroderma, or polymyositis. **sleep apnea s.,** sleep apnea. **Smith-Lemli-Opitz s.,** an autosomal recessive syndrome of microcephaly, mental retardation, hypotonia, incomplete development of male genitalia, short nose with anteverted nostrils, and syndactyly of second and third toes. **social breakdown s.,** deterioration of social and interpersonal skills, work habits, and behavior seen in chronically hospitalized psychiatric patients; due to the effects of long-term institutionalization rather than the primary illness. **stagnant loop s.,** stasis s. **staphylococcal scalded skin s.,** an infectious disease, usually affecting infants and young children, following infection with certain strains of *Staphylococcus aureus*, characterized by localized to widespread bullous eruption and exfoliation of the skin leaving raw, denuded areas that make the skin look scalded. **stasis s.,** overgrowth of bacteria in the small intestine secondary to various disorders causing stasis; it is characterized by malabsorption of vitamin B_{12}, steatorrhea, and anemia. **Steele-Richardson-Olszewski s.,** a progressive neurological disorder with onset during the sixth decade, characterized by supranuclear ophthalmoplegia, especially paralysis of the downward gaze, pseudobulbar palsy, dysarthria, dystonic rigidity of the neck and trunk, and dementia. **Stein-Leventhal s.,** polycystic ovary s. **Stevens-Johnson s.,** a sometimes fatal form of erythema multiforme presenting with a flulike prodrome and characterized by severe mucocutaneous lesions; pulmonary, gastrointestinal, cardiac, and renal involvement may occur. **Stewart-Treves s.,** lymphangiosarcoma occurring as a late complication of severe lymphedema of the arm after excision of the lymph nodes, usually in radical mastectomy. **stiff-man s.,** a condition of unknown etiology marked by progressive fluctuating rigidity of axial and limb muscles in the absence of signs of cerebral and spinal cord disease but with continuous electromyographic activity. **stroke s.,** stroke; a condition with sudden onset due to acute vascular lesions of the brain (hemorrhage, embolism, thrombosis, rupturing aneurysm), which may be marked by hemiplegia or hemiparesis, vertigo, numbness, aphasia, and dysarthria, and often followed by permanent neurologic damage. **Sturge's s., Sturge-Kalischer-Weber s., Sturge-Weber s.,** a congenital syndrome consisting of a port-wine stain type of nevus flammeus distributed over the trigeminal nerve accompanied by a similar vascular disorder of the underlying meninges and cerebral cortex. **subclavian steal s.,** cerebral or brain stem ischemia due to vertebrobasilar insufficiency in cases of subclavian steal. **sudden infant death s.,** sudden and unexpected death of an infant who had previously been apparently well, and which is unexplained by careful postmortem examination. **Swyer-James s.,** acquired unilateral hyperlucent lung, with severe airway obstruction during exhalation, oligemia, and a small hilum. **tarsal tunnel s.,** a complex of symptoms resulting from compression of the posterior tibial nerve or of the plantar nerves in the tarsal tunnel, with pain, numbness, and tingling paresthesia of the sole of the foot. **Taussig-Bing s.,** transposition of the great vessels of the heart and a ventricular septal defect straddled by a large pulmonary artery. **testicular feminization s.,** complete androgen resistance. **thoracic outlet s.,** any of several neurovascular syndromes due to compression of the brachial plexus nerve trunks, with pain, paresthesias, vasomotor symptoms, and weakness and small muscle wasting in upper limbs; causes include drooping shoulder girdle, a cervical rib or fibrous band, an abnormal first rib, limb hyperabduction (as during sleep), or compression of the edge of the scalenus anterior muscle. **Tolosa-Hunt s.,** unilateral ophthalmoplegia associated with pain behind the orbit and in the area supplied by the first division of the trigeminal nerve; it is thought to be due to nonspecific inflammation and granulation tissue in the superior orbital fissure or cavernous sinus. **TORCH s.,** (*t*oxoplasmosis, *o*ther agents, *r*ubella, *c*ytomegalovirus, *h*erpes simplex) any of a group of infections seen in neonates as a result of the infectious agent having crossed the placental barrier. **Tourette's s.,** Gilles de la Tourette's s. **Townes' s.,** an inherited disorder of auricular anomalies, anal defects, limb and digit anomalies, and renal deficiencies, occasionally including cardiac disease, deafness, or cystic ovary. **toxic shock s.,** a severe illness with sudden high fever, vomiting, diarrhea, and myalgia, followed by hypotension and, in severe cases, shock; a sunburn-like rash with skin peeling, especially on palms and soles, occurs during the acute phase. It primarily affects menstruating women using tampons, although a few women not using tampons and a few males have been affected. It is thought to be caused by infection with *Staphylococcus aureus.* **Treacher Collins s.,** the incomplete form of mandibulofacial dysostosis. **trisomy 8 s.,** a syndrome due to an extra chromosome 8, usually mosaic (trisomy 8/normal), with mild to severe mental retardation, prominent forehead, deep-set eyes, thick lips, prominent ears, and camptodactyly. **trisomy 11q s.,** a variable syndrome due to an extra long arm of chromosome 11, possibly including preauricular fistulas, hypoplasia of the gallbladder, micropenis, bicornuate uterus, microphthalmos, malformations of the heart, lungs, and brain, seizures, and recurrent infection. **trisomy 13 s.,** holoprosencephaly due to an extra chromosome 13, in which central nervous system defects are associated with mental retardation, along with cleft lip and palate, polydactyly, and dermal pattern anomalies, and abnormalities of the heart, viscera, and genitalia. **trisomy 18 s.,** neonatal hepatitis, mental retardation, scaphocephaly or other skull abnormality, micrognathia, blepharoptosis, low-set ears, corneal opacities, deafness, webbed neck, short digits, ventricular septal defects, Meckel's diverticulum, and other deformities. It is due to an extra chromosome 18. **trisomy 21 s.,** Down s. **Trousseau's s.,** spontaneous venous thrombosis of upper and lower limbs associated with visceral carcinoma. **tumor lysis s.,** severe hyperphosphatemia, hyperkalemia, hyperuricemia, and hypocalcemia after effective induction chemotherapy of rapidly growing malignant neoplasms. **Turcot's s.,** familial polyposis of the colon associated with gliomas of the central nervous sytem. **Turner's s.,** gonadal dysgenesis with short stature, undifferentiated (streak) gonads, and variable abnormalities such as webbing of neck, low posterior hair line, increased carrying angle of elbow, cubitus valgus, and cardiac defects. The genotype is XO (45, X) or X/XX or X/XXX mosaic. The phenotype is female. **twiddler's s.,** dislodgement, breakdown, or other malfunction of an implanted diagnostic device as a result of unconscious or habitual manipulation by the patient. **twin transfusion s., twin–twin transfusion s.,** one caused by twin-to-twin transfusion (q.v.); the donor twin is small, pale, and anemic, while the recipient is large and polycythemic, with an overloaded cardiovascular system. **urethral s.,** symptoms associated with a urethral problem other than infection, including suprapubic aching and cramping, urinary frequency, and bladder complaints such as dysuria, tenesmus, and low back pain. **Usher's s.,** an inherited syndrome of congenital deafness with retinitis pigmentosa, often ending in blindness; mental retardation and gait disturbances may also occur. **velo-cardiofacial s.,** an inherited syndrome of cardiac defects and craniofacial anomalies, often with abnormalities of chromosome 22; learning disabilities often occur, and less often other abnormalities. **Vernet's s.,** paralysis of the glossopharyngeal, vagus, and spinal accessory nerves due to a lesion in the region of the jugular foramen. **Vogt-Koyanagi-Harada s.,** bilateral uveitis with iridocyclitis, exudative choroiditis, meningism, and retinal detachment, accompanied by alopecia, vitiligo, poliosis, loss of visual acuity, headache, vomiting, and deafness; possibly an inflammatory autoimmune disorder. **Waardenburg's s.,** a hereditary, autosomal dominant disorder characterized by wide bridge of the nose due to lateral displacement of the inner canthi and puncta, pigmentary disturbances, including white forelock, heterochromia iridis, white eyelashes, leukoderma, and sometimes cochlear hearing loss. **WAGR s.,** a syndrome of Wilms' tumor, aniridia, genitourinary abnormalities or gonadoblastoma, and mental retardation, due to a deletion in chromosome 11. **Walker-Warburg s., Warburg's s.,** a usually fatal congenital syndrome of hydrocephalus, agyria, various ocular anomalies, and sometimes encephalocele. **Waterhouse-Friderichsen s.,** the malignant or fulminating form of epidemic cerebrospinal meningitis, with sudden onset, short course, fever, collapse, coma, cyanosis, petechiae on the skin and mucous membranes, and bilateral adrenal hemorrhage. **Weber's s.,** paralysis of the oculomotor nerve on the same side as the lesion, causing ptosis, strabismus, and loss of light reflex and accommodation; also spastic hemiplegia on the side opposite the lesion with increased reflexes and loss of superficial reflexes. **Weil's s.,** a severe form of leptospirosis, marked by jaundice usually accompanied by azotemia, hemorrhage, anemia, disturbances of consciousness, and continued fever. **Werner's s.,** premature aging of an adult, with early graying and some hair loss, cataracts, hyperkeratinization, muscular atrophy, scleroderma-like changes in the skin of the limbs, and a high incidence of neoplasm. **Wernicke-Korsakoff s.,** a neuropsychiatric disorder caused by thiamine deficiency, most often due to alcohol abuse, combining the features of Wernicke's encephalopathy and Korsakoff's syndrome. **whiplash shake s.,** subdural hematomas, retinal hemorrhage, and sometimes cerebral contusions caused by the stretching and tearing of cerebral vessels and brain substance, sometimes seen when a very young child is shaken vigorously by the limbs or trunk with the head unsupported; paralysis, visual disturbances, blindness, convulsions, and death may result. **Wilson-Mikity s.,** a rare form of pulmonary insufficiency in low-birth-weight infants, with hyperpnea and cyanosis during the first month of life, sometimes ending in death; there are also radiologic abnormalities. **Wiskott-Aldrich s.,** chronic eczema with chronic suppurative otitis media, anemia, and thrombocytopenic purpura, an immunodeficiency syndrome transmitted as an X-linked recessive trait, with poor antibody response to polysaccharide antigens and dysfunction of cell-mediated immunity. **withdrawal s.,** substance withdrawal. **Wolf-Hirschhorn s.,** a syndrome due to partial deletion of the short arm of chromosome 4, with microcephaly, ocular hypertelorism, epicanthus, cleft palate, micrognathia, low-set ears simplified in form, cryptorchidism, and hypospadias. **Wolff-Parkinson-White (WPW) s.,** the association of paroxysmal tachycardia (or atrial fibrillation) and pre-excitation, in which the electrocardiogram displays a short P–R interval and a wide QRS complex which characteristically shows an early QRS vector (delta wave). **Wyburn-Mason's s.,** arteriovenous aneurysms on one or both sides of the brain, with ocular anomalies, facial nevi, and sometimes mental retardation. **s. X,** angina pectoris or angina-like chest pain associated with normal arteriographic appearance of the coronary arteries. **Zollinger-Ellison s.,** the association of atypical, intractable, sometimes fulminating, peptic ulcers with extreme gastric hyperacidity and benign or malignant gastrinomas in the pancreas.

syn·drom·ic (sin-drom′ik) occurring as a syndrome.

syn·drom·ol·o·gy (sin″drom-ol′ah-je) the field concerned with the taxonomy, etiology, and patterns of congenital malformations.

syn·ech·ia (sĭ-nek′e-ah) pl. *syne′chiae.* [Gr.] adhesion, as of the iris to the cornea or lens. **s. vul′vae,** a congenital condition in which the labia minora are sealed in the midline, with only a small opening below the clitoris through which urination and menstruation may occur.

syn·echot·o·my (sin″ĕ-kot′ah-me) incision of a synechia.

syn·er·e·sis (sĭ-ner′ĕ-sis) a drawing together of the particles of the dispersed phase of a gel, with separation of some of the disperse medium and shrinkage of the gel.

syn·er·get·ic (sin″er-jet′ik) synergic.

syn·er·gic (sin-er′jik) acting together or in harmony.

syn·er·gism (sin′er-jizm) synergy.

syn·er·gist (-er-jist) a muscle or agent which acts with another.

syn·er·gis·tic (sin″er-jis′tik) 1. acting together. 2. enhancing the effect of another force or agent.

syn·er·gy (-er-je) 1. correlated action or cooperation on the part of two or more structures or drugs. 2. in neurology, the faculty by which movements are properly grouped for the performance of acts requiring special adjustments.

syn·es·the·sia (sin″es-the′zhah) 1. a secondary sensation accompanying an actual perception. 2. a dysesthesia in which a stimulus of one sense is perceived as sensation of a different sense, as when a sound produces a sensation of color. 3. a dysesthesia in which a stimulus to one part of the body is experienced as being at a different location.

syn·es·the·si·al·gia (-es-the″ze-al′jah) a painful synesthesia.

syn·ga·my (sing′gah-me) 1. sexual reproduction. 2. the union of two gametes to form a zygote in fertilization. **syn′gamous,** adj.

syn·ge·ne·ic (sin″jĕ-ne′ik) denoting individuals or tissues that have identical genotypes and thus could participate in a syngraft.

syn·gen·e·sis (sin-jen′ĕ-sis) 1. the origin of an individual from a germ cell derived from both parents and not from either one alone. 2. the state of having descended from a common ancestor.

syn·graft (sin′graft) isograft; a graft between genetically identical individuals, typically between identical twins or between animals of a single highly inbred strain.

syn·i·ze·sis (sin″ĭ-ze′sis) 1. occlusion. 2. a mitotic stage in which the nuclear chromatin is massed.

syn·ki·ne·sis (-kĭ-ne′sis) an involuntary movement accompanying a volitional movement. **synkinet′ic,** adj.

syn·ne·cro·sis (-nĕ-kro′sis) symbiosis in which the relationship between populations (or individuals) is mutually detrimental.

syn·oph·thal·mia (-of-thal′me-ah) the usual form of cyclopia, in which the two eyes are more or less completely fused into one.

syn·os·che·os (sin-os′ke-us) adhesion between the penis and scrotum.

syn·os·te·ot·o·my (sin″os-te-ot′ah-me) dissection of the joints.

syn·os·to·sis (-os-to′sis) pl. *synosto′ses.* 1. A union between adjacent bones or parts of a single bone formed by osseous material. 2. the osseous union of bones that are normally distinct. **synostot′ic,** adj.

sy·no·tia (sĭ-no′shah) persistence of the ears in their initial fetal position (horizontal, beneath the mandible).

syn·o·vec·to·my (sin″o-vek′tah-me) excision of a synovial membrane. **radiation s.,** synoviorthesis.

sy·no·via (sĭ-no′ve-ah) synovial fluid.

sy·no·vi·al (-al) 1. pertaining to a synovial membrane. 2. pertaining to or secreting synovia.

sy·no·vi·a·lis (sĭ-no″ve-a′lis) [L.] synovial.

sy·no·vi·o·ma (sĭ-no″ve-o′mah) a tumor of synovial membrane origin.

sy·no·vi·or·the·sis (sĭ-no″ve-or-the′sis) irradiation of a synovial membrane by intra-articular injection of radiocolloids to destroy inflamed synovial tissue.

syno·vi·tis (sin″o-vi′tis) inflammation of a synovial membrane, usually painful, particularly on motion, and characterized by fluctuating swelling, due to effusion in a synovial sac. **dry s., s. sic′ca,** that with little effusion. **simple s.,** that with clear or but slightly turbid effusion. **tendinous s.,** tenosynovitis. **villonodular s.,** proliferation of synovial tissue, especially of the knee joint, composed of synovial villi and fibrous nodules infiltrated by giant cells and macrophages.

sy·no·vi·um (sǐ-no′ve-um) synovial membrane.

syn·te·ny (sin′tĕ-ne) the presence together on the same chromosome of two or more gene loci whether or not in such proximity that they may be subject to linkage. **synten′ic**, adj.

syn·thase (-thās) a term used in the names of some enzymes, particularly lyases, when the synthetic aspect of the reaction is dominant or emphasized.

syn·the·sis (-thĕ-sis) 1. the creation of an integrated whole by the combining of simpler parts or entities. 2. the formation of a chemical compound by the union of its elements or from other suitable components. 3. in psychiatry, the integration of the various elements of the personality. **synthet′ic**, adj.

syn·the·tase (-thĕ-tās) a term used in the names of some of the ligases, no longer favored because of its similarity to synthase and its emphasis on reaction products.

syn·tro·pho·blast (sin-tro′fo-blast) syncytiotrophoblast.

syn·tro·pic (-tro′pik) 1. turning or pointing in the same direction. 2. denoting correlation of several factors, as the relation of one disease to the development or incidence of another.

syn·tro·py (sin′trah-pe) the state of being syntropic.

syph·i·lid (sif′ĭ-lid) any of the skin lesions of secondary syphilis.

syph·i·lis (sif′ĭ-lis) a venereal disease caused by *Treponema pallidum*, leading to many structural and cutaneous lesions, transmitted by direct sexual contact or in utero. See *primary s.*, *secondary s.*, and *tertiary s.* **syphilit′ic**, adj. **congenital s.**, syphilis acquired in utero, manifested by any of several characteristic malformations of teeth or bones and by active mucocutaneous syphilis at birth or shortly thereafter, and by ocular or neurologic changes. **endemic s.**, **nonvenereal s.**, a chronic inflammatory infection caused by a treponema morphologically indistinguishable from *Treponema pallidum*, transmitted nonsexually; the early stage is marked by mucous patches and by moist papules in the axillae and skin folds; a latent stage and finally late complications, including gummata, follow. **primary s.**, syphilis in its first stage, the primary lesion being a chancre, which is infectious and painless; the nearby lymph nodes become hard and swollen. **secondary s.**, syphilis in the second of three stages, with fever, multiform skin eruptions (syphilids), iritis, alopecia, mucous patches, and severe pain in the head, joints, and periosteum. **tertiary s.**, late generalized syphilis, with involvement of many organs and tissues, including skin, bones, joints, and cardiovascular and central nervous systems; see also *tabes dorsalis*.

syph·i·lo·ma (sif″ĭ-lo′mah) a tumor of syphilitic origin; a gumma.

sy·ringe (sǐ-rinj′, sir′inj) an instrument for injecting liquids into or withdrawing them from any vessel or cavity. **air s.**, **chip s.**, a small, fine-nozzled syringe, used to direct an air current into a tooth cavity being excavated, to remove small fragments, or to dry the cavity. **dental s.**, a small syringe used in operative dentistry, containing an anesthetic solution. **hypodermic s.**, one for introduction of liquids through a hollow needle into subcutaneous tissues. **Luer's s.**, **Luer-Lok s.**, a glass syringe for intravenous and hypodermic use.

syr·in·gec·to·my (sir″in-jek′tah-me) excision of the walls of a fistula.

syr·in·gi·tis (sir″in-ji′tis) inflammation of the auditory tube.

syring(o)- word element [Gr.], *tube; fistula.*

sy·rin·go·ad·e·no·ma (sǐ-ring″go-ad″e-no′mah) syringocystadenoma.

sy·rin·go·bul·bia (-bul′be-ah) the presence of cavities in the medulla oblongata.

sy·rin·go·car·ci·no·ma (-kahr″sǐ-no′mah) cancer of a sweat gland.

sy·rin·go·cele (sǐ-ring′go-sēl) 1. a cystlike swelling in a tubular structure of the body. 2. myelocele.

sy·rin·go·coele (sǐ-ring′go-sēl) the central canal of the spinal cord.

sy·rin·go·cys·tad·e·no·ma (sǐ-ring″go-sis″tad-ĕ-no′mah) a benign cystic tumor of the sweat glands.

sy·rin·go·cys·to·ma (-sis-to′mah) syringocystadenoma.

sy·rin·go·ma (sir″ing-go′mah) a benign tumor believed to originate from the ductal portion of the eccrine sweat glands, characterized by dilated cystic sweat ducts in a fibrous stroma.

sy·rin·go·my·elia (sǐ-ring″go mi e′le-ah) a slowly progressive syndrome of varying etiology, in which cavitation occurs in the central segments of the spinal cord, generally in the cervical region, with resulting neurologic defects; thoracic scoliosis is often present.

sy·rin·got·o·my (sir″ing-got′ah-me) fistulotomy.

syr·inx (sir′inks) [Gr.] 1. a tube or pipe. 2. fistula.

syr·up (sir′up) a concentrated solution of a sugar, such as sucrose, in water or other aqueous liquid, sometimes with a medicinal agent added; usually used as a flavored vehicle for drugs. It is commonly expanded to include any liquid dosage form (e.g., oral suspension) in a sweet and viscid vehicle.

sys·tal·tic (sis-tahl′tik) alternately contracting and dilating; pulsating.

sys·tem (sis′tim) 1. a set or series of interconnected or interdependent parts or entities (objects, organs, or organisms) that act together in a common purpose or produce results impossible by action of one alone. 2. a school or method of practice based on a specific set of principles. **alimentary s.,** digestive s. **auditory s.,** the series of structures by which sounds are received from the environment and conveyed as signals to the central nervous system; it consists of the outer, middle, and inner ear and the tracts in the auditory pathways. **autonomic nervous s.,** the portion of the nervous system concerned with regulation of activity of cardiac muscle, smooth muscle, and glands, usually restricted to the sympathetic and parasympathetic nervous systems. **Bethesda S.,** a classification of cervical and vaginal cytology used in cytopathologic diagnosis. **cardiovascular s.,** the heart and blood vessels, by which blood is pumped and circulated through the body. See Plates 15–24. **CD s.** [cluster *designation*], a system for classifying cell surface markers expressed by lymphocytes based on a computer analysis grouping similar monoclonal antibodies raised against human leukocyte antigens. **centimetergram-second s. (CGS, cgs),** a system of measurements in which the units are based on the centimeter as the unit of length, the gram as the unit of mass, and the second as the unit of time. **central nervous s. (CNS),** the brain and spinal cord. **centrencephalic s.,** the neurons in the central core of the brain stem from the thalamus to the medulla oblongata, connecting the two hemispheres. **chromaffin s.,** the chromaffin cells of the body considered collectively. **circulatory s.,** channels through which nutrient fluids of the body flow; often restricted to the vessels conveying blood. **colloid s., colloidal s.,** see *colloid* (2). **conduction s. of heart,** a system of specialized muscle fibers that generate and transmit cardiac impulses and coordinate contractions, comprising the sinoatrial and atrioventricular nodes, bundle of His and its bundle branches, and subendocardial branches of Purkinje fibers. **digestive s.,** the organs concerned with ingestion, digestion, and absorption of food or nutritional elements. **endocrine s.,** the glands and other structures that elaborate and secrete hormones that are released directly into the circulatory system, influencing metabolism and other body processes; included are the pituitary, thyroid, parathyroid, and adrenal glands, pineal body, gonads, pancreas, and paraganglia. **enteric nervous s.,** the enteric plexus, sometimes considered separately from the autonomic nervous system because it has independent local reflex activity. **extrapyramidal s.,** a functional, rather than anatomical, unit comprising the nuclei and fibers (excluding those of the pyramidal tract) involved in motor activities; they control and coordinate especially the postural, static, supporting, and locomotor mechanisms. It includes the corpus striatum, subthalamic nucleus, substantia nigra, and red nucleus, along with their interconnections with the reticular formation, cerebellum, and cerebrum. **genitourinary s.,** urogenital s. **haversian s.,** a haversian canal and its concentrically arranged lamellae, constituting the basic unit of structure in compact bone (osteon). **heterogeneous s.,** a system or structure made up of mechanically separable parts, as an emulsion or a suspension. **His-Purkinje s.,** a portion of the conducting system of the heart, usually referring specifically to the segment beginning with the bundle of His and ending at the terminus of the Purkinje fiber network within the ventricles. **homogeneous s.,** a system or structure made up of parts which cannot be mechanically separated, as a solution. **hypophysioportal s., hypothalamo-hypophysial portal s.,** the venules connecting the capillaries (gomitoli) in the median eminence of the hypothalamus with the sinusoidal capillaries of the adenohypophysis. **immune s.,** a complex system of cellular and molecular components having the primary functions of distinguishing self from not self and of defense against foreign organisms or substances. **International S. of Units,** see *SI unit,* under *unit.* **keratinizing s.,** the cells composing the bulk of the epithelium of the epidermis, which are of ectodermal origin and undergo keratinization and form the dead superficial layers of the skin. **limbic s.,** a group of brain structures (including the hippocampus, gyrus fornicatus, and amygdala) common to all mammals; it is associated with olfaction, autonomic functions, and certain aspects of emotion and behavior. **locomotor s.,** the structures in a living organism responsible for locomotion, in humans consisting of the muscles, joints, and ligaments of the lower limbs as well as the arteries and nerves that supply them. **lymphatic s.,** the lymphatic vessels and lymphoid tissue, considered collectively. **lymphoid s.,** the lymphoid tissue of the body, collectively; it consists of (a) a central component, including the bone marrow, thymus, and an unidentified portion called bursal equivalent tissue; and (b) a peripheral component consisting of lymph nodes, spleen, and gut-associated lymphoid tissue (tonsils, Peyer's patches). **lympho-reticular s.,** the tissues of the lymphoid and reticuloendothelial systems considered together as one system. **masticatory s.,** the bony and soft structures of the face and mouth involved in mastication, and the vessels and nerves supplying them. **metric s.,** a decimal system of weights and measures based on the meter; see *Table of Weights and Measures.* **mononuclear phagocyte s. (MPS),** the set of cells consisting of macrophages and their precursors (blood monocytes and their precursor cells in bone marrow). The term has been proposed to replace reticuloendothelial system, which does not include all macrophages and does include other unrelated cell types. **muscular s.,** the muscles of the body considered collectively; generally restricted to the voluntary, skeletal muscles. **nervous s.,** the organ system which, along with the endocrine system, correlates the adjustments and reactions of the organism to its internal and external environment, comprising the central and peripheral nervous systems. See Plates 8–14. **parasympathetic nervous s.,** the craniosacral portion of the autonomic nervous system, its preganglionic fibers traveling with cranial nerves III, VII, IX, X, and XI, and with the second to fourth sacral ventral roots; it innervates the heart, smooth muscle and glands of the head and neck, and thoracic, abdominal, and pelvic viscera. **peripheral nervous s.,** all elements of the nervous system (nerves and ganglia) outside the brain and spinal cord. **portal s.,** an arrangement by which blood collected from one set of capillaries passes through a large vessel or vessels and another set of capillaries before returning to the systemic circulation, as in the pituitary gland and liver. **Purkinje s.,** a portion of the conducting system of the heart, usually referring specifically to the Purkinje network. **respiratory s.,** respiratory tract; the tubular and cavernous organs that allow atmospheric air to reach the membranes across which gases are exchanged with the blood. See Plates 25

and 26. **reticular activating s.,** the system of cells of the reticular formation of the medulla oblongata that receive collaterals from the ascending sensory pathways and project to higher centers; they control the overall degree of central nervous system activity, including wakefulness, attentiveness, and sleep; abbreviated RAS. **reticulo-endothelial s. (RES),** a group of cells having the ability to take up and sequester inert particles and vital dyes, including macrophages and macrophage precursors, specialized endothelial cells lining the sinusoids of the liver, spleen, and bone marrow, and reticular cells of lymphatic tissue (macrophages) and bone marrow (fibroblasts). See also *mononuclear phagocyte s.* **SI s.,** see under *unit.* **stomatognathic s.,** structures of the mouth and jaws, considered collectively, as they subserve the functions of mastication, deglutition, respiration, and speech. **sympathetic nervous s. (SNS),** the thoracolumbar part of the autonomic nervous system, the preganglionic fibers of which arise from cell bodies in the thoracic and first three lumbar segments of the spinal cord; postganglionic fibers are distributed to the heart, smooth muscle, and glands of the entire body. **urogenital s.,** the urinary system considered together with the organs of reproduction. See Plate 28. **vascular s.,** circulatory s. **visual s.,** the series of structures by which visual sensations are received from the environment and conveyed as signals to the central nervous system; it consists of the photoreceptors in the retina and the afferent fibers in the optic nerve, chiasm, and tract.

sys·te·ma (sis-te′mah) [Gr.] system.

sys·tem·ic (sis-tem′ik) pertaining to or affecting the body as a whole.

sys·to·le (sis′to-le) the contraction, or period of contraction, of the heart, especially of the ventricles. **systol′ic,** adj. **aborted s.,** a weak systole, usually premature, not associated with pulsation of a peripheral artery. **atrial s.,** the contraction of the atria by which blood is propelled from them into the ventricles. **extra s.,** extrasystole. **ventricular s.,** the contraction of the cardiac ventricles by which blood is forced into the aorta and pulmonary artery.

sys·trem·ma (sis-trem′ah) a cramp in the muscles of the calf of the leg.

syz·y·gy (siz′ĭ-je) the conjunction and fusion of organs without the loss of identity. **syzyg′ial,** adj.

T

T tera-; tesla; threonine; thymine or thymidine; tetanus toxoid; thoracic vertebrae (T1–T12); intraocular tension (see under *pressure*.)

2,4,5-T a toxic chlorphenoxy herbicide (2,4,5-trichlorophenoxyacetic acid), a component of Agent Orange.

T absolute temperature.

$T_{1/2}$ half-life.

T_3 triiodothyronine.

T_4 thyroxine.

T_m transport maximum. In kidney function tests, it is expressed as T_m with inferior letters representing the substance used in the test; e.g., $T_{m_{PAH}}$ for *p*-aminohippuric acid.

t translocation.

t time; temperature.

$t_{1/2}$ half-life.

TA *Terminologia Anatomica*; toxin-antitoxin.

Ta tantalum.

tab·a·nid (tab'ah-nid) any gadfly of the family Tabanidae, including the horseflies and deerflies.

Ta·ba·nus (tah-ba'nus) a genus of biting, bloodsucking horse flies that transmit trypanosomes and anthrax to various animals.

ta·bes (ta'bēz) 1. wasting of the body or a part of it. 2. t. dorsalis. **t. dorsa'lis,** parenchymatous neurosyphilis marked by degeneration of the posterior columns and posterior roots and ganglion of the spinal cord, with muscular incoordination, paroxysms of intense pain, visceral crises, disturbances of sensation, and various trophic disturbances, especially of bones and joints. **t. mesente'rica,** tuberculosis of mesenteric glands in children.

ta·bes·cent (tah-bes'ent) wasting away.

ta·bet·ic (tah-bet'ik) pertaining to or affected with tabes.

ta·bet·i·form (tah-bet'ĭ-form) resembling tabes.

tab·la·ture (tab'lah-chur) separation of the chief cranial bones into inner and outer tables, separated by a diploë.

ta·ble (ta'b'l) a flat layer or surface. **inner t. of skull,** the inner compact layer of the bones covering the brain. **outer t. of skull,** the outer compact layer of the bones covering the brain. **vitreous t.,** inner t. of skull.

tab·let (tab'let) a solid dosage form containing a medicinal substance with or without a suitable diluent. **buccal t.,** one that dissolves when held between the cheek and gum, permitting direct absorption of the active ingredient through the oral mucosa. **enteric-coated t.,** one coated with material that delays release of the medication until after it leaves the stomach. **sublingual t.,** one that dissolves when held beneath the tongue, permitting direct absorption of the active ingredient by the oral mucosa.

ta·bo·pa·re·sis (ta″bo-pah-re'sis) general paresis occurring concomitantly with tabes dorsalis.

tache (tahsh) [Fr.] a spot or blemish. **tachet'ic,** adj. **t. blanche** (blahnsh), a white spot on the liver in certain infectious diseases. **t's bleuâtres** (blōō-ahtr'), maculae caeruleae. **t. cérébrale** (sa-ra-brahl'), a congested streak produced by drawing the nail across the skin; a concomitant of various nervous or cerebral diseases. **t. motrice** (mo-trēs'), motor end plate. **t. noire** (nwahr), an ulcer covered with a black crust, a characteristic local reaction at the presumed site of the infective bite in certain tickborne rickettsioses.

tach·og·ra·phy (tah-kog'rah-fe) the recording of the movement and speed of the blood current.

tachy- word element [Gr.], *rapid; swift.*

tachy·ar·rhyth·mia (tak″e-ah-rith'me-ah) any disturbance of the heart rhythm in which the heart rate is abnormally increased.

tachy·car·dia (-kahr'de-ah) abnormally rapid heart rate. **tachycar'diac,** adj. **atrial t.,** a rapid cardiac rate, usually 160–190 per minute, originating from an atrial locus. **atrioventricular (AV) junctional t., atrioventricular (AV) nodal t.,** junctional t. **atrioventricular nodal reentrant t.,** that resulting from reentry in or around the atrioventricular node; it may be *antidromic*, in which conduction is anterograde over the accessory pathway and retrograde over the normal conduction pathway or *orthodromic*, in which conduction is anterograde over the normal conduction pathway and retrograde over the accessory pathway. **atrioventricular reciprocating t. (AVRT),** a reentrant tachycardia in which the reentrant circuit contains both the normal conduction pathway and an accessory pathway as integral parts. **chaotic atrial t.,** that characterized by atrial rates of 100 to 130 beats per minute, markedly variable P wave morphology, and irregular P–P intervals, often leading to atrial fibrillation. **circus movement t.,** reentrant t. **ectopic t.,** rapid heart action in response to impulses arising outside the sinoatrial node. **junctional t.,** that arising in response to impulses originating in the atrioventricular junction, i.e., in the atrioventricular node, with a heart rate greater than 75 beats per minute. **multifocal atrial t. (MAT),** chaotic atrial t. **nonparoxysmal junctional t.,** a junctional tachycardia of slow onset, with a heart rate of 70 to 130 beats per minute; due to enhanced automaticity of the atrioventricular junctional tissue, often secondary to disease or trauma. **paroxysmal t.,** rapid heart action that starts and stops abruptly. **paroxysmal supraventricular t. (PSVT),** supraventricular tachycardia occurring in attacks of rapid onset and cessation, usually due to a reentrant circuit. **reciprocating t.,** a tachycardia due to a reentrant mechanism and characterized by a reciprocating rhythm. **reentrant t.,** any tachycardia characterized by a reentrant circuit. **sinus t. (ST),** tachycardia originating in the sinus node; normal during exercise or anxiety but also associated with shock, hypotension, hypoxia, congestive heart failure, fever, and various high output states. **supraventricular t. (SVT),** any regular tachycardia in which the point of stimulation is above the bundle branches; it may also include those arising from large reentrant circuits that encompass both atrial and ventricular sites. **ventricular t.,** an abnormally rapid ventricular rhythm with aberrant ventricular excitation, usually above 150 beats per minute, generated within the ventricle, and most often associated with atrioventricular dissociation.

tachy·dys·rhyth·mia (-dis-rith′me-ah) an abnormal heart rhythm with a rate greater than 100 beats per minute in an adult; the term *tachyarrhythmia* is usually used instead.

tachy·gas·tria (-gas′tre-ah) a sequence of electric potentials at abnormally high frequencies in the gastric antrum.

tachy·ki·nin (-ki′nin) any of a family of peptides structurally and functionally similar to substance P; all are potent, rapidly acting secretagogues and cause smooth muscle contraction and vasodilation.

tachy·pha·gia (-fa′jah) rapid eating.

tachy·phy·lax·is (-fĭ-lak′sis) 1. rapid immunization against the effect of toxic doses of an extract or serum by previous injection of small doses of it. 2. rapidly decreasing response to a drug or physiologically active

agent after administration of a few doses. **tachyphylac′tic,** adj.

tach·yp·nea (tak″ip-ne′ah) very rapid respiration.

tachy·rhyth·mia (tak″e-rith′me-ah) tachycardia.

tach·ys·te·rol (tak-is′ter-ol) an isomer of ergosterol produced by irradiation.

tac·rine (tak′rēn) a cholinesterase inhibitor used to improve cognitive performance in dementia of the Alzheimer type; used as the hydrochloride salt.

tac·ro·li·mus (tak″ro-li′mus) a macrolide immunosuppressant having actions similar to those of cyclosporine; used to prevent rejection of organ transplants; also used topically to treat moderate to severe atopic dermatitis.

tac·tile (tak′til) pertaining to touch.

tac·tom·e·ter (tak-tom′ĕ-ter) an instrument for measuring tactile sensibility.

Tae·nia (te′ne-ah) a genus of tapeworms. **T. echinococ′cus,** *Echinococcus granulosus.* **T. sagina′ta,** a species 4–8 meters long, found in the adult form in the human intestine and in the larval state in muscles and other tissues of cattle and other ruminants; human infection usually results from eating inadequately cooked beef. **T. so′lium,** a species 1–2 meters long, found in the adult intestine; the larval form most often is found in muscle and other tissues of the pig; human infection results from eating inadequately cooked pork.

tae·nia (te′ne-ah) pl. *tae′niae.* [L.] 1. a flat band or strip of soft tissue. 2. a tapeworm of the genus *Taenia.* **tae′niae co′li,** three thickened bands formed by the longitudinal fibers in the muscular tunic of the large intestine and extending from the vermiform appendix to the rectum.

tae·ni·a·cide (-sīd″) 1. destruction of tapeworms. 2. an agent lethal to tapeworms.

tae·ni·a·fuge (-fūj″) an agent that expels tapeworms. **taeniafu′gal,** adj.

tae·ni·a·sis (te-ni′ah-sis) infection with tapeworms of the genus *Taenia.*

tai chi (ti′ che′) [Chinese] a system of postures linked by elegant and graceful movements, originating in China, whose purpose is to balance yin and yang, creating inner and outer harmony. It improves cardiovascular, musculoskeletal, and respiratory function and increases central nervous system function, and can be used for treating various conditions.

tail (tāl) any slender appendage. **t. of spermatozoon,** the flagellum of a spermatozoon, which contains the axonema; it has four regions: the neck, middle piece, principal piece, and end piece.

talc (talk) a native hydrous magnesium silicate, sometimes with a small amount of aluminum silicate; in purified form, used as a dusting powder and pharmaceutic aid.

tal·co·sis (tal-ko'sis) talc pneumoconiosis.

tal·i·pes (tal'ĭ-pēz) a congenital deformity in which the foot is twisted out of shape or position; it may be in dorsiflexion (*t. calca'neus*), in plantar flexion (*t. equi'nus*), abducted and everted (*t. val'gus* or *flatfoot*), abducted and inverted (*t. va'rus*), or various combinations (*t. calcaneoval'gus, t. calcaneo-va'rus, t. equinoval'gus,* or *t. equinova'rus*).

tal·i·pom·a·nus (tal'ĭ-pom'ah-nus) club-hand.

ta·lo·cal·ca·ne·al (ta"lo-kal-ka'ne-al) per-taining to the talus and calcaneus.

ta·lo·cru·ral (-krōōr'al) pertaining to the talus and the leg bones.

ta·lo·fib·u·lar (-fib'u-ler) pertaining to the talus and fibula.

ta·lo·na·vic·u·lar (-nah-vik'u-ler) pertaining to the talus and navicular bone.

ta·lus (ta'lus) pl. *ta'li.* [L.] see *Table of Bones.*

ta·mas (tah-mus') [Sanskrit] according to ayurveda, one of the three gunas, character-ized by inertia and responsible for stability, lethargy, and retentiveness in the mind and body.

tam·bour (tam-boor') a drum-shaped appli-ance used in transmitting movements in a recording instrument.

ta·mox·i·fen (tah-mok'sĭ-fen) a nonsteroidal antiestrogen used as the citrate salt in the prophylaxis and treatment of breast cancer.

tam·pon (tam'pon) [Fr.] a pack, pad, or plug made of cotton, sponge, or other material, variously used in surgery to plug the nose, vagina, etc., for the control of hemorrhage or the absorption of secretions.

tam·pon·ade (tam"po-nād') 1. surgical use of a tampon. 2. pathologic compression of a part. **balloon t.**, esophagogastric tampo-nade by means of a device with a triple-lumen tube and two inflatable balloons, the third lumen providing for aspiration of blood clots. **cardiac t.**, compression of the heart caused by increased intrapericardial pressure due to collection of blood or fluid in the pericardium. **esophagogastric t.**, the exer-tion of direct pressure against bleeding esophageal varices by insertion of a tube with a balloon in the esophagus and one in the stomach and inflating them.

tam·su·lo·sin (tam-soo'lo-sin) an α_1-ad-renergic blocking agent specific for the receptors in the prostate; used as the hydro-chloride salt in the treatment of benign prostatic hyperplasia.

tan·gen·ti·al·i·ty (tan-jen"she-al'ĭ-te) a pattern of speech characterized by oblique, digressive, or irrelevant replies to questions; the responses never approach the point of the questions.

tan·nate (tan'āt) any of the salts of tannic acid, all of which are astringent.

tan·nic ac·id (-ik) a substance obtained from nutgalls, used as an ingredient of derma-tologic preparations and formerly used as an astringent.

tan·nin (-in) tannic acid.

tan·ta·lum (tan'tah-lum) chemical element (see *Table of Elements*), at. no. 73, symbol Ta; a noncorrosive and malleable metal that has been used for plates or disks to replace cranial defects, for wire sutures, and for making prosthetic appliances.

tan·y·cyte (tan'ĭ-sīt) a modified cell of the ependyma of the infundibulum of the hypothalamus; its function is unknown, but it may transport hormones from the cer-ebrospinal fluid into the hypophyseal circula-tion or from the hypothalamic neurons to the cerebrospinal fluid.

tap (tap) 1. a quick, light blow. 2. to drain off fluid by paracentesis. **spinal t.**, lumbar puncture.

tape (tāp) a long, narrow strip of fabric or other flexible material. **adhesive t.**, a strip of fabric or other material evenly coated on one side with a pressure-sensitive adhesive material.

tap·ei·no·ceph·a·ly (tap"ĭ-no-sef'ah-le) flatness of the skull, with a vertical index below 72. **tapeinocephal'ic**, adj.

ta·pe·to·ret·i·nal (tah-pe"to-ret'ĭ-n'l) per-taining to the pigmented layer of the retina.

ta·pe·tum (tah-pe'tum) pl. *tape'ta.* [L.] 1. a covering structure or layer of cells. 2. a stratum of fibers of the corpus callosum on the superolateral aspect of the occipital horn of the lateral ventricle.

tape·worm (tāp'werm) cestode; a parasitic intestinal worm with a flattened, bandlike form. **armed t.**, *Taenia solium.* **beef t.**, *Taenia saginata.* **broad t.**, *Diphyllobothrium latum.* **dog t.**, *Dipylidium caninum.* **fish t.**, *Diphyllobothrium latum.* **hydatid t.**, *Echino-coccus granulosus.* **pork t.**, *Taenia solium.* **unarmed t.**, *Taenia saginata.*

ta·pote·ment (tah-pōt-maw') [Fr.] a tap-ping or percussing movement in massage.

tar (tahr) a dark-brown or black, viscid liquid obtained from various species of pine or from bituminous coal (*coal t.*). It is used for topical treatment of skin conditions, including eczema, psoriasis, and dandruff, but is toxic and carcinogenic by inhalation or ingestion.

ta·ran·tu·la (tah-ran'chu-lah) a venomous spider whose bite causes local inflammation and pain, usually not to a severe extent, including *Eurypelma hentzii* (American t.), *Sericopelma communis* (black t.) of Panama, and *Lycosa tarentula* (European wolf spider).

tar·dive (tahr'div) [Fr.] tardy; late.

tare (tār) 1. the weight of the vessel in which a substance is weighed. 2. to weigh a vessel in order to allow for its weight when the vessel and a substance are weighed together.

tar·get (tahr'gĕt) 1. an object or area toward which something is directed, such as the area of the anode of an x-ray tube where the electron beam collides, causing the emission of x-rays. 2. a cell or organ that is affected by a particular agent, e.g., a hormone or drug.

tar·ich·a·tox·in (tar'ik-ah-tok″sin) name given to the lethal neurotoxin tetrodotoxin when it comes from the newt *Taricha*.

tar·ry (tahr'e) 1. filled with or covered by tar. 2. thick, dark; resembling tar.

tar·sad·e·ni·tis (tahr″sad-ĕ-ni'tis) inflammation of the meibomian glands and tarsus.

tar·sal (tahr's'l) pertaining to a tarsus.

tar·sal·gia (tahr-sal'jah) pain in a tarsus.

tar·sa·lia (tahr-sa'le-ah) the bones of the tarsus.

tar·sa·lis (tahr-sa'lis) [L.] tarsal.

tar·sec·to·my (tahr-sek'tah-me) 1. excision of one or more bones of the tarsus. 2. excision of a portion of the tarsus of an eyelid.

tar·si·tis (tahr-si'tis) blepharitis.

tars(o)- word element [Gr.], *edge of eyelid; tarsus of the foot; instep.*

tar·soc·la·sis (tahr-sok'lah-sis) surgical fracturing of the tarsus of the foot.

tar·so·con·junc·ti·val (tahr″so-kon-junk'tĭ-v'l) pertaining to the tarsus of an eyelid and the conjunctiva.

tar·so·ma·la·cia (-mah-la'shah) softening of the tarsus of an eyelid.

tar·so·meta·tar·sal (-met″ah-tar'sal) pertaining to the tarsus and metatarsus.

tar·so·plas·ty (tahr'so-plas″te) blepharoplasty.

tar·sop·to·sis (tahr″sop-to'sis) flatfoot.

tar·sor·rha·phy (tahr-sor'ah-fe) suture of a portion of or the entire upper and lower eyelids together; done to shorten or entirely close the palpebral fissure.

tar·sot·o·my (tahr-sot'ah-me) blepharotomy.

tar·sus (tahr'sus) 1. ankle; the seven bones (talus, calcaneus, navicular, medial, intermediate and lateral cuneiform, and cuboid) composing the joint between the foot and

leg. 2. the plate of connective tissue forming the framework of an eyelid.

tar·tar (tahr'ter) dental calculus.

tar·tar·ic ac·id (tahr-tar'ik) any of several isomers of the dicarboxylic acid $HOOC(CHOH)_2COOH$, occurring especially in grapes.

tar·trate (tahr'trāt) a salt of tartaric acid.

tas·tant (tās'tant) any substance, e.g., salt, capable of eliciting gustatory excitation, i.e., stimulating the sense of taste.

taste (tāst) 1. the sense effected by the gustatory receptors in the tongue. Four qualities are distinguished: sweet, sour, salty, and bitter. 2. the act of perceiving by this sense.

tast·er (tās'ter) an individual capable of tasting a particular test substance (e.g., phenylthiourea, used in genetic studies).

Tat·lock·ia mic·da·dei (tat-lok'e-ah mik-da'de-i) Pittsburgh pneumonia agent; a waterborne legionella-like organism implicated as a cause of pneumonia.

tat·too·ing (tah-too'ing) the introduction, by punctures, of permanent colors in the skin. **t. of cornea,** permanent coloring of the cornea, chiefly to conceal leukomatous spots.

tau·rine (taw'rēn) an oxidized sulfur-containing amine occurring conjugated in the bile, usually as cholyltaurine or chenodeoxycholyltaurine; it may also be a central nervous system neurotransmitter or neuromodulator.

tau·ro·cho·late (taw″ro-ko'lāt) a salt of taurocholic acid.

tau·to·mer (taw'to-mer) a chemical compound exhibiting, or capable of exhibiting, tautomerism.

tau·tom·er·al (taw-tom'er-al) pertaining to the same part; said especially of neurons and neuroblasts sending processes to aid in formation of the white matter in the same side of the spinal cord.

tau·tom·er·ase (-ās) any enzyme catalyzing the interconversion of tautomers.

tau·tom·er·ism (-izm) the relationship that exists between two constitutional isomers (those having the same atoms linked in different structures) that are in chemical equilibrium and freely change from one to the other. **tautomer'ic,** adj.

tax·is (tak'sis) [Gr.] 1. an orientation movement of a motile organism in response to a stimulus, either toward (positive) or away from (negative) the source of the stimulus. 2. exertion of force in manual replacement of a displaced organ or part.

-taxis word element [Gr.], *movement* of an organism in response to an external stimulus.

tax·on (tak'son) pl. *tax'a.* 1. A particular taxonomic grouping, e.g., a species, genus, family, order, class, phylum, or kingdom. 2. the name applied to a taxonomic grouping.

tax·on·o·my (tak-son'ah-me) the orderly classification of organisms into appropriate categories (taxa), with application of suitable and correct names. **taxonom′ic,** adj. **numerical t.,** a method of classifying organisms solely on the basis of the number of shared phenotypic characters, each character usually being given equal weight; used primarily in bacteriology.

ta·zar·o·tene (tah-zar'o-tēn) a retinoid prodrug used topically in the treatment of acne vulgaris and psoriasis.

taz·o·bac·tam (taz″o-bak'tam) a β-lactamase inhibitor having antibacterial actions and uses similar to those of sulbactam; used as the sodium salt.

Tb terbium.

Tc technetium.

TCM traditional Chinese medicine.

TD₅₀ median toxic dose.

Td tetanus and diphtheria toxoids, adult use; see *diphtheria toxoid,* under *toxoid.*

Te tellurium.

tea (te) 1. *Camellia sinensis* or its dried leaves, which contain caffeine, theophylline, tannic acid, and a volatile oil. Tea is either *green* or *black* depending on the curing method. 2. a decoction of these leaves, used as a stimulating beverage or soothing drink for various abdominal discomforts. Green tea has been used for prevention of dental caries and is also used in traditional Chinese medicine, ayurveda, and homeopathy. 3. any decoction or infusion.

tears (tērz) the watery, slightly alkaline and saline secretion of the lacrimal glands, which moistens the conjunctiva.

tease (tēz) to pull apart gently with fine needles to permit microscopic examination.

teat (tēt) nipple (1).

tea tree (te′ tre″) a tree, *Melaleuca alternifolia,* native to eastern Australia, from whose leaves and branches tea tree oil is obtained.

teb·u·tate (teb'u-tāt) USAN contraction for tertiary butyl acetate.

tech·ne·ti·um (tek-ne'she-um) chemical element (see *Table of Elements*), at. no. 43, symbol Tc. **t. 99m,** the most frequently used radioisotope in nuclear medicine, a gamma emitter (0.141 MeV) having a half-life of 6.01 hours.

tech·ni·cian (tek-nish'un) a person skilled in the performance of the technical or procedural aspects of a health care profession, usually with at least an associate degree, working under the supervision of a physician, therapist, technologist, or other health care professional.

tech·nique (tek-nēk′) a maneuver, method, or procedure. **dot blot t.,** a technique for protein detection, analysis, and identification that is similar to the Western blot technique but in which the samples are merely spotted directly onto the membrane through circular templates. **fluorescent antibody t.,** an immunofluorescence technique in which antigen in tissue sections is located by homologous antibody labeled with fluorochrome or by treating the antigen with unlabeled antibody followed by a second layer of labeled antiglobulin which is reactive with the unlabeled antibody. **isolation-perfusion t.,** a technique for administering high doses of a chemotherapy agent to a region while protecting the patient from toxicity; the region is isolated and perfused with the drug by means of a pump-oxygenator. **Jerne plaque t.,** a hemolytic technique for detecting antibody-producing cells: a suspension of presensitized lymphocytes is mixed in an agar gel with erythrocytes; after a period of incubation, complement is added and a clear area of lysis of red cells can be seen around each of the antibody-producing cells. **Mohs′ t.,** microscopically controlled excision of skin cancers in which the tissue to be excised is first fixed in situ with zinc chloride paste *(Mohs′ chemosurgery),* or in which only serial excisions of fresh tissue are used for microscopic analysis *(Mohs′ surgery).* **Northern blot t.,** a technique analagous to a Southern blot technique but performed on fragments of RNA. **Pomeroy t.,** sterilization by ligation of a loop of fallopian tube and resection of the tied loop. **Southern blot t.,** a technique for transferring DNA fragments separated by electrophoresis onto a filter, on which specific fragments can then be detected by their hybridization to defined probes. **Southwestern blot t.,** a technique analagous to a Southern blot technique but in which proteins are separated by electrophoresis, transferred to a filter, and probed with DNA fragments to identify expression of specific DNA binding proteins. **Western blot t.,** a technique for analyzing proteins by separating them by electrophoresis, transferring them in place to a filter or membrane, and probing with specific antibodies.

tech·nol·o·gist (tek-nol'ah-jist) a person skilled in the theory and practice of a technical profession, usually with at least a baccalaureate degree; in several allied health fields, technologist is the highest professional rank.

tech·nol·o·gy (-je) scientific knowledge; the sum of the study of a technique. **assisted reproductive t. (ART),** any procedure involving the manipulation of eggs or sperm to establish pregnancy in the treatment of infertility.

tec·ton·ic (tek-ton′ik) pertaining to construction.

tec·to·ri·al (tek-tor′e-al) of the nature of a roof or covering.

tec·to·ri·um (-um) pl. *tecto′ria.* [L.] Corti's membrane.

tec·to·spi·nal (tek″to-spi′n'l) extending from the tectum of the midbrain to the spinal cord.

tec·tum (tek′tum) a rooflike structure. **t. of mesencephalon, t. of midbrain,** the dorsal portion of the midbrain.

TEE transesophageal echocardiography.

teeth·ing (tēth′ing) the entire process resulting in eruption of the teeth.

Tef·lon (tef′lon) trademark for preparations of polytef (polytetrafluoroethylene).

teg·men (teg′men) pl. *teg′mina.* [L.] a covering structure or roof. **t. tym′pani,** the thin layer of bone that forms the roof of the tympanic cavity, separating it from the cranial cavity.

teg·men·tal (teg-men′t'l) pertaining to or of the nature of a tegmen or tegmentum.

teg·men·tum (-tum) pl. *tegmen′ta.* [L.] 1. a covering. 2. tegmentum of mesencephalon. 3. the dorsal part of each cerebral peduncle. **t. of mesencephalon,** the dorsal part of the mesencephalon, formed by continuation of the dorsal parts of the cerebral peduncles across the median plane, and extending on each side from the substantia nigra to the level of the mesencephalic aqueduct.

tei·cho·ic ac·id (ti-ko′ik) any of a diverse group of antigenic polymers of glycerol or ribitol phosphates found attached to the cell walls or in intracellular association with membranes of gram-positive bacteria; they determine group specificity of some species, e.g., the staphylococci.

tei·chop·sia (ti-kop′se-ah) the sensation of a luminous appearance before the eyes, with a zigzag, wall-like outline. It may be a migraine aura.

tei·co·pla·nin (ti-ko-pla′nin) a glycopeptide antibiotic used as a less toxic alternative to vancomycin in the treatment of infections caused by gram-positive bacteria.

te·la (te′lah) pl. *te′lae.* [L.] any weblike tissue. **t. elas′tica,** elastic tissue. **t. subcuta′nea,** subcutaneous tissue.

tel·al·gia (tel-al′jah) referred pain.

tel·an·gi·ec·ta·sia (tel-an″je-ek-ta′zhah) permanent dilation of preexisting small blood vessels, creating focal red lesions. **hereditary hemorrhagic t.,** a hereditary condition marked by multiple small telangiectases of the skin, mucous membranes, and other organs, associated with recurrent episodes of bleeding from affected sites and gross or occult melena. **spider t.,** vascular spider.

tel·an·gi·ec·ta·sis (-ek′tah-sis) pl. *telangiec′tases.* 1. The lesion produced by telangiectasia, which may present as a coarse or fine red line or as a punctum with radiating limbs (spider). 2. telangiectasia.

tel·an·gi·o·sis (-o′sis) any disease of the capillaries.

tele- word element [Gr.], *operating at a distance; far away.*

tele·can·thus (tel″ĕ-kan′thus) abnormally increased distance between the medial canthi of the eyelids.

tele·car·di·og·ra·phy (-kahr″de-og′rah-fe) the recording of an electrocardiogram by transmission of impulses to a site at a distance from the patient.

tele·car·dio·phone (-kahr′de-o-fōn″) an apparatus for making heart sounds audible at a distance from the patient.

tele·cep·tor (tel′ĕ-sep″ter) a sensory nerve terminal, such as those in the eyes, ears, and nose, that is sensitive to distant stimuli.

tele·di·ag·no·sis (tel″ĕ-di″ag-no′sis) determination of the nature of a disease at a site remote from the patient on the basis of transmitted telemonitoring data or closed-circuit television consultation.

tele·flu·o·ros·co·py (-floor-os′ko-pe) television transmission of fluoroscopic images for study at a distant location.

tele·ki·ne·sis (-kĭ-ne′sis) 1. movement of an object produced without contact. 2. the ability to produce such movement. **telekinet′ic,** adj.

tele·med·i·cine (-med′ĭ-sin) the provision of consultant services by off-site physicians to health care professionals on the scene, as by means of closed-circuit television.

te·lem·e·try (tĕ-lem′ĕ-tre) the making of measurements at a distance from the subject, the measurable evidence of phenomena under investigation being transmitted by radio signals, wires, or other means.

tel·en·ceph·a·lon (tel″en-sef′ah-lon) endbrain. 1. one of the two divisions of the prosencephalon, composing the cerebrum (q.v.). 2. the anterior of the two vesicles formed by specialization of the prosencephalon in embryonic development; from it the cerebral hemispheres are derived. **telen-cephal'ic,** adj.

tele·neu·rite (tel''ĕ-noor'īt) an end expansion of an axon.

tele·neu·ron (-noor'on) a nerve ending.

tele(o)- word element [Gr.], *an end.*

te·le·ol·o·gy (te''le-ol'ah-je) the doctrine of final causes or of adaptation to a definite purpose.

te·leo·mi·to·sis (tel''e-o-mi-to'sis) completed mitosis.

tele·op·sia (-op'se-ah) a visual disturbance in which objects appear to be farther away than they actually are.

te·le·or·gan·ic (-or-gan'ik) necessary to life.

Tele·paque (tel'ĕ-pāk) trademark for a preparation of iopanoic acid.

tele·pa·thol·o·gy (tel''ĕ-pah-thol'ŏ-je) the practice of pathology at a remote location by means of video cameras, monitors, and a remote-controlled microscope.

tele·ra·di·og·ra·phy (-ra''de-og'rah-fe) 1. interpretation of images transmitted over telephone lines or by satellite. 2. radiography with the radiation source 6.5 to 7 feet from the subject to maximize the parallelism of the rays and minimize distortion.

tele·ther·a·py (-ther'ah-pe) treatment in which the source of the therapeutic agent, e.g., radiation, is at a distance from the body.

tel·lu·ric (tĕ-lu'rik) 1. pertaining to tellurium. 2. pertaining to or originating from the earth.

tel·lu·ri·um (-re-um) chemical element (see *Table of Elements*), at. no. 52, symbol Te.

tel·mi·sar·tan (tel''mĭ-sahr'tan) an angiotensin II antagonist used as an antihypertensive.

tel(o)- word element [Gr.], *end.*

telo·den·dron (tel''o-den'dron) any of the fine terminal branches of an axon.

tel·o·gen (tel'o-jen) the quiescent or resting phase of the hair cycle, following catagen; the hair has become a club hair and does not grow further.

tel·og·no·sis (tel''og-no'sis) diagnosis based on interpretation of radiographs transmitted by *teleradiography.*

telo·lec·i·thal (tel''o-les'ĭ-thal) having a medium to large amount of yolk, with the yolk concentrated toward one pole (the vegetal pole); as in the eggs of fish, amphibians, birds, and reptiles.

telo·mer·ase (tĕ-lo'mer-ās) a DNA polymerase involved in the formation of telomeres and the maintenance of telomere sequences during replication.

telo·mere (tel'o-mēr) an extremity of a chromosome, which has specific properties,

one of which is a polarity that prevents reunion with any fragment after a chromosome has been broken.

telo·phase (-fāz) the last of the four stages of mitosis and of the two divisions of meiosis, in which the chromosomes arrive at the poles of the cell and the cytoplasm divides; in plants, the cell wall also forms.

te·maz·e·pam (tĕ-maz'ĕ-pam) a benzodiazepine used as a sedative and hypnotic in the treatment of insomnia.

te·mo·zo·lo·mide (tem''ah-zo'lah-mīd) a cytotoxic alkylating agent used as an antineoplastic in the treatment of refractory anaplastic astrocytoma.

tem·per·ate (tem'per-at) restrained; characterized by moderation; as a temperate bacteriophage, which infects but does not lyse its host.

tem·per·a·ture (tem'per-ah-chur) 1. an expression of heat or coldness in terms of a specific scale; a measure of the average kinetic energy due to thermal agitation of the particles in a system. Symbol *t.* See accompanying tables. 2. the level of heat natural to a living being. 3. colloquial term for *fever.* **absolute t.** (*T*), that reckoned from absolute zero (−273.15°C or −459.67°F), expressed on an absolute scale. **basal body t.** (**BBT**), the temperature of the body under conditions of absolute rest. **core t.,** the temperature of structures deep within the body, as opposed to peripheral temperature such as that of the skin. **critical t.,** that below which a gas may be converted to a liquid by increased pressure. **normal t.,** that of the human body in health, about 98.6°F or 37°C when measured orally.

tem·plate (tem'plit) 1. a pattern or mold. 2. in genetics, a strand of DNA or RNA (mRNA) that specifies the base sequence of a newly synthesized strand of DNA or RNA. 3. in dentistry, a curved or flat plate used as an aid in setting teeth in a denture.

tem·ple (tem'p'l) the lateral region on either side of the head, above the zygomatic arch.

tem·po·ra (tem'pŏ-rah) [L.] the temples.

tem·po·ral (-ral) 1. pertaining to the temple. 2. pertaining to time; limited as to time; temporary.

tem·po·ro·man·dib·u·lar (tem''pah-ro-man-dib'u-ler) pertaining to the temporal bone and mandible.

tem·po·ro·max·il·lary (-mak'sĭ-lar''e) pertaining to the temporal bone and maxilla.

tem·po·ro·oc·cip·i·tal (-ok-sip'ĭ-t'l) pertaining to the temporal and occipital bones.

tem·po·ro·sphe·noid (-sfe'noid) pertaining to the temporal and sphenoid bones.

TEMPERATURE EQUIVALENTS: CELSIUS TO FAHRENHEIT

°C	°F	°C	°F	°C	°F	°C	°F
−40	−40.0	−3	26.6	34	93.2	71	159.8
−39	−38.2	−2	28.4	35	95.0	72	161.6
−38	−36.4	−1	30.2	36	96.8	73	163.4
−37	−34.6	0	32.0	37	98.6	74	165.2
−36	−32.8	+1	33.8	38	100.4	75	167.0
−35	−31.0	2	35.6	39	102.2	76	168.8
−34	−29.2	3	37.4	40	104.0	77	170.6
−33	−27.4	4	39.2	41	105.8	78	172.4
−32	−25.6	5	41.0	42	107.6	79	174.2
−31	−23.8	6	42.8	43	109.4	80	176.0
−30	−22.0	7	44.6	44	111.2	81	177.8
−29	−20.2	8	46.4	45	113.0	82	179.6
−28	−18.4	9	48.2	46	114.8	83	181.4
−27	−16.6	10	50.0	47	116.6	84	183.2
−26	−14.8	11	51.8	48	118.4	85	185.0
−25	−13.0	12	53.6	49	120.2	86	186.8
−24	−11.2	13	55.4	50	122.0	87	188.6
−23	−9.4	14	57.2	51	123.8	88	190.4
−22	−7.6	15	59.0	52	125.6	89	192.2
−21	−5.8	16	60.8	53	127.4	90	194.0
−20	−4.0	17	62.6	54	129.2	91	195.8
−19	−2.2	18	64.4	55	131.0	92	197.6
−18	−0.4	19	66.2	56	132.8	93	199.4
−17	+1.4	20	68.0	57	134.6	94	201.2
−16	3.2	21	69.8	58	136.4	95	203.0
−15	5.0	22	71.6	59	138.2	96	204.8
−14	6.8	23	73.4	60	140.0	97	206.6
−13	8.6	24	75.2	61	141.8	98	208.4
−12	10.4	25	77.0	62	143.6	99	210.2
−11	12.2	26	78.8	63	145.4	100	212.0
−10	14.0	27	80.6	64	147.2	101	213.8
−9	15.8	28	82.4	65	149.0	102	215.6
−8	17.6	29	84.2	66	150.8	103	217.4
−7	19.4	30	86.0	67	152.6	104	219.2
−6	21.2	31	87.8	68	154.4	105	221.0
−5	23.0	32	89.6	69	156.2	106	222.8
−4	24.8	33	91.4	70	158.0		

te·nac·u·lum (tĕ-nak′u-lum) a hooklike surgical instrument for grasping and holding parts.

te·nal·gia (ten-al′jah) pain in a tendon.

te·nas·cin (ten′ah-sin) a glycoprotein of the extracellular matrix, isolated from a variety of embryo and adult tissues, including epithelial sites, smooth muscles, and some tumors.

ten·der·ness (ten′der-nes) a state of unusual sensitivity to touch or pressure. **rebound t.,** a state in which pain is felt on the release of pressure over a part.

ten·di·ni·tis (ten″dĭ-ni′tis) inflammation of tendons and of tendon-muscle attachments. **calcific t.,** inflammation and calcification of the subacromial or subdeltoid bursa, resulting in pain, tenderness, and limitation of motion in the shoulder.

tendin(o)- word element [L.], *tendon.*

ten·di·no·plas·ty (ten′dĭ-no-plas″te) tenoplasty.

TEMPERATURE EQUIVALENTS: FAHRENHEIT TO CELSIUS

°F	°C	°F	°C	°F	°C	°F	°C
−40	−40.0	34	1.1	112	44.4	163	72.7
−39	−39.4	35	1.6	113	45.0	164	73.3
−38	−38.9	36	2.2	114	45.5	165	73.8
−37	−38.3	37	2.7	115	46.1	166	74.4
−36	−37.8	38	3.3	116	46.6	167	75.0
−35	−37.2	39	3.8	117	47.2	168	75.5
−34	−36.7	40	4.4	118	47.7	169	76.1
−33	−36.1	41	5.0	119	48.3	170	76.6
−32	−35.6	42	5.5	120	48.8	171	77.2
−31	−35.0	43	6.1	121	49.4	172	77.7
−30	−34.4	44	6.6	122	50.0	173	78.3
−29	−33.9	45	7.2	123	50.5	174	78.8
−28	−33.3	46	7.7	124	51.1	175	79.4
−27	−32.8	47	8.3	125	51.6	176	80.0
−26	−32.2	48	8.8	126	52.2	177	80.5
−25	−31.7	49	9.4	127	52.7	178	81.1
−24	−31.1	50	10.0	128	53.3	179	81.6
−23	−30.6	55	12.7	129	53.8	180	82.2
−22	−30.0	60	15.5	130	54.4	181	82.7
−21	−29.4	65	18.3	131	55.0	182	83.3
−20	−28.9	70	21.1	132	55.5	183	83.8
−19	−28.3	75	23.8	133	56.1	184	84.4
−18	−27.8	80	26.6	134	56.6	185	85.0
−17	−27.2	85	29.4	135	57.2	186	85.5
−16	−26.7	86	30.0	136	57.7	187	86.1
−15	−26.1	87	30.5	137	58.3	188	86.6
−14	−25.6	88	31.0	138	58.8	189	87.2
−13	−25.0	89	31.6	139	59.4	190	87.7
−12	−24.4	90	32.2	140	60.0	191	88.3
−11	−23.9	91	32.7	141	60.5	192	88.8
−10	−23.3	92	33.3	142	61.1	193	89.4
−9	−22.8	93	33.8	143	61.6	194	90.0
−8	−22.2	94	34.4	144	62.2	195	90.5
−7	−21.7	95	35.0	145	62.7	196	91.1
−6	−21.1	96	35.5	146	63.3	197	91.6
−5	−20.6	97	36.1	147	63.8	198	92.2
−4	−20.0	98	36.6	148	64.4	199	92.7
−3	−19.4	98.6	37.0	149	65.0	200	93.3
−2	−18.9	99	37.2	150	65.5	201	93.8
−1	−18.3	100	37.7	151	66.1	202	94.4
0	−17.8	101	38.3	152	66.6	203	95.0
+1	−17.2	102	38.8	153	67.2	204	95.5
5	−15.0	103	39.4	154	67.7	205	96.1
10	−12.2	104	40.0	155	68.3	206	96.6
15	−9.4	105	40.5	156	68.8	207	97.2
20	−6.6	106	41.1	157	69.4	208	97.7
25	−3.8	107	41.6	158	70.0	209	98.3
30	−1.1	108	42.2	159	70.5	210	98.8
31	−0.5	109	42.7	160	71.1	211	99.4
32	0	110	43.3	161	71.6	212	100.0
33	+0.5	111	43.8	162	72.2	213	100.5

ten·di·no·su·ture (ten″dĭ-no-soo′chur) tenorrhaphy.

ten·di·nous (ten′dĭ-nus) pertaining to, resembling, or of the nature of a tendon.

ten·do (ten′do) pl. *ten′dines*. [L.] tendon. **t. Achil′lis, t. calca′neus,** Achilles tendon.

ten·don (ten′don) a fibrous cord of connective tissue continuous with the fibers of a muscle and attaching the muscle to bone or cartilage. **Achilles t., calcaneal t.,** the powerful tendon at the back of the heel, attaching the triceps surae muscle to the calcaneus. **t. of conus, t. of infundibulum,** a collagenous band connecting the posterior surface of the pulmonary annulus and the muscular infundibulum with the root of the aorta.

ten·do·ni·tis (ten″do-ni′tis) tendinitis.

ten·do·vag·i·nal (-vaj′ĭ-n′l) pertaining to a tendon and its sheath.

te·nec·te·plase (tĕ-nek′tĕ-plās) a modified form of human tissue plasminogen activator produced by recombinant DNA technology; used as a thrombolytic agent in the treatment of myocardial infarction.

te·nec·to·my (tĕ-nek′tah-me) excision of a lesion of a tendon or of a tendon sheath.

te·nes·mus (tĕ-nez′mus) straining, especially ineffectual and painful straining at stool or urination. **tenes′mic,** adj.

te·nia (te′ne-ah) pl. *te′niae*. Taenia.

te·ni·a·cide (-sīd″) taeniacide.

ten·i·a·fuge (-fūj″) taeniafuge.

te·nia·my·ot·o·my (te″ne-ah-mi-ot′ah-me) an operation involving a series of transverse incisions of the taeniae coli; done in diverticular disease.

te·ni·a·sis (te-ni′ah-sis) taeniasis.

ten·i·po·side (ten-ĭ-po′sīd) a semisynthetic antineoplastic used in the treatment of neuroblastoma, non-Hodgkin's lymphoma, and acute lymphoblastic leukemia.

ten(o)- word element [Gr.], *tendon*.

te·nod·e·sis (ten-od′ĕ-sis) suture of the end of a tendon to a bone.

ten·odyn·ia (ten″o-din′e-ah) tenalgia.

te·no·fo·vir (tĕ-no′fo-vir″) an antiretroviral agent that inhibits reverse transcriptase; used as *t. disoproxil fumarate* in the treatment of HIV-1 (human immunodeficiency virus-1) infection.

te·nol·y·sis (ten-ol′ĭ-sis) the operation of freeing a tendon from adhesions.

teno·myo·plas·ty (ten″o-mi′o-plas″te) plastic repair of a tendon and muscle.

teno·my·ot·o·my (-mi-ot′ah-me) excision of a portion of a tendon and muscle.

teno·nec·to·my (-nek′tah-me) excision of part of a tendon to shorten it.

teno·ni·tis (-ni′tis) 1. tendinitis. 2. inflammation of Tenon's capsule.

tenont(o)- word element [Gr.], *tendon*.

ten·on·tog·ra·phy (ten″on-tog′rah-fe) a written description or delineation of the tendons.

ten·on·tol·o·gy (ten″on-tol′ah-je) sum of what is known about the tendons.

teno·phyte (ten′o-fīt) a growth or concretion in a tendon.

teno·plas·ty (-plas″te) plastic repair of a tendon. **tenoplas′tic,** adj.

teno·re·cep·tor (ten″o-re-sep′ter) a proprioceptor in a tendon.

te·nor·rha·phy (tĕ-nor′ah-fe) suture of a tendon.

ten·os·to·sis (ten″os-to′sis) conversion of a tendon into bone.

teno·su·ture (ten″o-soo′chur) tenorrhaphy.

teno·syn·o·vec·to·my (-sin″o-vek′tah-me) excision or resection of a tendon sheath.

teno·syn·o·vi·tis (-sin″o-vi′tis) inflammation of a tendon sheath. **villonodular t.,** a condition marked by exaggerated proliferation of synovial membrane cells, producing a solid tumor-like mass, commonly occurring in periarticular soft tissues and less frequently in joints.

te·not·o·my (ten-ot′ah-me) transection of a tendon.

teno·vag·i·ni·tis (ten″o-vaj″ĭ-ni′tis) tenosynovitis.

TENS transcutaneous electrical nerve stimulation.

ten·sion (ten′shun) 1. the act of stretching. 2. the condition of being stretched or strained. 3. the partial pressure of a component of a gas mixture. 4. mental, emotional, or nervous strain. 5. hostility between two or more individuals or groups. **arterial t.,** blood pressure within an artery. **intraocular t. (T),** see under *pressure*. **intravenous t.,** venous pressure. **surface t.,** tension or resistance which acts to preserve the integrity of a surface. **tissue t.,** a state of equilibrium between tissues and cells which prevents overaction of any part.

ten·sor (ten′ser) any muscle that stretches or makes tense.

tent (tent) 1. a fabric covering for enclosing an open space. 2. a conical, expansible plug of soft material for dilating an orifice, or keeping a wound open to prevent its healing except at the bottom. **oxygen t.,** one above a patient's bed for administering oxygen by inhalation. **sponge t.,** a conical plug made of compressed sponge used to dilate the os uteri.

ten·to·ri·um (ten-tor'e-um) pl. *tento'ria*. [L.] an anatomical part resembling a tent or covering. **tento'rial**, adj. **t. cerebel'li, t. of cerebellum**, the process of the dura mater supporting the occipital lobes and covering the cerebellum.

tera- word element [Gr.] *monster*; used in naming units of measurement (symbol T) to designate a quantity one trillion (10^{12}) times the unit specified by the root to which it is joined, as teracurie.

ter·a·tism (ter'ah-tizm) an anomaly of formation or development. **terat'ic, ter'atoid**, adj.

terat(o)- word element [Gr.], *monster; monstrosity.*

ter·a·to·blas·to·ma (ter″ah-to-blas-to′mah) teratoma.

ter·a·to·car·ci·no·ma (-kahr″si-no′mah) a malignant neoplasm consisting of elements of teratoma with those of embryonal carcinoma or choriocarcinoma, or both; occurring most often in the testis.

ter·a·to·gen (ter'ah-to-jen) any agent or factor that induces or increases the incidence of abnormal prenatal development. **teratogen'ic**, adj.

ter·a·to·gen·e·sis (ter″ah-to-jen′ĕ-sis) the production of birth defects in embryos and fetuses. **teratogenet'ic**, adj.

ter·a·tog·e·nous (ter″ah-toj′ĕ-nus) developed from fetal remains.

ter·a·toid (ter'ah-toid) characterized by teratism.

ter·a·tol·o·gy (ter″ah-tol′ah-je) that division of embryology and pathology dealing with abnormal development and the production of congenital anomalies. **teratolog'ic**, adj.

ter·a·to·ma (ter″ah-to′mah) pl. *terato'mata, teratomas*. A true neoplasm made up of different types of tissue, none of which is native to the area in which it occurs; usually found in the ovary or testis. **teratom'atous**, adj. **malignant t.**, 1. a solid, malignant ovarian tumor resembling a dermoid cyst but composed of immature embryonal and/or extraembryonic elements derived from all three germ layers. 2. teratocarcinoma.

ter·a·to·sis (-sis) teratism.

ter·a·zo·sin (ter-a′zo-sin) an alpha₁-adrenergic blocking agent used as the hydrochloride salt in the treatment of hypertension and of benign prostatic hyperplasia.

ter·bin·a·fine (ter′bĭ-nah-fēn″) a synthetic antifungal used as the hydrochloride salt in the treatment of tinea and onychomycosis.

ter·bi·um (ter′be-um) chemical element (see *Table of Elements*), at. no. 65, symbol Tb.

ter·bu·ta·line (ter-bu′tah-lēn) a β_2-adrenergic receptor agonist; used as the sulfate salt

as a bronchodilator and as a tocolytic in the prevention of premature labor.

ter·co·na·zole (ter-kon′ah-zōl) an imidazole antifungal used in the treatment of vulvovaginal candidiasis.

ter·e·bra·tion (ter″ĕ-bra′shun) a boring pain.

te·res (te′rēz) [L.] long and round.

term (term) a definite period, especially the period of gestation, or pregnancy.

ter·mi·nal (ter′mĭ-n'l) 1. forming or pertaining to an end; placed at the end. 2. a termination, end, or extremity.

ter·mi·na·tio (ter″mĭ-na′she-o) pl. *terminatio'nes*. [L.] an ending; the site of discontinuation of a structure, as the free nerve endings (*terminatio'nes nervo'rum li'berae*), in which the peripheral fiber divides into fine branches that terminate freely in connective tissue or epithelium.

Ter·mi·no·lo·gia Ana·to·mi·ca (TA) (-no-lo′je-ah an″ah-tom′ĭ-kah) [L.] *International Anatomical Terminology:* the internationally approved official body of anatomical nomenclature, superseding the *Nomina Anatomica* (NA).

ter·mi·nol·o·gy (ter″mĭ-nol′ah-je) 1. the vocabulary of an art or science. 2. the science which deals with the investigation, arrangement, and construction of terms. **International Anatomical T.,** *Terminologia Anatomica.*

ter·mi·nus (ter′mĭ-nus) pl. *ter'mini*. [L.] an ending.

ter·na·ry (ter′nah-re) 1. third in order. 2. made up of three distinct chemical elements.

ter·pene (ter′pēn) any hydrocarbon of the formula $C_{10}H_{16}$.

ter·ror (ter′er) intense fright. **night t's,** pavor nocturnus.

ter·tian (ter′shun) recurring every third day (counting the day of occurrence as the first day); see under *malaria.*

ter·ti·ary (ter′she-ar″e) third in order.

ter·ti·grav·i·da (ter″tĭ-grav′ĭ-dah) a woman pregnant for the third time; gravida III.

ter·tip·a·ra (ter-tip′ah-rah) a woman who has had three pregnancies which resulted in viable offspring; para III.

tes·la (T) (tes′lah) the SI unit of magnetic flux density, a vector quantity that measures the magnitude of a magnetic field. It is equal to 1 weber per square meter.

tes·sel·lat·ed (tes′ah-lāt″ed) divided into squares, like a checker board.

test (test) 1. an examination or trial. 2. a significant chemical reaction. 3. a reagent. **abortus Bang ring t., ABR t.,** an agglutination test for brucellosis in cattle, performed by mixing a drop of stained brucellae with 1 mL of milk and incubating for 1 hour at 37°C; agglutinated bacteria rise to the surface to form a colored ring. **acid elution t.,** air-dried blood smears are fixed in 80 per cent methanol and immersed in a pH 3.3 buffer; all hemoglobins are eluted except fetal hemoglobin, which is seen in red cells after staining. **acidified serum t.,** incubation of red cells in acidified serum; after centrifugation, the supernatant is examined by colorimetry for hemolysis, which indicates paroxysmal nocturnal hemoglobinuria. **acoustic reflex t.,** measurement of the acoustic reflex threshold; used to differentiate between conductive and sensorineural deafness and to diagnose acoustic neuroma. **Adson's t.,** one for thoracic outlet syndrome; with the patient in a sitting position, hands on thighs, the examiner palpates both radial pulses as the patient rapidly fills the lungs by deep inhalation and, holding breath, hyperextends the neck, turning the head toward the affected side. If the radial pulse on that side is markedly or completely obliterated, the result is positive. **agglutination t.,** cells containing antigens to a given antibody are mixed into the solution being tested for a particular antibody, with agglutination indicative of antibody presence. **alkali denaturation t.,** a spectrophotometric method for determining the concentration of fetal (F) hemoglobin. **Ames t.,** a strain of *Salmonella typhimurium* that lacks the enzyme necessary for histidine synthesis is cultured in the absence of histidine and in the presence of the suspected mutagen and certain enzymes known to activate procarcinogens. If the substance causes DNA damage resulting in mutations, some of the bacteria will regain the ability to synthesize histidine and will proliferate to form colonies; almost all of the mutagenic substances are also carcinogenic. **anti-DNA t., anti-double-stranded DNA t.,** an immunoassay that uses native double-stranded DNA as an antigen to detect and monitor increased serum levels of anti-DNA antibodies; used in the detection and management of systemic lupus erythematosus. **antiglobulin t. (AGT),** a test for nonagglutinating antibodies against red cells, using antihuman globulin antibody to agglutinate red cells coated with the nonagglutinating antibody. The *direct antiglobulin test* detects antibodies bound to circulating red cells in vivo. It is used in the evaluation of autoimmune and drug-induced hemolytic anemia and hemolytic disease of the newborn. The *indirect antiglobulin test* detects serum antibodies that bind to red cells in an in vitro

incubation step. It is used in typing of erythrocyte antigens and in compatibility testing (cross-match). **aptitude t's,** tests designed to determine ability to undertake study or training in a particular field. **association t.,** one based on associative reaction, usually by mentioning words to a patient and noting what other words the patient will think of and give in reply. **automated reagin t. (ART),** a modification of the rapid plasma reagin (RPR) test for use with automated analyzers used in clinical chemistry. **basophil degranulation t.,** an in vitro procedure testing allergic sensitivity to a specific allergen at the cellular level by measuring staining of basophils after exposure to the allergen; a reduced number of granular cells is a positive result. **Benedict's t.,** a qualitative or quantitative test for the determination of glucose content of urine. **Binet's t., Binet-Simon t.,** a method of ascertaining a child's or youth's mental age by asking a series of questions adapted to, and standardized on, the capacity of normal children at various ages. **Bing t.,** a vibrating tuning fork is held to the mastoid process and the auditory meatus is alternately occluded and left open; an increase and decrease in loudness is perceived by the normal ear and in sensorineural hearing loss, whereas the hearing of no difference occurs in conductive hearing loss. **caloric t.,** irrigation of the normal ear with warm water produces a rotatory nystagmus toward that side; irrigation with cold water produces a rotatory nystagmus away from that side. **chi-square t.,** any statistical hypothesis test employing the chi-square (χ^2) distribution, measuring the difference between theoretical and observed frequencies and hypothesized to approach the χ^2-distribution as the sample size increases. **chromatin t.,** determination of genetic sex of an individual by examination of somatic cells for the presence of sex chromatin. **cis-trans t.,** a test in microbial genetics to determine whether two mutations that have the phenotypic effect, in a haploid cell or a cell with single phage infection, are located in the same gene or in different genes; the test depends on the independent behavior of two alleles of a gene in a diploid cell or in a cell infected with two phages carrying different alleles. **clomiphene citrate challenge t.,** measurement of fertility potential in a woman by examination of the response of follicle-stimulating hormone level to administration of clomiphene citrate early in the menstrual cycle. **complement fixation t.,** see under *fixation.* **contraction stress t. (CST),** the monitoring of the response of the fetal heart rate to spontaneous or induced uterine contractions by cardiotocography, with deceleration indicating possible fetal hypoxia. **Coombs' t.**, antiglobulin t. **Denver Developmental Screening t.**, a test for identification of infants and preschool children with developmental delay. **DFA-TP t.**, direct fluorescent antibody–*Treponema pallidum* t. **Dick t.**, an intracutaneous test for determination of susceptibility to scarlet fever. **direct fluorescent antibody–*Treponema pallidum* t.**, DFA-TP t.; a serologic test for syphilis using direct immunofluorescence. **disk diffusion t.**, a test for antibiotic sensitivity in bacteria; agar plates are inoculated with a standardized suspension of a microorganism. Antibiotic-containing disks are applied to the agar surface. Following overnight incubation, the diameters of the zones of inhibition are interpreted as sensitive (susceptible), indeterminate (intermediate), or resistant. **drawer t's**, tests for the integrity of the cruciate ligaments of the knee; with the knee flexed 90 degrees, if the tibia can be drawn too far forward there is rupture of the anterior ligaments (*anterior drawer t.*), if too far back then the rupture is of the posterior ligaments (*posterior drawer t.*). **early pregnancy t.**, a do-it-yourself immunological test for pregnancy, performed as early as one day after menstruation was expected (missed period); a variety of tests exist, all based on an increase in urinary levels of human chorionic gonadotropin after fertilization. **EP t., erythrocyte protoporphyrin t.**, determination of erythrocyte protoporphyrin levels as a screening test for lead toxicity; levels are increased in lead poisoning and iron deficiency. **exercise t's, exercise stress t's**, any of various stress tests in which exercise is used in the electrocardiographic assessment of cardiovascular health and function, particularly in the diagnosis of myocardial ischemia. The most widely used forms are the treadmill and bicycle ergometer exercise tests; they are usually graded, consisting of a series of incrementally increasing workloads sustained for defined intervals. **FAB t.**, fluorescent antibody t. **Fe$_{Na}$ t.**, excreted fraction of filtered sodium test, a measure of renal tubular reabsorption of sodium, calculated as (urine Na × plasma Cr) ÷ (urine Cr × plasma Na) × 100. **finger-nose t.**, one for coordinated limb movements; with upper limb extended to one side the patient is asked to try to touch the end of the nose with the tip of the index finger. **Finn chamber t.**, a type of patch test in which the materials being tested are held in shallow aluminum cups (Finn chambers) that are taped against the skin, usually for a few days. **Fishberg concentration t.**, determination of the ability of the kidneys to maintain excretion of solids under conditions of reduced water intake and a high protein diet, in which urine samples are collected and tested for specific gravity. **flocculation t.**, any serologic test in which a flocculent agglomerate is formed; usually applied to a variant form of the precipitin reaction. **fluorescent antibody t., FAB t.**; a test for the distribution of cells expressing a specific protein by binding antibody specific for the protein and detecting complexes by fluorescent labeling of the antibody. **fluorescent treponemal antibody absorption t., FTA-ABS t.**, the standard treponemal antigen serologic test for syphilis, using fluorescein-labeled antihuman globulin to demonstrate specific treponemal antibodies in patient serum. **gel diffusion t.**, see *immunodiffusion*. **glucose tolerance t.**, a test of the body's ability to utilize carbohydrates by measuring the plasma glucose level at stated intervals after ingestion or intravenous injection of a large quantity of glucose. **glycosylated hemoglobin t.**, measurement of the percentage of hemoglobin A molecules that have formed a stable keto–amine linkage between their terminal amino acid position of the β-chains and a glucose group; in normal persons this is about 7 per cent of the total, in diabetics about 14.5 per cent. **guaiac t.**, one for occult blood; glacial acetic acid and a solution of gum guaiac are mixed with the specimen; on addition of hydrogen peroxide, the presence of blood is indicated by a blue tint. **Ham's t.**, acidified serum t. **histamine t.**, 1. subcutaneous injection of 0.1 per cent solution of histamine to stimulate gastric secretion. 2. after rapid intravenous injection of histamine phosphate, normal persons experience a brief fall in blood pressure, but in those with pheochromocytoma, after the fall, there is a marked rise in blood pressure. **horse cell t.**, a modification of the Paul-Bunnell-Davidsohn test for antibodies associated with infectious mononucleosis, using horse erythrocytes instead of sheep erythrocytes. **Huhner t.**, postcoital t. **hydrogen breath t.**, a test for deficiency of lactase or other hydrolases or for colonic overgrowth of bacteria, in which the exhalations are trapped and measured after administration of carbohydrate, with excess carbohydrate fermentation in the colon resulting in high levels of exhaled hydrogen. **hypo-osmotic swelling t.**, determination of sperm viability by placing a sample in a hypo-osmotic solution, which causes swelling and curling of the tails of spermatozoa with normal plasma membranes. **immobilization t.,** detection of antibody based on its ability to inhibit the motility of a bacterial cell or protozoan. **inkblot t.,** Rorschach t. **intelligence t.,** a set of problems or tasks posed to assess an individual's innate ability to judge, comprehend, and reason. **intracutaneous t., intradermal t.,** skin test in which the antigen is injected intradermally. **Kveim t.,** an intradermal test for the diagnosis of sarcoidosis. **latex agglutination t., latex fixation t.,** a type of agglutination test in which antigen to a given antibody is adsorbed to latex particles and mixed with a test solution to observe for agglutination of the latex. **limulus t.,** an extract of blood cells from the horseshoe crab (*Limulus polyphemus*) is exposed to a blood sample from a patient; if gram-negative endotoxin is present in the sample, it will produce gelation of the extract of blood cells. **Lundh t.,** a test for pancreatic function in which trypsin concentrations in the duodenum after a test meal are measured, with lowered levels of trypsin indicating low pancreatic secretion. **lupus band t.,** an immunofluorescence test to determine the presence and extent of immunoglobulin and complement deposits at the dermal-epidermal junction of skin specimens from patients with systemic lupus erythematosus. **McMurray's t.,** as the patient lies supine with one knee fully flexed, the examiner rotates the patient's foot fully outward and the knee is slowly extended; a painful "click" indicates a tear of the medial meniscus of the knee joint; if the click occurs when the foot is rotated inward, the tear is in the lateral meniscus. **Mantoux t.,** an intracutaneous tuberculin test. **Master "two-step" exercise t.,** an early exercise test for coronary insufficiency in which electrocardiograms were recorded while and after the subject repeatedly ascended and descended two steps. **MIF t., migration inhibitory factor t.,** an in vitro test for production of MIF by lymphocytes in response to specific antigens; used for evaluation of cell-mediated immunity. MIF production is absent in certain immunodeficiency diseases. **Moloney t.,** one for detection of delayed hypersensitivity to diphtheria toxoid. **multiple-puncture t.,** a skin test in which the material used (e.g., tuberculin) is introduced into the skin by pressure of several needles or pointed tines or prongs. **neostigmine t.,** on injection of neostigmine methylsulfate mixed with atropine sulfate,

lessening of myasthenic symptoms indicates myasthenia gravis. **neutralization t.,** one for the neutralization power of an antiserum or other substance by testing its action on the pathogenic properties of a microorganism, toxin, virus, bacteriophage, or toxic substance. **nocturnal penile tumescence t.,** monitoring of erections occurring during sleep; used in the differential diagnosis of psychogenic and organic impotence. **nonstress t. (NST),** the monitoring of the response of the fetal heart rate to fetal movements by cardiotocography. **nontreponemal antigen t.,** any of various tests detecting serum antibodies to reagin (cardiolipin and lecithin) derived from host tissues in the diagnosis of the *Treponema pallidum* infection of syphilis. **NPT t.,** nocturnal penile tumescence t. **osmotic fragility t.,** heparinized or defibrinated blood is placed in sodium chloride solutions of varying concentrations; increased fragility, measured as hemolysis, indicates spherocytosis. **oxytocin challenge t. (OCT),** a contraction stress test in which the uterine contractions are stimulated by intravenous infusion of oxytocin. **Pap t., Papanicolaou t.,** an exfoliative cytological staining procedure for detection and diagnosis of various conditions, particularly malignant and premalignant conditions of the female genital tract; also used in evaluating endocrine function and in the diagnosis of malignancies of other organs. **patch t's,** tests for hypersensitivity, performed by observing the reaction to application to the skin of filter paper or gauze saturated with the substance in question. **Patrick's t.,** thigh and knee of the supine patient are flexed, the external malleolus rests on the patella on the opposite leg, and the knee is depressed; production of pain indicates arthritis of the hip. Also known as *fabere sign*, from the first letters of movements that elicit it (*f*lexion, *ab*duction, external *r*otation, *e*xtension). **Paul-Bunnell t.,** determination of the highest dilution of the patient's serum that will agglutinate sheep erythrocytes; used to detect serum heterophile antibodies in the diagnosis of infectious mononucleosis. **Paul-Bunnell-Davidsohn t.,** a modification of the Paul-Bunnell test that differentiates among three types of heterophile sheep agglutinins: those associated with infectious mononucleosis and serum sickness, and natural antibodies against Forssman antigen. **postcoital t.,** determination of the number and condition of spermatozoa in mucus aspirated from the cervical canal soon after intercourse. **precipitin t.,** any serologic test based on a precipitin reaction.

projective t., any of various tests in which an individual interprets ambiguous stimulus situations according to their own unconscious dispositions, yielding information about their personality and possible psychopathology. **psychological t.,** any test to measure a subject's development, achievement, personality, intelligence, thought processes, etc. **psychomotor t.,** a test that assesses the subject's ability to perceive instructions and perform motor responses. **Queckenstedt's t.,** see under *sign.* **Quick's t.,** 1. a test for liver function based on excretion of hippuric acid after administration of sodium benzoate. 2. prothrombin time. **radioallergosorbent t. (RAST),** a radioimmunoassay test for the measurement of specific IgE antibody in serum, using allergen extract antigens fixed in a solid-phase matrix and radiolabeled anti-human IgE. **radioimmunosorbent t. (RIST),** a radioimmunoassay technique for measuring serum IgE concentration, using radiolabeled IgE and anti-human IgE bound to an insoluble matrix. **rapid plasma reagin t.,** RPR test; a screening flocculation test for syphilis, using a modified VDRL antigen. **Rinne t.,** a test of hearing made with tuning forks of 256, 512, and 1024 Hz, comparing the duration of perception by bone and by air conduction. **rollover t.,** comparison of the blood pressure of a pregnant woman lying on her back versus on her side; an excessive increase when she rolls to the supine postion indicates increased risk of preeclampsia. **Rorschach t.,** an association technique for personality testing based on the patient's response to a series of inkblot designs. **RPR t.,** rapid plasma reagin test. **Rubin's t.,** one for patency of the uterine tubes, performed by transuterine inflation with carbon dioxide gas. **Schick t.,** an intradermal test for determination of susceptibility to diphtheria. **Schiller's t.,** one for early squamous cell carcinoma of the cervix, performed by painting the uterine cervix with a solution of iodine and potassium iodide, diseased areas being revealed by a failure to take the stain. **Schilling t.,** a test for vitamin B_{12} absorption employing cyanocobalamin tagged with Co-57; used in the diagnosis of pernicious anemia and other disorders of vitamin B_{12} metabolism. **Schirmer's t.,** a test of tear production in keratoconjunctivitis sicca, performed by measuring the area of moisture on a piece of filter paper inserted over the conjunctival sac of the lower lid, with the end of the paper hanging down on the outside. **Schwabach's t.,** a hearing test made, with the opposite ear masked, placing the stems of vibrating tuning forks on the mastoid process first of the patient and then of the examiner. If heard longer by the patient it indicates conductive hearing loss and if heard longer by the examiner it indicates sensorineural hearing loss in the patient. **scratch t.,** a skin test in which the antigen is applied to a superficial scratch. **sheep cell agglutination t. (SCAT),** any agglutination test using sheep erythrocytes. **sickling t.,** one for demonstration of abnormal hemoglobin and the sickling phenomenon in erythrocytes. **skin t.,** any test in which an antigen is applied to the skin in order to observe the patient's reaction; used to determine exposure or immunity to infectious diseases, to identify allergens producing allergic reactions, and to assess ability to mount a cellular immune response. **sperm agglutination t.,** any of various tests for the presence of antisperm antibodies as a cause of infertility, based on the ability of large multivalent isotypes such as IgM or secretory IgA to cross-link and agglutinate spermatozoa with such antibodies. **stress t's,** any of various tests that assess cardiovascular health and function after application of a stress, usually exercise, to the heart. **swinging flashlight t.,** with the eyes fixed at a distance and a strong light shining before the intact eye, a crisp bilateral contraction of the pupil is noted; on moving the light to the affected eye, both pupils dilate for a short period, and on moving it back to the intact eye, both pupils contract promptly and remain contracted; indicative of minimal damage to the optic nerve or retina. **Thematic Apperception T. (TAT),** a projective test in which the subject tells a story based on each of a series of standard ambiguous pictures, so that the responses reflect a projection of some aspect of the subject's personality and current psychological preoccupations and conflicts. **thyroid suppression t.,** after administration of liothyronine for several days, radioactive iodine uptake is decreased in normal persons but not in those with hyperthyroidism. **tine t.,** four tines or prongs, 2 mm long, attached to a handle and coated with dip-dried PPD or Old tuberculin (OT) are pressed into the skin of the volar surface of the forearm; 48 to 72 hours later the skin is checked for palpable induration around the wounds. **treponemal antigen t.,** any of various tests detecting specific antitreponemal antibodies in serum in the diagnosis of the *Treponema pallidum* infection of syphilis. **tuberculin t.,** any of a number of skin tests for tuberculosis using a variety of different types of tuberculin and methods of application. **unheated serum**

reagin t., USR t., a modification of the VDRL test using unheated serum; used primarily for screening. VDRL t. [*Venereal Disease Research Laboratory*], a flocculation test for syphilis using VDRL antigen, which contains cardiolipin, cholesterol, and lecithin, to test heat-inactivated serum. Weber's t., the stem of a vibrating tuning fork is placed on the vertex or midline of the forehead. If the sound is heard best in the affected ear, it suggests conductive hearing loss; if heard best in the normal ear, it suggests sensorineural hearing loss. Widal's t., a test for agglutinins to O and H antigens of *Salmonella typhi* and *Salmonella paratyphi* in the serum of patients with suspected *Salmonella* infection.

tes·tal·gia (tes-tal′jah) orchialgia.

test card a card printed with various letters or symbols, used in testing vision.

tes·tes (tes′tēz) [L.] plural of *testis*.

tes·ti·cle (tes′tĭ-k'l) testis.

tes·tic·u·lar (tes-tik′u-lar) pertaining to a testis.

tes·tis (tes′tis) pl. *tes′tes*. [L.] the male gonad; either of the paired egg-shaped glands normally situated in the scrotum, in which the spermatozoa develop. Specialized interstitial cells (Leydig cells) secrete testosterone. **abdominal t.,** an undescended testis in the abdominal cavity. **ectopic t.,** one outside the normal pathway of descent. **obstructed t.,** one whose normal descent is blocked, so that it goes into an inguinal pouch. **retained t.,** undescended t. **retractile t.,** one that can descend fully into the scrotum but then moves freely up into the inguinal canal. **undescended t.,** one that has failed to descend into the scrotum, as in cryptorchidism.

tes·ti·tis (tes-ti′tis) orchitis.

test meal (test mēl) see under *meal*.

tes·tos·te·rone (tes-tos′tĕ-rōn″) the principal androgenic hormone, produced by the interstitial (Leydig) cells of the testes in response to stimulation by the luteinizing hormone of the anterior pituitary gland; it is thought to be responsible for regulation of gonadotropic secretion, spermatogenesis, and wolffian duct differentiation. It is also responsible for other male characteristics after its conversion to dihydrotestosterone. In addition, testosterone possesses protein anabolic properties. It is used as replacement therapy for androgen deficiency in males, in the treatment of delayed male puberty or hypogonadism, and in the palliation of certain breast cancers in females; used as the base or various esters (e.g., cypionate, enanthate, propionate).

test type (test tīp) printed letters of varying size, used in the testing of visual acuity.

TET treadmill exercise test; tubal embryo transfer.

te·tan·ic (tĕ-tan′ik) pertaining to tetanus.

te·tan·i·form (tĕ-tan′ĭ-form) resembling tetanus.

tet·a·nig·e·nous (tet″ah-nij′ĕ-nus) producing tetanic spasms.

tet·a·nize (tet′ah-nīz) to induce tetanic convulsions or symptoms.

tet·a·node (tet′ah-nōd) the unexcited stage occurring between the tetanic contractions in tetanus.

tet·a·noid (tet′ah-noid) resembling tetanus.

tet·a·nol·y·sin (tet″ah-nol′ĭ-sin) the hemolytic fraction of the exotoxin formed by the tetanus bacillus (*Clostridium tetani*).

tet·a·no·spas·min (tet″ah-no-spaz′min) the neurotoxic component of the exotoxin (tetanus toxin) produced by *Clostridium tetani*, which causes the typical muscle spasms of tetanus.

tet·a·nus (tet′ah-nus) 1. an acute, often fatal, infectious disease caused by a neurotoxin (tetanospasmin) produced by *Clostridium tetani*, whose spores enter the body through wounds. There are two forms: *generalized tetanus*, marked by tetanic muscular contractions and hyperreflexia, resulting in trismus (lockjaw), glottal spasm, generalized muscle spasm, opisthotonos, respiratory spasm, seizures, and paralysis; and *localized tetanus*, marked by localized muscular twitching and spasm, which may progress to the generalized form. 2. a state of muscular contraction without periods of relaxation. **neonatal t., t. neonato′rum,** tetanus of very young infants, usually due to umbilical infection.

tet·a·ny (-ne) a syndrome of sharp flexion of the wrist and ankle joints (carpopedal spasm), muscle twitching, cramps, and convulsions, sometimes with attacks of stridor; due to hyperexcitability of nerves and muscles caused by decreased extracellular ionized calcium in parathyroid hypofunction, vitamin D deficiency, or alkalosis, or following ingestion of alkaline salts. **duration t.,** a continuous tetanic contraction in response to a strong continuous current, seen especially in degenerated muscles. **gastric t.,** a severe form due to disease of the stomach, with difficult respiration and painful tonic spasms of limbs. **hyperventilation t.,** tetany produced by forced inhalation and exhalation over a period of time. **latent t.,** tetany elicited by the application of electrical and mechanical stimulation. **neonatal t., t. of newborn,**

hypocalcemic tetany in the first few days of life, often marked by irritability, muscle twitchings, jitteriness, tremors, and convulsions, and less often by laryngospasm and carpopedal spasm. **parathyroid t., parathyroprival t.,** tetany due to removal or hypofunction of the parathyroids.

tet·ar·ta·no·pia (tet″ahr-tah-no′pe-ah) 1. quadrantanopia. 2. a rare type of dichromatic vision of doubtful existence, characterized by perception of red and green only, with blue and yellow perceived as an achromatic (gray) band.

tet·ar·ta·nop·sia (-nop′se-ah) tetartanopia.

tetr(a)- word element [Gr.], *four*.

tet·ra·caine (tet′rah-kān) a local, topical, and spinal anesthetic, used as the base or the hydrochloride salt.

tet·ra·chlo·ro·eth·y·lene (tet″rah-klōr″o-eth′ĭ-lēn) a moderately toxic chlorinated hydrocarbon used as a dry-cleaning solvent and for other industrial uses.

tet·ra·crot·ic (-krot′ik) having four sphygmographic elevations to one beat of the pulse.

tet·ra·cyc·lic (tet″rah-sik′lik) containing four fused rings or closed chains in the molecular structure.

tet·ra·cy·cline (-si′klēn) 1. any of a group of related broad-spectrum antibiotics, isolated from species of *Streptomyces* or produced semisynthetically. 2. a semisynthetic antibiotic produced semisynthetically from chlortetracycline, having the same wide spectrum of antimicrobial activity as other members of the tetracycline group; used as the base or the hydrochloride salt.

tet·rad (tet′rad) a group of four similar or related entities, as (1) any element or radical having a valence, or combining power, of four; (2) a group of four chromosomal elements formed in the pachytene stage of the first meiotic prophase; (3) a square of cells produced by division into two planes of certain cocci (*Sarcina*). **Fallot's t.,** tetralogy of Fallot.

tet·ra·dac·ty·ly (tet″rah-dak′tĭ-le) the presence of four digits on the hand or foot.

tet·ra·go·num (-go′num) [L.] a quadrilateral. **t. lumba′le,** the area bounded by the four lumbar muscles.

tet·ra·hy·dro·can·nab·i·nol (THC) (-hi″dro-kah-nab′ĭ-nol) the active principle of cannabis, occurring in two isomeric forms, both considered psychomimetically active.

tet·ra·hy·dro·fo·lic ac·id (-hi″dro-fo′lik) a form of folic acid in which the pteridine ring is fully reduced; it is the parent compound of a variety of coenzymes that serve as carriers of one-carbon groups in metabolic reactions; in dissociated form, called *tetrahydrofolate*. Abbreviated THF.

tet·ra·hy·droz·o·line (-hi-droz′ah-lēn) an adrenergic applied topically as the hydrochloride salt to the nasal mucosa and to the conjunctiva to produce vasoconstriction.

te·tral·o·gy (tĕ-tral′ah-je) a group or series of four. **t. of Fallot,** a complex of congenital heart defects consisting of pulmonary stenosis, interventricular septal defect, hypertrophy of right ventricle, and dextroposition of the aorta.

tet·ra·mer·ic (tet″rah-mer′ik) having four parts.

tet·ra·nop·sia (-nop′se-ah) quadrantanopia.

tet·ra·pa·re·sis (-pah-re′sis) muscular weakness of all four limbs.

tet·ra·pep·tide (-pep′tīd) a peptide which, on hydrolysis, yields four amino acids.

tet·ra·ple·gia (-ple′jah) quadriplegia.

tet·ra·ploid (tet′rah-ploid) 1. characterized by tetraploidy. 2. an individual or cell having four sets of chromosomes.

tet·ra·pus (-pus) a human fetus having four feet.

tet·ra·pyr·role (-pĭ-rōl″) a compound containing four pyrrole rings, e.g., heme or chlorophyll.

te·tras·ce·lus (tĕ-tras′ah-lus) a human fetus with four lower limbs.

tet·ra·so·my (tet′rah-so″me) the presence of two extra chromosomes of one type in an otherwise diploid cell. **tetraso′mic,** adj.

tet·ra·va·lent (tet″rah-va′lent) having a valence of four.

tet·ro·do·tox·in (tet′ro-do-tok″sin) a highly lethal neurotoxin present in numerous species of puffer fish and in certain newts (in which it is called *tarichatoxin*); ingestion rapidly causes malaise, dizziness, and tingling about the mouth, which may be followed by ataxia, convulsions, respiratory paralysis, and death.

tex·ti·form (teks′tĭ-form) formed like a network.

TGF transforming growth factor.

Th thorium.

thal·a·men·ceph·a·lon (thal″ah-men-sef′ah-lon) the part of the diencephalon comprising the thalamus, metathalamus, and epithalamus.

tha·lam·ic (thah-lam′ik) pertaining to the thalamus.

thal·a·mo·cor·ti·cal (thal″ah-mo-kor′tĭ-k′l) pertaining to the thalamus and cerebral cortex.

thal·a·mo·len·tic·u·lar (-len-tik′u-ler) pertaining to the thalamus and lenticular nucleus.

thal·a·mot·o·my (thal″ah-mot′ah-me) a stereotaxic surgical technique for the discrete destruction of specific groups of cells within the thalamus, as for the relief of pain, for relief of tremor and rigidity in paralysis agitans, or in the treatment of certain psychiatric disorders.

thal·a·mus (thal'ah-mus) pl. *thal'ami.* [L.] either of two large ovoid masses, consisting chiefly of gray substance, situated one on either side of and forming part of the lateral wall of the third ventricle. Each is divided into dorsal and ventral parts; the term *thalamus* without a modifier usually refers to the dorsal thalamus, which functions as a relay center for sensory impulses to the cerebral cortex.   **optic t.,** lateral geniculate body.

thal·as·se·mia (thal″ah-se′me-ah) a heterogeneous group of hereditary hemolytic anemias marked by a decreased rate of synthesis of one or more hemoglobin polypeptide chains, classified according to the chain involved (α, β, δ); the two major categories are α- and β-thalassemia.   **α-t.,** that caused by diminished synthesis of alpha chains of hemoglobin. The *homozygous* form is incompatible with life, the stillborn infant displaying severe hydrops fetalis. The *heterozygous* form may be asymptomatic or marked by mild anemia.   **β-t.,** that caused by diminished synthesis of beta chains of hemoglobin. The homozygous form is called *t. major* and the heterozygous form is called *t. minor.*   **t. ma′jor,** the homozygous form of β-thalassemia, in which hemoglobin A is completely absent; it appears in the newborn period and is marked by hemolytic, hypochromic, microcytic anemia, hepatosplenomegaly, skeletal deformation, mongoloid facies, and cardiac enlargement.   **t. mi′nor,** the heterozygous form of β-thalassemia, usually asymptomatic, although there is sometimes mild anemia.   **sickle cell–t.,** a hereditary anemia involving simultaneous heterozygosity for hemoglobin S and thalassemia.

tha·lid·o·mide (thah-lid′o-mīd) a sedative and hypnotic, commonly used in Europe in the early 1960's, and discovered to cause serious congenital anomalies in the fetus, notably amelia and phocomelia, when taken during early pregnancy; now used in the treatment of erythema nodosum leprosum.

thal·li·um (thal′e-um) chemical element (see *Table of Elements*), at. no. 81, symbol Tl. It may be absorbed from the gut and from the intact skin, causing a variety of neurologic and psychic symptoms and liver and kidney damage.   **t. 201,** a radioactive isotope of thallium having a half-life of 3.05 days and decaying by electron capture with emission of

gamma rays (0.135, 0.167 MeV); it is used as a diagnostic aid in the form of thallous chloride Tl 201.

thal·lous (thal′us) of, pertaining to, or containing thallium.   **t. chloride Tl 201,** the form in which thallium-201 in solution is injected intravenously for imaging of myocardial disease, parathyroid disorder, or neoplastic disease.

thanat(o)- word element [Gr.], *death.*

than·a·to·gno·mon·ic (than″ah-to″no-mon′ik) indicating the approach of death.

than·a·to·pho·ric (-for′ik) deadly; lethal.

THC tetrahydrocannabinol.

thea·ism (the′ah-izm) caffeinism resulting from ingestion of excessive quantities of tea.

the·baine (the-ba′in) a crystalline, poisonous, and anodyne alkaloid from opium, having properties similar to those of strychnine.

the·ca (the′kah) pl. *the′cae.* [L.] a case or sheath.   **the′cal,** adj.   **t. folli′culi,** an envelope of condensed connective tissue surrounding a vesicular ovarian follicle, comprising an internal vascular layer *(tunica interna)* and an external fibrous layer *(tunica externa).*

the·co·ma (the-ko′mah) theca cell tumor.

the·co·steg·no·sis (the″ko-steg-no′sis) contraction of a tendon sheath.

the·lal·gia (the-lal′jah) pain in the nipples.

the·lar·che (the-lahr′ke) the beginning of development of the breasts at puberty.

The·la·zia (the-la′zhah) a genus of nematode worms parasitic in the eyes of mammals, including, rarely, humans.

the·la·zi·a·sis (the″lah-zi′ah-sis) infection of the eye with *Thelazia.*

the·le·plas·ty (the′lĕ-plas″te) a plastic operation on the nipple.

the·ler·e·thism (thĕ-ler′ĕ-thizm) erection of the nipple.

the·li·tis (the-li′tis) inflammation of a nipple.

the·lor·rha·gia (the″lo-ra′jah) hemorrhage from the nipple.

the·nar (the′ner) 1. the fleshy part of the hand at the base of the thumb.   2. pertaining to the palm.

the·oph·yl·line (the-of′ĭ-lin) a xanthine derivative found in tea leaves and prepared synthetically; its salts and derivatives act as smooth muscle relaxants, central nervous system and cardiac muscle stimulants, and bronchodilators; used as a bronchodilator in asthma and in bronchitis, emphysema, or other chronic obstructive pulmonary disease. Its choline salt is oxtriphylline.

the·o·ry (the′o-re) 1. the doctrine or the principles underlying an art as distinguished from the practice of that particular art.   2. a formulated hypothesis or, loosely speaking, any hypothesis or opinion not based upon actual knowledge. **cell t.,** all organic matter consists of cells, and cell activity is the essential process of life. **clonal deletion t.,** a theory of immunologic self-tolerance according to which "forbidden clones" of immunocytes, those reactive with self antigens, are eliminated on contact with antigen during fetal life. **clonal selection t.,** there are several million clones of antibody-producing cells in each adult, each programmed to make an antibody of a single specificity and carrying cell-surface receptors for specific antigens; exposure to antigen induces cells with receptors for that antigen to proliferate and produce large quantities of specific antibody. **information t.,** a system for analyzing, chiefly by statistical methods, the characteristics of communicated messages and the systems that encode, transmit, distort, receive, and decode them. **overflow t.,** one similar to the underfilling theory but which proposes that the primary event in ascites formation is sodium and water retention with portal hypertension resulting; plasma volume expansion to the point of overflow from the hepatic sinusoids then causes ascites formation. **quantum t.,** radiation and absorption of energy occur in quantities (quanta) which vary in size with the frequency of the radiation. **recapitulation t.,** ontogeny recapitulates phylogeny, i.e., an organism in the course of its development goes through the same successive stages (in abbreviated form) as did the species in its evolutionary development. **underfilling t.,** a theory that ascites associated with portal hypertension causes hypovolemia and so both a lowering of portal pressure and retention of sodium and water. The higher sodium concentration causes increases in the plasma volume and portal pressure, and the subsequent formation of ascites renews the cycle. **Young-Helmholtz t.,** color vision depends on three sets of retinal receptors, corresponding to the colors red, green, and violet.

theque (tĕk) [Fr.] a round or oval collection, or nest, of melanin-containing nevus cells occurring at the dermoepidermal junction of the skin or in the dermis proper.

ther·a·peu·tic (ther″ah-pu′tik) 1. pertaining to therapy. 2. tending to overcome disease and promote recovery.

ther·a·pist (ther′ah-pist) a person skilled in the treatment of disease or other disorder. **physical t.,** a person skilled in the techniques of physical therapy and qualified to administer treatment prescribed by a physician. **speech t.,** a person specially trained and qualified to assist patients in overcoming speech and language disorders.

ther·a·py (-pe) the treatment of disease; see also *treatment*. **ablation t.,** the destruction of small areas of myocardial tissue, usually by application of electrical or chemical energy, in the treatment of some tachyarrhythmias. **adjuvant t.,** the use of chemotherapy or radiotherapy in addition to surgical resection in the treatment of cancer. **antiplatelet t.,** the use of platelet-modifying agents to inhibit platelet adhesion or aggregation and so prevent thrombosis, alter the course of atherosclerosis, or prolong vascular graft patency. **art t.,** the use of art, the creative process, and patient response to the products created for the treatment of psychiatric and psychologic conditions and for rehabilitation. **aversion t., aversive t.,** that using aversive conditioning to reduce or eliminate undesirable behavior or symptoms; sometimes used synonymously with *aversive conditioning.* **behavior t.,** a therapeutic approach that focuses on modifying the patient's observable behavior, rather than on the conflicts and unconscious processes presumed to underlie the behavior. **biological t.,** treatment of disease by injection of substances that produce a biological reaction in the organism. **chelation t.,** the use of a chelating agent to remove toxic metals from the body, used in the treatment of heavy metal poisoning. In complementary medicine, also used for the treatment of atherosclerosis and other disorders. **cognitive t., cognitive-behavioral t.,** that based on the theory that emotional problems result from distorted attitudes and ways of thinking that can be corrected, the therapist guiding the patient to do so. **convulsive t.,** treatment of mental disorders, primarily depression, by induction of convulsions; now it is virtually always by electric shock (*electroconvulsive t.*). **couples t.,** marital t. **dance t.,** the therapeutic use of movement to further the emotional, social, cognitive, and physical integration of the individual in the treatment of a variety of social, emotional, cognitive, and physical disorders. **electroconvulsive t. (ECT),** a treatment for mental disorders, primarily depression, in which convulsions and loss of consciousness are induced by application of brief pulses of low-voltage alternating current to the brain via scalp electrodes. **electroshock t. (EST),** electroconvulsive t. **endocrine t.,** treatment of disease by the use of hormones. **estrogen replacement t.,** administration of an estrogen to treat estrogen deficiency, as that following menopause; in women with a uterus, a progestational agent is usually included to prevent endometrial hyperplasia. **enzyme t.**, in complementary medicine, the oral administration of proteolytic enzymes to improve immune system function; used for a wide variety of disorders and as adjunctive therapy in cancer treatment. **family t.**, group therapy of the members of a family, exploring and improving family relationships and processes and thus the mental health of the collective unit and of individual members. **fibrinolytic t.**, the use of fibrinolytic agents (e.g., prourokinase) to lyse thrombi in patients with acute peripheral arterial occlusion, deep venous thrombosis, pulmonary embolism, or acute myocardial infarction. **gene t.**, manipulation of the genome of an individual to prevent, mask, or lessen the effects of a genetic disorder. **group t.**, psychotherapy carried out regularly with a group of patients under the guidance of a group leader, usually a therapist. **highly active antiretroviral t. (HAART)**, the aggressive use of extremely potent antiretroviral agents in the treatment of human immunodeficiency virus infection. **hormonal t., hormone t.**, endocrine t. **hormone replacement t.**, the administration of hormones to correct a deficiency, such as postmenopausal estrogen replacement therapy. **immunosuppressive t.**, treatment with agents, such as x-rays, corticosteroids, or cytotoxic chemicals, that suppress the immune response to antigen(s); used in conditions such as organ transplantation, autoimmune disease, allergy, multiple myeloma, and chronic nephritis. **inhalation t.**, former name for *respiratory care* (2). **light t.**, 1. phototherapy (def. 1). 2. photodynamic t. **marital t.**, a type of family therapy aimed at understanding and treating one or both members of a couple in the context of a distressed relationship, but not necessarily addressing the discordant relationship itself; sometimes used more restrictively as a synonym of *marriage therapy*. **marriage t.**, a subset of marital therapy (q.v.) that focuses specifically on the bond of marriage between two people, enhancing and preserving it. **massage t.**, the manipulation of the soft tissues of the body for the purpose of normalizing them, thereby enhancing health and healing. **milieu t.**, treatment, usually in a psychiatric hospital, that emphasizes the provision of an environment and activities appropriate to the patient's emotional and interpersonal needs. **music t.**, the use of music to effect positive changes in the psychological, physical, cognitive, or social functioning of individuals with health or educational problems. **occupational t.**, the therapeutic use of self-care, work, and play activities to increase function, enhance development, and prevent disabilities. **oral rehydration t. (ORT)**, oral administration of a solution of electrolytes and carbohydrates in the treatment of dehydration. **orthomolecular t.**, treatment of disease based on the theory that restoration of optimal concentrations of substances normally present in the body, such as vitamins, trace elements, and amino acids, will effect a cure. **photodynamic t.**, intravenous administration of hematoporphyrin derivative, which concentrates selectively in metabolically active tumor tissue, followed by exposure of the tumor tissue to red laser light to produce cytotoxic free radicals that destroy hematoporphyrin-containing tissue. **physical t.**, 1. treatment by physical means. 2. the health profession concerned with the promotion of health, the prevention of disability, and the evaluation and rehabilitation of patients disabled by pain, disease, or injury, and with treatment by physical therapeutic measures as opposed to medical, surgical, or radiologic measures. **poetry t.**, a form of bibliotherapy in which a selected poem, which may be created by the patient, is used to evoke feelings and responses for discussion in a therapeutic setting. **PUVA t.**, a form of photochemotherapy for skin disorders such as psoriasis and vitiligo; oral psoralen administration is followed two hours later by exposure to ultraviolet light. **radiation t.**, radiotherapy. **relaxation t.**, any of a number of techniques for inducing the relaxation response, used for the reduction of stress; useful in the management of a wide variety of chronic illnesses caused or exacerbated by stress. **replacement t.**, 1. treatment to replace deficiencies in body products by administration of natural or synthetic substitutes. 2. treatment that replaces or compensates for a nonfunctioning organ, e.g., hemodialysis. **respiratory t.**, see under *care*. **substitution t.**, the administration of a hormone to compensate for glandular deficiency. **thrombolytic t.**, fibrinolytic t. **thyroid replacement t.**, treatment with a preparation of a thyroid hormone.

therm (therm) a unit of heat. The word has been used as equivalent to (a) large calorie; (b) small calorie; (c) 1000 large calories; (d) 100,000 British thermal units.

ther·mal (ther'm'l) pertaining to or characterized by heat.

ther·mal·ge·sia (ther″mal-je′zhah) a dysesthesia in which application of heat causes pain.

ther·mal·gia (ther-mal′jah) causalgia.

therm·an·al·ge·sia (therm″an-al-je′ze-ah) thermoanesthesia.

therm·an·es·the·sia (-an-es-the′zhah) thermoanesthesia.

therm·es·the·sia (-es-the′zhah) temperature sense.

therm·es·the·si·om·e·ter (-es-the″ze-om′ĕ-ter) an instrument for measuring sensibility to heat.

therm·hy·per·es·the·sia (-hi″per-es-the′zhah) thermohyperesthesia.

therm·hy·pes·the·sia (-hi-pes-the′zhah) thermohypesthesia.

ther·mic (ther′mik) pertaining to heat.

therm(o)- word element [Gr.], *heat.*

ther·mo·an·es·the·sia (ther″mo-an″es-the′zhah) inability to recognize sensations of heat and cold; loss or lack of temperature sense.

ther·mo·cau·tery (-kaw′ter-e) cauterization by a heated wire or point.

ther·mo·chem·is·try (-kem′is-tre) the aspect of physical chemistry dealing with heat changes that accompany chemical reactions.

ther·mo·co·ag·u·la·tion (-ko-ag″u-la′shun) tissue coagulation with high-frequency currents.

ther·mo·dif·fu·sion (-dĭ-fu′zhun) diffusion due to a temperature gradient.

ther·mo·dy·nam·ics (-di-nam′iks) the branch of science dealing with heat, work, and energy, their interconversion, and problems related thereto.

ther·mo·ex·ci·to·ry (-ek-si′ter-e) stimulating production of bodily heat.

ther·mo·gen·e·sis (-jen′ĕ-sis) the production of heat, especially within the animal body. **thermogenet′ic, thermogen′ic,** adj.

ther·mo·gram (ther′mo-gram) 1. a graphic record of temperature variations. 2. the visual record obtained by thermography.

ther·mo·graph (-graf) 1. an instrument for recording temperature variations. 2. thermogram (2). 3. the apparatus used in thermography.

ther·mog·ra·phy (ther-mog′rah-fe) a technique wherein an infrared camera photographically portrays the body's surface temperature, based on self-emanating infrared radiation; sometimes used as a means of diagnosing underlying pathologic conditions, such as breast tumors.

ther·mo·hy·per·al·ge·sia (ther″mo-hi″per-al-je′ze-ah) extreme thermalgesia.

ther·mo·hy·per·es·the·sia (-hi″per-es-the′zhah) a dysesthesia with increased sensibility to heat and cold.

ther·mo·hy·pes·the·sia (-hi″pes-the′zhah) a dysesthesia with decreased sensibility to heat and cold.

ther·mo·in·hib·i·to·ry (-in-hib′ĭ-tor″e) retarding generation of bodily heat.

ther·mo·la·bile (-la′bīl) easily affected by heat.

ther·mol·y·sis (ther-mol′ĭ-sis) 1. chemical dissociation by means of heat. 2. dissipation of bodily heat by radiation, evaporation, etc. **thermolyt′ic,** adj.

ther·mo·mas·sage (ther″mo-mah-sahzh′) massage with heat.

ther·mom·e·ter (ther-mom′ĕ-ter) an instrument for determining temperatures, in principle making use of a substance with a physical property that varies with temperature and is susceptible of measurement on some defined scale (see table accompanying *temperature*). **clinical t.,** one used to determine the temperature of the human body. **infrared tympanic t.,** a clinical thermometer inserted into the external acoustic meatus to determine the body temperature by measuring the infrared radiation emanating from the tympanic membrane. **oral t.,** a clinical thermometer that is placed under the tongue. **recording t.,** a temperature-sensitive instrument by which the temperature to which it is exposed is continuously recorded. **rectal t.,** a clinical thermometer that is inserted into the rectum. **tympanic t.,** infrared tympanic t.

ther·mo·phile (ther′mo-fīl) an organism that grows best at elevated temperatures. **thermophil′ic,** adj.

ther·mo·phore (-for) a device or apparatus for retaining heat, used in therapeutic local application.

ther·mo·plac·en·tog·ra·phy (ther″mo-plas″en-tog′rah-fe) use of thermography for determination of the site of placental attachment.

ther·mo·ple·gia (-ple′jah) heat stroke or sunstroke.

ther·mo·re·cep·tor (-re-sep′ter) a nerve ending sensitive to stimulation by heat.

ther·mo·reg·u·la·tion (-reg″u-la′shun) the regulation of heat, as of the body heat of a warm-blooded animal. **thermoreg′ulatory,** adj.

ther·mo·sta·bile (-sta′bīl) not affected by heat.

ther·mo·sys·tal·tic (-sis-tahl′tik) contracting under the stimulus of heat.

ther·mo·tax·is (-tak′sis) 1. normal adjustment of bodily temperature. 2. movement of an organism in response to an increase in temperature. **thermotac′tic, thermotax′ic,** adj.

ther·mo·to·nom·e·ter (-to-nom′ĕ-ter) an instrument for measuring the amount of muscular contraction produced by heat.

ther·mot·ro·pism (ther-mot′rah-pizm) tropism in response to an increase in temperature. **thermotrop′ic,** adj.

THF tetrahydrofolic acid.

thi·a·ben·da·zole (thi″ah-ben′dah-zōl) a broad-spectrum anthelmintic used in the treatment of strongyloidiasis, trichinosis, and cutaneous or visceral larva migrans.

thi·a·mine (thi′ah-min) vitamin B_1; a water-soluble component of the B vitamin complex, found particularly in pork, organ meats, legumes, nuts, and whole grain or enriched breads and cereals. The active form is *thiamine pyrophosphate (TPP)*, which serves as a coenzyme in various reactions. Deficiency can result in beriberi and is a factor in alcoholic neuritis and Wernicke-Korsakoff syndrome. Written also *thiamin.* **t. pyrophosphate (TPP),** the active form of thiamine, serving as a coenzyme in a variety of reactions, particularly in carbohydrate metabolism.

thi·a·zide (thi′ah-zīd) any of a group of diuretics that act by inhibiting the reabsorption of sodium in the proximal renal tubule and stimulating chloride excretion, with resultant increase in excretion of water.

thickness (thik′nes) a measurement across the smallest dimension of an object. **triceps skinfold (TSF) t.,** a measurement of subcutaneous fat taken by measuring a fold of skin running parallel to the length of the arm over the triceps muscle midway between the acromion and olecranon.

thi·emia (thi-e′me-ah) sulfur in the blood.

thi·eth·yl·per·a·zine (thi-eth″il-par′ah-zēn) an antiemetic, used as the malate or maleate salt in the treatment and prophylaxis of nausea and vomiting.

thigh (thi) femur; the portion of the leg above the knee.

thig·mes·the·sia (thig″mes-the′zhah) touch (1).

thig·mo·tax·is (thig″mo-tak′sis) taxis of an organism in response to contact or touch. **thigmotac′tic, thigmotax′ic,** adj.

thig·mot·ro·pism (thig-mot′rah-pizm) tropism of an organism elicited by touch or by contact with a solid or rigid surface. **thigmotrop′ic,** adj.

thi·mero·sal (thi-mer′o-sal) an organomercurial antiseptic that is antifungal and bacteriostatic for many nonsporulating bacteria, used as a topical antiinfective and as a pharmaceutical preservative.

think·ing (thingk′ing) ideational mental activity (as opposed to emotional activity). **autistic t.,** preoccupation with inner thoughts, daydreams, fantasies, private logic; egocentric, subjective thinking lacking objectivity and connection with external reality. **dereistic t.,** thinking not in accordance with the facts of reality and experience and following illogical, idiosyncratic reasoning. **magical t.,** that characterized by the belief that thinking or wishing something can cause it to occur.

thi(o)- a word element [Gr.], *sulfur.*

thio·bar·bi·tu·ric ac·id (thi″o-bahr″bĭ-tu′rik) a condensation of malonic acid and thiourea, closely related to barbituric acid. It is the parent compound of a class of drugs, the thiobarbiturates, which are analogous in their effects to barbiturates.

thio·cy·a·nate (-si′ah-nāt) a salt analogous in composition to a cyanate, but containing sulfur instead of oxygen.

thio·es·ter (-es′ter) a carboxylic acid and a thiol group in ester linkage, e.g., acetyl coenzyme A.

thio·gua·nine (-gwah′nēn) an antineoplastic derived from mercaptopurine; used in the treatment of acute myelogenous leukemia.

thio·ki·nase (-ki′nās) any of the ligases that catalyze the formation of a thioester in a reaction coupled to cleavage of a high-energy phosphate bond.

thi·ol (thi′ol) 1. sulfhydryl. 2. any organic compound containing the —SH group.

thi·o·nine (thi′o-nēn) a dark-green powder, purple in solution, used as a metachromatic stain in microscopy.

thio·pen·tal (thi″o-pen′tal) an ultrashort-acting barbiturate; the sodium salt is used intravenously to induce general anesthesia, as an adjunct to general or local anesthesia, and as an anticonvulsant.

thi·o·rid·a·zine (-rid′ah-zēn) a tranquilizer with antipsychotic and sedative effects, used as the base or hydrochloride salt.

thio·sul·fate (-sul′fāt) the $S_2O_3^{2-}$ anion, or a salt containing this ion; produced in cysteine metabolism.

thio·tepa (-tep′ah) a cytotoxic alkylating agent, used as an antineoplastic in the treatment of breast, ovarian, or bladder cancer, Hodgkin's disease, and malignant pleural or pericardial effusion.

thio·thix·ene (-thik′sēn) a thioxanthene derivative, used as the base or the hydrochloride salt for the treatment of psychotic disorders.

thio·xan·thene (-zan'thēn) 1. a three-ring compound structurally related to phenothiazine. 2. any of a class of structurally related antipsychotic agents, e.g., thiothixene.

thirst (therst) a sensation, often referred to the mouth and throat, associated with a craving for drink; ordinarily interpreted as a desire for water.

this·tle (this'l) any of a number of weedy plants of the family Compositae, having spiny leaves and flower heads surrounded by spiny bracts. **blessed t.,** the thistlelike herb *Cnicus benedictus,* or its dried flowers, leaves, and upper stems; used for dyspepsia and loss of appetite; used also in folk medicine for fever and colds and as a diuretic. **milk t.,** the thistle, *Silybum marianum,* or its dried ripe fruit; used for loss of appetite and for supportive treatment in gallbladder and liver disorders.

thix·ot·ro·pism (thik-sot'rah-pizm) thixotropy.

thix·ot·ro·py (thik-sot'rah-pe) the property of certain gels of becoming fluid when shaken and then becoming semisolid again. **thixotrop'ic,** adj.

tho·ra·cal·gia (thor"ah-kal'jah) thoracodynia; pain in the chest.

tho·ra·cec·to·my (-sek'tah-me) thoracotomy with resection of part of a rib.

tho·ra·cen·te·sis (-sen-te'sis) pleurocentesis; surgical puncture of the chest wall into the parietal cavity for aspiration of fluids.

tho·ra·ces (tho'rah-sēz) [Gr.] plural of *thorax.*

tho·rac·ic (thah-ras'ik) pectoral; pertaining to the thorax (chest).

thorac(o)- word element [Gr.], *chest.*

tho·ra·co·acro·mi·al (thor"ah-ko-ah-kro'me-al) pertaining to the chest and acromion.

tho·ra·co·cyl·lo·sis (-sǐ-lo'sis) deformity of the thorax.

tho·ra·co·cyr·to·sis (-sir-to'sis) abnormal curvature of the thorax or unusual prominence of the chest.

tho·ra·co·dyn·ia (-din'e-ah) thoracalgia.

tho·ra·co·gas·tros·chi·sis (-gas-tros'kǐ-sis) congenital fissure of the thorax and abdomen.

tho·ra·co·lum·bar (-lum'bar) pertaining to thoracic and lumbar vertebrae.

tho·ra·col·y·sis (thor"ah-kol'ǐ-sis) the freeing of adhesions of the chest wall.

tho·ra·com·e·ter (-kom'ah-ter) stethometer.

tho·ra·cop·a·gus (-kop'ah-gus) conjoined twins united in or near the sternal region.

tho·ra·cop·a·thy (-kop'ah-the) any disease of the thoracic organs or tissues.

tho·ra·co·plas·ty (thor'ah-ko-plas"te) surgical removal of ribs to gain access during surgery or to collapse the chest wall and a diseased lung.

tho·ra·cos·chi·sis (thor"ah-kos'kǐ-sis) congenital fissure of the thorax.

tho·ra·co·scope (thŏ-rak'o-skōp) an endoscope for examining the pleural cavity through an intercostal space.

tho·ra·co·ste·no·sis (thor"ah-ko-stě-no'sis) abnormal contraction of the thorax.

tho·ra·cos·to·my (-kos'tah-me) 1. incision of the chest wall, with maintenance of the opening for drainage. 2. the incision so created.

tho·ra·cot·o·my (-kot'ah-me) pleurotomy; incision of the chest wall.

tho·rax (tho'raks) pl. *tho'races.* [Gr.] chest; the part of the body between the neck and diaphragm, encased by the ribs. **Peyrot's t.,** an obliquely oval thorax associated with massive pleural effusions.

tho·ri·um (thor'e-um) chemical element (see *Table of Elements*), at. no. 90, symbol Th.

thought broad·cast·ing (thawt brawd'kasting) the feeling that one's thoughts are being broadcast to the environment.

thought in·ser·tion (in-ser'shun) the delusion that thoughts that are not one's own are being inserted into one's mind.

thought with·draw·al (with-draw'al) the delusion that someone or something is removing thoughts from one's mind.

Thr threonine.

thread·worm (thred'werm) any long slender nematode, especially *Enterobius vermicularis.*

thready (thred'e) weak, thin; shallow.

thre·o·nine (Thr, T) (thre'o-nēn) a naturally occurring amino acid essential for human metabolism.

thresh·old (thresh'old) the level that must be reached for an effect to be produced, as the degree of intensity of a stimulus that just produces a sensation, or the concentration that must be present in the blood before certain substances are excreted by the kidney (*renal t.*).

thrill (thril) a vibration felt by the examiner on palpation. **diastolic t.,** one felt over the precordium during ventricular diastole in advanced aortic insufficiency. **hydatid t.,** one sometimes felt on percussing over a hydatid cyst. **presystolic t.,** one felt just before the systole over the apex of the heart. **systolic t.,** one felt over the precordium during systole in aortic stenosis, pulmonary stenosis, and ventricular septal defect.

-thrix word element [Gr.], *hair.*

throat (thrōt) 1. pharynx. 2. fauces. 3. anterior aspect of the neck. **sore t.,** 1. faucitis. 2. pharyngitis. **streptococcal sore t.,** septic sore throat; severe sore throat occurring in epidemics, usually caused by *Streptococcus pyogenes*, with local hyperemia and sometimes a gray exudate and enlargement of cervical lymph nodes.

throm·bas·the·nia (throm″bas-the′ne-ah) a platelet abnormality characterized by defective clot retraction and impaired ADP-induced platelet aggregation; clinically manifested by epistaxis, inappropriate bruising, and excessive posttraumatic bleeding. **Glanzmann t.,** thrombasthenia.

throm·bec·to·my (throm-bek′tah-me) surgical removal of a clot from a blood vessel.

throm·bi (throm′bi) plural of *thrombus.*

throm·bin (throm′bin) 1. the activated form of coagulation factor II (prothrombin); it catalyzes the conversion of fibrinogen to fibrin. 2. a preparation derived from prothrombin of bovine origin together with thromboplastin and calcium; used therapeutically as a local hemostatic.

thromb(o)- word element [Gr.], *clot; thrombus.*

throm·bo·an·gi·itis (throm″bo-an″je-i′tis) inflammation of a blood vessel, with thrombosis. **t. obli′terans,** Buerger's disease; an inflammatory and obliterative disease of the blood vessels of the limbs, primarily the legs, leading to ischemia and gangrene.

throm·bo·ar·ter·i·tis (-ar″ter-i′tis) thrombosis associated with arteritis.

throm·boc·la·sis (throm-bok′lah-sis) the dissolution of a thrombus. **thromboclas′tic,** adj.

throm·bo·cyst (throm′bo-sist) a chronic sac formed around a thrombus in a hematoma.

throm·bo·cys·tis (throm″bo-sis′tis) thrombocyst.

throm·bo·cy·ta·phe·re·sis (-si″tah-fĕ-re′sis) the selective separation and removal of platelets from withdrawn blood, the remainder of the blood then being retransfused into the donor.

throm·bo·cyte (throm′bo-sīt) platelet.

throm·bo·cy·the·mia (throm″bo-si-the′me-ah) thrombocytosis. **essential t.,** hemorrhagic t., a syndrome of repeated spontaneous hemorrhages, either external or into the tissues, and greatly increased number of circulating platelets.

throm·bo·cyt·ic (-sit′ik) 1. pertaining to, characterized by, or of the nature of a platelet (thrombocyte). 2. pertaining to the thrombocytic series.

throm·bo·cy·tol·y·sis (-si-tol′ĭ-sis) destruction of platelets.

throm·bo·cy·top·a·thy (-si-top′ah-the) any qualitative disorder of platelets.

throm·bo·cy·to·pe·nia (-si″to-pe′ne-ah) decrease in number of platelets in circulating blood. **thrombocytope′nic,** adj. **immune t.,** that associated with the presence of antiplatelet antibodies (IgG).

throm·bo·cy·to·poi·e·sis (-si″to-poi-e′sis) the production of platelets. **thrombocytopoiet′ic,** adj.

throm·bo·cy·to·sis (-si-to′sis) thrombocythemia; an increase in the number of circulating platelets.

throm·bo·em·bo·lism (-em′bo-lizm) obstruction of a blood vessel with thrombotic material carried by the blood from the site of origin to plug another vessel.

throm·bo·end·ar·ter·ec·to·my (-end″ahr-ter-ek′tah-me) excision of an obstructing thrombus together with a portion of the inner lining of the obstructed artery.

throm·bo·end·ar·ter·i·tis (-end″ahr-ter-i′tis) inflammation of the innermost coat of an artery, with thrombus formation.

throm·bo·en·do·car·di·tis (-en″do-kahr-di′tis) a term formerly used for nonbacterial thrombotic endocarditis or sometimes incorrectly for nonbacterial verrucous endocarditis.

throm·bo·gen·e·sis (-jen′ĕ-sis) clot formation. **thrombogen′ic,** adj.

β-throm·bo·glob·u·lin (-glob′u-lin) a platelet-specific protein released with platelet factor 4 on platelet activation; it mediates several reactions of the inflammatory response, binds and inactivates heparin, and blocks endothelial cell release of prostacyclin.

throm·boid (throm′boid) resembling a thrombus.

throm·bo·ki·nase (throm″bo-ki′nās) activated factor X; see *coagulation factors,* under *factor.*

throm·bo·ki·net·ics (-kĭ-net′iks) the dynamics of blood coagulation.

throm·bo·lym·phan·gi·tis (-lim″fan-ji′tis) inflammation of a lymph vessel due to a thrombus.

throm·bol·y·sis (throm-bol′ĭ-sis) dissolution of a thrombus.

throm·bo·lyt·ic (throm″bo-lit′ik) dissolving or splitting up a thrombus, or an agent that so acts.

throm·bo·phil·ia (throm″bo-fil′e-ah) a tendency to the occurrence of thrombosis.

throm·bo·phle·bi·tis (-flĕ-bi′tis) inflammation of a vein (phlebitis) associated with thrombus formation (thrombosis).

t. mi'grans, a recurring thrombophlebitis involving different vessels simultaneously or at intervals. **postpartum iliofemoral t.,** thrombophlebitis of the iliofemoral vein following childbirth.

throm·bo·plas·tic (-plas'tik) causing or accelerating clot formation in the blood.

throm·bo·plas·tin (-plas'tin) coagulation factor III. **tissue t.,** coagulation factor III.

throm·bo·poi·e·sis (-poi-e'sis) 1. thrombogenesis. 2. thrombocytopoiesis. **thrombopoiet'ic,** adj.

throm·bo·re·sis·tance (-re-zis'tans) resistance by a blood vessel to thrombus formation.

throm·bosed (throm'bōzd) affected with thrombosis.

throm·bo·sis (throm-bo'sis) the formation or presence of a thrombus. **thrombot'ic,** adj. **cerebral t.,** thrombosis of a cerebral vessel, which may result in cerebral infarction. **coronary t.,** thrombosis of a coronary artery, usually associated with atherosclerosis and often causing sudden death or myocardial infarction. **deep venous t.,** thrombosis of one or more of the deep veins of the lower limb, with swelling, warmth, and erythema, frequently a precursor of a pulmonary embolism.

throm·bo·spon·din (throm″bo-spon'din) a glycoprotein that interacts with a wide variety of molecules, including heparin, fibrin, fibrinogen, platelet cell membrane receptors, collagen, and fibronectin, and plays a role in platelet aggregation, tumor metastasis, adhesion of *Plasmodium falciparum,* vascular smooth muscle growth, and tissue repair in skeletal muscle following crush injury.

throm·bos·ta·sis (throm-bos'tah-sis) stasis of blood in a part with formation of a thrombus.

throm·bot·ic (-bot'ik) pertaining to or affected with thrombosis.

throm·box·ane (-bok'sān) either of two compounds, one designated A_2 and the other B_2. Thromboxane A_2 is synthesized by platelets and is an inducer of platelet aggregation and platelet release functions and is a vasoconstrictor; it is very unstable and is hydrolyzed to thromboxane B_2.

throm·bus (throm'bus) pl. *throm'bi.* A stationary blood clot along the wall of a blood vessel, frequently causing vascular obstruction. Some authorities differentiate thrombus formation from simple coagulation or clot formation. **mural t.,** one attached to the wall of the endocardium in a diseased area or to the aortic wall overlying an intimal

lesion. **occluding t., occlusive t.,** one that occupies the entire lumen of a vessel and obstructs blood flow. **parietal t.,** one attached to a vessel or heart wall.

thrush (thrush) candidiasis of the oral mucous membranes, usually seen in sick, weak infants, or persons who are debilitated or immunocompromised, characterized by creamy white plaques resembling milk curds, which if stripped away leave raw bleeding surfaces.

thryp·sis (thrip'sis) comminuted fracture.

thu·ja (thu'jah) the fresh tops of *Thuja occidentalis* (arbor vitae); used in some topical dermatologic preparations and also in homeopathy.

thu·li·um (thoo'le-um) chemical element (see *Table of Elements*), at. no. 69, symbol Tm.

thumb (thum) the radial or first digit of the hand. **tennis t.,** tendinitis of the tendon of the long flexor muscle of the thumb, with calcification.

thumb·print·ing (thum'print-ing) a radiographic sign appearing as smooth indentations on the barium-filled colon, as though made by depression with the thumb.

thump·ver·sion (thump-ver'zhun) delivery of one or two blows to the chest in initiating cardiopulmonary resuscitation, in order to initiate a pulse or to convert ventricular fibrillation to a normal rhythm.

thyme (tīm) 1. any plant of the genus *Thymus.* 2. a preparation of the leaves and flowers of garden thyme (*T. vulgaris*), used as an antitussive and expectorant.

thy·mec·to·mize (thi-mek'tah-mīz) to excise the thymus.

thy·mec·to·my (-me) excision of the thymus.

-thymia word element [Gr.], *condition of mind.* **-thy'mic,** adj.

thy·mic (thi'mik) pertaining to the thymus.

thy·mi·co·lym·phat·ic (thi″mĭ-ko-limfat'ik) pertaining to the thymus and lymphatic nodes.

thy·mi·dine (thi'mĭ-dēn) thymine linked to ribose, a rarely occurring base in rRNA and tRNA; frequently used incorrectly to denote deoxythymidine. Symbol T.

thy·min (thi'min) thymopoietin.

thy·mine (thi'mēn) a pyrimidine base, in animal cells usually occurring condensed with deoxyribose to form deoxythymidine, a component of DNA. The corresponding compound with ribose, thymidine, is a rare constituent of RNA. Symbol T.

thy·mi·tis (thi-mi'tis) inflammation of the thymus.

thym(o)- word element [Gr.], *thymus; mind, soul,* or *emotions.*

thy·mo·cyte (thi′mo-sīt) a lymphocyte arising in the thymus.

thy·mo·ki·net·ic (thi″mo-kĭ-net′ik) tending to stimulate the thymus.

thy·mo·lep·tic (-lep′tik) any drug that favorably modifies mood in serious affective disorders such as depression or mania; categories include tricyclic antidepressants, monoamine oxidase inhibitors, and lithium compounds.

thy·mo·ma (thi-mo′mah) a tumor derived from the epithelial or lymphoid elements of the thymus.

thy·mop·a·thy (thi-mop′ah-the) any disease of the thymus. **thymopath′ic,** adj.

thy·mo·poi·e·tin (thi″mo-poi′ĕ-tin) a polypeptide hormone secreted by thymic epithelial cells that induces differentiation of precursor lymphocytes into thymocytes.

thy·mo·priv·ic (-priv′ik) thymoprivous.

thy·mop·ri·vous (thi-mop′rĭ-vus) pertaining to or resulting from removal or atrophy of the thymus.

thy·mo·sin (thi′mo-sin) a humoral factor secreted by the thymus, which promotes the maturation of T lymphocytes.

thy·mus (thi′mus) a bilaterally symmetrical lymphoid organ consisting of two pyramidal lobules situated in the anterior superior mediastinum, each lobule consisting of an outer cortex, rich in lymphocytes (thymocytes) and an inner medulla, rich in epithelial cells. The thymus is the site of production of T lymphocytes: precursor cells migrate to the outer cortex, where they proliferate, then move through the inner cortex, where T-cell surface markers are acquired, and finally into the medulla, where they become mature T cells; maturation is controlled by hormones produced by the thymus, including thymopoietin and thymosin. The thymus reaches maximal development at about puberty and then undergoes gradual involution.

thyr(o)- word element [Gr.], *thyroid.*

thy·ro·ad·e·ni·tis (thi″ro-ad″ĕ-ni′tis) thyroiditis.

thy·ro·apla·sia (-ah-pla′zhah) defective development of the thyroid gland with hypothyroidism.

thy·ro·ar·y·te·noid (-ar″ĭ-te′noid) pertaining to the thyroid and arytenoid cartilages.

thy·ro·car·di·ac (-kahr′de-ak) pertaining to the thyroid gland and heart.

thy·ro·cele (thi′ro-sēl) goiter.

thy·ro·chon·drot·o·my (thi″ro-kon-drot′ah-me) median laryngotomy.

thy·ro·cri·cot·o·my (-kri-kot′ah-me) incision of the cricothyroid membrane.

thy·ro·epi·glot·tic (-ep″ĭ-glot′ik) pertaining to the thyroid gland and epiglottis.

thy·ro·gen·ic (-jen′ik) thyrogenous.

thy·rog·e·nous (thi-roj′ĕ-nus) originating in the thyroid gland.

thy·ro·glob·u·lin (thi″ro-glob′u-lin) an iodine-containing glycoprotein of high molecular weight, occurring in the colloid of the follicles of the thyroid gland; the iodinated tyrosine moieties of thyroglobulin form the active hormones thyroxine and triiodothyronine.

thy·ro·glos·sal (-glos′al) pertaining to the thyroid gland and tongue.

thy·ro·hy·al (-hi′al) pertaining to the thyroid cartilage and the hyoid bone.

thy·ro·hy·oid (-hi′oid) pertaining to the thyroid gland or cartilage and the hyoid bone.

thy·roid (thi′roid) 1. the thyroid gland; see under *gland.* 2. pertaining to the thyroid gland. 3. scutiform. 4. a preparation of thyroid gland from domesticated food animals, containing levothyroxine and liothyronine and used as replacement therapy in the diagnosis and treatment of hypothyroidism and the prophylaxis and treatment of goiter and thyroid carcinoma.

thy·roid·ec·to·mize (thi″roid-ek′tah-mīz) to excise the thyroid gland.

thy·roid·ec·to·my (-ek′tah-me) excision of the thyroid gland.

thy·roid·itis (-i′tis) inflammation of the thyroid gland. **atrophic t.,** a type of autoimmune thyroiditis with atrophy of the follicles and without goiter. **autoimmune t.,** any of various types characterized by autoantibodies against the thyroid, resulting in hypothyroidism; the two major types are Hashimoto's disease and atrophic thyroiditis; Riedel's thyroiditis is a less common type. **Hashimoto's t.,** see under *disease.* **Riedel's t.,** a chronic type of autoimmune thyroiditis with a proliferating, fibrosing, inflammatory process involving usually one but sometimes both lobes of the thyroid gland, as well as the trachea and other adjacent structures.

thy·roid·ot·o·my (-ot′ah-me) median laryngotomy.

thy·ro·lin·gual (thi″ro-ling′gw'l) thyroglossal.

thy·ro·meg·a·ly (-meg′ah-le) goiter.

thy·ro·mi·met·ic (-mi-met′ik) producing effects similar to those of thyroid hormones or the thyroid gland.

thy·ro·para·thy·roid·ec·to·my (-par″thi″roi-dek′tah-me) excision of thyroid and parathyroids.

thy·rop·to·sis (thi″rop-to′sis) downward displacement of the thyroid gland into the thorax.

thy·ro·ther·a·py (thi″ro-ther′ah-pe) thyroid replacement therapy.

thy·rot·o·my (thi-rot′ah-me) 1. median laryngotomy. 2. the operation of cutting the thyroid gland. 3. biopsy of the thyroid gland.

thy·ro·tox·ic (thi′ro-tok″sik) 1. pertaining to the effects of thyroid hormone excess. 2. describing a patient suffering from thyrotoxicosis.

thy·ro·tox·i·co·sis (thi″ro-tok″sĭ-ko′sis) a morbid condition due to overactivity of the thyroid gland; see *Graves' disease.*

thy·ro·trope (thi′ro-trōp) thyrotroph.

thy·ro·troph (-trōf) a type of basophil found in the adenohypophysis that secretes thyrotropin.

thy·ro·tro·phic (thi″ro-tro′fik) thyrotropic.

thy·ro·troph·in (-tro″fin) thyrotropin.

thy·ro·tro·pic (-tro′pik) 1. pertaining to or marked by thyrotropism. 2. having an influence on the thyroid gland.

thy·ro·tro·pin (thi-rot′rah-pin) thyroid-stimulating hormone; a hormone of the anterior pituitary gland having an affinity for and specifically stimulating the thyroid gland. **t. alfa,** a recombinant form of thyrotropin used as a diagnostic adjunct in serum thyroglobulin testing in followup of patients with thyroid cancer.

thy·rox·ine (T₄) (thi-rok′sin) an iodine-containing hormone secreted by the thyroid gland, occurring naturally as L-thyroxine; its chief function is to increase the rate of cell metabolism. It is deiodinated in peripheral tissues to form triiodothyronine, which has greater biological activity. A preparation of thyroxine, levothyroxine, is used pharmaceutically.

Ti titanium.

TIA transient ischemic attack.

ti·ag·a·bine (ti-ag′ah-bēn) an anticonvulsant agent used as the hydrochloride salt as an adjunct in the treatment of partial seizures.

tib·ia (tib′e-ah) see *Table of Bones.* **tib′ial,** adj. **t. val′ga,** bowing of the leg in which the angulation is away from the midline. **t. va′ra,** medial angulation of the tibia in the metaphyseal region, due to a growth disturbance of the medial aspect of the proximal tibial epiphysis.

tib·i·a·lis (tib″e-a′lis) [L.] tibial.

tib·io·fem·or·al (tib″e-o-fem′o-ral) pertaining to the tibia and femur.

tib·io·fib·u·lar (-fib′u-ler) pertaining to the tibia and fibula.

tib·io·tar·sal (-tahr′s'l) pertaining to the tibia and tarsus.

tic (tik) [Fr.] an involuntary, compulsive, rapid, repetitive, stereotyped movement or vocalization, experienced as irresistible although it can be suppressed for some length of time. **t. douloureux** (doo-loo-roo′), trigeminal neuralgia. **facial t.,** see under *spasm.* **habit t.,** any tic that is psychogenic in origin.

ti·car·cil·lin (ti″kahr-sil′in) a semisynthetic broad-spectrum penicillin effective against both gram-negative and gram-positive organisms; used as the disodium salt.

tick (tik) a bloodsucking acarid parasite of the superfamily Ixodoidea, divided into *soft-bodied ticks* and *hard-bodied ticks.* Some ticks are vectors and reservoirs of disease-causing agents.

ti·clo·pi·dine (ti-klo′pĭ-dēn) a platelet inhibitor used as the hydrochloride salt in the prophylaxis of stroke syndrome.

t.i.d. [L.] ter in di′e (three times a day).

ti·dal (ti′d'l) ebbing and flowing like the waters of the oceans.

tide (tīd) a physiological variation or increase of a certain constituent in body fluids. **acid t.,** temporary increase in the acidity of the urine which sometimes follows fasting. **alkaline t.,** temporary increase in the alkalinity of the urine during gastric digestion. **fat t.,** the increase of fat in the lymph and blood after a meal.

ti·lu·dro·nate (ti-loo′drah-nāt) an inhibitor of bone resorption, used as the disodium salt in the treatment of osteitis deformans.

tim·bre (tam′ber) [Fr.] musical quality of a tone or sound.

time (tīm) a measure of duration. Symbol *t.* **activated partial thromboplastin t. (APTT, aPTT, PTT),** the period required for clot formation in recalcified blood plasma after contact activation and the addition of platelet substitutes; used to address the intrinsic and common pathways of coagulation. **bleeding t.,** the duration of bleeding after controlled, standardized puncture of the earlobe or forearm; a relatively inconsistent measure of capillary and platelet function. **circulation t.,** the time required for blood to flow between two given points. **clotting t., coagulation t.,** the time required for blood to clot in a glass tube. **inertia t.,** the time required to overcome the inertia of a muscle after reception of a stimulus from a nerve. **one-stage prothrombin t.,** prothrombin t. **prothrombin t. (PT),** the rate at which prothrombin is converted to thrombin in citrated blood with added calcium; used to assess the extrinsic coagulation system of the blood. **reaction t.,** the time elapsing between the application of a stimulus and the resulting reaction. **stimulus-response t.,** reaction t. **thrombin t. (TT),** the time required for plasma fibrinogen to form thrombin, measured as the time for clot formation after exogenous thrombin is added to citrated plasma.

ti·mo·lol (ti′mo-lol) a nonselective beta-adrenergic blocking agent used as the maleate salt in the treatment of hypertension, the treatment and prophylaxis of recurrent myocardial infarction and the prophylaxis of migraine; also used as the hemihydrate or the maleate salt in the treatment of glaucoma and ocular hypertension.

tin (tin) chemical element (see *Table of Elements*), at. no. 50, symbol Sn.

tinct. [L.] tinctura (tincture).

tinc·to·ri·al (tingk-tor′e-al) pertaining to dyeing or staining.

tinc·ture (tingk′chur) an alcoholic or hydro-alcoholic solution prepared from vegetable materials or chemical substances. **iodine t.,** a preparation of iodine and sodium iodide in diluted alcohol, used as a topical antiinfective.

tine (tīn) a prong or pointed projection on an implement, as on a fork.

tin·ea (tin′e-ah) ringworm; any of numerous different superficial fungal infections of the skin, types being defined according to appearance, etiology, or site. **t. bar′bae,** tinea of bearded parts of the face and neck caused by species of *Trichophyton.* **t. ca′pitis,** tinea of the scalp, due to species of *Trichophyton* or *Microsporum.* **t. circina′ta, t. cor′poris,** tinea of glabrous skin, usually due to species of *Trichophyton* or *Microsporum.* **t. cru′ris,** tinea of the groin, perineum, or perineal regions, sometimes spreading to contiguous areas; it often accompanies tinea pedis and has the same causative organism. **t. fa′ciei,** tinea of the face, other than the bearded area. **t. ni′gra,** a minor fungal infection caused by *Hortaea werneckii,* having dark lesions with the appearance of spattered silver nitrate on the skin of the hands or occasionally other areas. **t. imbrica′ta,** a form of tinea corporis seen in the tropics, due to *Trichophyton concentricum;* the early lesion is annular with a circle of scales at the periphery. **t. pe′dis,** athlete's foot; a chronic superficial type on the skin of the foot, especially between toes or on the soles, due to species of *Trichophyton* or to *Epidermophyton floccosum.* **t. profun′da,** trichophytic granuloma. **t. syco′sis,** an inflammatory, deep type of tinea barbae, due to *Trichophyton violaceum* or *T. rubrum.* **t. un′guium,** tinea of the nails, first the surface and lateral and distal edges and later the part beneath the nail plate. **t. versi′color,** a chronic, noninflammatory, usually asymptomatic type with

multiple macular patches, seen in tropical regions and caused by *Malassezia furfur.*

tin·ni·tus (tin′ĭ-tus, tĭ-ni′tus) [L.] a noise in the ears, such as ringing, buzzing, roaring, or clicking.

tin·zap·a·rin (tin-zap′ah-rin) a low-molecular-weight heparin of porcine origin, having antithrombotic activity and used with warfarin in the treatment of deep venous thrombosis with or without pulmonary embolism.

ti·o·co·na·zole (ti″o-kon′ah-zōl) an imidazole antifungal used in the treatment of vulvovaginal candidiasis.

ti·o·pro·nin (ti-o′pro-nin) a thiol compound used in the treatment of cystinuria and the prophylaxis of cystine renal calculi.

ti·ro·fi·ban (ti″ro-fi′ban) a platelet inhibitor, used as the hydrochloride salt in prophylaxis of thrombosis in unstable angina or in myocardial infarction that is not characterized by abnormal Q waves.

tis·sue (tish′u) an aggregation of similarly specialized cells which together perform certain special functions. **adenoid t.,** lymphoid t. **adipose t.,** connective tissue made of fat cells in meshwork of areolar tissue. **areolar t.,** connective tissue made up largely of interlacing fibers. **bony t.,** bone. **brown adipose t.,** a thermogenic type of adipose tissue containing a dark pigment, and arising during embryonic life in certain specific areas in many mammals, including humans; it is prominent in the newborn. **cancellous t.,** the spongy tissue of bone. **cartilaginous t.,** the substance of cartilage. **chromaffin t.,** a tissue composed largely of chromaffin cells, well supplied with nerves and vessels; it occurs in the adrenal medulla and also forms the paraganglia of the body. **cicatricial t.,** the dense fibrous tissue forming a cicatrix, derived directly from granulation tissue. **connective t.,** the stromatous or nonparenchymatous tissues of the body; that which binds together and is the ground substance of the various parts and organs of the body. **elastic t., elastic t., yellow,** connective tissue made up of yellow elastic fibers, frequently massed into sheets. **endothelial t.,** endothelium. **epithelial t.,** epithelium. **erectile t.,** spongy tissue that expands and becomes hard when filled with blood. **extracellular t.,** the total of tissues and body fluids outside the cells. **fatty t.,** adipose t. **fibrous t.,** the common connective tissue of the body, composed of yellow or white parallel fibers. **gelatinous t., mucous t. glandular t.,** an aggregation of epithelial cells that elaborate secretions. **granulation t.,** the newly formed vascular tissue normally produced in healing of wounds of soft tissue, ultimately forming the cicatrix. **gut-associated lymphoid t.** (GALT), lymphoid tissue associated with the gut, including the tonsils, Peyer's patches, lamina propria of the gastrointestinal tract, and appendix. **indifferent t.,** undifferentiated embryonic tissue. **interstitial t.,** connective tissue between the cellular elements of a structure. **lymphadenoid t.,** tissue resembling that of lymph nodes, found in the spleen, bone marrow, tonsils, and other organs. **lymphoid t.,** a latticework of reticular tissue, the interspaces of which contain lymphocytes. **mesenchymal t.,** mesenchyme. **mucous t.,** a jellylike connective tissue, as occurs in the umbilical cord. **muscle t., muscular t.,** the substance of muscle, consisting of muscle fibers, muscle cells, connective tissue, and extracellular material. **myeloid t.,** red bone marrow. **nerve t., nervous t.,** the specialized tissue making up the central and peripheral nervous systems, consisting of neurons with their processes, other specialized or supporting cells, and extracellular material. **osseous t.,** the specialized tissue forming the bones. **reticular t., reticulated t.,** connective tissue consisting of reticular cells and fibers. **scar t.,** cicatricial t. **sclerous t's,** the cartilaginous, fibrous, and osseous tissue. **skeletal t.,** the bony, ligamentous, fibrous, and cartilaginous tissue forming the skeleton and its attachments. **subcutaneous t.,** the layer of loose connective tissue directly under the skin. **white adipose t., yellow adipose t.,** the adipose tissue comprising the bulk of the body fat.

ti·ta·ni·um (ti-ta′ne-um) chemical element (see *Table of Elements*), at. no. 22, symbol Ti; used for fixation of fractures and for dental implants. **t. dioxide,** a white powder used as a topical protectant against sunburn, in other protectant preparations, and as a pigment in the manufacture of artificial teeth.

ti·ter (ti′ter) the quantity of a substance required to react with or to correspond to a given amount of another substance. **agglutination t.,** the highest dilution of a serum which causes clumping of microorganisms or other particulate antigens.

ti·tra·tion (ti-tra′shun) determination of a given component in solution by addition of a liquid reagent of known strength until the endpoint is reached when the component has been consumed by reaction with the reagent.

tit·u·ba·tion (tit″u-ba′shun) 1. the act of staggering or reeling. 2. a tremor of the head and sometimes trunk, commonly seen in cerebellar disease.

ti·zan·i·dine (ti-zan′ĭ-dēn″) an antispastic used as the hydrochloride salt in the treatment of spasticity related to multiple sclerosis or spinal cord injury.

Tl thallium.

TLC total lung capacity; thin-layer chromatography.

Tm thulium.

TNM tumor-nodes-metastasis; see under *staging*.

TNT trinitrotoluene.

to·bac·co (tah-bak′o) 1. any of various plants of the genus *Nicotiana*, especially *N. tabacum*. 2. the dried prepared leaves of *N. tabacum*, the source of various alkaloids, principally nicotine; it is sedative and narcotic, emetic and diuretic, antispasmodic, and a cardiac depressant. **mountain t.,** arnica.

to·bra·my·cin (to″brah-mi′sin) an aminoglycoside antibiotic derived from a complex produced by *Streptomyces tenebrarius*, bactericidal against many gram-negative and some gram-positive organisms; also used as the sulfate salt.

to·cai·nide (to-ka′nīd) an antiarrhythmic agent, used as the hydrochloride salt in the treatment of ventricular arrhythmias.

toc(o)- word element [Gr.], *childbirth; labor.* See also words beginning *tok(o)-*.

to·col (to′kol) the basic unit of the tocopherols and tocotrienols, hydroquinone with a saturated side chain; it is an antioxidant.

to·col·y·sis (to-kol′ĭ-sis) inhibition of uterine contractions.

to·co·lyt·ic (to″ko-lit′ik) 1. pertaining to or causing tocolysis. 2. an agent having such an action.

to·com·e·ter (to-kom′ĕ-ter) tokodynamometer.

to·coph·er·ol (to-kof′er-ol) any of a series of structurally similar compounds, some of which have biological vitamin E activity. **α-t., alpha t.,** the most prevalent form of vitamin E in the body and that administered as a supplement; often used synonymously with vitamin E. Also used as the acetate and acid succinate esters.

to·co·pho·bia (to″ko-fo′be-ah) irrational fear of childbirth.

toe (to) a digit of the foot. **claw t.,** dorsal subluxation of toes 2 through 5, the metatarsal heads bearing weight and becoming painful when walking, resulting in a shuffling gait; occurring in rheumatoid arthritis. **hammer t.,** deformity of a toe, most often the second, in which the proximal phalanx is extended and the second and distal phalanges are flexed, giving a clawlike appearance.

Morton's t., see under *neuralgia*. **pigeon t.,** permanent toeing-in position of the feet. **tennis t.,** painful great toe associated with subungual hematoma; so called because it develops usually after vigorous tennis playing. **webbed t's,** syndactyly of the toes.

toe·nail (to'nāl) the nail on any of the digits of the foot. **ingrown t.,** see under *nail*.

to·ga·vi·rus (to''gah-vi'rus) a subgroup of arboviruses, including mosquito-borne and tickborne viruses that cause hemorrhagic fever; they are RNA viruses with envelopes (or "togas").

toi·let (toi'lit) the cleansing and dressing of a wound.

tok(o)- word element [Gr.], *childbirth; labor.* See also words beginning *toc(o)-*.

to·ko·dy·na·graph (to''ko-di'nah-graf) a tracing obtained by the tokodynamometer.

to·ko·dy·na·mom·e·ter (-di''nah-mom'ĕ-ter) an instrument for measuring and recording the expulsive force of uterine contractions.

tol·az·amide (tol-az'ah-mīd) a sulfonylurea used as a hypoglycemic in the treatment of type 2 diabetes mellitus.

tol·az·o·line (tol-az'o-lēn) an adrenergic blocking agent and peripheral vasodilator; used as the hydrochloride salt in the treatment of peripheral vascular disorders due to vasospasm and as a vasodilator in pharmacoangiography.

tol·bu·ta·mide (tol-bu'tah-mīd) a sulfonylurea used as a hypoglycemic in the treatment of type 2 diabetes mellitus; the monosodium salt is used to test for insulinoma and diabetes mellitus.

tol·ca·pone (tōl'kah-pōn'') an antidyskinetic used as an adjunct to levodopa and carbidopa in the treatment of Parkinson's disease.

tol·er·ance (tol'er-ans) 1. diminution of response to a stimulus after prolonged exposure. 2. the ability to endure unusually large doses of a poison or toxin. 3. drug t. 4. immunologic t. **tol'erant,** adj. **drug t.,** decrease in susceptibility to the effects of a drug due to its continued administration. **immunologic t.,** the development of specific nonreactivity of lymphoid tissues to a particular antigen capable under other conditions of inducing immunity, resulting from previous contact with the antigen and having no effect on the response to non-cross-reacting antigens. **impaired glucose t. (IGT),** a term denoting values of fasting plasma glucose or results of an oral glucose tolerance test that are abnormal but not high enough to be diagnostic of diabetes mellitus.

tol·ero·gen (tol'er-o-jen) an antigen that induces a state of specific immunological unresponsiveness to subsequent challenging doses of the antigen.

tol·le cau·sam (tol'ĕ kaw'zam) [L. "remove the cause"] a principle of naturopathic medicine, stating that the goal of treatment is to identify and remove the cause of the disease, often involving the removal of multiple causes in the proper order.

tol·met·in (tol'met-in) a nonsteroidal anti-inflammatory drug used as the sodium salt in the treatment of various rheumatic inflammatory disorders.

tol·naf·tate (tol-naf'tāt) a synthetic topical antifungal, used in the treatment of tinea.

tol·ter·o·dine (tol-ter'ah-dēn) an antispasmodic used in the treatment of bladder hyperactivity.

tol·u·ene (tol'u-ēn) the hydrocarbon C_7H_8; it is an organic solvent that can cause poisoning by ingestion or by inhalation of its vapors.

to·mac·u·lous (to-mak'u-lus) resembling a sausage, usually because of swelling.

-tome word element [Gr.], *an instrument for cutting; a segment.*

tom(o)- word element [Gr.], *a section; a cutting.*

to·mo·gram (to'mo-gram) an image of a tissue section produced by tomography.

to·mo·graph (-graf) an apparatus for moving an x-ray source in one direction as the film is moved in the opposite direction, thus showing in detail a predetermined plane of tissue while blurring or eliminating detail in other planes.

to·mog·ra·phy (to-mog'rah-fe) the recording of internal body images at a predetermined plane by means of the tomograph. **computed t. (CT), computerized axial t. (CAT),** an imaging method in which a cross-sectional image of the structures in a body plane is reconstructed by a computer program from the x-ray absorption of beams projected through the body in the image plane. **positron emission t. (PET),** a nuclear medicine imaging method similar to computed tomography, except that the image shows the tissue concentration of a positron-emitting radioisotope. **single-photon emission computed t. (SPECT),** a type in which gamma photon–emitting radionuclides are administered and then detected by one or more gamma cameras rotated around the patient, using the series of two-dimensional images to recreate a three-dimensional view. **ultrasonic t.,** the ultrasonographic visualization of a cross-section of a predetermined plane of the body.

-tomy word element [Gr.], *incision; cutting.*

tone (tōn) 1. normal degree of vigor and tension; in muscle, the resistance to passive elongation or stretch. 2. a healthy state of a part; tonus. 3. a particular quality of sound or of voice.

tongue (tung) the movable muscular organ on the floor of the mouth; it is the chief organ of taste, and aids in mastication, swallowing, and speech. **bifid t.,** one with an anterior lengthwise cleft. **black t., black hairy t.,** hairy tongue in which the papillae are brown or black. **cleft t.,** bifid t. **coated t.,** one covered with a whitish or yellowish layer consisting of desquamated epithelium, debris, bacteria, fungi, etc. **fissured t., furrowed t.,** a tongue with numerous furrows or grooves on the dorsal surface, often radiating from a groove on the midline; it is sometimes a familial condition. **geographic t.,** benign migratory glossitis. **hairy t.,** one with the papillae elongated and hairlike. **raspberry t.,** a red, uncoated tongue, with elevated papillae, as seen a few days after the onset of the rash in scarlet fever. **red strawberry t.,** raspberry t. **scrotal t.,** fissured t. **white strawberry t.,** the white-coated tongue with prominent red papillae characteristic of the early stage of scarlet fever.

tongue-tie (tung′ti) abnormal shortness of the frenum of the tongue, interfering with its motion; ankyloglossia.

ton·ic (ton′ik) 1. producing and restoring normal tone. 2. characterized by continuous tension.

to·nic·i·ty (to-nis′ĭ-te) the state of tissue tone or tension; in body fluid physiology, the effective osmotic pressure equivalent.

ton·i·co·clon·ic (ton″ĭ-ko-klon′ik) both tonic and clonic; said of a spasm or seizure consisting of a convulsive twitching of muscles.

ton(o)- word element [Gr.], *tone; tension.*

tono·clon·ic (ton″o-klon′ik) tonicoclonic.

tono·fi·bril (ton′o-fi″bril) a bundle of fine filaments (tonofilaments) in certain cells, especially epithelial cells, the individual strands of which traverse the cytoplasm in all directions and extend into the cell processes to converge and insert on the desmosomes.

to·nog·ra·phy (to-nog′rah-fe) recording of changes in intraocular pressure due to sustained pressure on the eyeball. **carotid compression t.,** a test for occlusion of the carotid artery by measuring ocular pressure and pulse before, during, and after the proximal portion of the carotid artery is compressed by the fingers.

to·nom·e·ter (to-nom′ĕ-ter) an instrument for measuring tension or pressure, particularly intraocular pressure. **air-puff t.,** an instrument for measuring intraocular pressure by sensing deflections of the cornea in reaction to a puff of pressurized air. **applanation t.,** an instrument that measures intraocular pressure by determination of the force necessary to flatten a corneal surface of constant size. **impression t., indentation t.,** an instrument that measures intraocular pressure by direct pressure on the eyeball.

to·nom·e·try (-ĕ-tre) measurement of tension or pressure, particularly intraocular pressure. **digital t.,** estimation of the degree of intraocular pressure by pressure exerted on the eyeball by the examiner's finger.

tono·plast (ton′o-plast) the limiting membrane of an intracellular vacuole.

ton·sil (ton′sil) a small, rounded mass of tissue, especially of lymphoid tissue; generally used alone to designate the palatine tonsil. **t. of cerebellum,** a rounded mass of tissue forming part of the caudal lobe of the hemisphere of the cerebellum. **faucial t.,** palatine t. **lingual t.,** an aggregation of lymph follicles at the root of the tongue. **Luschka's t.,** pharyngeal t. **palatine t.,** a small mass of lymphoid tissue between the pillars of the fauces on either side of the pharynx. **pharyngeal t.,** the diffuse lymphoid tissue and follicles in the roof and posterior wall of the nasopharynx.

ton·sil·la (ton-sil′ah) pl. *tonsil′lae.* [L.] tonsil.

ton·sil·lar (ton′sĭ-lar) of or pertaining to a tonsil.

ton·sil·lec·to·my (ton″sĭ-lek′tah-me) excision of a tonsil.

ton·sil·li·tis (-li′tis) inflammation of the tonsils, especially the palatine tonsils. **follicular t.,** tonsillitis especially affecting the crypts.

ton·sil·lo·lith (ton-sil′o-lith) a calculus in a tonsil.

ton·sil·lot·o·my (-lot′ah-me) incision of a tonsil.

to·nus (to′nus) tone or tonicity; the slight, continuous contraction of a muscle, which in skeletal muscles aids in the maintenance of posture and in the return of blood to the heart.

tooth (tooth) pl. *teeth.* One of the hard, calcified structures set in the alveolar processes of the jaws for the biting and mastication of food. **accessional teeth,** those having no deciduous predecessors: the permanent molars. **artificial t.,** one made of porcelain or other synthetic compound in imitation of a natural tooth. **auditory teeth of Huschke,** toothlike projections in the cochlea. **bicuspid t.,** premolar t. **canine t., cuspid t.,** the third tooth on either side from the midline in each jaw. Symbol C. **deciduous teeth,** primary teeth; the 20 teeth of the first dentition, which are shed and replaced by the permanent teeth. **eye t.,** a canine tooth of the upper jaw. **Hutchinson's teeth,** notched, narrow-edged permanent incisors, sometimes but not always a sign of congenital syphilis. **impacted t.,** one prevented from erupting by a physical barrier. **incisor t.,** one of the four front teeth, two on each side of the midline, in each jaw; see Plate 31. Symbol I. **milk teeth,** deciduous teeth. **molar t.,** any of the posterior teeth on either side in each jaw, numbering three in the permanent dentition and two in the deciduous; see Plate 31. Symbol M. **peg t.,** peg-shaped t., a tooth whose sides converge or taper together incisally. **permanent teeth,** the 32 teeth of the second dentition. **premolar t.,** bicuspid tooth; either of two permanent teeth found between the canine and molar teeth. Symbol P. **primary teeth,** deciduous teeth. **stomach t.,** a canine tooth of the lower jaw. **successional teeth,** the permanent teeth that have deciduous predecessors. **temporary teeth,** deciduous teeth. **wisdom t.,** the last molar tooth on either side in each jaw.

tooth·ache (tōōth′āk) pain in a tooth.

top·ag·no·sia (top″ag-no′zhah) 1. atopognosia. 2. loss of ability to recognize familiar surroundings.

to·pal·gia (to-pal′jah) pain localized or fixed in one spot; often a symptom of conversion disorder.

to·pec·to·my (tah-pek′tah-me) ablation of a small and specific area of the frontal cortex in the treatment of certain forms of epilepsy and psychiatric disorders.

top·es·the·sia (top″es-the′zhah) ability to recognize the location of a tactile stimulus.

to·pha·ceous (tah-fa′shus) gritty or sandy; pertaining to tophi.

to·phus (to′fus) pl. *to′phi.* [L.] a deposit of sodium urate in the tissues about the joints in gout, producing a chronic, foreign-body inflammatory response.

top·i·cal (top′ĭ-k′l) pertaining to a particular area, as a topical antiinfective applied to a certain area of the skin and affecting only the area to which it is applied.

to·pi·ra·mate (to-pi′rah-māt) a substituted monosaccharide used as an anticonvulsant in the treatment of partial seizures.

top(o)- word element [Gr.], *particular place* or *area.*

topo·an·es·the·sia (top″o-an″es-the′zhah) atopognosia.

to·pog·ra·phy (tah-pog′rah-fe) the description of an anatomic region or a special part. **topograph′ic,** adj.

topo·scop·ic (to″po-skop′ik) pertaining to endoscopic delivery to a specific site.

to·po·te·can (to″po-te′kan) an antineoplastic that inhibits DNA topoisomerase; used as the hydrochloride salt in the treatment of metastatic ovarian carcinoma and small cell lung carcinoma.

to·re·mi·fene (tor′ĕ-mĭ-fēn″) an analogue of tamoxifen that acts as an estrogen antagonist; used as the citrate salt in the palliative treatment of metastatic breast carcinoma.

tor·por (tor′per) [L.] sluggishness. **tor′pid,** adj. **t. re′tinae,** sluggish response of the retina to the stimulus of light.

torque (tork) 1. a rotary force causing part of a structure to twist about an axis. Symbol τ. 2. in dentistry, the rotation of a tooth on its long axis, especially the movement of the apical portions of the teeth by use of orthodontic appliances.

tor·se·mide (tor′sĕ-mīd) a diuretic related to sulfonylurea, used in the treatment of edema and hypertension.

tor·sion (tor′-shun) 1. the act or process of being twisted or rotated about an axis. 2. a type of mechanical stress, whereby the external forces twist an object about its axis. 3. in ophthalmology, any rotation of the vertical corneal meridians. **tor′sional, tor′sive,** adj.

tor·si·ver·sion (tor″sĭ-ver′zhun) turning of a tooth on its long axis out of normal position.

tor·so (tor′so) trunk (1).

tor·ti·col·lis (tor″tĭ-kol′is) wryneck; a contracted state of the cervical muscles, with torsion of the neck.

tor·ti·pel·vis (-pel′vis) dystonia musculorum deformans.

tor·u·lus (tor′u-lus) pl. *tor′uli.* [L.] a small elevation; a papilla. **to′ruli tac′tiles,** small tactile elevations in the skin of the palms and soles.

to·rus (tor′us) pl. *to′ri.* [L.] a swelling or bulging projection.

to·sy·late (to′sĭ-lāt) USAN contraction for *p*-toluenesulfonate.

to·ti·po·ten·cy (to″tĭ-po′ten-se) the ability to differentiate along any line or into any type of cell. **totip′otent, totipoten′tial,** adj.

to·ti·po·ten·ti·al·i·ty (-po-ten″she-al′ĭ-te) totipotency.

touch (tuch) 1. the sense by which contact with objects gives evidence as to certain of their qualities. 2. palpation with the finger.

therapeutic t. (TT), a healing method based on the premise that the body possesses an energy field that can be affected by the focused intention of the healer. The practitioner uses the hands to assess the patient's energy field, to release areas where the free flow of energy is blocked, and to balance the patient's energy, by transferring energy from a universal life energy force to the patient.

tour·ni·quet (toor´nĭ-ket) a band to be drawn tightly around a limb for the temporary arrest of circulation in the distal area.

tox·emia (tok-se´me-ah) 1. the condition resulting from the spread of bacterial products (toxins) by the bloodstream. 2. a condition resulting from metabolic disturbances, e.g., toxemia of pregnancy. **toxe´mic,** adj.

tox·ic (tok´sik) 1. poisonous. 2. manifesting the symptoms of severe poisoning.

tox·i·cant (tok´sĭ-kant) 1. poisonous. 2. poison.

tox·ic·i·ty (tok-sis´ĭ-te) the quality of being poisonous, especially the degree of virulence of a toxic microbe or of a poison. **O₂ t., oxygen t.,** serious, sometimes irreversible, damage to the pulmonary capillary endothelium associated with breathing high partial pressures of oxygen for prolonged periods.

toxic(o)- word element [Gr.], *poison; poisonous.*

tox·i·co·gen·ic (tok˝sĭ-ko-jen´ik) toxigenic.

tox·i·col·o·gy (tok˝sĭ-kol´ah-je) the science or study of poisons. **toxicolog´ic,** adj.

tox·i·cop·a·thy (tok˝sĭ-kop´ah-the) toxicosis. **toxicopath´ic,** adj.

tox·i·co·pex·is (tok˝sĭ-ko-pek´sis) the fixation or neutralization of a poison in the body. **toxicopec´tic, toxicopex´ic,** adj.

tox·i·co·pho·bia (-fo´be-ah) irrational fear of being poisoned.

tox·i·co·sis (tok˝sĭ-ko´sis) any diseased condition due to poisoning.

tox·if·er·ous (tok-sif´er-us) conveying or producing a poison.

tox·i·gen·ic (tok˝sĭ-jen´ik) 1. producing or elaborating toxins. 2. derived from or containing toxins.

tox·i·ge·nic·i·ty (tok˝sĭ-jĕ-nis´ĭ-te) the property of producing toxins.

tox·in (tok´sin) a poison, especially a protein or conjugated protein produced by some higher plants, certain animals, and pathogenic bacteria, that is highly poisonous for other living organisms. **bacterial t's,** toxins produced by bacteria, including exotoxins, endotoxins, and toxic enzymes. **botulinal t., botulinum t., botulinus t.,** an exotoxin produced by *Clostridium botulinum* that produces paralysis by blocking the release of acetylcholine in the central nervous system;

there are seven immunologically distinct types (A–G). Type A is used therapeutically to inhibit muscular spasm in the treatment of dystonic disorders such as blepharospasm and strabismus, as well as to treat wrinkles of the upper face; type B is used to treat cervical dystonia. **clostridial t.,** one produced by species of *Clostridium,* including those causing botulism, gas gangrene, and tetanus. **Dick t.,** streptococcal pyrogenic exotoxin. **diphtheria t.,** a protein exotoxin produced by *Corynebacterium diphtheriae* that is primarily responsible for the pathogenesis of diphtheritic infection; it is an enzyme that inhibits protein synthesis. **erythrogenic t.,** streptococcal pyrogenic exotoxin. **extracellular t.,** exotoxin. **gas gangrene t.,** an exotoxin produced by *Clostridium perfringens* that causes gas gangrene; at least 10 types have been identified. **intracellular t.,** endotoxin. **tetanus t.,** the potent exotoxin produced by *Clostridium tetani,* consisting of two components, one a neurotoxin (*tetanospasmin*) and the other a hemolysin (*tetanolysin*).

tox·in·an·ti·tox·in (TA) (tok´sin-an´tĭ-tok´sin) a nearly neutral mixture of diphtheria toxin with its antitoxin; used for diphtheria immunization.

tox·in·ol·o·gy (-ol´ah-je) the science dealing with the toxins produced by certain higher plants and animals and by pathogenic bacteria.

tox·ip·a·thy (tok-sip´ah-the) toxicosis.

tox(o)- word element [Gr.; L.], *poison; poisonous.*

Tox·o·ca·ra (tok˝so-kar´ah) a genus of nematode parasites found in the dog (*T. ca´nis*) and cat (*T. ca´ti*); both species are sometimes found in humans.

tox·o·car·i·a·sis (-kah-ri´ah-sis) infection by worms of the genus *Toxocara.*

tox·oid (tok´soid) a modified or inactivated exotoxin that has lost toxicity but retains the ability to combine with, or stimulate the production of, antitoxin. **diphtheria t.,** the formaldehyde-inactivated toxin of *Corynebacterium diphtheriae,* used as an active immunizing agent against diphtheria, usually in mixtures with tetanus toxoid and pertussis vaccine (DTP or DTaP) or with tetanus toxoid alone (DT for pediatric use and Td, which contains less diphtheria toxoid, for adult use). **tetanus t.,** the formaldehyde-inactivated toxins of *Clostridium tetani,* used as an active immunizing agent, usually in mixtures with diphtheria toxoid and pertussis vaccine.

tox·o·phil·ic (tok˝so-fil´ik) easily susceptible to poison; having affinity for toxins.

toxo·phore (tok'so-for) the group of atoms in a toxin molecule which produces the toxic effect. **toxoph'orous**, adj.

Toxo·plas·ma (tok"so-plaz'mah) a genus of sporozoa that are intracellular parasites of many organs and tissues of birds and mammals, including humans. *T. gon'dii* is the etiologic agent of toxoplasmosis.

toxo·plas·mic (-plaz'mik) pertaining to Toxoplasma or to toxoplasmosis.

tox·o·plas·mo·sis (-plaz-mo'sis) an acute or chronic, widespread disease of animals and humans caused by *Toxoplasma gondii* and transmitted by oocysts in the feces of cats. Most human infections are asymptomatic; when symptoms occur, they range from a mild, self-limited disease resembling mononucleosis to a disseminated, fulminating disease that may damage the brain, eyes, muscles, liver, and lungs. Severe manifestations are seen principally in immunocompromised patients and in fetuses infected transplacentally as a result of maternal infection. Chorioretinitis may be associated with all forms, but it is usually a late sequel of congenital disease.

TPA, t-PA tissue plasminogen activator.

t-plas·min·o·gen ac·ti·va·tor (plaz-min'o-jen" ak'tĭ-va-ter) see under *activator*.

TPN total parenteral nutrition.

TPP thiamine pyrophosphate.

tra·be·cu·la (trah-bek'u-lah) pl. *trabe'culae*. [L.] a little beam; in anatomy, a general term for a supporting or anchoring strand of connective tissue, e.g., a strand extending from a capsule into the substance of the enclosed organ. **trabe'cular**, adj. **trabeculae of bone,** anastomosing bony spicules in cancellous bone which form a meshwork of intercommunicating spaces that are filled with bone marrow. **fleshy trabeculae of heart,** irregular bundles and bands of muscle projecting from a great part of the interior walls of the ventricles of the heart. **septomarginal t.,** a bundle of muscle at the apical end of the right cardiac ventricle, connecting the base of the anterior papillary muscle to the interventricular septum.

tra·bec·u·late (-lāt) marked with transverse or radiating bars or trabeculae.

tra·bec·u·lo·plas·ty (trah-bek"u-lo-plas'te) plastic surgery of a trabecula. **laser t.,** the placing of surface burns in the trabecular network of the eye to lower intraocular pressure in open-angle glaucoma.

trac·er (trās'er) 1. a dissecting instrument for isolating vessels and nerves. 2. a mechanical device for graphically recording the outline of an object or the direction and extent of movement of a part. 3. a means or agent by which certain substances or structures can be identified or followed. **radioactive t.,** a radioactive isotope replacing a stable chemical element in a compound and so able to be followed or tracked through one or more reactions or systems; generally one that is introduced into and followed through the body.

tra·chea (tra'ke-ah) pl. *tra'cheae*. [L.] windpipe; the cartilaginous and membranous tube descending from the larynx and branching into the left and right main bronchi. **tra'cheal,** adj.

tra·che·al·gia (tra"ke-al'jah) pain in the trachea.

tra·che·itis (-i'tis) inflammation of the trachea. **bacterial t.,** membranous or pseudomembranous croup; an acute crouplike bacterial infection of the upper airway in children, with coughing and high fever.

tra·che·lec·to·my (-lek'tah-me) cervicectomy.

tra·che·lism (tra'kah-lizm) spasm of the neck muscles; spasmodic retraction of the head in epilepsy.

tra·che·lis·mus (tra"kah-liz'mus) trachelism.

tra·che·li·tis (tra"kĕ-li'tis) cervicitis.

trachel(o)- word element [Gr.], *neck; necklike structure*, especially the uterine cervix.

tra·che·lo·pexy (tra'kĕ-lo-pek"se) fixation of the uterine cervix.

tra·che·lo·plas·ty (-plas"te) plastic repair of the uterine cervix.

tra·che·lor·rha·phy (tra"kĕ-lor'ah-fe) suture of the uterine cervix.

tra·che·lot·o·my (-lot'ah-me) incision of the uterine cervix.

trache(o)- word element [Gr.], *trachea*.

tra·cheo·aero·cele (tra"ke-o-ār'-o-sēl") a tracheal hernia containing air.

tra·cheo·bron·chi·al (-brong'ke-al) pertaining to the trachea and bronchi.

tra·cheo·bron·chi·tis (-brong-ki'tis) inflammation of the trachea and bronchi.

tra·cheo·bron·chos·co·py (-brong-kos'kah-pe) inspection of the interior of the trachea and bronchi.

tra·cheo·cele (tra'ke-o-sēl") hernial protrusion of tracheal mucous membrane.

tra·cheo·esoph·a·ge·al (tra"ke-o-e-sof"ah-je'al) pertaining to the trachea and esophagus.

tra·cheo·la·ryn·ge·al (-lah-rin'je-al) pertaining to the trachea and larynx.

tra·cheo·ma·la·cia (-mah-la'shah) softening of the tracheal cartilages.

tra·che·op·a·thy (tra"ke-op'ah-the) disease of the trachea.

tra·cheo·pha·ryn·ge·al (tra"ke-o-fah-rin'je-al) pertaining to the trachea and pharynx.

tra·che·oph·o·ny (tra″ke-of'o-ne) a voice sound heard over the trachea.

tra·cheo·plas·ty (tra'ke-o-plas″te) plastic repair of the trachea.

tra·che·or·rha·gia (-ra'jah) hemorrhage from the trachea.

tra·che·os·chi·sis (tra″ke-os'kĭ-sis) fissure of the trachea.

tra·che·os·co·py (-os'kah-pe) inspection of interior of the trachea. **tracheoscop'ic**, adj.

tra·cheo·ste·no·sis (tra″ke-o-stĕ-no'sis) constriction of the trachea.

tra·che·os·to·my (tra″ke-os'tah-me) creation of an opening into the trachea through the neck, with the tracheal mucosa being brought into continuity with the skin; also, the opening so created.

tra·che·ot·o·my (-ot'ah-me) incision of the trachea through the skin and muscles of the neck. **inferior t.,** that performed below the isthmus of the thyroid. **superior t.,** that performd above the isthmus of the thyroid.

tra·cho·ma (trah-ko'mah) pl. *tracho'mata.* [Gr.] a contagious disease of the conjunctiva and cornea, producing photophobia, pain, and lacrimation, caused by a strain of *Chlamydia trachomatis.* It progresses from a mild infection with tiny follicles on the eyelid conjunctiva to invasion of the cornea, with scarring and contraction that may end in blindness. **tracho'matous,** adj.

tra·chy·onych·ia (trak″e-o-ni'ke-ah) roughness of nails, with brittleness and splitting.

tract (trakt) 1. a region, principally one of some length. 2. a bundle of nerve fibers having a common origin, function, and termination. 3. a number of organs, arranged in series and serving a common function. **alimentary t.,** see under *canal.* **atriohisian t's,** myocardial fibers that bypass the physiologic delay of the atrioventricular node and connect the atrium directly to the bundle of His, allowing preexcitation of the ventricle. **biliary t.,** the organs, ducts, etc., participating in secretion (the liver), storage (the gallbladder), and delivery (hepatic and bile ducts) of bile into the duodenum. **digestive t.,** alimentary canal. **dorsolateral t.,** a group of nerve fibers in the lateral funiculus of the spinal cord dorsal to the posterior column. **extracorticospinal t., extrapyramidal t.,** extrapyramidal system. **Flechsig's t.,** posterior spinocerebellar t. **gastrointestinal t.,** the stomach and intestine in continuity. **genito-urinary t.,** urogenital system. **Gowers' t.,** anterior spinocerebellar t. **iliotibial t.,** a thickened longitudinal band of fascia lata extending from the tensor muscle downward to the lateral condyle of the tibia. **intestinal t.,** the small and large intestines in continuity. **nigrostriatal t.,** a bundle of nerve fibers extending from the substantia nigra to the globus pallidus and putamen in the corpus striatum; injury to it may be a cause of parkinsonism. **optic t.,** the nerve tract proceeding backward from the optic chiasm, around the cerebral peduncle, and dividing into a lateral and medial root, which end in the superior colliculus and lateral geniculate body, respectively. **pyramidal t.,** two groups of nerve fibers arising in the brain and passing down through the spinal cord to motor cells in the anterior horns. **respiratory t.,** see under *system.* **reticulospinal t.,** a group of fibers arising mostly from the reticular formation of the pons and medulla oblongata; chiefly homolateral, the fibers descend in the ventral and lateral funiculi to most levels of the spinal cord. **spinocerebellar t., anterior,** a group of nerve fibers in the lateral funiculus of the spinal cord, arising mostly in the gray matter of the opposite side, and ascending to the cerebellum through the superior cerebellar peduncle. **spino-cerebellar t., posterior,** a group of nerve fibers in the lateral funiculus of the spinal cord, arising mostly from the nucleus thoracicus, and ascending to the cerebellum through the inferior cerebellar peduncle. **spinothalamic t.,** a group of nerve fibers in the lateral funiculus of the spinal cord that arise in the opposite gray matter and ascend to the thalamus, carrying the sensory impulses activated by pain and temperature. **urinary t.,** 1. see under *system.* 2. sometimes more specifically the conduits leading from the pelvis of the kidneys to the urinary meatus. **urogenital t.,** see under *system.* **uveal t.,** the vascular tunic of the eye, comprising the choroid, ciliary body, and iris.

trac·tion (trak'shun) the act of drawing or pulling. **axis t.,** traction along an axis, as of the pelvis in obstetrics. **elastic t.,** traction by an elastic force or by means of an elastic appliance. **skeletal t.,** traction applied directly upon long bones by means of pins, wires, etc., **skin t.,** traction on a body part maintained by an apparatus affixed by dressings to the body surface.

trac·tot·o·my (trak-tot'ah-me) surgical severing or incising of a nerve tract.

trac·tus (trak'tus) pl. *trac'tus.* [L.] tract.

tra·gus (tra'gus) pl. *tra'gi.* [L.] the cartilaginous projection anterior to the external opening of the ear; used also in the plural to designate hairs growing on the pinna of the external ear, especially on the tragus. **tra'gal,** adj.

train·a·ble (tra'nah-b'l) capable of being trained; formerly used to refer to persons with moderate mental retardation (I.Q. approximately 36–51).

train·ing (trān'ing) a system of instruction or teaching; preparation by instruction and practice. **assertiveness t.,** a form of behavior therapy in which individuals are taught appropriate interpersonal responses, involving direct expression of their feelings, both negative and positive. **bladder t.,** the training of a child or an incontinent adult in habits of urinary continence. **bowel t.,** the training of a child or incontinent adult in the habits of fecal continence.

trait (trāt) 1. any genetically determined characteristic; also, the condition prevailing in the heterozygous state of a recessive disorder, as the sickle cell trait. 2. a distinctive behavior pattern. **sickle cell t.,** the condition, usually asymptomatic, due to heterozygosity for hemoglobin S.

tra·ma·dol (tram'ah-dol″) an opioid analgesic used as the hydrochloride salt for the treatment of pain following surgical procedures and oral surgery.

trance (trans) a sleeplike state of altered consciousness marked by heightened focal awareness and reduced peripheral awareness.

tran·do·la·pril (tran-do'lah-pril″) an angiotensin-converting enzyme inhibitor used in the treatment of hypertension and post–myocardial infarction congestive heart failure or left ventricular dysfunction.

tran·ex·am·ic ac·id (tran″ek-sam'ik) an antifibrinolytic that competitively inhibits activation of plasminogen; used as a hemostatic in the prophylaxis and treatment of severe hemorrhage associated with excessive fibrinolysis.

tran·quil·iz·er (tran'kwĭ-li″zer) a drug with a calming, soothing effect; usually a *minor tranquilizer*. **major t.,** former name for antipsychotic agent; see *antipsychotic*. **minor t.,** antianxiety agent; see *antianxiety*.

trans (tranz) 1. in organic chemistry, having certain atoms or radicals on opposite sides of a nonrotatable parent structure. 2. in genetics, denoting two or more loci occurring on opposite chromosomes of a homologous pair. Cf. *cis*.

trans- word element [L.], *through; across; beyond*.

trans·ab·dom·i·nal (trans″ab-dom'ĭ-nal) across the abdominal wall or through the abdominal cavity.

trans·ac·e·tyl·a·tion (trans″-ah-set″ĭ-la'shun) a chemical reaction involving the transfer of the acetyl radical.

trans·ac·y·lase (trans-a'sĭ-lās) an enzyme that catalyzes transacylation.

trans·ac·y·la·tion (-a″sĭ-la'shun) a chemical reaction involving the transfer of an acyl radical.

trans·am·i·nase (-am'ĭ-nās) aminotransferase.

trans·am·i·na·tion (-am″ĭ-na'shun) the reversible exchange of amino groups between different amino acids.

trans·an·tral (-an'tr'l) performed across or through an antrum.

trans·aor·tic (trans″a-or'tik) performed through the aorta.

trans·au·di·ent (trans-aw'de-ent) penetrable by sound waves.

trans·ax·i·al (-ak'se-al) directed at right angles to the long axis of the body or a part.

trans·ba·sal (-ba's'l) through the base, as a surgical approach through the base of the skull.

trans·cal·lo·sal (trans″kah-lo's'l) performed across or through the corpus callosum.

trans·cal·var·i·al (-kal-var'e-al) through or across the calvaria.

trans·cath·e·ter (trans-kath'ĕ-ter) performed through the lumen of a catheter.

trans·co·bal·a·min (trans″ko-bal'ah-min) any of three plasma proteins (transcobalamins I, II, and III) that bind and transport cobalamin (vitamin B_{12}). Abbreviated TC.

trans·cor·ti·cal (trans-kor'tĭ-k'l) connecting two parts of the cerebral cortex.

trans·cor·tin (-kor'tin) an α-globulin that binds and transports biologically active, unconjugated cortisol in plasma.

trans·cra·ni·al (-kra'ne-al) performed through the cranium.

trans·crip·tase (-krip'tās) a DNA-directed RNA polymerase; an enzyme that catalyzes the synthesis (polymerization) of RNA from ribonucleoside triphosphates, with DNA serving as a template. **reverse t.,** see at *R*.

trans·crip·tion (-krip'shun) the synthesis of RNA using a DNA template catalyzed by RNA polymerase; the base sequences of the RNA and DNA are complementary.

trans·cu·ta·ne·ous (-ku-ta'ne-us) transdermal.

trans·der·mal (-der'm'l) entering through the dermis, or skin, as in administration of a drug via ointment or patch.

trans·du·cer (-doo'ser) a device that translates one form of energy to another, e.g., the pressure, temperature, or pulse to an electrical signal. **neuroendocrine t.,** a neuron, such as a neurohypophyseal neuron, that on stimulation secretes a hormone, thereby translating neural information into hormonal information.

trans·du·cin (trans-doo'sin) a G protein of the disk membrane of the retinal rods that interacts with activated rhodopsin and participates in the triggering of a nerve impulse in vision.

trans·duc·tion (-duk'shun) 1. a method of genetic recombination in bacteria, in which DNA is transferred between bacteria via bacteriophages. 2. the transforming of one form of energy into another, as by the sensory mechanisms of the body. **sensory t.,** the process by which a sensory receptor converts a stimulus from the environment to an action potential for transmission to the brain.

trans·du·ral (-door'al) through or across the dura mater.

tran·sec·tion (tran-sek'shun) a cross section; division by cutting transversely.

trans·esoph·a·ge·al (ĕ-sof"ah-je'al) through or across the esophagus.

trans·eth·moi·dal (-eth-moi'd'l) performed across or through the ethmoid bone.

trans·fem·o·ral (-fem'or-al) 1. across or through the femur. 2. through the femoral artery.

trans·fer (trans'fer) the taking or moving of something from one place to another. **gamete intrafallopian t. (GIFT),** retrieval of oocytes from the ovary, followed by laparoscopic placement of the oocytes and sperm in the fallopian tubes; used in the treatment of infertility. **passive t.,** the conferring of immunity to a nonimmune host by injection of antibody or lymphocytes from an immune or sensitized donor. **tubal embryo t. (TET),** 1. retrieval of oocytes from the ovary, fertilization and culture in vitro, then laparoscopic placement of resulting embryos in the fallopian tubes more than 24 hours after oocyte retrieval; used in the treatment of infertility. 2. laparoscopic transfer of cryopreserved embryos to the fallopian tubes. **zygote intrafallopian t. (ZIFT),** retrieval of oocytes from the ovary, fertilization and culture in vitro, then laparoscopic placement of the resulting zygotes in the fallopian tubes 24 hours after oocyte retrieval; used in the treatment of infertility.

trans·fer·ase (trans'fer-ās) a class of enzymes that transfer a chemical group from one compound to another.

trans·fer·ence (trans-fer'ens) in psychotherapy, the unconscious tendency to assign to others in one's present environment feelings and attitudes associated with significance in one's early life, especially the patient's transfer to the therapist of feelings and attitudes associated with a parent. **counter t.,** see *countertransference.*

trans·fer·rin (-fer'in) a glycoprotein mainly produced in the liver, binding and transporting iron, closely related to the *apoferritin* of the intestinal mucosa.

trans·fix·ion (-fik'shun) a cutting through from within outward, as in amputation.

trans·for·ma·tion (trans"for-ma'shun) 1. change of form or structure; conversion from one form to another. 2. in oncology, the change that a normal cell undergoes as it becomes malignant. **bacterial t.,** the exchange of genetic material between strains of bacteria by the transfer of a fragment of naked DNA from a donor cell to a recipient cell, followed by recombination in the recipient chromosome.

trans·fron·tal (trans-frun'tal) through the frontal bone.

trans·fu·sion (-fu'zhun) the introduction of whole blood or blood components directly into the bloodstream. **direct t.,** immediate t. **exchange t.,** repetitive withdrawal of small amounts of blood and replacement with donor blood, until a large proportion of the original volume has been replaced. **immediate t.,** transfer of blood directly from a vessel of the donor to a vessel of the recipient. **indirect t., mediate t.,** introduction of blood which has been stored in a suitable container after withdrawal from the donor. **placental t.,** return to an infant after birth, through the intact umbilical cord, of the blood contained in the placenta. **replacement t., substitution t.,** exchange t. **twin-to-twin t.,** an intrauterine abnormality of fetal circulation in monozygotic twins, in which blood is shunted directly from one twin to the other.

trans·glu·tam·in·ase (trans"gloo-tam'in-ās) an enzyme, formed by cleavage and activation of protransglutaminase, which forms stabilizing covalent bonds within fibrin strands. It is the activated form of coagulation factor XIII.

trans·il·i·ac (trans-il'e-ak) across the two ilia.

trans·il·lu·mi·na·tion (trans"ĭ-loo"mĭ-na'shun) the passage of strong light through a body structure, to permit inspection by an observer on the opposite side.

tran·si·tion (tran-zĭ'shun) 1. a passage or change from one state or condition to another. 2. in molecular genetics, a point mutation in which a purine base replaces a pyrimidine base or vice versa. **transi'tional,** adj.

trans·la·tion (trans-la'shun) in genetics, the process by which polypeptide chains are synthesized, the sequence of amino acids being determined by the sequence of bases in a messenger RNA, which in turn is determined by the sequence of bases in the DNA of the gene from which it was transcribed. **nick t.,** a process by which labeled nucleotides are incorporated into duplex DNA at single strand nicks or cleavage points created enzymatically along its two strands.

trans·lo·case (trans-lo′kās) transport protein.

trans·lo·ca·tion (trans″lo-ka′shun) the attachment of a fragment of one chromosome to a nonhomologous chromosome. Abbreviated t. **reciprocal t.,** the complete exchange of fragments between two broken nonhomologous chromosomes, one part of one uniting with part of the other, with no fragments left over. Abbreviated rcp. **robertsonian t.,** translocation involving two acrocentric chromosomes, which fuse at the centromere region and lose their short arms.

trans·lu·mi·nal (trans-loo′mĭ-n′l) through or across a lumen, particularly of a blood vessel.

trans·man·dib·u·lar (trans″man-dib′u-lar) through or across the mandible.

trans·mem·brane (trans-mem′brān) extending across a membrane, usually referring to a protein subunit that is exposed on both sides of a cell membrane.

trans·meth·y·la·tion (trans″meth-ĭ-la′shun) the transfer of a methyl group (CH_3—) from one compound to another.

trans·mis·si·ble (trans-mis′ĭ-b′l) capable of being transmitted.

trans·mis·sion (-mish′un) the transfer, as of a disease, from one person to another.

trans·mu·co·sal (trans″mu-ko′s′l) entering through, or across, a mucous membrane.

trans·mu·ral (trans-mu′ral) through the wall of an organ; extending through or affecting the entire thickness of the wall of an organ or cavity.

trans·mu·ta·tion (trans″mu-ta′shun) 1. evolutionary change of one species into another. 2. the change of one chemical element into another.

trans·neu·ro·nal (trans-noor′ŏ-n′l) between or across neurons.

trans·par·ent (-par′ent) permitting the passage of rays of light, so that objects may be seen through the substance.

trans·phos·phor·y·la·tion (trans″fos-for″ĭ-la′shun) the exchange of phosphate groups between organic phosphates, without their going through the stage of inorganic phosphates.

tran·spi·ra·tion (tran″spĭ-ra′shun) discharge of air, vapor, or sweat through the skin.

trans·pla·cen·tal (-plah-sen′tal) through the placenta.

trans·plant¹ (trans′plant) 1. graft: an organ or tissue taken from the body for grafting into another area of the same body or into another individual. 2. the process of removing and grafting such an organ or tissue.

trans·plant² (trans-plant′) to transfer tissue from one part to another.

trans·plan·ta·tion (trans″plan-ta′shun) the grafting of tissues taken from the patient's own body or from another. **allogeneic t.,** allotransplantation; transplantation of an allograft; it may be from a cadaveric, living related, or living unrelated donor. **bone marrow t. (BMT),** intravenous infusion of autologous, syngeneic, or allogeneic bone marrow or stem cells. **heterotopic t.,** transplantation of tissue typical of one area to a different recipient site. **homotopic t., orthotopic t.,** transplantation of tissue from a donor into its normal anatomical position in the recipient. **syngeneic t.,** transplantation of a syngraft. **xenogeneic t.,** transplantation of a xenograft.

trans·port (trans′port) movement of materials in biological systems, particularly into and out of cells and across epithelial layers. **active t.,** movement of materials in biological systems resulting directly from expenditure of metabolic energy. **bulk t.,** the uptake by or extrusion from a cell of fluid or particles, accomplished by invagination and vacuole formation (uptake) or by evagination (extrusion); it includes endocytosis, phagocytosis, pinocytosis, and exocytosis.

trans·pos·a·ble (trans-poz′ah-b′l) capable of being interchanged or put in a different place or order.

trans·po·si·tion (trans″po-zish′un) 1. displacement of a viscus to the opposite side. 2. the operation of carrying a tissue flap from one situation to another without severing its connection entirely until it is united at its new location. 3. the exchange of position of two atoms within a molecule. **t. of great vessels,** a congenital cardiovascular malformation in which the position of the chief blood vessels of the heart is reversed. Life then depends on a crossflow of blood between the right and left sides of the heart, as through a ventricular septal defect.

trans·po·son (trans-po′zon) a small mobile genetic (DNA) element that moves around the genome or to other genomes within the same cell, usually by copying itself to a second site but sometimes by splicing itself out of its original site and inserting in a new location. Eukaryotic transposons are sometimes called *transposable elements.*

trans·pu·bic (-pu'bik) performed through the pubic bone after removal of a segment of the bone.

trans·sa·cral (tran-sa'kral) through or across the sacrum.

trans·seg·men·tal (trans"seg-men'tal) extending across segments.

trans·sep·tal (trans-sep'tal) extending or performed through or across a septum.

trans·sex·u·al·ism (-sek'shoo-al-izm") 1. the most severe manifestation of gender identity disorder in adults, being a prolonged, persistent desire to relinquish their primary and secondary sex characteristics and acquire those of the opposite sex. 2. the state of being a transsexual.

trans·tha·lam·ic (trans"thah-lam'ik) across the thalamus.

trans·tho·rac·ic (-thah-ras'ik) through the thoracic cavity or across the chest wall.

trans·tib·i·al (trans-tib'e-al) across or through the tibia.

trans·tym·pan·ic (-tim-pan'ik) across the tympanic membrane or cavity.

tran·su·date (tran'su-dāt) a fluid substance that has passed through a membrane or has been extruded from a tissue; in contrast to an exudate, it is of high fluidity and has a low content of protein, cells, or solid materials derived from cells.

trans·ure·thral (trans"u-re'thral) performed through the urethra.

trans·vag·i·nal (trans-vaj'ĭ-nal) through the vagina.

trans·ve·nous (trans-ve'nus) performed or inserted through a vein.

trans·ver·sa·lis (trans"ver-sa'lis) [L.] transverse.

trans·verse (trans-vers') extending from side to side; at right angles to the long axis.

trans·ver·sec·to·my (trans"ver-sek'tah-me) excision of a transverse process of a vertebra.

trans·ver·sus (trans-ver'sus) [L.] transverse.

trans·ves·i·cal (-ves'ĭ-k'l) through the bladder.

trans·ves·tism (-ves'tizm) 1. the practice of wearing articles of clothing and assuming the appearance, manner, or roles of the opposite sex. 2. transvestic fetishism.

tran·yl·cy·pro·mine (tran"il-si'pro-mēn) a monoamine oxidase inhibitor; the sulfate salt is used as an antidepressant and in the prophylaxis of migraine.

tra·pe·zi·al (trah-pe'ze-al) pertaining to a trapezium.

tra·pe·zi·um (-um) [L.] 1. an irregular, four-sided figure. 2. see *Table of Bones.*

trap·e·zoid (trap'ĕ-zoid) 1. having the shape of a four-sided plane, with two sides parallel and two diverging. 2. trapezoid bone; see *Table of Bones.*

tras·tuz·u·mab (tras-tuz'u-mab) a monoclonal antibody that binds to a protein overexpressed in some breast cancers; used as an antineoplastic in the treatment of metastatic breast cancer with such overexpression.

trau·ma (traw'mah, trou'mah) pl. *traumas, trau'mata.* [Gr.] 1. injury. 2. psychological or emotional damage. **traumat'ic,** adj. **birth t.,** 1. an injury to the infant during the process of being born. 2. the psychic shock produced in an infant by the experience of being born. **psychic t.,** a psychologically upsetting experience that produces a mental disorder or otherwise has lasting negative effects on a person's thoughts, feelings, or behavior.

trau·ma·tism (traw'mah-tizm) 1. the physical or psychic state resulting from an injury or wound. 2. a wound or injury.

traumat(o)- word element [Gr.], *trauma.*

trau·ma·tol·o·gy (-tol'o-je) the branch of surgery dealing with wounds and disability from injuries.

trav·o·prost (trav'o-prost) a synthetic prostaglandin analogue used in the treatment of elevated intraocular pressure in open-angle glaucoma or ocular hypertension.

tray (tra) a flat-surfaced utensil for the conveyance of various objects or material. **impression t.,** a contoured container to hold the material for making an impression of the teeth and associated structures.

tra·zo·done (tra'zo-dōn) an antidepressant, used as the hydrochloride salt to treat major depressive episodes with or without prominent anxiety.

treat·ment (trēt'ment) management and care of a patient or the combating of disease or disorder. **active t.,** that directed immediately to the cure of the disease or injury. **causal t.,** treatment directed against the cause of a disease. **conservative t.,** that designed to avoid radical medical therapeutic measures or operative procedures. **empiric t.,** treatment by means which experience has proved to be beneficial. **expectant t.,** treatment directed toward relief of untoward symptoms, leaving cure of the disease to natural forces. **palliative t.,** treatment designed to relieve pain and distress with no attempt to cure. **preventive t., prophylactic t.,** that in which the aim is to prevent the occurrence of the disease; prophylaxis. **rational t.,** that based upon knowledge of disease and the action of the remedies given. **shock t.,** obsolete term for *electroconvulsive therapy.* **specific t.,**

treatment particularly adapted to the disease being treated. **supporting t., supportive t.,** that which is mainly directed to sustaining the strength of the patient. **symptomatic t.,** expectant t.

tree (tre) an anatomic structure with branches resembling a tree. **bronchial t.,** the bronchi and their branching structures. **dendritic t.,** the branching arrangement of a dendrite. **tracheobronchial t.,** the trachea, bronchi, and their branching structures.

Trem·a·to·da (trem″ah-to′dah) the flukes, a class of Platyhelminthes; they are parasitic in humans and other animals, infection usually resulting from ingestion of inadequately cooked fish, crustaceans, or vegetation containing their larvae.

trem·a·tode (trem′ah-tōd) an individual of the class Trematoda.

trem·or (trem′er) an involuntary trembling or quivering. **action t.,** rhythmic, oscillatory, involuntary movements of the outstretched upper limb; it may also affect the voice and other parts. **coarse t.,** one in which the vibrations are slow. **essential t.,** a hereditary tremor with onset usually at about 50 years of age, beginning with a fine rapid tremor of the hands, followed by tremor of the head, tongue, limbs, and trunk. **fine t.,** one in which the vibrations are rapid. **flapping t.,** asterixis. **intention t.,** action t. **parkinsonian t.,** the resting tremor seen with parkinsonism, consisting of slow regular movements of the hands and sometimes the legs, neck, face, or jaw; it typically stops upon voluntary movement of the part and is intensified by stimuli such as cold, fatigue, and strong emotions. **physiologic t.,** a rapid tremor of extremely low amplitude found in the legs and sometimes the neck or face of normal individuals; it may become accentuated and visible under certain conditions. **pill-rolling t.,** a parkinsonian tremor of the hand consisting of flexion and extension of the fingers in connection with adduction and abduction of the thumb. **resting t.,** tremor occurring in a relaxed and supported limb or other bodily part; it is sometimes abnormal, as in parkinsonism. **senile t.,** that due to the infirmities of old age. **volitional t.,** action t.

trem·u·lous (-u-lus) pertaining to or characterized by tremors.

treph·i·na·tion (tref″ĭ-na′shun) the operation of trephining.

tre·phine (trah-fīn′, trah-fēn′) 1. a crown saw for removing a disk of bone, chiefly from the skull. 2. an instrument for removing a circular area of cornea. 3. to remove with a trephine.

trep·i·dant (trep′ĭ-dant) tremulous.

trep·i·da·tion (trep″ĭ-da′shun) 1. tremor. 2. nervous anxiety and fear. **trep′idant,** adj.

Trep·o·ne·ma (trep″o-ne′mah) a genus of bacteria (family Spirochaetaceae), often pathogenic and parasitic; it includes the etiologic agents of pinta (*T. cara′teum*), syphilis (*T. pal′lidum* subspecies *pal′lidum*), and yaws (*T. pal′lidum* subspecies *perte′nue*).

trep·o·ne·ma (trep″o-ne′mah) an organism of the genus *Treponema.* **trepone′mal,** adj.

trep·o·ne·ma·to·sis (-ne″mah-to′sis) infection with organisms of the genus *Treponema.*

trep·o·ne·mi·ci·dal (-ne″mĭ-si′dal) destroying treponemas.

tre·pop·nea (tre″pop-ne′ah) dyspnea that is relieved when the patient is in lateral recumbent position.

trep·pe (trep′ĕ) [Ger.] the gradual increase in muscular contraction following rapidly repeated stimulation.

tret·i·noin (tret′ĭ-noin″) the all-*trans* stereoisomer of retinoic acid, used as a topical keratolytic in the treatment of acne vulgaris and disorders of keratinization and administered orally in the treatment of acute promyelocytic leukemia.

TRH thyrotropin-releasing hormone.

tri- word element [Gr.], *three.*

tri·ac·e·tin (tri-as′ĕ-tin) an antifungal agent used topically in the treatment of superficial fungal infections of the skin.

tri·ad (tri′ad) 1. any trivalent element. 2. a group of three associated entities or objects. **Beck's t.,** rising venous pressure, falling arterial pressure, and small quiet heart; characteristic of cardiac compression. **Currarino's t.,** a complex of congenital anomalies in the anococcygeal region, in varying combinations and degrees, with scimitar sacrum; presacral anterior meningocele, teratoma or cyst; and rectal malformations. **Hutchinson's t.,** diffuse interstitial keratitis, labyrinthine disease, and Hutchinson's teeth, seen in congenital syphilis. **Saint's t.,** hiatus hernia, colonic diverticula, and cholelithiasis.

tri·age (tre-ahzh′) [Fr.] 1. the sorting out of casualties of war or other disaster to determine priority of need and proper place of treatment. 2. by extension, the sorting and prioritizing of nonemergency patients for treatment.

tri·al (tri′al, trīl) a test or experiment. **clinical t.,** an experiment performed on human beings in order to evaluate the comparative efficacy of two or more therapies.

tri·am·cin·o·lone (tri″am-sin′o-lōn) a synthetic glucocorticoid used in replacement therapy for adrenocortical insufficiency and as an antiinflammatory and immunosuppressant in a wide variety of disorders.

tri·am·ter·ene (tri-am′ter-ēn) a potassium-sparing diuretic that blocks the reabsorption of sodium in the distal convoluted tubules; used in the treatment of edema and hypertension.

tri·an·gle (tri′ang-g′l) trigone; a three-cornered figure or area, such as on the surface of the body. **anal t.**, the portion of the perineal region surrounding the anus. **carotid t., inferior,** the part of the carotid trigone medial to the omohyoid muscle. **carotid t., superior,** carotid trigone. **cephalic t.**, one on the anteroposterior plane of skull, between lines from the occiput to the forehead and to the chin, and from the chin to the forehead. **Codman's t.**, a triangular area visible radiographically where the periosteum, elevated by a bone tumor, rejoins the cortex of normal bone. **digastric t.**, submandibular t. **t. of elbow,** in front, the supinator longus on the outside and pronator teres inside, the base toward the humerus. **facial t.**, a triangle whose points are the basion, and alveolar and nasal points. **Farabeuf's t.**, one in the upper part of the neck bound by the internal jugular vein, the facial nerve, and the hypoglossal nerve. **femoral t.**, 1. the area formed superiorly by the inguinal ligament, laterally by the sartorius muscle, and medially by the adductor longus muscle. 2. the surface area of the thigh overlying this area. **frontal t.**, one bounded by the maximum frontal diameter and the lines to the glabella. **Hesselbach's t.**, inguinal t. (1). **iliofemoral t.**, one formed by Nélaton's line, another line through the superior iliac spine, and a third from this to the greater trochanter. **infraclavicular t.**, one formed by the clavicle above, upper border of the pectoralis major on the inside, and the anterior border of the deltoid on the outside. **inguinal t.**, 1. the area on the inferoanterior abdominal wall bounded by the rectus abdominis muscle, the inguinal ligament, and inferior epigastric vessels. 2. femoral t. (1). **t. of Koch,** a roughly triangular area on the septal wall of the right atrium, between the tricuspid valve, coronary sinus orifice, and tendon of Todaro, that marks the site of the atrioventricular node. **Langenbeck's t.**, one whose apex is the anterior superior iliac spine, its base the anatomic neck of the femur, and its external side the external base of the greater trochanter. **Lesser's t.**, one formed by the hypoglossal nerve above, and the two bellies of the digastricus on the two sides. **lumbar t.**, Petit's t. **lumbocostoabdominal t.**, one

between the obliquus externus, the serratus posterior inferior, the erector spinae, and the obliquus internus. **Macewen's t.**, mastoid fossa. **occipital t.**, one having the sternomastoid in front, the trapezius behind, and the omohyoid below. **occipital t., inferior,** one having a line between the two mastoid processes as its base and the inion its apex. **omoclavicular t.**, subclavian t. **Pawlik's t.**, an area on the anterior vaginal wall corresponding to the trigone of the bladder. **Petit's t.**, the inferolateral margin of the latissimus dorsi and the external oblique muscle of the abdomen. **Scarpa's t.**, femoral t. (1). **subclavian t.**, a deep region of the neck: the triangular area bounded by the clavicle, sternocleidomastoid, and omohyoid. **submandibular t., submaxillary t.**, the triangular region of the neck bounded by the mandible, the stylohyoid muscle and posterior belly of the digastric muscle, and the anterior belly of the digastric muscle. **suboccipital t.**, one between the rectus capitis posterior major and superior and inferior oblique muscles. **supraclavicular t.**, subclavian t. **suprameatal t.**, mastoid fossa.

tri·an·gu·la·ris (-ang″gu-lar′is) [L.] triangular.

Tri·at·o·ma (tri″ah-to′mah) a genus of bugs (order Hemiptera), the cone-nosed bugs, important in medicine as vectors of *Trypanosoma cruzi.*

tri·atom·ic (-ah-tom′ik) containing three atoms.

tri·a·zo·lam (tri-a′zo-lam) a benzodiazepine used as a sedative and hypnotic in the treatment of insomnia.

tri·a·zole (tri′ah-zōl, tri-a′zōl) 1. a five-membered heterocyclic ring containing two carbon and three nitrogen atoms. 2. any of a class of antifungal compounds containing this structure.

tribe (trīb) a taxonomic category subordinate to a family (or subfamily) and superior to a genus (or subtribe).

tri·bra·chi·us (tri-bra′ke-us) 1. a fetus having three upper limbs. 2. conjoined twins having only three upper limbs.

tri·ceph·a·lus (tri-sef′ah-lus) a fetus with three heads.

tri·ceps (tri′seps) three-headed, as a triceps muscle. **t. su′rae,** see *Table of Muscles.*

tri·chi·a·sis (trī-ki′ah-sis) 1. a condition of ingrowing hairs about an orifice, or ingrowing eyelashes. 2. appearance of hairlike filaments in the urine.

trich·i·lem·mal (trik″ĭ-lem′al) pertaining to the root sheath of the hair.

trich·i·lem·mo·ma (-lem-o′mah) a benign neoplasm of the lower outer root sheath of the hair.

tri·chi·na (trĭ-ki′nah) pl. *trichi′nae.* An individual organism of the genus *Trichinella.*

Trich·i·nel·la (trik″ĭ-nel′ah) a genus of nematode parasites, including *T. spira′lis,* the etiologic agent of trichinosis, found in the muscles of rats, pigs, and humans.

trich·i·no·sis (-no′sis) a disease due to eating inadequately cooked meat infected with *Trichinella spiralis,* attended by diarrhea, nausea, colic, and fever, and later by stiffness, pain, muscle swelling, fever, sweating, eosinophilia, circumorbital edema, and splinter hemorrhages.

trich·i·nous (trik′ĭ-nus) affected with or containing trichinae.

tri·chlor·me·thi·a·zide (tri-klor″mĕ-thi′ah-zĭd) a thiazide diuretic used in the treatment of hypertension and edema.

tri·chlo·ro·ace·tic ac·id (tri-klor″o-ah-se′tik) an extremely caustic acid, used in clinical chemistry to precipitate proteins and applied topically in chemabrasion and to remove warts.

tri·chlo·ro·eth·y·lene (-eth′ĭ-lĕn) a clear, mobile liquid used as an industrial solvent; formerly used as an inhalant anesthetic.

trich(o)- word element [Gr.], *hair.*

tricho·ad·e·no·ma (trik″o-ad″ĕ-no′mah) a benign follicular tumor occurring on the face or trunk, with large cystic spaces lined by squamous epithelium and squamous cells.

tricho·be·zoar (-be′zor) a bezoar composed of hair.

tricho·dis·co·ma (-dis-ko′mah) a hamartoma of the mesodermal portion of the hair disk, usually occurring as multiple small papules that histologically resemble acrochordons.

tricho·epi·the·li·o·ma (-ep″ĭ-the″le-o′mah) a benign skin tumor originating in the follicles of the lanugo, usually on the face; it may occur as an inherited condition marked by multiple tumors *(multiple t.)* but also may occur as a noninherited solitary lesion *(solitary t.).*

tricho·es·the·sia (-es-the′zhah) the perception that one of the hairs of the skin has been touched, caused by stimulation of a hair follicle receptor.

tricho·fol·lic·u·lo·ma (-fŏ-lik″u-lo′mah) a benign usually solitary dome-shaped nodular lesion with a central pore that frequently contains a woolly hair-like tuft; usually occurring on the head or neck and derived from a hair follicle.

tricho·glos·sia (-glos′e-ah) hairy tongue.

tri·chome (tri′kōm) a filamentous or hairlike structure.

tricho·meg·a·ly (trik″o-meg′ah-le) a congenital syndrome consisting of excessive growth of the eyelashes and brow hair associated with dwarfism, mental retardation, and pigmentary degeneration of the retina.

tricho·mo·na·cide (-mo′nah-sīd) an agent destructive to trichomonads.

tricho·mo·nad (-mo′nad) a parasite of the genus *Trichomonas.*

Tricho·mo·nas (-mo′nas) a genus of flagellate protozoa. It includes *T. ho′minis,* a nonpathogenic human intestinal parasite, *T. te′nax,* a nonpathogenic species found in the human mouth, and *T. vagina′lis,* the cause of trichomoniasis. **trichomo′nal,** adj.

tricho·mo·ni·a·sis (-mo-ni′ah-sis) infection of the vagina or male genital tract by species of *Trichomonas vaginalis,* with pruritus and a refractory discharge.

tricho·my·co·sis (-mi-ko′sis) any disease of the hair caused by fungi. **t. axilla′ris,** infection of the axillary and sometimes of the pubic hair, due to *Corynebacterium tenuis,* a nocardia-like microorganism of uncertain affiliation, with development of clumps of bacteria on the hairs, appearing as red, yellow, or black nodules.

tricho·no·do·sis (-no-do′sis) a condition characterized by apparent or actual knotting of the hair.

tricho·pa·thy (trĭ-kop′ah-the) disease of the hair.

tricho·phyt·ic (trik″o-fit′ik) pertaining to trichophytosis.

tri·choph·y·tid (trĭ-kof′ĭ-tid) a dermophytid associated with trichophytosis; applied especially to the allergic manifestations of ringworm.

tri·choph·y·tin (trĭ-kof′ĭ-tin) a filtrate from cultures of *Trichophyton;* used in testing for trichophytosis.

tricho·phy·to·be·zoar (trik″o-fi″to-be′zor) a bezoar composed of animal hair and vegetable fiber.

Tri·choph·y·ton (trĭ-kof′ĭ-ton) a genus of fungi, species of which attack skin, hair, and nails.

tricho·phy·to·sis (trik″o-fi-to′sis) infection with fungi of the genus *Trichophyton.*

trich·op·ti·lo·sis (-tĭ-lo′sis) splitting of hairs at the end.

trich·or·rhex·is (-rek′sis) the condition in which the hairs break. **t. nodo′sa,** a condition marked by fracture and splitting of the cortex of a hair into strands, giving the appearance of white nodes at which the hair is easily broken.

trich·os·chi·sis (trĭ-kos′kĭ-sis) trichoptilosis.

tri·chos·co·py (trĭ-kos′kah-pe) examination of the hair.

tri·cho·sis (trĭ-ko′sis) any disease or abnormal growth of the hair.

Tri·chos·po·ron (trĭ-kos′po-ron) a genus of fungi that are normal flora of the respiratory and digestive tracts of humans and other animals, and may infect the hair.

tricho·spo·ro·sis (trik″o-spah-ro′sis) infection with *Trichosporon*; see *piedra*.

tri·chos·ta·sis spin·u·lo·sa (trĭ-kos′tah-sis spin″u-lo′sah) a condition in which the hair follicles contain a dark, horny plug that contains a bundle of vellus hair.

tricho·stron·gy·li·a·sis (trik″o-stron″jĭ-li′ah-sis) infection with *Trichostrongylus*.

Tricho·stron·gy·lus (-stron′jĭ-lus) a genus of nematodes parasitic in animals and humans.

tricho·thio·dys·tro·phy (-thi″o-dis′trah-fe) sparse, brittle hair with an unusually low sulfur content and a banded appearance under polarized light, often accompanied by short stature and mental retardation.

tricho·til·lo·ma·nia (-til″o-ma′ne-ah) compulsive pulling out of one's hair.

tri·chot·o·mous (trĭ-kot′ah-mus) divided into three parts.

tri·chro·ism (tri′kro-izm) the exhibition of three different colors in three different aspects. **trichro′ic**, adj.

tri·chro·ma·cy trichromatic vision.

tri·chro·mat·ic (tri″kro-mat′ik) 1. pertaining to or exhibiting three colors. 2. able to distinguish three colors.

tri·chro·mic (tri-kro′mik) trichromatic.

trich·u·ri·a·sis (trik″u-ri′ah-sis) infection with *Trichuris*, often asymptomatic in adults but with gastrointestinal symptoms in children.

Tri·chu·ris (trĭ-ku′ris) the whipworms, a genus of intestinal nematode parasites. *T. trichiu′ra* causes trichuriasis in humans.

tri·cip·i·tal (tri-sip′ĭ-tal) 1. three-headed. 2. relating to the triceps muscle.

tri·cit·rates (-sit′rāts) a solution of sodium citrate, potassium citrate, and citric acid; used as a systemic or urinary alkalizer, antiurolithic, and neutralizing buffer.

tri·cor·nute (-kor′nūt) having three horns, cornua, or processes.

tri·cro·tism (tri′krot-izm) quality of having three sphygmographic waves or elevations to one beat of the pulse. **tricrot′ic**, adj.

tri·cus·pid (tri-kus′pid) having three points or cusps, as a valve of the heart.

tri·cyc·lic (-sik′lik) containing three fused rings or closed chains in the molecular structure; see also under *antidepressant*.

tri·dac·ty·lism (-dak′tĭ-lizm) presence of only three digits on the hand or foot.

tri·den·tate (-den′tāt) having three prongs.

tri·der·mic (-der′mik) derived from all three germ layers (ectoderm, endoderm, and mesoderm).

tri·en·tene (tri′en-tēn) a chelating agent used as the hydrochloride salt for chelation of copper in the treatment of Wilson's disease.

tri·fa·cial (tri-fa′shul) designating the trigeminal (fifth cranial) nerve.

tri·fas·cic·u·lar (tri″fah-sik′u-lar) pertaining to three bundles, or fasciculi.

tri·fid (tri′fid) split into three parts.

tri·flu·o·per·a·zine (tri-floo-o-per′ah-zēn) a phenothiazine derivative used as the hydrochloride salt as an antipsychotic.

tri·flu·pro·ma·zine (-floo-pro′mah-zēn) a phenothiazine derivative; its hydrochloride salt is used as an antipsychotic and as an antiemetic.

tri·flur·i·dine (-floor′ĭ-dēn) an antiviral compound that interferes with viral DNA synthesis, used topically in the treatment of keratitis and keratoconjunctivitis caused by human herpesviruses 1 and 2.

tri·fo·cal (tri-fo′-, tri′fo-k′l) 1. having three foci. 2. containing one part for near vision, one for intermediate, and a third for distant vision, as a trifocal lens.

tri·fo·cals (tri′fo-k′lz) trifocal glasses.

tri·fur·ca·tion (tri″fur-ka′shun) division, or the site of separation, into three branches.

tri·gem·i·nal (tri-jem′ĭ-n′l) 1. triple. 2. pertaining to the trigeminal (fifth cranial) nerve; see *Table of Nerves*. 3. pertaining to trigeminy.

tri·gem·i·ny (tri-jem′ĭ-ne) 1. occurrence in threes. 2. the occurrence of a trigeminal pulse. **ventricular t.,** an arrhythmia consisting of the repetitive sequence of one ventricular premature complex followed by two normal beats.

tri·glyc·er·ide (-glis′er-īd) a compound consisting of three molecules of fatty acid esterified to glycerol; a neutral fat that is the usual storage form of lipids in animals.

tri·go·nal (tri′go-nal) 1. triangular. 2. pertaining to a trigone.

tri·gone (tri′gōn) 1. triangle. 2. the first three cusps of an upper molar tooth. **t. of bladder,** vesical t. **carotid t.,** the triangular area bounded by the posterior belly of the digastric muscle, the sternocleidomastoid muscle, and the anterior midline of the neck. **olfactory t.,** the triangular area of gray matter between the roots of the olfactory tract. **vesical t.,** the smooth triangular portion of the mucosa at the base of the bladder, bounded behind by the interureteric fold, ending in front in the uvula of the bladder.

trig·o·ni·tis (trig″o-ni′tis) inflammation or localized hyperemia of the vesical trigone.

trig·o·no·ceph·a·lus (trig″o-no-sef′ah-lus) an individual exhibiting trigonocephaly.

trig·o·no·ceph·a·ly (-le) triangular shape of the head due to sharp forward angulation at the midline of the frontal bone. **trigono·ceph·al′ic**, adj.

tri·go·num (tri-go′num) pl. *trigo′na*. [L.] triangle.

tri·hex·y·phen·i·dyl (tri-hek″si-fen′ĭ-dil) an antidyskinetic used as the hydrochloride salt in the treatment of parkinsonism and for the control of drug-induced extrapyramidal reactions.

tri·io·do·thy·ro·nine (tri″i-o″do-thi′ro-nēn) one of the thyroid hormones, an organic iodine-containing compound liberated from thyroglobulin by hydrolysis. It has several times the biological activity of thyroxine. Symbol T_3.

tri·kates (tri′kāts) a combination of potassium acetate, potassium bicarbonate, and potassium citrate used in the treatment and prophylaxis of hypokalemia.

tri·lam·i·nar (tri-lam′ĭ-ner) three-layered.

tri·lo·bate (-lo′bāt) having three lobes.

tri·loc·u·lar (-lok′u-ler) having three compartments or cells.

tril·o·gy (tril′o-je) a group or series of three. **t. of Fallot,** a term sometimes applied to concurrent pulmonic stenosis, atrial septal defect, and right ventricular hypertrophy.

tri·mep·ra·zine (tri-mep′rah-zēn) a phenothiazine derivative antihistamine; used as the tartrate salt as an antipruritic.

tri·mes·ter (-mes′ter) a period of three months.

tri·meth·a·di·one (tri″meth-ah-di′ōn) an anticonvulsant with analgesic properties, used for the control of petit mal seizures.

tri·meth·a·phan (tri-meth′ah-fan) a short-acting ganglionic blocking agent, used as the camsylate ester to produce controlled hypotension during surgery and for the emergency treatment of hypertensive crises and pulmonary edema due to hypertension.

tri·meth·o·ben·za·mide (-meth″o-ben′zah-mīd) an antiemetic, used as the hydrochloride salt.

tri·meth·o·prim (-meth′o-prim) an antibacterial closely related to pyrimethamine; almost always used in combination with a sulfonamide, primarily for the treatment of urinary tract infections. The sulfate salt is used in combination with polymyxin B sulfate in the topical treatment of ocular infections.

tri·me·trex·ate (tri″-mĕ-trek′sāt) a folic acid antagonist structurally related to methotrexate, used as the glucuronate salt, in combination with leukovorin, to treat *Pneumocystis carinii* pneumonia in AIDS.

tri·mip·ra·mine (tri-mip′rah-mēn) a tricyclic antidepressant of the dibenzazepine class; used as the maleate salt in the treatment of depression as well as peptic ulcer and severe chronic pain.

tri·mor·phous (tri-mor′fus) existing in three different forms.

tri·ni·tro·phe·nol (-ni″tro-fe′nol) a yellow substance used as dye and a tissue fixative; it can be detonated on percussion or by heating above 300°C.

tri·ni·tro·tol·u·ene (TNT) (-tol′u-ēn) a high explosive derived from toluene; it sometimes causes poisoning in those who work with it, marked by dermatitis, gastritis, abdominal pain, vomiting, constipation, and flatulence.

tri·or·chi·dism (tri-or′kĭ-dizm) the condition of having three testes. **trior′chid,** adj.

tri·ose (tri′ōs) a monosaccharide containing three carbon atoms in the molecule.

tri·ox·sa·len (tri-ok′sah-len) a psoralen used in conjunction with ultraviolet exposure in the treatment of vitiligo.

tri·pe·len·na·mine (tri″pĕ-len′ah-min) an antihistamine with anticholinergic and sedative effects, used as the citrate and hydrochloride salts.

tri·pep·tide (tri-pep′tīd) a peptide that on hydrolysis yields three amino acids.

tri·phal·an·gism (-fal′an-jizm) three phalanges in a digit normally having only two.

tri·pha·sic (-fa′zik) having three phases.

tri·phen·yl·meth·ane (-fen″il-meth′ān) a substance from coal tar, the basis of various dyes and stains, including rosaniline, basic fuchsin, and gentian violet.

tri·phos·phate (tri-fos′fāt) a salt containing three phosphate radicals.

trip·le blind (trip′l blind) pertaining to an experiment in which neither the subject nor the person administering the treatment nor the person evaluating the response to treatment knows which treatment any particular subject is receiving.

tri·ple·gia (tri-ple′jah) paralysis of three limbs.

trip·let (trip′let) 1. one of three offspring produced at one birth. 2. a combination of three objects or entities acting together, as three lenses or three nucleotides. 3. a triple discharge.

tri·plex (tri′pleks) triple or threefold.

trip·loid (trip′loid) having triple the haploid number of chromosomes (3n).

trip·lo·pia (trĭ-plo'pe-ah) the perception of three images of a single object.

tri·pro·li·dine (tri-pro'lĭ-dēn) an antihistamine with anticholinergic and sedative effects, used as the hydrochloride salt.

-tripsy word element [Gr.], *crushing;* used to designate a surgical procedure in which a structure is intentionally crushed.

trip·to·rel·in (trĭp″to-rel'in) a synthetic gonadorelin analogue that on prolonged administration suppresses gonadotropin release; used as *t. pamoate* as an antineoplastic in the treatment of prostatic carcinoma.

tri·pus (tri'pus) conjoined twins with tripodial symmelia.

TRIS tromethamine.

tris (tris) 1. tromethamine. 2. tris(2,3-dibromopropyl) phosphate.

tri·sal·i·cyl·ate (tri″sah-lis'ĭ-lāt) a compound containing three salicylate ions. **choline magnesium t.,** a combination of choline and magnesium salicylates, used as an analgesic, antipyretic, antiinflammatory, and antirheumatic.

tris·(2,3-di·bro·mo·pro·pyl) phos·phate (tris″di-bro″mo-pro'p'l fos'fāt) a yellow liquid flame retardant, formerly used in children's clothing but now restricted in use because it is carcinogenic.

tris·mus (triz'mus) motor disturbance of the trigeminal nerve, especially spasm of the masticatory muscles, with difficulty in opening the mouth (lockjaw); a characteristic early symptom of tetanus.

tri·so·my (tri'so-me) the presence of an additional (third) chromosome of one type in an otherwise diploid cell (2n + 1). See also entries under *syndrome.* **triso'mic,** adj.

tri·splanch·nic (tri-splangk'nik) pertaining to the three great visceral cavities.

tri·sul·cate (-sul'kāt) having three furrows.

tri·sul·fide (-sul'fid) a sulfur compound containing three atoms of sulfur to one of the base.

tri·ta·nom·a·ly (tri″tah-nom'ah-le) a rare type of anomalous trichromatic vision in which the third, blue-sensitive, cones have decreased sensitivity.

tri·ta·nope (trit'ah-nōp″) a person exhibiting tritanopia.

tri·ta·no·pia (tri″tah-no'pe-ah) a rare type of dichromatic vision marked by retention of the sensory mechanism for two hues only (red and green), with blue and yellow being absent. **tritanop'ic,** adj.

tri·ti·ceous (tri-tish'us) resembling a grain of wheat.

trit·i·um (trit'e-um) see *hydrogen.*

trit·ur·a·tion (trich″ĕ-ra'shun) 1. reduction to powder by friction or grinding. 2. a drug so created, especially one rubbed up with lactose. 3. the creation of a homogeneous whole by mixing, as the combining of particles of an alloy with mercury to form dental amalgam.

tri·va·lent (tri-va'lent) having a valence of three.

tRNA transfer RNA.

tro·car (tro'kahr) a sharp-pointed instrument equipped with a cannula, used to puncture the wall of a body cavity and withdraw fluid.

tro·chan·ter (tro-kan'ter) a broad, flat process on the femur, at the upper end of its lateral surface (*greater t.*), or a short conical process on the posterior border of the base of its neck (*lesser t.*). **trochanter'ic, trochanter'ian,** adj.

tro·che (tro'ke) lozenge (1).

troch·lea (trok'le-ah) pl. *troch'leae.* [L.] a pulley-shaped part or structure; used in anatomic nomenclature to designate a bony or fibrous structure through which a tendon passes or with which other structures articulate. **troch'lear,** adj.

tro·cho·ceph·a·ly (tro″ko-sef'ah-le) a rounded appearance of the head due to synostosis of the frontal and parietal bones.

tro·choid (tro'koid) pivot-like, or pulley-shaped.

tro·choi·des (tro-koi'dēz) a pivot joint.

Trog·lo·tre·ma (trog″lo-tre'mah) a genus of flukes, including *T. salmin'cola* (salmon fluke), a parasite of various fish, especially salmon and trout, which is a vector of *Neorickettsia helminthoeca.*

tro·le·an·do·my·cin (tro″le-an-do-mi'sin) a macrolide antibiotic used in the treatment of pneumococcal pneumonia and Group A β-hemolytic streptococcal infections.

Trom·bic·u·la (trom-bik'u-lah) a genus of acarine mites (family Trombiculidae), including *T. akamu'shi, T. delien'sis, T. fletch'eri, T. interme'dia, T. pal'lida,* and *T. scutella'ris,* whose larvae (chiggers) are vectors of *Rickettsia tsutsugamushi,* the cause of scrub typhus.

trom·bic·u·li·a·sis (trom-bik″u-li'ah-sis) infestation with mites of the genus *Trombicula.*

Trom·bic·u·li·dae (-de) a family of mites cosmopolitan in distribution, whose parasitic larvae (chiggers) infest vertebrates.

tro·meth·amine (tro-meth'ah-mēn) a proton acceptor used as an alkalizer in the treatment of metabolic acidosis; also used to make buffer solutions.

troph·ede·ma (trof″ĕ-de′mah) a chronic disease with permanent edema of the feet or legs.

tro·phic (tro′fik, trof′ik) pertaining to nutrition.

-trophic word element [Gr.], *nourishing; stimulating.*

troph(o)- word element [Gr.], *food; nourishment.*

tro·pho·blast (tro′fo-blast) the peripheral cells of the blastocyst, which attach the blastocyst to the uterine wall and become the placenta and the membranes that nourish and protect the developing organism. **trophoblas′tic,** adj.

tro·pho·neu·ro·sis (-noo-ro′sis) any functional disease due to failure of nutrition in a part because its nerve supply is defective. **trophoneurot′ic,** adj.

tro·phont (tro′font) the active, motile, feeding stage in the life cycle of certain ciliate protozoa.

tropho·plast (trof″o-plast) a granular placenta body.

tropho·tax·is (trof″o-tak′sis) taxis in response to nutritive materials.

tropho·zo·ite (-zo′īt) the active, motile feeding stage of a sporozoan parasite.

tro·pia (tro′pe-ah) strabismus.

-tropic word element [Gr.], *turning toward; changing; tending to turn or change.*

trop·i·cal (trop′ĭ-k′l) pertaining to the regions of the earth bounded by the parallels of latitude 23° 27′ north and south of the equator.

tro·pism (tro′pizm) the turning, bending, movement, or growth of an organism or part of an organism elicited by an external stimulus, either toward (*positive t.*) or away from (*negative t.*) the stimulus; used as a word element combined with a stem indicating the nature of the stimulus (e.g., phototropism) or material or entity for which an organism (or substance) shows a special affinity (e.g., neurotropism). Usually applied to nonmotile organisms.

trop(o)- word element [Gr.] *turn; reaction; change.*

tro·po·col·la·gen (tro″po-kol′ah-jen) the basic structural unit of all forms of collagen; it is a helical structure of three polypeptides wound around each other.

tro·po·my·o·sin (-mi′o-sin) a muscle protein of the I band that inhibits contraction by blocking the interaction of actin and myosin, except when influenced by troponin.

tro·po·nin (tro′po-nin) a complex of muscle proteins which, when combined with Ca^{2+}, influence tropomyosin to initiate contraction.

-tropy word element [Gr.], *a turn, turning, change in response to a stimulus.*

trough (trof) a shallow longtudinal depression. **synaptic t.,** an invagination of the membrane of a striated muscle fiber, surrounding a motor end plate at a neuromuscular junction.

tro·va·flox·a·cin (tro″vah-flok′sah-sin) an antibacterial effective against a broad spectrum of gram-positive and gram-negative organisms; used as the mesylate salt.

Trp tryptophan.

trun·cal (trung′k′l) pertaining to the trunk.

trun·cate (trung′kāt) 1. to amputate; to deprive of limbs. 2. having the end cut squarely off.

trun·cus (-kus) pl. *trun′ci.* [L.] trunk. **t. arterio′sus,** an arterial trunk, especially the artery connected with the embryonic heart, which gives off the aortic arches and develops into the aortic and pulmonary arteries.

trunk (trungk) 1. torso; the main part of the body, to which head and limbs are attached. 2. a major, undivided and often short, part of a nerve, vessel, or duct. **brachiocephalic t.,** a vessel arising from the arch of the aorta and giving rise to the right common carotid and right subclavian arteries. **celiac t.,** the arterial trunk arising from the abdominal aorta and giving origin to the left gastric, common hepatic, and splenic arteries. **lumbosacral t.,** a trunk formed by union of the lower part of the anterior branch of the fourth lumbar nerve with the anterior branch of the fifth lumbar nerve. **lymphatic t's,** the lymphatic vessels that drain lymph from the various regions of the body into the right lymphatic or the thoracic duct. **pulmonary t.,** a vessel arising from the conus arteriosus of the right ventricle and bifurcating into the right and left pulmonary arteries. **sympathetic t.,** two long ganglionated nerve strands, one on each side of the vertebral column, extending from the base of the skull to the coccyx.

truss (trus) an elastic, canvas, or metallic device for retaining a reduced hernia within the abdominal cavity.

try·pano·ci·dal (tri-pan″o-si′dal) destructive to trypanosomes.

try·pano·cide (tri-pan′o-sīd) an agent lethal to trypanosomes; called also trypanosomicide.

try·pan·ol·y·sis (tri″pan-ol′ĭ-sis) the destruction of trypanosomes. **trypanolyt′ic,** adj.

Try·pano·so·ma (tri″pan-o-so′mah) a genus of protozoa parasitic in the blood and lymph of invertebrates and vertebrates, including humans. *T. bru′cei gambien′se* and *T. bru′cei rhodesien′se* cause types of African trypanosomiasis and *T. cru'zi* causes Chagas' disease.

try·pano·some (tri-pan'o-sōm) an individual of the genus *Trypanosoma*. **trypanoso'mal,** adj.

try·pano·so·mi·a·sis (tri-pan″o-so-mi'ah-sis) infection with trypanosomes. **African t.,** human trypanosomiasis endemic in areas of tropical Africa, due to infection with *Trypanosoma gambiense* (Gambian t.) or *T. rhodesiense* (Rhodesian t.); it is transmitted by the bite of species of *Glossina* (tsetse flies) and in advanced stage attacks the central nervous system, resulting in meningoencephalitis that leads to lethargy, tremors, convulsions, and eventually coma and death. **South American t.,** Chagas' disease.

try·pano·so·mi·cide (-so'mĭ-sīd) trypanocide.

try·pano·so·mid (-so'mid) a skin eruption occurring in trypanosomiasis.

tryp·sin (trip'sin) an enzyme of the hydrolase class, secreted as trypsinogen by the pancreas and converted to the active form in the small intestine, that catalyzes the cleavage of peptide linkages involving the carboxyl group of either lysine or arginine; a purified preparation derived from ox pancreas is used for its proteolytic effect in débridement and in the treatment of empyema. **tryp'tic,** adj.

tryp·sin·o·gen (trip-sin'o-jen) the inactive precursor of trypsin, secreted by the pancreas and activated in the duodenum by cleavage by enteropeptidase.

tryp·ta·mine (trip'tah-mēn) a product of the decarboxylation of tryptophan, occurring in plants and certain foods such as cheese; it raises blood pressure via vasoconstriction by causing the release of norepinephrine at postganglionic nerve endings.

tryp·to·phan (Trp, W) (trip'to-fan) a naturally occurring amino acid, existing in proteins and essential for human metabolism. It is a precursor of serotonin. Adequate levels may mitigate pellagra by compensating for deficiencies of niacin.

tryp·to·phan·uria (trip″to-fan-ūr'e-ah) excessive urinary excretion of tryptophan.

TS tricuspid stenosis.

TSA tumor-specific antigen.

TSD Tay-Sachs disease.

tset·se (tset'se) an African fly of the genus *Glossina*, which transmits trypanosomiasis.

TSH thyroid-stimulating hormone; see *thyrotropin*.

T-spine thoracic spine.

TT therapeutic touch; thrombin time.

tu·ba (too'bah) pl. *tu'bae*. [L.] tube.

tu·bal (too'b'l) pertaining to or occurring in a tube.

tube (toob) a hollow cylindrical organ or instrument. **auditory t.,** eustachian tube; the narrow channel connecting the middle ear and the nasopharynx. **drainage t.,** a tube used in surgery to facilitate escape of fluids. **Durham's t.,** a jointed tracheotomy tube. **endobronchial t.,** a double-lumen tube inserted into the bronchus of one lung to deflate the other lung for anesthesia or thoracic surgery. **endotracheal t.,** an airway catheter inserted in the trachea in endotracheal intubation. **esophageal t.,** stomach t. **eustachian t.,** auditory t. **fallopian t.,** uterine t. **feeding t.,** one for introducing high-caloric fluids into the stomach. **Miller-Abbott t.,** a double-channel intestinal tube with an inflatable balloon at its distal end, for use in treatment of obstruction of the small intestine, and occasionally as a diagnostic aid. **nasogastric t.,** a soft tube to be inserted through a nostril and into the stomach, for instilling liquids or other substances, or for withdrawing gastric contents. **nasotracheal t.,** an endotracheal tube that passes through the nose. **neural t.,** the epithelial tube developed from the neural plate and forming the central nervous system of the embryo. **orotracheal t.,** an endotracheal tube that passes through the mouth. **otopharyngeal t., pharyngotympanic t.,** auditory t. **Sengstaken-Blakemore t.,** a multilumen tube used for tamponade of bleeding esophageal varices. **stomach t.,** a tube for feeding or for stomach irrigation; the most common kind is the nasogastric tube. **test t.,** a tube of thin glass, closed at one end; used in chemical tests and other laboratory procedures. **tracheal t.,** endotracheal t. **tracheostomy t.,** a curved endotracheal tube that is inserted into the trachea through a tracheostomy. **uterine t.,** fallopian tube; a slender tube extending from the uterus toward the ovary on the same side, for passage of oocytes to the cavity of the uterus and the usual site of fertilization. **Wangensteen t.,** a small nasogastric tube connected with a special suction apparatus to maintain gastric and duodenal decompression. **x-ray t.,** a vacuum tube used for the production of x-rays; when a suitable current is applied, high-speed electrons travel from the cathode to the anode, where they are suddenly arrested, giving rise to x-rays.

tu·bec·to·my (too-bek'tah-me) salpingectomy.

tu·ber (too'ber) pl. *tu'bera*, tubers. [L.] 1. a swelling or protuberance. 2. the essential lesion of tuberous sclerosis, presenting as a pale, firm, nodular, phakomalike glial hamartomatous brain lesion. **t. cine′reum,** a layer of gray matter forming part of the floor of the third ventricle, to which the infundibulum of the hypothalamus is attached.

tu·ber·cle (-k′l) 1. any small, rounded mass produced by infection with *Mycobacterium tuberculosis.* 2. a nodule or small eminence, especially one on a bone for attachment of a tendon. 3. the cusp of a tooth. **anatomical t.,** tuberculosis verrucosa cutis. **auricular t., auricular t. of Darwin, darwinian t.,** a small projection sometimes found on the edge of the helix; conjectured by some to be a relic of simioid ancestry. **Farre's t's,** masses beneath the capsule of the liver in some cases of hepatocellular carcinoma. **fibrous t.,** one of bacillary origin which contains connective-tissue elements. **genial t., inferior,** inferior mental spine. **genial t., superior,** superior mental spine. **genital t.,** an eminence ventral to the cloaca in the early embryo; the primordium of the penis or clitoris. **Ghon t.,** see under *focus.* **gracile t.,** an enlargement of the fasciculus gracilis in the medulla oblongata, produced by the underlying nucleus gracilis. **intervenous t.,** a ridge across the inner surface of the right atrium between the openings of the venae cavae. **Lisfranc's t.,** an eminence on the first rib, for attachment of the anterior scalene muscle. **Lower's t.,** intervenous t. **mental t.,** a prominence on the inner border of either side of the mental protuberance of the mandible. **miliary t.,** one of the many minute tubercles formed in many organs in acute miliary tuberculosis. **pubic t. of pubic bone,** a prominent tubercle at the lateral end of the pubic crest. **scalene t.,** Lisfranc's t. **supraglenoid t.,** one on the scapula for attachment of the long head of the biceps.

tu·ber·cu·lar (too-ber′ku-lar) 1. pertaining to or resembling tubercles. 2. tuberculous.

tu·ber·cu·late (too-ber′ku-lāt″) having tubercles.

tu·ber·cu·lat·ed (-ed) tuberculate.

tu·ber·cu·lid (-lid) recurrent eruptions of the skin usually characterized by spontaneous involution; considered by some authorities to be hyperergic reactions to mycobacteria or their antigens. **papulonecrotic t.,** a grouped, symmetric eruption of symptomless papules, appearing in successive crops and healing spontaneously with superficially depressed scars.

tu·ber·cu·lin (-lin) a sterile solution containing the growth products of, or specific substances extracted from, the tubercle bacillus; used in various forms in the diagnosis of tuberculosis; see also under *test.* **Old t. (OT),** a sterile solution of a heat-concentrated filtrate of tubercle bacillus culture grown on a special medium; used for tuberculin tests. **PPD t., purified protein derivative t.,** a sterile solution of a purified protein fraction precipitated from a filtrate of tubercle bacillus grown on a special medium; used in tuberculin tests.

tu·ber·cu·li·tis (too-ber″ku-li′tis) inflammation of or near a tubercle.

tu·ber·cu·loid (too-ber′ku-loid) resembling a tubercle or tuberculosis.

tu·ber·cu·lo·ma (too-ber″ku-lo′mah) a tumor-like mass resulting from enlargement of a caseous tubercle.

tu·ber·cu·lo·sis (-sis) any of the infectious diseases of humans and other animals due to species of *Mycobacterium* and marked by formation of tubercles and caseous necrosis in tissues of any organ; in humans the lung is the major seat of infection and the usual portal through which infection reaches other organs. **avian t.,** a form affecting various birds, due to *Mycobacterium avium,* which may be communicated to humans and other animals. **bovine t.,** an infection of cattle due to *Mycobacterium bovis,* transmissible to humans and other animals. **disseminated t.,** an acute form of miliary t. **genital t.,** tuberculosis of the genital tract, e.g., tuberculous endometritis. **t. of lungs,** pulmonary t. **miliary t.,** a form varying in severity, in which minute tubercles form in different organs due to dissemination of bacilli through the body by the blood stream. **open t.,** 1. that in which there are lesions from which tubercle bacilli are discharged out of the body. 2. pulmonary tuberculosis with cavitation. **pulmonary t.,** tuberculosis of lungs; infection of the lungs by *Mycobacterium tuberculosis,* with tuberculous pneumonia, formation of tuberculous granulation tissue, caseous necrosis, calcification, and cavity formation. Symptoms include weight loss, fatigue, night sweats, purulent sputum, hemoptysis, and chest pain. **renal t.,** renal disease due to *Mycobacterium tuberculosis.* **spinal t.,** osteitis or caries of vertebrae, usually as a complication of pulmonary tuberculosis. **t. verruco′sa cu′tis, warty t.,** a condition usually due to external inoculation of tubercle bacilli into the skin, with wartlike patches having an inflammatory, erythematous border.

tu·ber·cu·lo·stat·ic (too-ber″ku-lo-stat′ik) 1. inhibiting the growth of *Mycobacterium tuberculosis.* 2. an agent that so acts.

tu·ber·cu·lot·ic (too-ber″ku-lot′ik) pertaining to or affected with tuberculosis.

tu·ber·cu·lous (too-ber′ku-lus) pertaining to or affected with tuberculosis; caused by *Mycobacterium tuberculosis.*

tu·ber·cu·lum (-lum) pl. *tuber′cula.* [L.] tubercle (2). **t. arthri′ticum,** a gouty concretion in a joint. **t. doloro′sum,** a painful nodule or tubercle.

tu·ber·o·sis (too-ber-o′sis) a condition characterized by the presence of nodules.

tu·be·ros·i·tas (too″bĕ-ros′ĭ-tas) pl. *tuberosita′tes.* [L.] tuberosity.

tu·be·ros·i·ty (-te) an elevation or protuberance, especially one on a bone where a muscle is attached.

tu·ber·ous (too″ber-us) covered with tubers; knobby. See also under *sclerosis.*

tubo- word element [L.], *tube.*

tu·bo·ab·dom·i·nal (too″bo-ab-dom′ĭ-n′l) pertaining to the uterine tube and the abdomen.

tu·bo·cu·ra·rine (-ku-rah′rēn) an alkaloid from the bark and stems of *Chondrodendron tomentosum;* it is the active principle of curare and is a nondepolarizing neuromuscular blocking agent; used as the chloride salt as a skeletal muscle relaxant and as an aid in the diagnosis of myasthenia gravis.

tu·bo·lig·a·men·tous (-lig′ah-men′tus) pertaining to the uterine tube and broad ligament.

tu·bo·ovar·i·an (-o-var′e-an) of or pertaining to a uterine tube and ovary.

tu·bo·peri·to·ne·al (-per″ĭ-tah-ne′al) pertaining to the uterine tube and the peritoneum.

tu·bo·plas·ty (too′bo-plas″te) plastic repair of a tube, such as the uterine tube or auditory tube.

tu·bo·tym·pa·num (too″bo-tim′pah-num) the auditory tube and tympanic cavity considered together.

tu·bo·uter·ine (-u′ter-in) pertaining to a uterine tube and the uterus.

tu·bu·lar (too′bu-lar) 1. shaped like a tube. 2. of or pertaining to a tubule.

tu·bule (too′būl) a small tube. **collecting t.,** one of the terminal channels of the nephrons which open on the summits of the renal pyramids in the renal papillae. **connecting t.,** junctional t. **dental t's, dentinal t's,** dental canaliculi. **distal convoluted t.,** a distal, convoluted part of the ascending limb of the renal tubule, extending from the distal straight tubule to the junctional tubule. **distal straight t.,** part of the renal tubule primarily on the ascending limb, extending from the thin tubule to the distal convoluted tubule.

Henle's t., see under *loop.* **junctional t.,** a short, curved part of the distal end of the renal tubule, extending from the distal convoluted tubule to a collecting duct. **mesonephric t's,** those constituting the mesonephros of the embryo of an amniote. **metanephric t's,** those constituting the metanephros of an amniote. **pronephric t's,** the rudimentary tubules constituting the pronephros of an amniote. **proximal convoluted t.,** the most proximal part of the renal tubule, extending from the glomerular capsule to the proximal straight tubule. **proximal straight t.,** part of the descending limb of the renal tubule, extending from the proximal convoluted tubule to the thin tubule. **renal t.,** the minute reabsorptive canals made up of basement membrane and lined with epithelium, composing the substance of the kidney and secreting, collecting, and conducting the urine; see also *nephron.* **seminiferous t's,** channels in the testis in which the spermatozoa develop and through which they leave the gland, each comprising a convoluted portion and a straight terminal portion. **T t's,** the transverse intracellular tubules invaginating from the cell membrane and surrounding the myofibrils of the T system of skeletal and cardiac muscle, serving as a pathway for the spread of electrical excitation within a muscle cell. **thin t.,** part of the renal tubule where the walls are especially thin, extending from the proximal straight tubule to the distal straight tubule. **uriniferous t.,** renal t's.

tu·bu·lin (too′bu-lin) the constituent protein of microtubules.

tu·bu·lo·in·ter·sti·tial (too″bu-lo-in″ter-sti′shal) pertaining to the renal tubules and interstitial tubules.

tu·bu·lor·rhex·is (-rek′sis) rupture of the renal tubules.

tu·bu·lo·ve·sic·u·lar (-vĕ-sik′u-lar) composed of small tubes and sacs; used particularly of the cytoplasmic membranes of the resting parietal cell.

tu·bu·lus (too′bu-lus) pl. *tu′buli.* [L.] tubule; a minute canal.

tuft (tuft) a small clump or cluster; a coil.

tuft·sin (tuft′sin) a tetrapeptide cleaved from IgG that stimulates phagocytosis by neutrophils.

tug·ging (tug′ing) a pulling sensation, as a pulling sensation in the trachea *(tracheal t.),* due to aneurysm of the arch of the aorta.

tui na (too′e nah′) [Chinese] a Chinese system of massage, acupoint stimulation, and manipulation using forceful maneuvers, including pushing, rolling, kneading, rubbing, and grasping, sometimes in conjunction with acupuncture.

tu·la·re·mia (too″lah-re′me-ah) a plaguelike disease of rodents, caused by *Francisella tularensis* and transmissible to humans. **oculoglandular t.,** that in which the primary site of infection is the conjunctival sac, with conjunctivitis, corneal lesions, and enlargement of preauricular lymph nodes. **pulmonary t., pulmonic t.,** that with involvement of the lungs by spread of primary infection or inhalation of the pathogen, with cough, fever, chest pain, and bloody sputum. **typhoidal t.,** the most serious type, caused by swallowing the pathogen; symptoms are similar to those of typhoid. **ulceroglandular t.,** the most common type in humans, beginning with a painful red papule at the point of inoculation, later forming a shallow ulcer; lymphadenopathy, hepatosplenomegaly, and pneumonia may also occur.

tul·si (tool′se) a type of basil, *Ocimum sanctum,* considered sacred in India and having immunostimulant, antibacterial, antifungal, and antiviral properties, used in ayurvedic medicine.

tu·me·fa·cient (too″mah-fa′shent) producing swelling.

tu·me·fac·tion (-fak′shun) swelling.

tu·mes·cence (too-mes′ens) swelling.

tu·mid (too′mid) swollen; edematous.

tu·mor (too′mer) 1. swelling, one of the cardinal signs of inflammation; morbid enlargement. 2. neoplasm; a new growth of tissue in which cell multiplication is uncontrolled and progressive. **adenomatoid odontogenic t.,** a benign odontogenic tumor with ductlike or glandlike arrangements of columnar epithelial cells, usually occurring in the anterior jaw region. **Askin's t.,** a malignant small-cell tumor of soft tissue in the thoracopulmonary region in children; one of the peripheral neuroectodermal tumors. **benign t.,** one lacking the properties of invasion and metastasis and showing a lesser degree of anaplasia than do malignant tumors; it is usually surrounded by a fibrous capsule. **Brenner t.,** a rare, usually benign, tumor of the ovary characterized by groups of epithelial cells lying in a fibrous connective tissue stroma. **brown t.,** a giant-cell granuloma produced in and replacing bone, occurring in osteitis fibrosa cystica and due to hyperparathyroidism. **Buschke-Löwenstein t.,** a large, destructive, penetrating, cauliflower-like mass on the prepuce, especially in uncircumcised males, and also in the perianal region. **carcinoid t.,** carcinoid. **carcinoma ex mixed t.,** carcinoma

ex pleomorphic adenoma. **carotid body t.,** a chemodectoma of the carotid body, a firm, round mass at the bifurcation of the common carotid artery. **dermal duct t.,** a small, intradermal, papular, eccrine lesion occurring on the head and neck in older adults. **desmoid t.,** an unencapsulated locally invasive fibromatous tumor arising in the musculoaponeurotic tissue, usually the abdominal wall, and often resembling fibrosarcoma. **diarrheogenic t.,** VIPoma. **endodermal sinus t.,** yolk sac t. **erectile t.,** cavernous hemangioma. **Ewing's t.,** see under *sarcoma.* **false t.,** structural enlargement due to extravasation, exudation, echinococcus, or retained sebaceous matter. **feminizing t.,** a functional tumor that produces feminization in boys and men or precocious sexual development in girls, e.g., germinoma. **fibrohistiocytic t.,** a tumor containing cells resembling histiocytes and others resembling fibroblasts; often used to denote the most general meaning of benign or malignant fibrous histiocytoma. **functional t., functioning t.,** a hormone-secreting tumor in an endocrine gland. **germ cell t.,** any of a group of tumors arising from primitive germ cells, usually of the testis or ovary. **giant cell t.,** 1. a bone tumor, ranging from benign to frankly malignant, composed of cellular spindle cell stroma containing multinucleated giant cells resembling osteoclasts. 2. a benign, small, yellow, tumor-like nodule of tendon sheath origin, most often of the wrist and fingers or ankle and toes, laden with lipophages and containing multinucleated giant cells. **glomus t.,** 1. a benign, blue-red, painful tumor involving a glomeriform arteriovenous anastomosis (glomus body). 2. chemodectoma. **glomus jugulare t.,** a chemodectoma involving the tympanic body (glomus jugulare). **granular cell t.,** a usually benign, circumscribed, tumor-like lesion of soft tissue, particularly of the tongue, composed of large cells with prominent granular cytoplasm; the histiogenesis is uncertain, but Schwann cell derivation is favored. **granulosa t., granulosa cell t.,** an ovarian tumor originating in the cells of the membrana granulosa. **granulosa-theca cell t.,** an ovarian tumor composed of granulosa (follicular) cells and theca cells; either form may predominate. **heterologous t., heterotypic t.,** one made up of tissue differing from that in which it grows. **hilar cell t.,** a rare benign neoplasm of the hilus of the ovary, histologically resembling Leydig cell tumor of the testis. **homologous t.,** one resembling the surrounding parts in its structure. **Hürthle**

cell t., new growth of the thyroid gland composed predominantly of Hürthle cells; it is usually benign (Hürthle cell adenoma) but may be locally invasive or metastasize (Hürthle cell carcinoma or malignant Hürthle cell tumor). **islet cell t.,** a tumor of the pancreatic islets; many secrete excessive amounts of hormones. Types include gastrinoma, glucagonoma, insulinoma, somatostatinoma, and VIPoma. **Krukenberg's t.,** carcinoma of the ovary, usually metastatic from gastrointestinal cancer, marked by areas of mucoid degeneration and by the presence of signet-ring–like cells. **Leydig cell t.,** 1. a usually benign, nongerminal tumor of the Leydig cells of the testis. 2. hilar cell t. **lipoid cell t. of ovary,** a usually benign ovarian tumor composed of eosinophilic cells or cells with lipoid vacuoles; it causes masculinization. **malignant t.,** one having the properties of invasion and metastasis and showing a high degree of anaplasia. **mast cell t.,** mastocytosis. **melanotic neuroectodermal t.,** a benign, rapidly growing, dark tumor of the jaw and occasionally of other sites; seen almost exclusively in infants. **mixed t.,** a tumor composed of more than one type of neoplastic tissue. **müllerian mixed t.,** a malignant mixed tumor of the uterus containing both endometrial adenocarcinoma and sarcomatous cells that may be either of uterine or extrauterine origin. **neuroendocrine t., neuroendocrine cell t.,** any of a diverse group of tumors containing neurosecretory cells that cause endocrine dysfunction; most are carcinoids or carcinomas. **nonfunctional t., nonfunctioning t.,** a tumor located in an endocrine gland but not secreting hormones. **odontogenic t.,** a lesion derived from mesenchymal or epithelial elements, or both, that are associated with the development of the teeth; it occurs in the mandible or maxilla, or occasionally the gingiva. **papillary t.,** papilloma. **pearl t., pearly t.,** cholesteatoma. **peripheral neuroectodermal t.,** a primitive neuroectodermal tumor occurring outside of the central nervous system in a site such as the pelvis, a limb, or the chest wall. **phyllodes t.,** a large, locally aggressive, sometimes metastatic fibroadenoma in the breast, with an unusually cellular, sarcomalike stroma. **primitive neuroectodermal t. (PNET),** proposed name for a heterogeneous group of neoplasms thought to derive from undifferentiated cells of the neural crest. **proliferating trichilemmal t.,** a large, solitary, multilobulated lesion of the hair follicle, occurring on the scalp, usually in middle-aged or older women; often confused

with squamous cell carcinoma. **sand t.,** psammoma. **squamous odontogenic t.,** a benign odontogenic epithelial neoplasm occurring in the mandible or maxilla and believed to derive from transformation of the rests of Malassez. **stromal t's,** a diverse group of tumors derived from the ovarian stroma, many of which secrete sex hormones. **teratoid t.,** teratoma. **testicular t.,** a general term for any tumor of the testes; in adults these are almost always malignant germinomas, whereas in children many are yolk sac tumors or benign varieties such as teratomas or androblastomas. **theca cell t.,** a fibroid-like ovarian tumor containing yellow areas of lipoid material derived from theca cells. **turban t.,** a term used to describe the gross appearance of multiple cutaneous cylindromas of the scalp. **virilizing t.,** a functional tumor that produces virilization in girls and women or precocious sexual development in boys. **Warthin's t.,** adenolymphoma. **Wilms' t.,** a rapidly developing malignant mixed tumor of the kidneys, made up of embryonal elements, usually affecting children before the fifth year. **yolk sac t.,** a germ cell tumor that represents a proliferation of both yolk sac endoderm and extraembryonic mesenchyme; it produces α-fetoprotein and is usually in the testes.

tu·mor·i·ci·dal (too″mer-ĭ-si′dal) oncolytic.

tu·mor·i·gen·e·sis (-jen′ĕ-sis) oncogenesis.

tu·mor·let (too′mer-let) a type of tiny, often microscopic, benign neoplasm occurring singly or multiply in bronchial and bronchiolar mucosa of middle-aged to elderly people, often in areas of scarring.

Tun·ga (tun′gah) a genus of fleas, including *T. pe′netrans,* the chigoe (q.v.).

tung·sten (tung′sten) chemical element (see *Table of Elements*), at. no. 74, symbol W.

tu·ni·ca (too′nĭ-kah) pl. *tu′nicae.* [L.] a tunic; in anatomy, a general term for a membrane or other structure covering or lining a body part or organ. **t. adven′tia,** the outer coat of various tubular structures, made up of connective tissue and elastic fibers. **t. adventi′tia vaso′rum,** t. externa vasorum. **t. albugi′nea,** a dense, white, fibrous sheath enclosing a part or organ. **t. conjuncti′va,** the conjunctiva. **t. dar′tos,** the thin layer of subcutaneous tissue underlying the skin of the scrotum, consisting mainly of the dartos muscle. **t. exter′na,** an outer coat or layer. **t. exter′na vaso′rum,** the outer, fibroelastic coat of the blood vessels. **t. fibro′sa,** fibrous coat; an enveloping fibrous membrane. **t. inter′na,** an inner coat or layer. **t. in′tima vaso′rum,** the innermost coat of blood vessels. **t. me′dia vaso′rum,** the middle coat of blood vessels. **t. muco′sa,** the mucous membrane lining of various tubular structures. **t. muscula′ris,** the muscular coat or layer surrounding the tela submucosa in most portions of the digestive, respiratory, urinary, and genital tracts. **t. pro′pria,** a proper coat or layer of a part, as distinguished from an investing membrane. **t. sero′sa,** the membrane lining the external walls of the body cavities and reflected over the surfaces of protruding organs; it secretes a watery exudate. **t. vagina′lis tes′tis,** the serous membrane covering the front and sides of the testis and epididymis. **t. vasculo′sa,** a vascular coat, or a layer well supplied with blood vessels.

tun·nel (tun′el) a passageway of varying length through a solid body, completely enclosed except for the open ends, permitting entrance and exit. **carpal t.,** the osseofibrous passage for the median nerve and the flexor tendons, formed by the flexor retinaculum and the carpal bones. **Corti's t., inner t. flexor t.,** carpal t. **inner t.,** a canal extending the length of the cochlea, formed by the pillar cells of the organ of Corti. **tarsal t.,** the osseofibrous passage for the posterior tibial vessels, tibial nerve, and flexor tendons, formed by the flexor retinaculum and the tarsal bones.

tur·bi·dim·e·ter (ter″bĭ-dim′ĕ-ter) an apparatus for measuring turbidity of a solution.

tur·bid·i·ty (ter-bid′ĭ-te) cloudiness; disturbance of solids (sediment) in a solution, so that it is not clear. **tur′bid,** adj.

tur·bi·nal (ter′bĭ-n′l) turbinate.

tur·bi·nate (-nāt) 1. shaped like a top. 2. any of the nasal conchae.

tur·bi·nec·to·my (-nek′tah-me) excision of a turbinate bone (nasal concha).

tur·bi·not·o·my (-not′ah-me) incision of a turbinate bone.

tur·ges·cence (ter-jes′ens) swelling.

tur·gid (ter′jid) swollen and congested.

tur·gor (-ger) condition of being turgid; normal, or other fullness.

tu·ris·ta (too-rēs′tah) Mexican name for *traveler's diarrhea.*

tur·mer·ic (tur′mer-ik) *Curcuma longa* or its rhizome, which is used to treat dyspepsia and anorexia, and has a wide variety of uses in traditional Chinese medicine, ayurveda, and folk medicine.

turm·schä·del (toorm′sha-del) [Ger.] a developmental anomaly in which the head is high and rounded, due to early synostosis of the three major sutures of the skull.

turn·over (tern′o-ver) the movement of something into, through, and out of a place; the rate at which a thing is depleted and replaced. **erythrocyte iron t. (EIT),** the rate at which iron moves from the bone marrow into circulating red cells. **plasma iron t. (PIT),** the rate at which iron moves from the blood plasma to the bone marrow or other tissues.

TURP transurethral resection of the prostate.

tur·ri·ceph·a·ly (tur″ĭ-sef′ah-le) oxycephaly.

tus·si·gen·ic (tus″ĭ-jen′ik) causing cough.

tus·sis (tus′is) [L.] cough. **tus′sal, tus′sive,** adj.

tu·ta·men (too-ta′men) pl. *tu′tamina.* [L.] a protective covering or structure. **tuta′mina o′culi,** the protecting appendages of the eye, as the lids, lashes, etc.

twig (twig) a final ramification, as of branches of a nerve or blood vessel.

twin (twin) one of two offspring produced in the same pregnancy and developed from one oocyte (monozygotic) or from two oocytes (dizygotic) fertilized at the same time. **allantoidoangiopagous t's,** twins united by the umbilical vessels only. **conjoined t's,** monozygotic twins whose bodies are joined to a varying extent. **diamniotic t's,** twins developing within separate amniotic cavities; they may be monochorionic or dichorionic. **dichorionic t's,** twins having distinct chorions, including monozygotic twins separated within 72 hours of fertilization and all dizygotic twins. **dizygotic t's, fraternal t's, heterologous t's,** twins developed from two separate oocytes fertilized at the same time. **identical t's,** monozygotic t's. **impacted t's,** twins so situated during delivery that the pressure of one against the other prevents simultaneous engagement of both. **mono-amniotic t's,** twins developing within a single amniotic cavity; they are always monozygotic and monochorionic. **monochorionic t's,** twins developing with a single chorion; they are always monozygotic and may be monoamniotic or diamniotic. **monozygotic t's,** two individuals developed from one fertilized oocyte; they have identical genomes. **omphaloangiopagous t's,** allantoidoangiopagous t's. **Siamese t's,** conjoined t's. **similar t's,** monozygotic t's.

twin·ning (twin′ing) 1. the production of symmetrical structures or parts by division. 2. the simultaneous intrauterine production of two or more embryos.

twitch (twich) a brief, contractile response of a skeletal muscle elicited by a single maximal volley of impulses in the neurons supplying it.

ty·lec·to·my (ti-lek′tah-me) lumpectomy.

tyl·i·on (til′e-on) a point on anterior edge of the optic groove in the median line.

ty·lo·ma (ti-lo′ma) a callus or callosity.

ty·lo·sis (-sis) formation of callosities. **tylot′ic**, adj.

ty·lox·a·pol (ti-loks′ah-pol) a nonionic liquid polymer used as a surfactant to aid liquefaction and removal of mucopurulent bronchopulmonary secretions, administered by inhalation.

tym·pa·nal (tim′pah-n′l) tympanic.

tym·pa·nec·to·my (tim″pah-nek′tah-me) myringectomy; excision of the tympanic membrane.

tym·pan·ic (tim-pan′ik) 1. tympanal; of or pertaining to the tympanum. 2. bell-like; resonant.

tym·pa·nism (tim′pah-nizm) tympanites.

tym·pa·ni·tes (tim″pah-ni′tēz) abnormal distention due to the presence of gas or air in the intestine or the peritoneal cavity.

tym·pa·nit·ic (-nit′ik) 1. pertaining to or affected with tympanites. 2. bell-like; tympanic.

tympan(o)- word element [Gr.], *tympanic cavity; tympanic membrane.*

tym·pa·no·cen·te·sis (tim″pah-no-sen-te′sis) surgical puncture of the tympanic membrane or tympanum.

tym·pa·no·gen·ic (-jen′ik) arising from the tympanum or middle ear.

tym·pa·no·gram (tim′pah-no-gram″) a graphic representation of the relative compliance and impedance of the tympanic membrane and ossicles of the middle ear obtained by tympanometry.

tym·pa·no·mas·toid·itis (tim″pah-no-mas″toi-di′tis) inflammation of the middle ear and the mastoid air cells.

tym·pa·nom·e·try (tim″pah-nom′ĕ-tre) indirect measurement of the compliance (mobility) and impedance of the tympanic membrane and ossicles of the middle ear.

tym·pa·no·plas·ty (tim″pah-no-plas″te) surgical reconstruction of the tympanic membrane and establishment of ossicular continuity from the tympanic membrane to the oval window. **tympanoplas′tic**, adj.

tym·pa·no·scle·ro·sis (tim″pah-no-sklĕ-ro′sis) a condition characterized by the presence of masses of hard, dense connective tissue around the auditory ossicles in the tympanic cavity. **tympanosclerot′ic**, adj.

tym·pa·not·o·my (tim″pah-not′ah-me) myringotomy.

tym·pa·nous (tim′pah-nus) distended with gas.

tym·pa·num (-num) 1. tympanic membrane. 2. tympanic cavity.

tym·pa·ny (-ne) 1. tympanites. 2. a tympanic, or bell-like, percussion note.

type (tīp) the general or prevailing character of any particular case of disease, person, substance, etc. **blood t.**, see *blood group.* **constitutional t.**, a constellation of traits related to body build. **mating t.**, in ciliate protozoa, certain bacteria, and certain fungi, the equivalent of a sex. **phage t.**, an intraspecies type of bacterium demonstrated by phage typing. **wild t.**, in genetics, the standard phenotype for any experimental organism; also a gene that determines a standard phenotypic trait.

typh·lec·ta·sis (tif-lek′tah-sis) distention of the cecum.

typhl(o)- word element [Gr.], *cecum; blindness.*

typh·lo·dic·li·di·tis (tif″lo-dik″li-di′tis) inflammation of the ileocecal valve.

typh·lot·o·my (tif-lot′ah-me) cecotomy.

ty·phoid (ti′foid) 1. resembling typhus. 2. typhoid fever. 3. typhoidal.

ty·phoid·al (ti-foi′dal) resembling typhoid fever.

ty·phus (ti′fus) a group of closely related, acute, arthropod-borne rickettsial diseases that differ in the intensity of certain signs and symptoms, severity, and fatality rate; all are characterized by headache, chills, fever, stupor, and a macular, maculopapular, petechial, or papulovesicular eruption. Often used alone in English-speaking countries to refer to epidemic typhus, and in several European languages to refer to typhoid fever. **ty′phous**, adj. **endemic t.**, murine t. **epidemic t.**, the classic form, due to *Rickettsia prowazekii* and transmitted between humans by body lice. **flying squirrel t.**, an acute infectious disease similar to epidemic typhus, occurring in the southeastern United States; it is caused by *Rickettsia prowazekii* and is transmitted by the fleas and lice of the flying squirrel. **Kenya tick t.**, boutonneuse fever. **murine t.**, an infectious disease, clinically similar to epidemic typhus but milder, due to *Rickettsia typhi*, transmitted from rat to human by the rat flea and rat louse. **recrudescent t.**, Brill's disease. **scrub t.**, an acute, typhus-like infectious disease caused by *Rickettsia tsutsugamushi* and transmitted by chiggers, characterized by a primary skin lesion at the site of inoculation and development of a rash, regional lymphadenopathy, and fever. **tropical t.**, scrub t.

ty·pol·o·gy (ti-pol′ah-je) the study of types; the science of classifying, as bacteria according to type.

Tyr tyrosine.

ty·ro·ma·to·sis (ti″ro-mah-to′sis) a condition characterized by caseous degeneration.

ty·ro·pa·no·ate (-pah-no'āt) a radiopaque medium used as the sodium salt in oral cholecystography.

ty·ro·sine (Tyr, Y) (ti'ro-sēn) a naturally occurring, nonessential amino acid present in most proteins; it is a product of phenyl-alanine metabolism and a precursor of thyroid hormones, catecholamines, and melanin.

ty·ro·sin·e·mia (ti″ro-sĭ-ne′me-ah) an aminoacidopathy of tyrosine metabolism with elevated blood levels of tyrosine and urinary excretion of tyrosine and related metabolites. *Type I* shows inhibition of some liver enzymes and renal tubular function. *Type II* is marked by crystallization of the accumulated tyrosine in the epidermis and cornea and is frequently accompanied by mental retardation. *Neonatal t.* is asymptomatic, transitory, and may result in mild mental retardation. The fourth type is *hawkinsinuria.*

ty·ro·sin·uria (-nu're-ah) excessive tyrosine in the urine.

ty·ro·syl·uria (ti″ro-sil-u′re-ah) increased urinary secretion of para-hydroxyphenyl compounds derived from tyrosine, as in tyrosinemia.

ty·vel·ose (ti'vel-ōs) an unusual sugar that is a polysaccharide somatic antigen of certain *Salmonella* serotypes.

tzet·ze (tset'se) tsetse.

U uranium; uracil or uridine; international unit of enzyme activity; unit.

u atomic mass unit.

ubi·qui·nol (u″bĭ-kwĭ-nol′) the reduced form of ubiquinone.

ubi·qui·none (Q, Q₁₀) (u″bĭ-kwĭ-nōn′) a quinone derivative with an unsaturated branched hydrocarbon side chain occurring in the lipid core of inner mitochondrial membranes and functioning in the electron transport chain. In naturopathic practice it is used for a wide variety of indications; also used as a dietary supplement for its anti-oxidant properties.

UDP uridine diphosphate.

UK urokinase.

ul·cer (ul'ser) a local defect, or excavation of the surface, of an organ or tissue, produced by sloughing of necrotic inflammatory tissue. **corneal u.**, ulcerative keratitis. **decubital u., decubitus u.**, bedsore; an ulceration due to an arterial occlusion or prolonged pressure, as when a patient is confined to a bed or a wheelchair. **duodenal u.**, a peptic ulcer situated in the duodenum. **gastric u.**, an ulcer of the gastric mucosa. **Hunner's u.**, one involving all layers of the bladder wall, occurring in chronic interstitial cystitis. **jejunal u.**, an ulcer of the jejunum; such an ulcer following surgery is called a *secondary jejunal u.* **marginal u.**, a gastric ulcer in the jejunal mucosa near the site of a gastrojejunostomy. **peptic u.**, an ulceration of the mucous membrane of the esophagus, stomach, or duodenum, due to action of the acid gastric juice. **perforating u.**, one involving the entire thickness of an organ or of the wall of an organ creating an opening on both surfaces. **phagedenic u.**, 1. a necrotic lesion associated with prominent tissue destruction, due to secondary bacterial invasion of an existing cutaneous lesion or of intact skin in a person with impaired resistance as the result of systemic disease. 2. tropical phagedenic u. **plantar u.**, a deep neurotrophic ulcer of the sole of the foot, resulting from repeated injury because of lack of sensation in the part; seen with diseases such as diabetes mellitus and leprosy. **rodent u.**, ulcerating basal cell carcinoma of the skin. **stercoraceous u., stercoral u.**, one caused by pressure of impacted feces; also, a fistulous ulcer through which fecal matter escapes. **stress u.**, peptic ulcer, usually gastric, resulting from stress. **trophic u.**, one due to imperfect nutrition of the part. **tropical u.**, 1. a lesion of cutaneous leishmaniasis. 2. tropical phagedenic u. **tropical phagedenic u.**, a chronic, painful, phagedenic ulcer of unknown cause, usually on the lower limbs of malnourished children in the tropics. **varicose u.**, an ulcer due to varicose veins. **venereal u.**, a nonspecific term referring to the formation of ulcers resembling chancre or chancroid about the external genitalia.

ul·cer·ate (ul'ser-āt) to undergo ulceration.

ul·cer·a·tion (ul″ser-a′shun) 1. the formation or development of an ulcer. 2. an ulcer.

ul·cer·a·tive (ul'sĕ-ra″tiv, ul'ser-ah-tiv) pertaining to or characterized by ulceration.

ul·cer·o·gen·ic (ul″ser-o-jen′ik) causing ulceration; leading to the production of ulcers.

ul·cero·mem·bra·nous (-mem′brah-nus) characterized by ulceration and a membranous exudation.

ul·cer·ous (ul′ser-us) 1. of the nature of an ulcer. 2. affected with ulceration.

ul·cus (ul′kus) pl. *ul′cera.* [L.] ulcer.

ulec·to·my (u-lek′tah-me) 1. excision of scar tissue. 2. gingivectomy.

uler·y·the·ma (u″ler-ĭ-the′mah) an erythematous skin disease with formation of cicatrices and atrophy. **u. ophryo′genes,** a hereditary form in which keratosis pilaris involves the hair follicles of the eyebrows.

ul·na (ul′nah) pl. *ul′nae.* [L.] the inner and larger bone of the forearm; see *Table of Bones.*

ul·nad (ul′nad) toward the ulna.

ul·nar (ul′ner) pertaining to the ulna or to the ulnar (medial) aspect of the arm as compared to the radial (lateral) aspect.

ul·na·ris (ul-na′ris) [L.] ulnar.

ul·no·car·pal (ul″no-kahr′p′l) pertaining to the ulna and carpus.

ul·no·ra·di·al (-ra′de-al) pertaining to the ulna and radius.

ul(o)- word element [Gr.], (1) *scar;* (2) *gingiva.*

ulor·rha·gia (u″lo-ra′jah) a sudden or free discharge of blood from the gums.

-ulose a suffix denoting a ketose.

ulot·o·my (u-lot′ah-me) 1. incision of scar tissue. 2. incision of the gums.

ultra- word element [L.], *beyond; excess.*

ul·tra·cen·trif·u·ga·tion (ul″trah-sen-trif″u-ga′shun) subjection of material to an exceedingly high centrifugal force, which will separate and sediment the molecules of a substance.

ul·tra·di·an (ul-trah′de-an) pertaining to a period of less than 24 hours; applied to the rhythmic repetition of certain phenomena in living organisms occurring in cycles of less than a day *(ultradian rhythm).*

ul·tra·fil·tra·tion (ul″trah-fil-tra′shun) filtration through a filter capable of removing very minute (ultramicroscopic) particles.

ul·tra·mi·cro·scope (-mi′kro-skōp″) a special darkfield microscope for the examination of particles of colloidal size. **ultramicroscop′ic,** adj.

ul·tra·son·ic (-son′ik) beyond the upper limit of perception by the human ear; relating to sound waves having a frequency of more than 20,000 Hz.

ul·tra·son·ics (-son′iks) the science dealing with ultrasonic sound waves.

ul·tra·so·nog·ra·phy (ul″trah-sŏ-nog′rah-fe) the imaging of deep structures of the body by recording the echoes of pulses of ultrasonic waves directed into the tissues and reflected by tissue planes where there is a change in density. Diagnostic ultrasonography uses 1–10 megahertz waves. **ultrasonograph′ic,** adj. **Doppler u.,** that in which the shifts in frequency between emitted ultrasonic waves and their echoes are used to measure the velocities of moving objects, based on the principle of the Doppler effect. The waves may be continuous or pulsed; the technique is frequently used to examine cardiovascular blood flow (Doppler echocardiography). **gray-scale u.,** a B-scan technique in which the strength of echoes is indicated by a proportional brightness of the displayed dots.

ul·tra·sound (ul′trah-sound) 1. sound waves of a frequency greater than 20,000 Hz. 2. ultrasonography.

ul·tra·struc·ture (-struk″chur) the structure beyond the resolution power of the light microscope, i.e., visible only under the ultramicroscope and electron microscope.

ul·tra·vi·o·let (UV) (ul″trah-vi′o-let) denoting electromagnetic radiation between violet light and x-rays, having wavelengths of 200 to 400 nanometers. UVA is that from 320 to 400 nm, UVB is that from 290 to 320 nm, and UVC is that from 200 to 290 nm. **u. A (UVA),** ultraviolet radiation with wavelengths between 320 and 400 nm, comprising over 99 per cent of that reaching the surface of the earth. It enhances the harmful effects of UVB, is responsible for some photosensitivity reactions, and is used therapeutically in the treatment of various skin disorders. **u. B (UVB),** ultraviolet radiation with wavelengths between 290 and 320 nm, comprising 1 per cent of that reaching the surface of the earth. It causes sunburn and a number of damaging photochemical changes within cells, including damage to DNA leading to premature aging of the skin, premalignant and malignant changes, and various photosensitivity reactions; it is also used therapeutically in the treatment of skin disorders. **u. C (UVC),** ultraviolet radiation with wavelengths between 200 and 290 nm, all of which is filtered out by the ozone layer and does not reach the surface of the earth; it is germicidal and is also used in ultraviolet phototherapy.

um·bil·i·cal (um-bil′ĭ-k′l) pertaining to the umbilicus.

um·bil·i·ca·tion (um-bil″ĭ-ka′shun) a depression resembling the umbilicus.

um·bil·i·cus (um-bil′ĭ-kus) [L.] the navel; the scar marking the site of attachment of the umbilical cord in the fetus.

um·bo (um′bo) pl. *umbo′nes*. [L.] 1. a rounded elevation. 2. the slight projection at the center of the outer surface of the tympanic membrane.

UMP uridine monophosphate.

uña de ga·to (oo′nyah da gah′to) [Sp.] cat's claw.

un·cal (un′kal) of or pertaining to the uncus.

un·ci·form (un′sĭ-form) uncinate (1).

un·ci·na·ri·al (un″sĭ-nar′e-al) of, pertaining to, or caused by a hookworm.

un·ci·nate (un′sĭ-nāt) 1. shaped like a hook. 2. relating to or affecting the uncinate gyrus.

un·ci·pres·sure (-presh″ur) pressure with a hook to stop hemorrhage.

un·con·di·tion·ed (un″kon-dish′und) not a result of conditioning; unlearned; occurring naturally or spontaneously.

un·con·scious (un-kon′shus) 1. insensible; incapable of responding to sensory stimuli and of having subjective experiences. 2. the part of the mind not readily accessible to conscious awareness but whose existence may be manifested in symptom formation, in dreams, or under the influence of drugs. **collective u.,** the elements of the unconscious that are theoretically common to mankind.

un·co·ver·te·bral (ung″ko-ver′tah-bral) pertaining to the uncinate processes of a vertebra.

un·cus (ung′kus) 1. hook. 2. the medially curved anterior end of the parahippocampal gyrus. **un′cal,** adj.

un·dec·yl·en·ic ac·id (un-des″ĭ-len′ik) an unsaturated fatty acid used as a topical antifungal agent.

un·der·bite (un′der-bīt) retrognathism.

un·der·drive (-drīv″) pertaining to a rate less than normal; see under *pacing.*

un·der·sens·ing (-sens″ing) missed sensing of cardiac electrical signals by an artificial pacemaker, resulting in too frequent or irregular delivery of stimuli.

un·dif·fer·en·ti·at·ed (un-dif″er-en′she-āt-ed) anaplastic.

un·dine (un′dēn) a small glass flask for irrigating the eye; a vibration.

un·du·lant (un′jŭ-, un′dyŭ-lant) characterized by wavelike fluctuations.

un·du·late (-lāt) 1. to move in waves or in a wavelike motion. 2. to have a wavelike appearance, outline, or form. **un′dulatory,** adj.

un·du·la·tion (un″jŭ-, un″dyŭ-la′shun) 1. a wavelike motion; see also *pulsation.* 2. a wavelike appearance, outline, or form.

ung. [L.] unguen′tum (ointment).

un·gual (ung′gwal) pertaining to the nails.

un·guent (ung′gwent) ointment.

un·guic·u·late (ung-gwik′u-lāt) having claws or nails; clawlike.

un·guis (ung′gwis) pl. *un′gues*. [L.] nail (1).

uni- word element [L.], *one.*

uni·ax·i·al (u″ne-ak′se-al) 1. having only one axis. 2. developing in an axial direction only.

uni·cam·er·al (u″nĭ-kam′er-al) having only one cavity or compartment.

uni·cel·lu·lar (-sel′u-ler) made up of a single cell, as the bacteria.

uni·cor·nu·ate (-kor′nu-āt) having only one horn or cornu.

uni·fas·cic·u·lar (-fah-sik′u-lar) pertaining to a single bundle, or fasciculus.

uni·glan·du·lar (-glan′du-ler) affecting only one gland.

uni·lat·er·al (-lat′er-al) affecting only one side.

uni·loc·u·lar (-lok′u-ler) having but one cavity or compartment.

un·in·hib·it·ed (un″in-hib′ĭ-ted) free from usual constraints; not subject to normal inhibitory mechanisms.

uni·nu·cle·at·ed (u″nĭ-noo′kle-āt″ed) mononuclear (1).

uni·oc·u·lar (u″ne-ok′u-ler) monocular.

un·ion (ūn′yun) the renewal of continuity in a broken bone or between the edges of a wound.

uni·ov·u·lar (u″ne-ov′u-lar) 1. monozygotic. 2. monovular.

uni·p·a·rous (u-nip′ah-rus) 1. producing only one offspring or egg at one time. 2. primiparous; see *primipara.*

uni·po·lar (u″nĭ-po′ler) 1. having a single pole or process, as a nerve cell. 2. pertaining to mood disorders in which only depressive episodes occur.

uni·po·ten·cy (-po′ten-se) the ability of a part to develop in one manner only, or of a cell to develop into only one type of cell. **unip′otent, unipoten′tial,** adj.

unit (u′nit) 1. a single thing. 2. a quantity assumed as a standard of measurement. Symbol U. **Angström u.,** angstrom. **atomic mass u. (u, amu),** the unit mass equal to $\frac{1}{12}$ the mass of the nuclide of carbon-12. Called also *dalton.* **Bethesda u.,** a measure of the level of inhibitor to coagulation factor VIII; equal to the amount of inhibitor in patient plasma that will inactivate 50 per cent of factor VIII in an equal volume of normal plasma following a 2-hour incubation period. **Bodansky u.,** the quantity of alkaline phosphatase that liberates 1 mg of phosphate ion from glycerol 2-phosphate in 1 hour under standard conditions. **British thermal u. (BTU),** the amount of heat necessary to raise the temperature of one pound of water

SI UNITS

Quantity	Unit	Symbol	Pronunciation	Derivation
Base Units				
length	meter	m	me′ter	
mass	kilogram	kg	kil′o-gram	
time	second	s	sek′und	
electric current	ampere	A	am′pēr	
temperature	kelvin	K	kel′vin	
luminous intensity	candela	cd	kan-del′ah	
amount of substance	mole	mol	mōl	
Supplementary Units				
plane angle	radian	rad	ra′de-an	
solid angle	steradian	sr	stĕ-ra′de-an	
Derived Units				
force	newton	N	noo′ton	$kg \cdot m/s^2$
pressure	pascal	Pa	pas′kal	N/m^2
energy, work	joule	J	jōōl	$N \cdot m$
power	watt	W	waht	J/s
electric charge	coulomb	C	koo′lom	$A \cdot s$
electric potential	volt	V	volt	J/C
electric capacitance	farad	F	far′ad	C/V
electric resistance	ohm	Ω	ōm	V/A
electric conductance	siemens	S	se′menz	$Ω^{-1}$
magnetic flux	weber	Wb	web′er	$V \cdot s$
magnetic flux density	tesla	T	tes′la	Wb/m^2
inductance	henry	H	hen′re	Wb/A
frequency	hertz	Hz	hertz	s^{-1}
luminous flux	lumen	lm	loo′men	$cd \cdot sr$
illumination	lux	lx	luks	lm/m^2
temperature	degree celsius	°C	sel′se-us	$K - 273.15$
radioactivity	becquerel	Bq	bek-rel′	s^{-1}
absorbed dose	gray	Gy	gra	J/kg
absorbed dose equivalent	sievert	Sv	se′vert	J/kg

MULTIPLES AND SUBMULTIPLES OF THE METRIC SYSTEM

Multiples and Submultiples		Prefix	Symbol
1,000,000,000,000	(10^{12})	tera-	T
1,000,000,000	(10^{9})	giga-	G
1,000,000	(10^{6})	mega-	M
1,000	(10^{3})	kilo-	k
100	(10^{2})	hecto-	h
10	(10)	deka-	da
0.1	(10^{-1})	deci-	d
0.01	(10^{-2})	centi-	c
0.001	(10^{-3})	milli-	m
0.000 001	(10^{-6})	micro-	μ
0.000 000 001	(10^{-9})	nano-	n
0.000 000 000 001	(10^{-12})	pico-	p
0.000 000 000 000 001	(10^{-15})	femto-	f
0.000 000 000 000 000 001	(10^{-18})	atto-	a

one degree Fahrenheit, usually from 39°F to 40°F. **CGS u.,** any unit in the centimeter-gram-second system. **CH50 u.,** the amount of complement that will lyse 50 per cent of a standard preparation of sheep red blood cells coated with antisheep erythrocyte antibody. **coronary care u.,** a specially designed and equipped hospital area containing a small number of private rooms, with all facilities necessary for constant observation and possible emergency treatment of patients with severe heart disease. **intensive care u.,** a hospital unit in which are concentrated special equipment and skilled personnel for the care of seriously ill patients requiring immediate and continuous attention; abbreviated ICU. **International u. (IU),** a unit of biological material, as of enzymes, hormones, vitamins, etc., established by the International Conference for the Unification of Formulas. **motor u.,** the unit of motor activity formed by a motor nerve cell and its many innervated muscle fibers. **SI u.,** any of the units of the Système International d'Unités (International System of Units) adopted in 1960 at the Eleventh General Conference of Weights and Measures. See accompanying tables. **Somogyi u.,** that amount of amylase which will liberate reducing equivalents equal to 1 mg of glucose per 30 minutes under defined conditions. **Svedberg u. (S),** a unit equal to 10^{-13} second used for expressing sedimentation coefficients of macromolecules. **terminal respiratory u.,** the anatomical and functional unit of the lung, including a respiratory bronchiole, alveolar ducts and sacs, and alveoli. See Plate 25. **toxic u., toxin u.,** the smallest dose of a toxin which will kill a guinea pig weighing about 250 gm in three to four days. **USP u.,** one used in the United States Pharmacopeia in expressing potency of drugs and other preparations.

Unit·ed States Phar·ma·co·peia (USP) a legally recognized compendium of standards for drugs, published by The United States Pharmacopeial Convention, Inc., and revised periodically. It includes also assays and tests for the determination of strength, quality, and purity.

uni·va·lent (u″nĭ-va′lent) having a valence of one.

un·my·eli·nat·ed (un-mi′ĕ-lĭ-nāt″ed) not having a myelin sheath; said of a nerve fiber.

uno·pros·tone (u″no-pros′tōn) an antiglaucoma agent that decreases elevated intraocular pressure; used as *u. isopropyl* in the treatment of open-angle glaucoma and ocular hypertension.

un·phys·i·o·log·ic (un″fiz-e-o-loj′ik) not physiologic in character.

un·sat·u·rat·ed (un-sach′ur-āt″ed) 1. not holding all of a solute which can be held in solution by the solvent. 2. denoting compounds in which two or more atoms are united by double or triple bonds.

un·stri·at·ed (-stri′āt-ed) having no striations, as smooth muscle.

upa·dha·tu (oo″pah-thŭ′too) according to ayurveda, secondary, temporary tissue that arises from the metabolism and waste of primary tissues (dhatus).

u·plas·min·o·gen ac·ti·va·tor (plaz-min′o-jen ak′tĭ-va-ter) formal name for *urokinase.*

UPPP uvulopalatopharyngoplasty.

up·reg·u·la·tion (up reg-u-la′shun) increase in expression of a gene; most narrowly, that due to increased transcription of a specific mRNA, but also used more broadly for increase in mRNA levels for the gene by any means.

up·take (up′tāk) absorption and incorporation of a substance by living tissue.

ura·chus (u′rah-kus) a fetal canal connecting the bladder with the allantois, persisting throughout life as a cord (median umbilical ligament). **u′rachal,** adj.

ura·cil (ūr′ah-sil) a pyrimidine base, in animal cells usually occurring condensed with ribose to form the ribonucleoside uridine; the corresponding deoxyribonucleoside is deoxyuridine. Symbol U.

ura·ni·um (u-ra′ne-um) chemical element (see *Table of Elements*), at. no. 92, symbol U.

uran(o)- word element [Gr.], *palate.*

ura·nor·rha·phy (u″rah-nor′ah-fe) palatorrhaphy.

ura·no·staph·y·los·chi·sis (u″rah-no-staf″ĭ-los′kĭ-sis) cleft of both soft and hard palates.

urar·thri·tis (u″rahr-thri′tis) gouty arthritis.

urate (ūr′āt) any salt or anion of uric acid (q.v.).

ura·to·ma (u″rah-to′mah) a concretion made up of urates; tophus.

ura·tu·ria (u″rah-tu′re-ah) hyperuricosuria.

ur·ce·i·form (er-se′ĭ-form) pitcher-shaped.

urea (u-re′ah) 1. the chief nitrogenous end-product of protein metabolism, formed in the liver from amino acids and from ammonia compounds; found in urine, blood, and lymph. 2. a pharmaceutical preparation of urea used to lower intracranial or intraocular pressure, to induce abortion, and as a topical skin moisturizer. **ure′al,** adj. **u. nitrogen,** the urea concentration of serum or plasma, conventionally specified in terms of nitrogen content and called *blood urea nitrogen (BUN)*; an important indicator of renal function.

urea·gen·e·sis formation of urea. **ureagen·et′ic,** adj.

Urea·plas·ma (-plaz′mah) a genus of nonmotile pleomorphic, gram-negative bacteria (family Mycoplasmataceae) lacking a cell wall and hydrolyzing urea; *U. urealyt′icum* is associated with nonspecific urethritis in males and genital tract infections in females.

urea·poi·e·sis (u-re″ah-poi-e′sis) ureagenesis. **ureapoiet′ic,** adj.

ure·ase (u′re-ās) an enzyme that catalyzes the hydrolysis of urea to ammonia and carbon dioxide; it is a nickel protein of microorganisms and plants that is used in clinical assays of plasma urea concentrations.

ure·de·ma (u-rĕ-de′mah) swelling from extravasated urine.

ure·mia (u-re′me-ah) 1. azotemia; an excess of the nitrogenous end products of protein and amino acid metabolism in the blood. 2. the entire constellation of signs and symptoms of chronic renal failure. **ure′mic,** adj.

ure·mi·gen·ic (u-re″mĭ-jen′ik) 1. caused by uremia. 2. causing uremia.

ureo·tel·ic (u″re-o-tel′ik) having urea as the chief excretory product of nitrogen metabolism.

-uresis word element [Gr.], *urinary excretion of.* **-uret′ic,** adj.

ure·ter (u-re′ter) the fibromuscular tube through which urine passes from kidney to bladder. **ure′teral, ureter′ic,** adj.

ure·ter·al·gia (u-re″ter-al′jah) pain in the ureter.

ure·ter·ec·ta·sis (-ek′tah-sis) distention of the ureter.

ure·ter·ec·to·my (-ek′tah-me) excision of a ureter.

ure·ter·itis (-i′tis) inflammation of a ureter.

ureter(o)- word element [Gr.], *ureter.*

ure·tero·cele (u-re′ter-o-sēl″) sacculation of the terminal portion of the ureter into the bladder, as a result of stenosis of the ureteral meatus.

ure·tero·ce·lec·to·my (u-re″ter-o-se-lek′tah-me) excision of a ureterocele.

ure·tero·co·los·to·my (-kah-los′tah-me) anastomosis of a ureter to the colon.

ure·tero·cys·tos·to·my (-sis-tos′tah-me) ureteroneocystostomy.

ure·tero·en·ter·os·to·my (-en″ter-os′tah-me) anastomosis of one or both ureters to the wall of the intestine.

ure·ter·og·ra·phy (u-re″ter-og′rah-fe) radiography of the ureter after injection of a contrast medium.

ure·tero·il·e·os·to·my (u-re″ter-o-il″e-os′tah-me) anastomosis of the ureters to an isolated loop of the ileum drained through a stoma on the abdominal wall.

ure·tero·lith (u-re′ter-o-lith″) a calculus in the ureter.

ure·tero·li·thi·a·sis (u-re″ter-o-lĭ-thi′ah-sis) formation or presence of calculi in the ureter.

ure·tero·li·thot·o·my (-lĭ-thot′ah-me) incision of a ureter for removal of calculus.

ure·ter·ol·y·sis (u-re″ter-ol′ĭ-sis) 1. the operation of freeing the ureter from adhesions. 2. rupture of the ureter.

ure·tero·neo·cys·tos·to·my (u-re″ter-o-ne″o-sis-tos′tah-me) surgical transplantation of a ureter to a different site in the bladder.

ure·ter·o·ne·phrec·to·my (-nĕ-frek′tah-me) nephroureterectomy.

ure·ter·op·a·thy (u-re″ter-op′ah-the) any disease of the ureter.

ure·tero·pel·vic (-pel′vik) pertaining to or affecting the ureter and the renal pelvis.

ure·tero·pel·vio·plas·ty (u-re″ter-o-pel′ve-o-plas″-te) ureteropyelostomy.

ure·tero·plas·ty (u-re′ter-o-plas″te) plastic surgery of a ureter.

ure·tero·py·elog·ra·phy (u-re″ter-o-pi-ĕ-log′rah-fe) radiography of the ureter and renal pelvis.

ure·tero·py·elo·plas·ty (-pi′ĕ-lo-plas″te) ureteropyelostomy.

ure·tero·py·elos·to·my (u-re″ter-o-pi″ĕ-los′tah-me) surgical creation of a new communication between a ureter and the renal pelvis.

ure·tero·py·o·sis (-pi-o′sis) pyoureter.

ure·tero·re·nos·co·py (-re-nos′kah-pe) visual inspection of the interior of the ureter and kidney by means of a fiberoptic endoscope (ureterorenoscope), as for biopsy or removal or crushing of stones.

ure·ter·or·rha·gia (-ra′jah) discharge of blood from a ureter.

ure·ter·or·rha·phy (u-re″ter-or′ah-fe) suture of a ureter.

ure·ter·os·copy (u-re″ter-os′kah-pe) examination of the ureter by means of a fiberoptic endoscope (ureteroscope).

ure·tero·sig·moi·dos·to·my (u-re″ter-o-sig″moid-os′tah-me) anastomosis of a ureter to the sigmoid colon.

ure·ter·os·to·my (u-re″ter-os′tah-me) creation of a new outlet for a ureter.

ure·ter·ot·o·my (u-re″ter-ot′ah-me) incision of a ureter.

ure·tero·ure·ter·os·to·my (u-re″ter-o-u-re″ter-os′tah-me) end-to-end anastomosis of the two portions of a transected ureter.

ure·tero·vag·i·nal (-vaj′ĭ-n'l) pertaining to or communicating with a ureter and the vagina.

ure·tero·ves·i·cal (-ves′ĭ-k'l) pertaining to a ureter and the bladder.

ure·thra (u-re′thrah) the membranous canal through which urine is discharged from the bladder to the exterior of the body. **ure′thral,** adj. **membranous u.,** a short portion of the urethra between the prostatic urethra and spongy urethra. **prostatic u.,** that part of the urethra passing through the prostate. **spongy u.,** the portion of the urethra within the corpus spongiosum penis.

ure·thral·gia (u″re-thral′jah) pain in the urethra.

ure·thra·tre·sia (u-re″thrah-tre′zhah) urethral atresia.

ure·threc·to·my (u″re-threk′tah-me) surgical removal of all or part of the urethra.

ure·thri·tis (u″re-thri′tis) inflammation of the urethra. **u. cys′tica,** urethritis with formation of multiple submucosal cysts. **nongonococcal u., nonspecific u.,** urethritis without evidence of gonococcal infection. **simple u.,** nongonococcal u.

urethr(o)- word element [Gr.], *urethra*.

ure·thro·bul·bar (u-re″thro-bul′ber) bulbourethral.

ure·thro·cele (u-re′thro-sēl) prolapse of the female urethra.

ure·thro·cys·ti·tis (u-re″thro-sis-ti′tis) inflammation of the urethra and bladder.

ure·thro·dyn·ia (-din′e-ah) urethralgia.

ure·throg·ra·phy (u″re-throg′rah-fe) radiography of the urethra.

ure·throm·e·try (u″re-throm′ĕ-tre) 1. determination of the resistance of various segments of the urethra to retrograde flow of fluid. 2. measurement of the urethra.

ure·thro·pe·nile (u-re″thro-pe′nīl) pertaining to the urethra and penis.

ure·thro·peri·ne·al (-per″ĭ-ne′al) pertaining to the urethra and perineum.

ure·thro·peri·neo·scro·tal (-per″ĭ-ne″o-skro′t'l) pertaining to the urethra, perineum, and scrotum.

ure·thro·pexy (-pek′se) bladder neck suspension.

ure·thro·plas·ty (u-re′thro-plas″te) plastic surgery of the urethra.

ure·thro·pros·tat·ic (u-re″thro-pros-tat′ik) pertaining to the urethra and prostate.

ure·thro·rec·tal (-rek′t'l) rectourethral.

ure·thror·rha·gia (-ra′jah) flow of blood from the urethra.

ure·thror·rha·phy (u″re-thror′ah-fe) suture of the urethra.

ure·thror·rhea (u-re″thro-re′ah) abnormal discharge from the urethra.

ure·thro·scope (u-re′thro-skōp) an endoscope for viewing the interior of the urethra.

ure·thro·scop·ic (u-re″thro-skop′ik) 1. pertaining to a urethroscope. 2. pertaining to urethroscopy.

ure·thros·co·py (u″re-thros′ko-pe) inspection of the interior of the urethra with a urethroscope.

ure·thro·stax·is (u-re″thro-stak′sis) oozing of blood from the urethra.

ure·thro·ste·no·sis (-stĕ-no′sis) stricture or stenosis of the urethra.

ure·thros·to·my (u″re-thros′tah-me) surgical formation of a permanent opening of the urethra at the perineal surface.

ure·thro·tome (u-re′thro-tōm) an instrument for cutting a urethral stricture.

ure·throt·o·my (u″re-throt′ah-me) incision of the urethra, either through the perineum (*external u.*) or from within (*internal u.*).

ure·thro·tri·go·ni·tis (u-re″thro-tri″go-ni′tis) inflammation of the urethra and trigone of the bladder.

ure·thro·vag·i·nal (-vaj′ĭ-n'l) pertaining to the urethra and vagina.

ure·thro·ves·i·cal (-ves′ĭ-k'l) vesicourethral.

ur·gen·cy (ur′jen-se) a sudden compelling need to do something. **bowel u.,** the sudden need to defecate. **urinary u.,** the sudden need to urinate.

ur·hid·ro·sis (ūr″hĭ-dro′sis) the presence in the sweat of urinous materials, chiefly uric acid and urea.

-uria word element [Gr.], *characteristic or constituent of the urine*. **-u′ric,** adj.

uric ac·id (u′rik) the water-insoluble end product of primate purine metabolism; deposition of it as crystals in the joints and kidneys causes gout.

uric·ac·i·de·mia (u″rik-as″ĭ-de′me-ah) hyperuricemia.

uric·ac·i·du·ria (-as″ĭ-du′re-ah) hyperuricosuria.

uri·ce·mia (u″rĭ-se′me-ah) hyperuricemia.

uri·com·e·ter (u″rĭ-kom′ĕ-ter) an instrument for measuring uric acid in urine.

uri·co·su·ria (u″rĭ-ko-su′re-ah) hyperuricosuria.

uri·co·su·ric (u″rĭ-ko-su′rik) 1. pertaining to, characterized by, or promoting uricosuria. 2. an agent that so acts.

uri·dine (ūr′ĭ-dēn) a pyrimidine nucleoside containing uracil and ribose; it is a component of nucleic acid and its nucleosides are involved in the biosynthesis of polysaccharides.

Symbol U. **u. diphosphate (UDP),** a pyrophosphate-containing nucleotide that serves as a carrier for hexoses, hexosamines, and hexuronic acids in the synthesis of glycogen, glycoproteins, and glycosaminoglycans. **u. monophosphate (UMP),** uridylic acid; a nucleotide, uridine 5′-phosphate. **u. triphosphate (UTP),** a nucleotide involved in RNA synthesis.

uri·dyl·ic ac·id (u″rĭ-dil′ik) phosphorylated uridine; uridine monophosphate unless otherwise specified.

uri·nal (u″rĭ-n′l) a receptacle for urine.

uri·nal·y·sis (u″rĭ-nal′ĭ-sis) analysis of the urine.

uri·nary (u′rĭ-nar″e) pertaining to, containing, or secreting urine.

uri·nate (u′rĭ-nāt) to discharge urine.

uri·na·tion (u″rĭ-na′shun) the discharge of urine.

urine (u′rin) the fluid excreted by the kidneys, stored in the bladder, and discharged through the urethra. **residual u.,** urine remaining in the bladder after urination.

uri·nif·er·ous (u″rĭ-nif′er-us) transporting or conveying urine.

urin(o)- word element [L.], *urine.*

uri·nog·e·nous (u″rĭ-noj′ĕ-nus) of urinary origin.

uri·no·ma (u″rĭ-no′mah) 1. a cyst containing urine. 2. a collection of urine surrounded by fibrous tissue, from leakage through a tear in the ureter, renal pelvis, or renal calix due to obstruction, or from trauma.

uri·nom·e·ter (u″rĭ-nom′ĕ-ter) an instrument for determining the specific gravity of urine.

uri·nom·e·try (u″rĭ-nom′ĕ-tre) determination of the specific gravity of urine.

ur(o)- word element [Gr.], *urine; urinary tract; urination.*

uro·bi·lin (u″ro-bi′lin) a brownish pigment formed by oxidation of urobilinogen, found in feces.

uro·bil·in·emia (-bil″ĭ-ne′me-ah) urobilin in the blood.

uro·bi·lino·gen (-bi-lin′o-jen) a colorless compound formed in the intestines by reduction of bilirubin.

uro·can·ic ac·id (-kan′ik) an intermediate metabolite of histamine, convertible normally to glutamic acid.

uro·cele (u′ro-sēl) distention of the scrotum with extravasated urine.

uro·che·zia (u″ro-ke′zhah) the discharge of urine in the feces.

uro·chrome (u′ro-krōm) the end product of hemoglobin breakdown, found in the urine and responsible for its yellow color.

uro·cys·ti·tis (u″ro-sis-ti′tis) cystitis.

uro·dy·nam·ics (-di-nam′iks) the dynamics of the propulsion and flow of urine in the urinary tract. **urodynam′ic,** adj.

uro·dyn·ia (-din′e-ah) pain accompanying urination.

uro·ede·ma (-ĕ-de′mah) edema due to infiltration of urine.

uro·flow·me·ter (-flo′me-ter) a device for the continuous recording of urine flow in milliliters per second.

uro·fol·li·tro·pin (-fol′ĭ-tro″pin) a preparation of gonadotropins from the urine of postmenopausal women, containing follicle-stimulating hormone and used in conjunction with human chorionic gonadotropin to induce ovulation.

uro·gas·trone (-gas′trōn) a urinary peptide derived from epidermal growth factor, with which it shares substantial homology and similar effects on the stomach.

uro·gen·i·tal (-jen′ĭ-tal) genitourinary.

urog·e·nous (u-roj′ĕ-nus) 1. producing urine. 2. produced from or in the urine.

uro·gram (u′ro-gram) a film obtained by urography.

urog·ra·phy (u-rog′rah-fe) radiography of any part of the urinary tract. **ascending u., cystoscopic u.,** retrograde u. **descending u., excretion u., excretory u., intravenous u.,** urography after intravenous injection of an opaque medium which is rapidly excreted in the urine. **retrograde u.,** urography after injection of a contrast medium into the bladder through the urethra.

uro·ki·nase (UK) (u″ro-ki′nās) u-plasminogen activator; an enzyme in the urine of humans and other mammals, elaborated by the parenchymal cells of the human kidney and acting as a plasminogen activator. It is used as a therapeutic thrombolytic agent.

uro·lith (u′ro-lith) urinary calculus. **urolith′ic,** adj.

uro·li·thi·a·sis (u″ro-lĭ-thi′ah-sis) the formation of urinary calculi, or the condition associated with urinary calculi.

urol·o·gy (u-rol′ah-je) the medical specialty concerned with the urinary system in the male and female and genital organs in the male. **urolog′ic, urolog′ical,** adj.

uron·cus (u-rong′kus) urinoma.

urop·a·thy (u-rop′ah-the) any disease or other pathologic change in the urinary tract.

uro·poi·e·sis (-poi-e′sis) the formation of urine. **uropoiet′ic,** adj.

uro·por·phyr·ia (-por-fir′e-ah) porphyria with excessive excretion of uroporphyrin.

uro·por·phy·rin (-por′fĭ-rin) any of several porphyrins produced by oxidation of uroporphyrinogen; one or more are excreted in excess in the urine in several of the porphyrias.

uro·por·phy·rin·o·gen (-por″fĭ-rin′o-jen) a porphyrinogen formed from porphobilinogen; it is a precursor of uroporphyrin and coproporphyrinogen.

uro·pro·tec·tion (-pro-tek′shun) protection of the urinary tract, especially against urotoxic chemicals. **uroprotec′tive,** adj.

uro·psam·mus (-sam′us) sediment or gravel in the urine.

uro·ra·di·ol·o·gy (-ra″de-ol′ah-je) radiology of the urinary tract.

uros·co·py (u-ros′kah-pe) diagnostic examination of the urine. **uroscop′ic,** adj.

uro·sep·sis (u″ro-sep′sis) a term used imprecisely to denote infection ranging from urinary tract infection to generalized sepsis which may result from such infection. **urosep′tic,** adj.

uro·tox·ic (u′ro-tok″sik) pertaining to that which is harmful to the bladder.

ur·so·di·ol (ur″so-di′ol) the secondary bile acid ursodeoxycholic acid used as an anticholelithic to dissolve radiolucent, noncalcified gallstones.

Ur·ti·ca (ur-ti′kah) [L.] see *nettle.*

ur·ti·cant (ur′tĭ-kant) producing urticaria.

ur·ti·ca·ria (ur″tĭ-kar′e-ah) hives; a vascular reaction of the upper dermis marked by transient appearance of slightly elevated patches (wheals) which are redder or paler than the surrounding skin and often attended by severe itching; the exciting cause may be certain foods or drugs, infection, or emotional stress. **urticar′ial,** adj. **u. bullo′sa, bullous u.,** that in which bullae are superimposed on the wheals. **cold u.,** urticaria precipitated by cold air, water, or objects, occurring in a hereditary and an acquired form. **giant u.,** angioedema. **u. medicamento′sa,** that due to use of a drug. **papular u.,** a hypersensitivity reaction to insect bites, manifested by crops of small papules and wheals, which may become infected or lichenified because of rubbing and excoriation. **u. pigmento′sa,** the most common form of mastocytosis, characterized by small, reddish brown macules or papules that occur mainly on the trunk and tend to urtication upon mild mechanical trauma or chemical irritation.

ur·ti·ca·tion (ur″tĭ-ka′shun) 1. the development or formation of urticaria. 2. a burning sensation as of stinging with nettles.

uru·shi·ol (u-roo′she-ol) the toxic irritant principle of poison ivy and various related plants.

US ultrasound.

USAN United States Adopted Name.

USP *United States Pharmacopeia.*

USPHS United States Public Health Service.

us·ti·lag·i·nism (us′tĭ-laj′ĭ-nizm) a condition resembling ergotism due to ingestion of maize containing *Ustilago maydis,* the corn smut fungus.

uter·al·gia (u″ter-al′jah) hysteralgia.

uter·ine (u′ter-in) pertaining to the uterus.

uter(o)- word element [L.], *uterus.*

utero·ab·dom·i·nal (u″ter-o-ab-dom′ĭ-n′l) pertaining to the uterus and abdomen.

utero·cer·vi·cal (-ser′vĭ-k′l) pertaining to the uterus and cervix uteri.

utero·lith (u′ter-o-lith″) uterine calculus.

uter·om·e·ter (u″ter-om′ĕ-ter) an instrument for measuring the uterus.

utero·ovar·i·an (u″ter-o-o-var′e-an) pertaining to the uterus and ovary.

utero·pel·vic (-pel′vik) pertaining to or connecting the uterus and the pelvis.

utero·pla·cen·tal (-plah-sen′tal) pertaining to the placenta and uterus.

utero·rec·tal (u″ter-o-rek′t′l) rectouterine.

utero·sa·cral (-sa′kr′l) pertaining to the uterus and sacrum.

utero·ton·ic (-ton′ik) 1. increasing the tone of uterine muscle. 2. an agent that so acts.

utero·tu·bal (-too′b′l) tubouterine.

utero·vag·i·nal (-vaj′ĭ-n′l) pertaining to the uterus and vagina.

uter·o·ves·i·cal (-ves′ĭ-k′l) vesicouterine.

uter·us (u′ter-us) pl. *u′teri.* [L.] the hollow muscular organ in female mammals in which the blastocyst normally becomes embedded and in which the developing embryo and fetus is nourished. Its cavity opens into the vagina below and into a uterine tube on either side. **bicornuate u.,** one with two horns, or cornua. **u. didel′phys,** the existence of two distinct uteri in the same individual. **gravid u.,** one containing a developing fetus. **septate u.,** a uterus whose cavity is divided into two parts by a septum. **unicornuate u.,** one with a single horn, or cornu.

UTI urinary tract infection.

UTP uridine triphosphate.

utri·cle (u′tri-k′l) 1. any small sac. 2. the larger of the two divisions of the membranous labyrinth of the internal ear. **prostatic u., urethral u.,** a small blind pouch in the substance of the prostate.

utric·u·lar (u-trik′u-ler) 1. pertaining to the utricle. 2. bladderlike.

utric·u·li·tis (u-trik″u-li′tis) inflammation of the prostatic utricle or the utricle of the ear.

utric·u·lo·sac·cu·lar (u-trik″u-lo-sak′u-ler) pertaining to utricle and saccule of the labyrinth.

utric·u·lus (u-trik'u-lus) pl. *utri'culi*. [L.] utricle. **u. masculi'nus, u. prosta'ticus,** prostatic utricle.

UV ultraviolet.

UVA ultraviolet A; see *ultraviolet*.

uva ur·si (u'vah ur'se) *Arctostaphylos uva-ursi* or its leaves, which are used medicinally and homeopathically for urinary tract inflammation.

UVB ultraviolet B; see *ultraviolet*.

UVC ultraviolet C; see *ultraviolet*.

uvea (u've-ah) the tunica vasculosa of the eyeball, consisting of the iris, ciliary body, and choroid. **u'veal,** adj.

uve·itis (u"ve-i'tis) inflammation of all or part of the uvea. **uveit'ic,** adj. **heterochromic u.,** see under *iridocyclitis*. **sympathetic u.,** see under *ophthalmia*.

uveo·scle·ri·tis (u"ve-o-sklĕ-ri'tis) scleritis due to extension of uveitis.

uvi·form (u'vĭ-form) shaped like a grape.

uvu·la (u'vu-lah) pl. *u'vulae*. [L.] 1. a pendant, fleshy mass. 2. palatine u. **u'vular,** adj. **u. of bladder,** a rounded elevation at the bladder neck, formed by convergence of muscle fibers terminating in the urethra. **u. of cerebellum,** u. vermis. **palatine u.,** the small, fleshy mass hanging from the soft palate above the root of the tongue. **u. ver'mis,** the part of the vermis of the cerebellum between the pyramid and nodule.

uvu·lec·to·my (u"vu-lek'tah-me) excision of the uvula.

uvu·li·tis (u"vu-li'tis) inflammation of the uvula.

uvu·lo·pal·a·to·phar·yn·go·plas·ty (UPPP) (u"vu-lo-pal"ah-to-fah-ring'go-plas"te) an operation performed on the soft tissues of the soft palate and pharyngeal area in the treatment of sleep apnea.

uvu·lop·to·sis (u"vu-lop-to'sis) a relaxed, pendulous state of the uvula.

uvu·lot·o·my (u"vu-lot'ah-me) the cutting off of the uvula or a part of it.

V valine; vanadium; vision; volt; volume.

v. [L.] ve'na (vein).

VAC a regimen of vincristine, dactinomycin, and cyclophosphamide, used in cancer therapy.

vac·ci·nal (vak'sĭ-n'l) 1. pertaining to vaccine or to vaccination. 2. having protective qualities when used by way of inoculation.

vac·ci·na·tion (vak"sĭ-na'shun) the introduction of vaccine into the body to produce immunity.

vac·cine (vak'sēn) a suspension of attenuated or killed microorganisms (viruses, bacteria, or rickettsiae), or of antigenic proteins derived from them, administered for prevention, amelioration, or treatment of infectious diseases. **acellular v.,** a cell-free vaccine prepared from purified antigenic components of cell-free microorganisms, carrying less risk than whole-cell preparations. **anthrax v.,** a cell-free protein extract of cultures of *Bacillus anthracis*, used for immunization against anthrax. **attenuated v.,** a vaccine prepared from live microorganisms or viruses cultured under adverse conditions leading to loss of their virulence but retention of their ability to induce protective immunity. **autogenous v.,** a vaccine prepared from microorganisms which have been freshly isolated from the lesion of the patient who is to be treated with it. **BCG v.,** a preparation used as an active immunizing agent against tuberculosis and in treatment of bladder cancer, consisting of a dried, living, avirulent culture of the Calmette-Guérin strain of *Mycobacterium bovis*. **cholera v.,** a preparation of killed *Vibrio cholerae*, used in immunization against cholera. **diphtheria and tetanus toxoids and pertussis v. (DTP),** a combination of diphtheria and tetanus toxoids and pertussis vaccine; used for simultaneous immunization against diphtheria, tetanus, and whooping cough. When the pertussis vaccine is an acellular form, the combination may be abbreviated DTaP. **diphtheria and tetanus toxoids and pertussis v. adsorbed and Haemophilus b conjugate v.,** a combination of diphtheria toxoid, tetanus toxoid, pertussis vaccine, and *Haemophilus* b conjugate vaccine; used for simultaneous immunization against diphtheria, tetanus, pertussis, and infection by *Haemophilus influenzae* type b. **Haemophilus b conjugate v. (HbCV),** a preparation of *Haemophilus influenzae* type b capsular polysaccharide covalently bound to diphtheria toxoid or to a specific diphtheria, meningococcal, or tetanus protein; it stimulates both B and T lymphocyte responses and is used as an immunizing agent in infants and young children. **Haemophilus b polysaccharide v. (HbPV),** a preparation of highly purified capsular polysaccharide derived from *Haemophilus influenzae* type b, which stimulates an immune response in B lymphocytes only; used as an immunizing agent in children. **hepatitis A v. inactivated,** an inactivated whole virus vaccine derived from an attenuated strain of hepatitis A virus grown in cell culture. **hepatitis B v.,** a preparation of hepatitis B surface antigen, derived either from human plasma of carriers of hepatitis B (*hepatitis B v. inactivated*) or from cloning in yeast cells (*hepatitis B v. [recombinant]*). **heterologous v.,** a vaccine that confers protective immunity against a pathogen that shares cross-reacting antigens with the microorganisms in the vaccine. **human diploid cell v. (HDCV),** see *rabies v.* **influenza virus v.,** a killed virus vaccine used in immunization against influenza; it is trivalent, usually containing two influenza A virus strains and one influenza B virus strain. **live v.,** one prepared from live microorganisms that have been attenuated but that retain their immunogenic properties. **Lyme disease v. (recombinant OspA),** a preparation of outer surface protein A (OspA), a cell surface lipoprotein of *Borrelia burgdorferi*, produced by recombinant technology; used for active immunization against Lyme disease. **measles, mumps, and rubella virus v. live (MMR),** a combination of live attenuated measles, mumps, and rubella viruses, used for simultaneous immunization against measles, mumps, and rubella. **measles and rubella virus v. live,** a combination of live attenuated measles and rubella viruses, used for simultaneous immunization against measles and rubella. **measles virus v. live,** a live attenuated virus vaccine used for immunization against measles, although it is generally administered as the combination measles, mumps, and rubella virus vaccine. **meningococcal polysaccharide v.,** a preparation of capsular polysaccharide antigen of *Neisseria meningitidis*, used to provide immunity to meningitis. **mixed v.,** polyvalent v. **mumps virus v. live,** a live attenuated virus vaccine used in immunization against mumps; usually administered as the combination measles, mumps, and rubella virus vaccine. **pertussis v.,** a preparation of killed *Bordetella pertussis* bacilli (whole-cell vaccine) or of purified antigenic components thereof (acellular vaccine), used to immunize against pertussis; generally used in combination with diphtheria and tetanus toxoids (DTP or DTaP). **plague v.,** a preparation of killed *Yersinia pestis* bacilli, used as an active immunizing agent. **pneumococcal heptavalent conjugate v.,** a preparation of capsular polysaccharides from the seven serotypes of *Streptococcus pneumoniae* most commonly isolated from young children, coupled to a nontoxic variant of diphtheria toxin; used as an active immunizing agent. **pneumococcal v. polyvalent,** a preparation of purified capsular polysaccharides from the 23 serotypes of *Streptococcus pneumoniae* causing the majority of pneumococcal disease; used as an active immunizing agent. **poliovirus v. inactivated (IPV),** Salk v.; a suspension of formalin-inactivated polioviruses used for immunization against poliomyelitis. **poliovirus v. live oral (OPV),** Sabin v.; a preparation of a combination of the three types of live, attenuated polioviruses used as an active immunizing agent against poliomyelitis. **polyvalent v.,** one prepared from cultures or antigens of more than one strain or species. **purified chick embryo cell v.,** a preparation of inactivated rabies virus grown in cultures of chicken fibroblasts; used for pre- and postexposure rabies immunization. **rabies v.,** an inactivated virus vaccine used for pre- and postexposure immunization against rabies; it may be prepared from virus grown in human diploid cell culture (*human diploid cell v.*), that grown in cultures of chicken fibroblasts (*purified chick embryo cell v.*), or that grown in cultures of fetal rhesus lung and concentrated by adsorption to aluminum phosphate (*rabies v. adsorbed*). **replicative v.,** any vaccine containing organisms that are able to reproduce, including live and attenuated viruses and bacteria. **rotavirus v. live oral,** a live virus vaccine produced from a mixture of four rotavirus types grown in fetal rhesus diploid cells; used to immunize infants against rotaviral gastroenteritis. **rubella and mumps virus v. live,** a combination of live attenuated rubella and mumps viruses, used for simultaneous immunization against rubella and mumps. **rubella virus v. live,** a live attenuated virus vaccine used for immunization against rubella, usually administered as the combination measles, mumps, and rubella virus vaccine. **Sabin v.,** poliovirus v. live oral. **Salk v.,** poliovirus v. inactivated. **subunit v.,** a vaccine produced from specific protein subunits of a virus and thus having less risk of adverse reactions than whole virus vaccines. **typhoid v.**, any of several preparations of *Salmonella typhi* used for immunization against typhoid fever, including a parenteral heat- and phenol-inactivated bacteria vaccine, an oral live vaccine prepared from the attenuated strain Ty21a, and a parenteral vaccine prepared from typhoid Vi capsular polysaccharide. **varicella virus v. live,** a preparation of live, attenuated human herpesvirus 3 (varicella-zoster virus) used for production of immunity to varicella and herpes zoster. **yellow fever v.,** a preparation of attenuated yellow fever virus, used to immunize against yellow fever.

vac·u·o·lar (vak′u-o″lar) containing, or of the nature of, vacuoles.

vac·u·o·lat·ed (vak′u-o-lāt″ed) containing vacuoles.

vac·u·o·la·tion (vak″u-o-la′shun) the process of forming vacuoles; the condition of being vacuolated.

vac·u·ole (vak′u-ōl) a space or cavity in the protoplasm of a cell.

vac·u·um (vak′ūm) [L.] a space devoid of air or of other gas; a space from which the air has been exhausted.

VAD ventricular assist device.

va·gal (va′gal) pertaining to the vagus nerve.

va·gi·na (vah-ji′nah) pl. *vagi′nae*. [L.] 1. a sheath or sheathlike structure. 2. the canal in the female, from the vulva to the cervix uteri, that receives the penis in copulation. **vag′inal**, adj.

va·gi·nate (vaj′ĭ-nāt) enclosed in a sheath.

vag·i·nec·to·my (vaj″ĭ-nek′tah-me) excision of the vagina.

vag·i·nis·mus (vaj″ĭ-niz′mus) painful spasm of the vagina due to involuntary muscular contraction, usually severe enough to prevent intercourse; the cause may be organic or psychogenic.

vag·i·ni·tis (vaj″ĭ-ni′tis) 1. inflammation of the vagina. 2. inflammation of a sheath. **adhesive v.,** a form of atrophic vaginitis marked by formation of superficial erosions, which often adhere to opposing surfaces, obliterating the vaginal canal. **atrophic v.,** vaginitis with tissue atrophy occurring in postmenopausal women and associated with estrogen deficiency. **candidal v.,** vulvovaginal candidiasis. **desquamative inflammatory v.,** a form resembling atrophic vaginitis but affecting women with normal estrogen levels. **emphysematous v.,** inflammation of the vagina and adjacent cervix, characterized by numerous, asymptomatic, gas-filled cystlike lesions. **senile v.,** atrophic v.

vag·i·no·ab·dom·i·nal (vaj″ĭ-no-ab-dom′ĭ-nal) pertaining to the vagina and abdomen.

vag·i·no·cele (vaj′ĭ-no-sēl″) 1. vaginal hernia. 2. prolapse of the vagina.

vag·in·odyn·ia (vaj″ĭ-no-din′e-ah) pain in the vagina.

vag·i·no·fix·a·tion (-fik-sa′shun) suture of the vagina to the abdominal wall.

vag·i·no·la·bi·al (-la′be-al) pertaining to the vagina and labia.

vag·i·no·my·co·sis (-mi-ko′sis) any fungal disease of the vagina.

vag·i·nop·a·thy (vaj″ĭ-nop′ah-the) any disease of the vagina.

vag·i·no·per·i·ne·al (vaj″ĭ-no-per″ĭ-ne′al) pertaining to the vagina and perineum.

vag·i·no·peri·ne·or·rha·phy (-per″ĭ-ne-or′ah-fe) suture repair of the vagina and perineum.

vag·i·no·peri·ne·ot·o·my (-per″ĭ-ne-ot′ah-me) paravaginal incision.

vag·i·no·peri·to·ne·al (-per″ĭ-to-ne′al) pertaining to the vagina and peritoneum.

vag·i·no·pexy (vah-ji′no-pek″se) vagino-fixation.

vag·i·no·plas·ty (-plas″te) plastic surgery of the vagina.

vag·i·no·scope (vaj′ĭ-no-skōp) colposcope.

vag·i·not·o·my (vaj″ĭ-not′ah-me) colpotomy.

vag·i·no·ves·i·cal (vaj″ĭ-no-ves′ĭ-k'l) vesicovaginal.

va·gi·tus (vah-ji′tus) [L.] the cry of an infant. **v. uteri′nus,** the cry of an infant in the uterus.

va·gol·y·sis (va-gol′ĭ-sis) surgical destruction of the vagus nerve.

va·go·lyt·ic (va″go-lit′ik) 1. pertaining to or caused by vagolysis. 2. having an effect resembling that produced by interruption of impulses transmitted by the vagus nerve.

va·go·mi·met·ic (-mi-met′ik) having an effect resembling that produced by stimulation of the vagus nerve.

va·got·o·my (va-got′ah-me) interruption of the impulses carried by the vagus nerve or nerves. **highly selective v.,** division of only those vagal fibers supplying the acid-secreting glands of the stomach, with preservation of those supplying the antrum as well as the hepatic and celiac branches. **medical v.,** that accomplished by administration of suitable drugs. **parietal cell v.,** selective severing of the vagus nerve fibers supplying the proximal two-thirds (parietal area) of the stomach; done for duodenal ulcer. **selective v.,** division of the vagal fibers to the stomach with preservation of the hepatic and celiac branches. **truncal v.,** surgical division of the two main trunks of the abdominal vagus nerve.

va·go·to·nia (va″go-to′ne-ah) hyperexcitability of the vagus nerve, particularly with respect to its parasympathetic effects on body organs, resulting in vasomotor instability, sweating, constipation, and involuntary motor spasms with pain. **vagoton′ic,** adj.

va·go·tro·pic (va″go-tro′pik) having an effect on the vagus nerve.

va·go·va·gal (-va′gal) arising as a result of afferent and efferent impulses mediated through the vagus nerve.

va·gus (va′gus) pl. *va′gi.* [L.] the vagus nerve; see *Table of Nerves.*

vai·dya (vī′dyah) [Sanskrit "one who knows"] in ayurveda, a physician.

Val valine.

val·a·cy·clo·vir (val″a-si′klo-vir) an ester of acyclovir, to which it is metabolized; used as the hydrochloride salt as an antiviral agent in the treatment of genital herpes and herpes zoster in immunocompetent adults.

val·de·cox·ib (val″dě-kok′sib) a nonsteroidal antiinflammatory drug of the COX-2 inhibitors group, used for the treatment of osteoarthritis, rheumatoid arthritis, and primary dysmenorrhea.

va·lence (va′lens) 1. a positive number that represents the number of bonds that each atom of an element makes in a chemical compound; now replaced by the concept "oxidation number" but still used to denote (*a*) the number of covalent bonds formed by an atom in a covalent compound or (*b*) the charge on a monatomic or polyatomic molecule. 2. in immunology, the number of antigen binding sites possessed by an antibody molecule.

va·le·ri·an (vah-lēr′e-an) 1. a plant of the genus *Valeriana.* 2. the dried roots, rhizome, and stolons of *V. officinalis,* which are antispasmodic and sedative and are used for nervousness and insomnia.

val·gan·ci·clo·vir (val″gan-si′klo-vir) a prodrug of ganciclovir, used as the hydrochloride salt in the treatment of cytomegalovirus retinitis in patients with AIDS.

val·gus (val′gus) [L.] bent out, twisted; denoting a deformity in which the angulation is away from the midline of the body, as in talipes valgus. The meanings of valgus and varus are often reversed.

val·ine (Val, V) (va′lēn) a naturally occurring amino acid, essential for human metabolism.

val·in·emia (val″ĭ-ne′me-ah) hypervalinemia.

Val·i·um (val′e-um) trademark for preparations of diazepam.

val·late (val′āt) having a wall or rim; cup-shaped.

val·lec·u·la (vah-lek′u-lah) pl. *valle′culae.* [L.] a depression or furrow. **vallec′ular,** adj. **v. cerebel′li,** the longitudinal fissure on the inferior cerebellum, in which the medulla oblongata rests. **v. un′guis,** the sulcus of the matrix of the nail.

val·pro·ate (val-pro′āt) a salt of valproic acid; the sodium salt has the same uses as the acid.

val·pro·ic ac·id (-ik) an anticonvulsant used particularly for the control of absence seizures.

val·ru·bi·cin (val-roo′bĭ-sin″) an antineoplastic that interferes with nucleic acid metabolism and other related biological functions; used intravesically for treatment of bladder carcinoma.

val·sar·tan (-sahr′tan) an angiotensin II antagonist used as an antihypertensive.

val·ue (val′u) a measure of worth or efficiency or of the activity, concentration, etc., of something. **normal v's,** the range in concentration of specific substances found in normal healthy tissues, secretions, etc. *P* **v.,** *p* **v.,** the probability of obtaining by chance a result at least as extreme as that observed, even when the null hypothesis is true and no real difference exists; if it is ≤ 0.05 the sample results are usually deemed statistically significant and the null hypothesis rejected. **reference v's,** a set of values of a quantity measured in the clinical laboratory that characterize a specified population in a defined state of health.

val·va (val′vah) pl. *val′vae.* [L.] a valve.

valve (valv) a membranous fold in a canal or passage that prevents backward flow of material passing through it. **aortic v.,** that guarding the entrance to the aorta from the left ventricle. **artificial cardiac v.,** a substitute, mechanical or composed of tissue, for a cardiac valve. **atrioventricular v's,** the valves between the right atrium and right ventricle (*tricuspid v.*) and the left atrium and left ventricle (*mitral v.*). **Béraud's v.,** a fold of mucous membrane sometimes occurring at the beginning of the nasolacrimal duct. **bicuspid v.,** mitral v. **bileaflet v.,** a heart valve prosthesis consisting of a circular sewing ring to which are attached two semicircular occluding disks that swing open and closed to regulate blood flow. **bioprosthetic v.,** an artificial cardiac valve composed of biological tissue, usually porcine. **caged-ball v.,** a heart valve prosthesis comprising a sewing ring attached to a cage composed of curved struts that contains a free-floating ball. **cardiac v's,** those controlling the flow of blood through and from the heart. **coronary v.,**

that at the entrance of the coronary sinus into the right atrium. **flail mitral v.,** a cardiac valve having a cusp that has lost its normal support (as in ruptured chordae tendineae) and flutters in the blood stream. **Houston's v's,** permanent transverse folds, usually numbering three, in the rectum. **ileocecal v., ileocolic v.,** that guarding the opening between the ileum and cecum. **mitral v.,** that between the left atrium and left ventricle, usually having two cusps (anterior and posterior). **pulmonary v.,** that at the entrance of the pulmonary trunk from the right ventricle. **pyloric v.,** a prominent fold of mucous membrane at the pyloric orifice of the stomach. **semilunar v.,** one having semilunar cusps, i.e., the aortic and pulmonary valves; sometimes used to designate the semilunar cusps composing these valves. **thebesian v.,** coronary v. **tilting-disk v.,** a heart valve prosthesis consisting of a sewing ring and a valve housing containing a suspended disk that swings between open and closed positions. **tricuspid v.,** that guarding the opening between the right atrium and right ventricle. **ureteral v.,** a congenital transverse fold across the lumen of the ureter, composed of redundant mucosa made prominent by circular muscle fibers; it usually disappears in time but may rarely cause urinary obstruction.

val·vot·o·my (val-vot′ah-me) incision of a valve.

val·vu·la (val′vu-lah) pl. *val′vulae.* [L.] valvule; a small valve; formerly used in official nomenclature for any valve, but now restricted to certain small valves and cusps of heart valves.

val·vu·lar (val′vu-ler) pertaining to, affecting, or of the nature of a valve.

val·vule (val′vūl) see *valvula.*

val·vu·li·tis (val-vu-li′tis) inflammation of a valve, especially of a heart valve.

val·vu·lo·plas·ty (val′vu-lo-plas″te) plastic repair of a valve, especially a heart valve. **balloon v.,** dilation of a stenotic cardiac valve by means of a balloon-tipped catheter that is introduced into the valve and inflated.

val·vu·lo·tome (-tōm) an instrument for cutting a valve.

va·na·di·um (vah-na′de-um) chemical element (see *Table of Elements*), at. no. 23, symbol V. Its salts have been used in treating various diseases. Absorption of its compounds, usually via the lungs, causes chronic intoxication, the symptoms of which include respiratory tract irritation, pneumonitis, conjunctivitis, and anemia.

van·co·my·cin (van″ko-mi′sin) an antibiotic produced by *Streptomyces orientalis*, highly effective against gram-positive bacteria, especially against staphylococci; used as the hydrochloride salt.

va·nil·lism (vah-nil′izm) dermatitis, coryza, and malaise seen in handlers of raw vanilla, caused by the mite *Acarus siro*.

va·nil·lyl·man·del·ic ac·id (vah-nil″il-mandel′ik) an excretory product of the catecholamines; urinary levels are used in screening patients for pheochromocytoma. Abbreviated VMA.

va·por (va′por) pl. *vapo′res, vapors.* [L.] 1. steam, gas, or exhalation. 2. an atmospheric dispersion of a substance that in its normal state is liquid or solid.

va·por·iza·tion (va″por-ĭ-za′shun) 1. the conversion of a solid or liquid into a vapor without chemical change. See also *nebulization.* 2. distillation.

var·i·a·ble (var′e-ah-b′l) 1. changing from time to time. 2. in mathematics, a symbol that represents an arbitrary number or an arbitrary element of a set.

var·i·ance (var′e-ans) a measure of the variation shown by a set of observations: the average of the squared deviations from the mean; it is the square of the standard deviation.

var·i·ant (var′e-ant) 1. something that differs in some characteristic from the class to which it belongs. 2. exhibiting such variation.

var·i·a·tion (var″e-a′shun) the act or process of changing; in genetics, deviation in characters in an individual from the group to which it belongs or deviation in characters of the offspring from those of its parents. **antigenic v.,** a mechanism by which parasites can escape the immune surveillance of a host by modifying or completely altering their surface antigens. **microbial v.,** the range of characteristics within a species used in identification and differentiation. **phenotypic v.,** the total variation, for whatever cause, observed in one character.

var·i·ca·tion (var″ĭ-ka′shun) 1. formation of a varix. 2. varicosity (1).

var·i·ce·al (var″ĭ-ce′al) varicose.

var·i·cel·la (var″ĭ-sel′ah) [L.] chickenpox.

Var·i·cel·lo·vi·rus (var″ĭ-sel′o-vi″rus) varicella and pseudorabies-like viruses; a genus of viruses of the subfamily Alphaherpesvirinae (family Herpesviridae), including human herpesvirus 3, pseudorabies virus, and bovine and equid herpesviruses.

var·i·cel·li·form (var″i-sel′ĭ-form) resembling varicella.

var·i·ces (var′ĭ-sēz) [L.] plural of *varix.*

var·ic·i·form (vah-ris'ĭ-form) varicose.

varic(o)- word element [L.], *varix; swollen.*

var·i·co·bleph·a·ron (var"ĭ-ko-blef'ah-ron) a varicose swelling of the eyelid.

var·i·co·cele (var'ĭ-ko-sēl) 1. varicosity of the pampiniform plexus of the spermatic cord, forming a scrotal swelling that feels like a "bag of worms." 2. a similar condition in females, with varicosity of the veins of the broad ligament of the uterus.

var·i·co·ce·lec·to·my (var"ĭ-ko-se-lek'tah-me) ligation and excision of a varicocele.

var·i·cog·ra·phy (var"ĭ-kog'rah-fe) x-ray visualization of varicose veins.

var·i·com·pha·lus (var"ĭ-kom'fah-lus) a varicose tumor of the umbilicus.

var·i·co·phle·bi·tis (var"ĭ-ko-flĕ-bi'tis) varicose veins with inflammation.

var·i·cose (var'ĭ-kōs) variceal or variciform; of the nature of or pertaining to a varix; unnaturally and permanently distended.

var·i·cos·i·ty (var"ĭ-kos'ĭ-te) 1. the quality or fact of being varicose. 2. varix. 3. varicose vein.

var·i·cot·o·my (var"ĭ-kot'ah-me) excision of a varix or of a varicose vein.

va·ric·u·la (vah-rik'u-lah) a varix of the conjunctiva.

var·i·e·gate (var'e-ĭ-gāt") 1. marked by variety; diversified. 2. having patchy spots or streaks of different colors.

va·ri·e·ty (vah-ri'ĕ-te) in taxonomy, a subcategory of a species.

va·ri·o·la (vah-ri'o-lah) smallpox. **vari'olar, vari'olous,** adj.

va·ri·o·late (var'e-o-lāt) 1. having the nature or appearance of smallpox. 2. to inoculate with smallpox virus.

va·ri·ol·i·form (var"e-o'lĭ-form) resembling smallpox.

va·rix (var'iks) pl. *va'rices.* [L.] an enlarged tortuous vein, artery, or lymphatic vessel. **aneurysmal v.,** a markedly dilated tortuous vessel. **arterial v.,** a racemose aneurysm or varicose artery. **esophageal v.,** varicosities of branches of the azygos vein which anastomose with tributaries of the portal vein in the lower esophagus, due to portal hypertension in cirrhosis. **lymph v., v. lympha'ticus,** a soft, lobulated swelling of a lymph node, due to obstruction of lymphatic vessels.

va·ro·li·an (vah-ro'le-an) pertaining to the pons.

va·rus (var'us) [L.] bent inward; denoting a deformity in which the angulation of the part is toward the midline of the body, as in talipes varus. The meanings of *varus* and *valgus* are often reversed.

vas (vas) pl. *va'sa.* [L.] vessel. **va'sal,** adj. **v. aber'rans,** 1. a blind tubule sometimes connected with the epididymis; a vestigial mesonephric tubule. 2. any anomalous or unusual vessel. **va'sa affferen'tia,** vessels that convey fluid to a structure or part. **va'sa bre'via,** short gastric arteries. **v. capilla're,** a capillary. **v. de'ferens,** ductus deferens. **va'sa efferen'tia,** vessels that convey fluid away from a structure or part. **va'sa lympha'tica,** lymphatic vessels. **va'sa prae'via,** presentation, in front of the fetal head during labor, of the blood vessels of the umbilical cord where they enter the placenta. **va'sa rec'ta re'nis,** straight arterioles of kidney; see *Table of Arteries.* **va'sa vaso'rum,** the small nutrient arteries and veins in the walls of the larger blood vessels. **va'sa vortico'sa,** vorticose veins.

vas·cu·lar (vas'ku-ler) 1. pertaining to vessels, particularly blood vessels. 2. indicative of a copious blood supply.

vas·cu·lar·iza·tion (vas"ku-ler-ĭ-za'shun) 1. the process of becoming vascular. 2. angiogenesis. 3. the surgically induced development of vessels in a tissue.

vas·cu·la·ture (vas'ku-lah-chur) 1. circulatory system. 2. any part of the circulatory system.

vas·cu·li·tis (vas"ku-li'tis) inflammation of a blood or lymph vessel. **vasculit'ic,** adj. **systemic necrotizing v.,** any of a group of disorders characterized by inflammation and necrosis of blood vessel walls.

vas·cu·lo·gen·e·sis (vas"ku-lo-jen'ĕ-sis) angiogenesis.

vas·cu·lo·gen·ic (vas"ku-lo-jen'ik) angiogenic (1).

vas·cu·lop·a·thy (vas"ku-lop'ah-the) any disorder of blood vessels.

va·sec·to·my (vah-sek'tah-me) surgical removal of all or part of the ductus (vas) deferens.

vas·i·form (vas'ĭ-form) resembling a vessel.

va·si·tis (vah-si'tis) deferentitis.

vas(o)- word element [L.], *vessel; duct.*

vaso·ac·tive (va"zo-, vas"o-ak'tiv) exerting an effect upon the caliber of blood vessels.

vaso·con·stric·tion (-kon-strik'shun) decrease in the caliber of blood vessels. **vasoconstric'tive,** adj.

vaso·con·stric·tor (-kon-strik'ter) 1. causing constriction of blood vessels. 2. a nerve or agent that does this.

vaso·de·pres·sion (-de-presh'un) decrease in vascular resistance with hypotension.

vaso·de·pres·sor (-de-pres'er) 1. having the effect of lowering the blood pressure through reduction in peripheral resistance. 2. an agent that causes vasodepression.

vaso·di·la·ta·tion (-dī″lah-ta′shun) vasodilation.

vaso·di·la·tion (-di-la′shun) 1. increase in caliber of blood vessels. 2. a state of increased caliber of blood vessels. **vasodi′lative,** adj.

vaso·di·la·tor (-di-la′ter) 1. causing dilatation of blood vessels. 2. a nerve or agent that does this.

vaso·epi·did·y·mog·ra·phy (-ep″ĭ-did″ĭ-mog′rah-fe) radiography of the vas deferens and epididymis after injection of a contrast medium.

vaso·epi·did·y·mos·to·my (-ep″ĭ-did″ĭ-mos′tah-me) anastomosis of the ductus (vas) deferens and the epididymis.

vaso·for·ma·tive (-for′mah-tiv) angiogenic (1).

vaso·gan·gli·on (-gang′gle-on) a vascular ganglion or rete.

vaso·gen·ic (va″zo-jen′ik) originating in the blood vessels.

va·sog·ra·phy (va-zog′rah-fe) angiography.

vaso·hy·per·ton·ic (va″zo-, vas″o-hi″per-ton′ik) vasoconstrictor (1).

vaso·hy·po·ton·ic (-hi″po-ton′ik) vasodilator (1).

vaso·in·hib·i·tor (-in-hib′ĭ-ter) an agent that inhibits the action of the vasomotor nerves. **vasoinhib′itory,** adj.

vaso·li·ga·tion (-li-ga′shun) ligation of the ductus (vas) deferens.

vaso·mo·tor (-mo′tor) 1. affecting the caliber of blood vessels. 2. a vasomotor agent or nerve.

vaso·neu·rop·a·thy (-noo-rop′ah-the) a condition caused by combined vascular and neurologic defect.

vaso·neu·ro·sis (-noo-ro′sis) angioneuropathy.

vaso·oc·clu·sion (-ŏ-kloo′zhun) occlusion of a blood vessel or vessels. **vasoocclu′sive,** adj.

vaso·pa·re·sis (-pah-re′sis) partial paralysis of vasomotor nerves.

vaso·per·me·a·bil·i·ty (-per″me-ah-bil′ĭ-te) the extent to which a blood vessel is permeable.

vaso·pres·sin (-pres′in) a hormone secreted by cells of the hypothalamic nuclei and stored in the posterior pituitary for release as necessary; it constricts blood vessels, raising the blood pressure, and increases peristalsis, exerts some influence on the uterus, and influences resorption of water by the kidney tubules, resulting in concentration of urine. In most mammals, including humans, it exists

as the arginine form, a synthetic preparation of which is used as an antidiuretic and in tests of hypothalamo-neurohypophysial-renal function in the diagnosis of central diabetes insipidus. A lysine form occurs in pigs; the synthetic pharmaceutical preparation is lypressin.

vaso·pres·sor (-pres′er) 1. stimulating contraction of the muscular tissue of the capillaries and arteries. 2. an agent that so acts.

vaso·re·flex (-re′fleks) a reflex involving a blood vessel.

vaso·re·lax·a·tion (-re″lak-sa′shun) decrease of vascular pressure.

vaso·sec·tion (-sek′shun) severing of a vessel or vessels.

vaso·sen·so·ry (-sen′sor-e) supplying sensory filaments to the vessels.

vaso·spasm (va′zo-, vas′o-spazm) angiospasm; spasm of blood vessels, causing vasoconstriction. **vasospas′tic,** adj.

vaso·stim·u·lant (va″zo-, vas″o-stim′u-lant) stimulating vasomotor action.

va·sos·to·my (vah-sos′tah-me) 1. surgical formation of an opening into the ductus (vas) deferens. 2. vasotomy.

va·sot·o·my (vah-sot′ah-me) incision of the ductus (vas) deferens.

vaso·to·nia (va″zo-, vas″o-to′ne-ah) tone or tension of the vessels. **vasoton′ic,** adj.

vaso·tro·phic (-tro′fik) pertaining to the nutrition of blood vessels.

vaso·tro·pic (-tro′pik) tending to act on blood vessels.

vaso·va·gal (-va′gal) vascular and vagal; see also under *attack.*

vaso·va·sos·to·my (-vah-sos′tah-me) reanastomosis of the ends of the severed ductus (vas) deferens.

vaso·ve·sic·u·lec·to·my (-vĕ-sik″u-lek′tah-me) excision of the ductus (vas) deferens and seminal vesicles.

vas·tu (vahs′too) [Sanskrit] a traditional Hindu system of space design whose purpose is to promote well-being by constructing buildings in harmony with natural forces.

vas·tus (vas′tus) [L.] great; describes muscles.

va·ta (vah′tah) [Sanskrit] in ayurveda, one of the three doshas, condensed from the elements air and space. It is the principle of kinetic energy in the body, is concerned with the nervous system and with circulation, movement, and pathology, and is eliminated from the body through defecation.

VC vital capacity.

VCG vectorcardiogram.

VD venereal disease.

VDH valvular disease of the heart.

VDRL Venereal Disease Research Laboratory.

vec·tion (vek'shun) the carrying of disease germs from an infected person to a well person.

vec·tor (vek'ter) 1. a carrier, especially the animal (usually an arthropod) that transfers an infective agent from one host to another. 2. a plasmid or viral chromosome into whose genome a fragment of foreign DNA is inserted; used to introduce foreign DNA into a host cell in the cloning of DNA. 3. a quantity possessing magnitude, direction, and sense (positivity or negativity). **vecto'rial,** adj. **biological v.,** an arthropod vector in whose body the infecting organism develops or multiplies before becoming infective to the recipient individual. **mechanical v.,** an arthropod vector which transmits an infective organism from one host to another but which is not essential to the life cycle of the parasite.

vec·tor·car·dio·gram (VCG) (vek''ter-kahr'de-o-gram'') the record, usually a photograph, of the loop formed on the oscilloscope in vectorcardiography.

vec·tor·car·di·og·ra·phy (-kahr''de-og'rah-fe) the registration, usually by formation of a loop display on an oscilloscope, of the direction and magnitude (vector) of the moment-to-moment electromotive forces of the heart during one complete cycle. **vectorcardiograph'ic,** adj.

ve·cu·ro·ni·um (vek''u-ro'ne-um) a nondepolarizing neuromuscular blocking agent used as the bromide salt as an adjunct to anesthesia.

VEE Venezuelan equine encephalomyelitis.

veg·an (ve'gan, vej'an) a vegetarian whose diet excludes all food of animal origin.

veg·e·tal (vej'ĕ-t'l) vegetative (defs. 1, 2, and 3).

veg·e·tar·i·an (vej''ĕ-tar'e-an) 1. one who practices vegetarianism. 2. pertaining to vegetarianism.

veg·e·tar·i·an·ism (-tar'e-ah-nizm'') restriction of the diet to disallow some or all foods of animal origin, consuming mainly or wholly foods of plant origin.

veg·e·ta·tion (vej''ĕ-ta'shun) any plantlike fungoid neoplasm or growth; a luxuriant fungus-like growth of pathologic tissue. **marantic v's,** small, sterile, verrucous, fibrinous excrescences occurring in the left-side heart valves in nonbacterial thrombotic (marantic) endocarditis.

veg·e·ta·tive (vej''ĕ-ta''tiv) 1. of, pertaining to, or characteristic of plants. 2. concerned with growth and nutrition, as opposed to reproduction. 3. of or pertaining to asexual reproduction, as by budding or fission.

4. functioning involuntarily or unconsciously. 5. resting; denoting the portion of a cell during which the cell is not replicating.

VEGF vascular endothelial growth factor.

ve·hi·cle (ve'ĭ-k'l) excipient.

veil (vāl) 1. a covering structure. 2. a caul or piece of amniotic sac occasionally covering the face of a newborn child.

Veil·lon·el·la (va''yon-el'ah) a genus of gram-negative bacteria (family Veillonellaceae), found as nonpathogenic parasites in the mouth, intestines, and urogenital and respiratory tracts of humans and other animals.

vein (vān) a vessel in which blood flows toward the heart, in the systemic circulation carrying blood that has given up most of its oxygen. For names of veins of the body, see Table of Veins, and see Plates 20–23. **accompanying v.,** a vein that closely follows the artery of the same name, seen especially in limbs. **afferent v's,** veins that carry blood to an organ. **allantoic v's,** paired vessels that accompany the allantois; they enter the body stalk of the early embryo with the allantois and later form the umbilical veins. **cardinal v's,** embryonic vessels that include the precardinal and postcardinal veins and the ducts of Cuvier (*common cardinal v's*). **central v.,** one that occupies the axis of an organ. **deep v's of lower limb,** veins that drain the lower limb, found accompanying homonymous arteries, and anastomosing freely with the superficial veins; the principal ones are the femoral and popliteal veins. **deep v's of upper limb,** veins that drain the upper limb, found accompanying homonymous arteries, and anastomosing freely with the superficial veins; they include the brachial, ulnar, and radial veins, and their tributaries, all of which ultimately drain into the axillary vein. **diploic v's,** veins of the skull, including the frontal, occipital, anterior temporal, and posterior temporal diploic veins, which form sinuses in the cancellous tissue between the laminae of the cranial bones and communicate with meningeal veins, dural sinuses, pericranial veins, and each other. **emissary v.,** one passing through a foramen of the skull and draining blood from a cerebral sinus into a vessel outside the skull. **gonadal v's,** the ovarian veins and testicular veins. **intrarenal v's,** the veins within the kidney, including the interlobar, arcuate, interlobular, and stellate veins, and the straight venules. **v's of orbit,** the veins that drain the orbit and its structures, including the superior ophthalmic vein and its tributaries and the inferior ophthalmic vein. **postcardinal v's,** paired vessels in the early embryo caudal to the heart.

TABLE OF VEINS

Common Name*	TA Term†	Region*	Receives Blood From*	Drains Into*
accompanying v. of hypoglossal nerve	v. comitans nervi hypoglossi	accompanies hypoglossal nerve	formed by union of deep lingual v. and sublingual v.	facial, lingual, or internal jugular v.
anastomotic v., inferior	v. anastomotica inferior	interconnects superficial middle cerebral v. and transverse sinus		continues inferiorly as facial v.
anastomotic v., superior	v. anastomotica superior	interconnects superficial middle cerebral v. and superior sagittal sinus		
angular v.	v. angularis	between eye and root of nose	formed by union of supratrochlear v. and supraorbital v.	cephalic v. and/or basilic v., or median cubital v.
antebrachial v., median	v. mediana antebrachii	forearm between cephalic v. and basilic v.	a palmar venous plexus	
anterior v's of right ventricle. *See* cardiac v's, anterior				
anterior v. of septum pellucidum	v. anterior septi pellucidi		anterior septum pellucidum	superior thalamostriate v.
apical v. *See* segmental v's, apical				
apicoposterior v. *See* segmental v's, apicoposterior				
appendicular v.	v. appendicularis	accompanies appendicular artery		joins anterior and posterior cecal v's to form ileocolic v.
v. of aqueduct of cochlea	v. aqueductus cochleae	along aqueduct of cochlea	cochlea	superior bulb of internal jugular v.
v. of aqueduct of vestibule	v. aqueductus vestibuli	passes through aqueduct of vestibule	internal ear	superior petrosal sinus
arcuate v's of kidney	vv. arcuatae renis	a series of complete arches across the bases of the renal pyramids, formed by union of interlobular v's and straight venules of kidney		interlobar v's
articular v's	vv. articulares		plexus around temporo-mandibular joint	retromandibular v.
auditory v's, internal. *See* labyrinthine v's				
auricular v's, anterior	vv. auriculares anteriores	anterior part of auricle	external ear	superficial temporal v.
auricular v., posterior	v. auricularis posterior	passes down behind auricle	a plexus on side of head	joins retromandibular v. to form external jugular v.
axillary v.	v. axillaris	the upper limb	formed at lower border of teres major muscle by junction of basilic v. and brachial v.	at lateral border of first rib is continuous with subclavian v.
azygos v.	v. azygos	intercepting trunk for right inter-costal v's as well as connecting branch between superior and inferior venae cavae; it ascends in front of and on right side of vertebrae	ascending lumbar v.	superior vena cava

912

basal v.	v. basalis	passes from anterior perforated substance backward and around cerebral peduncle	anterior perforated substance	internal cerebral v.
basal v., anterior	v. basalis anterior	either of two veins, each draining the anterior basal segment of the inferior lobe of a lung and emptying into the corresponding superior basal v.		
basal v., common	v. basalis communis	either of two veins, each draining the inferior lobe of a lung, via the superior and inferior basal veins, and emptying into the corresponding inferior pulmonary v.		
basal v., inferior	v. basalis inferior	either of two veins, each draining the medial and posterior basal segments of the inferior lobe of a lung and emptying into the corresponding common basal v.		
basal v., superior	v. basalis superior	either of two veins, each draining the lateral and anterior basal segments of the inferior lobe of a lung and emptying into the corresponding common basal v.		
basilic v.	v. basilica	forearm, superficially	ulnar side of dorsal rete of hand	joins brachial v's to form axillary v.
basilic v., median		sometimes present as medial branch of a bifurcation of median antebrachial v.		basilic v.
basivertebral v's	vv. basivertebrales	venous sinuses in cancellous tissue of bodies of vertebrae, which communicate with venous plexus on anterior surface of vertebrae and with anterior external and anterior internal vertebral plexuses		
brachial v's	vv. brachiales	accompany brachial artery		joins basilic v. to form axillary v.
brachiocephalic v.	v. brachiocephalica	either of two veins (right and left) that drain blood from the head, neck, and upper limbs. Each is formed at the root of the neck by union of the ipsilateral internal jugular and subclavian v's. The right passes vertically downward in front of the brachiocephalic artery and the left passes from left to right behind the upper part of the sternum		right and left unite to form superior vena cava
bronchial v's	vv. bronchiales	larger subdivisions of bronchi		azygos v. on left; hemiazygos or superior intercostal v. on right
v. of bulb of penis	v. bulbi penis	bulb of penis		internal pudendal v.
v. of bulb of vestibule	v. bulbi vestibuli	bulb of vestibule of vagina		internal pudendal v.
cardiac v's, anterior	vv. ventriculi dextri anteriores	ascend in subepicardial tissue to cross right part of atrioventricular sulcus	anterior aspect of right ventricle	right atrium of heart
cardiac v., great	v. cardiaca magna	follows anterior longitudinal sulcus	anterior surface of ventricles	coronary sinus
cardiac v., middle	v. cardiaca media	follows posterior longitudinal sulcus	diaphragmatic surface of ventricles	coronary sinus
cardiac v., small	v. cardiaca parva	follows coronary sulcus to left heart	right atrium and ventricle	coronary sinus

*v. = vein; v's = (pl.) veins.

†v. = [L.] vena; vv. = ([L.] pl.) venae.

913

TABLE OF VEINS *Continued*

Common Name*	TA Term†	Region*	Receives Blood From*	Drains Into*
cardiac v's, smallest	vv. cardiacae minimae	numerous small veins arising in myocardium, draining independently into cavities of heart and most readily seen in the atria		right atrium of heart
v's of caudate nucleus	vv. nuclei caudati	the veins of the caudate nucleus, which drain into the superior thalamostriate v.		
vena cava, inferior	vena cava inferior	the venous trunk for the lower limbs and for pelvic and abdominal viscera; it begins at level of fifth lumbar vertebra by union of common iliac v's and ascends on right of aorta		right atrium of heart
vena cava, superior	vena cava superior	the venous trunk draining blood from head, neck, upper limbs, and thorax; it begins by union of 2 brachiocephalic v's and passes directly downward		right atrium of heart
cavernous v's of penis	vv. cavernosae penis		corpora cavernosa	deep v's and dorsal v. of penis
central v's of liver	vv. centrales hepatis	in middle of hepatic lobules	liver substance	hepatic v.
central v. of retina	v. centralis retinae	eyeball	retinal v's	superior ophthalmic v.
central v. of suprarenal gland	v. centralis glandulae suprarenalis	the large single vein into which the various veins within the substance of the gland empty, and which continues at the hilum as the suprarenal v.		
cephalic v.	v. cephalica	winds anteriorly to pass along anterior border of brachioradial muscle; above elbow, ascends along lateral border of biceps and pectoral border of deltoid muscles	radial side of dorsal rete of hand	axillary v.
cephalic v., accessory	v. cephalica accessoria	forearm	dorsal rete of hand	joins cephalic v. just above elbow
cephalic v., median	v. cephalica antebrachii	sometimes present as lateral branch formed by bifurcation of median antebrachial v.		cephalic v.
cerebellar v's, inferior	vv. inferiores cerebelli		inferior surface of cerebellum	straight or sigmoid sinus, or inferior petrosal and occipital sinuses
cerebellar v., precentral	v. precentralis cerebelli	arises in precentral cerebellar fissure, passes anterior and superior to culmen		great cerebral v.
cerebellar v's, superior	vv. superiores cerebelli		superior surface of cerebellum	straight sinus or great cerebral v., or transverse and superior petrosal sinuses
cerebral v's, anterior	vv. anteriores cerebri	accompany anterior cerebral artery		basal v.
cerebral v., deep middle	v. media profunda cerebri	accompanies middle cerebral artery in floor of lateral sulcus		basal v.
cerebral v., great	v. magna cerebri	curves around splenium of corpus callosum	formed by union of the 2 internal cerebral veins	continues as or drains into straight sinus

cerebral v's, inferior	vv. inferiores cerebri	veins that ramify on base and inferolateral surface of brain, those on inferior surface of frontal lobe draining into inferior sagittal sinus and cavernous sinus; those on temporal lobe into superior petrosal sinus and transverse sinus; and those on occipital lobe into straight sinus	
cerebral v's, internal (2)	vv. internae cerebri	formed by union of thalamostriate v. and choroid v.; collect blood from basal nuclei	unite at splenium of corpus callosum to form great cerebral v.
cerebral v., superficial middle	v. media superficialis cerebri	follows lateral cerebral fissure	cavernous sinus
cerebral v's, superior	vv. superiores cerebri	the 8 to 12 veins draining superolateral and medial surfaces of cerebrum toward longitudinal fissure	superior sagittal sinus
cervical v., deep	v. cervicalis profunda	accompanies deep cervical artery down neck	vertebral v. or brachiocephalic v.
cervical v's, transverse	vv. transversae cervicis	accompany transverse cervical artery	subclavian v.
choroid v., inferior	v. choroidea inferior	inferior choroid plexus	basal v.
choroid v., superior	v. choroidea superior	runs whole length of choroid plexus	joins superior thalamostriate v. to form internal cerebral v.
ciliary v's	vv. ciliares	anterior vessels follow anterior ciliary arteries; posterior follow posterior ciliary arteries	choroid plexus, hippocampus, fornix, corpus callosum
		arise in eyeball by branches from ciliary muscle; anterior ciliary v's also receive branches from sinus venosus, sclerae, episcleral v's, and conjunctiva of eyeball	superior ophthalmic v; posterior ciliary v's empty also into inferior ophthalmic v.
circumflex femoral v's, lateral	vv. circumflexae femoris laterales	accompany lateral circumflex femoral artery	femoral v. or deep femoral v.
circumflex femoral v's, medial	vv. circumflexae femoris mediales	accompany medial circumflex femoral artery	femoral v. or deep femoral v.
circumflex iliac v's, deep	v. circumflexa ilium profunda	a common trunk formed by veins accompanying deep circumflex iliac artery	external iliac v.
circumflex iliac v's, superficial	v. circumflexa ilium superficialis	accompanies superficial circumflex iliac artery	great saphenous v.
v. of cochlear caniculus. See v. of aqueduct of cochlea			
colic v., left	v. colica sinistra	accompanies left colic artery	inferior mesenteric v.
colic v., middle	v. colica media	accompanies middle colic artery	superior mesenteric v.
colic v., right	v. colica dextra	accompanies right colic artery	superior mesenteric v.
communicating v's. See perforating v's			
conjunctival v's	vv. conjunctivales	conjunctiva	superior ophthalmic v.

915

TABLE OF VEINS *Continued*

Common Name*	TA Term†	Region*	Receives Blood From*	Drains Into*
coronary v., left		the portion of the great cardiac v. lying in the coronary sulcus	anterior interventricular v.	coronary sinus
coronary v., right			posterior interventricular v.	coronary sinus
costoaxillary v's	vv. costoaxillares	anastomose with upper 6 or 7 posterior intercostal v's	areolar venous plexus	axillary v.
cubital v., median	v. mediana cubiti	the large connecting branch passing obliquely upward across cubital fossa	cephalic v., below elbow	basilic v.
cutaneous v.	v. cutanea	one of the small veins that begin in papillae of skin, form subpapillary plexuses, and open into the subcutaneous veins		
cystic v.	v. cystica	within substance of liver	gallbladder	right branch of portal v.
deep v's of clitoris	vv. profundae clitoridis		clitoris	vesical venous plexus
deep v's of penis	vv. profundae penis	accompany deep artery of penis	penis	dorsal v. of penis
digital v's, palmar	vv. digitales palmares	accompany proper and common palmar digital arteries		superficial palmar venous arch
digital v's, plantar	vv. digitales plantares	plantar surfaces of toes		unite at clefts to form plantar metatarsal v's
digital v's of foot, dorsal	vv. digitales dorsales pedis	dorsal surfaces of toes		unite at clefts to form dorsal metatarsal v's
diploic v., anterior temporal	v. diploica temporalis anterior		lateral portion of frontal bone, anterior part of parietal bone	sphenoparietal sinus internally, and a deep temporal v. externally
diploic v., frontal	v. diploica frontalis		frontal bone	supraorbital v. externally, and superior sagittal sinus internally
diploic v., occipital	v. diploica occipitalis		occipital bone	occipital v. or transverse sinus
diploic v., posterior temporal	v. diploica temporalis posterior		parietal bone	transverse sinus
dorsal v. of clitoris, deep	v. dorsalis profunda clitoridis	accompanies dorsal artery of clitoris		vesical venous plexus
dorsal v's of clitoris, superficial	vv. dorsales superficiales clitoridis		clitoris, subcutaneously	external pudendal v.
dorsal v. of corpus callosum	v. dorsalis corporis callosi		superior surface of corpus callosum	great cerebral v.
dorsal v. of penis, deep	v. dorsalis profunda penis	the single median vein lying subfascially in penis between the dorsal arteries; it begins in small veins around corona of glans, is joined by deep v's of penis as it passes proximally, and passes between arcuate pubic and transverse perineal ligaments, where it divides into a left and a right vein to join prostatic plexus		

dorsal v's of penis, superficial	vv. dorsales superficiales penis		penis, subcutaneously	external pudendal v.
dorsal v's of tongue. *See* lingual v's, dorsal				
emissary v.	vv. emissaria	foramina of skull	dural venous sinuses	scalp v's, deep v's below base of skull
emissary v's, condylar	v. emissaria condylaris	a small vein running through condylar canal of skull connecting sigmoid sinus with vertebral v. or internal jugular v.		
emissary v., mastoid	v. emissaria mastoidea	a small vein passing through mastoid foramen of skull, connecting sigmoid sinus with occipital v. or posterior auricular v.		
emissary v., occipital	v. emissaria occipitalis	an occasional small vein running through a minute foramen in occipital protuberance of skull, connecting confluence of sinuses with occipital v.		
emissary v's, parietal	v. emissaria parietalis	a small vein passing through parietal foramen of skull, connecting superior sagittal sinus with superficial temporal v's		
epigastric v., inferior	v. epigastrica inferior	accompanies inferior epigastric artery		external iliac v.
epigastric v's, superficial	v. epigastrica superficialis	accompanies superficial epigastric artery		great saphenous v. or femoral v.
epigastric v's, superior	vv. epigastricae superiores	accompany superior epigastric artery		internal thoracic v.
episcleral v's	vv. episclerales	around cornea		vorticose v's and ciliary v's
esophageal v's	vv. oesophageales		esophagus	hemiazygos v. and azygos v., or left brachiocephalic v.
ethmoidal v's	vv. ethmoidales	accompany anterior and posterior ethmoidal arteries and emerge from ethmoidal foramina		superior ophthalmic v.
facial v.	v. facialis	the vein beginning at medial angle of eye as angular v., descending behind facial artery, and usually ending in internal jugular v.; sometimes joins retromandibular v. to form a common trunk		
facial v., deep	v. profunda faciei		pterygoid plexus	facial v.
facial v., posterior. *See* retromandibular v.				
facial v., transverse	v. transversa faciei	passes backward with transverse facial artery just below zygomatic arch		retromandibular v.
femoral v.	v. femoralis	follows course of femoral artery in proximal two-thirds of thigh	continuation of popliteal v.	at inguinal ligament becomes external iliac v.
femoral v., deep	v. profunda femoris	accompanies deep femoral artery		femoral v.
fibular v's. *See* peroneal v's				
frontal v's	vv. frontales	superficial superior cerebral veins that drain the frontal cortex		

TABLE OF VEINS *Continued*

Common Name*	TA Term†	Region*	Receives Blood From*	Drains Into*
gastric v., left	v. gastrica sinistra	accompanies left gastric artery		portal v.
gastric v., right	v. gastrica dextra	accompanies right gastric artery		portal v.
gastric v's, short	vv. gastricae breves		left portion of greater curvature of stomach	splenic v.
gastroepiploic v's. *See* gastroomental v's				
gastroomental v., left	v. gastroomentalis sinistra	accompanies left gastroomental artery		splenic v.
gastroomental v., right	v. gastroomentalis dextra	accompanies right gastroomental artery		superior mesenteric v.
genicular v's	vv. geniculares	accompany genicular arteries		popliteal v.
gluteal v's, inferior	vv. gluteae inferiores	accompany inferior gluteal artery; unite into a single vessel after passing through greater sciatic foramen	subcutaneous tissue of back of thigh, muscles of buttock	internal iliac v.
gluteal v's, superior	vv. gluteae superiores	accompany superior gluteal artery and pass through greater sciatic foramen	muscles of buttock	internal iliac v.
hemiazygos v.	v. hemiazygos	an intercepting trunk for lower left posterior intercostal v's; ascends on left side of vertebrae to eighth thoracic vertebra, where it may receive accessory branch, and crosses vertebral column	ascending lumbar v.	azygos v.
hemiazygos v., accessory	v. hemiazygos accessoria	the descending intercepting trunk for upper, often fourth through eighth, left posterior intercostal v's; it lies on left side and at eighth thoracic vertebra joins hemiazygos v. or crosses to right side to join azygos v. directly; above, it may communicate with left superior intercostal v.		azygos v.
hemorrhoidal v's. *See* rectal v's				
hepatic v's	vv. hepaticae	3 large veins (left, middle, right) in an upper group and 6 to 20 small veins (coming from right and caudate lobes) in a lower group	central v's of liver	inferior vena cava on posterior aspect of liver
hepatic v., left	v. hepatica sinistra		central v's on left side of liver	inferior vena cava
hepatic v., middle	v. hepatica intermedia		central v's in middle of liver	inferior vena cava
hepatic v., right	v. hepatica dextra		central v's on right side of liver	inferior vena cava

918

hypophysioportal v's	vv. portales hypophysiales	a system of venules connecting capillaries in the hypothalamus with sinusoidal capillaries in the anterior lobe of the hypophysis	
ileal v's	vv. ileales	ileum	superior mesenteric v.
ileocolic v.	v. ileocolica	accompanies ileocolic artery	superior mesenteric v.
iliac v., common	v. iliaca communis	arises at sacroiliac joint by union of external and internal iliac v's	unites with fellow of opposite side to form inferior vena cava
iliac v., external	v. iliaca externa	continuation of femoral v.	joins internal iliac v. to form common iliac v.
iliac v., internal	v. iliaca interna	formed by union of parietal branches	joins external iliac v. to form common iliac v.
iliolumbar v.	v. iliolumbalis	accompanies iliolumbar artery	internal iliac v. and/or common iliac v.
inferior v. of vermis	v. inferior vermis	inferior surface of cerebellum	straight sinus or one of the sigmoid sinuses
innominate v. *See* brachiocephalic v.			
insular v's	vv. insulares	insula	deep middle cerebral v.
intercapitular v's of foot	vv. intercapitulares pedis	veins at clefts of toes that pass between heads of metatarsal bones and establish communication between dorsal and plantar venous systems of foot	
intercapitular v's of hand	vv. intercapitulares manus	veins at clefts of fingers that pass between heads of metacarpal bones and establish communication between dorsal and palmar venous systems of hand	
intercostal v's, anterior (12 pairs)	vv. intercostales anteriores	accompany anterior thoracic arteries	internal thoracic v's
intercostal v., highest	v. intercostalis suprema	first posterior intercostal v. of either side, which passes over apex of lung	brachiocephalic, vertebral, or superior intercostal v.
intercostal v., left superior	v. intercostalis superior sinistra	crosses arch of aorta	left brachiocephalic v.
intercostal v's, posterior	vv. intercostales posteriores	accompany posterior intercostal arteries	formed by union of second, third, and sometimes fourth posterior intercostal v's
intercostal v., right superior	v. intercostalis superior dextra	intercostal spaces	1: brachiocephalic or vertebral v.; 2,3: superior intercostal v'; 4–11: azygos v. on right; hemiazygos or accessory hemiazygos v. on left
		formed by union of second, third, and sometimes fourth posterior intercostal v's	azygos v.
interlobar v's of kidney	vv. interlobares renis	arcuate v's	unite to form renal v.
interlobular v's of kidney	vv. interlobulares renis	capillary network of renal cortex	arcuate v's
interlobular v's of liver	vv. interlobulares hepatis	pass down between renal pyramids	portal v.
		arise between hepatic lobules	

919

Common Name*	TA Term†	Region*	Receives Blood From*	Drains Into*
interosseous v's, anterior	vv. interosseae anteriores	accompany anterior interosseous artery		ulnar v's
interosseous v's, posterior	vv. interosseae posteriores	accompany posterior interosseous artery		ulnar v's
interventricular v., anterior	v. interventricularis anterior	the portion of the great cardiac v. ascending in the anterior interventricular sulcus		left coronary v.
interventricular v., posterior. *See cardiac v., middle*				
intervertebral v.	v. intervertebralis	vertebral column, passing out through intervertebral foramina	vertebral venous plexuses	in neck, vertebral v.; in thorax, intercostal v's; in abdomen, lumbar v's; in pelvis, lateral sacral v's
jejunal v's	vv. jejunales		jejunum	superior mesenteric v.
jugular v., anterior	v. jugularis anterior	arises under chin and passes down neck		external jugular v., subclavian v., or jugular venous arch
jugular v., external	v. jugularis externa	begins in parotid gland behind angle of jaw and passes down neck	formed by union of retromandibular v. and posterior auricular v.	subclavian v., internal jugular v., or brachiocephalic v.
jugular v., internal	v. jugularis interna	from jugular fossa, descends in neck with internal carotid artery and then with common carotid artery	begins as superior bulb, draining much of head and neck	joins subclavian v. to form brachiocephalic v.
labial v's, anterior	vv. labiales anteriores		anterior aspect of labia in female	external pudendal v.
labial v's, inferior	vv. labiales inferiores		region of lower lip	facial v.
labial v's, posterior	vv. labiales posteriores		labia in female	vesical venous plexus
labial v., superior	v. labialis superior		region of upper lip	facial v.
labyrinthine v's	vv. labyrinthi	pass through internal acoustic meatus	cochlea	inferior petrosal sinus or transverse sinus
lacrimal v.	v. lacrimalis		lacrimal gland	superior ophthalmic v.
laryngeal v., inferior	v. laryngea inferior		larynx	inferior thyroid v.
laryngeal v., superior	v. laryngea superior		larynx	superior thyroid v.
lateral direct v's	vv. directae laterales			
v. of lateral recess of fourth ventricle	v. recessus lateralis ventriculi quarti	passes lateral recess of fourth ventricle	lateral ventricle	great cerebral v.
v. of lateral ventricle, lateral	v. lateralis ventriculi lateralis	passes through lateral wall of lateral ventricle	tonsil of cerebellum	petrosal v.
			temporal and parietal lobes	superior thalamostriate v.

v. of lateral ventricle, medial	v. medialis ventriculi lateralis	passes through medial wall of lateral ventricle	parietal and occipital lobes	internal cerebral v. or great cerebral v.
lingual v.	v. lingualis	a deep vein, following distribution of lingual artery		internal jugular v.
lingual v., deep	v. profunda linguae		deep aspect of tongue	joins sublingual v. to form accompanying v. of hypoglossal nerve
lingual v's, dorsal	vv. dorsales linguae	veins that unite with a small vein accompanying lingual artery and join main lingual trunk		
lingular v.	v. lingularis			a vein draining the lingular segments of the superior lobe of the left lung, emptying into the left superior pulmonary v. and formed by the union of superior and inferior parts
lumbar v's	vv. lumbales	4 or 5 veins on each side accompanying corresponding lumbar arteries and draining posterior wall of abdomen, vertebral canal, spinal cord, and meninges; first 4 usually end in inferior vena cava, although first may end in ascending lumbar v.; fifth is a tributary of common iliac v. or iliolumbar v.; and all are generally united by ascending iliac v.		
lumbar v., ascending	v. lumbalis ascendens	an ascending intercepting vein for lumbar v's on either side; it begins in lateral sacral region and ascends to first lumbar vertebra, where by union with subcostal v. it becomes on right side the azygos v. and on left side the hemiazygos v.		
marginal v., lateral	v. marginalis lateralis	dorsal venous arch, dorsal venous network, superficial v's of sole	lateral side of foot	small saphenous v.
marginal v., left		ascends along left margin of heart	left ventricle	great cardiac v.
marginal v., medial	v. marginalis medialis	dorsal venous arch, dorsal venous network, superficial v's of sole	medial side of foot	great saphenous v.
marginal v., right	v. marginalis dextra	ascends along right margin of heart	right ventricle	right atrium or anterior cardiac v's
masseteric v's			masseter muscle	facial v.
maxillary v's	vv. maxillares	from pterygoid plexus, usually forming a single short trunk		join superficial temporal v. in parotid gland to form retromandibular v.
mediastinal v's	vv. mediastinales		anterior mediastinum	brachiocephalic v., azygos v., or superior vena cava
v's of medulla oblongata	vv. medullae oblongatae		medulla oblongata	v's of spinal cord, dural venous sinuses, inferior petrosal sinus, superior bulb of jugular v.
meningeal v's	vv. meningeae	accompany meningeal arteries	dura mater (also communicate with lateral lacunae)	regional sinuses and veins
meningeal v's, middle	vv. meningeae mediae	accompany middle meningeal artery		pterygoid venous plexus
mesenteric v., inferior	v. mesenterica inferior	follows distribution of inferior mesenteric artery		splenic v.

TABLE OF VEINS *Continued*

Common Name*	TA Term†	Region*	Receives Blood From*	Drains Into*
mesenteric v., superior	v. mesenterica superior	follows distribution of superior mesenteric artery		joins splenic v. to form portal v.
metacarpal v's, dorsal	vv. metacarpales dorsales	veins arising from union of dorsal veins of adjacent fingers and passing proximally to join in forming dorsal venous network of hand		deep palmar venous arch
metacarpal v's, palmar	vv. metacarpales palmares	accompany palmar metacarpal arteries		dorsal venous arch
metatarsal v's, dorsal	vv. metatarsales dorsales		arise from dorsal digital v's of toes at clefts of toes	dorsal venous arch
metatarsal v's, plantar	vv. metatarsales plantares	deep veins of foot	arise from plantar digital v's at clefts of toes	plantar venous arch
middle lobe v.	v. lobi medii		a vein draining the middle lobe of the right lung, emptying into the right superior pulmonary v. and formed by the union of lateral and medial parts	
musculophrenic v's	vv. musculophrenicae	accompany musculophrenic artery	parts of diaphragm and wall of thorax and abdomen	internal thoracic v's
nasal v's, external	vv. nasales externae	small ascending branches from nose	supraorbital v.	angular v., facial v.
nasofrontal v.	v. nasofrontalis	enters orbit		superior ophthalmic v.
oblique v. of left atrium	v. obliqua atrii sinistri	left atrium of heart		coronary sinus
obturator v's	vv. obturatoriae	enter pelvis through obturator canal	hip joint and regional muscles	internal iliac v. and/or inferior epigastric v.
occipital v.	v. occipitalis	scalp; follows distribution of occipital artery		opens under trapezius muscle into suboccipital venous plexus, or accompanies occipital artery to end in internal jugular v.
v. of olfactory gyrus	v. gyri olfactorii		olfactory gyrus	basal v.
ophthalmic v., inferior	v. ophthalmica inferior	a vein formed by confluence of muscular and ciliary branches, and running backward either to join superior ophthalmic v. or to open directly into cavernous sinus; it sends a communicating branch through inferior orbital fissure to join pterygoid venous plexus		
ophthalmic v., superior	v. ophthalmica superior	a vein beginning at medial angle of eye, where it communicates with frontal, supraorbital, and angular v's; it follows distribution of ophthalmic artery, and may be joined by inferior ophthalmic v. at superior orbital fissure before opening into cavernous sinus		
ovarian v., left	v. ovarica sinistra		pampiniform plexus of broad ligament on left	left renal v.
ovarian v., right	v. ovarica dextra		pampiniform plexus of broad ligament on right	inferior vena cava

922

	Latin (NA)	Description	Drains into / becomes
palatine v., external	v. palatina externa	tonsils and soft palate	facial v.
palpebral v's	vv. palpebrales	small branches from eyelids	superior ophthalmic v.
palpebral v's, inferior	vv. palpebrales inferiores	lower eyelid	facial v.
palpebral v's, superior	vv. palpebrales superiores	upper eyelid	angular v.,
pancreatic v's	vv. pancreaticae	pancreas	splenic v., superior mesenteric v.
pancreaticoduodenal v's	vv. pancreaticoduodenales	4 veins that drain blood from pancreas and duodenum, closely following pancreaticoduodenal arteries, a superior and an inferior vein originating from an anterior and a posterior venous arcade; anterior superior v. joins right gastroomental v., and posterior superior v. joins portal v.; anterior and posterior inferior v's join, sometimes as one trunk, uppermost jejunal v. or superior mesenteric v.	
paraumbilical v's	vv. paraumbilicales	veins that communicate with portal v. above and descend to anterior abdominal wall to anastomose with superior and inferior epigastric and superior vesical v's in region of umbilicus; they form a significant part of collateral circulation of portal v. in event of hepatic obstruction	
parotid v's	vv. parotideae	parotid gland	superficial temporal v.
pectoral v's	vv. pectorales	pectoral region	subclavian v.
peduncular v's	vv. pedunculares	cerebral peduncle	basal v.
perforating v's	vv. perforantes	valved veins that drain blood from the superficial to the deep veins in the leg and foot	
pericardiacophrenic v's	vv. pericardiacophrenicae	pericardium and diaphragm	left brachiocephalic v.
pericardial v's	vv. pericardiacae		brachiocephalic, inferior thyroid, and azygos v's, superior vena cava
peroneal v.	vv. fibulares	accompany peroneal artery	posterior tibial v.
petrosal v.	v. petrosa	a short trunk arising from the union of 4 or 5 cerebellar and pontine v's and terminating in the superior petrosal sinus	
pharyngeal v's	vv. pharyngeae	pharyngeal plexus	internal jugular v.
phrenic v's, inferior	vv. phrenicae inferiores	accompany inferior phrenic arteries	on right, enters inferior vena cava; on left, enters left suprarenal or renal v., or inferior vena cava
phrenic v's, superior	vv. phrenicae superiores	superior surface of diaphragm	azygos v., hemiazygos v.
v's of pons	vv. pontis	pons	basal v., cerebellar v's, petrosal or venous sinuses, or venous plexus of foramen ovale
pontomesencephalic v., anterior	v. pontomesencephalica anterior	superior and anterior aspects of pons in midline of interpeduncular fossa	basal v., petrosal v.
popliteal v.	v. poplitea	follows popliteal artery; formed by union of anterior and posterior tibial v's	at adductor hiatus becomes femoral v.

Common Name*	TA Term†	Region*	Receives Blood From*	Drains Into*
portal v.	v. portae hepatis	a short, thick trunk formed by union of superior mesenteric and splenic v's behind neck of pancreas; it ascends to right end of porta hepatis, where it divides into successively smaller branches, following branches of hepatic artery, until it forms a capillarylike system of sinusoids that permeates entire substance of liver		
posterior v. of corpus callosum	v. posterior corporis callosi		posterior surface of corpus callosum	great cerebral v.
posterior v. of left ventricle	v. ventriculi sinistri posterior		posterior surface of left ventricle	coronary sinus
posterior v. of septum pellucidum	v. posterior septi pellucidi		septum pellucidum	superior thalamostriate v.
prepyloric v.	v. prepylorica	accompanies prepyloric artery, passing upward over anterior surface of junction between pylorus and duodenum		right gastric v.
profunda femoris v. *See* femoral v., deep				
profunda linguae v. *See* lingual v., deep				
v. of pterygoid canal	v. canalis pterygoidei	passes through pterygoid canal		pterygoid plexus
pudendal v's, external	vv. pudendae externae	follow distribution of external pudendal artery		great saphenous v.
pudendal v., internal	v. pudenda interna	follows course of internal pudendal artery		internal iliac v.
pulmonary v., left inferior	v. pulmonalis sinistra inferior		lower lobe of left lung (superior segmental and common basal v's)	left atrium of heart
pulmonary v., left superior	v. pulmonalis sinistra superior		upper lobe of left lung (apicoposterior, anterior segmental, and lingular v's)	left atrium of heart
pulmonary v., right inferior	v. pulmonalis dextra inferior		lower lobe of right lung (superior segmental and common basal v's)	left atrium of heart
pulmonary v., right superior	v. pulmonalis dextra superior		upper and middle lobes of right lung (middle lobe, apical, anterior segmental, and posterior segmental v's)	left atrium of heart
pyloric v. *See* gastric v., right				

radial v's	vv. radiales	accompany radial artery	brachial v's
ranine v. *See* sublingual v.			
rectal v's, inferior	vv. rectales inferiores	rectal plexus	internal pudendal v.
rectal v's, middle	vv. rectales mediae	rectal plexus	internal iliac and superior rectal v's
rectal v., superior	v. rectalis superior	upper part of rectal plexus	inferior mesenteric v.
renal v's	vv. renales		inferior vena cava at level of second lumbar vertebra
		interlobar v's; left also drains left testicular (ovarian), left suprarenal, and (sometimes) inferior phrenic v's	
retromandibular v.	v. retromandibularis	the vein formed in upper part of parotid gland behind neck of mandible by union of maxillary and superficial temporal v's; it passes downward through the gland, communicates with facial v. and, emerging from the gland, joins with posterior auricular v. to form external jugular v.	
sacral v's, lateral	vv. sacrales laterales	follow lateral sacral arteries	help form lateral sacral plexus; empty into internal iliac v. or superior gluteal v's
sacral v., median	v. sacralis mediana	follows median sacral artery	common iliac v.
saphenous v., accessory	v. saphena accessoria	when present, medial and posterior superficial parts of thigh	great saphenous v.
saphenous v., great	v. saphena magna	extends from dorsum of foot to just below inguinal ligament	femoral v.
saphenous v., small	v. saphena parva	drains foot and leg via numerous tributaries	popliteal v.
		from behind ankle passes up back of leg to knee	
scleral v's	vv. sclerales	sclera	anterior ciliary v's
scrotal v's, anterior	vv. scrotales anteriores	anterior aspect of scrotum	external pudendal v.
scrotal v's, posterior	vv. scrotales posteriores	posterior aspect of scrotum	vesical venous plexus
segmental v., anterior	v. anterior lobi superioris	either of two veins, each draining the anterior segment of the superior lobe of a lung and emptying into the corresponding superior pulmonary v.	
segmental v., apical	v. apicalis	apical segment of superior lobe of right lung	right superior pulmonary v.
segmental v., apicoposterior	v. apicoposterior	apicoposterior segment of superior lobe of left lung	left superior pulmonary v.
segmental v., posterior	v. posterior lobi superioris pulmonis dextri	posterior segment of superior lobe of right lung	right superior pulmonary v.
segmental v., superior	v. superior lobi inferioris	either of two veins, each draining the superior segment of the inferior lobe of a lung and emptying into the corresponding inferior pulmonary v.	
sigmoid v's	vv. sigmoideae	sigmoid colon	inferior mesenteric v.

925

TABLE OF VEINS *Continued*

Common Name*	TA Term†	Region*	Receives Blood From*	Drains Into*
spinal v's, anterior and posterior spiral v. of modiolus	{ vv. spinales anteriores vv. spinales posteriores	anastomosing networks of small veins that drain blood from spinal cord and its pia mater into internal vertebral venous plexuses modiolus		labyrinthine v's
splenic v.	v. splenica	passes from left to right of neck of pancreas	formed by union of several branches at hilum of spleen	joins superior mesenteric v. to form portal v.
stellate v's of kidney	vv. stellatae renis	surface of kidney	superficial parts of renal cortex	interlobular v's of kidney
sternocleidomastoid v.	v. sternocleidomastoidea	follows course of sternocleidomastoid artery		internal jugular v.
stylomastoid v.	v. stylomastoidea	follows stylomastoid artery		retromandibular v.
subclavian v.	v. subclavia	follows subclavian artery		joins internal jugular v. to form brachiocephalic v.
subcostal v.	v. subcostalis	accompanies subcostal artery		joins ascending lumbar v. to form azygos v. on right, hemiazygos v. on left
subcutaneous v's of abdomen	vv. subcutaneae abdominis	superficial layers of abdominal wall		
sublingual v.	v. sublingualis	follows sublingual artery		lingual v.
submental v.	v. submentalis	follows submental artery		facial v.
superior v. of vermis	v. superior vermis	runs forward and medially across superior vermis	superior surface of cerebellum	straight sinus or great cerebral v.
supraorbital v.	v. supraorbitalis	passes down forehead lateral to supratrochlear v.		joins supratrochlear v. at root of nose to form angular v.
suprarenal v., left	v. suprarenalis sinistra		left suprarenal gland	left renal v.
suprarenal v., right	v. suprarenalis dextra		right suprarenal gland	inferior vena cava
suprascapular v.	v. suprascapularis	accompanies suprascapular artery		usually into external jugular v., occasionally into subclavian v.
supratrochlear v's (2)	vv. supratrochleares	descend to root of nose		each joins supraorbital v. at root of nose to form angular v.
sural v's	vv. surales	accompany sural arteries	calf	popliteal v.
temporal v's, deep	vv. temporales profundae	descends under fascia to zygoma	deep portions of temporal muscle arises in substance of temporal muscle	pterygoid plexus
temporal v., middle	v. temporalis media			joins superficial temporal v.
temporal v's, superficial	vv. temporales superficiales	veins that drain lateral part of scalp frontal and parietal regions, the branches forming a single superficial temporal v. in front of ear, just above zygoma; this descending vein receives middle temporal and transverse facial v's and, entering parotid gland, unites with maxillary v. deep to neck of mandible to form retromandibular v.		

testicular v., left	v. testicularis sinistra		left pampiniform plexus	left renal v.
testicular v., right	v. testicularis dextra		right pampiniform plexus	inferior vena cava
thalamostriate v's, inferior	vv. thalamostriatae inferiores		anterior perforated substance of brain	join deep middle cerebral and anterior cerebral v's to form basal v.
thalamostriate v., superior	v. thalamostriata superior		corpus striatum and thalamus	joins choroid v. to form internal cerebral v.
thoracic v's, internal	vv. thoracicae internae	2 veins formed by junction of the veins accompanying internal thoracic artery of either side; each continues along the artery to open into brachiocephalic v.		brachiocephalic v.
thoracic v., lateral	v. thoracica lateralis	accompanies lateral thoracic artery		axillary v.
thoracoacromial v.	v. thoracoacromialis	follows thoracoacromial artery		subclavian v.
thoracoepigastric v's	vv. thoracoepigastricae	long, longitudinal, superficial veins in anterolateral subcutaneous tissue of trunk		superiorly into lateral thoracic v.; inferiorly into femoral v.
thymic v's	vv. thymicae		thymus	left brachiocephalic v.
thyroid v., inferior	v. thyroidea inferioris	either of two veins, left and right, that drain thyroid plexus into left and right brachiocephalic v's; occasionally they may unite into a common trunk to empty, usually into left brachiocephalic v.		left brachiocephalic v.
thyroid v's, middle	vv. thyroideae mediae		thyroid gland	internal jugular v.
thyroid v., superior	v. thyroidea superior	arises from side of upper part of thyroid gland	thyroid gland	internal jugular v., occasionally in common with facial v.
tibial v's, anterior	vv. tibiales anteriores	accompany anterior tibial artery		join posterior tibial v's to form popliteal v.
tibial v's, posterior	vv. tibiales posteriores	accompany posterior tibial artery		join anterior tibial v's to form popliteal v.
tracheal v's	vv. tracheales		trachea	brachiocephalic v.
tympanic v's	vv. tympanicae	small veins from middle ear that pass through petrotympanic fissure and open into the plexus around temporomandibular joint		retromandibular v.
ulnar v's	vv. ulnares	accompany ulnar artery		join radial v's at elbow to form brachial v's
v. of uncus	v. uncalis		uncus	ipsilateral inferior cerebral v.
uterine v's	vv. uterinae		uterine plexus	internal iliac v's
ventricular v., inferior	v. ventricularis inferior		temporal lobe	basal v.
vertebral v.	v. vertebralis	passes with vertebral artery through foramina of transverse processes of upper to cervical vertebrae	suboccipital plexus	brachiocephalic v.
vertebral v's, accessory	v. vertebralis accessoria	descends with vertebral v. and emerges through transverse foramen of cervical vertebra C7	plexus formed around vertebral artery by vertebral v.	brachiocephalic v.

TABLE OF VEINS *Continued*

Common Name*	TA Term†	Region*	Receives Blood From*	Drains Into*
vertebral v., anterior	v. vertebralis anterior	accompanies ascending cervical artery	venous plexus adjacent to more cranial cervical transverse processes	vertebral v.
v's of vertebral column	vv. columnae vertebralis	a plexiform venous network extending the length of the vertebral column, outside or inside the vertebral canal; the anterior and posterior external and anterior and posterior internal groups freely anastomose		intervertebral v's
vesical v's	vv. vesicales		vesical plexus	internal iliac v.
vestibular v's	vv. vestibulares		vestibule	labyrinthine v's
v's of Vieussens. *See* cardiac v's, anterior				
vorticose v's	vv. vorticosae	4 veins piercing sclera	choroid	superior ophthalmic vein

precardinal v's, paired venous trunks in the embryo cranial to the heart. **pulmonary v's,** the four veins, right and left superior and right and left inferior, that return aerated blood from the lungs to the left atrium of the heart. **pulp v's,** vessels draining the venous sinuses of the spleen. **renal v's,** 1. see *Table of Veins.* 2. intrarenal v's. **subcardinal v's,** paired vessels in the embryo, replacing the postcardinal veins and persisting to some degree as definitive vessels. **sublobular v's,** tributaries of the hepatic veins that receive the central veins of hepatic lobules. **superficial v's of lower limb,** veins that drain the lower limb, found immediately beneath the skin, and anastomosing freely with the deep veins; the principal ones are the great and small saphenous veins. **superficial v's of upper limb,** veins that drain the upper limb, found immediately beneath the skin, and anastomosing freely with the deep veins; they include the cephalic, basilic, and median cubital and antebrachial veins, and their tributaries, all of which ultimately drain into the axillary vein. **supracardinal v's,** paired vessels in the embryo, developing later than the subcardinal veins and persisting chiefly as the lower segment of the inferior vena cava. **trabecular v's,** vessels coursing in splenic trabeculae, formed by tributary pulp veins. **umbilical v's,** the two veins *(left umbilical v.* and *right umbilical v.)* that carry blood from the placenta to the sinus venosus of the heart in the early embryo; the right later degenerates, leaving the left as a single umbilical vein which carries the blood from the placenta to the ductus venosus. **varicose v.,** a dilated, tortuous vein, usually in the subcutaneous tissues of the leg; incompetency of the venous valve is associated. **vesalian v.,** an emissary vein connecting the cavernous sinus with the pterygoid venous plexus. **vitelline v's,** veins that return the blood from the yolk sac to the primordial heart of the early embryo.

ve·la·men (ve-la'men) pl. *vela'mina.* [L.] a membrane, meninx, or velum.

vel·a·men·tous (vel″ah-men'tus) membranous and pendent; like a veil.

vel·lus (vel'us) [L.] 1. the fine hair that succeeds the lanugo over most of the body. 2. a structure resembling this fine hair.

ve·lo·pha·ryn·ge·al (vel″o-fah-rin'je-al) pertaining to the soft palate and pharynx.

ve·lum (ve'lum) pl. *ve'la.* [L.] a covering structure or veil. **ve'lar,** adj. **v. inter·po′situm ce'rebri,** membranous roof of the third ventricle. **medullary v.,** one of the two portions *(superior medullary v.* and *inferior*

medullary v.) of the white substance that form the roof of the fourth ventricle. **v. pala·ti′num,** soft palate.

ve·na (ve'nah) pl. *ve'nae.* [L.] vein. **ve'nae ca'vae,** see *Table of Veins.* **ve'nae vaso′rum,** small veins that return blood from the tissues making up the walls of the blood vessels themselves.

ve·na·ca·vo·gram (ve″nah-ka'vo-gram) a film obtained by venacavography.

ve·na·ca·vog·ra·phy (-ka-vog′rah-fe) radiography of a vena cava, usually the inferior vena cava.

ve·nec·ta·sia (ve″nek-ta'zhah) a varicosity of a vein.

ve·nec·to·my (ve-nek′tah-me) phlebectomy.

ve·ne·re·al (vĕ-nēr′e-al) due to or propagated by sexual intercourse.

ve·ne·re·ol·o·gist (vĕ-nēr″e-ol'ah-jist) a specialist in venereology.

ve·ne·re·ol·o·gy (-ol'ah-je) the study and treatment of venereal diseases.

vene·sec·tion (ven″ĕ-sek'shun) phlebotomy.

veni·punc·ture (ven″ĭ-pungk'chur) surgical puncture of a vein.

veni·su·ture (-soo'chur) phleborrhaphy.

ven·la·fax·ine (ven″lah-fak'sēn) an inhibitor of serotonin and norepinephrine reuptake that potentiates neurotransmitter activity in the central nervous system; used as the hydrochloride salt as an antidepressant and antianxiety agent.

ven(o)- word element [L.], *vein.*

ve·nog·ra·phy (ve-nog′rah-fe) phlebography.

ven·om (ven'om) a poison, especially one normally secreted by a serpent, insect, or other animal.

ve·no·mo·tor (ve″no-mo′ter) controlling dilation or constriction of the veins.

ve·no·oc·clu·sive (-ŏ-kloo′siv) characterized by obstruction of the veins.

ve·no·peri·to·ne·os·to·my (-per″ĭ-to″ne-os′tah-me) anastomosis of the saphenous vein with the peritoneum for drainage of ascites.

ve·no·pres·sor (-pres′er) 1. pertaining to venous blood pressure. 2. an agent that causes venous constriction.

ve·nor·rha·phy (ve-nor′ah-fe) suture of a vein.

ve·no·scle·ro·sis (-sklĕ-ro′sis) phlebosclerosis.

ve·nos·i·ty (ve-nos′ĭ-te) 1. the condition of being venous. 2. excess of venous blood in a part. 3. a plentiful supply of veins.

ve·no·sta·sis (ve″no-sta'sis) venous stasis.

ve·not·o·my (ve-not′ah-me) phlebotomy.

ve·nous (ve'nus) pertaining to the veins.

ve·no·ve·nos·to·my (ve″no-ve-nos′tah-me) phlebophlebostomy.

vent (vent) an opening or outlet, such as an opening that discharges pus, or the anus.

ven·ter (ven'ter) pl. *ven'tres.* [L.] 1. a fleshy contractile part of a muscle. 2. abdomen. 3. a hollowed part or cavity.

ven·ti·la·tion (ven″tĭ-la'shun) 1. breathing; the exchange of air between the lungs and the environment, including inhalation and exhalation. 2. circulation, replacement, or purification of the air or other gas in a space. 3. the equipment with which this is done. 4. verbalization of one's problems, emotions, or feelings. **alveolar v.,** the amount of air that reaches the alveoli and is available for gas exchange with the blood per unit time. **high-frequency v.,** mechanical ventilation in which small tidal volumes are delivered at a high respiration rate. **maximum voluntary v.,** maximal breathing capacity; the greatest volume of gas that can be breathed per minute by voluntary effort. **mechanical v.,** that accomplished by extrinsic means; usually either *negative pressure v.* or *positive pressure v.* **minute v.,** total v.; the total volume of gas in liters exhaled from the lungs per minute. **negative pressure v.,** mechanical ventilation in which negative pressure is generated on the outside of the patient's chest and transmitted to the interior to expand the lungs and allow air to flow in; used with weak or paralyzed patients. **positive pressure v.,** mechanical ventilation in which air is delivered into the airways and lungs under positive pressure, usually via an endotracheal tube, producing positive airway pressure during inspiration. **pulmonary v.,** a measure of the rate of ventilation, referring to the total exchange of air between the lungs and the ambient air. **total v.,** minute v.

ven·ti·la·tor (ven'tĭ-la-tor) 1. an apparatus for qualifying the air breathed through it. 2. a device for giving artificial respiration or aiding in pulmonary ventilation. **cuirass v.,** one applied only to the chest, either completely surrounding the trunk or only on the front of the chest and abdomen.

ven·ti·la·to·ry (-lah-tor″e) pertaining to ventilation.

ven·trad (ven'trad) toward a belly, venter, or ventral aspect.

ven·tral (ven'tral) 1. pertaining to the abdomen or to any venter. 2. directed toward or situated on the belly surface; opposite of dorsal.

ven·tra·lis (ven-tra'lis) [L.] ventral.

ventri- see *ventr(o)-.*

ven·tri·cle (ven'trĭ-k'l) a small cavity or chamber, as in the brain or heart. **ventric′ular,** adj. **v. of Arantius,** the rhomboid fossa, especially its lower end. **double-inlet v.,** a congenital anomaly in which both atrioventricular valves, or a single common atrioventricular valve, open into a single ventricle, which usually resembles the left ventricle morphologically (*double-inlet left v.*) but may resemble the right (*double-inlet right v.*) or neither or both ventricles. **double-outlet left v.,** a rare anomaly in which both great arteries arise from the left ventricle, often associated with a hypoplastic right ventricle, ventricular septal defect, and other cardiac malformations. **double-outlet right v.,** incomplete transposition of the great ventricles in which both the aorta and the pulmonary artery arise from the right ventricle, associated with a ventricular septal defect. **fifth v.,** the median cleft between the two laminae of the septum pellucidum. **fourth v. of cerebrum,** a median cavity in the hindbrain, containing cerebrospinal fluid. **v. of larynx,** the space between the true and false vocal cords. **lateral v. of cerebrum,** the cavity in each cerebral hemisphere, derived from the cavity of the embryonic tube, containing cerebrospinal fluid. **left v. of heart,** the lower chamber of the left side of the heart, which pumps oxygenated blood out through the aorta to all the tissues of the body. **Morgagni's v.,** v. of larynx. **pineal v.,** an extension of the third ventricle into the stalk of the pineal body. **right v. of heart,** the lower chamber of the right side of the heart, which pumps venous blood through the pulmonary trunk and arteries to the capillaries of the lungs. **third v. of cerebrum,** a narrow cleft below the corpus callosum, within the diencephalon between the two thalami. **Verga's v.,** an occasional space between the corpus callosum and fornix.

ven·tric·u·li·tis (ven-trik″u-li'tis) inflammation of a ventricle, especially a cerebral ventricle.

ventricul(o)- word element [L.], *ventricle* (of heart or brain).

ven·tric·u·lo·atri·al (ven-trik″u-lo-a'tre-al) connecting a cerebral ventricle with a cardiac atrium, as a shunt in the treatment of hydrocephalus.

ven·tric·u·lo·atri·os·to·my (-a″tre-os'tah-me) ventriculoatrial shunt.

ven·tric·u·lo·en·ceph·a·li·tis (-en-sef″ah-li'tis) ventriculitis accompanied by encephalitis.

ven·tric·u·log·ra·phy (ven-trik″u-log'rah-fe) 1. radiography of the cerebral ventricles after introduction of air or other contrast medium. 2. radiography of a ventricle of the heart after injection of a contrast medium.

first pass v., see under *angiocardiography.*
gated blood pool v., equilibrium radionuclide angiocardiography. **radionuclide v.,**
see under *angiocardiography.*

ven·tric·u·lom·e·try (ven-trik″u-lom′ĕ-tre)
measurement of intracranial pressure.

ven·tric·u·lo·peri·to·ne·al (ven-trik″u-lo-
per″ĭ-to-ne′al) connecting a cerebral ventricle
with the peritoneum, as a shunt in the treatment of hydrocephalus.

ven·tric·u·lo·punc·ture (-pungk′chur) ventricular puncture.

ven·tric·u·los·co·py (ven-trik″u-los′kah-pe)
endoscopic or cystoscopic examination of
cerebral ventricles.

ven·tric·u·los·to·my (ven-trik″u-los′tah-me)
surgical creation of a free communication
or shunt between the third ventricle and the
interpeduncular cistern for relief of hydrocephalus.

ven·tric·u·lo·sub·arach·noid (ven-trik″u-
lo-sub″ah-rak′noid) pertaining to the cerebral
ventricles and subarachnoid space.

ven·tric·u·lot·o·my (ven-trik″u-lot′ah-me)
incision of a ventricle of the brain or heart.

ven·tric·u·lus (ven-trik′u-lus) pl. *ventri′culi.*
[L.] 1. ventricle. 2. stomach.

ven·tri·duct (ven′trĭ-dukt) to bring or carry
ventrad.

ventr(o)- word element [L.], *belly; front (anterior) aspect of the body; ventral aspect.*

ven·tro·fix·a·tion (ven″tro-fik-sa′shun) fixation of a viscus, e.g., the uterus, to the abdominal wall.

ven·tro·hys·tero·pexy (-his′ter-o-pek″se)
ventrofixation of the uterus.

ven·tro·lat·er·al (-lat′er-al) both ventral and
lateral.

ven·tro·me·di·an (-me′de-an) both ventral
and median.

ven·tro·pos·te·ri·or (-pos-tēr′e-or) both
ventral and posterior (caudal).

ven·trose (ven′trōs) having a bellylike expansion.

ven·tro·sus·pen·sion (ven″tro-sus-pen′-
shun) ventrofixation.

ven·trot·o·my (ven-trot′ah-me) celiotomy.

ven·u·la (ven′u-lah) pl. *ve′nulae.* [L.] venule.

ven·ule (ven′ūl) any of the small vessels that
collect blood from the capillary plexuses and
join to form veins. **ven′ular,** adj. **postcapillary v.,** venous capillary. **stellate v's of
kidney,** stellate veins of kidney; see *Table of
Veins.* **straight v's of kidney,** venules that
drain the papillary part of the kidney and
empty into the arcuate veins.

ven·u·li·tis (ven″u-li′tis) inflammation of the
venules.

ve·rap·a·mil (vĕ-rap′ah-mil) a calcium channel blocker that dilates coronary arteries and
decreases myocardial oxygen demand, used as
the hydrochloride salt in the treatment of
angina pectoris and of hypertension and the
treatment and prophylaxis of supraventricular
tachyarrhythmias.

ver·big·er·a·tion (ver-bij″er-a′shun) stereotyped and meaningless repetition of words
and phrases.

verge (verj) a circumference or ring. **anal v.,**
the opening of the anus on the surface of the
body.

ver·gence (ver′jens) a disjunctive reciprocal
rotation of both eyes so that the axes of
fixation are not parallel; the kind of vergence
is indicated by a prefix, e.g., convergence,
divergence.

ver·mi·cide (ver′mĭ-sīd) anthelmintic (2).

ver·mic·u·lar (ver-mik′u-ler) wormlike in
shape or appearance.

ver·mic·u·la·tion (ver-mik″u-la′shun)
1. wormlike movement. 2. peristalsis.

ver·mic·u·lous (ver-mik′u-lus) 1. wormlike.
2. infested with worms.

ver·mi·form (ver′mĭ-form) vermicular.

ver·mi·fuge (ver′mĭ-fūj) anthelmintic (2).
vermifu′gal, adj.

ver·mil·ion·ec·to·my (ver-mil″yon-ek′-
tah-me) excision of the vermilion border of
the lip.

ver·min (ver′min) 1. an external animal
parasite. 2. such parasites collectively.
ver′minous, adj.

ver·mis (ver′mis) [L.] a wormlike structure,
particularly the vermis cerebelli. **v. cere-
bel′li,** the median part of the cerebellum,
between the two lateral hemispheres.

ver·nal (ver′n'l) pertaining to or occurring in
the spring.

ver·nix (ver′niks) [L.] varnish. **v. caseo′sa,**
an unctuous substance composed of sebum
and desquamated epithelial cells, which covers
the skin of the fetus.

ver·ru·ca (vĕ-roo′kah) pl. *verru′cae.* [L.] 1. a
common wart; a lobulated hyperplastic epidermal lesion with a horny surface, caused by
a human papillomavirus, transmitted by contact or autoinoculation, and usually occurring
on the dorsa of the hands and fingers. 2. any
of various nonviral, wartlike epidermal proliferations. **v. pla′na,** flat wart. **v. vulga′ris,**
verruca (1).

ver·ru·ci·form (vĕ-roo′sĭ-form) wartlike.

ver·ru·cose (vĕ-roo′kōs) verrucous.

ver·ru·cous (vĕ-roo′kus) rough; warty.

ver·ru·ga (vĕ-roo′gah) [Sp.] wart. **v. peru-
a′na,** the second or chronic stage of bartonellosis.

ver·si·co·lor (ver″si-kol′er) variegated; having a variety of colors, or changing in color.

ver·sion (ver′zhun) 1. the act or process of turning or changing direction. 2. the situation of an organ or part in relation to an established normal position. 3. in gynecology, misalignment or tilting of the uterus. 4. in obstetrics, the manual turning of the fetus. 5. in opthalmology, rotation of the eyes in the same direction. **bimanual v.,** version by combined external and internal manipulation. **bipolar v.,** turning effected by acting upon both poles of the fetus, either by external or combined version. **cephalic v.,** turning of the fetus so that the head presents. **combined v.,** bimanual v. **external v.,** turning effected by outside manipulation. **internal v.,** turning effected by the hand or fingers inserted through the dilated cervix. **pelvic v.,** version by manipulation of the breech. **podalic v.,** conversion of a more unfavorable presentation into a footing presentation. **spontaneous v.,** one which occurs without aid from any extraneous force.

ver·te·bra (ver′tĕ-brah) pl. *ver′tebrae*. [L.] any of the 33 bones of the vertebral (spinal) column, comprising 7 *cervical*, 12 *thoracic*, 5 *lumbar*, 5 *sacral*, and 4 *coccygeal vertebrae*. See *Table of Bones*. **ver′tebral,** adj. **basilar v.,** the lowest lumbar vertebra. **cervical vertebrae,** the seven vertebrae closest to the skull, constituting the skeleton of the neck. Symbols C1–C7. **coccygeal vertebrae,** the three to five rudimentary segments of the vertebral column most distant from the skull, which fuse to form the coccyx. **cranial vertebrae,** the segments of the skull and facial bones, regarded by some as modified vertebrae. **dorsal vertebrae,** thoracic vertebrae. **false vertebrae,** those vertebrae which normally fuse with adjoining segments; the sacral and coccygeal vertebrae. **lumbar vertebrae,** the five segments of the vertebral column between the twelfth thoracic vertebra and the sacrum. Symbols L1–L5. **odontoid v.,** the second cervical vertebra (axis). **v. pla′na,** a condition of spondylitis in which the body of the vertebra is reduced to a sclerotic disk. **sacral vertebrae,** the segments (usually five) below the lumbar vertebrae, which normally fuse to form the sacrum. Symbols S1–S5. **sternal v.,** sternebra. **thoracic vertebrae,** the 12 segments of the vertebral column between the cervical and the lumbar vertebrae, giving attachment to the ribs and forming part of the posterior wall of the thorax. Symbols T1–T12. **true vertebrae,** those segments of the vertebral column that normally remain unfused throughout life: the cervical, thoracic, and lumbar vertebrae.

Ver·te·bra·ta (ver″tĕ-bra′tah) a subphylum of the Chordata, comprising all animals having a vertebral column, including mammals, birds, reptiles, amphibians, and fishes.

ver·te·brate (ver′tĕ-brāt) 1. having a spinal column (vertebrae). 2. an animal with a vertebral column; any member of the Vertebrata.

ver·te·brec·to·my (ver″tĕ-brek′tah-me) excision of a vertebra.

vertebr(o)- word element [L.], *vertebra; spine*.

ver·te·bro·bas·i·lar (ver″tĕ-bro-bas′ĭ-ler) pertaining to or affecting the vertebral and basilar arteries.

ver·te·bro·chon·dral (-kon′dral) pertaining to a vertebra and a costal cartilage.

ver·te·bro·cos·tal (-kos′t'l) pertaining to a vertebra and a rib.

ver·te·bro·gen·ic (-jen′ik) arising in a vertebra or in the vertebral column.

ver·te·bro·ster·nal (-ster′n'l) pertaining to a vertebra and the sternum.

ver·te·por·fin (ver″tĕ-por′fin) a photosensitizing agent that accumulates preferentially in neovasculature, including that in the choroid; used, together with appropriate laser irradiation of the lesion, in the treatment of neovascularization due to disciform macular degeneration, to presumed ocular histoplasmosis, or to pathologic myopia.

ver·tex (ver′teks) pl. *ver′tices*. [L.] the summit or top, especially the top of the head (*v. cra′nii*). **ver′tical,** adj.

ver·ti·cal (ver′tĭ-k'l) 1. perpendicular to the plane of the horizon. 2. relating to the vertex. 3. relating to or occupying different levels in a hierarchy, as the spread from one generation to another in vertical transmission.

ver·ti·ca·lis (ver″tĭ-ka′lis) [L.] vertical; denoting relationship to this orientation when the body is in the anatomical position.

ver·tic·il·late (ver-tis′ĭ-lāt) arranged in whorls.

ver·ti·go (ver′tĭ-go) [L.] a sensation of rotation or movement of one's self (*subjective v.*) or of one's surroundings (*objective v.*) in any plane; sometimes used erroneously to mean any form of dizziness. **vertig′inous,** adj. **alternobaric v.,** a transient, true, whirling vertigo sometimes affecting those subjected to large, rapid variations in barometric pressure. **benign paroxysmal postural v.,** recurrent vertigo and nystagmus occurring when the head is placed in certain positions, usually not associated with lesions of the central nervous system. **cerebral v.,** a type resulting from a brain lesion. **cervical v.,**

vertigo after injury to the neck such as whiplash. **disabling positional v.,** constant positional vertigo or dysequilibrium and nausea with the head in the upright position, without hearing disturbance or loss of vestibular function. **labyrinthine v.,** Meniere's disease. **objective v.,** see *vertigo.* **ocular v.,** a form due to eye disease. **organic v.,** cerebral v. **positional v., postural v.,** that associated with a specific position of the head in space or with changes in position of the head in space. **subjective v.,** see *vertigo.* **vestibular v.,** vertigo due to disturbances of the vestibular system.

ve·ru·mon·ta·num   (ver″u-mon-ta′num) seminal colliculus.

ve·sa·li·a·num (vĕ-sa″le-a′num) a sesamoid bone in the tendon of origin of the gastrocnemius muscle, or in the angle between the cuboid and fifth metatarsal.

ve·si·ca (vĕ-si′kah) pl. *vesi′cae.* [L.] bladder. **v. bilia′ris, v. fel′lea,** gallbladder. **v. urina′ria,** urinary bladder.

ves·i·cal (ves′ĭ-k′l) pertaining to the urinary bladder. Cf. *cystic.*

ves·i·cant (ves′ĭ-kant) 1. producing blisters. 2. an agent that so acts.

ves·i·ca·tion (ves″ĭ-ka′shun) 1. the process of blistering. 2. a blistered spot or surface.

ves·i·cle (ves′ĭ-k′l) 1. a small bladder or sac containing liquid. 2. a small circumscribed elevation of the epidermis containing a serous fluid; a small blister. **acrosomal v.,** a membrane-bounded vacuolelike structure which spreads over the upper two-thirds of the head of a spermatozoon to form the head cap. **auditory v., otic v. blastodermic v.,** blastocyst. **brain v's, cephalic v's, cerebral v's,** the five divisions of the closed neural tube in the head of the developing embryo, including the telencephalon, diencephalon, mesencephalon, metencephalon, and myelencephalon. **chorionic v.,** see under *sac.* **encephalic v's,** brain v's. **germinal v.,** the fluid-filled nucleus of an oocyte toward the end of prophase of its first meiotic division. **lens v.,** a vesicle formed from the lens pit of the embryo, developing into the crystalline lens. **matrix v's,** small membrane-limited structures at sites of calcification of the cartilage matrix. **olfactory v.,** 1. the vesicle in the embryo that later develops into the olfactory bulb and tract. 2. a bulbous expansion at the distal end of an olfactory cell, from which the olfactory hairs project. **optic v.,** an evagination on either side of the forebrain of the early embryo, from which the percipient parts of the eye develop. **otic v.,** a detached ovoid sac

formed by closure of the otic pit in embryonic development of the external ear. **primary brain v's,** the three earliest subdivisions of the embryonic neural tube, including the prosencephalon, mesencephalon, and rhombencephalon. **secondary brain v's,** the five brain vesicles formed by specialization of the prosencephalon (telencephalon and diencephalon), mesencephalon, and rhombencephalon (metencephalon and myelencephalon) in later embryonic development. **seminal v.,** either of the paired sacculated pouches attached to the posterior urinary bladder; the duct of each joins the ipsilateral ductus deferens to form the ejaculatory duct. **umbilical v.,** the pear-shaped expansion of the mammalian yolk sac growing out into the cavity of the chorion, joined to the midgut by the yolk stalk.

vesic(o)- word element [L.], *blister; bladder.*

ves·i·co·cele (ves′ĭ-ko-sēl″) cystocele.

ves·i·co·cer·vi·cal (ves″ĭ-ko-ser′vĭ-k′l) pertaining to the bladder and cervix uteri, or communicating with the bladder and cervical canal.

ves·i·co·en·ter·ic (-en-ter′ik) enterovesical.

ves·i·co·in·tes·ti·nal (-in-tes′tĭ-n′l) enterovesical.

ves·i·co·pros·tat·ic (-pros-tat′ik) pertaining to the urinary bladder and the prostate.

ves·i·co·pu·bic (-pu′bik) pubovesical; pertaining to the urinary bladder and the pubic region.

ves·i·co·sig·moid·os·to·my (-sig″moidos′tah-me) surgical creation of an opening between the urinary bladder and the sigmoid colon.

ves·i·co·spi·nal (-spi′nal) pertaining to the urinary bladder and the spinal cord.

ves·i·cos·to·my (ves″ĭ-kos′tah-me) cystostomy. **cutaneous v.,** surgical anastomosis of the bladder mucosa to an opening in the skin below the umbilicus, creating a stoma for bladder drainage.

ves·i·cot·o·my (ves″ĭ-kot′ah-me) cystotomy.

ves·i·co·um·bil·i·cal (ves″ĭ-ko-um-bil′ĭ-k′l) pertaining to the urinary bladder and the umbilicus.

ves·i·co·ure·ter·al (-u-re′ter-al) ureterovesical.

ves·i·co·ure·ter·ic (-u-re′ter-ik) ureterovesical.

ves·i·co·ure·thral (-u-re′thral) pertaining to the urinary bladder and urethra.

ves·i·co·uter·ine (-u′ter-in) pertaining to or connecting the bladder and uterus.

ves·i·co·vag·i·nal (-vaj′ĭ-n′l) pertaining to or connecting the bladder and vagina.

ve·sic·u·la (vě-sik′u-lah) pl. *vesi′culae*. [L.] vesicle.

ve·sic·u·lar (vě-sik′u-ler) 1. composed of or relating to small, saclike bodies. 2. pertaining to or made up of vesicles on the skin. 3. having a low pitch, such as the normal breath sound over the lung during ventilation.

ve·sic·u·lec·to·my (vě-sik″u-lek′tah-me) excision of a vesicle, especially the seminal vesicles.

ve·sic·u·li·form (vě-sik′u-lĭ-form″) shaped like a vesicle.

ve·sic·u·li·tis (vě-sik″u-li′tis) inflammation of a vesicle, especially a seminal vesicle (*seminal v.*).

ve·sic·u·lo·cav·er·nous (vě-sik″u-lo-kav′er-nus) both vesicular and cavernous.

ve·sic·u·log·ra·phy (vě-sik″u-log′rah-fe) radiography of the seminal vesicles.

ve·sic·u·lo·pap·u·lar (vě-sik″u-lo-pap′u-ler) both vesicular and papular.

ve·sic·u·lo·pus·tu·lar (-pus′tu-ler) both vesicular and pustular.

ve·sic·u·lot·o·my (vě-sik″u-lot′ah-me) incision into a vesicle, especially the seminal vesicles.

Ves·ic·u·lo·vi·rus (vě-sik′u-lo-vi″rus) vesicular stomatitis-like viruses; a genus of viruses of the family Rhabdoviridae that includes viruses that cause vesicular stomatitis in swine, cattle, and horses and related viruses that infect humans and other animals.

ves·sel (ves″l) any channel for carrying a fluid, such as blood or lymph. **blood v.**, one of the vessels conveying the blood, comprising arteries, capillaries, and veins. **chyliferous v.**, lacteal (2). **collateral v.**, 1. a vessel that parallels another vessel, nerve, or other structure. 2. a vessel important in establishing and maintaining a collateral circulation. **great v's**, the large vessels entering the heart, including the aorta, the pulmonary arteries and veins, and the venae cavae. **lacteal v.**, lacteal (2). **lymphatic v's**, the capillaries, collecting vessels, and trunks that collect lymph from the tissues and carry it to the blood stream. **nutrient v's**, vessels supplying nutritive elements to special tissues, as arteries entering the substance of bone or the walls of large blood vessels.

ves·ti·bule (ves′tĭ-būl) a space or cavity at the entrance to a canal. **vestib′ular**, adj. **v. of aorta**, a small space at root of the aorta. **v. of ear**, an oval cavity in the middle of the bony labyrinth. **v. of mouth**, the portion of the oral cavity bounded on the one side by teeth and gingivae, or residual alveolar ridges, and on the other by the lips (*labial v.*) and cheeks (*buccal v.*). **nasal v.**, **v. of nose**, the anterior part of the nasal cavity. **v. of vagina**, **v. of vulva**, the space between the labia minora into which the urethra and vagina open.

ves·tib·u·li·tis (ves-tib″u-li′tis) inflammation of the vulvar vestibule and the periglandular and subepithelial stroma, resulting in a burning sensation and dyspareunia.

ves·tib·u·lo·gen·ic (ves-tib″u-lo-jen′ik) arising in a vestibule, as that of the ear.

ves·tib·u·lo·oc·u·lar (-ok′u-ler) 1. pertaining to the vestibular and oculomotor nerves. 2. pertaining to the maintenance of visual stability during head movements.

ves·tib·u·lo·plas·ty (ves-tib′u-lo-plas″te) surgical modification of gingival–mucous membrane relationships in the vestibule of the mouth.

ves·tib·u·lot·o·my (ves-tib″u-lot′ah-me) surgical opening of the vestibule of the ear.

ves·tib·u·lo·ure·thral (ves-tib″u-lo-u-re′thral) pertaining to the vestibule of the vagina and the urethra.

ves·tib·u·lo·vag·i·nal (-vaj′ĭ-n′l) pertaining to the vestibule of the vagina.

ves·ti·bu·lum (ves-tib′u-lum) pl. *vesti′bula*. [L.] vestibule.

ves·tige (ves′tij) the remnant of a structure that functioned in a previous stage of species or individual development. **vestig′ial**, adj.

ves·ti·gi·um (ves-tĭ′je-um) pl. *vesti′gia*. [L.] vestige.

vet·er·i·nar·i·an (vet″er-ĭ-nar′e-an) a person trained and authorized to practice veterinary medicine and surgery; a doctor of veterinary medicine.

vet·er·i·nary (vet′er-ĭ-nar″e) 1. pertaining to domestic animals and their diseases. 2. veterinarian.

VF vocal fremitus.

vf visual field.

VFib ventricular fibrillation.

VFl ventricular flutter.

VHDL very-high-density lipoprotein.

vi·a·ble (vi′ah-b′l) able to maintain an independent existence; able to live after birth.

vi·bex (vi′beks) pl. *vi′bices*. A narrow linear mark or streak; a linear subcutaneous effusion of blood.

vi·bra·tion (vi-bra′shun) 1. a rapid movement to and fro. 2. massage with a light, rhythmic, quivering motion; often performed with a mechanical device (electrovibratory massage).

vi·bra·tor (vi′bra-tor) an instrument for producing vibrations.

vi·bra·to·ry (vi′brah-tor″e) vibrating or causing vibration.

Vib·rio (vib′re-o) a genus of gram-negative bacteria (family Spirillaceae). *V. cho′lerae*

(*V. com'ma*), or cholera vibrio, is the cause of Asiatic cholera; *V. metschniko'vii* causes gastroenteritis; *V. parahaemoly'ticus* causes gastroenteritis due to consumption of raw or undercooked seafood; and *V. vulni'ficus* causes septicemia and cellulitis in persons who have consumed raw seafood.

vib·rio (vib're-o) pl. *vibrio'nes, vibrios.* An organism of the genus *Vibrio* or other spiral motile organism. **cholera v.,** *Vibrio cholerae;* see *Vibrio.* **El Tor v.,** a biotype of *Vibrio cholerae;* see *Vibrio.*

vib·rio·ci·dal (vib″re-o-si′dal) destructive to organisms of the genus *Vibrio,* especially *V. cholerae.*

vi·bris·sa (vi-bris′ah) [L.] a long coarse hair, such as those growing in the vestibule of the nose.

vi·car·i·ous (vi-kar′e-us) 1. acting in the place of another or of something else. 2. occurring at an abnormal site.

Vic·ia (vish′e-ah) a genus of herbs, including *V. fa'ba* (*V. fa'va*), the fava or broad bean, whose beans or pollen contain a component capable of causing favism in susceptible persons.

vi·cine (vi′sin) a pyrimidine-based glycoside occurring in species of *Vicia;* in fava beans it is cleaved to form the toxic compound divicine.

vi·dar·a·bine (vi-dar′ah-bēn) adenine arabinoside (ara-A), a purine analogue that preferentially inhibits viral DNA synthesis; used as an antiviral agent to treat herpes simplex keratitis or keratoconjunctivitis.

vid·eo·den·si·tom·e·try (vid″e-o-den″si-tom′ĕ-tre) densitometry using a video camera to record the images to be analyzed.

vid·eo·en·dos·co·py (-en-dos′kah-pe) endoscopy aided by a video camera in the tip of the endoscope.

vid·eo·lap·a·ros·co·py (-lap″ah-ros′kah-pe) laparoscopic surgery aided by a video camera in the tip of the laparoscope.

vid·eo·flu·o·ros·co·py (-floo-ros′kah-pe) the recording on videotape of the images appearing on a fluoroscopic screen.

vid·eo·la·ser·os·co·py (-la-zer-os′kah-pe) a modification of laser laparoscopy in which the inside of the cavity is visualized through a video camera that projects an enlarged image onto a video monitor.

vi·kri·ti (vik′rĭ-te) in ayurveda, a disordered physical constitution, resulting from an imbalance of the doshas.

vil·li (vil′i) plural of *villus.*

vil·lo·ma (vĭ-lo′mah) papilloma.

vil·lo·nod·u·lar (vil″o-nod′u-lar) characterized by villous and nodular thickening.

vil·lose (vil′ōs) shaggy with soft hairs; covered with villi.

vil·lo·si·tis (vil″o-si′tis) a bacterial disease with alterations in the villi of the placenta.

vil·los·i·ty (vĭ-los′ĭ-te) 1. condition of being covered with villi. 2. a villus.

vil·lous (vil′us) villose.

vil·lus (vil′us) pl. *vil'li.* [L.] a small vascular process or protrusion, especially from the free surface of a membrane. **arachnoid villi,** 1. microscopic projections of the arachnoid into some of the venous sinuses. 2. arachnoidal granulations. **chorionic v.,** one of the threadlike projections growing in tufts on the external surface of the chorion. **intestinal villi,** multitudinous threadlike projections covering the surface of the mucous membrane lining the small intestine, serving as the sites of absorption of fluids and nutrients. **synovial villi,** slender projections of the synovial membrane from its free inner surface into the joint cavity.

vil·lus·ec·to·my (vil″us-ek′tah-me) synovectomy.

vi·men·tin (vĭ-men′tin) a protein forming the vimentin filaments, a common type of intermediate filament; used as a marker for cells derived from embryonic mesenchyme.

vin·blas·tine (vin-blas′tēn) an antineoplastic vinca alkaloid used as the sulfate salt in the palliative treatment of a variety of malignancies.

vin·cris·tine (vin-kris′tēn) an antineoplastic vinca alkaloid; used as the sulfate salt in the treatment of various neoplasms, including Hodgkin's disease, acute lymphocytic leukemia, non-Hodgkin's lymphoma, Kaposi's sarcoma associated with AIDS, and neuroblastoma.

vin·cu·lum (ving′ku-lum) pl. *vin'cula.* [L.] a band or bandlike structure. **vin'cula ten'dinum,** filaments which connect the phalanges and interphalangeal articulations with the flexor tendons.

vi·nor·el·bine (vĭ-nor′el-bēn″) an antineoplastic vinca alkaloid used as the tartrate salt in the treatment of advanced non–small cell lung carcinoma.

vi·nyl (vi′nil) the univalent group $CH_2=CH-$. **v. chloride,** a vinyl group to which an atom of chlorine is attached; the monomer which polymerizes to polyvinyl chloride; it is toxic and carcinogenic.

vi·o·la·ceous (vi″o-la′shus) having a violet color, usually describing a discoloration of the skin.

vi·o·let (vi′o-let) 1. the color produced by the shortest waves of the visible spectrum, beyond indigo, approximately 380 to 420 nm. 2. a dye or stain with this color. **crystal v., gentian v., methyl v.,** gentian violet; see under *gentian.*

vi·per (vi′per) any venomous snake, especially any member of the families Viperidae (true vipers) and Crotalidae (pit vipers). **European v.,** *Vipera berus,* a venomous snake native to Europe, North America, and the Middle East. **Gaboon v.,** *Bitis gabonica,* a deadly, brightly marked, viperine snake found in tropical West Africa. **pit v.,** crotalid (1). **rhinoceros v.,** *Bitis nasicornis,* a venomous, brightly colored, viperine snake found in tropical Africa, having a pair of hornlike growths on its snout. **Russell's v.,** *Vipera russelli,* an extremely venomous, brightly colored, viperine snake of southeastern Asia and Indonesia. **sand v.,** *Vipera ammodytes,* a venomous snake found in southern Europe and Turkey that has a hornlike protuberance on its snout for burrowing. **true v.,** any of the snakes of the family Viperidae.

Vi·pera (vi′per-ah) a genus of venomous snakes of the family Viperidae. *V. ammody′tes* is the sand viper; *V. be′rus* is the adder or European viper; and *V. rus′selli* is Russell's viper.

VIP·oma (vĭ-po′mah) an endocrine tumor, usually an islet cell tumor, that produces vasoactive intestinal polypeptide, causing a syndrome of watery diarrhea, hypokalemia, and hypochlorhydria, leading to potentially fatal renal failure. Alternatively, vipoma.

vip·oma (vĭ-po′mah) VIPoma.

vi·ral (vi′ral) pertaining to or caused by a virus.

vi·re·mia (vi-re′me-ah) the presence of viruses in the blood.

vir·gin (vir′jin) 1. a person who has not had sexual intercourse. 2. a laboratory animal that has been kept free from sexual intercourse.

vir·ile (vir′il) 1. masculine. 2. specifically, having male copulative power.

vir·i·lism (vir′ĭ-lizm) the development or possession of male secondary sex characters in a female or prepubertal male. **adrenal v.,** that due to inappropriate adrenal cortical androgen production.

vi·ril·i·ty (vĭ-ril′ĭ-te) masculinity.

vir·il·iza·tion (vir″ĭ-lĭ-za′shun) masculinization; usually used for that occurring in a female or prepubertal male.

vir·il·iz·ing (vir′ĭ-līz″ing) producing virilization.

vi·ri·on (vi′re-on) the complete viral particle, found extracellularly and capable of surviving in crystalline form and infecting a living cell; it

comprises the nucleoid (genetic material) and the capsid.

vi·ro·lac·tia (vi″ro-lak′she-ah) secretion of viruses in the milk.

vi·rol·o·gy (vi-rol′ah-je) the study of viruses and virus diseases.

vir·tu·al (vir′choo-al) 1. having the essence or effect, although not the actual fact or form. 2. created by, carried on, or performed by means of computers.

vi·ru·cide (vi′rŭ-sīd) an agent which neutralizes or destroys a virus. **viruci′dal,** adj.

vir·u·lence (vir′u-lens) the degree of pathogenicity of a microorganism as indicated by the severity of disease produced and the ability to invade the tissues of the host; by extension, the competence of any infectious agent to produce pathologic effects. **vir′ulent,** adj.

vir·u·lif·er·ous (vir″u-lif′er-us) conveying or producing a virus or other noxious agent.

vir·uria (vi-roo′re-ah) viruses in the urine.

vi·rus (vi′rus) [L.] a minute infectious agent which, with certain exceptions, is not resolved by the light microscope, lacks independent metabolism and is able to replicate only within a living host cell; the individual particle (virion) consists of nucleic acid (nucleoid)—DNA or RNA (but not both)—and a protein shell (capsid), which contains and protects the nucleic acid and which may be multilayered. **attenuated v.,** one whose pathogenicity has been reduced by serial passage or other means. **Bayou v.,** a virus of the genus *Hantavirus* that causes hantavirus pulmonary syndrome in the southwestern United States. **BK v. (BKV),** a human polyomavirus that causes widespread infection in childhood and remains latent in the host; it is believed to cause hemorrhagic cystitis and nephritis in immunocompromised patients. **Central European encephalitis v.,** a species of tick-borne viruses of the genus *Flavivirus* that includes the agents of Central European encephalitis and the Russian spring-summer encephalitis virus. **cowpox v.,** a virus of the genus *Orthopoxvirus* that is the etiologic agent of cowpox. **Coxsackie v.,** coxsackievirus. **defective v.,** one that cannot be completely replicated or cannot form a protein coat; in some cases replication can proceed if missing gene functions are supplied by other viruses; see *helper v.* **dengue v.,** a flavivirus existing as four distinct types (designated 1, 2, 3, and 4) that causes dengue. **DNA v.,** one whose genome consists of DNA. **eastern equine encephalomyelitis v.,** see *equine encephalomyelitis v.* **EB v.,** Epstein-Barr v. **Ebola v.,** 1. an RNA virus almost identical to the Marburg virus but serologically distinct;

it causes a similar disease. **2.** a virus of the genus *Filovirus* that is the etiologic agent of Ebola virus disease. **EEE v.,** eastern equine encephalomyelitis v.; see *equine encephalomyelitis v.* **encephalomyocarditis v.,** an enterovirus that causes mild aseptic meningitis and encephalomyocarditis. **enteric v's,** an epidemiologic class of viruses that are normally acquired by ingestion and replicate in the intestinal tract, causing local rather than generalized infection. **enveloped v.,** a virus having an outer lipoprotein bilayer acquired by budding through the host cell membrane. **Epstein-Barr v. (EBV),** human herpesvirus 4; a virus that causes infectious mononucleosis and is associated with Burkitt's lymphoma and nasopharyngeal carcinoma. **equine encephalomyelitis v.,** a group of arbovirus species of the genus *Alphavirus* that cause encephalomyelitis in horses, mules, and humans, transmitted by mosquitoes; there are three strains: *eastern, western,* and *Venezuelan.* **fixed v.,** one whose virulence and incubation period have been stabilized by serial passage and remained fixed during further transmission. **foamy v's,** *Spumavirus.* **helper v.,** one that aids in the development of a defective virus by supplying or restoring the activity of the viral gene or enabling it to form a protein coat. **hepatitis v.,** the etiologic agent of viral hepatitis. Six types are recognized: *hepatitis A virus,* the agent causing infectious hepatitis, acquired by parenteral inoculation or by ingestion; *hepatitis B virus,* the agent causing serum hepatitis, transmitted by inadequately sterilized syringes and needles, or through infectious blood plasma, or certain blood products; *hepatitis C virus,* which causes hepatitis C; *hepatitis D virus,* a defective RNA viral agent that can replicate only in the presence of hepatitis B virus and is transmitted with it and causes hepatitis D; *hepatitis E virus,* a calicivirus transmitting hepatitis E; and *hepatitis G virus,* flavivirus isolated from patients with hepatitis but whose etiologic role is uncertain. **hepatitis B–like v's,** Hepadnaviridae. **herpes v.,** herpesvirus. **herpes simplex v. (HSV),** a virus of the genus *Simplexvirus* that is the etiologic agent of herpes simplex in humans. It is separable into two serotypes, designated 1 and 2 (called also *human herpesvirus 1* and *human herpesvirus 2*); type 1 is transmitted by infected saliva and causes primarily nongenital lesions, and type 2 is sexually transmitted and causes primarily genital lesions. **human immunodeficiency v. (HIV),** a human T-cell leukemia/lymphoma virus, of the genus *Lentivirus,* with a selective affinity for helper T cells that is the agent of the acquired immunodeficiency syndrome. **human T-cell leukemia v.,** human T-lymphotropic v. **human T-lymphotropic v. 1 (HTLV-1),** a species of retroviruses of worldwide distribution, having an affinity for helper/inducer T lymphocytes; it causes chronic infection and is associated with adult T-cell leukemia/lymphoma and chronic progressive myelopathy. **human T-lymphotropic v. 2 (HTLV-2),** a species of retroviruses having extensive serologic cross-reactivity with HTLV-1; no clear association with disease has been established. **igbo-ora v.,** an arbovirus of the genus *Alphavirus* that has been associated with a dengue-like disease in Nigeria, the Central African Republic, and the Ivory Coast. **influenza v.,** any of a group of orthomyxoviruses that cause influenza, including at least three genera: Influenzavirus A, Influenzavirus B, and Influenzavirus C. Serotype A viruses are subject to major antigenic changes (antigenic shifts) as well as minor gradual antigenic changes (antigenic drift) and cause the major pandemics. **influenza A v., influenza B v., influenza C v.,** species in the genera *Influenzavirus A, Influenzavirus B,* and *Influenzavirus C;* see *influenza v.* **Jamestown Canyon v.,** a virus of the genus *Bunyavirus,* serologically related to California encephalitis virus, that occasionally causes encephalitis. **JC v. (JCV),** a polyomavirus that causes widespread infection in childhood and remains latent in the host; it is the cause of progressive multifocal leukoencephalopathy. **La Crosse v.,** a virus of the California serogroup of the genus *Bunyavirus,* the etiologic agent of La Crosse encephalitis. **lymphocyte-associated v.,** any virus of the subfamily Gammaherpesviridae, members of which are specific for either B or T lymphocytes; infection is often arrested at a lytic or prelytic stage without production of infectious virions, and latent virus may frequently be demonstrated in lymphoid tissue. **lytic v.,** one that is replicated in the host cell and causes death and lysis of the cell. **Marburg v.,** an RNA virus occurring in Africa, transmitted by insect bite and causing Marburg disease. **masked v.,** a virus that ordinarily occurs in a noninfective state and is demonstrable by indirect methods which activate it, as by blind passage in experimental animals. **measles v.,** a paramyxovirus that is the cause of measles. **measles-like v's,** *Morbillivirus.* **monkeypox v.,** an orthopoxvirus that produces mild exanthematous disease in monkeys and a smallpox-like disease in humans. **mumps v.,** a virus of the genus

Rubulavirus that causes mumps and sometimes tenderness and swelling of the testes, pancreas, ovaries, or other organs. **naked v., nonenveloped v.,** a virus lacking an outer lipoprotein bilayer. **neurotropic v.,** one that has a predilection for and causes infection in nervous tissues, e.g., the rabies virus. **Norwalk v.,** a calicivirus that is a common agent of epidemics of acute gastroenteritis. **oncogenic v's,** an epidemiologic class of viruses that are acquired by close contact or injection and cause usually persistent infection; they may induce cell transformation and malignancy. **Oropouche v.,** a virus of the genus *Bunyavirus* that causes illness in Brazil; infection is characterized by fever, chills, malaise, headache, myalgia, and arthralgia, sometimes nausea and vomiting, and occasionally central nervous system involvement. **orphan v's,** viruses isolated in tissue culture but not found specifically associated with any illness. **papilloma v.,** papillomavirus. **parainfluenza v.,** a group of viruses of the family Paramyxoviridae that cause upper respiratory tract disease in humans and other animals. **paravaccinia v.,** pseudocowpox v. **Powassan v.,** a tickborne virus of the genus *Flavivirus* that causes encephalitis in the eastern United States and Canada. **pox v.,** poxvirus. **pseudocowpox v.,** a virus of the genus *Parapoxvirus* that produces nodular lesions similar to those of cowpox and orf on the udders and teats of milk cows and the oral mucosa of suckling calves (paravaccinia), which can be transmitted to humans during milking. **Puumala v.,** see *Hantavirus.* **rabies v.,** an RNA virus of the rhabdovirus group that causes rabies. **rabies-like v's,** *Lyssavirus.* **respiratory v's,** an epidemiologic class of viruses that are acquired by inhalation of fomites and replicate in the respiratory tract, causing local rather than generalized infection; they are included in the families Adenoviridae, Coronaviridae, Orthomyxoviridae, Paramyxoviridae, and Picornaviridae. **respiratory syncytial v's (RSV),** viruses belonging to the genus *Pneumovirus,* causing respiratory disease that is particularly severe in infants, and in tissue causing syncytium formation. **RNA v.,** one whose genome consists of RNA. **Rous-associated v. (RAV),** a helper virus in whose presence a defective Rous sarcoma virus is able to form a protein coat. **Rous sarcoma v. (RSV),** see *Rous sarcoma,* under *sarcoma.* **rubella v.,** the sole species of the genus *Rubivirus,* the etiologic agent of rubella. **St. Louis encephalitis v.,** a virus of the genus *Flavivirus,* that is the etiologic agent of St. Louis

encephalitis; transmitted by mosquitoes. **sandfly fever v's,** *Phlebovirus.* **satellite v.,** a strain of virus unable to replicate except in the presence of helper virus; considered to be deficient in coding for capsid formation. **Seoul v.,** see *Hantavirus.* **simian immunodeficiency v. (SIV),** a virus of the genus *Lentivirus,* closely related to human immunodeficiency virus, that causes inapparent infection in African green monkeys and a disease resembling acquired immunodeficiency syndrome in macaques. **Sin Nombre v.,** a virus of the genus *Hantavirus* that causes hantavirus pulmonary syndrome in the western United States. **slow v.,** any virus causing a disease characterized by a long preclinical course and gradual progression once the symptoms appear. **street v.,** virus from a naturally infected animal, as opposed to a laboratory-adapted strain of the virus. **tanapox v.,** a virus of the genus *Yatapoxvirus* that is the etiologic agent of tanapox. **Toscana v.,** a virus of the Naples serogroup of the genus *Phlebovirus,* an etiologic agent of phlebotomus fever. **varicella-zoster v.,** human herpesvirus 3; see table at *herpesvirus.* **variola v.,** the virtually extinct virus, belonging to the genus *Orthopoxvirus,* that is the etiologic agent of smallpox. No natural infection has occurred since 1977 and no reservoir of the virus now exists. **VEE v., Venezuelan equine encephalomyelitis v.,** see *equine encephalomyelitis v.* **WEE v., western equine encephalomyelitis v.,** see *equine encephalomyelitis v.* **West Nile v.,** a virus of the genus *Flavivirus* that causes West Nile encephalitis; it is transmitted by *Culex* mosquitoes, with wild birds serving as the reservoir. **Yaba monkey tumor v.,** a virus of the genus *Yatapoxvirus* that is the etiologic agent of yabapox. **yellow fever v.,** a mosquito-borne species of the genus *Flavivirus* that causes yellow fever in Central and South America and Africa.

vis·ce·ra (vis′er-ah) plural of *viscus.*

vis·cer·ad (vis′er-ad) toward the viscera.

vis·cer·al (vis′er-al) pertaining to a viscus.

vis·cer·al·gia (vis″er-al′jah) pain in any viscera.

viscer(o)- word element [L.], *viscera.*

vis·cero·meg·a·ly (vis″er-o-meg′ah-le) organomegaly; enlargement of the viscera.

vis·cero·mo·tor (-mo′ter) conveying or concerned with motor impulses to the viscera.

vis·cero·pa·ri·e·tal (-pah-ri′ah-tal) pertaining to the viscera and the abdominal wall.

vis·cero·peri·to·ne·al (-per″ĭ-to-ne′al) pertaining to the viscera and peritoneum.

vis·cero·pleu·ral (-ploor′al) pertaining to the viscera and the pleura.

vis·cero·skel·e·tal (-skel′ah-tal) pertaining to the visceral skeleton.

vis·cer·o·tro·pic (-tro′pik) primarily acting on the viscera; having a predilection for the abdominal or thoracic viscera.

vis·cid (vis′id) glutinous or sticky.

vis·cos·i·ty (vis-kos′ĭ-te) resistance to flow; a physical property of a substance that is dependent on the friction of its component molecules as they slide by one another.

vis·cous (vis′kus) sticky or gummy; having a high degree of viscosity.

vis·cus (vis′kus) pl. *vis′cera*. [L.] any large interior organ in any of the three great body cavities, especially those in the abdomen.

vi·sion (vizh′un) 1. the sense by which objects in the external environment are perceived by means of the light they give off or reflect. 2. the act of seeing. 3. an apparition; a subjective sensation of seeing not elicited by actual visual stimuli. 4. visual acuity. **achromatic v.,** monochromatic vision. **anomalous trichromatic v.,** defective color vision in which a person has all three cone pigments but one is deficient or anomalous but not absent. **binocular v.,** the use of both eyes together without diplopia. **central v.,** that produced by stimuli impinging directly on the macula retinae. **chromatic v.,** color v. **color v.,** 1. perception of the different colors making up the spectrum of visible light. 2. chromatopsia. **day v.,** visual perception in the daylight or under conditions of bright illumination. **dichromatic v.,** defective color vision in which one of the three cone pigments is missing; the two types are *protanopia* and *deuteranopia*. **direct v.,** central v. **double v.,** diplopia. **indirect v.,** peripheral v. **low v.,** impairment of vision such that there is significant visual handicap but also significant usable residual vision. **monochromatic v.,** complete color blindness; inability to discriminate hues, all colors of the spectrum appearing as neutral grays with varying shades of light and dark. **monocular v.,** vision with one eye. **multiple v.,** polyopia. **night v.,** visual perception in the darkness of night or under conditions of reduced illumination. **oscillating v.,** oscillopsia. **peripheral v.,** that produced by stimuli falling on areas of the retina distant from the macula. **solid v., stereoscopic v.,** perception of the relief of objects or of their depth; vision in which objects are perceived as having three dimensions. **trichromatic v.,** 1. any ability to distinguish the three primary colors of light and mixtures of them.

2. normal color vision. **tunnel v.,** 1. that in which the visual field is severely constricted. 2. in psychiatry, restriction of psychological or emotional perception to a limited range.

vis·u·al (vizh′oo-al) pertaining to vision or sight.

vis·u·al·iza·tion (vizh″oo-al-ĭ-za′shun) 1. the act of viewing or of achieving a complete visual impression of an object. 2. the process of forming a mental picture of something.

vis·uo·au·di·to·ry (vizh″oo-o-aw′dĭ-tor″e) simultaneously stimulating, or pertaining to simultaneous stimulation of, the senses of both hearing and sight.

vis·uo·mo·tor (-mo′ter) pertaining to connections between visual and motor processes.

vis·uo·sen·so·ry (-sen′sor-e) pertaining to perception of stimuli giving rise to visual impressions.

vis·uo·spa·tial (-spa′shal) pertaining to the ability to understand visual representations and their spatial relationships.

vi·tal (vi′t'l) necessary to or pertaining to life.

Vi·tal·li·um (vi-tal′e-um) trademark for a cobalt-chromium alloy used for cast dentures and surgical appliances.

vi·ta·min (vi′tah-min) any of a group of unrelated organic substances occurring in many foods in small amounts and necessary in trace amounts for the normal metabolic functioning of the body; they may be water- or fat-soluble. **v. A,** retinol or any of several fat-soluble compounds with similar biological activity; the vitamin acts in numerous capacities, particularly in the functioning of the retina, the growth and differentiation of epithelial tissue, the growth of bone, reproduction, and the immune response. Deficiency causes skin disorders, increased susceptibility to infection, nyctalopia, xerophthalmia and other eye disorders, anorexia, and sterility. As vitamin A it is mostly found in liver, egg yolks, and the fat component of dairy products; its other major dietary source is the provitamin A carotenoids of plants. It is toxic when taken in excess; see *hypervitaminosis A*. **v. A_1,** retinol. **v. A_2,** dehydroretinol. **v. B_1,** thiamine. **v. B_2,** riboflavin. **v. B_6,** any of a group of water-soluble substances (including pyridoxine, pyridoxal, and pyridoxamine) found in most foods, especially meats, liver, vegetables, whole grains, cereals, and egg yolk, and concerned in the metabolism of amino acids, in the degradation of tryptophan, and in the metabolism of glycogen. **v. B_{12},** cyanocobalamin by chemical definition, but generally any substituted cobalamin derivative with similar biological activity; it is a water-soluble hematopoietic vitamin occurring in meats and animal products. It is necessary for the growth and replication of all body cells and the functioning of the nervous system, and deficiency causes pernicious anemia and other forms of megaloblastic anemia, and neurologic lesions. **v. B complex,** a group of water-soluble substances including thiamine, riboflavin, niacin (nicotinic acid), niacinamide (nicotinamide), the vitamin B_6 group, biotin, pantothenic acid, and folic acid, and sometimes including p-aminobenzoic acid, inositol, vitamin B_{12}, and choline. **v. C,** ascorbic acid. **v. D,** either of two fat-soluble compounds with antirachitic activity or both collectively: cholecalciferol, which is synthesized in the skin and is considered a hormone, and ergocalciferol, which is the form generally used as a dietary supplement. Dietary sources include some fish liver oils, egg yolks, and fortified dairy products. Deficiency can result in rickets in children and osteomalacia in adults, while excessive ingestion can cause hypercalcemia, mobilization of calcium from bone, and renal dysfunction. **v. D_2,** ergocalciferol. **v. D_3,** cholecalciferol. **v. E,** any of a group of at least eight related fat-soluble compounds with similar biological antioxidant activity, particularly α-tocopherol but also including other isomers of tocopherol and the related compound tocotrienol. It is found in wheat germ oil, cereal germs, liver, egg yolk, green plants, milk fat, and vegetable oils and is also prepared synthetically. In various species it is important for normal reproduction, muscle development, and resistance of erythrocytes to hemolysis. **fat-soluble v's,** those (vitamins A, D, E, and K) that are soluble in fat solvents and are absorbed along with dietary fats; they are not normally excreted in the urine and tend to be stored in the body in moderate amounts. **v. K,** any of a group of structurally similar fat-soluble compounds that promote blood clotting. Two forms, phytonadione and menaquinone, exist naturally, and there is one synthetic provitamin form, menadione. The best sources are leafy green vegetables, butter, cheese, and egg yolk. Deficiency, usually seen only in neonates, in disorders of absorption, or during antibiotic therapy, is characterized by hemorrhage. **v. K_1,** phytonadione. **v. K_2,** menaquinone. **v. K_3,** menadione. **water-soluble v's,** the vitamins soluble in water (i.e., all but vitamins A, D, E, and K); they are excreted in the urine and are not stored in the body in appreciable quantities.

vi·tel·line (vi-tel'in) pertaining to or resembling a yolk.

vi·tel·lus (vi-tel'us) [L.] yolk.

vit·i·lig·i·nes (vit″ĭ-lij'ĭ-nēz) depigmented areas of the skin.

vit·i·li·go (vit″ĭ-li'go) a usually progressive, chronic pigmentary anomaly of the skin manifested by depigmented white patches that may be surrounded by a hyperpigmented border. **vitilig'inous,** adj.

vi·trec·to·my (vĭ-trek'tah-me) surgical extraction, usually via the pars plana, of the contents of the vitreous chamber of the eye.

vit·reo·ret·i·nal (vit″re-o-ret'ĭ-n'l) of or pertaining to the vitreous and retina.

vit·re·ous (vit're-us) 1. glasslike or hyaline. 2. vitreous body. **primary persistent hyperplastic v.,** a congenital anomaly, usually unilateral, due to persistence of embryonic remnants of the fibromuscular tunic of the eye and part of the hyaloid vascular system. Clinically, there is a white pupil, elongated ciliary processes, and often microphthalmia; the lens, although clear initially, may become completely opaque.

vit·ro·nec·tin (vit″ro-nek'tin) an adhesive glycoprotein whose many functions include regulation of the coagulation, fibrinolytic, and complement cascades, also playing a role in hemostasis, wound healing, tissue remodeling, and cancer, and promoting adhesion, spreading, and migration of cells. It has been shown to be identical to *S protein,* which was identified as a complement inhibitor acting to prevent insertion of the membrane attack complex into the membrane.

vivi- word element [L.], *alive; life.*

vi·vip·a·rous (vi-vip'ah-rus) giving birth to living young which develop within the maternal body.

vivi·sec·tion (viv″ĭ-sek'shun) surgical procedures performed upon a living animal for purpose of physiologic or pathologic investigation.

VLDL very-low-density lipoprotein. **β-VLDL, beta VLDL,** a mixture of lipoproteins with diffuse electrophoretic mobility approximately that of β-lipoproteins but having lower density; they are remnants derived from mutant chylomicrons and very-low-density lipoproteins that cannot be metabolized completely and accumulate in plasma. **pre-β-VLDL,** very-low-density lipoprotein, emphasizing its electrophoretic mobility.

VMA vanillylmandelic acid.

VMD [L.] Veterina'riae Medici'nae Doc'tor (Doctor of Veterinary Medicine).

voice (vois) sound produced by the speech organs and uttered by the mouth. **vo'cal,** adj.

void (void) excrete.

vo·la (vo'lah) pl. *vo'lae*. [L.] a concave or hollow surface. **v. ma'nus,** the palm. **v. pe'dis,** the sole.

vo·lar (vo'lar) pertaining to sole or palm; indicating the flexor surface of the forearm, wrist, or hand.

vo·la·ris (vo-lar'is) palmar.

vol·a·tile (vol'ah-til) evaporating rapidly; vaporizing readily.

vol·a·til·iza·tion (vol"ah-til-ĭ-za'shun) conversion into vapor or gas without chemical change.

vol·ley (vol'e) a number of simultaneous muscle twitches or nerve impulses all caused by the same stimulus.

vol·sel·la (vol-sel'ah) vulsella.

volt (V) (vōlt) the SI unit of electric potential or electromotive force, equal to 1 watt per ampere, or 1 joule per coulomb. **electron v. (eV),** a unit of energy equal to the energy acquired by an electron accelerated through a potential difference of 1 volt; equal to 1.602×10^{-19} joule.

vol·ume (vol'ūm) the measure of the quantity or capacity of a substance. Symbol V or *V*. **end-diastolic v. (EDV),** the volume of blood in each ventricle at the end of diastole, usually about 120–130 mL but sometimes reaching 200–250 mL in the normal heart. **end-systolic v. (ESV),** the volume of blood remaining in each ventricle at the end of systole, usually about 50–60 mL but sometimes as little as 10–30 mL in the normal heart. **expiratory reserve v.,** the maximal amount of gas that can be exhaled from the resting end-expiratory level. Abbreviated ERV. **forced expiratory v.,** the fraction of the forced vital capacity that is exhaled in a specific number of seconds. Abbreviated FEV with a subscript indicating how many seconds the measurement lasted. **inspiratory reserve v.,** the maximal amount of gas that can be inhaled from the end-inspiratory position. **mean corpuscular v.,** the average volume of erythrocytes, conventionally expressed in cubic micrometers or femtoliters per red cell. **minute v. (MV),** the quantity of gas exhaled from the lungs per minute; tidal volume multiplied by respiratory rate. **packed-cell v. (PCV), v. of packed red cells (VPRC),** hematocrit. **residual v.,** the amount of gas remaining in the lung at the end of a maximal exhalation. **stroke v.,** the volume of blood ejected from a ventricle at each beat of the heart, equal to the difference between the end-diastolic volume and the end-systolic volume. **tidal v.,** the volume of gas inhaled and exhaled during one respiratory cycle.

vol·u·met·ric (vol"u-met'rik) pertaining to or accompanied by measurement in volumes.

vol·un·tary (vol'un-tar"e) accomplished in accordance with the will.

vo·lute (vo-lūt') rolled up.

vol·vu·lo·sis (vol"vu-lo'sis) onchocerciasis due to *Onchocerca volvulus*.

vol·vu·lus (vol'vu-lus) [L.] torsion of a loop of intestine, causing obstruction.

vo·mer (vo'mer) [L.] see *Table of Bones*. **vo'merine,** adj.

vo·mero·na·sal (vo"mer-o-na'z'l) pertaining to the vomer and the nasal bone.

vom·it (vom'it) 1. to eject stomach contents through the mouth. 2. matter expelled from the stomach by the mouth. **black v.,** vomit consisting of blood which has been acted upon by the gastric juice, seen in yellow fever and other conditions in which blood collects in the stomach. **coffee-ground v.,** vomit consisting of dark altered blood mixed with stomach contents.

vom·it·ing (-ing) forcible ejection of contents of stomach through the mouth. **cyclic v.,** recurring attacks of vomiting. **dry v.,** attempts at vomiting, with the ejection of nothing but gas. **pernicious v.,** vomiting in pregnancy so severe as to threaten life. **v. of pregnancy,** that occurring in pregnancy, especially early morning vomiting (morning sickness). **projectile v.,** vomiting with the material ejected with great force. **stercoraceous v.,** vomiting of fecal matter.

vom·i·to·ry (vom'i-tor"e) emetic.

vom·i·tu·ri·tion (vom"it-u-rish'un) repeated ineffectual attempts to vomit; retching.

vom·i·tus (vom'ĭ-tus) [L.] 1. vomiting. 2. matter vomited.

v-onc (viral *onc*ogene) a nucleic acid sequence in a virus responsible for the oncogenicity of the virus; it is derived from the cellular proto-oncogene and acquired from the host by recombination. Cf. *c*-onc.

vor·tex (vor'teks) pl. *vor'tices*. [L.] a whorled or spiral arrangement or pattern, as of muscle fibers, or of the ridges or hairs of the skin.

vo·yeur·ism (voi'yer-izm) a paraphilia characterized by recurrent, intense sexual urges or arousal involving real or fantasized observation of unsuspecting people who are naked, disrobing, or engaging in sexual activity.

VP variegate porphyria.

VPB ventricular premature beat; see *ventricular premature complex*, under *complex*.

VPC ventricular premature complex.

VPD ventricular premature depolarization; see *ventricular premature complex*, under *complex*.

VPF vascular permeability factor; see *vascular endothelial growth factor*, under *factor*.

VR vocal resonance.

VS volumetric solution.

VT ventricular tachycardia.

vu·er·om·e·ter (vu″er-om′ĕ-ter) an instrument for measuring distance between the pupils.

vul·ga·ris (vul-ga′ris) [L.] ordinary; common.

vul·nus (vul′nus) pl. *vul′nera*. [L.] a wound.

vul·sel·la (vul-sel′ah) [L.] a forceps with clawlike hooks at the end of each blade.

vul·sel·lum (-sel′um) [L.] vulsella.

vul·va (vul′vah) [L.] the external genital organs of the female, including the mons pubis, labia majora and minora, clitoris, and vestibule of the vagina. **vul′val, vul′var,** adj. **fused v.,** synechia vulvae.

vul·vec·to·my (vul-vek′tah-me) excision of the vulva.

vul·vi·tis (vul-vi′tis) inflammation of the vulva. **atrophic v.,** lichen sclerosus in females.

vul·vo·uter·ine (vul″vo-u′ter-in) pertaining to the vulva and uterus.

vul·vo·vag·i·nal (-vaj′ĭ-n′l) pertaining to the vulva and vagina.

vul·vo·vag·i·ni·tis (-vaj″ĭ-ni′tis) inflammation of the vulva and vagina. **candidal v.,** vulvovaginal candidiasis.

vv. [L. pl.] ve′nae (veins).

v/v volume (of solute) per volume (of solvent).

vWF von Willebrand's factor.

W

W tryptophan; tungsten (Ger. *Wolfram*); watt.

waist (wāst) the portion of the body between the thorax and the hips.

walk·er (wawk′er) an enclosing framework of lightweight metal tubing, sometimes with wheels, for patients who need more support in walking than that given by a crutch or cane.

walk·ing (wawk′ing) 1. progressing on foot. 2. gait. **sleep w.,** somnambulism.

wall (wawl) paries; a structure bounding or limiting a space or a definitive mass of material. **cell w.,** a rigid structure that lies just outside of and is joined to the plasma membrane of plant cells and most prokaryotic cells, which protects the cell and maintains its shape. **chest w.,** the bony and muscular structures that form the outer framework of the thorax and move during breathing. **nail w.,** a fold of skin overlapping the sides and proximal end of a fingernail or toenail. **parietal w.,** somatopleure. **splanchnic w.,** splanchnopleure.

wall·eye (wawl′i) 1. leukoma of the cornea. 2. exotropia.

wan·der·ing (wahn′der-ing) 1. moving about freely. 2. abnormally movable; too loosely attached.

ward (word) 1. a large room in a hospital for the accommodation of several patients. 2. a division within a hospital for the care of numerous patients having the same condition.

war·fa·rin (wor′fah-rin) a synthetic coumarin anticoagulant administered as the sodium salt; it is also used as a rodenticide, causing fatal hemorrhaging in any mammal consuming a sufficient dose.

wart (wort) verruca; a hyperplastic epidermal lesion with a horny surface, caused by a human papillomavirus; also loosely applied to any of various wartlike, epidermal proliferations of nonviral origin. **wart′y,** adj. **anatomical w.,** tuberculosis verrucosa cutis. **flat w.,** a small, smooth, usually skin-colored or light brown, slightly raised wart sometimes occurring in great numbers; seen most often in children. **genital w.,** condyloma acuminatum. **juvenile w.,** flat w. **moist w.,** condyloma latum. **mosaic w.,** an irregularly shaped lesion on the sole, with a granular surface, formed by an aggregation of contiguous plantar warts. **necrogenic w.,** tuberculosis verrucosa cutis. **Peruvian w.,** verruga peruana. **pitch w's,** precancerous, keratotic, epidermal tumors occurring in those working with pitch and coal tar derivatives. **plantar w.,** a viral epidermal tumor on the sole of the foot. **pointed w.,** condyloma acuminatum. **postmortem w., prosector's w.,** tuberculosis verrucosa cutis. **soot w.,** a sign of chimney-sweeps' cancer, which occurs beneath the wart. **venereal w.,** condyloma acuminatum.

wash (wosh) 1. to clean or bathe. 2. a solution used for cleansing or bathing a part.

wast·ing gradual loss or decay, with emaciation.

wa·ter (waw′ter, wah′ter) 1. clear, colorless, odorless, tasteless liquid, H_2O. 2. an aqueous solution of a medicinal substance; called also *aromatic w.* 3. purified w. **bound w.,** water in the tissues of the body bound to macromolecules or organelles. **distilled w.,** water purified by distillation. **free w.,** that portion of the water in body tissues which is not bound by macromolecules or organelles. **w. for injection,** water for parenteral use, prepared by distillation or reverse osmosis and meeting certain standards for sterility and clarity; it may be specified as sterile if it has been sterilized and as bacteriostatic if suitable antimicrobial agents have been added. **purified w.,** water obtained by either distillation or deionization; used when mineral-free water is required.

wa·ters (waw′terz) popular name for *amniotic fluid.*

watt (W) (waht) the SI unit of power, being the work done at the rate of 1 joule per second. In electric power, it is equivalent to a current of 1 ampere under a pressure of 1 volt.

wave (wāv) a uniformly advancing disturbance in which the parts moved undergo a double oscillation; any wavelike pattern. **alpha w's,** see under *rhythm.* **beta w's,** see under *rhythm.* **brain w's,** the fluctuations of electric potential in the brain, as recorded by electroencephalography. **delta w.,** 1. an early QRS vector in the electrocardiogram in preexcitation. 2. (pl.) electroencephalographic waves with a frequency below 3.5 per second, typical in deep sleep, infancy, and serious brain disorders. **electromagnetic w's,** the spectrum of waves propagated by an electromagnetic field, having a velocity of 3×10^8 m/s in a vacuum and including, in order of decreasing wavelength, radio waves, microwaves, infrared, visible, and ultraviolet light, x-rays, gamma rays, and cosmic rays. **F w's,** 1. flutter w's; rapid sawtooth-edged atrial waves without isoelectric intervals between them; seen in the electrocardiogram in atrial flutter. Written also *f w's.* 2. f w's (1). **f w's,** 1. fibrillary w's; small, irregular, rapid deflections in the electrocardiogram in atrial fibrillation. Written also *F w's.* 2. F w's (1). **fibrillary w's,** f w's (1). **flutter w's,** F w's (1). **J w.,** a deflection occurring in the electrocardiogram between the QRS complex and the onset of the ST segment, occurring prominently in hypothermia and in hypocalcemia. **P w.,** a deflection in the electrocardiogram produced by excitation of the atria. **pulse w.,** the elevation of the pulse felt by the finger or shown graphically in a recording of pulse pressure. **Q w.,** in the QRS complex, the initial downward (negative) deflection, related to the initial phase of

depolarization of the ventricular myocardium, the depolarization of the interventricular septum. **R w.,** the initial upward deflection of the QRS complex, following the Q wave in the normal electrocardiogram and representing early depolarization of the ventricles. **S w.,** a downward deflection of the QRS complex following the R wave in the normal electrocardiogram and representing late depolarization of the ventricles. **T w.,** the deflection of the normal electrocardiogram following the QRS complex; it represents repolarization or recovery of the ventricles. **Ta w.,** a small asymmetric wave, of opposite polarity to the P wave, representing atrial repolarization; together with the P wave it defines atrial systole. **theta w's,** brain waves in the electroencephalogram with a frequency of 4 to 7 per second, mainly seen in children and emotionally stressed adults. **U w.,** a potential undulation of unknown origin immediately following the T wave and often concealed by it; seen in the normal electrocardiogram and accentuated in tachyarrhythmias and electrolyte disturbances.

wave·length (λ) (wāv′length) the distance between the top of one wave and the identical phase of the succeeding one

wax (waks) a low-melting, high-molecular-weight, organic mixture or compound, similar to fats and oils but lacking glycerides; it may be deposited by insects, obtained from plants, or prepared synthetically. **dental w.,** a mixture of two or more waxes with other additives, used in dentistry for casts, construction of nonmetallic denture bases, registering of jaw relations, and laboratory work. **ear w.,** cerumen. **white w.,** bleached beeswax; bleached, purified wax from the honeycomb of the bee, *Apis mellifera;* used as a pharmaceutical stiffening agent. **yellow w.,** beeswax; purified wax from the honeycomb of the bee, *Apis mellifera;* used as a pharmaceutical stiffening agent.

waxy (wak′se) 1. composed of or covered by wax. 2. resembling wax, especially denoting some combination of pliability, paleness, and smoothness and luster.

wax·ing (wak′sing) the shaping of a wax pattern or the wax base of a trial denture into the contours desired.

Wb weber.

WBC white blood cell; see *leukocyte.*

wean (wēn) to discontinue breast feeding and substitute other feeding habits.

wean·ling (wēn′ling) 1. recently weaned. 2. a recently weaned infant.

web (web) a tissue or membrane. **laryngeal w.,** a web spread between the vocal folds near the anterior commissure; the most common congenital malformation of the larynx. **terminal w.,** a feltwork of fine filaments in the cytoplasm immediately beneath the free surface of certain epithelial cells; it is thought to have a supportive or cytoskeletal function.

webbed (webd) connected by a membrane.

web·er (Wb) (web′er) the SI unit of magnetic flux which, linking a circuit of one turn, produces in it an electromotive force of one volt as it is reduced to zero at a uniform rate in one second.

wedge (wej) 1. a piece of material thick at one end and tapering to a thin edge at the other end. 2. to force something into a space of limited size. **step w.,** a block of absorber, usually aluminum, machined in steps of increasing thickness, used to measure the penetrating power of x-rays.

WEE western equine encephalomyelitis.

weep (wēp) 1. to shed tears. 2. to ooze serum.

weight (wāt) 1. heaviness; the degree to which a body is drawn toward the earth by gravity. See *Table of Weights and Measures.* Abbreviated wt. 2. in statistics, the process of assigning greater importance to some observations than to others, or a mathematical factor used to apply such a process. **apothecaries' w.,** a system of weights used in compounding prescriptions, based on the grain (64.8 mg). Its units are the scruple (20 grains), dram (3 scruples), ounce (8 drams), and pound (12 ounces). **atomic w.,** the sum of the masses of the constituents of an atom; it can be expressed in atomic mass units, SI units, or as a dimensionless ratio based on its value relative to the ^{12}C isotope of carbon, defined as 12.00000. Abbreviated At wt. **avoirdupois w.,** the system of weight commonly used for ordinary commodities in English-speaking countries; its units are the grain, dram (27.344 grains), ounce (16 drams), and pound (16 ounces). **equivalent w.,** the amount of a substance that combines with or displaces 8.0 g of oxygen (or 1.008 g of hydrogen); it is the ratio of the molecular weight to the number of protons (acid/base reactions) or electrons (redox reactions) involved in the reaction. **molecular w.,** the weight of a molecule of a substance as compared with that of an atom of carbon-12; it is equal to the sum of the atomic weights of its constituent atoms and is dimensionless. Abbreviated Mol wt or MW. Although widely used, it is not technically correct; relative molecular mass (M_r) is preferable.

wen (wen) 1. a sebaceous or epidermal inclusion cyst. 2. pilar cyst.

wheal (hwēl) a localized area of edema on the body surface, often attended with severe itching and usually evanescent; it is the typical lesion of urticaria.

wheeze (hwēz) a whistling type of continuous sound.

whip·lash (hwip′lash) see under *injury.*

whip·worm (-werm) any nematode of the genus *Trichuris.*

white·head (hwīt′hed) 1. milium. 2. closed comedo.

whit·low (hwit′lo) felon. **herpetic w.,** primary herpes simplex infection of the terminal segment of a finger, with extensive tissue destruction, sometimes accompanied by systemic symptoms. **melanotic w.,** subungual melanoma.

WHO World Health Organization, an international agency associated with the United Nations and based in Geneva.

whoop (hōōp) the sonorous and convulsive inhalation of whooping cough.

wild-type (wīld′tīp) that occurring in a natural population or in the standard laboratory stock, as a strain, phenotype, or gene, and therefore designated as representative of the group.

wil·low (wil′o) any plant of the genus *Salix.* White willow bark (q.v.) contains a precursor of salicylic acid and is used as an herbal remedy.

win·dow (win′do) 1. a circumscribed opening in a plane surface. 2. the voltage limits that determine which pulses will be allowed to pass on. **aortic w.,** a transparent region below the aortic arch, formed by the bifurcation of the trachea, visible in the left anterior oblique radiograph of the heart and great vessels. **oval w.,** fenestra vestibuli. **round w.,** fenestra cochleae.

wind·pipe (wind′pīp) the trachea.

wink·ing (wingk′ing) quick opening and closing of the eyelids. **jaw w.,** Gunn's syndrome.

wire (wīr) a slender, elongated, flexible structure of metal. **Kirschner w.,** a steel wire for skeletal transfixion of fractured bones and for obtaining skeletal traction in fractures.

witch ha·zel (wich′ ha′z'l) the deciduous bush *Hamamelis virginiana,* or any of various preparations of its twigs, leaves, or bark, which are used topically for their astringent effects and also have various uses in folk medicine and in homeopathy.

with·draw·al (with-drawl′) 1. pathological retreat from interpersonal contact and social involvement. 2. substance w. **substance w.,** a substance-specific mental disorder that

TABLES OF WEIGHTS AND MEASURES

MEASURES OF MASS

Avoirdupois Weight

Grains	Drams	Ounces	Pounds	Metric Equivalents (grams)
1	0.0366	0.0023	0.00014	0.0647989
27.34	1	0.0625	0.0039	1.772
437.5	16	1	0.0625	28.350
7000	256	16	1	453.5924277

Apothecaries' Weight

Grains	Scruples (℈)	Drams (ʒ)	Ounces (℥)	Pounds (£)	Metric Equivalents (grams)
1	0.05	0.0167	0.0021	0.00017	0.0647989
20	1	0.333	0.042	0.0035	1.296
60	3	1	0.125	0.0104	3.888
480	24	8	1	0.0833	31.103
5760	288	96	12	1	373.24177

Metric Weight

Microgram	Milligram	Centigram	Decigram	Gram	Decagram	Hectogram	Kilogram	Metric Ton
1	—	—	—	—	—	—	—	—
10^3	1	—	—	—	—	—	—	—
10^4	10	1	—	—	—	—	—	—
10^5	100	10	1	—	—	—	—	—
10^6	1000	100	10	1	—	—	—	—
10^7	10^4	1000	100	10	1	—	—	—
10^8	10^5	10^4	1000	100	10	1	—	—
10^9	10^6	10^5	10^4	1000	100	10	1	—
10^{12}	10^9	10^8	10^7	10^6	10^5	10^4	1000	1

Equivalents

	Avoirdupois	Apothecaries'
		0.000015 gr
		0.015432 gr
		0.154323 gr
		1.543235 gr
		15.432356 gr
	5.6438 dr	7.7162 scr
	3.527 oz	3.215 oz
	2.2046 lb	2.6792 lb
	2204.6223 lb	2679.2285 lb

Troy Weight

Grains	Pennyweights	Ounces	Pounds	Metric Equivalents (grams)
1	0.042	0.002	0.00017	1.0647989
24	1	0.05	0.0042	1.555
480	20	1	0.083	31.103
		12	1	373.24177

MEASURES OF CAPACITY

Apothecaries' (Wine) Measure

Minims	Fluid Drams	Fluid Ounces	Gills	Pints	Quarts	Gallons	Cubic Inches	Equivalents Milliliters	Cubic Centimeters
1	0.0166	0.002	0.0005	0.00013	—	—	0.00376	0.06161	0.06161
60	1	0.125	0.0312	0.0078	0.0039	—	0.22558	3.6967	3.6967
480	8	1	0.25	0.0625	0.0312	0.0078	1.80468	29.5737	29.5737
1920	32	4	1	0.25	0.125	0.0312	7.21875	118.2948	118.2948
7680	128	16	4	1	0.5	0.125	28.875	473.179	473.179
15360	256	32	8	2	1	0.25	57.75	946.358	946.358
61440	1024	128	32	8	4	1	231	3785.434	3785.434

Metric Measure

Microliter	Milliliter	Centiliter	Deciliter	Liter	Decaliter	Hectoliter	Kiloliter	Megaliter	Equivalents (Apothecaries' Fluid)
1	—	—	—	—	—	—	—	—	0.01623108 min
10^3	1	—	—	—	—	—	—	—	16.23 min
10^4	10	1	—	—	—	—	—	—	2.7 fl dr
10^5	100	10	1	—	—	—	—	—	3.38 fl oz
10^6	10^3	100	10	1	—	—	—	—	2.11 pt
10^7	10^4	10^3	100	10	1	—	—	—	2.64 gal
10^8	10^5	10^4	10^3	100	10	1	—	—	26.418 gal
10^9	10^6	10^5	10^4	10^3	100	10	1	—	264.18 gal
10^{12}	10^9	10^8	10^7	10^6	10^5	10^4	10^3	1	26418 gal

1 liter = 2.113363738 pints (Apothecaries')

MEASURES OF LENGTH

Metric Measure

Micrometer	Millimeter	Centimeter	Decimeter	Meter	Decameter	Hectometer	Kilometer	Megameter	Equivalents
1	0.001	10^{-4}	—	—	—	—	—	—	0.000039 inch
10^3	1	10^{-1}	—	—	—	—	—	—	0.03937 inch
10^4	10	1	—	—	—	—	—	—	0.3937 inch
10^5	100	10	1	—	—	—	—	—	3.937 inches
10^6	1000	100	10	1	—	—	—	—	39.37 inches
10^7	10^4	1000	100	10	1	—	—	—	10.9361 yards
10^8	10^5	10^4	1000	100	10	1	—	—	109.3612 yards
10^9	10^6	10^5	10^4	1000	100	10	1	—	1093.6121 yards
10^{10}	10^7	10^6	10^5	10^4	1000	100	10	—	6.2137 miles
10^{12}	10^9	10^8	10^7	10^6	10^5	10^4	1000	1	621.370 miles

CONVERSION TABLES

Avoirdupois—Metric Weights

Ounces	Grams	Pounds	Grams	Kilograms
1/16	1.772	1 (16 oz)	453.59	
1/8	3.544	2	907.18	
1/4	7.088	3	1360.78	1.36
1/2	14.175	4	1814.37	1.81
1	28.350	5	2267.96	2.27
2	56.699	6	2721.55	2.72
3	85.049	7	3175.15	3.18
4	113.398	8	3628.74	3.63
5	141.748	9	4082.33	4.08
6	170.097	10	4535.92	4.54
7	198.447			
8	226.796			
9	255.146			
10	283.495			
11	311.845			
12	340.194			
13	368.544			
14	396.893			
15	425.243			
16 (1 lb)	453.59			

Metric—Avoirdupois Weight

Grams	Ounces	Grams	Ounces	Grams	Pounds
0.001 (1 mg)	0.00035274	1	0.035274	1000 (1 kg)	2.2046

Apothecaries'—Metric Weight

Grains	Grams		Grains	Grams		Scruples	Grams
1/150	0.0004		2/5	0.03		1	1.296 (1.3)
1/120	0.0005		1/2	0.032		2	2.592 (2.6)
1/100	0.0006		3/5	0.04		3 (1 ℨ)	3.888 (3.9)
1/90	0.0007		2/3	0.043			
1/80	0.0008		3/4	0.05		**Drams**	**Grams**
1/64	0.001		7/8	0.057		1	3.888
1/60	0.0011		1	0.065		2	7.776
1/50	0.0013		1 1/2	0.097 (0.1)		3	11.664
1/48	0.0014		2	0.12		4	15.552
1/40	0.0016		3	0.20		5	19.440
1/36	0.0018		4	0.24		6	23.328
1/32	0.002		5	0.30		7	27.216
1/30	0.0022		6	0.40		8 (1 ℥)	31.103
1/25	0.0026		7	0.45			
1/20	0.003		8	0.50		**Ounces**	**Grams**
1/16	0.004		9	0.60		1	31.103
1/12	0.005		10	0.65		2	62.207
1/10	0.006		15	1.00		3	93.310
1/9	0.007		20 (1 ℈)	1.30		4	124.414
1/8	0.008		30	2.00		5	155.517
1/7	0.009					6	186.621
1/6	0.01					7	217.724
1/5	0.013					8	248.828
1/4	0.016					9	279.931
1/3	0.02					10	311.035
						11	342.138
						12 (1 ℔)	373.242

Metric—Apothecaries' Weight

Milligrams	Grains	Grams	Grains	Grams	Equivalents
1	0.015432	0.1	1.5432	10	2.572 drams
2	0.030864	0.2	3.0864	15	3.858 "
3	0.046296	0.3	4.6296	20	5.144 "
4	0.061728	0.4	6.1728	25	6.430 "
5	0.077160	0.5	7.7160	30	7.716 "
6	0.092592	0.6	9.2592	40	1.286 oz
7	0.108024	0.7	10.8024	45	1.447"
8	0.123456	0.8	12.3456	50	1.607"
9	0.138888	0.9	13.8888	100	3.215 "
10	0.154320	1.0	15.4320	200	6.430"
15	0.231480	1.5	23.1480	300	9.644"
20	0.308640	2.0	30.8640	400	12.859"
25	0.385800	2.5	38.5800	500	1.34 lb
30	0.462960	3.0	46.2900	600	1.61"
35	0.540120	3.5	54.0120	700	1.88"
40	0.617280	4.0	61.728	800	2.14"
45	0.694440	4.5	69.444	900	2.41"
50	0.771600	5.0	77.162	1000	2.68"
100	1.543240	10.0	154.324		

Apothecaries'—Metric Liquid Measure

Minims	Milliliters	Fluid Drams	Milliliters	Fluid Ounces	Milliliters
1	0.06	1	3.70	1	29.57
2	0.12	2	7.39	2	59.15
3	0.19	3	11.09	3	88.72
4	0.25	4	14.79	4	118.29
5	0.31	5	18.48	5	147.87
10	0.62	6	22.18	6	177.44
15	0.92	7	25.88	7	207.01
20	1.23	8 (1 fl oz)	29.57	8	236.58
25	1.54			9	266.16
30	1.85			10	295.73
35	2.16			11	325.30
40	2.46			12	354.88
45	2.77			13	384.45
50	3.08			14	414.02
55	3.39			15	443.59
60 (1 fl dr)	3.70			16 (1 pt)	473.17
				32 (1 qt)	946.33
				128 (1 gal)	3785.32

Metric—Apothecaries' Liquid Measure

Milliliters	Minims	Milliliters	Fluid Drams	Milliliters	Fluid Ounces
1	16.231	5	1.35	30	1.01
2	32.5	10	2.71	40	1.35
3	48.7	15	4.06	50	1.69
4	64.9	20	5.4	500	16.91
5	81.1	25	6.76	1000 (1 L)	33.815
		30	7.1		

U.S. and British—Metric Length

Inches	Millimeters	Centimeters	Meters
1/25	1.00	0.1	0.001
1/8	3.18	0.318	0.00318
1/4	6.35	0.635	0.00635
1/2	12.70	1.27	0.00127
1	25.40	2.54	0.0254
12 (1 foot)	304.80	30.48	0.3048

follows the cessation of use or reduction in intake of a psychoactive substance that had been regularly used to induce a state of intoxication.

wob·ble (wob''l) to move unsteadily or unsurely back and forth or from side to side. See under *hypothesis.*

Wohl·fahr·tia (võl-fahr'te-ah) a genus of flies. The larvae of *W. magnif'ica* produce wound myiasis; those of *W. o'paca* and *W. vig'il* cause cutaneous myiasis.

Wol·bach·ia (wol-bak'e-ah) a genus of bacteria that infect a wide variety of invertebrates, including insects, spiders, crustaceans, and nematodes.

wolfs·bane (woolfs'bān) 1. arnica. 2. aconite.

word sal·ad (werd sal'ad) a meaningless mixture of words and phrases characteristic of advanced schizophrenia.

work·up (werk'up) the procedures done to arrive at a diagnosis, including history taking, laboratory tests, x-rays, and so on.

worm (werm) 1. any of the soft-bodied, naked, elongated invertebrates of the phyla Annelida, Acanthocephala, Aschelminthes, and Platyhelminthes. 2. vermis. flat w., any of the Platyhelminthes. guinea w., *Dracunculus medinensis.* heart w., heartworm. round w., nematode. spinyheaded w., thorny-headed w., an individual of the phylum Acanthocephala.

worm·wood (werm'wood) a plant of the genus *Artemisia,* especially *A. absinthium* (common wormwood), which is used to make the liqueur absinthe.

wound (woōnd) trauma; an injury, usually restricted to a physical one with disruption of normal continuity of structures. contused w., one in which the skin is unbroken. incised w., one caused by a cutting instrument. lacerated w., one in which the tissues are torn. open w., one having a free outward opening. penetrating w., one caused by a sharp, usually slender object, which passes through the skin into the underlying tissues. perforating w., a penetrating wound that extends into a viscus or body cavity. puncture w., penetrating w.

wrist (rist) the region of the joint between the forearm and hand; the carpus.

wrist·drop (rist'drop) a condition resulting from paralysis of the extensor muscles of the hand and fingers.

wry (ri) abnormally twisted; bent to one side; crooked or contorted.

wry·neck (ri'nek) torticollis.

wt weight.

Wu·cher·e·ria (voo''ker-e're-ah) a genus of nematodes of the superfamily Filarioidea that affect mainly humans in warmer regions of the world. *W. bancrof'ti* causes elephantiasis, lymphangitis, and chyluria by interfering with the lymphatic circulation.

wu·cher·e·ri·a·sis (voo''ker-e-ri'ah-sis) infestation with species of *Wuchereria.*

w/v weight (of solute) per volume (of solvent).

X xanthine or xanthosine.

x abscissa.

xan·thel·as·ma (zan''thē-laz'mah) planar xanthoma affecting the eyelids.

xan·thic (zan'thik) 1. yellow. 2. pertaining to xanthine.

xan·thine (-thēn) a purine base found in most body tissues and fluids, certain plants, and some urinary calculi; it is an intermediate in the degradation of AMP to uric acid. Methylated xanthine compounds (e.g., caffeine, theobromine, theophylline) are used for their bronchodilator effect. Abbreviated X.

xan·thine ox·i·dase (ok'sĭ-dās) a flavoprotein enzyme that catalyzes the oxidation of hypoxanthine to xanthine and then to uric acid, the final steps in the degradation of purines; deficiency, an autosomal recessive trait, causes xanthinuria.

xan·thin·uria (zan''thin-ūr'e-ah) 1. excretion of xanthine in the urine. 2. a hereditary disorder of purine metabolism due to a deficiency of the enzyme xanthine oxidase, with excessive xanthine and hypoxanthine in urine and sometimes xanthine calculi in the urinary tract.

xanth(o)- word element [Gr.], *yellow.*

xan·tho·chro·mat·ic (zan''tho-kro-mat'ik) yellow-colored.

xan·tho·chro·mia (-kro'me-ah) yellowish discoloration, as of the skin or spinal fluid.

xan·tho·chro·mic (-kro'mik) having a yellow discoloration; said of cerebrospinal fluid.

xan·tho·cy·a·nop·sia (-si″ah-nop′se-ah) ability to discern yellow and blue tints, but not red or green.

xan·tho·der·ma (-der′mah) any yellowish discoloration of the skin.

xan·tho·gran·u·lo·ma (-gran″u-lo′mah) a tumor having histologic characteristics of both granuloma and xanthoma. **juvenile x.,** a benign, self-limited disorder of infants and children, with single or multiple yellow, pink, orange, or reddish brown papules or nodules on the scalp, face, proximal limb, or trunk, sometimes with involvement of mucous membranes, viscera, eye, and other organs.

xan·tho·ma (zan-tho′mah) a tumor composed of lipid-laden foam cells, which are histiocytes containing cytoplasmic lipid material. **diabetic x.,** x. diabetico′rum, eruptive x. **disseminated x.,** x. dissemina′tum, a rare, normolipoproteinemic form manifested by the development of reddish yellow to brown papules and nodules that may coalesce to form plaques, chiefly involving flexural ureases, the mucous membranes of the mouth and respiratory tract, cornea, sclera, and central nervous system. **eruptive x.,** x. erupti′vum, a form marked by sudden eruption of crops of small, yellow or yellowish orange papules encircled by an erythematous halo, especially on the buttocks, posterior thighs, and elbows, and caused by high concentrations of plasma triglycerides, especially that associated with uncontrolled diabetes mellitus. **fibrous x.,** benign fibrous histiocytoma. **x. mul′tiplex,** disseminated x **planar x., plane x.,** x. pla′num, a form manifested as soft yellowish, tannish, or dark red flat macules or slightly elevated plaques, sometimes having a central white area, which may be localized or generalized, often occurring in association with other xanthomas and certain hyperlipoproteinemias. **x. tendino′sum, tendinous x.,** a form manifested by free movable papules or nodules in the tendons, ligaments, fascia, and periosteum, especially on the backs of the hands, fingers, elbows, knees, and heels, in association with some hyperlipoproteinemias and certain other xanthomas. **x. tubero′sum, tuberous x.,** a form manifested by groups of flat, or elevated and rounded, yellowish or orangish nodules on the skin over joints, especially on elbows and knees; it may be associated with certain types of hyperlipoproteinemia, biliary cirrhosis, and myxedema.

xan·tho·ma·to·sis (zan″tho-mah-to′sis) a condition marked by the presence of xanthomas. **x. bul′bi,** fatty degeneration of the cornea.

xan·tho·ma·tous (zan-tho′mah-tus) pertaining to xanthoma.

xan·thop·sia (zan-thop′se-ah) chromatopsia in which objects are seen as yellow.

xan·tho·sine (zan′tho-sēn) a nucleoside composed of xanthine and ribose. Symbol X.

xan·tho·sis (zan-tho′sis) yellowish discoloration; degeneration with yellowish pigmentation.

xanth·u·ren·ic ac·id (zanth″u-ren′ik) a bicyclic aromatic compound formed as a minor catabolite of tryptophan and present in increased amounts in urine in vitamin B_6 deficiency and some disorders of tryptophan catabolism.

Xe xenon.

xen(o)- word element [Gr.], *strange; foreign.*

xeno·an·ti·gen (zen″o-an′ti-jen) an antigen occurring in organisms of more than one species.

xeno·di·ag·no·sis (-di″ag-no′sis) a method of animal inoculation using laboratory-bred bugs and animals in the diagnosis of certain parasitic infections when the infecting organism cannot be demonstrated in blood films; used in Chagas' disease (examination of the feces of clean bugs fed on the patient's blood) and trichinosis (examination of rats to which the patient's muscle tissue has been fed). **xenodiagnos′tic,** adj.

xeno·ge·ne·ic (-jen-e′ik) in transplantation biology, denoting individuals or tissues from individuals of different species and hence of disparate cell type.

xeno·gen·e·sis (-jen′ĕ-sis) 1. heterogenesis (1). 2. the hypothetical production of offspring unlike either parent.

xen·og·e·nous (ze-noj′ĕ-nus) caused by a foreign body, or originating outside the organism.

xeno·graft (zen′o-graft) a graft of tissue transplanted between animals of different species; it may be *concordant*, occurring between closely related species, in which the recipient lacks natural antibodies specific for the transplanted tissue, or *discordant*, occurring between members of distantly related species, in which the recipient has natural antibodies specific for the transplanted tissue.

xe·non (ze′non) chemical element (see *Table of Elements*), at. no. 54, symbol Xe. The radioactive isotope ^{133}Xe is used in assessment of pulmonary function, lung imaging, and cerebral blood flow studies.

xeno·para·site (zen″o-par′ah-sīt) an organism not usually parasitic on a particular species, but which becomes so because of a weakened condition of the host.

xeno·pho·bia (-fo′be-ah) irrational fear of strangers.

xeno·pho·nia (-fo′ne-ah) alteration in the quality of the voice.

xen·oph·thal·mia (zen″of-thal′me-ah) ophthalmia caused by a foreign body in the eye.

Xen·op·syl·la (zen″op-sil′ah) a genus of fleas, many species of which transmit pathogens; *X. che′opis*, the rat flea, transmits plague and murine typhus.

xeno·tro·pic (zen″o-tro′pik) pertaining to a virus that is found benignly in cells of one animal species but that will replicate into complete virus particles only when it infects cells of a different species.

xer(o)- word element [Gr.], *dry; dryness*.

xe·ro·der·ma (zēr″o-der′mah) a mild form of ichthyosis, marked by a dry, rough, discolored state of the skin. **xerodermat′ic**, adj.
    x. pigmento′sum, a rare pigmentary and atrophic autosomal recessive disease in which extreme cutaneous sensitivity to ultraviolet light results from an enzyme deficiency in the repair of DNA damaged by ultraviolet light. It begins in childhood, with early development of excessive freckling, telangiectases, keratomas, papillomas, and malignancies in sun-exposed skin, severe opthalmologic abnormalities, and, in some cases, neurological disorders.

xe·rog·ra·phy (ze-rog′rah-fe) xeroradiography.

xe·ro·ma (ze-ro′mah) abnormal dryness of the conjunctiva; xerophthalmia.

xe·ro·mam·mog·ra·phy (zēr″o-mah-mog′-rah-fe) xeroradiography of the breast.

xe·ro·me·nia (-me′ne-ah) the appearance of constitutional symptoms at the menstrual period without any flow of blood.

xe·roph·thal·mia (zēr″of-thal′me-ah) abnormal dryness and thickening of the conjunctiva and cornea due to vitamin A deficiency.

xe·ro·ra·di·og·ra·phy (zēr″o-ra″de-og′rah-fe) the making of radiographs by a dry, totally photoelectric process, using metal plates coated with a semiconductor, such as selenium.

xe·ro·si·a·log·ra·phy (-si″ah-log′rah-fe) sialography in which the images are recorded by xerography.

xe·ro·sis (ze-ro′sis) abnormal dryness, as of the eye, skin, or mouth. **xerot′ic**, adj. **x. generalisa′ta**, dryness of the skin, with pruritus and branny scaling, seen in patients with acquired immunodeficiency syndrome.

xe·ro·sto·mia (zēr″o-sto′me-ah) dryness of the mouth due to salivary gland dysfunction.

xe·rot·ic (zēr-ot′ik) characterized by xerosis or dryness.

xe·ro·to·mog·ra·phy (zēr″o-to-mog′rah-fe) tomography in which the images are recorded by xeroradiography.

xiphi·ster·num (zif″ĭ-ster′num) xiphoid process. **xiphister′nal**, adj.

xiph(o)- word element [Gr.], *xiphoid process*.

xipho·cos·tal (zif″o-kos′tal) pertaining to the xiphoid process and ribs.

xiph·oid (zif′oid, zi′foid) 1. ensiform; sword-shaped. 2. xiphoid process.

xiph·oi·di·tis (zif″oi-di′tis) inflammation of the xiphoid process.

xi·phop·a·gus (zĭ-fop′ah-gus) symmetrical conjoined twins fused in the region of the xiphoid process.

X-linked (eks′linkt) transmitted by genes on the X chromosome; sex-linked.

x-ray (eks′ra) see under *ray*.

xy·lan (zi′lan) any of a group of pentosans composed of xylose residues; major structural constituents of wood, straw, and bran.

xy·lene (zi′lēn) 1. dimethylbenzene; any of three isomeric hydrocarbons, $C_6H_4(CH_3)_2$, from methyl alcohol or coal tar. 2. a mixture of all three isomers, with uses including solvent and clarifier, protective coating, and in various syntheses.

xy·li·tol (zi′lĭ-tol) a five-carbon sugar alcohol derived from xylose and as sweet as sucrose; used as a noncariogenic sweetener and also as a sugar substitute in diabetic diets.

Xy·lo·caine (zi′lo-kān) trademark for preparations of lidocaine.

xy·lo·met·a·zo·line (zi″lo-met″ah-zo′lēn) an adrenergic used as the hydrochloride salt as a topical nasal decongestant.

xy·lose (zi′lōs) a pentose found in plants in the form of xylans; it is used in a diagnostic test of intestinal absorption.

xy·lu·lose (zi′lu-lōs) a pentose epimeric with ribulose, occurring naturally as both L- and D-isomers. The latter is excreted in the urine in essential pentosuria; the former, in phosphorylated form, is an intermediate in the pentose phosphate pathway.

xys·ma (zis′mah) material resembling bits of membrane in stools of diarrhea.

xys·ter (zis′ter) rasp (1).

Y

Y tyrosine; yttrium.

y ordinate.

yab·a·pox (yab′ah-poks) a viral disease caused by a poxvirus that causes subcutaneous tumor-like growths in African monkeys; accidental human infection has occurred, characterized by localized skin nodules that resolve spontaneously.

yang (yang) [Chinese] in Chinese philosophy, the active, positive, masculine principle that is complementary to yin; see *yin/yang principle*, under *principle*.

yar·row (yar′o) 1. any of several plants of the genus *Achillea*, especially *A. millefolium*. 2. a preparation of the above-ground parts of *A. millefolium*, used for anorexia and dyspepsia and for liver and gallbladder complaints; also used in homeopathy.

Yat·a·pox·vi·rus (yat′ah-poks-vi″rus) a genus of viruses of the subfamily Chordopoxvirinae (family Poxviridae) comprising tanapox virus and Yaba monkey tumor virus.

yaw (yaw) a lesion of yaws. **mother y.**, the initial cutaneous lesion of yaws.

yaws (yawz) an endemic infectious tropical disease caused by *Treponema pertenue*, usually affecting persons under 15 years of age, spread by direct contact with skin lesions or by contaminated fomites. It is initially manifested by the appearance of a papilloma at the site of inoculation; this heals, leaving a scar, and is followed by crops of generalized granulomatous lesions that may relapse repeatedly. There may be bone and joint involvement.

Yb ytterbium.

yeast (yēst) a general term including single-celled, usually rounded fungi that produce by budding; some yeasts transform to a mycelial stage under certain environmental conditions, while others remain single-celled. They are fermenters of carbohydrates, and a few are pathogenic for humans. **bakers′ y., brewers′ y.,** *Saccharomyces cerevisiae*, used in brewing beer, making alcoholic liquors, and baking bread. **dried y.,** dried cells of any suitable strain of *Saccharomyces cerevisiae*, usually a by-product of the brewing industry; used as a natural source of protein and B-complex vitamins.

yel·low (yel′o) 1. a color between orange and green, produced by energy of wavelengths between 570 and 590 nm. 2. a dye or stain with this color.

Yer·sin·ia (yer-sin′e-ah) a genus of nonmotile, ovoid or rod-shaped, nonencapsulated, gram-negative bacteria (family Enterobacteriaceae); *Y. enterocoli′tica* is a ubiquitous species that causes acute gastroenteritis and mesenteric lymphadenitis in children and arthritis, septicemia, and erythema nodosum in adults; *Y. pes′tis* causes plague in humans and rodents, transmitted from rats to humans by the rat flea, and from person to person by the human body louse; *Y. pseudotuberculo′sis* causes disease in rodents and mesenteric lymphadenitis in humans.

yin (yin) [Chinese] in Chinese philosophy, the passive, negative, feminine principle that is complementary to yang; see *yin/yang principle*, under *principle*.

yo·ga (yo′gah) [Sanskrit] an ancient system of Indian philosophy incorporated into the ayurvedic system of medicine and well-being, whose goal is the attainment of ultimate balance of mind and body, or self-realization. The different systems of yoga all share certain basic principles: control of the body through correct posture and breathing, control of the emotions and mind, and meditation. In the West, yoga is often used for healing and well-being without attention to the larger philosophy. **ashtanga y.,** a physically demanding style, based in hatha yoga, in which breathing is synchronized with movement between asanas (postures); it encourages profuse sweating to purify and detoxify and it produces strength, flexibility, and stamina. **hatha y.,** a path of yoga based on physical purification and strengthening as a means of self-transformation. It encompasses a system of asanas (postures), designed to promote mental and physical well-being and to allow the mind to focus and become free from distraction for long periods of meditation, along with pranayama (breath control). **Iyengar y.,** a style, based in hatha yoga, that emphasizes correct body alignment in the asanas (postures) and holding the asanas for extended periods of time, using props to help achieve and support them. **kundalini y.,** a style, based in hatha yoga, whose purpose is controlled release of latent kundalini energy.

yo·him·bine (yo-him′bēn) an alkaloid chemically similar to reserpine, from the bark of the yohimbe tree; it possesses alpha-adrenergic blocking properties and is used as the hydrochloride as a sympatholytic and mydriatic, and for the treatment of impotence.

yoke (yōk) 1. a connecting structure. 2. jugum.

yoked (yōkd) joined together, and so acting in concert.

yolk (yōk) the stored nutrient of an oocyte or ovum.

yt·ter·bi·um (ĭ-ter′be-um) chemical element (see *Table of Elements*), at no. 70, symbol Yb.

yt·tri·um (ĭ′tre-um) chemical element (see *Table of Elements*), at. no. 39, symbol Y. The radioisotope ^{90}Y emits high energy beta particles, localizes predominantly in bone, and has been used in radiotherapy.

Z

Z atomic number; impedance.

za·fir·lu·kast (zah-fir′loo-kast) a leukotriene receptor antagonist used as an antiasthmatic agent.

zal·ci·ta·bine (zal-si′tah-bēn) 2′3′-dideoxycytidine, an antiretroviral agent that inhibits the action of reverse transcriptase; used in the treatment of HIV infection.

zal·e·plon (zal′ĕ-plon) a nonbenzodiazepine sedative and hypnotic used in the short term treatment of insomnia.

za·nam·i·vir (zah-nam′ĭ-vir) an inhibitor of viral neuraminidase used for the prophylaxis and treatment of influenza A and B.

ze·ro (zēr′o) 1. the absence of all quantity or magnitude; naught. 2. the point on a thermometer scale at which the graduation begins; the ice point on the Celsius scale and 32° below the ice point on the Fahrenheit. **absolute z.,** the lowest possible temperature, designated as 0 on the Kelvin or Rankine scale; the equivalent of −273.15°C or −459.67°F.

zi·do·vu·dine (zi-do′vu-dēn) a synthetic nucleoside (thymidine) analogue that inhibits replication of some retroviruses, including the human immunodeficiency virus; used in the treatment of HIV infection and AIDS.

ZIFT zygote intrafallopian transfer.

zig·zag·plas·ty (zig′zag-plas″te) the surgical technique of minimizing the visual impact of a long linear scar by breaking it up into short irregular segments at right or acute angles to each another.

zi·leu·ton (zi-loo′ton) an inhibitor of leukotriene formation, used as an antiasthmatic.

zinc (zingk) chemical element (see *Table of Elements*), at. no. 30, symbol Zn; it is an essential micronutrient present in many enzymes, but is toxic on excessive exposure, as by ingestion or inhalation (e.g., *metal fume fever*). **z. acetate,** an astringent and styptic. **z.**

chloride, a salt used as a nutritional supplement in total parenteral nutrition and applied topically as an astringent and a desensitizer for dentin. **z. oxide,** a topical astringent and protectant; also a sunscreen. **z. sulfate,** a topical astringent for mucous membranes, especially those of the eye. **z. undecylenate,** the zinc salt of undecylenic acid; it is a topical antifungal.

zi·pra·si·done (zĭ-pra′sĭ-dōn) an antipsychotic used as the hydrochloride salt in the treatment of schizophrenia.

zir·co·ni·um (zir-ko′ne-um) chemical element (see *Table of Elements*), at. no. 40, symbol Zr.

Zn zinc.

zo·ac·an·tho·sis (zo″ak-an-tho′sis) dermatitis caused by animal structures, such as bristles, sting, or hairs.

zo·an·thro·py (zo-an′thro-pe) delusion that one has become an animal. **zoanthrop′ic,** adj.

zo·le·dron·ic ac·id (zo′lĕ-dron″ik) a bisphosphonate inhibitor of osteoclastic bone resorption, used for the treatment of hypercalcemia of malignancy.

zol·mi·trip·tan (zōl″mĭ-trip′tan) a selective serotonin receptor agonist used to relieve acute migraine.

zol·pi·dem (zōl-pi′dem) a non-benzodiazepine sedative-hypnotic; used as the tartrate salt in the short term treatment of insomnia.

zo·na (zo′nah) pl. *zo′nae.* [L.] 1. zone. 2. herpes zoster. **z. arcua′ta,** inner tunnel. **z. cilia′ris,** ciliary zone. **z. denticula′ta,** the inner zone of the lamina basilaris of the cochlear duct with the limbus of the osseous spiral lamina. **z. fascicula′ta,** the thick middle layer of the adrenal cortex. **z. glomerulo′sa,** the thin outermost layer of the adrenal cortex. **z. hemorrhoida′lis,** that part of the anal canal extending from the anal valves to the anus and containing the rectal venous plexus. **z. incer′ta,** a narrow band of gray matter between the subthalamic nucleus and thalamic fasciculus. **z. ophthal′mica,** herpetic infection of the cornea. **z. orbicula′ris articulatio′nis cox′ae,** a ring around the neck of the femur formed by circular fibers of the articular capsule of the hip joint. **z. pectina′ta,** the outer part of the lamina basilaris of the cochlear duct running from the rods of Corti to the spiral ligament. **z. pellu′cida,** the transparent, noncellular secreted layer surrounding an oocyte. **z. perfora′ta,** the inner portion of the lamina basilaris of the cochlear duct. **z. reticula′ris,** the innermost layer of the adrenal cortex. **z. tec′ta,** inner tunnel. **z. vasculo′sa,** a region in the supramastoid fossa containing many foramina for the passage of blood vessels.

zone (zōn) an encircling region or area; by extension, any area with specific characteristics or boundary. **zo′nal,** adj. **ciliary z.,** the outer of the two regions into which the anterior surface of the iris is divided by the collarette. **comfort z.,** an environmental temperature between 13° and 21°C (55°–70°F) with a humidity of 30 to 55 per cent. **epileptogenic z.,** see under *focus.* **erogenous z., erotogenic z.,** an area of the body whose stimulation produces erotic excitation. **inner z. of renal medulla,** the part of the medulla farthest from the cortex, containing ascending and descending limbs of the thin tubule as well as the inner part of the medullary collecting duct. **Lissauer's marginal z.,** a bridge of white substance between the apex of the posterior horn and the periphery of the spinal cord. **outer z. of renal medulla,** the part of the medulla nearest to the cortex; containing the medullary part of the distal straight tubule as well as the outer part of the medullary collecting duct. **z. of partial preservation,** in spinal cord injury, a region where there may be only partial damage to nerves, including one to three spinal segments below the level of the injury. **pellucid z.,** zona pellucida. **pupillary z.,** the inner of the two regions into which the anterior surface of the iris is divided by the collarette. **transitional z.,** any anatomical region that marks the point at which the constituents of a structure change from one type to another.

zo·nes·the·sia (zo″nes-the′zhah) a dysesthesia consisting of a sensation of constriction, as by a girdle.

zo·nif·u·gal (zo-nif′u-g′l) passing outward from a zone or region.

zo·nip·e·tal (zo-nip′ah-t′l) passing toward a zone or region.

zo·nis·am·ide (zo-nis′ah-mīd″) a sulfonamide that acts as an anticonvulsant, used in the treatment of partial seizures in adults.

zo·nu·la (zo′nu-lah) pl. *zo′nulae.* [L.] zonule.

zo·nule (zōn′ūl) a small zone. **zon′ular,** adj. **ciliary z., z. of Zinn,** a series of fibers connecting the ciliary body and lens of the eye.

zo·nu·li·tis (zo″nu-li′tis) inflammation of the ciliary zonule.

zo·nu·lol·y·sis (zōn″u-lol′ĭ-sis) dissolution of the ciliary zonule by use of enzymes to permit surgical removal of the lens.

zon·u·lot·o·my (zōn″u-lot′ah-me) incision of the ciliary zonule.

zo(o)- word element [Gr.], *animal.*

zoo·der·mic (zo″o-der′mik) performed with the skin of an animal, as in skin grafting.

zo·og·e·nous (zo-oj′ĕ-nus) 1. acquired from animals. 2. viviparous.

zoo·glea (zo″o-gle′ah) pl. *zoogle′ae.* A colony of bacteria embedded in a gelatinous matrix.

zo·og·o·ny (zo-og′ah-ne) the production of living young from within the body. **zoog′onous,** adj.

zoo·graft·ing (zo′o-graf″ting) the grafting of animal tissue.

zo·oid (zo′oid) 1. animal-like. 2. an animal-like object or form. 3. an individual in a united colony of animals.

zoo·lag·nia (zo″o-lag′ne-ah) sexual attraction toward animals.

zo·ol·o·gy (zo-ol′o-je) the biology of animals.

Zoo·mas·ti·go·pho·rea (zo″o-mas″tĭ-go-for′e-ah) a class of protozoa (subphylum Mastigophora), including all the animal-like, as opposed to plantlike, protozoa.

zoo·no·sis (-no′sis, zo-on′ĕ-sis) pl. *zoono′ses.* Disease of animals transmissible to humans. **zoonot′ic,** adj.

zoo·para·site (zo″o-par′ah-sīt) any parasitic animal organism or species. **zooparasit′ic,** adj.

zoo·oph·a·gous (zo-of′ah-gus) carnivorous.

zoo·phil·ia (zo″o-fil′e-ah) 1. abnormal fondness for animals. 2. bestiality; a paraphilia in which intercourse or other sexual activity with animals is the preferred method of achieving sexual excitement.

zoo·pho·bia (-fo′be-ah) irrational fear of animals.

zoo·plas·ty (zo′o-plas″te) zoografting.

zoo·sper·mia (zo″o-sper′me-ah) the presence of live spermatozoa in the ejaculated semen.

zoo·spore (zo′o-spor) a motile, flagellated, sexual or asexual spore, as produced by certain algae, fungi, and protozoa.

zoo·tox·in (-tok″sin) a toxic substance of animal origin, e.g., venom of snakes, spiders, and scorpions.

zos·ter (zos″ter) herpes zoster.

zos·ter·i·form (zos-ter′ĭ-form) resembling herpes zoster.

zos·ter·oid (zos′ter-oid) zosteriform.

Z-plas·ty (ze′plas-te) repair of a skin defect by the transposition of two triangular flaps, for relaxation of scar contractures.

Zr zirconium.

zwit·ter·ion (tsvit′er-i″on) an ion that has both positive and negative regions of charge.

zy·gal (zi′g′l) shaped like a yoke.

zy·ga·poph·y·sis (zi″gah-pof′ĭ-sis) pl. *zygapoph′yses.* The articular process of a vertebra.

zyg·i·on (zij′e-on) pl. *zyg′ia.* [Gr.] the most lateral point on the zygomatic arch.

zyg(o)- word element [Gr.], *yoked; joined; a junction.*

zy·go·dac·ty·ly (zi″go-dak′tĭ-le) union of digits by soft tissues (skin), without bony fusion of the phalanges.

zy·go·ma (zi-go′mah) 1. the zygomatic process of the temporal bone. 2. zygomatic arch. 3. a term sometimes applied to the zygomatic bone.

zy·go·mat·ic (zi″go-mat′ik) pertaining to, connecting with, or in the region of the zygomatic bone.

zy·go·mat·i·co·fa·cial (zi″go-mat″ĭ-ko-fa′-shul) pertaining to the zygomatic process or bone and the face.

zy·go·mat·i·co·tem·po·ral (-tem′pah-rul) pertaining to the zygomatic process or bone and the temporal bone.

zy·go·my·co·sis (zi″go-mi-ko′sis) 1. an infectious disease of humans or animals caused by fungi of the division Zygomycota. 2. mucormycosis.

Zy·go·my·co·ta (zi″go-mi-ko′tah) a division of the soil fungi consisting of soil saprobes and invertebrate parasites. Organisms may cause human or animal infection in debilitated or highly stressed individuals. In some systems of classification, the Zygomycota are treated as a subdivision, Zygomycotina, which is classified under the division Eumycota.

zy·gon (zi′gon) the stem connecting the two branches of a zygal fissure.

zy·gos·i·ty (zi-gos′ĭ-te) the condition relating to conjugation, or to the zygote, as *(a)* the state of a cell or individual in regard to the alleles determining a specific character, whether identical (homozygosity) or different (heterozygosity); or *(b)* in the case of twins, whether developing from one zygote (monozygosity) or two (dizygosity).

zy·gote (zi′gōt) the diploid cell resulting from union of a male and a female gamete. More precisely, the cell after synapsis at the completion of fertilization until first cleavage. **zygot′ic,** adj.

zy·go·tene (zi′go-tēn) the synaptic stage of the first meiotic prophase in which the two leptotene chromosomes undergo pairing by the formation of synaptonemal complexes to form a bivalent structure.